Pediatric Emergency Medicine

Pediatric Emergency Medicine

Third Edition

Gary R. Strange, MD
Chairman, Department of Emergency Medicine
University of Illinois at Chicago
Chicago, Illinois

William R. Ahrens, MD
Associate Professor Clinical Emergency Medicine
University of Illinois at Chicago
Chicago, Illinois

Robert W. Schafermeyer, MD, FACEP, FAAP
Chief and Associate Chair, Department of Emergency Medicine
Carolinas Medical Center, Charlotte, North Carolina
Clinical Professor of Emergency Medicine and Pediatrics
University of North Carolina School of Medicine
Chapel Hill, North Carolina

Robert A. Wiebe, MD, FAAP, FACEP
Professor, Division of Pediatric Emergency Medicine
University of Texas Southwestern Medical Center
Dallas, Texas

McGraw Hill Medical

New York   Chicago   San Francisco   Lisbon   London   Madrid   Mexico City   Milan
New Delhi   San Juan   Seoul   Singapore   Sydney   Toronto

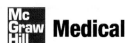

Pediatric Emergency Medicine, 3rd Edition

1 2 3 4 5 6 7 8 9 0   CTP/CTP   12 11 10 9

ISBN 978-0-07-159737-1
MHID 0-07-159737-9

This book was set in Garamond by Aptara®, Inc.
The editors were Anne Sydor and Karen G. Edmonson.
The production supervisor was Catherine Saggese.
The cover designer was Mary McKeon.
Project management was provided by Satvinder Kaur at Aptara®, Inc.
China Translation and Printing Services was printer and binder.

This book is printed on acid-free paper.

Library of Congress Cataloging-in-Publication Data

Pediatric emergency medicine / [edited by] Gary R. Strange . . . [et al.].
– 3rd ed.
     p. ; cm.
  Includes bibliographical references and index.
  ISBN 978-0-07-159737-1 (alk. paper)
  1. Pediatric emergencies–Handbooks, manuals, etc. I. Strange, Gary
R., 1947-
  [DNLM: 1. Emergencies–Handbooks. 2. Child. 3. Infant. WS 39
P37125 2009]
  RJ370.P4523 2009
  618.92′0025–dc22   2009019854

The first and second editions were dedicated to my parents, my teachers, and my family; those who prepared me for and supported me during my career. I now dedicate this work to the future generations who will pick up our work, maintain the dedication, and expand it beyond all that we might imagine. Along with the many students, residents, fellows, and junior faculty who will study pediatric emergency medicine, I want to include the newest generation of my own family, my grandchildren, Jacob Ryan Dominguez and Jackson Paul Dominguez, who are just beginning their journey. May the road be rich, exciting, challenging, and meaningful.
— Gary R. Strange —

To the Children of Chicago
— William R. Ahrens —

Caring for sick and injured children has been a privilege that I will never forget. They have taught me many things during my career, as have the many residents whom I have had the opportunity to teach. I also dedicate this work to the future practitioners who will provide the care, teaching, and research to further our ability to treat our young patients. I thank my many teachers, colleagues, and mentors, including Dr. John Marx, who have helped me be a better physician. I thank my parents, William and Virginia for their love, encouragement, and support. I also thank my wife, An Ping, and our children, Christina, David, Matthew, and Joseph for their love and support and wish them success as they pursue their dreams.
— Robert W. Schafermeyer —

To the fellows and residents that I have had the privilege of working with over the years. I have always gotten more from them than I have given. To my wife, Jacqueline, who's tolerance, patience, and support is limitless.
— Robert A. Wiebe —

CONTENTS

Preface ....*xvi*

Contributors...*xvii*

SECTION I: **CARDINAL PRESENTATIONS**

Chapter 1.   Approach to the Child in the Emergency Department 3
Valerie McDougall Kestner

Chapter 2.   The Febrile- or Septic-Appearing Neonate 9
Robert A. Felter and Ron D. Waldrop

Chapter 3.   The Febrile- or Septic-Appearing Infant or Child.. 15
Ron D. Waldrop and Robert A. Felter

Chapter 4.   Respiratory Distress.. 23
Joanna Cohen and Kathleen M. Brown

Chapter 5.   Sudden Infant Death Syndrome and Apparent Life-Threatening Event 27
Collin S. Goto and Sing-Yi Feng

Chapter 6.   Altered Mental Status and Coma.. 33
Susan Fuchs

Chapter 7.   Seizures 39
Susan Fuchs

Chapter 8.   Chest Pain.. 51
Wendy C. Matsuno

Chapter 9.   Acute Abdominal Conditions 57
Jonathan Singer

Chapter 10.   Vomiting, Diarrhea, and Gastroenteritis.. 73
William R. Ahrens

Chapter 11.   Feeding Disorders... 79
William R. Ahrens

Chapter 12.   Jaundice... 83
Anjali Singh and William R. Ahrens

Chapter 13.   The Crying Infant 91
Joan M. Mavrinac

Chapter 14.   Limping Child 97
Isabel A. Barata

Chapter 15.   Mild Head Injury in Children 105
Eustacia Su

Chapter 16.   Approach to the Patient with Rash..113
Elizabeth Turner and Gregory Garra

Chapter 17.   Neck Masses...121
Raemma Paredes Luck

Chapter 18.   Neonatal Emergencies..129
Alfred Sacchetti

Chapter 19.   The Transplant Patient in the ED..135
Neil A. Evans and Susan M. Scott

SECTION II: SEDATION, ANALGESIA, AND IMAGING

Chapter 20.   Procedural Sedation and Analgesia 143
Amy L. Baxter

Chapter 21.   Pain Management..155
Amy L. Baxter and Lindsey L. Cohen

Chapter 22.   Imaging 165
Wendy C. Matsuno

SECTION III: RESUSCITATION

Chapter 23.   Airway Management...177
Loren G. Yamamoto

Chapter 24.   Respiratory Failure..189
Lynette L. Young

Chapter 25.   Shock..195
Jonathan K. Marr

Chapter 26.   Cardiopulmonary Resuscitation..203
Alson S. Inaba

Chapter 27.   Neonatal Resuscitation...211
Paul Jeremy Eakin

SECTION IV: TRAUMA

Chapter 28.   Evaluation and Management of the Multiple Trauma Patient...........................221
Michael J. Gerardi

Chapter 29.   Head Trauma 237
Kimberly S. Quayle

Chapter 30. Pediatric Cervical Spine Injury 245
          Julie Leonard and Jeffrey Russell Leonard

Chapter 31. Thoracic Trauma 259
          Karen O'Connell, Wendy Ann Lucid, and Todd Brian Taylor

Chapter 32. Abdominal Trauma 273
          Shireen M. Atabaki, Wendy Ann Lucid, and Todd Brian Taylor

Chapter 33. Genitourinary Trauma 281
          Joyce C. Arpilleda

Chapter 34. Maxillofacial Trauma 289
          Joanna York and Stephen A. Colucciello

Chapter 35. Orthopedic Injuries 297
          Greg Canty

Chapter 36. Pediatric Sports Injuries in the ED 305
          Greg Canty

Chapter 37. Injuries of the Upper Extremities 309
          Jim R. Harley

Chapter 38. Injuries of the Pelvis and Lower Extremities 323
          Greg Canty

Chapter 39. Soft Tissue Injury and Wound Repair 333
          D. Matthew Sullivan

SECTION V: **RESPIRATORY EMERGENCIES**

Chapter 40. Upper Airway Emergencies 353
          Richard M. Cantor and Linnea Wittick

Chapter 41. Asthma 361
          Kathleen M. Brown

Chapter 42. Bronchiolitis 373
          Kathleen M. Brown

Chapter 43. Pneumonia 379
          Sharon E. Mace

Chapter 44. Pertussis 395
          Sharon E. Mace

Chapter 45. Bronchopulmonary Dysplasia 401
          Madeline Matar Joseph

Chapter 46. Cystic Fibrosis 405
          Sabah F. Iqbal, Kathleen M. Brown, and Bruce L. Klein

SECTION VI: CARDIOVASCULAR EMERGENCIES

Chapter 47. Congenital Heart Disease...413
Timothy Horeczko and Kelly D. Young

Chapter 48. Congestive Heart Failure 431
Donna M. Moro-Sutherland, William C. Toepper, and Joilo Barbosa

Chapter 49. Inflammatory and Infectious Heart Disease 439
William T. Tsai

Chapter 50. Dysrhythmias in Children 445
Ghazala Q. Sharieff and Stephanie Donige

Chapter 51. Pediatric Hypertension 455
Emily C. MacNeill

Chapter 52. Thromboembolic Disease 461
Lee S. Benjamin

SECTION VII: NEUROLOGIC EMERGENCIES

Chapter 53. Syncope...469
Susan Fuchs

Chapter 54. Ataxia...475
Susan Fuchs

Chapter 55. Weakness 481
Susan Fuchs

Chapter 56. Headache 489
Susan Fuchs

Chapter 57. Hydrocephalus 495
Susan Fuchs

Chapter 58. Cerebral Palsy 499
Susan Fuchs

Chapter 59. Cerebrovascular Syndromes...501
Susan Fuchs

SECTION VIII: INFECTIOUS EMERGENCIES

Chapter 60. Influenza...509
Karen C. Hayani and Arthur L. Frank

Chapter 61. Meningitis...519
Steven Lelyveld and Gary R. Strange

Chapter 62. Toxic Shock Syndrome...525
Shabnam Jain and Anthony Cooley

Chapter 63.   Kawasaki Disease 531
Anthony Cooley and Shabnam Jain

Chapter 64.   The Pediatric HIV Patient in the ED 537
John F. Marcinak

Chapter 65.   Tick-Borne Infections 545
Scott A. Heinrich, Marcie Stoshak-Chavez, and Kemedy K. McQuillen

Chapter 66.   Common Parasitic Infestations 553
Steven Lelyveld and Gary R. Strange

Chapter 67.   Imported Diseases/Diseases in the Traveling Child 563
Thomas L. Hurt

Chapter 68.   Bioterrorism: A Pediatric Perspective 575
Janet Lin and Timothy B. Erickson

SECTION IX: **IMMUNOLOGIC EMERGENCIES**

Chapter 69.   Common Allergic Presentations: Allergic Conjunctivitis/Rhinitis 585
William R. Ahrens

Chapter 70.   Anaphylaxis 589
E. Bradshaw Bunney

SECTION X: **GASTROINTESTINAL EMERGENCIES**

Chapter 71.   Abdominal Pain 595
Philip H. Ewing

Chapter 72.   Gastrointestinal Bleeding 601
Rebecca L. Partridge

Chapter 73.   Gastroesophageal Reflux 609
Jamie N. Deis and Thomas J. Abramo

Chapter 74.   Gastrointestinal Foreign Bodies 615
Philip H. Ewing

Chapter 75.   Liver and Gallbladder 619
Ashley Kumar and Susan M. Scott

SECTION XI: **ENDOCRINE EMERGENCIES**

Chapter 76.   Disorders of Glucose Metabolism 629
Nicholas Furtado

Chapter 77.   Adrenal Insufficiency 639
Nicholas Furtado

Chapter 78.   Hyperthyroidism 645
Nicholas Furtado

Chapter 79. Rickets..649
Carla Minutti

Chapter 80. Fluid and Electrolyte Disorders...657
Susan A. Kecskes

Chapter 81. Inborn Errors of Metabolism..669
George E. Hoganson

SECTION XII: GENITOURINARY EMERGENCIES

Chapter 82. Male Genitourinary Problems..677
John W. Williams and Marianne Gausche-Hill

Chapter 83. Urinary Tract Diseases..687
John W. Williams and Marianne Gausche-Hill

Chapter 84. Specific Renal Syndromes...693
Roger M. Barkin

SECTION XIII: DERMATOLOGIC EMERGENCIES

Chapter 85. Petechiae and Purpura..701
Malee V. Shah and Robert A. Wiebe

Chapter 86. Pruritic Rashes...707
Malee V. Shah and Robert A. Wiebe

Chapter 87. Superficial Skin Infections...713
Malee V. Shah and Robert A. Wiebe

Chapter 88. Exanthems..717
Robert A. Wiebe and Malee V. Shah

Chapter 89. Infant Rashes...727
Robert A. Wiebe and Malee V. Shah

SECTION XIV: OTOLARYNGOLOGIC EMERGENCIES

Chapter 90. Ear and Nose Emergencies...733
Raemma Paredes Luck and Evan J. Weiner

Chapter 91. Emergencies of the Oral Cavity and Neck 741
Daryl Williams and Gregory Garra

SECTION XV: OPHTHALMOLOGIC EMERGENCIES

Chapter 92. Eye Trauma..753
Jeremiah J. Johnson and Stephen A. Coluicciello

Chapter 93. Eye Emergencies in Childhood..761
Lauren P. Ortega, Katherine M. Konzen, and Ghazala Q. Sharieff

SECTION XVI: GYNECOLOGIC EMERGENCIES

Chapter 94. The Adolescent Pregnant Patient...779
Adriana M. Rodriguez, Pamela J. Okada, and Jeanne S. Sheffield

Chapter 95. Gynecologic Disorders of Infancy, Childhood, and Adolescence......................785
Geetha M. Devdas and Maria Stephan

Chapter 96. Vaginitis...793
Geetha M. Devdas and Maria Stephan

Chapter 97. Sexually Transmitted Diseases..797
Geetha M. Devdas and Maria Stephan

Chapter 98. Dysmenorrhea and Dysfunctional Uterine Bleeding.......................................807
Mercedes Uribe and Pamela J. Okada

SECTION XVII: HEMATOLOGIC AND ONCOLOGIC EMERGENCIES

Chapter 99. Anemia...817
Audra L. McCreight and Jonathan E Wickiser

Chapter 100. Sickle Cell Disease..821
Audra L. McCreight and Jonathan E. Wickiser

Chapter 101. Bleeding Disorders..827
Audra L. McCreight and Jonathan E. Wickiser

Chapter 102. Blood Component Therapy..833
Audra L. McCreight and Jonathan E. Wickiser

Chapter 103. Oncologic Emergencies..837
Audra L. McCreight and Jonathan E. Wickiser

SECTION XVIII: NON-TRAUMATIC BONE AND JOINT DISORDERS

Chapter 104. Infectious Musculoskeletal Disorders...851
Kemedy K. McQuillen

Chapter 105. Inflammatory Musculoskeletal Disorders...859
Kemedy K. McQuillen

Chapter 106. Nonmalignant Tumors of Bone..869
Kemedy K. McQuillen

SECTION XIX: TOXICOLOGIC EMERGENCIES

Chapter 107. General Approach to the Poisoned Pediatric Patient....................................877
Timothy B. Erickson

Part 1: Antipyretic Analgesics

Chapter 108. Acetaminophen..887
Leon Gussow

Chapter 109. Aspirin...893
Michele Zell-Kanter

Chapter 110. Nonsteroidal Anti-inflammatory Drugs..................................895
Michele Zell-Kanter

Part 2: Household Chemicals
Chapter 111. Toxic Alcohols..897
Timothy B. Erickson

Chapter 112. Organophosphates and Carbamates 903
Leon Gussow

Chapter 113. Caustics 907
Jenny J. Lu and Trevonne M. Thompson

Chapter 114. Hydrocarbons 913
Trevonne M. Thompson

Chapter 115. Rodenticides..915
Michael S. Wahl and Anthony Burda

Part 3: Prescription Drugs
Chapter 116. Cardiotoxins 923
Allan R. Mottram and Jerrold B. Leikin

Chapter 117. Antidepressants...931
Timothy Meehan and Steven E. Aks

Chapter 118. Neuroleptics 933
Timothy B. Erickson

Chapter 119. Isoniazid Toxicity 937
Jenny J. Lu and Theodore Toerne

Chapter 120. Carbon Monoxide Poisoning...941
Sean M. Bryant

Part 4: Drugs of Abuse
Chapter 121. Opioids...945
Timothy B. Erickson

Chapter 122. Cocaine Toxicity..951
Steven E. Aks

Chapter 123. Phencyclidine and Ketamine Toxicity...................................953
Christopher Hoyte and Steven E. Aks

Chapter 124. Amphetamines...955
James W. Rhee

Chapter 125. Gamma-Hydroxybutyrate 959
Jenny J. Lu and Timothy B. Erickson

Chapter 126. Lead Poisoning 963
Mark B. Mycyk

Chapter 127. Iron Poisoning...969
Steven E. Aks

Part 5: Environmental Poisons

Chapter 128. Cyanide Poisoning...973
Mark B. Mycyk

Chapter 129. Mushroom Poisoning..977
Steven E. Aks

Chapter 130. Poisonous Plants..981
Ejaaz A. Kalimullah and Andrea G. Carlson

Chapter 131. Lethal Toxins in Small Doses 989
Leon Gussow

Chapter 132. Chemical Weapons: Nerve Agents and Vesicants 993
Leon Gussow

SECTION XX: ENVIRONMENTAL EMERGENCIES

Chapter 133. Human and Animal Bites...999
David A. Townes

Chapter 134. Snake Envenomations 1003
Timothy B. Erickson and Andrew Zinkel

Chapter 135. Spider and Arthropod Bites...1009
Timothy B. Erickson and Renee King

Chapter 136. Marine Envenomations..1017
Timothy B. Erickson and Armando Marquez

Chapter 137. Drowning 1025
Julie Martino and Mark Mackey

Chapter 138. Pediatric Burns 1029
Kavitha Reddy and Lisa Parke Maier

Chapter 139. Electrical and Lightning Injuries 1035
Mary Ann Cooper

Chapter 140. Heat and Cold Illness...1045
Heather M. Prendergast and Gary R. Strange

Chapter 141. High-Altitude Illness 1059
Ira J. Blumen and Janis Tupesis

Chapter 142. Dysbaric Injuries 1073
Ira J. Blumen and Lisa Rapoport

Chapter 143. Radiation Emergencies...1081
Ira J. Blumen and James W. Rhee

SECTION XXI: **PSYCHOSOCIAL EMERGENCIES**

Chapter 144. Sexual Abuse 1101
  Sara L. Beers and Matthew Cox

Chapter 145. Abuse and Neglect.. 1109
  Matthew Cox and Sara L. Beers

Chapter 146. Psychiatric Emergencies.. 1117
  Catherine Porter Moore

Chapter 147. Death of a Child in the Emergency Department.. 1123
  William R. Ahrens

SECTION XXII: **EMERGENCY MEDICAL SERVICES AND MASS CASUALTY INCIDENTS**

Chapter 148. Pediatric Prehospital Care... 1129
  Craig J. Huang and Maeve Sheehan

Chapter 149. Interfacility Transport.. 1141
  Maeve Sheehan and Craig J. Huang

Chapter 150. Mass Casualty Management.. 1149
  Janet Lin

SECTION XXIII: **MEDICOLEGAL AND ADMINISTRATIVE ISSUES**

Chapter 151. Medico-Legal Considerations 1157
  William R. Ahrens

Chapter 152. Ethical Considerations 1161
  Alan Johnson

Chapter 153. Withholding or Terminating Resuscitation and Brain Death........................ 1167
  Howard Hast

Index *1169*

PREFACE

Since we started work on the first edition 14 years ago, much has changed in our specialty and indeed in the world around us. We have seen the subspecialty of *Pediatric Emergency Medicine* continue to mature and develop during those years and we have seen exemplary collaboration between the specialties of Pediatrics and Emergency Medicine as we work together to improve the care of children in the nation's emergency departments. We hope the first and second editions of our text have assisted in this effort.

The specialty of *Pediatric Emergency Medicine* has changed over these years as new knowledge from research, new pharmaceuticals, and new technology have shaped how we evaluate and treat our young patients. For the third edition, we have again worked to create a resource for clinicians who regularly provide pediatric emergency care as well as for those who only occasionally are called upon to care for a sick or injured child. The third edition is a significant update of the material, which we believe will allow this text to serve as a key resource at the bedside as well as at the desk.

For the most part, we have maintained the organization by body systems used in the first two editions. But we have added a large section at the beginning of the book to cover cardinal presentations in the pediatric emergency department. In this section, we have split the discussion of fever and sepsis into two chapters to differentiate the approach for neonates from that for infants and children and to acknowledge the changing approach to this complex presentation with the advent of modern immunization practices. The content pertinent to the management of neonates has also been expanded with chapters on feeding problems, jaundice, and common neonatal presentations. Also to reflect the increasing complexity of patients seen in our pediatric emergency departments, we have added a chapter on emergency management of the transplant patient.

The infectious disease section has been markedly expanded to include topics that have taken on new or expanded significance in the 21st century. These include influenza, im- ported diseases, bioterrorism, and HIV. The endocrine/metabolic section has been enhanced with the addition of chapters on rickets and inborn errors of metabolism. New chapters on chemical terrorism and mass casualty management have also been added.

Essentially, every chapter has been enhanced to facilitate access of information and ease of use. The use of photographs, figures, diagrams, tables, and algorithms has been maximized where appropriate.

Clearly, we are very proud of our product and hope the students, residents, fellows, pediatricians, emergency physicians, and others that use it will find it a useful adjunct to their practice. We are sensitive as well to the evolving use of reference material in the practice of modern medicine and this work will be available online via McGraw-Hill's AccessEM as well as in print.

The editorial team would like to welcome our new coeditor, Robert Wiebe. Bob has been a key contributor to the first two editions and we are fortunate to have him join the editorial team this time around. In addition, we have a new executive editor at McGraw-Hill, Anne M. Sydor, who has facilitated the completion of the third edition with exceptional advice, assistance, and attention to detail. We are also pleased to welcome those who are new authors for the third edition and to thank the many returning authors. The excellence of our authors has made the editorial process a real pleasure and of course is the key to the quality of the finished product. We also thank the many authors who helped make the first two editions useful to you.

Gary R. Strange

William R. Ahrens

Robert W. Schafermeyer

Robert A. Wiebe

CONTRIBUTORS

Thomas J. Abramo, MD, FAAP, FACEP
Professor of Emergency Medicine & Pediatrics
Director, Pediatric Emergency Department
Medical Director of Pediatric Transport
Pediatric Emergency Physician-in-Chief
Department of Emergency Medicine
Vanderbilt University Medical Center
Attending Physician, Monroe Carell Jr. Children's
    Hospital at Vanderbilt
Nashville, Tennessee

William R. Ahrens, MD
Associate Professor Clinical Emergency Medicine
Director, Pediatric Emergency Medicine
University of Illinois at Chicago
Chicago, Illinois

Steven E. Aks, DO, FACMT, FACEP
Associate Professor
Department of Medicine
Rush Medical College
Director, The Toxikon Consortium, Division
    of Toxicology
Department of Emergency Medicine
Cook County Hospital
Chicago, Illinois

Joyce C. Arpilleda, MD, FAAP
Associate Professor
Department of Pediatrics
University of California, San Diego
San Diego, California

Shireen M. Atabaki, MD, MPH
Assistant Professor of Pediatrics and Emergency
    Medicine
The George Washington University School of Medicine
    and Health Sciences
Attending Physician
Division of Emergency Medicine
Children's National Medical Center
Washington, DC

Isabel A. Barata, MS, MD
Assistant Professor
Department of Pediatrics
New York University School of Medicine
New York, New York

Roger M. Barkin, MD
Clinical Professor
Department of Pediatrics
University of Colorado at Denver
Denver, Colorado

Amy L. Baxter, MD
Clinical Associate Professor
Emergency Medicine Department
Medical College of Georgia
Augusta, Georgia

Sara L. Beers, MD
Assistant Professor
Division of Pediatric Emergency Medicine
Department of Pediatrics
University of Texas Southwestern Medical Center
Dallas, Texas

Lee S. Benjamin, MD
Assistant Professor
Duke University School of Medicine
Duke University Medical Center
Durham, North Carolina

Ira J. Blumen, MD
Clinical Associate Professor of Medicine
    and Pediatrics
University of Chicago
Chicago, Illinois

Kathleen M. Brown, MD
Associate Professor of Pediatrics
The George Washington School of Medicine
    and Health Sciences
Medical Director, Emergency Department
Children's National Medical Center
Washington, DC

Sean M. Bryant, MD
Assistant Professor
Cook County-Stroger Hospital
Rush Medical College
Department of Emergency Medicine
Associate Medical Director
Illinois Poison Center
Chicago, Illinois

E. Bradshaw Bunney, MD
Associate Professor, Residency Director
Department of Emergency Medicine
University of Illinois at Chicago
Chicago, Illinois

Richard M. Cantor, MD, FAAP, FACEP
Associate Professor
Department of Emergency Medicine
  and Pediatrics
Upstate Medical University
Syracuse, New York

Greg Canty, MD
Fellow
Department of Pediatric Emergency Medicine
University of Missouri-Kansas City
Kansas City, Missouri

Lindsey L. Cohen, PhD
Associate Professor
Department of Psychology
Georgia State University
Atlanta, Georgia

Stephan Colucciello, MD
Associate Chair and Vice Chief
Department of Emergency Medicine
Carolinas Medical Center
Charlotte, North Carolina

Karen O'Connell, MD, FACEP
Assistant Professor of Pediatrics and Emergency
  Medicine
The George Washington University School of Medicine
  and Health Sciences
Attending Physician, Pediatric Emergency Medicine
Children's National Medical Center
Washington, DC

Mary Ann Cooper
Professor of Emergency Medicine
University of Illinois
Chicago, Illinois

Matthew Cox, MD
Assistant Professor
Department of Pediatrics
University of Texas Southwestern Medical Center
Dallas, Texas

Jamie N. Deis, MD
Clinical Fellow, Pediatric Emergency Medicine
Monroe Carell Jr. Children's Hospital at
  Vanderbilt
Nashville, Tennessee

Geetha M. Devdas, MD
Pediatric Emergency Medicine Fellow
University of Texas Southwestern
Pediatric Emergency Medicine Fellow
Dallas Children's Medical Center
Dallas, Texas

Stephanie Doniger, MD
Rady Children's Hospital Emergency
  Care Center
University of California
Palomar- Pomerado Health System
California Emergency Physicians
San Diego, California

Paul Jeremy Eakin, MD, FAAP
Associate Professor
University of Hawaii John A. Burns School
  of Medicine
Emergency Department
Attending Physician
Kapi'olani Medical Specialists
Honolulu, Hawaii

Timothy B. Erickson, MD, FACEP, FAACT, FACMT
Professor, University of Illinois at Chicago
Associate Head, Department of Emergency Medicine
Director, Division of Clinical Toxicology
Chicago, Illinois

Cristina M. Estrada, MD
Assistant Professor
Department of Emergency Medicine and Pediatrics
Vanderbilt University Medical Center
Nashville, Tennessee

Neil A. Evans, MD
Fellow
Department of Pediatric Emergency Medicine
University of Texas Southwestern Children's
  Medical Center
Dallas, Texas

Philip H. Ewing
Pediatric Emergency Medicine Fellow
University of Texas Southwestern Medical Center
Children's Medical Center of Dallas
Dallas, Texas

Robert A. Felter
Professor of Pediatrics
Georgetown University School of Medicine
Medical Director
Pediatric Emergency Medicine
INWA Loudon Hospital
Washington, DC

Sing-Yi Feng, MD
Assistant Professor
Department of Pediatrics
University of Texas Southwestern Medical Center
   of Dallas
Dallas, Texas

Arthur L. Frank, MD
Associate Professor of Pediatrics
University of Illinois at Chicago
Chicago, Illinois

Susan Fuchs
Division of Pediatric Emergency Medicine
Children's Memorial Hospital
Chicago, Illinois

Nicholas Furtado, MD, FAAP
Assistant Professor
Department of Emergency Medicine
University of Illinois
Chicago, Illinois

Gregory Garra, DO
Clinical Assistant Professor
Department of Emergency Medicine
Stony Brook University
Stony Brook, New York

Michael J. Gerardi
Director, Pediatric Emergency Medicine
Goryeb Children's Hospital
Department of Emergency Medicine
Morristown Memorial Hospital
Morristown, New Jersey

Collin S. Goto
Children's Medical Center of Dallas
Emergency Center
Dallas, Texas

Leon Gussow, MD, FACMT
Lecturer
Department of Emergency Medicine
University of Illinois Hospital
Chicago, Illinois

Jim R. Harley, MD, MPH
Medical Director
Division of Pediatric Emergency Medicine UCSD
   Department of Pediatrics
Rady Children's Hospital
San Diego, California

Howard Hast, MD
Assistant Professor of Clinical Pediatrics
Division of Pediatric Critical Care Medicine
The University of Illinois at Chicago
Chicago, Illinois

Karen C. Hayani, MD
Associate Professor of Pediatrics
Division of Pediatric Infectious Diseases
University of Illinois at Chicago
Chicago, Illinois

Scott A. Heinrich, MS, MD
Attending Physician
Department of Emergency Medicine
Mercy Hospital and Medical Center
Chicago, Illinois

George E. Hoganson, MD
Associate Professor of Pediatrics
Division of Genetics, University of Illinois
Chicago, Illinois

Timothy Horeczko, MD
Clinical Instructor of Medicine
David Geffen School of Medicine at UCLA
Harbor-UCLA Medical Center
Department of Emergency Medicine
Torrance, California

Craig J. Huang, MD
Assistant Professor
University of Texas Southwestern Medical Center
   at Dallas
Attending Physician
Children's Medical Center of Dallas
Dallas, Texas

Thomas L. Hurt, MD
Medical Director
Emergency Department
Mary Bridge Children's Hospital
Tacoma, Washington

Alson S. Inaba, MD, FAAP
Associate Professor of Pediatrics
University of Hawaii John A. Burns
    School of Medicine
Kapi'olani Medical Center for Women & Children
Honolulu, Hawaii

Sabah F. Iqbal, MD
Fellow
Pediatric Emergency Medicine
Children's National Medical Center
Washington, DC

Shabnam Jain, MD
Assistant Professor
Department of Pediatrics and Emregency Medicine
Emory University
Atlanta, Georgia

Alan Johnson, MD
Attending Physician
Department of Pediatric Emergency Medicine
Children's Hospital and Research Center at Oakland
Oakland, California

Jeremiah J. Johnson, MD
Pediatric Emergency Medicine Fellow
Department of Emergency Medicine
Carolinas Medical Center
Charlotte, North Carolina

Madeline Matar Joseph, MD, FACEP, FAAP
Associate Professor of Emergency Medicine
    and Pediatrics
Chief, Pediatric Emergency Medicine Division
Medical Director
Pediatric Emergency Department
University of Florida Health Science Center
Jacksonville, Florida

Ejaaz A. Kalimullah, MD
Medical Toxicology Fellow
Department of Emergency Medicine
John H. Stroger Jr. Hospital of Cook County
Chicago, Illinois

Susan A. Kecskes, MD
Clinical Associate Professor of Pediatrics
University of Illinois
Chicago, Illinois

Renee A. King, MD, MPH
Senior Instructor
Division of Emergency Medicine
University of Colorado
Aurora, Colorado

Bruce L. Klein, MD
Associate Professor of Pediatrics and Emergency
    Medicine
George Washington University School of Medicine
    and Health Sciences
Chief, Division of Transport Medicine
Children's National Medical Center
Washington, DC

Katherine M. Konzen, MD, MPH
Assistant Professor
UCSD Department of Pediatrics
Medical Director, Urgent Care
Rady Children's Hospital
San Diego, California

Ashley Kumar, DO, MPH
Senior Fellow
Pediatric Emergency Medicine
Childrens Medical Center Dallas
Dallas, Texas

Jerrold B. Leikin, MD
Professor
Department of Medicine
Rush Medical College
Chicago, Illinois

Steven Lelyveld, MD, FAAP, FACEP
Associate Professor
Departments of Medicine and Pediatrics
University of Chicago Pritzker School of Medicine
Chicago, Illinois

Jeffrey Russell Leonard, MD
Assistant Professor
Washington University School of Medicine in St. Louis
Physician
St. Louis Children's Hospital
St. Louis, Missouri

Julie Leonard, MD, MPH
Assistant Professor
Washington University School of Medicine in St. Louis
Physician
St. Louis Children's Hospital
St. Louis, Missouri

Janet Lin
Assistant Professor of Emergency Medicine
University of Illinois
Chicago, Illinois

Jenny J. Lu, MD, MS
Assistant Professor
Department of Emergency Medicine, Division
    of Toxicology
Cook County-Stroger Hospital
Chicago, Illinois

Sharon E. Mace, MD, FACEP, FAAP
Professor, Department of Medicine
Cleveland Clinic Lerner College of Medicine of Case
    Western Reserve University
Faculty, MetroHealth Medical Center
Emergency Medicine Residency
Director, Pediatric Education/Quality Improvement
Emergency Services Institute
Cleveland Clinic
Cleveland, Ohio

Mark Mackey, MD, MBA
Assistant Professor, Clinical Medicine
University of Illinois at Chicago
Chicago, Illinois

Emily C. MacNeill, MD
Program Director, Pediatric Emergency Medicine
    Fellowship Program
Department of Emergency Medicine
Carolinas Medical Center
Charlotte, North Carolina

Lisa Parke Maier, MD
Clinical Instructor
Department of Emergency
University of Illinois at Chicago
Chicago, Illinois

John F. Marcinak, MD
Associate Professor of Pediatrics
University of Chicago
Chicago, Illinois

Armando Marquez
Assistant Professor of Clinical Emergency Medicine
University of Illinois
Chicago, Illinois

Jonathan K. Marr, MD
Assistant Professor
Department of Pediatrics
University of Hawaii John A. Burns School of Medicine
Honolulu, Hawaii

Julie Martino, MD
Resident Physician
University of Illinois at Chicago
Chicago, Illinois

Wendy C. Matsuno, MD
Pediatric Emergency Medicine Fellow
University of Texas Southwestern Medical Center
Fellow, Children's Medical Center of Dallas
Dallax, Texas

Joan M. Mavrinac, MD, MPH, FACEP
Clinical Assistant Professor
Department of Emergency Medicine
University of Pittsburgh
Pittsburgh, Pennsylvania

Audra L. McCreight, MD
Assistant Professor
Department of Pediatrics
University of Texas Southwestern Medical Center
Dallas, Texas

Valerie McDougall Kestner, MD
Assistant Professor
Department of Pediatrics
University of Missouri-Kansas City School of Medicine
Kansas City, Missouri

Kemedy K. McQuillen, MD
Attending Physician
Central Maine Medical Center
Lewiston, Maine

Carla Minutti, MD
Assistant Professor
Department of Pediatrics
Loyola University School of Medicine
Maywood, Illinois

Catherine Porter Moore, MD, PhD
Pediatric Emergency Medicine Fellow
Emergency Department
University of Texas Southwestern Children's
    Medical Center
Dallas, Texas

Allan R. Mottram
Fellow, Clinical Toxicology
Stroger-Cook County Hospital
Chicago, Illinois

Mark B. Mycyk, MD
Associate Professor
Department of Emergency Medicine
Boston University School of Medicine
Boston, Massachusetts

Pamela J. Okada, MD, FAAP, FACEP
Associate Professor
University of Texas Southwestern Medical Center
Attending Physician
Children's Medical Center at Dallas
Dallas, Texas

Lauren P. Ortega, MD
Faculty-Neonatology-UCSD
UC San Diego and Rady Children's Hospital
    San Diego
Attending-Newborn Nursery, University of California,
    San Diego
Urgent Care Physician University of California,
    San Diego
Children's Hospital San Diego
San Diego, California

Frank Paloucek, PharmD
Clinical Associate Professor of Pharmacy Practice
University of Illinois
Chicago, Illinois

Raemma Paredes Luck, MD, MBA
Associate Professor
Department of Pediatrics and Emergency
    Medicine
Temple University School of Medicine
Philadelphia, Pennsylvania

Rebecca L. Partridge, MD
Clinical Fellow
Department of Pediatric Emergency Medicine
Vanderbilt University Medical Center
Nashville, Tennessee

Heather M. Prendergast, MD, MPH, FACEP
Associate Professor
Department of Emergency Medicine
University of Illinois
Chicago, Illinois

Kimberly S. Quayle, MD
Associate Professor of Pediatrics
Washington University School of Medicine
Attending Physician, St. Louis Children's
    Hospital
Chicago, Illinois

Kavitha Reddy, MD
Faculty Physician
University of Illinois, Chicago
Faculty, Mercy Hospital
Chicago, Illinois

James W. Rhee, MD
Assistant Professor
Department of Medicine and Pediatrics
The University of Chicago
Chicago, Illinois

Adriana M. Rodriguez, MD
Fellow
Department of Pediatric Emergency Medicine
University of Texas, Southwestern
Dallas, Texas

Alfred Sacchetti, MD
Chief Emergency Services
Department of Emergency Medicine
Our Lady of Lourdes Medical Center
Camden, New Jersey

Robert W. Schafermeyer, MD, FACEP, FAAP
Associate Chair, Department of Emergency Medicine
Carolinas Medical Center
Charlotte, North Carolina
Adjunct Clinical Professor of Emergency Medicine and
    Clinical Professor of Pediatrics
UNC School of Medicine
Chapel Hill, North Carolina

Susan M. Scott, MD
Associate Professor
Division of Pediatric Emergency Medicine
Department of Pediatrics
University of Texas Southwestern Medical Center
Dallas, Texas

Malee V. Shah, MD
Assistant Professor
Department of Emergency Medicine
Vanderbilt University School of Medicine
Nashville, Tennessee

Ghazala Q. Sharieff, MD, FACEP, FAAEM, FAAP
Associate Clinical Professor
Rady Children's Hospital Emergency Care Center/
    Univeristy of California, San Diego
Director of Pediatric Emergency Medicine, Palomar-
    Pomerado Health System/California
Emergency Physicians
San Diego, California

Maeve Sheehan, MD
Assistant Professor
UT Southwestern Medical Center
Medical Director of Transport Services
Children's Medical Center
Dallas, Texas

Jeanne S. Sheffield, MD
Associate Professor
University of Texas Southwestern Medical Center
Dallas, Texas

Jonathan Singer, MD
Professor of Emergency Medicine & Pediatrics
Boonshoft School of Medicine
Staff Physician
Wright State University
Children's Medical Center,
Dayton, Ohio

Anjali Singh, MD
Pediatric Emergency Medicine Fellow
Department of Pediatrics, Division of Emergency
   Services
University of Tennessee Health Sciences Center
Le Bonheur Children's Medical Center
Memphis, Tennessee

Maria Stephan, MD
Associate Professor
Division of Pediatric Emergency Medicine
University of Texas Southwestern Medical Center
Dallas, Texas

Marcie Stoshak-Chavez, MD
Clinical Assistant Professor of Emergency Medicine
University of Illinois
Chicago, Illinois

Gary R. Strange, MD
Chairman, Department of Emergency Medicine
University of Illinois at Chicago
Chicago, Illinois

Eustacia Su, MD
Staff Physician
Portland VA Medical Center
Portland, Oregon

D. Matthew Sullivan, MD
Associate Director of Operations
Department of Emergency Medicine
Carolinas Medical Center
Charlotte, North Carolina

Donna M. Moro-Sutherland, MD
Assistant Professor
Department of Emergency Medicine
University of North Carolina at Chapel Hill
Chapel Hill, North Carolina

Trevonne M. Thompson, MD
Assistant Professor
The University of Chicago
Attending Physician/Emergency Medicine
Associate Director of Medical Toxicology
The University of Chicago Medical Center
Chicago, Illinois

David A. Townes, MD
Associate Professor of Emergency Medicine
University of Washington
Seattle, Washington

William T. Tsai, MD
Attending Physician
Department of Critical Care
Levine Children's Hospital at Carolinas Medical Center
Charlotte, North Carolina

Elizabeth Turner, MD
Department of Emergency Medicine
Stony Brook University
Stony Brook, New York
Attending Physician
Brookhaven Memorial Hospital
Patchogue, New York

Mercedes Uribe, MD, FAAP
Pediatric Emergency Medicine Fellow
Department of Pediatrics
UT Southwestern/Children's Medical Center
Dallas, Texas

Michael S. Wahl, MD
Clinical Instructor
Division of Emergency Medicine
University of Chicago
Chicago, Illinois

Ron D. Waldrop, MD
Pediatric Emergency Medicine Attending
INOVA Loudoun Hospital
Leesburg, Virginia

Evan J. Weiner, MD, FAAP
Assistant Professor
Department of Pediatrics and Emergency Medicine
Drexel University College of Medicine
Attending
St. Christopher's Hospital for Children
Philadelphia, Pennsylvania

Jonathan E. Wickiser, MD
Assistant Professor
Department of Pediatrics
University of Texas Southwestern Medical Center
  at Dallas
Dallas, Texas

Robert A. Wiebe, MD, FAAP, FACEP
Professor, Division of Pediatric Emergency Medicine
University of Texas Southwestern Medical Center
Dallas, Texas

Daryl Williams, MD
Department of Emergency Medicine
Stony Brook University
Stony Brook, New York

John W. Williams, MD
Assistant Professor of Clinical Emergency Medicine
University of Illinois
Chicago, Illinois

Linea Wittick, MD
Department of Emergency Medicine and Pediatrics
Upstate Medical University
Syracuse, New York

Loren G. Yamamoto, MD, MPH, MBA
Professor of Pediatrics
Department of Pediatrics
University of Hawaii John A. Burns School
  of Medicine
Honolulu, Hawaii

Joanna York, MD
Pediatirc Emergency Medicine Fellow
Emergency Medicine
Carolinas Medical Center
Charlotte, North Carolina

Lynette L. Young, MD
Assistant Professor
Department of Pediatrics
University of Hawaii
Honolulu, Hawaii

Kelly D. Young, MD, MS
Associate Clinical Professor of Pediatrics
David Geffen School of Medicine at UCLA
  Department of Emergency Medicine
Harbor-UCLA Medical Center
Torrance, California

Michele Zell-Kanter
Coordinator, TOXIKON Consortium
Emergency Medicine Department
Cook County Hospital
Chicago, Illinois

Andrew Zinkel, MD
Attending Physician
Emergency Medicine
Regions Hospital
St. Paul, Minnesota

SECTION I

CARDINAL PRESENTATIONS

CHAPTER 1

Approach to the Child in the Emergency Department

Valerie McDougall Kestner

▶ HIGH-YIELD FACTS

- The clinician must have a reasonable knowledge of the developmental stages so that one can identify abnormal or delayed development.
- Simply observing the child play or watch TV can tell the physician many things. Often, the best examination occurs while the parent is holding the child in her lap or arms.
- Good history taking can minimize the need for blood work as the child's age, immunization status, and past medical history all impact the need for them.
- The "as low as reasonably achievable" (ALARA) radiation concept is ever-important in pediatrics.

The game plan for approaching children in the emergency department (ED) is completely different than for the adult. The physician gets one attempt to engage the patient, greet the parent, perform the examination, and formulate a treatment plan.

Children present to the ED for a variety of reasons (Table 1–1).[1] This chapter focuses on deconstructing the visit and empowering the emergency physician to be comfortable with and competently treat the child.

Tables 1–2 to 1–5[2–5] provide quick reference for normal pediatric respiratory rate, heart rate, blood pressure, and weight. Figure 1–1[6] references the Pediatric Assessment Triangle (PAT), which was popularized in Advanced Pediatric Life Support (APLS) by Ronald Dieckmann, MD. The PAT can help the provider establish a quick initial assessment of the patient. The components of the PAT are appearance, effort of breathing, and circulation to skin.

In general, the ED itself must be prepared for the pediatric patient. The American Academy of Pediatrics and the American College of Emergency Physicians have established a list of recommended pediatric resuscitation equipment and emergency medications.[7] Dosing medication for children is challenging, especially in a dire situation. There are several tools available to help a provider with weight-based dosing. These available items range from low to high tech and include the following: the length-based Broselow tape and chart with corresponding colors for dosing, computer support programs such as the PEMSOFT calculator software package with dosing calculators and algorithms, and Pediatric Advanced Life Support (PALS) or regional children's hospital code cards. Having a clinical pharmacologist or pharmacist present at pediatric codes also can be invaluable to one's practice.

▶ PREPARING FOR THE EXAMINATION

Consider this: The first-time parents of a 7-day-old baby are in the waiting room of a busy ED; with little sleep, their baby has been crying for 2 hours and has fed poorly today. They are referred to the ED. Once back to the waiting room, they wait for the nurse, then the physician, and then repeat their story again. The element of time inherent in the ED visit is not easily palatable by parents of a sick child. The repetition and waiting game can turn into fear and anger.

After ensuring that the child does not have an impending emergency that requires immediate treatment, conduct a quick chart review. It is crucial to know if there is a chronic illness or if it is rare or a genetic syndrome. A basic text review or Internet search can prepare the physician for what may be normal for the child or what special problems the child may have. Remember, to the parents, syndrome X is their life and they may know more on the topic than the physician. Listen to the parents, as the child more than likely had an exacerbation like this before and the treatment was the same.

Next, is the right equipment available in the room? There is nothing worse than a child having a sore throat, and no light source or throat swab in the room. Children have high anxiety, and when the physician leaves the room, the child thinks the anxiety-provoking things are done. When that turns out not to be true, the child may be more uncooperative.

Talk with the parents and figure out what is their main concern. One must also expect to patiently relay information to multiple concerned parties. For example, the physician talks to the father and is then handed the cell phone to repeat the same information to the mother.

Finally, the emergency physician should consider what the young patient's role should be during the history taking and physical examination. This is where the dreaded developmental stages of children come into play. There are several charts and tables regarding month-by-month development of children.[8,9] Table 1–6[10] is included for reference of developmental milestones. These have relatively large standard deviations, and thus should be considered in the broader spectrum.

▶ TABLE 1–1. **MOST COMMON DIAGNOSES FOR CHILDREN PRESENTING TO EMERGENCY DEPARTMENT**

<1 y	1–12 y	13–21 y
Acute upper respiratory infection	Acute upper respiratory infections	Contusion with intact skin surface
Pyrexia of unknown origin	Otitis media and eustachian tube dysfunction	Open wound, excluding head
Otitis media and eustachian tube dysfunction	Open wound of head	Abdominal pain
Unspecified viral and chlamydial infections	Contusion with intact skin surface	Fractures, excluding lower limb
Noninfectious enteritis and colitis	Pyrexia of unknown origin	Acute upper respiratory infection, excluding pharyngitis

With permission from Nawar EW, Niska RW, Xu J. *National Hospital Ambulatory Medical Care Survey: 2005 Emergency Department Summary. Advance Data from Vital and Health Statistics; No. 386*. Hyattsville, MD: National Center for Health Statistics; 2007. http://www.cdc.gov/nchs/data/ad/ad386.pdf (Table 12).

▶ TABLE 1–2. **NORMAL RESPIRATORY RATES FOR CHILDREN**

Age (y)	Respiratory Rate/min
<1	24–38
1–3	22–30
4–6	20–24
7–9	18–24
10–14	16–22
15–18	14–20

With permission from Bardella IJ. Pediatric advanced life support: a review of the AHA recommendations. *Am Fam Physician*. 1999;60(6):1743–1750. http://www.aafp.org/afp/991015ap/1743.htm.

▶ TABLE 1–3. **NORMAL HEART RATES FOR CHILDREN**

Age (y)	Heart Rate (beats/min)
<1	100–160
1–10	70–120
>10	60–100

With permission from A.D.A.M., Inc. *Medical Encyclopedia of MedlinePlus 2007*. http://www.nlm.nih.gov/medlineplus/ency/article/003399.htm.

▶ TABLE 1–4. **NORMAL BLOOD PRESSURE FOR CHILDREN**

Age	Systolic BP (mm Hg)
0–28 d (full-term)	>60
1–12 mo	>70
1–10 y	>70 + 2x age in y
>10 y	>90

American Heart Association. Part 12: Pediatric advanced life support. *Circulation*. 2005;112(24)(suppl I):IV-167–IV-187.

▶ TABLE 1–5. **ESTIMATION OF CHILDREN'S WEIGHTS**

Age	Weight (kg)
Neonate (term)	3.5
6 mo	8
1 y	10
2 y	13
3 y	15
4 y	17
5 y	20
6 y	22
8 y	27
10 y	30
12 y	38
14 y	50

City of Frankfort Fire and Emergency Medical Services. Frankfort Regional Medical Center. *Medical Protocols* 2005. http://www.frankfortfireandems.com/EMSprotocolsWebpage.htm.

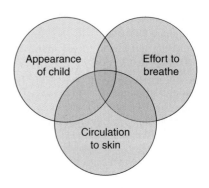

Figure 1–1. Three Components of Pediatric Assessment.

▶ TABLE 1–6. DEVELOPMENTAL MILESTONES

Age	Gross Motor	Visual-Motor/Problem Solving	Language	Social/Adaptive
1 mo	Raises head from prone position	*Birth:* Visually fixes *1 mo:* Has tight grasp, follows to midline	Alerts to sound	Regards face
2 mo	Holds head in midline, lifts chest off table	No longer clenches fists tightly, follows object past midline	Smiles socially (after being stroked or talked to)	Recognizes parent
3 mo	Supports on forearms in prone position, holds head up steadily	Holds hands open at rest, follows in circular fashion, responds to visual threat	Coos (produces long vowel sounds in musical fashion)	Reaches for familiar people or objects, anticipates feeding
4 mo	Rolls over, supports on wrists, and shifts weight	Reaches with arms in unison, brings hands to midline	Laughs, orients to voice	Enjoys looking around
6 mo	Sits unsupported, puts feed in mouth in supine position	Unilateral reach, uses raking grasp, transfers objects	Babbles, ah-goo, razz, lateral orientation to bell	Recognizes that someone is a stranger
9 mo	Pivots when sitting, crawls well, pulls to stand, cruises	Uses immature pincer grasp, probes with forefinger, holds bottle, throws objects	Says "mama, dad" indiscriminately, gestures, waves bye-bye, understands "no"	Starts exploring environment, plays gesture games (e.g., pat-a-cake)
12 mo	Walks alone	Uses mature pincer grasp, can make a crayon mark, releases voluntarily	Uses two words other than mama/dad or proper nouns, jargoning (runs several unintelligible words together with tone or inflection), one-step command with gesture	Imitates actions, comes when called, cooperates with dressing
15 mo	Creeps up stairs, walks backward independently	Scribbles in imitation, builds tower of two blocks in imitation	Uses four to six words, follows one-step command without gesture	15–18 mo: Uses spoon and cup
18 mo	Runs, throws objects from standing without falling	Scribbles spontaneously, builds tower of three blocks, turns two to three pages at a time	Mature jargoning (includes intelligible words), 7–10 word vocabulary, knows five body parts	Copies parents in tasks (sweeping, dusting), plays in company of other children
24 mo	Walks up and down steps without help	Imitates stroke with pencil, builds tower of seven blocks, turns pages one at a time, removes shoes, pants, etc	Uses pronouns (I, you, me) inappropriately, follows two-step commands, has a 50-word vocabulary, uses two-word sentences	Parallel play
3 y	Can alternate feet when going up steps, pedals tricycle	Copies a circle, undresses completely, dresses partially, dries hands if reminded, unbuttons	Uses a minimum of 250 words, three-word sentences, uses plurals, knows all pronouns, repeats two digits	Group play, shares toys, takes turns, plays well with others, knows full name, age, gender
4 y	Hops, skips, alternates feet going down steps	Copies a square, buttons clothing, dresses self completely, catches ball	Knows colors, says song or poem from memory, asks questions	Tells "tall tales," plays cooperatively with a group of children
5 y	Skips alternating feet, jumps over low obstacles	Copies triangle, ties shoes, spreads with knife	Prints first name, asks what a word means	Plays competitive games, abides by rules, likes to help in household tasks

With permission from Capute AJ, Biehl RF. *Pediatr Clin Nort Am.* 1973;20:3; Capute AJ, Accardo PJ. *Clin Pediatr.* 1978;17:847; and Capute AJ et al. *Am J Dis Child.* 1986;140:694. Rounded norms from Capute AJ et al. *Dev Med Child Neurol* 1986;28:762. Jordan LC. Development and behavior. In: Gunn VL, Nechyba C, Barone MA, eds. *Harriet Lane Handbook: A Manual for Pediatric House Officers.* 16th ed. Philadelpha, PA: Mosby, 2002:230–232.

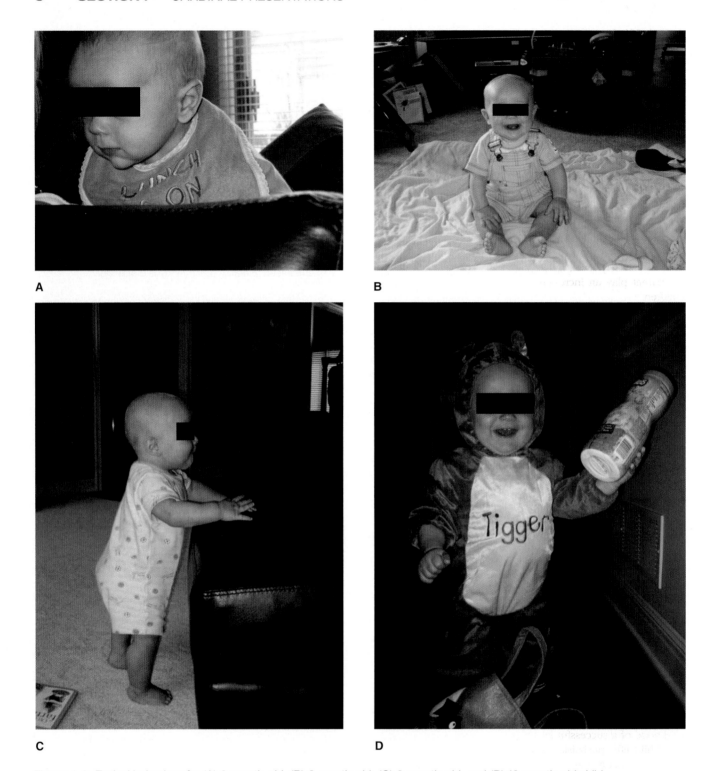

A

B

C

D

Figure 1–2. Typical behavior of a (A) 3-month-old, (B) 6-month-old, (C) 9-month-old, and (D) 12-month-old child.

▶ DEVELOPMENTAL STAGES AND ACTIVITY LEVEL

It helps to have a mental image of the child one is about to examine. The neonate is active, vigorously sucking on a pacifier. The baby opens his eyes briefly, actively moves all extremities. This movement is frequently interrupted by the Moro (startle) reflex.

By 3 months, this baby will smile at the examiner and track light or movements. The baby will lift his head with good strength (Fig. 1–2A). At 6 months, the baby can sit up with his parent's support; holds his head up well, as well as babbles (Fig. 1–2B).

At 9 months, the baby is curious and wants to explore his surroundings and pulls to stand (Fig. 1–2C). He is attentive, grabs with the fingers bent at the metacarpals, using the index through fifth fingers instead of a pincer grasp. By 1 year, the child is crawling well (Fig. 1–2D). He attempts to take independent steps, maybe walking. This baby says at least a word or two.

The 18-month-old child is a more active, if that is possible. He is more independent, but also will cling to his mother. The 2-year-old child has an expanding vocabulary, and will put two words together, and may or may not cooperate.

The 3-year-old child is generally cooperative. He may be a chatterbox or may be quiet, but this child is at an age where the examiner has a fair chance at a structured examination. The 4-year-old child is a joy to examine. He is more cooperative and can relay some history. Children aging 5 years and older continue in their development as already established with increasing independence. There are some 3-year-olds who are more cooperative than 10-year-olds, and vice versa. The child's maturity, anxiety level, intelligence level, and the vibe set by the parent play an increasingly larger role with school-aged children.

▶ THE HISTORY AND PHYSICAL

There are several principles that will make this visit more productive for the physician. First, the physician's general approach should be flexible. Start interviewing the parent while the child plays. Children are fickle creatures, but they can be examined. Simply observing the child play or watch TV can tell the physician many things. Often, the best examination occurs while the parent is holding the child in her lap or arms.

If the patient has a respiratory or cardiac complaint, examine the child's lungs and heart first before the history taking. Again, if the child is screaming, it's hard to listen for that heart murmur or crackles. If the child is very resistant to the examination, showing him the process on a parent, sibling, or stuffed animal can decrease anxiety. Let the child know what to expect during the examination: scratch his hand with the ear curette or blow a puff of air from the otoscope insufflator onto his face so that he knows what his eardrum will feel like.

Usually, it is best to examine the painful or injured part last. If the child has a painful ear, and the physician looks at that first, the rest of the examination may be a struggle because of the child's uncomfortable disposition. The child may cry during the entire examination. In these cases, the examiner has to rely on differential crying, or comparing crying when touching one region versus another location. This is extremely important in toddlers. Special mention should be made of the child with fever. If this can be treated in triage, it will help increase the likelihood of a successful examination as well.

Child life specialists are extremely adept and helpful at the role of distraction. Dedicated child life personnel can be invaluable during procedures as well. They bring their arsenal of age-appropriate books, spinning toys, DVDs, and a calming third-party presence to the room. They can minimize the need for sedation in many patients.

Honesty is very important and there is a delicate balance of enough information with too much information. The setting of laceration repair illustrates this dilemma. Show the child the saline, let him feel it, and show him how the irrigation works. Telling the child "OK, now a big bee sting" is counterproductive. She knows that they hurt. A better choice is to tell the child: "Some kids think the medicine feels hot and some thinks

it feels cold, what do you think it feels like?" Talk to the child during the procedure—about school, her brother or sister, or her pet, anything but the pain.

The emergency physician has to gauge the parents' attitude. Will the parent be a help or a hindrance? The parent can be the best ally, explaining the process and steps to the child. However, the parent can also be an obstacle. An example is in the setting of laceration repair—if the parent is in tears and visibly upset, the child will be more distressed. This parent can be coached, however, outside of the room as to the counterproductive nature of her behavior—often being able to return to the room or send another family member in for the procedure.

Ask parents the important questions in repetition. For example, not simply "Does your child have asthma?" but also "Has he ever used albuterol?" and "Do you give breathing treatments at home?" Repetition will often remind the parents that the child does in fact have asthma. The same is true with immunization status: not "Are her immunizations up to date?" but also "Did she get her 6 month shots yet?"

In school-aged and adolescent patients, the child's personal input is needed. If the parent is dominating the conversation, a gentle "And what do you think about all of this?" to the patient is necessary. A parent, especially of teenagers, doing all of the talking is a red flag. Get the parent out of the room to conduct a sensitive and thorough interview. This is mandatory in any teenager with abdominal pain, back pain, fever, or vomiting, and highly recommended in all other situations. Having the parent leave the room can be a difficult scenario but focusing on the patient's right to autonomy and its impact on the care of the child is enough to achieve this goal.

A unique situation in pediatrics is the presence of siblings. The energy level in the room is highly palpable. Keys for a successful examination are as follows: turn down the TV, ask one adult to step out with the other children, or give them something to do.

▶ ASSESSMENT AND PLAN

There are several considerations to be made at this stage: ordering diagnostic blood work, performing radiographic studies, answering the parents' questions, and making a proper treatment plan.

Good history taking can minimize the need for blood work as the child's age, immunization status, and past medical history all impact the need for them. Children's smaller blood volume, tiny blood vessels, and subsequent propensity for clotted or hemolyzed specimens all are reasons to make the clinician stop and think before ordering tests.

The next consideration is the ordering of imaging studies. Increasingly evident is the detrimental effect of radiation on anyone, let alone young children with developing brains and reproductive organs. The "as low as reasonably achievable" (ALARA) radiation concept is ever-important in pediatrics.[11] One should strongly consider whether that closed head injury really merits a CT scan. Could that abdominal pain be addressed by a radiation-free modality such as ultrasound?

Consider the parents' role in the child's treatment. Is the treatment plan reasonable for a parent to follow or is there an easier way to achieve the same goal? The physician must listen to what the parent is saying. Is it possible to prescribe a medication once a day instead of twice a day? Is it possible to teach the parent how to use an inhaler instead of a cumbersome nebulizer? Can the physician prescribe an Epi-pen for both mom and dad's individual houses?

Enlisting the support of the parent in the child's care is important for education, clear discharge instructions, and answering questions. Adult learners use several modalities to learn, so visual teaching, written instructions, and verbal review of the plan all increase the chance of compliance. The discharge instructions must be clear and written out for the parent. Leave follow-up phone numbers, names of subspecialists, if appropriate, and a time frame for follow-up. Give the parent symptoms to look for as reasons to return to the ED. Finally, allow the parents a final chance to ask their remaining questions.

Finally, address any remaining concerns and reward the child. It can be a material reward such as a sticker or stuffed animal, a pat on the back for being such a good patient, or simply a statement complimenting the child's maturity level or behavior. The ED is a scary place for a child, and a reward lets her know that the physicians are here to help her.

▶ SUMMARY

Pediatric patients in the ED present a wonderful, yet challenging opportunity. Breaking down the visit into components, consider the challenges the physician will face during preparation, history and physical, and assessment and plan. Preparation for the examination of the child, enlisting the role of the parent, decreasing anxiety of all parties, and educating with clear instructions will make the encounter a successful one.

REFERENCES

1. Nawar EW, Niska RW, Xu J. *National Hospital Ambulatory Medical Care Survey: 2005 Emergency Department Summary. Advance Data from Vital and Health Statistics; No. 386.* Hyattsville, MD: National Center for Health Statistics; 2007. http://www.cdc.gov/nchs/data/ad/ad386.pdf (Table 12). Accessed April 12, 2008.
2. Bardella IJ. Pediatric advanced life support: a review of the AHA recommendations. *Am Fam Physician.* 1999;60(6):1743–1750. http://www.aafp.org/afp/991015ap/1743.html. Accessed April 12, 2008.
3. A.D.A.M., Inc. *Medical Encyclopedia of Medline Plus 2007.* http://www.nlm.nih.gov/medlineplus/ency/article/003399.html. Accessed April 12, 2008.
4. American Heart Association. Part 12: Pediatric advanced life support. *Circulation.* 2005;112(24)(suppl I):IV-167–IV-187.
5. City of Frankfort Fire and Emergency Medical Services. Frankfort Regional Medical Center. *Medical Protocols* 2005. http://www.frankfortfireandems.com/EMSprotocolsWebpage.html. Accessed April 12, 2008.
6. American Academy of Pediatrics and the American College of Emergency Physicians. *Textbook for APLS: The Pediatric Emergency Medicine Resource.* 4th ed. Sudbury, MA: Jones and Bartlett Publishers; 2004.
7. American Academy of Pediatrics, Committee on Pediatric Emergency Medicine and American College of Emergency Physicians, Pediatric Committee. Care of children in the emergency department: guidelines for preparedness. *Pediatrics.* 2001;107(4):777–781.
8. Needleman RD. Growth and development. In: Behrman RE, Kliegman RM, Jenson HB, eds. *Nelson Textbook of Pediatrics.* 17th ed. Philadelphia, PA: Saunders; 2004:23–57.
9. American Academy of Pediatrics. *Children's Health Topics.* Elk Grove Village, IL; 2004. http://www.aap.org/topics.html. Accessed April 12, 2008.
10. Capute AJ, Biehl RF, Accardo PJ, et al. Development and behavior. In: Gunn VL, Nechyba C, Barone MA, eds. *Harriet Lane Handbook: A Manual for Pediatric House Officers.* 16th ed. Philadelpha, PA: Mosby; 2002:230–232.
11. Frush DP, Donnelly LF, Rosen NS. Computed tomography and radiation risks: what pediatric health care providers should know. *Pediatrics.* 2003;112(4):951–957.

CHAPTER 2

The Febrile- or Septic-Appearing Neonate

Robert A. Felter and Ron D. Waldrop

▶ HIGH-YIELD FACTS

- The risk of serious bacterial infection (SBI) is greatest during the neonatal period, defined as birth to 28 days of life. Some authorities recommend that a child born prematurely should have the degree of immaturity subtracted from the child's chronological age for this consideration.
- It is generally accepted that a fever is a temperature of ≥38°C or 100.4°F taken with a rectal thermometer.
- A neonate who had a documented fever by any method but is afebrile on admission to the ED should be treated as a febrile neonate whether or not antipyretics have been given.
- The most frequent bacterial pathogens in the neonatal period are group B *Streptococcus* (GSB), *Escherichia coli*, and *Listeria monocytogenes*.
- Hypothermia is a rectal temperature less than 36°C or 96.8°F and, in the neonatal period, may actually be a more common presentation than elevated temperature. All neonates with hypothermia should be treated as septic.
- Causes other than SBI, especially herpes simplex virus (HSV) infection, should be considered and, if suspected, treated expectantly.
- Noninfectious problems, such as congenital heart disease (CHD) and inborn errors of metabolism, may present in a similar way and must always be on the list of potential causes of the septic-appearing infant.
- If the child is exhibiting signs of shock, such as tachycardia, mottling, apnea or prolonged capillary refill time, aggressive fluid resuscitation must be immediate.
- Antibiotics should be started after cultures have been obtained.
- If the child is unstable, the lumbar puncture may need to be postponed.

The risk of serious bacterial infection (SBI) is greatest during the neonatal period, defined as birth to 28 days of life. Some authorities recommend that a child born prematurely should have the degree of immaturity subtracted from the child's chronological age for this consideration. Since the initial publication of practice guidelines in 1993, many advances have occurred in the management of neonates with fever without source.[1] Hematogenous spread is most frequent in neonates, resulting from colonization of the nasopharynx, which occurs early in life. Bacteria can enter the blood stream from the pharynx at any time, but more frequently following a viral prodrome. There is general consensus among emergency physicians regarding the management of the febrile neonate. With a documented history of a fever, infants will undergo a sepsis workup (Table 2–1) and be admitted to the hospital for 48 to 72 hours of antibiotic coverage. The length of treatment will depend on the findings of the initial workup and the child's clinical condition.[2] Because of the increasing problem with drug resistance, iatrogenic problems, and the relatively low incidence of SBIs in febrile neonates, efforts are underway to see if any specific tests can allow febrile neonates with low-risk factors to be observed without use of antibiotics and hospitalization.[3] Although some studies have shown that febrile neonates who fit low-risk criteria (Table 2–2) can be managed without antibiotics, hospitalization and close observation are still required at a minimum.[4] A recent consensus conference on pediatric sepsis has suggested dividing the neonatal period into the newborn (0–7 days) and neonate (7–30 days) for purposes of future studies and recommendations.[5]

Specific causes of the febrile- or septic-appearing neonate include infections, such as meningitis, urinary tract infection, pneumonia, and septicemia. The most frequent bacterial pathogens in the neonatal period are GBS, *E. coli*, and *L. monocytogenes*. Other bacterial causes include *Hemophilus influenza*, *Staphylococcus aureus*, *Neisseria meningitidis*, and *Salmonella*. Of the numerous viral agents, *Herpes simplex* (HSV) and nonpolio enterovirus are the most common causes of serious illness in the neonate. In the past year, this author has seen numerous cases of influenza causing a septic appearance in children younger than 4 weeks. Noninfectious causes include CHD and inborn errors of metabolism.

The etiology, presentation, and ED management of the febrile neonate will be discussed. The ED physician is faced with several significant decisions in the management of patients in this period of life.

▶ FEVER

It is generally accepted that a fever is a temperature of ≥38°C or 100.4°F taken with a rectal thermometer. Although not as accurate, temperature may be taken by the axillary or otic routes and elevated temperatures taken by these routes must also be considered a fever. A normal temperature taken by either of these methods must be repeated. A frequent dilemma is encountered when a parent presents with an infant who felt warm to the parent or was given an antipyretic and is afebrile at the time of examination. A neonate who had a documented

▶ **TABLE 2-1. POTENTIAL EVALUATION OF THE FEBRILE NEONATE**

Complete blood count (CBC)
Blood culture
Urinalysis and culture (regardless of U/A results)—catheterized specimen
Lumbar puncture with cell count and differential, culture, protein, glucose
CSF-PCR for herpes and enterovirus
Chest radiograph (when indicated)
Complete metabolic panel (electrolytes, glucose, liver function tests)
Stool culture and leukocyte count (with diarrhea)
C-reactive protein
Procalcitonin

fever by any method but is afebrile on admission to the ED should be treated as a febrile neonate whether or not antipyretics have been given. Often, a minimally elevated temperature is attributed to "bundling" of the child. Accepting this reason and not observing or evaluating the child is risky.

Hypothermia in the neonatal period may actually be a more common presentation than elevated temperature.[3] All neonates with hypothermia should be treated as septic.[1] Hypothermia is a rectal temperature less than 36°C or 96.8°F.

▶ CLINICAL PRESENTATION

The first step in the assessment of the neonate is review of the vital signs (Table 2–3). The presence of fever is obvious but the septic neonate can present with a wide variety of signs and symptoms which may be due to serious infection. Hypothermia may be present and when noted in the ED must never be discounted unless there is a definite exposure to a cold environment. All vital signs are important. Persistent tachycardia or any bradycardia may be a sign of sepsis.

Either irritability or lethargy may be present and the parent's complaint about a change in the child's behavior must be taken seriously even if the child appears in no distress at the time of examination in the ED. Children who do not exhibit normal patterns of hunger and interest in feeding must also be presumed to be at risk for serious illness. Abdominal distension, vomiting, or diarrhea may also presage an underlying infection. Many illnesses will present with respiratory symptoms such as cough, tachypnea, wheezing, grunting, or apnea. The child may also present with a variety of skin findings, some of which represent the presence or potential of underlying illness.

▶ **TABLE 2-2. LOW-RISK CRITERIA FOR FEBRILE NEONATES[3]**

Unremarkable medical history
Good appearance
No focal physical signs of infection
Erythrocyte sedimentation rate (ESR) <30 at the end of the first hour
White blood cell (WBC) count 5000–15 000
Normal urinalysis by dipstick

▶ **TABLE 2-3. NORMAL VITAL SIGNS FOR THE NEONATAL PERIOD[5]**

Vital sign parameter	0–7 d	7–30 d
Heart rate	100–180	100–180
Respiratory rate	<50	<40
Blood pressure (systolic)	>65	>75

▶ SPECIFIC BACTERIAL ETIOLOGIES

The most common bacterial causes of infections in the neonate are GBS, *E. coli*, and other gram-negative enteric organisms, *L. monocytogenes*, *Streptococcus pneumoniae*, *H. influenza*, *S. aureus*, *Neisseria meningitis*, and *Salmonella*. GBS has been the most common gram-positive organism causing sepsis and meningitis in the United States since the 1970s.[6] Up to 30% of pregnant women are colonized with GBS in the vagina or rectum. Although up to 50% of newborns born to infected mothers are colonized with GBS, only 1% develop serious bacterial illness (sepsis, meningitis, pneumonia, or urinary tract infection). GBS disease has been classified into early onset (first week of life) and late onset (after the first week). Intrapartum prophylaxis of infected mothers has reduced the incidence of early-onset GBS disease but not eradicated it. Early-onset GBS disease presents with nonspecific symptoms, while fever is more common in late-onset disease. *E. coli* is the second most common cause of bacterial meningitis in the neonate. More frequently, it causes a urinary tract infection in the neonate. *L. monocytogenes* is the third most frequent cause of bacterial infection in the neonate. The fatality rate can be as high as 45%. Although any of the physical signs and symptoms of sepsis may be present, respiratory distress was the most common initial presentation in one study followed by fever, seizure, apnea, and skin rash or mottling.[7] Listeriosis, like GBS, has an early- and late-onset form. Early onset occurs within the first week of life and is often associated with maternal illness and preterm delivery. Because of the possibility of *Listeria* infection, ampicillin remains one of the empiric antibiotics.

▶ SPECIFIC VIRAL ETIOLOGIES

The two most frequent causes of viral meningitis and sepsis in the neonatal period are herpes (HSV-2, although HSV-1 is becoming more frequent)[8] and enterovirus. Contact with HSV in the maternal genital tract at the time of labor accounts for 90% of the causes of neonatal herpes.[9] Clinical presentation of HSV disease in the neonate is nonspecific. Vesicular skin lesions are the most indicative finding of HSV disease but are absent in up to 40% of cases.[10] HSV infection has three occasionally overlapping presentations: meningitis, disseminated and localized infection of skin, eyes, or mouth. Hepatitis and coagulopathy may be present but fever is often absent. Disseminated herpes infection accounts for 25% of cases, usually occurs during the first week of life and has the highest mortality (85%). Mortality is 50% with meningitis and the majority of survivors have neurological deficits. Although new antiviral drugs are being studied, acyclovir remains the drug of choice against HSV 1 and 2 and *Varicella zoster*. The recommended dose is 60 mg/kg/d for 14 days in disseminated infection and 21 days with CNS disease.[10]

Nonpolio enterovirus also causes infection in the first month of life. Neonates with this infection may present anywhere from asymptomatic-to-severe meningoencephalitis or sepsis. Enterovirus infections were the most frequently identified pathogen in neonates from 8 to 29 days of age in one study. There may be a history of post- or peripartum fever in the mother or in other members of the family. Symptoms are nonspecific. Fever or hypothermia may be present as well as a nonspecific rash. A biphasic disease with initial mild symptoms, recovery followed by more severe symptoms is also common with enteroviral infection. Severe disease may include sepsis, meningoencephalitis, myocarditis, pneumonia, hepatitis, or coagulopathy.[11] Diagnosis of enteroviral infection is done by enterovirus PCR assays. Patients with enteroviral disease are initially treated as other febrile/septic neonates including acyclovir. Immunoglobulin therapy has also been used. Specific antiviral therapy is currently in development. General supportive care is provided as outlined above.

▶ EVALUATION

Evaluation of the neonate begins with assessment of the child's general condition. In the hemodynamically stable child, a systematic examination is performed looking for any obvious signs of infection (e.g., otitis media, and pneumonia). As these are often absent, the physical examination must look for the more subtle findings of early infection. These include general interaction with environment, interest in feeding, tone, and irritability with motion. All neonates should have a thorough evaluation of the skin. Early petechiae may appear on the buttocks and can be missed. Rashes are usually nonspecific blanching, maculopapular blanching, and generalized blanching. Vesicular rashes may indicate a herpetic infection. Bullae may represent impetigo. Any cellulitis or abscess is a potentially serious finding. Petechiae and purpura are ominous signs. Mottling of the extremities may also be an early sign of sepsis.

For the febrile but well-appearing neonate, the evaluation is outlined in Table 2–1. The basic laboratory evaluations have remained standard. A complete blood count and blood cultures should be obtained. Urine must be collected in a sterile fashion (catheterization or suprapubic aspirate). A bag-collected specimen is never acceptable for a culture. Regardless of the results of the urinalysis, a culture should be obtained, as neonates may have a normal urinalysis and still have a urinary tract infection.

A lumbar puncture should be obtained. If the specimen is contaminated with blood, the same tests should be performed, especially the culture. One must be certain, however, that it is a specimen of cerebral spinal fluid and not just blood obtained during the procedure by penetration of venous vessels. This is usually obvious but a simple test of letting a drop of the fluid fall on the sterile paper will give a double ring sign if it contains both blood and CSF. Because these children will receive empiric antibiotics, the debate regarding how to evaluate a bloody tap is not as important as in the older child. Of significant concern however is the question of ordering CSF-HSV-PCR to diagnose HSV disease. While it is not recommended that every neonate who has a lumbar puncture should have the fluid examined for HSV, there are some neonates who should be tested for HSV. These include those with seizure activity, bloody lumbar puncture (especially with a mononuclear CSF pleocytosis), afebrile septic-appearing infants, those with elevated serum transaminases, and those with a rash consistent with herpetic lesions.[12]

A chest radiograph is indicated if there are signs or symptoms of a respiratory infection or if another cause of septic appearance is considered (EG and CHD).

Tests for other viral pathogens (enterovirus, influenza A and B, rotavirus, and RSV) have been recommended in the appropriate season and presentation. It has been suggested that febrile infants with confirmed viral infections are at lower risk for SBI than those in whom a viral illness is not identified.[13]

Several other tests have been recommended but are of more use in deciding whether or not a patient needs admission and antibiotic therapy. As this is not as much an issue in the neonate, their importance may not be as great. C-reactive protein (CRP) is an acute phase protein synthesized in the liver in response to increases in interleukin-6, interleukin-1b, and tumor necrosis factor. It starts being formed approximately 6 hours after the beginning of an infection and peaks around 36 hours. It has been recommended to distinguish between viral and bacterial infections early in the course of an illness.[14] While the CRP may not be useful in the decision to start antibiotics, it may play a role in the length of therapy in a neonate if the cultures recommended above are not useful because of pretreatment with antibiotics. This would be especially true if the WBC count and CRP are both elevated.[15] A recent study, which included neonates, found the CRP useful in distinguishing between bacterial and viral gastroenteritis.[16] Other early-phase reactants are being investigated in the evaluation of neonatal sepsis. These include procalcitonin, interleukin-6 and -8, tumor necrosis factor-alpha, and some leukocyte surface antigens.[17]

▶ TREATMENT

The first priority in the febrile- or septic-appearing neonate is assuring hemodynamic stability, adequate ventilation, and temperature control (for the hypothermic child). Some of the initial testing can be done simultaneously, but other tests, especially the lumbar puncture, may need to be delayed until the child is stabilized. An intravenous line should be placed and an immediate check of the blood glucose performed. If hypoglycemia is detected, it should be corrected immediately since hypoglycemia is a stress to the infant and can mimic shock. The remainder of the laboratory tests are listed in Table 2–1. During this period, it is critical to maintain the infant's temperature. While reducing an elevated temperature is not a critical factor, hypothermia, either pathogenic or iatrogenic, must be avoided by appropriate use of warmers. Hypothermia adds an additional, unnecessary stress to the neonate and can mimic signs of shock.

If the child is exhibiting signs of shock, such as tachycardia, mottling, apnea, or prolonged capillary refill time, aggressive fluid resuscitation must be immediate. If rehydration fails to reestablish hemodynamic stability, pressor agents should be started. Antibiotics should be started after cultures have been obtained. If the child is unstable, the lumbar puncture may need to be postponed (Table 2–4).

▶ **TABLE 2–4. ANTIBIOTIC THERAPY FOR THE FEBRILE- OR SEPTIC-APPEARING NEONATE**[21]

	BW 1200–2000 g	BW >2000 g
Infants Younger Than 1 wk (mg/kg)		
Gentamicin IV, IM	2.5 q 12 h	2.5 q 12 h
Cefotaxime IV, IM	50 q 12 h	50 q 8 or 12 h
Cefrtriaxone IV, IM	50 q 24 h	50 q 24 h
Ampicillin IV, IM	25–50 q 12 h	25–50 q 8 h
Vancomycin IV	10–15 q 12–18 h	10–15 q 8–12 h
Clindamycin IV, IM, PO	5 q 12 h	5 q 8 h
Erythromycin PO	10 q 12 h	10 q 12 h
Infants Aged 7 to 28 d (mg/kg)		
Gentamicin IV, IM	2.5 q 8 or 12 h	2.5 q 8
Cefotaxime IV, IM	50 q 8 h	50 q 8 or 12 h
Ceftriaxone IV, IM	50 q 24 h	50–75 q 24 h
Ampicillin IV, IM	25–50 q 8 h	25–50 q 6 h
Vancomycin IV	10–15 q 8–12 h	10–15 q 6–8 h
Clindamycin IV, IM, PO	5 q 8 h	5–7.5 q 6 h
Erythromycin PO	10 q 8 h	10 q 8 h

▶ SPECIFIC CONDITIONS THAT MAY PRESENT AS OR LIKE NEONATAL SEPSIS

PERTUSSIS

Although there is widespread immunization against pertussis, it is still present. Neonates have the highest risk of morbidity and mortality and present with atypical signs and symptoms. In 2000, infants younger than 4 months accounted for all of the mortality from pertussis. High-risk factors include preterm delivery and teenage mothers. Pertussis is caused by *Bordatella pertussis*, a gram-negative bacillus whose only host is humans. Transmission is spread by respiratory secretions. Classically, there are three stages: catarrhal, paroxysmal, and convalescent. Because the symptoms of the catarrhal phase may be mild and it is often shorter in neonates, the diagnosis is usually not suspected. During the paroxysmal stage, the characteristic "whoop" may be absent. Patients may become dehydrated because of posttussive emesis. Physical signs and symptoms are often nonspecific and include hypoxia, poor feeding, apnea, and seizures.[18] Characteristic laboratory tests such as leukocytosis with lymphocyte predominance may not be present. Classically, the diagnosis is by nasopharyngeal culture but these are most frequently positive in the early catarrhal stage and because this stage may be brief in the neonate, the opportunity for positive culture is brief. Additional tests include direct immunofluoresence assay and PCR of nasopharyngeal specimens. PCR tests may be more reliable. Chest radiographs can have a wide variety of findings. Treatment, in addition to those items mentioned above, should include the addition of erythromycin to the antibiotic therapy. Respiratory support may be required.

CONGENITAL HEART DISEASE

Congenital heart disease (CHD) may present at any time after birth and may present with similar signs and symptoms to those of sepsis. A detailed discussion of CHD is provided in Chapter 46.

INBORN ERRORS OF METABOLISM

Inborn errors of metabolism consist of more than 400 currently known conditions. See Chapter 80 for discussion.

CHLAMYDIA INFECTIONS

Although not usually causing serious infection, *Chlamydia trachomatis* infection can occur in the first month of life. In addition to *Neisseria gonorrhea*, *C. trachomatis* is one of the causes of ophthalmia neonatorum. The patient presents with copious purulent discharge and requires aggressive IV antibiotic therapy. Ophthalmia neonatorum can be followed by *Chlamydia* pneumonia, which usually presents with staccato cough, tachypnea, and rales, but without fever. Chest radiographs typically show bilateral interstitial infiltrates and hyperinflation. A CBC may show eosinophilia. Diagnosis can be made by antigen test performed by ELISA and direct detection of *C. trachomatis* IgM and IgG.[19] Treatment is 14 days of erythromycin or 5 days of azithromycin. This infection is often misdiagnosed as bronchiolitis.

OMPHALITIS

Because of the neonates relative inability to localize and fight infection, several conditions in which the neonate is neither febrile nor septic-appearing require the same aggressive management. Omphalitis is an infection of the area around the umbilicus with the potential for vascular and abdominal extension. With the recent increase in MRSA infections, antibiotic coverage should be directed against this organism until culture and sensitivities are available.

CEPHALOHEMATOMAS

Infected cephalohematomas, although uncommon, do occur usually in association with vacuum extraction, amnionitis, instrumental delivery, electronic fetal monitoring, prolonged delivery, or prolonged rupture of membranes. Because these infections are usually polymicrobial, broad-spectrum antibiotics are indicated.[20]

REFERENCES

1. Baraff LJ, Schriger DL, Bass JW, et al. Practice guideline for the management of infants and children 0 to 36 months with fever without source. *Pediatrics.* 1993;92:1–12.
2. Kourtis A, Sullivan D, Sathian U. Practice guidelines for the management of febrile infants less than 90 days of age at the ambulatory network of a large pediatric health care system

in the United States: summary of new evidence. *Clin Pediatr (Phila).* 2004;43(1):11–16.

3. Marom R, Sakran W, Antonelli J, et al. Quick identification of febrile neonates with low risk for serious bacterial infection: an observational study. *Arch Dis Child Fetal Neonatal ED.* 2007;92:15–18.

4. Rudd P. Is there a place for "drive thru" management of neonatal fever? Not yet! *Arch Dis Child Fetal Neonatal ED.* 2007;92: 2–3.

5. Goldstein B, Giror B, Randolph A, et al. International pediatric sepsis consensus conference: definitions for sepsis organ dysfunction in pediatrics. *Pediat Crit Care Med.* 2005;6(1):2–8.

6. Chung M, Ko D, Chen C, et al. Neonatal group B streptococcal infection: a 7-year experience. *Chang Gung Med J.* 2004;27(7): 501–508.

7. Chen S, Leigh F, Lee P. Neonatal listeriosis. *J Formos Med Assoc.* 2007;106(2):161–164.

8. Handsfield H, Waldo A, Brown Z, et al. Neonatal herpes should be a reportable disease. *Sex Transm Dis.* 2008;35(1):22–24.

9. Kimberlin D. Neonatal herpes simplex infections. *Clin Microbiol Rev.* 2004;17:1–13.

10. Luck S, Sharland M, Griffiths P, et al. Advances in the antiviral therapy of herpes virus infection in children. *Expert Rev Anti Infect Ther.* 2006;4(6):1005–1020.

11. Abzug MJ. Presentation, diagnosis, and management of enterovirus infections in neonates. *Pediatr Drugs.* 2004;6(1):1–10.

12. Cohen D, Lorch S, King R, et al. Factors influencing the decision to test young infants for herpes simplex virus infection. *Ped Infect Dis J.* 2004;26(12):1156–1158.

13. Byington C, Enriquez F, Hoff C, et al. Serious bacterial infections in febrile infants 1 to 90 days old with and without viral infections. *Pediatrics.* 2004;113:1662–1666.

14. Papaevangelou V, Papassotiriou I, Sakou I, et al. Evaluation of a quick test for C-reactive protein in an emergency department. *Scan J Clin Lab Invest.* 2006;66:717–722.

15. Peltola V, Toikka P, Irjala K, et al. Discrepancy between total white blood cell counts and serum C-reactive protein levels in febrile children. *Scan J Infect Dis.* 2007;39:560–565.

16. Marcus N, Mor M, Amir L, et al. The quick read C-reactive protein test for the prediction of bacterial gastroenteritis in the pediatric emergency department. *Ped Emerg Care.* 2007;23(9): 634–637.

17. Kocabas E, Sarikcioglu A, Aksaray N, et al. Role of procalcitonin, C-reactive protein, interleukin-6, interleukin-8 and tumor necrosis factor-alpha in the diagnosis of neonatal sepsis. *Turk J Pediatr.* 2007;49:7–20.

18. Colletti J, Homme J, Woodridge D. Unsuspected neonatal killers in emergency medicine. *Emerg Med Clin North Am.* 2004;22:929–960.

19. Chen C, Wu K, Tand R, et al. Characteristics of Chlamydia trachomatis infection in hospitalized infants with lower respiratory tract infection. *J Micrbiol Immunol Infect.* 2007;40:255–259.

20. Brook I. Infected neonatal cephalohematomas caused by anaerobic bacteria. *J Perinat Med.* 2005;33:255–258.

21. American Academy of Pediatrics. Tables of antibacterial drug dosages. In: Pickering LK, Baker GJ, Long SS, et al, eds. *Red Book: 2006 Report of the Committee on Infectious Disease.* 27th ed. Elk Grove Village, IL: American Academy of Pediatrics; 2006:751–752.

CHAPTER 3

The Febrile- or Septic-Appearing Infant or Child

Ron D. Waldrop and Robert A. Felter

► HIGH-YIELD FACTS

- The risk of bacteremia appears to have been modified dramatically by the use of more advanced broad-spectrum antibiotics, advanced diagnostic testing, and immunization against *Hemophilus influenza* and *Streptococcus pneumoniae*. A positive blood culture is nearly as likely to be due to a contaminant as to a real pathogen.
- Given the extremely low risk of bacteremia and its sequelae, the best expectant therapy in the well-appearing child is close observation and follow-up pending culture results.
- Tachycardia and tachypnea may be the only indications of a serious illness in an otherwise well-appearing febrile child.
- Signs of clinical toxicity include altered or decreased mental status; significantly abnormal vital signs; dyspnea; color changes, such as cyanosis and pallor; and hypoxia, as measured by pulse oximetry. These children require immediate stabilization including airway management, oxygen, intravenous access and administration of saline fluid bolus, temperature management, rapid examination, laboratory evaluation and immediate empiric antibiotic therapy, pending further diagnosis.
- Well-appearing febrile infants who have no identifiable source and normal leukocyte count, chest radiograph and urinalysis, and who are fully immunized may be safely discharged with symptomatic care for close follow-up of cultures without presumptive antibiotic therapy.
- In the nontoxic child with no obvious clinical syndrome, risk factors for serious bacterial infection need to be determined, including fever greater than 39°C; age <2 months; unimmunized status; chronic diseases such as asthma, congenital heart disease, and CSF shunts; and immunocompromised patients.
- When risk factors are present, a workup should be performed including a complete blood count with leukocyte and immature neutrophil count and markers of inflammation including C-reactive protein, blood culture, and urinalysis and urine culture in established risk groups. Lumbar puncture and spinal fluid analysis should be performed in those children who appear to have or are at risk for meningitis.
- In those with no identified source, the chart should clearly reflect cardiorespiratory stability, adequate feeding behavior, adequate urine output, and alertness at the time of discharge. Follow-up must be arranged before discharge with symptomatic care only.

Fever is the most common complaint for children presenting to the emergency department (ED), representing more than 20% of all presenting complaints annually.[1] The evaluation of fever in the pediatric patient is complicated by age-related variations such as patient's ability to communicate, immune system development, immunization status, the presence of fever in both minor and serious illness, and parental perception of seriousness. Similarly, advances in the understanding of clinical assessment, diagnostic modalities, and treatment regimens are ongoing. As a result, the classic approach to febrile children by age group is under constant revision.[2–6] While little disagreement exists regarding the management of neonates younger than 30 days, considerable disagreement and practice variation exists for children 30 days to 36 months of age. In children older than 36 months, there are more reliable clinical findings and the risk of disseminated bacterial infection is low. As a result, clinical evaluation, diagnostic testing, and treatment focus on a specific source of infection and therefore there is greater agreement among practitioners. In addition, older febrile patients who have a viral illness require no further workup. This chapter deals specifically with the infant and young child between the ages of 1 and 36 months.

► THERMOREGULATION

Humans maintain body temperature at a level that is within two standard deviations above or below the mean. Variations above and below this range are termed hyperthermia or fever and hypothermia. Maintenance of body temperature involves a complex interplay of physiologic heat loss by radiation, evaporation, convection, and conduction; heat gain by metabolic and physiologic activity; and variations in ambient temperature. Examples of heat exchange mechanisms include sweating and hyperventilation for losses, shivering and catabolism for heat gain, and swaddling for ambient temperature changes.

The thermoregulatory center is located in the preoptic region of the hypothalamus and damage to this area may result in extreme body temperature variations. The immature thermoregulatory mechanisms in young infants and children may result in susceptibility to temperature extremes due to either physiologic or external reasons.

Significant variation may occur between temperatures measured externally (axillary) and those measured in core areas (rectal) with core temperatures more accurately and consistently reflecting overall body temperature status. Therefore, the gold standard for measuring core body temperature in the noncritical care setting is rectally by either glass mercury thermometer or electronic probe. Other sites, such as axillary, oral, tympanic, or skin, and other devices, such as infrared or liquid crystal, may serve as effective screening tools but are less accurate in the young infant and child.[7,8]

► FEVER

Fever in young infants and children is defined as a body temperature greater than 100.4°F (38°C).[4,5] Fever may occur in association with infection, immune-related illness including response to immunizations, collagen vascular disease, heat illness, and malignancy.[9,10] Infections result in fever due to a complex cascade of cell mediators released during the immune system response. Therefore, fever represents the normal response to infection and has many beneficial effects on immune function. The vast majority of febrile children have benign self-limited viral illnesses or simple bacterial infections, although a small but significant number may have an SBI (Table 3–1). Nonetheless, fever may cause any child to appear ill due to increased metabolic rate, decreased peripheral vascular resistance, and increased tissue demand leading to tachypnea, tachycardia, diaphoresis, and chills.[11] In addition, there is no reliable relationship between fever height and the clinical response to antipyretics in predicting serious illness.[2] The most important consideration is merely the presence of any fever.

Hyperpyrexia is defined as an extreme body temperature elevation above 106°F (41.1°C).[12,13] Hyperpyrexia is associated with a significant increased risk of serious infection, but is also associated with central nervous system abnormalities, medication toxicity, as with psychotropic drugs and neuroleptic malignant syndrome from anesthetics, and heat stroke (Table 3–2). Hyperpyrexia is associated with an increased incidence of febrile seizures and rhabdomyolysis.

Parents often panic at the presence of fever, fearing seizures or brain damage, and do not understand the beneficial aspects. Parental education should attempt to provide

► TABLE 3–1. FEBRILE ILLNESSES IN CHILDREN YOUNGER THAN 36 MONTHS

Viral	Bacterial
Croup	Pharyngitis (Strep)
Stomatitis	Otitis media
Roseola	Sinusitis
Influenza	Lymphadenitis
Bronchiolitis	UTI
Gastroenteritis	Abscess
Influenza	Consolidated pneumonia
Pharyngitis (viral)	Meningitis
Upper respiratory infection	Osteomyelitis
Interstitial pneumonia	Septic arthritis
Varicella	

► TABLE 3–2. NONINFECTIOUS CAUSES OF FEVER

Excessive clothing
Ambient hyperthermia
Medications
    Side effects, as with psychotropics
    Overdose, EG, aspirin
    Interaction, EG, anesthetic agents (neuroleptic malignant syndrome)
Central nervous system abnormalities
    Congenital malformations
    Trauma

parents with an understanding of the use of antipyretics to treat symptoms and not to cure the disease. When possible, parents should also be brought to understand the recurrent nature of fever and the lack of relationship of height of temperature to the presence of serious illness. The likelihood of a benign viral illness as the cause for most febrile illness in infants and children should be stressed.[2,3,14] Significant parental coaching is often warranted to avoid over- or underevaluation and treatment.

► SEPSIS

Pediatric sepsis is the most common cause of death in infants and children worldwide and may be caused by bacterial, viral, parasitic, or fungal organisms.[15] Sepsis is more correctly termed systemic immune response syndrome (SIRS) and is defined by temperature instability, age inappropriate tachycardia or tachypnea, as well as an abnormal leukocyte count (Table 3–3).[16] SIRS represents one step in the continuum from infection to occult bacteremia, SIRS, severe sepsis, septic shock, and finally multiorgan dysfunction syndrome (MODS). When managing fever in young infants and children, the goal is to clinically distinguish those children having SIRS (toxic-appearing) and needing immediate evaluation and intervention from those who are nontoxic but have an increased risk of bacteremia with SIRS or those who have a self-limited viral illness.[17] Much of the research in this area over the last 35 years has dealt with the selection of febrile children at risk for bacteremia and SBI that are not clinically apparent.

► BACTEREMIA

Early studies on bacteremia in young infants and children demonstrated a correlation between fever and likelihood of bacteremia. In these early studies, fevers of 100.5°F were associated with approximately 1% risk of bacteremia, 102.2°F with a 3% to 11% risk, and 104°F with a 4% to 11% risk.[2,3,6,8] Up to 80% of bacteria isolated in these studies were represented by *H. influenzae*, *S. pneumoniae*, and *Nisseria meningitides*. Bacteremia from such organisms results in significant risk of end organ damage including meningitis, osteomyelitis, urinary tract infection (UTI), and pneumonia, all of which are potentially fatal. Each of these will be discussed in depth in other

▶ **TABLE 3-3. DEFINITIONS FOR THE CONTINUUM OF PEDIATRIC SEPSIS**

Infection
  A suspected or proven infection caused by any pathogen or a clinical syndrome associated with a high probability of infection

Bacteremia
  Presence of a bacterial pathogen in the circulatory system and demonstrated by blood culture which may or may not be causing overt illness

Systemic immune response syndrome (SIRS)
  The presence of two of the following four criteria with one being abnormal temperature or leukocyte count:
  a. Temperature >38.5°C or <36°C
  b. Age inappropriate tachycardia or bradycardia in the absence of other modifying stimuli such as medications, fever, or stress
  c. Age inappropriate tachypnea in the absence of modifying medication or neuromuscular disease
  d. Abnormal leukocyte count or >10% immature neutrophils

Sepsis
  SIRS in the presence of, or as result of, a suspected or proven infection

Severe sepsis
  Sepsis plus one of the following: cardiovascular dysfunction, respiratory distress, or two other organ dysfunctions

Septic shock
  Sepsis and cardiovascular dysfunction such as age inappropriate hypotension, need for vasoactive drugs, metabolic acidosis, lactic acidosis, oliguria, poor capillary refill, or core to peripheral temperature gap of >3°C

Multiorgan dysfunction syndrome (MODS)
  Sepsis with more than two organ systems impaired including cardiovascular, respiratory, neurologic, hematologic, renal, and hepatic

chapters. Infections with these organisms can present in the same way as common benign childhood illnesses.[3,4,6,18]

In more recent studies, the risk of bacteremia appears to have been modified dramatically by the use of more advanced broad-spectrum antibiotics, advanced diagnostic testing, and immunization first against *H. influenzae* and subsequently against *S. pneumoniae*.[3,18–20] A summary of current literature estimates that the risk of *H. influenzae* is negligible and the risk of *S. pneumoniae* is less than 1% to 2%. This means a positive blood culture is nearly as likely to be due to a contaminant as to a real pathogen.[20]

Unfortunately, new and more resistant bacteria, such as methicillin-resistant *Staphylococcus aureus* (with skin and soft tissue infections) and *Escherichia coli* (with UTI) are now the most common causes of bacteremia and are equally capable of being invasive or leading to fulminant infection and sepsis. In the well-appearing febrile child who has no source but laboratory evidence of infection, such as an abnormal leukocyte count, elevated immature neutrophil percentage, or ele-

vated inflammatory markers, such as C-reactive protein (CRP), some have suggested expectant therapy with a single parenteral dose of ceftriaxone pending culture results.[4,6] However, presumptive antibiotic therapy has not been shown to prevent bacteremia.[21] In addition, antibiotic therapy may have significant side effects, including promotion of bacterial resistance, gastrointestinal symptoms, and allergies. Reports of interaction between ceftriaxone and calcium-containing intravenous fluids, leading to lethal precipitation of crystalline material in the lungs and kidneys of neonates, have led to warnings against concomitant use of these two agents for all age groups. Antibiotics may also cloud further evaluation for serious illnesses such as meningitis. Given the extremely low risk of bacteremia and its sequelae, the best expectant therapy in the well-appearing child is close observation and follow-up pending culture results.

▶ **PRESENTATION AND HISTORY**

Careful history is one of the keys to accurate diagnosis in young infants and children. The primary caretaker should be asked about methods of fever measurement as well as fever onset, timing, height, and response to antipyretics. Lack of caretaker familiarity with thermometers and pretreatment of fever before arrival may result in misleading information and inaccurate conclusions.

The caretaker's perception of illness is vitally important as a background description of normal and abnormal behavior in the patient.[22] Specific observations include activity level, feeding behavior, and interactive behavior. It is important to use common terms familiar to parents, such as fussiness and drowsiness, rather than medical terms such as irritability or lethargy, which may be misunderstood.

An extensive discussion of symptoms from head to toe may elicit important diagnostic clues. Respiratory tract symptoms are common and may include upper respiratory tract complaints, such as congestion, cough, sore throat, or ear pain, while lower respiratory tract symptoms may include cough, wheezing, noisy breathing, or shortness of breath with increased work. Ominous symptoms of respiratory tract disease include difficulty feeding, cyanotic color changes, grunting, and apneic episodes. Because of physiologic reserve in young infants and children, symptoms described by the parents may be intermittent with intervening periods of relatively normal behavior. A history of ill-appearance should be treated with the same concern as ill-appearance in the ED.

Gastrointestinal symptoms are common in the febrile patient. These may include vomiting, diarrhea, or feeding refusal and may be found in both minor or serious and viral or bacterial illnesses. Gastrointestinal symptoms can be among the presenting complaints of SBI, such as meningitis, UTI, pneumonia, and sepsis. In vomiting patients, the character of the emesis, whether bilious or nonbilious and whether projectile or nonprojectile, may be informative. Similarly, the presence of blood in diarrheal stools may indicate serious infection.

Skin and musculoskeletal symptoms may also be important clinical cues. Certain illnesses, such as roseola, Fifth's disease, or scarlet fever, have characteristic appearances. The timing of the appearance of a rash as it relates to the onset of fever can be an important observation. The most ominous skin symptom or sign is the presence of petechiae or purpura, which may indicate disseminated intravascular coagulation (DIC) and potential life-threatening sepsis.

Musculoskeletal symptoms may include limp or refusal to walk and arthritis or arthralgia. Musculoskeletal symptoms may be intermittent.

Many infectious diseases are highly contagious. These range from minor illnesses such as colds to serious infections such as tuberculosis. Exposures from family members or friends or day care exposures may provide important clues to diagnosis.

Proper immunization significantly reduces the likelihood of SBI caused by *H. influenzae* and *S. pneumoniae*, as well as the classic childhood illnesses of diphtheria, pertussis, polio, and varicella. In addition, a history of recent immunization adds the possibility of febrile reaction to the differential and may prevent unnecessary evaluation and treatment.

Finally, medication history is vital in properly evaluating fever. Antipyretics may improve a child's symptoms and provide a false sense of security on presentation. Antibiotic treatment may cause false negative culture evaluation of a patient and result in either undertreatment of a serious illness such as meningitis or result in overtreatment of an illness due to the inability to rule out such an illness.

▶ PHYSICAL EXAMINATION

The physical examination is of paramount importance in evaluating a febrile infant or child and remains the most useful tool in determining risk of SBI and the need for antibiotic therapy.[22,23] Skill at determining risk for SBI on physical examination results from a combination of careful observation, training, experience, and clinical judgment. Despite variability and subjectivity, some important reproducible principles do exist.

Often, the first clues to significant illness are abnormal vital signs. Vital signs should be compared with published age-appropriate norms for heart and respiratory rate. Heart rate is known to be affected by many factors, including fever, which may elevate the pulse rate up to 10 beats per minute per degree.[11] However, tachycardia may also indicate hypoperfusion and septic shock. Bradycardia is an ominous sign, potentially indicating impending cardiorespiratory arrest. Tachypnea may be the result of fever, hypoxia, or acidosis associated with serious illness. Bradypnea is also a cardinal sign of impending respiratory arrest and mandates immediate airway stabilization. Tachycardia and tachypnea may be the only indications of a serious illness in an otherwise well-appearing febrile child.

In the unstable child, signs of clinical toxicity include altered or decreased mental status, significantly abnormal vital signs, dyspnea, color changes such as cyanosis and pallor, and hypoxia as measured by pulse oximetry. These children require immediate stabilization including airway management, oxygen, intravenous access and administration of saline fluid bolus, temperature management, rapid examination, laboratory evaluation, and immediate empiric antibiotic therapy pending further diagnosis.

Examination of the clinically stable child should include an assessment of mental status, including activity level and in-

teraction with parents, as well as interaction with the health care provider. In the young infant, poor feeding behavior and poor consolability may be important clues to serious illness. In the older child, anxiety may be normal but should be lessened when the child is consoled in the parent's arms. The presence of a social smile is an important indicator of wellness. Decreased activity or lethargy is always a sign of serious illness. Finally, character of the cry may be informative, with a lusty loud cry suggesting a healthy child and a weak, high-pitched cry or absent cry suggesting a child who is seriously ill.

Assessment of perfusion is invaluable in determining the risk of serious illness. Normal peripheral perfusion is indicated by capillary refill of less than 3 seconds in a warm extremity. In the presence of dehydration or septic shock, perfusion will be delayed. Another hallmark of poor perfusion is decreased mental status. Reassessment of perfusion and mental status is mandatory as clinical condition may wax and wane in young infants and children due to cardiovascular reserve, but when the reserve is exhausted, sudden vascular collapse can occur. A hallmark of impending collapse is an ashen or mottled appearance of the skin. Any child with even a momentary decrease in mental status by history or examination should be considered seriously ill until proven otherwise.

A thorough head to toe examination for a source of fever should be performed. Skin findings may include rashes, redness associated with cellulitis, or pain associated with subcutaneous infections. Petechiae and purpura should always alert the practitioner to the possibility of meningococcal disease or sepsis, especially in the ill-appearing child. Petechiae distributed on the face and chest may also suggest intense vasalva maneuvers associated with vomiting or severe cough.

Head examination should include fontanel examination for fullness or pulsation, which may indicate meningitis, or depression, which may indicate dehydration. The eyes are examined for erythema and discharge as well as for periorbital swelling and redness. All patients should have a thorough examination of the ears, as otitis media is the most common bacterial illness diagnosed in childhood. The nose is examined for purulent discharge and the oropharyngeal cavity is examined for lesions, erythema, exudates, and swelling.

The neck is palpated for lymphadenopathy and localized swelling. Localized swelling may be associated with congenital anomalies, such as brachial cleft and thyroglossal duct cysts, which may become obstructed and secondarily infected. It is important to note that the absence of neck stiffness does not reliably exclude meningitis in the young infant and child.

The chest is evaluated for the presence of airway obstruction or lower respiratory tract pathology. Observation of increased work of breathing and stridor may indicate serious illness resulting from upper airway obstruction (retropharyngeal abscess, epiglottitis, or croup). Auscultation may reveal wheezes or rales from the lower respiratory tract or rhonchi referred from the upper respiratory tract.

Cardiac examination includes palpation of pulses for rate and strength as well as auscultation. Rubs or new murmurs may be findings of serious illnesses, such as infective endocarditis or rheumatic fever. This is especially true in children with a history of congenital heart disease.[24]

The abdomen is evaluated for tenderness, guarding, or rebound, which may indicate surgical illnesses, such as appendicitis. The presence of hepatosplenomegaly is associated

▶ TABLE 3-4. DECISION SCALES FOR PREDICTING FEBRILE PEDIATRIC PATIENTS AT LOW RISK FOR SERIOUS BACTERIAL ILLNESS

Scale	Year	Discussion	Age	Clinical Appearance	Laboratory
Yale	1982	2.7% risk of SBI	1–24 mo	Scale based on lusty cry, consolability, response to parents, alertness, pink color, perfusion.	None
Rochester	1985	Negative predictive value 98.5%	<60 d	Well-appearing; no source	Normal WBC, Bands <1500; normal urine and stool
Boston	1992	All given ceftriaxone, 50 mg/kg; 5.4% SBI	1–3 mo	Well-appearing (not well-defined); no source; temperature >38°C	Normal WBC (<20 000); normal urine, CSF, CXR, and stool
Philadelphia	1999	Correctly identified all SBI	29–56 d	Well-appearing (Yale scale <10); no source; temperature >38°C	Normal WBC (<15 000); bands <20%; normal urine, CSF, CXR, and stool

with many viral infections. A mass in the region of the kidney or suprapubic tenderness may indicate a significant UTI.

Finally, extremities are examined for movement, range of motion, swelling, and pain. Pain in an extremity or joint, especially with a limp, may be associated with septic arthritis and osteomyelitis.

▶ RISK OF SERIOUS BACTERIAL ILLNESS

In an attempt to identify infants and young children who are at low risk for clinically unapparent SBI, numerous studies have evaluated clinical findings and diagnostic tests. The Yale, Rochester, Boston, and Philadelphia criteria have been developed for this use (Table 3–4).[6,18,23] To summarize, well-appearing febrile infants who have no identifiable source and normal leukocyte count, chest radiograph, and urinalysis and are fully immunized may be safely discharged with symptomatic care for close follow-up of cultures without presumptive antibiotic therapy. It is important, however, to reiterate that no constellation of clinical findings has 100% sensitivity for selecting infants at low risk of SBI.

Numerous diagnostic tests, such as leukocyte count, immature neutrophil percentage, and CRP, have been evaluated for predicting risk of SBI either alone or in combination with clinical scales.[6,18,25] None of these alone have proven to be sufficiently sensitive for selecting children with SBI; however, they do have excellent negative predictive value when combined with predictive clinical findings[3,6,18] (Table 3–4). By considering the high risk of groups, such as unimmunized infants and immunocompromised patients (Table 3–5), and combining that with predictive constellations of clinical and laboratory findings, the clinician may make a superior assessment of SBI risk.[26–28]

▶ RISK OF SBI IN PATIENTS WITH VIRAL INFECTIONS

The majority of febrile infants and children have self-limited viral infections, although viral sepsis also may rarely result in life-threatening illness.[29] Viral illnesses may also mimic either minor or serious bacterial illnesses. The prevalence of common

viral infections is often predictable based on clinical presentation and season (Table 3–6).[30,31] The introduction of rapid viral testing for organisms, such as respiratory syncitial virus, influenza and rotavirus, has led to a decreased need for extensive laboratory workup.[6,18,32–35] The risk of SBI in the presence of these identifiable viral infections is significantly less; however, a small but significant group of febrile infants will still have either a concomitant or secondary SBI. The most common SBI diagnosed is UTI. The pattern of these UTIs is similar to that described in the general population of febrile infants and young children and warrants laboratory screening despite a positive viral antigen screen.

▶ MANAGEMENT

The management of febrile children between 1 and 36 months of age is dependent on clinical appearance, risk factors for bacterial illness, and the presence or absence of an identifiable source (Fig. 3–1). Meta-analysis of studies regarding the evaluation of febrile children between 1 and 36 months of age suggests the differences in management based on age may no longer be as applicable as they were before the development of modern bacterial immunizations.[2] For children who are clinically unstable, stabilization, including airway management, intravenous fluids, and oxygen administration, takes precedence.

▶ TABLE 3-5. PEDIATRIC PATIENTS INDEPENDENTLY AT HIGH RISK FOR SBI

Unimmunized
Immunocompromised
   Acquired or congenital neutropenia
   HIV
   Debilitated state
   Splenectomy
   Sickle cell disease
Congenital heart disease
Lung disease
   Bronchpulmonary dysplasia
   Cystic fibrosis
Central nervous system abnormality
   Trauma
   Cerebrospinal fluid shunts

▶ **TABLE 3–6. COMMON SEASONAL VIRAL ILLNESSES IN INFANTS AND CHILDREN CAUSING FEVER IN THE UNITED STATES**

Organism	Symptoms	Season
Adenovirus	Pharyngitis, conjunctivitis, croup, bronchiolitis, gastroenteritis	Winter–early spring
Influenza A/B	Croup, bronchiolitis, pneumonia, myalgias	Winter
Parainfluenza type 1–3	Pharyngitis, croup, bronchiolitis	Summer–autumn
Respiratory syncitial virus	URI, croup, bronchiolitis, pneumonia	Fall–winter
Rotavirus	Gastroenteritis	Winter–spring
Rhinovirus	URI, bronchiolitis	Fall–spring

If a source is identified, such as UTI, pneumonia, or skin/soft tissue/bone infection, then directed antibiotic therapy is initiated. For those children who are septic or at risk for SBI, empiric antibiotic therapy should begin as soon as possible, preferably within 1 hour of arrival.

In the nontoxic child who appears to have a specific clinical syndrome, rapid antigen testing may be invaluable and prevent unnecessary excessive workup. These tests include screening for influenza, streptococcal antigen, rotavirus, and respiratory syncitial virus. UTI should still be ruled out in established risk groups.

In the nontoxic child with no obvious clinical syndrome, risk factors for SBI need to be determined. Risk factors include fever greater than 39°C; age <2 months; unimmunized state; those with chronic diseases, such as asthma, congenital heart disease, or conditions requiring CSF shunts; and immunocompromised patients. When risk factors are present, a workup should be performed including a complete blood count with leukocyte and immature neutrophil count and markers of in-

flammation including CRP, blood culture as well as urinalysis and urine culture when indicated. Lumbar puncture for spinal fluid should be performed in those children who appear to have or are at risk for meningitis. Imaging for pneumonia may also be indicated. Additional imaging in search of sources of infection will be based on clinical and laboratory findings and may include computed tomography for sinusitis, mastoiditis, neck abscesses, or appendicitis. In the well-appearing child with no risk factors and no illness warranting rapid screening, no workup of any kind may be warranted. The diagnosis of presumptive viral syndrome may be made, followed by discharge with close follow-up. Fever alone may result in patient discomfort and the use of antipyretics is therefore recommended. Both acetaminophen (15 mg/kg every 4 hours) and ibuprofen (10 mg/kg every 6 hours) are effective antipyretics.[36] In febrile infants younger than 2 months, a medical evaluation should be performed prior to the use of acetaminophen since fever may be the only evidence of a serious infection in this age group. In older infants and children,

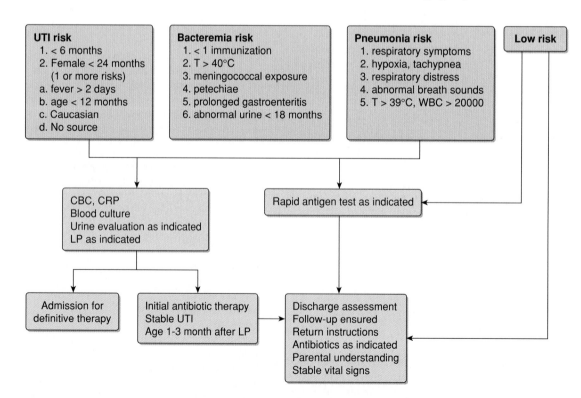

Figure 3–1. Management of nontoxic febrile child (29 days to 36 months).

acetaminophen may be used empirically to treat documented fever causing discomfort. Ibuprofen may be used in febrile children older than 6 months. Recent studies suggest not using acetaminophen and ibuprofen simultaneously for extended periods due to increased risk of renal injury.[37]

Disposition of clinically unstable patients with the presence or risk of SBI should be admission for stabilization and empiric or directed antibiotic therapy. In well-appearing infants and young children with an identified source, symptomatic and directed care may be initiated outpatient with close follow-up. In those with no identified source, the chart should clearly reflect cardiorespiratory stability, adequate feeding behavior, urine output, and alertness at the time of discharge. Follow-up must be arranged before discharge with symptomatic care only.

REFERENCES

1. Nelson DS, Walsh K, Fleisher GR. Spectrum and frequency of pediatric illness presenting to a general community hospital emergency department. *Pediatrics.* 1992;90(1)(Part 1):5–10.
2. American College of Emergency Physicians. Clinical policy for children younger than 3 years presenting to the emergency department with fever. *Ann Emerg Med.* 2003;42(4):530–545.
3. American College of Emergency Physicians. Clinical policy for the initial approach to children under the age of 2 years presenting with fever. *Ann Emerg Med.* 1993;22:628–637.
4. Baraff LJ, Bass JW, Fleisher GR, et al. Practice guidelines for the management of infants and children 0–36 months of age with fever without source. Agency for Health Care Policy and Research. *Ann Emerg Med.* 1993;22:1198–1210.
5. Kourtis AP, Sullivan DT, Sathian U. Practice Guidelines for the management of febrile infants less than 90 days of age at the ambulatory network of a large pediatric healthcare system in the United States: summary of new evidence. *Clin Pediatr (Phila).* 2004;43:11–16.
6. Ishimine P. The evolving approach to the young child who has fever and no obvious source. *Emerg Med Clin North Am.* 2007;25:1087–1115.
7. Dodd SR, Lancaster GA, Craig JV, et al. In a systematic review, infrared thermometry for fever diagnosis in children finds poor sensitivity. *J Clin Epidem.* 2006;59:354–357.
8. Devrim I, Kara A, Ceyhan M, et al. Measurement accuracy of fever by tympanic and axillary thermometry. *Ped Emerg Care.* 2007;23(1):16–19.
9. Ellison VJ, Davis PG, Doyle CW. Adverse reactions to immunizations with newer vaccines in the very preterm infant. *J Pediatr Child Health.* 2005;41:441–443.
10. Adam HM. Fever and host responses. *Pediatr Rev.* 1996;17:330–331.
11. Hanna CM, Greenes DS. How much tachycardia can be attributed to fever? *Ann Emerg Med.* 2004;43:699–705.
12. Trautner BW, Caviness AC, Gerlacher GR, et al. Prospective evaluation of the risk of serious bacterial infection in children who present to the emergency department with hyperpyrexia (temperature of 106 degrees F or higher). *Pediatrics.* 2006;118(1):34–40.
13. Stanley R, Pagon Z, Bachur R. Hyperpyrexia among infants younger than 3 months. *Ped Emerg Care.* 2005;21(5):291–294.
14. Betz MG, Grunfeld AF. "Fever phobia" in the emergency department: a survey of children's caregivers. *Eur J Emerg Med.* 2006;13:129–133.
15. Watson SR, Carcillo JA. Scope and epidemiology of pediatric sepsis. *Pediatr Crit Care Med.* 2005;6(3):S3–S5.
16. Goldstein B, Giroir B, Randolph A, et al. International pediatric sepsis conference: definitions for sepsis and organ dysfunction in pediatrics. *Pediatr Crit Care Med.* 2005;6(1):2–8.
17. Huang H, Chen H, Chu S. Clinical spectrum of meningococcal infections in infants younger than 6 months of age. *Chang Gung Med J.* 2006;29:107–113.
18. Givens TG. Fever caused by occult infections in the 3–36 month child. *Pediatr Emerg Med Prac.* 2007;4(7):1–24.
19. Herz M, Arnd M. Changing epidemiology of outpatient bacteremia in 3–36 months old children after introduction of the heptavalent conjugated pneumococcal vaccine. *PCD Inf Dis J.* 2006;25(4):293–300.
20. Sard B, Bailey M, Vinci R. An analysis of pediatric blood culture in the postpneumococcal conjugate vaccine era in a community hospital emergency department. *Ped Emerg Care.* 2006;22(5):295–300.
21. Fleisher GR, Rosenberg N, Vinci R, et al. Intramuscular *versus* oral antibiotic therapy for the prevention of meningitis and other bacterial sequelae in young, febrile children at risk for occult bacteremia. *J Pediatr.* 1994;42:104–110.
22. Van der Bruel A, Bruyinckx R, Vermeire E, et al. Signs and symptoms in children with serious infection: a qualitative study. *BMC Fam Pract.* 2005;6:36–39.
23. McCarthy PL. Observation scales to identify serious bacterial illness in febrile children. *Pediatrics.* 1985;70(5):802–809.
24. Liew WK, Wong KY. Infective endocarditis in childhood: a seven year experience. *Singapore Med J.* 2004;45(11):525–529.
25. Pratt A, Attia M. Duration of fever and markers of serious bacterial infection in young febrile children. *Pediatr Int.* 2007;49:31–35.
26. Wang K, Chang W, Shih T, et al. Infection of cerebrospinal fluid shunts: causative pathogens, clinical features, and outcomes. *Jpn J Infect Dis.* 2004;57:44–48.
27. Lodha R, Upadhyay A, Kapoor V, et al. Clinical profile and natural history of children with HIV infection. *Indian J Pediatr.* 2006;73(3):201–204.
28. Hijhuis CO, Kamps WA, Daenen SM, et al. Feasibility of withholding antibiotics in selected febrile neutropenic cancer patients. *J Clin Oncol.* 2005;23:7437–7444.
29. Abzug MJ. Presentation, diagnosis, and management of enterovirus infections in neonates. *Pediatr Drugs.* 2004;6(1):1–10.
30. Bonner AB. Winter viral illness in infants and children. *Pediatr Emerg Med Rep.* 2006;11(1):1–12.
31. Miller EK, Lu X, Erdman DD, et al. Rhinovirus-associated hospitalizations in young children. *JID.* 2007;195(15):773–781.
32. Smitherman HF, Caviness AC, Macias CG. Retrospective review of serious bacterial infections in infants 0–36 months of age and having influenza A infection. *Pediatrics.* 2005;115:110–115.
33. Melendez E, Harper MH. Utility of sepsis evaluation in infants 90 days of age or younger with fever and clinical bronchiolitis. *Pediatr Infect Dis J.* 2003;22(12):1053–1056.
34. Titus MO, Wright SW. Prevalence of serious bacterial infection in febrile infants with RSV infection. *Pediatrics.* 2003;112:282–284.
35. Oray-Schrom P, Phoenix C, St. Martin D. Sepsis workup in febrile infants 0–90 days of age with respiratory syncytial virus infection. *Ped Emerg Care.* 2003;19(5):314–319.
36. Goldman RD, Ko K, Linett LJ, et al. Antipyretic efficacy and safety of ibuprofen and acetaminophen in children. *Ann Pharm Fr.* 2004;38:146–150.
37. Mayoral CE, Marino RV, Rosenfeld W, Greensher J. Alternating antipyretics: is this an alternative? *Pediatrics.* 2000;105(5):1009–1012.

CHAPTER 4

Respiratory Distress

Joanna Cohen and Kathleen M. Brown

▶ HIGH-YIELD FACTS

- Tachypnea, hyperpnea, nasal flaring, and retractions are the key features of respiratory distress.
- Respiratory distress is the most common precipitating cause of cardiopulmonary arrest in pediatrics.
- Effective bag-mask ventilation is the single most important skill for managing a patient with respiratory failure.

Respiratory distress is one of the most common complaints in children who present to an emergency department (ED). Respiratory distress is characterized by increased respiratory effort, rate or work of breathing as manifested by tachypnea, hyperpnea, nasal flaring, and inspiratory retractions.

The primary function of respiration is to oxygenate tissues and to remove carbon dioxide produced from metabolism. Respiratory distress can progress to respiratory failure, which results in inadequate oxygenation or ventilation or both. In children, respiratory failure is the most common precipitating cause of in-hospital cardiopulmonary arrest necessitating cardiopulmonary resuscitation. Therefore, early recognition and management of respiratory distress is critical for the physician.

▶ PATHOPHYSIOLOGY

The respiratory system functions primarily to oxygenate the tissues and eliminate carbon dioxide and secondarily to provide immunologic defense and acid–base balance. Control of gas exchange is maintained through a well-coordinated interaction of the respiratory system, the central and peripheral nervous systems, the diaphragm, the chest wall, and the circulatory system.

The respiratory system can be divided into the upper airway which includes the nose, nasopharynx, oropharynx, larynx, trachea, and bronchi and the lower airway consisting of bronchioles, alveoli, and interstitium. Disruption anywhere along this anatomic pathway can produce respiratory distress. For instance, airway obstruction secondary to croup or a foreign body in the larynx will produce respiratory distress originating from the upper airway, while pulmonary edema, fibrosis, or pneumonia will produce respiratory distress originating from the lower airway.

CNS control of respiration lies in the respiratory centers of the medulla. Central chemoreceptors in the medulla respond to changes in the pH of CSF. Peripheral chemoreceptors, located in the aortic and carotid bodies, send afferent signals via the vagus nerve and the glossopharyngeal nerve respec-

tively regarding changes in oxygen, carbon dioxide, and pH in the arterial blood. Disruption of the CNS control of respiration, such as in hydrocephalus or CNS immaturity in the case of premature infants, can produce respiratory distress. The peripheral nervous system provides innervation to the muscles of respiration and can be disrupted in diseases of the peripheral motor nerve, neuromuscular junction, or the muscle itself.

The diaphragm is the principal muscle of inspiration, while the intercostal muscles help to lower the ribs. The accessory muscles, such as the sternocleidomastoid, come into play when respiratory effort is increased. In infants, the chest wall is more compliant than in adults so that during inspiration the lower ribs descend rather than elevate. This provides for less efficient expansion of the lungs, meaning that the diaphragm needs to do more work to achieve good tidal volumes than in the adult.[1] This predisposes infants to more rapidly progressing and severe respiratory distress.

Oxygen and carbon dioxide exchange at the alveolo-capillary membrane depends on adequate ventilation and perfusion (V/Q) matching. Any process that compromises the delivery of oxygen to the alveoli or blood to the capillaries will cause a V/Q mismatch and lead to respiratory distress. Increased metabolic demands, such as in exercise or illness, can also produce respiratory distress, as can states that affect the blood's ability to deliver oxygen to the tissues, such as anemia or abnormal hemoglobin states (methemoglobinemia or carboxyhemoglobinemia). Decreased blood flow to the lungs secondary to poor cardiac output or shock can also cause respiratory distress.

▶ CLINICAL PRESENTATION

The pediatric patient in respiratory distress may present with an altered respiratory rate, increased work of breathing (including the use of accessory muscles; abnormal breath sounds, such as stridor or wheezing; altered level of consciousness or changes in the color of the skin and mucous membranes). The respiratory rate should be visually evaluated before the patient is physically examined by the provider because anxiety and agitation commonly cause tachypnea. Quiet tachypnea is usually an attempt to increase minute ventilation to blow off carbon dioxide from nonpulmonary diseases such as DKA or shock, whereas tachypnea with grunting, stridor, or wheezing suggests airway obstruction. A slow or irregular respiratory rate may indicate fatigue, CNS depression, or hypothermia. A child in respiratory distress whose respiratory rate goes from rapid to normal may be improving; however, if the child's level of consciousness is waning, this improvement in respiratory rate may actually indicate fatigue and a deterioration in the child's clinical condition.

Increased respiratory effort, as with nasal flaring, retractions, and use of accessory muscles, increases oxygen demand of the respiratory muscles and produces more carbon dioxide. Stridor is a high-pitched inspiratory noise that suggests an extrathoracic airway obstructing mechanism, such as foreign body or croup, while wheezing during exhalation suggests an intrathoracic airway obstruction etiology, such as asthma. Grunting occurs during expiration and is an effort to increase airway pressure and maintain patency of the small airways and alveoli during collapse that can occur with pulmonary edema, pneumonia, or atelectasis. Decreased breath sounds suggest airflow obstruction, parenchymal lung disease, or poor respiratory effort. Seesaw respiration or abdominal breathing with chest wall retractions and abdominal expansion during diaphragmatic contraction during inspiration indicate upper airway obstruction.[2]

▶ LABORATORY AND RADIOGRAPHIC FINDINGS

Pulse oximetry should be used to assess oxygen tissue saturation. End-tidal carbon dioxide monitoring can help assess ventilation. Capnography is a graphic display of exhaled carbon dioxide that can be measured by the placement of a probe in the nostril of a spontaneously breathing patient or in line with an endotracheal tube in the intubated patient. The use of capnography has been increasing in pediatric emergency medicine and is currently used for endotracheal tube confirmation, moderate sedation, trauma, and acid–base disturbances.[3] An arterial blood gas can be used to assess blood gas exchange in the lungs, the acid–base balance of the body, and electrolyte levels. A basic metabolic panel to calculate the anion gap in a patient with a metabolic acidosis aids in diagnosis. An elevated anion gap in a patient with a metabolic acidosis could be indicative of diarrheal dehydration, diabetic ketoacidosis, an inborn error of metabolism, sepsis, or toxin ingestion, while a metabolic acidosis with a normal anion gap is more likely to be from hypernatremic dehydration, renal tubular acidosis, or rapid volume expansion. An ammonia level may also be useful diagnostically for a patient with metabolic acidosis when a metabolic or hepatic disease is in the differential diagnosis of a patient with metabolic acidosis. A bedside dextrose test and urine toxicologic screen can help evaluate patients with altered mental status.

The chest radiograph is the most frequent test ordered when a patient presents with respiratory distress. Usually, a routine chest radiograph consists of two images, a posteroanterior (PA) frontal view and a left lateral view. In the case of respiratory distress, a chest radiograph may show the presence of a radiopaque foreign body, lobar pneumonia, pneumothorax, atelectasis, hyperinflation, or cardiac enlargement, in addition to a number of other indicators that may help with the diagnosis.

Other radiographic studies may be helpful in certain situations. A lateral neck radiograph may show a retropharyngeal abscess or a radiopaque foreign body that has been aspirated. In children with a suspected pulmonary foreign body who cannot cooperate for inspiratory and expiratory radiographs, lateral decubitis films may help make the diagnosis. Foreign

bodies may also be identified on fluoroscopy or computed tomography (CT). While the best method to diagnose pulmonary embolism in children has not been established, CT scan, MRA, and V/Q scans have all been used.[4] Imaging studies of other organ systems may be useful depending on the clinical evaluation. For instance, an echocardiogram will identify patients with myocarditis and a creatinine phosphokinase level is useful to screen for suspected muscle diseases.

▶ **TABLE 4–1. MAJOR CAUSES OF RESPIRATORY DISTRESS IN NEWBORNS**

Upper airway	Lower airway
Craniofacial anomalies	Neonatal respiratory distress syndrome
Laryngomalacia	
Laryngeal webs	Bronchopulmonary dysplasia
Vascular rings	Gastroesophageal reflux
	Meconium aspiration
	Diaphragmatic hernia
Cardiac	Nervous system
Congenital heart disease	Congenital CNS anomalies
	Neonatal apnea
Metabolic	Seizure
Inborn errors of metabolism	

▶ **TABLE 4–2. MAJOR CAUSES OF RESPIRATORY DISTRESS IN INFANTS AND CHILDREN**

Upper airway	Lower airway
Craniofacial anomalies	Asthma
Foreign body	Bronchiolitis
Facial or neck trauma	Aspiration of emesis
Tonsillitis/peritonsillar abscess	Foreign body
Ludwig's angina	Near-drowning
Burns	Gastroesophageal reflux
Epiglottitis	Pneumonia
Croup	Cystic fibrosis
Retropharyngeal abscess	Pertussis
Tracheitis	Pulmonary edema
Anaphylaxis	Pulmonary contusion
Angioedema	Pulmonary embolism
	Smoke inhalation
	Pneumothorax Tension pneumothorax
	Pleural effusion/empyema
	Hemothorax
	Rib fractures/flail chest
Cardiac	Nervous system
Myocarditis	Intoxication
Acute decompensated heart failure	Seizure
	Tetanus
Metabolic	Myelitis
Hyperventilation	Guillian–Barré syndrome
Diabetic ketoacidosis	Botulism
Other causes of acidosis	Tick paralysis

▶ DIFFERENTIAL DIAGNOSIS

A differential diagnosis for respiratory distress can be organized by age and the anatomic location of the source of the distress. It is useful to think of the respiratory system as consisting of an upper airway and a lower airway. In addition to originating directly from the respiratory system, respiratory distress can be caused by problems in the muscles that perform the work of breathing or the central or peripheral nervous system which controls respiration. Metabolic, cardiac, gastrointestinal, and hematologic causes must also be considered (Tables 4–1 and 4–2).

▶ TREATMENT

The goals of treating respiratory distress are to provide adequate ventilation and oxygenation. Each child in respiratory distress must first be evaluated for impending respiratory failure. Airway, breathing, and circulation should be assessed rapidly and conditions requiring immediate lifesaving interventions, such as upper airway obstruction, tension pneumothorax, cardiac tamponade, and respiratory failure, must be identified and treated. Airway patency must be established. A patient with complete upper airway obstruction will have no air movement and may present with gagging or choking. With partial airway obstruction the patient may present with stridor. An alert child will assume a position of comfort and agitation should be minimized, since it increases minute ventilation and often worsens upper airway obstruction. A child who is obtunded may have soft tissue obstruction of the airway, which can be relieved by positioning the airway with a chin-lift or jaw thrust. The mouth and nose should be suctioned and any foreign body that is visualized should be removed. An oropharyngeal airway or nasopharyngeal airway may be indicated to maintain patency of the airway. In extreme cases, a surgical airway may be needed.

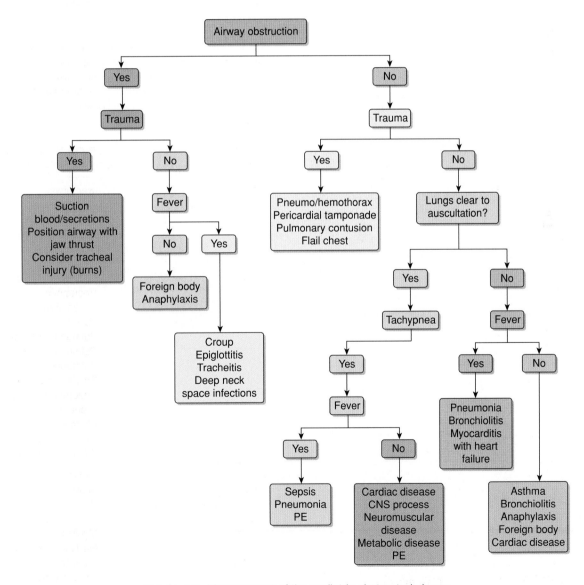

Figure 4–1. Management of the pediatric obstructed airway.

In the pediatric trauma patient with respiratory distress, the differential diagnosis of upper airway obstruction should include blunt or penetrating injury to the trachea. Endotracheal intubation or cricothyrotomy may be required and the most skilled provider available should manage the airway. Trauma patients might also have respiratory distress secondary to a tension pneumothorax, which requires immediate decompression via needle thoracentesis (Fig. 4–1).

Once an airway is established, attention should be turned to breathing. For patients with severe respiratory distress or impending failure, high-concentration humidified oxygen should be delivered to maintain cerebral and myocardial oxygenation. Effective bag-velve-mask (BVM) ventilation is still the single most important intervention in managing a patient with respiratory failure. Children with out-of-hospital respiratory arrest who received BVM and endotracheal tube placement did not have better outcomes than those who received BVM alone.[5] However, in the ED, endotracheal intubation may be indicated and one should be prepared to intubate when required.

Medications to address specific causes of respiratory distress should be given if the cause can be identified or if there is a suspicion based on the history. Croup can be treated with nebulized racemic epinephrine and dexamethasone. Anaphylaxis can be treated with IM epinephrine, diphenhydramine, H2-blockers, methylprednisolone, and an isotonic crystalloid fluid bolus. Albuterol and steroids should be given for asthma. See later chapters for further information on treatment of specific diseases.

▶ DISPOSITION/OUTCOME

Many pediatric patients presenting to the ED with respiratory distress can be treated and discharged. Patient with asthma who respond to steroids and inhaled bronchodilators can be safely discharged after being observed off treatment for a reasonable amount of time. Patients who have had foreign bodies successfully removed and patients with intoxication who recover can probably be discharged home after a period of observation.

Indications for admission to the hospital include, but are not limited to a persistent increased work of breathing, hypoxia requiring oxygen administration, and a concern for rebound of symptoms, for example the late phase response to anaphylaxis. Patients who require further workup may also be admitted to facilitate the workup. For example, an infant with persistent stridor may be admitted for bronchoscopy with general anesthesia. Patients who require endotracheal intubation or have severe respiratory distress with impending respiratory failure should be admitted to an intensive care unit.

Respiratory distress can lead to respiratory failure. Fortunately, pediatric cardiopulmonary arrest is a rare event. However, outcome studies examining inpatient pediatric cardiopulmonary resuscitation show 24-hour survival rates only around 35%.[6,7] In pediatric patients, respiratory distress is the number one cause of cardiopulmonary arrest and is associated with better 24-hour survival when compared to shock, the second leading cause of cardiopulmonary arrest.[7] For this reason, a thorough understanding and ability to manage respiratory distress in children is critical to the emergency medicine provider.

REFERENCES

1. Heulitt MJ, Ouellet P. Pediatric critical care medicine. In: Slonim AD, Pollack MM, eds. *Respiratory System Physiology.* Philadelphia, PA: Lippincott Williams & Wilkins; 2006:264.
2. Ralston M. et al., eds. *Pediatric Advanced Life Support Provider Manual.* Dallas, TX: American Heart Association, Subcommittee on Pediatric Resuscitation; 2006, ch 2.
3. Langhan ML, Chen L. Current utilization of continuous end-tidal carbon dioxide monitoring in pediatric emergency departments. *Pediatr Emerg Care.* 2008;24(4):211–213.
4. Chn AK, Deveber G, Monagle P, et al. Venous thrombosis in children. *J Thromb Haemost.* 2003;1(7):1143–1155.
5. Gausche M, Lewis RJ, Stratton SJ, et al. Effect of out-of-hospital pediatric endotracheal intubation on survival and neurological outcome: a controlled clinical trial. *JAMA.* 2000;283(6):783–790.
6. Torres A Jr, Pickert CB, Firestone J, et al. Long-term functional outcome of inpatient pediatric cardiopulmonary resuscitation. *Pediatr Emerg Care.* 1997;13:369–373.
7. Reis AG, Nadkarni V, Perondi MB, et al. A prospective investigation into the epidemiology of in-hospital pediatric cardopulmonary resuscitation using the international Utstein reporting style. *Pediatrics.* 2002;109:200–209.

CHAPTER 5

Sudden Infant Death Syndrome and Apparent Life-Threatening Event

Collin S. Goto and Sing-Yi Feng

▶ HIGH-YIELD FACTS

- Sudden infant death syndrome (SIDS) is defined as the sudden death of an infant younger than 1 year which remains unexplained after a thorough case investigation, including a complete autopsy, examination of the death scene, and review of the clinical history.
- Typically, the SIDS victim is brought to the emergency department by ambulance after a caregiver finds the unresponsive infant. The child has usually been asleep for a variable length of time and it is unclear how long the infant has been pulseless and apneic.
- As soon as possible, the parents should be informed of the resuscitation and interviewed regarding the events leading up to the discovery of the infant. Information solicited should include past medical history, present illnesses, current medications, and any history of trauma.
- Prevention is the key to reducing mortality secondary to SIDS and risk reduction is the most important measure in preventing SIDS. Parents should be given specific risk reduction strategies such as nonprone sleeping, avoiding maternal smoking in pregnancy, decreasing environmental smoke exposure, maintaining comfortable ambient temperature, providing a safe sleep environment, and fully immunizing the child.
- To help with the grieving process, the parents should be allowed to see and hold the baby and details of the resuscitation should be explained. Immediate social work and pastoral support will help the family to cope with the difficult and confusing situation.
- An apparent life-threatening event (ALTE) is defined as an episode that is frightening to the observer and is characterized by some combination of apnea (central or obstructive), color change (cyanosis, pallor, erythema, or plethora), marked change in muscle tone (rigidity or limpness), or unexplained choking or gagging.
- The differential diagnosis is extensive because ALTE is primarily a historic description of the event rather than a single, unifying pathophysiologic process. Even after a thorough evaluation, a definitive diagnosis of the ALTE is found in only approximately 50% of patients.
- The history often provides the most important information in the evaluation of an ALTE, especially when the infant appears well and has a normal physical examination. The first step is to determine whether a true ALTE has occurred.

- True apnea must be distinguished from the normal periodicity of breathing that occurs during infancy. Normal periodic breathing is not associated with skin color changes.
- An infant may be discharged from the emergency department if a detailed history and physical examination do not indicate that a true ALTE has occurred, provided the infant continues to do well and the parents are comfortable with the situation and capable of observing the infant at home.
- Any infant with a history of apnea, pallor, cyanosis, limpness or unresponsiveness requiring vigorous physical stimulation, or cardiopulmonary resuscitation is excluded from outpatient consideration.

▶ SUDDEN INFANT DEATH SYNDROME

SIDS is defined as the sudden death of an infant younger than 1 year which remains unexplained after a thorough case investigation, including a complete autopsy, examination of the death scene, and review of the clinical history.[1] The emergency department physician should be prepared to manage the infant who presents with SIDS and give a thorough, well-informed, and compassionate explanation of the situation to the parents, who will undoubtedly be anxious and distressed.

EPIDEMIOLOGY AND PATHOPHYSIOLOGY

Despite declines in SIDS rates following risk-reduction campaigns, SIDS remains the most common cause of death for children aged 1 month to 1 year in developed countries. Approximately 2500 infants die from SIDS every year in the United States.[2] The peak incidence is between 2 and 4 months of age and 90% of SIDS deaths occur in the first 6 months of life. Boys are more likely to die than girls at a ratio of 60:40. Younger maternal age, lack of prenatal care, low birth weight, prone sleeping position, overheating, and preterm birth are all risk factors for SIDS.[3] In the United States, African Americans and Native Americans have SIDS rates that are two to three times the national average irrespective of socioeconomic status.[4]

The pathophysiology of SIDS is polygenic and multifactorial with medical, genetic, environmental, and behavioral/sociocultural factors (Table 5–1). Abnormalities of arousal are

▶ **TABLE 5-1. FACTORS ASSOCIATED WITH SUDDEN INFANT DEATH SYNDROME**

Medical/Genetic	Environmental/Behavioral/ Sociocultural
Congenital defects	Bed sharing
Low birth weight	Head covering
Preterm infant	Higher ambient temperature
Polymorphisms	Low socioeconomic status
causing impaired	Maternal smoking
autonomic	Multiple layers of clothing
regulation and	Soft sleeping surfaces
arousal	Smoke exposure
	Supine sleep position

now thought to be involved in the pathogenesis of SIDS. Multiple studies have shown that SIDS risk factors alter sleep patterns and impair infant arousal responses. Prone sleeping has been shown to increase the time infants spend in a state of reduced spontaneous arousability.[5] Infants who lie prone are more likely to rebreathe the carbon dioxide trapped around their face which can lead to hypercarbia and death.[6,7] In 1992, the American Academy of Pediatrics first published its recommendation that infants should sleep in a nonprone position and started the "Back to Sleep" campaign in 1994.[8] The percentage of infants sleeping prone has changed from 70% in 1994 to less than 15% in 2002. The SIDS rate in the United States has decreased from 1.2 deaths per 1000 at the initiation of the "Back to Sleep" campaign in 1994 to 0.57 deaths per 1000 in 2002.[2]

EVALUATION AND MANAGEMENT

Typically, the SIDS victim is brought to the emergency department by ambulance after a caregiver finds the unresponsive infant. The child has usually been asleep for a variable length of time and it is unclear how long the infant has been pulseless and apneic. In the absence of dependent lividity or rigor mortis, resuscitation is indicated and should follow the guidelines set forth in Chapter 26.

As soon as possible, the parents should be informed of the resuscitation and interviewed regarding the events leading up to the discovery of the infant. Information solicited should include past medical history, present illnesses, current medications, and any history of trauma. The child should be thoroughly examined for any congenital abnormalities, signs of concurrent illness, or evidence of physical abuse.

In SIDS cases, resuscitation is unsuccessful. In an event in which a perfusing rhythm is restored, the child should be admitted to the pediatric intensive care unit. Further interventions and diagnostic evaluation depend on the patient's condition and the possible etiology of the event. The family should be counseled on the situation and the likelihood of demise despite return of spontaneous circulation. Often, cardiovascular status deteriorates or multiple organ failure develops. Spontaneous circulation may persist, but the child may be declared brain dead because of severe hypoxic-ischemic insult (Fig. 5–1).

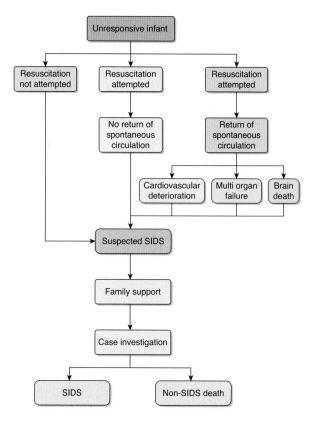

Figure 5-1. Management of sudden infant death syndrome.

SIDS is a diagnosis of exclusion. The differential diagnosis of sudden infant death includes sepsis, pneumonia, myocarditis, congenital heart defect, cardiomyopathy, arrhythmia, prolonged QT syndrome, accidental or nonaccidental trauma, suffocation, adrenal hyperplasia, and inherited metabolic disorders such as fatty acid oxidation disorders.[2,9–18] Autopsies and death scene investigations are warranted to help determine the cause of death and provide valuable information and closure for the family.[9]

Prevention is the key to reducing mortality secondary to SIDS and risk reduction is the most important measure in preventing SIDS. Parents should be given specific risk reduction strategies such as nonprone sleeping, avoiding maternal smoking in pregnancy, decreasing environmental smoke exposure, maintaining comfortable ambient temperature, providing a safe sleep environment, and fully immunizing the child.[19]

DISPOSITION

The loss of a child is a devastating event. When an infant dies of SIDS, families face the shock of the sudden loss, the stress of an investigation, and long wait times for autopsy results which are often inconclusive. To help with the grieving process, the parents should be allowed to see and hold the baby and details of the resuscitation should be explained. Immediate social work and pastoral support will help the family to cope with the difficult and confusing situation. Parental grief and guilt is universal in this situation. Surviving siblings and other family members also need age-appropriate support.

▶ THE APPARENT LIFE-THREATENING EVENT

ALTE is defined as an episode that is frightening to the observer and is characterized by some combination of apnea (central or obstructive), color change (cyanosis, pallor, erythema, or plethora), marked change in muscle tone (rigidity or limpness), or unexplained choking or gagging.[20] The infant often receives some degree of stimulation or resuscitation at home, but occasionally recovers spontaneously and is subsequently brought to medical attention. Any infant with an ALTE who has cardiopulmonary compromise upon arrival to the emergency department should be appropriately resuscitated, stabilized, evaluated, and admitted to the hospital. However, the majority will appear well, and the challenge for the emergency physician is to determine whether a true life-threatening event has occurred so that decisions can be made regarding evaluation and hospitalization.

EPIDEMIOLOGY

Although the true incidence of ALTE is unknown, it is estimated to occur in 0.5% to 6% of all children during the first year of life and is more common in boys and premature infants.[21] The peak incidence is in infants younger than 2 months.[22] Although there is some overlap of epidemiologic risk factors, the exact relationship between ALTE and SIDS is not clear.[23] Therefore, older terms for ALTE such as "near-miss SIDS" and "aborted SIDS" are misleading and no longer appropriate.

ETIOLOGY

When evaluating the infant presenting with ALTE, the clinician must consider many possible causes of the event (Table 5–2). The differential diagnosis is extensive because ALTE is primarily a historic description of the event rather than a single, unifying pathophysiologic process. Apnea is a common presentation but is also the final common pathway for many disease processes seen in infants. Even after a thorough evaluation, a definitive diagnosis of the ALTE is found in only approximately 50% of patients.[21]

INITIAL ASSESSMENT AND STABILIZATION

The initial evaluation of the unstable or ill-appearing infant is directed at identifying and stabilizing immediate life-threatening conditions (Fig. 5–2). Attention is focused on establishing a patent airway and assuring adequate breathing and circulation. Vital signs are obtained, cardiac monitors are placed, and intravenous access is established. Pulse oximetry and rapid bedside glucose determination, electrolyte, hemoglobin, and blood gas analysis may identify physiologic disturbances requiring immediate intervention. Once the patient has been stabilized, a more thorough secondary survey is performed to identify any physical findings that may elucidate the etiology of the ALTE.

▶ TABLE 5–2. DIFFERENTIAL DIAGNOSIS OF AN APPARENT LIFE-THREATENING EVENT

Cardiovascular System
Anemia
Cardiomyopathy
Congenital heart disease
Dysrhythmia (prolonged QT syndrome, Wolff-Parkinson-White syndrome)
Hemorrhage (child abuse)
Myocarditis
Vascular rings and slings

Central Nervous System
Apnea of prematurity
Congenital brain malformation
Head trauma (child abuse)
Idiopathic central apnea
Increased intracranial pressure (congenital hydrocephalus, tumor)
Meningitis/encephalitis
Seizure

Respiratory System
Breath-holding spell
Bronchiolitis (respiratory syncytial virus)
Congenital malformation (choanal atresia, laryngeal cleft, tracheoesophageal fistula)
Foreign body
Laryngomalacia/tracheomalacia
Laryngospasm (choking spell, gastroesophageal reflux)
Obstructive sleep apnea
Periodic breathing of infancy
Pertussis
Pneumonia
Smothering (intentional or unintentional)
Upper airway obstruction (nasal congestion)

Systemic/Metabolic/Other
Dehydration
Electrolyte abnormality (hyponatremia, hypocalcemia, congenital adrenal hyperplasia)
Factitious (Munchausen's syndrome by proxy)
Hypoglycemia
Hypothermia
Inborn errors of metabolism
Sepsis
Toxins/drugs

HISTORY

The history often provides the most important information in the evaluation of an ALTE, especially when the infant appears well and has a normal physical examination. The first step is to determine whether a true ALTE has occurred. The parents should be questioned closely about the details of the event, including the infant's respiratory effort, skin color, mental status, muscle tone, the duration of the event, and the degree of resuscitation required prior to evaluation in the emergency department. An accurate history may be difficult to obtain

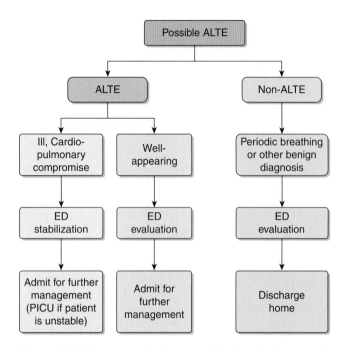

Figure 5–2. Management of apparent life-threatening event.

because of parental anxiety surrounding the event, as well as other factors that inhibit accurate observation, such as home lighting conditions and the amount of clothes or bedding covering the infant.[24]

True apnea must be distinguished from the normal periodicity of breathing that occurs during infancy. The parents are often unable to accurately estimate the duration of the ALTE; therefore, the association of apnea or respiratory difficulty with pallor or cyanosis is significant. Normal periodic breathing is not associated with skin color changes. Central apnea is characterized by an absence of respiratory effort, whereas, during obstructive apnea, the infant typically appears to be struggling to breathe with choking, gasping, or gagging. Facial color changes are common in infants with a history of choking or gagging and it is important to distinguish the more common facial redness and flushing from true cyanosis, which indicates significant hypoxia. The infant's mental status during the event is also important. An infant who remains awake and alert during an event is unlikely to have suffered prolonged hypoxia or an acute neurologic event such as a seizure. Likewise, the history of muscle tone can provide important information. Hypotonia associated with apnea or color change implies significant hypoxia or decreased cerebral perfusion, while hypertonicity is characteristic of seizures. A history of apnea that required vigorous physical stimulation or cardiopulmonary resuscitation is ominous and implies a true life-threatening event.

Information is also gathered concerning past medical history and any recent illness that may have contributed to the ALTE. A history of fever alerts the physician to the possibility of sepsis or meningitis. A preceding respiratory illness implies the possibility of apnea because of upper respiratory obstruction, bronchiolitis, or pneumonia. Vomiting and diarrhea can lead to hypoglycemia or significant electrolyte abnormalities. A history of regurgitation with feedings suggests the possibility of laryngospasm secondary to gastroesophageal reflux. The infant with a preexisting neurologic disorder may be at increased

risk of seizures. The possibility of intentional or unintentional trauma should also be explored.

A family history of other infants with sudden death alerts the physician to the possibility of inherited disorders, such as inborn errors of metabolism or the prolonged QT syndrome. A history of a sibling with SIDS is a recognized risk factor for sudden death. In addition, cases of multiple infant deaths because of child abuse within a family have been reported. Finally, the possibility of factitious ALTE because of Munchausen's syndrome by proxy must be considered in the infant who repeatedly presents with an ALTE or other unexplained illnesses. The physician should be alerted to the possibility of child abuse or Munchausen's syndrome by proxy if the history is inconsistent, the parents' reaction to the situation is abnormal, or other signs of abuse or neglect are present.

PHYSICAL EXAMINATION

A thorough head-to-toe examination of the infant may provide clues to the etiology of the ALTE. Particular attention should be paid to the respiratory, cardiovascular, and neurologic systems. In addition, evidence of infection, trauma, neglect, or congenital malformations should be sought. Even in the infant with a normal physical examination, continuous monitoring in the emergency department may provide the opportunity to observe events such as gastroesophageal reflux, choking, cyanosis, or apnea. It is important to monitor the infant over a period of time during a variety of activities such feeding and sleeping and to observe whether the events result in hypoxia or bradycardia.

EVALUATION AND MANAGEMENT

The challenge for the emergency clinician is to be selective in choosing those studies that will impact immediate decision-making, including determining the severity of the event and stability of the infant (Fig. 5–2). In addition, a possible diagnosis should be sought, especially with respect to those conditions that require immediate intervention. The studies should also help to determine the disposition of the patient (i.e., discharge home versus admit to monitored ward or intensive care setting). Once stability of the infant and hospitalization have been determined, further studies can be performed after admission even if a definitive diagnosis has not been established.

The many diagnostic studies to be considered in the evaluation of an ALTE reflect the diverse differential diagnosis. Selection should be guided by the presentation of the infant. For example, if a serious bacterial infection is suspected, a complete blood count, blood culture, urinalysis with urine culture, and lumbar puncture are performed prior to initiation of age-appropriate antibiotics. Nasopharyngeal swabs for viral identification are considered when a viral respiratory infection is suspected, especially respiratory syncytial virus. A chest radiograph is obtained for any infant with respiratory or cardiac abnormalities. In addition, a bedside electrocardiogram is useful to assess for cardiac pathology, including prolonged QT syndrome, Wolff-Parkinson-White syndrome, myocarditis, or anomalous left coronary artery with myocardial ischemia.

If the history suggests a seizure, serum electrolytes, glucose, blood urea nitrogen, serum creatinine, calcium, magnesium, and phosphorus are obtained. If child abuse is suspected, consideration is given to obtaining a computed axial tomography scan of the head, skeletal survey, and drug screen. Other studies may be indicated, depending on the clinical scenario. Once the infant is admitted to the hospital, further evaluation may include sleep studies, pH probe testing, electroencephalography, and other studies that are beyond the scope of the emergency department.

DISPOSITION

An infant may be discharged from the emergency department if a detailed history and physical examination do not indicate that a true ALTE has occurred, provided the infant continues to do well and the parents are comfortable with the situation and capable of observing the infant at home. Examples of such a situation include periodic breathing mistaken for apnea or a minor coughing or gagging episode. A reasonable period of observation in the emergency department during which the infant is asymptomatic while sleeping and feeding is important, but does not prove that the prior event was insignificant and does not rule out recurrence. After parental education, the infant may be discharged home with specific instructions for follow-up in 24 hours with a primary care provider or return to the emergency department sooner if any problems occur.

Any infant with a history of apnea, pallor, cyanosis, limpness or unresponsiveness requiring vigorous physical stimulation, or cardiopulmonary resuscitation is excluded from outpatient consideration. If there is any question about the nature of the event, the parents' ability to care for the infant at home or the adequacy of follow-up, it is best to err on the side of caution and admit the infant for observation and monitoring.

Any infant with a true life-threatening event is placed on a cardiopulmonary monitor and admitted to the hospital after emergency department evaluation. Any infant who is unstable is admitted to the pediatric intensive care unit.

REFERENCES

1. Willinger M, James LS, Catz C. Defining the sudden infant death syndrome (SIDS): deliberations of an expert panel convened by the National Institute of Child Health and Human Development. *Pediatr Pathol.* 1991;11(5):677–684.
2. Moon RY, Fu LY. Sudden infant death syndrome. *Pediatr Rev.* 2007;28(6):209–214.
3. American Academy of Pediatrics, Task Force on Sudden Infant Death Syndrome. The changing concept of sudden infant death syndrome: diagnostic coding shifts, controversies regarding the sleeping environment, and new variables to consider in reducing risk. *Pediatrics.* 2005;116(5):1245–1255.
4. Moon RY, Horne RS, Hauck FR. Sudden infant death syndrome. *Lancet.* 2007;370(9598):1578–1587.
5. Bhat RY, Hannam S, Pressler R, Rafferty GF, Peacock JL, Greenough A. Effect of prone and supine position on sleep, apneas, and arousal in preterm infants. *Pediatrics.* 2006;118(1):101–107.
6. Hunt CE, Lesko SM, Vezina RM, et al. Infant sleep position and associated health outcomes. *Arch Pediatr Adolesc Med.* 2003;157(5):469–474.
7. Kinney HC. Abnormalities of the brainstem serotonergic system in the sudden infant death syndrome: a review. *Pediatr Dev Pathol.* 2005;8(5):507–524.
8. American Academy of Pediatrics. Changing concepts of sudden infant death syndrome: implications for infant sleeping environment and sleep position. American Academy of Pediatrics. Task Force on Infant Sleep Position and Sudden Infant Death Syndrome. *Pediatrics.* 2000;105(3)(pt 1):650–656.
9. Bajanowski T, Vege A, Byard RW, et al. Sudden infant death syndrome (SIDS)—standardised investigations and classification: recommendations. *Forensic Sci Int.* 2007;165(2–3):129–143.
10. Beeber B, Cunningham N. Fatal child abuse and sudden infant death syndrome (SIDS): a critical diagnostic decision. *Pediatrics.* 1994;93(3):539–540.
11. Blair PS, Platt MW, Smith IJ, Fleming PJ. Sudden Infant Death Syndrome and the time of death: factors associated with nighttime and day-time deaths. *Int J Epidemiol.* 2006;35(6):1563–1569.
12. Border WL, Benson DW. Sudden infant death syndrome and long QT syndrome: the zealots versus the naysayers. *Heart Rhythm.* 2007;4(2):167–169.
13. Reece RM. Fatal child abuse and sudden infant death syndrome: a critical diagnostic decision. *Pediatrics.* 1993;91(2):423–429.
14. Schwartz PJ, Stramba-Badiale M, Segantini A, et al. Prolongation of the QT interval and the sudden infant death syndrome. *N Engl J Med.* 1998;338(24):1709–1714.
15. Valdes-Dapena M, Gilbert-Barness E. Cardiovascular causes for sudden infant death. *Pediatr Pathol Mol Med.* 2002;21(2):195–211.
16. Wedekind H, Bajanowski T, Friederich P, et al. Sudden infant death syndrome and long QT syndrome: an epidemiological and genetic study. *Int J Legal Med.* 2006;120(3):129–137.
17. Emery JL, Howat AJ, Variend S, Vawter GF. Investigation of inborn errors of metabolism in unexpected infant deaths. *Lancet.* 1988;2(8601):29–31.
18. Lundemose JB, Kolvraa S, Gregersen N, Christensen E, Gregersen M. Fatty acid oxidation disorders as primary cause of sudden and unexpected death in infants and young children: an investigation performed on cultured fibroblasts from 79 children who died aged between 0–4 years. *Mol Pathol.* 1997;50(4):212–217.
19. Mitchell EA. Recommendations for sudden infant death syndrome prevention: a discussion document. *Arch Dis Child.* 2007;92(2):155–159.
20. National Institutes of Health Consensus Development Conference on Infantile Apnea and Home Monitoring, Sept 29 to Oct 1, 1986. *Pediatrics.* 1987;79(2):292–299.
21. Brooks JG. Apparent life-threatening events and apnea of infancy. *Clin Perinatol.* 1992;19(4):809–838.
22. Davies F, Gupta R. Apparent life threatening events in infants presenting to an emergency department. *Emerg Med J.* 2002;19(1):11–16.
23. Esani N, Hodgman JE, Ehsani N, Hoppenbrouwers T. Apparent life-threatening events and sudden infant death syndrome: comparison of risk factors. *J Pediatr.* 2008;152(3):365–370.
24. Dewolfe CC. Apparent life-threatening event: a review. *Pediatr Clin North Am.* 2005;52(4):1127–1146, ix.

CHAPTER 6

Altered Mental Status and Coma

Susan Fuchs

▶ HIGH-YIELD FACTS

- For coma to occur, there must be an insult to both cerebral hemispheres or to the reticular activating system.
- Decorticate posturing signifies dysfunction of the cerebral hemispheres with an intact brain stem.
- Decerebrate posturing signifies a lesion of the midbrain.
- Intussuception can have a "neurologic" presentation ranging from lethargy to obtundation.

The term *altered mental status* refers to an aberration in a patient's level of consciousness. It always implies serious pathology and mandates an aggressive search for the underlying disorder. More precise terminology describes the degree of altered mental status and has important implications for differential diagnosis and management:

- *Lethargy* is a state of reduced wakefulness in which the patient displays disinterest in the environment and is easily distracted but is easily arouseable and can communicate.
- *Delirium* is characterized by disorientation, delusions, hallucinations, fearful responses, irritability, and sensory misperception.
- *Obtundation* is severe blunting of alertness with a decreased response to stimuli.
- *Stupor* exists when the patient can only be aroused by extremely vigorous and repeated stimulation.
- *Coma* occurs when a profound reduction in neuronal function results in unresponsiveness to sensory stimuli. It constitutes the most severe manifestation of altered mental status. Coma is further categorized depending on the area of the brain affected.[1,2]

Several scoring systems exist that permit objective and reproducible assessment of the degree of altered mental status and allow effective communication among health care providers. The most widely used is the Glasgow Coma Scale (GCS), which scores three responses with a range from 3 to 15.[2,3] The GCS has been modified so that it can be applied to infants and children. The main difference is the verbal response (Table 6–1).[2,4]

▶ PATHOPHYSIOLOGY

In general, patients with altered mental status have suffered a diffuse insult to the brain. For patients with no history of trauma, the most common causes are metabolic abnormalities, toxic ingestions, and infectious etiologies, such as meningitis and encephalitis. The more severe the insult, the greater the alteration in mental status.

For coma to occur, the underlying abnormality must involve damage to either both cerebral hemispheres or to the ascending reticular activating system, which transverses the brain stem through the upper pons, midbrain, and diencephalon, and plays a fundamental role in arousal. Coma does not result from isolated injury to one cerebral hemisphere but can result from damage to the reticular activating system despite a normally functioning cerebral cortex.[2]

Coma can result from structural damage to tissue, infectious processes, metabolic derangements, toxic ingestions, and inadequate cerebral perfusion. Metabolic, infectious, and toxic etiologies tend to produce diffuse but symmetric deficits, such as confusion, that precede other abnormalities, such as motor deficits. Structural lesions result in focal deficits that progress in a predictable pattern. Supratentorial lesions produce focal findings that progress in a rostral-caudal fashion, whereas subtentorial lesions result in brain stem dysfunction followed by a sudden onset of coma, cranial nerve palsies, and respiratory disturbances. The causes of coma are listed in Tables 6–2 and 6–3.[5,6]

▶ HISTORY

The history of a patient with altered mental status focuses on identifying the underlying abnormality. Events prior to the onset of mental status changes are elicited, including headache, febrile illness, trauma, and drug ingestion. Associated symptoms such as vomiting, diarrhea, or respiratory difficulties are important clues. Past medical history including diabetes, seizure disorder, or underlying heart or kidney disease is elicited. A prior history of similar episodes may imply an underlying metabolic abnormality, such as an inborn error of metabolism.

▶ PHYSICAL EXAMINATION

The physical examination focuses on assessing the degree of neurologic impairment and localizing the lesion responsible for the patient's altered mental status. Particular attention is paid to the vital signs, including temperature. Many systemic illnesses that result in central nervous system dysfunction are associated with profound abnormalities in basic physiologic parameters.

▶ TABLE 6-1. GLASGOW AND CHILDREN'S COMA SCALE

Glasgow	Children's	Score
Eye opening		
Spontaneous	Spontaneous	4
To command	To speech	3
To pain	To pain	2
None	None	1
Motor response		
Follows command	Spontaneous	6
Localizes pain	Withdraws to touch	5
Withdraws to pain	Withdraws to pain	4
Abnormal flexion (decorticate)	Abnormal flexion	3
Abnormal extension (decerebrate)	Abnormal extension	2
No response	No response	1
Verbal response		
Oriented	Coos, babbles, age-appropriate verbalizations	5
Confused	Irritable cry	4
Inappropriate words	Cries to pain	3
Incomprehensible	Moans, grunts	2
No response	No response	1 (Modified from Taylor, APLS)

▶ TABLE 6-2. ETIOLOGY OF ALTERED MENTAL STATUS BASED ON THE MNEMONIC "TIPS FROM THE VOWELS"

Mnemonic Device	Category	Cause
A	Abuse	Head trauma
		Shock
E	Epilepsy (and other causes of seizures)	Hypernatremia
		Hypocalcemia
		Hypoglycemia
		Hyponatremia
		Postictal state
		Status epilepticus
	Endocrine	Addison's disease
		Hyperthyroidism
		Hypothyroidism
		Inborn errors of metabolism
	Electrolyte disorders	Hypercalcemia
		Hypernatremia
		Hyponatremia
I	Infection	Brain abscess
		Encephalitis
		Meningitis
		Sepsis
		Subdural empyema
	Intussusception	Neurologic presentation
O	Overdose	Alcohol
		Carbon monoxide
		Lead
		Opiates
		Salicylates
		Sedatives
U	Uremia (and other metabolic causes)	Hemolytic uremic syndrome
		Hepatic encephalopathy
		Hypoxia
		Renal failure
		Reye's syndrome
T	Trauma	Child abuse
		Head trauma
		Hemorrhage
	Tumor	
I	Insulin-related problems	Diabetic ketoacidosis (DKA)
		Hyperglycemia
		Hypoglycemia
		Ketotic hypoglycemia
		Nonketotic hypoglycemia
P	Psychogenic	Diagnosis of exclusion
S	Shock	Anaphylactic
		Cardiogenic
		Hemorrhagic
		Hypovolemic
		Neurogenic
		Septic
	Stroke (and other CNS lesions)	Arteriovenous malformations
		Hemorrhage
	Shunt-related problems	Hydrocephalus
		Shunt dysfunction

Conversely, primary central nervous system pathology often affects cardiovascular and respiratory status. Airway, breathing, and circulation must be evaluated and managed prior to completing the examination. Important parameters of the general physical examination in patients with altered mental status are outlined in Table 6–4.[2]

The general neurologic evaluation focuses on an exact description of the patient's mental status, which provides a baseline for comparison during the course of illness. Cranial nerves and motor function are assessed for potentially localizing findings, which may indicate a mass lesion. For patients with severely depressed mental status, it is especially important to evaluate the response of the extremities to a painful stimulus. The biceps, triceps, patellar, and Achilles reflexes are tested for strength and symmetry and the patient is evaluated for the presence of a Babinski response, which indicates an upper motor neuron lesion.

For patients in coma, the area of the brain involved can be localized by considering physical examination findings (Table 6–5).[2,5,7]

▶ DIAGNOSTIC TESTING

All patients with altered mental status should have a bedside glucose determination and the serum glucose should

► **TABLE 6-3. MNEMONIC FOR COMA USING CHILDHOOD IMMUNIZATIONS**

DPT	**HIB**
Dehydration	Hypoxia, hypothermia
Poisoning	Intussusception
Trauma	Brain tumor
OPV	**MMR**
Occult trauma (child abuse), overdose	Meningitis
Postictal	Metabolic
Ventriculoperitoneal shunt problem	Reye's syndrome
IPV	**Hep B**
Infection	Hyperthermia
Postanoxia	Electrolyte, endocrine
Viral encephalitis	Psychogenic
	Bleeding

be checked. Other helpful studies include complete blood count with differential and platelets, electrolytes, calcium, renal functions, and urinalysis. In some cases, arterial blood gas and serum ammonia are indicated. Patients who may have ingested a toxin require a urine drug screen, as well as blood levels for suspected toxins such as aspirin or alcohol. Infants suspected of suffering from inborn errors of metabolism require testing for urine and serum, amino and organic acids, ammonia, liver function, thyroid function, plasma free fatty acids, and serum carnitine. If infection is suspected, cultures are obtained from the blood, urine, and cerebrospinal fluid. Lumbar puncture is withheld until increased intracranial pressure (ICP) is excluded (Fig. 6–1).[2,5,7,8]

Radiographic examination of the cervical spine is performed if there is any suspicion of trauma. If physical examination findings suggest a structural lesion, herniation, or increased ICP, a computed tomography (CT) scan should be performed. Although magnetic resonance imaging (MRI) may provide more information for certain etiologies of coma, a CT scan can provide useful initial information. An electroencephalogram is useful to diagnose seizures and some metabolic and infectious disorders but is not an emergency department procedure unless needed to diagnose nonconvulsive status epilepticus.[2,5,7–9]

► **THERAPY**

The first priority in the emergency department management of a patient with altered mental status is stabilization of the airway, breathing, and circulation. Intubation is required for patients with altered mental status who have lost protective airway reflexes and who are at risk for aspiration. Intubation is also indicated for patients with evidence of critically increased ICP.

All patients should receive oxygen and, if hypoglycemia is suspected, 0.5 to 1.0 g/kg of glucose. If an ingestion is suspected, a trial of naloxone may prove useful. Patients who are hypotensive are resuscitated with crystalloids. Fluids are titrated carefully for patients who may have increased ICP, in whom overaggressive hydration can precipitate herniation. Yet, hypotension is avoided, since it can result in cerebral hypoperfusion and ischemia.[2,7–9]

Hypertension can be secondary to increased ICP, but can also be due to hypertensive encephalopathy. If the etiology is the later, the blood pressure should be lowered slowly. The goal is to lower the diastolic blood pressure to 100 to 110 mm Hg or a maximum of 25% over 2 to 6 hours.[8,10]

Hyperventilation produces vasoconstriction of the cerebral arteries and has been used as the treatment for impending herniation due to elevated ICP. If there are no signs of impending herniation, it is best not to reduce the P_{CO_2} below 35 torr because severe vasoconstriction and cerebral ischemia can result. Elevating the head of the bed to 30 degrees may also be beneficial.[4,11] Mannitol or furosemide may be useful adjuncts for patients with severely increased ICP, but hypotension must be avoided and a neurosurgeon should be consulted.

► **TABLE 6-4. IMPORTANT PARAMETERS OF THE GENERAL PHYSICAL EXAMINATION OF PATIENTS WITH ALTERED MENTAL STATUS**

Body Area	Technique	Findings
Head	Palpation	Hematoma, fracture
	Fontanelle palpation (in infants)	Fullness, depression, pulsations (reflects ICP)
Eyes	Eye position	Midposition, deviated
	Reactivity of the pupils	Constricted, dilated
	Funduscopic examination	Papilledema, retinal hemorrhages
Ears	Inspection	Bleeding, CSF drainage
Nose	Inspection	Bleeding, CSF drainage
Neck	Palpation	Tenderness, spasm, stepoff
	Auscultation	Bruits
Breath	Check for odor	DKA: fruity smell
		Hepatic coma: musty smell
		Uremia: urine smell
Skin	Inspection	Jaundice, petichiae, purpura
Chest	Auscultation	Signs of respiratory pathology
Abdomen	Palpation	Hepatosplenomegaly, masses, evidence of intussusception

▶ **TABLE 6-5. LOCALIZATION OF THE AREA OF BRAIN DYSFUNCTION USING PHYSICAL FINDINGS**

Finding	Description	Significance
Patient Posture	Decorticate: arms flexed, legs extended	Dysfunction of the cerebral hemispheres with intact brain stem
	Decerebrate: extension and internal rotation of the upper and lower extremities (spontaneous or in response to examination or pain)	Lesion of the midbrain, toxic, or metabolic etiology
	Unilateral decerebrate posturing	Uncal herniation
	Flaccid paralysis	Diffuse lesions of both hemispheres and brain stem
Respiratory Pattern	Consistent hyperventilation	Compensation for metabolic acidosis, e.g., DKA, or salicylate intoxication; lesions of the midbrain or low pons
	Cheyne-Stokes (periods of tachypnea followed by apnea)	Bilateral hemispheric abnormality with intact brain stem; impending temporal lobe herniation
	Ataxic breathing (irregular rate and depth)	Lesions of the pons or upper medulla
	Irregular breathing	Lesion at the level of the medulla
Pupils	Small, reactive pupils	Lesions affecting the cerebral hemispheres or intoxication
	Pinpoint, nonreactive pupils	Metabolic derangement
	Midposition, fixed pupils	Lesions of the midbrain or upper pons
	Unilateral dilated pupil (in the presence of coma)	Third nerve compression, as with uncal herniation; in the late phase the pupil is nonreactive
	Bilateral fixed pupils	Tectal herniation; severe hypothermia; may imply severe permanent brain damage
Reflex Eye Movements	Oculocephalic (doll's eye) reflex—contraindicated with suspicion of neck trauma	Passively move head from side to side: if eyes move together toward the side opposite that to which the head is turned (+), brain stem function is intact. Impairment indicates a lesion at the midbrain or upper pons, sedation, toxic or metabolic encephalopathy Absence indicates lesion at the lower pons or medulla
	Oculovestibular response—contraindicated with suspicion of neck trauma	Elevate the head to 30 degrees and irrigate one of both ear canals with ice water. Normal: slow deviation of the eyes toward the irrigated side with lateral nystagmus away from the irrigated ear Asymmetric response indicates brain stem lesion Bilateral loss indicates metabolic or structural brain stem lesion In the unconscious patient, only slow deviation to the irrigated ear is seen If warm water is used, the quick phase is toward the irrigated ear. COWS = cold, opposite, warm, same
	Corneal reflex (touch the cornea with a small piece of cotton)	Normal: close/blink both eyes simultaneously Bilateral absence: pontine lesion, intoxication, metabolic disorder, or paralysis

Additional therapy is directed at maintaining normal body temperature, controlling seizures and correcting acid–base or electrolyte abnormalities. Further management in the emergency department may include the administration of antibiotics or antidote therapy for toxins.[2]

▶ **DISPOSITION**

Patients with significant alteration in mental status are best managed in an intensive care unit. For patients with milder disease, the decision to admit to the hospital or discharge from the emergency department largely depends on the etiology of the problem.

▶ **SPECIAL CONSIDERATIONS**

Several causes of altered mental status and coma are characteristic of the pediatric population and deserve special mention. None are common, but all represent serious problems that confront the emergency physician.

LEAD ENCEPHALOPATHY

Although lead toxicity severe enough to cause encephalopathy is now uncommon, it is a consideration in the differential diagnosis of any child with profoundly altered mental status or coma. Lead encephalopathy can be associated with increased

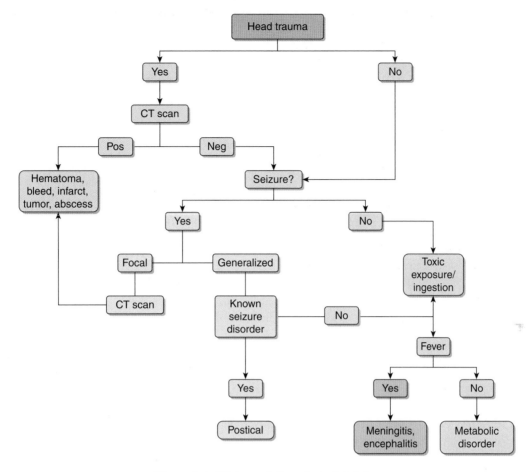

Figure 6–1. Etiology of altered mental status.

ICP and seizures. Patients with lead encephalopathy often have a history of pica and parents may have noted abdominal pain, constipation, or vomiting prior to the development of encephalopathy.[5] The evaluation and management of lead encephalopathy is discussed in Chapter 113.

INTUSSUSCEPTION

Intussusception is a fairly common gastrointestinal emergency in children younger than 3 years. Although this entity commonly presents with episodes of intermittent abdominal pain and vomiting, there is a "neurologic presentation" in which the child manifests a depressed level of consciousness that can range from lethargy to obtundation. The overall appearance of the patient can mimic shock, with fulminant sepsis a consideration. In some cases the abdominal examination may reveal a mass and rectal examination shows heme-positive or "currant jelly" stools.[5,9] Intussusception is discussed in detail in Chapter 9.

REYE'S SYNDROME

Reye's syndrome is a disorder characterized by the acute onset of encephalopathy, often developing approximately 2 weeks following a viral infection. The diagnosis is based on the presence of encephalopathy, elevated liver enzymes, and the pres-

ence of microvesicular fatty changes in the liver. The exact pathophysiology is unknown, but it may involve the interaction of salicylates and certain viruses, especially influenza and varicella.[12,13] The decreased use of aspirin in the treatment of these illnesses may have contributed to the decline in the incidence of Reye's syndrome. However, the decline also may be due to advances in diagnosis of inborn errors of metabolism (especially medium-chain acyl-CoA dehydrogenase [MCAD] deficiency).[12]

The syndrome begins with unremitting vomiting and can progress from lethargy to disorientation, combativeness, and coma.[13] The encephalopathy is characterized by increased ICP, which at high levels can lead to cardiovascular and respiratory instability and death. The increased ICP appears to be the predominant factor in influencing outcome. The mechanism resulting in encephalopathy is unknown.

Reye's syndrome in the United States occurred mainly in children younger than 12 to 13 years, but, especially in the United Kingdom, it has been described in patients younger than 1 year. In infants, vomiting may be less prominent and seizures more common.

The encephalopathy is associated with elevated liver function tests and serum ammonia is generally three times normal. Characteristically, serum bilirubin is only slightly elevated and jaundice is absent. Hypoglycemia is common in infants and in patients with severe encephalopathy. Fatty microvesicular metamorphosis of the liver can be confirmed by biopsy. At an ultrastructural level, mitochondrial abnormalities may be present and may reflect a fundamental lesion in the syndrome.[12]

If the diagnosis of Reye's syndrome is entertained, aggressive management is indicated. To avoid overhydration and worsening of cerebral edema, intravenous fluids are administered at or slightly below maintenance requirements. Hypoglycemic patients may require 10% or 15% dextrose. Patients who are not arouseable to voice or light pain are candidates for elective intubation and ventilation. Mannitol may be required for control of ICP.[14] Some centers institute ICP monitoring to guide therapy. In some cases, barbiturate coma and decompressive craniotomy have been used, but their efficacy is unknown. The need for a liver biopsy to confirm the diagnosis is controversial.

Early intervention can potentially avert the progression of encephalopathy and avoid serious morbidity and mortality. Patients with lethargy only usually recover completely. Patients who recover from more severe encephalopathy can suffer permanent neuropsychiatric impairment.

INBORN ERRORS OF METABOLISM

Numerous inborn errors of metabolism can present early in life with vomiting, seizures, and altered mental status. These disorders are discussed in Chapter 80.

HYPOGLYCEMIA

In any patient with altered mental status, hypoglycemia is a consideration. See Chapter 75 for further discussion.

Congenital Adrenal Hyperplasia

In a child with congenital adrenal hyperplasia, hypoglycemia may result from the absence of cortisol. A constellation of symptoms such as lethargy, vomiting, dehydration, and altered mental status should suggest this disorder. See Chapter 76 for further discussion.

REFERENCES

1. Plum F, Posner JB. *The Diagnosis of Stupor and Coma.* 3rd ed. Philadelphia, PA: FA Davis; 1980.
2. Taylor DA, Ashwal S. Impairment of consciousness and coma. In: Swaiman KF, Ashwal S, Ferriero DM, eds. *Pediatric Neurology: Principles and Practice.* 4th ed. Philadelphia, PA: Mosby/Elsevier; 2006:1377–1400.
3. Jennet B, Teasdale G. Aspects of coma after severe head injury. *Lancet.* 1977;1:878.
4. Tepas JJ, Fallat ME, Moriarty TM. Trauma. In: Gausche-Hill M, Fuchs S, Yamamoto L, eds. *APLS, The Pediatric Emergency Medicine Resource.* 4th ed. Sudbury, MA: Jones and Bartlett Publishers; 2004:282, 295–298.
5. Isaacman DJ, Trainor JL, Rothrock SG. Central nervous system. In: Gausche-Hill M, Fuchs S, Yamamoto L, eds. *APLS, The Pediatric Emergency Medicine Resource.* 4th ed. Sudbury, MA: Jones and Bartlett Publishers; 2004:146–153.
6. Schunk JE. The pediatric patient with altered level of consciousness; remember your "immuzations". *J Emerg Nurs.* 1992;18:419–421.
7. Michelson D, Thompson L, Williams E. Evaluation of stupor and coma. UpToDate Rose ed. Waltham, MA 2006.
8. Thompson L, Williams E. Treatment and prognosis of coma in children. UpToDate Rose ed. Waltham, MA 2006.
9. Nelson DS. Coma and altered level of consciousness. In: Fleisher GR, Ludwig S, Henretig FM, eds. *Textbook of Pediatric Emergency Medicine.* 5th ed. Philadelphia, PA: Lippincott, Williams & Wilkins; 2006:201–212.
10. Williams O, Brust JC. Hypertensive encephalopathy. *Curr Treat Options Cardiovasc Med.* 2004;6:209.
11. American Heart Association guidelines for cardiopulmonary resuscitation and emergency cardiovascular care, part 12: pediatric advanced life support. *Circulation.* 2005;112(suppl IV):IV-181.
12. Orlowski JP. Whatever happened to Reye's syndrome? Did it ever really exist? *Crit Care Med.* 1999;27:1582–1587.
13. Sarnaik AP. Reye's syndrome: Hold the obituary. *Crit Care Med.* 1999;27:1674–1676.
14. Durbin DR, Liacouras CA. Gastrointestinal emergencies. In: Fleisher GR, Ludwig S, Henretig FM, eds. *Textbook of Pediatric Emergency Medicine.* 5th ed. Philadelphia, PA: Lippincott, Williams & Wilkins; 2006:1101–1103.

CHAPTER 7

Seizures

Susan Fuchs

► HIGH-YIELD FACTS

- For febrile patients, the etiology of the fever should be investigated if it has not been determined on physical examination. A lumbar puncture is performed in any patient suspected of having a central nervous system infection.
- Neuroimaging should be reserved for those with a postictal focal deficit (Todd's paralysis) that does not quickly resolve: a child whose level of consciousness remains depressed or who has not returned to baseline mental status within several hours.
- A nonemergent magnetic resonance imaging (MRI) (several days later) should be considered in a child with an afebrile focal seizure that does not generalize: one with unexplained abnormalities on neurologic examination, unexplained cognitive or motor impairment, children younger than 1 year, and those who have had an electroencephalogram (EEG) that does not demonstrate a benign partial epilepsy or primary generalized epilepsy.
- The MRI is preferable to a computed tomography (CT) scan in most cases as it can better demonstrate small tumors, vascular malformations, atrophy, infarction, and cortical dysplasia. If trauma is suspected, a CT scan is preferred so that an acute hemorrhage can be detected, but MRI is preferred for brain damage and old hemorrhage detection.
- Any child who experiences a first focal seizure or who has an abnormal neurologic examination should be considered for hospital admission, with neurologic consultation. If the child has a first focal seizure, a nonfocal neurologic examination, and a negative emergency department (ED) workup and is stable, further workup can be performed on an outpatient basis in consultation with the child's primary physician, neurologist, and the parents or caretakers.
- Neonatal seizures are commonly related to perinatal asphyxia, intracranial hemorrhage, central nervous system infections, cerebral infraction, metabolic abnormalities, especially hypoglycemia and hypocalcemia, and congenital abnormalities of the brain. Less commonly, seizures are related to inherited metabolic abnormalities, including urea cycle defects and abnormalities in amino acid metabolism.
- For patients in whom an inherited metabolic defect is considered, serum ammonia is measured, as are serum and urine amino acids. Some defects are associated with a metabolic acidosis; therefore, arterial blood gas and, if possible, serum lactate are indicated.
- Phenobarbital (20 mg/kg intravenously) is the drug of choice for neonatal seizures, with phenytoin (20 mg/kg) the second choice. In refractory seizures, pyridoxine (100 mg intravenously) is indicated, to treat for potential pyridoxine-dependent seizures.
- For the first simple febrile seizure, there are no required laboratory studies other than a bedside glucose determination.
- Benzodiazepines are usually effective treatment of actively seizing patients but are not useful for long-term seizure control. The administration of a long-acting antiseizure medication is indicated after seizures are controlled with benzodiazepines.

A seizure results from the abnormal, excessive, paroxysmal electrical discharge of neurons within the brain, primarily within the cerebral cortex.[1] These discharges occur in various locations and may spread in different directions and at different speeds, resulting in several types of seizures, each with its own clinical manifestation.[2] Epilepsy is defined as seizures that occur over a period of time without an obvious precipitant.[1] The incidence of childhood epilepsy in the United States is 4 to 9 cases per 1000 children, but 1% of children will experience an afebrile seizure by age 14, and 5% of children will experience a febrile seizure by age 6.[1,2]

► CLASSIFICATION

The international classification of epilepsies, epileptic syndromes, and related seizure disorders was developed in 1989 and serves to classify seizure types.[1,2] Seizures are classified as location-related (partial, focal, and local), generalized, undetermined, and special syndromes.[2,3] The major categories are also subdivided into whether the seizure is idiopathic (primary), where no identifiable cause is found and the child has normal development; symptomatic (secondary), when an identifiable brain lesion is found or the cause is inherited/genetic (metabolic disorders, neurocutaneous disorders, and chromosomal abnormalities), congenital (vascular malformations and prenatal injury), acquired (e.g., trauma, tumors, and infection), or cryptogenic.[2]

Partial seizures are caused by the electrical discharge of a limited number of neurons in one hemisphere; their signs and symptoms often allow localization of the epileptic focus.[1,2] A partial seizure is also classified based on whether consciousness is lost. A simple partial seizure results in no impairment in consciousness. A complex partial seizure results in impaired consciousness and involves both sides of the brain. There can also be partial seizures that evolve into secondary generalized seizures.[1,2]

Partial seizures are further subdivided based on their clinical signs and symptoms. Motor seizures can have motor manifestations that include jerking of an extremity, but this can spread (march) to another area. They can also occur without motor involvement but with complex somatosensory symptoms such as numbness, tingling or paresthesias of an extremity, or visual phenomena. Autonomic symptoms include sweating, change in heart rate, pupil size, and piloerection; psychic symptoms include aphasia, déjà vu or jamias vu experiences, and illusions of perception (size and sound); and affective symptoms include such as fear, anger or depression, and even hallucinations.[1,2]

In addition to differing from simple partial seizures by alteration in consciousness, a predominant aspect of complex partial seizures is the presence of psychomotor automatisms, which are activities that occur during the seizure and for which the patient is amnestic. They can include such activities as chewing or swallowing, gestures such as clapping, or repetitive verbalizations.[1]

Generalized seizures involve both hemispheres of the brain. They impair consciousness and motor symptoms are bilateral. Generalized seizures can be convulsive or nonconvulsive, depending upon motor involvement.[1,2] Absence (petit mal) seizures are nonconvulsive and are characterized by an abrupt and brief loss of awareness (<15 seconds), which may include staring or eye blinking, without postictal confusion. It is often possible to induce these seizures by hyperventilation or photic stimulation.[2]

There are multiple manifestations of generalized seizures characterized by convulsions. Myoclonic seizures consist of brief muscle contractions of one or several muscles. Clonic seizures are characterized by jerking and flexor spasms of muscles that can be irregular and asymmetric. Tonic seizures are due to sustained muscle contraction resulting in rigidity, and tonic–clonic seizures (grand mal) combine the tonic, clonic movements, and a postictal phase.[2] Atonic seizures (drop attacks) involve a loss of muscle tone, which causes the child to fall to the floor.[4]

Several distinct types of epileptic syndromes occur only in children. Benign childhood epilepsy with centrotemporal spikes, also known as benign rolandic epilepsy, has an onset between 3 and 13 years of age. It is the most common partial epilepsy syndrome in children, and often occurs upon awakening, and consists of facial movements, grimacing, drooling, and vocalizations. It can also occur during sleep as tonic or clonic muscle activity. Diagnosis is based on finding midtemporal or centrotemporal spikes on an EEG. Most seizures resolve by adolescence, and no treatment is the usual approach due to its benign course and prognosis.[2,5]

Juvenile myoclonic epilepsy (Janz syndrome) is characterized by myoclonic jerks or the arm that occur after awakening, but can also include some generalized tonic–clonic seizures and absence seizures. It begins between 8 and 18 years of age, and there is a strong family history of seizures. Sleep deprivation, hyperventilation, photosensitivity, and alcohol can trigger a seizure. The EEG shows generalized 4 to 6 hertz polyspikes and spike and wave discharges.[2,5]

West syndrome (infantile spasms), is characterized by sudden symmetric bilateral tonic contractions of the extremities, head, and trunk. The onset is at 5 to 12 months of life, with spasms occurring upon falling asleep or after awakening, with occurrences a few times to hundreds of times a day.

Tuberous sclerosis is the most common cause. The classic EEG finding is hypsarrhythmia. Although the spasms tend to resolve by age 3, many children with West syndrome develop other seizures and epileptic syndromes, and most have neurocognitive delay.[2]

Lennox–Gastaut syndrome has its onset at 1 to 8 years of age and consists of multiple seizure types. These children often have seizures every day, and there is an associated deterioration in intelligence, as well as behavior disorders. Diagnosis is by the EEG finding of diffuse spikes and slow waves. The etiology can be secondary to infections, hypoxia, ischemia, intracranial hemorrhage, degenerative disorders, and neurocutaneous syndromes (tuberous sclerosis). Most children have neurocognitive delay, and difficult to control seizures.[2,5]

Benign neonatal convulsions, other neonatal seizures, febrile seizures, and status epilepticus are discussed in detail in the following sections.

▶ THE FIRST AFEBRILE SEIZURE

The majority of children who present to the ED with seizures have suffered from a febrile seizure or an exacerbation of a known seizure disorder. However, on occasion a patient may have experienced a first afebrile seizure, or may be experiencing recurrent manifestations of an atypical, undiagnosed seizure disorder. Aside from fever, the most common causes of seizures in children include infections, trauma, toxic exposures, metabolic disorders, and failure to take prescribed anticonvulsants.[6,7] In addition, childhood seizures are often idiopathic. A more thorough list is included in Table 7–1.

HISTORY

In a patient with a suspected seizure, it is necessary to elicit detailed information regarding the episode itself, as well as preceding events. A clear description of the patient's level of consciousness during the episode, memory of the event, duration, and any postictal phenomena is important in categorizing the seizure. Abnormal motor movements are noted and characterized as localized or generalized. Information regarding abnormal eye movements, facial grimacing, lip movements, and urinary or fecal incontinence is elicited. It is important to document the duration of the episode. Patients are questioned regarding the presence of any associated aura or somatosensory manifestations, such as visual or auditory hallucinations. If there have been recurrent episodes, a pattern may be evident, such as a predilection for the event to occur upon wakening or when the patient is fatigued. A history of fever, trauma, prior seizures, drug use or withdrawal, underlying medical disorders, perinatal problems, developmental milestones, and a family history of seizures will help direct further evaluation.[2,7,8]

A key question is whether the event was truly a seizure or another paroxysmal event. The differential diagnosis of seizures includes syncope, gastroesophageal reflux, breath-holding spells, migraine headache, sleep disorders (sleep myoclonus and night terrors), behavioral disorders (daydreaming), movement disorders (tics), and psychogenic (pseudoseizures, panic attacks).[2,7,9] Syncopal episodes are usually preceded by blurred vision, dizziness, and pallor.[2] Gastroesophageal reflux usually results in an arched back position

Infections	Hypernatremia
Meningitis	Hypocalcemia
Meningoencephalitis	Hypomagnesemia
Brain abscess	Pyridoxine deficiency
Parasites	Inborn errors of metabolism
Trauma	Vascular
Hemorrhage: epidural, subdural	Intracranial hematoma
	Embolism
Posttraumatic	Infarction
Intoxication	Hypertensive encephalopathy
Lead	Tumor
Cocaine	Psychological
PCP	Hyperventilation
Amphetamine	Breath-holding spells
Aspirin	Congenital
Carbon monoxide	Malformations
Isoniazid	Birth asphyxia
Organophosphates	Neurocutaneous syndromes
Theophylline	Other
Lidocaine	S/P DPT immunization
Lindane	Seizure disorder
Drug withdrawal (anticonvulsants)	Noncompliance
Metabolic	Inadequate drug level
Hypoglycemia	
Hyponatremia	

With permission from Isaacman DJ, Trainor JL, Rothrock SG. Central nervous system. In: Gausche-Hill M, Fuchs S, Yamamoto L, eds. *APLS: The Pediatric Emergency Medicine Course.* Sudbury, MA: Jones and Bartlett Publishers; 2004:168–182; Chiang VW. Seizures. In: Fleisher GR, Ludwig S, Henretig FM, eds. *Textbook of Pediatric Emergency Medicine.* 5th ed. Philadelphia, PA: Lippincott Williams & Wilkins; 2006:629–636.

with crying, no loss of consciousness, and is usually associated with feeding. Cyanotic breath-holding spells usually occur after a crying episode, and result in limpness and loss of consciousness, occasionally with posturing.[9] With a pallid breath-holding spell, the infant often sustains minor head trauma, loses consciousness, stops breathing, becomes pale, and limps. They may develop generalized increased muscle tone with incontinence, and have a postictal period.[9] A child who is daydreaming maintains his or her posture and head control, and can be interrupted by name calling or touch.[1,7] During a pseudoseizure, the patient often keeps his or her eyes tightly closed, resists eye opening, and avoids painful stimuli, and afterwards there is rapid return to a normal level of consciousness.[2,7,9]

PHYSICAL EXAMINATION

If the child is actively seizing, stabilization of airway, breathing, and circulation are priorities. However, most children will have stopped seizing by the time of evaluation, and a thorough physical examination is required. Complete vital signs including temperature, heart rate, respiratory rate, and blood pressure are obtained. Determining the child's level of con-

sciousness is important, as in the postictal period he or she may be sleepy or confused; if the level of consciousness does not return to normal within 1 hour after the seizure, additional studies may be needed. The head circumference is measured in a young infant to detect micro- or macrocephaly, and the head is palpated in any child with trauma to detect hematomas or skull fractures. Examination of the eyes includes an assessment of pupillary reactivity, establishing whether gaze is conjugate or disconjugate, and a funduscopic examination to detect papilledema or retinal hemorrhages. The presence or absence of meningismus and photophobia should be documented. The skin should be examined for petechiae and signs of neurocutaneous syndromes such as café au lait spots, ash leaf spots, and adenoma sebaceum.[7,10]

A thorough neurologic examination is performed. In some patients, examination may reveal Todd's paresis, a transient paralysis that can follow a seizure. It is usually unilateral and may involve both the face and extremities.

LABORATORY EVALUATION

A bedside glucose check should be performed on all patients to detect hypoglycemia. Other laboratory studies are based on the type of seizure, history, and likely etiologies.[8] If there is a history of drug exposure or substance abuse, a toxicology screen may be considered.[8] Other studies such as electrolytes, liver function tests, lead level, ammonia, urine amino acids, and organic acids should be individualized.[10] If the child has been on antiseizure medication, a drug level is obtained, if available.

For febrile patients, etiology of the fever should be investigated if not determined on physical examination. A lumbar puncture should be performed in any patient suspected of having a central nervous system infection. However, if there are focal findings on physical examination or suspicion of a mass lesion or increased intracranial pressure, the lumbar puncture is delayed pending CT scan of the brain.[8] In infants younger than 6 months with a first afebrile seizure, with no etiology, and persistent decreased level of consciousness, a lumbar puncture should be performed.[8,11]

RADIOLOGIC EVALUATION

For most patients with a generalized seizure, no focal findings on physical examination, and no history of trauma, there is little use for a CT scan or MRI. Neuroimaging should be reserved for those with a postictal focal deficit (Todd's paralysis) that does not quickly resolve, a child whose level of consciousness remains decreased, or who has not returned to baseline mental status within several hours.[8] A nonemergent MRI (several days later) should be considered in a child with an afebrile focal seizure that does not generalize: one with unexplained abnormalities on neurologic examination, unexplained cognitive or motor impairment, children younger than 1 year, and those who have had an EEG that does not demonstrate a benign partial epilepsy or primary generalized epilepsy.[8] MRI is preferable to a CT scan in these cases as it can better demonstrate small tumors, vascular malformations, atrophy, infarction, and cortical dysplasia.[8,12] If trauma is suspected, a CT scan is preferred as an acute hemorrhage can be detected, but MRI is preferred for brain damage and old hemorrhage detection.

ELECTROENCEPHALOGRAM

An EEG is the study of choice in the evaluation of childhood afebrile seizures.[8] The most beneficial one is during a seizure (ictal EEG), but this is rarely possible. An EEG performed 24 to 48 hours after a seizure will probably show diffuse slowing, so it should be performed a few days to weeks after the seizure.[8] The EEG helps to confirm if the event was a seizure, classify the seizure type, or epilepsy syndrome, predicts recurrence, and guide therapy.[7,8,10,12] Unfortunately, a normal EEG occurs in 10% to 20% of children with epilepsy.[12] If the suspicion of epilepsy is high, activation methods such as hyperventilation, photic stimulation, or sleep deprivation can be useful.[7,10,12] In addition, up to 5% of normal children without a seizure disorder will have an abnormal EEG.[10]

DISPOSITION

Any child who has an abnormal neurologic examination should be considered for hospital admission, with neurologic consultation. If the child has a first afebrile seizure, a non-focal neurologic examination, a negative ED workup, and is stable, further workup can be performed on an outpatient basis, in consultation with the child's primary physician, neurologist, and the parents/caretakers. A child with a first generalized seizure does not necessarily need to be admitted and, depending on the type of seizure and etiology, may not require treatment until an EEG is performed. See Figure 7–1 for seizure algorithm.[2,13]

Many parents will be uncomfortable taking their child home due to fear of another seizure. It is important to stress

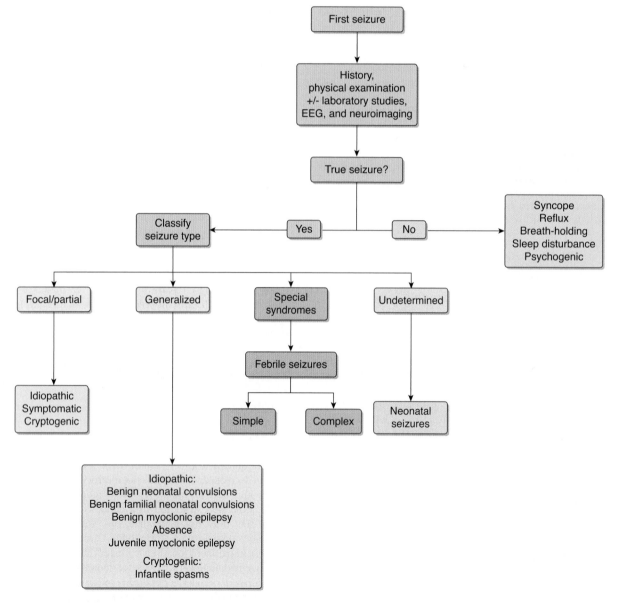

Figure 7–1. Seizure algorithm. (With permission from Major P, Thiele EA. Seizures in children: determining the variation. *Pediatr Rev.* 2007;28:363–371; LaRoche SM, Helmers SL. The new antiepileptic drugs: clinical applications. *JAMA.* 2004;291:615–620.)

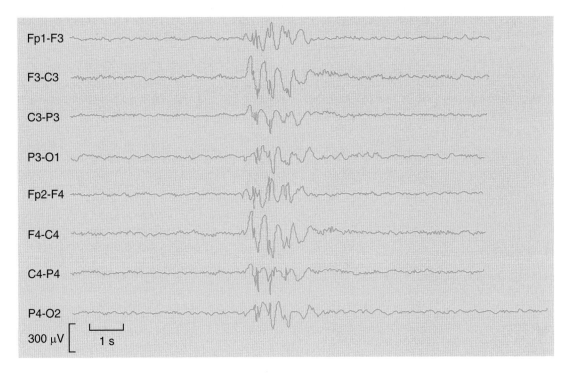

Figure 7–2. EEG of a patient with idiopathic (primary generalized) epilepsy. A burst of generalized epileptiform activity (**center**) is seen on a relatively normal background. These findings, obtained at a time when the patient was not experiencing **seizures**, support the clinical diagnosis of epilepsy. Odd-numbered leads indicate electrode placements over the left side of the head; even numbers, those over the right side. (With permission from Aminoff MJ, Greenberg DA, Simon RP. *Clinical Neurology*. 6th ed. New York: McGraw-Hill;2005.)

to parents that there is no evidence that a single seizure damages the brain. There is no way to absolutely predict seizure recurrence, but the majority of recurrences occur within 1 to 2 years.[14] The overall 3 to 5 years recurrence risk is 40% to 50%.[14,15] This drops to a 1-year recurrence of 24% if the child is neurologically normal, has no history of prior neurologic problems, and had an unprovoked seizure.[16] The recurrence rate is increased when there is an underlying neurologic problem, an abnormal EEG (Fig. 7–2), or a sleep-associated seizure.[15] The duration of seizure, occurrence of status epilepticus, and even treatment after a first seizure have no bearing on recurrence.[14] While treatment with an antiepileptic drug (AED) may reduce the risk of recurrence, withholding treatment does not change the long-term prognosis.[14,16] The decision to begin AED therapy should weigh the recurrence rate versus the behavioral and cognitive side effects of the specific medication chosen, such as drowsiness, blood dyscrasias, rash, or ataxia.[14]

Some of the most important information to provide the patient and parents involves addressing the anxiety of the parents; providing safety considerations such as not bathing or swimming alone, but avoidance of unnecessary restrictions (children can participate in sports); and a discussion about rescue medications such as rectal diazepam.[15] Rectal diazepam comes in a premeasured gel formulation in a prefilled special tip syringe that is useful for children with prolonged seizures and those far from medical care. While rectal administration has a slower absorption and response rate than intravenous use, the medication has a low risk of respiratory depression, and does not require refrigeration.[15,16] The dose is 0.2 to 0.5 mg/kg with a maximum dose of 5 mg for those <5 years, and 10 mg for those ≥5 years.[4,15,17]

▶ ANTIEPILEPTIC DRUGS

Many anticonvulsants are available, some of which have efficacy for certain types of seizures (Tables 7–2 and 7–3). The decision to initiate therapy should be made in conjunction with a pediatric neurologist. The various medications have various dosing forms and schedules, side effects, and drug interactions which must be taken into account. (Table 7–4) Therapeutic drug levels are available for some AEDs, but serious side effects tend to be idiosyncratic (Table 7–5).

▶ NEONATAL SEIZURES

These are seizures that occur during the first 28 days of life, although most occur shortly after birth. Because the cerebral cortex is immature, seizures in neonates can be convulsive (asymmetric or bilateral posturing of the trunk or extremities and eye deviation), or nonconvulsive (motor automatisms such as of lip smacking, tongue movements, random eye movement, and pedaling movements of legs).[21]

Neonatal seizures are commonly related to perinatal asphyxia; intracranial hemorrhage; central nervous system

▶ **TABLE 7–2. ANTIEPILEPSY DRUGS (AEDs) USED FOR SPECIFIC SEIZURE TYPES**

Partial/Focal Seizure	Focal or Generalized	Syndrome Specific
Carbamazepine	Valproic acid	Ethosuxmide (absence)
Fos/Phenytoin	Felbamate	ACTH (infantile spasms)
Phenobarbital	Lamotrigine	Viagbatrin (infantile spasms)*
Primidone	Topiramate	Valproic acid (Lennox-Gastaut)
Gabapentin	Levetiracetam	
Tiagabine	Zonisamide	
Oxcarbazepine		
Pregabalin		

*Not available in the United States.
With permission from Major P, Thiele EA. Seizures in children: Laboratory diagnosis and management. *Pediatr Rev.* 2007;28:405–414; Wilfong A. Treatment of seizures and epileptic syndromes in children. In: Rose BD, ed. *UpToDate.* Waltham, MA: UpToDate; 2007; Chapman K. *Controversies in the Treatment of Epilepsy. Seizure Medications, the Old and the New.* San Francisco, CA: American Academy of Pediatrics, National Conference and Exhibition; 2007.

▶ **TABLE 7–3. ANTICONVULSANT CHOICE—DAILY ORAL MEDICATIONS**

Seizure Type	Drug of Choice
Absence	Ethosuximide (Zarontin) 15–30 mg/kg/d
	Valproic acid (Depakene) or divalproex (Depakote) 15–60 mg/kg/d
	Lamotrigine (Lamictal) 10–12 mg/kg/d if given alone; 2–5 mg/kg/d when given with valproic acid
Atonic	Benzodiazepines, Valproic acid, clonazepam (Klonopin) 0.2 mg/kg/d, ethosuximide
Myoclonic	Valproic acid, clonazepam, lamotrigine
Partial	Carbamazepine (Tegretol/Carbatrol) 10–40 mg/kg/d bid or qid
	Felbamate 45–60 mg/kg/d
	Levetiracetam (Keppra) 10–60 mg/kg/d
	Phenytoin/fosphenytoin 4–8 mg/kg/d
	Valproic acid
	Phenobarbital 4–6 mg/kg/d
	Primidone (Mysoline) 10–20 mg/kg/d
	Gabapentin (Neurontin) 40–80 mg/kg/d
	Oxcarbazepine (Trileptal) 20–40 mg/kg/d
	Tiagabine (Gabatril) < 12 y 0.5 mg/kg/d, ≥12 y 4 mg/kg/d
Generalized, tonic–clonic	Carbamazepine, phenytoin, phenobarbital, primidone, valproic acid, lamotrigine, topiramate (Topamax)* 4–10 mg/kg/d)
Infantile spasms	ACTH, benzodiazepines, valproic acid, topiramate, ketogenic diet

*Not available in the United States.
With permission from Wilfong A. Treatment of seizures and epileptic syndromes in children. In: Rose BD, ed. *UpToDate.* Waltham, MA: UpToDate; 2007; Friedman MJ, Sharieff GQ. Seizures in children. *Pediatr Clin Nroth Am.* 2006;53:257–277.

infections; cerebral infraction; metabolic abnormalities, especially hypoglycemia and hypocalcemia; and congenital abnormalities of the brain.[22,23] Less commonly, seizures are related to inherited metabolic abnormalities, including urea cycle defects and abnormalities in amino acid metabolism. These defects often become apparent after the infant begins feeding and usually cause lethargy, vomiting, and poor feeding as well as seizures. A rare cause of refractory seizures in neonates is inherited pyridoxine deficiency, which is inherited as an autosomal recessive trait. Specific neonatal epileptic syndromes are listed in Table 7–6.[22] Important aspects of the history for patients with neonatal seizures are listed in Table 7–7.

NEONATAL EPILEPTIC SYNDROMES

Benign neonatal convulsions ("fifth day fits") begin between days 2 and 5 of life in neurologically normal infants, with no family history of seizures. They consist of short tonic or apneic episodes and usually recur during a 24- to 48-hour period. Although the outcome for most is good, 15% develop epilepsy in the future.[2,23]

Benign familial neonatal convulsions are an autosomal dominant channelopathy that results in focal or multifocal tonic or clonic seizures in the first week of life. There is a family history of neonatal seizures, but the infants have no neurologic abnormalities. The seizures may occur up to 2 to 3 months of life, and some infants will develop epilepsy later in life.[23]

Early myoclonic encephalopathy consists of segmental or erratic myoclonus in a neonate with an altered level of consciousness. It begins within the first few hours of life. Partial motor or focal clonic seizures develop later, and often extend to generalized myoclonus. Most cases are due to inborn errors of metabolism such as propionic acidemia, nonketotic hyperglycemia, or methylmalonic academia. The EEG is suppression-burst and assists in the diagnosis. The prognosis

is poor as although the myoclonus resolves, the focal motor seizures are difficult to control. There is neurologic delay and 50% die within 1 year of life.[23]

Early infantile epileptic encephalopathy (Ohtahara's syndrome) has its onset in the first 3 months of life. It is characterized by frequent tonic seizures, abnormal neurologic examination, spasticity, and severe developmental delay. Brain abnormalities that have been associated with this syndrome include porencephaly, cerebral atrophy, and migrational defects. EEG shows a suppression-burst pattern both when awake and asleep. Approximately 50% of infants die, and those who survive develop hypsarrhythmia or other seizures and have severe neurologic impairment.[5,23]

LABORATORY EVALUATION

Bedside glucose determination, serum glucose, electrolytes, calcium, and magnesium are obtained. In most instances, a lumbar puncture for bacterial and viral cultures, cell count, protein, glucose, and Gram stain is performed as soon as possible.

▶ TABLE 7–4. ADVERSE EFFECTS OF AEDs

AED	Adverse Events
Carbamazepine	Blood dyscrasia, elevated liver functions, rash
Ethosuximide	Blood dyscrasia, somnolence, rash
Felbamate	Aplastic anemia, severe hepatic toxicity
Gabapentin	Fatigue, ataxia, weight gain
Lamotrigine	Rash, TEN, SJS
Levetiracetam	Ataxia, behavioral changes
Oxcarbazepine	Hypo Na, hepatic or blood dyscrasia
Phenobarbital/primidone	Somnolence, cognitive impairment, rash
Phenytoin/fosphenytoin	Ataxia, rash, somnolence
Pregabalin	Ataxia, fatigue
Tiagabine	Spike wave stupor, weakness
Topiramate	Renal calculi, glaucoma, weight loss, metabolic acidosis
Valproic Acid	Drowsiness, thrombocytopenia, hepatic necrosis
Vigabatrin*	Dizziness, retinal degeneration
Zonisamide	Rash, renal calculi, photosensitivity

SJS, Steven's Johnson Syndrome; TEN, Toxic epidermal necrolysis.
*Not available in the United States.
With permission from Major P, Thiele EA. Seizures in children: laboratory diagnosis and management. *Pediatr Rev.* 2007;28:405–414; Wilfong A. Treatment of seizures and epileptic syndromes in children. In: Rose BD, ed. *UpToDate.* Waltham, MA: UpToDate; 2007; Chapman K. *Controversies in the Treatment of Epilepsy. Seizure Medications, the Old and the New.* San Francisco, CA: American Academy of Pediatrics, National Conference and Exhibition; 2007; LaRoche SM, Helmers SL. The new antiepileptic drugs: scientific review. *JAMA.* 2004;291:605–614.

For patients in whom an inherited metabolic defect is considered, serum ammonia is measured, as are serum and urine amino acids. Some defects are associated with a metabolic acidosis; therefore, arterial blood gas and, if possible, serum lactate are indicated. Cranial ultrasound or CT scan can be useful to diagnose hemorrhage.[24]

TREATMENT

The initial treatment is aimed at securing an adequate airway and ensuring oxygenation. If hypoglycemia (<40 mg/dL) is found, 2 mL/kg of D_{10} W is administered intravenously, followed by an infusion of D_{10} W. Phenobarbital (20 mg/kg intravenously) is the drug of choice for neonatal seizures, with phenytoin (20 mg/kg) the second choice. In refractory seizures, pyridoxine (100 mg intravenously) is indicated to treat the potential for pyridoxine-dependent seizures. Other metabolic abnormalities such as hypocalcemia (<7 mg/dL) and hypomagnesemia are corrected. Hypomagnesemia may be made worse by giving calcium.[24]

▶ TABLE 7–5. THERAPEUTIC MONITORING

AED	Monitoring
Carbamezepine	4–12 µg/mL
Ethosuximide	40–100 µg/mL
Felbamate	40–100 µg/mL
Phenobarbital	10–40 µg/mL
Phenytoin	10–20 µg/mL
Valproic acid	50–100 µg/mL
Gabapentin (Neurontin)	None
Lamotrigine (Lamictal)	None
Levetiracetam (Keppra)	None
Oxcarbazepine (Trileptal)	None
Pregablin (Lyrica)	None
Tiagabine (Gabatril)	None
Topiramate (Topamax)	None
Zonisamide (Zonegran)	None

With permission from Wilfong A. Treatment of seizures and epileptic syndromes in children. In: Rose BD, ed. *UpToDate.* Waltham, MA: UpToDate; 2007; Conway JM, Kriel RL, Birnbaum AK. Antiepileptic drug therapy in children. In: Swaiman KF, Ashwal S, Ferriero DM, eds. *Pediatric Neurology: Principles and Practice.* 4th ed. Philadelphia, PA: Mosby/ Elsevier; 2006:1105–1130; Chapman K. *Controversies in the Treatment of Epilepsy. Seizure Medications, the Old and the New.* San Francisco, CA: American Academy of Pediatrics, National Conference and Exhibition; 2007.

▶ TABLE 7–6. CAUSES OF NEONATAL SEIZURES

Hypoxia/anoxia (intrauterine or perinatal)

Cerebral ischemia (secondary to hypoxia/anoxia)

Hemorrhage
  Subarachnoid (birth trauma)
  Subdural (birth trauma)
  Intraventricular/intracerebral (prematurity)

Infection
  Meningitis: group B streptococci, *Escherichia coli*
  Meningoencephalitis: herpes, cytomegalovirus, toxoplasmosis

Metabolic
  Hypoglycemia (especially first day of life)
  Hypocalcemia (days 3–14)
  Pyridoxine (vitamin B_6) deficiency

Inborn errors of metabolism (days 4–7)
  Aminoacidurias
    Maple syrup urine disease
    Phenylketonuria
  Urea cycle defects: citrullinemia
  Organic acidurias: proprionic academia

Structural anomalies
  Lissencephaly

Hereditary disorders
  Tuberous sclerosis

Drug withdrawal
  Narcotics
  Neonatal epileptic syndromes

▶ **TABLE 7–7. IMPORTANT ASPECTS OF THE HISTORY FOR PATIENTS WITH NEONATAL SEIZURES**

Gestational age of the infant
History of maternal infections
Maternal drug use during pregnancy
Maternal fever during labor
Premature rupture of membranes
Duration of labor
Method of delivery
Complications during delivery
Need for the newborn to be aggressively resuscitated, which may indicate perinatal asphyxia
Feeding pattern and the type of formula (important for a child who has a seizure after 3 d of age, when inherited metabolic defects become more likely)

▶ FEBRILE SEIZURES

A febrile seizure is a seizure accompanied by a fever without evidence of intracranial infection, intracranial abnormality, metabolic abnormality, toxins, or an endotoxin, such as *Shigella* neurotoxin.[11,25–27] Febrile seizures usually occur between 6 months and 5 years of age. Most febrile seizures are self-limited, generalized, last for less than 15 minutes, and occur once in a 24-hour period, in which case they are classified as simple. A complex febrile seizure lasts more than 15 minutes, occurs more than once in a 24-hour period, or has a focal component.[4,25–27] Following a febrile seizure, children will usually have a postictal period during which they are lethargic, irritable, or confused, and may have a brief period of hemiparesis.[26]

Approximately 2% to 5% of all children will have a febrile seizure. They occur most commonly in children younger than 2 years. Twenty-five to thirty percent of children who have one febrile seizure will have a recurrence. The rate of recurrence is increased if the first seizure occurs before 1 year of age (50% recurrence, vs. 30% recurrence if >1 year of age), is most likely in the first 6 to 12 months after the first seizure, and is not affected by the height of the fever or duration of the original seizure.[25] Risk factors that correlate with an increased risk of subsequent epilepsy include a prolonged or unilateral seizure, a prior neurologic deficit, and a family history of epilepsy.[25,26]

Any illness that causes fever can provoke a febrile seizure. The seizure usually occurs during the early phase of the infectious illness. Commonly implicated etiologies include upper respiratory tract infections, viral syndrome, pharyngitis, otitis media, pneumonia, gastroenteritis, urinary tract infections, and roseola.[4] Febrile seizures can also occur after immunizations.[26]

The history should focus on the presence of a preceding febrile illness. A description of the seizure and its duration is obtained from a witness. Preexisting neurologic abnormalities, developmental delay, and a family history of seizures are obtained to provide information regarding the risk of recurrence.

In most cases, the seizure will have terminated upon arrival in the ED, but the child may still be postictal. If the child continues to seize, anticonvulsant therapy as described in the section on status epilepticus is indicated. A complete physical examination focuses on determining the etiology of the fever, with particular attention to excluding central nervous system infection. In a febrile seizure, the neurologic examination is normal. If a neurologic deficit exists, consider another etiology for the fever.

LABORATORY EVALUATION

A bedside glucose determination is done on all patients. For the first simple febrile seizure, there are no required laboratory studies.[4,11,26] Complete blood count may be helpful for children with complex febrile seizures or if history or physical examination warrants it. It should be understood that the complete blood count may not be reliable, since the seizure may result in an elevated white blood cell count. If no source of fever has been determined by physical examination, a blood culture, urinalysis, and urine culture may be helpful. Electrolytes, calcium, and glucose are usually normal but may be useful if the history is compatible with an electrolyte imbalance or vomiting. For example, a child with gastroenteritis in whom hyponatremia is a possibility will require electrolyte determination. The greatest controversy surrounds the need to perform a lumbar puncture in a child who has had a febrile convulsion. A child older than 18 months who is nontoxic, with a normal mental status, and who has no evidence of neck pain or stiffness does not require a lumbar puncture. In a child who is still postictal or noncommunicative (younger than 12 months) or who has received prior antibiotics, detecting meningismus may be difficult. In this situation, a lumbar puncture should be strongly considered.[4,11,26]

Other studies such as skull radiographs, CT scan, and even EEG are rarely helpful and not warranted after the first simple febrile seizure, unless history or physical findings suggests some underlying pathology.[4,11,26]

THERAPY

The initial management of the patient with a febrile seizure includes stabilizing the airway and ensuring adequate oxygenation. If the seizure persists for more than 5 minutes, anticonvulsant therapy is indicated (see status epilepticus). Acetaminophen, 15 mg/kg po or pr or ibuprofen, 10 mg/kg po is administered to reduce the fever.

The benign nature of febrile seizures, even considering the risk of recurrence, outweighs the benefits of the medications used, given their side effects. The risk of death from a febrile seizure due to aspiration, injury, or arrhythmia is theoretical and has not been documented.[25] The medication commonly used in the past was phenobarbital, which has been associated with undesirable side effects on behavior and mood.[25] Valproic acid is an alternative; however, it can cause gastrointestinal upset, thrombocytopenia, liver dysfunction, and pancreatitis. Primidone has been used and has reduced the recurrence rate, but also has some undesirable side effects such as irritability and behavioral disturbances.[25] Carbamazepine and phenytoin have not been effective in preventing recurrence.[25] The use of oral or rectal diazepam prophylaxis at the time of fever has been studied and was found to be effective in reducing the risk of recurrence, but it also results in side effects including ataxia, lethargy, and irritability.[25] Unfortunately, the use of antipyretic agents without concurrent anticonvulsants is not useful to prevent recurrent febrile seizures.[25,26,28]

DISPOSITION

Patients who have had a febrile seizure may be discharged, with follow-up by their primary care provider, unless an underlying infection precludes discharge. If a bacterial infection is the etiology of the fever, it is treated with appropriate antibiotics. Parental reassurance and education regarding the benign nature of febrile seizures, the low risk of recurrence, and the low incidence of subsequent epilepsy are part of the discharge instructions.[26,28]

▶ STATUS EPILEPTICUS

Status epilepticus is a seizure lasting 30 minutes or longer or two or more seizures without recovery of consciousness in between.[29,30] Status can present in several forms, including generalized (convulsive and nonconvulsive) and partial seizures (convulsive and nonconvulsive). More than 50% of cases of status occur in children younger than 3 years, with the most in the first year of life.[29] Approximately one-third of cases of status epilepticus are the initial presentation of epilepsy, one-third occur in patients with known epilepsy, and one-third occur due to an isolated brain injury/insult.[4]

Etiologies for status epilepticus overlap those for a first seizure and include non-CNS fever or infection, central nervous system infection, medication change or noncompliance in children on anticonvulsant therapy, head trauma, hypoxia, metabolic disorders, toxic ingestions, ethanol, tumor, vascular lesions, and progressive neurologic disorders.[4]

Initial therapy consists of meticulous attention to maintaining patency of the airway and adequacy of oxygenation and ventilation. Venous access is secured as soon as possible.[4,31] Head positioning, using the chin lift and jaw thrust, may open the airway, and an oral or nasal airway can be inserted. Oral suctioning may be required, so this should be available. High-flow oxygen (15 L) is administered to all patients via non-rebreather mask or bag-mask ventilation, and cardiac status and pulse oximetry are monitored continuously. Intubation may be necessary to oxygenate and ventilate the patient adequately. In addition, when administering anticonvulsants, especially benzodiazepines, intubation may be necessary because of respiratory depression.[4]

After intravenous access is obtained, a bedside glucose determination is performed.[4,29,31] Blood should be drawn for complete blood count, electrolytes, BUN, glucose, calcium, and magnesium.[31] For patients on anticonvulsant therapy, drug levels are obtained, and in some patients a toxicology screen may be indicated.[25] If the glucose is <60 mg/dL, 0.5 to 1.0 g/kg of dextrose is given as $D_{25}W$, 2 to 4 mL/kg or $D_{50}W$ 1 to 2 mL/kg.[4] In adolescents and adults, thiamine 100 mg intravenously is also given.

If vascular access cannot be obtained, intraosseous access is an acceptable alternative, although some of the initial AED medications can be administered rectally, or via the intranasal or intramuscular route.[31]

Drug therapy requires a clear plan, prompt administration of anticonvulsants in adequate doses, and with attention to side effects, such as hypoventilation or apnea. The use of medications should begin within 5 to 10 minutes of status onset, as there is a risk of mortality or 1% to 3% related to prolonged seizures.[4,15] Benzodiazepines are effective for treatment of an actively seizing patient. Lorazepam (Ativan) has an onset of action of 2 to 3 minutes and a relatively long half-life of 12 to 24 hours. Side effects, although less frequent and of shorter duration than those of diazepam, include respiratory depression and sedation. The dose is 0.10 mg/kg, up to a maximum of 4 mg per dose.[4,31] Diazepam (Valium) is useful for control of seizures. It has an onset of action of 1 to 3 minutes, but its half-life of 15 to 20 minutes means that repeated doses are often required. The dose is 0.1 to 0.3 mg/kg, administered slowly by intravenous push. Side effects include respiratory depression, hypotension, sedation, and bradycardia. Diazepam can also be given rectally, using the intravenous formulation in a dose of 0.5 mg/kg for the first dose and 0.25 mg/kg for any subsequent dose, to a maximum of 20 mg. With rectal administration, the onset of action is usually within 5 to 10 minutes.[4] There is also a rectal gel form of diazepam (Diastat) available, with the dose via this formulation of 0.2 to 0.5 mg/kg with a maximum dose of 5 mg for those <5 years, and 10 mg for those ≥5 years. It is available in several premeasured sizes: 2.5, 5.0, and 10 mg.[4,15,17] Midazolam (Versed) is a benzodiazepine that is rapidly absorbed after intramuscular injection and is an alternative to other benzodiazepines when it is impossible to obtain intravenous or intraosseous access. The intravenous dose is 0.1 mg/kg, and the intramuscular dose is 0.2 mg/kg with an onset of action in approximately 2 to 3 minutes IV and 15 minutes IM.[4,31] It has also been used via buccal administration, using the 5 mg/mL IV solution, squirting it into the buccal pocket of the mouth at a dose approximately 0.5 mg/kg (2.5 mg for children 6–12 months, 5 mg for 1–4 years, 7.5 mg for 5–9 years, and 10 mg for those 10 years and older).[15,16,32]

Because benzodiazepines are not useful for long-term seizure control, the administration of a long-acting antiseizure medication is indicated after seizures are controlled with benzodiazepines.[4]

Fosphenytoin is a new water-soluble prodrug of phenytoin. The conversion is 1.5 mg fosphenytoin = 1 mg phenytoin = 1 mg phenytoin equivalents (PE). (Therefore, 150 mg fosphenytoin = 100 mg phenytoin = 100 mg PE, and all doses listed below are in PE.) The intravenous loading dose is 20 mg PE/kg, which can be given at a rate of 3 mg PE/kg/min up to 150 mg PE/min. (It can also be given IM.) The only side effects are pruritus and paresthesias (groin). Because it is in a neutral solution and does not contain propylene glycol, it can also be given intramuscularly (same dose as intravenously); however, peak levels are reached in 3 hours.[4,18,31]

Phenytoin, when given intravenously, has rapid brain deposition but takes longer to control the seizure than a benzodiazepine (10 to 30 minutes). The loading dose is 20 mg/kg, which must be given slowly, 50 mg/min in adults or 1 mg/kg/min in children <50 kg. Side effects include hypotension and cardiac conduction disturbances (widened QT interval and arrhythmias), which if they occur should prompt a slower infusion or stopping the medication. Phenytoin will precipitate in glucose solutions, so it should be given directly into the vein, or in saline. Long-term seizure control can be accomplished by repeating half of the initial dose in 2 to 3 hours (intravenously or po) and then continuing the medication on a bid schedule (4–8 mg/kg), following serum levels.[4,18,31]

Phenobarbital is still a useful drug for treating status epilepticus, and it remains the drug of choice for neonatal seizures. Peak brain levels are reached in 10 to 20 minutes, and its duration of action is > 48 hours. The loading dose is 20 mg/kg IV given slowly at 100 mg/min. Side effects include respiratory depression (additive with benzodiazepines), sedation, and occasionally hypotension. If seizures stop before the entire loading dose is given, the remainder can be given intravenously or even orally within 1 to 2 hours. Long-term therapy can be initiated in 24 hours using 4 to 6 mg/kg/d, monitoring drug levels to avoid oversedation.[4,19,31]

If status persists after giving one dose of a benzodiazepine followed by phenytoin or phenobarbital, an additional dose of benzodiazepine can be given. If the seizure persists after phenytoin or phenobarbital is given, the alternate drug of the two can be administered. In such cases, the risk of apnea is high, so assisted ventilation and possibly intubation may be required.[4]

For refractory status, midazolam, pentobarbital, propofol or valproic acid may be given as continuous infusions. Pentobarbital is given as a loading dose of 5 to 15 mg/kg intravenously followed by an infusion of 0.5 to 5 mg/kg/h, to keep the level between 20 and 50 μg/mL and to produce burst suppression on the EEG, or cessation of epileptic activity. Vasopressors are often needed with pentobarbital coma, and the patient should be weaned off of the infusion to determine whether status has stopped.[4,31]

Midazolam is given as a 0.2 mg/kg load followed by and infusion of 1 μg/kg/min, and titrated upward (up to 4 μg/kg/min) over 60 minutes until there is cessation of seizures or burst suppression on the EEG.[4,31] Other options include the use of intravenous propofol (1–3 mg/kg load followed by 2–10 mg/kg/h). However, side effects include hypotension with rapid infusion, as well as fatal acidosis and rhabdomyolysis with maintenance infusions.[31] It is also contraindicated in children on a ketogenic diet.[31] Valproic acid can also be given IV (Depacon) as a 15 to 20 mg/kg load, and repeated every 10 to 15 minutes to a maximum of 40 mg/kg, followed by an infusion of 5 mg/kg/h.[4,31]

Therapy of nonconvulsive status epilepticus is similar to that of convulsive status, using a benzodiazepine, fosphenytoin, or phenytoin. For absence status, a benzodiazepine can be followed by oral or nasogastric ethosuximide. Although unlabeled for use in absence status, valproic acid (IV 15–25 mg/kg over 5–10 minutes, but at a rate <6 mg/kg/min) has been successful.[33] Valproic acid can also be used rectally, orally, or via a nasogastric tube (5–25 mg/kg of the liquid formulation). Oral clonazepam is another alternative but do not give both valproic acid and clonazepam.[17,31,33]

DISPOSITION

Any child who has received lorazepam or a long-acting anticonvulsant medication should be admitted to the hospital. Since diazepam is short acting, if no other drugs have been given, admission decisions can be individualized. Intensive care admission is obviously needed for any child still in status, requiring assisted or mechanical ventilation, or in whom the evaluation has revealed an etiology requiring close monitoring.[4]

REFERENCES

1. Wilfong A. Overview of the classification, etiology, and clinical features of pediatric seizures and epilepsy. In: Rose BD, ed. *UpToDate*. Waltham, MA: UpToDate; 2007.
2. Major P, Thiele EA. Seizures in children: determining the variation. *Pediatr Rev*. 2007;28:363–371.
3. Commission on Classification and Terminology of the International League Against Epilepsy. Proposal for revised classification of epilepsies and epileptic syndromes. *Epilepsia*. 1989;30:389–399.
4. Isaacman DJ, Trainor JL, Rothrock SG. Central nervous system. In: Gausche-Hill M, Fuchs S, Yamamoto L, eds. *APLS: The Pediatric Emergency Medicine Course*. Sudbury, MA: Jones and Bartlett Publishers; 2004:168–182.
5. Wilfong A. Epilepsy syndromes in children. In: Rose BD, ed. *UpToDate*. Waltham, MA: UpToDate; 2007.
6. Chiang VW. Seizures. In: Fleisher GR, Ludwig S, Henretig FM, eds. *Textbook of Pediatric Emergency Medicine*. 5th ed. Philadelphia, PA: Lippincott Williams & Wilkins; 2006:629–636.
7. Chapman K. *Controversies in the Treatment of Epilepsy. Epilepsy-Making the Diagnosis*. San Francisco, CA: American Academy of Pediatrics, National Conference and Exhibition; 2007.
8. Hirtz D, Ashwal S, Berg A, et al. Practice parameter: evaluating a first nonfebrile seizure in children. Report of the quality standards subcommittee of the American Academy of Neurology, the Child Neurology Society, and the American Epilepsy Society. *Neurology*. 2000;55:616–623.
9. Wilfong A. Differential diagnosis of seizures in children. In: Rose BD, ed. *UpToDate*. Waltham, MA: UpToDate; 2007.
10. Wilfong A. Clinical and laboratory diagnosis of seizures in infants and children. In: Rose BD, ed. *UpToDate*. Waltham, MA: UpToDate; 2007.
11. American Academy of Pediatrics: Provisional Committee on Quality Improvement, Subcommittee on Febrile Seizures. Practice parameter: the neurodiagnostic evaluation of the child with a first simple febrile seizure. *Pediatrics*. 1996;97:769–775.
12. Major P, Thiele EA. Seizures in children: laboratory diagnosis and management. *Pediatr Rev*. 2007;28:405–414.
13. LaRoche SM, Helmers SL. The new antiepileptic drugs: clinical applications. *JAMA*. 2004;291:615–620.
14. Hirtz D, Berg A, Bettis D, et al. Practice parameter: treatment of the child with a first unprovoked seizure; Report of the quality standards committee of the American Academy of Neurology and the practice committee of the Child Neurology Society. *Neurology*. 2003;60:166–175.
15. Roberts C. *Controversies in the Treatment of Epilepsy. Part 2: When to Treat, When not to Treat*. San Francisco, CA: American Academy of Pediatrics, National Conference and Exhibition; 2007.
16. Wilfong A. Treatment of seizures and epileptic syndromes in children. In: Rose BD, ed. *UpToDate*. Waltham, MA: UpToDate; 2007.
17. Conway JM, Kriel RL, Birnbaum AK. Antiepileptic drug therapy in children. In: Swaiman KF, Ashwal S, Ferriero DM, eds. *Pediatric Neurology: Principles and Practice*. 4th ed. Philadelphia, PA: Mosby/Elsevier; 2006:1105–1130.

18. Chapman K. Controversies in the Treatment of Epilepsy. Seizure Medications, the Old and the New. San Francisco, CA: American Academy of Pediatrics, National Conference and Exhibition; 2007.

19. Friedman MJ, Sharieff GQ. Seizures in children. *Pediatr Clin North Am.* 2006;53:257–277.

20. LaRoche SM, Helmers SL. The new antiepileptic drugs: scientific review. *JAMA.* 2004;291:605–614.

21. Mizrahi EM. Clinical features and electrodiagnosis of neonatal seizures. In: Rose BD, ed. *UpToDate.* Waltham, MA: UpToDate; 2007.

22. Mizrahi EM. Etiology and prognosis of neonatal seizures. In: Rose BD, ed. *UpToDate,* Waltham, MA: UpToDate; 2007.

23. Mizrahi EM. Neonatal epileptic syndromes. In: Rose BD, ed. *UpToDate.* Waltham, MA: UpToDate; 2007.

24. Mizrahi EM. Treatment of neonatal seizures. In: Rose BD, ed. *UpToDate.* Waltham, MA: UpToDate; 2006.

25. American Academy of Pediatrics, Steering Committee on Quality Improvement and Management, Subcommittee on Febrile Seizures. Febrile Seizures: clinical practice guideline for the long-term management of the child with simple febrile seizures. *Pediatrics.* 2008;121:1281–1286.

26. Fishman M. Febrile seizures. In: Rose BD, ed. *UpToDate.* Waltham, MA: UpToDate; 2007.

27. Nelson KB, Ellenberg JH. Prognosis in children with febrile seizures. *Pediatrics.* 1978;61:720–726.

28. Fishman M. Patient information: febrile seizures. In: Rose BD, ed. *UpToDate.* Waltham, MA: UpToDate; 2007.

29. Riviello JJ, Ashwal S, Hirtz D, et al. Practice parameter: diagnostic assessment of the child with status epilepticus (an evidence-based review). Report of the Quality Standards Committee of the American Academy of Neurology and the Practice Committee of the Child Neurology Society. *Neurology.* 2006;67: 1542–1550.

30. Wilfong A. Clinical features and complications of status epilepticus in children. In: Rose BD, ed. *UpToDate.* Waltham, MA: UpToDate; 2007.

31. Wilfong A. Management of status epilepticus in children. In: Rose BD, ed. *UpToDate.* Waltham, MA: UpToDate; 2007.

32. McIntyre J, Robertson S, Norris E, et al. Safety and efficacy of buccal midazolam versus rectal diazepam for emergency treatment of seizures in children; a randomized controlled trial. *Lancet.* 2005;366:205–210.

33. Morton LD, Pellock JM. Status epilepticus. In: Swaiman KF, Ashwal S, Ferriero DM, eds. *Pediatric Neurology: Principles and Practice.* 4th ed. Philadelphia, PA: Mosby/Elsevier; 2006:1100.

CHAPTER 8

Chest Pain

Wendy C. Matsuno

▶ HIGH-YIELD FACTS

- Chest pain in children is usually benign, but preadolescent children are more likely to have a cardiorespiratory source.
- Chest pain with fever, dyspnea with exertion, fatigue, and an examination that reveals distant heart sounds or a friction rub should alert the physician to consider myocarditis or pericarditis.
- Asthma and pneumonia are common causes of chest pain in children.
- Electrocardiogram, chest radiographs, and cardiac enzymes should only be ordered when there is a history or physical examination suggesting a cardiopulmonary etiology for chest pain in children.

Chest pain is a worrisome symptom that often causes parents to bring their child to the emergency department (ED) for evaluation. The rate of pediatric patients presenting to the ED with a complaint of chest pain is 3 to 6 for every 1000 patient visits.[1,2] In the majority of cases, the etiology of the chest pain is benign, but symptoms are distressing enough to cause 27% to 30% of children to miss school.[2,3]

▶ CLINICAL PRESENTATION

The clinical presentation of the pediatric patient with chest pain varies greatly. The average age of presentation is 10 to 12 years, with an equal distribution between sexes.[1–4] Younger children are more likely to have a cardiorespiratory source for their chest pain, whereas the chest pain of an adolescent patient is more likely to be of psychogenic origin.[1,3]

The duration of the chest pain in the majority of patients is either acute or subacute in onset.[1,3] Patients that present with a complaint of chronic chest pain (>6 months duration) usually have idiopathic or psychogenic chest pain.[3,4]

Children often have difficulty localizing and qualifying their pain. In instances where the child is able to indicate a location for their chest pain (e.g., right-sided, left-sided, and sternal), no specific relationship to a particular diagnosis or diagnostic category has been found.[1–3] The description of the pain (e.g., sharp, dull, and aching) also shows no relationship to the actual diagnosis.[3]

▶ DIFFERENTIAL DIAGNOSIS

The differential diagnosis for pediatric chest pain is extensive. The diagnostic categories with precipitating clinical causes are listed in Table 8–1.

CARDIAC

A cardiac cause for pediatric chest pain is found in 4% to 5% of cases presenting to the ED.[1,3] Myocardial infarction is rare in the pediatric population, but has been reported in the literature in previously healthy adolescents.[5] These patients usually present with the classic severe, substernal chest pain with radiation to the left arm or jaw; however, it is important to note that the location and severity of a child's chest pain is not specific to myocardial infarction or a cardiac etiology.[1–3,5] Patients are at greater risk for myocardial ischemia if they have a history of congenital heart disease, acquired heart disease (e.g., Kawasaki disease), or drug abuse (e.g., cocaine), thus a thorough history and physical is imperative.

Pericarditis and myocarditis are cardiac diseases that cause chest pain. Both conditions can present with fever and chest pain, although myocarditis usually has a more insidious onset. Pericarditis usually presents with sharp, substernal chest pain that is alleviated by leaning forward. On physical examination, the patient classically has distant heart sounds, a friction rub, and signs of congestive heart failure. Myocarditis patients often have vague symptoms including chest pain, dyspnea, dizziness, nausea, vomiting, and fatigue. Physical examination usually reveals a gallop, signs of congestive heart failure, and tachycardia unresponsive to fluids. A concerning history and physical examination should prompt the practitioner to consider myocarditis and pericarditis (see Chapter 48).

Structural abnormalities of the heart and vessels can cause chest pain. Hypertrophic cardiomyopathy patients usually give a history of increased chest pain with exertion. Aortic stenosis, pulmonary stenosis, abnormal coronary arteries, and mitral valve prolapse, depending on the severity, can lead to ischemia of the heart and papillary muscles. History and physical examination of these patients typically reveal a heart murmur associated with the lesion.

Arrhythmias can cause chest pain in the pediatric patient. Premature ventricular tachycardia can present as a fleeting, sharp pain, or palpations. Supraventricular tachycardia (SVT) is usually described as a rapid heartbeat. Physical examination should cue the physician to the possibility of supraventricular tachycardia (SVT) (see Chapter 50).

RESPIRATORY

Pediatric chest pain attributed to a pulmonary etiology was found in 12.5% to 19% of cases.[1,2,4] Patients presenting with a history of asthma or reactive airway disease should prompt the physician to assess for the possibility of chest pain secondary to

▶ **TABLE 8–1. DIFFERENTIAL DIAGNOSIS OF CHEST PAIN**

Diagnostic Categories	Diagnostic Considerations
Cardiac	Myocardial infarction or ischemia
	Myocarditis
	Pericarditis
	Structural abnormalities
	Arrhythmia
Pulmonary	Asthma exacerbation
	Pneumonia ± pleural effusion
	Pneumothorax
	Pneumomediastinum
	Hemothorax
	Pulmonary embolism
Gastrointestinal	Gastroesophageal reflux
	Esophageal foreign body
Musculoskeletal	Rib fracture
	Muscle strain
	Costochondritis
	Tietze's syndrome
	Slipping rib syndrome
	Precordial catch syndrome (Texidor's twinge)
Psychogenic	Anxiety
	Depression
	Stress
Idiopathic	No organic or psychologic cause identified

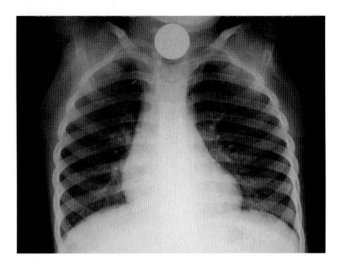

Figure 8–1. Foreign body in esophagus.

causes a burning, substernal type of pain because of the resulting gastritis and esophagitis. Epigastric tenderness on physical examination and the association of the pain with eating food is suggestive of a gastrointestinal origin of the chest pain and should be further investigated.[1,6]

Children that have ingested a foreign body that is lodged in the esophagus can have chest pain (Fig. 8–1). Patients may have dysphagia depending on the location of the foreign body. A careful history usually reveals the diagnosis.

MUSCULOSKELETAL

A musculoskeletal etiology for chest pain is found in 32.5% to 43% of ED visits.[2,4] Trauma can cause fractures and contusions that may result in chest pain. Overuse or overexertion of the chest wall muscles may cause muscle strain.

Costochondritis is a common condition recognized by the practitioner when chest pain is elicited by palpating the costochondral joints. The etiology of costochondritis is unknown, but it is considered to be a benign, inflammatory condition. A similar disease, Tietze's syndrome, also occurs at the costochondral junctions, but has the associated findings of swelling, redness, and warmth. Like costochondritis, Tietze's syndrome is thought to be a self-limited inflammatory condition.

Slipping rib syndrome usually occurs at the false or floating ribs. The patient usually describes a sharp, intermittent pain that lasts a few minutes and settles to a dull ache. There may be a history of trauma and aggravation with movement. The etiology of the pain is thought to result from the anterior end of the rib, slipping out of place and aggravating the adjacent intercostal nerve. The "hooking maneuver" can be used to help diagnose this condition. The patient is instructed to lie on the unaffected side and the practitioner reaches under the lower costal margin and pulls the rib anteriorly. A positive test results is the reproduction of the patient's pain and a click sensation.

Precordial catch syndrome, or Texidor's twinge, is a benign condition that causes a brief, sharp pain to the left chest without radiation. The pain may occur with exercise or when the patient is at rest in a slouched position. The etiology is unclear, but is thought to occur from the parietal pleura,

an asthma exacerbation. Bronchospasm and persistent coughing can lead to excess use of the chest wall muscles and is a common cause of chest pain.

Pneumonia with or without pleural effusion can also cause chest pain. Presenting signs and symptoms would usually include fever, tachypnea, and upper respiratory symptoms. Physical examination may reveal decreased breath sounds or rales.

Patients who report acute pain and subsequent respiratory distress should raise suspicion for a spontaneous pneumothorax or pneumomediastinum. Patients with asthma, Marfan's syndrome, or cystic fibrosis are at increased risk for developing pneumothoraces. Physical examination may reveal decreased breath sounds on the affected side and crepitus depending on the extent of the pathology. A hemothorax should also be considered if there is a history of trauma.

Pulmonary embolism is rare in pediatrics, but should be considered in adolescents who complain of dyspnea, pleuritic chest pain, hemoptysis, and low-grade fever. Risk factors for a pulmonary embolism are the use of birth control pills, recent abortion, prolonged immobility, inherited hypercoagulable disorders, indwelling central lines, and major trauma, particularly to the lower extremities.

GASTROINTESTINAL

Gastrointestinal causes for pediatric chest pain make up 3% to 4% of ED visits.[1,3] Gastroesophageal reflux disease often intercostal nerves, or from the stretching of the supporting ligaments of the heart.

Chest wall pain that follows a dermatome should raise the physician's suspicion for a herpes zoster infection. This is not a musculoskeletal condition, but deserves mentioning as the patient's pain may precede the skin lesions.

PSYCHOGENIC

A psychogenic source for chest pain accounts for 5% to 9% of ED visits.[1–3] Pediatric patients experiencing anxiety, depression, or stress can have symptoms manifesting as chest pain. The history usually reveals a major stressful event in the child or adolescent's life that has recently occurred. A concomitant organic cause for the chest pain should also be explored.

IDIOPATHIC

Idiopathic chest pain is diagnosed in 12% to 45% of cases.[2–4] A thorough history and physical examination is essential to look for a possible etiology before this diagnosis is made.

▶ DIAGNOSTIC EVALUATION

The diagnostic evaluation of pediatric patients presenting with chest pain includes a thorough history and physical examination. Further diagnostic studies may be needed (Fig. 8–2).

A chest radiograph can be a useful diagnostic study in patients presenting with chest pain. A chest film can reveal a cardiac process leading to the appearance of an enlarged heart or pulmonary edema resulting from congestive heart failure. A pulmonary etiology such as pneumonia (Fig. 8–3), pleural effusion, pneumothorax (Fig. 8–4), hemothorax, and

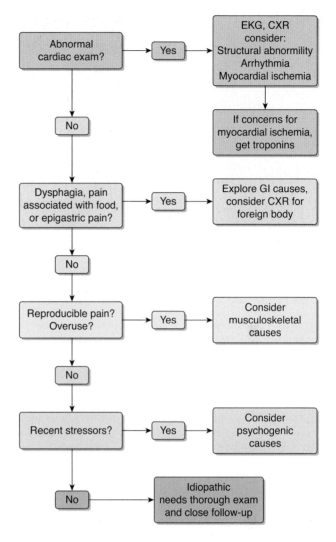

Figure 8–2. (Continued)

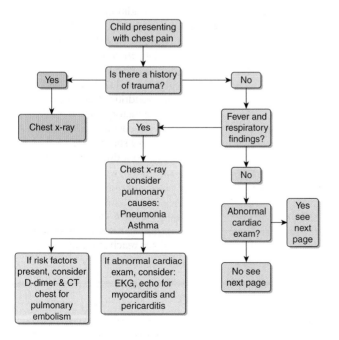

Figure 8–2. Chest pain diagnostic algorithm.

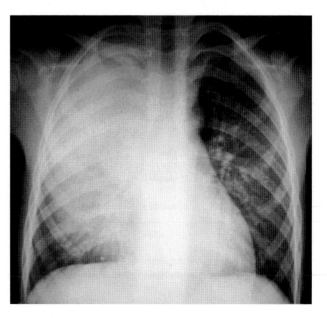

Figure 8–3. Pneumonia. Chest x-ray with right upper and middle lobe pneumonia.

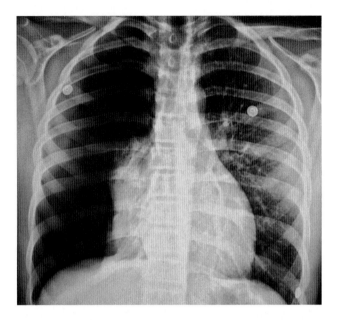

Figure 8–4. Pneumothorax. Patient presented with an acute onset chest pain. Note large pneumothorax on right.

pneumomediastinum can also be confirmed by chest radiograph. An esophageal foreign body may be visible on the film depending on the composition of the foreign body. Most musculosketetal causes of chest pain would not have noticeable changes on a chest film, except for a rib or sternum fracture (Fig. 8–5). Chest x-rays are not required in every pediatric patient with chest pain, but should be ordered when there is suspicion for one of the aforementioned conditions.[1–3]

Electrocardiograms (ECG) are frequently used in adults with chest pain to evaluate for an acute myocardial infarction. In children, myocardial ischemia is rare, thus routine ECG is not required on every patient. Patients with a concerning history or physical examination, however, merit evaluation with an ECG.

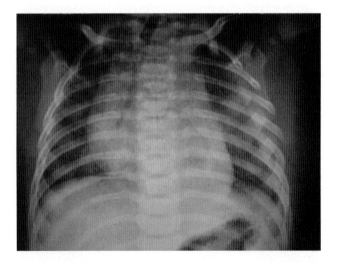

Figure 8–5. Rib fracture. Patient presented with irritability and was noted crying with chest palpation. Note nondisplaced rib fractures on ribs 3 to 6 on the right, and 2, 6, and 7 on the left. There are displaced rib fractures on the right to ribs 3, 4, and 5.

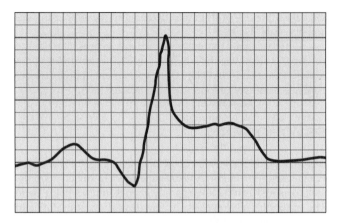

Figure 8–6. ECG illustrating common findings in pediatric myocardial infarction. Note the wide Q wave (>35 ms), ST segment elevation (≥2 ms), and prolonged calculated QT interval >440 ms (not shown) (7).

Common ECG findings with childhood myocardial infarction include Q waves greater than 35 ms, ST segment elevation greater than or equal to 2 mm, and prolonged calculated QT interval greater than 440 ms (Fig. 8–6).[7]

An ECG can alert the physician to conduction and structural heart defects. Myocardial and pericardial disease can also be revealed on ECG. The initial ECG interpretation is often done by the emergency physician, and careful review is imperative. When the interpretation of ECGs by pediatric ED physicians was compared to that of pediatric cardiologists, there was a high rate of concordance. The pediatric emergency physicians' interpretations had a positive predictive value of 88.3% and a negative predictive value of 96.3%.[8]

Laboratory studies can assist with the identification of certain causes of chest pain. For example, an elevated white blood cell count may indicate an infectious etiology, such as pneumonia. A D-dimer can be helpful to rule out the likelihood of a pulmonary embolism in low to intermediate risk patients.[9] Blood gases may not determine a cause, but they can be helpful in managing patients with chest pain and respiratory distress.

Cardiac enzyme levels may help to recognize myocardial injury. Creatine kinase (CK) and troponin levels are widely accepted in the adult population, and can be utilized in the pediatric population to diagnose myocardial necrosis.[5,10,11] CK can be released by skeletal muscle as well as heart muscle, thus a more specific CK-MB fraction is a better indicator of myocardial damage. Troponin I is found only in the myocardium and can be detected within 3 to 6 hours after the onset of ischemia.[5] Troponin I levels may persist for up to 5 to 8 days.[5] Troponin T is also found in the cardiac myocytes and is a very sensitive marker of cardiac damage. Troponin T can be present in the serum within 3 hours, depending on the severity of the injury, and can persists for 6 to 14 days.[11,12] Troponin I and T are more sensitive and specific than CK and CK-MB, and are the preferred method of detecting myocardial injury.[5,11,13]

▶ MANAGEMENT

The management of patients with chest pain is dependent upon the underlying cause. Appropriate therapy should be initiated in the ED with specialty consultation and referrals as needed. Cardiac causes of chest pain generally require cardiology consultation. Depending on the clinical severity of the patient and diagnosis, the patient may require immediate consultation or outpatient referral.

Pulmonary causes such as asthma and pneumonia should be treated with standard medications. Pneumothorax and hemothorax may require emergent intervention with a needle decompression or chest tube placement, but that would depend on the size of the lesion and patient status. Patients with a pulmonary embolism require admission and anticoagulation therapy similar to adults (see Chapter 52).

Gastrointestinal causes of chest pain can usually be treated as an outpatient. Patients with gastroesophageal reflux disease can have medication therapy initiated and subsequent follow-up with either a gastroenterologist or pediatrician. Patients with an esophageal foreign body will usually be able to pass it through the gastrointestinal tract, but if concerned because of the size or other factors, a consultation to remove the foreign body can be made (see Chapter 74).

Musculoskeletal causes of chest pain can generally be treated with rest and nonsteroidal anti-inflammatory agents. The slipping rib syndrome can be treated with education and avoidance of the offending movements. Local nerve blocks and corticosteroid injections are sometimes necessary. A surgical alternative is to have the anterior end of the rib and costal cartilage removed, but this is usually done after failure of medical management. Precordial catch syndrome is a self-limiting condition that requires only education and supportive care.

Psychogenic causes of chest pain usually require outpatient follow-up by the patient's pediatrician or psychiatrist. If the anxiety, depression, or stress is severe, then psychiatric consultation and medical management should be considered.

In cases of idiopathic chest pain, no specific therapy is needed, but follow-up is essential. Emergency follow-up recommendations should also be given to the patient and family.

REFERENCES

1. Massin MM, Bourguignont A, Coremans C, et al. Chest pain in pediatric patients presenting to an emergency department or to a cardiac clinic. *Clin Pediatr (Phila).* 2004;43:231.
2. Rowe BH, Dulberg CS, Peterson RG, et al. Characteristics of children presenting with chest pain to a pediatric emergency department. *Can Med Assoc J.* 1990;143:388.
3. Selbst SM, Ruddy RM, Clark BJ, et al. Pediatric chest pain: a prospective study. *Pediatr.* 1998;82:319.
4. Driscoll DJ, Glicklich LB, Gallen WJ. Chest pain in children: a prospective study. *Pediatr.* 1976;57:648.
5. Lane JR, Ben-Shachar G. Myocardial infarction in healthy adolescents. *Pediatr.* 2007;120:e948.
6. Sabri MR, Ghavanini AA, Haghighat M, et al. Chest pain in children and adolescents: epigastric tenderness as a guide to reduce unnecessary work-up. *Pediatr Cardiol.* 2003; 24:3.
7. Towbin JA, Bricker JT, Garson A Jr. Electrocardiographic criteria for diagnosis of acute myocardial infarction in childhood. *Am J Cardiol.* 1992;69:1545.
8. Wathen JE, Rewers AB, Yetman AT, et al. Accuracy of ECG interpretation in the pediatric emergency department. *Pediatr.* 2005;46:507.
9. Stein PD, Woodard PK, Weg JG, et al. Diagnostic pathways in acute pulmonary embolism: recommendations of the PIOPED II investigators. *Am J Med.* 2006;119:1048.
10. Hirsch R, Landt Y, Porter S, et al. Cardiac Troponin I in pediatrics: normal values and potential use in the assessment of cardiac injury. *J Pediatr.* 1997;130:872.
11. Soongswang J, Durongpisitkul K, Nana A, et al. Cardiac troponin T: a marker in the diagnosis of acute myocarditis in children. *Pediatr Cardiol.* 2005;26:45.
12. Katus HA, Remppis A, Neumann FJ, et al. Diagnostic efficiency for troponin T measurements in acute myocardial infarction. *Circulation.* 1991;83:902.
13. Lauer B, Niederau C, Kuhl U, et al. Cardiac troponin T in patients with clinically suspected myocarditis. *J Am Coll Cardiol.* 1997;30:1354.

CHAPTER 9

Acute Abdominal Conditions

Jonathan Singer

▶ HIGH-YIELD FACTS

- Infants with an abrupt onset of bilious vomiting are likely to have a midgut volvulus complicating malrotation.
- In the first few months of life, infants with persistent, painless, and forceful vomiting should be evaluated for upper intestinal tract obstruction. Pyloric stenosis is far more common than are congenital bands, antral webs, intestinal duplication, or annular pancreas.
- Intussusception should be the provisional diagnosis for a child with severe, episodic abdominal pain associated with vomiting.
- Failure to remove the diaper of infants with deceptively benign vomiting may preclude the diagnosis of incarcerated inguinal hernia.
- Enterocolitis is a potentially deadly complication of Hirschsprung's disease. It can develop before the diagnosis of Hirschsprung's disease is established or present years after surgical repair.
- Inflammatory bowel disease should be suspected in any infants or children with prolonged gastrointestinal symptoms. This is especially true when stomatitis or perianal disease is present.
- The most likely diagnosis of an abdominal catastrophe presenting as peritonitis is appendicitis.

There are a large number of disorders that are associated with abdominal complaints. These include diseases unrelated to the alimentary canal as well as gastrointestinal disorders. A large number of gastrointestinal disease states can lead to an emergency department (ED) visit. It is the responsibility of the emergency physician to accurately assess these patients and establish a working diagnosis. A detailed inquiry that characterizes the nature and course of recent events and elicits the contributing symptoms, as well as past medical history, will usually lead to an appropriate provisional diagnosis for those children beyond infancy. For younger patients without a wide verbal repertoire, observations of the caretaker are of no less importance but may be misinterpreted. Thus, the essential tetrad of the abdominal examination (inspection, auscultation, percussion, and palpation) assumes greater importance in preverbal children.[1]

There are a small number of nontraumatic abdominal disease states that may present as an "abdominal emergency." The treating physician must emergently recognize these surgical conditions. The physician must initiate treatment, and in certain circumstances, acquire laboratory studies, including imaging. These may confirm clinical suspicion and provide baseline parameters for surgical consultants.[2]

The acute abdominal conditions that may require surgical intervention share common historic features and physical examination findings. Vomiting may be the presenting feature and dominant concern to both caretaker and emergency physician in circumstances of an abdominal emergency. The appearance of the emesis (blood tinged, bilious, feculent) is a defining historic feature. The presence or apparent absence of abdominal pain narrows the differential diagnosis. The general appearance of the patient and specific abdominal examination findings from inspection, auscultation, palpation, and percussion are priorities for refining the differential diagnosis. Of the available bedside findings, the presence or absence of abdominal distention further narrows the differential diagnosis. This algorithmic approach to selected abdominal emergencies is depicted in Figure 9–1. An expansion of these entities can be found under headings The Obstructions, Intra-Abdominal Sepsis, Gastrointestinal Foreign Bodies, and Megacolon.

▶ THE OBSTRUCTIONS

MALROTATION WITH MIDGUT VOLVULUS

An arrest of the normal embryonic rotation of the alimentary tract may result in suspension of sections of bowel, including the vascular supply, by a narrow pedicle. Three outcomes are possible. Least likely (<10% of all patients with malrotation) is the lifelong absence of symptoms. More likely, a rotational anomaly will create a vague gastrointestinal symptom such as failure to thrive, chronic recurrent abdominal distension, pain-free episodic vomiting, or persistent unexplained diarrhea. Most likely, especially with malrotations about the duodenum, small bowel, and colon up to the midtransverse portion (the midgut), a strangulating twist affects dramatic symptomatology.[3] Males are affected twice as often as females. Nearly half of all patients present within the first week of life, two-thirds present within the first month, and more than 90% present within the first year of life.[4]

Neonates and young infants with midgut volvulus uniformly present with vomiting, which is characteristically bilious.[5] Some infants seem to have no abdominal discomfort, whereas others have episodic crying that may be intense.[6] Failure to pass stools or constipated stools is present in a majority of infants. Rarely, when the superior mesenteric artery has been compromised, gangrenous bowel is associated with hematochezia.[5]

The physical examination features with volvulus are variable and age dependent. Almost 90% of newborns evaluated

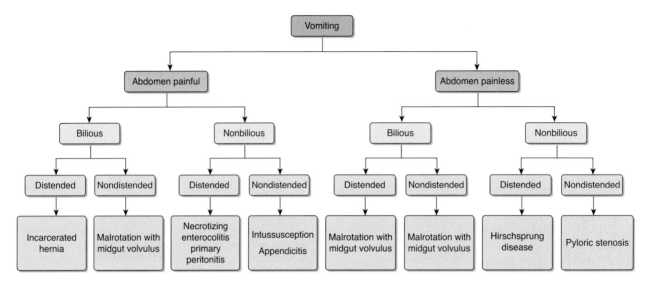

Figure 9–1. Approach to selected abdominal emergencies in childhood.

shortly after the onset of vomiting appear well. They have a soft, nondistended, nontender abdomen. In 10% of cases where vasculature to the bowel is compromised, the infants will appear ill and distressed. They will exhibit pallor and poor perfusion. Abdominal distention may be prominent. Gangrenous bowel loops may be transabdominally visualized as a discolored mass. Children of all ages with longer-standing ischemia and children with volvulus beyond early infancy will more often have distended bowel loops, voluntary guarding of the abdomen and diffuse abdominal tenderness.[7] Stool from the rectal examination may be positive for occult blood.

Plain radiographs of the abdomen, with two views, may exhibit a normal bowel gas pattern. More often, radiographs will demonstrate the presence and general level of obstruction (Fig. 9–2).

Duodenal obstruction yields air–fluid levels in the dilated stomach and duodenum with little air (doubled bubble) or no gas in the remainder of the bowel.

More distal complete obstruction typically creates numerous loops of dilated bowel and air–fluid levels with a paucity of intraluminal air beyond the obstruction. With incomplete obstructions, the bowel gas pattern may appear relatively normal and further imaging is required. Ultrasonography may demonstrate an abnormal anatomic relationship between the superior mesenteric artery and vein,[8] or may reveal a circle of vascularity representing the superior mesenteric vein twisting around the superior mesenteric artery, forming a "whirlpool" sign.[9] Ultrasonography of the abdomen may additionally provide supporting evidence of obstruction, such as bowel wall edema and intraluminal fluid. However, contrast studies provide conclusive diagnostic evidence. Since the cecum may be upwardly or medially displaced in early infancy, a barium enema may not differentiate a normally mobile cecum from malrotation. Thus, the upper gastrointestinal series is preferred. The findings of midgut volvulus include obstruction of the duodenum at its third portion and an associated inability to locate the normal ligament of Treitz to the left of the spine. Intestinal obstruction of the descending duodenum, just over the right of the spine, is pathognomonic. Also, with midgut volvulus the intestine dis-

tal to the obstruction wraps around the superior mesenteric vessels and creates a corkscrew appearance[3] (Fig. 9–3).

Obstructed children require intestinal intubation and decompression. Volume depletion necessitates fluid resuscitation. In selected circumstances, blood replacement may be needed in the preoperative period. Prophylactic antibiotics are preferred in toxic patients. Prompt laparotomy, the definitive care, is necessary to preserve the bowel.

PYLORIC STENOSIS

Pyloric stenosis is the most common cause of intestinal obstruction after the first month of life. Affected patients may present as early as 1 week or as late as 3 months of age. The typical infant becomes symptomatic between the second and sixth week of life. Symptoms in preterm infants are delayed.[10] Males are four times more likely to be affected than are females, with first-born males being especially prone to develop pyloric stenosis. Symptoms of gastric outlet obstruction are produced by hypertrophy of circular fibers about the pylorus.[11]

The initial symptom is unpredictable, infrequent projectile vomiting. The vomiting becomes more frequent, more forceful, and eventually incessant. Within a week, nonbilious, postprandial, projectile vomiting is uniformly encountered. If gastritis is also present, the stomach contents may contain blood. Anorexia is absent. Stools are generally small and infrequent in nature. Urination may decrease in frequency secondary to dehydration. The antecedent history of a steady weight gain is replaced by weight deceleration as formula retention is compromised.[11]

The physical examination generally reveals alert infants with good nutritional status. However, adipose tissue may be reduced and there may be decreased elasticity of the skin, particularly if dehydration is present. The hydration status may be severely compromised if vomiting has been of a prolonged duration. Unless significantly electrolyte or volume depleted, infants appear healthy, suck eagerly and, if fed, swallow without difficulty. A midabdominal peristaltic wave may be

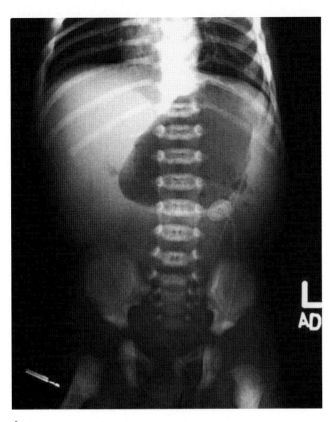

A

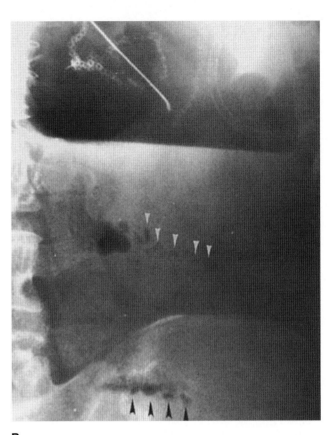

B

Figure 9–2. (A) Abdominal x-ray of a 10-day-old infant with bilious emesis. Note the dilated proximal bowel and the paucity of distal bowel gas, characteristic of volvulus. (B) Small bowel obstruction. Two rows of air bubbles (arrowheads) with fluid levels in the left midabdomen are indicative of mechanical obstruction in the small intestine.

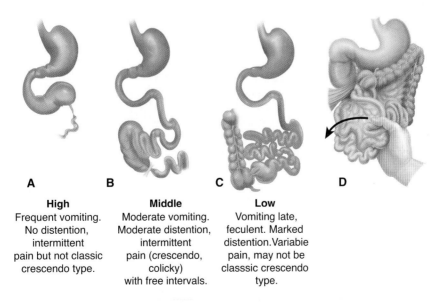

A	**B**	**C**	**D**
High	**Middle**	**Low**	
Frequent vomiting. No distention, intermittent pain but not classic crescendo type.	Moderate vomiting. Moderate distention, intermittent pain (crescendo, colicky) with free intervals.	Vomiting late, feculent. Marked distention. Variabie pain, may not be classsic crescendo type.	

Figure 9–3. Malrotation of the midgut with volvulus. Note cecum at the origin of the superior mesenteric vessels. Fibrous bands cross and obstruct the duodenum as they adhere to the cecum. Volvulus is untwisted in a counterclockwise direction.

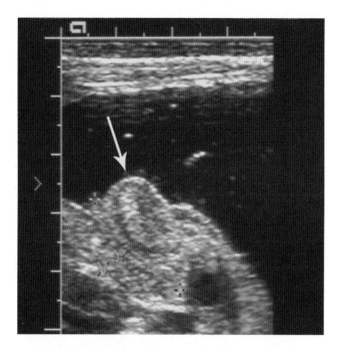

Figure 9–4. Antral nipple sign. The nipple-shaped mass (arrow) protruding into the fluid-filled gastric antrum is formed by thickened gastric mucosa adjacent to the pylorus.

seen prior to the eventual regurgitant event.[12] An epigastric, rounded mass, traditionally described as olive-like, is found in a quarter to a half of cases.[13] Gastric distension may displace the pyloris posteriorly and prevent palpation of the mass, which may be more successful after children vomit, following decompression of the stomach with a feeding tube or by placing infants in a decubitus position.[14] In circumstances where an abdominal mass cannot be palpated, imaging may establish the diagnosis.

A plain abdominal radiograph may demonstrate a dilated stomach and hypertrophic walls.

An ultrasound allows for direct visualization and measurement of the pyloric muscle. An ultrasound study will reveal an elongated and hypertrophied pyloric sphincter, and thickened mucosa may be seen protruding into the gastric antrum (antral nipple sign) (Fig. 9–4).[15,16] If ultrasonography is not available, or if the ultrasound is inconclusive, then an upper gastrointestinal study can be performed. A barium feeding reveals curvature, elongation, and narrowing of the pyloric channel (string sign).[17]

Loss of both potassium and hydrogen ions from vomiting infrequently results in a characteristic hypokalemic, hypochloremic, and metabolic alkalosis.[18] When infants have pyloric stenosis, a nasogastric tube should be placed and volume and electrolyte replacement initiated. Once a diagnosis is confirmed, surgical intervention with a pyloromyotomy constitutes definitive care.

INTUSSUSCEPTION

Intussusception is an invagination of a proximal portion of the intestine into a distal adjacent part. Intussusception is the most frequent cause of intestinal obstruction between the ages of

3 months and 5 years. Cases have been described in preterm infants, throughout childhood, and into adulthood. More than 60% of cases occur in the first year of life, with most of these occurring between the fifth and ninth month. Of late, more cases have been depicted in children beyond the fifth year of age. Classically, it occurs in well-nourished children. Males are affected twice as often as females, and this difference becomes more pronounced in children older than 4 years, rising to an 8:1 ratio.[19]

Intussusception classically creates a triad of clinical symptoms: colicky pain, vomiting, and bloody stools. In a typical case, there is a sudden onset of severe abdominal pain that may last several minutes. After an asymptomatic interval, repeated paroxysms will cause children to cry out again. Children may be impossible to console or may seem comfortable only in a knee–chest position on the floor or in the arms of an attendant. The intermittent nature of the pain with the children appearing quite well between bouts is a significant clue that should be given weight when considering the diagnosis.[20] Pain is the initial manifestation of intussusception in over half of the patients. Vomiting may occur either with the initial painful episode or soon after. Concurrent with vomiting, children typically have several bowel movements, which vary from formed stools to thin liquid. Within 12 to 24 hours, stool is passed that has a gelatinous, mucous-like consistency. The presence of blood in fecal material may be trace to copious.[21]

The classic triad of colicky, intermittent, and obviously extreme abdominal pain, vomiting, and proctorrhea is found in less than one-third of all patients. Between 85% and 92% of children manifest colicky abdominal pain and 60% to 80% of patients experience vomiting.[22,23] Rectal bleeding may be found in 40% to 50% of patients. "Currant jelly" stools, which are bloody, maroon-colored, mucous-laden stools (Fig. 9–5), are seen late and account for a minority of bloody stools.[21]

Associated findings can occur in combination with the classic triad, or they may occur alone, contributing to diagnostic error. Anorexia is an almost universal but nonspecific symptom. Diarrhea may be seen in approximately 7% to 10% of cases where there is complete intestinal obstruction and may be found in up to 40% of cases where there is an incomplete bowel obstruction.[24] There is increasing appreciation that apathy or listlessness may occasionally be the dominant manifestation. This altered sensorium with intussusception may be seen in the context of prolonged symptomatology or as the initial complaint. Mental status changes may be accompanied by pronounced pallor, mimicking shock.[25]

The general appearance of children may vary from cheerful and interactive to lethargic and poorly perfused.[20] Not uncommonly, those with advanced disease complicated by either fluid or electrolyte imbalance or blood loss may appear less responsive. However, children with a very brief history of enteric manifestations may be obtunded at presentation.[25] Unless patients have an underlying disease such as anaphylactoid purpura or cystic fibrosis, positive physical findings are typically limited to the abdominal examination. On inspection, the abdomen may appear scaphoid and the right lower quadrant may seem empty (Dance's sign). Guarding or distension is uncommon. Bowel sounds may be normal, decreased, or absent. A sausage-shaped mass may be found. The advancing mass, typically ill defined and variably tender, may be palpated in any quadrant or on rectal examination.[26] Grossly bloody stool

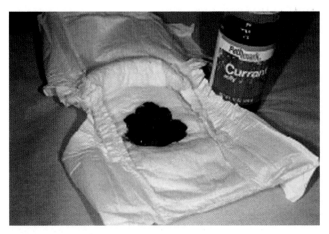

A

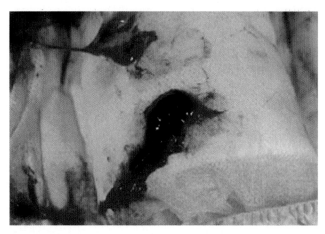

B

Figure 9–5. (A) Commercially available currant jelly. (B) Diarrhea containing mucus and blood constitutes the classic currant-jelly stool seen in a minority of patients with intussusception.

may be found on the withdrawn examining finger, or normal-appearing stool may be positive for occult blood.

Plain abdominal radiographs, in two views, should be obtained for two reasons. One function of plain radiographs is to see if intussusception is likely. The radiographic finding suggestive of intussusception include localized air–fluid levels, di-

lated small bowel loops, reduced intestinal air, minimal fecal content in the colon, inability to visualize the liver tip or mass lesion[27] (Fig. 9–6A).

Occasionally, the diagnosis can be confirmed when the plain film exhibits the visible head of the intussusception in the bowel lumen.[28] A normal plain abdominal radiograph cannot

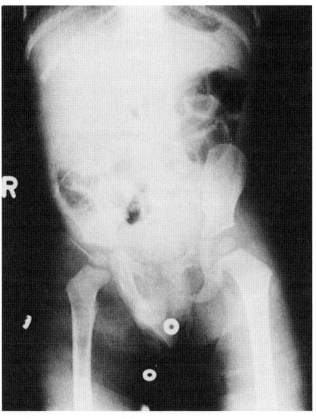

A

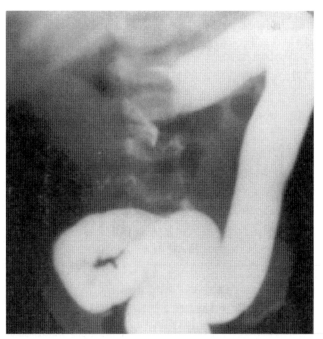

B

Figure 9–6. (A) Intussusception. Plain film with loss of bowel pattern in the right upper quadrant. (B) Contrast enema demonstrating obstruction to retrograde flow of barium by a filling defect (intussusceptum) in the midtransverse colon.

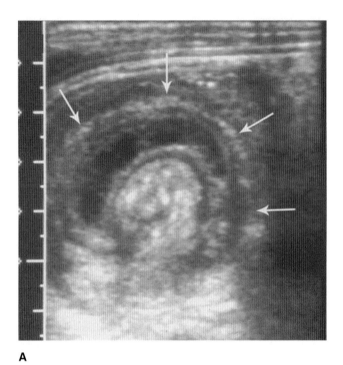

A

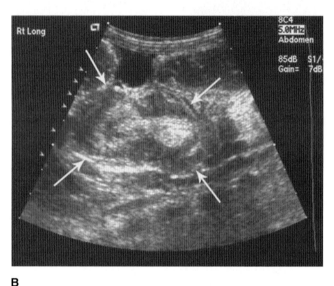

B

Figure 9–7. (A) Doughnut sign. (B) Pseudokidney sign.

exclude the diagnosis of intussusception; plain films may be normal in 25% to 30% of cases.[29] The second role of plain abdominal radiography is to uncover contraindications to contrast enema. Patients with radiographic evidence of complete bowel obstruction, intraperitoneal air, ascites, or pneumatosis intestinalis should not be subject to contrast enema (Fig. 9–6B).

Ultrasonography is useful in establishing the diagnosis of intussusception, and when uncovered, may dictate the optimum mode of reduction. Ultrasonography tends to be of greater utility in patients with a nonspecific history, normal physical examination, or atypical clinical pattern. Sonographic findings of intussusception include a large sonographic target, bull's eye, or doughnut sign on the transverse or cross section, and a sleeve or pseudokidney sign on the longitudinal section (Fig. 9–7). The rim in either case represents the head of the intussusception.[30]

Spiral computed tomography (CT) scan can also be employed to diagnose equivocal cases. Findings are a distended bowel loop with a thickened, edematous wall, and an eccentrically crescentic or wedge-shaped, low-density intraluminal mass that represents the invaginated mesentery.[31]

Nontoxic, hydrated children with a provisional diagnosis of intussusception should be given nothing by mouth (npo). Those who appear dehydrated are given a normal saline bolus, followed by polyionic intravenous fluid pending serum electrolytes. A nasogastric tube may be inserted. A decision must be made concerning whether there are contraindications to nonoperative attempts at reduction of the intussusception. For patients without contraindications, the radiologist and surgical consultant can determine whether air insufflation or barium should be employed.[32] If pneumatic or hydrostatic pressure techniques fail to reduce the intussusception, a repeat effort

at nonoperative reduction is one option.[33] Should reduction techniques fail, operative therapy is necessary.

INCARCERATED HERNIAS

Hernias are protrusions of tissue through an abnormal opening. In children, they occur with descending frequency at the umbilicus, inguinal and scrotal regions, midline epigastrium, and lateral border of the rectus sheath. Because of attenuation of musculofascial layers, preperitoneal fat, abdominal, or pelvic viscus (including small bowel, large bowel, ovary, fallopian tube, testicle, or testicular appendages) may become entrapped.[34] When the incarcerated sac contents cannot be reduced into the peritoneal cavity, strangulation and necrosis of tissues may result. Male children with hernias outnumber female children by an 8:1 to 10:1 ratio. Both sexes have the greatest risk for incarceration during the first 6 months of life. With advancing age, incarceration becomes less likely. There is a very low incidence of incarceration after 8 years of age.[35]

The hallmark of childhood hernias is an asymptomatic bulge that becomes more prominent with increased abdominal pressure, such as straining at defecation, crying, coughing, or laughing. Usually the hernia has been long-standing and recognized both by the parent and primary physician prior to incarceration. On rare occasion, the initial clinical presentation is one of abrupt appearance of the hernia with incarceration.[36]

The first symptom of incarceration in infancy is the abrupt onset of irritability. Expressive children indicate crampy abdominal pain that does not necessarily localize to the hernia site. Poor rooting and refusal to feed is seen in infancy shortly after incarceration. Anorexia or nausea may be expressed in older children. Infrequent nonbilious vomiting may rapidly

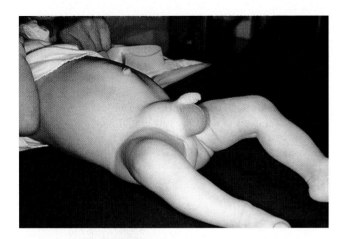

Figure 9–8. This infant presented with inconsolable crying and a few episodes of vomiting. Inguinal hernia may be either unilateral or bilateral. This patient's hernia (hernial sac contents) could not be reduced into the abdominal cavity and the patient required surgical repair.

progress to bilious vomiting.[37] If the incarceration is long-standing, feculent vomiting may be seen as the bowel strangulates.

The diagnosis of incarcerated hernia is not difficult if children are completely undressed. All children with incarceration appear uncomfortable. The abdominal findings vary depending upon the site of incarceration. The omental, reproductive, or intestinal masses are usually nontender and fluctuant at onset. They become firm and tender with passage of time and when viability of the viscus is compromised.[37]

The diagnosis of incarcerated hernia is obvious upon inspection (Fig. 9–8).

Radiographic confirmation is rarely necessary. Plain films of the abdomen may reveal partial or complete bowel obstruction. With inguinal hernias, gas-containing soft tissue masses may be noted within the scrotum. Ultrasonography may be used in infants born prematurely to discriminate the contents of an incarcerated sac.

Nonoperative reduction of a strangulated hernia can often be achieved by the emergency physician.[38] Greatest success follows a period of withheld oral intake, application of ice to the hernia sac, and sedation followed by continuous bimanual pressure.[39] Suspected strangulation or unsuccessful reduction by the emergency physician mandates surgical consultation.

▶ INTRA-ABDOMINAL SEPSIS

ACUTE APPENDICITIS WITHOUT PERFORATION

Appendicitis is a disease of all ages, but the late elementary school age population has the highest incidence of appendicitis in childhood. There is a gradual reduction in frequency of acute appendicitis in younger children, with a precipitous drop (<2% of all patient encounters) in children younger than 2 years.[40] Acute appendicitis without perforation is encountered equally in both sexes. Transmural bacterial invasion of

the appendix may begin as an intraluminal infection or result from obstruction of the appendiceal lumen by enlarged lymphatic tissue, intestinal parasites, foreign bodies, or fecalith. Irrespective of the precipitating factor, the inflammatory process gives rise to a clinical picture that is "classic" in 60% to 75% of cases.[41]

The triad of abdominal pain, vomiting, and low-grade fever is highly suggestive of appendicitis.[42] Abdominal pain is the first manifestation of the disease. The pain is epigastric or periumbilical. At onset, the pain is described as a dull, aching sensation. As the obstruction in the appendix maximizes, pain becomes more intense and constant. As the inflammation proceeds to include the parietal peritoneum of the cecum over a 1- to 12-hour time frame, pain migrates and localizes. In most cases, the pain is maximal at 3 to 5 cm from the anterosuperior iliac spine on a straight line drawn from that process to the umbilicus (McBurney's point). Pain may radiate to the flank or back with retrocecal appendicitis or the suprapubic region with a pelvic appendicitis, and to the testicle with a retroileal appendicitis. The inflammatory process causes reflex pylorospasm, and patients will vomit. At least one to two episodes of nonbilious vomiting occur in more than 90% of cases.[43] On occasion, parents may not be aware of the abdominal pain that precedes the vomiting or they may not consider their child's discomfort significant until vomiting ensues. Temperature elevation is a noted feature in 75% to 80% of patients. Review of systems may be positive for upper respiratory tract symptoms, anorexia, nausea, or constipation in 15% to 50% of affected children. An inflamed appendix, particularly if retrocecal, may cause fecal urgency, tenesmus, and frequent passage of a small volume of stool in approximately 15% of children. Dysuria may be experienced by 5% to 15% of children with an inflamed appendix in proximity to the ureter. The latter two atypical symptoms are more often clinical features in misdiagnosed cases.[44]

With the exception of low-grade fever, typically in a 38°C (100.4°F) to 39°C (102.2°F) range, patients with nonperforated appendicitis will have minimal alteration of their vital signs. They are ambulatory, but they may walk slowly or limp favoring the right leg and climb upon the examining table only with assistance. If the appendix is in a retrocecal position or in contact with pelvic musculature, elevation and extension of the right leg against pressure of the examiner's hand causes pain (iliopsoas sign). Alternately, when the flexed right thigh is held at right angles to the trunk and internally rotated, hypogastric pain may result (obturator sign). Increased abdominal pain with a heel strike is variably present. Bowel sounds may be normal or diminished. Abdominal distension is absent. Patients may voluntarily guard the entire abdomen or only the right lower quadrant. Exquisite tenderness is often noted directly over McBurney's point. Pressure applied to the descending colon may cause referred pain at the McBurney's point (Rovsing's sign). No abdominal masses are palpated. A rectal examination is unnecessary in children with obvious appendicitis. With appendicitis, the rectal examination reveals right lower quadrant tenderness but no masses.[45]

A complete blood count is unnecessary in the patient with obvious appendicitis. Complete blood counts are frequently ordered in children whose clinical diagnosis is less secure. Their value in the decision-making process is unclear. In a majority

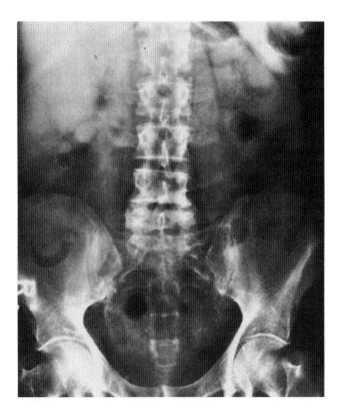

Figure 9–9. Acute appendicitis. An oval calcification measuring 0.8 cm in diameter projects over the iliac bone and laterally to the right sacroiliac joint with a distended appendiceal lumen filled with gas.

of children with appendicitis, the total white blood cell count is elevated beyond 15 000 cells/mm³ or the total neutrophil count is elevated beyond 10 000 cells/mm³. This holds, especially in the patients who have been symptomatic ≥48 hours at the time of phlebotomy.[46] A normal white blood cell count is seen in approximately 7% of pediatric patients with appendicitis.[47]

Radiologic studies and other imaging techniques are not necessary with clear-cut appendicitis. However, imaging studies may be helpful in equivocal cases.

Flat plate and upright abdominal radiographs are frequently the first imaging studies obtained. Plain radiographic findings suggestive, but not pathognomic, of appendicitis include protective scoliosis of the lumbar spine, localized air–fluid levels in the region of the cecum and terminal ileum, obliteration of the right properitoneal fat stripe, haziness over the right sacroiliac joint, and loss of the right-sided psoas shadow and fecalith (Fig. 9–9).[48] Sonography is considered by some as the examination of choice in patients with equivocal clinical findings of appendicitis (Fig. 9–10). Ultrasonography in the evaluation of pediatric appendicitis is highly operator dependent. However, sounding has reported sensitivity between 75% and 89% and specificity between 86% and 100%.[49] With ultrasonography, the appendix is visualized on longitudinal imaging as a hypoechogenic, tubular structure in continuity with the cecum and having a blind distal end. The appendix appears as a target lesion on transverse sections. With appendicitis, the organ is enlarged, exhibiting >2-mm thickness or an outer wall-to-wall diameter >6 mm.

Conventional CT scan utilizing intravenous and oral contrast is another technique that may be employed for patients in whom the diagnosis of appendicitis is uncertain (Fig. 9–11). Sensitivity ranges from 53% to 100% and specificity from 83% to 100%.[50,51] The highest accuracy has been achieved with focused helical appendiceal CT scan.[50] For this imaging, a water-soluble contrast is administered rectally and followed by contiguous 5-mm cuts of the right lower quadrant.

The goal of the emergency physician in managing a child with suspected appendicitis is to facilitate appendectomy prior to rupture. Timely consultation, access to the operating room, or transfer to another health care facility are key. Surgical consultation should be obtained immediately when appendicitis is the primary diagnosis after completion of the history and physical examination.[52] When the emergency physician is in doubt regarding the diagnosis, nonoperative diagnostic modalities may be chosen and consultation delayed.[53]

ACUTE APPENDICITIS WITH PERFORATION

Age is the single most important factor in determining the likelihood of perforation in the course of acute appendicitis. In younger patients, particularly in those <2 years of age, the anticipated sequence of migratory and advancing abdominal pain may not occur. Symptoms in the very young also may be misleading.[44] Irritability, lethargy, refusal to be handled, diarrhea, apparently painless vomiting, anorexia, or unexplained grunting or abdominal distension may overshadow the anticipated symptoms of acute appendicitis.[54] As a result of these ambiguous features, nearly 100% of patients in the first year of life will have perforated appendixes at the time of diagnosis, 94% of those >2 years of age, 60% to 65% of those <6 years of age, and 30% to 40% of those >6 years of age. Younger patients have an appendix that is relatively thin walled and the cecum may fail to distend and ineffectively decompress an inflamed appendix. Necrosis, gangrene, and perforation may therefore result with greater rapidity than they will in those who are older. Rapid progression with perforation has been described in preschool-age children in as little as 6 to 12 hours from onset of symptoms.

Classically, patients experience increasingly severe abdominal pain until the appendix perforates. Pain may then lessen or cease.[55] Once the perforation has occurred, age may also influence the subsequent clinical course. After the appendix ruptures, a small amount of pus is extruded. In the first year of life, a short, thin omentum has little capacity to wall off infection. Diffuse peritonitis within hours to days is anticipated rather than focal abscess. Older children tend to isolate an expanding collection of pus. Children who have appendixes that have perforated may encounter vague abdominal complaints for days to weeks after the intraperitoneal event.[56] There may be periods of remissions interspersed with exacerbations. The abscesses that develop are most common in the periappendiceal region, although subphrenic abscess or empyema has been described.[57,58] The specific signs with perforated appendicitis may therefore vary.

Patients with perforated appendicitis appear acutely ill and their vital signs are abnormal. Tachycardia and fever are common. The temperatures tend to be higher with perforation,

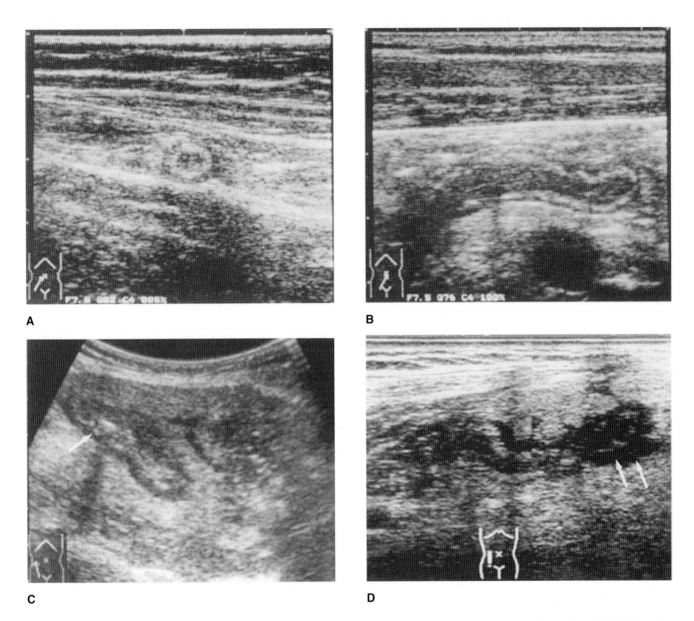

Figure 9-10. Acute appendicitis. A noncompressible, inflamed appendix is shown in (A) a cross-sectional view (7.5 MHz) and (B) a longitudinal section (7.5 MHz). Mural lamination of the swollen appendix is maintained in the early stages of acute appendicitis. (C) An appendicolith (arrow) with acoustic shadowing is demonstrated (5 MHz). (D) A focal loss of mural lamination in the appendiceal tip (arrows) is demonstrated as a result of gangrene (9 MHz).

typically in the range of 39°C (102.2°F) to 40°C (104°F).[56] Extreme tachycardia, hypotension, and altered tissue perfusion may be found with severe dehydration or superimposed sepsis. Patients with perforation experience great discomfort with all bumps in the road en route to the ED. They plead to be carried from their vehicle to the examining table. If forced to ambulate, the children will shuffle forward, severely bent at the waist. They cannot climb onto the examining table, and when placed supine, they will remain motionless with the right leg flexed. Abdominal distension may be prominent, especially in infancy. Bowel sounds are diminished or absent. Children will voluntarily and involuntarily guard the abdomen. A mass, even if present, may therefore be difficult to discern. Palpation of the abdomen in any quadrant may be painful. Rebound tenderness is most prominent in the right lower quadrant. Iliopsoas and obturator signs are variable. Rectal tenderness is noted, but a mass is an inconstant finding.

The hematologic profile for a patient with perforated appendicitis resembles the patient with appendicitis without perforation. An elevated white blood cell count is seen in approximately 75% of patients.[59] Patients with perforation have a greater proportion of band counts.[56] Despite this finding, the differential cannot discriminate between perforated and nonperforated appendicitis.[46]

Imaging studies may be performed as long as they do not impede the preparation of patients for exploratory laparotomy. Scoliosis, appendicolithiasis, obliteration of the right psoas margin, interruption of the properitoneal fat line, and

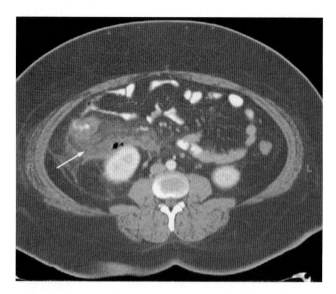

Figure 9–11. CT scan with oral and intravenous contrast of acute appendicitis. There is thickening of the wall of the appendix and periappendiceal stranding (arrow).

abnormal intestinal gas patterns may be seen on plain films as in nonperforated appendicitis. Signs that suggest appendicitis with perforation include a focal increase in thickness of the lateral abdominal wall, the presence of a single gas bubble at the inferior portion of the right lower abdominal quadrant, free intraperitoneal fluid, or pneumoperitoneum. Ultrasonography, in addition to revealing an enlarged, edematous appendix, may demonstrate a periappendiceal fluid collection.[60]

An oral, intravenous, or focused rectal contrast CT scan may be equally satisfactory in diagnosing complications associated with perforated appendix, including the extent and progression of an abscess. Abdominal CT scan may have equal ability for diagnosing complications associated with perforated appendicitis, including the extent and progression of an abscess.

The preferred preoperative management of patients with perforated appendicitis includes the following:

- 45 to 60 degrees elevation of the head of the bed
- npo status
- Nasogastric suction
- Sedation
- Intravenous hydration
- Broad-spectrum antibiotics
- Blood
- Supplemental oxygen (as necessary)
- Mechanical reduction of fever, with tepid water sponging, fans, or cooling blanket

SPONTANEOUS PERITONITIS

The most common childhood conditions leading to peritonitis, in descending order, are the following:

- Perforated appendicitis
- Intestinal obstruction
- Incarcerated hernia
- Inflammatory bowel disease
- Hirschsprung's disease
- Posttraumatic (including instrumentation and foreign body)
- Spontaneously ruptured viscus (including Meckel's diverticulum, bile duct, and inflamed colon or ileum)
- Necrotizing enterocolitis (NEC)

In cases with the preceding conditions, the normally sterile peritoneal cavity is contaminated from an intra-abdominal source. In 10% to 15% of cases, pyoperitoneum results from a focus outside of the abdominal cavity. The bacterial access is postulated to result from bacteremia or extension of a urogenital infection.[61] This spontaneous peritonitis may occur in previously healthy children, but patients with ventriculoperitoneal shunt, immunodeficiency (including splenectomy and HIV infection), and ascites from cirrhosis or nephrosis are at increased risk.[62] Rarely, a spontaneous bacterial peritonitis may be the presenting feature of unrecognized nephrotic syndrome.[63] Whatever the inciting condition, primary peritonitis tends to occur more often in females, with peak incidence between the ages of 5 and 10 years.

Patients with spontaneous peritonitis have an acute to insidious onset of diffuse abdominal pain. The pain does not localize and increases in intensity over hours to days. Nonbilious vomiting, diarrhea, and fever follow the abdominal pain.[64]

Affected children are anxious and acutely ill. Vital signs are typically abnormal. Temperature elevations are noted in the 39°C (102.2°F) to 40.5°C (104.9°F) range; tachycardia is prominent. The respirations are rapid and shallow and may be accompanied by a terminal expiratory grunt. Bowel sounds are diminished. The abdomen is diffusely distended, and when ascites is present, evidence of free fluid will be evident. The abdomen is diffusely tender and guarded. Rebound tenderness may be generalized. Rectal examination reveals tenderness without mass.[65]

Plain radiographic features of peritonitis include marked gaseous distension of the large and small intestines. Multiple air–fluid levels may be present. Intestinal loops may become separated, and the more dependent portions become more opaque. In circumstances where peritoneal exudate localizes into a large abscess, intestinal coils may be displaced away from the inflammatory mass.[66]

If a spontaneous peritonitis is suspected preoperatively, abdominal paracentesis with Gram stain and culture of the fluid may obviate the need for exploratory laparotomy. If the diagnosis cannot be established preoperatively, laparotomy is necessary.

NECROTIZING ENTEROCOLITIS

Diverse events in the perinatal period may lead to gastric dilatation, functional ileus, and erosive intestinal mucosal injury, all of which are characteristic of NEC. The terminal ileum and colon are the most common sites of histologic changes.[67] The pathologic findings range from mucosal edema to full-thickness necrosis with perforation. Premature infants who have sustained any of multiple stresses to their cardiovascular system such as acute blood loss, transient hypotension, and birth asphyxia or who require central vascular instrumentation are at increased risk for NEC. Approximately 10% of cases occur in term infants.[68] Most infants are diagnosed prior to their initial hospital discharge, but the emergency physician may encounter infants affected with NEC within the first month of life.[69]

NEC represents a spectrum of illness that varies from a self-limited, transient process to a potentially fatal disease. The symptoms range from isolated gastrointestinal upset to systemic manifestations. Anorexia and gastric distension, followed by nonbilious vomiting, abdominal distension, or diarrhea are seen at the onset. Hemochezia may develop. Those who do not spontaneously recover may develop altered mental status and profound alteration of all vital signs. Apnea, bradycardia, hypotension, and vascular instability may all occur.[68,70]

Affected infants are pale and often septic-appearing. Abdominal distension may be generalized, or a single segment of colon may dilate to striking proportions. Multiple dilated loops of bowel or a localized dilated loop of bowel may be palpated. Abdominal tenderness and guarding are highly variable. Bowel sounds are diminished. Rectal examination reveals grossly bloody stool or seedy stool that is guaiac positive.[71]

On abdominal flat plate, bowel distension is the most common finding. The dilatation may occur in an isolated, diseased, unobstructed colonic segment. Alternately, multiple loops of distal small and large bowel exhibit dilatation suggesting partial obstruction. Concentric loops, centrally located, and associated with increased opacity in the flanks may be seen with ascites. Intraluminal air (pneumatosis intestinalis) may be limited to scattered colonic segments or be generalized. Intrahepatic portal vein gas and pneumoperitoneum are ominous findings (Fig. 9–12).[72]

The documentation of either is enhanced with cross-table lateral, decubitus, or erect views. When the clinical picture or radiographic signs are ambiguous, barium enema may provide evidence of colitis, including small ulcerations, mucosal irregularity, and intraluminal extravasation of barium.[73] Ultrasonography in NEC has proved to be of benefit only to detect and track the passage of air through the portal vein system.

Treatment includes withholding feedings, initiating parenteral nutrition, nasogastric decompression, and parenteral as well as intraluminal antibiotics. In the absence of perforation, obvious peritonitis, and gangrenous bowel, surgery is withheld.[70,74]

HIRSCHSPRUNG'S DISEASE

Hirschsprung's disease is characterized by the absence of intramural ganglion cells. The histologic deficit is usually limited to a segment of bowel in the rectosigmoid region. The functional abnormality with Hirschsprung's disease is an increase in muscular tone and contractility of the aganglionic segment. Relaxation needed to facilitate the onward movement of stool does not occur. This disease is four times more frequent in males than females.[75,76]

The pattern of presentation of Hirschsprung's disease is extremely variable.[77] The diagnosis may be suspected within the first few days of birth or not entertained until late childhood. Newborns with aganglionosis may have delayed passage of the first meconium stool. Infants have diminished stool frequency. If undiagnosed, the clinical course in the first year of life is one of gradually increasing fecal retention, obstipation, constipation, and sporadic abdominal distention. Diminished appetite and extended periods of failure to thrive are often noted. Intermittent vomiting and unexplained bouts of nonbloody diarrhea may be encountered.[75] Patients with previously undiagnosed Hirschsprung's disease may present with rectal prolapse.

Parents frustrated by repeated therapeutic failures for chronic constipation are likely to seek ED attention. Examination of affected children reveal a variable nutrition status. There may be mild to moderate abdominal distention. The abdomen is soft, and nontender, mobile fecal masses may be palpable in the left lower quadrant. Children's underwear is not soiled from overflow, as is typically the case with children who have functional constipation. Rectal examination reveals an empty vault that is not dilated. Withdrawal of the examining finger may result in an explosive release of stool. This "squirt" in the correct historic context suggests the diagnosis of aganglionosis. If the diagnosis is not entertained, patients may precipitously develop a potentially fatal enterocolitis.[78]

Enterocolitis with Hirschsprung's disease is more common in the newborn period, but can occur at any age. It can occur preoperatively and postoperatively.[79] The enterocolitis is characterized by sudden abdominal distention, generalized abdominal discomfort, and explosive diarrhea that rapidly becomes bloody. Temperature elevation, volume depletion, and altered mental status are typically noted. With the most severe cases, a denudation of the intestinal mucosa predisposes to colonic perforation, peritonitis, and gram-negative septicemia.[79,80]

Progressively confirmatory steps for diagnosing Hirschsprung's disease in children with chronic constipation include plain abdominal films, barium enema, anal rectal manometry, and pathologic examination of rectal tissue.[81] The latter two diagnostic modalities require equipment and personnel

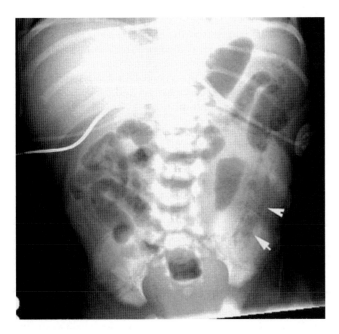

Figure 9–12. Abdominal radiograph of infant with NEC. Arrows point to area of pneumatosis intestinalis.

that are typically unavailable in an ED. With aganglionosis, the abdominal flat plate may be normal or demonstrate dilated colon proximal to the aganglionic segment. Barium enema confirms a normal caliber of the rectum and dilatation of the proximal colon. A cone-shaped transition zone in between is pathognomonic.[82]

In the presence of enterocolitis, plain abdominal radiographs show variable distention of multiple intestinal loops and air–fluid levels. The sigmoid or descending colon may be massively dilated. Pneumoperitoneum may be present if spontaneous perforation of the colon has occurred.[75] ED intervention for enterocolitis includes gastric decompression, use of a rectal tube, fluid resuscitation, parenteral antibiotics, and keeping patients npo.

▶ GASTROINTESTINAL FOREIGN BODIES

The size, configuration, consistency, and chemistry of an ingested object, when coupled with children's age and personal anatomy, determines whether the children remain asymptomatic or if they develop clinical manifestations. Small (<15–20 mm), round, oval, and cuboid objects without sharp edges or projections cause the least difficulty. Rigid, elongated, slender objects may also traverse the intestinal tract without difficulty, but are more inclined to cause complications. A single ingested magnet causes no problems, but multiple magnet ingestions may attract through the bowel wall causing pressure necrosis or bowel perforation.[83] Medicamental concretions or repeated ingestion of hair or vegetable matter, such as seeds, leaves, roots, stems, and fiber, can lead to bezoars. These compact masses of foreign material can create havoc anywhere within the intestinal tract.[84] Ingested batteries retained within the esophagus, stomach, or lodged in the appendix or a Meckel's diverticulum can lead to tragedy. Children with underlying congenital, anastomotic, or inflammatory diseases of mediastinal structures are at increased risk of gastrointestinal foreign body impaction. Children <1 year of age, those most likely to inappropriately mouth objects, are at increased risk for complications because of the diminutive caliber of their digestive system.[85]

Complications of gastrointestinal foreign bodies may occur rapidly after inadvertent ingestion or be delayed for months. They include obstruction within the gastrointestinal tract and perforation anywhere within the gut, with subsequent peritonitis, intraperitoneal, hepatic, or extraperitoneal abscess. Other gastrointestinal complications include gut fistulization or hemorrhage. Less common, but with higher mortality, are complications of prolonged esophageal foreign bodies that include obstruction of the airway, mediastinitis, and erosion into the major vessels.[86,87]

The symptoms exhibited by individual patients who have ingested a foreign body are therefore myriad. Those who become obstructed typically do so at the hypopharynx, thoracic inlet, and the cardioesophageal junction (Fig. 9–13).

Patients with a hypopharyngeal foreign body have persistent gagging and pooling of oral secretions, extreme pain localized to the superior neck, and are unable to swallow or speak. Those who have a foreign body lodged at the aortic arch may localize pain to the area of the sternal notch. They

too have dysphagia and drooling, but lack dysphonia. Foreign bodies retained at the distal esophagus create vague chest discomfort as well as dysphagia and odynophagia. Obstruction lower down in the intestinal tract causes intermittent abdominal pain with or without vomiting. Distal problem sites include the pylorus, the loop of the duodenum, the ligament of Treitz, and the ileocecal valve.

Physical findings are limited when an ingested foreign body has caused isolated obstruction in the gastrointestinal tract. Vital signs are normal, the abdomen is generally soft and nontender, and, with the exception of bezoars, a mass is absent. Bowel sounds are normal or high pitched; crescendo sounds may be heard coincident with colicky abdominal pain and separated by periods of silence. A metal detector (used by even a novice examiner) is an effective, radiation-free diagnostic tool for locating ingested metallic bodies.[88] If patients are found to have a metallic foreign body below the diaphragm, there is no need for radiography. If a handheld unit is unavailable, the mainstay for locating metallic foreign bodies remains anteroposterior films of the chest and abdomen. A lateral neck film should be reserved for children with retained esophageal coins in order to determine the number of coins present. Sounding or CT scan is of benefit only in patients who have perforated organs.

Children without underlying esophageal disease who have a single coin lodged for <24 hours in any portion of the esophagus are likely to have spontaneous passage of the coin into the stomach. If there is no respiratory compromise, they may be kept npo and provided intravenous hydration for 12 hours while awaiting spontaneous passage. Children with proximal or middle esophageal impaction may require sedation while waiting for passage of the object. Alternative management to watchful waiting includes balloon extraction and esophagoscopy.[89] One of these active methods should be employed for batteries with corrosive potential regardless of the level point of esophageal impaction.[90] Active retrieval may also be required for objects that are pointed or elongated.[91]

In cases where patients with a history of foreign body ingestion are discharged from the ED, the parents should *not* be instructed to examine fecal contents. This recommendation is unnecessarily burdensome and typically unrewarding. Parents *do* need to be advised of the potential for delayed obstruction anywhere in the gastrointestinal tract and made aware of the signs and symptoms of obstruction.

▶ MEGACOLON

Inflammatory bowel disease in late childhood or early adolescence may be caused by ulcerative colitis, primarily a disease of the rectal and colonic mucosa, or Crohn's disease, a transmural disease primarily restricted to the distal ileum.[7] The risk of acquiring either disease is similar in both sexes. Extraintestinal manifestations such as growth retardation, fever, anemia, arthritis, arthralgia, mouth ulcerations, erythema nodosum, pyogenic gangrenosa, liver dysfunction, and uveitis are common to both disorders and may precede the onset of the gastrointestinal complaints. In most children with these two conditions, the overriding concern is persistent diarrhea followed by the appearance of mucus and blood admixed in the stools. In the majority of cases the diarrhea begins insidiously,

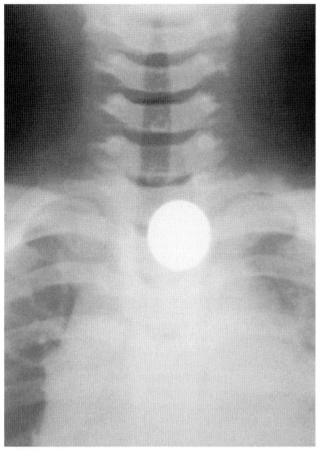

A

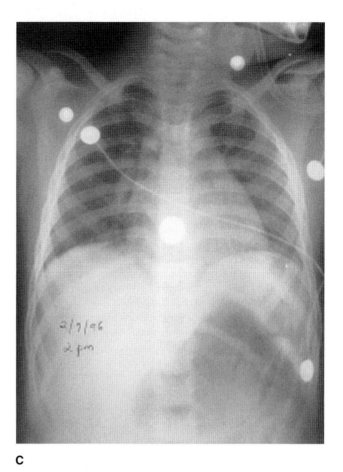

C

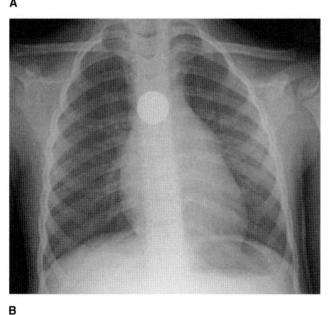

B

Figure 9–13. The three most common places an ingested foreign body becomes lodged.

but a small percentage may have an acute, fulminant course with apparent bacterial sepsis and profuse, bloody diarrhea.[92]

Either as an exacerbation of long-standing disease or as the precipitating event of the disease, patients with either condition may develop a toxic dilatation of the colon (megacolon). The transverse colon is typically involved. A transmural inflam-

matory process occurs, and the segment of colon massively dilates. Peristalsis ceases. Significant hemorrhage and multiple areas of microperforation may be preludes to peritonitis and overwhelming sepsis.[93]

Patients with megacolon develop a temperature spike and experience malaise and anorexia. Abdominal pain and distension will occur over a period of a few hours to a day. Abundant, grossly bloody stools will be passed. Lethargy may develop.[94]

Physical examination is remarkable for toxicity and apparent volume depletion. Temperature elevation and tachycardia are noted. Bowel sounds are diminished. The abdomen is distended, tympanitic, and tender. Guarding and rebound may occur with frank perforation. Rectal examination is painless and reveals no masses, sinuses, or fistulas unless the inflammatory bowel disease has been long-standing. Stool is grossly bloody.[95]

The hallmark radiologic feature of toxic megacolon, seen on a supine abdominal film, is dilatation of the transverse colon ≥6 to 7 cm in diameter.

As perforation may complicate megacolon, an upright or decubitus view should be obtained to search for free air. Ultrasonography is more useful following perforation. However, edema and inflammatory infiltration of the colon wall may be determined by sounding the transverse colon.[92,96] Computerized tomography scans may be diagnostic.[97]

Initial treatment for toxic megacolon involves fluid resuscitation, with added albumin or blood as necessary. High-dose corticosteroids are required for patients on maintenance steroids. Pending surgical consultation, a nasogastric tube should be passed and parenteral antibiotics begun.[98]

REFERENCES

1. Brown L, Jones J. Acute abdominal pain in children: "classic" presentations versus reality. *Emerg Med Prac.* 2000;2:1.
2. Heller RM, Hernanz-Schulman M. Applications of new imaging modalities to the evaluation of common pediatric conditions. *J Pediatr.* 1999;135:632.
3. Pollack ES. Pediatric abdominal surgical emergencies. *Pediatr Ann.* 1996;25:448.
4. Irish MS, Pearl RH, Caty MG, Glick PL. The approach to common abdominal diagnosis in infants and children. *Pediatr Clin North Am.* 1998;45:729.
5. Bonadio WA, Clarkson T, Naus J. The clinical features of children with malrotation of the intestine. *Pediatr Emerg Care.* 1991;7:348.
6. Andrassy RJ, Mahour GH. Malrotation of the midgut in infants and children: a 25-year review. *Arch Surg.* 1981;116:158.
7. Velez LI, Benitez FL, Villanueva SE. Acute abdominal pain in special populations, part I: pediatric patients. *Emerg Med Rep.* 2004;25:273.
8. Weinberger E, Winters WD. Abdominal pain and vomiting in infants and children: imaging evaluation. *Compr Ther.* 1997;23:679.
9. Pracros JP, Sann L, Genin G, et al. Ultrasound diagnosis of midgut volvulus: the "whirlpool" sign. *Pediatr Radiol.* 1992;22:18.
10. Janik JS, Wayne ER, Janik JP. Pyloric stenosis in premature infants. *Arch Pediatr Adolesc Med.* 1996;150:223.
11. Letton RW Jr. Pyloric stenosis. *Pediatr Ann.* 2001;30:745.
12. Knoop KJ, Dillon EC. Pediatric vomiting. *Acad Emerg Med.* 1996;3:77.
13. Hulka F, Campbell TJ, Campbell JR, Harrison MW. Evolution in the recognition of infantile hypertrophic pyloric stenosis. *Pediatrics.* 1997;100:E9.
14. Senquiz AL. Use of decubitus position for finding the "olive" of pyloric stenosis. *Pediatrics.* 1991;87:266.
15. Hernanz-Schulman M, Sells LL, Ambrosino MM, et al. Hypertrophic pyloric stenosis in the infant without a palpable olive: accuracy of sonographic diagnosis. *Radiology.* 1994;193:771.
16. Neilson D, Hollman AS. The ultrasonic diagnosis of infantile hypertrophic pyloric stenosis: technique and accuracy. *Clin Radiol.* 1994;49:246.
17. Hulka F, Campbell JR, Harrison MW, Campbell TJ. Cost-effectiveness in diagnosing infantile hypertrophic pyloric stenosis. *J Pediatr Surg.* 1997;32:1604.
18. Papadakis K, Chen EA, Luks FI, et al. The changing presentation of pyloric stenosis. *Am J Emerg Med.* 1999;17:67.
19. Orenstein J. Update on intussusception. *Contemp Pediatr.* 2000;17:180.
20. Fanconi S, Berger D, Rickham PP. Acute intussusception: a classic clinical picture? *Helv Paediatr Acta.* 1982;37:345.
21. Yamamoto LG, Morita SY, Boychuk RB, et al. Stool appearance in intussusception: assessing the value of the term "currant jelly". *Am J Emerg Med.* 1997;15:293.
22. Bergdahl S, Hugosson C, Lauren T, Soderlund S. Atypical intussusception. *J Pediatr Surg.* 1972;7:700.
23. Luks FI, Yazbeck S, Perreault G, Desjardins JG. Changes in the presentation of intussusception. *Am J Emerg Med.* 1992;10:574.
24. Ein SH, Stephens CA. Intussusception: 354 cases in 10 years. *J Pediatr Surg.* 1971;6:16.
25. Singer J. Altered consciousness as an early manifestation of intussusception. *Pediatrics.* 1979;64:93.
26. Ravitch MM. Consideration of errors in the diagnosis of intussusception. *AMA Am J Dis Child.* 1952;84:17.
27. Daneman A, Alton DJ. Intussusception. Issues and controversies related to diagnosis and reduction. *Radiol Clin North Am.* 1996;34:743.
28. Lazar L, Rathaus V, Erez I, Katz S. Interrupted air column in the large bowel on plain abdominal film: a new radiological sign of intussusception. *J Pediatr Surg.* 1995;30:1551.
29. Eklof O, Hartelius H. Reliability of the abdominal plain film diagnosis in pediatric patients with suspected intussusception. *Pediatr Radiol.* 1980;9:199.
30. Harrington L, Connolly B, Hu X, et al. Ultrasonographic and clinical predictors of intussusception. *J Pediatr.* 1998;132:836.
31. Schulman H, Laufer L, Kurzbert E, et al. Chronic intussusception in childhood. *Eur Radiol.* 1998;8:1455.
32. Daneman A, Navarro O. Intussusception. Part 2: an update on the evolution of management. *Pediatr Radiol.* 2004;34:97.
33. Sandler AD, Ein SH, Connolly B, et al. Unsuccessful air–enema reduction of intussusception: is a second attempt worthwhile? *Pediatr Surg Int.* 1999;15:214.
34. George EK, Oudesluys-Murphy AM, Madern GC, et al. Inguinal hernias containing the uterus, fallopian tube, and ovary in premature female infants. *J Pediatr.* 2000;136:696.
35. Katz DA. Evaluation and management of inguinal and umbilical hernias. *Pediatr Ann.* 2001;30:729.
36. Stylianos S, Jacir NN, Harris BH. Incarceration of inguinal hernia in infants prior to elective repair. *J Pediatr Surg.* 1993;28:582.
37. Hamilton RS, Mardoum RM. Radiological case of the month. Inguinal hernia presenting as an intestinal obstruction. *Arch Pediatr Adolesc Med.* 1997;151:1159.
38. Davies N, Najmaldin A, Burge DM. Irreducible inguinal hernia in children below two years of age. *Br J Surg.* 1990;77:1291.
39. Rowe MI, Marchildon MB. Inguinal hernia and hydrocele in infants and children. *Surg Clin North Am.* 1981;61:1137.
40. Kokoska ER, Minkes RK, Silen ML, et al. Effect of pediatric surgical practice on the treatment of children with appendicitis. *Pediatrics.* 2001;107:1298.

41. Mannenbach MS. Appendicitis in the young child: making the right diagnosis. *Ped Emerg Med Rep.* 2005;10:117.
42. Bundy DG, Byerley JS, Liles EA, et al. Does this child have appendicitis? *JAMA.* 2007;298:438.
43. Blair GL, Gaisford WD. Acute appendicitis in children under six years. *J Pediatr Surg.* 1969;4:445.
44. Rothrock SG, Skeoch G, Rush JJ, Johnson NE. Clinical features of misdiagnosed appendicitis in children. *Ann Emerg Med.* 1991;20:45.
45. Dickson AP, MacKinlay GA. Rectal examination and acute appendicitis. *Arch Dis Child.* 1985;60:666.
46. Rothrock SG, Pagane J. Acute appendicitis in children: emergency department diagnosis and management. *Ann Emerg Med.* 2000;36:39.
47. Gronroos JM. Do normal leucocyte count and C-reactive protein value exclude acute appendicitis in children? *Acta Paediatr.* 2001;90:649.
48. Wilkinson RH, Bartlett RH, Eraklis AJ. Diagnosis of appendicitis in infancy. The value of abdominal radiographs. *Am J Dis Child.* 1969;118:687.
49. Crady SK, Jones JS, Wyn T, Luttenton CR. Clinical validity of ultrasound in children with suspected appendicitis. *Ann Emerg Med.* 1993;22:1125.
50. Pena BM, Taylor GA, Lund DP, Mandl KD. Effect of computed tomography on patient management and costs in children with suspected appendicitis. *Pediatrics.* 1999;104:440.
51. Reich JD, Brogdon B, Ray WE, et al. Use of CT scan in the diagnosis of pediatric acute appendicitis. *Pediatr Emerg Care.* 2000;16:241.
52. Kosloske AM, Love CL, Rohrer JE, et al. The diagnosis of appendicitis in children: outcomes of a strategy based on pediatric surgical evaluation. *Pediatrics.* 2004;113:29.
53. Garcia Pena BM, Cook EF, Mandl KD. Selective imaging strategies for the diagnosis of appendicitis in children. *Pediatrics.* 2004;113:24.
54. Hayden S, Dorfman D. Grunting, hot and vomiting: what's the bother in baby's belly? *Contemp Pediatr.* 2002;19:21.
55. Swischuk LE. Abdominal pain for 3 days, but now the patient is feeling better. *Pediatr Emerg Care.* 2002;18:105.
56. Nelson DS, Bateman B, Bolte RG. Appendiceal perforation in children diagnosed in a pediatric emergency department. *Pediatr Emerg Care.* 2000;16:233.
57. Law DK, Murr P, Bailey WC. Empyema. A rare presentation of perforated appendicitis. *JAMA.* 1978;240:2566.
58. Bechtel K. Appendicitis: an unusual cause of pneumonia and impending shock in a toddler. *Pediatr Emerg Care.* 1997;13:342.
59. Nance ML, Adamson WT, Hedrick HL. Appendicitis in the young child: a continuing diagnostic challenge. *Pediatr Emerg Care.* 2000;16:160.
60. Quillin SP, Siegel MJ, Coffin CM. Acute appendicitis in children: value of sonography in detecting perforation. *AJR Am J Roentgenol.* 1992;159:1265.
61. Leggiadro RJ, Lazar LF. Spontaneous bacterial peritonitis due to Neisseria meningitidis serogroup Z in an infant with liver failure. *Clin Pediatr (Phila).* 1991;30:350.
62. Woods CR, Mason CS. Primary group A streptococcal peritonitis in a human immunodeficiency virus-infected patient. *Pediatr Infect Dis J.* 1997;16:1185.
63. Markenson DS, Levine D, Schacht R. Primary peritonitis as a presenting feature of nephrotic syndrome: a case report and review of the literature. *Pediatr Emerg Care.* 1999;15:407.
64. Gorensek MJ, Lebel MH, Nelson JD. Peritonitis in children with nephrotic syndrome. *Pediatrics.* 1988;81:849.
65. Kimber CP, Hutson JM. Primary peritonitis in children. *Aust N Z J Surg.* 1996;66:169.
66. Clark JH, Fitzgerald JF, Kleiman MB. Spontaneous bacterial peritonitis. *J Pediatr.* 1984;104:495.
67. Coit AK. Necrotizing enterocolitis. *J Perinat Neonatal Nurs.* 1999;12:53.
68. Madi K, Mattos EA, Fernandez ET. Necrotizing enterocolitis in term infants and older children. *Intl Pediatr.* 1994;9:37.
69. Turner LM, Miller RF. Necrotizing enterocolitis: an unusual cause of rectal bleeding in a term infant. *Ann Emerg Med.* 1986;15:742.
70. Wheeler DS. Radiological case of the month. Necrotizing enterocolitis in a term infant. *Arch Pediatr Adolesc Med.* 1999;153:199.
71. Santulli TV, Schullinger JN, Heird WC, et al. Acute necrotizing enterocolitis in infancy: a review of 64 cases. *Pediatrics.* 1975;55:376.
72. O'Kada PS, Hicks B. Neonatal surgical emergencies. *Clin Pediatr Emerg Med.* 2002;3:3.
73. Buonomo C. The radiology of necrotizing enterocolitis. *Radiol Clin North Am.* 1999;37:1187.
74. Hostetler MA, Schulman M. Necrotizing enterocolitis presenting in the emergency department: case report and review of differential considerations for vomiting in the neonate. *J Emerg Med.* 2001;21:165.
75. Okada PJ, Hicks B. Neonatal surgical emergencies. *Clin Pediatr Emerg Med.* 2002;3:3.
76. Pearl RH, Irish MS, Caty MG, Glick PL. The approach to common abdominal diagnoses in infants and children. Part II. *Pediatr Clin North Am.* 1998;45:1287.
77. Carty HM. Paediatric emergencies: non-traumatic abdominal emergencies. *Eur Radiol.* 2002;12:2835.
78. Bill JAH, Chapman ND. The enterocolitis of Hirschsprung's disease: it's natural history and treatment. *Am J Surg.* 1962;103:70.
79. Marty TL, Matlak ME, Hendrickson M, et al. Unexpected death from enterocolitis after surgery for Hirschsprung's disease. *Pediatrics.* 1995;96:118.
80. Fraser GC, Barry C. Mortality in neonatal Hirschsprung's disease: with particular reference to enterocolitis. *J Pediatr Surg.* 1967;2:205.
81. Mason JD. The evaluation of acute abdominal pain in children. *Emerg Med Clin North Am.* 1996;14:629.
82. Franken EA Jr, Smith WL, Frey EE, et al. Intestinal motility disorders of infants and children: classification, clinical manifestations and roentgenology. *Crit Rev Diagn Imaging.* 1987;27:203.
83. Chung JH, Kim JS, Song YT. Small bowel complication caused by magnetic foreign body ingestion of children: two case reports. *J Pediatr Surg.* 2003;38:1548.
84. Faria AP, Silva IZ, Santos A, et al. The Rapunzel syndrome—a case report: trichobezoar as a cause of intestinal perforation. *J Pediatr (Rio J).* 2000;76:83.
85. Al-Qudah A, Daradkeh S, Abu-Khalaf M. Esophageal foreign bodies. *Eur J Cardiothorac Surg.* 1998;13:494.
86. Lai AT, Chow TL, Lee DT, Kwok SP. Risk factors predicting the development of complications after foreign body ingestion. *Br J Surg.* 2003;90:1531.
87. Kerschner JE, Beste DJ, Conley SF, et al. Mediastinitis associated with foreign body erosion of the esophagus in children. *Int J Pediatr Otorhinolaryngol.* 2001;59:89.
88. Schalamon J, Haxhija EQ, Ainoedhofer H, et al. The use of a hand-held metal detector for localisation of ingested metallic foreign bodies – a critical investigation. *Eur J Pediatr.* 2004;163:257.
89. Vargas EJ, Mody AP, Kim TY, et al. The removal of coins from the upper esophageal tract of children by emergency physicians: a pilot study. *CJEM.* 2004;6:434.

90. Yardeni D, Yardeni H, Coran AG, Golladay ES. Severe esophageal damage due to button battery ingestion: can it be prevented? *Pediatr Surg Int.* 2004;20:496.

91. Kim JK, Kim SS, Kim JI, et al. Management of foreign bodies in the gastrointestinal tract: an analysis of 104 cases in children. *Endoscopy.* 1999;31:302.

92. Roy MA. Inflammatory bowel disease. *Surg Clin North Am.* 1997;77:1419.

93. Greenstein AJ, Sachar DB, Gibas A, et al. Outcome of toxic dilatation in ulcerative and Crohn's colitis. *J Clin Gastroenterol.* 1985;7:137.

94. Strauss RJ, Flint GW, Platt N, et al. The surgical management of toxic dilatation of the colon: a report of 28 cases and review of the literature. *Ann Surg.* 1976;184:682.

95. Caprilli R, Vernia P, Latella G, Torsoli A. Early recognition of toxic megacolon. *J Clin Gastroenterol.* 1987;9:160.

96. Levine MS. Crohn's disease of the upper gastrointestinal tract. *Radiol Clin North Am.* 1987;25:79.

97. Bitton A, Peppercorn MA. Emergencies in inflammatory bowel disease. *Crit Care Clin.* 1995;11:513.

98. Farthing MJ. Severe inflammatory bowel disease: medical management. *Dig Dis.* 2003;21:46.

CHAPTER 10

Vomiting, Diarrhea, and Gastroenteritis

William R. Ahrens

▶ HIGH-YIELD FACTS

- Most of the time vomiting and/or diarrhea are caused by gastroenteritis.
- Life-threatening causes of vomiting include bowel obstructions, increased intracranial pressure, diabetic ketoacidosis, and inborn errors of metabolism.
- Life-threatening causes of diarrhea include toxic megacolon, *Escherichia coli* 0157, and pseudomembranous enterocolitis.
- Most dehydrated patients with gastroenteritis can be treated with oral rehydrating solutions.
- Most cases of gastroenteritis resolve without antibiotic therapy.
- New vaccines against rotavirus have so far been found to be safe and effective.

Vomiting is the forceful expulsion of the contents of the stomach. Diarrhea is defined as frequent (three or more per day) loose or liquid bowel movements. There are several general classifications of diarrhea. In secretory diarrhea there is an increase in secretion or decrease in absorption of intestinal liquid; such diarrhea is often toxin mediated. In inflammatory diarrhea there is damage to the intestinal mucosa. Osmotic diarrhea occurs when liquid is lost accompanying a high intestinal osmotic load. Inappropriately increased intestinal motility can also cause diarrhea. Separately or in combination, vomiting and diarrhea constitute one of the most common manifestations of childhood illness. Diarrheal illnesses remain one of the most common causes of childhood death, especially in impoverished countries.[1,2]

By far the most common cause of vomiting and/or diarrhea is acute infectious gastroenteritis, which in the majority of cases resolves with minimal intervention. However, before the diagnosis of gastroenteritis is established, other potentially life-threatening illnesses that can present with vomiting and/or diarrhea must be excluded. For the most part, this can be accomplished by a careful history and physical examination.

The history regarding the patient who is vomiting focuses on the duration of the illness, the frequency of the vomiting, the character/color of the contents vomited, and associated abdominal pain. Most acute infectious illnesses result in frequent vomiting of a short duration; a history of protracted or intermittent vomiting can imply an underlying anatomic lesion. In infants of 2 to 6 weeks of age, pyloric stenosis should be considered. Bilious vomiting is rare in infants and children, and

always raises the suspicion of a bowel obstruction, especially a malrotation, with or without a volvulus. Vomiting associated with persistent, severe, or localized abdominal pain suggests peritonitis. Vomiting accompanied by a headache raises the possibility of increased intracranial pressure. The history regarding diarrhea focuses on the duration of the problem, the frequency of the stools, and the presence of blood or mucus in the stools. Most acute gastrointestinal infections in the developed world are caused by viruses, and result in frequent, watery stools; the presence of blood or mucus in the feces increases the possibility of a bacterial or inflammatory illness.[1-5] Frank rectal bleeding suggests an anatomic lesion, such as an intussusception, Meckel's diverticulum, or juvenile polyps. Protracted diarrhea (lasting weeks) suggests a malabsorption syndrome or inflammatory bowel disease.

The physical examination of the patient with vomiting and/or diarrhea focuses on excluding life-threatening illness and ascertaining that the diagnosis is indeed gastroenteritis. Perhaps the most important aspect of the physical examination of the patient with vomiting and diarrhea is mental status. A happy, playful infant or child is unlikely to have a life-threatening problem. A patient who is lethargic, on the other hand, is either significantly dehydrated or is at high risk for a significant metabolic or anatomic lesion. Vomiting and altered mental status can occur secondary to increased intracranial pressure; associated physical findings include splitting of the cranial sutures and/or a bulging anterior fontanelle. Metabolic abnormalities due to inborn errors of metabolism, diabetic ketoacidosis, uremia, and hyper- or hyponatremia can also present with vomiting and altered mental status. Inborn errors of metabolism usually present in infants. A rare cause of vomiting and altered mental status is Reye's syndrome. A child with intussusception can present with profound lethargy and there is usually an associated history of vomiting. Patients with a history of diarrhea who present with altered mental status are at risk for toxic megacolon. This can occur secondary to known or as yet undiagnosed Hirschsprung disease; a history of significant constipation might be obtained. Physical examination may reveal palpable stool throughout the abdomen and an empty rectal vault. Profound diarrhea, in which rapid losses of fluid and electrolytes occur, can cause altered mental status secondary to shock The classic example of this is cholera, although viral causes, such as rotavirus, are also implicated. Diarrheal illness secondary to shigella can be associated with altered mental status, although this is usually not life threatening. Bloody diarrhea can be caused by infection with *E. coli*

▶ **TABLE 10–1. LIFE-THREATENING CAUSES OF VOMITING**

Increased intracranial pressure
Bowel obstruction (malrotation, intussusception,
  incarcerated hernia, adhesions)
Inborn errors of metabolism
Diabetic ketoacidosis
Toxic ingestions
Reye's syndrome

0157; up to 10% of affected children will develop potentially life-threatening hemolytic uremic syndrome. Campylobacter is associated with Guillan–Barre syndrome.[6–8] Tables 10–1 and 10–2 list some life-threatening causes of vomiting and diarrhea.

▶ GASTROENTERITIS

Acute infectious gastroenteritis remains one of the most common health problems throughout the world. In the United States, it is responsible for an enormous number of emergency department visits and hospitalizations, especially in younger children; it may account for up to 300 deaths per year. In the developing world, it remains a common cause of mortality, especially in younger, malnourished children; it may be responsible for up to 1.8 million pediatric deaths per year. Especially in malnourished children, gastroenteritis is also a major cause of morbidity.[3,4] There is widespread agreement that the development of inexpensive oral rehydrating solutions has had a profound impact in decreasing mortality from diarrheal illnesses.

ETIOLOGY

In the United States and Europe, the majority of cases of gastroenteritis are caused by viral diseases that peak in the winter months. The most common of these is rotavirus, which remains the most common cause of infectious diarrhea in children worldwide. Other viral causes of acute infectious gastroenteritis include adenovirus serotypes 40 and 41, noroviruses (Norwalk like viruses) virus, calcivirus, and astrovirus. Noroviruses are responsible for a large number of food-borne outbreaks. Rotavirus and adenovirus predominantly infect children younger than the age of 3 years.[1–6]

In the developing world, bacterial infections account for a high percentage of diarrheal illnesses. Bacteria-mediated gastroenteritis is much less common in industrialized nations. Enterotoxogenic bacteria include enterotoxogenic *E. coli*, *Clostridium perfringens*, Cholera species, and Vibrio species;

▶ **TABLE 10–2. LIFE-THREATENING CAUSES OF DIARRHEA**

Toxic megacolon (Hirschsprung disease, ulcerative colitis)
E. coli 0157 (hemolytic uremic syndrome)
Pseudomembranous enterocolitis (antibiotic-associated
  diarrhea)

diarrhea is caused by the secretion of toxin. Enteroinvasive bacteria include enteroinvasive and enterohemorrhagic *E. coli*, Shigella species, Salmonella species, Campylobacter, Yersinia species, and Pleosiomonas species; diarrhea is associated with inflammatory changes in the small and/or large bowel. *Clostridium difficile*, an antibiotic-associated diarrhea, is toxin mediated. Although a fairly high percentage of infants are colonized with Clostridium difficile, it rarely causes disease. Noninvasive parasites that cause diarrhea include Giardia species and Cryptosporidium species. Giardia is a pathogen associated with children attending day care; it can cause acute and chronic diarrhea; it has a minimum infective dose of 10 to 100 cysts; in untreated children, cysts can be shed for months. An invasive parasitic cause of diarrhea is *Entameba histolytica*; it is especially common in the tropics during the rainy season.

PATHOPHYSIOLOGY

In acute infectious gastroenteritis, diarrhea occurs when intestinal output exceeds the ability of the gastrointestinal tract to reabsorb liquid. Viruses tend to directly damage the small intestinal villi, causing malabsorption of carbohydrates that results in watery osmotic diarrhea. Rotavirus may also secrete an enterotoxin that contributes to secretory diarrhea.[1] Bacteria produce diarrhea by a variety of mechanisms. Enterotoxogenic *E. coli* is the most common cause of traveler's diarrhea and the most common cause of bacterial diarrhea in children worldwide; it is uncommon in the United States. It infects the small intestine and causes noninvasive watery diarrhea via two major toxins.[8] Enteropathogenic *E. coli* are an important cause of diarrhea in infants in developing countries, especially diarrhea lasting more that 2 weeks; the mechanism by which diarrhea occurs is not known. Enterohemorrhagic *E. coli* 0157 is an invasive organism associated with hemorrhagic colitis that is complicated by hemolytic uremic syndrome in 5% to 10% of cases. The source of infection is cattle or sheep. Shigella can cause invasive diarrhea after exposure to as little as 10 organisms. Organisms tend to colonize the colonic epithelium, causing intestinal ulcerations, neutrophil infiltration, and bloody diarrhea, except in infants where diarrhea can be nonbloody. Organisms also secrete various toxins, including Shiga toxin, which has been also been implicated in hemolytic uremic syndrome. Shigella infection is associated with seizures in some children. Salmonella enteriditis is a common cause of self-limited, noninvasive diarrhea; it is commonly found in poultry and other farm animals, and has been associated with pet turtles. Infants younger than 1 year of age, patients with sickle cell disease, and immunocompromised patients are at risk for bacteremia from *S. enteriditis*. *Salmonella typhi* and paratyphi infect only humans and are capable of causing serious blood-borne disease, especially in infants and children; they remain a common cause of mortality in some parts of the world. Campylobacter are the most common cause of bacterial gastroenteritis in developed countries; transmission occurs via consumption of contaminated food or water. It can also be a cause of traveler's diarrhea. Infection causes inflammatory enteritis; abdominal pain and a flu-like syndrome are common, and diarrhea can be bloody. Campylobacter infection is associated with the development of Guillan–Barre syndrome.[5–8]

▶ TABLE 10–3. ASSESSMENT OF DEHYDRATION

Two of the following signs:	Severe dehydration
Lethargic or unconscious	
Sunken eyes	
Not able to drink or drinking	
poorly	
Skin pinch goes back very slowly	
Two of the following signs:	Some dehydration
Restless, irritable	
Sunken eyes	
Drinks eagerly, thirsty	
Skin pinch goes back slowly	
Not enough signs to classify as	No dehydration
some or severe dehydration	

DIAGNOSTIC EVALUATION

Physical Assessment

Once the diagnosis of gastroenteritis is assured, the main emphasis is on assessing hydration status (Table 10–3). All children with significant vomiting and diarrhea will have a deficit of fluids and electrolytes. Loss of total body water is calculated as a percentage of body weight: 3% to 5% is generally considered mild, 5% to 10% moderate, and greater than 10% severe. In point of fact, percent dehydration can only be estimated, since it is very unlikely that a baseline weight will be available. In addition, how "sick" the patient is will depend not only on the fluid deficit, but the rate at which it occurred. Fluid losses that occur slowly are compensated for by water in the intracellular and interstitial spaces that shifts to the intravascular space, protecting systemic perfusion. Fulminant losses from severe diarrhea are poorly compensated for, especially in infants, and can result in hypovolemic shock and death. Indeed, the degree of dehydration is notoriously difficult to assess in younger infants. There are a variety of established, teachable, and reproducible methods for estimating the extent to which a patient is dehydrated. Currently, the emphasis is on simplifying the assessment. As it can be difficult to distinguish between mild and moderate dehydration, the two can be grouped together. Important findings indicating the presence of significant dehydration are delayed capillary refill, abnormal skin turgor, and an abnormal respiratory pattern.[9] Other important findings include tachycardia, dry mucus membranes, and the absence or tears. The importance of assessing mental status cannot be overstated. Guidelines regarding the assessment and treatment of diarrhea in children from the World Health Organization (WHO) and UNICEF for physicians and nonphysician health care providers are available on the Internet.[3,4]

Diagnostic Studies

Most children with gastroenteritis do not require laboratory studies. If moderate or severe dehydration is present, it is reasonable to evaluate serum electrolytes. Most patients with significant diarrhea will have low serum bicarbonate. Hypoglycemia can complicate gastroenteritis; in patients with significant dehydration or altered mental status a bedside

glucose is indicated.[10] In patients with bloody diarrhea or protracted diarrhea, a stool sample for culture and ova/parasites should be sent. The presence of fecal leukocytes suggests colitis and the presence of an enteroinvasive infection. For infants, patients with sickle cell disease, and patients who are immunocompromised—in whom salmonella is suspected—a blood culture is indicated since they are at risk for bacteremia. Shigella infection is associated with bandemia. Rotavirus antigen can be detected in the stool via enzyme immunoassay and latex agglutination; there is a fairly high false-negative rate.[1,7,8]

Treatment

Oral Rehydration Therapy

Abundant literature makes it clear that oral rehydration therapy (ORT) is an effective treatment for the vast majority of patients with gastroenteritis-related dehydration. It is credited with saving literally millions of lives around the globe. It is also clear that it is underutilized in environments where intravenous therapy is available. The mechanism crucial to the efficacy of ORT is the coupled transport of sodium and glucose molecules at the intestinal brush border accompanied by free water (Fig. 10–1). There are a variety of oral hydration solutions (ORS) available; currently literature supports the use of formulas containing between 65–75 mg/L of sodium and 75–90 mmol/L of glucose. In the vast majority of cases, rehydration can be accomplished without risk of causing hypo- or hypernatremia.[11–15]

In infants and children with minimal dehydration, treatment is directed at maintaining nutrition and preventing dehydration. Fluid intake can be generally increased, or ORS can be administered at a volume of 10 mL/kg for each stool, or 2 mL/kg for each emesis. Diet should not be restricted.

Patients with mild-to-moderate dehydration should receive 50 to 100 mL/kg of ORS over 2 to 4 hours. Ongoing losses are also replaced. Caregivers can administer fluid with a syringe or teaspoon. Nasogastric administration of ORS is safe and effective, and may be especially useful in patients in whom intravenous access is difficult, or in infants who have difficulty swallowing.[16] Moderately dehydrated patients who require intravenous rehydration can be rehydrated over several hours in the emergency department.[17]

Patients in shock or with severe dehydration require intravenous therapy when it is available. An initial bolus of 20 mL/kg of 0.9 NS or Lactated Ringers is rapidly administered; it is repeated until adequate perfusion is restored. Once perfusion is restored, hydration can be continued intravenously or ORT initiated. Intravenous therapy, if utilized, consists of replacement of the estimated volume deficit along with maintenance fluid therapy. If ongoing fluid losses are severe, they need to be added to therapy. Intravenous rehydration is discussed further in the chapter "Fluid and Electrolyte Emergencies."

Adjunctive Therapy

Persistent vomiting can limit or delay oral rehydration. There are studies that show that oral ondansetron can facilitate oral therapy in children with persistent vomiting, and may decrease the number of children who require intravenous salvage therapy.[18,19]

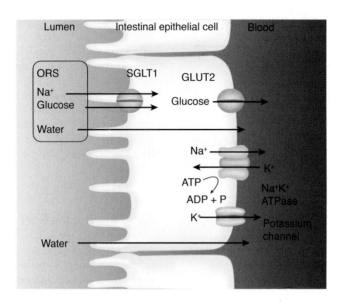

Figure 10–1. Oral rehydration therapy. (Reprinted with permission from Duggan C, Fontaine O, Pierce NF, et al. *JAMA.* 2004;291:2628).

▶ TABLE 10–4. **TREATMENT OF COMMON GASTROINTESTINAL INFECTIONS**

Cause	Antibiotic	Alternative Treatment	Comment
Cholera	Adults: Docycycline Tetracycline Children: Tetracycline	Erythromycin	
Shigella dysentery	Adults and children: Ciprofloxacin Levofloxacin	Trimethoprim/sulfamethoxazole Ampicillin Azithromycin Ceftriaxone Pivmecillinam	Treatment recommended for patients with dysentery; increasing resistance to commonly used antibiotics
Giardiasis	Adults and children: Metronidazole	Tinidazole Albendazole Mebendazole	Albendazole and mebendazole effective in children, also treat other parasitic infections
Amebiasis (dysentery)	Adults and children: Metronidazole	Tindazole	
Campylobacter	Adults and children: Azithromycin	Erythromycin Ciprofloxacin	Most cases self-limited and do not require therapy; treatment in severe cases shortens duration of symptoms
Enterotoxigenic *E. coli*	Levofloxacin Ciprofloxacin	Azithromycin Trimethoprim/sulfamethoxazole	Treatment is empiric; most cases self-limited
Salmonella (non-typhoid)	Ciprofloxacin	Azithromycin Trimethoprim/sulfamethoxazole Ampicillin Cefotaxime Ceftriaxone	Treatment recommended for patients at risk for invasive disease: infants younger than 3 mo of age, patients with sickle cell disease, patients with HIV or other forms of immunosuppression
E. coli 0157	none		Treatment with antibiotics may trigger or exacerbate hemolytic uremic syndrome (controversial)

Zinc deficiency is widespread in the developing world. Numerous studies have now shown that zinc supplementation reduces the severity and duration of diarrhea in children younger than 5 years. It also reduces the incidence of subsequent diarrhea in the next 2 months. The WHO recommends zinc supplementation (10–20 mg/d for 10–14 days) in children with diarrhea.[4]

It is vitally important to maintain the nutritional status of children with diarrhea, especially those who are malnourished. Breast-feeding should be continued, as should an age-appropriate diet, as soon as the patient can tolerate feeding without vomiting. There is insufficient evidence to support withholding lactose-containing formulas in patients with acute diarrhea. Liquids containing high sugar loads, such as colas and apple juice, can increase the intestinal osmotic load and worsen diarrhea; they are best avoided.[3,4]

Antibiotic therapy is not indicated in the majority of cases of diarrheal illness. Even patients with bloody diarrhea can still have a viral illness, such as rotavirus, or a bacterial illness that is self-limited, such as nontyphoidal salmonella. Antibiotic therapy is becoming increasingly complicated by the rapid development of resistance to commonly used medications. Ideally, therapy is directed by culture and sensitivity; these are of course unavailable in most places in the world where bacterial gastroenteritis is common (Tables 10–3 and 10–4).

PREVENTION

Prevention of gastroenteritis fundamentally depends on improving hygiene. In the industrialized world, attention to handwashing and improved handling of meat, poultry, and egg products is important. In the developing world, access to potable water is crucial; it does little good to tell families who cannot afford wood to boil their water. Access to latrines is also an important public health goal in developing nations where plumbing is nonexistent.[20]

Vaccines have been or are being developed for several of the most common causes of gastroenteritis. A vaccine licensed in 1998 for rotavirus was withdrawn within a year because it was associated with an increased risk of intussesception. Since then, two vaccines against rotavirus have been developed, and are currently in use.[21,22] Salmonella typhi, which is capable of causing fatal disease, especially in young children, is especially prevalent in Asia. There are now two vaccines—one oral and the other injectable—that have been show to be safe and efficacious, and are licensed for children older than 2 years of age.[23] Oral cholera vaccines have been developed that are effective in reducing incidence and severity of disease. Vaccines against shigella, campylobacter, and enterotoxigenic *E. coli* are in various stages of development.[24]

REFERENCES

1. Guandalini S, Frye RE. emedicine: Diarrhea. http://www.emedicine.com/ped/topic583.htm. Accessed April 25, 2008.
2. Levine A, Santucci KA. emedicine: Pediatrics, Gastroenteritis. http://www.emedicine.com/emerg/topic380.htm. Accessed April 25, 2008.
3. Centers for Disease Control and Prevention. *Managing Acute Gastroenteritis Among Children: Oral Rehydration, Maintenance, and Nutritional Therapy.* http://cdc.gov/mmwr/preview/mmwrhtml/rr521al.htm, Bethesda, MD: Centers for Disease Control and Prevention; 2003. Accessed April 25, 2008.
4. World Health Organization. *The Treatment of Diarrhoea: A Manual for Physicians and Other Health Care Providers.* 4th rev ed. 2005.
5. Dennehy PH. Acute diarrheal disease in children: epidemiology, prevention, and treatment. *Infect Dis Clin North Am.* 2005;19:585.
6. Podwils LJ, Mintz ED, Nataro JP, et al. Acute, infectious diarrhea among children in developing countries. *Semin Pediatr Infect Dis.* 2004;15:155.
7. Elliott EJ. Acute gastroenteritis in children. *BMJ.* 2007;6:35.
8. Amieva MR. Important bacterial gastrointestinal pathogens in children: a pathogenesis perspective. *Pediatr Clin North Am.* 2005;52:749.
9. Steiner JH, DeWalt DA, Byerley JS. Is this child dehydrated? *JAMA.* 2004;291:2746.
10. Reid SR, Losek JD. Hypoglycemia complicating dehydration in children with acute gastroenteritis. *J Emerg Med.* 2005;29:141.
11. Hartling L, Bellemare S, Wiebe N, et al. Oral versus intravenous rehydration for treating dehydration due to gastroenteritis in children. *Cochrane Database Syst Rev.* 2007;4.
12. Bellemare S, Hartling L, Wiebe N, et al. Oral rehydration versus intravenous therapy for treating dehydration due to gastroenteritis in children: a metanalysis of randomized controlled trials. *BMC Med.* 2004;2:11.
13. Spandorfer PR, Allesandri EA, Joffe MD, et al. Oral versus intravenous rehydration of moderately dehydrated children: a randomized, controlled trial. *Pediatrics.* 2005;115:295.
14. Duggan C, Fontaine O, Pierce N, et al. Scientific rationale for a change in the composition of oral rehydration solution. *JAMA.* 2004;291:269.
15. Boyd R, Busuttil M, Stuart P. Pilot study of a paediatric emergency department oral rehydration protocol. *Emerg Med J.* 2005;22:116.
16. Nager AL, Wang VJ. Comparison of nasogastric and intravenous methods of rehydration in pediatric patients with acute dehydration. *Pediatrics.* 2002;109:566.
17. Bender BJ, Ozuah PO. Intravenous rehydration for gastroenteritis: how long does it usually take? *Pediatr Emerg Care.* 2004;4:215.
18. Freedman SB, Adler M, Seshadri R, et al. Oral ondansetron for gastroenteritis in a pediatric emergency department. *N Engl J Med.* 2006;353:1698.
19. Quintana ED. Emergency department treatment of viral gastritis using intravenous ondansetron or dexamethasone in children. *Ann Emerg Med.* 2007;50:627.
20. Clasen T, Roberts I, Rabie T, et al. Interventions to improve water quality for preventing diarrhea. *Cochrane Database Syst Rev.* 2007;4.
21. Vesikari T, Matson DO, Dennehy P, et al. Safety and efficacy of a pentavalent human-bovine (WC3) reassortment rotavirus vaccine. *NEJM.* 2006;354:23.
22. Ruiz-Palacios, Perez-Schael I, Velazquez R, et al. Safety and efficacy of an attenuated vaccine against severe rotavirus gastroenteritis. *NEJM.* 2006;354:11.
23. World Health Organization. *Typhoid Vaccines: WHO position paper. Weekly Epidemiological Record.* 2008;6:49.
24. World Health Organization. *Initiative for Vaccine Research: Diarrheal Diseases.* 2007. http://www.who.int/vaccine_research/diseases/diarrheal/en/index7.html. Accessed April 25, 2008.

CHAPTER 11

Feeding Disorders

William R. Ahrens

▶ HIGH-YIELD FACTS

- Gastroesophageal reflux (GER) is a very common problem in young infants.
- Pathologic GER is associated with multiple medical problems.
- Most patients with GER respond to conservative treatment.
- Cow's milk protein allergy (CMPA) affects a significant percentage of infants. Many of these patients are also intolerant of Soy protein.
- Patients with CMPA should be switched to an extensively hydrolyzed- or amino acid–based formula.

▶ COMMON FEEDING PROBLEMS IN INFANTS

For the human infant, the first year of life, and especially the first 6 months, is a period of explosive growth. Sustaining normal weight gain and development require virtually continuous intake of a large amount of calories. For the first 4 months, this occurs almost exclusively via the intake of liquid, either as breast milk or formula. After 4 months, solid foods are gradually introduced. Problems related to feeding are common, especially in younger infants, many of whom will present to an emergency department (ED) for diagnosis and treatment. This chapter will focus on two feeding problems especially common in younger infants: gastroesophageal reflux and formula intolerance.

▶ GASTROESOPHAGEAL REFLUX

Gastroesophageal reflux (GER) occurs when there is retrograde flow of gastric contents into the esophagus. Some degree of GER is so common in infants that it can be considered a normal variant in the first year of life. It is thought to be due to immaturity of lower esophageal sphincter function that results in transient lower esophageal sphincter relaxations (tLSER). Less commonly, GER can be secondary to motility disorders or gastric outlet obstruction. Clinically, gastrointestinal reflux presents as regurgitation or vomiting of breast milk or formula. The vast majority of babies vomit during the first week of life; 60% to 70% suffer from some element GER at age 3 to 4 months.[1] Emesis can be forceful, or of the mild variety often referred to as "spitting up." The emesis usually occurs after feeding; it should never be bilious or bloody. Most cases of gas-

trointestinal reflux are physiologic, which implies that there is no associated underlying pathology, growth and development are normal, and there are no resultant medical complications. Physiologic reflux usually resolves by approximately 1 year of age. Pathologic GER is associated with multiple complications including poor weight gain or failure to thrive, esophagitis, and respiratory complications, including reactive airway disease and recurrent pneumonia, thought to be secondary to recurrent aspiration. In patients with severe GER, these complications can coexist. There may be a relationship between GER and acute life-threatening events. Risk factors for GER include prematurity and underlying neurologic disease. CMPA may also be implicated as a cause of GER.[1,2]

The history of the infant suspected of having GER includes determining the amount and frequency of feeding, especially in formula-fed infants, in whom overfeeding is common as well as noting whether the formula is cow's milk or soy based. Stooling pattern is evaluated, especially for the presence of bloody diarrhea that could indicate a formula allergy. Infants with pathologic or symptomatic GER often have a history of excessive crying or irritability, poor appetite, and "arching" of their back that may be related to pain secondary to erosive esophatitis.[1,2]

The physical examination in the infant with GER is most likely to be unremarkable, except in the patient with and underlying neurologic disorder or with severe GER that results in failure to thrive. No laboratory studies available in the ED are diagnostic. An upper GI barium study may be useful in the child with a history of repetitive vomiting, since it may reveal esophageal dysmotility or anatomic lesions that cause vomiting in young infants, especially pyloric stenosis and malrotation, but the test is not sensitive for reflux. A 24-pH probe study is currently the most sensitive test to evaluate the presence of GER; a catheter placed at the lower esophagael sphincter (LES) evaluates episodes of reflux over 24 hours, and a composite score is calculated based on the results. A pH probe study is predominantly useful when the diagnosis of GER is not clinically obvious.[1–3]

TREATMENT

The vast majority of infants with physiologic GER respond to very conservative measures. For the most part, reassuring parents that the child is basically well and that the regurgitation/vomiting will abate without therapy is all that is needed. Conservative measures include recommending smaller more frequent feeding, positioning the baby upright after feeding,

▶ **TABLE 11-1. THICKENED FORMULAS**

United States: Enfamil AR LIPIL
Canada: Enfamil A+ Thickened with rice starch

and thickening the formula with cereal. Formula can be thickened by adding one tablespoon (15 mL) of dry rice cereal per ounce of formula.[4] Premixed thickened formulas are also commercially available (Table 11-1). Prone positioning can reduce GER, but this is not recommended in infants younger than 6 months due to a possible increase in the risk of sudden infant death syndrome. Patients with GER thought to be secondary to CMPA may improve if switched to an extensively hydrolyzed or amino acid formula. Many patients with pathologic GER who have mild complications will also respond to conservative measures; however, some patients will benefit from medical treatment. Medical therapy is predominantly directed at reducing secretion of gastric acid and reducing gastric emptying time. For the most part, medical therapy for GER in infants should be directed by a pediatric gastroenterologist when possible. Medications used include H2 receptor blockers such as ranitidine and nizatidine and proton pump inhibitors such as omeprazole and lansoprazole. A small percentage of infants, especially those with neurologic disorders, will not improve with medical therapy, and is at risk for long-term complications of GER, especially involving the lungs. The majority of these patients will respond well to surgical intervention; the standard operation to correct GER is the Nissan Fundoplication.[1-4]

▶ FORMULA INTOLERANCE AND HYPERSENSITIVITY

Formula intolerance is a vague term that can generally be described as any adverse reaction to ingested formula. It can be allergic or nonallergic in nature—an example of non-allergy-mediated intolerance is lactose intolerance. Approximately 5% to 15% of infants are in some way intolerant of cow's milk. Of these, between 2% and 7.5% have CMPA. Given the fact that at any given moment there are literally millions of babies consuming any of the many varieties of infant formulas, there is surprising little information regarding the types of adverse events they experience from formula consumption. A couple of studies have shown that parents often change from one formula to another based on the belief that the infant is experiencing some difficulty or another; the change was often made without seeking medical consultation. Common reasons given for changing formula were colic, "spitting up," and diarrhea or constipation.[5,6] In some cases, tolerance may be associated with relatively subtle differences in the composition of two formulas.[7]

Formula hypersensitivity or allergy is a relatively common cause of formula intolerance. Food allergy affects approximately 6% to 8% of infants. It is more common in children with severe atopic dermatitis. In infants, the most common food allergens are cow's milk and soy protein. Many infants with CMPA are also soy protein intolerant. Breast-feeding reduces the incidence of CMPA; however, breast-fed babies can develop CMPA from antigens secreted in breast milk. Allergic symptoms can be IgE or non-IgE mediated. Manifestations of IgE sensitivity usually develop shortly after ingesting the offending allergen and include urticaria, angioedema, and wheezing; in its most severe form, an IgE-mediated reaction can result in anaphylaxis. Non-IgE-mediated hypersensitivity often presents in infants between 1 week and 3 months of age. Vomiting and diarrhea are common complaints; bloody stools are not uncommon. Poor weight gain and failure to thrive may be noted. GER can occur.[8-11] Specific diagnoses include allergic proctocolitis, enterocolitis, food protein–induced proctocolitis, and food protein-induced enteropathy syndromes.[9,11]

In the ED, diagnosis of formula intolerance, allergy, or specifically CMPA depends mainly on a careful history and high level of clinical suspicion; there is no diagnostic test available. In infants in whom formula intolerance or allergy is suspected, the potentially offending formula is withdrawn; if symptoms resolve, the patient can be rechallenged with the formula—return of symptoms is considered diagnostic. This will obviously be handled by the infant's pediatrician or an allergist.[8-13]

The ED management of infants with suspected formula intolerance/allergy will depend on the severity of symptoms and, in the case of a likely allergy, the type of reaction involved. The majority of infants are likely to be well-appearing; in these cases, it is the patient's pediatrician who should be involved in the decision to change formulas. Infants who are malnourished or dehydrated secondary to formula intolerance may require laboratory studies and possibly hospital admission. If an anaphylactic reaction is suspected, the offending formula should be immediately stopped and the patient referred to an allergist; consideration should be given to prescribing an epi-pen. Infants with lactose intolerance should be placed on a lactose free formula. Current recommendations are that infants with CMPA be changed to an extensively hydrolyzed or amino acid based formula; soy formulas are avoided because of cross-sensitization with cow's milk protein. Some infants will tolerate an extensively hydrolyzed formula.[13] Infants who do not tolerate a hydrolyzed formula should be placed on an amino acid formula. Those infants with CMPA who have symptoms such severe eczema, reflux esophagitis, or failure to thrive may benefit from an immediate introduction to an amino acid formula without a preceding trial of a extensively hydrolyzed formula[14] (Table 11-2). Breast-feeding mothers whose infants develop CMPA are advised to avoid consuming milk-based products. The natural history of CMPA is such that most affected infants will eventually tolerate cow's milk.[13,14]

▶ **TABLE 11-2. LACTOSE-FREE, EXTENSIVELY HYDROLYZED, AND AMINO ACID FORMULAS**

Lactose-free formulas
    United States: Enfamil LactoFree Lipil, Isomil DF, Similac
Lactose-free advance
    Canada: Enfalac LactoFree, Similac LF
Extensively hydrolyzed formulas
    United States: Nutramigin LIPIL, Pregestimil, Alimentum
Advance
    Canada: Nutramigin, Pregestimil, Alimentim
Amino acid formula
    Neocate

REFERENCES

1. Schwartz SM. Gastroesophageal Reflux. emedicine http://www.emedicine.com/PED/topic1177. Htm updated Jan 18, 2008.
2. Jaksic T. Gastroesophageal Reflux: Surgical Perspective Emedicine. http://www.emedicine.com/ped/TOPIC2957. HTM updated Mar 2008.
3. Rudolph CD, Mazur LJ, Liptak GS, et al. Pediatric GE reflux clinical practice guidelines. *J Pediatr Gastroenterol Nutr.* 2001;32(s2):51.
4. Orenstein SR, McGowan JD. Efficacy of conservative therapy as taught in the primary care setting for symptoms suggesting infant gastroesophageal reflux. *J Peds.* 2008;152:310.
5. Nevo N, Rubin L, Tamir A, et al. Infant feeding patterns I the first 6 months: an assessment in full term infants. *J Pediatr Gastroenterol Nutr.* 2007;45:234.
6. Polack FP, Khan Nafees, Maisels MJ. Changing partners: the dance of infant formula changes. *Clin Pediatr.* 1999;38:703.
7. Beate L, Halter RJ, Kuchan MH, et al. Formula tolerance in postbreast fed and exclusively formula fed infants. *Pediatrics.* 1999;103:e7. http://pediatrics.aapublications.org/cgi/content/full/103/1/e7.
8. Kvenshagen B, Halvorsen R, Jacobsen M. Adverse reactions to milk in infants. *Acta Paediatr.* 2008;97:196.
9. Nowack-Wegrzyn A, Sampson HA. Adverse reactions to foods. *Med Clin North Am.* 2006;90:97.
10. Vanderhoof JA. Food hypersensitivity in children. *Curr Opin Clin Nutr Metab Care.* 1998;1:419.
11. Atkins D. Food allergy: diagnosis and management. *Prim Care.* 2008;35:119.
12. Magazzu G, Scoglio R. Gastrointestinal manifestations of cow's milk allergy. *Ann Asthma Immunol.* 2002;89:65.
13. Vandenplas Y, Brueton M, Dupont C, et al. Guidelines for the diagnosis and management of cow's milk protein allergy in infants. *Arch Dis Child.* 2007;92:902.
14. Hill DJ, Murch SH, Rafferty K, et al. The efficacy of amino acid-based formulas in relieving the symptoms of cow's milk allergy: a systematic review. *Clin Exp Allergy.* 2007;37:808.

CHAPTER 12

Jaundice

Anjali Singh and William R. Ahrens

▶ HIGH-YIELD FACTS

- In the immediate neonatal period, unconjugated hyperbilirubinemia is associated with kernicterus, an irreversible neurologic disorder that occurs when unbound bilirubin is deposited in the brain.
- Visual assessment of jaundice is inaccurate, especially in darkly pigmented infants.
- Increased enterohepatic circulation is an important cause of neonatal jaundice.
- It is imperative to interpret bilirubin levels in terms of the infant's age in hours.
- Knowledge of risk factors for severe hyperbilirubinemia is necessary to initiate early treatment.
- Jaundice that persists longer than 2 weeks or appears beyond the immediate neonatal period is almost always a manifestation of pathology.
- Conjugated hyperbilirubinemia is virtually always pathologic.

Jaundice is a yellowish-green discoloration of the skin and sclera caused by hyperbilirubinemia. It is apparent when the serum bilirubin reaches 5 mg/dL.[1] In newborns, some degree of hyperbilirubinemia is virtually universal. Recent reviews demonstrate that hyperbilirubinemia remains one of the common reasons for readmission to the hospital in the neonatal period, especially with the advent of early newborn discharge.[1,2] Consequently, emergency department (ED) physicians must be familiar with the management of the jaundiced newborn.

Although sequelae from hyperbilirubinemia are relatively rare, unconjugated bilirubin is potentially toxic to the developing CNS. Cases of kernicterus continue to occur worldwide and provide a stark reminder of the importance of maintaining a healthy respect for the complications of hyperbilirubinemia. Conjugated hyperbilirubinemia, although not directly neurotoxic, is often a marker for serious underlying disease.[1–3]

▶ PATHOPHYSIOLOGY

Bilirubin is largely formed by the destruction of red blood cells and the catabolism of heme proteins. Heme is converted to biliverdin, which is converted to bilirubin by biliverdin reductase. Bilirubin is transported to the liver, where it undergoes enzymatic-mediated conversion from an insoluble unconjugated form to a water-soluble conjugate. The conjugating enzyme is uridine diphosphate glucuronosyltransferase (UGT), which is markedly diminished in the newborn infant. The insoluble form of bilirubin is indirect reacting, the water-soluble form direct reacting. After conjugation, bilirubin is excreted in the bile and from there into the intestinal tract. In the intestinal tract, some of the conjugated bilirubin is reconverted to the unconjugated variety by beta glucuronidase. This allows its reabsorption into the enterohepatic circulation. Bilirubin metabolism is summarized in Figure 12–1.[1–5]

At elevated levels, the unconjugated form is potentially neurotoxic in the newborn. Bilirubin enters the brain if it is unbound to albumin, unconjugated, or if the blood–brain barrier has been disrupted from a number of causes, including sepsis, acidosis, and prematurity. The concentration of bilirubin in the brain and the duration of exposure are important determinants of neurotoxicity.

The newborn is especially vulnerable to hyperbilirubinemia for several reasons. Increased hemolysis secondary to shortened red blood cell survival time or fetal–maternal blood group incompatibility can result in increased formation of bilirubin. Impaired hepatic uptake and inadequately developed enzymes delay its conjugation, and increased enterohepatic circulation results in inefficient excretion. At any given time after birth, the serum bilirubin reflects a combination of bilirubin production, conjugation, and enterohepatic circulation.

Hyperbilirubinemia is especially common in newborns and young infants, and it is helpful to consider this age group separately.[1–5]

▶ UNCONJUGATED HYPERBILIRUBINEMIA

NEWBORNS AND YOUNG INFANTS

Differential Diagnosis

Physiologic Jaundice

The most common cause of unconjugated hyperbilirubinemia in the neonatal period is physiologic jaundice. It is thought to result primarily from a sixfold increase in bilirubin load and a marked deficiency in uridine diphosphate glucuronosyltransferase (UGT) activity. In addition, the hepatic uptake and excretion of bilirubin is transiently impaired. Physiologic jaundice becomes visible on the second to third day of life and peaks around the fourth day. The maximum elevation is usually <6 mg/dL. In premature infants, jaundice both peaks and resolves somewhat later, and peak levels can reach 12 mg/dL. Lower levels of bilirubin may be associated with kernicterus in low-birth-weight, high-risk infants; therefore, any degree

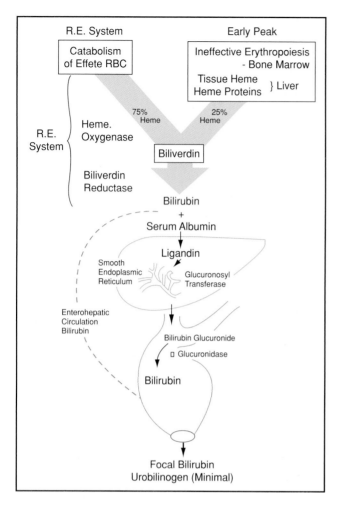

Figure 12–1. Neonatal bile pigment metabolism. RBC, erythrocytes; RE, reticuloendothelial.

of jaundice in a premature infant must be taken seriously. Physiologic jaundice is a nonpathologic condition, with no neurologic sequelae.[1–5]

Breast Milk Jaundice

In general, jaundice is more common in breast-fed infants than it is in bottle-fed infants. The early-onset jaundice is referred to as breast-feeding jaundice, which is akin to a relative starvation state, putting infants at risk for dehydration and increased enterohepatic reuptake of bilirubin. Effective early lactation is the key to its prevention. Breast milk jaundice typically occurs after the first 3 to 5 days of life and can persist for several weeks to a few months. This may be due in part to substances contained in breast milk that antagonize the conjugation and excretion of bilirubin. Rarely, breast-fed infants can develop elevations of unconjugated bilirubin starting in the first week of life, which can reach 15 to 27 mg per 100 mL by the second or third week. The hyperbilirubinemia resolves with the cessation of breast-feeding and does not recur when it is resumed. Interruption of breast-feeding is not recommended in all infants, but rather is reserved for infants with bilirubin levels that place the newborn at risk for kernicterus. A diagnosis of breast milk jaundice

assumes that other pathologic causes of hyperbilirubinemia have been considered and eliminated. It is important to note that although 50% of breast-fed infants develop jaundice, less than 1% develop bilirubin levels that are of concern.[1–5]

Increased Hemolysis

Increased hemolysis in newborn infants is the most common cause of hyperbilirubinemia severe enough to warrant phototherapy or exchange transfusion. It is usually secondary to maternal–fetal blood group incompatibility in either rhesus or ABO antigens. Jaundice usually appears in the first 24 hours of life. In addition to isoimmunization, erythrocyte enzymatic defects predispose erythrocytes to oxidative stress, leading to significant hyperbilirubinemia as seen in G6PD deficiency. Other causes of hemolysis include erythrocyte structural defects such as hereditary spherocytosis and elliptocytosis. Severe bruising or cephalohematoma secondary to trauma during delivery can also result in increased metabolism of heme proteins and unconjugated hyperbilirubinemia.[1–5]

Miscellaneous

Unconjugated hyperbilirubinemia can result from a variety of unusual causes. These include hypothyroidism, Down's syndrome, polycythemia, pyloric stenosis, or other high intestinal obstructions. Bacterial infections, including those from the urinary tract, can cause unconjugated hyperbilirubinemia, although there may also be a component of conjugated bilirubin. It is generally believed that neonatal sepsis causes hyperbilirubinemia by either hemolysis as a result of oxidative stress or bacterial endotoxins reducing bile flow.

Sequelae

In the immediate neonatal period, unconjugated hyperbilirubinemia is of great concern largely because of its association with kernicterus—an irreversible neurologic disorder that occurs when unbound bilirubin is deposited in the CNS, especially the basal ganglia and various brainstem nuclei. Unconjugated bilirubin has the potential to penetrate the nervous system and cause either transient bilirubin encephalopathy or the permanent sequelae of kernicterus. There have been conflicting published reports of the association between bilirubin levels and long-term neurocognitive outcomes, with most data from term neonates with bilirubin levels less than 25 mg/dL.

Acute Bilirubin Encephalopathy

Acute bilirubin encephalopathy can be categorized in phases, characterized clinically by lethargy that can progress to stupor and coma. Changes in the brainstem auditory evoked response have been noted, although the long-term consequences of these are unknown. There have been some reports that if emergent exchange transfusion is performed during the intermediate phase, the CNS changes may be reversible.

Chronic Bilirubin Encephalopathy (Kernicterus)

In its full-blown form, chronic bilirubin encephalopathy ultimately results in choreoathetosis or athetoid cerebral palsy, auditory dysfunction, dental enamel dysplasia, paralysis of upward gaze, extrapyramidal signs, and less often mental retardation. In full-term newborns, kernicterus is associated with levels of unconjugated serum bilirubin levels >20 mg/dL. In premature infants, lower levels can cause kernicterus.[1–5]

Evaluation and Management

The evaluation of unconjugated hyperbilirubinemia depends on the specific age at which hyperbilirubinemia is noted and the rate of rise of bilirubin. The American Academy of Pediatrics subcommittee on hyperbilirubinemia has put forth guidelines for the management of hyperbilirubinemia in infants older than 35 weeks gestation or more, which largely still serve as the cornerstone of management.[6,7]

History and Physical

Special attention should be given to whether the infant has accompanying poor feeding, lethargy, or fever. Sepsis is rare among jaundiced well-appearing infants. Other important considerations are feeding history and weight gain to help assess hydration status.

In neonates, jaundice progresses in a cephalocaudad direction. Blanching of skin with digital pressure for visual inspection of the skin alone is not an accurate method for estimating the degree of hyperbilirubinemia, especially in darkly pigmented infants. It is also important to look for a cephalohematoma or extensive bruising.

Laboratory Evaluation

Measurement of the serum bilirubin is the standard for accurate diagnosis. Various transcutaneous devices (TcB) are also available to measure bilirubin noninvasively. Transcutaneous devices (TcB) have been shown to correlate with serum bilirubin levels less than 12 to 15 mg/dL; however, it is less accurate in darkly pigmented babies, babies of lower gestational age, and babies undergoing phototherapy. When heme is catabolized, carbon monoxide (CO) is produced in equimolar quantities with bilirubin. Hence, end-tidal CO levels can be used in conjunction with serum bilirubin levels as an indicator of ongoing hemolysis and thus bilirubin production in hospitalized babies.[3]

Laboratory evaluation includes a complete blood cell count, type and screen, blood smear, reticulocyte count, and Coomb's test. If a bacterial infection is a consideration, cultures of blood, cerebrospinal fluid, and urine are obtained, in addition to a urinalysis. In infants with vomiting, a bowel obstruction must be ruled out. Further diagnostics should be based on information obtained from the history and physical and individualized to the infant in question.

Management Approach

A neonate who is likely to have physiologic jaundice does not need an extensive workup. Important considerations are rate of rise of bilirubin and identification of any risk factors, which must be applied in the context of the individual patient. The most important risk factors are breast-feeding, gestational age less than 38 weeks, significant jaundice noted in a sibling, and jaundice noted prior to discharge. Newborns with unconjugated bilirubin >5 to 6 mg/dL after 2 to 3 days of life merit investigation. In addition, further workup is indicated if cord blood bilirubin is 4 mg/dL or greater, increasing at a rate of 0.5 mg/dL over a 4- to 8- hour period or increasing greater than 5 mg/dL in the first 24 hours of life. Workup is also indicated if for bilirubin greater than 13 to 15 mg/dL in term infants, greater than 10 mg/dL in premature infants, and when jaundice persists beyond 10 days of life in term infants, or 21 days in premature infants. Any infant who is going to need phototherapy requires a workup to identify the cause of jaundice. Based on a study of healthy term and near-term infants, Bhutani and colleagues established a percentile based predictive nomogram using age-in-hours specific bilirubin levels to determine infants at risk of developing severe hyperbilirubinemia. It is imperative to always interpret bilirubin levels in terms of the infant's age in hours (Fig. 12–2).

Treatment of hyperbilirubinemia may consist of phototherapy, exchange transfusion, or pharmacologic agents. The criteria for initiating phototherapy are not completely clear, but largely depend on precise gestational age and birth weight. A serum bilirubin greater than 25 mg/dL is considered a medical emergency; affected newborns should be admitted directly to the hospital rather than directed to the ED, so that treatment is not delayed. Guidelines published by the AAP in 2004 can help direct the decision to begin initiate therapy (Fig. 12–3).[6,7]

Indirect bilirubin is reduced by exposure to high-intensity light with wavelength in the blue–green spectrum. Phototherapy principally acts by converting bilirubin into isomers which bypass hepatic conjugation and are excreted without further metabolism. It is the treatment of choice for most babies with moderate to severe elevation of indirect bilirubin.[8] It is recommended that intravenous γ-globulin should be administered if the bilirubin continues to rise in spite of intensive phototherapy, especially in infants with hemolytic disease.

Infants with rapidly rising serum bilirubin and no response to phototherapy may require exchange transfusion. Exchange transfusion should be performed in consultation with a neonatologist Figure 12–4. Phenobarbital and ursodeoxycholic acid have been shown to improve bile flow and potentially decrease bilirubin. Other agents such as tin mesoporphyrin inhibit heme oxygenase thereby reducing bilirubin production.

OLDER INFANTS AND CHILDREN

Differential Diagnosis

In older children, unconjugated hyperbilirubinemia is most likely the result of a hemolytic process or an inherited defect in the conjugation of bilirubin. Hemolytic anemia can be congenital, as in of sickle cell disease, thallasemia, hereditary spherocytosis, pyruvate kinase, or G6PD deficiency or can be acquired, as in drug-induced hemolysis.

Gilbert's syndrome results in mild, intermittent unconjugated hyperbilirubinemia resulting form partial deficiency of glucuronyl transferase. Symptoms are usually nonspecific abdominal pain and nausea with an elevated bilirubin up to 5 mg/dL. Crigler–Najjar syndrome is characterized by a partial (type II) or complete absence (type I) of glucuronyl transferase,

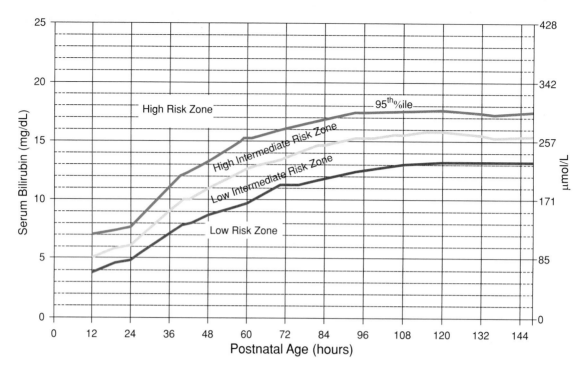

Figure 12–2. Nomogram of bilirubin serum levels in neonates older than 35-weeks gestation. (Reprinted with permission from American Academy of Pediatrics Subcommittee on Hyperbilirubinemia: Maisels MJ, Baltz RD, Bhutani VK, Newman TB, Palmer H, Rosenfeld W, et al. Clinical practice guideline: management of hyperbilirubinemia in the newborn infant ≥35 weeks of gestation. *Pediatrics.* 2004;114:297–316.)

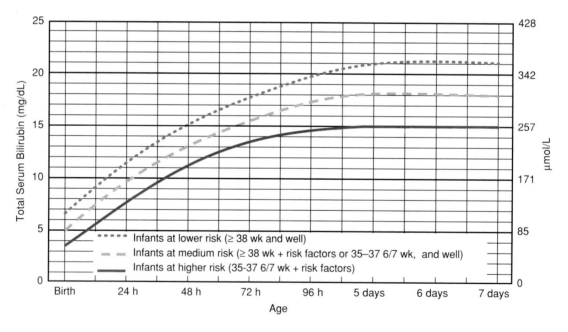

- Use total bilirubin. Do not subtract direct reacting or conjugated bilirubin.
- Risk factors = isoimmune hemolytic disease, G6PD deficiency, asphyxia, significant lethargy, temperature instability, sepsis, acidosis, or albumin < 3.0 g/dL (if measured).
- For well infants 35–37 6/7 wk can adjust TSB levels for intervention around the medium risk line. It is an option to intervene at lower TSB levels for infants closer to 35 wks and at higher TSB levels for those closer to 37 6/7 wk.
- It is an option to provide conventional phototherapy in hospital or at home at TSB levels 2–3 mg/dL (35-50 mmol/L) below those shown but home phototherapy should not be used in any infant with risk factors.

Figure 12–3. Guidelines for phototherapy in hospitalized infants older than 35-weeks gestational age. (Reprinted with permission from American Academy of Pediatrics Subcommittee on Hyperbilirubinemia: Maisels MJ, Baltz RD, Bhutani VK, Newman TB, Palmer H, Rosenfeld W, et al. Clinical practice guideline: management of hyperbilirubinemia in the newborn infant ≥35 weeks of gestation. *Pediatrics.* 2004;114:297–316.)

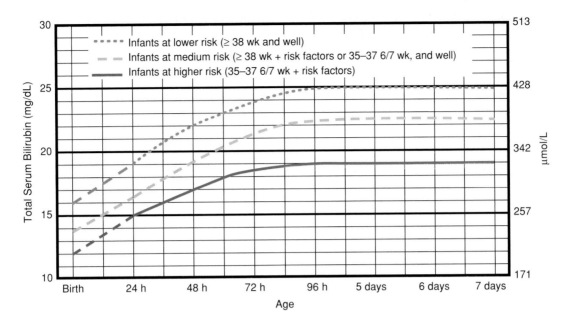

- The dashed lines for the first 24 hours indicate uncertainty due to a wide range of clinical circumstances and a range of responses to phototherapy.
- Immediate exchange transfusion is recommended if infant shows signs of acute bilirubin encephalopathy (hypertonia, arching, retrocollis, opisthotonos, fever, high pitched cry) or if TSB is ≥5 mg/dL (85 μmol/L) above these lines.
- Risk factors—isoimmune hemolytic disease, G6PD deficiency, asphyxia, significant lethargy, temperature instability, sepsis, acidosis.
- Measure serum albumin and calculate B/A ratio (see legend).
- Use total bilirubin. Do not subtract direct reacting or conjugated bilirubin.
- If infant is well and 35–37 6/7 wk (median risk) can individualize TSB levels for exchange based on actual gestational age.

Figure 12–4. Guidelines for exchange transfusion in hospitalized infants older than 35-weeks gestational age. (Reprinted with permission from American Academy of Pediatrics Subcommittee on Hyperbilirubinemia: Maisels MJ, Baltz RD, Bhutani VK, Newman TB, Palmer H, Rosenfeld W, et al. Clinical practice guideline: management of hyperbilirubinemia in the newborn infant ≥35 weeks of gestation. *Pediatrics.* 2004;114:297–316.)

with type II presenting later in childhood and amenable to treatment with phenobarbital.

Evaluation and Management

Hemolysis and Gilbert's syndrome are the most common cause of jaundice beyond the neonatal period. It is important to look for risk factors for jaundice such as family history, certain ethnic backgrounds such as African American (sickle cell disease and G6PD) and Mediterranean (G6PD), and drug ingestions.

History and Physical

Important considerations are general appearance, hepatomegaly, splenomegaly, or other signs of hemolysis.

Laboratory Evaluation

Workup begins with the serum bilirubin level. The workup for hemolytic anemia includes a complete blood cell and reticulocyte count and a serum haptoglobin level. If anemia is present, then a peripheral smear looking for abnormal cell morphology is also warranted. These include sickle cells, spherocytes, ellip-

tocytes, fragmented cells, and nucleated red cells. Additional testing includes Coombs test, G6PD level, and hemoglobin electrophoresis.

Management Approach

Besides serum bilirubin, CBC is the next most important test to aid in ascertaining the etiology of the jaundice and make management decisions. If anemia is present then, hemolytic causes should be considered. When the hematocrit is normal, liver function tests will differentiate hepatic disease from bilirubin metabolic disorders such as Gilbert's syndrome.

Etiology-specific treatment is the mainstay of therapy in this age group.

▶ CONJUGATED HYPERBILIRUBINEMIA

NEWBORN

Conjugated hyperbilirubinemia is present when the conjugated fraction of bilirubin exceeds 20% of the total bilirubin or is greater than 2 mg/dL. It is far less common in newborns and young infants than is unconjugated hyperbilirubinemia. It most commonly occurs secondary to intrahepatic cellular damage; less often it is because of obstruction of biliary flow. Conjugated hyperbilirubinemia is always pathologic. Most infants with conjugated hyperbilirubinemia will present within the first month of life.

Differential Diagnosis
Infectious Causes
Neonatal cholestasis can occur secondary to hepatic injury from a multitude of infectious causes. Cytomegalovirus, rubella, herpes simplex, varicella, coxsackie, and hepatitis B are common viral etiologies. Syphilis and toxoplasmosis are also implicated. Most of these diseases are present in utero, and are often associated with congenital anomalies and hepatosplenomegaly.

Bacterial sepsis can result in conjugated hyperbilirubinemia, although the unconjugated fraction is also usually increased. The urinary tract is a common site of infection and can involve gram-negative organisms such as *Escherichia coli*. Jaundice often starts at 3 to 4 days of age and, in some instances, is the only manifestation of infection.[1]

Metabolic Causes
Metabolic disorders that can cause conjugated hyperbilirubinemia include α_1-antitrypsin deficiency, cystic fibrosis, and galactosemia. Most metabolic disorders will have clinical manifestations other than jaundice that will lead to the diagnosis. Another hepatocellular cause of neonatal cholestasis is idiopathic neonatal hepatitis, which is characterized by prolonged jaundice and typical liver biopsy findings of "giant" hepatocytes. Alagille syndrome is an autosomal dominant syndromic paucity of the bile ducts, or arteriohepatic dysplasia, which presents with cholestatic jaundice in the first 3 postnatal months.[4,5]

Extrahepatic Diseases
The major extrahepatic cause of conjugated hyperbilirubinemia in infancy is biliary atresia—a syndrome characterized by absence of the bile ducts anywhere between the duodenum and hepatic ducts. Patients present with jaundice, dark urine, and often with acholic stools. Mild hepatomegaly may be present. The evaluation of patients with suspected biliary atresia usually includes a liver biopsy, which may help to exclude neonatal hepatitis. Depending on the location of the lesion in the biliary tree, the Kasai procedure, involving surgical anastamosis of the remaining bile ducts to the bowel, may be palliative. A major complication of the Kasai procedure is ascending cholangitis.

Another cause of extrahepatic biliary obstruction is choledochal cyst—a congenital saccular dilatation of the common bile duct. It can present with jaundice and a right upper quadrant mass or with symptoms of cholangitis, including fever and leukocytosis. A right upper quadrant ultrasound may facilitate the diagnosis.

Most patients with conjugated hyperbilirubinemia require referral to a pediatric gastroenterologist for definitive evaluation.[4,5]

OLDER CHILDREN
Differential Diagnosis
Conjugated hyperbilirubinemia in older children most commonly results from infectious hepatitis. Hepatitis A virus infection is the most common cause of acute jaundice in young children. Infants are typically asymptomatic, while older children exhibit a prodrome of fever and malaise followed by abdominal pain, nausea, vomiting, and jaundice with elevated hepatic enzymes. Hepatitis B virus infections typically have a more protracted course, with older children being jaundiced in the acute phase and typically asymptomatic in the chronic carrier stage. Epstein–Barr virus is another cause of jaundice in older children as part of the infectious mononucleosis syndrome.

Drug-induced liver injury is also fairly common. Acetaminophen overdose is one of the leading causes of fulminant hepatic failure in adolescents and young adults. Less commonly, genetic or metabolic disorders can present with jaundice and conjugated hyperbilirubinemia. Relatively common metabolic defects include α_1-antitrypsin deficiency and Wilson disease. Wilson disease is an autosomal recessive disorder of copper metabolism resulting in excess accumulation of copper in the liver, CNS, kidney, cornea, and heart. The liver involvement ranges from acute hepatitis with jaundice to fulminant liver failure with encephalopathy. Although α_1-antitrypsin deficiency commonly presents as neonatal cholestasis, new-onset jaundice can occur any age. It is the most common genetic cause of acute and chronic liver disease in children and the most common genetic disorder requiring liver transplantation in children. In addition, hepatobiliary disease is now assuming a greater role in older children with cystic fibrosis. Extrahepatic biliary tract disorders may present in older children with obstructive jaundice. Autoimmune hepatitis is a chronic progressive inflammatory disorder of possible autoimmune etiology. Type 1 disease affects adolescent females, causing abdominal pain, malaise, and jaundice. Type 2 causes a rapidly progressive illness in younger infants.

EVALUATION AND MANAGEMENT
Jaundice beyond the neonatal period is usually pathologic and requires investigation. Once a distinction is made between conjugated versus unconjugated hyperbilirubinemia, cholestatic versus noncholestatic causes should be explored. Historic clues are an important diagnostic tool, especially when features of specific disorders or a family history of jaundice are present. A review of medications and inquiring about risk factors for viral hepatitis are important. Physical examination should focus on signs that distinguish chronic from acute liver involvement. Important laboratory evaluations to consider are outlined in Table 12–1, but should be tailored to the individual child. A strong consideration should be given to an abdominal ultrasound in any child who presents with conjugated hyperbilirubinemia. Liver biopsy may ultimately lead to the definitive diagnosis. Treatment is directed to the specific underlying cause along with attention to nutrition and hydration. Most patients with conjugated hyperbilirubinemia require referral to a pediatric gastroenterologist for definitive evaluation[9] (Table 12–1).

► TABLE 12–1. **LABORATORY EVALUATION OF HYPERBILIRUBINEMIA IN OLDER CHILDREN**

Unconjugated Hyperbilirubinemia
   Complate blood count
   Reticulocyte count
   Blood smear
   Serum haptoglobins
   Direct and indirect Coombs test
   Hemoglobin electrophoresis
   Red cell enzyme assay
   Test for spherocytosis

Conjugated Hyperbilirubinemia
   Liver function test (AST, ALT, ALP, and GGT)
   Synthetic liver function (prothrombin time, total
      protein, albumin, glucose, cholesterol, ammonia)
   Abdominal ultrasonography
   HAV IgM, HBsAg, IgM-anti-HB score, anti-HCV,
      moniscopt/EBV titers
   Serum ceruloplasmin, 24-hour urinary copper
      excretion
   Serum IgG, autoantibodies (ANA, ASMA,
      anti-liver-kidney-microsomal antibody)
   Serum α_1-antitrypsin level and phenotype
   Liver biopsy

REFERENCES

1. Coletti JE, Kothari S, Jackson DM, Kilgore KP, Barringer K. An Emergency medicine approach to neonatal hyperbilirubinemia. *Emerg Med Clin N Amer.* 2007;25:1117.
2. Maisels MJ. Neonatal jaundice. *Pediatr Rev.* 2006;27(12):443.
3. Dennery PA, Seidman DS, Stevenson DK. Neonatal hyperbilirubinemia. *N Engl J Med.* 2001;344:581.
4. Wong RJ, DeSandre GH, Sibley E, Stevenson DK. Neonatal jaundice and liver disease. In: Martin RJ, Fanaroff AA, Walsh MC, eds. *Fanaroff and Martin's Neonatal-Perinatal Medicine: Diseases of the Fetus and Infant.* Philadelphia, PA: Mosby Elsevier; 2006:1419–1465.
5. Maisels MJ. Jaundice. In: MacDonald MG, Seshia MMK, Mullett MD, eds. *Avery's Neonatology: Pathophysiology and Management of the Newborn.* Philadelphia, PA: Lippincott Co; 2005:768–846.
6. Maisels MJ, Baltz RD, Bhutani VK, et al. Clinical practice guideline: management of hyperbilirubinemia in the newborn infant 35 or more weeks of gestation. *Pediatrics.* 2004;114:297.
7. Bhutani VK, Maisels MJ, Stark AR, et al. Management of jaundice and prevention of severe neonatal hyperbilirubinemia in infants >35 weeks of gestation. *Neonatology.* 2008;94;63.
8. Maisels MJ, McDonagh AF. Phototherapy for neonatal jaundice. *NEJM.* 2008;358;920.
9. Harb R, Thomas DW. Conjugated hyperbilirubinemia: screening and treatment in older infants and children. *Pediatr Rev.* 2007;28(3):83–91.

CHAPTER 13

The Crying Infant

Joan M. Mavrinac

▶ HIGH-YIELD FACTS

- The infant cry may signal hunger, an unmet need for attention, or a diaper change, or crying may signal distress or pain.
- An infant not interacting with the parents appropriately is toxic and has a serious reason for his or her crying. Note the pitch of the cry, as this is important and will help the clinician decide the direction of the assessment.
- It is important to observe the infant for at least 1 to 2 hours if one has not identified the cause. If after this period of observation, the crying abates, the infant may be sent home with close follow-up with the primary care physician. If the crying persists, the clinician should proceed with a more complete workup and have the infant admitted for observation.

▶ OVERVIEW

The assessment of the acutely crying infant in the emergency department (ED) is difficult because the infant can be disruptive as the parents are usually overwhelmed, and the crying is distractive to the ED staff. Given these challenges, the clinician must resist the urge to rush through the history and physical examination. Instead, the clinician must be deliberate in their search for the cause, since the clues to the diagnosis may be subtle. The clinician should perform serial observations and examinations until the cause is found or infants return to their normal baseline behavior. Fortunately, with a thorough history, a meticulous physical examination, limited diagnostic tests, and a period of observation in the ED, most of the diagnoses of the crying, irritable infant are identified.[1]

▶ NORMAL CRYING PATTERNS IN INFANCY AND COLIC DEFINED

To unravel the cause of acute, unexplained crying, it is important to know what normal infant crying encompasses and the definition of colic. Crying is part of normal psychomotor and psychosocial development and is the infant's source of communication. The infant cry may signal hunger, an unmet need for attention, or a diaper change, or crying may signal distress or pain.

The normal crying pattern in the first year of life has been described.[2] There is a progressive increase in crying, which peaks in the second month of life and then gradually decreases.[2,3] The peak crying time may be as much as 2 to 3 hours per day at 6 weeks of life.[4] When the infant has other ways to communicate, such as interacting with a social smile, the daily crying time decreases. Infant crying time has been reported to usually decrease to 1 hour a day by 14 weeks of age (3.5 months).[5]

Colic is a chronic crying syndrome in the first 3 months of life. Colic has been described as unexplained, paroxysmal crying in healthy, well-fed infants with normal weight gain. Colic starts around 3 weeks of age and continues till the infant is 3 months old. A typical colic episode is when infants suddenly flex their legs, their face turns red, and the parents report that the infant expels a lot of flatus. These episodes last for more than 3 hours per day on more than 3 days per week and usually take place in the early evening hours.[6] There are many theories regarding colic but the etiology remains undetermined.[4] Colic is a diagnosis of exclusion.

▶ APPROACH TO THE CRYING, IRRITABLE INFANT

Crying may also be a symptom of an underlying medical problem. The parents usually bring the infant to the ED because of the intensity and/or the duration of the crying and concern that their infant may be in pain. The clinician must differentiate between the benign and serious causes of crying. It is critical not to miss the serious causes because these may lead to untoward morbidity or death. Although the differential diagnosis is broad, a conservative, organized approach with a thorough history and examination will narrow the differential in the majority of cases.[1]

▶ HISTORY

As Sir William Osler reminds us, "Listen to the patient, he is telling you the diagnosis."[7]

Listen attentively to the history from the parents, since the clues to the diagnosis often lie in the history.[1] What elements should the history include? Crying should be investigated as a symptom. Questions should be directed to diagnose the symptoms: (1) When did it *start*? What time of day? How long? (2) What seems to *provoke* the crying? Was there any trauma? (3) What *alleviates* the crying? (4) What is the *quality* of the cry? Is it high-pitched or weak? (5) Are there any *related* symptoms such as fever, vomiting, diarrhea, constipation, cough, and nasal congestion? Any exposure to illness? (6) What is the *duration* of the crying? Is there a recurrent pattern?

Past medical history should include (1) *perinatal and birth history:* Is there any maternal history of herpes or recent cytomegalovirus (CMV) infection or of premature rupture of membranes? What is the mother's group B strep immunization status? Any history of maternal medication or drug abuse? If the infant is breast-feeding, maternal medication or drug intake is important. Were there any neonatal problems? (2) *Immunization history:* Has the infant had any immunizations? (3) *Growth and development:* Has there been normal weight gain? Has the infant reached the appropriate developmental milestones? (See Chapter 1.)

REVIEW OF SYSTEMS

Ask about the *activity* of the infant: if there was any *fever*, their *intake*, and *output*. How has the infant been acting other than this crying episode? Questions related to the infant's intake refer to the feeding history, medication history, and possible toxin ingestion. Questions related to the infant's output include the following: Is there any vomiting, diarrhea, constipation, hematochezia, or change in urination? Has the infant interacted normally with the parents prior to this episode of crying?

WHAT IS THE RELATIONSHIP OF CRYING TO FEEDING?

If the crying is only with feeding, consider oral pharyngeal pathology such as gingivostomatitis, herpangina, or even an oral burn. If the crying is only with a bowel movement, consider an anal fissure. If during feeding or after feeding infants arch their neck and upper back, consider gastroesophageal reflux. Also consider gastroesophageal reflux if there is any

Approach to the crying irritable infant

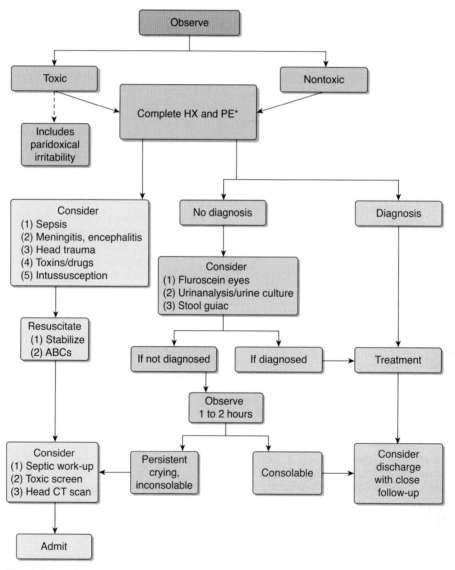

*If toxic infant obtain stool guiac during PE (physical examination)

Figure 13–1. Crying infant algorithm.

history of overfeeding. Milk allergy may present with vomiting and possibly stools with blood or mucous. If there is any blood in the stool also consider infectious enteritis.

▶ PHYSICAL EXAMINATION

"The whole art of medicine is in observation...but to educate the eye to see, the ear to hear and the finger to feel takes time, and to make a beginning, to start a man on the right path, is all that we can do."[8]

OBSERVATION

The clinician should observe the infant with attention to the infant's color, quality of respirations (specifically noting any retractions), the infant's attentiveness, and the infant–parent interaction. An infant not interacting with the parents appropriately is toxic and has a serious reason for their crying. Note the pitch of the cry, as this is important and will help the clinician decide the direction of the assessment. An infant with a high-pitched cry should be considered toxic until proven otherwise. If the infant is toxic appearing, the history, physical examination, and resuscitation will be occurring simultaneously (Fig. 13–1).

Initially, most of the physical examination of an infant can be done by observation with the infant in the parent's arms. The clinician should leave invasive examinations until last (otoscopy, fundoscopy, genital examination, and rectal examination). Completely undress the infant including the diaper. Lay infants on their back on the examination table to assess movement of the extremities (asymmetry of movement may be the clue to a fracture) and for an adequate abdominal and genital examination. Inspect the genital urinary area; look for symmetric testicles (testicular torsions) and abnormal masses (hernias) (Fig. 13–2).

Inspect the infant's complete skin surface. Hair tourniquets hide under clothing as can signs of child abuse (unusual bruising pattern) (Table 13–1; Fig. 13–3). In the retrospective review of infants who presented to the ED with excessive,

▶ **TABLE 13-1. PHYSICAL EXAMINATION TIPS**

Observe first, note the quality of the cry
Completely undress the infant (look under diaper)
Invasive examinations last (oral pharynx, otoscopy, fundoscopy, genital, and rectal examination)

prolonged crying, without fever and without a cause that was apparent to the parents, the physical examination revealed the diagnosis in a significant percentage of the cases.[1]

CLUES TO THE DIAGNOSIS IN THE PHYSICAL EXAMINATION

Vital Signs

Temperature: temperature instability, fever, or hypothermia may represent sepsis. Check the *pulse*: tachycardia or bradycardia may also signal sepsis, dehydration, or anemia. When observing *respirations*, note the rate, quality, and look for intercostals retractions. Capillary refill is used to assess hydration and perfusion status. *Pulse oximetry* may identify hypoxia and is useful if there are signs of any respiratory distress. *Weight* is an important "vital sign" in an infant. Normal weight gain is usually the sign of a healthy infant. Any acute illness in infancy, especially during the neonatal period, the first month of life, is likely to cause the infant to stop gaining weight.

Head

Look for signs of head trauma? If the anterior fontanelle is bulging, consider causes of increased intracranial pressure including meningitis, encephalitis, intracranial masses, or bleeding. If anterior fontanelle is depressed, consider dehydration.

Eyes

Consider corneal abrasion or a foreign body under lid (e.g., eyelash). Infants are more likely to open their eyes in a darkened room, which may help with the fundoscopic examination for retinal hemorrhages (Fig. 13–4).

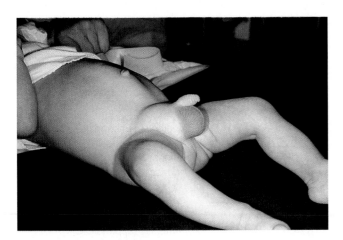

Figure 13–2. Inguinal Hernia. (Courtesy of Michael P. Hirsh, MD, FACS, FAAP, University of Massachusetts Memorial Children's Medical Center.)

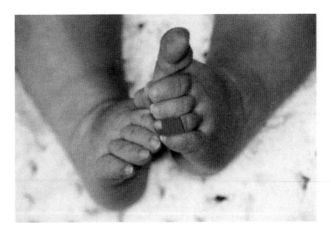

Figure 13–3. Hair tourniquet. (Courtesy of Roger Knapp, MD.)

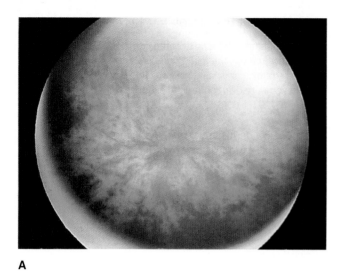
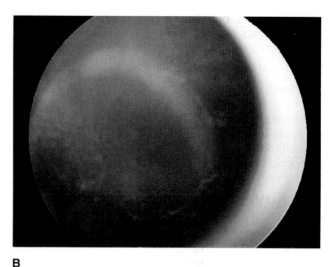

A   **B**

Figure 13–4. Retinal hemorrhages. (Courtesy of Joseph Paviglianiti, MD, Pittsburgh, PA.)

Nose

Obstruction secondary to upper respiratory tract infection (most infants are obligate nose breathers).

Cardiovascular

Evaluate pulse for supraventricular tachycardia (SVT).

Abdominal

Consider intussusception, peritoneal irritation, and constipation.

Genital–Urinary

Differential diagnoses include urinary tract infection, incarcerated hernias, testicular torsion, and hair tourniquets (penis or clitoral).

Musculoskeletal

Fractures (accidental, nonaccidental, and rare causes such as osteogenesis imperfecta). Consider child abuse if the injury pattern is not congruent with the history.[9] By becoming familiar with a few key developmental milestones in infants, it will be easier to recognize nonaccidental trauma. A fracture in a nonambulatory infant should raise suspicion of nonaccidental trauma. The infants with septic arthritis and osteomyelitis will be irritable when the involved extremity is moved.

Skin

Look for hair tourniquets, bruises (consider child abuse), and skin rashes (if petechial, consider meningococcemia).

Neurological

Paradoxical irritability is a dangerous sign. This occurs when the infant cries with holding and is calm when not touched. Consider meningeal irritation, such as meningitis and intracra-

nial bleeding. Paradoxical irritability may also herald peritoneal irritation, for example, early appendicitis.

Irritability may also be the sign of an electrolyte disturbance. Consider hyponatremia, hypernatremia, hypocalcemia, hypercalcemia, and hypoglycemia. Medication reactions from pseudephedrine (now off market for infants younger than 2 years) and antihistamines may present as irritability in the infant.[10]

Psychiatric

Child abuse must always be excluded. Colic, parental anxiety, overstimulation, and sensory integration problems (autism spectrum) are diagnoses of exclusion.

▶ TOXIC VERSUS NONTOXIC INFANT

In the **toxic** infant, the history and physical examination will be taking place simultaneously with the resuscitation. As always, start with the ABCs: airway, breathing, and circulation. The differential diagnosis includes severe infectious causes such

▶ **TABLE 13-2. CAUSES OF ACUTE CRYING IN TOXIC INFANTS**

Infectious	Sepsis
	Meningitis, Encephalitis
Trauma	Head trauma: accidental and nonaccidental
	Nonaccidental: Shaken Baby, subdural hematoma
Ingestions/poisonings	Toxins, drugs, medications
Abdominal process	Intussusception (late)
	Peritonitis (appendicitis)
*Paradoxical fussiness	Infant does not want to be held: consider meningeal irritation, peritoneal irritation, fractures

▶ TABLE 13-3. CAUSES OF ACUTE CRYING IN NONTOXIC INFANTS

HEENT	Otitis media, corneal abrasion, foreign body eye (e.g., eyelash)
Respiratory	Carbon monoxide poisoning
Cardiac	Supraventricular Tachycardia (SVT)
Gastrointestinal	Intussusception (early), GERD, milk allergy, constipation
Genitourinary	Urinary tract infection (UTI), incarcerated hernia, testicular torsion
Musculoskeletal	Fracture(s): accidental, nonaccidental, unusual causes (e.g., osteogenesis imperfecta)
Skin	Hair tourniquet (digit, penis, clitoris), burns
Other	Electrolyte disturbance: hypernatremia, hyponatremia, hypocalcemia, hypercalcemia,
	Immunization reaction
	Diagnoses of Exclusion
	Colic
	Parental anxiety
	Overstimulation
	Sensory integration problems (autism)

as sepsis,[11] meningitis, encephalitis, trauma which includes subdural hematomas from nonaccidental trauma (shaken infant syndrome)[12] as well as intracranial bleeding from accidental trauma, ingestions and poisonings, and intra-abdominal processes such as the advanced stage of intussusception or early appendicitis (Table 13–2).

In the **nontoxic** infant, the differential diagnosis is broad (Table 13–3). If a detailed history and meticulous physical examination do not offer an explanation, two additional procedures and two laboratory screening tests should be considered. First, consider fluroscein staining of the corneas to rule out corneal abrasion. If this is the cause of the crying, application of topical ophthalmic anesthetic alone will stop the crying. The second procedure is a stool guiac. In an infant, this is best obtained from stool sample on the rectal thermometer or a stool sample from the diaper. If positive, this may reflect milk protein allergy, anal fissure, or infectious enterocolitis. For screening tests, the urinalysis and urine culture should be obtained since occult urinary tract infections presenting without fever can occur.[1,13]

If a diagnosis has still not been obtained, it is necessary to observe the infant in the ED for at least 1 to 2 hours. During this period of observation, redirecting the history as well as repeating the physical examination may be helpful in elu-

cidating the diagnosis. If after this period of observation, the crying abates, the infant may be sent home with close follow-up with the primary care physician. Contact the primary care physician who will be doing the follow-up. On the other hand, if after this period of observation the crying persists in the nontoxic infant, the clinician should proceed with a more complete workup (consider obtaining a septic workup, toxin screen, and a head CT scan) and then have the infant admitted for observation.

▶ ACKNOWLEDGMENTS

The author wishes to thank Drs. Ingrid Henar, Michael P. Hirsh, Roger Knapp, Grace Nejman, Thomas P. Martin, Joseph Paviglianiti, Grace Walters and Ms. Elizabeth Meade.

REFERENCES

1. Poole SR. The infant with acute, unexplained, excessive crying. *Pediatrics.* 1991;88:450–455.
2. Barr RG. The normal crying curve: what do we really know? *Develop Med Child Neuro.* 1990;32:356–362.
3. Baildam EM, Hillier VF, Ward BS, et al. Duration and pattern of crying in the first year of life. *Develop Med Child Neuro.* 1995;37:345–353.
4. Barr RG. Changing our understanding of infant colic. *Arch Pediatr Adolesc Med.* 2002;156:1171–1174.
5. Mortimer EA. Drug toxicity from breast milk. *Pediatrics.* 1977;60:780–781.
6. Wessel MA, Cobb JC, Jackson EB, et al. Paroxysmal Fussing in Infancy, Sometimes called "Colic." *Pediatrics.* 1954;14:421–434.
7. Sakula A. *The Portraiture of Sir William Osler.* London; New York: Royal Society of Medicine; 1991:79–81.
8. Silverman ME, Murray TJ, Bryan CS, eds. *The Quotable Osler.* American College of Physicians-American Society of Internal Medicine; 2003 No. 277,281.
9. Pierce MC, Bertocci G. Fractures resulting from inflicted trauma: assessing injury and history compatibility. *Clin Pediatr Emerg Med.* 2006;7:143–148.
10. Mechcatie E. Interim ban expected on OTC cold products for tots. *Pediatr News.* November 2007.
11. Ruiz-Contreras J, Urquia L, Bastero R. Persistent crying as predominant manifestation of sepsis in infants and newborns. *Pediatr Emerg Care.* 1999;15:113–115.
12. Caffey J. The whiplash shaken infant syndrome: manual shaking by the extremities with whiplash-induced intracranial and intraocular bleedings, linked with residual permanent brain damage and mental retardation. *Pediatrics.* 1974;54:396–403.
13. Du JNH. Colic as the sole symptom of urinary tract infection in infants. *Can Med Assoc J.* 1976;115:334–337.

CHAPTER 14

Limping Child

Isabel A. Barata

▶ HIGH-YIELD FACTS

- A delay in diagnosis may be devastating in certain cases that cause a limp such as septic joint, bone tumors, and leukemia, as well as in the case of child abuse.
- Rule out bone tumors and leukemia as possible causes of a limp.
- Consider hip pathology in children presenting with knee or thigh pain.
- A septic hip causes increased intra-articular pressure and will compromise the blood supply to the femoral head, possibly resulting in avascular necrosis unless surgical decompression is performed emergently.

A limp is a common reason for a child to visit the emergency department and it has several serious causes.[1] The most common form of limp is an antalgic gait caused by pain. Gait reflects the coordinated action of the lower extremities. The body moves forward smoothly with economy of motion and energy. The stance phase (60% of the entire gait cycle) is the weight-bearing portion.[2] It is initiated by heel contact and ends with toe lift-off from the same foot. Swing phase is initiated with toe off and ends with heel strike. Limb advancement occurs during the swing phase (40% of normal gait cycle). During this phase, the foot pronates first and then supinates. Pronation shortens the foot, which helps it to clear the ground. Pronation also minimizes the energy expenditure necessary for ground clearance as the non-weight-bearing limb passes the weight-bearing limb.[2] Supination stabilizes the bony architecture of the foot thus preparing it for heel strike, when the foot must absorb the shock of striking the ground. In an antalgic gait, the gait is uneven because to minimize weight bearing on an injured limb, the time in stance phase is shortened in the painful limb with a resultant increase in swing phase.

The incidence of limp has been found to be 1.8 per thousand. The male-to-female ratio is 1.7:1 and the median age 4.35 years. Limp is mainly right-sided (54%) and painful (80%); 33.7% of the children have localized pain in the hip. A preceding illness has been found in 40%.[3]

An acute limp implies an underlying pathology that causes disruption of the standard gait pattern. The clinician must consider the spine, pelvis, and lower extremities for a possible etiology. A useful approach is to consider the causes of limping from head to foot to avoid overlooking common underlying conditions such as diskitis, psoas abscess, or septic hip, which are less obvious than conditions involving the lower extremities. In considering the differential diagnosis of an acutely limping child, the clinician should first consider broader categories of etiologies, such as traumatic, infectious, neoplastic, inflammatory, congenital, neuromuscular, or developmental causes (Table 14–1). You can further narrow the diagnosis by taking into account the age of the patient because certain diseases are more common in a given age group (Table 14–2).

▶ HISTORY

Question the child or caretaker about the onset and duration of the limp and the association of the limp with pain (Table 14–3).[4] Painless limp is likely to be the result of mechanical or neuromuscular disorders and seldom presents acutely. Acute onset of pain is more likely to be infectious, traumatic, or neoplastic in etiology. Younger children may not be able to verbalize the location of discomfort. A history of the way the child prefers to walk or crawl may be helpful. Usually, the older patient can localize a painful joint or focal area of pain, which is helpful in narrowing the differential diagnosis; however, consider referred pain patterns such as hip pathology causing knee pain.

A history of limp that appears worse in the morning suggests a rheumatologic process. Night pain, especially pain that wakes a child from sleep, is a worrisome indicator of a malignant process and warrants a rapid diagnostic approach.

Complete a review of systems to obtain any history of recent fever or other infections. A recent upper respiratory infection could be the instigating event to a septic process or raise the possibility of poststreptococcal reactive arthritis.[5]

Fever suggests an infection or an inflammatory condition. Also, weight loss or malaise suggests a systemic process. Abdominal pain, diarrhea, or urinary symptoms may suggest nonorthopedic etiologies such as appendicitis, psoas abscess, orchitis, or testicular torsion. Immunization history is important since Hemophilus influenza type B may cause both septic arthritis and osteomyelitis.[6] Also include in your history if the patient lives in an area endemic for Lyme disease or travels to such areas.[7]

Past medical history may be helpful since the history of endocrine problems such as hypothyroidism or delayed sexual development may be associated with slipped femoral capital epiphysis. A family history should also be obtained for rheumatologic or muscular diseases that may be inherited.

▶ PHYSICAL EXAMINATION

Vital signs, in particular the child's temperature, may help identify an infectious process. Among a series of 95 children with

▶ **TABLE 14–1. DIFFERENTIAL DIAGNOSIS OF AN ACUTELY LIMPING CHILD**

Trauma
 Fracture
 Stress fracture
 Upper femur, Salter–Harris type I fracture
 Upper femur impaction fracture
 Toddler's fracture (type I, minimally displaced spiral
  fracture of the tibia)
 Upper tibial fracture (type II, hyperextension-induced)
 Distal tibia and fibula buckle fractures
 "Bunk-bed foot" (type I, fracture, impaction-buckle fracture
  of the base of the first metatarsal)
 "Bunk-bed foot" (type II, fracture a compression fracture of
  the cuboid bone)
 Ankle fractures
 Plastic bending fractures of the fibula
 Soft-tissue contusion

Infection
 Cellulitis
 Osteomyelitis
 Septic arthritis
 Lyme disease
 Tuberculosis of bone
 Gonorrhea
 Postinfectious reactive arthritis

Tumor
 Spinal cord tumors
 Tumors of bone
 Benign: osteoid osteoma, osteoblastoma
 Malignant: osteosarcoma, Ewing's sarcoma
 Lymphoma
 Leukemia

Inflammatory
 Juvenile rheumatoid arthritis
 Transient synovitis
 Systemic lupus erythematosus

Congenital
 Developmental dysplasia of the hip
 Sickle cell
 Congenitally short femur
 Clubfoot

Developmental
 Legg-Calvé-Perthes disease
 Slipped capital femoral epiphysis
 Tarsal coalitions
 Osteochondritis dissecans (knee, talus)

Neurologic
 Cerebral palsy, especial mild hemiparesis
 Hereditary sensory motor neuropathies
 Physical evaluation

▶ **TABLE 14–2. DIFFERENTIAL DIAGNOSIS OF AN ACUTELY LIMPING CHILD BY AGE**

All ages
 Septic arthritis
 Osteomyelitis
 Cellulitis
 Stress fracture
 Neoplasm (including leukemia)
 Neuromuscular

Toddler (age 1–3)
 Septic hip
 Developmental dysplasia of the hip
 Occult fractures
 Leg-length discrepancy

Child (age 4–10)
 Legg-Calvé-Perthes disease
 Transient synovitis
 Juvenile rheumatoid arthritis

Adolescent (age 11–16)
 Slipped capital femoral epiphysis
 Avascular necrosis of femoral head
 Overuse syndromes
 Tarsal coalitions
 Gonococcal septic arthritis

toe, including examination of the abdomen and genitalia. Examine the feet looking for ingrown toenails and any evidence of puncture wounds. Observe the child's gait. In an antalgic gait, the child has asymmetrical cadence due to less time spent in the stance phase of the affected leg. A child who walks stiffly may be attempting to reduce pain in the spine, such as that occurring in diskitis. In addition, a child who walks with a Trendelburg gait, the torso shifts over the pathologic limb, may be an indication of hip inflammation or hip muscle weakness, such as Perthes' disease and transient synovitis.[9] Perform a focused neurologic examination by observing the child walking on the toes, walking on the heels, and hopping on one foot.

▶ **TABLE 14–3. HISTORY**

What is the duration and progression of limp?
Is there any recent trauma and mechanism of injury?
 (Beware of the limitations of pediatric history and
 possibility of unintentional trauma, such as child abuse.)
Associated pain and its characteristics?
Accompanying weakness?
Time of day when limp is worse?
Does the child have pain at night?
Can the child walk or bear weight?
Has the limp interfered with normal activities?
Are systemic symptoms such as fever, weight loss, and
 malaise present?
Do not forget the medical history, birth history, immunization
 history, nutritional history, and developmental history.
Also include the other essentials—drug history and allergies
 and family history.

septic arthritis, most had a low-grade fever but one-third were afebrile at presentation[8]; therefore the absence of fever should not sway the physician from the diagnosis. The generalized demeanor of the child, for example, a child with septic arthritis, may be quiet. Complete a thorough examination from head to

Also check the feet for clawing of the toes or cavus foot deformity, which are red flags for an underlying neurologic condition, especially if either condition is unilateral. The patient should be tested for deep tendon reflexes and clonus.

A careful musculoskeletal examination needs to be done with evaluation of the spine, sacroiliac joint, hip, knee, ankle, and foot. All joints should be taken through their full range of motion passively and actively and be palpated for tenderness and warmth. Loss of range of motion will help localize the site of pathology.

SPINE

Check the spine on flexion to identify an asymmetric turning of the spine, a sign of spinal cord pathology. With diskitis, there is limited spinal flexion accompanied by a stiff posture and local tenderness. Adolescents with spondylosis or spondylolisthesis experience an exacerbation of lumbosacral pain with spinal extension, so check the spine on extension as well by having the patient bend backward.

SACROILIAC JOINTS

Next evaluate the sacroiliac joints, which may be involved in infectious or inflammatory conditions such as juvenile ankylosing spondylitis. On physical examination, the flexion, abduction, and external rotation (FABER) test consisting of hip flexion, abduction, and external rotation if it causes groin pain indicates a hip problem rather than a spinal. However, when the physician presses firmly on the flexed knee and on the opposite anterosuperior iliac crest, pain in the sacroiliac area indicates a problem with sacroiliac joints (Fig. 14–1).

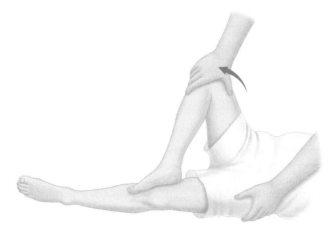

Figure 14–1. The flexion, abduction, and external rotation (FABER) test to detect hip problems. The test is performed by having the patient lie in a supine position and placing the foot of the affected side on the opposite knee; groin pain indicates a hip problem rather than a spinal problem. The physician then presses firmly on the flexed knee and on the opposite anterosuperior iliac crest; pain in the sacroiliac area indicates a problem with sacroiliac joints.

HIP JOINTS

Examination of the hip may be the most important part of the physical examination if the site of pathology cannot be easily identified since hip pathology often results in vague pain and many hip conditions require emergent treatment. While infection of other joints such as the knee or ankle may be readily apparent from swelling, tenderness, warmth, and erythema, the hip joint is not as easily visualized and the clinician must rely on indirect assessment on physical examination through range of motion.

To diagnose slipped capital femoral epiphysis, the examiner will observe obligate external rotation of the involved lower extremity when the hip is flexed. These rotational changes can occur when the radiographic findings are still quite minimal. Prompt referral for operative management is warranted.

Inflammatory conditions of the hip as well as developmental dysplasia of the hip present with asymmetry in hip abduction. Hip abduction is tested with the hips flexed and extended making certain the pelvis remains level. The Galeazzi test (Fig. 14–2) is performed by putting the child in a supine position and bringing the ankles to the buttocks with the hips and knees flexed. The test is positive when the knees are at different heights, suggesting developmental dysplasia or a leg-length discrepancy. In addition, measurement of thigh and calf circumference is important since atrophy (more than 1–2 cm

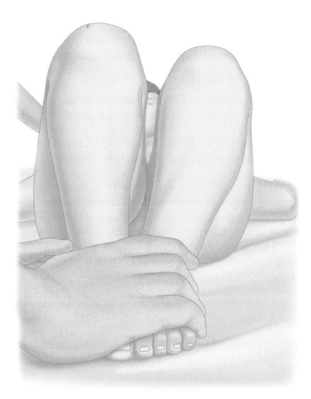

Figure 14–2. Galeazzi Test. A Galeazzi test suggesting developmental dysplasia of the hip or a leg-length discrepancy. The test is positive when the knees are at different heights as the patient lies supine with ankles to buttocks and hips and knees flexed.

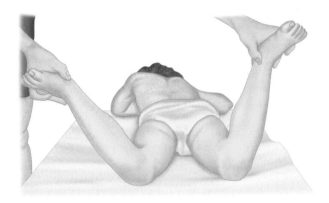

Figure 14–3. Prone internal rotation of the hip. This is the most sensitive test for intra-articular hip pathology. In this test, any inflammation of the hip manifests as decreased internal rotation of the hip.

of difference between sides) should be seen in a patient with any hip or knee condition that has limited function for more than 1 to 2 months.

A child with a septic hip keeps the hip in a position of flexion, abduction and external rotation. The reason being increased production of fluid within the joint capsule and increased intracapsular pressure,[9] since it has been shown in children with transient synovitis of the hip that the mean intracapsular pressure is only 18 mm Hg when the hip is in 45 degrees of flexion, but it increases to 178 mm Hg when the hip is in extension and internal rotation.[10] Conversely, the position of prone internal rotation is provocative in a child with hip pathology. Every child lacking a clear explanation for a limp should be placed prone, with the knees flexed and the ankles falling away from the body (Fig. 14–3), so that the physician can look for a difference in internal rotation between the hips. It is important that the pelvis be kept flat on the table or else the difference in internal rotation between the two sides may not be appreciated.

Differentiating transient synovitis from septic arthritis is particularly challenging, because both conditions present with decreased motion of the hip. A modified log-roll (Fig. 14–4). test may be helpful in differentiating the degree of hip irritation. While distracting the supine child by gently holding the big toe and pretending to examine the foot from different angles, significant hip rotation may be attempted. If an arc of 30 degrees or more of hip rotation is possible without complaints of pain, a diagnosis of transient synovitis is more likely than one of sepsis.

KNEE

The knee examination should include ballotment of the patella to identify an effusion or hemarthrosis (blood in the joint). Pain at extremes of flexion or extension can signal meniscal pathology; however, in an acute injury, the amount of fluid and pain in the knee joint often makes motion limited.

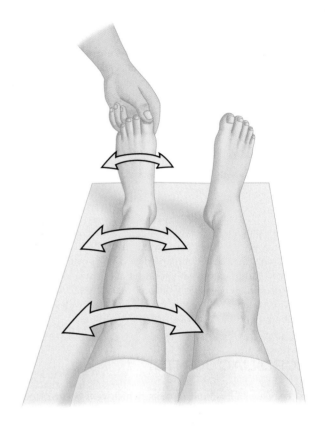

Figure 14–4. The modified log-roll test. The modified log-roll test may help determine the severity of hip irritation and aid in distinguishing between transient synovitis of the hip and septic arthritis. The diagnosis of transient synovitis is more likely if an arc of 30 degrees or more of hip rotation is possible without pain.

ANKLE/FOOT

Examination of the ankle should include careful palpation of the fibula and tibial physis, foot, and toes to identify possible occult fracture through the growth plate.

▶ EVALUATION

Evaluation of the child can be directed by presence or absence of systemic signs or symptoms as noted in the algorithm for the evaluation of a child with a limp (Fig. 14–5).

If the patient has systemic signs and symptoms and infection or neoplasia is being considered in the differential diagnosis, a complete blood count with differential, erythrocyte sedimentation rate (ESR) and C-reactive protein (CRP) level should be ordered. The platelet count may be low or the white cell count elevated in the child with leukemia. The CRP becomes elevated earlier than the sedimentation rate and is considered more sensitive for an infectious process. CRP, as compared to ESR, has a better negative predictive value than a positive predictor. If CRP is less than 1 mg/dL, the probability that the patient does not have septic arthritis is 87%.[11] In addition, having

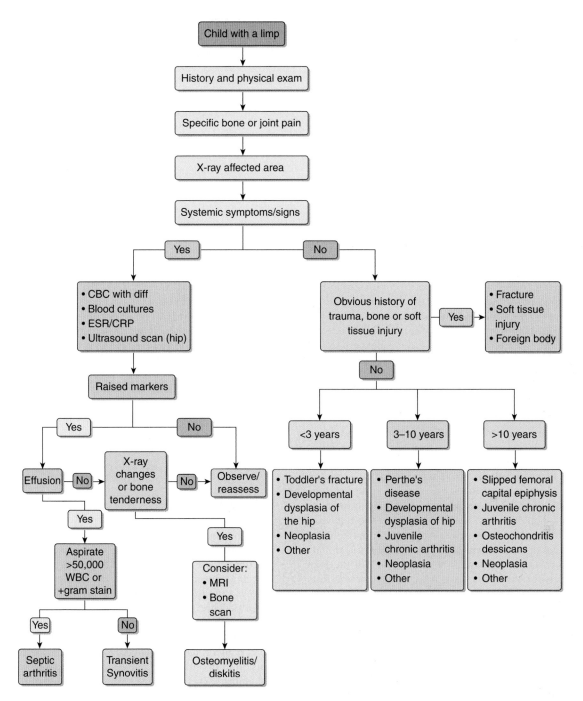

Figure 14–5. Algorithm for the diagnosis of child with limp. CRP, C-reactive protein; ESR, erythrocyte sedimentation rate; MRI, magnetic resonance imaging; WBC, white blood cell count.

a baseline ESR and CRP is helpful to monitor clinical improvement during antibiotic treatment.

Several studies have shown that a combination of laboratory and radiographic evaluation is helpful in identifying septic arthritis. When examined together, the combination of an ESR greater than 20 and a temperature more than 37.5°C (99.5°F) identified septic arthritis of the hip in 97% of patients presenting with a limp in one series.[12] Another study[13] showed that the probability of septic arthritis was 99.6% when all four of these clinical factors were present: history of fever, non-weight-bearing, ESR of at least 40 mg/h, and a serum white blood cell count greater than 12×10^9. In addition, according to a study by Jung, including radiographic and laboratory evaluation, plain radiographs showed a displacement or blurring of periarticular fat pads in all patients with acute septic arthritis, and additional multivariate regression analysis showed that body temperature >37°C, ESR >20 mm/h, CRP >1 mg/dL, WBC >11 000/mL, and an increased hip joint space of >2 mm were independent multivariate predictors of acute septic arthritis.[14] Another prospective study of children with findings that were highly suspicious for septic arthritis showed that an oral temperature >38.5°C was the best predictor of septic arthritis followed by an elevated CRP level, an elevated ESR, refusal to bear weight, and an elevated serum white blood cell count.[15] In this study,[15] a CRP level of >2.0 mg/dL (>20 mg/L) was a strong independent risk factor and a valuable tool for assessing and diagnosing children suspected of having septic arthritis of the hip. Further evidence indicates that duration of symptoms, constitutional symptoms, temperature, white cell count, and ESR were significantly different in children with musculoskeletal infection (p <0.05). Multivariate analysis demonstrated that when all three variables of duration of symptoms >1 and <5 days, temperature >37.0°C, and ESR >35 mm/h were present, the predicted probability of infection was 0.66, falling to 0.01 when none were present. This multivariate model enables us to rule out musculoskeletal infection with 99% certainty in limping children with none of these three presenting variables.[16]

If a septic process is suspected, the first priority should be to aspirate joints with effusion and evaluate the synovial fluid. The synovial fluid needs to be sent for cell count, Gram stain, anaerobic, and aerobic cultures. The evidence is not as strong on sending the synovial fluid for protein and glucose analyses.[17] While there is significant overlap of synovial white cell counts in infection and inflammatory conditions, synovial fluid white blood cell count and percentage of polymorphonuclear cells perform well as discriminators between inflammatory and noninflammatory disease; the sensitivity and specificity of white blood cell count in the synovial fluid above 40 000 per mm³ exceeded 90% in differentiating septic arthritis from other kinds of arthritis.[18] The white blood cell count in synovial fluid greater than 50 000 per mm³ is considered to be an indication of an infectious process. A septic joint partially treated with antibiotics may have a lower-than-expected white cell count. In addition, a negative culture does not rule out a septic joint; in approximately 33% of cases, the joint aspirate does not recover an organism in a septic joint.[19] If the joint in question is the knee in a sexually active patient, the fluid should be cultured for gonorrhea as well [20] by using a special media (Thayer-Martin) for growth. If the patient lives in an area that is endemic for Lyme disease, blood titers should be determined because acute Lyme disease can mimic a septic process.[7]

Serum rheumatoid factor antinuclear antibody and HLA typing should not be considered initially, because inflammatory diseases in children tend to be seronegative, making blood work less critical than the clinical history and physical examination.

▶ RADIOGRAPHIC ANALYSIS

Plain films of the areas in question should be the first radiographic studies ordered since they provide an excellent means of screening for fracture, joint effusion, lytic lesions, periosteal reaction, and avascular necrosis.[21–23] In the nonverbal patient, a screening anteroposterior film from hips to feet identifies a fracture in one-fifth of patients presenting with a limp.[22] It is useful to remember that the growth plate is weaker than the ligamentous attachments to the bone; occult fracture through

the growth plate is considerably more common than a ligamentous injury. If an area of pathology is localized by examination or history, anteroposterior and lateral views are indicated because a single view often misses pathology that is obvious in the second view. Especially in hip films, anteroposterior and frog-lateral views are necessary because the pathology is frequently best seen on lateral views.

The pelvic films should be examined for bone fragmentation (Perthes'), joint space widening (sepsis, Perthes'), and structural abnormalities (hip dysplasia). Fractures of the upper femur are rather uncommon, and if they occur in the young age group, they usually consist of a nondisplaced Salter–Harris type I fracture. Other fractures are also basically uncommon, but occasionally, one can encounter an impaction fracture of the upper femur.[24] For young children with point tenderness of the lower extremity, consider Toddler's fracture—a spiral fracture of the tibia first described by Dunbar et al.[25] The term "Toddler's fracture" has been synonymous with this fracture. However, there are other fractures that should be considered within this symptom complex. Toddler's fracture concept could be expanded to include other fractures[24,26] such as the original Toddler's fracture (type I), the hyperextension-induced upper tibial fracture (type II); various buckle fractures of the distal tibia and fibula; the so-called "bunk-bed foot" such as type I fracture, an impaction-buckle fracture of the base of the first metatarsal, and the type II fracture, a compression fracture of the cuboid bone as well as ankle fractures; and plastic bending fractures of the fibula. Child abuse should be considered with multiple fractures or a fracture of a suspicious nature.[27] Missing this diagnosis can put the child at high risk of mortality.

ULTRASOUND

Ultrasonography is useful to identify fluid in the hip joint in patients with a history and physical examination consistent with infection of the hip.[28,29] It was found to be 100% sensitive as well as specific for effusions of the hip joint in children. However, ultrasound cannot be used safely to distinguish between pediatric septic hip and transient synovitis.[30] Again, it may be helpful to the physician to do a bedside ultrasound to diagnose the presence of fluid in the joint.[31] Ultrasonography is much more sensitive than plain films, identifying an effusion in two-thirds of a series of 500 children with normal plain films.[29] The sonographic detection of hip effusion is better when the hip is in slight extension and abduction than in the neutral hip position.[32] Power Doppler does not seem to allow the exclusion of septic arthritis and should not be used to preclude aspiration when otherwise clinically indicated.[33] Ultrasound is also helpful in identifying fluid in the soft tissues consistent with a soft-tissue abscess.[28] Ultrasonography is noninvasive but highly dependent on the operator for an accurate result.

BONE SCAN/CT SCAN/MRI

When the cause of a child's limp cannot be localized by history or physical examination, a bone scan is an excellent way to help localize pathology.[34,35] The overall accuracy of bone scans

▶ TABLE 14–4. **CORRELATING HISTORY, EXAMINATION, AND DIAGNOSTIC STUDIES**

Category	History	Physical Examination May Show	Laboratory Studies	Radiology
Traumatic	Fall	Localized pain, swelling, loss of motion	None unless infection is possible	Plain films, bone scan
Infectious	Fever, chills, erythema, pain	Rigid guarding, warmth, erythema	CBC, ESR, CRP, joint aspirate	Plain films, MRI, bone scan
Neoplastic	Night pain, pain unrelated to activity	Mass	CBC, ESR, CRP, alkaline phosphatase, calcium, electrolytes, joint aspirate	Plain films, MRI/CT, bone scan, staging workup
Congenital	Problem since birth	Deformity, leg-length discrepancy, loss of ROM	None	Plain films
Neurologic	Ataxia, loss of balance, disorganized gait	High/low muscle tone, increased/decreased deep tendon reflexes, cavus foot or claw toes	Creatine kinase (if DMD is in differential diagnosis)	Plain films
Inflammatory	Pain >6 months, family history of rheumatoid arthritis	Warmth/erythema, one or more joints	CBC, ESR, CRP, joint aspiration	Plain films
Developmental	Painless limp (LCP disease) Knee pain (LCP disease, SCFE)	Loss of ROM in joints, asymmetric ROM, pain with ROM	None	Plain films

CBC, complete blood count; ESR, erythrocyte sedimentation rate; CRP, C-reactive protein; MRI, magnetic resonance imaging; CT, computed tomography; ROM, range of motion; DMD, Duchene's muscular dystrophy; LCP, Legg-Calvé-Perthes; SCFE, slipped capital femoral epiphysis.

was found to be 81%. The predictive value for a bone scan to be correct was 100% for a cold scan and 82% for a hot scan. The main reason for a false-positive scan was contiguous soft-tissue infection.[36] A negative bone scan makes an infection, a fracture, or most tumors less likely so that observation may be more safely pursued. An area that is bright on bone scan can be further evaluated with plain films, computed tomographic (CT) scan with bone windows, or magnetic resonance imaging (MRI) studies. CT scan best delineates bone structure, whereas MRI best highlights areas of pathology in the soft tissues as well as inflammation of bone.[37,38] Table 14–4 presents diagnostic criteria for various categories of limp.[39]

▶ MICROBIOLOGY

Microscopy of the joint fluid cannot be used to rule out septic arthritis. In one study, Gram stain was 100% specific but only 45% sensitive for septic arthritis. The incidence of elevated white blood cell count was higher in the group of patients with a positive Gram stain study (60%) as compared to patients with a negative Gram stain study (33%).[40] The authors concluded that Gram staining is an unreliable tool in early decision making in patients requiring urgent surgical drainage and washout. Parenteral antibiotics should be given only after synovial fluid has been obtained for Gram stain and culture.

▶ CONCLUSION

A child who limps often presents a diagnostic challenge. The differential diagnosis is extensive. Although the most common

cause is trauma, awareness of other potential causes is important. The age of the child and the pattern of the gait help narrow the differential diagnosis. In most cases, a diagnosis can be made from the history and physical examination. If the diagnosis is not obvious after a careful clinical evaluation, plain radiographs provide an excellent means of screening for fracture, joint effusion, lytic lesions, periosteal reaction, and avascular necrosis. Other tests should be ordered only when indicated.

REFERENCES

1. Flynn JM, Widmann RF. The limping child: evaluation and diagnosis. *J Am Acad Orthop Surg.* 2001;9:89–98.
2. Barkin RM, Barkin AZ, Barkin SZ. The limping child. *J Emerg Med.* 2000;18:331–339.
3. Fischer SU, Beattie TF. The limping child: epidemiology, assessment and outcome. *J Bone Joint Surg Br.* 1999;81(6):1029–1034.
4. MacEwen GD, Dehne R. The limping child. *Pediatr Rev.* 1991;12:268–274.
5. Birdi N, D'Astous J. Poststreptococcal reactive arthritis mimicking acute septic arthritis: a hospital-based study. *J Pediatr Orthop.* 1995;15:661–665.
6. Peltola H, Kallio MJ, Unkila-Kallio L. Reduced incidence of septic arthritis in children by Haemophilus influenzae type-b vaccination. Implications for treatment. *J Bone Joint Surg Br.* 1998;80(3):471–473.
7. Dabney KW, Lipton G. Evaluation of limp in children. *Curr Opin Pediatr.* 1995;7:88–94.
8. Welkon CJ, Long SS, Fisher MC, Alburger PD. Pyogenic arthritis in infants and children: a review of 95 cases. *Pediatr Infect Dis.* 1986;5(6):669–676.

9. Hensinger RN. Limp. *Pediatr Clin North Am.* 1986;33:1355–1364.
10. Kesteris U, Wingstrand H, Forsberg L, Egund N. The effect of arthrocentesis in transient synovitis of the hip in the child: a longitudinal sonographic study. *J Pediatr Orthop.* 1996;16:24–29.
11. Levine MJ, McGuire KJ, McGowan KL, Flynn JM. Assessment of the test characteristics of C-reactive protein for septic arthritis in children. *J Pediatr Orthop.* 2003;23(3):373–737.
12. Del Beccaro MA, Champoux AN, Bockers T, Mendelman PM. Septic arthritis versus transient synovitis of the hip: the value of screening laboratory tests. *Ann Emerg Med.* 1992;21:1418–422.
13. Kocher MS, Zurakowski D, Kasser JR. Differentiating between septic arthritis and transient synovitis of the hip in children: an evidence-based clinical prediction algorithm. *J Bone Joint Surg Am.* 1999;81(12):1662–1670.
14. Jung ST, Rowe SM, Moon ES, Song EK, Yoon TR, Seo HY. Significance of laboratory and radiologic findings for differentiating between septic arthritis and transient synovitis of the hip. *J Pediatr Orthop.* 2003;23(3):368–372.
15. Caird MS, Flynn JM, Leung YL, et al. Factors distinguishing septic arthritis from transient synovitis of the hip in children. A prospective study. *J Bone Joint Surg Am.* 2006;88(6):1251–1257.
16. Delaney RA, Lenehan B, O'sullivan L, McGuinness AJ, Street JT. The limping child: an algorithm to outrule musculoskeletal sepsis. *Ir J Med Sci.* 2007;176(3):181–187. Epub Jul 12, 2007.
17. Shmerling RH, Delbanco TL, Tosteson AN, Trentham DE. Synovial fluid tests. What should be ordered? *JAMA.* 1990;264(8):1009–1014.
18. Kunnamo I, Pelkonen P. Routine analysis of synovial fluid cells is of value in the differential diagnosis of arthritis in children. *J Rheumatol.* 1986;13(6):1076–1080.
19. Herndon WA, Knauer S, Sullivan JA, Gross RH. Management of septic arthritis in children. *J Pediatr Orthop.* 1986;6:576–578.
20. Renshaw TS. The child who has a limp. *Pediatr Rev.* 1995;16:458–465.
21. Blatt SD, Rosenthal BM, Barnhart DC. Diagnostic utility of lower extremity radiographs of young children with gait disturbances. *Pediatrics.* 1991;87:138–140.
22. Oudjhane K, Newman B, Oh KS, Young LW, Girdany BR. Occult fractures in preschool children. *J Trauma.* 1998;28:858–860.
23. Phillips WA. The child with a limp. *Orthop Clin North Am.* 1987;18:489–501.
24. Swischuk LE. The limping infant: imaging and clinical evaluation of trauma. *Emerg Radiol.* 2007;14:219–226.
25. Dunbar JS, Owen HF, Nogrady MB, et al. Obscure tibial fracture of infants—the toddler's fracture. *J Can Assoc Radiol.* 1964;5:136–144.
26. John SD, Moorthy CS, Swischuk LE. Expanding the concept of the toddler's fracture. *Radiographics.* 1997;17:367–376.
27. Leventhal JM, Thomas SA, Rosenfield NS, Markowitz RI. Fractures in young children. Distinguishing child abuse from unintentional injuries. *Am J Dis Child.* 1993;147:87–92.
28. Alexandra JE, Seibert JJ, Glasier CM, et al. High resolution hip ultrasound in the limping child. *J Clin Ultrasound.* 1989;17:19–24.
29. Miralles M, Gonzalez G, Pulpeiro JR, et al. Sonography of the painful hip in children: 500 consecutive cases. *AJR Am J Roentgenol.* 1989;152:579–582.
30. Zamzam MM. The role of ultrasound in differentiating septic arthritis from transient synovitis of the hip in children. *J Pediatr Orthop B.* 2006;15(6):418–422.
31. Shavit I, Eidelman M, Galbraith R. Sonography of the hip-joint by the emergency physician: its role in the evaluation of children presenting with acute limp. *Pediatr Emerg Care.* 2006;22(8):570–573.
32. Chan YL, Cheng JC, Metreweli C. Sonographic evaluation of hip effusion in children. Improved visualization with the hip in extension and abduction. *Acta Radiol.* 1997;38(5):867–869.
33. Strouse PJ, DiPietro MA, Adler RS. Pediatric hip effusions: evaluation with power Doppler sonography. *Radiology.* 1998;206(3):731–735.
34. Choban S, Killian JT. Evaluation of acute gait abnormalities in preschool children. *J Pediatr Orthop.* 1990;10:74–78.
35. Aronson J, Garvin K, Seibert J, Glasier C, Tursky EA. Efficiency of bone scan for occult limping toddlers. *J Pediatr Orthop.* 1992;12:38–44.
36. Tuson CE, Hoffman EB, Mann MD. Isotope bone scanning for acute osteomyelitis and septic arthritis in children. *J Bone Joint Surg Br.* 1994;76(2):306–310.
37. Yang WJ, Im SA, Lim GY, et al. MR imaging of transient synovitis: differentiation from septic arthritis. *Pediatr Radiol.* 2006;36(11):1154–1158. Epub Sep 20, 2006.
38. Kwack KS, Cho JH, Lee JH, Cho JH, Oh KK, Kim SY. Septic arthritis versus transient synovitis of the hip: gadolinium-enhanced MRI finding of decreased perfusion at the femoral epiphysis. *AJR Am J Roentgenol.* 2007;189(2):437–445.
39. Leet AI, Skaggs DL. Evaluation of the acutely limping child. *Am Fam Physician.* 2000;61:1011–1018.
40. Faraj AA, Omonbude OD, Godwin P. Gram staining in the diagnosis of acute septic arthritis. *Acta Orthop Belg.* 2002;68(4):388–391.

CHAPTER 15

Mild Head Injury in Children

Eustacia Su

▶ HIGH-YIELD FACTS

- Carefully rule out mild head injury in the context of other facial or scalp injuries.
- Suspect nonaccidental trauma in infants and toddlers, especially when the history is not consistent either with the child's developmental milestones or with the physical findings.
- Have a lower threshold for imaging younger children (<2 years old) because they are at greater risk of asymptomatic intracranial injury.
- Do not hesitate to observe the child for a few hours, especially if there is any discomfort on the part of the physician or the caregiver(s).
- Evaluate concussed athletes carefully: They are very motivated to hide their symptoms so that they can return to play. The player may not have had any loss of consciousness, but may still have sustained a significant concussion.
- Discharge instructions and counseling are critical, especially as to reasons to return to the emergency department, return to play criteria, and the possible duration of concussive symptoms.

Unintentional, blunt traumatic brain injury (TBI) is the leading cause of death and disability in the under-20 age group. There are 7440 deaths, 642000 emergency department (ED) visits, and 65000 hospitalizations annually because of TBI.[1] The majority (84%) of these head injuries is classified as mild traumatic brain injury (MTBI). Unfortunately, there is significant variability in how investigators define MTBI; they also disagree over whether any lasting effects may result (Tables 15–1 and 15–2).

Concussion is included in the spectrum of MTBI. Physicians have long regarded concussion to be a benign condition, but its role in long-term brain damage is being investigated and argued. The American Congress of Rehabilitation Medicine has a slightly different definition, based on the belief that the trauma has induced a physiologic disruption of brain function with possible prolonged or permanent sequelae. The inclusion criteria comprise at least one of the following.

▶ ANATOMY

The infant's head has a disproportionately large size and weight relative to the rest of the body, and is supported on a relatively short, weak, and flexible neck. Any forces on the head or body will result in more momentum on the head and with less restriction from the weaker neck muscles and cervical spinal ligaments, leading to increased likelihood of injury to the brain. In infancy, the open fontanelles and sutures provide more flexibility, which can absorb greater impact as well as provide an expandable intracranial volume. Incomplete myelinization makes for greater plasticity of the brain. This flexibility allows for more distortion between the container (the skull and dura) and its contents (the brain and the cerebral blood vessels), which results in increased susceptibility to hemorrhage. The brain is housed inside the skull and is protected by the cerebrospinal fluid, the pia mater, the arachnoid, the dura mater, and the calvarium. Beyond the bony layer lie the periosteum, subgaleal soft tissue, the galea, the subcutaneous soft tissue, and the skin (see Chapter 29 for further description).

▶ BIOMECHANICS

Most head trauma results from a combination of direct impact, acceleration/deceleration, or rotational shear forces. The more pliable skull of the younger child tends to bend inward on impact, putting pressure on the inner table and its underlying vessels in the epidural and subdural spaces. The surrounding areas bend outward, putting pressure on the outer table, producing a fracture which may or may not be proximate to the area of impact. Younger children and infants with isolated skull fractures tend to present with normal mental status unless there is a significant underlying brain injury with mass effect.[2]

▶ PATHOPHYSIOLOGY

Laboratory studies suggest that concussive brain injury (CBI) is characterized by transient, functional, cellular impairments, including abrupt neuronal depolarization, release of excitatory neurotransmitters, ionic shifts, changes in glucose metabolism, altered cerebral blood flow, and impaired axonal function.[3,4]

Any of these conditions may lead to a state of enhanced vulnerability, during which time the patient may have symptoms of confusion or headache. A second impact before the brain is fully recovered may result in a potentially fatal loss of cerebrovascular autoregulation resulting in vasoparalysis, brain swelling, increased intracranial pressure, and death (second impact syndrome [SIS]).[5] Research indicates that, after a single brain impact, this state of increased vulnerability can persist for 3 to 5 days but usually resolves within a week.[6]

In the patient with a mild head injury, a more prolonged "postconcussion syndrome" may occur, characterized by persistent alterations in cognition, behavior, and personality changes as well as emotional swings. This can affect interpersonal relationships, school, and work. Athletes reporting

▶ **TABLE 15–1. DEFINITION OF MTBI BY THE AMERICAN ACADEMY OF PEDIATRICS**

1. Normal mental status on initial examination.
2. No abnormal or focal neurologic findings.
3. No physical evidence of skull fracture.
4. LOC of <1 min.
5. May have had a seizure immediately after injury.
6. May have vomited after injury.
7. May exhibit other signs and symptoms, e.g., headache or lethargy.

Exclusion criteria:
1. Multiple trauma;
2. Unobserved LOC;
3. Known or suspected cervical spine injury;
4. Suspected intentional head trauma; and
5. History of bleeding diathesis or neurologic disorders.

posttraumatic headache up to 7 days after injury demonstrated significantly worse neurocognitive scores, possibly associated with incomplete recovery.[7]

Chronic cognitive impairments can occur in athletes who have sustained multiple, seemingly minor, head injuries are associated with accelerated or increased neurodegeneration in specific brain regions. Clinical symptoms of concussions (e.g., confusion, amnesia, headache, attention deficits, disorientation, and loss of motor coordination) are usually transient.[5]

▶ ASSESSMENT

Ensure that the patient is not in any danger and that the airway is patent, and that breathing and circulation are adequate. The primary injury can be exacerbated by hypotension and acidosis, leading to a secondary injury. Hypotension, which can result from a simple scalp laceration in the young child, disrupts cerebral autoregulation even more than hypertension.[8] Pay careful attention to the vital signs: A young infant may have an elevated blood pressure and a low heart rate with values that are close to normal numbers for adults or older children. Crying may result in hyperventilation, temporarily normalizing the vital signs, even though the intracranial pressure is increasing.

▶ **TABLE 15–2. DEFINITION OF MTBI BY AMERICAN CONGRESS OF REHABILITATION MEDICINE**

1. Any LOC.
2. Any loss of memory for events immediately before or after the injury.
3. Any alteration in mental state at the time of the injury.
4. Focal neurologic deficits that may or may not have resolved.

Exclusion criteria include:
1. LOC >30 min;
2. GCS score <13 after 30 min; and
3. Posttraumatic amnesia >24 h.

▶ HISTORY

A careful history should include the time and nature of the incident in particular the height of fall or force of impact. Ask about loss of consciousness (LOC), alteration of mental status, or change in neurologic function since the injury, their duration, and if the signs are ongoing. Also ask about any vomiting or seizures since the injury. Determine if the patient has any preexisting conditions that increase the risk of more serious intracranial injury, for example, bleeding diatheses, bony diseases, or developmental delay. With young infants, be especially alert to any features of the history that are inconsistent with the child's developmental milestones, since this is the age group at highest risk for nonaccidental trauma (NAT). The high-performing athlete may try to hide symptoms because of pressures to perform. Ask carefully about previous head injuries.

▶ PHYSICAL EXAMINATION

After completing the primary survey, and instituting any necessary resuscitative measures, a meticulous neurologic examination should be performed. The Glasgow Coma Scale (GCS) is helpful in communicating to a consultant how the child is functioning. In young children, the GCS has been validated, but is more difficult to use because of lack of verbal skills and cooperation (e.g., "6" on the motor scale is still defined as "follows commands," rare amongst toddlers). MTBI is usually defined as a GCS score of 13 to 15.

Examine the scalp for linear hematomas, especially over the temporal or occipital areas. Palpate carefully, looking for crepitus or depressions. In young infants, feel the fontanelle for fullness. Check for blood and cerebrospinal fluid leaking from the ears or the nose; look for ecchymoses around the eyes (raccoon sign) and behind the ears (Battle sign). Also look for blood behind the tympanic membrane (hemotympanum), another indicator of a basilar skull fracture, not to be confused with blood within the tympanic membrane.

Ensure that all cranial nerves are intact and that the child is not exhibiting any stereotyped posturing. Watch the child's movements to ensure that all extremities move equally. Observe how the child holds his head; if he moves his head about freely, it is unlikely that he has a neck injury. Palpate the neck for any step offs, swelling, or crepitus.

▶ THE INFANT OR TODDLER

Assess the child's interactions with caregivers and surroundings and ask the caregiver how the child's current status compares with the child's baseline. The infant should visually track to the caregiver and console easily. The toddler should show stranger anxiety but should gradually become more playful and start exploring the room. If the cervical spine has been cleared and the child seems interested and active enough, evaluate the gait. This is best done by moving the child a short distance from the caregiver and letting the child return to the caregiver.

► THE SCHOOL-AGED CHILD

The preverbal children can often show a finger count to indicate age and can correctly identify caregivers. They will usually overcome initial shyness and be very curious about equipment, posters, etc. The child with verbal abilities should be able to answer some mental status questions correctly, e.g., age, phone numbers, and do more complicated motor maneuvers, e.g., finger-to-nose test, tandem gait, one-legged balance, etc.

► ED MANAGEMENT

RESUSCITATION

As with all injuries, ensure that the airway is intact and that the ventilation and circulation are adequate. In very young children, make sure that the vital signs are appropriate for their age: Again, hypertension and bradycardia may easily be mistaken for normal vital signs. If there are any sources of bleeding, for example, a large scalp laceration, fluid resuscitation may be necessary to prevent hypotension and a possible secondary brain injury.

GUIDELINES FOR IMAGING

In Europe and Canada, physicians report greater use of plain skull films as a screen to help determine if there is a need for CAT scan. The Canadian Rule[9] and its offshoot, the NICE guidelines,[10] have been criticized for increasing threefold the number of head CT scans ordered in children with mild head injury.[11] In the United States, most practitioners start with the CAT scan if they are going to image at all, except in facilities where CT scan is not available and skull films may help to determine whether the child needs to be transferred for CT scan. One study[12] identified five clinical findings that were predictive of intracranial injury: abnormal mental status, clinical signs of skull fracture, scalp hematoma (in children <2 years of age), history of headache, and vomiting. The benefit of CT scan should be weighed against the risk of procedural sedation and the risk of radiation exposure.[13] However, imaging followed by discharge is reported as more cost-effective than observation without imaging, with no difference in outcome.[14,15]

The main guidelines used in the United States address the management of children younger than 2 years old and those between 2 and 20 years. These do not recommend plain skull radiography. MRI is usually more difficult to obtain, takes longer, and often requires sedation. Hence, only CT scans are included since neurosurgical management is usually determined by findings on these studies.

IMAGING IN CHILDREN YOUNGER THAN 2 YEARS

In 1991, the American Academy of Pediatrics (AAP) published "Evaluation and management of children younger than two years old with apparently minor head trauma: Proposed Guide-

lines," the work of a multidisciplinary panel comprising nine experts in pediatric head injury.[16] Younger children have a higher incidence of apparently asymptomatic intracranial injury. They also have a higher incidence of complications and are more difficult to assess clinically. Infants younger than 3 months are at the highest risk not only of occult head injury but also of NAT. They are less likely to need sedation than older infants and toddlers. The latter group is more likely to develop paradoxical hyperactivity reactions to midazolam. The guideline (Table 15–3) proposes that there are three main categories of presentation and offer recommendations for CT scan usage.

IMAGING IN PRESCHOOL AND SCHOOL-AGED CHILDREN

In 1999, the AAP and the AAFP published a practice parameter "The Management of Minor Closed Head Injury in Children"[17] (Table 15–4). In this age group, it is sometimes easier to obtain a history. However, many of them are in day care or school settings where witnesses to the event may not be available to give an account of the event. It is also easier to perform an accurate physical examination in these children. Unfortunately, children with intracranial lesions after MTBI are not distinguishable clinically from the large majority who has no intracranial injury.[18,19] Boran et al.,[20] in a study of 421 children in Turkey, rather strongly advocated routine CT scanning in all pediatric patients with any head injury. The risk of finding a significant lesion on head CT scan in children with mild head injury and a brief LOC ranges from 2% to 5% in some reports[21–23] to as low as 0.02%.[24]

The AAP recommends imaging in head-injured children (2–20 years old) if there is a LOC for more than 1 minute or ongoing symptoms. Observation at home by a reliable caregiver is recommended if neither of these conditions is present. However, their management algorithm is based almost entirely on whether or not there was LOC associated with the injury.[25] CT scanning should be done by ALARA standards (as low as reasonably achievable).

There is not a good correlation between presence of intracranial injury and persistent vomiting or posttraumatic seizure. However, parental anxiety in the context of the latter presentation may justify an overnight admission.

THE "HYPERACUTE" CT SCAN

There is a very small subset of patients who, on initial CT scan, have a normal scan, but who later deteriorate. They often present at the scene with or without a history of LOC and a worrisome, initial presentation with significant alteration of mental status. These patients would have been classified as "moderate" or even "severe" head injuries initially, but clear up almost completely by the time the ED assessment is completed. They often qualify for admission for overnight observation. The initial CT scan is obtained very promptly, usually within an hour, and looks normal. The child is then admitted to the regular ward and deteriorates several hours later, often fatally. Repeat CT scan shows either diffuse swelling or a large subdural hematoma.[26] Many trauma services will

▶ TABLE 15–3. **CLASSIFICATION OF HEAD INJURY RISK AND RECOMMENDATIONS FOR IMAGING STUDIES**

Risk	Recommendation

A. High risk:
  Depressed mental status
  Focal neurologic findings
  Depressed or basilar skull fractures
  Irritability
  Bulging fontanelle
  Seizure
  Vomiting >5 times or >6 h
  LOC >1 min
	Head CT scans should be obtained in these children.

B. Intermediate risk:
  B-1. Clinical indicators of possible brain injury:
    Transient LOC (<1 min)
    3 or more episodes of vomiting
    Period of irritability or lethargy, now resolved
    Alteration of LOC or not at baseline behavior according
      to caregivers
    Skull fracture >24 h ago
	If two or more of these risk factors are present, or if the duration and severity of the LOC or alteration of behavior is significant, CT scan should be more strongly considered.

B-2. Concerning or unknown mechanism of injury or suspicion
    of skull fracture on physical examination:
    Higher force mechanism
    Falls onto hard surfaces
    Unwitnessed trauma with the possibility of significant
      mechanism (e.g., finding child at bottom of stairs or wall)
    History inconsistent with the physical findings or the child's
      developmental status
	Consider CT scan or further observation (4–6 h), depending on the clinical situation.

C. Low risk:
  Low-energy mechanism (e.g., fall <3 ft)
  Asymptomatic for at least 2 h after injury
	This group may be observed at home.

routinely obtain follow-up head CT scans on these children who had moderate or severe symptoms when initially injured.

▶ SPECIAL SITUATIONS

CONCUSSION IN THE ATHLETE

There is growing evidence that even mild brain injury can result in memory and concentration problems and affect academic performance in children, especially those involved in competitive sports. Neuropsychologic testing is mandated by the National Hockey League and the majority of National Football League franchises, but seldom covered by standard health insurance policies and is not widely used in high school, where the largest majority of at-risk athletes is found.[27]

Experts disagree about whether cumulative concussions have an additive effect on behavioral, neuropsychologic or cognitive function, and academic performance. Unfortunately, the studies published on this topic have many methodological problems, in particular, lack of preinjury data and inadequate control subjects. Satz et al.[28] extensively reviewed all 40 studies of mild TBI in children and adolescents older than 25 years and found conflicting conclusions. In the academic and psychosocial domains, most studies reported a null outcome up

to 5 years after the injury; these studies were thought to be methodologically stronger than the studies that reported an adverse outcome.

In the area of neuropsychologic outcomes (language, memory, and hand–eye coordination), the stronger studies seemed to indicate that MTBI may be associated with alterations in neuropsychologic performance, but recovery usually occurred within 12 months. Ponsford et al.[29] and Bijur et al.[30] found that those patients (and parents) reporting persistent problems often had a history of previous head injury, learning difficulties, preexisting neurologic or psychiatric diagnoses, or family stressors. However, McKinlay et al.[31] prospectively studied a population of children born in mid-1977 whose families had been interviewed regularly since birth. They concluded that most cases of mild head injury in young children were benign, but that long-term problems in psychosocial function did occur in the more severe cases of MTBI, especially when it occurred during the preschool years.

SECOND IMPACT SYNDROME

SIS is the usually fatal result of a second concussive head injury before the brain has had time to recover and the patient is still symptomatic from the first impact.[32,33] The typical scenario

► **TABLE 15-4. EVALUATION OF CHILDREN AND ADOLESCENTS (2–20 YEARS OLD) WITH MINOR HEAD TRAUMA**

	Recommendation

Exclusion criteria:
  1. Multiple trauma
  2. Known or suspected C-spine injury
  3. Previous neurologic disorder
  4. Bleeding diathesis
  5. Suspicion for NAT
  6. Social factors (language barrier, distance from home, transportation, parental reliability, and intoxication of either patient or parents)	

A. Low-risk group:
  No LOC and low-risk mechanism.
  Normal examination includes:
  1. normal neurologic examination;
  2. normal fundoscopic examination;
  3. no significant skull trauma (parietal location, crepitus or depression, evidence of basilar skull fracture, and large linear hematoma);
  4. normal mental status (age appropriate); and
  5. no vomiting.
	Observe at home if parents understand instructions, are reliable, and transportation back is not a problem.

B. Intermediate-risk group:
  Brief LOC (<1 min)
  Amnesia for event itself, retrograde and/or antegrade
  Brief generalized posttraumatic seizure with brief postictal period, completely resolved
  Vomiting and/or headache
  Continued altered mental status or level of activity and interaction.
	CT scan of head:
	1. If positive for intracranial injury, consult appropriate specialist and admit.
	2. If normal, and child is now better, may observe at home if social situation is safe, and parents are comfortable and have good access to follow-up care.
	3. If normal, and child is still vomiting or confused, short stay admit advisable. Consider repeat head CT scan in 4–6 h.

is that of a football player who is "dinged" by a head impact. While still symptomatic, he reenters the game. The second impact is sometimes not even a direct impact to the head, but may just be a deceleration injury (e.g., if he is tackled and his body is stopped by his shoulder hitting the tackler's leg). He may get up again and even finish the play, but he collapses within a few minutes and then dies.

It is believed that the second impact to the brain causes severe loss of cerebrovascular autoregulation, resulting in massive brain swelling and almost inevitable death. Experts disagree on the actual existence of SIS,[34] but those who have witnessed these deaths are adamant that SIS exists and can be prevented by careful adherence to return-to-play guidelines.

The return-to-play guidelines are designed to try to prevent SIS. There is no evidence to support their use in preventing cumulative morbidity from repeated concussions. However, the physician should discuss the risks of SIS and possible cumulative brain damage with the patient and caregivers.

POSTCONCUSSION SYNDROME

A minority of head-injured patients go on to develop a persistent symptom complex that is called "postconcussion syndrome." There are three categories of complaints: Cognitive, somatic, and affective or emotional (Table 15–5). Most of these resolve over time. There is controversy over whether this is an organic (physiologic) or functional (psychogenesis) problem: Both processes may be involved.[35]

The occurrence of postconcussive symptoms after mild CHI may reflect premorbid vulnerability, postinjury child and family adjustment and postinjury changes in brain function. Ponsford et al.[36] found that providing an information booklet about expected symptoms and suggested coping strategies seemed to reduce the duration of symptoms, as well as the perception of stress, in the intervention group. By 3 months, the symptoms had resolved for most of the children in both groups.

► **TABLE 15-5. ICD-10 DIAGNOSTIC CRITERIA FOR POSTCONCUSSION SYNDROME**

History of head trauma with LOC with 4 wk of symptom onset;
Three or more symptom categories are:
  headache, dizziness, malaise, fatigue, and noise intolerance;
  irritability, depression, anxiety, and emotional lability;
  subjective concentration and memory or intellectual difficulties without neuropsychologic evidence of impairment;
  insomnia; and
  reduced alcohol intolerance.
Preoccupation with above symptoms, fear of brain damage with hypochondriacal concern and adoption of sick role.

A small group with a history of previous head injury or of learning or behavioral difficulties did report ongoing problems.[36]

▶ DISPOSITION AND DISCHARGE INSTRUCTIONS

Consider the following factors when planning a patient's disposition: What is the ability of the caregivers to understand discharge instructions; how reliable and comfortable are the caregivers; what is the distance of their home to the hospital; what is their access to transportation and telephone or EMS; and do they have access to reliable, early, outpatient follow-up? Many caregivers believe that it is dangerous to allow head-injured children to fall asleep. They should be reassured that these children can be allowed to fall asleep. Instructions should be easy to follow and not too burdensome.

Children should not participate in demanding physical activities over the first 24 to 48 hours following a head injury. However, toddlers and preschoolers will do whatever they wish, and trying to restrict their activities will prove futile. Caregivers should avoid putting the child into a stimulating environment for the next day or two. School-aged children would benefit from a day or two off school. Children are expected to perform well at school. Children who have sustained mild CHI often show no visible signs of incapacitation. Distractibility, restlessness, poor memory, or lack of concentration may be misinterpreted as sloth or deliberate misbehavior, resulting in criticism and punishment, rather than support and assistance. It is important to provide information about expected symptoms and duration and to suggest strategies for coping with them.[36]

▶ THE CONCUSSED ATHLETE AND RETURN TO PLAY

In the United States, 300 000 sport-related brain injuries occur in high school sports each year, most of which (~90%) are MTBIs or concussions. The highest number of sport-related head injuries has been reported in American football, but TBIs also occur in many other sports. The exact pathophysiologic changes to the brain following concussion are poorly understood, but they involve a graded set of clinical syndromes, which may or may not include LOC. The acute clinical symptoms reflect a functional disturbance rather than a structural injury; hence neuroimaging studies are usually normal.

▶ TABLE 15–6. **SIGNS AND SYMPTOMS OF ACUTE CONCUSSION***

1. Cognitive features:
   a. Unaware of period, opposition, score of game
   b. Confusion
   c. Amnesia
   d. LOC
   e. Unaware of time, date, place
2. Typical symptoms:
   a. Headache
   b. Dizziness
   c. Nausea
   d. Unsteadiness, loss of balance
   e. Feeling stunned or dazed, "having my bell rung"
   f. Seeing stars or flashing lights
   g. Double vision
   h. Sleepiness, fatigue, feeling of slowness
3. Physical signs:
   a. LOC or impaired state of consciousness
   b. Poor coordination or balance, gait unsteadiness
   c. Temporally associated seizure
   d. Slow to answer questions, follow directions or unable to concentrate or staring vacantly or slurred speech
   e. Displaying inappropriate emotions, personality changes
   f. Vomiting
   g. Inappropriate play behavior (e.g., running in wrong direction) or significantly decreased playing ability

*A head injury should be suspected and appropriate management instituted if any of these is present.

Athletes who have sustained a concussion are often evaluated in the ED. Some will come to the ED to get clearance to play from a different physician. It is important for emergency physicians to properly evaluate the athlete before clearing him or her to play. An approach to concussion management is the four "R"s: Recognition, response, rehabilitation, and return.

RECOGNITION

Recognition is "perhaps the most challenging aspect of managing sport-related concussion ... especially in athletes with no obvious signs that a concussion has actually occurred" (Table 15–6).[37] LOC should be viewed as one of a number of potential signs and not a requirement of diagnosis. Paradoxically, LOC is the most obvious presentation and the most likely to produce appropriate management for CBI.

▶ TABLE 15–7. **COMBINED CONCUSSION GRADING SYSTEM**

Grade 1	Grade 2	Grade 3
1. No LOC	1. No LOC	1. Any LOC
2. No posttraumatic amnesia (antegrade or retrograde) or transient memory loss with rapid recovery (<15 min)	2. Transient confusion lasting >15 min	2. Prolonged retrograde amnesia
3. Slight or transient confusion	3. Mild amnesia	3. Confusion with slow recovery
Return to play is allowed if asymptomatic for 15–20 min.	Return to play if asymptomatic for 1 wk.	Transport to a hospital ED. May return to play if asymptomatic for 2 wk.

▶ TABLE 15-8. GRADING SYSTEM FOR FIRST AND SUBSEQUENT CONCUSSION

Level of Concussion	Grade 1	Grade 2	Grade 3
First	Asymptomatic for 15–20 min	Asymptomatic × 1 wk	Asymptomatic × 2 wk
Second	Asymptomatic × 1 wk	Asymptomatic × 1 mo. Consider terminating season	Terminate season. RTP next season if asymptomatic
Third	Terminate season	Terminate season. May RTP next season if asymptomatic	Terminate season, strongly discourage contact/collision sports

RESPONSE

Any athlete who is suspected of having a concussion should be removed immediately from the game or practice.[38] Return to play (RTP) while still symptomatic greatly increases the risk of more severe symptoms and a longer postconcussive course. The athlete is obviously at greater risk for another injury if reaction time or coordination is impaired. SIS is an extremely rare, but usually fatal, sequela of RTP while still symptomatic.[39] Whether SIS exists is rather hotly debated.[40]

Multiple concussions also have a cumulative and deleterious effect on cognition and academic potential.[41,42] It is critical to let the young athlete's brain recover sufficiently before risking another concussion. The emergency physician should ensure that the parents and the athlete understand the risks. Close follow-up is essential to ensure that symptoms resolve fully prior to RTP.

REHABILITATION (REST)

Postconcussive symptoms are aggravated by both physical[43] and cognitive stressors.[44] Concentration, memorization, and learning (which are particularly stressed in school) can aggravate both the physical and the cognitive symptoms of the postconcussive period. Failure to rest until asymptomatic is the main reason that athletes have prolonged postconcussive symptoms. Unfortunately, it is not yet possible to predict how long an absence is required for a concussed individual; this, combined with the lack of outward physical signs of concussion, makes it difficult for teachers and employers to believe the seriousness of the athlete's condition, increasing stress at a time when stress reduction and cognitive rest are so important. Many athletes interpret "rest" from sporting activity to mean that they can still train with weights. Resistance (weight) training increases intracranial pressure and can exacerbate postconcussive symptoms.[45] It is critical to emphasize the importance of total rest to the athlete, the family, and the coach(es). Depression is common following a concussion; enforced rest, isolation from the rest of the team, and lack of endorphins may exacerbate depression in this setting. Support from the family, team, and peer group is very important during this time.

CONCUSSION GRADING SYSTEMS AND RETURN TO PLAY

It may be in the best interest of the athlete not to return to a collision or contact sport. In particular, some athletes seem to be at high risk of cumulative brain damage from multiple concussions. These include the athlete who has had numerous concussions, with progressively lesser mechanisms, or with symptoms that are more severe or last longer; the athlete who has residual neurocognitive problems persisting after the other symptoms have resolved; and the athlete with protracted, prolonged symptoms. There are multiple systems for grading concussions and determining RTP according to whether there have been other concussive injuries.[46] The major grading systems are the Cantu, Colorado Medical Society, American Academy of Neurology, and McGill systems (Table 15–7). Each investigative group seems to construct a new grading system. The emergency physician should be familiar with these systems when counseling player and parents.

▶ RETURN TO PLAY GUIDELINES

If there have been previous concussions, use the following guidelines (Table 15–8) to determine when the athlete might RTP. Use the highest-grade concussion to decide which recommendation to follow.

If there is any doubt, err on the side of caution and keep the athlete out of harm's way until completely asymptomatic, even with any exertion. The physician should also consider giving these instructions to the family of any child who has sustained a concussion, even outside of an athletic event.

REFERENCES

1. Rutland-Brown W, Langlois JA, Thomas KE, et al. Incidence of traumatic brain injury in the United States, 2003. *J Head Trauma Rehabil.* 2006;21(6):544–548.
2. Hymel KP, Bandak FA, Partington MD, et al. Abusive head trauma? A biomechanics based approach. *Child Maltreat.* 1998;3:116–128.
3. Yoshino A, Hovda DA, Kawamata T, et al. Dynamic changes in local cerebral glucose utilization following cerebral concussion in rats: evidence of hyper and subsequent hypometabolic state. *Brain Res.* 1991;561:106–119.
4. Hovda DA, Yoshino A, Kawamata T, et al. Diffuse prolonged depression of cerebral oxidative metabolism following concussive brain injury in the rat: a cytochrome oxidase histochemistry study. *Brain Res.* 1991;567:1–10.
5. Bailes JE, Cantu RC. Head injury in athletes. *Neurosurgery.* 2001;48:26–45.
6. Longhi L, Saatman KE, Fujimoto et al. Temporal window of vulnerability to repetitive experimental concussive brain injury. *Neurosurgery.* 2006;56(2):364–374.
7. Collins MW, Field M, Lovell MR, et al. Relationship between post concussion headache and neuropsychological

test performance in high school athletes. *Am J Sports Med.* 2003;31(2):168–173.

8. Bouma GJ, Muizelaar JP. Relationship between cardiac output and cerebral blood flow in patients with intact and with impaired autoregulation. *J Neurosurg.* 1990;73:368–374.

9. Stiell IG, Wells GA, Vandemheen K, et al. The Canadian CT Head Rule for patients with minor head injury. *Lancet.* 2001;357:1391–1396.

10. Shravat BP, Huseyin TS, Hynes KA. NICE guideline for the management of head injury: an audit demonstrating its impact on a district general hospital, with a cost analysis for England and Wales. *Emerg Med J.* 2006;23(2):109–113.

11. Willis AP, Latif SAA, Chandratre S, et al. Not a NICE CT protocol for the acutely head injured child. *Clin Radiol.* 2008;63:165–169.

12. Palchak MJ, Holmes JF, Vance CW, et al. A decision rule for identifying children at low risk for brain injuries after blunt head trauma. *Ann Emerg Med.* 2003;24:492–506.

13. Brody AS, Frush DP, Huda W, et al. Radiation risk to children from computed tomography. *Pediatrics.* 2007;120(3):677–682.

14. Norlund A, Marke L-A, af Geijerstam JL, et al. Immediate computed tomography or admission for observation after mild head injury: cost comparison in randomized, controlled trial. *BMJ.* 2006;333:469–471.

15. af Geijerstam JL, Oredsson S, Britton M, et al. Medical outcome after immediate computed tomography or admission for observation in patients with mild head injury: randomized controlled trial. *BMJ.* 2006;333:465.

16. Schutzman SA, Barnes P, Duhaime A-C, et al. Evaluation and management of children younger than two years old with apparently minor head trauma: proposed guidelines. *Pediatrics.* 2001;107(5):983–993.

17. Committee on Quality Improvement, American Academy of Pediatrics. The management of minor closed head injury in children. *Pediatrics.* 1999;104(6):1407–1415.

18. Rivara F, Taniguchi D, Parish RA, et al. Poor prediction of positive computed tomographic scans by clinical criteria in symptomatic pediatric head trauma. *Pediatrics.* 1987;80:579–584.

19. Davis RL, Mullen N, Makela M, et al. Cranial computed tomography scans in children after minimal head injury with loss of consciousness. *Ann Emerg Med.* 1994;24:640–645.

20. Boran BO, Boran P, Barut N, et al. Evaluation of mild head injury in a pediatric population. *Pediatr Neurosurg.* 2006;42:203–207.

21. Dacey RG Jr, Alves WM, Rimel RW, et al. Neurosurical complications after apparently minor head injury: assessment of risk in a series of 610 patients. *J Neurosurg.* 1986;65:203–210.

22. Hahn YS, McLone DG. Risk factors in the outcome of children with minor head injury. *Pediatr Neurosurg.* 1993;19:135–142.

23. Rosenthal BW, Bergman I. Intracranial injury after moderate head trauma in children. *J Pediatr.* 1989;115(3):346–350.

24. Teasdale GM, Murray G, Anderson E, et al. Risks of acute traumatic intracranial complications in hematoma in children and adults: implications for head injuries. *Br Med J.* 1990;300:363–367.

25. American Academy of Pediatrics. The management of minor closed head trauma in children. *Pediatrics.* 1999;104:1407–1415.

26. Hollingworth W, Vavilala MS, Jarvik FG, et al. The use of repeated head computed tomography in pediatric blunt head trauma: factors predicting new and worsening brain injury. *Pediatr Crit Care Med.* 2007;8(4):348–356.

27. Lovell MR, Collins MW, Iverson GL, et al. Recovery from mild concussion in high school athletes. *J Neurosurg.* 2003;98:296–301.

28. Satz P, Aucha K, McCleary C, et al. Mild head injury in children and adolescents: a review of studies (1970–1995). *Psychol Bull.* 1997;122(2):107–131.

29. Ponsford J, Wilmott C, Rothwell A, et al. cognitive and behavioral outcome following mild traumatic head injury in children. *J Head Trauma Rehabil.* 1999;14(4):360–372.

30. Bijur PE, Haslum M, Golding J. Cognitive outcomes of multiple mild head injuries in children. *J Dev Behav Pediatr.* 1996;17(3):143–148.

31. McKinlay A, Dalrymple-Alford JC, Horwood LJ, et al. Long term psychosocial outcomes after mild head injury in early childhood. *J Neurol Neurosurg Psychiatry.* 2002;73(3):281–288.

32. Cantu RC. Second impact syndrome: immediate management. *Phys Sports Med.* 1992;20:55–66.

33. Cantu RC, Voy R. Second Impact Syndrome: a risk in any contact sport. *Phys Sports Med.* 1995;23:27–34.

34. McCrory P, Johnston KM, Mohtadi, et al. Evidence-based review of sport-related concussion: basic science. *Clin J Sport Med.* 2001;11:160–165.

35. Yeates KO, Taylor HG. Neurobehavioral outcomes of mild head injury in children and adolescents. *Pediatr Rehabil.* 2005;8(1):5–16.

36. Ponsford J, Willmott C, Rothwell A, et al. Impact of early intervention on outcome after mild traumatic brain injury in children. *Pediatrics.* 2001;108(6):1297–1303.

37. Guskiewicz KM, Bruce SL, Cantu RC, et al. National Athletic Trainers' Association position statement: management of sport-related concussion. *J Athl Train.* 2004;39:280–297.

38. Canadian Academy of Sport Medicine Concussion Committee. Guidelines for assessment and management of sport-related concussion. *Clin J Sport Med.* 2000;209–211.

39. Cantu RC. Second-impact syndrome. *Clin Sports Med.* 1998;17:37–44.

40. McCrory P. Does second impact syndrome exist? *Clin J Sport Med.* 2001;11:144–149.

41. Robadi MH, Jordan BD. The cumulative effect of repetitive concussion in sports. *Clin J Sports Med.* 2001;11:194–198.

42. Guskiewicz KM, McCrea M, Marshall SW, et al. Cumulative effects associated with recurrent concussion in collegiate football players: the NCAA Concussion Study. *JAMA.* 2003;290:2549–2555.

43. Johnson KM, Bloom GA, Ramsay J, et al. Current concepts in concussion rehabilitation. *Curr Sports Med Rep.* 2004;3:316–323.

44. McCrory P, Johnston KM, Aubry M et al. Summary and agreement statement of the 2nd International Conference on Concussion in Sport, Prague 2004. *Clin J Sport Med.* 2005;15:48–55.

45. Haykowsky M, Eves N, Warburton D, et al. Resistance exercise, the Valsalva maneuver and cerebrovascular transmural pressure. *Med Sci Sports Exerc.* 2003;35:65–68.

46. Patel DR, Shivdasani V, Baker RJ. Management of sport-related concussion in young athletes. *Sports Med.* 2005;35(8):671–684.

CHAPTER 16

Approach to the Patient with Rash

Elizabeth Turner and Gregory Garra

▶ HIGH-YIELD FACTS

- Primary lesions are uncomplicated abnormalities which represent the initial pathologic change. Secondary changes reflect progression of disease such as excoriation, infection, or keratinization.
- The physician must search for the primary lesion, look at the morphology and grouping to reach a diagnosis, and must know the pattern of emergency dermatologic conditions.
- The clinician must recognize, and communicate to the patient, that there are times when it is difficult to narrow the final diagnosis to a single entity.

▶ GENERAL INTRODUCTION

An emergency physician may be faced with a vast range of dermatologic problems in a busy emergency department (ED). At any given time, there may be a case of simple urticaria or a more serious presentation of Stevens–Johnson syndrome (SJS) waiting to be seen. The role of the emergency physician is not necessarily to diagnose every dermatologic "zebra" but rather to distinguish the benign from the malignant and those conditions which need urgent care from those which do not. Recognizing these distinctions necessitates expertise and significant experience. In the following pages, we outline an approach that will assist the emergency physician in making these decisions. We hope to simplify an approach for the novice physician and expand the realm of diagnosable pathology for the more experienced physician.

▶ HISTORY AND PHYSICAL

HISTORY

Physicians are taught, early in training, that the key to any successful diagnosis is a thorough history and physical. One must have a systematic approach to provide appropriate care in a timely fashion. Any systematic approach is designed to be applied broadly knowing that certain patients will need additional evaluations. Sometimes, we visualize one problem and assume that it is the primary reason for the patient's visit to the ED. In fact, it is prudent to ask the patient specifically and not make assumptions as their concerns may be more

extensive or entirely different. The history component can be broken down to a series of questions including:

1. What specifically prompted the patient to seek medical care? What do they think is causing the rash?
2. Where are the lesions? Where did the lesions originate?
3. When did the lesions first develop and what has been the progression of the rash?
4. Was there any prodrome to the lesions? What are the associated symptoms?
5. How does it feel? Does it itch, hurt, sting, etc.?
6. What made it better or worse? What treatment was applied?
7. How is the patient's general health including allergies? What medications do they take regularly or intermittently?
8. What kind of exposures have they had, including occupation (applicable for adolescent population), travel, foods, and contacts?
9. Family history of any skin-related disorders?

PHYSICAL

Dermatology is a visual specialty and diagnosis relies heavily on careful inspection of the skin. The examination should be performed in a well-lit area where you can examine the entire skin surface including mouth, scalp, and nails. Physical examination depends largely on inspection. Palpation of the rash confirms consistency and depth. The entire eruption should be visualized to evaluate distribution and configuration. After evaluation of the eruption at a distance, individual lesions are examined. For purposes of this systematic approach, the most important objective of the physical examination is to characterize the morphology of the primary lesion. A thorough description of a rash should include morphology, color, configuration, and distribution.

MORPHOLOGY

Morphology describes the general appearance of a rash and can be described in terms of primary and secondary lesions.[1–3] Primary lesions are uncomplicated abnormalities which represent the initial pathologic change. Secondary changes reflect progression of disease such as excoriation, infection, or keratinization. The morphologic expression of a dermatologic condition is the basic entity on which all diagnoses are founded.

In some cases, the appearance is distinctive enough to make a diagnosis at a glance (i.e., the grouped vesicular lesions of herpes simplex). In other cases, the appearance may be modified by scratching, secondary infection, or prior treatment. Most importantly, it is important to recognize that skin disease may evolve overtime.

Primary Lesions

Macule: Circumscribed, flat discoloration <1 cm in diameter, examples include ash-leaf spots, flat nevi, and freckle. Macules may constitute the whole or part of a rash or may represent the early phase.

Patch: Flat discoloration that is >1 cm in diameter, circumscribed, flat discoloration, examples include vitiligo or tinea versicolor. Patches often have a very fine scale on the surface (i.e., pityriasis alba).

Papule: Circumscribed, superficial, solid elevated lesion <1 cm in diameter, examples include warts, elevated nevi, insect bites, and molluscum contagiosum.

Plaque: >1 cm elevated, flat top, superficial lesion, examples include psoriasis and pityriasis rosea.

Vesicle: Fluid-filled lesion <1 cm in diameter, examples include herpes simplex and varicella.

Bulla: Fluid-filled lesion >1 cm in diameter, examples include staph scalded skin syndrome and bullous impetigo.

Pustule: Vesicle with purulent exudate, examples include acne and folliculitis.

Nodule: Lesion <1 cm in diameter with depth, may be subsurface, suprasurface, or at level of surface, examples include secondary/tertiary syphilis.

Tumor: >1 cm solid lesion with depth, which may be subsurface, suprasurface, or at level of surface.

Petechiae: Pinpoint <1 cm flat, round red spots under the skin surface, because of deposits of blood and/or pigment, examples include drug eruption, Rocky Mountain spotted fever.

Purpura: >1 cm visible collection blood/pigment, examples include Henoch–Scholein purpura and idiopathic thrombocytopenia purpura.

Wheal: Transient, edematous papule, or plaque with pale center and pink margin, peripheral erythema, examples include hives and insect bites.

Secondary Lesions

Scale: Dry or greasy masses of keratin ranging from fine and delicate to coarse. Generally implies a pathologic process in the epidermis.

Crust: Dried exudate (serum, pus, or blood).

Excoriation: Punctate or linear abrasions generally caused by scratching.

Fissure: Linear crack or cleavage on skin, with sharply defined margins.

Ulcer: Depressed lesion because of epidermal or dermal tissue loss.

Scar: Permanent lesion results from process of repair by replacing connective tissue.

Lichenification: Area of increased epidermal thickness with accentuation of skin.

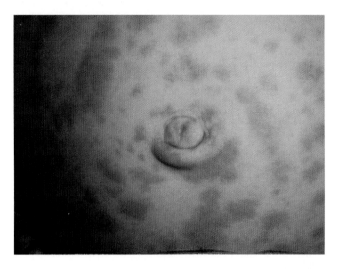

Figure 16–1. Coalescing papular lesions of a drug eruption.

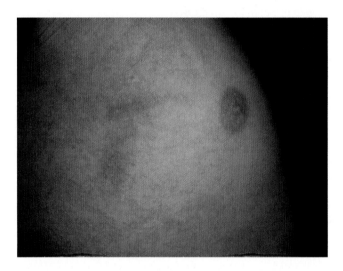

Figure 16–2. Sandpaper appearance (texture) of scarlet fever.

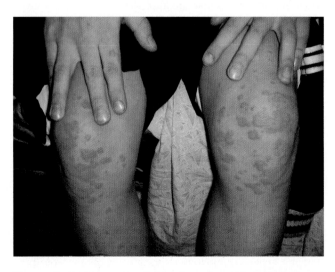

Figure 16–3. Symmetric distribution seen with erythema multiforme.

▶ DIAGNOSTIC FEATURES OF LESION

Rashes may present with few or numerous lesions. The primary morphologic lesion may be discrete or coalesce (Fig. 16–1). Distribution, configuration, and color are common diagnostic features. Additionally, findings such as the texture (i.e., the sandpaper texture of scarlet fever, Fig. 16–2) or other abnormalities such as a positive Nikolsky's sign (epithelial shearing caused by lateral pressure to unblistered skin) may assist in narrowing the diagnosis of a rash.

DISTRIBUTION

Many skin diseases have a preferential area of involvement. Eruptions may be widespread or may be localized to specific areas, for example, acne face; dermatophyte infection groin, foot, scalp; wrist scabies. Widespread lesions may demonstrate symmetry (Gianotti–Crosti syndrome or erythema multiforme, Fig. 16–3) or may be asymmetric distributed to different areas of the body (viral exanthema). Figure 16–4 illustrates common distributive patterns.

WIDESPREAD

SYMMETRICAL

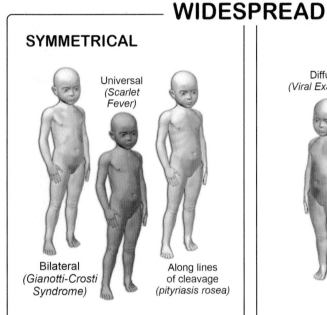

Universal
(Scarlet Fever)

Bilateral
(Gianotti-Crosti Syndrome)

Along lines of cleavage
(pityriasis rosea)

ASYMMETRICAL

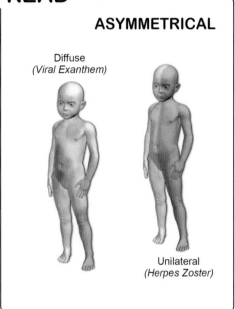

Diffuse
(Viral Exanthem)

Unilateral
(Herpes Zoster)

LOCALIZED

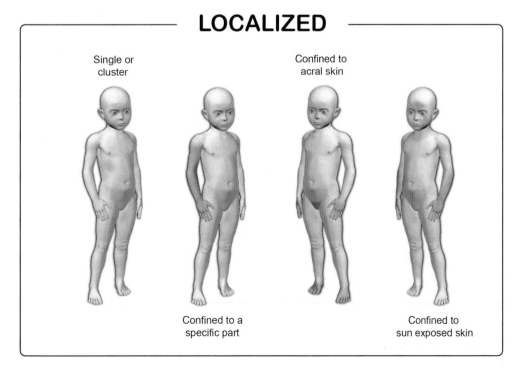

Single or cluster

Confined to acral skin

Confined to a specific part

Confined to sun exposed skin

Figure 16–4. Common distributions.

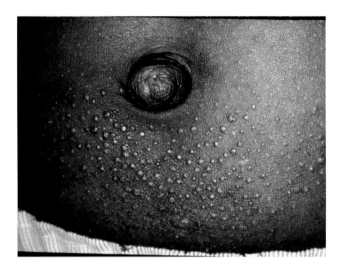

Figure 16–5. Grouped papules seen with molluscum contagiosum.

LINEAR

Rhus Dermatitis	Insect Bites	Herpes Zoster
Confluent	Discrete	Zosteriform

ARCIFORM

Bullous Impetigo	Granuloma Annular	Dermatophytosis	Cutaneous Larva Migrans
Arcuate	Annular	Polycyclic	Serpentine

CIRCULAR

Psoriasis	Eczema
Guttate	Nummular

GROUPED

Herpes Simplex	Spitz's Nevi	Verrucae	Candida
Herpetiform	Agminated	Corymbiform	Moniliform

Figure 16–6. Common configurations.

CONFIGURATION

Configuration is the general shape or pattern in which the lesions are arranged. Occasionally, the configuration is diagnostic of the disease. Lesions may be grouped into a pattern (i.e., grouped papules in molluscum contagiosum, Fig. 16–5) or form a specific shape (annular plaque of tinea corporis). Certain dermatologic conditions manifest in a typical configuration, for example, herpes simplex typically present with group vesicles. Figure 16–6 illustrates common configurations.

An Algorithmic Approach

Not uncommonly, the patient with a rash presents a diagnostic challenge to the emergency physician. Similar to the diagnosis of other conditions, a systematic approach to the disease may assist in narrowing the differential diagnosis. The approach described depends heavily on recognition of the primary lesion. Clinicians must be thorough in their attempt to identify the primary lesion. Once the primary lesion has been identified, diagnostic details should be sought; secondary changes, distribution, configuration. Lastly, historic features may help to further refine the diagnosis. Because of overlap of certain clinical conditions, the clinician must recognize (and communicate to the patient) that there are times when it is difficult to narrow the final diagnosis to a single entity. A common example is the febrile patient presenting with a generalized, confluent, erythematous papular rash who was placed on an antibiotic

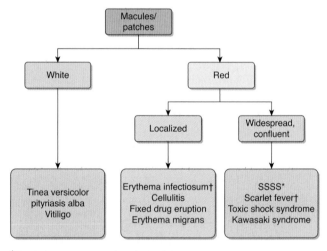

† Can appear as vesiculobullous disease in later stage
* May also present with papules and plaques

Tinea versicolor	Pink, tan or white, slighty scaling- KOH (+) is scraped
Pityriasis alba	poorly demarcated white, fine scale
Vitiligo	well demarcated, complete depigmentation
Erythema infectiosum	red cheeks followed by net like erythema on trunk
Cellulitis	cardinal signs of inflammation
Fixed drug eruption	violaceous, occuring within hours of offending drug ingestion
Erythema migrans	erythematous border with central clearing, lesion at least 5 cm

Figure 16–7. Algorithmic approach to a rash with macule/patch primary lesion.

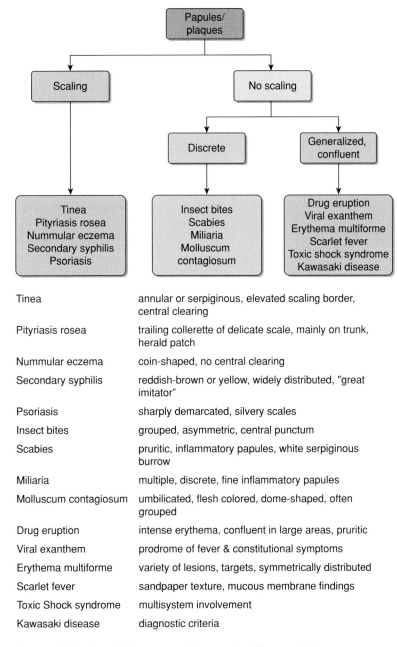

Figure 16–8. Algorithmic approach to a rash with papule/plaque primary lesion.

2 days prior to the eruption (viral exanthem versus drug eruption). Figures 16–7 to 16–11 illustrate an algorithmic approach to rashes based upon the primary lesion.

True Emergencies in the Pediatric Dermatologic Presentation

There are certain presentations which are imperative for the emergency physician to diagnose and initiate treatment. The following diseases are those that may result in significant morbidity and/or mortality if missed in the ED setting. We seek to provide only a brief summary of the red flag components of each disease that should alert the ED physician to institute management quickly.

Toxic epidermal necrolysis (TEN) and Stevens–Johnson syndrome (SJS). The typical presentation for each includes constitutional symptoms followed by skin lesions approximately 1 to 3 days later which are characterized by their mucosal membrane involvement. Patients are toxic appearing and this disease spectrum is notoriously rapid in its progression. The skin lesions generally begin as macules that eventually develop into blisters which may have a positive Nikolsky sign. History may be suggestive of recent or current pharmacologic exposures. Typical agents which have been known to cause TEN or SJS include the sulfa-containing drugs, aminopenicillins, quinolones, and cephalosporins. The rash tends to develop 1 to 3 weeks following initiation of drug.[4]

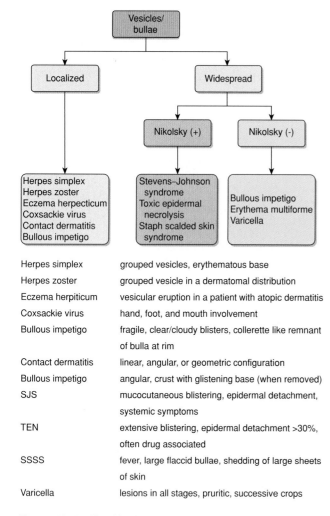

Herpes simplex	grouped vesicles, erythematous base
Herpes zoster	grouped vesicle in a dermatomal distribution
Eczema herpiticum	vesicular eruption in a patient with atopic dermatitis
Coxsackie virus	hand, foot, and mouth involvement
Bullous impetigo	fragile, clear/cloudy blisters, collerette like remnant of bulla at rim
Contact dermatitis	linear, angular, or geometric configuration
Bullous impetigo	angular, crust with glistening base (when removed)
SJS	mucocutaneous blistering, epidermal detachment, systemic symptoms
TEN	extensive blistering, epidermal detachment >30%, often drug associated
SSSS	fever, large flaccid bullae, shedding of large sheets of skin
Varicella	lesions in all stages, pruritic, successive crops

Figure 16–9. Algorithmic approach to a rash with vesicle/bulla primary lesion.

Staphylococcal scalded skin syndrome, an exfoliative dermatitis which often begins with constitutional symptoms followed by skin lesions that progress from generalized erythema to blisters that rupture leaving a painful red base. One key feature is perioral exudate. A Nikolsky sign is typically present.[5]

Toxic shock syndrome results from an exotoxin often linked to *Staphylococcus aureus* and presents with fever, headache, altered mental status, and scarletiniform skin lesions. GI symptoms including diarrhea and vomiting as well as hypotension are also often present.[6]

Kawasaki disease is a vasculitis which typically manifests in patients younger than 5 years, but may be seen in a child of any age. The disease process usually begins with a fever. The criteria for defining Kawasaki was recently revised and now includes: fever >5 days without another probable etiology as well as at least 4 of the following additional criteria:

– mucous membrane changes which may be injected pharynx, fissured lips, or the classic strawberry tongue.
– generalized erythema which evolves into a polymorphous rash.

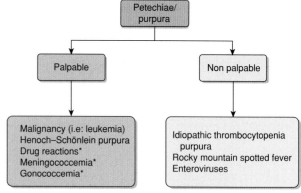

* may present as palpable or nonpalpable petechiae/purpura

Malignancy	systemic signs and symptoms
HSP	symmetric, acral distribution, abdominal or joint pain
Drug reactions	nontoxic appearance, history of exposure
Meningococcemia	influenza like illness with rapid progression
Gonococcemia	purpuric pustules, sparse, acral distribution, fever, arthralgia
ITP	pronounced on dependant areas, mucosal bleeding
RMSF	fever, headache, peripherally distributed
Enteroviruses	non toxic appearance, viral prodrome

Figure 16–10. Algorithmic approach to a rash with petechiae/purpura.

– cervical lymphadenopathy.
– bilateral conjunctival injection.
– edema (hands, feet).

There is no specific diagnostic test for Kawasaki; therefore, the clinical acumen of the practitioner is crucial in making this diagnosis.[7]

Meningococcemia. In the early stages, the pediatric patient with meningococcal disease can be difficult to differentiate from more benign disease processes. Meningeal infection often manifests as headache, fever, stiff neck, nausea,

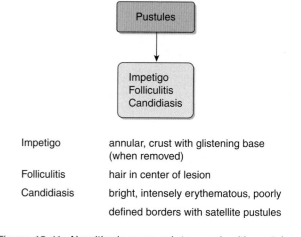

Impetigo	annular, crust with glistening base (when removed)
Folliculitis	hair in center of lesion
Candidiasis	bright, intensely erythematous, poorly defined borders with satellite pustules

Figure 16–11. Algorithmic approach to a rash with pustule primary lesion.

vomit, photophobia, and altered mental status. Infants are unable to communicate any of these clinical findings and clinical presentation may include flat fontanelles. The characterizing component of meningococcemia is sudden onset of fever and rash which is typically petechiae and purpura. Hypotension, adrenal failure, and multiorgan failure may be seen as well.[8]

Anaphylaxis, a life-threatening allergic reaction that manifests in the pediatric patient with urticaria, angioedema, wheezing, dyspnea, hypotension, as well as a myriad of other less common symptoms. Symptoms may develop within seconds to minutes of exposure.[9]

Purpura fulminans is a life-threatening disease that occurs abruptly. It is a hemorrhagic disease that is often seen in the setting of sepsis. The skin lesions ultimately result in perivascular hemorrhage and necrotic gangrene. The presentation typically includes fever, hypotension, and DIC.[10]

▶ CONCLUSION

In conclusion, the approach to the pediatric dermatology patient in the ED may appear daunting, however with a systematic approach, one can more readily and successfully arrive at a diagnosis and manage the patient effectively.

REFERENCES

1. MacKie RM. *Clinical Dermatology.* 4th ed. New York, NY: Oxford University Press; 1997:29–33.
2. Sauer GC, Hall JC. *Manual of Skin Diseases.* Philadelphia, PA: Lippincott-Raven Publishers; 1996:15–18.
3. Marks JG Jr, Miller JJ. *Lookinbill and Mark's Principles of Dermatology.* 4th ed. China: Saunders Elsevier; 2006:15–29.
4. Wolf R, Orion E, Marcos B, et al. Life-threatening acute adverse cutaneous drug reactions. *Clin Dermatol.* 2005;23:171.
5. Farrell AM. Staphylococcal scalded-skin syndrome. *Lancet.* 1999;354:880.
6. Ruocco E, Donnarumma G, Baroni A, et al. Bacterial and viral skin diseases. *Dermatol Clin.* 2007;25(4):663–676.
7. Burns JC, Glode MP. Kawasaki syndrome. *Lancet.* 2004;364: 533.
8. Rosenstein NE, Perkins BA, Stephens DA, et al. Meningococcal disease. *N Engl J Med.* 2001;344:1378–1388.
9. Zuberier T. Urticaria. *Allergy.* 2003;58:1224.
10. Leung AK, Chan KW. Evaluating the child with purpura. *Am Fam Physician.* 2001;64(3):419–425.

CHAPTER 17

Neck Masses

Raemma Paredes Luck

▶ HIGH-YIELD FACTS

- Reactive cervical lymphadenopathy and lymphadenitis are the most common causes of neck masses in children.
- Laboratory testing is often not necessary in the evaluation of cervical lymphadenopathy as the cause can usually be determined by the history and physical examination.
- An enlarged cervical mass that does not improve after 4 to 6 weeks needs to be referred to a subspecialist for further work-up.
- Congenital neck lesions can present even after the first decade of life often with an infection or obstruction.
- Supraclavicular lymphadenopathy in any age group is worrisome and should be investigated.

The emergency physician is often called upon to evaluate an infant or child with a neck mass. Most of these neck masses are benign and result from reactive lymph nodes caused by viral infections. On occasion, a patient can present with a significant neck mass of unknown etiology. The challenge is to distinguish between the pathologic lesions that need expeditious management versus those neck conditions that are benign but still cause a lot of parental anxiety. This chapter will discuss an approach to the pediatric patient presenting with a neck mass. Important elements of the history and physical examination will be highlighted and a discussion of the differential diagnoses and management options will be presented (see Fig. 17–1).

▶ ANATOMY

An understanding of the anatomy of the neck is important in generating a working differential diagnoses in a pediatric patient presenting with a neck mass. There are several anatomic classifications used in describing the location of neck lesions. A simple method is to divide the neck into two compartments or triangles with the sternocleidomastoid muscle as the common boundary (Fig. 17–1). The anterior compartment is defined by the anterior border of the sternocleidomastoid muscle, the lower border of the mandible, the sternum inferiorly, and a line extending from the submandibular symphysis to the sternal notch.[1] Vital structures located in this compartment include the larynx, trachea, esophagus, the thyroid and parathyroid glands, the carotid sheath, and the suprahyoid and infrahyoid muscles. Several lymph node chains are found in this area, including the jugulodigastric chain that lies anterior to the sternocleidomastoid muscle. The posterior compartment is defined inferiorly by the clavicle, laterally by the trapezius, and medially by the sternocleidomastoid muscle. Structures that are found in this area include the subclavian vessels, cervical roots of the brachial plexus, spinal accessory nerve, and also several lymph node chains.

Knowledge of the anatomy of the neck and the specific regions drained by the lymph node group will help the clinician in locating the primary infection. The posterior part of the tongue, tonsils, sinuses, nasopharynx, larynx, and pharyngeal regions drain into the superficial and deep anterior cervical lymph nodes. The anterior scalp, ear canal, pinna, and the conjunctiva drain into the preauricular lymph nodes; the temporal and parietal scalp regions drain into the postauricular nodes and the posterior scalp region drain into the occipital nodes. For example, scalp infections such as tinea capitis or folliculitis can cause occipital lymphadenopathy. Conjunctivitis can cause enlargement of the preauricular lymph nodes and when seen together is called the "oculoglandular syndrome." Infections of the cheek, anterior part of the nose, tongue, and buccal mucosa drain into the submandibular nodes. The right supraclavicular lymph nodes communicate with the lymphatics of the mediastinum while the left side communicates with the thoracic duct.[2]

The retropharyngeal, prevertebral, and parapharyngeal spaces are potential spaces extending from the base of the skull to the superior mediastinum, diaphragm, and to the hyoid cartilage, respectively.[3] An infection in one of these spaces can spread to the rest of the other spaces through the fascial planes.

Lastly, the short neck of a child relative to the large head makes it less susceptible to direct trauma. However, because a large number of vital structures are located in such a small area, even minor neck injuries can become potentially life-threatening.

▶ ASSESSMENT OF A PATIENT WITH A NECK MASS AND IN RESPIRATORY DISTRESS

An infant or a child presenting with a neck mass and respiratory distress should be managed according to the pediatric advanced life support (PALS) guidelines. Those with a history of a major traumatic injury should be managed according to the advanced trauma life support (ATLS) guidelines. A pediatric patient in respiratory distress who refuses to lie down should not be forced to do so, as it may precipitate cardiopulmonary arrest from a possible retropharyngeal or mediastinal mass compressing the trachea. Maintaining the airway is a top priority in a child with a neck mass and respiratory distress. Depending on the level of obstruction, administration of oxygen, a nasopharyngeal or oral airway, mask ventilation, or a

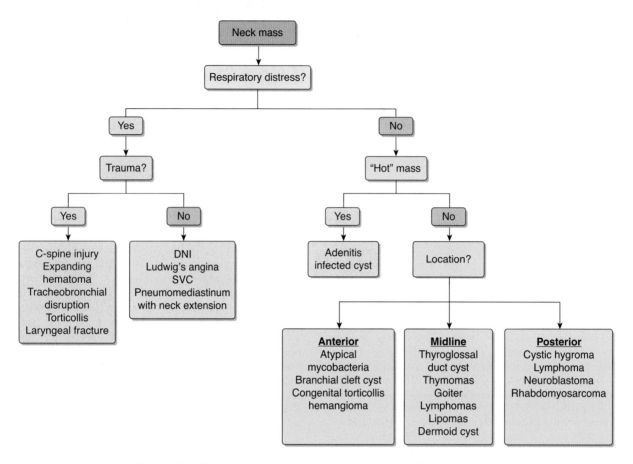

Figure 17–1. Algorithm on the management of a child with a neck mass.

laryngeal mask airway may be used to support a compromised airway. Endotracheal intubation may be necessary either using direct laryngoscopy or fiber-optic methods. A transtracheal jet ventilation may be lifesaving, although can be technically challenging in the young child. An urgent tracheotomy in an unsecured pediatric airway carries considerable risk and should be employed only when other methods fail.

Once the patient is stabilized, a brief history and a more detailed physical examination as to the cause of the patient's neck mass can be pursued. After a complete examination of the head region, note the consistency, size, and location of the neck mass, any deviation of the trachea, and presence of ecchymosis or subcutaneous emphysema. The progression of the neck mass and symptoms such as neck pain, dysphagia, stridor, drooling, hemoptysis or dysphonia should be noted. Also note any puncture wound, however minor, since this can be misleading and may result in a delay in diagnosis of significant injuries. A history of trauma to the neck in a child who is in distress should make the clinician entertain several possibilities including an expanding hematoma, tracheobronchial disruption, laryngeal injuries, or cervical spine injuries. These conditions are discussed more in depth in Chapter 30.

In the absence of trauma, a child presenting with dysphagia, stiff neck, trismus, stridor, or muffled speech should be suspected of having a deep neck infection. Deep neck space infections involving the retropharyngeal and parapharyngeal spaces are still potentially life-threatening conditions that continue to be seen despite the widespread use of antibiotics (Fig. 17–2).

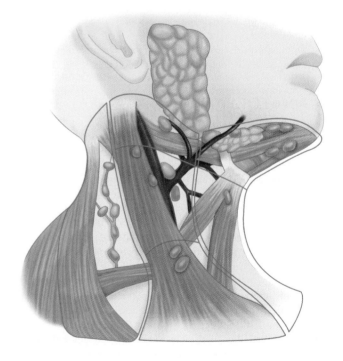

Figure 17–2. Triangles of the neck and location of lymph nodes.

▶ **TABLE 17-1. LIFE-THREATENING CAUSES OF NECK MASSES**

Traumatic	Inflammatory	Congenital	Neoplastic
Subcutaneous emphysema from tracheal/pulmonary injury Expanding hematoma	Deep neck infections Ludwig's angina Infected cysts	Large cystic hygroma	Hodgkin's lymphoma with mediastinal extension

These infections originate from a tonsillitis, pharyngitis, or sinusitis that had spread through the regional lymph nodes of the neck.[3,4] In a recent case series of patients with deep neck space infections, no etiology can be found in the majority of patients.[5] The usual organisms cultured are staphylococci, streptococci as well as anaerobic organisms. Complications of deep neck infections include spontaneous rupture into the pharynx, extension to the lateral side of the neck, or dissection into the mediastinum and prevertebral space leading to aspiration, airway obstruction, compression of major blood vessels, and death.[6] Therefore, a suspicion of a possible deep neck infection calls for early consultation with our surgical colleagues.

Other causes of respiratory distress in an infant with a neck mass are cystic hygromas and hemangiomas (Table 17–1). Cystic hygromas can extend from the tongue to the mediastinum and in rare cases, rapidly enlarge, causing extrinsic compression of the adjacent vital structures. Such rapid enlargement can occur secondary to trauma, infection, or hemorrhage into the cyst.[7]

▶ ASSESSMENT OF A PATIENT WITH A NECK MASS IN NO DISTRESS

The first critical step in the evaluation of a pediatric patient with a neck mass is a thorough history and physical examination. Details will help narrow the differential diagnoses. The age of the child is important because normal lymph node sizes vary with age. In the newborn period, lymph nodes are not palpable, as the infant has not yet been exposed to many antigens. Neck masses noted in this age group will be mostly congenital in origin. Over time, the size of the lymph nodes increases such that palpable or "shotty" nodes up to 1 cm in size in the cervical, axillary, and inguinal areas are considered normal and frequently seen without signs of infection.[2,8,9]

The duration of the neck mass is important. A painless mass noted since birth or shortly after birth suggests a congenital lesion. However, some congenital lesions may not be apparent until years later when there is an obstruction or infection causing it to mimic an inflammatory condition. Any history of neck pain, hoarseness, stridor, or dysphagia is worrisome and may be caused by a mass compressing on a nerve or a vital organ and therefore needs a more emergent workup. Presence of systemic symptoms such as fever, night sweats, fatigue, and weight loss is significant and suggests a systemic disease such as tuberculosis, sarcoidosis, or malignancy. A history of travel to another country or endemic area, exposure to animals, or ingestion of unpasteurized milk may also provide some clues to the cause of the neck mass.

Note any limitation in the range of motion of the neck as well as tilting toward one direction. Palpation may reveal crepitus suggesting leakage of air from the tracheobronchial tree. The size and consistency of the mass, its mobility, and location are important especially for congenital lesions that consistently appear at certain locations. For example, most branchial cleft sinuses or cysts are located in the lateral neck at the anterior border of the sternocleidomastoid muscle.[7,8,10] Thyroglossal duct cysts are usually located in the midline anywhere between the base of the tongue and the thyroid. These lesions move with tongue protusion. A soft, nontender, compressible mass in the posterior triangle of the neck is highly suggestive of a cystic hygroma while hemangiomas can be located anywhere in the neck.

Supraclavicular lymphadenopathy in any age group is a serious concern and should be promptly investigated for an underlying malignancy.[7,11] Other characteristics of a neck mass that should increase suspicion of a malignancy include the presence of irregular margins, hard consistency, size of more than 3 cm, adherence to surrounding areas and association with other systemic symptoms.[8,10,11]

Examination of the rest of the body is important to detect clues that will help in narrowing the differential diagnoses. For example, generalized lymphadenopathy is caused by a systemic illness such as human immunodeficiency virus (HIV) infection or tuberculosis. Splenomegaly in a child with exudative pharyngitis and enlarged cervical lymphadenopathy suggests infectious mononucleosis.

▶ DIFFERENTIAL DIAGNOSES

Adults who have an asymptomatic neck mass should be considered to have a malignancy until proven otherwise.[11] In contrast, majority of neck masses in children are benign in nature.[8,10,12] These neck masses can be classified into four general categories that include inflammatory, congenital, neoplastic, and traumatic conditions (Table 17–2).

INFLAMMATORY CONDITIONS

The vast majority of pediatric neck masses fall under this category. Viral upper respiratory tract infection is the most common cause of bilateral cervical lymph node enlargement. Other viral infections such as pharyngitis, conjunctivitis, and stomatitis are causes easily identified on physical examination. It is not unusual for viral infections to cause nodal enlargement in two or more noncontiguous sites. Most cases of cervical lymphadenopathy are reactive in nature, self-limited, and require no treatment.

Bacterial infections of the head and neck often cause unilateral lymph node enlargement. Cervical adenitis results when this enlargement is accompanied by local tenderness, redness,

▶ **TABLE 17-2. DIFFERENTIAL DIAGNOSES OF NECK MASSES BY LOCATION AND ETIOLOGY[8,11,13]**

	Anterior Triangle	Midline	Posterior Triangle
Inflammatory	Adenitis from various causes	Adenitis	Adenitis
	Reactive adenopathy	Thyroiditis	Sialadenitis
	Parotitis	Ludwig's angina	
	Atypical mycobacteria		
Congenital	Branchial cleft cyst	Thyroglossal duct cyst	Cystic hygroma
	Laryngocoele	Dermoid cyst	
	Congenital torticollis		
Neoplastic	Hemangioma	Thymomas	Lymphoma
	Neurogenic tumors	Lymphoma	Metastatic lesions
	Salivary gland tumors	Lipoma	Neuroblastoma
		Goiter	Rhabdomyosarcomas
Traumatic	Hematoma	Laryngeal fracture	Hematoma
	Acquired torticollis		Acquired torticollis

and warmth (Fig. 17–3). This is usually accompanied by systemic symptoms such as fever and irritability. Because 80% of all cases of acute adenitis are caused by *Streptococcus* and *Staphylococcus*, the antimicrobial therapy of choice is a first-generation cephalosporin, oxacillin, or clindamycin.[9] Anaerobic organisms should be considered when the cause of the adenitis is from an odontogenic infection. Failure to respond to oral antibiotics, abscess formation, concomitant cellulitis, or systemic toxicity necessitates hospitalization for intravenous antibiotics (Fig. 17–4). Computed tomography (CT) of the neck with contrast or ultrasonography is helpful in distinguishing a lesion that has progressed into an abscess that may require incision and drainage.

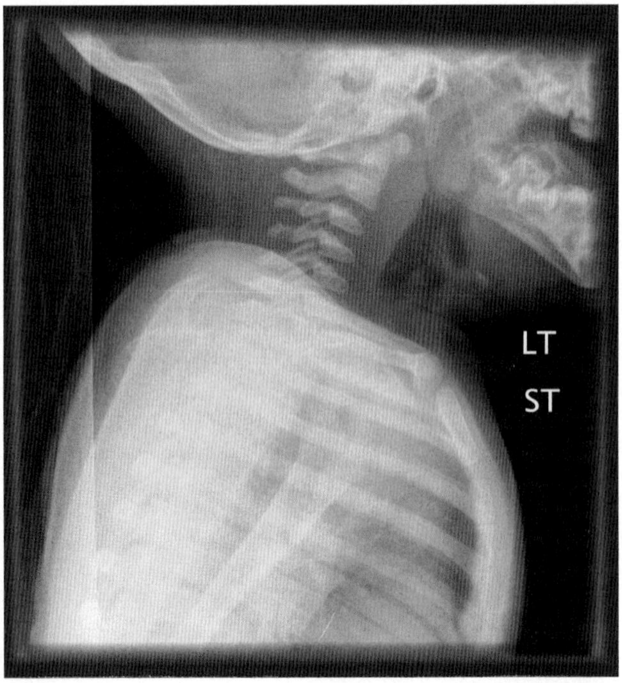

Occasionally, the emergency physician may encounter a patient with a neck mass that is minimally tender, nonfluctuant, slowly enlarging over a few days or weeks with no obvious source or systemic symptoms. The differential diagnoses of such a mass is wide and consideration should be given to atypical mycobacterium as well as mycobacterium tuberculosis infection, infectious mononucleosis, cat scratch disease, HIV infection, sarcoidosis, actinomycosis, and toxoplasmosis. If a patient has not been treated, a course of an appropriate oral antibiotic is indicated with close follow-up to assess response to treatment. Ancillary testing may be initiated depending on the history and physical examination. This may include a complete blood count and a chest radiograph to detect pulmonary infiltrates or mediastinal adenopathy. Persistence of the mass despite antibiotics, suspicion of malignancy, or other esoteric etiology necessitates a referral to an infectious disease specialist or to an otolaryngologist for a biopsy.

Figure 17–3. Lateral neck of a child with a retropharyngeal abscess showing widening of the retrophayngeal space.

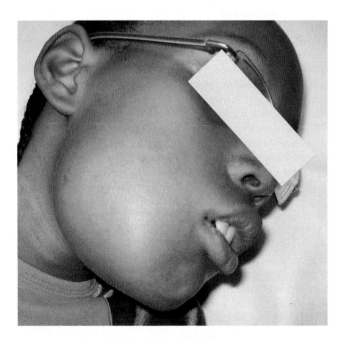

Figure 17–4. Right submandibular neck abscess.

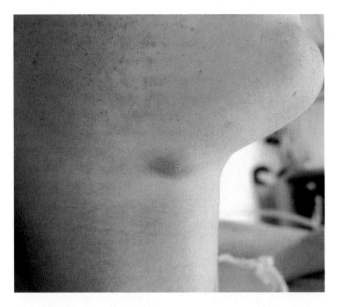

Figure 17–5. Atypical mycobacterial infection of the neck. (Courtesy of Glenn Issacson, MD, Temple University School of Medicine.)

Atypical mycobacteria also known as nontubercular mycobacteria (NTM) and in particular, mycobacterium avium complex (MAC), presents as a chronic cervical adenitis. This is usually seen in children between 1 and 5 years of age. The bacteria gain entry from a breakdown in the mucous membranes of the oropharynx and tonsils and then invade the regional lymph nodes. The usual presentation is that of an enlarged lymph node in the submandibular region that has a rubbery consistency, minimal tenderness, and a dull reddish color (Fig. 17–5). Occasionally, a draining sinus is present (Fig. 17–6). The treatment of choice is complete surgical resection or curettage of the node as most atypical mycobacteria respond poorly to antibiotics.[13]

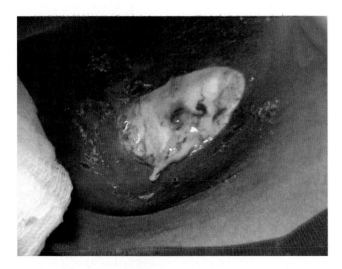

Figure 17–6. Draining sinus in atypical mycobacteria. (Courtesy of Christopher Russo, MD, St. Christopher's Hospital for Children.)

Bartonella henselae, the organism responsible for cat scratch disease, is a common cause of regional lymphadenopathy. The enlarged node usually involves the axillary area but occasionally can affect the cervical, epitrochlear, or inguinal nodes as well. Recent contact with a cat or kitten can be obtained in the majority of patients. A papule at the site of the inoculation is frequently noted, followed in 1 to 2 weeks by the development of tender, indurated, erythematous skin overlying the enlarged node in the lymphatic chain that drains the site of infection. Systemic symptoms such as fever and malaise are seen in about a third of the patients. Management consists of symptomatic relief, as the disease is usually self-limited, resolving spontaneously in 2 to 4 months. In patients with systemic involvement or painful adenitis, antibiotics such as trimethoprim-sulfamethoxazole, rifampin, azithromycin, ciprofloxacin, or parenteral gentamicin may be effective in ameliorating symptoms.[14]

Other inflammatory conditions to consider are infections of the salivary glands or sialadenitis. This can present as a tender and swollen mass in the area of the submandibular or parotid glands. Occasionally, the condition can be bilateral as in parotitis caused by the mumps virus. Majority can be treated with conservative measures such as hydration, pain relief, application of moist heat, and sialogogues. In those with bacterial superinfection, broad-spectrum antibiotics effective against staphylococcus, streptococcus, and anaerobic flora should be initiated.

TRAUMATIC CONDITIONS

Minor trauma to the neck and a variety of other conditions can cause spasm of the cervical muscles, primarily the sternocleidomastoid. Underlying etiologies of torticollis include upper respiratory infection, cervical adenitis, retropharyngeal abscess, atlantoaxial rotatory subluxation and rarely, dystonic reactions or intracranial and spinal cord tumors.[15,16] Major traumatic injuries to the neck are covered in Chapter 30.

Congenital torticollis is suspected when an infant, usually at 2 to 8 weeks of age, presents with an ipsilateral neck mass with the head tilted toward it and the chin in the opposite direction. The cause of congenital torticollis is still not clear, although it may be related to bleeding into the sternocleidomastoid muscle from a difficult delivery.[17] The onset of marked facial hypoplasia or asymmetry is an indication for surgical transection of the middle third of the affected sternocleidomastoid muscle.[18]

CONGENITAL MASSES

Hemangiomas are the most common congenital lesions of the head and neck. These lesions are red or purplish in color, flat or raised, and blanch with pressure. They grow rapidly in the first few months of life, slowly regress afterwards, and may even disappear with time. Close observation is the rule unless the lesions cause airway obstruction, high-output cardiac failure, thrombocytopenia or hemorrhage, and coagulopathy (Kasabach–Merritt syndrome).

Thyroglossal duct cysts arise from the vestiges of the thyroglossal duct that runs in the middle of the neck from the base

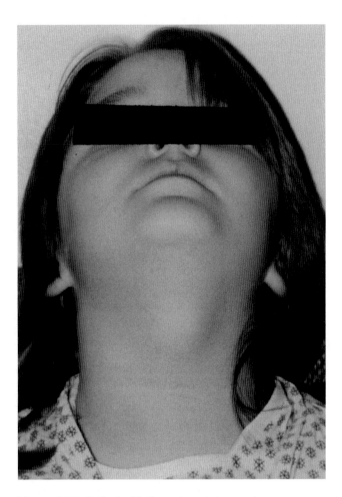

Figure 17–7. Patient with thyroglossal duct cyst.

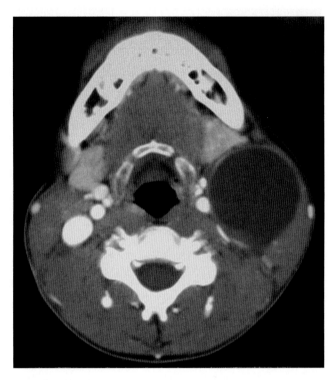

Figure 17–8. CT scan of an infected brachial cleft cyst. (Courtesy of William Collins, MD, University of Florida, Gainsville.)

of the tongue to the thyroid gland (Fig. 17–7). These cysts enlarge after bouts of upper respiratory infections. One clue that points toward a thyroglossal cyst aside from its midline location is that protusion of the tongue will retract the lesion. Majority of these cysts manifests between the age of 2 and 10 years, although a third do not become apparent until after the second decade of life.[8,19] Infection is common because of the persistent communication with the base of the tongue and the oral flora. Once the infection has been treated, surgical excision to remove the cyst and its entire tract can follow.

When primordial lymphatic ducts fail to establish drainage into the venous system, multiloculated cystic masses or cystic hygromas are formed. These lesions are found in areas where lymphatic ducts drain into large veins such as the neck, axilla, and mediastinum. The left side of the neck is frequently involved because it is where the thoracic duct enters the subclavian vein.[7] Majority of the lesions are identified at birth, although some may not be diagnosed until the second decade of life or unless they become infected. There is a strong association between congenital cystic hygromas of the neck and Turner syndrome.[20,21]

Anomalous development of the branchial arches and cleft produces brachial cysts, sinuses, fistulae, or skin tags in the neck. Most branchial cleft anomalies originate from the second cleft. These painless cysts or sinuses are usually seen at the anterior border of the middle to lower third of the sternocleidomastoid muscle. They can become secondarily infected (Fig. 17–8). Brachial cysts are more commonly diagnosed after the first decade of life while fistulas are usually diagnosed shortly after birth.[7,8]

NEOPLASTIC MASSES

Malignant neoplasms of the head and neck account for approximately 5% of all malignancies in childhood.[22] Ninety percent of neck cancers in children are mesenchymal in origin in contrast to adults where the squamous cell line is involved.[23] The most common malignancies of the neck are lymphomas (Hodgkin and non-Hodgkin lymphomas) and soft tissue sarcomas, primarily rhabdomyosarcoma. The neck is second to the orbit as a common site of rhabdomyosarcoma. The tumor presents as a rapidly enlarging, painless neck mass that is hard and immobile. Other tumors include neuroblastoma and lymph node metastasis from malignancies of the skin and thyroid. These masses tend to be hard and fixed to the underlying structures.

▶ ANCILLARY TESTING

The vast majority of neck masses are the result of inflammatory or infectious causes that are detected by history and physical examination. Therefore, laboratory testing is often not necessary. A neck mass that is rapidly enlarging does not respond to the standard antibiotic regimen or has been present for a few weeks needs further laboratory and radiographic evaluation to narrow the cause. A complete blood count with differential, and either erythrocyte sedimentation rate or C-reactive protein may be obtained.

Chest radiographs can detect pulmonary infiltrates or mediastinal involvement in patients suspected of having tuberculosis, sarcoidosis, or primary lung tumors. CT or magnetic resonance imaging (MRI) can help differentiate vascular, solid, or cystic lesions. They can delineate the location of a mass and its relation to other structures in the neck. Occasionally, the CT scan or MRI can identify a source of infection or the primary tumor. For deep pediatric neck infections, the accuracy of CT scans in differentiating between an abscess and a cellulitis has recently been questioned by several investigators, with one study showing an overall accuracy of only 63%.[24–26] Ultrasonography has also been used in differentiating solid from cystic lesions.

Children with chronic or subacute lymphadenopathy should have a purified protein derivative (PPD) tuberculin test done to exclude mycobacterial infections. However, in atypical mycobacterial infections, majority of the chest radiographs are normal and the PPD are usually negative or intermediate.

▶ DISPOSITION

When the history and physical examination point to a benign condition, the emergency physician should provide parental reassurance. Cervical lymphadenopathy in response to specific infections is the most common cause of neck masses. Treatment of the underlying cause is sufficient in most cases. A patient with an acute "hot" neck node deserves a trial of antibiotics with close follow-up. Indications for hospitalization include failure of oral antibiotics with progression of symptoms, suspicion of a deep neck infection, systemic toxicity, or respiratory distress. Indications for a surgical referral include persistence of the neck mass after 4 weeks; an increase in size during that time; mass size of more than 3 cm; supraclavicular location; and systemic signs and symptoms suggestive of a malignancy.[8,10,12]

REFERENCES

1. Lin D, Descher D. Neck masses. In: Lalwani A, ed. *Current Diagnosis & Treatment in Otolaryngology—Head and Neck Surgery*. 2nd ed. New York: McGraw-Hill; 2007.
2. Friedmann A. Evaluation and management of lymphadenopathy in children. *Pediatr Rev*. 2008;29:53–59.
3. Nagy M, Pizzuto M, Backstrom J, Brodsky L. Deep neck infections in children: a new approach to diagnosis and treatment. *Laryngoscope*. 1997;107:1627–1634.
4. Ungkanont K, Yellon RF, Weissman J, et al. Head and neck space infections in infants and children. *Otolaryngol Head Neck Surg*. 1995;112:375–382.
5. Ridder K, Technau-Ihling K, Sander A, Boedeker C. Spectrum and management of deep neck space infections: an 8-year ex-

perience of 234 cases. *Otolaryngol Head Neck Surg*. 2005;133: 709–714.
6. Brook I. Microbiology and management of peritonsillar, retropharyngeal, and parapharyngeal abscesses. *J Oral Maxillofac Surg*. 2004;62:1545–1550.
7. Brown R, Azizkhan R. Pediatric head and neck lesions. *Pediatr Clin North Am*. 1998;45:889–905.
8. Park Y. Evaluation of neck masses in children. *Am Fam Physician*. 1995;51:1904–1912.
9. Peters T, Edwards K. Cervical lymphadenopathy and adenitis. *Pediatr Rev*. 2000;21:399–404.
10. McGuirt WF. Differential Diagnosis of Neck Masses. In: Charles WC, et al. eds. *Cummings: Otolaryngology: Head and Neck Surgery*, 4th ed. Philadelphia, PA: Mosby, Inc. 2005.
11. Soldes OS, Younger JG, Hirschl RB. Predictors of malignancy in childhood peripheral lymphadenopathy. *J Pediatr Surg*. 1999;34:1447–1452.
12. Torsiglieri AJ Jr, Tom LW, Ross AJ III, et al. Pediatric neck masses: guidelines for evaluation. *Int J Pediatr Otorhinolaryngol*. 1988;16:199–210.
13. American Academy of Pediatrics. Diseases caused by nontuberculous mycobacteria. In: Pickering LK, ed. *Red Book: Report of the Committee on Infectious Diseases*. Elk Grove Village, IL: American Academy of Pediatrics; 2006:698–704.
14. American Academy of Pediatrics. Cat-scratch disease. In: Pickering LK, ed. *Red Book: Report of the Committee on Infectious Diseases*. Elk Grove Village, IL: American Academy of Pediatrics; 2006:246–248.
15. Bredenkamp JK, Maceri DR. Inflammatory torticollis in children. *Arch Otolaryngol Neck Head Surg*. 1990;116:310–313.
16. Muniz AC, Belfer RA. Atlantoaxial rotary subluxation in children. *Pediatr Emerg Care*. 1990;15:25–29.
17. Cheng JC, Au AW. Infantile torticollis: a review of 624 cases. *J Pediatr Orthop*. 1994;14:802–808.
18. Cheng JC, Tang SP, Chen TM. Sternocleidomastoid pseudotumor and congenital muscular torticollis in infants: a prospective study of 510 cases. *J Pediatr*. 1999;134:712–716.
19. Koeller KK, Alamo L, Adair CF. Congenital cystic masses of the neck: radiographic-pathologic correlation. *Radiographics*. 1999;19:121–146.
20. Baena N, De Vigan C, Cariati E, et al. Turner syndrome: evaluation of prenatal diagnosis in 19 European countries. *Am J Med Genet* (A). 2004;129:16–20.
21. Gedikbasi A, Gul A, Sarquin A, Ceylan Y. Cystic hygroma and lymphangioma: associated findings, perinatal outcomes and prognostic factors in live-born infants. *Arch Gynecol Obstet*. 2007;276:491–498.
22. Bonilla JA, Healy GB. Management of malignant head and neck tumors in children. *Pediatr Clin North Am*. 1989;36:1443–1450.
23. May M. Neck Masses in children: diagnosis and treatment. *Ear Nose Throat J*. 1978;57:136–158.
24. Vural C, Gungor A, Comerci S. Accuracy of computerized tomography in deep neck infections in the pediatric population. *Amer J Otolaryngol*. 2003;24:143–148.
25. Sichel JY, Gomori J, Saah D, Elidan J. Parapharyngeal abscess in children: the role of CT for diagnosis and treatment. *Int J Pediatr Otolaryngol*. 1996;35:213–222.
26. Stone et al. Correlation between computed tomography and surgical findings in retropharyngeal inflammatory processes in children. *Int J Pediatr Otorhinolaryngol*. 1999;49:121–125.

CHAPTER 18

Neonatal Emergencies

Alfred Sacchetti

▶ HIGH-YIELD FACTS

- Because of a neonate's limited number of activities, presenting symptoms are rather limited.
- Every sick neonate must have a bedside blood sugar checked as soon as possible and hypoglycemia treated immediately.
- Children with both pulmonary and cardiac defects can appear normal initially because of the existence of the foramen ovale and the ductus arteriosus, with symptoms appearing days after discharge when the right and left sides of the heart become completely isolated.
- Inborn errors of metabolism associated with well-defined clinical syndromes are generally identified early. In contrast, those conditions associated with a single hormone or enzyme defect may go undetected until a toxic metabolite accumulates or an electrolyte or endocrine catastrophe occurs.
- An ominous sign in any newborn is bilious emesis.

The first 30 days of the life of a child can be a very revealing time in the life of a child both for parents and for medical personnel. In utero, the fetus is protected from metabolic and anatomic anomalies by its relationship with the placenta and maternal circulation. Once delivery occurs, the child must be self-sustaining; and if a congenital problem exists, maternal compensatory effects are no longer available.

Aside from the expansion of the lungs, most of the physiologic changes associated with birth occur gradually. As such, many congenital problems will not become clinically evident until hours to weeks after birth and may not occur until after discharge from the nursery.

Because of a neonate's limited number of activities, presenting symptoms are rather limited. Changes in level of consciousness, respiratory distress, feeding or stooling difficulties, or abnormal motor activities are complaints that lead a parent to bring their infant to the emergency department (ED). Unfortunately, the specific cause of the presenting symptoms may have nothing to do with the origin of the child's pathology, and it is the emergency physicians' responsibility to discover the underlying cause of the concerning behavior. This chapter will discuss the ED presentation and management of these neonatal emergencies.

Because of the limited history and physical findings in this age group, much of the evaluation of ill-appearing neonates is protocol driven. All sick neonates should have a capillary glucose determination and pulse oximetry as part of their initial assessment on arrival to the ED. Other studies that should be included as part of the ED evaluation are complete blood count, electrolyte panel with sodium, potassium, bicarbonate, calcium, glucose, BUN and creatinine, blood cultures, urinalysis, urine culture, and chest x-ray. Lumbar punctures, electrocardiograms, electroencephalograms, and diagnoses-specific studies may also be ordered as the clinical scenario dictates. Sepsis is the primary cause of an ill-appearing neonate and is discussed at length in Chapter 2.

▶ CARDIORESPIRATORY PRESENTATIONS

In utero, all oxygen requirements are handled through the placenta. Anatomic problems in the lungs and heart are masked because in effect the fetus requires only a single heart chamber to circulate oxygenated blood. In addition, because of multiple internal shunts within the heart, there are redundant pathways to circulate this blood. Oxygenated blood from the placenta returns to the right atrium where it mixes with blood from the superior and inferior vena cava. Although not anatomically directed, the more oxygenated placental blood flows preferentially through the foramen ovale into the left atrium while caval blood tends to flow through the tricuspid valve into the right ventricle. Additional shunting and mixing of blood occurs between the pulmonary artery and the aorta through the ductus arteriosus—an aorta-sized vessel connecting these two arteries.

At birth the foramen ovale will functionally close and the ductus arteriosus will begin to anatomically close, although the actual completion of this process will not be complete for 7 to 10 days. Concomitant with this, the initially high pulmonary pressures will fall toward their normal low-pressure state. Because of the existence of the foramen ovale and the ductus arteriosus, it is possible for children with both pulmonary and cardiac defects to appear normal initially, with symptoms appearing days after discharge when the right and left sides of the heart completely isolate.

A myriad of anatomic descriptions, eponyms, and syndromes describe congenital cardiac defects. Although the specific anatomic problem is important for the ultimate management and repair of these children, in the ED, these children may be effectively described in terms of their oxygenation, pulmonary blood flow, and left ventricular function. Table 18–1 lists the more common cardiac lesions with their presentation patterns.

Children with cyanotic lesion tend to have obstruction to pulmonary blood flow or isolation of the pulmonary and systemic circulations. With the exception of children with D-transposition of the great vessels or total anomalous pulmonary venous return (TAPVR), most of these children will have

▶ **TABLE 18–1. CARDIAC LESIONS PRESENTING IN FIRST MONTH OF LIFE**

Presentation Type	Cardiac Lesion
Cyanotic lesions	Tetralogy of Fallot (TOF)
	Transposition of great arteries (TGA)
	Tricuspid atresia (TA)
	Total anomalous pulmonary venous return (TAPVR)
	Truncus arteriosus
	Pulmonary stenosis (PS)
Increased pulmonary blood flow	Atrial septal defect (ASD)
	Ventricular septal defect (VSD)
	Patent ductus arteriosus (PDA)
	Endocardial cushion defect (AV Canal)
Left ventricular outflow obstruction or ventricular artesia	Aortic stenosis (AS)
	Coarctation of aorta
	Hypoplastic left heart syndrome (HLHS)

decreased pulmonary blood flow. The addition of supplemental oxygenation will generally not improve the hypoxia in these patients and can often be used as a diagnostic maneuver to identify a newborn with a fixed cardiac lesion.[1] Termed the hyperoxygenation test, it is performed by obtaining a baseline arterial oxygen determination. The child is then placed on 100% oxygen for 10 minutes and a repeat arterial blood gas obtained. Pulmonary causes of hypoxia should result in at least a 10% rise in PaO_2 while cardiac lesions will show no improvement with the additional oxygen. To be performed correctly, the hyperoxia test requires an actual arterial puncture and direct arterial oxygen tension determination preferably from a sample site in the right arm. However, in the ED setting a lack of response to supplemental oxygen as determined by pulse oximetry readings in both upper extremities and a leg may be taken as presumptive evidence for a fixed cardiac lesion.

The next category of neonatal cardiac presentations involves children with increased pulmonary blood flow. Described as having left to right shunts, because of the shift of blood flow from the systemic to the pulmonary circulation, these children will present with symptoms of congestive heart failure (CHF). Although they may have low oxygen saturations secondary to pulmonary edema, most will improve with supplemental oxygen.

The final category of patients is those with left ventricular obstructive lesions or ventricular atresias. Lesions with limited obstruction such as coarctation of the aorta or aortic stenosis may present with CHF. Children with more severe obstructions or absent effective left ventricles will present with frank shock.

Although it is convenient to classify different cardiac lesions in this manner, many variations in the anatomy of these patients exist and similar lesions can present with any combination of signs and symptoms. For example, depending on the specifics of the lesion, a coarctation of the aorta and ventricular septal defect can present with either cyanosis, CHF, or shock depending on the status of the ductus arteriosus.

The behavioral complaints of children with cardiac lesions involve decreased activity, poor feeding, and possibly cyanosis.[2] Children with cyanotic lesions will appear dusky or frankly blue, although this color change may be difficult to recognize in members of dark skinned races. Regardless of skin pigmentation, all these children will be recognized if routine pulse oximetry is performed as part of the routine assessment of every ill-appearing neonate. Pulse oximetry should always be performed on the right upper extremity to obtain the best estimate of actual aortic root oxygen saturation. The right upper extremity readings can be compared to the left arm or toe readings to determine the impact of admixing of aortic and pulmonary blood through the ductus arteriosus. Children with CHF may have cyanosis, although more times than not they will present with low normal oximetry readings associated with tachypnea and tachycardia. On physical examination, classic rales are relatively rare, with wheezing or rhonchi being more common. Hepatomegaly is a common finding in these children as is jugular distention, although most neonates will have distended neck veins. Children with left ventricular outflow obstruction will appear in shock with pallor or an ashen color, slow or absent capillary refill, and low pulse oximetry.

Treatment of neonatal primary cardiac emergencies is generally empiric in the ED setting. It is not necessary for the emergency physician to know the specific lesion present in any child, since the resulting pathology is generally the same regardless of the specific anatomic problem. In cyanotic children and those in shock, treatment is dependent on restoration of the fetal circulation through reestablishment of a patent ductus arteriosus. Opening an anatomic/physiologic shunt between the pulmonary and systemic circulations will permit admixing of oxygenated and deoxygenated blood as well as allow blood to flow to both the circulatory beds. Restoration of the ductus arteriosus is accomplished through a continuous infusion of prostaglandin E_1 (PGE_1) (0.05–0.1 µg/kg/min).[1] Many neonatologists and pediatric cardiologists now strongly recommend empiric institution of a prostaglandin infusion in any child who fails a hyperoxia test or demonstrates severe acute CHF. The effect of the prostaglandin may be immediate but frequently takes at least 15 minutes to be seen. Apnea is a common side effect of this drug and prophylactic intubation is recommended in any department needing to transfer a patient. A very few lesions can be made worse with prostaglandin infusion, so the treating emergency physician needs to continuously monitor these children and discontinue this treatment should the oxygen saturation drop.

CHF in this age group will also benefit from restoration of a ductus arteriosus since most CHF causes in neonates are related to some form of fixed cardiac lesion such as a coarctation of the aorta. If the child does not respond to the PGE_1, then inotropic support with a drug like dopamine or dobutamine may be needed. There is some evidence that receptors for sympathomimetic amines are less available in this age group and the myocardial makeup of the neonatal heart makes them less responsive to these agents. For this reason, bipyridines agent such as milrinone may be a better choice for this age group.[1] Digoxin is a well-proven inotropic drug for the treatment of CHF in children; however, its time to clinical onset makes it of limited use in the ED setting.

Pulmonary emergencies: Most primary congenital pulmonary problems become symptomatic at or shortly after birth and are recognized prior to nursery discharge. Children with congenital lobar emphysema may occasionally be discharged only to become symptomatic when air trapping behind a mucus or mucous plug results in overdistention. This effect usually is the result of endotracheal intubation and appears in the nursery. Other overdistention lesions such as cystic adenomatoid malformations may also present in a similar delayed manner. Most commonly though, neonatal pulmonary problems will result from viral or bacterial infections, which lead to bronchiolitis or pneumonia. Management of these children is the same as for any infant with a suspected lower respiratory tract infection, including nasal viral screening for respiratory syncytial virus, pertussis, and chalymdia as well as blood cultures, pulse oximetry, and a chest x-ray. Unlike neonates with cardiac problems, these patients will respond to supplemental oxygen with an increase in oxygen saturation. Management is based on clinical progression with endotracheal intubation for neonates demonstrating signs of respiratory failure. Antibiotics selection in these patients may include ampicillin plus a third-generation cephalosporin or amino glycoside but will depend on the suspected etiology and results of viral tests.

▶ ENDOCRINE AND METABOLIC DISORDERS

Because the maternal circulation can compensate for most endocrine and metabolic abnormalities in a fetus, many defects in hormonal or enzyme systems will not become clinically evident until days to months after a child is delivered. Inborn errors of metabolism (IEMs) associated with well-defined clinical syndromes are generally identified early because of associated physical abnormalities. In contrast, those conditions associated with a single hormone or enzyme defect may go undetected until a toxic metabolite accumulates in the neonates system or an electrolyte or endocrine catastrophe occurs.

Congenital adrenal hyperplasia (CAH) is generally regarded as more of an endocrine problem than an IEM but it does result from a single enzyme defect in the adrenal steroid genesis pathway. The most common enzyme abnormality involves 21-hydroxylase and results in loss of both aldosterone and cortisol production. These patients have profound salt wasting leading to severe hyponatremia and hyperkalemia. Adrenogenic precursors accumulate in these patients, which results in ambiguous genitalia for genotypic females. Abnormalities in 11β-hydroxylase is the next most common form of CAH, but unlike the 21-hydroxylase patients does not produce symptomatic mineralocorticoid deficits. Other forms of CAH, which produce varying combinations of salt wasting and ambiguous genitalia, also exist.[3]

Initial stabilization of these children will require vascular access and routine laboratory studies. In addition, extra serum should be obtained for later specific IEM studies.

The most common emergency presentation for children with CAH involves symptomatic salt wasting including dehydration, hypoglycemia, hyponatremia, and hyperkalemia.[2] The hyperkalemia may be extreme, up to 10 mEq/L, but is remarkably well tolerated. Initial management includes rapid rehydration with normal saline solution, usually 20 mL/kg or more in the first hour. This hydration will generally be sufficient to treat the dramatic hyperkalemia found in these children. Hypoglycemia when present is treated with a 10% dextrose

slow bolus or infusion. Higher viscosity D_{50} and D_{25} solutions should be avoided in these children. Hyponatremia will generally correct with the saline infusions and subsequent mineralocorticoid replacement. If seizures or other CNS abnormalities are present, the serum sodium will need to be corrected with a slow infusion of 3% NaCl solution. An infusion of 1 mL/kg of this solution will generally raise the serum sodium 1 mEq/L. Emergent treatment with this therapy is generally aimed at resolution of seizure activity or serum sodium of 125 mEq/L. The osmotic demyelination syndrome can occur with too rapid correction of hyponatremia, so as gradual a correction as possible is preferred. Hydrocortisone at 25 mg/m² should also be initiated if possible.[2,4]

Inborn errors of metabolism: Although the prevalence of any individual IEM is rare, as a whole, IEMs occur in up to 1 per 2000 live births. Because of the wide variety of chemical pathways that can be affected, IEMs may produce symptoms at any time including the prenatal period, at birth, in the first few days of life, or into adulthood. Clinically these children appear septic, and infection is the most common misdiagnosis assigned.[5,6]

Multiple classification systems exist to organize IEMs; however, for emergency physicians, the system based on the patterns of deterioration appears to be the most appropriate. The associated findings for these disorders are summarized in Table 18–2. As a general rule those errors associated with accumulation of small molecules lead to CNS sequestration of molecules and acute metabolic encephalopathies. A small group of IEMs affects predominately the liver and present with jaundice, hepatomegaly, and clotting abnormalities. Disorders with long-chain fatty acid oxidation manifest as cardiolmyopathies, arrhythmias, and even sudden death. Another small set of IEMs present with encephalopathy but have seizures as a prominent finding. Classic syndromes associated with IEMs

▶ TABLE 18–2. INBORN ERRORS OF METABOLISM

Type	Characteristic Findings
Acute metabolic encephalopathy	Lactic acidosis
	Organic acidoses
	Hypoglycemia
	Hyperammonemia
	Amino acid disorders
Jaundice—severe liver dysfunction	Galatosemia
	Tyrosinemia type I
	Fructose intolerance
Cardiac disease	Long-chain fatty acid oxidation disorders
Encephalopathy with seizures	Nonketotic hyperglycinemia
Phenotypic distinctive disorders	Lysosomal disorders
	Glycosylation disorders
Severe hypotonia	Peroxisomal disorders
	Nonketotic hyperglycinemia
	Congenital lactic acidosis
	Congenital disorders of glycosylation
Nonimmune hydrops fetalis	Lysosomal storage disorders

frequently have distinctive phenotypes with facial dysmorphisms and congenital malformations. Neonates with disorders involving perixisome formation have profound hypotonia, neurologic impairment, and typical facial appearances. Finally, hydrops fetalis is generally associated with prenatal blood incompatibility but may also result from IEMs such as Gaucher disease type II or Niemann-Pick type C.[5,6]

Most of the problems with IEM stem from the catabolic state that develops in the child as a result of an inability to properly metabolize a given substrate. Despite more widespread screening for IEMs in the nursery, many of these children will become symptomatic and present to the ED before results of these studies are returned. As with cardiac presentations, the emergency physician will generally be forced to provide empiric therapy pending more sophisticated testing. In addition to those tests performed for a potentially septic neonate, specimens should be obtained for venous blood gas, liver function tests, and ammonia level. If available, Guthrie blood spot cards may be obtained from the nursery for amino acid and acylcarnitine analysis.

Immediate treatment of the IEM toxic neonate is aimed at rehydration and conversion from a catabolic to an anabolic state. Electrolyte solutions with 10% glucose should be started and all enteral feedings stopped. Metabolic acidosis should respond to hydration but some authors will recommend supplemental bicarbonate if the serum bicarbonate is less than 15 mEq/L. Sodium benzoate and sodium phenylbutyrate may be used in cases of hyperammonemia to divert ammonia to a more excretable form.[5,6]

▶ GASTROINTESTINAL

Any portion of the gastrointestinal (GI) tract from the esophagus to the anus is at risk for a congenital malformation or atresia. Most lesions will again be identified in the nursery, although a significant minority will not reveal themselves until after discharge.[7]

Vomiting is the most common presenting complaint of neonates with GI abnormalities. Although the vast majority of vomiting is simple spitting up secondary to overfeeding, true vomiting must be taken seriously in any neonate. An ominous sign in any newborn is bilious emesis. Children have rapid transit times so any child with bilious vomiting must be considered a true emergency until proven otherwise. More than 20% of these children will require immediate surgical interventions and early consultation should be placed even before a definitive diagnosis is identified.

The most serious potential abnormality in neonates with bilious vomiting is intestinal malrotation with or without volvulus.[8] In these patients, the intestines fail to negotiate their normal embryonic rotations and return to the abdominal cavity malpositioned and at risk for volvulus. If volvulus occurs, not only will the intestinal obstruction occur but the mesenteric blood supply will also be occluded leading to entire bowel ischemia and infarction. Other causes of bilious emesis include atresia of different levels of the GI tract, although these will generally declare themselves as soon as enteral feedings begin. Anomalies such as peritoneal bands, a preduodenal portal vein, annular pancreas, and Hirschsprung disease among many others can also lead to these symptoms.

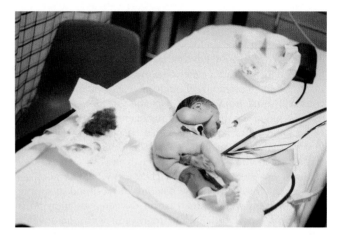

Figure 18–1. Bloody diarrhea in a 5-day-old infant secondary to malrotation and mid gut volvulus.

In addition to routine hydration and baseline blood studies, these children may require an immediate oral contrast study of the upper GI tract. Contrast that does not cross the midline is virtually diagnostic for malrotation. Additional ED management is generally at the discretion of the consultant, although most will recommend placement of a nasogastric tube for upper GL drainage.

Bloody emesis is another high-risk finding and should prompt the same aggressive management approach as bilious vomiting. Breast-fed neonates are the exception as they may simply be vomiting maternal blood from cracked or inflamed nipples. In these cases, fetal and maternal blood can be distinguished through an Apt test. To perform the test a small amount of the bloody material is mixed with 5 mL of water and centrifuge. One part of 0.25 N (1%) NaOH is added to five parts of the blood solution. Maternal blood turns brown when the NaOH is added while fetal blood remains pink.[7] Unless a maternal source of vomited blood is confirmed, a CBC, type and screen, and baseline electrolyte and liver tests should be obtained.

Bloody diarrhea may also indicate a potential GI emergency. The same etiologies that produce bloody emesis should be considered in children with bloody diarrhea, although benign causes such as food allergies may also lead to these findings. Figure 18–1 contains a photo of a 5-day-old infant with bloody diarrhea from infarcted bowel secondary to malrotation and volvulus.

Pyloric stenosis is unusual before the age of 5 weeks but can occur in the neonatal period. Persistent projectile vomiting is the typical presentation and the diagnosis is confirmed through ultrasonography. Children with pyloric stenosis will frequently demonstrate a classic electrolyte pattern with a hypochloremic, hypokalemic, and metabolic alkalosis in the face of pronounced dehydration.[8]

Jaundice is a very common neonatal presentation and is discussed in Chapter 12.

▶ SEIZURES

Seizures in the neonatal period are relatively common and may present in much more subtle patterns than in older children.[9,10]

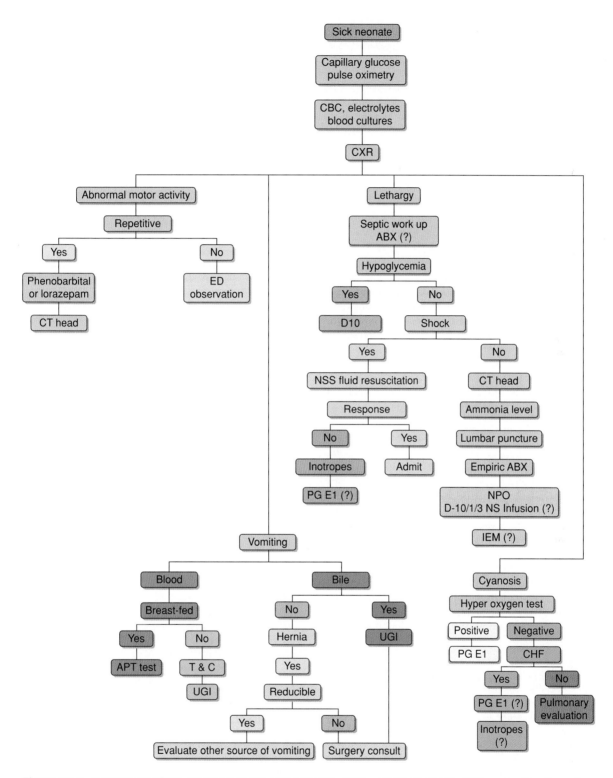

Figure 18–2. A summary of the approach to the sick neonate. PGE₁, prostaglandin E₁; UGI, upper GI with oral contrast; ABX, antibiotics; IEM, inborn error of metabolism.

In addition, neonates have much lower seizure thresholds because of a higher excitatory (glutamate) to inhibitory (GABA) receptor ratio.[11]

Neonatal seizures are frequently categorized into four subgroups: subtle seizures, clonic seizures, tonic seizures, and myoclonic seizures. Subtle seizures are the most common subtype

comprising almost 50% of all newborn seizures. These seizures may combine different actions involving different remote body parts. For example, a child may demonstrate lip smacking followed by pedaling-like motions of the legs followed by eye fixation. As a general rule, any consistent repetitive action on the part of a neonate should be considered a potential seizure until proven otherwise. Clonic seizures demonstrate repeated biphasic movements with a fast contraction followed by a slower relaxation. Tonic seizures are characterized by a sustained period of muscle contraction and are more common in premature than term infants. Finally, myoclonic seizures involve very quick nonrhythmic muscle actions. Because of their immature neurologic systems, neonates can demonstrate a large spectrum of motor actions that can closely mimic seizures including jitteriness, sleep myoclonus, and even transient sucking actions.[12]

The leading cause of neonatal seizures is cerebral hypoxia or ischemia. As would be expected, perinatal asphyxia is the most common cause of these insults. Stroke is the second most common cause of neonatal seizures accounting for up to 20% of all cases, while intracranial hemorrhages account for 10%. Most such hemorrhages in term neonates are subarachnoid in location compared to the intraventricular bleeds seen in premature infants.[11] Because of the large incidence of intracranial bleeding in neonates with seizures, a CT scan of the head should be obtained routinely prior to performance of any lumbar puncture. If the CT scan will be delayed, then empiric antibiotics to cover CNS bacterial and viral infections should be administered. Other causes of neonatal seizures include CNS infections, electrolyte abnormalities, and IEMs.

In addition to routine blood studies, urine drug screens should be considered in all seizure patients. Depending on the circumstances, screening of the mother may be required as well.

The ED management of neonatal seizures is directed at both seizure control and correction of any underlying metabolic abnormalities. Phenobarbital (20 mg/kg) is the initial drug treatment for neonatal seizures, although many clinicians prefer lorazepam (0.05 mg/kg) because of their greater experience with the medication. Phenytoin (20 mg/kg) may be considered in refractory cases. Close attention to respiratory status should be maintained in all these cases as most seizure therapies can produce respiratory depression. Hypoglycemia is managed with 2 to 4 mL/kg boluses of 10% dextrose, while hypocalcemia is treated with 4 mg/kg of 5% calcium gluconate and hypomagnesemia is managed with 50% magnesium sulfate at 0.2 mL/kg IM. Hyponatremia in the seizing neonate is best managed with 1 mL/kg aliquots of 3% saline until the seizure ceases.

▶ SURGICAL EMERGENCIES

Parents may notice a lump in the inguinal area of the child, particularly premature or male patients. Hernias are the most common source of masses occurring in 5% to 30% of low–birth-weight individuals.[7] The presence of a hernia in and of itself is not generally an issue—it is the ability of the hernia to be re-

duced that is important. Care should be taken in male neonates because the testicle itself may be located in the inguinal canal while in female patients the ovary is frequently contained in the hernia sac. Children in whom hernias are easily reduced may be referred for definitive out patient surgery.

Surprisingly, the neonatal period is a relatively common time for testicular torsion. If acute, these patients will present with a red tender swollen hemiscrotum. The swelling may extent to the inguinal canal making it difficult to distinguish from an inguinal hernia. Approximately 70% of testicular torsions occur in utero and will present as a firm, nontender scrotal mass.

The diagnosis of testicular torsion is confirmed through ultrasound examination. Acute torsions are surgical emergencies requiring immediate surgical interventions. In contrast, prenatal torsions generally involve necrotic testicles for which surgical intervention will be of no immediate value.[7,13]

A summary of the approach to the sick neonate is presented in Figure 18–2.

REFERENCES

1. Yee L. Cardiac emergencies in the first year of life. *Emerg Med Clin North Am.* 2007;25:981.
2. Brousseau T, Sharieff G. Newborn emergencies: the first 30 days of life. *Pediatr Clin North Am.* 2006;53:69.
3. Merke DP, Bornstein SR. Congenital adrenal hyperplasia. *Lancet.* 2005;365:2125.
4. Speiser PW. Congenital adrenal hyperplasia owing to 21-hydroxylase deficiency. *Endocrinol Metab Clin North Am.* 2001;30:31.
5. Leonard JV, Morris AA. Inborn errors of metabolism around the time of birth. *Lancet.* 2000;356:583.
6. Ogier de Baulny H. Management and emergency treatments of neonates with a suspicion of inborn errors of metabolism. *Semin Neonatol.* 2001;7:17.
7. Ringer SA, Hansen AR. Surgical emergencies in the newborn. In: Cloherty JP, Eichenwald EC, Stark AR, eds. *Manual of Neonatal Care.* 6th ed. Philadelphia, PA: Lippincott Williams & Wilkins; 2008:616.
8. Millar AJ, Rode H, Cywes S. Malrotation and volvulus in infancy and childhood. *Semin Pediatr Surg.* 2003;12:229.
9. eMedline. Pediatrics, Pyloric Stenosis. http://www.emedicine.com/EMERG/topic397.htm. Accessed December 22, 2008.
10. Nabbout R, Dulac O. Epileptic syndromes in infancy and childhood. *Curr Opin Neurol.* 2008;21:161.
11. Du Plessis AJ. Neonatal seizures. In: Cloherty JP, Eichenwald EC, Stark AR, eds. *Manual of Neonatal Care.* 6th ed. Philadelphia, PA: Lippincott Williams & Wilkins; 2008:616.
12. Korff CM, Nordli DR Jr. Epilepsy syndromes in infancy. *Pediatr Neurol.* 2006;34:253.
13. Chiang MC, Chen HW, Fu RH, Lien R, Wang TM, Hsu JF. Clinical features of testicular torsion and epididymo-orchitis in infants younger than 3 months. *J Pediatr Surg.* 2007;42:1574.

CHAPTER 19

The Transplant Patient in the ED

Neil A. Evans and Susan M. Scott

▶ HIGH-YIELD FACTS

- The most common presenting complaint by the transplant patient is fever. This can be due to infection in an immune compromised state, or to graft rejection.
- A febrile transplant patient should be carefully assessed for early signs of shock.
- Commonly used calcineurin inhibitors (e.g., tacrolimus) can place a transplant patient at risk for nephrotoxicity.
- Drugs commonly prescribed in the ED can interfere with the metabolism of potent immunosuppressive medications, causing adverse drug–drug interactions in transplant patients.

▶ INTRODUCTION

Over the past 10 years, the number of transplant recipients in the United States has increased from almost 20,000 to nearly 30,000 per year and the corresponding number in pediatric transplantation has also grown dramatically.[1] This increase has also accompanied improved outcomes and survival rates largely because of improved surgical techniques and immunosuppression drug regimens.[2–6] From a historical perspective, the developments in the field have been dramatic. A brief time line is given in Table 19–1 describing key milestones.

As advances in transplant medicine progress, more and more transplant patients will present to the emergency department (ED) and the pediatric emergency medicine provider should remain aware of the complexities involved in the care of the transplant patient. This includes an understanding of the usual presenting signs and symptoms, the common complications as well as the common medications used for immunosuppression, and their interactions.

▶ COMMON COMPLAINTS PRESENTING TO THE ED

The majority of transplant patients will likely require hospitalization sometime during the first 6 months after transplant. Some of the common reasons for presentation are fever, rejection, gastrointestinal symptoms, and neurological complaints.[7]

The most common presenting complaint by the transplant patient is fever, with other associated infectious symptoms. If the patient presents in extremis with hemodynamic instability, the usual priorities of resuscitation should be performed with the primary focus on patient survival, not graft survival. The transplant service or nearest transplant center should be involved in the patient's care early on during the ED visit. They can be an invaluable resource and aid in management and disposition.

Fever should be investigated and treated aggressively as most transplant patients are in an immunocompromised state, allowing for rapid deterioration if infection is not detected and treated quickly. Cultures of blood, urine, and when indicated cerebrospinal fluid should be obtained and broad-spectrum antibiotic coverage initiated. A careful history and physical examination must be obtained and any associated symptoms investigated further. Subtle signs of shock (tachycardia, bounding or weak peripheral pulses, and wide or narrow pulse pressure) should be recognized and treated aggressively. A history of cough, tachypnea, or cyanosis warrants pulse oximetry and chest radiography. Tests such as a complete blood count with differential, coagulation/DIC panel, urinalysis, and viral studies may also be helpful during the workup (see Table 19–2). Many transplant patients have central venous catheters and these should be considered a source of infection and cultures obtained followed by rapid administration of antibiotics.[8] Those transplant patients presenting with fever, who are found to have a source in the ED such as otitis media, viral upper respiratory infection, urinary tract infection, or other common causes of fever, should be treated appropriately and can be discharged home with notification sent to the transplant service and close follow-up arranged.

Fever may also be an indicator of graft rejection, which should always be a concern and in the differential of the transplant patient in the ED. For liver transplant patients, a screen of liver function tests and bilirubin levels can be of benefit in detecting graft rejection. If these screening tests are elevated above the patient's baseline values, further testing is required. This may include an ultrasound with Doppler to evaluate blood flow to the graft and status of the biliary system.[9] These patients may also require admission to the hospital for close monitoring. For renal transplant patients, a screen of serum creatinine and blood urea nitrogen may be an indicator of rejection as well as abnormalities of blood pressure, urine output, and pain over the engrafted kidney. Further workup should include admission, consultation with the transplant service, and other studies such as ultrasound, nuclear renal scans, and biopsy.

A wide range of GI symptoms may be encountered in the transplant patient including nausea, vomiting, diarrhea, abdominal pain, and bleeding. Liver transplant patients can develop GI symptoms from a wide range of causes including bile leakage or biliary stricture from the anastomosis site, which can

▶ **TABLE 19–1. ADVANCES IN TRANSPLANT MEDICINE**

Year	Event
1954	Dr. Joseph Murray at Peter Bent Brigham Hospital, Boston performs first successful twin to twin kidney transplant
1956	Dr. E. Donnall Thomas at Colombia University affiliated hospital, Cooperstown, New York, performs first bone marrow transplant using related donor
1967	Dr. Thomas Starzl at the University of Colorado Health Sciences Center, Denver, performs first successful liver transplant
1967	Dr. Christiaan Barnard at Groote Schur Hospital, Cape Town, South Africa, performs first successful heart transplant
1962	Introduction of antirejection drug azathioprine
1979	Dr. David Sutherland at the University of Minnesota, Minneapolis, performs first living-related pancreas transplant
1981	Dr. Bruce Reitz at Stanford University, California, performs first successful heart–lung transplant
1983	U.S. FDA approves use of cyclosporine as an immunosuppressant drug
1988	Dr. David Grant at the University Hospital of London Health Sciences Centre, London, Ontario, performs first successful liver–bowel transplant
1990	Tacrolimus (FK 506) becomes available as an immunosuppressant drug
1995	U.S. FDA approves use of mycophenolate mofetil to prevent organ rejection in kidney transplants
1995	Physicians at the University of Miami, Florida, perform first transplantation of all abdominal organs in a single patient
1998	Physicians at Emory University, Atlanta, perform first unrelated stem cell transplant
1999	U.S. FDA approves use of sirolimus to prevent organ rejection in adult renal transplant patients

▶ **TABLE 19–2. LABORATORY/IMAGING STUDIES FOR EVALUATION OF THE TRANSPLANT PATIENT WITH FEVER**

Complete blood count with differential
Blood cultures
Electrolytes
BUN/Creatinine
Serum glucose
Urinalysis
Urine culture
Sedimentation rate
C-reactive protein
Immunosuppressant drug levels
Chest x-ray as needed
Cerebrospinal fluid studies as needed
Viral studies as needed

Special Studies for:
Liver Transplant Patients
   Liver function tests (AST, ALT, GGT, alkaline phosphatase)
   Bilirubin levels (total and direct)
   Coagulation panel (PT, PTT, fibrinogen, INR)
   Albumin
   Liver sonogram as needed
Renal Transplant Patient
   Renal sonogram as needed
Heart Transplant Patient
   Echocardiogram as needed

ing cause of headache in immunocompromised individuals with or without associated neck pain or stiffness. Malignant hypertension can also be a concerning cause. One of the more common causes of headache is pseudotumor cerebri often associated with corticosteroid use. Evaluation of headache in the transplant patient may include appropriate imaging and evaluation of the cerebrospinal fluid and opening pressure.[10]

▶ COMMON COMPLICATIONS

The complications associated with surgery and postoperative care will not be discussed. This chapter will concentrate on complications which cause the transplant patient to visit the ED. One of the most common is immunosuppression from maintenance medications. An increased risk of infection is always associated with immunosuppression and can lead to fever, cough, congestion, vomiting, and other signs and symptoms of infection.[7] The transplant patient presenting with fever may have a minor or serious infection, or be rejecting a transplanted organ.

Other complications related to medication adverse effects can also lead to an ED visit. The commonly used calcineurin inhibitors like tacrolimus can place a patient at higher risk for nephrotoxicity. Combine this risk with nonsteroidal anti-inflammatory drug (NSAID) use, low cardiac output, or dehydration and renal dysfunction may develop. These patients will present with decreased urine output, edema, or complications from electrolyte imbalances. Kidney function and serum

lead to peritonitis. Variceal bleeding can occur from portal venous hypertension in the setting of portal venous thrombosis or stricture.[9] GI symptoms can also be caused by adverse effects of immunosuppressant medications (Table 19–3). For example, tacrolimus can cause diffuse abdominal pain; mycophenolate mofetil can cause colitis, gastritis, pancreatitis, and diarrhea; azathioprine can cause pancreatitis. Viral infection of the intestinal tract can also cause numerous GI symptoms. Other infectious etiologies that should also be considered are candidal esophagitis and *Clostridium difficile* colitis. Management of the GI symptoms for the transplant patient in the ED is the same as other patients and may include fluid resuscitation, nasogastric decompression, bowel rest, and further monitoring with hospital admission.

The most common neurological symptom encountered in the transplant patient is headache. Common causes of headache encountered in the transplant patient include migraine and tension headache, but it could also be an indicator of a more serious problem. Meningitis is a concern-

▶ TABLE 19–3. ADVERSE EFFECTS OF IMMUNOSUPPRESSANT DRUGS

Adverse Effect	Steroids	Azathioprine	Cyclosporine	Tacrolimus	Mycophenolate	Sirolimus
Immunologic						
Increased risk of infection	+	+	+	+	+	+
Myelosuppression		+	+	+	+	+
Increased risk of malignancy		+	+	+	+	+
Hypersensitivity reactions		+				
Cardiovascular						
Hypertension	+		+	+	+	+
Arrhythmia			+	+		
Cardiomyopathy				+		
Chest pain					+	+
Syncope						+
Respiratory						
Pulmonary fibrosis					+	+
Cough					+	
Endocrine						
Hyperglycemia	+			+	+	
Cushing's syndrome	+			+		+
Growth suppression	+					
Neurologic						
Headache	+		+	+	+	+
Seizures	+		+	+		
Depression			+	+		+
Tinnitus			+	+		
Encephalopathy				+		
Dermatologic						
Hirsutism			+			+
Acne			+			+
Rash				+	+	+
Renal						
Nephrotoxic			+	+		+
Electrolyte imbalances				+		+
Dysuria				+		
Hematuria					+	
Edema						+
Gastrointestinal						
Nausea/vomiting	+	+	+	+	+	+
Diarrhea		+	+	+	+	+
Hepatotoxicity		+	+	+		+
Pancreatitis		+	+	+	+	
Colitis					+	
Abdominal pain						+
Constitutional						
Weight gain	+					+
Weight loss			+			
Muscle weakness	+		+		+	
Arthralgias		+				
Gynecomastia	+		+			
Fever/chills						+

drug levels should be obtained and volume status carefully controlled. Transplant maintenance medications which have nephrotoxic effects, high serum levels, or are cleared by the kidney should not be administered until normal drug levels have again been established and the cause of the renal dysfunction has been identified and corrected. With early detection and proper therapy, the potential for severe kidney damage from an acute insult to a kidney with calcineurin inhibitor exposure is greatly diminished. Without early detection, the potential effects could lead to renal failure, requiring dialysis.[10]

Corticosteroids, another commonly used transplant maintenance medication, can cause other complications such as hypertension. Antihypertensive medications such as calcium channel blockers and angiotensin converting enzyme inhibitors can be used to control blood pressure in these patients.[11] In the event of a hypertensive urgency or emergency, the use of labetalol, nifedipine, or nicardipine is indicated (see Chapter 51).

▶ IMMUNOSUPPRESSIVE MEDICATIONS

CORTICOSTEROIDS

One of the main causes of immunosuppression in the transplant patient is the use of corticosteroids both to induce an immunosuppressed state and to treat acute episodes of rejection.[4] Corticosteroid therapy suppresses the migration of polymorphonuclear leukocytes and decreases capillary permeability, thus decreasing the body's inflammatory response. Often, IV doses of methylprednisolone are used initially after transplant with the patient transitioning to an oral prednisone regimen prior to discharge. Some common adverse effects of corticosteroids include hypertension, headache, psychoses, and hyperglycemia (Table 19–3).[12] Long-term use can also cause other adverse effects including Cushing's syndrome, growth suppression, decreased bone mineral density, adrenal suppression, glaucoma, and cataracts.[13]

Corticosteroids are still widely used today but new evidence continues to emerge supporting use of other newer immunosuppressive agents in order to avoid the long-term adverse effects of corticosteroids.

AZATHIOPRINE

Once used as a primary immunosuppressant along with corticosteroids, azathioprine now is used mainly as an adjunctive therapy.[14,15] Often, it is used in combination with corticosteroids or a calcineurin inhibitor such as tacrolimus. Azathioprine is converted to 6-mercaptopurine (6-MP), which then antagonizes purine synthesis and thus synthesis of DNA, RNA, and proteins decreasing lymphocytic proliferation. In order to monitor dosing and compliance, 6-mercaptopurine (6-MP) levels can be measured when concern for rejection arises in the ED. Common adverse effects of azathioprine include myelosuppression, hepatotoxicity, pancreatitis, and hypersensitivity reactions such as drug fever (Table 19–3). Long-term use can lead to increased risk of infection and neoplasm, particularly lymphoma and skin cancers.

▶ **TABLE 19–4. MEDICATIONS WITCH ALTER METABOLISM OF CYCLOSPORINE AND TACROLIMUS**

Increase Serum Drug Level (Decrease Drug Metabolism)	Decrease Serum Drug Level (Increase Drug Metabolism)	Synergistic Effect Causing Nephrotoxicity
Chloramphenicol	Antacids	Aminoglycosides
Cimetidine	Carbamazepine	Amphotericin B
Clarithromycin	Cholestyramine	Cisplatin
Clotrimazole	Isoniazid	NSAIDs
Cyclosporine	Nafcillin	Sulfonamides
Diltiazem	Phenobarbital	
Erythromycin	Phenytoin	
Fluconazole	Primidone	
Grapefruit	Rifabutin	
Itraconazole	Rifampin	
Ketoconazole	St. John's wort	
Methylprednisolone	Ticlopidine	
Metoclopramide	Trimethoprim	
Nicardipine		
Nifedipine		
Verapamil		

CYCLOSPORINE

Since the 1980s, cyclosporine has been used either alone or in combination with other medications as an effective prophylaxis for transplant rejection. Its mechanism of action involves the inhibition of production and release of interleukin-II and inhibits activation of resting T lymphocytes.[16] Serum drug levels can be obtained to monitor dosing. Monitoring drug levels is important when administering other medications as several drugs alter the metabolism of cyclosporine via the cytochrome P450 isoenzyme (Table 19–4).[17–19] Common adverse effects from the use of cyclosporine include hypertension, seizures, nephrotoxicity, hepatotoxitcity, and posttransplant lymphoproliferative disease (PTLD).[11] Frequently, hirsutism and gingival hyperplasia are seen with its use[20] (Table 19–3).

TACROLIMUS (FK 506)

Tacrolimus is a potent immunosuppressant in the class of calcineurin inhibitors useful in both the maintenance of immunosuppression and the treatment of acute or chronic rejection.[21, 22] It acts by inhibiting phosphatase activity of calcineurin and thus inhibition of T-cell activation.[23] Its oral bioavailability is erratic and serum drug levels are often needed, especially when adding other medicines which can alter metabolism via cytochrome P450[19] (Table 19–4). Some common adverse effects include hypertension, hyperglycemia, encephalopathy, headache, electrolyte imbalances (especially potassium and magnesium), and rashes. Less common side effects include cardiomyopathy, seizures, pancreatitis, hepatotoxicity, and nephrotoxicity[12] (Table 19–3). As with all immunosuppressed patients, the risk of infection is increased and with tacrolimus the risk of PTLD is increased as well.[24] Caution should be used with patients on both cyclosporine and tacrolimus as the agents are synergistic and can increase toxicities of both agents.[25,26]

MYCOPHENOLATE MOFETIL

Used as an adjunct to other immunosuppressants or for acute rejection, mycophenolate is hydrolyzed in the body to its active metabolite mycophenolic acid, which acts as a selective inhibitor of inosine monophosphate dehydrogenase in the purine biosynthesis pathway. It inhibits the production of the purine nucleotide guanosine which T and B lymphocytes are dependent on for proliferation. Other cell types can use alternative pathways to maintain purine biosynthesis. Therefore, mycophenolate selectively inhibits proliferation of T and B lymphocytes and antibody formation by B cells. Common adverse effects include hypertension, rash, pancreatitis, leukopenia, PTLD, and pulmonary fibrosis[27] (Table 19–3).

SIROLIMUS

Sirolimus can be used as a single agent or in combination with calcineurin inhibitor therapy for maintenance of immunosuppression or as a rescue agent for acute and chronic rejection. Its mechanism of action reduces T-cell activation by inhibiting cytokine-induced signal transduction pathways suppressing IL-2 and IL-4 driven T-cell proliferation.[28] Common adverse effects include hypertension, edema, syncope, hypercholesterolemia, acne, nephrotoxicity, and abdominal pain[12] (Table 19–3).

MUROMONAB-CD3 (OKT3)

OKT3 is a mouse antibody which attaches to the CD3 antigen receptor on circulating T lymphocytes.[29] It is useful in the treatment of acute rejection episodes resistant to conventional treatment.[30] By attaching to CD3 and modulating the antigen receptor complex, the CD3 molecules are removed from the T-cell surface, thus making the cell unable to function as a T lymphocyte.[29] The administration of OKT3, especially the first few doses, can lead to common adverse events attributable to a cytokine release syndrome including hyperpyrexia, shock, pulmonary edema, cardiovascular collapse, and cerebral edema. Initiation of therapy is usually performed in an intensive care unit for close monitoring and quick intervention if needed. Other associate side effects include aseptic meningitis, increased risk of sepsis, seizures, and PTLD.[31]

▶ INFECTION PROPHYLAXIS

Immunosuppression of the transplant patient leads to an increased risk of infection. Most transplant centers use a combination of prophylactic antibiotics, antifungals, and antiviral medications in the postoperative period.[9] As time from transplant increases, the level of prophylaxis decreases but still includes antiviral therapy for CMV such as acyclovir or ganciclovir. Bactrim is also commonly used to prevent *Pneumocystis carinii* infection. Monthly pentamidine is another option

sometimes used. Fungal infections are prophylaxed with the use of nystatin or other antifungal agents.[32]

Depending on the patient's age at transplantation, the number of vaccinations received can be quite varied. After recovery from transplant surgery and any associated complications, the immunization schedule should be continued with catch-up doses as needed according to current recommendations. The only type of vaccine that should not be given is a live virus vaccine. While on immunosuppressant therapy, a patient's level of seroconversion in response to a vaccine will be diminished. During the first year after transplant while immunosuppressant levels are high, vaccines may be deferred until lower levels of immune suppression can be reached in order to increase rates of seroconversion after immunization.[9]

▶ CONCLUSION

With the increased presence of the transplant patient in the emergency department, pediatric emergency care providers need to be aware of the complexities involved in the care of the immunosuppressed transplant patient. This includes an awareness of the common transplant immunosuppressant medications including their interactions with other drugs and adverse effects. Infection prophylaxis used in the transplant patient and common reasons for presentation to the ED along with the management of those complaints should be a part of the clinician's knowledge base.

REFERENCES

1. OPTN/SRTR 2006 Annual Report. [cited; Available from: www.ustransplant.org.]
2. Burckart GJ. Transplant pharmacy: 30 years of improving patient care. *Ann Pharmacother.* 2007;41(7):1261–1263.
3. Cronin DC, Faust TW, Brady L, et al. Modern immunosuppression. *Clin Liver Dis.* 2000;4(3):619–655, ix.
4. Murray JE, Merrill JP, Harrison JH, et al. Prolonged survival of human-kidney homografts by immunosuppressive drug therapy. *N Engl J Med.* 1963;268:1315–1323.
5. Sudan D, Bacha EA, John E, Bartholomew A. What's new in childhood organ transplantation. *Pediatr Rev.* 2007;28(12):439–453.
6. Lechler RI, Sykes M, Thomson AW, Turka LA. Organ transplantation—how much of the promise has been realized? *Nat Med.* 2005;11(6):605–613.
7. Zitelli BJ, Gartner JC, Malatack JJ, et al. Pediatric liver transplantation: patient evaluation and selection, infectious complications, and life-style after transplantation. *Transplant Proc.* 1987;19(4):3309–3316.
8. Crandall WV, Norlin C, Bullock EA, et al. Etiology and outcome of outpatient fevers in pediatric heart transplant patients. *Clin Pediatr (Phila).* 1996;35(9):437–442.
9. Alonso MH, Ryckman FC. Current concepts in pediatric liver transplant. *Semin Liver Dis.* 1998;18(3):295–307.
10. Fleisher GR, Ludwig S, Henretig FM. *Textbook of Pediatric Emergency Medicine.* 5th ed. Philadelphia, PA: Lippincott Williams & Wilkins; 2006:xxxv, 2052.
11. Kirk AJ, Omar I, Bateman DN, Dark JH. Cyclosporine-associated hypertension in cardiopulmonary transplantation. The beneficial effect of nifedipine on renal function. *Transplantation.* 1989;48(3):428–430.

12. Shapiro R, Scantlebury VP, Jordan ML, et al. A pilot trial of tacrolimus, sirolimus, and steroids in renal transplant recipients. *Transplant Proc.* 2002;34(5):1651–1652.

13. Roxane Laboratories, Inc. *Prednisone Tablets, Oral Solution, Prednisone Intensol Concentrated Soltuion Prescribing Information.* Columbus, OH: Boehringer Ingelheim Roxane Laboratories. 2002.

14. Leichter HE, Sheth KJ, Gerlach MJ, et al. Outcome of renal transplantation in children aged 1–5 and 6–18 years. *Child Nephrol Urol.* 1992;12(1):1–5.

15. Baum D, Bernstein D, Starnes VA, et al. Pediatric heart transplantation at Stanford: results of a 15-year experience. *Pediatrics.* 1991;88(2):203–214.

16. Kahan BD. Cyclosporine. *N Engl J Med.* 1989;321(25):1725–1738.

17. Baciewicz AM, Baciewicz FA Jr. Cyclosporine pharmacokinetic drug interactions. *Am J Surg.* 1989;157(2):264–271.

18. Wandstrat TL, Schroeder TJ, Myre SA. Cyclosporine pharmacokinetics in pediatric transplant recipients. *Ther Drug Monit.* 1989;11(5):493–496.

19. Yee GC. Pharmacokinetic interactions between cyclosporine and other drugs. *Transplant Proc.* 1990;22(3):1203–1207.

20. Yee GC. Clinical pharmacology of cyclosporine. *Int J Rad Appl Instrum B,* 1990;17(7):729–732.

21. Asante-Korang A, Boyle GJ, Webber SA, et al. Experience of FK506 immune suppression in pediatric heart transplantation: a study of long-term adverse effects. *J Heart Lung Transplant.* 1996;15(4):415–422.

22. McDiarmid SV. The use of tacrolimus in pediatric liver transplantation. *J Pediatr Gastroenterol Nutr.* 1998;26(1):90–102.

23. Kelly PA, Burckart GJ, Venkataramanan R. Tacrolimus: a new immunosuppressive agent. *Am J Health Syst Pharm.* 1995;52(14):1521–1535.

24. MacDonald AS, Sketris IS. Tacrolimus in transplantation. *Am J Health Syst Pharm.* 1995;52(14):1569–1571.

25. Starzl TE, Fung J, Jordan M, et al. Kidney transplantation under FK 506. *JAMA.* 1990;264(1):63–67.

26. Todo S, Fung JJ, Starzl TE, et al. Liver, kidney, and thoracic organ transplantation under FK 506. *Ann Surg.* 1990;212(3):295–305; discussion 306–307.

27. Lipsky JJ. Mycophenolate mofetil. *Lancet.* 1996;348(9038):1357–1359.

28. Kahan BD. Efficacy of sirolimus compared with azathioprine for reduction of acute renal allograft rejection: a randomised multicentre study. The Rapamune US Study Group. *Lancet.* 2000;356(9225):194–202.

29. Todd PA, Brogden RN. Muromonab CD3. A review of its pharmacology and therapeutic potential. *Drugs.* 1989;37(6):871–899.

30. Goldstein G, Kremer AB, Barnes L, Hirsch RL. et al. OKT3 monoclonal antibody reversal of renal and hepatic rejection in pediatric patients. *J Pediatr.* 1987;111(6)(Pt 2):1046–1050.

31. Hooks MA, Wade CS, Millikan WJ Jr. Muromonab CD-3: a review of its pharmacology, pharmacokinetics, and clinical use in transplantation. *Pharmacotherapy.* 1991;11(1):26–37.

32. Paya CV. Prevention of fungal infection in transplantation. *Transpl Infect Dis.* 2002;4(suppl 3):46–51.

SECTION II

SEDATION, ANALGESIA, AND IMAGING

CHAPTER 20

Procedural Sedation and Analgesia

Amy L. Baxter

▶ HIGH-YIELD FACTS

- Delaying sedation because of recent food/drink intake must be balanced by the urgency of the procedure and the risk to the patient imposed by such a delay.
- Any patient who could be a "difficult intubation" (craniofacial abnormalities, atlantoaxial instability, and prior tracheal reconstruction) merits consultation with anesthesia.
- Continuous monitoring of oxygen saturation and heart rate will identify the most common serious risk of sedation, hypoxia.
- Intravenous administration of sedative agents offers the greatest flexibility for titrating doses and for deep sedation.
- Infants younger than 3 months should not get ketamine due to the high risk of airway complications.
- Pressure applied to the "laryngospasm notch" (see Figure 20–3) may reverse laryngospasm.
- Emergence reactions associated with ketamine appear to be related to the pretreatment anxiety level of the patient.
- Deep sedation for painless procedures can be achieved by a variety of drugs; the clinician should become familiar with one or two and understand fully the risks and dosing.
- Etomidate as a sedative is associated with very few airway events, and can be used in the hypotensive patient.
- Combinations of drugs may potentiate desired properties of each, but it may also increase adverse effects such as respiratory depression.

Over the last two decades, acknowledgment of the presence[1] and importance of pediatric pain[2] has transformed the management of ill and injured patients. Procedural sedation and analgesia (PSA) are now an integral component of pediatric emergency care.[3] Increased availability of emergent imaging has expanded the emergency physician's role to include magnetic resonance imaging (MRI) and computed tomography (CT) scan sedation.[4] With the corresponding increase in research, the ability of emergency medicine practitioners to safely control pain and produce sedation is now established and expected.[5–7]

Sedatives with or without analgesics are given for tedious, precise, or painful procedures, resulting in a level of consciousness depressed enough to accomplish the procedure while maintaining respiratory drive. The previous misnomer *conscious sedation* has been replaced by four levels of procedural sedation, each with increasing risk of loss of protective and cardiorespiratory functions.[8] Anxiolysis or "Minimal Sedation" impairs coordination and cognitive function, but allows patients to respond appropriately to verbal stimuli. "Moderate sedation" retains purposeful response to verbal or light stimuli,

but with profound relaxation. Under "deep sedation," repeated painful stimulation yields purposeful response, at doses "not likely" to depress ventilatory function. "General anesthesia" is the state where painful stimuli do not evoke a response, thus the corresponding lack of tone can compromise both airway reflexes and cardiorespiratory function.

The Joint Commission and the American Academy of Pediatrics recognize that sedation is a continuum; therefore, safety and monitoring guidelines focus on the ability to rescue a patient from a deeper level of sedation than intended.[3,9] Cooperation for a painless diagnostic study, such as MRI, requires a different degree and duration of sedation than a painful fracture reduction. Safety guidelines encompass patient assessment, personnel and monitoring equipment, discharge criteria, and quality assurance. Knowledge of specific medications is critical, but guidelines leave specific requirements to individual hospital credentialing committees. As the specific intent of rapid sequence intubation (RSI) is to eliminate protective airway reflexes and respiratory drive, RSI is not considered procedural sedation and will not be discussed.

▶ PATIENT ASSESSMENT

The analgesic or sedative need is determined by the patient complaint, the status and responses of the child, the preference of the treating clinician, and, when appropriate, family. Not every child requires sedation for a laceration repair, and not every child can complete a fast CT scan awake.

Prior to moderate or deep procedural sedation, children should undergo a focused history pertinent to their chief complaint using a modified SAMPLE approach[10] (see Table 20–1).

In addition to obstructive airway concerns such as snoring, other factors which have been associated with an increased risk of adverse events or the need for intervention include recurrent or current stridor, obstructive sleep apnea, morbid obesity, symptomatic asthma or heart disease, gastroesophageal reflux, or swallowing problems.[11]

The importance of recent food intake is balanced in the emergency department (ED) by the urgency of the procedure and whether overall ED acuity will be unsafe with compromised flow (e.g., delaying sedation a full 6 hours after intake of a cracker when multiple high-acuity patients are waiting for rooms). A recent emergency clinical practice guideline takes urgency, sedative type, and recent literature into account to determine reasonable fasting times[12] (Fig. 20–1).

Vital signs including baseline blood pressure, oxygen saturation, and temperature should be documented, as well as a

► **TABLE 20–1. PEDIATRIC SAMPLE HISTORY FOR SEDATION**

- Signs/Symptoms: Respiratory infections or obstruction? Snoring? Sleep apnea? Stridor? Heart Disease? Gastroesophageal reflux? Swallowing problems?
- Allergies: Include egg, soy, and latex
- Medications: Particularly concurrent opioids, other analgesics
- Past medical and sedation history: Seizures? Family history of, or prior sedation problems?
- Last meal, liquid
- Events leading to need for sedation: Head injury? Previous failed sedation? Bad experiences with needles or health care?

brief examination of the oropharynx, posterior pharynx, and chest. Because of the relatively larger tongue and more reactive tonsils and adenoids in children, positional respiratory compromise is more of a concern in children undergoing PSA than adults. Larger tonsils or a history of snoring or apnea should guide a clinician to consider having a nasopharyngeal airway at the bedside, rather than across the department. Evaluate the airway using a Malampati score or other method to assess ease of emergent intubation[13] (Fig. 20–2). Any patient who could be dangerous or difficult to intubate, including those with craniofacial abnormalities, past reconstruction of the trachea, or atlantoaxial instability, merits careful risk-benefit consideration and consultation if general anesthesia may be more appropriate.

Assign any child undergoing PSA in the ED an American Society of Anesthesiologists (ASA) score. ASA 1 or 2 patients are generally healthy children who are good candidates for PSA in the ED; ASA 4 or 5 patients are generally better treated in a formal operating room or procedural unit. ASA 3 patients may be managed in either area depending on the nature of the problem and the capabilities of the treating physician. Rating of ASA category may be subjective even for anesthesiologists[14]; a low systemic risk score should not override a concerning airway evaluation.

Immediately prior to sedation, Joint Commission requirements state that patients must be reassessed to ensure that their physical condition has not deteriorated since the initial examination. The AAP guidelines call for a "time out," documenting the patient's name, procedure, and reason for procedure.[3]

► EQUIPMENT

The mnemonic "Soap Me!" includes all aspects of equipment that should be immediately available during deep sedation (Table 20–2). Of these, suction, oxygen, and monitoring equipment should be set up and running in the room prior to initiation of sedation, while an airway crash cart can be readily available but not opened. A bag-valve-mask setup may be left unopened in the room for moderate sedation, but should be open and ready to use for anticipated deep sedation.

Use of supplemental oxygen is surprisingly controversial, perhaps because of early association with adverse events in dental clinics where its use is routine.[15] While critics argue it may mask hypoventilation, studies of ED sedations where supplemental 02 is supplied have fewer hypoxia events than

when it is withheld. Rates of desaturation in ketamine and propofol studies without supplemental oxygen are provided for comparison in Table 20–3.[16–19]

► PATIENT MONITORING

The degree of monitoring required is determined by the intended depth of sedation and the procedure to be performed. Patients receiving analgesia alone for an acute painful condition or minimal sedation/anxiolysis generally do not require any additional monitoring. For example, a child with a clavicle fracture receiving oral acetaminophen with hydrocodone or a patient with abdominal pain receiving a standard dose of morphine generally will not require continuous monitoring beyond repeat vital signs. Likewise, anxiolysis alone does not require additional monitoring.

Single smaller doses of nonparenteral medications separated in time typically result in minimal sedation/anxiolysis. A child given hydrocodone in triage who then receives intranasal midazolam immediately prior to a procedure is unlikely to descend to deep sedation. The sedation level anticipated with combinations and dosages given concurrently is often addressed explicitly in individual hospital policies. When 0.1 mg/kg of morphine is inadequate for severe fractures,[20,21] or when adjunct parenteral benzodiazepines are needed (e.g., femur fractures), monitoring with a minimum of continuous pulse oximetry is warranted.

Patients undergoing moderate or deep procedural sedation require continuous cardiac and pulse oximetry monitoring, with intermittent blood pressure and respiratory rate checks. Generally, electronic monitoring should be in place prior to sedation initiation. In difficult circumstances, PSA may begin with bedside monitoring by an appropriately trained nurse or physician after a check to ensure the electronic equipment works. A child who continually screams and thrashes from the blood pressure cuff, oximetry, or an end-tidal monitor is in danger of laryngospasm or postsedation emergence.[22] After baseline vitals immediately prior to sedation, if necessary, remove the offending monitor and calm the child prior to induction, then replace when the child is asleep.

Deep sedation requires an additional person whose sole responsibility is to monitor the patient. Using moderate sedation, the seditionist can perform a procedure with a person monitoring who can intermittently assist with the procedure. The seditionist should understand monitoring equipment, recognize the signs and symptoms of respiratory depression, and be able to provide effective bag-valve-mask ventilation should apnea occur.

The most common serious risk of PSA is hypoxia from respiratory depression. For most patients, continuous pulse oximetry will provide both an ongoing assessment of oxygenation as well as a continuous display of heart rate. Clinicians should recognize that pulse oximetry may not reflect hypoventilation, particularly if supplemental oxygen is being provided. For children in whom it is important to maintain normal arterial CO_2 tensions, a continuous end-tidal capnometer (ETCO2) should be added to the monitoring equipment. In addition to providing information about apnea and obstruction well in advance of oximetry,[23] the ETCO2 wave form shows each exhalation, giving information about perfusion, shallow breathing,

Standard-risk patient[a]

Oral intake in the prior 3 h	Procedural urgency[b]			
	Emergent procedure	Urgent procedure	Semiurgent	Nonurgent
Nothing	All levels of sedation	All levels of sedation	All levels of sedation	All levels of sedation
Clear liquids only	All levels of sedation	All levels of sedation	Up to and including brief deep sedation	Up to and including extended moderate sedation
Light snack	All levels of sedation	Up to and including brief deep sedation	Up to and including dissociative sedation; nonextended moderate sedation	Minimal sedation only
Heavier snack or meal	All levels of sedation	Up to and including extended moderate sedation	Minimal sedation only	Minimal sedation only

Higher-risk patient[a]

Oral intake in the prior 3 h	Procedural urgency[b]			
	Emergent procedure	Urgent procedure	Semiurgent	Nonurgent
Nothing	All levels of sedation	All levels of sedation	All levels of sedation	All levels of sedation
Clear liquids only	All levels of sedation	Up to and including brief deep sedation	Up to and including extended moderate sedation	Minimal sedation only
Light snack	All levels of sedation	Up to and including dissociative sedation; nonextended moderate sedation	Minimal sedation only	Minimal sedation only
Heavier snack or meal	All levels of sedation	Up to and including dissociative sedation; nonextended moderate sedation	Minimal sedation only	Minimal sedation only

Procedural sedation and analgesia targeted depth and duration[c] (Increasing potential aspiration risk):

- Minimal sedation only
- Dissociative sedation; brief or intermediate-length moderate sedation
- Extended moderate sedation
- Brief-deep sedation
- Intermediate or extended-length deep sedation

Brief: < 10 min
Intermediate: 10–20 min
Extended: > 20 min

[a]Higher-risk patients are those with one or more of the following present to a degree individually or cumulativel judged clinically important by the treating physician:
- Potential for difficult-or prolonged-assisted ventilation should an airway-complication occur (e.g., short neck, small mandible/micrognathia, large tongue, tracheomalacia, laryngomalacia, history ofdifficult intubation, congential anomalies of the airway and neck, sleep apnea).
- Conditions predisposing to esophageal reflux (e.g., elevated intracranial pressure, esophageal disease, hiatal hernia, peptic ulcer disease, gastritis, bowel obstruction, ileus, tracheoesophageal fistula).
- Extremes of age (e.g., >70 y or <6 mo).
- Severe systemic disease with definite functional limitation (i.e., ASA physical status 3 or greater).
- Other clinical findings leading the EP to judge the patient to be at higher than standard risk (e.g., altered level of consciousness, frail appearance).

[b]Procedural urgency:
- Emergent (e.g., cardioversion for life-threatening dysrhythmia, reduction of markedly angulated fracture or dislocation with soft-tissue or vascular compromise, intractable pain or suffering).
- Urgent (e.g., care of dirty wounds and lacerations, animal and human bites, abscess incision and drainage, fracture reduction, hip reduction, lumbar puncture for suspected meningitis, arthrocentesis, neuroimaging for trauma).
- Semiurgent (e.g., care of clean wounds and lacerations, shoulder reduction, neuroimaging for new-onset seizure, foreign body removal, sexual assault examination).
- Nonurgent or elective (e.g., nonvegetable foreign body in external auditory canal, chronic embedded soft tissue foreign body, ingrown toenail).

[c]Procedural sedation and analgesia terminology and definitions:
- Minimal sedation (anxiolysis):[1,15] A drug-induced state during which patients respond normally to verbal commands. Although cognitive function and coordination may be impaired, ventilatory and cardiovascular functions are unaffected.
- Moderate sedation (formerly "conscious sedation"):[1,15] A drug-induced depression of consciousness during which patients respond purposefully to verbal commands, either alone or accompanied by light tactile stimulation. Reflex withdrawal from a painful stimulus is not considered a purposeful response. No interventions are required to maintain a patent airway, and spontaneous ventilation is adequate. Cardiovascular function is usually maintained.
- Dissociative sedation:[15,17] A trance-like cataleptic state induced by the dissociative agent ketamine characterized by profound analgesia and amnesia, with retention of protective airway reflexes, spontaneous respirations, and cardiopulmonary stability.
- Deep sedation:[1,15] A drug-induced depression of consciousness during which patients cannot be easily aroused but respond purposefully following repeated or painful stimulation. The ability to independently maintain ventilatory function may be impaired. Patients may require assistance in maintaining a patient airway and spontaneous ventilation may be inadequate. Cardiovascular function is usually maintained.
- General anesthesia:[1,15] A drug-induced loss of consciousness during which patients are not arousable, even by painful stimulation. The ability to independently maintain ventilatory function is often impaired. Patients often require assistance in maintaining a patent airway, and positive pressure ventilation may be required because of depressed spontaneous ventilation or drug-induced depression of neuromuscular function. Cardiovascular function may be impaired.

Figure 20–1. Prudent limits of targeted depth and length of ED procedural sedation and analgesia based on presedation assessment of aspiration risk. (With permission from Green SM, Roback M, Miner J, et al. Fasting and emergency department procedural sedation and analgesia: a consensus-based clinical practice advisory. *Ann Emerg Med*. 2007;49(4):454–461.)

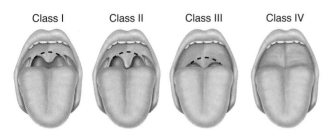

Figure 20-2. The Mallampati score. Mallampati I, if the examiner can see down to the tonsillar pillars; class II, if the examiner can visualize just the full uvula; class III, if only the soft palate can be seen; and class IV if the hard palate is all that is visualized. (With permission from Samsoon Y. Difficult tracheal intubation: a retrospective study. *Anaesthesia.* 1987;42:487.)

coughing, or erratic breaths suggesting waking or obstruction. While the AAP guidelines do not require ETCO2 monitoring for every sedation performed, whenever the patient is physically removed from the ED (as for an MRI), ETCO2 monitoring should be used. In cases where the patient's respiratory effort is difficult to assess even at the bedside, as in the obese patient with a gluteal abscess who will be sedated prone, ETCO2 may be useful.

The timing and duration of patient monitoring is determined by both the agent used and the procedure performed. At a minimum, any sedated children should have monitoring continued until the clinical effects of their drug therapy have dissipated, the pharmacologic peak is past, and the child's respiratory and mental status have approached baseline. This is extremely important in children undergoing acute painful procedures such as fracture reductions. The greatest risk of hypoventilation in these children may occur after the painful stimuli of the procedure have ceased. Conversely, children who initially present extremely agitated and crying vigorously may exhaust themselves and remain sleeping long after the pharmacologic effects of a sedative have passed. As a consequence, the duration of patient monitoring must be determined individually, but it should be maintained long enough to be certain that any clinically dangerous effects of administered drugs have resolved.

▶ **TABLE 20-2. EQUIPMENT FOR DEEP SEDATION (SOAP ME)**

- Suction: Appropriate size suction catheters connected and tested
- Oxygen: Appropriate size mask, bag, and sufficient oxygen flow to inflate anesthesia bag
- Airway: Nasopharyngeal, oropharyngeal airways, LMAs, laryngoscope, blades, endotracheal tubes
- Pharmacy: Advanced life support medications and reversal agents
- Monitors: Cardiac, respiratory, oxygen saturation, and ETCO2 when appropriate
- Equipment: Case appropriate special equipment (C-arm, defibrillator)

▶ **TABLE 20-3. RATES OF OXYGEN DESATURATION BY REGIMEN AND SUPPLEMENTAL O₂ USE**

Study	Medication	Supplemental O₂	Desaturation %
Godambe	Ketamine/Midazolam	N	4/54 (7%)
Kennedy	Ketamine/Midazolam	N	8/130 (6%)
Kennedy	Fentanyl/Midazolam	N	32/130 (25%)
Godambe	Propofol/Fentanyl	N	19/59 (30%)
Guenther	Propofol/Fentanyl	Y	20/291 (7%)
Bassett	Propofol/Fentanyl	Y	19/393 (5%)

Discharge of children undergoing PSA should not occur until the child has returned to an appropriate presedation mental and physical baseline. Children should demonstrate the ability to tolerate sips of fluids, and maintain head control if they are still in a child-seat. After-care instructions should reflect the fact that the child has received an agent that may alter mental status and must therefore receive close supervision. Caution caregivers to restrict play activities such as bike riding or climbing for 24 hours. Patients receiving long-acting medications, or for whom reversal agents were required, may require monitoring in a step-down unit until peak medication action has passed.

Properly staffed and prepared EDs have demonstrated low complication rates for all PSA patients, with no published aspirations or deaths. Implementation of current guidelines has further improved hospital sedation safety.[5,6,24–26]

▶ ROUTES OF ADMINISTRATION IV, IM, SQ, PO, TM

Intravenous (IV) administration offers the greatest flexibility in terms of titrating medications to a specific patient response. The most significant limitation to this approach is the problem that IV access may present in infants and agitated children. IV administration is also the preferred route for a child when medication titration is anticipated or deep sedation is planned.

Intramuscular (IM) and subcutaneous (SQ) injections provide reliable delivery but should be reserved for drugs with well-established dose–response relationships such as ketamine. Repeated administration of drugs via these routes is painful and places children in the position of deciding between the pain of their medical condition and the pain of another needle.

Oral (PO) administration should be reserved for drugs with predictable actions, or in cases when placement of an IV is not possible until oral sedatives take effect (such as strong, combative patients with autism or other psychiatric conditions). The timing of repeat doses can be difficult to determine due to delays in absorption and onset of action. PO administration does have the advantage of being the most comfortable of all routes of administration.

Transmucosal (TM) drug administration is rising in popularity. Quicker in onset than PO administrations, TM delivery still is slow enough to make titration of medications difficult. Sedative medications have been successfully delivered transmucosally through the oral, buccal, intranasal, and rectal routes, with the two best-researched being rectal methohexital,[27,28] midazolam,[29–31] and Fentanyl.[32]

Inhalation of nitrous oxide[33,34] and methoxyfluorane[35] has been described in children in the ED setting and is a relatively well-tolerated route of delivery. Advantages of this route include ease of delivery and painless administration; the disadvantages are the need for specialized equipment and patient cooperation.

▶ SEDATIVE AND ANALGESIC AGENTS

Medications most commonly used for PSA are listed in Table 20–4. Physicians intent on using these agents clinically must be familiar with their indications, all of their actions, relative contraindications, and potential alternatives. Physicians caring for children should have a working knowledge of multiple agents and be adept at choosing alternate drugs when their drug of choice is inappropriate in a given circumstance.

MINIMAL SEDATION/ANXIOLYSIS

Minimal sedation/anxiolysis in the ED is most commonly provided for laceration repair when a topical anesthetic will provide pain control, or when a patient is anxious about a brief painless procedure (e.g., a CT scan). Regimens which will not require an IV are preferred when an IV is not required for any other reason.

Benzodiazepines, the most commonly used sedative hypnotic agents for anxiolysis, act on γ-aminobutyric acid (GABA) receptors and are reversible with the competitive antagonist flumazenil if needed. Midazolam is a short-acting benzodiazepine commonly used for procedural sedation in the ED setting. Oral midazolam doses of 0.5 to 1 mg/kg as a single agent typically result in calmness within 15 to 30 minutes, while intranasal delivery at 0.3 mg/kg to 0.5 mg/kg takes effect in 5 to 15 minutes.[29,30] The medication may burn during nasal administration, and is more associated with paradoxical reactions and subsequent irritability at home than the oral route (6%).[31] Rectal doses of 0.45 mg/kg to 1 mg/kg have ranged in efficacy from 62%[36] to 93% for laceration repair, but result in up to 27% agitation.[37] IV administration results in a paradoxical reaction in 1.4% of patients, which can be reversed with flumazenil.[38,39]

The combination of oral midazolam and Fentanyl resulted in more vomiting during laceration repair,[40] but enteral hydrocodone and midazolam have not been adequately studied. Since the time of peak effect of hydrocodone is 1.3 hours, it may be more effective if given in triage rather than immediately before a procedure.

Nitrous oxide is an inhaled sedative analgesic that does not function through opioid receptor stimulation. Administered as an oxygen–nitrous oxide mixture, it has an onset of action of 2 to 3 minutes and a similar duration of action. This drug is not metabolized and is excreted only through exhalation by the lungs. The sedation and analgesia produced by this drug is dose dependent. The minimal concentration with any clinical efficacy is a 30% nitrous oxide to 70% oxygen mixture, typically

slowly dialed up to 50% to 50% mixture or delivered premixed in the 50:50 ratio. Considered "minimal sedation/anxiolysis" up to 50%, at concentrations of 51% to 70% it is considered moderate, and can become deep when adjunct opioids are given.[18]

Older demand-valve nitrous oxide systems designed for self-administration have been supplemented by continuous flow systems applicable to young children.[18,41] For laceration repair, N_2O delivered by a free flow system with a scavenger[18] was found to be more effective and associated with better caregiver satisfaction than midazolam or nitrous and midazolam in combination.[18] Because of its rapid diffusion, N_2O is contraindicated with trapped air (e.g., pneumocephalus or pneumothorax) and may cause ear pain in patients with otitis media. Vomiting is an issue with 10% to 20% of patients, but this can be lessened with a slow increase in percentage of N_2O. One study found that eating small amounts eliminated vomiting, which would contradict most hospital npo policies unless doses limited to anxiolysis were administered.[34]

MODERATE SEDATION

As the distinction between minimal and moderate sedation is clinically nuanced, institutional guidelines often arbitrarily define "moderate" based on types and doses of medications. Traditionally, combinations of IV opioid and benzodiazapines in variable doses are considered moderate sedation, resulting in profound relaxation during which a patient can still respond to verbal stimuli.

Multiple redoses may be needed before patients will tolerate painful procedures, however, and as noted in Table 20–3 adverse events may be more common than with "deep" sedatives due to synergistic respiratory depression. The Pitetti study found that 23% of the IV fentanyl/midazolam sedation regimens had complications, compared with 8.6% of the IV ketamine/midazolam group ($p < 0.001$). Roback et al. echoed these findings, reporting in 2005 that airway complications occurred in 6.1% of ketamine sedations, compared to 19.3% of those using fentanyl/midazolam.[24]

Ketamine has become the most commonly used sedative for painful emergency procedures. As a dissociative analgesic agent, it produces a trance-like cataleptic state through disruption of communications between the cortical and limbic systems. Within 2 minutes after induction, patients rarely respond to repeated painful stimulation. While this more closely matches the definition of "deep sedation" or even "general anesthesia," the safety profile is better than combinations of benzodiazepines and opioids, and spontaneous respiratory drive is maintained even with large doses. A clinical practice guideline recommended introducing a new category of sedation, "dissociative," be reserved just for this drug.[42] For induction, 4 to 5 mg/kg IM or 1.5 mg/kg IV have been found to be effective doses.[43,44]

Ketamine has mild sympathomimetic effects that can decrease bronchospasm, raise systemic blood pressure, and produce tachycardia. Ketamine does increase intracranial and intraocular pressure and should be avoided in children at risk for increased intracranial pressure. Transient apnea has been reported when the drug has been administered by rapid intravenous bolus, so administration over 60 seconds is prudent.[26] The ketamine clinical practice guideline cites numerous

▶ TABLE 20-4. COMMON PEDIATRIC PROCEDURAL SEDATION AND ANALGESIC AGENTS

Medication	Route	Dose (mg/kg)	*Typical Maximum	Onset in Minutes	Duration	Comments
			Sedative Analgesics			
Morphine	IV, IM, SQ	0.1–0.15	8	5	2–4 h	Treat itching with diphenydramine
Fentanyl	IV, IN	0.001–0.002 (1–2 µg/kg/dose)	0.075 (75 µg/dose)	1–2	20 min	Rigidity with rapid administration
	TM	0.010–0.015 (10–15 µg/kg/dose)		30		Increased vomiting when combined with midazolam, not recommended[40,77]
Hydromorphone	IV	0.01–0.02	2	30	4–6 h	
Hydrocodone	PO	0.2	10	30	4–6 h	
Codeine	PO	1–1.5	60	30	4–6 h	Up to 15% of children would not metabolize to effective metobolite
			Sedatives			
Midazolam	IV	0.05–0.1	2	2	30 min–2 h	
	IN	0.3–0.5	12	5–15	1–3 h	
	PR, PO	0.5–1 mg/kg		30	60–90	
Pentobarbital	IV	2.0–6.0	200	2–5	2–4 h	
Thiopental	IV	3.0–5.0	500	0.5	20 min	Intubation doses
	PR	15–40	1200	10–30	60–90	17% defecation
Methohexital	IV	1–3	100	1	20 min	
	PR	18.0–25.0		6–20	1–2 h	
Chloral Hydrate	PO	50–75	1000	60–90	10–24 h	Postdischarge deaths, not an ED drug
Propofol	IV	1–2	75	0.5	20 min	Egg/soy allergy
	Infusion	100 µg/kg/min			5 min	
Etomidate	IV	0.3	20	0.5	10 min	Do not use if septic
			Other Agents			
Ketamine	IV	1.0–1.5	60	2	45–90 min	
	IM	4–5	100	5	1–2 h	
	PO	10	250	35	3 h	
Nitrous Oxide	Inhalation	30–70%		1–2	1–2 min	
Diphenhydramine	PO	1.0–1.5	50	15	2–4 h	
Dexmedetomidine	IV	1–2 µg/kg over 10 min		5–6	45–85	Hypotension and bradycardia
	Infusion	1.5 µg/kg/h				
	Intranasal	1 µg/kg		45	90	
	Buccal	4 µg/kg		15	30	
Olanzapine (Zydis)	PO	Repeat of child's normal dose				Existing psychiatric history
Risperidone (M-Tabs)	PO	6 and up, 1 mg		15		Existing psychiatric history
Ziprasidone	IM	10 mg		15		Existing psychiatric history
			Reversal Agents			
Naloxone	IV, IM	0.1	2 mg	2 min	20 min	
Flumazenil	IV	0.01	0.2 mg	2 min	30 min	

*Typical maximum dose = effective in most patients. Since all patients respond differently, some patients may require more, in which case precautions in monitoring the patient should be taken.

references of airway complications in infants younger than 3 months, and considers this age to be an absolute contraindication with risks outweighing benefits.[42]

Ketamine increases protective airway reflexes. While protective against aspiration, a 0.4% to 0.9% incidence of transient laryngospasm has been reported[45,46] with rare reports of persistent laryngospasm after IM ketamine leading to intubation without cardiorespiratory sequellae.[40] This laryngospasm rate increased to 2.5% in a series of children receiving upper airway manipulation, although none required intubation.[47] Use of atropine has been shown to decrease hypersalivation, a theoretical risk factor, with a significantly decreased percentage of postsedation vomiting.[48]

Given the low incidence of laryngospasm, prospective randomized trials would need to be prohibitively large to demonstrate increased risk from upper airway infections, asthma, or secretions. Data extrapolated from anesthesia suggests all of these are risk factors,[49] but whether these conclusions apply to procedural sedation is debated. Given the risk, a useful location to know is the "laryngospasm notch" (Fig. 20–3). Described by Philip C. Larson, "pressure is applied with the thumbs or forefingers inwardly and anteriorly on each side of the head at the apex of the notch (see pressure point arrow)." Its effectiveness has been attributed to either pain from pushing the styloid process reversing supraglottic obstruction or an unknown physiologic response.

Two other complications associated with ketamine are emergence and vomiting. Emergent reactions range from confused agitation to vivid hallucinations to hours of screaming. The widely varying incidence reported in the literature reflects this spectrum of definitions, but is roughly 15% for mild and <2% for severe agitation. Emergence reactions appear to be related to the child's level of anxiety prior to the procedure, so pretreatment with a benzodiazepine may be helpful for the anxious child.[22] Midazolam after ketamine administration has not been shown to decrease emergence, but may cut the 20% rate of vomiting in half.[50]

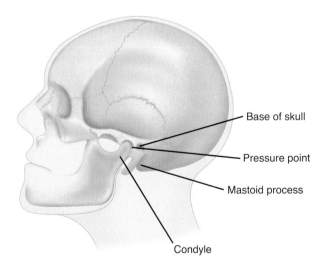

Figure 20–3. The Laryngospasm notch. "Digital pressure is applied firmly inwardly and anteriorly on each side of the head at the apex of the notch" (see pressure point arrow).

DEEP SEDATION

Medications in this group are also referred to as sedative hypnotic agents because of the ability to sedate patients and induce sleep. Most of the agents in this class exert their effect through the GABA receptor of central nervous system neurons. It is imperative to administer sufficient sedative hypnotic medications; delivery of subtherapeutic doses of any agents in this class will cause disinhibition in the child and may result in agitated, uncontrolled behavior with an increased risk of laryngospasm. Treatment of this state is through administration of more of the sedative hypnotic agent to take the child through the plane of disinhibition to one of somnolence.

Barbiturates are the classic pediatric sedative agents. All the medications in this class produce predictable sedation with variability in effects related to their lipid solubility and rate of central nervous system penetration. Drugs used for ED sedation include pentobarbital, thiopental, and methohexital.

Thiopental has largely been replaced by etomidate as an induction agent for rapid-sequence intubation protocols. Methohexital, however, has a similar onset and dosage as propofol (see below) when administered IV, and can be used as a continuous bolus for patients needing an MRI for whom propofol is contraindicated. Both rapidly penetrate the central nervous system and induce profound sedation within 30 seconds. Respiratory depression is a prominent feature of IV administration of these drugs at standard induction doses, and apnea should be anticipated in any child in whom these doses are used. Rectal administration of 25 to 30 mg/kg of methohexital has proved effective for sedation of children undergoing diagnostic radiology studies, with transient airway events in 4% to 10%.[27,28] Absorption via this route may be rapid, and parents holding a child after administration of the drug should be closely supervised, sitting down, and positioned as if the child is already sleeping.

Pentobarbital is a rapid-acting, less-potent sedative hypnotic used primarily in sedation for very brief diagnostic studies. Administered either IV or IM, this agent produces very predictable actions, with a success rate of 97% for diagnostic studies. Pentobarbital produces better, more reliable sedation than benzodiazepines alone, but is outperformed and has more complications than etomidate for CTs.[51] "Pentobarbital rage" can occur in up to 7% of patients, requiring time and input from ED staff. Most protocols give up to 6 mg/kg in two to three rapid push divided doses, stacking doses every 30 seconds if the preceding one does not result in sleep.

Barbiturates have the advantage of not burning with administration, but may be hyperalgesic, and should be avoided in patients with known temporal lobe seizures.

Propofol is an ultra–short-acting sedative hypnotic used for both RSI and PSA. Propofol's mechanism of action is unclear and may relate to both a GABA receptor effect and a direct neuronal membrane action. Propofol is a highly lipid soluble agent that produces clinical effects within 30 seconds (one arm brain circulation) with a duration of 6 to 8 minutes. Contraindications include allergies to egg, soy, or propofol.

For procedures such as fast CTs and lumbar punctures, recent studies use a 2 mg/kg bolus, with supplemental boluses of 1 to 2 mg/kg maintain the sedation during the procedure.[11] For prolonged sedation, a propofol bolus is generally followed by a continuous infusion of 100 to 150 μg /kg/min.[52] ED-only studies have started with 1 mg/kg when adjunctive opioids have been used.[17,53] Propofol burns with injection, which can be mitigated by a 1 mg/kg lidocaine mini-bier block applied with tourniquet for 1 minute prior to delivery. Pain is less of an issue in older patients, particularly when an anticubital vein is used.

Airway events are the most common complications, given the profound relaxation of tone seen with propofol. The need for repositioning of the head should be expected at induction, with jaw thrusts being required 3% to 4% of the time.[16,17] One study comparing methohexital and propofol in adults noted brief bag-valve-mask in 4/52 methohexital patients and 2/51 propofol.[54] Hypotension with good perfusion is common; one study found that supplemental IV fluids resulted in a mean change of systolic blood pressure of 22 mm Hg compared to 21 mm Hg in children who were not bolused.[16]

Supplemental 02 seems to decrease the incidence of the most common side effect, mild hypoxia. Despite the greater frequency of airway-related events with propofol, serious adverse events are rare when deep sedation guidelines are followed and ED practitioners trained in airway management administer the drug.[5] Given the growing ED popularity due to rapid resolution of effects and efficacy,[6,25] propofol clinical practice guidelines for ED use were published in 2007.[7]

Propofol can actually act as an antiemetic; the balancing side effects of propofol and ketamine have led to a spate of research combining the two.[55–57] One unique side effect of propofol is the blunting of sympathetic responses, particularly cardiac.[58] For this reason, patients are uniquely susceptible to vagal stimulation, resulting in rare bradycardia and deaths reported in anesthesia literature.[59] Adjunct atropine should be readily available, though is not required for routine use in children with normal cardiac function.

Etomidate is an imidazole sedative hypnotic agent that has found application in the ED care of children. Most commonly used as an induction agent for emergency intubations, etomidate has a flat cardiovascular curve and is appropriate for hypotensive patients. Dosing at 0.3 mg/kg in a fast push brings on sedation within 30 seconds.[60] In contrast to propofol, barbiturates, or opioid/benzodiazepine combinations, etomidate is associated with very few airway events in children, with only one reported case of apnea when used alone.[51]

Etomidate does not provide analgesia, and so for emergency department procedures such as fracture reductions, adjunct opioids are required. Studies evaluating its use for pediatric painful procedures have started at 0.2 to 0.3 mg/kg, with hypoxia noted in 0% to 2% and no reported apnea.[61–63]

Side effects include burning with injection and brief myoclonus up to 22% of the time. Smaller studies in adults suggest that myoclonus can be reduced by pushing more rapidly, or by giving small 0.015 mg/kg doses of midazolam prior to administration.[64,65] Sedation from etomidate in a single bolus wears off as or even more rapidly than with propofol, which may limit its applicability in the ED. Of note, the adrenal suppression reported with prolonged ICU use can occur transiently with even a single dose. Recent evaluation of ICU patients with meningococcemia found greater death rates in patients who were intubated with etomidate rather than other sedatives;[66] thus, it should not be used for procedures in potentially septic or critically ill patients.[67]

Dexmedetomidine, related to clonidine, is a central acting α2-adrenoceptor agonist with potent sedative, analgesic, and anxiolytic actions. This drug produces minimal respiratory depression and historically was used predominately for control of patients undergoing mechanical ventilation. Hypotension and bradycardia are potential side effects diminished by loading over 10 minutes, which may limit ED utility. Recovery is relatively slow, and most studies have evaluated the drug for noninvasive prolonged studies such as MRI scans.[68,69]

Studies in children during CT scans found a 2 μg/kg bolus over 10 minutes to be effective, with no adverse airway events in 62 children.[70] Combinations of dexmedetomidine and ketamine were less satisfactory than ketamine/propofol,[57] but buccal and intranasal routes of administration may be promising future applications for agitated children where an IV is not possible.[71]

► NONPHARMACOLOGIC SEDATION AND ANALGESIA

Because of their short attention spans and susceptibility to suggestion, children are excellent candidates for nonpharmacologic sedation and analgesia techniques. Distraction either through intensive conversation, story telling, or visual or tactile stimuli are all effective means of diverting a child's attention from a brief painful procedure such as a local infiltration or IV injection. Music via earphones or videos is another distraction that may be used to occupy a child for performance of a more prolonged procedure.

In newborns, a highly concentrated sugar solution has been shown to decrease observational scores during painful procedures, such as circumcisions. The mechanism of action for this effect appears to be related to induction of central nervous system encephalins. One to two milliliter of a 50% sucrose solution and sucrose-coated nipples have proved effective in decreasing crying in neonates undergoing heel sticks or venipunctures.

► SELECTION OF PSA AGENTS

Which PSA agent to employ in any given scenario should be left to the clinician caring for a particular child. Hospital or departmental policies that permit access to a complete choice of medications allow treating physicians to match a child more appropriately to the correct PSA agent. In a study of sedation preferences for posttraumatic head CT scans, more than 20 different regimens were described. Overly restrictive ED formularies may force performance of a procedure with a less-than-optimal drug and increase the possibilities of an injury or adverse advent.

PSA selection is also dictated by the intended effect on a child. If cooperation for a painless diagnostic procedure is desired, then a sedative hypnotic agent will be the drug of choice. Use of a narcotic analgesic to produce somnolence may require such a large dose that respiratory depression becomes a risk. For the same reasons, use of a pure sedative with no analgesic properties to provide cooperation for a painful procedure is equally inappropriate.

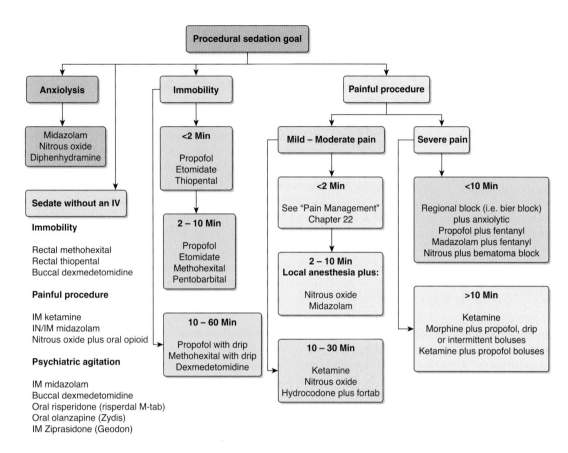

Figure 20–4. Regimens are given in order of decreasing efficacy based on prospective trials. When no evidence is available, the regimen with the fewest airway complications is listed first.

Combinations of different agents may be used to take advantage of the desired properties of each. The most frequent combinations pair short-acting sedatives with short-acting narcotics such as fentanyl/midazolam or fentanyl/propofol. Caution should be maintained with such combinations because not only will the desired effects be enhanced but adverse effects such as respiratory depression may also be increased. Doses lower than those of either agent alone should be used initially when combining potent agents.

Combining a local anesthetic with a sedative can also produce effective patient control. The regional anesthesia permits pain control, and the sedative produces anxiolysis and cooperation for the procedure. Procedures such as lumbar punctures and laceration repairs are examples of where this technique is applied.

Potential agents for different desired clinical outcomes are listed in Figure 20–4.

▶ CHILDREN WITH SPECIAL HEALTH CARE NEEDS

At times an emergency physician will be asked to provide sedation for an agitated or psychotic patient so that IV access can be obtained. For patients who already carry a psychiatric diagnosis (autism and schizophrenia), one option is orally dissolving tablets of atypical antipsychotics. These have been shown to be more effective than haloperidol, with less risk of extrapyramidal side effects.[72] Intramuscular midazolam has been proven more effective and safer than IM haloperidol as well.[73] Newer antipsychotics such as ziprasidone result in sedation in 15 minutes when given IM, but have largely been tested only in adults.[74,75] For pediatric patients, repeating an oral dose of medications the patient already takes is an option. For psychosis, starting with low doses and repeating in 20 minutes after consultation with a psychiatrist is recommended. For milder psychiatric disease, dexmedetomidine is a promising new option. One series of 122 patients, many with diagnoses of delay, autism, or psychiatric illness, found onset of sedation in a mean time of 27 minutes using 5 μg/kg of buccal dexmedetomidine.[76]

Children with underlying medical conditions, frequently referred to as children with special health care needs (CSHCN), are becoming more frequent visitors to community as well as academic EDs. These children will require PSA both for problems related to their underlying conditions and for acute problems common to all children. Often sedation or analgesic agents are withheld for fear of complications related to preexisting conditions. In reality, these patients are more appropriate candidates for PSA to avoid undue physiologic or psychological stresses.

The approach to PSA in this population is the same as for any other child, except that selection of the PSA agent must take into account not only the child's acute problem but also preexisting conditions. Whenever possible, coordination of sedation with a child's medication schedule should be attempted. A child on neuropsychiatric or seizure medications who becomes somnolent following routine dosing of the medication may undergo a painless diagnostic study a short time after receipt of their last medication dose. Children with cardiovascular problems should be managed with agents such as fentanyl, which have little blood pressure or heart rate effects. Children with respiratory pathology or anatomic upper airway difficulties may best be served with regional anesthesia or a drug with minimal ventilatory effects such as ketamine. Children with hepatic or renal failure may be more sensitive to barbiturate and other drugs, requiring prolonged postprocedure observation. Emergency physicians should also not hesitate to involve anesthesiology colleagues to help with these patients, particularly those who are ASA class 3 or above.

▶ SUMMARY

Safe, effective PSA is an integral part of any child's ED care. Emergency physicians have proved competent and reliable in the delivery of this treatment to ED patients, but they must remain vigilant throughout the administration and recovery from PSA to ensure patient safety and comfort.

REFERENCES

1. Anand KJ, Sippell WG, Aynsley-Green A. Randomised trial of fentanyl anaesthesia in preterm babies undergoing surgery: effects on the stress response. *Lancet.* 1987;1(8524): 62–66.
2. Weisman SJ, Bernstein B, Schechter NL. Consequences of inadequate analgesia during painful procedures in children. *Arch Pediatr Adolesc Med.* 1998;152(2):147–149.
3. Cote CJ, Wilson S. Guidelines for monitoring and management of pediatric patients during and after sedation for diagnostic and therapeutic procedures: an update. *Pediatrics.* 2006;118(6):2587–2602.
4. Sacchetti A, Carraccio C, Giardino A, Harris RH. Sedation for pediatric CT scanning: is radiology becoming a drug-free zone? *Pediatr Emerg Care.* 2005;21(5):295–297.
5. Cravero JP, Blike GT, Beach M, et al. Incidence and nature of adverse events during pediatric sedation/anesthesia for procedures outside the operating room: report from the Pediatric Sedation Research Consortium. *Pediatrics.* 2006;118(3):1087–1096.
6. Sacchetti A, Stander E, Ferguson N, Maniar G, Valko P. Pediatric procedural sedation in the community emergency department: results from the ProSCED registry. *Pediatr Emerg Care.* 2007;23(4):218–222.
7. Miner JR, Burton JH. Clinical practice advisory: emergency department procedural sedation with propofol. *Ann Emerg Med.* 2007;50(2):182–187.
8. Mace SE, Barata IA, Cravero JP, et al. Clinical policy: evidence-based approach to pharmacologic agents used in pediatric sedation and analgesia in the emergency department. *Ann Emerg Med.* 2004;44(4):342–377.
9. JCAHO. *Comprehensive Accreditation Manual for Hospitals (CAMH): The Official Handbook;* 2006:NPC41–PC43.
10. Dieckmann R, Brownstein D, Gausche-Hill M, eds. *Pediatric Education for Prehospital Professionals.* 2nd ed. Sudbury, MA: Jones and Bartlett Publishers; 2006.
11. Vespasiano M, Finkelstein M, Kurachek S. Propofol sedation: intensivists' experience with 7304 cases in a children's hospital. *Pediatrics.* 2007;120(6):e1411–e1417.
12. Green SM, Roback MG, Miner JR, Burton JH, Krauss B. Fasting and emergency department procedural sedation and analgesia: a consensus-based clinical practice advisory. *Ann Emerg Med.* 2007;49(4):454–461.
13. Mallampati SR. Clinical sign to predict difficult tracheal intubation (hypothesis). *Can Anaesth Soc J.* 1983;30(3)(Pt 1):316–317.
14. Burgoyne LL, Smeltzer MP, Pereiras LA, Norris AL, De Armendi AJ. How well do pediatric anesthesiologists agree when assigning ASA physical status classifications to their patients? *Paediatr Anaesth.* 2007;17(10):956–962.
15. Leelataweedwud P, Vann WF Jr. Adverse events and outcomes of conscious sedation for pediatric patients: study of an oral sedation regimen. *J Am Dent Assoc.* 2001;132(11):1531–1539; quiz 96.
16. Guenther E, Pribble CG, Junkins EP Jr, Kadish HA, Bassett KE, Nelson DS. Propofol sedation by emergency physicians for elective pediatric outpatient procedures. *Ann Emerg Med.* 2003;42(6):783–791.
17. Bassett KE, Anderson JL, Pribble CG, Guenther E. Propofol for procedural sedation in children in the emergency department. *Ann Emerg Med.* 2003;42(6):773–782.
18. Luhmann JD, Kennedy RM, Porter FL, Miller JP, Jaffe DM. A randomized clinical trial of continuous-flow nitrous oxide and midazolam for sedation of young children during laceration repair. *Ann Emerg Med.* 2001;37(1):20–27.
19. Godambe SA, Elliot V, Matheny D, Pershad J. Comparison of propofol/fentanyl versus ketamine/midazolam for brief orthopedic procedural sedation in a pediatric emergency department. *Pediatrics.* 2003;112(1)(Pt 1):116–123.
20. Birnbaum A, Esses D, Bijur PE, Holden L, Gallagher EJ. Randomized double-blind placebo-controlled trial of two intravenous morphine dosages (0.10 mg/kg and 0.15 mg/kg) in ED patients with moderate to severe acute pain. *Ann Emerg Med.* 2006.
21. Bijur PE, Kenny MK, Gallagher EJ. Intravenous morphine at 0.1 mg/kg is not effective for controlling severe acute pain in the majority of patients. *Ann Emerg Med.* 2005;46(4):362–367.
22. Sherwin TS, Green SM, Khan A, Chapman DS, Dannenberg B. Does adjunctive midazolam reduce recovery agitation after ketamine sedation for pediatric procedures? A randomized, double-blind, placebo-controlled trial. *Ann Emerg Med.* 2000;35(3):229–238.
23. Anderson JL, Junkins E, Pribble C, Guenther E. Capnography and depth of sedation during propofol sedation in children. *Ann Emerg Med.* 2007;49(1):9–13.
24. Roback MG, Wathen JE, Bajaj L, Bothner JP. Adverse events associated with procedural sedation and analgesia in a pediatric emergency department: a comparison of common parenteral drugs. *Acad Emerg Med.* 2005;12(6):508–513.
25. Sacchetti A, Senula G, Strickland J, Dubin R. Procedural sedation in the community emergency department: initial results of the ProSCED registry. *Acad Emerg Med.* 2007;14(1):41–46.
26. Pitetti R, Davis PJ, Redlinger R, White J, Wiener E, Calhoun KH. Effect on hospital-wide sedation practices after implementation of the 2001 JCAHO procedural sedation and analgesia guidelines. *Arch Pediatr Adolesc Med.* 2006;160(2):211–216.
27. Audenaert SM, Montgomery CL, Thompson DE, Sutherland J. A prospective study of rectal methohexital: efficacy and side effects in 648 cases. *Anesth Analg.* 1995;81(5):957–961.
28. Pomeranz ES, Chudnofsky CR, Deegan TJ, Lozon MM, Mitchiner JC, Weber JE. Rectal methohexital sedation for computed tomography imaging of stable pediatric emergency department patients. *Pediatrics.* 2000;105(5):1110–1114.

29. Acworth JP, Purdie D, Clark RC. Intravenous ketamine plus midazolam is superior to intranasal midazolam for emergency paediatric procedural sedation. *Emerg Med J.* 2001;18(1):39–45.

30. Connors K, Terndrup TE. Nasal versus oral midazolam for sedation of anxious children undergoing laceration repair. *Ann Emerg Med.* 1994;24(6):1074–1079.

31. Everitt IJ, Barnett P. Comparison of two benzodiazepines used for sedation of children undergoing suturing of a laceration in an emergency department. *Pediatr Emerg Care.* 2002;18(2):72–74.

32. Wolfe T. Intranasal fentanyl for acute pain: techniques to enhance efficacy. *Ann Emerg Med.* 2007;49(5):721–722.

33. Babl FE, Puspitadewi A, Barnett P, Oakley E, Spicer M. Preprocedural fasting state and adverse events in children receiving nitrous oxide for procedural sedation and analgesia. *Pediatr Emerg Care.* 2005;21(11):736–743.

34. Burnweit C, Diana-Zerpa JA, Nahmad MH, et al. Nitrous oxide analgesia for minor pediatric surgical procedures: an effective alternative to conscious sedation? *J Pediatr Surg.* 2004;39(3):495–499; discussion 9.

35. Babl F, Barnett P, Palmer G, Oakley E, Davidson A. A pilot study of inhaled methoxyflurane for procedural analgesia in children. *Paediatr Anaesth.* 2007;17(2):148–153.

36. Shane SA, Fuchs SM, Khine H. Efficacy of rectal midazolam for the sedation of preschool children undergoing laceration repair. *Ann Emerg Med.* 1994;24(6):1065–1073.

37. Kanegaye JT, Favela JL, Acosta M, Bank DE. High-dose rectal midazolam for pediatric procedures: a randomized trial of sedative efficacy and agitation. *Pediatr Emerg Care.* 2003;19(5):329–336.

38. Massanari M, Novitsky J, Reinstein LJ. Paradoxical reactions in children associated with midazolam use during endoscopy. *Clin Pediatr (Phila).* 1997;36(12):681–684.

39. Weinbroum AA, Szold O, Ogorek D, Flaishon R. The midazolam-induced paradox phenomenon is reversible by flumazenil. Epidemiology, patient characteristics and review of the literature. *Eur J Anaesthesiol.* 2001;18(12):789–797.

40. Klein EJ, Diekema DS, Paris CA, Quan L, Cohen M, Seidel KD. A randomized, clinical trial of oral midazolam plus placebo versus oral midazolam plus oral transmucosal fentanyl for sedation during laceration repair. *Pediatrics.* 2002;109(5):894–897.

41. Denman WT, Tuason PM, Ahmed MI, Brennen LM, Cepeda MS, Carr DB. The PediSedate device, a novel approach to pediatric sedation that provides distraction and inhaled nitrous oxide: clinical evaluation in a large case series. *Paediatr Anaesth.* 2007;17(2):162–166.

42. Green SM, Krauss B. Clinical practice guideline for emergency department ketamine dissociative sedation in children. *Ann Emerg Med.* 2004;44(5):460–471.

43. Green SM, Hummel CB, Wittlake WA, Rothrock SG, Hopkins GA, Garrett W. What is the optimal dose of intramuscular ketamine for pediatric sedation? *Acad Emerg Med.* 1999;6(1):21–26.

44. Krauss B, Green SM. Procedural sedation and analgesia in children. *Lancet.* 2006;367(9512):766–780.

45. Green SM, Rothrock SG, Lynch EL, et al. Intramuscular ketamine for pediatric sedation in the emergency department: safety profile in 1022 cases. *Ann Emerg Med.* 1998;31(6):688–697.

46. Roback MG, Wathen JE, MacKenzie T, Bajaj L. A randomized, controlled trial of i.v. versus i.m. ketamine for sedation of pediatric patients receiving emergency department orthopedic procedures. *Ann Emerg Med.* 2006;48(5):605–612.

47. Novak H, Karlsland Akeson P, Akeson J. Sedation with ketamine and low-dose midazolam for short-term procedures requiring pharyngeal manipulation in young children. *Paediatr Anaesth.* 2008;18(1):48–54.

48. Heinz P, Geelhoed GC, Wee C, Pascoe EM. Is atropine needed with ketamine sedation? A prospective, randomised, double blind study. *Emerg Med J.* 2006;23(3):206–209.

49. Olsson GL, Hallen B. Laryngospasm during anaesthesia. A computer-aided incidence study in 136,929 patients. *Acta Anaesthesiol Scand.* 1984;28(5):567–575.

50. Wathen JE, Roback MG, Mackenzie T, Bothner JP. Does midazolam alter the clinical effects of intravenous ketamine sedation in children? A double-blind, randomized, controlled, emergency department trial. *Ann Emerg Med.* 2000;36(6):579–588.

51. Baxter AL, Mallory MD, Spandorfer PR, Sharma S, Freilich SH, Cravero J. Etomidate versus pentobarbital for computed tomography sedations. A Report from the Pediatric Sedation Research Consortium. *Pediatr Emerg Care.* 2007;23(10):690–695.

52. Frankville DD, Spear RM, Dyck JB. The dose of propofol required to prevent children from moving during magnetic resonance imaging. *Anesthesiology.* 1993;79(5):953–958.

53. Miner JR, Danahy M, Moch A, Biros M. Randomized clinical trial of etomidate versus propofol for procedural sedation in the emergency department. *Ann Emerg Med.* 2007;49(1):15–22.

54. Miner JR, Biros M, Krieg S, Johnson C, Heegaard W, Plummer D. Randomized clinical trial of propofol versus methohexital for procedural sedation during fracture and dislocation reduction in the emergency department. *Acad Emerg Med.* 2003;10(9):931–937.

55. Willman EV, Andolfatto G. A prospective evaluation of "ketofol" (ketamine/propofol combination) for procedural sedation and analgesia in the emergency department. *Ann Emerg Med.* 2007;49(1):23–30.

56. Loh G, Dalen D. Low-dose ketamine in addition to propofol for procedural sedation and analgesia in the emergency department. *Ann Pharmacother* 2007;41(3):485–492.

57. Tosun Z, Akin A, Guler G, Esmaoglu A, Boyaci A. Dexmedetomidine-ketamine and propofol-ketamine combinations for anesthesia in spontaneously breathing pediatric patients undergoing cardiac catheterization. *J Cardiothorac Vasc Anesth.* 2006;20(4):515–519.

58. Wang X, Huang ZG, Gold A, et al. Propofol modulates gamma-aminobutyric acid-mediated inhibitory neurotransmission to cardiac vagal neurons in the nucleus ambiguus. *Anesthesiology.* 2004;100(5):1198–1205.

59. Musial KM, Wilson S, Preisch J, Weaver J. Comparison of the efficacy of oral midazolam alone versus midazolam and meperidine in the pediatric dental patient. *Pediatr Dent.* 2003;25(5):468–474.

60. Bergen JM, Smith DC. A review of etomidate for rapid sequence intubation in the emergency department. *J Emerg Med.* 1997;15(2):221–230.

61. Dickinson R, Singer AJ, Carrion W. Etomidate for pediatric sedation prior to fracture reduction. *Acad Emerg Med.* 2001;8(1):74–77.

62. Di Liddo L, D'Angelo A, Nguyen B, Bailey B, Amre D, Stanciu C. Etomidate versus midazolam for procedural sedation in pediatric outpatients: a randomized controlled trial. *Ann Emerg Med.* 2006;48(4):433–440, 40 e1.

63. McDowall RH, Scher CS, Barst SM. Total intravenous anesthesia for children undergoing brief diagnostic or therapeutic procedures. *J Clin Anesth.* 1995;7(4):273–280.

64. Schwarzkopf KR, Hueter L, Simon M, Fritz HG. Midazolam pretreatment reduces etomidate-induced myoclonic movements. *Anaesth Intensive Care.* 2003;31(1):18–20.

65. Gillies GW, Lees NW. The effects of speed of injection on induction with propofol. A comparison with etomidate. *Anaesthesia.* 1989;44(5):386–388.

66. den Brinker M, Hokken-Koelega AC, Hazelzet JA, de Jong FH, Hop WC, Joosten KF. One single dose of etomidate negatively

influences adrenocortical performance for at least 24[Symbol: see text]h in children with meningococcal sepsis. *Intensive Care Med.* 2008;34(1):163–168.

67. Cotton BA, Guillamondegui OD, Fleming SB, et al. Increased risk of adrenal insufficiency following etomidate exposure in critically injured patients. *Arch Surg.* 2008;143(1):62–67; discussion 7.

68. Rosen DA, Daume JT. Short duration large dose dexmedetomidine in a pediatric patient during procedural sedation. *Anesth Analg.* 2006;103(1):68–69, table of contents.

69. Berkenbosch JW, Wankum PC, Tobias JD. Prospective evaluation of dexmedetomidine for noninvasive procedural sedation in children. *Pediatr Crit Care Med.* 2005;6(4):435–439; quiz 40.

70. Mason KP, Zgleszewski SE, Dearden JL, et al. Dexmedetomidine for pediatric sedation for computed tomography imaging studies. *Anesth Analg.* 2006;103(1):57–62, table of contents.

71. Yuen VM, Irwin MG, Hui TW, Yuen MK, Lee LH. A double-blind, crossover assessment of the sedative and analgesic effects of intranasal dexmedetomidine. *Anesth Analg.* 2007; 105(2):374–380.

72. Allen MH, Currier GW, Carpenter D, Ross RW, Docherty JP. The expert consensus guideline series. Treatment of behavioral emergencies 2005. *J Psychiatr Pract.* 2005;11(suppl 1):5–108; quiz 110–112.

73. TREC Collaborative Group Rapid tranquillisation for agitated patients in emergency psychiatric rooms: a randomised trial of midazolam versus haloperidol plus promethazine. *BMJ.* 2003;327(7417):708–713.

74. Mendelowitz AJ. The utility of intramuscular ziprasidone in the management of acute psychotic agitation. *Ann Clin Psychiatry.* 2004;16(3):145–154.

75. Daniel DG, Potkin SG, Reeves KR, Swift RH, Harrigan EP. Intramuscular (IM) ziprasidone 20 mg is effective in reducing acute agitation associated with psychosis: a double-blind, randomized trial. *Psychopharmacology (Berl).* 2001;155(2):128–134.

76. Lubisch N, Tordella T, Roskos R. *Buccal Dexmedetomidine Is an Effective Alternative for Procedural Sedations in Pediatric Patients.* San Francisco, CA: American Academy of Pediatrics; 2007.

77. Schutzman SA, Burg J, Liebelt E, et al. Oral transmucosal fentanyl citrate for premedication of children undergoing laceration repair. *Ann Emerg Med.* 1994;24(6):1059–1064.

CHAPTER 21

Pain Management

Amy L. Baxter and Lindsey L. Cohen

▶ HIGH-YIELD FACTS

- Untreated, pain in children causes short and long-term consequences, and its monitoring in the emergency department should be considered a "fifth vital sign."
- The numbing effect of topical lidocaine and tetracaine preparations can be considered effective when there is visible blanching of surrounding tissue.
- Buffering intradermal lidocaine with 1:9 concentration of sodium bicarbonate will reduce pain from chemical irritation.
- When removing packing from an abscess, moisten the edges of the packing with lidocaine, epinephrine, and tetracaine to allow for more painless removal.
- Oral sucrose on a pacifier can provide pain relief for small infants during painful procedures.
- Children report the most painful part of fracture management is obtaining radiographs. This can be reduced by early splinting of the fracture site.
- Behavioral techniques for management of pain include relaxation exercises, deep breathing, distraction, and imagery.

Pain is the most common reason a patient presents for health care. The cost of pain to society is exorbitant, and can impact all aspects of life. The Joint Commission on Accreditation of Healthcare Organizations (JCAHO) directs that pain be considered the "fifth vital sign," and monitored with other vital signs in routine medical care. Recently, the International Association for the Study of Pain (IASP) and the World Health Organization (WHO) posited "the relief of pain should be a human right." Despite growing recognition of the importance of pain, it is often undertreated for children in emergency department (ED) settings.[1–3]

This chapter will review the physiologic and clinical research supporting adequate pain management for emergent procedures. Methods of assessing pain in the ED will be presented, along with supporting literature. Specific pain management options will be grouped by procedure or complaint—venipuncture, laceration repair, lumbar puncture (LP), catheterization, severe fracture, burn pain management, and sickle cell pain crisis—and by specific medications, including sucrose for infant pain. Finally, effective and counterproductive behavioral interventions will be discussed.

▶ OLIGOANALGESIA FOR PEDIATRIC EMERGENCY PATIENTS

Untreated pain in children causes short and long-term consequences. In 1987, Anand et al.[4] first demonstrated significant immediate morbidity from untreated pain in neonates undergoing PDA ligation, including bradycardia, increased ventilator time, and intraventricular hemorrhage. Pain in infants can have lasting negative effects on neuronal development, pain threshold and sensitivity, coping strategies, emotionality, and pain perceptions.[5]

While pain control for all emergency patients is often inadequate, children receive less pain medication than adults for the same emergent complaints.[3] The reasons for this "oligoanalgesia" include persistence of myths that children do not experience or remember pain,[6] fear of using opioids in younger patients, and difficulty assessing pediatric pain.

Concern for pain even in children too young to talk is not frivolous. The effects of untreated pain impact medical outcomes[4] and are remembered even by preverbal children.[5] These effects may amplify with age: Adolescents avoid medical treatment,[7] 16% to 75% of adults surveyed refuse to donate blood,[8–10] and geriatric patients refuse flu shots because of the fear of needle pain.[11] The health implications of needle phobia extend beyond the affected individuals; HIV patients continue to infect others while delaying blood tests[12] and needle-phobic parents are less likely to immunize their children.[13]

Children with a history of negative medical experiences show higher levels of anxiety prior to a venipuncture procedure and are less cooperative during the procedure. Further, high pain during medical visits predicts missed future medical appointments and poor health care follow-up. Older children also suffer sequellae from inadequate pain control: Weisman et al.[14] demonstrated that untreated pain from LPs increases pain response with subsequent procedures. Pain control should be an important goal for health care providers for compassionate and practical reasons, as both immediate and long-term patient health are affected by inappropriate analgesia.

▶ PAIN ASSESSMENT

In the ED, the periodic evaluation of pain using the Wong-Baker FACES scale has become routine for both staff and patients.[15] While most widely used in the United States, this scale suffers from two methodologic flaws and is rendering response distribution less parametric: The smiling anchor to the left is rarely appropriate for anyone in the ED, and cultural and concrete thinking biases may limit endorsement of the crying face (Fig. 21–1). Another more parametric scale is the Faces Pain Scale—Revised,[16,17] which is used more widely throughout the world (Fig. 21–2).

Other validated options include a vertical, graduated, and colored VAS scale to assess pain. Initially validated by McGrath

WHICH FACE SHOWS HOW MUCH HURT YOU HAVE NOW?

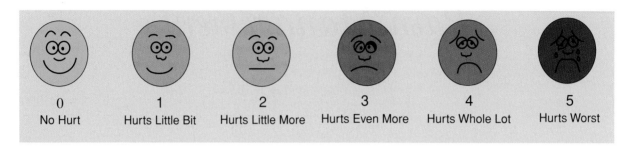

Figure 21–1. Wong Baker faces pain scale. With permission from Wong D.L. *Essentials of Pediatric Nursing.* 5th ed. 1997; 1215–1216.)

et al. in 1996, this scale appears as an upside down triangle with the topmost part being wide and red representing the worst pain and the bottom part being narrow and white representing no pain.[20] The scale has been found to be easier to administer than a standard VAS and avoids the most common problem seen with "face"-based scales, the choosing of higher numbers because of unhappiness rather than pain.[18,19]

The value of pain assessment has empiric support: Routine use of pain assessments improve treatment.[20] In a large review of ED visits by sickle cell patients, the change in self-reported pain after initial morphine dose was found to more accurately predict need for admission than absolute number of morphine doses.[21] Furthermore, incorporating pain assessment increases appropriate pain management in ED settings.

▶ PROCEDURAL PAIN MANAGEMENT

VENIPUNCTURE

Needle sticks are the most common and greatest source of procedural pain in the world. The American Academy of Pediatrics recommends pain control for venipuncture "whenever possible,"[22] and numerous modalities are effective even within the time constraints of the ED. Familiarity with and utilizing available methods to diminish needle pain for children can have far-reaching effects, including increasing parent's satisfaction with the ED experience.

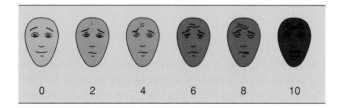

Figure 21–2. Faces Pain Scale—Revised. For correct use and translations, visit www.painsourcebook.ca. (With permission from Hicks CL, von Baeyer CL, Spafford PA, van Korlaar I, Goodenough B. The Faces Pain Scale–Revised: toward a common metric in pediatric pain measurement. *Pain.* 2001;93(2):173–183.)

Topical anesthetics (e.g., prilocaine, lidocaine, tetracaine) stop sodium transmission, raising the action potential threshold so the fast pain impulse cannot be conducted.[23] All local anesthetics contain hydrophilic and hydrophobic ends, the former being repelled by the oil layer of intact skin. Three common anesthetic formulations that overcome the skin barrier are EMLA (Astra-Zeneca), LMX-4 (Eloquest), and tetracaine (e.g., Ametop Gel, Smith & Nephew, Synera, Endo Pharmaceuticals).

Eutectic mixture of local anesthetics (EMLA) is the first and most studied topical cream: Prilocaine 2.5% and lidocaine 2.5%. Copious evidence supports reduction of pain with IV catheter insertion when applied for a minimum of 45 minutes.[6,21,24–27] In contrast to the other topical anesthetics, EMLA can be left on up to 4 hours with a depth of penetration up to 6 mm. Numbness lasts an hour after removal.[24] EMLA does cause vasoconstriction which theoretically can decrease venipuncture success, although most studies in children have shown either no difference[28] or improved procedure ease with EMLA.[26,29] Venipuncture success improves the longer EMLA is in place, up to 92% when left on 2 to 3 hours.[30]

Methemoglobinemia is rare side effect more likely in preterm infants lacking the enzyme necessary for reduction.[31] Current recommendations limit EMLA to infants of at least 37 weeks gestational age. A purpuric rash of presumed toxic origins has been described in 1% to 2%, particularly in atopic patients.

LMX-4 (previously called ELA-Max) places a 4% lidocaine preparation into liposomes for rapid absorption. Effective in 30 minutes, it works as well as EMLA for venipuncture pain.[32,33] The rapid absorption correlates with a rapid dissipation of the drug, with diminishing anesthesia approximately 40 to 60 minutes after application. LMX-4 improves cannulation success on the first attempt (74% vs. 55%, $p = 0.03$) when compared to placebo, and significantly lowers time of insertion and pain scores.[34] LMX-4 does not require a prescription and does not carry the risk of methemoglobinemia. Several products enhance absorption of LMX-4 to make it even more rapidly effective, including ultrasound devices and lasers.

Tetracaine gel, formerly known as amethocaine (Ametop Gel, Smith & Nephew Healthcare Limited, Hull, UK) is available alone and compounded with lidocaine. The 4% formulation works in 30 to 45 minutes, and lasts 4 to 6 hours with an efficacy similar to EMLA.[35,36]

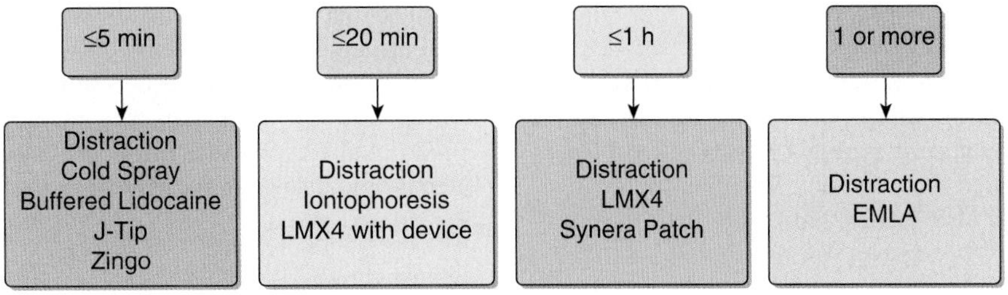

Figure 21–3. Options for venipuncture pain (in order of increasing cost).

For venipuncture, tetracaine and lidocaine mixed 7%/7% are available in a self-contained patch. Synera (Endo Pharmaceuticals) is designed to look like a child's bandage and is recommended for children three and older. The patch contains a heating element that decreases absorption time and causes local vasodilation. The mixture was tested as the S-Caine patch without the heating element, and showed good pain control and IV start success in children.[37]

Lidocaine Devices and Techniques

Iontophoresis uses a low-voltage electrical current to drive the positively charged end of lidocaine through the epidermis.[38] As the current flows to the negative reservoir, lidocaine is carried from the positive side into the skin. The current flow is noxious to some children, but those who tolerate the device may prefer it to EMLA. Time of application is at a minimum 10 minutes even with newer delivery systems.

Even the few minutes needed to apply creams or run current are a barrier to their use. One rapidly effective and well-tolerated pain relief method is simply to inject buffered lidocaine using a 30G needle prior to venipuncture. Use of this method is inexpensive, depending on bundled hospital charges for the extra needle, syringe, and buffered lidocaine.

A newer product, the J-tip (National Medical Products, Irvine, CA), puts lidocaine under the skin via a jet of compressed carbon dioxide. Early studies found the delivery method less painful than a 25G needle, and investigations in children show better pain relief from J-tip use than EMLA. Of note, 81% found J-tip lidocaine administration painless compared to 64% who felt pain with removal of EMLA's occlusive dressing.[39]

Finally, a disposable product approved for children in mid-2007 uses compressed helium to puff lidocaine through the skin in a 1-cm area.[40] As with the other devices, if the prepared area is not subsequently used, the cost recurs in a newly chosen site.

Cold Spray

The idea of cold for pain is as old as the ice pack. Applying cold spray (Pain Ease, ethyl chloride, Gebauer) directly to the penetration site has been used in hospitals for needle sticks, but placebo-controlled randomized trials have produced varying results for venipuncture. The cold can cause veins to shrink, making inserting an intravenous cannula difficult.[41] Because the spray is subfreezing and can injure children's more delicate tissues, cold spray may be more effective for children older

than 8 years. Cold spray is appealing, as it costs pennies per application and can be used at another site instantly if needed. Figure 21–3 provides an algorithm for balancing optimal pain control with time available.

LACERATIONS

Open lacerations permit easy drug absorption, rendering the hydrophilic ester issue irrelevant. The first combinations of tetracaine and cocaine mixed with "adrenaline" for vasoconstriction (TAC) were very effective. TAC had minimal toxicity when placed directly into the wound, and eliminated the need for injection for many pediatric cuts. The use of the controlled substance cocaine, however, increased the logistic difficulties of widespread availability. When lidocaine, epinephrine, and tetracaine (LET or LAT) were shown in 1995 to be just as effective,[14] LET became the standard of care for pediatric wound repair.

A shred of LET-soaked cotton or LET mixed with methylcellulose is placed directly in the wound before irrigation and repair. The solution or gel can be held in place with an occlusive dressing, tape, or bandage. Avoid placing gauze or other absorptive surfaces near the LET, which can draw the medication away from the wound. Numbness is present when the tissues blanch, usually after 20 minutes, and anesthesia lasts approximately 21 minutes after removal.[42] LET alone gives sufficient pain control for 70% to 90% of pediatric facial lacerations,[42] and can decrease length of stay by 30 minutes compared to traditional lidocaine injection.[43]

In extremities, LET has decreased efficacy (approximately 50%) but has not been shown to cause digital ischemia in two small studies. Mucous membrane absorption is a theoretic concern, but the primary reason to avoid LET for oral lacerations is loss of vermilion border landmarks because of the blanching effect. If LET is not available, EMLA has been used for laceration repair but has decreased numing effect.[44]

Infiltration

When local anesthetics are inadequate, unavailable, or inadvisable because of the location, local infiltration is needed and should be performed prior to cleaning. Both the tissue disruption from the volume of infiltrate and the acidic pH of lidocaine can cause increased pain. In adults, pain is diminished when lidocaine is injected slowly with the smallest gauge needle possible. Inject from within the wound rather than through the adjacent intact skin.[45] When possible, tapping, jiggling, or vibrating several centimeters proximal to the site of infiltration can distract the nerves and decrease the pain of injection.

The chemical irriation from lidocaine itself can be minimized by buffering with sodium bicarbonate in a 9:1 ratio in the same syringe. Premixed syringes typically keep for a week in an unrefrigerated environment. Warming the syringe to body temperature is also more comfortable than injecting refrigerated anesthetic.[46]

Several areas of the body are amenable to regional nerve blockade rather than direct local infiltration. For a simple digital laceration, local injection was not found to be superior to a digital block.[47] For foot lacerations, facial lacerations, and palmar lacerations regional nerve blockade can be considered, but with smaller lacerations local infiltration may be less painful.[48]

ABSCESS

Abscess management often required procedural sedation to adequately address the pain of incisions and drainage. The amount of sedative needed can be reduced; however, with adequate pain control. Using a combination of topical anesthetic over intact skin and local infiltration of lidocaine in a circular area prior to incision, pain may theoretically be reduced to an extent where parenteral pain medicine alone or with nitrous oxide would be sufficient.

When abscesses are packed with gauze, applying LET to the gauze for 20 minutes prior to removal moistens the retained edges of packing allowing for less painful removal.

LUMBAR PUNCTURE

Pain control for infant LPs has become commonplace. While in 1990, 100% of physicians reported performing LPs with no analgesia, by 2003 that number had dropped to 30%.[49] Since then, two studies have demonstrated improved success rates when topical anesthetics are applied, further supporting a practical as well as palliative role.[35,50] When placed prior to collection of blood and urine, the rapid efficacy of LMX-4 makes it a feasible option for a septic work-up. EMLA has been demonstrated to improve neonatal LP pain but the required hour to achieve efficacy may be impractical for a neonate with fever. When the LP needs to be performed emergently, as little as 0.1 mL of oral sucrose on a pacifier (e.g., Sweet-Ease, a 24% sucrose and water solution) provides pain relief during the procedure. The effectiveness of sucrose is most commonly cited for neonates younger than 2 months of age, although some literature supports pain relief in 6-month-old infants for less invasive procedures.

For older children, local anesthetics with or without an anxiolytic may be adequate. When a child is expected to require multiple LPs over the course of illness, as with leukemia or pseudotumor cerebri, providing deep sedation initially improves subsequent fear and posttraumatic stress surrounding the procedure. If this is not possible, providing optimal pain control will help avoid "hyperalgesia" and increased pain response with subsequent LPs.[14]

EMLA has been extensively demonstrated to decrease the pain of LPs in older children. When a CT or blood draw must be completed first, there is sufficient time for EMLA to become effective. By approximately 2 to 3 months, infants are large

enough that topical anesthetics will not penetrate far enough past the epidermis for optimal pain control. Infiltrating a generous amount of buffered lidocaine (approximately 1 mL per 10 kg of body weight up to a maximum of 5 mL) into the predural space provides improved pain relief. Adding a short acting opioid (e.g., fentanyl) can further improve comfort with the procedure.

PENILE PROCEDURES

Paraphimosis reduction is an extremely painful procedure, but occurs too rarely to have had definitive clinical studies on which to base pain control recommendations. Moderate or deep sedation, particularly with a rapid acting agent such as nitrous oxide, may be ideal. Local pain control could be either topical or regional. LMX-4 for 30 minutes was equivalent to EMLA for 45 minutes in the meatal region. Both may be even more rapidly effective given the friability of the skin in this context, and care should be taken not to leave either on too long to avoid toxic absorption. A dorsal penile nerve block could be considered and oral or IV opioids prior to the procedure will help.

URETHRAL CATHETERIZATION

For children undergoing urethral catheterization, 2% lidocaine jelly (available in a prefilled syringe Urolet) can be administered and allowed to sit for one to two minutes prior to catheterization. While effective at reducing pain in adult males, research to date in children has either been underpowered or has shown equivocal results. One study found decreased crying, but found no statistic change in observational pain scales or vital sign parameters. Some institutions use nitrous oxide for VCUG catheterization, an option impractical for catheterization in many EDs without additional equipment.

FRACTURES AND BURNS

The pain related to burns and fractures is similar in severity. Fracture reduction and burn debridement often require procedural sedation to accomplish, as opioid monotherapy can result in inadequate pain control or respiratory depression after procedure completion. For initial management, however, a narcotic as a single agent is the appropriate choice. Studies have found that the common initial parenteral dose of 0.1 mg/kg of morphine is often inadequate for extremely painful events, and 0.15 mg may be considered as an initial dose for injuries such as severe burns or displaced long bone fractures.[51,52] An initial dose of an oral opioid such as hydrocodone or oxycodone may speed pain relief if an IV has not yet been established. A faster option is intranasal fentanyl, which is as effective as IV morphine for pain relief in less time but may be associated with increased vomiting.

For fracture management, immobilization as quickly as possible improves pain relief. Temoprary splinting and providing analgesia prior to obtaining radiographs is recommended, as children report initial x-rays as the most painful part of emergency fracture treatment. After initial pain management and obtaining radiographs, regional pain control is an option for fracture reduction or burn debridement on extremities. A Bier block is a well-described technique used most commonly for forearm fracture reduction. An IV is placed on the affected side, and plain lidocaine and saline are administered after inflation of a double-blood pressure cuff to 250 mm Hg. Within 5 minutes, the extremity becomes mottled and completely numb, and procedures can be performed without pain.[53] This is an excellent option for children for whom a recent meal precludes sedation. The sight of their limb being manipulated may be disturbing, so a short-acting anxiolytic may be considered during the procedure itself regardless of npo times.

Another regional analgesic option which has been described favorably when compared to ketamine sedation is a hematoma block, concurrent with nitrous oxide. Femoral nerve blocks for fracture pain have been described, but require specific training to apply effectively.

▶ SICKLE CELL PAIN

Severe pain experienced during a vaso-occlusive episode (VOE) is the most common cause of acute morbidity in patients with sickle cell disease (SCD), and in adults has been linked with increased mortality. Patients with sickle cell anemia will average 0.8 painful episodes annually and 60% will require hospital based care, with as many as 42% of children requiring inpatient treatment.[54] Interventions such as IV placement, intravenous fluids, laboratory tests, and analgesic choice including combinations and methods of delivery are not well studied.

VOE incidence rate increases over time, especially in patients younger than 20 years of age, with those 10 to 30 years old experiencing the highest rates. Adolescents with sickle cell pain report greater pain intensity from crisis than from postoperative pain. More recent descriptive studies have found that sickle cell patients experience pain to a greater extent on a more frequent basis than previously reported.[55] This frequency can dull the tachycardia and hypertension response seen with acute injury, causing caregivers to erroneously judge that patients are not in pain "because they are not tachycardic." Likewise, the myth that a sleeping sickle cell patient is not in pain results in oligoanalgesia; a pain crisis typically lasts 3 to 5 days, and patients must sleep at some time regardless of pain control. Anxiety from untreated pain increases pain perception, so scheduled pain medicine should be maintained even to the point of waking these patients if in an observational ED bed.

Current management of patients failing outpatient pain management include liberal use of parenteral opioids, typically morphine, with early transition to patient-controlled analgesia (PCA) when appropriate. Patients may develop tolerance to opioids very early in their administration and experience hyperalgesia, or extreme sensitivity to painful stimuli, and allodynia, or pain with stimuli that are not usually painful, secondary to activation of the N-methyl-D-aspartate (NMDA) receptor. Morphine is a mild NMDA agonist, resulting in increased pain sensitivity, but adjunctive use of an NMDA blocker with initial opioid therapy is in the research stages.

The decision to admit a patient with VOE for further management in the hospital is multifactorial. In a survey of ED physicians treating both pediatric and adult sickle cell patients, pain was considered refractory to outpatient therapy after two doses of intravenous opioids in 23% of respondents and after three doses in 53%. However, in the largest series, a substan-

tial number of patients receiving two doses of IV opioid were still discharged without a subsequent ED return. In that group, lack of pain relief by self-report after the first opioid dose was most predictive of need for admission.[20]

▶ ANALGESIC AGENTS

The medications in the class of pure analgesic agents include acetaminophen and nonsteroidal anti-inflammatory drugs (NSAIDs).

These agents are commonly used as antipyretics and for treatment of minor extremity pain. Of note, in dosing acetaminophen one study found that rectal adminstration required 40 mg/kg as a loading dose to achieve sufficient analgesic blood levels after surgery. Rectal doses of 20 mg/kg are required for subsequent pain relief.

Ketorolac, the only parenteral NSAID available in the United States, has proved particularly effective in prostaglandin-mediated conditions, such as biliary or renal colic, although its use in other painful conditions generally requires addition of a supplemental narcotic. Many of the pure analgesics are also combined with opioid agents for synergistic effects in oral combination therapies.

Synthetic and naturally occurring narcotic analgesics all produce their effect through stimulation of opioid receptor sites in the central nervous system. Differences in the effects of the various clinically used agents result from differential binding preferences for these receptor sites. Opioid analgesics create dose-dependent pain relief with mild sedative effects. Cardiovascular and respiratory depression may be seen at any dose, although it is generally not clinically significant at standard dosages. More minor adverse effects include nausea and transient itching or urticaria from histamine release. The side effect of oversedation can be reversed through administration of a competitive antagonist such as naloxone or nalmephine.

Morphine, the classic narcotic analgesic, is generally employed to treat moderate to severe pain, as an adjunct for painful procedures, and occasionally as a sedative hypnotic. For patients with a history of itching, it may be administered with diphenhydramine or hydroxazine. In contrast to many medications which are more rapidly metabolized, neonates and younger patients may need less per kilogram than patients older than 6 months. After this age, children younger than 11 years metabolize morphine more rapidly than adults, and may need more frequent redosing.

Meperidine is another analgesic with clinical characteristics very similar to those of morphine. Unlike morphine, meperidine is metabolized to an active metabolite, normeperidine, which has a longer serum half-life than that of its parent compound. If allowed to accumulate in a child, normeperidine can result in seizures thus it should not be used in children who will require multiple doses of a narcotic over an extended period.

Hydromorphone is a more potent semisynthetic narcotic analgesic similar to morphine and meperidine and is frequently used in pain management protocols for renal colic pain, abdominal pain, or sickle cell anemia patients.

Fentanyl citrate is a synthetic short-acting narcotic approximately 100 times more potent than morphine. It has a rapid onset and 20-minute duration of action, making it ideal

▶ **TABLE 21–1. COMMON PEDIATRIC ANALGESIC AGENTS**

Medication	Route	Dose (mg/kg)	Typical Maximum*	Duration	Comments
Sedative analgesics					
Meperidine	IV, IM	1.0–2.0	100 mg/kg	3–4 h	Chronic accumulation risk
Morphine	IV, IM, SQ	0.1–0.15	10 mg/kg	2–4 h	
Fentanyl	IV	0.001–0.002	0.05 mg/kg	20 min	Rigidity, apnea, lower dose <6 mo
	TM	0.005–0.010			
Remifentanil	IV	0.001	0.05 mg/kg	4–6 min	Rigidity, apnea
Hydromorphone	IV	0.01–0.02	2 mg/kg		
Hydrocodone	PO	0.2	10 mg/kg	4–6 h	
Codeine	PO	1–1.5	60 mg/kg	4–6 h	
Reversal agents					
Naloxone	IV, IM	0.1	2 mg	20 min	
Flumazenil	IV	0.01	0.2 mg	30 min	

*Typical maximum dose represents dose that is effective in most patients. Since all patients respond differently, it is possible that for some patients a dose in excess of this dose may be required. If such a higher dose is utilized, precautions in monitoring the patient should be taken.

for brief painful procedures. Unlike other narcotics, fentanyl has few cardiovascular effects, making it attractive in hypovolemic or cardiac patients. One unique side effect of fentanyl is chest wall rigidity, which can occur if the drug is administered too rapidly, particularly in infants. This side effect may be reversed with naloxone, although on occasion endotracheal intubation and skeletal muscle paralysis may be required. Fentanyl is also unique in that it is the only narcotic administered through transmucosal routes. Initially provided as a "lollipop," early studies found it effective as an analgesic and sedative, but overdosing and emesis have caused this form to be removed from the market. Current studies with intranasal routes use the standard IV formulation. Reduced doses should be used in neonates and very young infants, as they are more sensitive to the respiratory depressant effects.

Codeine, hydrocodone, and *oxycodone* are less potent narcotic analgesics generally administered orally in combination with a pure analgesic, such as acetaminophen or ibuprofen. Codeine is used as a classic example in the field of pharmacogenetics, as races have differing abilities to metabolize the drug to the active form. Up to 15% of Asian patients and 7% to 10% of Caucasian patients have decreased ability to complete O-methylation which renders the codeine into the active morphine analog. Thus, these patients may experience no additional pain relief from the addition of codeine to the pure analgesic, which could explain small studies finding no statistic improvement comparing acetaminophen with and without codeine.[56] While the other two opioids are structurally similar, they appear to better metabolized into the active morphine.[57] Table 21–1 summarizes dosing of common pediatric analgesic agents.

▶ BEHAVIORAL PEDIATRIC PAIN MANAGEMENT

There is an arsenal of evidence-based behavioral strategies that mitigate the anxiety and discomfort associated with pediatric pain. Whereas anxiety might heighten pain experience, relaxation or focusing elsewhere can decrease pain. Accordingly, behavioral recommendations often include coping skills training or providing distraction. Behavioral interventions can be organized as those done to prepare the patient for medical procedures and those implemented during the painful medical events.

PREPARATION

Research suggests that preparation is beneficial to pediatric patients facing a range of medical stressors. While advanced preparation is in order for more complex procedures (e.g., surgery), same-day preparation is sufficient for minor medical events (e.g., venipuncture) and can be done in the ED setting. Preparation might include videos, written summaries, or other aids depending on availability. It is beneficial if the information combines diversion with didactic information. Allowing patients and their parents to ask questions may alleviate any fears or inaccurate expectations. Content should be clear and concise, presented in a nonemotive manner, age-appropriate, and contain details about what the child should expect in terms of procedural steps and physical sensations. Preparation should include training in coping skills, such as relaxation techniques (e.g., deep breathing, progressive muscle relaxation) or distraction (e.g., imagery, watching a movie, solving mental mathematics problems). In addition to adequately preparing the pediatric patients, it is helpful to prepare the parents.[58] This is especially pertinent given parents' own anxiety[59,60] which is strongly predictive of their children's medical distress.[61] In addition to knowing exactly what to expect for the procedure, parents should learn how to best assist their child during painful medical procedures. Specifically, parents should learn that coaching in distraction and encouraging coping is beneficial and that excessive reassurance, criticism, or apologizing might exacerbate child distress. Educating parents that self-blame increases the pain response,[62] while focused distraction or hypnosis decreases it, which may enable them to provide proper support.

PROCEDURAL INTERVENTIONS

Behavioral interventions implemented during painful medical procedures are strongly supported in the literature.[63] These intervention packages often include relaxation, praise, and other reinforcement for appropriate behavior, imagery, and distraction. Distraction stimuli vary and include movies, interactive toys, virtual reality, music, bubbles, and short stories. Clinical and functional MRI evidence suggest that the brain has a limited attention capacity—if focused on a distracting task, there may be few resources remaining to attend to painful stimuli. One potential mechanism is that distraction alters nociceptive functions by initiating an internal pain-suppressing system. Behaviorally, distraction diverts attention away from stimuli that have been classically conditioned to produce anxiety (e.g., medical equipment).[61] In addition, some distracting stimuli may induce behaviors that are incompatible with distress, such as laughing while watching a funny movie.

A meta-analysis suggested that distraction was equally effective across gender and ethnic groups, but was most effective for children younger than 7 years of age. Other ages still benefit—one study in adults found less venipuncture pain when patients were instructed to cough while the needle went in.[64] The idea distraction stimulus likely varies by individual: One study found an interactive robot to be more effective than a story book, while another showed movies to be better than an interactive toy. Ideally, distraction should involve multiple sensory modalities (e.g., vision, hearing, touch) and produce positive emotions that are inconsistent with pain. Stimuli that might include parents as coaches is helpful, as research suggests that children engage in little coping without adults coaching them. Research has consistently shown that distraction should be done prior to, during, and following the procedure.

BEHAVIORAL INTERVENTIONS FOR INFANTS

Data suggest that distraction might benefit children down to 1 to 24 months of age,[65] but is not as effective as for older patients. Recommended behavioral interventions for young infants include sucrose, nonnutritive sucking, and skin-to-skin contact. Sucrose water given immediately prior to an acute painful procedure has been found to decrease pain in neonates and infants up to approximately 4 to 6 months of age. Mild activation of endogenous opioids[66] is likely enhanced by other stress-relieving factors.[67] Sucrose is usually given by dipping a pacifier into a solution or instilling it directly into the mouth with a syringe.

Other modalities for infant pain relief include nonnutritive sucking, breast-feeding[68,69] and skin-to-skin contact ("kangaroo care"). Applying these techniques to the ED environment, allowing parents to cuddle children in a "position of comfort" has diminished procedural pain.

In summary, behavioral approaches have been shown to be effective at minimizing children's medical pain and distress and parents' anxiety. Preparation prior to medical procedures should benefit the patient and parents and research provides details regarding specific behavioral interventions that can be conducted during the painful medical events. Given the minimal side effects and low cost of most behavioral interventions, they should be consistently implemented to help minimize pain and suffering in ED.

REFERENCES

1. Jones JS, Johnson K, McNinch M. Age as a risk factor for inadequate emergency department analgesia. *Am J Emerg Med.* 1996;14(2):157–160.
2. Rupp T, Delaney KA. Inadequate analgesia in emergency medicine. *Ann Emerg Med.* 2004;43(4):494–503.
3. Selbst SM, Clark M. Analgesic use in the emergency department. *Ann Emerg Med.* 1990;19(9):1010–1013.
4. Anand KJ, Sippell WG, Aynsley-Green A. Randomised trial of fentanyl anaesthesia in preterm babies undergoing surgery: effects on the stress response. *Lancet.* 1987;1(8524):62–66.
5. Taddio A, Katz J, Ilersich AL, Koren G. Effect of neonatal circumcision on pain response during subsequent routine vaccination. *Lancet.* 1997;349(9052):599–603.
6. Young KD. Pediatric procedural pain. *Ann Emerg Med.* 2005;45(2):160–171.
7. Vika M, Raadal M, Skaret E, Kvale G. Dental and medical injections: prevalence of self-reported problems among 18-yr-old subjects in Norway. *Eur J Oral Sci.* 2006;114(2):122–127.
8. Harrington M, Sweeney MR, Bailie K, Morris K, Kennedy A, Boilson A, et al. What would encourage blood donation in Ireland? *Vox Sang.* 2007;92(4):361–367.
9. Grossman B, Watkins AR, Fleming F, Debaun MR. Barriers and motivators to blood and cord blood donations in young African-American women. *Am J Hematol.* 2005;78(3):198–202.
10. Wiwanitkit V. Knowledge about blood donation among a sample of Thai university students. *Vox Sang.* 2002;83(2):97–99.
11. Allsup SJ, Gosney MA. Difficulties of recruitment for a randomized controlled trial involving influenza vaccination in healthy older people. *Gerontology.* 2002;48(3):170–173.
12. Spielberg F, Branson BM, Goldbaum GM, Lockhart D, Kurth A, Celum CL, et al. Overcoming barriers to HIV testing: preferences for new strategies among clients of a needle exchange, a sexually transmitted disease clinic, and sex venues for men who have sex with men. *J Acquir Immune Defic Syndr.* 2003;32(3):318–327.
13. Froehlich H, West DJ. Compliance with hepatitis B virus vaccination in a high-risk population. *Ethn Dis.* 2001;11(3):548–553.
14. Weisman SJ, Bernstein B, Schechter NL. Consequences of inadequate analgesia during painful procedures in children. *Arch Pediatr Adolesc Med.* 1998;152(2):147–149.
15. Wong ML, Chia KS, Yam WM, Teodoro GR, Lau KW. Willingness to donate blood samples for genetic research: a survey from a community in Singapore. *Clin Genet.* 2004;65(1):45–51.
16. Bieri D, Reeve RA, Champion GD, Addicoat L, Ziegler JB. The Faces Pain Scale for the self-assessment of the severity of pain experienced by children: development, initial validation, and preliminary investigation for ratio scale properties. *Pain.* 1990;41(2):139–150.
17. Hicks CL, von Baeyer CL, Spafford PA, van Korlaar I, Goodenough B. The Faces Pain Scale-Revised: toward a common metric in pediatric pain measurement. *Pain.* 2001;93(2):173–183.
18. Chambers CT, Hardial J, Craig KD, Court C, Montgomery C. Faces scales for the measurement of postoperative pain intensity in children following minor surgery. *Clin J Pain.* 2005;21(3):277–285.
19. Bulloch B, Tenenbein M. Validation of 2 pain scales for use in the pediatric emergency department. *Pediatrics* 2002;110(3):e33.

20. Homer JJ, Frewer JD, Swallow J, Semple P. An audit of post-operative analgesia in children following tonsillectomy. *J Laryngol Otol.* 2002;116(5):367–370.

21. Frei-Jones MJ, Baxter AL, Rogers ZR, Buchanan GR. Vaso-occlusive episodes in older children with sickle cell disease: emergency department management and pain assessment. *J Pediatr.* 2008;152(2):281–285.

22. American Academy of Pediatrics, Committee on Psychosocial Aspects of Child and Family Health, and American Pain Society, Task Force on Pain in Infants, Children, and Adolescents. The assessment and management of acute pain in infants, children, and adolescents. *Pediatrics.* 2001;108(3):793–797.

23. Gilman AG, Rall TW, Nies AS, Taylor P, eds. *The Pharmacological Basis of Therapeutics.* 8th ed. New York, NY: Pergamon Press; 1990.

24. Evans JK, Buckley SL, Alexander AH, Gilpin AT. Analgesia for the reduction of fractures in children: a comparison of nitrous oxide with intramuscular sedation. *J Pediatr Orthop.* 1995;15(1):73–77.

25. Chen BK, Cunningham BB. Topical anesthetics in children: agents and techniques that equally comfort patients, parents, and clinicians. *Curr Opin Pediatr.* 2001;13(4):324–330.

26. Cooper JA, Bromley LM, Baranowski AP, Barker SG. Evaluation of a needle-free injection system for local anaesthesia prior to venous cannulation. *Anaesthesia.* 2000;55(3):247–250.

27. Fetzer SJ. Reducing the pain of venipuncture. *J Perianesth Nurs.* 1999;14(2):95–101, 112.

28. Hallen B, Uppfeldt A. Does lidocaine-prilocaine cream permit painfree insertion of IV catheters in children? *Anesthesiology.* 1982;57(4):340–342.

29. Moller C. A lignocaine-prilocaine cream reduces venipuncture pain. *Ups J Med Sci.* 1985;90(3):293–298.

30. Baxter AL, Ewing PH, Evans NRM, Ware A, Mix A. EMLA application in ED triage increases venipuncture success. *Pediatr Emerg Care.* 2005.

31. Taddio A, Ohlsson A, Einarson TR, Stevens B, Koren G. A systematic review of lidocaine-prilocaine cream (EMLA) in the treatment of acute pain in neonates. *Pediatrics.* 1998;101(2):E1.

32. Eichenfield LF, Funk A, Fallon-Friedlander S, Cunningham BB. A clinical study to evaluate the efficacy of ELA-Max (4% liposomal lidocaine) as compared with eutectic mixture of local anesthetics cream for pain reduction of venipuncture in children. *Pediatrics.* 2002;109(6):1093–1099.

33. Koh JL, Harrison D, Myers R, Dembinski R, Turner H, McGraw T. A randomized, double-blind comparison study of EMLA and ELA-Max for topical anesthesia in children undergoing intravenous insertion. *Paediatr Anaesth.* 2004;14(12):977–982.

34. Taddio A, Soin HK, Schuh S, Koren G, Scolnik D. Liposomal lidocaine to improve procedural success rates and reduce procedural pain among children: a randomized controlled trial. *CMAJ.* 2005;172(13):1691–1695.

35. Baxter AL, Fisher RG, Burke BL, Goldblatt SS, Isaacman DJ, Lawson ML. Local anesthetic and stylet styles: factors associated with resident lumbar puncture success. *Pediatrics.* 2006;117(3):876–881.

36. O'Brien L, Taddio A, Lyszkiewicz DA, Koren G. A critical review of the topical local anesthetic amethocaine (Ametop) for pediatric pain. *Paediatr Drugs.* 2005;7(1):41–54.

37. Sethna NF, Verghese ST, Hannallah RS, Solodiuk JC, Zurakowski D, Berde CB. A randomized controlled trial to evaluate S-Caine patch for reducing pain associated with vascular access in children. *Anesthesiology.* 2005;102(2):403–408.

38. Zempsky WT, Parkinson TM. Lidocaine iontophoresis for topical anesthesia before dermatologic procedures in children: a randomized controlled trial. *Pediatr Dermatol.* 2003;20(4):364–368.

39. Jimenez N, Bradford H, Seidel KD, Sousa M, Lynn AM. A comparison of a needle-free injection system for local anesthesia versus EMLA for intravenous catheter insertion in the pediatric patient. *Anesth Analg.* 2006;102(2):41141–4.

40. Tansey B. Needle Pain device OKd for Children. *San Francisco Chronicle.* August 18, 2007;18.

41. Ramsook C, Kozinetz CA, Moro-Sutherland D. Efficacy of ethyl chloride as a local anesthetic for venipuncture and intravenous cannula insertion in a pediatric emergency department. *Pediatr Emerg Care.* 2001;17(5):341–343.

42. Resch K, Schilling C, Borchert BD, Klatzko M, Uden D. Topical anesthesia for pediatric lacerations: a randomized trial of lidocaine-epinephrine-tetracaine solution versus gel. *Ann Emerg Med.* 1998;32(6):693–697.

43. Priestley S, Kelly AM, Chow L, Powell C, Williams A. Application of topical local anesthetic at triage reduces treatment time for children with lacerations: a randomized controlled trial. *Ann Emerg Med.* 2003;42(1):34–40.

44. Singer AJ, Stark MJ. LET versus EMLA for pretreating lacerations: a randomized trial. *Acad Emerg Med.* 2001;8(3):223–230.

45. Bartfield JM, Sokaris SJ, Raccio-Robak N. Local anesthesia for lacerations: pain of infiltration inside vs outside the wound. *Acad Emerg Med.* 1998;5(2):100–104.

46. Colaric KB, Overton DT, Moore K. Pain reduction in lidocaine administration through buffering and warming. *Am J Emerg Med.* 1998;16(4):353–356.

47. Chale S, Singer AJ, Marchini S, McBride MJ, Kennedy D. Digital versus local anesthesia for finger lacerations: a randomized controlled trial. *Acad Emerg Med.* 2006;13(10):1046–1050.

48. Tarsia V, Singer AJ, Cassara GA, Hein MT. Percutaneous regional compared with local anaesthesia for facial lacerations: a randomised controlled trial. *Emerg Med J.* 2005;22(1):37–40.

49. Baxter AL, Welch JC, Burke BL, Isaacman DJ. Pain, position, and stylet styles: infant lumbar puncture practices of pediatric emergency attending physicians. *Pediatr Emerg Care.* 2004;20(12):816–820.

50. Nigrovic LE, Kuppermann N, Neuman MI. Risk factors for traumatic or unsuccessful lumbar punctures in children. *Ann Emerg Med.* 2007;49(6):762–771.

51. Bijur PE, Kenny MK, Gallagher EJ. Intravenous morphine at 0.1 mg/kg is not effective for controlling severe acute pain in the majority of patients. *Ann Emerg Med.* 2005;46(4):362–367.

52. Birnbaum A, Esses D, Bijur PE, Holden L, Gallagher EJ. Randomized double-blind placebo-controlled trial of two intravenous morphine dosages (0.10 mg/kg and 0.15 mg/kg) in ED patients with moderate to severe acute pain. *Ann Emerg Med.* 2007;49(4):445–453.

53. Mohr B. Safety and effectiveness of intravenous regional anesthesia (Bier block) for outpatient management of forearm trauma. *CJEM.* 2006;8(4):247–250.

54. Meyerhoff AS, Weniger BG, Jacobs RJ. Economic value to parents of reducing the pain and emotional distress of childhood vaccine injections. *Pediatr Infect Dis J.* 2001;20(11 Suppl):S57-S62.

55. Dampier C, Setty BNY, Eggleston B, Brodecki D, O'Neal P, Stuart M. Vaso-occlusion in children with sickle cell disease: clinical characteristics and biologic correlates. *J Pediatr Hematol Oncol.* 2004;26(1077–4114):785–790.

56. Moir MS, Bair E, Shinnick P, Messner A. Acetaminophen versus acetaminophen with codeine after pediatric tonsillectomy. *Laryngoscope.* 2000;110(11):1824–1827.

57. Caraco Y, Sheller J, Wood AJ. Impact of ethnic origin and quinidine coadministration on codeine's disposition and pharmacodynamic effects. *J Pharmacol Exp Ther.* 1999;290(1):413–422.

58. Jay SM, Elliott CH. A stress inoculation program for parents whose children are undergoing painful medical procedures. *J Consult Clin Psychol.* 1990;58(6):799–804.

59. Bernard RS, Cohen LL, McClellan CB, MacLaren JE. Pediatric procedural approach-avoidance coping and distress: a multitrait-multimethod analysis. *J Pediatr Psychol.* 2004;29(2): 131–141.

60. Lamontagne LL, Hepworth JT, Byington KC, Chang CY. Child and parent emotional responses during hospitalization for orthopaedic surgery. *MCN Am J Matern Child Nurs.* 1997;22(6): 299–303.

61. Cohen LL. Reducing infant immunization distress through distraction. *Health Psychol.* 2002;21(2):207–211.

62. Langer DA, Chen E, Luhmann JD. Attributions and coping in children's pain experiences. *J Pediatr Psychol.* 2005;30(7):615– 622.

63. Powers SW. Empirically supported treatments in pediatric psychology: procedure-related pain. *J Pediatr Psychol.* 1999;24(2): 131–145.

64. Usichenko TI, Pavlovic D, Foellner S, Wendt M. Reducing venipuncture pain by a cough trick: a randomized crossover volunteer study. *Anesth Analg.* 2004;98(2):343–345, table of contents.

65. Cohen LL, MacLaren JE, Fortson BL, Friedman A, DeMore M, Lim CS, et al. Randomized clinical trial of distraction for infant immunization pain. *Pain.* 2006;125(1–2):165–171.

66. Segato FN, Castro-Souza C, Segato EN, Morato S, Coimbra NC. Sucrose ingestion causes opioid analgesia. *Braz J Med Biol Res.* 1997;30(8):981–984.

67. Hatfield LA, Gusic ME, Dyer AM, Polomano RC. Analgesic properties of oral sucrose during routine immunizations at 2 and 4 months of age. *Pediatrics.* 2008;121(2):e327– e334.

68. Taddio A, Manley J, Potash L, Ipp M, Sgro M, Shah V. Routine immunization practices: use of topical anesthetics and oral analgesics. *Pediatrics.* 2007;120(3):e637–e643.

69. Gray L, Miller LW, Philipp BL, Blass EM. Breastfeeding is analgesic in healthy newborns. *Pediatrics.* 2002;109(4):590– 593.

CHAPTER 22

Imaging

Wendy C. Matsuno

▶ HIGH-YIELD FACTS

- Ultrasonography is the imaging of choice for confirmation of pyloric stenosis, testicular torsion, ectopic pregnancy, ovarian torsion, and appendicitis.
- High clinical suspicion for testicular torsion or ovarian torsion should not be ignored when not confirmed by ultrasonography. Sensitivity and specificity is limited.
- Successful diagnosis with ultrasonography may be limited in obese children.
- Computed tomography is an extremely valuable imaging tool, but the risk of ionizing radiation exposure should be considered when ordering this test in young children.
- MRI in the ED is usually reserved for emergent conditions such as cord compression and stroke.

▶ INTRODUCTION

The practice of emergency medicine brings patients with a variety of complaints to our doorstep. In deciphering the many signs and symptoms, the art of medicine comes into play when trying to reach a diagnosis. Technology has allowed us a more innovative method to confirm a diagnosis with various imaging studies. This chapter will review the most commonly available imaging modalities and discuss the various considerations for optimal visualization and patient safety.

▶ ULTRASOUND

Ultrasound technology was first commercially available in the late 1960s as a rigid contact B-mode machine.[1] These early machines were able to take still pictures only, thus had limited usefulness in the emergency department due to the time and labor-intensive nature of the equipment. In the late 1970s, the first real-time ultrasonography machine was introduced, and by the mid-1980s ultrasound machines started to be used in the emergency department (Fig. 22–1).[1,2] By 1996, the American College of Emergency Physicians founded the Section of Emergency Ultrasound to promote further advancement in this field.[2] Figures 22–2 and 22–3 provide an approach to the use of imaging for pediatric trauma victims and medical diagnosis in children.

PHYSICS AND PATHOPHYSIOLOGY

Ultrasound employs sound waves, a form of nonionizing radiation, to visualize internal structures. As sound travels through the tissue, the molecules are compressed and decompressed. An isolated compression and decompression event is defined as one cycle. The number of cycles that occur over time is termed the frequency. Frequency is measured in hertz (Hz), where one hertz equals one cycle per second. Diagnostic ultrasound uses frequencies from 2 to 10 MHz (2–10 million cycles per second), which is considerably above the threshold that human ears can hear.[2]

The picture generated by the ultrasound machine is a result of various elements working together. The transducer, also known as the probe, is the portion of the machine that is held by the examiner to the patient's body. A linear probe emits sound waves at a higher frequency, which makes it ideal for viewing superficial structures (Fig. 22–4). In contrast, the curved probe emits sound waves at a lower frequency, which allows deeper penetration and is useful for deep structures (e.g., organs). The sound waves from the transducer are affected by the density of the tissue and the resulting impedance on the sound wave.

As sound waves travel through the body, the sound wave may be affected in different ways depending on the tissue and tissue planes. The sound wave can be reflected back to the transducer if it meets with an object that is very dense and has a high impedance value. A dense object (e.g., gallstone) is referred to as being echogenic and appears white on the image screen (Fig. 22–5). The surrounding fluid filled areas, which do not reflect the sound wave, appears black on the ultrasound image. The black, nonreflecting medium is labeled as being anechoic. Objects that strongly reflect the sound wave produce a shadow effect on distal structures as seen in by the gallstone in Figure 22–5.

Other factors that affect how a sound wave travels through the body are refraction, attenuation, and scatter. These factors can affect the quality of the ultrasound image, thus diminishing these effects is very important for optimal viewing. Refraction occurs when the sound wave hits a tissue plane at an angle and part of the reflected wave is lost due to being angled away from the transducer. To prevent the loss of signal, the transducer should be perpendicular to the area of interest to lessen the degree of refraction. Sound waves can also be attenuated, where it is difficult for the sound wave to pass through a given tissue to see distant objects. Sound waves can also be scattered in various directions by irregular, small material (e.g., gas) that make good visualization difficult. Thus to prevent attenuation

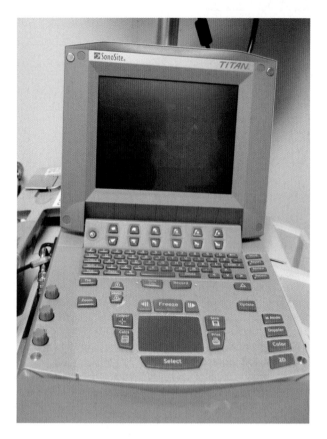

Figure 22–1. Picture of typical ultrasound machine.

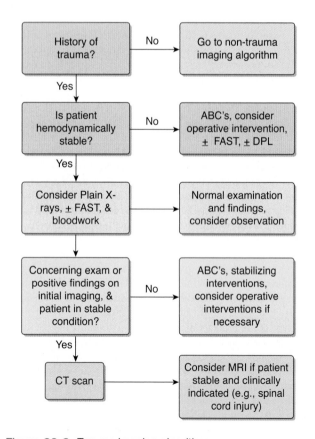

Figure 22–2. Trauma imaging algorithm.

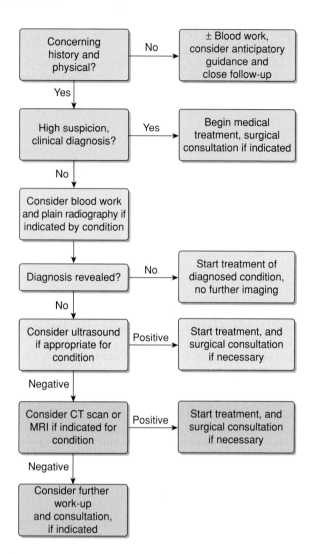

Figure 22–3. Medical imaging algorithm.

and scatter an acoustic window is often used, whereby visualization of distant structures is done through an area of good penetration (e.g., full bladder).

Current ultrasound machines in the emergency department are able to provide real time ultrasonography. Many are also equipped with the ability to provide concurrent Doppler imaging. Doppler works by registering the sound waves that return to the transducer off of a moving object (e.g., red blood cells). The reflected sound waves are registered and the calculated change in frequency relates to the amount and speed of the particles. Doppler by itself does not provide structural information, thus it is most helpful when used concurrently with real-time ultrasonography.

SAFETY CONSIDERATIONS

Ultrasound is a relatively new medical technique. There are a few hypothetical risks that have been raised regarding ultrasonography. The following is a discussion of the potential hazards.

Two means by which ultrasound may have a deleterious effect on tissue are by a thermal and cavitation mechanism.[3,4]

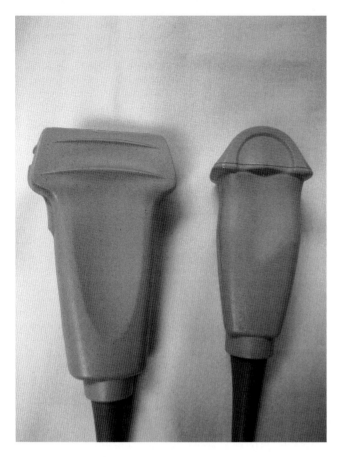

Figure 22–4. Ultrasound probes. Linear probe on left and curved probe on the right.

The thermal mechanism postulates that as heat is produced by the absorption of ultrasound by the tissues, the increase in the temperature may cause tissue damage. Thermal damage is unlikely to occur with diagnostic ultrasonography, as the intensity and time of exposure needed to produce such a tem-

perature change is significantly greater than is currently used for imaging.

The cavitation mechanism can be divided into transient and stable cavitation. Transient cavitation occurs at high intensities where gas-filled bubbles enlarge, then suddenly collapse resulting in a localized temperature change, thermal decomposition of water, and release of free radicals. In stable cavitation, which occurs at low intensities, the gas-filled bubbles vibrate and may cause shearing stress to surrounding tissue. The low intensity level and short duration of ultrasound exposure that occurs with modern diagnostic ultrasonography makes the occurrence of cavitation unlikely. These phenomena are theoretical risks, and current diagnostic ultrasonography is considered safe without proof of risk.

BENEFITS AND LIMITATIONS

Ultrasound is a very useful tool in the pediatric emergency department. As discussed above, ultrasound does not use ionizing radiation and is considered safe at current diagnostic settings. Ultrasound is a noninvasive, painless procedure that does not require the patient to be completely still, thus sedation is not needed. With the advent of portable machines, it is easily accessible at the bedside and can be performed quickly. Furthermore, the lean body habitus of most pediatric patients makes visualization of internal structures relatively easy. For these reasons, many emergency department physicians have embraced the use of ultrasound for select common emergency department conditions and procedures.

Ultrasound does have some limitations. One limitation of ultrasound is that it is operator-dependent. The skill of the person operating the ultrasound machine can greatly affect the quality of the image and the ease by which structures are identified. Furthermore, most diagnostic ultrasound studies are performed in the radiology department by ultrasound technologists. The availability of ultrasound technologists may be limited in the late night hours, limiting the accessibility of ultrasound by emergency department patients.

DIAGNOSTIC AND PROCEDURAL CONSIDERATIONS

There are several circumstances that occur in the emergency department that can benefit from the use of ultrasonography. In most cases when ultrasound is being used to diagnose a condition, the procedure is carried out in the radiology department. With the increased availability of ultrasound machines, emergency physicians have been utilizing ultrasound for procedures and limited diagnostic uses. The following is a brief discussion of common circumstances that utilize ultrasound technology.

Pyloric stenosis occurs in 1 in 250 births, where there is hypertrophy of the pylorus muscle.[5] The diagnosis can be confirmed by the finding of a thickened pylorus muscle of 0.3 cm or greater, or by an elongation of the pylorus to 1.4 cm or greater (Fig. 22–6).[5] The sensitivity of ultrasound for pyloric stenosis is reported to be 97% to 100% and with a specificity of 99% to 100%.[6,7]

Testicular torsion is a surgical emergency and an accurate diagnosis is critical. In cases where the diagnosis is not made

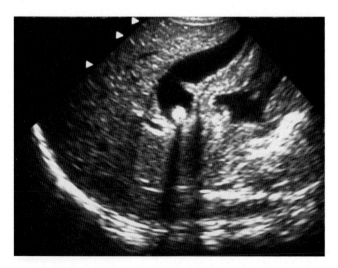

Figure 22–5. Ultrasound image of gallstone. Notice the bright white appearance of the echogenic gallstone and the shadow it casts distally.

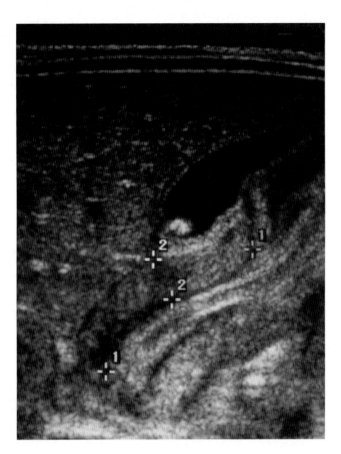

Figure 22–6. Ultrasound positive for pyloric stenosis. Elongated pyloric channel of 2.13 cm (see 1 in image) and increased muscular wall thickness of 0.49 cm (see 2 in image).

clinically, an ultrasound may be obtained. The sensitivity of ultrasound for testicular torsion is 78% with a specificity of 97%.[8] In comparison, the sensitivity and specificity of nuclear medicine scintigraphy is 79% and 91%, respectively.[8] With the similar diagnostic capabilities of the two studies, ultrasound should be the first choice because it can be obtained quickly and does not use ionizing radiation. In cases of high clinical suspicion, a negative study should not rule out torsion.

Ectopic pregnancy can be detected through transabdominal or transvaginal techniques. With transabdominal ultrasound, an intrauterine pregnancy can be detected as early as 5 weeks of gestation.[2,9] The timeline for development and visualization allows the gestational sac to be seen at 5 to 6 weeks, the fetal pole at 6 to 7 weeks, and the embryo with cardiac movement at 7 to 8 weeks.[2,9] The use of the transvaginal method allows detection of these structures approximately a week earlier. An ectopic pregnancy is visualized as a mass in the cul-de-sac area.[1] The sensitivity of emergency physicians to detect an ectopic pregnancy by the transvaginal technique ranges from 90% to 100%.[2,9] The specificity of transvaginal ultrasonography for an ectopic pregnancy is from 88% to 95%.[2,9]

Ultrasonography for ovarian torsion is primarily carried out in the radiology department. The finding of an enlarged ovary with a heterogeneous appearance or a whirl sign, consisting of the twisted vascular structures, is suggestive of ovarian pathology[10,11] Color Doppler flow can be seen in 57% to 62% of torsed ovaries, thus the presence of flow is does not rule out ovarian torsion.[10,11] The sensitivity and specificity of transabdominal and transvaginal ultrasound to diagnose ovarian torsion is 88% and 87%, respectively.[11]

The evaluation for acute appendicitis by ultrasound is complex, thus it is generally carried out by the radiology department. Appendicitis is determined on transabdominal ultrasound by the presence of a noncompressible, tubular structure that measures longer than 6 mm in diameter.[1] The presence of increased color Doppler flow can add to the confirmation of the diagnosis by suggesting inflammation. The presence of fluid around the appendix may suggest a perforated appendix with subsequent abscess formation. The sensitivity and specificity of ultrasound to diagnose appendicitis in children is 80% to 92% and 86% to 98%, respectively.[5,12,13]

Focused abdominal sonography for trauma (FAST) has been used in adult trauma patients to evaluate for intra-abdominal injury. FAST is based on the concept that free fluid (e.g., blood) collects in the dependent portions of the supine trauma patient.[9] The four areas that are evaluated are the pericardial sac, Morrison's pouch, splenorenal recess, and the pelvis. In adult patients, a positive FAST is determined when there is more than 150 mL of intraperitoneal blood.[9] A modified FAST can also be performed, which looks at the four areas mentioned above, plus the paracolic gutters bilaterally.[2]

The utility of the FAST examination in children has been debated. One benefit of the FAST is the ability to perform the examination at the bedside in 5 minutes or less depending on the experience of the operator.[2] FAST is less invasive than a diagnostic peritoneal lavage and may yield more information about which organs are injured. Unlike computed tomography (CT), FAST uses no radiation or contrast and does not require patient transport.

The limitation of the pediatric FAST scan is the difficulty in determining what a positive finding is in a child. Another limitation to consider is that 26% to 34% of patients with intra-abdominal traumatic injuries do not have hemoperitoneum.[14] Furthermore, in pediatric patients with hemoperitoneum, 14% are treated conservatively without surgery.[2]

The usefulness of FAST in pediatric trauma needs further investigation. The sensitivity and specificity for FAST to detect hemoperitoneum is 80% and 96%, respectively.[14] The interpretation of detecting intra-abdominal fluid is more complicated. FAST is useful as a screening tool for intra-abdominal injury, but further studies are needed to better define its role in pediatric trauma patients.

▶ DIAGNOSTIC RADIOGRAPHS (X-RAYS)

The discovery of x-rays was made by Roentgen in 1895.[15] He used a photographic plate to record the appearance of platinum as radiation was projected onto it. Roentgen noted that the platinum absorbed the radiation, thus appeared white on the photographic plate. He further went on to test this phenomenon on his wife's hand, and found that the bones were bright white while the surrounding tissue was darker in appearance. Report of these findings prompted use of diagnostic radiology in the medical community.

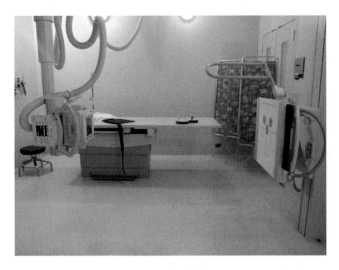

Figure 22–7. Picture of a plain x-ray machine where the x-ray source is located on the left and the film is located on the right.

PHYSICS AND PATHOPHYSIOLOGY

Plain radiography accounts for approximately 80% of all imaging studies.[16] The image obtained from plain radiography is acquired with the aid of an x-ray, which is a collection of electromagnetic energy called a photon. Electromagnetic energy travels at the speed of light at different frequencies, where the higher the frequency, the more energy it possesses. For example, the low frequency of a light photon has 1 eV of energy, compared to the high frequency of an x-ray photon that has 30 keV of energy.[17] The large amount of energy that x-rays contain allows them to ionize atoms that they encounter, hence labeling x-rays as a form of ionizing radiation.

Approximately 1% of x-rays navigate all the way through the patient to the film (Fig. 22–7).[17] The remainder of the x-rays are either absorbed or scattered. Absorption of an x-ray results in a white appearance on the film because the x-ray does not penetrate through the given object onto the film. Objects that have a high atomic number (e.g., bone) are more likely to absorb the x-ray and appear white on the image. Absorption is inversely proportional to the voltage, thus when the voltage is decreased, absorption increases causing the contrast between different substances to be enhanced on the developed image. However, the decreased x-ray voltage means a higher radiation dose is required to get a sufficient amount of x-rays to penetrate through to the film.

Approximately one-third of the x-rays reaching the film are primary x-rays, which travel directly through the patient in a straight line.[17] The other x-rays are the result of scattering, which occurs when an x-ray encounters an atom and bounces off in another direction. The scattered x-rays that reach the film appear as a gray color, which decreases the quality of the image. To remove the scattered x-rays, an antiscatter grid is often used, which consists of thin lead strips with intermingled radiolucent bands. The scattered x-rays are absorbed by the lead while the primary x-rays are allowed to reach to the film. The grid usually slides over a little during the exposure process to prevent gridlines. The drawback of the antiscatter grid is that it may eliminate too much x-rays from reaching the film, resulting in an underpenetrated film. To fix this problem, a higher x-ray exposure is usually required. The techniques to decrease scatter and to increase absorption must be carefully balanced to provide the best image with the lowest radiation dose.

SAFETY CONSIDERATIONS

X-rays can cause damage to biologic tissue. This occurs when the x-ray is either absorbed or scattered by its encounter with an atom causing electrons to shoot off and ionize surrounding atoms.[17] Because of the damage x-rays can cause, lead shields are often used to protect body parts that are not being imaged. The high atomic number of lead prevents x-rays from penetrating through it, thus making it a good shield.

BENEFITS AND LIMITATIONS

The benefit of using diagnostic radiography is that one is able to get a quick view of a large area with a relatively low amount of radiation. The images can be interpreted by emergency physicians for acute pathology. Portable x-ray devices make it available at the bedside limiting the need for transport to the radiology department.

One limitation of x-ray is that it is a two-dimensional image of a three-dimensional subject. This makes interpretation difficult and often necessitates the need to obtain multiple views. Another limitation is that radiolucent objects cannot be seen on film (e.g., plastic). Thus when dealing with foreign bodies, the utility of x-rays may be limited depending on the suspected object (Fig. 22–8).

DIAGNOSTIC AND PROCEDURAL CONSIDERATIONS

Diagnostic x-rays are the most commonly ordered imaging study in the emergency department setting. It is the standard for diagnosing fractures and is generally used to evaluate for chest and abdominal pathology. Diagnostic x-rays also have the benefit of allowing the practitioner to assess for multiple causes for the patient's symptoms at the same time (Fig. 22–9).

Procedures are usually not done by using diagnostic x-rays, but can be done with fluoroscopy. Fluoroscopy is similar to diagnostic x-rays except that the fluorescent screen is viewed directly with the help of an image intensifier.[17] Fluoroscopic procedures allow the practitioner to view real-time images, but the drawback is that the image quality is poorer and the patient is exposed to more radiation. Common fluoroscopic procedures include fracture reductions and contrast studies.

▶ COMPUTED TOMOGRAPHY

Computed tomography (CT) was developed in the late 1960s by the British engineer Geoffry Hounsfield.[17] Hounsfield

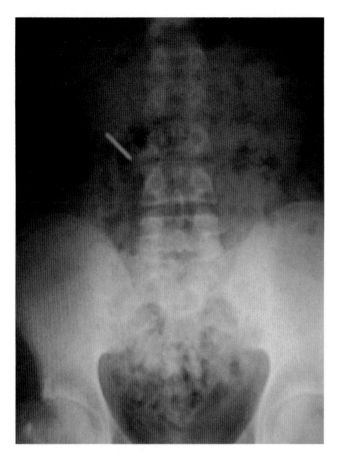

Figure 22–8. Plain x-ray revealing a radio-opaque foreign body. Patient had reported accidentally swallowing a screwdriver.

recognized that by compiling image data from numerous different angles, the attenuation properties of each object could be determined. A computer was used to accumulate the data and to compose a cross-sectional image.

There are approximately 62 million CT scans performed in the United States annually, with 2 to 4 million CT scans

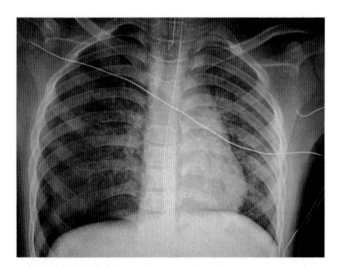

Figure 22–9. X-ray of a trauma patient. Note rib fractures on the right with pneumothorax.

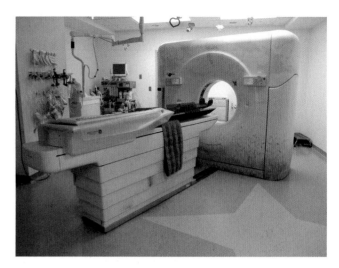

Figure 22–10. Picture of a typical CT scanner.

performed in children.[18,19] This reflects an increase in the utilization of CT scans over the last 10 years, where the use of CT in adults and children has risen 7- to 10-fold.[18] It is hypothesized that the increased usage is attributed to increased availability and improved technology.

PHYSICS AND PATHOPHYSIOLOGY

The basic principle of CT scans is similar to plain radiography as x-rays are used to visualize different densities within the body of interest. The patient lies on a table that slides through the CT machine (Fig. 22–10). Within the CT machine, there is a narrow opening where the x-ray source emits a thin, fan-shaped beam. Instead of film, the x-rays are received by x-ray detectors, which are located on the opposite side of the patient. The x-ray source and detectors rotate simultaneously around the patient during the examination. The information from the detectors is processed by a computer to create a three-dimensional image.

Recent advances in CT scanners have allowed CT to be done more rapidly. Axial CT scans are done where the table moves intermittently between rotations of the x-ray source and detectors. Helical CT scanners, which were developed in the 1990s, allow the table to move the patient continually through the examination, and not have to wait for each rotation.[20] Multidetector, also known as multislice CT scanners, now have multiple rows of x-ray detectors that rotate next to each other allowing multiple slices to be processed concurrently. This further decreases the time needed to perform a CT scan.

X-rays, as noted above, are a form of ionizing radiation that can release electrons from atoms and molecules. In the case of water molecules, hydroxy radicals are released that can damage deoxyribonucleic acid (DNA) causing strands to break and bases to be harmed. DNA can also be directly ionized by x-rays. The damage to DNA can be fixed by the cell in most cases, but the double-strand breaks are less easily mended. During the repair of double strand breaks, there can be incorrect repairs that can lead to point mutations, translocations, gene fusions, and ultimately cancers.[19] Because of the serious side effects brought about by ionizing radiation, the safety of radiologic studies has been brought into question.

SAFETY CONSIDERATIONS

Ionizing radiation is present in the environment from natural sources in addition to man-made sources. Natural sources of radiation include cosmic rays, terrestrial rocks, and mountains. For people living in the United States the average background radiation is estimated to be 3 mSv per year.[20,21] Man-made sources of radiation include those from diagnostic x-rays and CT scans. Ionizing radiation can alter biologic tissues and thus cause a safety hazard.

In considering the safety of CT scans, there are some terms that should be defined. The absorbed dose is the radiation dose delivered to an organ. It is measured in grays (Gy), where 1 Gy is equal to 1 joule of absorbed radiation energy per kilogram.[19] The organ dose represents the deposition of the radiation within the organ. The effective dose is used when calculating the risk to nonhomogenous tissues (e.g., different organs in an abdominal CT). The effective dose takes into account the amount of radiation each organ receives as well as the radiosensitivity of the specific organs. The effective dose is measured in mSv. For x-ray radiation, a whole-body radiation dose of 1 mGy is the same as an effective dose of 1 mSv.

CT scans provide a significantly higher organ dose than a plain radiograph. For example, with anterior-posterior abdominal x-ray, the stomach receives an organ dose of approximately 0.25 mGy, which is 50 times less than what the stomach would get from an abdominal CT.[19] The Food and Drug Administration (FDA) estimates that a CT scan with an effective dose of 10 mSv (e.g., abdominal CT) increases the chance of a person dying from a fatal cancer to 1 in 2000.[22] The lifetime cancer mortality risk to a child from an abdominal CT scan is estimated to be 1 in 550.[22] The increase in radiation induced cancer mortality risk is alarming, but it is also important to keep this in perspective with the overall cancer mortality risk from all causes, which is approximately one in five individuals.[21]

The increase in cancer mortality risk is relatively small compared to the overall cancer risk, but with the increased utilization of CT scans, especially in children, there is greater concern for the consequences in the future. Children are more vulnerable to ionizing radiation from CT scans than adults for three reasons. The first is that the tissues and organs of children are more radiosensitive, because they are still developing. Thus, given the same radiation dose, the child's organs would be more susceptible to the ionizing effects. The second reason is that since there is a latent period between the time of exposure and the development of cancer, a child who presumably has a longer life expectancy would have more time for the cancer to become evident. The latent period for leukemia is the shortest at 2 to 5 years postradiation exposure, and solid malignancies have the longest latent period of 10 to 20 years.[22] The third reason children are more susceptible is that when children undergo a CT scan, they are often exposed to adult parameters. This is commonly seen in adult institutions where parameters may not be adjusted to children. Radiologists and CT technicians should adjust parameters to use the radiation dose that is as low as reasonably achievable (ALARA) to get an adequate scan.[21]

Decreasing ionizing radiation to children should follow the ALARA principle. The CT parameters should be adjusted to the individual patient. By decreasing the CT radiation dose, there may be a more speckled appearance to the scan, but this usually does not sacrifice the diagnostic accuracy. A 50% to 90% decrease in the radiation dose from adult to child parameters has been used without any compromise to the interpretation of the scan.[21] For the practitioner, it is essential for the reason for the scan to be indicated so that the CT parameters can be tailored to the indication. Secondly, CT as well as other diagnostic x-ray studies should only be done when entirely necessary. In some cases, alternative studies such as ultrasound and magnetic resonance imaging (MRI) can be used as an alternative means of imaging to avoid unnecessary ionizing radiation.

BENEFITS AND LIMITATIONS

CT scans are readily available to most emergency medicine practitioners. The main benefit of CT is its ability to provide useful information quickly. Since most CT scans are performed rapidly, many can be done without the need for sedation.

The main limitation of CT is that it provides a significant radiation exposure, especially in the pediatric age group. Secondly, the interpretation of CT in many cases must be by a trained radiologist. Thirdly, in order to obtain a CT scan the patient needs to be transported to the radiology department, which may limit its use in unstable patients. Lastly, contrast is sometimes needed to better visualize structures, but has some notable side effects. Approximately 5% of patients will have mild reaction such as nausea, vomiting, rash, or a metallic taste.[16] Approximately 1 in 1000 patients will have a severe reaction including hypotension, laryngeal edema, and possibly cardiac arrest.[16] Contrast can cause impairment of renal function, thus cannot be used in patients with renal dysfunction or multiple myeloma.

DIAGNOSTIC AND PROCEDURAL CONSIDERATIONS

Overall, the benefits, limitations, and safety considerations must be weighed carefully with the clinical picture to determine the best diagnostic option. Common conditions that utilize CT scans are discussed below.

The diagnosis of appendicitis can be made based on clinical examination. As discussed previously, ultrasound can be used to diagnose appendicitis and should be used as the first diagnostic option when available. When ultrasound cannot determine the diagnosis, abdominal CT scan can be obtained with a sensitivity and specificity of 87% to 100% and 83% to 97%, respectively.[5,12]

In pediatric trauma patients, CT scans can provide a great deal of information quickly. The information can be used to prompt or obviate the need for surgical intervention. Also, the need for airway intervention may remove the ability of the practitioner to clinically assess and monitor the patient, thus CT scans are the practical approach to diagnose suspected intracranial and intra-abdominal injury.

In the unstable trauma patient, CT often has the disadvantage of requiring transport to the radiology department. It also may require moving the patient from the gurney onto the scanner bed, which can be labor-intensive. Furthermore, in cases where a patient is unstable and needs operative intervention, an abdominal CT scan has little to add to the management.

► MAGNETIC RESONANCE IMAGING

MRI was developed in the 1980s.[15] Since then, it has become available in most institutions. MRI provides better evaluation of soft-tissue and organs, but is generally not considered to be a routine emergency department study. There are conditions that require emergent MRI, thus a brief summary will be included.

PHYSICS AND PATHOPHYSIOLOGY

MRI uses radiofrequency energy, which is a type of non-ionizing radiation. This energy is absorbed by tissue and is expressed as the specific absorption rate (SAR). The SAR is usually averaged for the whole-body and is measured in watts per kilogram (W/kg). Radiofrequency energy can cause an increase in body temperature, which in certain patients with medical challenges (e.g., fever, obesity, hypertension, etc.) can theoretically cause tissue damage. In studies of whole-body SARs of 4 to 6 W/kg, which is higher than usual MRI levels, normal healthy individuals had no deleterious effects.[23]

MRI systems also employ a static magnetic field usually in the range of 0.2 to 3 Teslas (T).[23] The FDA states that clinical MRI machines that use a static magnetic field up to 8 T can be used without significant risk to the patient.[23]

SAFETY CONSIDERATIONS

Overall, MRI is considered a safe imaging modality. The biggest safety hazard is the risk for ferromagnetic objects to be brought into the MRI magnetic field. There are two regions within the magnetic field that should be mentioned. Region one comprises the spatial area in the isocenter of the magnet that exerts a constant force.[24] A ferromagnetic object in this area will be subject to a rotational force, which can destroy adjacent tissue. Region two is the spatial area outside the magnet that exerts a gradient field where the greatest force is closer to the magnet and decreases further out from the magnet.[24] In this area, ferromagnetic objects are subjected to a translational force in the direction of the magnet. Due to the forces subject to ferromagnetic objects, a careful history must be done to be sure the patient does not have any metallic clips or coils, internal defibrillators/pacemakers, ferromagnetic foreign bodies or foil containing medicine patches.

There has been some controversy over whether tattoos with metal-based pigments should exclude a patient from getting an MRI. There have been reports of local irritation and heating sensations in 1.5% of patients who underwent MRI with a cosmetic tattoo.[23] With relatively minor adverse effects, the FDA states that the risk of not having an MRI done when it is indicated is likely greater than the risk of the potential complications.[23]

MRI can subject the patient to high levels of acoustic noise. To be consistent with Occupational Safety and Health Administration guidelines for industrial workers, the noise level should be kept below 100 decibels when protective gear is in place.[24] Thus, whether high levels of noise are expected or not, it is generally accepted that patients should receive ear protection (e.g., ear plugs).

BENEFITS AND LIMITATIONS

The benefit of MRI is that it provides a more detailed image for most organs and soft tissue than a CT scan. Also, MRI does not use ionizing radiation thereby making it a safer alternative. Finally, MRI uses gadolinium-based contrast agents, which are safer than the iodine contrast agents used for CT.[15]

The limitation of MRI is that it cannot be used in patients with ferromagnetic objects. MRI cannot be performed at the bedside and requires a significantly longer time to complete the study compared to a CT. This delays the diagnosis and is often not feasible in critically ill patients. In children, MRI scans often require the use of sedation, which adds other potential safety risks. In addition, MRI requires radiology interpretation and due to the labor and time intensive nature of MRI, it is usually not readily available to emergency department patients in many institutions.

DIAGNOSTIC AND PROCEDURAL CONSIDERATIONS

MRI in the emergency department setting is usually reserved for emergent conditions, such as cord compression and strokes. Further MRI studies are usually carried out in the inpatient or outpatient setting, depending on the urgency of the medical condition. Discussion of detailed MRI use is beyond the scope of this chapter.

► CONCLUSION

Diagnostic imaging is vital to the practice of pediatric emergency medicine. The familiarity and accessibility of x-rays and CT scans make it the usual first choice study. As practitioners are becoming more aware of the radiation risk of x-ray and CT studies and nonionizing radiation modalities become more available, we will likely see a shift in diagnostic imaging selections.

REFERENCES

1. Cohen HL, Moore WM. History of emergency ultrasound. *J Ultrasound Med.* 2004;23:451.
2. Yen K, Gorelick MH. Ultrasound applications for the pediatric emergency department: a review of the current literature. *Pediatr Emerg Care.* 2002;18:226.
3. Meyer RA. Interaction of ultrasound and biologic tissues—potential hazards. *Pediatrics.* 1974;54:266.

4. Brown BSJ. How safe is diagnostic ultrasonography? *Can Med Assoc J.* 1984;131:307.

5. Bachur RG. Abdominal emergencies. In: Fleisher GR, Ludwig S, et al., eds. *Textbook of Pediatric Emergency Medicine.* 5th ed. Philadelphia, PA: Lippincott Williams & Wilkins; 2006:1605

6. Neilson D, Hollman AS. The ultrasonic diagnosis of infantile hypertrophic pyloric stenosis: technique and accuracy. *Clin Radiol.* 1994;49:246.

7. Hernanz-Schulman M, Sells LL, Ambrosino MM, et al. Hypertrophic pyloric stenosis in the infant without a palpable olive: accuracy of sonographic diagnosis. *Pediatr Radiol.* 1994;193:771.

8. Nussbaum Blask AR, Bulas D, Shalaby-Rana E, et al. Color Doppler sonography and scintigraphy of the testis: a prospective, comparative analysis in children with acute scrotal pain. *Pediatr Emerg Care.* 2002;18:67.

9. Chen L, Baker MD. Novel applications of ultrasound in pediatric emergency medicine. *Pediatr Emerg Care.* 2007;23:115.

10. Servaes S, Zurakowski D, Laufer MR, et al. Sonographic findings of ovarian torsion in children. *Pediatr Radiol.* 2007;37:446.

11. Lee EJ, Kwon HC, Joo HJ, et al. Diagnosis of ovarian torsion with color Doppler sonography: depiction of twisted vascular pedicle. *J Ultrasound Med.* 1998;17:83.

12. Dorias AS, Moineddin R, Kellenberger CJ, et al. US or CT for diagnosis of appendicitis in children and adults? A meta-analysis. *Radiology.* 2006;241:83.

13. Kaiser S, Frenckner B, Jorulf HK. Suspected appendicitis in children: US and CT—a prospective randomized study. *Radiology.* 2002;223:633.

14. Holmes JF, Gladman A, Chang CH. Performance of abdominal ultrasonography in pediatric blunt trauma patients: a meta-analysis. *J Pediatr Surg.* 2007;42:1588.

15. Chen MYM, Bradbury MS. Scope of diagnostic imaging. In: Chen MYM, Pope TL Jr, Ott DJ, eds. *Basic Radiology.* New York, NY: McGraw-Hill; 2004:chap 1. http://www.accessmedicine.com. Accessed February 15, 2008.

16. Mettler FA Jr.: X-ray: In: Mettler FA Jr, ed. *Essentials of Radiology.* 2nd ed. Philadelphia, PA: Elsevier; 2005:2.

17. Dixon RL. The physical basis of diagnostic imaging. In: Chen MYM, Pope TL Jr, Ott DJ, eds. *Basic Radiology.* New York, NY: McGraw-Hill; 2004:chap 2. http://www.accessmedicine.com. Accessed February 15, 2008.

18. National Cancer Institute. Radiation and pediatric computed tomography: a guide for health care providers. Rockville, MD: National Cancer Institute; 2002 http://www.cancer.gov/cancertopics/causes/radiation-risks-pediatric-CT. Accessed February 15, 2008.

19. Brenner DJ, Hall EJ, Phil D. Computed tomography—an increasing source of radiation exposure. *NEJM.* 2007;357:2277.

20. Frush DP, Donnelly LF, Rosen NS. Computed tomography and radiation risks: what pediatric health care providers should know. *Pediatrics.* 2003;112:951.

21. Brody AS, Frush DP, Huda W, et al. Radiation risk to children from computed tomography. *Pediatrics.*2007;120:677.

22. Semelka RC, Armao DM, Junior JE, et al. Imaging strategies to reduce the risk of radiation in CT studies, including selective substitution with MRI. *J Magn Reson Imaging.* 2007;25:900.

23. Shellock FG, Crues JV. MR procedures: biologic effects, safety, and patient care. *Radiology.* 2004;232:635.

24. Price RR. The AAPM/RSNA physics tutorial for residents. *Radiographics.* 1999;19:1641.

SECTION III

RESUSCITATION

CHAPTER 23

Airway Management

Loren G. Yamamoto

► HIGH-YIELD FACTS

- The relatively large tongue in an unconscious infant is the most common cause of airway obstruction. An oral or nasopharyngeal airway can resolve the problem.
- Overinflation with bag-mask ventilation can result in gastric distention and restrict lung expansion. This can be resolved by placing a nasogastric tube.
- A self-inflating bag does not deliver blow-by oxygen when it is not being compressed.
- Before using sedatives and paralytics for tracheal intubation, be sure to assess for conditions that may be associated with a "difficult airway."
- Selection of a sedating agent for tracheal intubation is based on recognition of three specific clinical conditions: head trauma (increased intracranial pressure), asthma, and hypotension.
- Confirmation of tracheal intubation should always include use of an $ETCO_2$ device.

► AIRWAY ANATOMY

Appreciation of pediatric airway conditions is based on the anatomy of the airway. Figures 23–1A and B are lateral neck x-rays of a child with croup. The patient's nose (anterior) is on the right and the occiput (posterior) is on the left. Note the lordotic (extended) cervical spine vertebral bodies.

PEDIATRIC AIRWAY DIFFERENCES

Physical factors that differ between adults and children account for the airway differences that are clinically important. The most important of these is a smaller airway diameter. Smaller airways with the same degree of airway edema result in proportionately greater obstruction (Fig. 23–2). Some textbooks have quoted Poiseuille's equation describing airflow resistance is proportional to the fourth power of the radius. This is not quite correct under conditions of respiratory distress since Poiseuille's law describes laminar flow, and during respiratory distress, nonlaminar flow dominates; however, airway resistance is proportionately greater and coupled with a weaker patient, the degree of ventilation compromise is greater.

The tongue of children is relatively larger.[1] The posterior portion of the tongue can easily fall backward in the supine position, compromising the upper airway. Some patients have a particularly large tongue, amplifying this factor. The narrow-est point of the child's upper airway is the cricoid ring (which is below the vocal cords), while the narrowest portion of the adult airway is the vocal cords.[1] This is important because occasionally, an endotracheal tube (ETT) will pass through the cords, but it cannot be advanced further because the cricoid region is too narrow for this tube, in which case a smaller tube should be used. The larynx in children is more cephalad, the epiglottis is softer and more curved, and the airways are less rigid.[1] This is especially noticeable in patients with tracheomalacia and laryngomalacia.

RECOGNIZING CONDITIONS ASSOCIATED WITH A DIFFICULT AIRWAY

An airway emergency will present with an acute process that adversely affects a normal airway, or an exacerbation of a chronic airway condition. Some children have airway conditions that place them at higher risk of airway obstruction, other children have airway conditions that make intubation and visualization of the airway more difficult, and some children have both. Children with chronic airway conditions include those with Down's syndrome, Pierre Robin syndrome, and other congenital conditions and malformations that affect the tongue, mandible, and neck. Tumors, masses, swelling, and edema (e.g., burns, chemical inhalations, and allergic reactions) in this area can also lead to airway compromise and difficult intubation.[1] Laryngomalacia and tracheomalacia place patients at higher risk for airway obstruction. Head trauma, neck trauma, and multiple trauma require cervical spine immobilization making visualization of the larynx potentially more difficult. Trauma of the face, mouth, neck, and airway structures can directly injure the airway resulting in airway compromise. Infections such as croup, epiglottitis, bacterial tracheitis, and retropharyngeal abscess can narrow the airway, with epiglottitis and bacterial tracheitis presenting with the most serious degree of airway obstruction. Patients with an altered sensorium and patients who are pharmacologically sedated are at higher risk for airway compromise as the oral structures relax and fall posteriorly over the airway when the patient is in a supine position.

► CLINICAL ASSESSMENT

Air exchange and the degree of airway obstruction can be assessed by observation, auscultation, and technology, but preferably by all three.

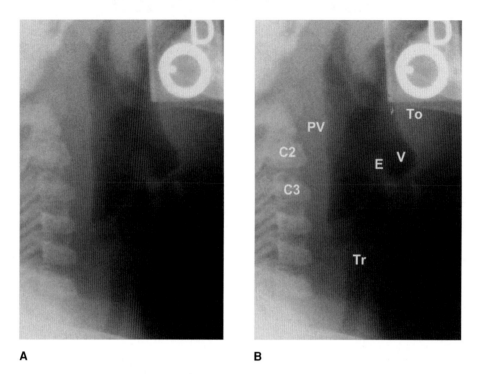

A   B

Figure 23–1. (**A**) Lateral neck of a child with croup. (**B**) Labeled version of
Figure 23-1-1 A. Identify the following structures. To: Tongue (posterior portion). The
laryngoscope blade slides over this portion to visualize the airway. V: Valeculla, also
called the preepiglottic space. The tip of the laryngoscope blade can be directed into
this space to lift the epiglottis anteriorly. E: Epiglottis. This stucture is a curved paddle
(an elongated spoon). Understanding this structure in 3 dimensions helps to
understand its radiographic appearance depending on the angle of the x-ray beam.
Note that the hinge of the epiglottis is anterior. Gravity causes the epiglottis to fall
posteriorly and inferiorly (downward) to cover the opening to the airway. Tr: Trachea.
The Tr label is in the superior aspect of the trachea. The portion of the airway between
the upper trachea and the epiglottis is the larynx which contains the vocal chords. In
this particular x-ray, the trachea narrows inferiorly due to subglottic edema (croup). PV:
Prevertebral soft tissue, also called the retropharyngeal soft tissue because it is behind
the pharynx. This tissue should be approximately the width of half a vertebral body. C2
and C3: Cervical spine vertebral bodies C2 and C3. (With permission from Boychuk RB.
Drooling, stridor, and a barking cough: croup?? In: Yamamoto LG, Inaba AS, DiMauro
R, eds. *Radiology Cases in Pediatric Emergency Medicine*. 1994:1(10).
www.hawaii.edu/medicine/pediatrics/pemxray/v1c10.html. Accessed January 2, 2008.)

A patient with an airway obstruction might have visibly abnormal chest movements with retractions and exaggerated respiratory efforts. A gentle rise and fall of the chest suggests good air exchange. If the patient is wearing an oxygen mask, you might be able to see condensation on the mask with each breath, which suggests significant exhaling (a good sign).

A patient with an airway obstruction might have noisy breathing. More severe obstruction might have no noise if all air movement has ceased. Auscultation of the chest can usually assess the degree of air exchange. Noisy environments and obese individuals can make auscultation difficult.

End-tidal CO_2 (ETCO$_2$) monitoring is useful to confirm the degree of air exchange. While monitors are often used in-line on a ventilator for intubated patients, they can also be used near the patient's mouth or nose to partially assess air exchange. Colorimetric ETCO$_2$ detectors are less sensitive for this purpose. Pulse oximetry does not measure air exchange

directly, but the presence of hypoxia suggests that air exchange might be poor.

▶ AIRWAY MANAGEMENT

The ability to rescue a patient from an airway emergency in order to maintain oxygenation is a vital skill that emergency physicians must possess.

MANUAL MANIPULATION OF THE AIRWAY

Most airway repositioning maneuvers work by moving the posterior portion of the tongue to a more anterior location so that

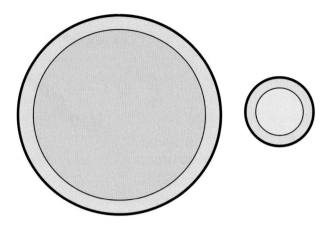

Figure 23–2. Similar degrees of edema result in proportionately greater degrees of narrowing in smaller airways compared to larger airways.

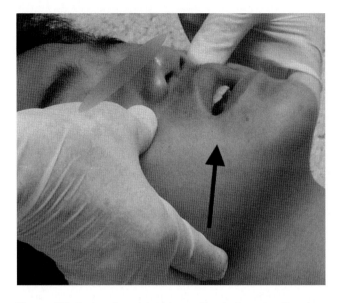

Figure 23–4. Jaw thrust maneuver. By placing your thumbs on the patient's maxilla or zygoma, grasp the mandibular angle with your fingers and pull the mandible forward (black arrow) to open the airway. This can be done without cervical spine movement.

it does not block the airway. Figure 23–3A and B demonstrates how the jaw thrust maneuver opens the airway. Note that this maneuver should not move the cervical spine if immobilization is required. While placing your thumbs on the patient's zygoma or maxilla, grasp the mandibular angle with your fingers and pull it anteriorly (Fig. 23–4). The chin-lift maneuver is similar but if the head is tilted, this could move the cervical spine. If cervical spine movement is not a concern, then other maneuvers that can be attempted with varying degrees of success include the following:

1. Raising the patient's occiput (putting a thick towel underneath it) into the sniffing position. This brings the tongue more anterior, opening the airway and improving the angle of view for laryngoscopy and intubation.
2. Placing a towel roll under the patient's scapulae and upper thoracic spine while permitting the head to tilt

backward. This essentially does the opposite of raising the occiput, but the backward tilt of the head can often raise the posterior portion of the tongue. An excessive head tilt can stretch and compress the airway.
3. Placing the patient on his/her side with the face slightly downward. This permits gravity to move the tongue forward.
4. Placing the patient prone. While this position permits gravity to move the tongue forward and secretions

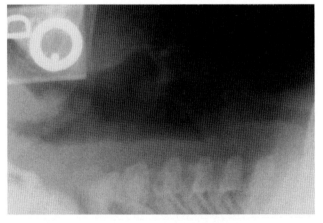

A

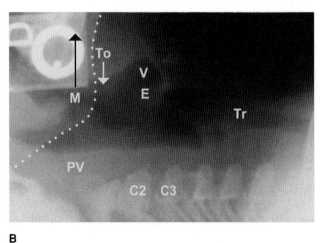

B

Figure 23–3. (**A**) This is the same lateral neck x-ray in Figure 23–1 A, except that the image is now rotated to the supine position. The nose is pointing upward, and the occiput is down below. (**B**) Labeled version of Figure 23–3 A. Note that gravity will move the tongue (To) downward (white arrow) to narrow the airway opening. The dotted line is the angle of the mandible (M). By pushing the angle of the mandible anteriorly (upward in this position, black arrow), this will move the tongue (To) anteriorly (upward) to open the airway. (With permission from Boychuk RB. Drooling, stridor, and a barking cough: croup?? In: Yamamoto LG, Inaba AS, DiMauro R, eds. *Radiology Cases in Pediatric Emergency Medicine*. 1994;1(10). www.hawaii.edu/medicine/pediatrics/pemxray/v1c10.html.)

drain out of the mouth, it does not permit easy access to the airway for other manipulations such as laryngoscopy. However, bag-mask ventilation (BMV) can be done in this position. This position might be especially optimal for a patient with epiglottitis in respiratory failure. The large inflamed epiglottis in the prone position falls backward obstructing the airway. The patient prefers to be in the "tripodding" position (erect, leaning forward), to keep the epiglottis off the airway. As the patient tires and succumbs to respiratory failure, placing the patient in the prone position utilizes gravity such that the epiglottis falls anteriorly, opening the airway and permitting BMV, which should optimally be performed using the two rescuer method.

PHARMACOLOGIC TREATMENT OF THE AIRWAY

Aerosolized epinephrine can improve air exchange in croup and other conditions resulting from upper airway edema. Note that the standard dose of 0.5 mL of 2.25% racemic epinephrine is equal to 5.5 mg (5.5 mL of 1:1000) epinephrine. Aerosolized and systemic corticosteroids can also reduce airway swelling caused by inflammation. Anticholinergics (atropine, ipratropium) and albuterol can reduce airway resistance in some instances.

OXYGEN ADMINISTRATION

For spontaneously breathing patients, supplemental oxygen can be delivered via nasal cannula, blow-by, oxygen mask, non-rebreather oxygen mask or Rusch bag and mask (Fig. 23–5). Nasal cannula and blow-by oxygen enrich the oxygen concentration in the oral-nasal area to improve the inspired fraction of oxygen depending on the flow rate. Even at high flow rates, this enrichment is modest. Conventional oxygen masks leak and entrain substantial amounts of room air. Non-rebreather oxygen masks have a reservoir bag that should be inflated with pure oxygen such that when the patient inhales, pure oxygen from the reservoir bag is inhaled. A Rusch bag and mask is a closed circuit so that with a tight mask seal, close to 100% FIO_2 can be delivered. Additionally continuous positive airway pressure (CPAP) and positive pressure ventilation can be administered with a Rusch bag and mask.

RESCUE BREATHING AND BAG-MASK VENTILATION

BMV is a vital skill that must be practiced for proficiency. Airway repositioning is generally required simultaneously. The two-rescuer technique is easier (Fig. 23–6). One rescuer uses both hands to apply a properly fitting mask seal covering the patient's mouth and nose, while simultaneously optimizing the patient's airway position. The second rescuer squeezes the bag to provide positive pressure, while ideally checking the chest rise. A third rescuer if available can auscultate the chest to confirm air exchange and/or assist with airway repositioning to optimize ventilation.

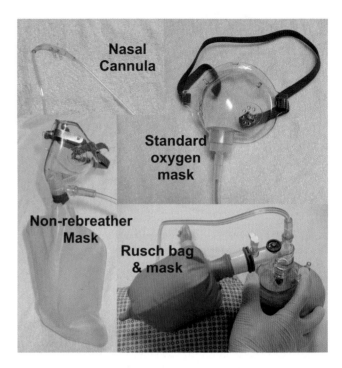

Figure 23–5. Different types of oxygen delivery devices. Nasal cannula, standard oxygen mask, non-rebreather mask, Rusch bag & mask.

The single rescuer technique is more difficult to perform optimally (Fig. 23–7). With one hand, the rescuer holds the mask with the thumb and index finger, while using the other three fingers to grasp the patient's mandible. This is called the E-C (or CE) method because the thumb and index finger form the letter C, while the other three fingers form the letter E. This hand must also position the airway properly to optimize ventilation. The other hand must be used to squeeze the bag. Rescuers with large hands can squeeze the bag directly, while those with smaller hands can squeeze the bag against their thigh.

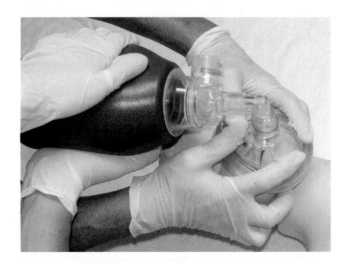

Figure 23–6. Two-rescuer method of BMV. Note that one rescuer uses both hands to secure a mask seal, while a second rescuer squeezes the bag.

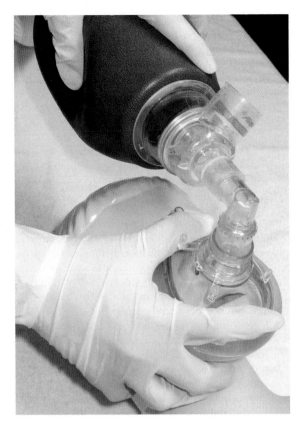

Figure 23-7. Single rescuer method of BMV. Note the E-C method of holding the mask against the child's face. The thumb and index finger apply pressure on the mask, while the other three fingers are used to "hook" the patient's mandible. The bag can either be squeezed with a large hand, or it can be squeezed against the rescuer's thigh as shown in this photo.

Over inflation by BMV can result in gastric distention, which can restrict lung expansion and place the patient at risk for gastric regurgitation. Applying cricoid pressure (the Sellick maneuver) can reduce gastric inflation to some degree. Excessive ventilation volumes and pressures can also increase intrathoracic pressure impeding venous return.[2]

VENTILATION BAG TYPES

There are basically two different bag types. The self-inflating bag is stiffer (Fig. 23–8). The Rusch bag (also called anesthesia bag) is more floppy and it normally collapses (Figs. 23–5 and 23–9). The term "ambu" bag can refer to both types of bags. The self-inflating bag (Fig. 23–8) does not require a positive pressure gas source. Since it inflates spontaneously, it can entrain room air and ventilate the patient with room air without an oxygen tank. If the tail of the bag is attached to a high flow oxygen source, the patient will be ventilated with an oxygen rich mixture than can approach 100% FiO_2. This type of bag should not be used in conjunction with a mask to deliver blow-by or mask oxygen to a spontaneously breathing patient because oxygen does not flow through the bag unless the bag is squeezed. The manikin in Figure 23–7 is receiving room air

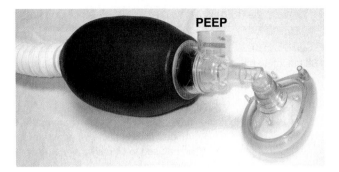

Figure 23-8. Self-inflating bag. The tail is on the left. High flow oxygen entering the tail increases the FiO_2 entering the bag. This particular model has an opening for an optional PEEP valve.

unless the bag is squeezed, regardless of how much oxygen is flowing into the tail of the bag.

The Rusch bag (Fig. 23–9) is a closed circuit system. Oxygen flows into one end inflating the bag, and it is squeezed out the other end. No outside air is entrained if a proper mask seal is maintained, so 100% oxygen can be easily delivered if 100% oxygen enters the bag. If the patient is spontaneously breathing, this differs from the self-inflating bag in that the Rusch bag mask setup functions as an oxygen flow mask because oxygen flows into the mask even if the bag is not squeezed. Another useful application of the Rusch bag and mask is that it can be used to visibly monitor ventilation. If the gas flow is adjusted optimally with a proper mask seal, the bag will collapse partially as the patient inhales, and the bag will fill as the patient exhales. This visible bag movement is an indicator of air exchange.

Both bag types can deliver positive end-expiratory pressure (PEEP), which is useful and sometimes essential for pulmonary edema and some other respiratory failure conditions. The Rusch bag delivers PEEP more routinely by simply increasing the gas flow, so that during exhalation, the bag is still full (exerting some positive pressure even during the exhalation phase). Most Rusch bags have a controlled leak valve and a visible pressure gauge or a pressure gauge connector to measure inspiratory and expiratory pressures. This also permits CPAP for spontaneously breathing patients. The self-inflating bag normally does not provide positive pressure during exhalation (PEEP); however, the addition of a PEEP valve attached to the

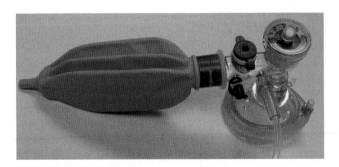

Figure 23-9. Rusch bag and mask. Note the built-in manometer.

▶ **TABLE 23–1. ADVANTAGES AND DISADVANTAGES OF SELF-INFLATING BAG VERSUS RUSCH BAG**

	Advantages	Disadvantages
Self-inflating bag	Does not require pressurized gas source	Does not deliver oxygen blow-by or CPAP
	Stiffer bag permits higher inflation pressures, especially during transtracheal ventilation	Does not routinely have PEEP, but PEEP valve can be added
Rusch bag	Can deliver blow-by oxygen, CPAP, and PEEP	Requires pressurized gas source
	More easily attached to a manometer, with some models having built-in manometers	Bag is often flimsy making it difficult to deliver high inspiratory pressures such as during transtracheal ventilation
	Can be used to visually monitor spontaneous ventilation	

exhalation port (Fig. 23–8) provides resistance during exhalation so that PEEP is provided. Both bag types have advantages and disadvantages. Know how to use both types properly. Table 23–1 summarizes the differences.

The laryngeal mask airway is an alternative to endotracheal intubation. As with any airway device, training and practice is required for proficient use. When endotracheal intubation is not possible, the laryngeal mask airway is an acceptable adjunct, but it is associated with a higher incidence of complications in young children.[2]

TRACHEAL INTUBATION

Tracheal intubation is best accomplished via the rapid sequence intubation (RSI) method with direct visualization using a laryngoscope. Other techniques that have been described are blind nasal tracheal intubation, blind oral intubation via palpation, and intubation via fiberoptic laryngoscopy visualization and guidance. These techniques have been less well described and hence the experience level amongst practitioners is not as extensive. Under the stress of an airway emergency, the likelihood of success is greatest with the technique that the practitioner has the greatest skill, expertise, and experience with. In teaching centers, another factor is the requirement that the procedures is supervisable and confirmable by the teaching physician.

RSI is described in a series of the following steps (a sequence):

1. Patient assessment, preparation, resuscitation
2. Premedications
3. Hyperoxygenation
4. Cricoid pressure (Sellick maneuver)
5. Paralyzing agent
6. Sedation agent
7. Intubation
8. Confirmation of intubation

Step 1. Assess the patient and perform immediate resuscitation measures such as mask ventilation, if necessary. Patient assessment includes determining the need and priority for intubation. Decompressing the stomach with a nasogastric tube can be helpful to improve ventilation; however, it makes the maintenance of a mask seal more difficult if BMV is necessary, it can be noxious triggering movement, which would be adverse to patients with cervical spine injuries, and it can interfere with gastroesophageal sphincter function increasing the risk of gastric regurgitation. In most instances, it is better

to pass a nasogastric tube after intubation.[2] Clinical assessment includes the determination of whether a nasogastric tube should be inserted prior to intubation or after intubation is confirmed. Preparation includes procuring the supplies necessary for the procedure (suction, laryngoscope, ventilation devices, ETT, tracheal intubation confirmation devices, etc.) as well as the practice sessions and creating an environment conducive to optimally performing RSI. The latter of which must in be place prior to the presentation of the emergency case requiring RSI. Posting Table 23–2 would be part of basic preparation.[3]

Step 2. Premedications depend on the clinical circumstances and practitioner preference. An abbreviated list of these includes atropine and lidocaine. Atropine potentially reduces oral secretions and the risk for laryngoscopy-induced bradycardia. Lidocaine potentially blunts the rise in intracranial pressure (ICP) during laryngoscopy, which is more important for patients with elevated ICP.

Step 3. RSI includes a brief period of apnea during intubation, which is best tolerated if the patient can maintain oxygenation during this period. Thus is best accomplished with hyperoxygenation prior to intubation. For patients who are breathing spontaneously, applying 100% F_{IO_2} by high flow non-rebreathing mask or Rusch bag and mask, maximizes oxygen hemoglobin saturation which is measurable via pulse oximetry, and additionally, it saturates the nonhemoglobin (plasma) oxygen content which is not measurable via pulse oximetry but can increase oxygen content by approximately 20%. Hypoxic patients and patients who are not spontaneously breathing sufficiently should be mask ventilated via BMV (PEEP may be necessary in many of these patients) to maximally oxygenate the patient prior to intubation. Patients who are still hypoxic despite rescue measures, are at high risk for worsening hypoxia and deterioration during intubation. However, such scenarios are commonly encountered in the emergency department, and they must still be intubated to take resuscitation to the next step.

Step 4. Cricoid pressure occludes the esophagus. This is known as the Sellick maneuver and it reduces the risk of passive regurgitation. It can also push the larynx more posteriorly to facilitate visualization during laryngoscopy. Cricoid pressure should be applied by a single dedicated person who should not be distracted by other tasks. Unfortunately, this person is perceived as doing very little during RSI so this person is commonly asked to do other tasks, which results in a prompt release of cricoid pressure and a loss of its advantages. While cricoid pressure reduces the risk of passive gastric regurgitation, it does not prevent vomiting if the patient is actively retching.

▶ TABLE 23-2. RSI DRUGS, DOSES (mg/kg), SIZES, DISTANCES

Age	2 mo	6 mo	1 y	3 y	5 y	7 y	9 y	11 y	12 y	14 y	16 y	Adult
Average weight (kg)	5	8	10	15	19	23	29	36	44	50	58	65
Preoxygenation												
Adjunctive agents (optional):												
Atropine (0.01–0.02 mg/kg): Use in all children or with ketamine.	0.1	0.15	0.2	0.3	0.3	0.4	0.5	0.5	0.5	0.5	0.5	0.5
Lidocaine (1.5 mg/kg): Lowers ICP	8	12	15	22	28	35	44	54	66	75	90	100
Sellick maneuver												
Sedative												
Hypotension												
Etomidate (0.3 mg/kg):	1.5	2.4	3.0	4.5	6	7	9	11	13	15	17	20
Head trauma without hypotension												
Etomidate (see above) or												
Thiopental (3–5 mg/kg):	15–25	24–40	30–50	45–75	57–95	70–115	90–145	110–180	130–220	150–250	170–290	195–325
Status asthmaticus:												
Ketamine (1–2 mg/kg):	5–7	8–16	10–20	15–30	19–38	23–46	29–58	36–72	44–88	50–100	58–100	65–100
Paralyzing agent:												
Succinylcholine (1.0–1.5 mg/kg):	8	12	15	25	30	40	50	55	60	65	70	80
Rocuronium (0.6–1.0 mg/kg):	4	6	9	12	15	20	25	30	40	45	50	60
Intubate (tube size):	3.5	3.5	4.0	4.5	5.0	5.5	6.0	6.5	7.0	7.0 female, 8.0 male		
Tube depth at lip (cm):	11	12	13	14	15	16	18	19	20	22	22	22
Laryngoscope blade size:	1	1	1	2	2	2	2	2	3	3	3	3–4

With permission from Gausche-Hill M, Fuchs S, Yamamoto L, eds. *Instructor's Toolkit to Accompany APLS the Pediatric Emergency Medicine Resource.* 4th rev ed. Sudbury, MA: Jones and Bartlett Publishers; 2008.

Step 5. Selecting a paralyzing agent is controversial. The two common choices are succinylcholine and rocuronium. A detailed discussion of the differences between these two are beyond the scope of this chapter. The basic differences are that succinylcholine has a shorter duration, but a higher risk of adverse reactions that include malignant hyperthermia, and hyperkalemia, while rocuronium has a longer duration of paralysis but a lower risk of adverse reactions. The onset of paralysis by using agents such as vecuronium and pancuronium is slower than the onset of succinylcholine. The onset time of rocuronium is similar to the onset time of succinylcholine.

Further reading about RSI will reveal principles known as priming and defasciculation. Many experts recommend these; however, this practice prolongs the time to intubation. While these principles fit best with anesthesia practices for stable patients, the typical emergency department patient requires emergent intubation. "Priming" is the principle of giving a small dose of rocuronium 1 to 2 minutes prior to the full dose of rocuronium. Priming reduces the paralysis onset time of the full dose of rocuronium by a few seconds, but it prolongs the RSI procedure by 1 to 2 minutes. "Defasciculation" is the practice of administering a small dose of rocuronium 1 to 2 minutes prior to administering succinylcholine. Succinylcholine typically results in brief muscle contractions prior to the onset of paralysis known as fasciculations, which are sometimes associated with muscle pain (in muscular patients), movement, and hyperkalemia. Defasciculation prevents these fasciculations. Both priming and defasciculation have minimal benefit or no benefit, while delaying the intubation itself.

Step 6. Selection of a sedation agent is similarly controversial. A detailed discussion of this is beyond the scope of this chapter. Table 23–2 describes a basic method of selecting a sedation agent.[3] Selection criteria may be separated into patients with head trauma (or increased ICP), hypotension, and respiratory failure due to asthma. Considering these three factors permits the selection of a sedative. Thiopental has cerebroprotective properties, but it is a myocardial depressant and can lower blood pressure. Ketamine increases blood pressure and bronchodilation, but it also increases ICP. Etomidate is a more intermediate agent, and is purported to be a universal RSI sedative because of less adverse effects. Benzodiazepines are moderate sedatives, require titration (not feasible in RSI) and most often do not result in sedation deep enough for intubation. However, they have few adverse side effects and are used by some practitioners for RSI. Propofol has also been added to the list of possible sedatives with RSI; however, it does not have substantial advantages over the agents listed in Table 23–2. Another option is to use no sedative at all. This is a serious consideration in hypotensive patients or those at risk for septic shock. Any agent administered to patients under significant cardiovascular stress (including benzodiazepines, ketamine, and etomidate) could result in acute deterioration such as cardiac arrest, and thus the benefit of a sedative must be considered against this risk for severe patients.

Another issue of controversy is whether to give the sedative before the paralyzing agent or vice versa. Giving the paralyzing agent first reduces the time to intubation. Since the paralyzing agent takes 60 to 90 seconds to achieve sufficient paralysis, the sedation agent can be given during this waiting time. Giving the sedation agent first (as listed in Table 23–2) permits the patient to avoid the sensation of becoming paralyzed. These differences have different priorities in various clinical circumstances. Giving the paralyzing agent first makes more sense in severe patients in need of immediate intubation. Giving the sedation agent first makes more sense if the patient is conscious and the patient is less seriously in need of immediate intubation. Regardless of which is given first, the paralyzing agent and the sedation agent should be given in "rapid sequence."

Step 7. ETT size selection is critical in children. The common formula cited is 4 + (age ÷ 4). Thus a 6-year-old would need a 5.5 ETT. Newborns should be intubated with a 3.0 or

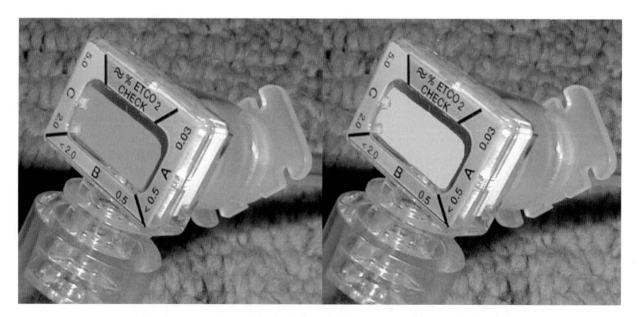

Figure 23–10. ETCO$_2$ colorimetric detector. This particular model is small, made for neonates. Color changes from purple to yellow if CO$_2$ is detected. (With permission from Gausche-Hill M, Fuchs S, Yamamoto L, eds. *Instructor's Toolkit to Accompany APLS the Pediatric Emergency Medicine Resource.* 4th rev ed. Sudbury, MA: Jones and Bartlett Publishers; 2008.)

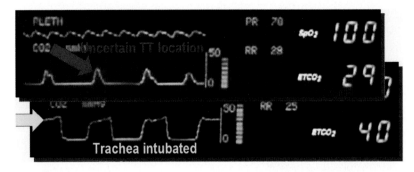

Figure 23–11. $ETCO_2$ monitor wave forms. This tracing shows a pulse oximeter waveform on the top. The upper pair of tracings shows an irregular peaked $ETCO_2$ waveform (red arrow), which does not confirm tracheal intubation. The lower tracing (yellow arrow) shows a regular square wave $ETCO_2$ waveform that confirms tracheal intubation. (With permission from Gausche-Hill M, Fuchs S, Yamamoto L, eds. *Instructor's Toolkit to Accompany APLS the Pediatric Emergency Medicine Resource.* 4th rev ed. Sudbury, MA: Jones and Bartlett Publishers; 2008.)

3.5 ETT (smaller for premature infants). However, memorizing a formula may risk error. Using a length-based resuscitation system or posting Table 23–2 in the resuscitation room would be more reliable. Posting Table 23–2 has the added advantage of including drug doses, drug selection criteria, and the depth of the ETT. Selection of a laryngoscope blade type is a matter of personal preference. The classic teaching is that straight blades are better for young children, and curved blades are better for older children; however, both blade types are available in all sizes and are really a matter of personal preference. Visualization of the larynx can be facilitated by adjusting the degree of cricoid pressure. Repeating the fact that the narrowest point of the airway is the cricoid (below the cords) is useful because advancing the ETT through the cords will sometimes stop at the cricoid. ETTs can be cuffed or uncuffed. A cuffed ETT provides better airway protection and a tighter seal, which is beneficial when higher ventilation pressure is required. However, with small ETTs, the deflated cuff significantly increases the size of the ETT making it more difficult to advance. A commonly cited cutoff in the past was age 9 (size 6 ETT), below which uncuffed ETTs were recommended. However, current recommendations permit the option of cuffed ETTs to all children except for neonates.[2] Cuff inflation pressures should be measured and kept below 20 cm H_2O.[2]

Step 8. Confirmation of tracheal intubation should be confirmed with more than one method and one of these methods should be a carbon dioxide detection device. Colorimetric $ETCO_2$ indicators that visibly change color during ventilation (Fig. 23–10) reliably confirm that the trachea is intubated in most instances. These colorimetric $ETCO_2$ indicators come in different sizes. Using an adult sized unit for a newborn will not work since the volume of CO_2 produced by the newborn will be insufficient to change its color. Additionally, many colorimetric $ETCO_2$ indicators will eventually become disabled due to water vapor saturation. An $ETCO_2$ monitor quantifies the $ETCO_2$ (which can be correlated to the patient's venous or arterial PCO_2), displays the actual waveform of $ETCO_2$ production, and it can be used continuously and indefinitely. A typical square waveform reliably confirms tracheal intubation, while a nonsquare waveform raises concerns that the trachea is not intubated (Fig. 23–11).

$ETCO_2$ is not produced in the absence of pulmonary perfusion. Inadequate CPR will result in no $ETCO_2$. CPR is a known false-negative (i.e., the trachea is intubated, but $ETCO_2$ is negative). The presence of an $ETCO_2$ square waveform

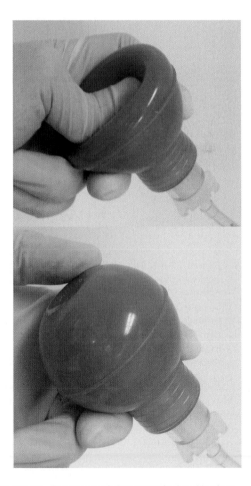

Figure 23–12. Esophageal detector device ("turkey baster"). This bulb attaches to the ETT. By squeezing the bulb, it should rapidly inflate if the trachea is intubated. Slow inflation indicates that the esophagus is intubated.

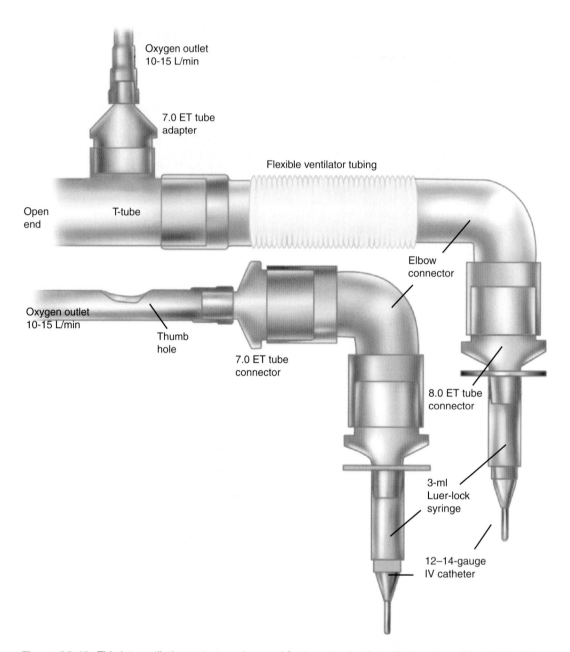

Figure 23–13. This jet ventilation setup can be used for transtracheal ventilation via an IV catheter. By occluding the open end or the thumbhole, high-pressure oxygen is forced through the transtracheal catheter. Releasing this results in passive exhalation. This diagram shows connection to the IV catheter using a 3 mL syringe and an 8.0 ETT connector. Instead, a 3.0 ETT connector can connect directly into the hub of the IV catheters. However, the connector has no Luer lock onto the catheter hub, and under high inflation pressures, this could pop off. (With permission from Yamamoto LG. Emergency airway management—rapid sequence intubation. In: Fleisher GR, Ludwig S, Henretig FM, eds. *Textbook of Pediatric Emergency Medicine*. 5th ed. Philadelphia, PA: Lippincott Williams & Wilkins; 2006:89.)

during CPR confirms tracheal intubation and pulmonary perfusion, confirming effective chest compressions.

Auscultation can confirm equal chest aeration, and the absence of gastric breath sounds. Visualization can confirm chest rise and fall with ventilation, and condensation visible in the ETT. Improvements in oxygenation and resuscitation parameters are consistent with tracheal intubation. None of these definitively confirm tracheal intubation; however collectively, the presence of all of these highly support successful tracheal intubation. The esophageal detector bulb (also known as the "turkey baster") method utilizes a rubber bulb attached to an ETT connector (Fig. 23–12). Squeeze the bulb, then apply it to the ETT. If the bulb inflates rapidly, this suggests that the tube is in the trachea or the pharynx. If the bulb inflates slowly or it does not inflate, this suggests that the tube is in a collapsible tube such as the esophagus.

If tracheal intubation is in doubt, direct visual confirmation with the laryngoscope should be attempted. Once tracheal confirmation is confirmed, the ETT depth needs to be optimized based on the clinician's visual intubation depth (during laryngoscopy) and the ETT depth guidelines in Table 23–2. The ETT should be secured. There are several ways to do this using tape, and there are commercial products designed for securing the ETT. A chest x-ray is useful to confirm the placement of the tip of the ETT, which should be within the trachea, above the tracheal bifurcation. The ETT position can be readjusted if needed, being careful not to extubate the patient.

CAN'T VENTILATE, CAN'T INTUBATE SCENARIO

Preparing for this difficult scenario requires preparation to initiate airway access through the anterior neck. Cricothyrotomy (also known as cricothyroidotomy and transtracheal ventilation) is one of these options. The cricothyroid membrane is punctured with a large IV catheter or an airway quick catheter. Most large bore IV catheters are placed by puncturing the cricothyroid membrane aiming in an inferior (caudal) direction. The catheter is advanced and the catheter hub is attached to a 3.0 ETT connector. Holding the catheter hub in place is critical since the catheter can be easily kinked, which would narrow it substantially. If a bag is used, substantial effort is required to squeeze the bag to deliver a sufficient tidal volume (a self-inflating bag accomplishes this better than a Rusch bag). A jet ventilation setup (Fig. 23–13) can deliver greater tidal volumes through an IV catheter.

Having a commercially configured quick airway kit in the resuscitation room is better since the airway diameter provided is larger. Many airway kits puncture the cricothyroid membrane and utilize a dilator and a wire similar to the Seldinger vascular access technique. The specifics of each kit should be reviewed prior to the presentation of an airway emergency in which it is needed. In smaller children, the cricothyroid membrane cannot be easily identified. Estimating its location is essential to these interventions.

An emergency surgical airway such as a tracheostomy or surgical cricothytomy is complication prone, but in the "can't intubate, can't ventilate" scenario, this might be the only option to oxygenate the patient.[3] The actual procedure is beyond the scope of this chapter. If this is to be attempted, a surgical airway kit should be available at all times and the procedure should be reviewed ahead of time.

A complication to avoid is explosive combustion. The patient is likely being ventilated with high-flow oxygen during this procedure. The use of electrocautery or heat cautery must be avoided since this can trigger explosive combustion.

REFERENCES

1. Stenklyft PH, Cataletto ME, Lee BS. The pediatric airway in health and disease. In: Gausche-Hill M, Fuchs S, Yamamoto L, eds. *APLS The Pediatric Emergency Medicine Resource.* 4th rev ed. Sudbury, MA: Jones and Bartlett Publishers; 2006, :52–106.
2. 2005 American Hear Association Guidelines for Cardiopulmonary Resuscitation and Emergency Cardiovascular Care. Part 12: Pediatric Advanced Life Support. *Circulation.* 2005;112(24, suppl):IV-167–187.
3. King BR, King C, Coates WC. Critical procedures. In: Gausche-Hill M, Fuchs S, Yamamoto L, eds. *APLS The Pediatric Emergency Medicine Resource.* 4th rev ed. Sudbury, MA: Jones and Bartlett Publishers; 2006:674–767.

CHAPTER 24

Respiratory Failure

Lynette L. Young

► HIGH-YIELD FACTS

- Tachypnea is a universal finding in infants with respiratory distress; the increased muscle exertion can result in fatigue and respiratory failure.
- Children have twice the oxygen consumption rate compared to adults and smaller functional residual capacity. During intubation they may desaturate rapidly.
- A well-positioned and proper-sized endotracheal tube will have an air leak when ventilation is applied at 15 to 20 cm water level.
- For older infants and children requiring ventilator assistance, a volume-controlled ventilator is usually preferred with a tidal volume of 8 to 10 mL/kg.
- Use of modest positive end-expiratory pressure (PEEP) (3–5 cm H_2O) will help maintain lung volume and reduce the risk of barotrauma associated with high tidal volumes.
- When managing ventilator care, pH and Pco_2 can be adjusted by manipulating minute ventilation; Po_2 can be adjusted by manipulating Fio_2 and PEEP.
- Noninvasive mechanical ventilation techniques such as continuous positive airway pressure (CPAP), bimodal positive airway pressure (BiPAP), and Vapotherm are finding their way into the emergency department (ED) as alternatives to avoid intubation.

Respiratory failure is the most common cause of cardiac arrest in pediatric patients. It is important to recognize respiratory distress early so that actions can be taken to avoid respiratory failure whenever possible. If respiratory failure does occur, prompt intervention will give the patient the best chance for survival with the least neurologic sequelae. Young children have less physiologic reserve and can deteriorate very rapidly. In a critical situation, the emergency physician has the task of not only making quick resuscitation management decisions but must also consider age-related anatomic differences, appropriate equipment (Table 24–1), and drug-dosage differences when caring for infants and children.

► ANATOMY AND PHYSIOLOGY

Children have anatomic and physiologic differences that should be considered when evaluating a pediatric patient presenting in respiratory distress. Young infants may be obligate nose breathers, and any degree of obstruction of the nasal passages can produce respiratory difficulty.

The chest wall of children is more flexible and the muscles are less developed compared to adults. The diaphragm is more prone to fatigue. The limitation of diaphragmatic movement by gastric distention, increased residual capacity from air trapping from asthma, bronchiolitis, or foreign body obstruction can result in reduction of tidal volume, which may produce respiratory failure. The relatively smaller lower airways are especially vulnerable to mucus plugging and ventilation–perfusion mismatch associated with common diseases of the lower airways, such as asthma and bronchiolitis.

The actual area available for gas exchange in infants and young children is relatively limited. Alveolar space doubles by 18 months of age and triples by 3 years of age. The limited ability to recruit additional alveoli makes the infant dependent on increasing the respiratory rate to augment minute ventilation and eliminate carbon dioxide. Tachypnea, therefore, is a universal finding in infants and young children in respiratory distress. The combination of increased muscle exertion and the need to sustain a rapid respiratory rate can result in progressive muscle fatigue and respiratory failure. This is especially true in young infants, who have a limited metabolic reserve. Children have about twice the oxygen consumption rate compared to adults, and they have proportionally smaller functional residual capacity. With intubation of an infant or child, it is important to remember that they have the potential to desaturate more quickly than adults (see Chapter 23 for airway differences between infants and children).

► PERTINENT HISTORY

Most commonly, a patient in respiratory distress will present to the ED with a history of difficulty breathing. Parents may note coughing, rapid noisy breathing, or a change in behavior. Feeding problems are often a sign of respiratory compromise in infants. In older children, wheezing or decreased physical activity may be presenting complaints.

The past medical history is essential in determining the etiology of the acute problem. Infants with a history of significant prematurity may have bronchopulmonary dysplasia, a syndrome characterized by varying degrees of hypoxia, hypercarbia, reactive airway disease, and a heightened susceptibility to respiratory infections. Infants with a history of sweating during bottle-feedings may have undiagnosed congestive heart failure. For patients with a history of asthma, information regarding the frequency and severity of past exacerbations is important in determining both the acute treatment and disposition. A patient with a history of a chronic cough or recurrent pneumonia may have an underlying disorder, such as reactive

▶ **TABLE 24–1. ENDOTRACHEAL TUBE SIZE AND LENGTH AND SIZE OF LARYNGOSCOPE BLADES BY AGE*,†**

Age	Size (mm)	Type
Endotracheal Tubes		
Newborn	3.0	Uncuffed
Newborn–6 mo	3.5	Uncuffed or cuffed (not in newborn)
6–18 mo	3.5–4.0	Uncuffed or cuffed
18 mo–3 y	4.0–4.5	Uncuffed or cuffed
3–5 y	4.5	Uncuffed or cuffed
5–6 y	5.0	Uncuffed or cuffed
6–8 y	5.5–6.0	Uncuffed or cuffed
8–10 y	6.0	Cuffed
10–12 y	6.0–6.5	Cuffed
12–14 y	6.5–7.0	Cuffed
Laryngoscope Blades		
<2.5 kg	0	Straight
0–3 mo	1.0	Straight
3 mo–3 y	1.5	Straight
3 yr–12 y	2.0	Straight or curved
Adolescent	3.0	Straight or curved

*Uncuffed tracheal tube size (mm) = (age in years/4) + 4 = internal diameter of endotracheal tube or patient's fifth digit.
†Cuffed tube size (mm) = (age in years)/4 + 3 = internal diameter of cuffed endotracheal tube. Depth can be calculated by taking the internal diameter and multiplying by 3.

airway disease, cystic fibrosis, or a retained foreign body. Respiratory symptoms can also be caused by systemic disorders. Effortless tachypnea and hyperpnea accompany disorders such as diabetic ketoacidosis and sepsis, as an attempt to compensate for metabolic acidosis.

▶ PHYSICAL EXAMINATION

Simply observing the patient yields a wealth of information regarding the degree of respiratory distress. Mental status is the first and foremost factor to evaluate. Infants and young children with mild respiratory difficulty will have normal mental status. Patients with more severe disease become irritable or anxious and can appear restless and unable to assume a comfortable position. Older patients in extreme distress are usually unable to lie supine and may exhibit head-bobbing. Young infants in severe distress will appear anxious, will often not make eye contact, and usually will not smile. If feeding is attempted, they will refuse the bottle, since the work of breathing precludes the exertion of sucking. Incipient respiratory failure is heralded by extreme agitation, and finally by lethargy or somnolence. Cyanosis is an ominous finding.

Observing the patient's chest will add to the assessment of the degree of respiratory distress. Patients with significant respiratory distress will virtually always be tachypneic. However, because respiratory rate is age dependent and can be influenced by underlying medical conditions, it must be viewed in the context of the overall clinical picture. Visual inspection of the chest wall may reveal retractions, which signify the use

of accessory muscles of respiration. Retractions are seen in the supraclavicular and subcostal areas. In more severe cases, nasal flaring is seen. Retractions imply a significant degree of respiratory distress and must never be overlooked.

Listening to grossly audible breath sounds will help to localize the pathology. Stridor is generally heard on inspiration, but with severe obstruction, it can be present on both inspiration and expiration. Stridor suggests upper airway pathology, such as croup, epiglottitis, or foreign body obstruction. Grossly audible wheezing usually indicates obstruction of the lower airways. Lower airway disease resulting in alveolar collapse can also be associated with grunting, which is caused by premature closure of the glottis during expiration. Grunting increases airway pressure and can help prevent further alveolar collapse and thus preserve functional residual capacity. Grunting is most often seen in infants and always indicated severe respiratory distress, whether from primary lung disease or a systemic illness, such as sepsis.

Auscultation of the chest supplements the information gained from observation of the patient. The first factor to assess is air exchange. Upper airway obstruction predominantly affects the inhalation of air, whereas lower airway obstruction predominantly affects exhalation. Patients who appear to be struggling to breathe and have limited air exchange appreciated on auscultation are in imminent danger of respiratory failure.

▶ LABORATORY STUDIES

Laboratory studies are useful in assessing the degree of respiratory compromise. The advent of a reliable measurement of oxygen saturation via percutaneous pulse oximetry has made it possible to evaluate a patient's blood oxygen-carrying status quickly and painlessly. Pulse oximetry is especially useful in infants, in whom the physical findings may be difficult to assess and an arterial blood gas difficult to obtain. However, pulse oximetry provides only limited information regarding overall pulmonary physiology. The slope of the oxygen–hemoglobin dissociation curve is such that patients with marginal oxygen saturations may have significant hypoxemia. The pulse oximeter does not measure the arterial carbon dioxide tension ($Paco_2$) or acid–base status, and therefore careful clinical correlation is necessary in many situations, such as asthma and bronchiolitis, in which CO_2 retention and respiratory acidosis are possible. Pulse oximetry is also unreliable for patients with low-perfusion states, carbon monoxide toxicity, and methemoglobinemia.

For patients with moderate to severe respiratory distress, pulse oximetry cannot replace the information obtained by an arterial blood gas. Respiratory failure is often defined as arterial oxygen tension (Pao_2) <60 mm Hg despite supplemental inhaled oxygen of 60% or arterial carbon dioxide tension ($Paco_2$) >60 mm Hg. However, absolute values of arterial oxygen and carbon dioxide tension must be viewed in the context of the clinical situation, as well as the patient's baseline pulmonary status. A patient may not meet strict criteria for respiratory failure but may develop muscle fatigue such that the work of breathing cannot be sustained despite blood gas values that appear adequate. Conversely, a patient with severe underlying lung disease, such as bronchopulmonary dysplasia or cystic fibrosis, may be well adjusted to chronic hypercarbia; in this case the clinical assessment of the work of breathing supplants the laboratory data. In most children with severe lung disease, parents are aware of baseline information that can aid the physician in interpreting percutaneous oxygen saturation and the arterial blood gas values.

▶ INDICATIONS FOR ASSISTED VENTILATION

In the event that respiratory failure occurs, assisted ventilation is indicated. The most common indication for assisted ventilation in a pediatric patient in respiratory distress is progressive muscle fatigue. In this situation, laboratory parameters will often reveal hypoxemia refractory to supplemental oxygen and a rising $Paco_2$. Other indications for assisted ventilation are apnea, inadequate respiratory effort, and conditions in which it is desirable to reduce the work of breathing, such as refractory shock or increased intracranial pressure that requires controlled ventilation.[1] For patients with altered mental status, when the ability to maintain an adequate airway is in question, assisted ventilation is also indicated, although pulmonary function may be normal.

The initial treatment of hypoxemia is administration of oxygen. Supplemental oxygen can be delivered by nasal cannula, simple mask, non-rebreather mask, and bag-mask. Ventilatory assistance begins with establishing a patent airway (see Chapter 23 for airway management).

VENTILATION

Effective bag-valve-mask (BVM) ventilation of infants and children is a vital skill (Fig. 24–1). In the out-of-hospital setting, it has been shown that endotracheal intubation by paramedics compared to BVM ventilation did not improve survival or neurologic outcome in the pediatric patient.[2] The 2005 American Heart Association (AHA) guidelines recommends BVM ventilation for infants and children in the prehospital setting especially if there is a short transport time.[3] A transparent mask should

fit snugly from the bridge of the nose to the prominence of the symphysis of the mandible. Circular masks with seals are more effective in infants and in small children than triangular masks that attempt to duplicate the shape of the face (see Chapter 23 for a detailed description of equipment and technique for BVM ventilation of infants and children).

▶ ADVANCED AIRWAY MANAGEMENT

In most situations that require BVM ventilation, insertion of an endotracheal tube is necessary to establish an adequate airway and allow optimal management. Successful intubation of the trachea depends on adequate preparation of personnel, medications, and equipment.

Preoxygenation displaces nitrogen from the lungs and provides a physiologic reservoir of oxygen that protects the patient from anoxic injury during the process of intubation. In spontaneously breathing patients, 3 to 5 minutes of 100% O_2 delivered by a non-rebreather mask provides the patient with 3 to 4 minutes of adequate oxygenation even in the face of apnea. For patients receiving assisted ventilation, minimizing the time of bagging is important in reducing the possibility of gastric distention and aspiration during intubation. In this situation, several breaths with 100% O_2 provides an adequate reservoir of oxygen. The Sellick maneuver may be used to reduce gastric distention and emesis (Fig. 24–2). The technique for tracheal intubation can be reviewed in Chapter 23.

The correct endotracheal tube size can be determined by using a length-based system or formula based on age (Table 24–1). With a well-positioned endotracheal tube of the proper size, an audible air leak is heard when ventilation is applied at a pressure of 15 to 20 cm H_2O. If no air leak is audible, the tube is too tight. Conversely, if the air leak is too large, it will impair

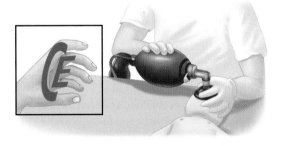

Figure 24–1. In the proper placement of the bag-mask ventilator, the thumb and forefinger form a "C" shape to tightly seal the mask onto the face while the remaining fingers of the same hand form an "E" shape to lift the jaw, pulling the face toward the mask. (With permission from Goodman et al. *Current Procedures Pediatrics.* New York: McGraw-Hill; 2007.)

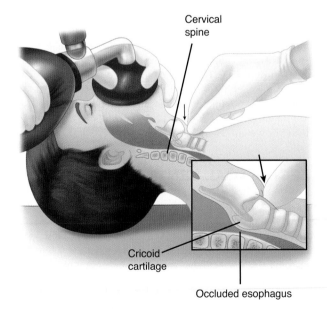

Figure 24–2. Sellick maneuver. (With permission from Goodman et al. *Current Procedures Pediatrics.* New York: McGraw-Hill; 2007.)

ventilation since insufficient tidal volume is generated. Cuffed endotracheal tubes have been shown to be safely used in the operating room and intensive care unit in children. With the 2005 AHA updates cuffed endotracheal tube are noted to be as safe as uncuffed tubes and may be used in the hospital for infants past the newborn period and children.[3] Using a cuffed endotracheal tube might be beneficial in certain situations such as poor lung compliance, high airway resistance, and large glottic air leak.

Correct endotracheal tube placement is confirmed clinically by observing adequate chest wall expansion and auscultating bilateral breath sounds. Asymmetric breath sounds imply that the tube is too far down the trachea and has lodged in either the right or left mainstem bronchus. The anatomic vectors are such that the right mainstem bronchus is more likely to be intubated, and breath sounds are heard louder on the right side. In young infants, however, the airway vectors are such that intubation of the left mainstem bronchus may occur. This situation is corrected by slowly withdrawing the tube until equal breath sounds are heard. If unilateral breath sounds persist despite withdrawal of the tube, a pneumothorax is possible. The laryngeal mask airway (LMA) is a tube with a deflatable masklike projection at the distal end. The LMA is an alternative to the endotracheal tube for a patient with a difficult airway.[4] The LMA is passed through the pharynx and advanced until resistance is felt when the mask is over the epiglottis/tracheal opening. The inflation of the cuff occludes the hypopharynx but leaves the distal end open over the glottic opening, providing a clear secure airway. The LMA has been demonstrated in numerous studies as a successful airway management tool in the hospital and in out-of-hospital settings. Numerous studies have shown that the LMA is effective in pediatrics, but proper training and supervision is required to master correct LMA placement. LMA is contraindicated in the infant or child with a gag response or with the potential for excessive patient movement. There is a risk of aspiration that must be considered when using LMA. LMA may be an alternative if endotracheal intubation is not possible in pediatric cardiac arrest, although there is no data about its routine use in this scenario. The Combitube and the laryngeal tube airway (King LT Airway) are two other airway devices. The Combitube comes in two sizes. The smaller size tube is for patients over 4 ft and thus cannot be used in many pediatric patients. The King LT-D (disposable) is now available in pediatric sizes (size 2 for height 35–45″ or weight 12–25 kg and size 2.5 for height 41–51″ or weight 25–35 kg).

MECHANICAL VENTILATION

It is occasionally necessary to provide mechanical ventilation for intubated patients in the ED while awaiting transport or intensive care unit admission. Although a thorough discussion of ventilators is beyond the scope of this chapter, a few facts regarding the use of these machines are important. The two major types of mechanical ventilators are pressure and volume ventilators. Both assist the patient by delivering compressed gases with positive pressure; however, they differ in the method that terminates the inspiratory phase of the breathing cycle.

A volume ventilator delivers a preset volume of gas during each mechanical inspiration. This type of ventilator compen-

sates for all changes in resistance and is therefore useful for patients with decreased lung compliance. The danger of volume ventilators is that they generate high airway pressures that can result in barotrauma. Currently they are used for children and older infants. The usual tidal volume in an infant or child is 8 to 10 mL/kg. Previously higher volumes were used, but using PEEP to maintain lung volume will reduce the risk of barotrauma associated with higher volumes. The rate depends on the patient's age and the clinical condition.

Pressure ventilators terminate inspiration when a preset pressure is reached and therefore avoid excessive inflating pressures. With pressure ventilators, it is possible to control the inspiratory time, and exhalation is allowed when the preset pressure is reached. They do not compensate for changes in lung compliance, and they deliver a variable amount of gas with each breath. Currently pressure ventilators are used mainly in neonates and young infants. The inspiratory pressure used is the lowest pressure that attains adequate chest expansion and ventilation. This is best determined by observing a manometer while the patient is being bagged.

Both volume and pressure ventilators have the ability to provide PEEP, which is added to prevent alveolar collapse during exhalation and to preserve functional residual capacity. This can alleviate ventilation–perfusion mismatch and consequent hypoxemia and is especially important in situations in which there is decreased lung compliance. The major side effect of excessive PEEP is decreased venous return to the right side of the heart and decreased cardiac output. In the ED setting, PEEP is usually set at 3 to 5 cm H_2O.

Despite the widespread availability of pulse oximetry and end-tidal CO_2 monitoring, most patients on ventilators will require serial arterial blood gases until the optimal parameters for ventilating the patient are determined. Adjusting pH and P_{CO_2} can be done by manipulating minute ventilation, adjusting respiratory rate, and tidal volume. Controlling P_{O_2} is done by adjusting F_{IO_2} and PEEP.

NONINVASIVE MECHANICAL VENTILATION

Noninvasive mechanical ventilation has been used to provide respiratory support without the risks associated with tracheal intubation.[5–7] The benefits may include improved oxygenation and ventilation with decreased muscle fatigue. The modalities of aiding the patient's own spontaneous respiratory efforts includes CPAP, BiPAP, and high-flow nasal cannula.

With CPAP, there is continuous pressure delivered through the entire respiratory cycle. Generally, positive airway pressures are delivered at 4 to 10 cm water level. CPAP can be delivered by face mask in children, and with the use of binasal prongs for small infants where it is difficult to fit a mask. Nasal CPAP has been successfully studied in prematures, neonates, and infants with improvement of oxygenation and reduction of respiratory distress.[8–10] The infant with bronchiolitis may benefit from this mode of respiratory support.

BiPAP cycles between a higher inspiratory positive airway pressure (IPAP) and the lower expiratory positive airway pressure (EPAP). When initiating BiPAP, start with small initial pressure settings and increase gradually over time. IPAP is usually set at 8 to 10 cm H_2O and increased to 16 cm or more to achieve a decrease in the work of breathing, decrease in respiratory rate, and improved oxygenation. The EPAP is used to improve functional residual capacity and is usually started at 4 to 10 cm H_2O. Successful use of BiPAP requires a cooperative patient and a good-fitting mask.[11] A retrospective study reviewed the use of BiPAP to treat status asthmaticus in a pediatric ED in 83 patients who were refractory to conventional medical therapy.[12] It was tolerated by 88% of patients and with an age range of 2 to 17 years. All of these patients had been planned PICU admissions. Sixteen patients (22%) had improved in the ED and were weaned off BiPAP. They were subsequently admitted to the wards.

Humidified high-flow nasal cannulae have been used to provide CPAP mainly in newborns. Vapotherm is an example of this where warm and humidified gases are delivered by nasal canula at up to 8 L/min and well tolerated.[13,14]

Most of the experience using noninvasive positive pressure ventilation (NIPPV) in pediatric patients comes from the pediatric intensive care unit.[15] These modalities have also been used in the home for children with obstructive sleep apnea and neuromuscular diseases. With newer technology and more experience being obtained, NIPPV may be considered for use in the ED also.[16] NIPPV could be beneficial in the acute management of children with asthma, cystic fibrosis, and neuromuscular disease presenting in respiratory distress. NIPPV should not be used in patients who are obtunded, vomiting, hypotensive, or have cardiac dysrhythmias. Clinical improvement is usually seen in several hours. Any patient who is receiving NIPPV acutely in the ED is critically ill and must therefore be watched very closely for deterioration. The emergency physicians must be prepared for tracheal intubation of the child if necessary.

▶ ACKNOWLEDGMENT

Thomas J. Abramo and Michael Cowan who authored the 1st and 2nd edition of this chapter.

REFERENCES

1. Cheifetz IM. Invasive and noninvasive pediatric mechanical ventilation. *Respi Care.* 2003;48(4):442–458.

2. Gausche M, Lewis RJ, Stratton SJ, et al. A prospective randomized study of the effect of out of hospital pediatric endotracheal intubation on survival and neurological outcome. *JAMA.* 2000;283:783–790.

3. ECC Committee, Subcommittees and Task Forces of the American Heart Association. American Heart Association guidelines for cardiopulmonary resuscitation and emergency cardiovascular care. Pediatric advanced life support (Part 12). *Circulation.* 2005;112(24):IV-167–IV-187.

4. Berry AM, Brimacombe JR, Verghese C. The laryngeal mask airway in emergency medicine, neonatal resuscitation and intensive care medicine. *Int Anesthesiol Clin.* 1998;36:91–109.

5. Ganesan R, Watts KD, Lestrud S. Noninvasive mechanical ventilation. *Clin Pediatr Emerg Med.* 2007;8:139–144.

6. Essouri S, Chevret L, Durand P, et al. Noninvasive positive pressure ventilation: five years of experience in a pediatric intensive care unit. *Pediatr Crit Care Med.* 2006;7:329–334.

7. Courtney SE, Barrington KJ. Continuous positive airway pressure and noninvasive ventilation. *Clin Perinatol.* 2007;34:73–92.

8. Krouskop RW, Brown EG, Sweet AY. The early use of continuous positive airway pressure in the treatment of idiopathic respiratory distress syndrome. *J Pediatr.* 1975;87:263–267.

9. Miller MJ, DiFiore JM. Effects of nasal CPAP on supraglottic and total pulmonary resistance in preterm infants. *J Appl Physiol.* 1990;68:141–146.

10. Gaon P, Lee S, Hannan S, et al. Assessment of effect of nasal continuous positive airway pressure on laryngeal opening using fibre optic laryngoscopy. *Arch Dis Child.* 1999;80:230–232.

11. Akingbola OA, Hopkins RL. Pediatric noninvasive positive pressure ventilation. *Pediatr Crit Care Med.* 2001;2:164–169.

12. Beers SL, Abramo TJ, Bracken A, et al. Bilevel positive airway pressure in the treatment of status asthmaticus in pediatrics. *Am J Emerg Med.* 2007;25:6–9.

13. Saslow JG, Aghai ZH, Nakhla TA, et al. Work of breathing using high-flow nasal canula in preterm infants. *J Perinatol.* 2006;26(8):476–480.

14. Spence KL, Murphy D, Kilian C, et al. High-flow nasal canula as a device to provide continuous positive airway pressure in infants. *J Perinatol.* 2007;27(12):772–775.

15. Lemyre B, Davis PG, De Paoli AG. Nasal intermittent positive pressure ventilation (NIPPV) verses nasal continuous positive airway pressure (NCPAP) for apnea of prematurity (Cochrane Review). In: *The Cochrane Library.* Issue 4. Chichester, UK: John Wiley & Sons; 2003.

16. Deis JN, Abramo TJ, Crawley L. Noninvasive respiratory support. *Pediatr Emerg Care.* 2008;24(5):331–338.

CHAPTER 25

Shock

Jonathan K. Marr

▶ HIGH-YIELD FACTS

- Tachycardia and pallor must be considered "shock" until proven otherwise.
- Decompensated shock with hypotension can be clinically recognized by altered mental status. Hypotension is an ominous sign and heralds cardiac arrest.
- Hypovolemia is the most common cause of shock worldwide.
- Although septic shock is categorized as "distributive," it also has a component of cardiac dysfunction and hypovolemia.
- Congenital cardiac lesions that are dependent on a patent ductus arteriosus for survival include those with left ventricular outflow obstruction such as coarctation of the aorta, critical aortic stenosis, and hypoplastic left heart.
- Effortless tachypnea may be an attempt to correct for the metabolic acidosis caused by anaerobic metabolism from shock.
- Tissue perfusion (capillary refill) can be used as a surrogate marker for cardiac output.
- Early, aggressive therapy for shock is necessary to restore tissue perfusion and oxygenation.
- If a patient in shock has no hepatomegaly, no rales on auscultation of the lungs, and clear and distinct heart sounds, early and aggressive isotonic fluid delivery with 20 mL/kg boluses to 60 mL/kg or more is the first line of therapy.

Shock is a reflection of acute depletion of energy (ATP) secondary to inadequate oxygen and substrate delivery to cells relative to metabolic demand. Oxygen delivery depends on multiple variables and includes heart rate, preload, contractility, afterload, hemoglobin content, oxygen saturation, and dissolved oxygen in blood (Fig. 25–1). Disease processes creates alterations in the above variables and the body has developed compensatory mechanisms to adjust. When the ability to adjust is exceeded, there is progression to impairment of organ function, irreversible organ failure, and death.

Children differ from adults with respect to anatomy and physiology. In infants, cardiac output is dependent on heart rate since stroke volume is relatively fixed. In children, low cardiac output is often due to low stroke volume. In order to maintain oxygen delivery to tissues, compensatory mechanisms are activated. The first line of defense in maintaining cardiac output is tachycardia and this is the first subtle sign of shock.[1] Other common reasons for tachycardia in the emergency department other than shock include fever, pain, anxiety, hypoxia, and medications (i.e., albuterol).

The next compensatory mechanism is the redirection of blood from nonvital to vital organs through increasing systemic vascular resistance. Blood is shunted away from the skin, gut, kidneys, and muscle and this is clinically reflected by cool extremities, delayed capillary refill, and decreased urine output. Other mechanisms such as increase in contractility and increasing smooth muscle tone to move blood from the venous system to the heart are other ways to augment increases in cardiac output.

The physiologic "fight or flight" response to stress involves central and sympathetic nervous system activation. Adrenocorticotropic hormone is released from the central nervous system to produce cortisol while the sympathetic nervous system releases epinephrine and norepinephrine from the adrenal gland. These catecholamines increase cardiac output by increasing heart rate and stroke volume and the result is an increase in blood pressure. Glucagon is also released to provide glucose via glycogenolysis and gluconeogenesis. Glucose is used as substrate and flows through the Krebs cycle to produce ATP.

The shock response results from decreased oxygen delivery and low ATP rather than stress. The levels of cortisol and catecholamines are more than 5 to 10 times higher in the shock state compared to the stress response.[2] Intravascular volume is preserved with activation of the angiotensin/aldosterone-antidiuretic hormone/vasopressin system and oliguria results. Finally, superphysiologic levels of cortisol and catecholamines with glucagon cause hyperglycemia; this is due to a combination of increased glucose production and insulin-resistance. Ironically, hyperglycemia in sepsis is considered potentially harmful since research suggests that it impairs neutrophil function, acts as a procoagulant, induces cellular apoptosis, increases risk of infection, and impairs wound healing.[3, 4]

Shock can be subcategorized into compensated and hypotensive shock. Presence of inadequate perfusion with normal systolic blood pressure maintained by compensatory mechanisms delineates compensated shock. Signs of inadequate perfusion include tachycardia, delayed capillary refill, cool pale skin, and weak pulses. Once the body is unable to physiologically maintain normal systolic blood pressure, hypotension results and heralds impending cardiac arrest. The transition from compensated to hypotensive shock progresses along a physiologic continuum. Deterioration in mental status is a clinical observation that is indicative of compromised perfusion to the brain.

Shock can be subdivided into four general categories: hypovolemic, distributive, cardiogenic, and obstructive (Table 25–1). These subcategories of shock have pathophysiologic etiologies related to components of stroke volume—preload, contractility, and afterload. Preload is the volume of blood

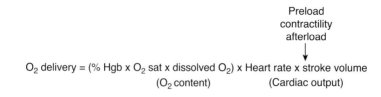

Figure 25–1. Factors influencing oxygen delivery.

present in the ventricle before contraction and is estimated by the central venous pressure (CVP). CVP is not equivalent to total blood volume. Total blood volume in a newborn is estimated at 85 mL/kg while in infants it is estimated to be 65 mL/kg. Distribution of blood in the arteries, veins, and capillaries is estimated to be 8%, 70%, and 12%, respectively.[2] Contractility is defined as the strength of cardiac contraction. Finally, afterload is the resistance against which the ventricle is contracting. Together, these components affect the volume of blood distributed by the heart with each beat.

► HYPOVOLEMIC SHOCK

Hypovolemia is the most common cause of shock in children worldwide.[1] Fluid losses due to diarrhea and electrolyte abnormalities are a major cause of infant mortality in Third World countries. Other causes of hypovolemic shock include acute hemorrhage following trauma, burns, and osmotic diuresis from diabetic ketoacidosis.

Volume depletion results in reduced preload and stroke volume with compensatory tachycardia. In acute hemorrhage

from trauma, the reduction in blood volume is further complicated by a concomitant reduction in hemoglobin. Decreased cardiac output and oxygen content decreases oxygen delivery. Compensatory mechanisms such as the release of catecholamines increase heart rate, contractility, and systemic vascular resistance, while the neuroendocrine system facilitates retention of sodium and water. Failure to correct volume depletion and oxygen-carrying capacity will progress into organ dysfunction, circulatory failure, and death.

► DISTRIBUTIVE SHOCK

Distributive shock is characterized by inappropriate distribution of blood volume causing inadequate organ and tissue perfusion. The three types of distributive shock include septic shock, anaphylactic shock, and neurogenic shock. All three have common features that include dysfunction of vascular tone and integrity. Distributive shock is further unique since the high cardiac output and low systemic vascular resistance is in contrast to the low cardiac output and high systemic vascular resistance found in hypovolemic, cardiogenic, and obstructive shock.[1]

An international consensus definition of sepsis is infection plus systemic manifestations of infection (i.e., fever, tachycardia, tachypnea, or leukocytosis). Severe sepsis is sepsis with sepsis-induced organ dysfunction or tissue hypoperfusion (i.e., hypotension, hypoxemia, oliguria, metabolic acidosis, thrombocytopenia, or obtundation). Finally, septic shock is defined as sepsis-induced hypotension despite adequate fluid resuscitation.[3,5]

Sepsis is the culmination of complex interactions between infecting organisms and host immune, inflammatory, and coagulation responses. The theory that sepsis was due to an uncontrolled inflammatory state has been recently challenged after multiple studies looking at blocking inflammation were not successful in reducing mortality. Existing research suggests that although early sepsis may be characterized by increases in proinflammatory mediators, as sepsis persists, there is a shift toward an anti-inflammatory *immunosuppressive* state.[3,4] Furthermore, research suggests that specific cell types (B cells, CD4 T cells, and follicular dendritic cells) are dying by apoptosis rather than necrosis; apoptotic cells induce anergy or anti-inflammatory cytokines that impair the response to pathogens. Finally, the profound, progressive, apoptosis-induced loss of B cells, CD4 T cells, and follicular dendritic cells are all part of the adaptive immune system, which constrains antibody production, macrophage activation, and antigen presentation. Although septic shock is usually categorized as a form of *distributive shock*, it usually has components of cardiac dysfunction, and hypovolemia as well.

► TABLE 25–1. **CAUSES OF SHOCK**

Components of Stroke Volume	Type of Shock	Examples
Preload	Hypovolemic	Gastroenteritis Dehydration Trauma/blood loss
	Distributive	Septic Anaphylactic Neurogenic
Contractility	Cardiogenic	Myocarditis Congestive heart failure Cardiomyopathy Toxicologic ingestion Blunt trauma
Afterload	Obstructive	Cardiac tamponade Pneumothorax Pulmonary embolism Coarctation of aorta Interrupted aortic arch Hypoplastic Left Heart Syndrome

Anaphylaxis is a type I immunoglobulin E (IgE-) mediated immediate hypersensitivity reaction resulting in the release of chemical mediators from mast cells and basophils, including histamine, prostaglandin D2, leukotrienes, platelet-activating factor, and tryptase.[6] These mediators cause increased vascular permeability, bronchospasm, vasodilation, and an alteration in smooth muscle tone. This acute multisystem allergic response is characterized by venodilation, systemic vasodilation, increased capillary permeability, and pulmonary vasoconstriction.[1] The most common causes of anaphylaxis in children are from foods, medications, Hymenoptera (wasps, bees, and ants) envenomations, blood products, latex, vaccines, and radiographic contrast media.[6]

Neurogenic shock is often due to acute spinal cord injury with resultant disruption of sympathetic control of blood vessels and the heart. Commonly caused by cervical trauma, injuries to the thoracic spine above T6 can result in failure of sympathetic tone and subsequent neurogenic shock. The balance between vasodilator and vasoconstrictor influences on arterioles and venules are disrupted leading to decreased peripheral resistance, hypotension, bradycardia, and decreased cardiac output.[7]

▶ CARDIOGENIC SHOCK

Cardiogenic shock is defined as persistent hypotension and tissue hypoperfusion due to cardiac dysfunction in the presence of adequate intravascular volume and left ventricular filling pressure.[8] Cardiac dysfunction can be associated with poor contractility (myocarditis, cardiomyopathy, sepsis, infarction, trauma, poisoning, or toxicity), structural abnormalities (congenital heart disease), and rhythm disturbances (arrhythmia). The hallmark of cardiogenic shock is low cardiac output and high systemic vascular resistance.[1]

Cardiac muscle fibers have the ability to increase contractility when stretched as long as the fibers are not overstretched; this was illustrated by pioneering research by Otto Frank and Ernest Starling. Increased venous return and preload cause a greater force of ventricular contraction resulting in increased stroke volume and cardiac output. When the fibers are overstretched, however, contractility decreases and heart failure occurs. Dysfunctional cardiac contractility results in poor cardiac output and blood pressure. The compensatory neurohormonal response activates catecholamines and the renin-angiotensin systems leading to tachycardia, systemic vasoconstriction, and fluid retention. This response is harmful in cardiogenic shock since tachycardia increases myocardial oxygen demand shifting aerobic to anaerobic metabolism with resultant lactic acid production. Additionally, increased vasoconstriction increases afterload and leads to decreased stroke volume and compromises cardiac output further.

▶ OBSTRUCTIVE SHOCK

Obstructive shock occurs when cardiac output is compromised by physical obstruction of blood flow. Types of obstructive shock include cardiac tamponade, tension pneumothorax, ductal-dependent congenital heart lesions, and massive pulmonary embolism.[1] Obstruction leads to diminished cardiac output and compensatory mechanisms, which cause tachycardia and increased systemic vascular resistance.

Cardiac tamponade occurs when fluid or air accumulates within the pericardial space. Increased intrapericardial pressure and compression of the heart prevents venous and pulmonary venous return, reduces ventricular filling, and creates a fall in cardiac output.[1] Risk factors include trauma, cardiac surgery, infection, and other inflammatory disorders.

Tension pneumothorax occurs when air progressively accumulates in the pleural space to create positive intrathoracic pressure. The result is compression of lung tissue and mediastinal structures to the contralateral side that leads to respiratory failure and impaired return of blood to the heart. Risk factors include penetrating chest trauma and positive-pressure ventilation.

Fetal circulation bypasses the pulmonary system in utero since oxygenated blood comes from the mother via the placenta. This diversion from the pulmonary circuit is a right-to-left shunt through the *patent ductus arteriosus* that allows systemic perfusion. Closure of the ductus arteriosus occurs during the first few weeks after delivery. During this transition, certain structural anomalies of the cardiac system may be dependent on a patent ductus for systemic perfusion. These are also known as left-ventricular outflow tract obstructive lesions and include coarctation of the aorta, interrupted aortic arch, critical aortic stenosis, and hypoplastic left heart syndrome.[1] With closure of the ductus, blood flow bypassing the left-sided obstruction is no longer possible. Systemic vascular resistance increases with closure of the ductus and stroke volume decreases along with cardiac output. Patency of the ductus arteriosus is critical for survival in these patients.

Pulmonary embolism is the partial or total obstruction of flow to the pulmonary artery from thrombus, fat, air, amniotic fluid, or catheter fragments. Although rare in pediatrics, predisposing factors include indwelling central venous catheters, sickle cell disease, malignancy, connective tissue disorders, and hypercoagulable states (i.e., antithrombin III, protein C, and protein S deficiencies).

▶ RECOGNITION

Pediatric physiology is unique since progressive decline in cardiac output is masked by tachycardia. Early recognition of compensated shock is imperative so that interventions can be directed to preventing progression to decompensated shock. Hypotension is an ominous sign and heralds impending cardiac arrest.

Historical events preceding the presentation to the emergency department can provide important clues to the etiology of the disease process. Progressive vomiting and diarrhea in an infant or significant femur deformity in a child after an all terrain vehicle (ATV) crash represents likely mechanisms for the development of hypovolemia. Fever and purpura in a teen or tachycardia in a child with leukemia and central venous line after induction chemotherapy have a high likelihood for sepsis. Similarly, urticaria, vomiting, facial swelling, and difficulty breathing within minutes of IV contrast or after eating peanuts are consistent with anaphylaxis. Likewise, trauma with bradycardia, flaccid paralysis, and priapism are indicative of a spinal cord injury. Ingestions of calcium or beta-blockers are toxic to the cardiac myocyte and will progress to cardiogenic shock. Diaphoresis with feeding, difficulty breathing with feeds, poor weight gain, or cyanosis suggests a structural cardiac lesion. Often the etiology is not clear; the 2-week-old infant with lethargy, poor feeding, and poor perfusion can be hypovolemia, hypoglycemia, sepsis, an inborn error of metabolism, or an undiagnosed cardiac lesion in failure.

The physical examination of children in an emergency department can be challenging especially when volume is high. Hidden within the steady flow of visits for minor problems are a few disasters waiting to happen. Recognition of the obtunded, pale, and poorly perfused patient in hypotensive shock is obvious. The challenge is to discern which febrile and tachycardic patients are in early stages of shock. A crying or frightened child may be tachycardic and tachypneic. Many children are evaluated for fever in the emergency department. Cool ambient temperatures and the early stages of fever cause vasoconstriction and diminished peripheral perfusion. These factors make the physical examination a challenge to distinguish the minor problems from true impending disasters.

Tachycardia remains the most consistent sign of circulatory compromise in children. The subcategories of shock all commonly end up with decreased stroke volume, and the first compensatory mechanism to maintain cardiac output is tachycardia. The exception is neurogenic shock or cardiogenic shock secondary to toxicologic mechanisms that "poison" the cardiac myocyte (i.e., calcium-channel or beta-blocker toxic ingestions). Persistent tachycardia in a calm, afebrile child reflects a metabolic abnormality. Tachypnea can be observed in two forms: effortless or with distress. Effortless tachypnea, also referred to as quiet tachypnea, is the respiratory compensation for metabolic acidosis. There is minimal accessory muscle use and is classically described for children in early sepsis. Respiratory distress with tachypnea implies lung pathology from V/Q mismatch, hypoxemia, pulmonary edema, or heart failure. Classically described with cardiogenic shock, it is also found in patients with obstructive shock.

Blood pressure is used to distinguish between compensated and hypotensive shock. Normal blood pressure is maintained by increased vascular resistance in early shock states. Widened pulse pressure, or the difference between systolic and diastolic pressures, is consistent with low systemic vascular resistance, suggestive of distributive shock. As compensatory mechanisms fail, hypotension occurs and heralds impending cardiac arrest. Tissue perfusion can be used as a surrogate marker for cardiac output and when capillary refill is greater than 2 seconds, this suggests that cardiac output is compromised.[9,10] Warm skin and bounding pulses in a febrile child with borderline hypotension is consistent with *warm shock*. Cold skin and weak pulses in a febrile child with borderline hypotension *is cold shock*. Other clinical markers suggestive of compromised perfusion include altered mental status, diminished peripheral pulses, and mottled extremities. The diagnosis of shock can be difficult and all information available needs to be carefully and repeatedly considered to reach the correct diagnosis.

Although shock is a clinical diagnosis, laboratory evaluation can aid in determining severity of disease. Rapid tests that are helpful in delineating treatment include bedside glucose, ionized calcium, and blood gas. For trauma, serial hemoglobin measurements may indicate ongoing blood loss as the ini-

tial hemoglobin may not reliably indicate degree of hemorrhage. Lactate is often used as a biochemical marker for anaerobic metabolism and may predict mortality in cardiogenic shock,[2] trauma,[11] and septic shock.[12] Lactate can be elevated in metabolic disorders, lymphoproliferative disorders, and liver failure. Serum electrolyte allows calculation of the anion gap and values greater than 16 mEq/L are used as a surrogate marker for lactic acidosis.[2] Other considerations include uremia, diabetic ketoacidosis, alcohol ketoacidosis, and acute ingestions of aspirin, ethylene glycol, methanol, and paraldehyde. Leukocytosis is common in sepsis while neutropenia and lymphopenia indicate overwhelming infection and immunosuppression in septic shock preceding death.[3,4] Renal dysfunction and failure result from the release of renal tubular cells into the tubules after persistent shock. Low-flow shock states provide conditions conducive for coagulation within vessels. The systemic inflammatory response to infection activates the vascular endothelium to a procoagulant and antifibrinolytic state causing consumption of proteins in platelet and fibrin thrombi. The result is the prolongation of prothrombin and plasma thromboplastin time.

▶ TREATMENT/INTERVENTIONS

Early and aggressive intervention is crucial for management of shock. Intervention strategies for shock are twofold. First, restore oxygen delivery to tissues by optimizing oxygen content of the blood. Second, improve tissue perfusion by increasing vascular volume and distribution of cardiac output.[13]

Oxygen content is influenced by oxygen-carrying capacity (hemoglobin) and percentage of hemoglobin that is saturated with oxygen (O_2 saturation). Administration of 100% oxygen to increase bound and dissolved oxygen in blood is imperative. Airway maintenance is critical and providing a secure airway via intubation should be performed if necessary. With intubation and pharmacologic paralysis, the work of breathing is reduced while simultaneously decreasing oxygen demand. Improving ventilation/perfusion (V/Q) abnormalities using continuous positive airway pressure (CPAP) and positive endexpiratory pressure (PEEP) helps to correct V/Q abnormalities. Correction of anemia can dramatically increase oxygencarrying capacity. Less often considered, but causes of reduced oxygen delivery are abnormal hemoglobin states from carbon monoxide or nitrites exposure creating carboxyhemoglobin or methemoglobinemia, respectively. Also consider exposure to toxins that induce cellular hypoxia despite adequate oxygenation supply such as cyanide and hydrogen sulfide.[13]

In most cases, fluid resuscitation is critical to improving cardiac output. The only contraindication to aggressive fluid management is congestive heart failure. Dehydration and the maldistribution of blood volume can create challenges for vascular access. If intravenous access is difficult, early establishment of intraosseous access is encouraged.[14] Provided there is no hepatomegaly or rales to suggest heart failure, rapid and successive 20 mL/kg boluses of fluid up to 60 mL/kg or more are warranted until perfusion is restored. In severe sepsis, persistent capillary leak from the systemic inflammatory response syndrome (SIRS) can result in persistent maldistribution of blood volume and significant pulmonary edema. If blood loss is the etiology of shock, it is sensible to replenish

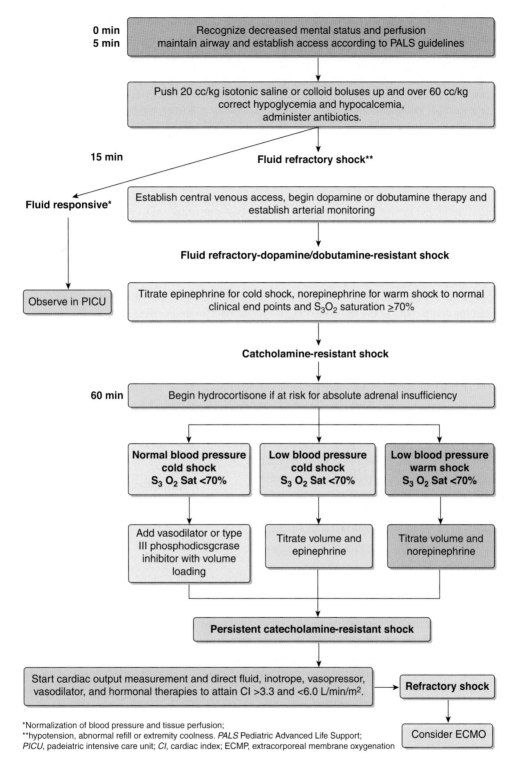

| 0 min | Recognize decreased mental status and perfusion |
| 5 min | maintain airway and establish access according to PALS guidelines |

Push 20 cc/kg isotonic saline or colloid boluses up and over 60 cc/kg
correct hypoglycemia and hypocalcemia,
administer antibiotics.

15 min   **Fluid refractory shock****

Fluid responsive*   Establish central venous access, begin dopamine or dobutamine therapy and establish arterial monitoring

Fluid refractory-dopamine/dobutamine-resistant shock

Observe in PICU   Titrate epinephrine for cold shock, norepinephrine for warm shock to normal clinical end points and S_3O_2 saturation $\geq$70%

Catcholamine-resistant shock

60 min   Begin hydrocortisone if at risk for absolute adrenal insufficiency

| **Normal blood pressure cold shock** $S_3 O_2$ Sat <70% | **Low blood pressure cold shock** $S_3 O_2$ Sat <70% | **Low blood pressure warm shock** $S_3 O_2$ Sat <70% |
| Add vasodilator or type III phosphodicsgcrase inhibitor with volume loading | Titrate volume and epinephrine | Titrate volume and norepinephrine |

Persistent catecholamine-resistant shock

Start cardiac output measurement and direct fluid, inotrope, vasopressor, vasodilator, and hormonal therapies to attain CI >3.3 and <6.0 L/min/m². → **Refractory shock**

Consider ECMO

*Normalization of blood pressure and tissue perfusion;
**hypotension, abnormal refill or extremity coolness. *PALS* Pediatric Advanced Life Support;
PICU, padeiatric intensive care unit; *CI*, cardiac index; *ECMP*, extracorporeal membrane oxygenation

Figure 25–2. Approach to management of pediatric septic shock. (With permission from Dellinger RP, Levy MM, Carlet JM, et al. Surviving sepsis campaign: international guidelines for management of severe sepsis and septic shock: 2008. *Crit Care Med*. 2008;36:296.)

the vascular space with blood, as two goals will be accomplished: restoration of intravascular volume and increased oxygen-carrying capacity of the circulating blood volume.

The outcome in adult septic shock is critically dependent on early aggressive goal-directed therapy.[5] This includes monitoring central mixed venous oxygen saturation (>70%), mean arterial pressure (>65 mm Hg), central venous pressure (CVP) (between 8 and 12 mm Hg), and hematocrit (>30%).[15] Studies in pediatrics are limited, but two studies support early goal-directed therapy for septic shock in children.[9, 10] Perfusion represented by capillary refill was used as a surrogate marker for cardiac output.

In 2008, an international consortium developed guidelines for the management of severe sepsis and septic shock in adult and pediatric patients.[5] A proposed approach to pediatric septic shock is referenced in Figure 25–2. Therapeutic end points for resuscitation of septic shock include normalization of heart rate, capillary refill <2 seconds, normal pulses, warm extremities, urine output >1 mL/kg/h, and normal mental status. A summary of pediatric considerations in sepsis were addressed in 2008 (Table 25-2). Other goal-directed management of pediatric shock is referenced in Table 25–3.

Anaphylactic shock has the potential for airway obstruction due to swelling of the upper airway so that early airway intervention may be warranted. Fluid resuscitation is needed to compensate for the vasodilation related to histamine release. Epinephrine (1:1000) administration intramuscularly to the anterolateral thigh is critical for decreasing morbidity and mortality. Epinephrine promotes vasoconstriction and decreases mucosal edema through α_1 effects. In addition, increases in heart rate and strength of contractility occur through beta effects along with bronchodilation and stabilization of histamine-releasing mast cells and basophils.[6] Repeated doses may be needed and when hypotension is persistent an epinephrine drip (1:10000) should be started. Other adjunctive therapies include corticosteroids, H1 and H2 blockers, and nebulized albuterol.

Neurogenic shock results primarily through loss of sympathetic innervation from the central nervous system. The hypotension from the loss of vasomotor tone is not always responsive to fluid administration, but does respond to α_1 stimulation from norepinephrine and epinephrine.[13] Warming measures may be needed since the vasodilation increases insensible heat loss. Bradycardia from loss of sympathetic input to the heart can be improved with epinephrine.

Cardiogenic shock requires therapies that increase the contractility of the heart while reducing the resistance that the heart is working against. Overzealous fluid administration can result in decreased cardiac function and pulmonary edema. Tachycardia and respiratory distress increases oxygen demand on a heart that is already compromised in delivering oxygen to the body. Goals of therapy are to reduce oxygen demand by reducing the work of breathing. This can be accomplished by rapid sequence intubation, paralysis, sedation, and control of pain. Reduction of systemic vascular resistance allows for an increase in stroke volume and cardiac output. A consequence of this therapy is the compensatory tachycardia that unfortunately increases cardiac oxygen demand. Buffering metabolic acidosis with bicarbonate is thought to improve myocardial depression that occurs when the pH is less than

► TABLE 25-2. **SUMMARY OF PEDIATRIC CONSIDERATIONS IN SEPSIS 2008**

Category	Recommendations	Notes
Antibiotics	Within 1 h	
Mechanical ventilation	None	Caution with etomidate due to adrenal suppression
Fluid resuscitation	Crystalloid	20 mL/kg titrate to clinical monitors
Vasopressors/inotropes	Dopamine first choice	If dopamine refractory consider epinephrine or norepinephrine ↓ CO, ↑ SVR, consider dobutamine
Therapeutic end points	Heart rate Capillary refill <2 s Normal pulses Warm extremities Urine output >1 mL/kg/h Normal mental status	
Steroids	Only for catecholamine-resistant shock or proven adrenal insufficiency	High risk for adrenal insufficiency: severe shock and purpura, recent steroid for chronic illness, pituitary or adrenal abnormalities.
Activated protein C	Not recommended	
Glycemic control	None	Insulin helpful in adults; benefits in pediatrics unknown.
Sedation/analgesia	Recommended	Avoid propofol
Blood products	None	Hemoglobin recommended to be >7 g/L in adults. Pediatric data limited.
Intravenous immunoglobulin	Consider in severe sepsis	Reduced mortality in neonate and pediatric septic shock.
Extracorporeal membrane oxygenation (ECMO)	Only if conventional methods fail	

CO, cardiac output; SVR, systemic vascular resistance.
With permission from Dellinger RP, Levy MM, Carlet JM, et al. Surviving sepsis campaign: international guidelines for management of severe sepsis and septic shock: 2008. *Crit Care Med.* 2008;36:296.

▶ TABLE 25–3. GOAL-DIRECTED MANAGEMENT OF PEDIATRIC SHOCK

1. Recognize shock at time of triage
   a. Hypotension alone with bounding pulses in warm shock
   b. Diminished peripheral perfusion alone (diminished peripheral compared with central pulses and capillary refill >2 s) in compensated cold shock
   c. Combination of hypotension with diminished peripheral perfusion in decompensated cold shock
2. Transfer patient immediately to shock/trauma room and amass resuscitation team
3. Begin nasal oxygen and establish intravenous access using 90 s for peripheral attempts
4. If unsuccessful after 2 peripheral attempts, consider intraosseus access
5. Palpate for hepatomegaly; auscultate for rales
6a. If liver is up and if no rales are present, push 20 mL/kg boluses of isotonic saline or 5% albumin up to 60 mL/kg in 15 min until improved perfusion or liver comes down or patient develops rales. Give 20 mL/kg pRBCs if unresponsive hemorrhagic shock [18]
6b. If liver is down, beware of cardiogenic shock, and give only 10 mL/kg bolus of isotonic crystalloid. Begin PGE₁ to maintain ductus arteriosus in all neonates
7. If capillary refill >2 s and/or hypotension persists during fluid resuscitation, begin IO/peripheral epinephrine at 0.05 μg/kg/min
8. If at risk for adrenal insufficiency (e.g., previous steroid exposure, Waterhouse Friderichsen, or pituitary anomaly) give hydrocortisone as bolus (50 mg/kg) and then as infusion titrating between 2 and 50 mg/kg/d
9. If continued shock, use atropine (0.2 mg/kg) plus ketamine (2 mg/kg) for sedation for central line placement. If mechanical ventilation is required, use atropine plus ketamine plus neuromuscular blocker (in skilled hands) for induction for intubation
10. Direct therapy to goals
    a. Capillary refill <3 s (e.g., ≤2 s)
    b. Normal blood pressure for age
    c. Improving shock index (HR/SBP)

pRBC, packed red blood cells; PGE1, prostaglandin E1; IO, intraosseous.
With permission from Carcillo JA, Han K, Lin J, et al. Goal-directed management of pediatric shock in the emergency department. *Clin Ped Emerg Med.* 2007;8:165.

7.2. In patients with evidence of pulmonary edema and volume overload, furosemide and other diuretics should be instituted upon diagnosis. Finally, consultation with pediatric critical care and cardiology should be initiated at the earliest opportunity.

Physical obstructions that impede cardiac output such as tension pneumothorax and cardiac tamponade can be improved with needle thoracentesis and pericardiocentesis, respectively. Outcomes are improved with early diagnosis and treatment. For congenital left-ventricular outflow tract lesions that are dependent on the ductus arteriosus for systemic per-

fusion, prostaglandin E₁ continuous infusion restores patency of the ductus by vasodilation.[13] Other interventions include ventilatory support, inotropic agents to improve contractility, echocardiography to direct therapy, and correction of metabolic abnormalities (acidosis, hypocalcemia, and hypoglycemia) that impair cardiac function. Pulmonary embolism is rare in the pediatric population unless risk factors are present. Therapy primarily includes anticoagulation with heparin and early consultation with pediatric critical care and hematology.

▶ PHARMACOLOGIC AGENTS

Vasoactive agents are indicated for shock after adequate volume resuscitation has optimized preload.[13] These are adjunctive agents that stimulate adrenergic receptors in cardiac, pulmonary, and vascular beds. Table 25–4 reviews tissue effects after stimulation of the adrenergic receptors.

Drugs that increase heart rate and cardiac contractility are known as inotropes and do so via the β₁ receptor. Examples include dopamine, dobutamine, epinephrine, and norepinephrine. Other drugs increase peripheral vascular resistance via the α₁ receptor and examples are epinephrine, norepinephrine, phenylephrine, and vasopressin. Finally, there are phosphodiesterase inhibitors that are unique because they have both inotrope and vasodilatory properties. Drugs in this class include milrinone, amrinone, enoximone, and pentoxyfilline.[2] Table 25–5 lists common vasoactive agents used in pediatric shock and their clinical effects.

Dopamine is also referred to as an *indirect* vasoactive agent since the α₁ and β₁ adrenergic effects are mediated through endogenous release of norepinephrine from sympathetic vesicles. Infants younger than 6 months appear to have decreased response and this is postulated to be related to inadequate numbers of sympathetic vesicles.[2] This phenomenon is also seen in older children and adults who have exhausted their catecholamine reserves. Dobutamine has similar age-specific insensitivity in children younger than 2 years.[16] Unlike catecholamines, which are metabolized in minutes, phosphodiesterase inhibitors breakdown occurs over hours.

▶ TABLE 25–4. ADRENERGIC RECEPTORS

Receptors	Tissue Effect
Alpha (α)	Peripheral vasoconstriction (α₁)
	Dilation of the iris (α₁)
	Intestinal smooth muscle relaxation (α₁)
	Increased bladder and intestinal sphincter tone (α₁)
	Prevent release of endogenous norepinephrine (α₂)
Beta-1 (β₁)	Increased heart rate
	Improved myocardial contractility
	Peripheral vasodilation
Beta-2 (β₂)	Bronchodilation
	Bladder, uterine, and intestinal smooth muscle relaxation

▶ **TABLE 25-5. VASOACTIVE AGENTS**

Drug	Dose	Mechanism	Clinical Effect
Dopamine	2–20 μg/kg/min	β_1 stimulation α_1 stimulation at >10 μg/kg/min	↑ HR and contractility ↑ SVR
Epinephrine	0.05–1 μg/kg/min	β_1 stimulation at 0.05 μg/kg/min α_1 stimulation when >0.3 μg/kg/min	↑ HR and contractility ↑ SVR
Norepinephrine	0.05–1 μg/kg/min	α_1 stimulation predominates β_1 stimulation	↑ SVR ↑ HR and contractility
Dobutamine	2–20 μg/kg/min	β_1 stimulation α_2 stimulation	↑ HR and contractility ↓ SVR

Milrinone	50–75 μg/kg load
	0.5–1 μg/kg/min
		↑ cAMP by inhibiting
		  phosphodiesterase
			↑ contractility
			Vasodilation of pulmonary
			  and arterial vessels

HR, heart rate; SVR, systemic vascular resistance; cAMP, cyclic AMP.
Carcillo JA, Han K, Lin J, et al. Goal-directed management of pediatric shock in the emergency department. *Clin Ped Emerg Med.* 2007;8:165.

When organ dysfunction is present, drug metabolism can be prolonged and may add to the duration of toxicities should they develop.

In summary, there are a myriad of causes of shock in pediatric patients and some causes are unique compared to the adult population. Early recognition is paramount and research has expanded our knowledge of therapies that are helpful and those that are not.

Fluid resuscitation with crystalloid, colloid, or blood is crucial for increasing preload and cardiac output. Once this is optimized, cardiac output can be augmented with vasopressors. Each shock state is unique and requires individualized combinations of therapies.

REFERENCES

1. Ralston M, Hazinski MF, Zaritsky AL, et al., eds. *Recognition of Shock in Pediatric Advanced Life Support.* American Heart Association; 2006:61, chap 4.
2. Carcillo JA, Han K, Lin J, et al. Goal-directed management of pediatric shock in the emergency department. *Clin Ped Emerg Med.* 2007;8:165.
3. Russell JA. Management of sepsis. *N Engl J Med.* 2006;355:1699.
4. Hotchkiss RS, Karl IE. The pathophysiology and treatment of sepsis. *N Engl J Med.* 2003;348:138.
5. Dellinger RP, Levy MM, Carlet JM, et al. Surviving sepsis campaign: international guidelines for management of severe sepsis and septic shock: 2008. *Crit Care Med.* 2008;36:296.
6. Lane RD, Bolte RG. Pediatric anaphylaxis. *Ped Emerg Care.* 2007;23:49.
7. Dumont RJ, Okonkwo DO, Verma S, et al. Acute spinal cord injury, part I: pathophysiological mechanisms. *Clin Neuropharmacol.* 2001;24:254.
8. Topalian S, Ginsberg F, Parrillo JE. Cardiogenic shock. *Crit Care Med.* 2008;36:S66.
9. Han YY, Carcillo JA, Dragotta MA, et al. Early reversal of pediatric-neonatal septic shock by community physicians is associated with improved outcome. *Pediatrics.* 2003;112:793.
10. Orr RA, Kuch B, Carcillo J, et al. Shock is under-reported in children transported for respiratory distress: a multi-center study. *Crit Care Med.* 2003;31:A18.
11. Kaplan LJ, Kellum JA. Comparison of acid-base models for prediction of hospital mortality after trauma. *Shock.* 2008;29:662.
12. Ramzi J, Mohamed Z, Yosr B, et al. Predictive factors of septic shock and mortality in neutropenic patients. *Hematology.* 2007;12:543.
13. Ralston M, Hazinski MF, Zaritsky AL, et al., eds. *Management of Shock in Pediatric Advanced Life Support.* American Heart Association; 2006:Chap 5.
14. Kanter RK, Zimmerman JJ, Strauss RH, et al.: Pediatric emergency intravenous access: Evaluation of a protocol. *Am J Dis Child.* 1986;140:132.
15. Rivers E, Nguyen B, Havstad S, et al. Early goal-directed therapy in the treatment of severe sepsis and septic shock. *N Engl J Med.* 2001;345:1368.
16. Perkins RM, Levin DL, Webb R, et al. Dobutamine: a hemodynamic evaluation in children with shock. *J Pediatr.* 1982;100:977.

CHAPTER 26

Cardiopulmonary Resuscitation

Alson S. Inaba

▶ HIGH-YIELD FACTS

- Primary cardiac arrest is rare in children. Early recognition and prompt treatment of respiratory distress and shock are essential to prevent the progression to cardiopulmonary arrest.
- High-quality cardiopulmonary resuscitation (CPR) must be integrated into advanced life-support measures in order to ensure a good outcome during resuscitation. The code leader must therefore continually monitor the quality of chest compressions during the entire resuscitation.
- When two or more health care providers are performing CPR in an infant or child the correct compression to ventilation ratio is 15:2 (15 compressions followed by 2 ventilations). In all other circumstances, the new universal 30:2 compression to ventilation ratio should be used.
- Minimizing interruptions of chest compressions provides for better myocardial perfusion during CPR. Two-minute cycles of CPR should be performed before stopping compressions to reassess the child.
- Automated external defibrillators can be safely and effectively used in children older than 1 year. If at all possible a pediatric attenuator device should be used if the automated external defibrillator is being used in a child younger than 8 years of age or less than 25 kg.
- Overzealous ventilations via an advanced airway can impede venous return to the heart and thus potentially decrease cardiac output during CPR.
- Ventricular fibrillation and pulseless ventricular tachycardia are now treated with single shocks followed immediately by 2-minute cycles of CPR in order to maintain myocardial perfusion after each defibrillation.
- The use of length-based tapes are encouraged during resuscitations in order to more accurately calculate proper doses of medications and select the appropriate size equipment.
- Intraosseous (IO) lines can be safely and effectively used in victims of any age. Anything that can be administered through an intravenous (IV) line can also be given via an IO line.
- Medication administration via vascular access (IV or IO) is highly preferred over endotracheal administration because of an unreliable absorption of medications via the endotracheal route.
- High-dose epinephrine is no longer routinely recommended in the Pediatric Advanced Life Support guidelines.
- Always remember to consider the possibility of paroxysmal supraventricular tachycardia in any infant who presents with lethargy, fussiness, poor feeding, pallor, tachypnea, or shock.

- The key to treating a child with pulseless electrical activity (PEA) is to quickly search for and correct any reversible causes. The most common cause of PEA in children is hypovolemia so always consider a rapid fluid bolus in any child presenting in a PEA rhythm.

The primary etiology of cardiopulmonary arrest in children differs from that in adult patients. Sudden cardiac arrest because of a primary cardiac dysrhythmia is rare in children.[1] Unrecognized respiratory distress and shock are the most common etiologies of cardiopulmonary arrest in children. Once cardiopulmonary arrest has occurred in an out-of-hospital setting, the outcome generally remains poor with only 5% to 12% of children surviving to hospital discharge. The survival rate for children who experience cardiopulmonary arrest in an in-hospital setting has a slightly better survival rate to discharge of approximately 27%.[2] Therefore, early recognition of a child in respiratory distress and/or compensated shock is essential to prevent the progression to cardiopulmonary arrest. The recognition and management of respiratory distress, respiratory failure, and shock are addressed in Chapters 23, 24, and 25.

▶ THE IMPORTANCE OF INCORPORATING HIGH-QUALITY BASIC LIFE SUPPORT INTO ADVANCED LIFE-SUPPORT MEASURES

Once cardiopulmonary arrest occurs, the resuscitation team must integrate the most up-to-date guidelines in basic pediatric life support with their assessment and management skills in advanced pediatric life support. The updated 2005 American Heart Association's (AHA) Pediatric Advanced Life Support (PALS) guidelines are based on an international consensus of the largest review of the resuscitation literature.[3] One of the essential points in the 2005 AHA guidelines is an emphasis on high-quality CPR by lay rescuers and by health care providers. Because there are many barriers to lay rescuers being willing to perform bystander CPR, the 2005 guidelines have simplified the process in hopes that more victims of cardiac arrest will receive immediate bystander CPR. The five essential components of high-quality chest compressions are listed in Table 26–1.[4] The "5 & 2" rule for high-quality CPR reminds the code leader to closely monitor the five components of high-quality chest compressions and to continue CPR in 2-minute intervals before

▶ **TABLE 26–1. DR. AL'S "5 & 2" RULE FOR HIGH-QUALITY CPR.**[4]

Five critical components when performing chest compressions:

1. Correct hand position—the heel of one hand placed over the sternum at the nipple line in children and one finger breath below the nipple line in infants. When two-rescuer CPR is performed in infants, use the two-thumb-encircling hands technique to compress the sternum with the thumbs and squeeze the infant's chest with the encircling fingers.
2. Push hard—compress the chest 1/3 to 1/2 the depth of the chest.
3. Push fast—compress at a rate of 100 compressions per min. *Note*: If you perform chest compressions at the same beat as the popular Bee Gee's song Stayin Alive, you will achieve the correct rate of 100 compressions/min.[5]
4. Allow complete recoil of the chest in order to allow the heart to refill with blood before the next compression.
5. Minimize interruption of chest compressions; perform uninterrupted CPR in 2-min intervals before reassessing the patient.

stopping compressions to reassess the patient. The universal compression to ventilation ratio for one-rescuer CPR in any age victim is 30:2. When there are two health care providers performing CPR, the compression to ventilation ratio for infants and children is 15:2. The effectiveness of CPR is measured by palpable pulses during cardiac compressions. Overzealous ventilations during CPR may be harmful by decreasing venous return to the heart and limiting cardiac output. Major changes in CPR guidelines from the 2005 PALS are reviewed in Table 26–2.

▶ **TABLE 26–2. KEY CHANGES AND MAJOR POINTS OF EMPHASIS IN THE 2005 PALS GUIDELINES**

1. Ventilation to compression ratios for infant and child CPR:
   Lone rescuer: 30:2.
   Two-rescuer: 15:2.
   CPR with an advanced airway in place: 8–10 breaths/min, and compressions at 100/min.
   Apnea with a pulse: 12–20 breaths/min.
2. Palpable pulses during compressions assesses quality of CPR.
3. Avoid overzealous ventilations during CPR.
4. AEDs can be safely and effectively used in infants and children older than 1 year.
5. Cuffed ETTs may be used under certain circumstances; however, the cuff pressure must be kept <20 cm H_2O.
6. The vascular route (IV or IO) for medication administration is highly preferred over endotracheal administration.
7. High-dose epinephrine is no longer routinely recommended and may be harmful.[3]
8. VF and PVT (pulseles ventricular tachycardia) are now treated with single defibrillations followed immediately by 2-min cycles of high-quality CPR.
9. Minimize interruptions of chest compression.

▶ AIRWAY AND VENTILATION

A detailed discussion of the assessment and management of respiratory distress, respiratory failure, and advanced airway management are covered in other chapters within this book. Although uncuffed endotracheal tubes (ETTs) have traditionally been used in pediatric patients, the 2005 PALS guidelines also approves the use of cuffed ETTs in children younger than 8 years (except for the newly born). Cuffed ETTs may be safely used in the in-hospital setting in children under certain circumstances such as poor lung compliance, high airway resistance, or a large glottic leak.[3] If a cuffed ETT is used, the cuff pressure must be closely monitored and kept <20 cm H_2O.

Although laryngeal mask airways (LMAs) have been extensively used by pediatric anesthesiologist in the operating room, there is currently insufficient evidence to the recommend the routine use of LMAs in children during cardiac arrest.[3] However, if a child in cardiopulmonary arrest cannot be adequately ventilated and oxygenated via bag-mask techniques and if attempts of an ETT insertion have failed, an LMA can be used as an alternate adjunct of advanced airway management during CPR.

Once an advanced airway has been inserted, confirm proper tube placement and proper ventilation by clinical assessment and confirmatory devices. The best way to determine whether the correct sized advanced airway is properly placed and that the patient is being effectively ventilated is to observe for adequate and symmetric rise and fall of the chest. The most commonly used confirmatory device in both the out-of-hospital and in-hospital setting is the colorimetric carbon dioxide detector device. Although one of the more common colorimetric capnometers registers the presence of carbon dioxide by changing from its initial purple color to yellow, there are many other similar devices on the market by different manufacturers which use different color schemes to detect exhaled carbon dioxide. The clinician should remember that there are various false-positive and false-negative results that may occur when using a colorimetric carbon dioxide detector device. During cardiopulmonary arrest, the lungs are poorly perfused and therefore the colorimetric capnometer device may not detect sufficient amounts of carbon dioxide despite the advanced airway being correctly positioned within the trachea. If the standard size capnometer is used in smaller infants, carbon dioxide may not be detected by the device (despite proper placement of the advanced airway) because of low lung volumes in infants and smaller children. Therefore, be sure to check the manufacturer's specifications and weight limitations for the various capnometer devices. As an example, one of the manufacturers of a capnometer device recommends that their neonatal/infant device be used if the patient is <15 kg (otherwise the standard adult-sized capnometer device should be sufficient if the patient is >15 kg). A false-positive result (i.e., apparent detection of exhaled carbon dioxide even though the advanced airway was not actually inserted into the trachea) may occur if the capnometer device is contaminated by gastric acid and/or contaminated by acidic medications such as epinephrine that were instilled into the advanced airway. Children who have consumed carbonated beverages just prior to intubation may have enough carbon dioxide present in their stomachs to produce a color change during an accidental esophageal intubation. Therefore to avoid this false-positive result of an esophageal intubation, provide six ventilations prior to attaching a capnometer device to check for the presence of exhaled carbon dioxide.

Once the patient is intubated, avoid hyperventilation by providing 8 to 10 ventilations per minute during CPR.[6] Excessive ventilations during CPR can impede venous return to the heart and thus potentially compromise cardiac output during CPR.[7]

During the resuscitation, the clinician must continuously reassess the adequacy of ventilations via the ETT. ETT complications should always be considered whenever an intubated patient suddenly deteriorates during the resuscitation or during the postresuscitation stages. The complications of ETT intubation can be quickly and systematically assessed via the "DOPE" mnemonic.[8]

D = Dislodged or displaced ETT (esophageal intubation or right mainstem displacement)

O= Obstructed ETT (kinked tube or internal obstruction with blood, mucus, and/or emesis)

P = Pneumothorax (tension)

E = Equipment failure (disconnected tubing, too small ETT with air leak, and/or inadequate volume of ventilations)

▶ VASCULAR ACCESS PRIORITIES FOR MEDICATION ADMINISTRATION

Intravenous (IV) or intraosseous (IO) access is the preferred method of medication administration during any resuscitation. Although a few lipid-soluble medications (i.e., "L-A-N-E" = lidocaine, atropine, naloxone, and epinephrine) can be administered via the ETT during a resuscitation, a review of several human and animal studies have demonstrated lower blood concentrations of medications that were administered via the ETT as compared which the same medication dose administered intravenously. Some animal studies have even suggested that the lower blood epinephrine concentrations that are achieved when the medication is given into the trachea may produce transient β-effects which can produce detrimental effects of hypotension and lowering of the coronary perfusion pressure.[3] Therefore, the IV or IO route is highly preferred over the ETT route for medication administration during a resuscitation. There is no age restriction for placement of an IO line. In infants and younger children the preferred site is the flat-medial portion of the proximal tibia (i.e., 2–3 cm below the tibial tuberosity). An alternative site for IO placement in older children is the distal tibia (i.e., 2–3 cm proximal to the medial malleous). Any medication that can be given via the IV route can also be administrated via the IO route.

ESTIMATION OF A CHILD'S WEIGHT FOR MEDICATION ADMINISTRATION

Difficulties encountered during a pediatric resuscitation include medication calculations, which are always based on a child's weight, and selection of appropriate size equipment (i.e., ETT, IV catheter sizes, chest tube sizes, etc.). During the stressful situation of a resuscitation, parents may not be able

▶ **TABLE 26-3. ESTIMATING A CHILD'S WEIGHT BASED ON THE CHILD'S AGE[9]**

Full-term neonate = 3–3.5 kg.
Doubles birth weight by 4–6 mo.
Triples birth weight by 1 year of age (1-year-old child = ~10 kg).
The target ages according to this formula are the odd numbered years. Start at 10 kg for the 1-year-old and simply increase the weight in increments of 5 kg for each subsequent odd numbered target year until age 11 years. After 11 years of age, increase the weight in 10-kg increments in order to compensate for the rapid growth spurt during the adolescent period.

Age = weight:

1 year old	= 10 kg
3 years old	= 15 kg
5 years old	= 20 kg
7 years old	= 25 kg
9 years old	= 30 kg
11 years old	= 35 kg
13 years old	= 45 kg
15 years old	= 55 kg
17 years old	= 65 kg

to accurately recall their child's weight and therefore the emergency physician is often faced with the daunting task of estimating the child's weight in order to calculate the correct dose of resuscitation medications. One quick method for estimating a child's weight is based on the child's age and can be reviewed in Table 26–3.[9]

Length-based tapes (i.e., Broselow tape) are recommended by the PALS guidelines in order to estimate a child's weight during a resuscitation. These length-based tapes also precalculate the appropriate doses of various resuscitation medications and appropriate equipment sizes based on the child's length. The validity of length-based tapes has been reverified in recent studies.[10,11] However, there is no perfect method to accurately estimate a child's weight and the limitation of the currently available length-based tapes is that they do not take the child's body habitus into account. A recent study claims that a length-based tape inaccurately estimated the actual weight in up to one-third of children.[12] Although length-based resuscitation systems have reduced the potential for equipment and medication dosing errors, weight estimate error concerns have been raised with regard to the obese child and the cachectic child. Currently, the length-based tapes only take into account the length of the patient and do not take into account the overall body habitus. The addition of body habitus assessments in addition to length-based systems has demonstrated a more accurate means of estimating a child's true weight.[13]

▶ A SYSTEMATIC APPROACH TO ARREST AND PREARREST DYSRHYTHMIAS

A systematic approach to pediatric dysrhythmia stabilization and management depends on two key clinical factors:

1. Does the child have a pulse?

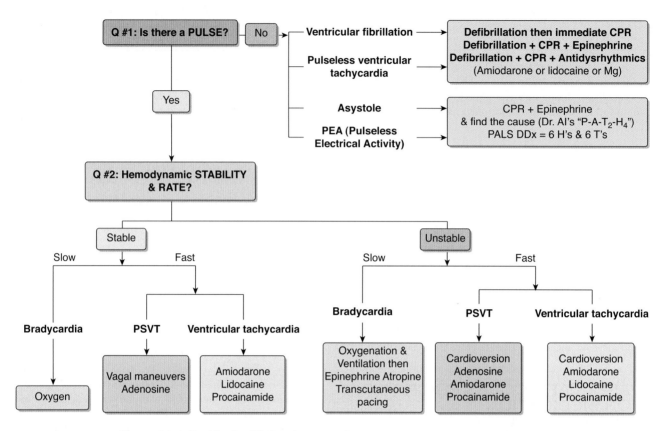

Figure 26–1. Dr. Al's simplified and systematic approach to pediatric dysrhythmias.

2. If a pulse is present, is the child hemodynamically stable or unstable and what is the child's heart rate?

All of the 2005 PALS dysrhythmia treatment algorithms can be summarized into one treatment algorithm. Refer to Figure 26–1 for a simplified and systematic approach to pediatric dysrhythmias. Children who present with a dysrhythmia but who exhibit good perfusion parameters including strong distal pulses, brisk capillary refill and warm extremities, may not require any emergent interventions unless the presenting rhythm has the potential to degenerate into a more serious condition. Children who exhibit ECG evidence of conduction abnormalities (i.e., Mobitz type II second-degree heart blocks, complete heart blocks, prolonged QT intervals or aberrant conduction such as the Wolff–Parkinson–White syndrome) may also warrant more emergent treatment.[14] In infants, prearrest rhythm disturbances can manifest as fussiness, lethargy, poor feeding, pallor, respiratory distress, or as cardiogenic shock. In older children, it may present as chest pain, palpitations, difficulty breathing, or syncope.

The most common pediatric arrest rhythms that will confront the emergency physician are asystole and bradyasystole. Ventricular fibrillation (VF) and ventricular tachycardia (VT) are not as common in children as they are in adults. However, the emergency physician must also be aware of a select group of infants and children who are at a higher risk of developing various primary cardiac dysrhythmias[14] (Table 26–4).

The four pulseless rhythms that will be addressed in this chapter can be clinically divided into two general categories based on their similar treatment approaches:

1. Shockable rhythms: VF and pulseless ventricular tachycardia (PVT).
2. Nonshockable rhythms: Asystole and pulseless electrical activity (PEA).

▶ **TABLE 26–4. CLINICAL CONDITIONS ASSOCIATED WITH A HIGH RISK FOR DEVELOPING DYSRHYTHMIAS[14]**

Congenital heart defects (uncorrected defects and postoperative complications)
Congenital complete heart blocks (i.e., maternal systemic lupus erythematosus)
Myocarditis
Rheumatic heart disease
Kawasaki disease with coronary artery involvement
Prolonged QT syndrome (familial or drug-induced)
Aberrant AV conduction pathways
Commotio cordis
Severe hypoxia
Profound hypothermia
Electrolyte abnormalities (potassium, calcium magnesium disturbances)

► TABLE 26-5. **REVERSIBLE CAUSES OF CARDIOPULMONARY ARREST IN CHILDREN**

"P-A-T2-H4"[14]:

When confronted with a child in PEA, use the asystole treatment algorithm and "head down the right PATH in the algorithm":

P = **P**neumothoarx
A = **A**cidosis
T = **T**amponade
T = **T**oxins
H = **H**ypovolemia
H = **H**ypoxemia
H = **H**yper/**H**ypokalemia
H = **H**ypothermia

Note: The most common cause of PEA in children is hypovolemia. Myocardial and pulmonary thromboses are rare in children.

The treatment approach and management priorities for VF and PVT are the same and require defibrillation followed immediately by CPR, while the treatment approach for asystole and PEA will require CPR, epinephrine, and a search for the reversible causes. Regardless of the presenting arrest rhythm, the emergency physician must also place a high priority on finding the underlying etiology or etiologies which may have lead to the arrest rhythm. The 12 reversible causes of cardiopulmonary arrest that are emphasized in the PALS guidelines can remembered as the "six Hs and six Ts".[15] Another useful mnemonic to rapidly remember the most common reversible causes of PEA in children is "P-A-T2-H4"[14] (Table 26-5).

Because atrial fibrillation and atrial flutter are not very common in children, the other dysrhythmias that will be addressed will be limited to paroxysmal supraventricular tachycardia (PSVT), bradycardia and VT. For a more detailed discussion of pediatric dysrhythmias, refer to Chapter 50.

► PAROXYSMAL SUPRAVENTRICULAR TACHYCARDIA

PSVT is the most common symptomatic dysrhythmia in infants and children. Infants with PSVT typically present with nonspecific symptoms such as fussiness, lethargy, tachypnea, pallor, and/or difficulty feeding. Although infants can generally tolerate PSVT episodes with heart rates in the 200 to 300 beats/min range, if left untreated they may present with signs and symptoms of congestive heart failure and/or shock. Older children with PSVT typically complain of palpitations, difficulty breathing, and/or vague chest discomfort. The QRS width in pediatric PSVT is most commonly of a narrow complex. Wide complex PSVT is less common but may be seen in a child with a preexisting bundle branch block or in a child with an antidromic reentry phenomenon, in which the conduction from the atria initially goes down to the ventricles via an accessory pathway and then returns retrograde from the ventricles back to the atria from the atrioventricular (AV) node.

The management of PSVT depends on the child's hemodynamic stability and availability of IV access. Refer to Tables

26–6 and 26–7 for the management and medication doses for PSVT. During any conversion attempt such as vagal maneuvers, adenosine or cardioversion, a continuous rhythm strip should be used to monitor and document the response to each conversion attempt and also to capture the initial resulting rhythm after a conversion. Hemodynamically stable PSVT in infants and young children can be initially treated with ice applied to the face. A plastic bag or surgical glove filled with a slurry of crushed ice and water can be applied over the infant's forehead, eyes, and bridge of the nose for approximately 10 to 15 seconds. Care must be taken to avoid occluding the infant's nostril and mouth during this maneuver. Older children may be asked to submerge their face in a basin of cold water in addition to trying other vagal maneuvers listed in Table 26–6.

Patients with hemodynamically stable PSVT who fail to convert after several appropriately administered doses of adenosine may require a pediatric cardiology consultation, elective cardioversion, and/or other medications such as amiodarone or procainamide to convert the PSVT. Verapamil should be avoided in infants and younger children because of the high incidence of profound hypotension and cardiovascular collapse when this medication is administered in this age group. Immediate cardioversion should be performed in any infant or child who exhibits PSVT with significant hemodynamic instability.

SYMPTOMATIC BRADYCARDIA

Bradydysrhythmias are the most common prearrest rhythms in children and are usually associated with severe hypoxemia, hypotension, and metabolic acidosis.[16] Bradycardia is poorly tolerated in infants and children because they are not physiologically capable of increasing their stroke volume to maintain an adequate cardiac output. Clinically significant bradycardia is defined as a heart rate lower than the normal rate for age associated with signs of poor systemic perfusion. Chest compressions should be initiated for an absolute heart rate <60 beats/min that is associated with signs of poor systemic perfusion.

The first step in the management of symptomatic bradycardia is to ensure adequate oxygenation and ventilation because hypoxia is the most common etiology of bradycardia in children. Children who remain symptomatic despite adequate oxygenation and ventilation will require chest compressions and medications to convert the bradycardia. In contrast to adult where atropine is the first-line medication to treat symptomatic bradycardia, epinephrine is the first medication of choice to treat children. Because the efficacy of epinephrine is reduced in the face of hypoxia and acidosis, ensure adequate ventilation, oxygenation, and chest compressions/perfusion[17] (Tables 26–6 and 26–7). Atropine would be indicated before epinephrine if the etiology of the child's bradycardia was felt to be because of an increase in vagal tone, cholinergic toxicity, or AV blocks.[17] Although hypoxia is the most common cause of bradycardia in children other etiologies to consider include hypothermia, increased intracranial pressure, heart blocks (congenital and acquired), a denervated heart status–postcardiac transplant, hypothyroidism, sick sinus syndrome, and various medications and toxins such as digoxin, β-blockers, calcium

▶ TABLE 26–6. **SUMMARY OF PEDIATRIC DYSRHYTHMIA MANAGEMENT**

Asystole and PEA:
    CPR (reassess after 2-min intervals).
    Epinephrine (q 3–5 min).
    Treat the underlying cause of PEA (Table 26–5).

VF and PVT:
    Defibrillation followed immediately by 2 min of CPR.
    Defibrillation followed immediately by 2 min of CPR + epinephrine (q 3–5 min).
    Defibrillation followed immediately by 2 min of CPR + (amiodarone or lidocaine or magnesium).

VT (with a pulse):
    Unstable: Immediate cardioversion.
    Stable: Amiodarone or lidocaine or procainamide (*Note:* Avoid concurrent use of amiodarone and procainamide).

PSVT:
    Unstable: If IV access is immediately available administer adenosine while preparing for cardioversion if adenosine fails to convert
        the PSVT. If IV access is not immediately available and/or if the patient is hemodynamically unstable, perform immediate
        cardioversion.
    Stable: Various vagal maneuvers (valsalva maneuver, ice water slurry in a bag applied to the face, blowing on an occluded straw,
        and/or blowing on the distal end of a syringe in an attempt to blow out the plunger).
    Adenosine if vagal maneuvers fail to convert the PSVT.

Bradycardia:
    Unstable: Ensure adequate ventilation and oxygenation.
    CPR (reassess after 2-min intervals).
    Epinephrine.
        Atropine if suspect an increase in vagal tone or cholinergic poisoning.
        Cardiac pacing.
    Stable: No emergent treatment is required.

channel blockers, and cholinergic toxicity. Consider emergency pacing for Mobitz type II second-degree AV blocks, complete AV blocks, or sick sinus syndrome.

▶ VENTRICULAR TACHYCARDIA (WITH A PULSE)

VT is an uncommon pediatric dysrhythmia. The majority of children with VT have underlying conditions that predispose them to developing VT such as, postcardiac surgery, myocarditis, cardiomyopathies, and prolonged QT syndrome. Electrolyte abnormalities (hyperkalemia, hypocalcemia, and hypomagnesemia), and drug toxicities (cyclic antidepressants and cocaine) must also be considered.[14] The treatment of a child with VT and a pulse will be dependent on the child's hemodynamic stability (Tables 26–6 and 26–7). Torsades de pointes is a unique type of polymorphic VT that deserves special consideration. Prolonged QT syndrome, hypomagnesemia, underlying cardiac defects, and various medications (cyclic antidepressants and calcium channel blockers) have all been implicated as known causes of torsades de pointes. Procainamide and amiodarone are both contraindicated in the treatment of torsades because both of these antidysrhythmic agents are capable of prolonging the QT interval, which could then cause a further deterioration of the torsades rhythm. Lidocaine may be the preferred medication to treat VT that is caused by a drug-induced prolongation of the QT interval.

VENTRICULAR FIBRILLATION AND PVT

VF and PVT were previously thought to occur very rarely in pediatric cardiopulmonary arrest cases. However, in a recent study of in-hospital cardiac arrest, a shockable rhythm was present during some point of the resuscitation in 25% of the cases.[2] VF and PVT should also be suspected as the initial arrest rhythm in cases of commotio cordis and in cases of witnessed sudden cardiac arrest in children. The treatment approach to VF and PVT has been drastically revised in the 2005 PALS guidelines. Once VF or PVT is detected, defibrillation maneuvers are now immediately followed by 2-minute cycles of CPR.[19] Rhythm checks and pulse checks are now only performed after 2-minute cycles of CPR. Although a single shock by a biphasic defibrillator has a high likelihood of terminating VF, the resulting rhythm is typically a nonperfusing rhythm that therefore requires CPR in order to maintain perfusion to the heart and brain until normal cardiac contractility can resume.[19,20.] Based on the new 2005 guidelines, epinephrine is administered with the second defibrillation maneuver (and can be repeated every 3–5 minutes), and an antidysrhythmic agent is administered with the third defibrillation maneuver.

▶ ASYSTOLE AND PEA

Asystole is the most common pulseless arrest rhythm presenting to the emergency department (ED). The survival rate for children who present to the ED in asystole is dismal.

► **TABLE 26–7. RESUSCITATION MEDICATIONS—DEFIBRILLATION AND CARDIOVERSION DOSES**

Epinephrine:
  IV or IO dose (Standard Dose = SD) = 0.01 mg/kg (which equals 0.1 ml/kg of the 1:10,000 epinephrine solution)
    PEDS = SD stands for Pediatric Epinephrine Dosing Story = Slide the Decimals[18]
    Starting with the patient's weight in kg slide the decimal point one spot over to the left to determine the correct volume (milliliters) of the 1:10,000 epinephrine solution to draw up. Then after that volume (milliliters) of epinephrine is administered, slide the decimal point one more spot over to the left to document the correct amount (milligram dose) of the 1:10,000 epinephrine that was given.
  ETT dose (High Dose = HD) = 0.1 mg/kg (which equals 0.1 ml/kg of the 1:1,000 epinephrine solution)

Adenosine:
  First dose = 0.1 mg/kg IV/IO (maximum = 6 mg/dose).
  Second and subsequent doses = 0.2 mg/kg IV/IO (maximum = 12 mg/dose).
Note: Because of the extremely short half-life of adenosine, all doses must be rapidly administered followed by 10–20 mL of NS flush to rapidly get the medication into the central circulation. A proximal vein is preferred over a distal IV site.

Amiodarone (maximum = 300 mg/dose):
  VF and PVT = 5 mg/kg rapid IV/IO bolus.
  Stable VT = 5 mg/kg IV/IO slowly over 20–60 min to avoid the hypotensive effects of amiodarone.
  PSVT unresponsive to adenosine = 5 mg/kg IV/IO slowly over 20–60 min to avoid the hypotensive effects of amiodarone.
Note: Avoid the concurrent use of other medications that can also prolong the QT interval (i.e., procainamide).

Lidocaine (does not cause QT prolongation like amiodarone and procainamide):
  1 mg/kg IV/IO.

Atropine:
  0.02 mg/kg IV/IO (minimum of 0.1 mg/dose to avoid paradoxic bradycardia). Maximum single dose of 0.5 mg for a child and 1 mg for an adolescent. May repeat to a total maximum dose of 1 mg in a child and 2 mg in an adolescent.

Dextrose:
  0.5 g/kg IV/IO (Table 26–8)

Sodium bicarbonate:
  1 mEq/kg IV/IO (for severe metabolic acidosis, hyperkalemia or cyclic antidepressant toxicity).

Magnesium sulfate (maximum = 2 g/dose):
  25–50 mg/kg (rapid IV/IO push for PVT because of torsades or slowly over 10–20 min for VT with a pulse because of torsades).

Calcium chloride (10% solution = 100 mg/mL):
  20 mg/kg IV/IO (equals 0.2 mL/kg of the 10% solution) over 30–60 min.
Note: When calcium and bicarbonate are being infused in an emergent situation flush the IV line with NS after each medication to avoid the formation of an insoluble precipitate in the IV line.

Procainamide:
  15 mg/kg IV/IO over 30–60 min for stable VT or for PSVT unresponsive to adenosine.

Defibrillation:
  Start at 2 J/kg then double to 4 J/kg for second and subsequent doses.

Cardioversion:
  Start at 0.5–1 J/kg then may increase up to 2 J/kg.

Tables 26–6 and 26–7 summarize the treatment of asystole and PEA. Children who present to the ED in PEA have a slightly higher chance of survival compared to those children who present in asystole. The key management issue when confronted with a child in PEA is to rapidly and systematically identify and then correct the underlying cause of PEA. If the underlying cause of PEA is not identified and corrected, the child will not survive. The most common etiology of PEA in children is profound hypovolemia. Therefore, one should always consider a rapid fluid bolus when confronted with a child in PEA. The various etiologies of PEA are listed in Table 26–5. In addition to a much focused history and physical examination, a bedside measurement of pH, Pao_2, potassium, ion-ized calcium, and hematocrit can quickly assist the emergency physician in ruling out various etiologies of PEA.

► **SPECIAL ETIOLOGIES OF CARDIOPULMONARY ARREST AND POSTRESUSCITATION CONSIDERATIONS**

Special circumstances such as trauma, drowning, toxins, and anaphylaxis can all precipitate cardiopulmonary arrest in children. The specific management issues in these special circumstances are covered in other chapters throughout this book.

▶ **TABLE 26–8. DR. AL'S "HAWAII FIVE-O" RULE FOR THE TREATMENT OF HYPOGLYCEMIA:**[21]

A bolus of 0.5 g/kg of dextrose will raise the patient's serum glucose by approximately 60–100 mg/dL. If the child remains symptomatic after the first dose of 0.5 g/kg, the same dose may be repeated. Although $D_{10}W$ is the most commonly used dextrose solution in pediatrics, a simple method to quickly draw up 0.5 g/kg of dextrose using any of the four available dextrose solutions is as follows: (The numeric concentration of the dextrose solution) × (The number of mL/kg of that particular dextrose solution) = the number 50 always.

(Dextrose solution concentration) × (mL/kg of that solution) = 50:

    5% × 10 mL/kg

    10% × 5 mL/kg

    25% × 2 mL/kg

    50% × 1 mL/kg

Note: $D_{50}W$ solutions should first be diluted to a less concentrated solution before administration to infants and younger children.

Although a detailed description of postresuscitation care is beyond the scope of this chapter, several key points should be kept in mind. Avoid hyperthermia and treat fever aggressively. Consider the use of vasoactive medications in the postresuscitation phase because myocardial depression commonly exists in those children who survive the initial resuscitation. Avoid the routine use of hyperventilation in the postresuscitation phase unless the patient is exhibiting signs of impending cerebral herniation. Treat postresuscitation seizures aggressively and search for an underlying etiology such as hypoglycemia and various other electrolyte disturbances. Patients who remain comatose during the postresuscitation period may neurologically benefit from a brief period of hypothermia at 32°C to 34°C for 12 to 24 hours.[8] Hypoglycemia is another common problem encountered in the postresuscitation phase. Because glucose is the major metabolic substrate for the neonatal myocardium, untreated hypoglycemia can depress neonatal myocardial function.[15] A quick and easy method to rapidly calculate 0.5 g/kg of IV dextrose is listed in Table 26–7 and 26–8.[21]

REFERENCES

1. Young KD, Seidel JS. Pediatric cardiopulmonary resuscitation: a collective review. *Ann Emerg Med.* 1999;25(4):492–494.
2. Nadkarni VM, Larkin GL, Peberdy MA, et al. First documented rhythm and clinical outcome from in-hospital cardiac arrest among children and adults. *JAMA.* 2006;295:50–57.
3. International Liaison Committee on Resuscitation. 2005 International consensus on cardiopulmonary resuscitation and emergency cardiovascular care science with treatment recommendations, Part 6: pediatric basic and advanced life support. *Circulation.* 2005;112(22)(suppl 3);73–90.
4. Inaba AS. Five fingers and the five components of high quality CPR. *J Emerg Med Services.* 2006;30(11):online issue.
5. Inaba AS. Perfect teaching tool for timing compressions and it's disco! *AHA Currents in Emerg Cardiovascular Care.* 2006;17(3):7.
6. Ralston M, Hazinski MF, Zaritsky AL, et al. Recognition and management of cardiac arrest. In: *American Heart Association's PALS Provider Manual.* 2006:167.
7. Aufderheide TP, Sigurdsson G, Pirrallo RG, et al. Hyperventilation-induced hypotension during cardiopulmonary resuscitation. *Circulation.* 2004;109(16):1960–1965.
8. 2005 American Heart Association Guidelines for Cardiopulmonary Resuscitation and Emergency Cardiovascular Care. Part 12: Pediatric advanced life support. *Circulation.* 2005; 112(24)(suppl IV); 169–187.
9. Inaba AS. Wait . . . what's the weight? *Contemp Pediatr.* 1999; 16(10):193.
10. Varghese A, Vasudevan VK, Lewin S, et al. Do the length-based (Broselow) tape, APLS, Argall and Nelson's formulae accurately estimate weight of Indian children? *Indian Pediatr.* 2006;43:889–894.
11. Hofer CK, Ganter M, Tucci M, et al. How reliable is length-based determination of body weight and tracheal tube size in the pediatric age group? The Broselow tape reconsidered. *Br J Anaesth.* 2002;88(2):283–285.
12. Nieman CT, Manacci CF, Super DM, et al. Use of the Broselow tape may result in underresuscitation of children. *Acad Emerg Med.* 2006;13(10):1011–1019.
13. Yamamoto LG, Inaba AS, Young LL. Improving length-based weight estimates by adding a body habitus (obesity) icon. *Ann Emerg Med.* 2007;50(3):S61–S62.
14. Inaba AS. Cardiac disorders. In: Marx JA, Hockberger RS, Walls RM, eds. *Rosen's Emergency Medicine Concepts and Clinical Practice,* 6th ed. Philadelphia, PA: Mosby Elsevier; 2006:2584–2590.
15. Ralston M, Hazinski MF, Zaritsky AL, et al. Recognition and management of cardiac arrest. In: *American Heart Association's PALS Provider Manual.* 2006:178.
16. Ralston M, Hazinski MF, Zaritsky AL, et al. Recognition and management of bradyarrhythmias and tachyarrhythmias. In: *American Heart Association's PALS Provider Manual.* 2006:116.
17. Ralston M, Hazinski MF, Zaritsky AL, et al. Recognition and management of bradyarrhythmias and tachyarrhythmias. In: *American Heart Association's PALS Provider Manual.* 2006:124.
18. Inaba AS. PEDS = SD (Pediatric Epinephrine Dosing Story = Slide the Decimals). *AHA Currents in Emerg Cardiovascular Care.* 2008;19(30):4.
19. Ralston M, Hazinski MF, Zaritsky AL, et al. Recognition and management of cardiac arrest. In: *American Heart Association's PALS Provider Manual.* 2006:175.
20. Berg M, Clark LL, Valenzuela TD, et al. Post-shock chest compression delays with automated external defibrillator usage. *Resuscitation.* 2005;64:287–291.
21. Inaba AS. The "Hawaii Five-O" rule for IV hypoglycemia. *Contemp Pediatr.* 1999;16(10):189.

CHAPTER 27

Neonatal Resuscitation

Paul Jeremy Eakin

▶ HIGH-YIELD FACTS

- Most newly born infants will respond to adequate stimulation and warming. Very few will require advanced life support.
- Chest compressions are only initiated if there is no pulse or if the heart rate remains <60 beats/min after adequate assisted ventilation for 30 seconds.
- Only isotonic crystalloid or packed red blood cells should be used for initial volume resuscitation. Albumin-containing solutions are not recommended.
- The dose of epinephrine for the newly born infant should be 0.1 to 0.3 mL/kg of 1:10 000 solution. Higher doses of epinephrine are *not* recommended.
- When meconium-stained amniotic fluid is present, mouth and nasal suctioning after delivery of the head is no longer recommended. Intratracheal suctioning should only be performed if after delivery the infant has absent or depressed respirations, decreased muscle tone, or a heart rate <100 beats/min.
- Laryngeal mask airways may be considered for assisted ventilation in the hands of experienced providers.
- The best site to palpate for pulses in the newly born infant is the umbilicus.
- The umbilical vein is the best site for intravenous access.
- The ratio of chest compressions to ventilations in the newly born infant should be 3:1, with 90 compressions and 30 ventilations per minute.
- The recommended technique for chest compression in the newly born infant is the two-thumb-encircling hands technique.
- Epinephrine is indicated for asystole or a heart rate <60 beats/min after 30 seconds of adequate ventilation and chest compressions.

Of the nearly 4 million infants that are born in the United States each year, more than 90% will successfully transition from intrauterine life with little or no intervention. Roughly 10% will require some assistance and 1% will require more extensive resuscitation.[1] This is greatly influenced by factors such as prematurity, since premature infants are at a much higher risk for requiring resuscitation. Because of the large number of births, it is inevitable that the emergency medicine practitioner will be faced with a newly born infant in their emergency department and therefore needs to understand neonatal resuscitation. As in any critical situation in medicine, preparation and anticipation play a key role in neonatal resuscitation. This includes equipment (Table 27–1) and personnel to be ready as soon as a newly born infant presents to the emergency department. Current American Heart Association (AHA) guidelines recommend that at least one skilled provider should attend every birth in the delivery room.[2] For deliveries in the emergency department, it is preferable that at least three providers who are experienced in neonatal resuscitation should be present.[2]

▶ PHYSIOLOGY OF THE NEWLY BORN INFANT

The transition from the intrauterine environment to spontaneous breathing is a complex and dynamic physiologic event, which entails multiple cardiac and respiratory changes. During intrauterine development, the fetus has two large right-to-left shunts, one from the pulmonary artery to the aorta via the ductus arteriosus and from the right atrium to the left atrium through the patent foramen ovale. Little blood circulates through the lungs, which are fluid filled, and the fetus receives oxygen rich blood from the low resistance placenta. After birth and clamping of the umbilical cord, the infant is no longer connected to the placenta and the lungs become the only source of oxygen. Systemic blood flow increases as the pulmonary artery pressure decreases. As the infant cries and the lungs are filled with air, the amniotic fluid is absorbed into lung tissue and perfusion of the lungs is established. The ductus arteriosus begins closing stimulated by rising blood oxygen levels and more blood is shunted into the lungs.

▶ MATERNAL RISK FACTORS

Successful neonatal resuscitation depends on anticipation, preparation, and immediate support of infants who are not successfully transitioning to life outside of the womb.[1] Because births that occur outside of the delivery room are often complicated by lack of prenatal care, trauma, or prematurity, it is vital to take a focused history to guide the level of expected resuscitation.[2] Key antepartum factors to focus on include the gestation of the pregnancy, the last menstrual period, multiple gestation, and history of previous fetal or neonatal death. Maternal diabetes or hypertension also have been associated with increased perinatal morbidity. If a history of drug abuse is suspected or elicited, the practitioner can be aware of the possibility of narcotic respiratory depression or withdrawal syndrome. Intrapartum risk factors that should be addressed include prolonged rupture of membranes (>18 hours), prolonged labor

▶ TABLE 27–1. **SUPPLIES FOR NEONATAL RESUSCITATION**[3]

Resuscitation Tray (Sterile)	Resuscitation Equipment
Bulb syringe	Radiant warmer
DeLee suction trap	Wall suction with manometer
Endotracheal tubes (2.0, 2.5, 3.0, 3.5, and 4.0 mm)	Oxygen source with flow meter
Suction catheters (6, 8, 10, and 12F catheter)	Resuscitation bag (250–500 mL) with manometer
Endotracheal tube stylet	Laryngoscope
Umbilical catheter (3.5, 5F catheter)	Laryngoscope blades (Miller 0 and 1)
Syringes (5, 10, and 20 mL)	Charts with proper drug doses and equipment sizes for various sized neonates.
Three-way stopcock	Warmed linens
Feeding tubes (5, 8F catheter)	
Towels	
Umbilical cord clamps	
Scissors	

(>24 hours), meconium stained or foul smelling amniotic fluid, bleeding, and prolapsed umbilical cord.[2]

▶ NEWLY BORN INFANTS REQUIRING RESUSCITATION

The current AHA neonatal resuscitation guidelines describes a rapid observational tool, which can be used to identify which newly born infants will not need to be resuscitated.[1] This tool consists of four questions:

- Was the baby born after a full-term gestation?
- Is the amniotic fluid clear of meconium and without evidence of infection?
- Is the baby breathing and crying?
- Does the baby have good muscle tone?

If the answer to all of the questions is yes, the infant will likely not require significant resuscitation. If the answer to any of these questions is no, then resuscitation may be required.

The actions undertaken during resuscitation should occur in an orderly manner as described by the AHA (Fig. 27–1). These include initial steps in stabilization, ventilation, chest compressions, and administration of epinephrine or volume expansion. The heart rate, respiratory effort, and color are monitored closely and guide the decision to escalate the level of resuscitation.

▶ ASSESSMENT OF NEWLY BORN INFANT

The Apgar score is a method of objectively measuring the newborn's condition and response to resuscitation. The Apgar

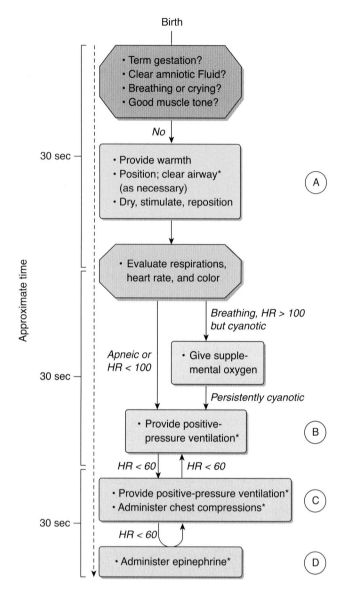

* Endotracheal intubation may be considered at several steps.

Figure 27–1. Algorithm for neonatal resuscitation. (With permission from *Textbook of Neonatal Resuscitation*. 5th ed. American Academy of Pediatrics and American Heart Assocation; 2006.)

score is normally assigned at 1 minute and again at 5 minutes, based on the infant's respirations, heart rate (best evaluated by palpating the umbilicus), color, muscle tone, and reflex irritability (Table 27–2). Each category receives a score of 0 to 2 and the five categories are summed to give a maximum score of 10. If the 5-minute Apgar score is less than 7, then additional scores should be made every 5 minutes up to 20 minutes. It is very important to note that the Apgar score is not used to determine the need for resuscitation or to guide the resuscitation efforts and the resuscitation must not be delayed for the purpose of tabulating the Apgar score. Neonates with a 1-minute Apgar score >7 require minimal resuscitation other than drying and stimulation. Scores between 4 to 6

▶ TABLE 27–2. **THE APGAR SCORE**[3]

Parameter	Score 0	Score 1	Score 2
Color	Blue, pale	Body pink, extremities blue	Totally pink
Muscle tone	None, limp	Slight flexion	Active, good flexion
Heart rate (beats/min)	0	<100	>100
Respiration	Absent	Slow, irregular	Strong, regular
Reflex irritability (response to nasal catheter)	None	Some grimace	Good grimace, crying

To calculate Apgar score, add numbers for all parameters together.

indicate that mild to moderate asphyxia has occurred and more vigorous resuscitation may be needed, including supplemental oxygen and vigorous stimulation. One-minute Apgar scores <3 indicated moderate to severe asphyxia and aggressive resuscitation should be started immediately.[3]

▶ RESUSCITATION

POSITIONING OF THE NEWBORN

After delivery, the infant should be dried with warm towels and placed supine under a radiant warmer. The head should be put into a "sniffing" position and oral and nasal suctioning should be performed with a bulb syringe or suction catheter (Fig. 27–2). This position aligns the posterior pharynx, larynx, and trachea and allows for unimpeded air entry. Excessive extension or flexion of the neck may result in airway occlusion.

TEMPERATURE CONTROL

Newborns are at risk for hypothermia following delivery because of their large surface area to mass ratio as well as evaporative heat loss. Hypothermia can lead to hypoglycemia, increased oxygen consumption and if severe, respiratory depression, and acidosis. This can be avoided by careful drying of the infant with warm towels and placing the infant under a radiant heat source. Very low-birth-weight infants (<1500 g)

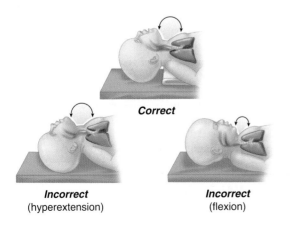

Correct

Incorrect
(hyperextension)

Incorrect
(flexion)

Figure 27–2. Sniffing position.

are particularly prone to hypothermia and may need to be placed under plastic wrapping to avoid evaporative loss.[1] Continual monitoring of temperature is very important, because hyperthermia can have deleterious effects such as worsening ischemic brain injury. Some research suggests that modest cerebral hypothermia may be beneficial in patients with suspected asphyxia, but more research is needed to determine the scope of potential benefit.[1]

STIMULATION

For vigorous newborns, drying and suctioning of the mouth is usually adequate stimulation as evidenced by increased heart rate and respiratory effort. If the infant does not have adequate respirations, flicking the soles of the feet or rubbing the infant's trunk may be needed.[1] If the newborn does not respond to this tactile stimulation, positive pressure breaths (PPV) may be initiated.

OXYGEN

Free-flow oxygen should be provided to all infants with central cyanosis (evidenced by cyanosis of the mouth and tongue) even mild respiratory distress.[1] Acrocyanosis, which is cyanosis of the hands and feet, represents peripheral vasoconstriction and is not an indication for oxygen. Oxygen is administered at 5 L/min using a face mask or flow inflating bag mask held over the infant's nose and mouth. Research has raised concerns about the possible toxicity of 100% oxygen administered to neonates.[4] Until further research clarifies this toxicity, 100% oxygen should be used during neonatal resuscitation.[1]

VENTILATION

The normal newborn breathes spontaneously within seconds of birth and establishes regular respirations within the first minute of life. PPV is indicated if the infant remains apneic or gasping, the heart rate is <100 beats/min after 30 seconds of initial resuscitation, or has central cyanosis despite supplemental oxygen.[1]

Ventilation is performed using either cushioned mask with a flow inflating bag or a T-piece connector. 100% oxygen is utilized for PPV, although some studies have shown that room air PPV may be just as effective. If only room air PPV is available, this should be initiated until an oxygen source can be

▶ **TABLE 27–3. ENDOTRACHEAL TUBE SIZING[1]**

Tube Size (mm) (Internal Diameter)	Weight (g)	Gestational Age (wk)
2.5	Below 1000	Below 28
3.0	1000–2000	28–34
3.5	2000–3000	34–38
3.5–4.0	Above 3000	Above 38

From *Textbook of Neonatal Resuscitation*. American Academy of Pediatrics and American Heart Assocation. 5th ed. 2006.

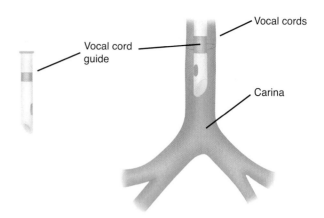

Figure 27–3. Vocal cord guide for correct intubation depth.

provided. The mask must make a tight seal over the nose and mouth and the pop-off valve may need to be bypassed because of the high peak inspiratory pressures needed for the initial breaths. Peak pressures up to 40 cm H_2O may be necessary because of the "stiff" fluid filled lungs of newborns. After the initial breaths, the fluid will begin to be expressed from the lungs and lower pressures can be utilized. It is important to use the lowest pressure that will adequately give chest rise to avoid iatrogenic pneumothorax. Bag-mask ventilation at 40 to 60 breaths/min is continued for 30 seconds and the infant is then reassessed. Assisted ventilation can be discontinued once the heart rate is >100 beats/min, the infant is breathing spontaneously and improvements in color and tone are seen. If the heart rate remains <100 beats/min, assisted ventilation is continued. If the heart rate remains <60 beats/min, despite assisted ventilation, chest compressions are initiated and the infant should be intubated.[1]

ENDOTRACHEAL INTUBATION

There are several indications for endotracheal intubation during neonatal resuscitation.[1] These include poor response to or the inability to provide adequate PPV, the need for endotracheal suctioning or chest compressions, extreme prematurity, or suspected diaphragmatic hernia. The size of the endotracheal tube depends on the weight or gestation of the newly born infant (Table 27–3). A laryngoscope with a straight blade is utilized, using a 0 or 1 blade. Successful endotracheal intubation is evidenced by bilateral chest rise and improvement in heart rate, color, and muscle tone. The use of an end tidal carbon dioxide monitor can assist with confirmation of proper tube placement, even in very low-birth-weight infants. Care must be made not to advance the ET tube too far, which will result in mainstem bronchus intubation. If this occurs, the result will be diminished breath sounds over half of the chest. The tube should be slowly withdrawn, until equal bilateral breath sounds are auscultated. Most endotracheal tubes have a black guide line that should be place adjacent to the vocal cords, resulting in proper depth of intubation (Fig. 27–3). A rough formula[2] for depth of intubation is as follows:

Depth of tube insertion at gums (in cm) = 6 + infant's weight (in kg)

The oxygen saturation should be monitored after intubation, as well observing for any evidence of pneumothorax.

LARYNGEAL MASK AIRWAYS

Laryngeal mask airways (LMA) are ventilation devices that are placed into the infant's airway and fit over the laryngeal inlet. They have been shown to be effective for ventilation of term or near-term newborns. They may be considered for assisted ventilation of infants, where bag-mask ventilation or intubation have been unsuccessful. LMAs should only be used by providers experienced in their use.[1]

CHEST COMPRESSIONS

Chest compressions are rarely needed in the resuscitation of all but the most critical of newly born infants. They are indicated when the heart rate remains <60 beats/min, despite 30 seconds of effective positive pressure ventilation.[1] Practitioners much ensure that adequate ventilation is occurring while chest compressions are being given. There are two different techniques for administering chest compressions (Fig. 27–4). One is the two finger technique, where two fingers (usually the middle and ring finger) are used to deliver the compression while the other hand supports the back. The more effective technique is the two thumb-circling hand technique. Here, two thumbs deliver the compression, with the provider's hands encircling the infant and supporting the back. This technique is recommended because it may deliver higher peak systolic and coronary perfusion pressure.[1] Compressions should be given over the lower third of the sternum to a depth of roughly one-third the diameter of the chest cavity (Fig. 27–5). There should be a 3:1 compression to ventilation ratio with ventilation and compression coordinated to avoid simultaneous delivery There should be 120 events/min (90 compressions and 30 ventilations) resulting in an event roughly twice a second. Every 30 seconds, respiratory effort, color, pulse, and muscle tone should be reassessed. Chest compressions and ventilations can be discontinued when the heart rate is >60 beats/min.

INTRAVENOUS ACCESS

For infants who require volume expansion or epinephrine, intravenous access is necessary. The umbilical vein is the

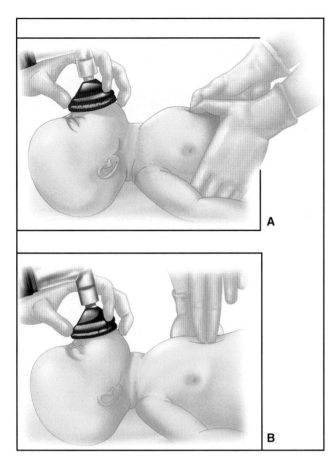

Figure 27–4. Chest compression techniques. (A) Thumb-circling hand technique and (B) two-finger technique.

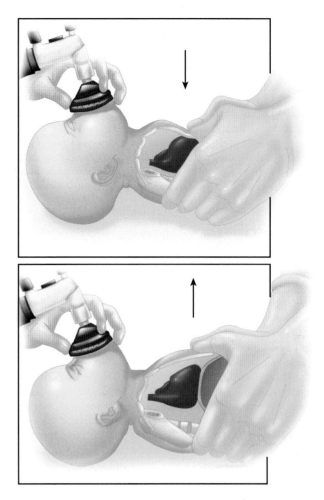

Figure 27–5. Correct depth of chest compressions.

preferred route for intravenous access in the newly born, because it is easily identified and large enough for rapid catheter insertion.[2] The umbilical vein can be identified as a thin walled structure usually in the 11- or 12-o'clock position in the umbilical cord. Conversely, the umbilical arteries are two thicker walled vessels lying in the 4- to 8-o'clock position (rarely will a neonate have only one umbilical artery). After cleaning the umbilical cord and using aseptic technique, the cord is cut 1 to 2 cm above the skin line, perpendicular to the cord. A 3.5 or 5F umbilical catheter can be advanced 2 to 4 cm or until blood can be easily aspirated from the catheter (Fig. 27–6). Deeper

advancement of the catheter should be avoided because of the risk of infusing hypertonic solution into the liver. Once the line is adequately in place, it should be sutured to avoid accidental removal. Intraosseous line placement may be pursued if other attempts at access have been unsuccessful.[2] The site for placement is the medial aspect of the proximal tibia, just distal to the tibial tuberosity. Because the neonatal intraosseous space is quite small, it might be useful to attempt access with a 20- or 22-gauge spinal needle.

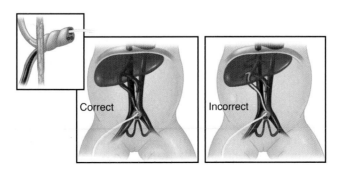

Figure 27–6. Correct placement of umbilical venous catheter.

► MEDICATIONS

Medications are rarely needed in the resuscitation of newborn infants. One large series demonstrated that medications were required in only 0.15% of 15 000 deliveries.[6] Bradycardia in the newly born is usually secondary to inadequate ventilation or hypoxemia and establishing effective ventilation should be the focus during resuscitation. If the heart rate remains <60 beats/min despite effective ventilation and chest compressions, then epinephrine or volume expansion may be indicated. Other agents including bicarbonate or narcotic antagonists may rarely be used during prolonged resuscitation.

EPINEPHRINE

Epinephrine is the most important drug used in infant resuscitation.[1] It is indicated in asystole and in bradycardia with a heart rate less than 60 after 30 seconds of effective ventilation with 100% oxygen and chest compressions. The recommended IV dose is 0.1 to 0.3 mL/kg (0.01 to 0.03 mg/kg) per dose of 1:10 000 solution. Higher IV doses are not recommended from studies in animals that showed exaggerated hypertension, decreased myocardial function and worse neurologic function after doses in the range of 0.1 mg/kg.[7] The preferred route is IV, although the endotracheal route can be used if IV access has not been established. There is evidence that the standard IV dose given endotracheally is likely inadequate. If the endotracheal route is used, a higher dose may be considered (up to 0.1 mg/kg) but this has not been studied in human subjects and the safety and efficacy are unknown.[8] Epinephrine can be repeated every 3 to 5 minutes, reassessing the patient carefully between doses.

VOLUME EXPANSION

The indication for using volume expansion in neonatal resuscitation is hypovolemia or hypovolemic shock.[1] Some of the conditions that may lead to hypovolemic shock include placental abruption, placenta previa, trauma, avulsed umbilical cord, or premature cord clamping. Babies in shock appear pale, have weak pulses, and delayed capillary refill. Often, they will not respond adequately to well-administered resuscitation and have persistent bradycardia. Volume expansion is given in aliquots of 10 mL/kg over 5 to 10 minutes. The acute treatment of hypovolemia is initiated with normal saline or lactated Ringer's solution, followed by packed red blood cells if there is a large volume blood loss or a poor response to the crystalloid solution. Uncross-matched O-negative blood should be administered if a full type and cross-match cannot be obtained in a timely fashion.

GLUCOSE

Low blood glucose has been associated with adverse neurologic events in animal models of asphyxia and resuscitation.[1] Hypoglycemia is often seen in premature infants and infants born to diabetic mothers. Acute signs of hypoglycemia include jitteriness, seizures, and decreased level of consciousness.[3] Infants who are symptomatic or require significant resuscitation should have their glucose levels monitored and glucose should be administered to maintain normoglycemia (>50 mg/dL). The dose of glucose is 2 to 4 mL/kg of $D_{10}W$ given intravenously. Higher concentrations should be avoided because they may lead to hyperosmolality and increased risk of intraventricular hemorrhage.[2] Until the infant is stabilized and feedings are established, glucose should be infused at a rate of 6 to 8 mg/kg/min.

SODIUM BICARBONATE

Sodium bicarbonate is a hydrogen ion buffer that aids in the reversal of metabolic acidosis, but it plays a limited role in acute neonatal resuscitation as it may contribute to respiratory acidosis.[3] It may be helpful during prolonged resuscitation for the treatment of hyperkalemia or metabolic acidosis after adequate ventilation has been established. The dose of sodium bicarbonate is 1 to 2 mEq/kg (4.2% solution) given slowly IV over 2 minutes.

NALOXONE

Naloxone is a direct narcotic antagonist used to reverse respiratory depression because of narcotic exposure.[1] This effect can be observed if maternal narcotics were administered within 4 hours of delivery. The current dosing recommendation for naloxone is 0.1 mg/kg given either intravenously or intramuscularly.[1] Intratracheal administration of naloxone is not supported by current recommendations[1] Naloxone should not be given if there is maternal history of long-term narcotic abuse because severe acute withdrawal syndrome and seizures can occur.[3]

ATROPINE

Atropine is not indicated for neonatal resuscitation.[2] The mechanism of atropine is to block parasympathetic mediated vagal reflex and bradycardia. Because this is not the cause of bradycardia in neonatal resuscitation, the use of atropine is not recommended.

► SPECIAL SITUATIONS

MECONIUM

Meconium stained amniotic fluids complicates approximately 13% of live born births.[9] A smaller percentage (5%–12%) of these infants go on to develop meconium aspiration syndrome, which ranges in severity from mild respiratory distress to respiratory arrest and severe pulmonary hypertension.[9] The likelihood of meconium stained fluid is much higher in infants who are postmature or have in utero fetal distress.

The management of infants born through meconium stained fluids underwent a major paradigm shift based on a multicenter study in 2000, which demonstrated that endotracheal suction of meconium was not helpful for vigorous infants (strong respiratory effort, HR >100, and good muscle

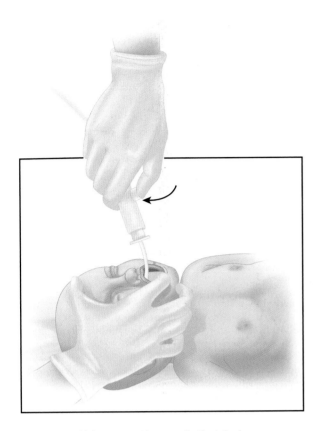

Figure 27-7. Using meconium aspiration device.

tone).[8] Recent recommendations no longer advise routine obstetrical suctioning of the oropharynx and nasopharynx after deliver of the head for infants born through meconium stained fluid. Further management following delivery is based on the activity of the infant, not the consistency of the meconium. Vigorous newly born infants do not require endotracheal suctioning of meconium.[9] This should be performed only on depressed infants (absent or depressed respirations, heart rate <100 beats/min, and poor muscle tone). The technique is to visualize the trachea using a laryngoscope, intubate the trachea and then suction the meconium by attaching the ET tube to wall suction (Fig. 27–7). Multiple attempts and fresh ET tubes may be necessary if the meconium is especially thick or adherent. The infant's clinical status needs to be monitored very closely during these attempts and positive pressure ventilation should be instituted if the infant becomes severely depressed or bradycardic.[1]

PREMATURITY

The definition of prematurity is up to 37 weeks of gestation. The premature infant represents a unique challenge in resuscitation because of multiple differences in their physiology and development.[1] Close involvement with skilled neonatology providers is crucial to providing good outcomes in resuscitation. Their lungs are often undeveloped and as a result of lack of surfactant may be very difficult to ventilate. The chest wall is very compliant and with less muscle mass, the premature infant will fatigue rapidly as they try to maintain their respiratory status. Often, intubation is needed to support ventilation and to provide a route to administer surfactant. Premature infants are particularly prone to hypothermia and cold stress because of their immature skin and larger surface area to body–mass ratio. Great care must be taken to minimize heat loss with radiant heaters, warm blankets, and plastic membranes. They are also very prone to intraventricular hemorrhage because of the extremely fragile nature of the subependymal germinal matrix. Rapid changes in blood pressure, intravascular volume, and osmolality should be avoided to minimize the risk of intraventricular hemorrhage.

Medical technology has pushed the limits of viability for premature infants to never-before-seen levels. However, the decision to withhold resuscitation is a very complex issue, both medically and ethically even when all information is readily available. Unfortunately, this is often not an option for the emergency medicine practitioner. Resuscitation should be pursued when an infant is born with spontaneous heart rate and respirations. The decision to withdraw care can be considered if there are no signs of life (no heart beat or respiratory effort) after 10 minutes of continuous and adequate resuscitation.[1]

DIAPHRAGMATIC HERNIA

Diaphragmatic hernia occurs when there is a defect in the diaphragm (usually on the left side), giving rise to displacement of the lung by abdominal contents entering the chest cavity. The infant with this condition will be in respiratory distress, cyanotic, and often has a scaphoid abdomen. This is a true neonatal emergency and needs to be addressed promptly. A gastric tube should be placed to decompress the stomach and oxygen should be administered. Prompt intubation and positive pressure ventilation is usually required and bag-mask ventilation should be avoided because it will lead to gastric distension and respiratory compromise.

OMPHALOCELE/GASTROSCHISIS

Congenital defects of the umbilical ring result in herniation of abdominal contents into the amniotic fluid and can be identified on prenatal ultrasound. Omphalocele describes herniation within the umbilical cord where intestinal contents may be covered by a thin layer of peritoneum. Cardiovascular malformations are often seen with this disorder. Gastroschisis describes a herniation adjacent to the umbilical cord (usually to the right) and the abdominal contents will easily be visualized outside of the newborn's body. Both of these conditions are very prone to evaporative fluid and heat loss, which may result in hypovolemic shock. To prevent this, saline-soaked gauze and a sterile plastic bag should be placed over the protruded abdominal contents. Intravenous access should be obtained and fluid resuscitation initiated. A gastric tube should be placed and pediatric surgery should be consulted. The patient should be transferred to a tertiary center with a neonatal intensive care unit. The repair is a staged procedure to allow for adequate intra-abdominal space to accommodate the protruded abdominal contents.

PNEUMOTHORAX

Pneumothorax is reported to occur in 1% to 2% of term newborns and is often asymptomatic. In the context of neonatal resuscitation and positive pressure ventilation, pneumothorax can rapidly lead to tension pneumothorax and potentially lethal cardiorespiratory compromise. Premature infants and infants with meconium aspiration syndrome are at a higher risk for pneumothorax. Infants with this condition will be tachypneic, retracting, grunting, and tachycardic. As the tension pneumothorax progresses, the infant may become bradycardic and have symptoms of shock. It may be difficult to localize the affected lung based on auscultation, but illumination may be helpful. If this condition is suspected and significant respiratory distress is present, needle decompression is indicated. This can be performed using a 20-gauge needle antiseptically advanced into the affected lung field either in the fourth intercostal space in the anterior axillary line or the second intercostal space in the midclavicular line. This will decompress pressure in the pleural cavity and should result in relief of the cardiorespiratory compromise.[2]

INFANT OF A DIABETIC MOTHER

Infants born to a mother with glucose intolerance are exposed in utero to increased glucose levels, and respond accordingly with elevated insulin production. This makes the infant prone to multiple complications including hypoglycemia, polycythemia, respiratory distress, intrapartum asphyxia, birth defects, and large for gestational age. Cesarean section is often necessary because of the infant's macrosomia. Following delivery, these infants need to be monitored very closely for hypoglycemia and respiratory distress.

REFERENCES

1. 2005 American Heart Association. Guidelines for cardiopulmonary resuscitation and emergency cardiovascular care. Part 13: Neonatal resuscitation guidelines. *Circulation.* 2005; 112(24)(suppl 4):188–195.
2. Alessandrini EA. Neonatal resuscitation. In: Fleisher GR, Ludwig S, Henretig FM, eds. *Textbook of Pediatric Emergency Medicine.* Philadelphia, PA: Lippincott Williams & Wilkins; 2006:35–49.
3. Goto CG, Bates B. Resuscitation of the newly born infant. In: Strange GR, Ahrens WR, Lelyveld S, Schafermeyer RW, eds. *Pediatric Emergency Medicine: A Comprehensive Study Guide.* New York, NY: McGraw-Hill; 2002:37–44.
4. Richmond S, Goldsmith JP. Air or 100% Oxygen in Neonatal Resuscitation? *Clin Perinatol.* 2006;33:11–27.
5. American Academy of Pediatrics and American Heart Assocation. *Textbook of Neonatal Resuscitation.* 5th ed.2006.
6. Perlman JM, Risser R. Cardiopulmonary resuscitation in the delivery room. *Arch Pediatr Adolesc Med.* 1995;149:20–25.
7. Wyckoff MH, Perlman JM. Use of High-Dose epinephrine and sodium bicarbonate during neonatal resuscitation: is there proven benefit? *Clin Perinatol.* 2006;33:141–151.
8. Wyckoff MH, Wyllie J. Endotracheal delivery of medications during neonatal resuscitation. *Clin Perinatol.* 206;33:153–160.
9. Wiswell TE, Gannon CM, Jacob J, et al. Delivery room management of the apparently vigorous meconium-stained neonate: results of the multicenter, international collaborative trial. *Pediatrics.* 2000;105:1–7.

SECTION IV

TRAUMA

CHAPTER 28

Evaluation and Management of the Multiple Trauma Patient

Michael J. Gerardi

▶ HIGH-YIELD FACTS

- Injury is the leading cause of death of children in the United States.
- Children have physiologic and psychologic responses to trauma that are different from those seen in adults.
- The airway is secured while concomitantly stabilizing the neck. The jaw thrust maneuver is used to open the airway and the oropharynx is cleared of debris and secretions.
- Orotracheal intubation is the most reliable means of securing an airway. An uncuffed tube should be used in children <8 years of age.
- *Hypovolemic shock* is caused by blood loss, which makes up 8% to 9% of the body weight of a child. Determining the extent of volume depletion and shock is difficult in children and multiple parameters must be used.
- Vascular access is difficult under the best of circumstances and can be a reason for delay in transport of a critically ill child. Attempt vascular access en route to avoid prolonged stay at the scene. Intraosseous infusion should be used as a quick access for crystalloid infusion if attempts at intravenous cannulation are unsuccessful after 90 seconds.
- For shock, the initial resuscitative fluid is isotonic crystalloid solution, such as normal saline or Ringer's lactate. Give an initial infusion of 20 mL/kg as rapidly as possible.
- Urinary output may help assess perfusion and intravascular status. Insert a Foley catheter and monitor urinary output as follows: 1 mL/kg/h for children >1 year of age and 2 mL/kg/h for children <1 year of age.
- Unique characteristics of the pediatric cervical spine predispose it to ligamentous disruption and dislocation injuries without radiographic evidence of bone injury.

Injury is the leading cause of death in children in the United States and causes more deaths than all other causes combined.[1] In 2004, trauma accounted for 59.5% of all deaths in children younger than 18 years and those caused by injuries, intentional or unintentional, account for more years of potential life lost than do deaths attributable to sudden infant death syndrome, cancer, and infectious diseases combined.[2] Overall, mortality from pediatric trauma occurs at one-third of the rate of adult trauma deaths, pediatric case–fatality rates are higher when compared with adults who have similar injuries. Eighty percent of their trauma deaths occur either at the scene or prior to admission.

Mortality data alone does not reveal the profound impact of trauma. Each year, 20% of American children receive medical care for an injury. For children <14 years of age, injuries are the leading cause of visits to emergency departments (EDs), numbering 7.9 million, and the second leading cause of hospitalization, accounting for >200 000 admissions. The health care costs for injury are staggering. Unintentional injuries resulted in an estimated $14 billion in lifetime medical spending, $1 billion in other resource costs, and $66 billion in present and future work losses.[3] Even minor injuries can have lasting effects causing functional impairment or subtle cognitive or behavioral deficits years after the acute traumatic event. Therefore, physical, emotional, and psychologic needs of the child and family must be considered.

▶ NATURE OF INJURIES AND UNIQUE PEDIATRIC ASPECTS

The blunt trauma is the predominant mechanism in children, with only 10% to 20% suffering a penetrating injury. Motor vehicle crashes (MVCs) account for as many as half of all childhood trauma deaths. These MVC death rates begin to climb steeply at 13 years and peak at 18 years. Falls from heights and falls against fixed objects account for 25% to 30% of deaths; drowning, 10% to 15%; and burns, 5% to 10%. Boys are injured twice as frequently as girls. Other major causes of death are homicide, suicide, drowning, pedestrian/motor vehicle collisions, and burns, with the relative risk for each type of injury varying by age group (Table 28–1).

Infants (birth to 12 months), toddlers (1–3 years), and preschoolers (3–5 years) are at greatest risk from falls. They have a proportionally larger head and a higher center of gravity. They sustain a higher proportion of isolated closed-head injuries. Infants and toddlers are also at risk of child abuse.

School-age children (6–12 years of age) are most commonly victims of unintentional trauma, especially motor vehicle-related trauma, as pedestrians, bicyclists, or unrestrained passengers. They also sustain a large number of closed-head injuries, often in association with other injuries. Adolescents (13–19 years of age) engage in many risk-taking behaviors, and are at risk for homicide and suicide. They require treatment considerations that combine psychologic requirements of a child with the physical needs of an adult.

▶ TABLE 28–1. LEADING CAUSES OF TRAUMA IN CHILDREN BY AGE GROUP

<1 y	1–4 y	5–9 y	10–14 y
Suffocation	Motor vehicle traffic	Motor vehicle traffic	Motor vehicle traffic
Motor vehicle traffic	Drowning and submersion	Drowning and submersion	Drowning and submersion
Drowning and submersion	Fire and burn	Fire and burn	Fire and burn
Fire and burn	Suffocation	Suffocation	Suffocation

Children have physiologic and psychologic responses to trauma that are different from those seen in adults. An understanding of these anatomic, physiologic, and psychologic differences is a fundamental tenet in providing appropriate, expert care for children. Kinetic energy from injury is distributed over a smaller area and impacts a greater proportion of the total body volume. Musculoskeletal compliance is greater in children and they have less protective muscle and subcutaneous tissue. The increased flexibility and resilience of the pediatric skeleton and surrounding tissues permits external forces to be transmitted to the deeper internal structures. Always consider the possibility of internal injury, even in the absence of external signs of trauma.

Since a child's head represents a larger percentage of total body mass than that of an adult, head injuries are common in children and account for a large percentage of serious morbidity and mortality. The head is also a major source of heat loss in a child. The occiput is more prominent in young children and decrease in prominence from birth until approximately 10 years of age. Take this into account when positioning the head for intubation and airway management. The bony sutures are open at birth—they gradually fuse by 18 to 24 months of age. Palpation of the fontanels can provide useful information regarding intracranial pressure (ICP). The child's brain, having a higher percentage of white matter than gray matter, may have greater resilience in withstanding blunt trauma. However, it is more susceptible to axonal shearing forces and cerebral edema.

A child's neck is shorter and supports a relatively heavier weight than an adult's, making it especially vulnerable to forces of trauma and sudden movements. A younger child's short, fat neck makes it difficult to evaluate neck veins and tracheal position.

The most dramatic and critical differences between children and adults are in the airway (Table 28–2). A child's larynx is located in a more cephalad and anterior position. In addition, the epiglottis is tilted almost 45 degrees in a child and is more floppy, making manipulation and visualization for intubation more difficult. Unlike the adult, where the glottis is the narrowest portion of the upper airway, the cricoid cartilage is the narrowest portion of the child's airway. This fact, plus the abundant loose columnar epithelium, limits the size of the endotracheal tube and is the reason that uncuffed tubes are frequently used in children younger than 8 years of age.

The pediatric thorax is more pliable because of flexible ribs and cartilage and there is less overlying fat and muscle. This allows a greater amount of blunt force to be transmitted to underlying tissues. The diaphragmatic muscle is much more distensible in a child. A child's mediastinum is also very mobile. Therefore, the mediastinum and abdominal organs are subject to sudden, wide excursions that can be dramatically seen, such as in tension pneumothorax.

The diaphragm inserts at a nearly horizontal angle from birth until approximately 12 years of age, in contrast to the oblique insertion in the adult. This, in effect, causes abdominal organs to be more exposed and less protected by ribs and muscle. Therefore, apparent insignificant forces can cause serious internal injury. Young children are primarily diaphragmatic or "belly" breathers, making them dependent on diaphragmatic excursion for ventilation.

The spleen and the liver are in a more caudal and anterior position. Even though the increased elasticity and compliance of a child's connective tissue and suspensory ligaments should protect these organs, they are actually more subject to injury because of the increased motion at impact.

▶ TABLE 28–2. COMPARISON OF INFANT AND ADULT AIRWAYS

	Infant	Adult
Head	Large, prominent occiput, assumes sniffing position when supine	Flat occiput
Tongue	Relatively larger	Relatively smaller
Larynx	Cephalad position, opposite C2–3	Opposite C4–6
Epiglottis	"Ω" or "U" shaped, soft	Flat, flexible
Vocal cords	Short, concave	Horizontal
Smallest diameter	Cricoid ring, below cords	Vocal cords
Cartilage	Soft	Firm
Lower airways	Smaller, less developed	Larger, more cartilage

Source: Used with permission from Gausche M, Yamamoto L, eds. *APLS: The Pediatric Emergency Medicine Resource.* Elk Grove Village, IL; Dallas, TX: American Academy of Pediatrics; American College of Emergency Physicians; 2005.

Long bones in children differ from the adult because of the presence of growth plates or epiphyses and increased compliance (see Chapter 35). The epiphyseal–metaphyseal junctions are relatively weak and ligaments are stronger than the growth plate. This weakness predisposes a child to disturbances of the growth plate. The Salter–Harris classification system was created to assist in the diagnosis and management of such injuries. Increased compliance of bone results in significant absorption of energy without radiographic signs of fracture even though there is bony damage. Therefore, the physical examination is often more sensitive than radiographs for growth plate and long bone fractures. Blood supply to bones can also be easily disrupted, resulting in limb length disparity.

▶ PEDIATRIC TRAUMA SYSTEMS

The differences in mechanisms and patterns of injury observed in early childhood, late childhood, and adolescence, together with immature anatomic features and the developing physiologic functions of the pediatric patient, result in unique responses to major trauma, which in turn drive the need for specialized pediatric resources. Therefore, the injured pediatric patient has special needs that may be provided optimally at a children's hospital with demonstrated expertise in and commitment to both pediatric and trauma care. Geographic areas with access to a pediatric trauma center should integrate them into the regional trauma system through invited participation, appropriate field triage, and interfacility transport of the most critically injured children. When a pediatric trauma center, whether freestanding or affiliated with an adult trauma center, is not available, this role should be fulfilled by the adult trauma center with the largest volume of pediatric patients.[4-6]

▶ PREHOSPITAL CARE ISSUES

Considerations in the field care of the traumatized child include endotracheal intubation, IV access, immobilization, and rapid transport. Which procedures should be attempted in the field is controversial. The prehospital success rate for endotracheal intubation varies from 48% to 89%. It has been demonstrated that trauma deaths can be reduced by 25% when a system provides personnel trained to perform airway management and develops guidelines for ground versus aeromedical transport. Rural systems may require more aggressive initial treatment in the field because of transport times that are three to four times greater than those in urban areas. Regionalized trauma care is generally believed to confer benefits to the injured patients.

Vascular access is a difficult procedure under the best of circumstances and is often a reason for delay in transport of a critically ill child. It is reasonable for traumatized children to be transported immediately without vascular access if a short transport time is expected. Vascular access can be attempted en route to avoid prolonged scene time. Intraosseous (IO) infusion (Fig. 28–1) should be used as a quick access for crystalloid infusion if attempts at intravenous cannulation are unsuccess-

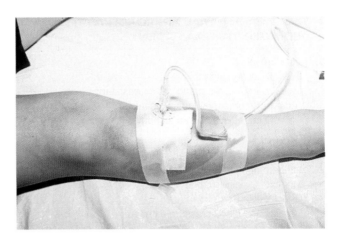

Figure 28–1. IO lines can be used to ensure adequate oxygenation.

ful after 90 seconds. IO lines can be placed successfully in the field 80% of the time.[7]

▶ INITIAL ASSESSMENT AND MANAGEMENT GUIDELINES FOR THE INJURED CHILD

The highest priority in caring for an injured child is identifying and treating life-threatening injuries immediately. The next priority is identifying injuries requiring operative intervention. Finally, the child is examined for non–life-threatening injuries and initiating specific therapy (Table 28–3). Because of the closing of many hospitals in the United States, the remaining EDs will receive an increased volume trauma. Thus, emergency physicians must be well versed in the initial care of these patients and work closely with their surgical colleagues (Fig. 28–2). There are recognized criteria for transferring a patient to a trauma center or activating an in-house trauma team (Tables 28–4 and 28–5).

Equipment tables should be readily available in the resuscitation room as an aid in determining tube and catheter sizes. As an alternative, the Broselow tape or similar system can be used to ensure the use of properly sized equipment.

The *primary survey* and initial *resuscitation,* occurs simultaneously, usually during the first 5 to 10 minutes and focuses on diagnosing and treating life-threatening disorders.[7,8] The *secondary survey* continues with a more thorough physical examination and diagnostic testing. It is an anatomic survey that evaluates in a timely, directed fashion, each body area from head to toe. In this fashion, life-threatening injuries are promptly recognized before proceeding to less urgent problems. Children with serious injuries require continual reassessment. Repeat vital signs should be performed every 5 minutes during the primary survey and every 15 minutes while in the ED awaiting transfer or operative intervention.

PRIMARY SURVEY[9,10]

The primary survey includes evaluation of the airway, stabilization of the cervical spine (C-spine), adequacy of breathing,

▶ **TABLE 28-3. INITIAL APPROACH TO THE PEDIATRIC TRAUMA PATIENT**

1. Before arrival
    Prepare all equipment
    Mobilize trauma team and call for assistance (respiratory therapy, nurses, radiology technician)
    Have O-negative blood on standby

2. First 5 min
    Assess respiration, oxygenation; ventilate if necessary
    Intubate or attain surgical airway if indicated
    Maintain C-spine immobilization
    Check pulse oximetry reading
    Cardiac and blood pressure monitoring
    Consider end-tidal CO_2 monitoring if available
    Perform needle or tube thoracostomy if tension pneumothorax suspected
    Treat obvious wounds: Apply pressure to external hemorrhage; dressing to sucking chest wound

3. Second 5 min
    Reassess airway, ventilation, oxygenation, temperature
    Evaluate level of consciousness/neurologic status
    Assess perfusion
    Volume resuscitation: 20 mL/kg with crystalloid and repeat as necessary
    Consider uncross-matched or O-negative blood
    Send laboratory specimens: Type and cross, CBC, amylase, liver transaminases, BUN, creatinine, glucose, electrolytes, ABG, urinalysis
    Needle pericardiocentesis, thoracotomy, and aortic clamping if indicated
    Nasogastric tube, urinary catheter

4. Next 10 min/secondary survey
    Reassess airway, ventilation, oxygenation, perfusion, neurologic status, and disability
    Assess head, neck, chest, abdomen, pelvis, neurologic examination, extremities
    Tube thoracostomy if indicated
    Reduce vascular-compromising dislocations
    Administer drugs: Tetanus toxoid, antibiotics, analgesics, sedatives
    Lateral neck, chest, and pelvis radiographs
    ECG
    Start to make arrangements for transfer, admission, and movement to operating room or ICU

5. Next 10 min
    Reassess airway, ventilation, oxygenation, perfusion, neurologic status, and disability
    Document resuscitation; talk to family
    Splint fractures; dress wounds
    Ultrasound, CT scan, IVP, DPL, as indicated
    Consider more invasive monitoring devices central venous line, arterial line

and ventilatory effort. Next, the clinician must evaluate the circulatory status and control hemorrhage then evaluate for disability (neurologic screening examination). This is followed by exposure and thorough examination. Remember to avoid hypothermia by keeping the child warm. The primary survey and

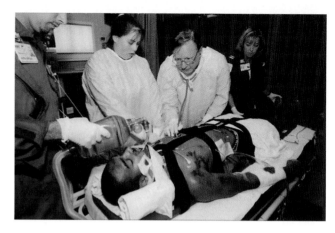

Figure 28-2. A team approach is required for management of multisystem trauma.

resuscitation is carried on simultaneously. Airway management will be described in this section. Vital signs vary by age and one should have access to a table or chart with them (Table 28–6).

▶ **TABLE 28-4. CRITERIA FOR TRAUMA ACTIVATION**

Trauma team to ED

Physiologic
    Cardiopulmonary arrest
    Respiratory arrest
    Hypotension
    Neurologic failure (Glasgow Coma Scale score <8)
    Trauma score <12

Anatomic
    Penetrating (gunshot or stab) wound to head, chest, or abdomen
    Facial/tracheal injury with potential airway compromise
    Burn >30% body surface area (BSA); Inhalation airway burn
    Major electrical injury

Trauma alert
    Mechanism
    Ejected from motor vehicle
    Extrication time of >20 min
    Fatality of another passenger in MVC
    Intrusion of vehicle >20 inch by collision
    Vehicle traveling >20 mph in pedestrian accident or passenger unrestrained in MVC (>35 mph restrained)
    Fall >20 ft
    Run over by vehicle
    Lightning

Anatomic
    Significant injuries both above and below the diaphragm
    Two or more proximal long bone fractures
    Burn of 15%–30% BSA (second/third degree)
    Traumatic amputation of limb proximal to wrist or ankle
    Crush injury of torso
    Spinal injury with paralysis

▶ **TABLE 28-5. REASONS FOR TRANSFER OF PEDIATRIC TRAUMA PATIENTS FOR TERTIARY CARE**

I. Mechanism of trauma
  A. Falls
    1. Falls >10 ft involving patients <14 y old
    2. Falls from second floor or higher
  B. Motor vehicle–crash passenger
    1. Evidence of high-impact velocity motor vehicle accident
      a. Shattered windshield
      b. Evidence of intrusion into the passenger compartment
      c. Bent steering wheel
    2. Rollover incident with unrestrained victim
    3. Ejection of the patient from the vehicle
    4. Death of an occupant within the same passenger compartment
    5. Extraction time >20 min
  C. Auto vs. pedestrian incident at >20 mph and victim <15 y old
  D. Major burns
  E. Blast injuries
II. Physiology
  A. Total trauma score of ≤12
  B. Pediatric trauma score ≤8
  C. Unstable vital signs (age appropriate)
  D. Compromise of airway, breathing, or circulation, or need for protracted ventilation
  E. Severely compromised neurologic status (Glasgow Coma Scale of ≤8)
III. Injuries
  A. Penetrating injuries involving the head, neck, chest, and abdomen or groin
  B. Two or more proximal long bone fractures
  C. Traumatic amputation proximal to either the wrist or the ankle
  D. Evidence of neurologic deficit because of spinal cord injury
  E. Flail chest, major chest wall injury, or pulmonary contusion
  F. Penetrating head injury, open-head injury, or CSF leak
  G. Suspicion of vascular or cardiac injury
  H. Severe maxillofacial injuries
  I. Depressed skull fracture

▶ **TABLE 28-6. PEDIATRIC VITAL SIGNS[21]**

Age	Weight,* kg	Respiratory Rate	Heart Rate	Systolic BP†
Preterm	2	55–65	120–180	40–60
Term newborn	3	40–60	90–170	52–92
1 mo	4	30–50	110–180	60–104
6 mo–1 y	8–10	25–35	120–140	65–125
2–4 y	12–16	20–30	100–110	80–95
5–8 y	18–26	4–20	90–100	85–100
8–12 y	26–50	12–20	60–110	90–115
>12 y	>40	12–16	60–100	100–130

*Weight estimate: $8 + [2 \times$ age (in y)] = weight (in kg).
†Blood pressure minimum $70 + [2 \times$ age (in y)] = systolic blood pressure; $\frac{2}{3} \times$ systolic pressure = diastolic pressure.

controlled mild hyperventilation in patients with serious head injuries. It should also be considered for flail chest with pulmonary contusion and in patients with shock that is unresponsive to fluid volume.

Orotracheal intubation is the most reliable means of securing an airway. An uncuffed tube should be used in children <8 years of age. Appropriate tube size is approximated by the diameter of the nostril or the diameter of the child's fifth finger (Table 28–7). Emergency intubation should always be accomplished via the oral approach. Nasotracheal intubation should not be preformed in a child younger than age 9. Besides being extremely difficult in an acutely injured child, it is relatively contraindicated because of the acute angle of the posterior pharynx, the necessity of additional tube manipulation, and the probability of causing or increasing pharyngeal bleeding. Preparation should always precede intubation and includes guaranteeing the presence of all equipment and drugs necessary to adequately manage an acute airway. This should be accomplished even before an injured child arrives.

Intubation may be necessary to maintain an adequate airway. However, intubation may be difficult because of poor airway visualization, seizures, agitation, or combativeness. Prolonged intubation procedures can lead to ICP elevation, pain, bradycardia, regurgitation, and hypoxemia. Rapid sequence induction (RSI) can greatly facilitate intubation and reduce adverse effects significantly (see Chapter 23).

Emergency physicians must be able to secure an airway when unable to perform orotracheal or nasotracheal intubation. There are several options:

- *Cricothyrotomy* has a role for patients in whom there is extensive central facial or upper airway injury or when there have been unsuccessful attempts at orotracheal intubation. However, it is difficult and hazardous in children. It is not recommended in children younger than the age of 10 and complication rates are as high as 10% to 40%.
- *Tracheostomy* is time consuming and hazardous in the ED, in addition to requiring surgical skill.
- *Needle cricothyrotomy with transtracheal jet ventilation (TTJV)* currently is the preferred surgical method of choice to secure an emergency airway in children.

Airway

The airway is secured while concomitantly stabilizing the neck. The jaw thrust maneuver is used to open the airway and the oropharynx is cleared of debris and secretions. Although bony C-spine injuries are less common in children, they are at high risk for cervical cord injuries. Cervical spine injury should be assumed until a normal examination and an adequate C-spine series is obtained.

Indications for endotracheal intubation in the trauma patient include the inability to ventilate the child by bag-valve-mask methods, the need for prolonged control of the airway, prevention of aspiration in a comatose child, or the need for

▲ TABLE 28–7. EQUIPMENT SIZES FOR PEDIATRIC TRAUMA

Age	Mask Size	Oral Airway	Nasal Airway	Laryngoscope Blade	Endotracheal Tube (mm)	Foley Catheter	Orogastric Tube (F)	Suction Catheter	Chest Tube	Vascular Catheter	IO Needle (G)
Newborn	Infant	0		0	3–3.5	5–8	5 or 8 feeding	8	12–18	20–22	
6 mo	Infant/child	1	12	1	3.5	8	8	8	14–20	20–22	17
1 y	Child (s)	1–2	12	1	4.0	8	10	8	14–24	20–22	17
3 y	Child (s)	2	16	2	4.5	10	10	10	16–28	18–22	15
5 y	Child (m)	3	16	2	5.0	10	10–12	10	20–32	18–20	15
6 y	Child (m)	3	16	2–3	5.5	10–12	12	10	20–32	18–20	
8 y	Sm med	4	20	2–3	6.0	12	14	12	24–32	16–20	
12 y	Med lg	4–5	24–28	3	6.5	12–16	14	12	28–36	16–20	
16 y	Med lg	5	28–30	3–4	7.0–8.0	14–18	16–18	12–14	28–40	14–18	

Permission granted from W.B. Saunders. Schafermeyer RW. Pediatric trauma in advances in trauma. *Emerg Med Clin North Am.* 1993;11:187–205.

A percutaneous technique and TTJV has several advantages over a surgical cricothyrotomy in the ED because it is done in a straightforward technique, allows adequate ventilation for at least 45 to 60 minutes, which allows time for definitive airway placement. It plays a central role in those patients in whom intubation is not possible.

However, advantages over traditional surgical methodologies have not been scientifically demonstrated, despite being inherently obvious. Some expertise and/or practice are required and the airway is not protected from aspiration. Complications include subcutaneous emphysema, bleeding, and catheter dislodgment. However, the issue of CO_2 retention, although controversial, is overstated and of relative unimportance when airway access and oxygenation are critical. TTJV undoubtedly provides a lifesaving and temporary airway, which should be adequate for 45 minutes to 2 hours, until endotracheal intubation can be achieved.

The procedure for TTJV is as follows. A 14-gauge angiocatheter or a TTJV needle is connected to a 5-mL syringe with 3 mL of saline. The trachea is stabilized with the nondominant hand and, after the region is prepped, the cricothyroid membrane is punctured at a 30-to 45-degree angle caudally. Special care is required to avoid puncturing the posterior wall of the trachea. Placement is verified with aspiration of air. Slide the catheter off the needle and reconfirm placement with the syringe. The catheter must be held constantly or secured in place and the jet ventilation tubing is attached to the O_2 source. This O_2 source *must be a high-pressure* source directly from the wall and not from a regulator valve. The psi (pounds per square inch) can then be adjusted on the pressure gauge. There are no well-studied guidelines for psi settings for TTJV in children. However, parameters are recommended by practitioners familiar with this technique. A low psi must be used initially in children and the provider should look for adequate chest excursion. The psi can be adjusted upward until adequate chest rise is observed and is the best indicator of adequate tidal volume. The inspiration:expiration ratio is 1:3 or 1:4 (Table 28–8).

Breathing

Acceptable ventilation only occurs if there is adequate spontaneous air exchange with normal O_2 saturation and CO_2 levels. Pulse oximetry is mandatory and end-tidal CO_2 monitoring should be used to confirm and monitor endotracheal tube placement. Hypoxemia may manifest as any combination of and degree of agitation, altered mental status, cyanosis, poor end-organ function, poor capillary refill, and desaturation on pulse oximetry. Children with respiratory failure must have positive pressure ventilation (PPV) started immediately.

▶ **TABLE 28-8. PARAMETERS FOR TRANSTRACHEAL JET VENTILATION**

	Initial psi	Estimated Tidal Volume
Adult	30–50	700–1000 mL
8 y to young teens	10–25	340–625
5–8 y	5–10	240–340
<5 y	5	100

Signs that indicate that a child has inadequate ventilation include tachypnea, nasal flaring, grunting, retractions, stridor, and wheezing. Reasons for compromised ventilatory function include depressed sensorium, airway occlusion, restriction of lung expansion, and direct pulmonary injury. Restriction of lung expansion by gastric distention is more likely to occur in young children because of the limitation of diaphragmatic excursion. This problem is addressed by early placement of an oro- or nasogastric tube.

Ventilation with a bag-valve-mask device is initiated to treat inadequate ventilation. Cricoid pressure must be applied when ventilating a patient with a bag and mask to prevent gastric insufflation.

At this phase of the resuscitation, immediate attention and treatment of tension or hemopneumothorax is required, if present or suspected. The classic presentation for tension pneumothorax of absent breath sounds, tympany, hypotension, and jugular venous distention because of high intrathoracic pressures, is rare in children. Children are especially sensitive to mediastinal shift in tension pneumothorax and needle decompression should be performed immediately if any of the following are present: Decreased breath sounds, refractory hypotension, hypoxia, or radiographically confirmed hemopneumothoraces. Massive hemothorax may present as absent breath sounds, dullness to percussion on the affected side of the chest, and hypotension. Jugular venous distention is not seen because of slow circulatory volume. Operative thoracotomy should be considered when the initial drainage is greater than 15 mL/kg or the chest tube output exceeds 4 mL/kg/h.

For an open pneumothorax, place an occlusive dressing (petrolatum gauze or plastic sheet) that is secured by tape on three sides, leaving one side of the dressing open to act as a flutter valve to minimize the risk for development of a tension pneumothorax. A tube thoracostomy can wait until completion of the primary survey.

Circulation

The initial circulatory assessment and treatment includes identifying and controlling both external and internal hemorrhage and assessing perfusion. Vascular access for fluid infusion and phlebotomy are additional goals. The child's volume status and perfusion are estimated by assessment of pulse, skin color, and capillary refill time and obtaining a blood pressure. A palpable peripheral pulse correlates with a blood pressure above 80 mm Hg, and a palpable central pulse indicates a pressure above 50 to 60 mm Hg. A euvolemic, euthermic patient's capillary refilling time, assessed after blanching, will be 2 to 3 seconds. Control external hemorrhage by direct pressure. Application of extremity tourniquets or hemostats to bleeding vessels should be avoided. Application and inflation of a pneumatic anti-shock garment is controversial but may control bleeding in the pelvis or lower extremities, although a properly applied external pelvic wrap is preferred for pelvic fractures. As in adults, Trendelenburg position may be of benefit in low perfusion states to maintain central circulation.

Absent pulses or cardiac arrest in a child with traumatic injuries portends a poor outcome. In children with penetrating chest or abdominal trauma, a resuscitative thoracotomy can be lifesaving if vital signs were recently lost. In children with

▶ TABLE 28-9. PEDIATRIC GLASGOW COMA SCALE

Score	0–1 (y)	>1 (y)	0–2 (y)	2–5 (y)	>5 (y)
Eye opening					
4	Spontaneously	Spontaneously			
3	To shout	To verbal command			
2	To pain	To pain			
1	No response	No response			
Best motor response					
6		Obeys command			
5	Localizes pain	Localizes pain			
4	Flexion withdrawal	Flexion withdrawal			
3	Decorticate	Decorticate			
2	Decerebrate	Decerebrate			
1	No response	No response			
Best verbal response					
5			Appropriate cry, smiles, coos	Appropriate words and phrases	Oriented, converses
4			Cries	Inappropriate words	Disoriented, converses
3			Inappropriate cry	Cries/screams	Inappropriate words
2			Grunts	Grunts	Incomprehensible sound
1			No response	No response	No response

Note: A score is given in each category. The individual scores are then added to give a total of 3–15. A score of <8 indicates severe neurologic injury.

traumatic arrest from blunt trauma, the outcome is invariably death. During resuscitation of traumatic arrest, standard advanced cardiac life-support algorithms should be followed and there should be early administration of blood products. If chest trauma is present or there has been a deceleration injury, as with an automobile crash or fall, consider the presence of cardiac tamponade, a rare condition in children. Although echocardiography is diagnostic, look for Beck's triad, which consists of hypotension, muffled heart sounds, and jugular venous distention. Fluid boluses should be administered early and may temporize until periocardiocentesis and resuscitative thoracotomy is undertaken.

Obtain vascular access in a rapid and safe manner, with a capability to infuse the greatest possible volume of fluid. Attaining vascular access is difficult in children so one functioning intravenous line is all that may be readily achieved and is usually adequate. Two lines are placed in the more severely injured child, so blood, fluids, and medications can be given simultaneously. Consider an IO line in a severely injured child if vascular access is difficult. Any fluids, medications, or blood products can be given through this line. If central venous access is desired, the femoral vein is the easiest site because of identifiable landmarks and relative ease of the procedure compared to other sites in children. Ultrasound guided placement of central lines has improved safety and ease of inserting them.

Administer fluid boluses in aliquots of 20 mL/kg and repeat as necessary until perfusion improves.[11] Since traumatic shock is caused by blood loss, packed red blood cells should be used without hesitation when it becomes apparent that there is significant blood loss and crystalloids are inadequate for volume replacement.

Outcomes research may support "low-volume" fluid resuscitation (LVFR) in select patients with uncontrolled hemorrhagic shock, that is, an injury that can only be managed operatively. The reasoning for this approach is that internal hemorrhage cannot be controlled by external means and the body effectively tamponades hemorrhage, but probably more so with venous injuries. IV fluid boluses, under these circumstances, will raise the central venous pressure, which could disrupt a clot and cause a dilution effect of the clotting factors that would ultimately worsen hemorrhage.[12,13] Further study is needed.

Disability

Disability is assessed by performing a rapid neurologic examination to determine level of consciousness and pupil size and reaction to light. The Glasgow Coma Scale is a more quantitative measure of level of consciousness (Table 28–9). Although recently noted to be less predictive of overall outcomes in children with trauma, it is extremely useful to identify improvement or deterioration. However, in the midst of a trauma resuscitation, the AVPU system (Table 28–10) is helpful in following mental status changes.

▶ TABLE 28-10. AVPU METHOD FOR ASSESSING LEVEL OF CONSCIOUSNESS

A	Alert
V	Vocal stimuli: Responds
P	Painful stimuli: Responds
U	Unresponsive

▶ TABLE 28–11. **THERAPEUTIC CLASSIFICATION OF HEMORRHAGIC SHOCK IN THE PEDIATRIC PATIENT**

	Blood Loss Percent of Blood Volume*			
	Up to 15	15–30	30–40	≥40
Pulse rate	Normal	Mild tachycardia	Moderate tachycardia	Severe tachycardia
Blood pressure	Normal or increased	Decreased	Decreased	Decreased
Capillary refill	Normal	Positive	Positive	Positive
Respiratory rate	Normal	Mild tachypnea	Moderate tachypnea	Severe tachypnea
Urinary output	1–2 mL/kg/h	0.5–1.0 mL/kg/h	0.25–0.5 mL/kg/h	Negligible
Mental status	Slightly anxious	Mildly anxious	Anxious and confused	Confused and lethargic
Fluid replacement (3:1 rule)	Crystalloid	Crystalloid	Crystalloid + blood	Crystalloid + blood

*Assume blood volume to be 8%–9% of body weight (80–90 mL/kg).

Exposure

Completely undress the patient in order to perform a thorough assessment. Children have a larger body surface area:weight ratio so preventing hypothermia is a constant concern.

▶ RESUSCITATION

This phase occurs simultaneously with the primary survey, but it is separated in presentation for clarity and organization.[14-16]

Ensure adequate oxygenation and ventilation of all trauma victims as discussed above. Vascular access is the next priority via percutaneous or cutdown cannulation of the upper or lower extremity veins. Establish two large bore intravenous lines, with size guided by the size of available veins. The highest success rate is obtained at the antecubital fossae or the saphenous veins at the ankle (anterior to the medial maleolus). Veins are often visibly absent, difficult to cannulate with an appropriately sized catheter, or collapsed in the face of hypovolemia. In these situations, femoral vein central line or IO infusion into the tibia marrow space are reasonable lifesaving alternatives. A third option is rapid venous cut down performed on an antecubital vein or the saphenous vein at either the ankle or in the groin.

Send blood for type and cross-match, complete blood count, serum electrolytes, liver transaminases, and amylase. Liver transaminase elevation in the acute trauma setting serves as a marker of liver injury that might not be clinically apparent. Send a blood gas for any patient who may have significant volume loss, respiratory compromise, or concomitant toxic exposure (e.g., carbon monoxide poisoning in a burn patient).

Perform an assessment for shock and determine whether or not adequate organ perfusion exists. Shock after trauma is usually hypovolemic. Cardiogenic shock and neurogenic shock are less likely but need to be considered. Isolated head trauma, except in infancy, is not a cause of shock in children.

Hypovolemic shock occurs most commonly after major trauma and is caused by blood loss (Table 28–11). The blood volume of the child makes up 8% to 9% of the total body weight. Determination of volume depletion and shock is difficult in children, and multiple parameters must be used. Hematocrit can be normal in the face of acute blood loss—and blood pressure alone is an insensitive indicator of shock, especially when determining treatment priorities. Pulse and respiratory rate and mental status are more sensitive in identifying early stages of shock.

Cardiogenic shock after a major childhood injury is rare but could occur because of cardiac tamponade or direct cardiac contusion. It should be suspected if there are dilated neck veins in a patient with decelerating injury, penetrating chest trauma, or sternal contusion. Neurogenic shock presents with hypotension without tachycardia or vasoconstriction and is usually because of spinal cord injury. Isolated head injury does not produce shock unless there is significant intracerebral hemorrhage in an infant. Distributive or septic shock is not a consideration immediately after trauma, even if there is contamination of the abdominal cavity.

Normal saline (NS) or Ringer's lactate (LR) is the fluid of choice for initial resuscitation of the pediatric trauma victim. Fluid replacement can be divided into two phases: (1) Initial therapy and (2) total replacement (Tables 28–12 and 28–13). The initial resuscitative fluid should be isotonic crystalloid solution. Give an initial infusion of 20 mL/kg as rapidly as possible.

▶ TABLE 28–12. **CLASSIFICATION FOR FLUID RESUSCITATION IN SHOCK**

	Class I	Class II	Class III	Class IV
Blood loss%/blood volume	Up to 15%	15%–30%	30%–40%	40% or more
Pulse rate	Normal	Mild tachycardia	Moderate tachycardia	Severe tachycardia
Blood pressure	Normal/increased	Normal/decreased	Decreased	Decreased
Capillary blanch test	Normal	Positive	Positive	Positive
Respiratory rate	Normal	Mild tachypnea	Moderate tachypnea	Severe tachypnea
Urine output	1–2 mL/kg/h	0.5–1 mL/kg/h	0.25–0.5 mL/kg/h	Negligible
Mental status	Slightly anxious	Mildly anxious	Anxious/confused	Confused/lethargic
Fluid replacement	Crystalloid	Crystalloid	Crystalloid + blood	Crystalloid + blood

▶ **TABLE 28–13. GUIDELINES FOR FLUID RESUSCITATION IN SHOCK**

Mild shock (15%–25% of blood volume loss)
  Initial volume:
    20 mL/kg LR or NS
    If no improvement, repeat 20 mL/kg LR or NS
  Total volume:
    If improved, run LR or NS at 5 mL/kg/h for several hours
    If child remains stable, adjust intravenous rate downward
      toward maintenance levels
  Maintenance after volume is restored:
    10 kg: 100 mL/kg/24 h
    10–20 kg: 1000 mL 50 mL/kg/24 h
    20 kg: 1500 mL 20 mL/kg/24 h

Moderate shock (25%–40% of blood volume loss)
  Initial volume:
    20 mL/kg/LR or NS; repeat immediately if not improved
  If no improvement, alternative therapy includes:
    20–40 mL/kg LR, or NS again, *or* 10–20 mL/kg packed red
      blood cells, *or* operative intervention
    10–20 mL/kg packed red blood cells if initial Hgb < 7.0
  Total volume:
    If improved, run LR or NS at 5 mL/kg/h for several hours
    If a child remains stable, adjust intravenous rate toward
      maintenance levels
    May need transfusion depending on clinical response and
      hematocrit

Severe shock (>40% of blood volume loss)
  Initial volume:
    Push LR or NS until colloid available
    Push packed red blood cells or whole blood
    Surgery
  Total volume:
    Replace loss with type-specific blood

This is best accomplished by using a 3-way stopcock and pushing boluses rather than trying to infuse via a pump or gravity, especially if the vein cannulation device is smaller than 18-gauge. After a rapid 20-mL/kg bolus over 10 minutes, the child should be reassessed. Repeat fluid boluses up to four times if necessary. If the child continues to be unstable, 10 to 20 mL/kg packed red blood cells or whole blood need to be infused urgently. The 3:1 rule is commonly used in replacing lost blood with crystalloid as follows: 300 mL of crystalloid for each 100 mL of blood loss. If the initial hemoglobin value is <7, blood should be given immediately since this level of hemoglobin overwhelms compensatory mechanisms and increases cellular hypoxia.

Clinically assess volume and perfusion status during resuscitation. Vital signs are checked before and after bolus therapy. If a child is not responding, suspect continued bleeding and look for other causes of refractory shock, such as tension pneumothorax or hypoxemia. Insert a Foley catheter and use urinary output as a straightforward, readily available monitor as directed: 1 mL/kg/h for children >1 year of age and 2 mL/kg/h for children <1 year of age. Urinary output may help assess perfusion and intravascular status.

While restoring or immediately after attaining adequate perfusion, place a urinary and gastric catheter. Blood at the urethral meatus or in the scrotum or abnormal placement of prostate on rectal examination prohibit urinary catheterization until a retrograde urethrogram (RUG) proves that the urethra is intact. This is done by instilling gastrograffin into a partially inserted Foley catheter. Nasogastric tube insertion should be avoided or performed with the utmost care to avoid passage into the brain via a cribiform plate fracture when a patient has blood coming from the ears, nose, or mouth.

Measure and monitor the patient's body temperature. Hypothermia must be avoided and/or corrected. Use radiant warmers, warmed IV fluids, cover exposed body parts, and raise the room temperature.

Obtain radiographs at this time, but limit them to C-spine, chest, and pelvic films until the patient is initially resuscitated.

It is important to obtain surgical consultation in any significantly injured child as early in the evaluation as possible. If notified by EMS of a severely injured child coming to the facility, contact the surgeon on call for trauma or contact the referral center to prepare for early transfer of the critically injured child. Initiation of a transfer protocol, if warranted, should be activated at this time (Table 28–5).

▶ **SECONDARY SURVEY AND DEFINITIVE CARE**

Once life-threatening conditions identified in the primary survey are stabilized, perform a timely, directed evaluation of each body area, proceeding from head to toe.[10,14] Continuously reassess vital signs and abnormal conditions identified in the primary survey at a minimum of every 15 minutes. The components of the secondary survey include a history, a complete head to toe examination, laboratory studies, radiographic studies, and problem identification. Use an AMPLE history to determine the mechanism of injury, time, status at scene, changes in status, and complaints that the child may have. This includes **A**llergies, **M**edications, **P**ast medical and surgical history, **L**ast meal time, and **E**vents preceding the injury. Complete laboratory and radiologic studies that were not done during the initial resuscitation. A decision regarding disposition can probably be made at this point during most resuscitations.

HEAD EXAMINATION

Reevaluate pupil size and reactivity. Perform a conjunctival and fundal examination for hemorrhage or penetrating injury. Assess visual acuity by determining if the patient can read, see faces, recognize movement, and distinguish light versus dark.

Palpate the skull and mandible looking for fractures or dislocations. Although relatively uncommon, infants may become hypotensive from blood loss into either the subgaleal or epidural space. An infant with an open fontanelle is more tolerant of an expanding intracranial mass lesions and signs of this may be hidden until rapid decompensation occurs. Unlike adults, vomiting and altered mental status, such as amnesia, commonly occur in head injured children and do not necessarily imply increased ICP. However, persistent vomiting, progressive headache, palpable skull defect, or an inability to observe a patient's mental status (e.g., they are going to the operating room) are some of the indications for a head CT scan immediately. If airway is secure, maxillofacial trauma is a lower priority and the physician should move on quickly.

CERVICAL SPINE

Injuries of the C-spine are not common in children but the presence of one or more of several injuries increases the risk. These include injuries above the clavicles, injuries from falling >1 floor, motor vehicle–pedestrian crash at >30 mph, unrestrained or poorly restrained occupant of a MVC, sports injuries, etc. Children tend to have injuries of the upper C-spine and cord.

In very low-risk injuries, the C-spine can usually be cleared in the ED with a normal C-spine films and a normal clinical examination. Caveats are that C-spine film must show all seven C-spine vertebrae and that the patient should be awake, cooperative, and free of other distracting painful injuries before ruling out a cervical injury. The child, performing the movements voluntarily, should actively flex, extend, and rotate the neck with no symptoms or signs of spasm, guarding, pain, or tenderness.

Unique characteristics of the pediatric C-spine predispose it to ligamentous disruption and dislocation injuries without radiographic evidence of bone injury. The incomplete development of the bony spine, the relatively large size of the head, and the weakness of the soft tissue of the neck predispose to spinal cord injury without radiographic abnormality (SCIWORA). Children with high-risk mechanisms of injury should have three views: Anteroposterior (AP), an odontoid, and lateral views. Patients with altered sensorium cannot be cleared despite negative films and the collar should remain in place while further testing and imaging studies are completed (see Chapter 30).

Special considerations are required in four situations:

- The child who requires immediate intubation because of airway compromise should not have airway management delayed waiting for C-spine film(s). The safety of oral intubation with in-line C-spine immobilization has been demonstrated in multiple studies.
- If such a child who is intubated is at high risk for C-spine injury, then a CT scan of the upper cervical vertebrae should be done when a head CT scan is performed.
- If an injured patient arrives with a helmet in place and does not require immediate airway intervention, then lateral C-spine can be done prior to removing the helmet. There should be careful attention to maintaining C-spine immobilization while removing the helmet.
- Penetrating injuries to the neck requiring operative intervention should have entry and exit sites noted with opaque markers on AP and lateral films of the C-spine.

CHEST

Expose and visually inspect the chest for wounds requiring immediate attention. Sucking chest wounds require a sterile occlusive dressing. A flail chest component could be splinted but the patient may need intubation to do so. Roll the patient, keeping in-line spine immobilization, and look for posterior wounds. Auscultate the chest and evaluate for pneumothorax, hemothorax, or cardiac tamponade. Tension pneumothorax may be manifested by contralateral tracheal shift, distended neck veins, and diminished breath sounds. However, a child's small chest size facilitates the contralateral lung's transmission of breath sounds that makes auscultation an insensitive marker for pneumothorax. Neck vein distention is difficult to appreciate and an insensitive marker when assessing for tension pneumothorax. Therefore, a hemodynamically unstable child should undergo immediate needle decompression thoracentesis if there is reason to suspect blunt or penetrating injury to the thorax. After thoracentesis, tube thoracostomy(ies) should be done. Impaled objects protruding from the chest should be left in place until the child undergoes surgery.

If the chest radiograph reveals a widened mediastinum or apical cap, or other signs suggesting aortic injury or there is a history of significant deceleration injury, CT angiography of the chest is indicated. Aortography may be needed in select circumstances. Although first or second rib fractures increase the likelihood of a vascular injury, their absence does not preclude an aortic injury.[15]

Air lucencies on chest radiography appearing to be of intestinal origin should be considered evidence of a diaphragmatic injury. Any penetrating injury to abdomen or lower chest carries a risk of diaphragmatic injury.

ABDOMEN

During the secondary survey, determining the exact etiology of an abdominal injury is secondary to determining whether or not an injury is present. Retroperitoneal injuries are difficult to identify, unless there is a high index of suspicion. Signs suggesting abdominal injury include abdominal wall contusion, distention, abdominal or shoulder pain, and signs of peritoneal irritation and shock. Penetrating wounds to the abdomen usually need immediate operative intervention.[16, 17]

Controversies arise in diagnosing and managing blunt abdominal injuries. CT scan with IV, oral, and colonic contrast may be the most sensitive and useful diagnostic modality (see below under heading Imaging). Diagnostic peritoneal lavage (DPL) provides rapid, objective evaluation of possible intraperitoneal injury, especially involving the liver, spleen, and bowel. It can be considered more sensitive than a CT scan in diagnosing hollow viscous injuries, especially early in the evaluation of a child who is a victim of a deceleration injury while wearing a seatbelt (Fig. 28–3). It is much less sensitive than CT scan in diagnosing injuries to the pancreas, duodenum, genitourinary tract, aorta, vena cava, and diaphragm.

The role of the Focused Assessment Sonography in Trauma (FAST) in pediatric trauma remains to be seen. In children, FAST may identify intra-abdominal blood but this is not enough information to dictate management. However, finding blood on a FAST examination in a patient who is hypotensive and is not responding adequately to crystalloid and packed red blood cell expansion would indicate a need for immediate laparotomy.[18]

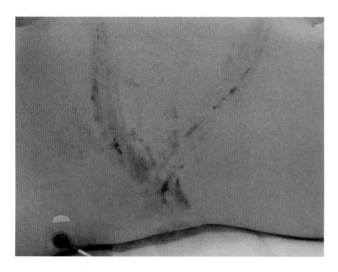

Figure 28–3. Children with bruises from seatbelts should be checked for deceleration injuries.

DPL, although rarely done, may have a role in the hypotensive, injured child because it is valuable in deciding whether or not a patient needs immediate laparotomy. Consider performing DPL in the patient requiring urgent anesthesia and nonabdominal surgery, such as evacuation of an epidural hematoma or treatment of a penetrating upper chest injury.

In children, after emptying the bladder with a Foley catheter, use a midline approach above or below the umbilicus. Instill 10 mL/kg of LR if the initial aspirate is not grossly bloody. An aspirate is considered positive if it has >100 000 red blood cells/μL, >500 white blood cells (WBCs)/μL, a spun effluent hematocrit >2%, bile, bacteria, or fecal material are found. False-positive tests most commonly occur in the face of a pelvic fracture. A positive DPL >100 000 RBCs may be due to a laceration of the liver or spleen but this would not be an indication for surgery. Greater than 80% of these patients will stop bleeding under observation without an operative intervention. In these cases, a CT scan is more valuable for evaluating and assessing damage and determining a treatment plan in the stable patient.

PELVIS

Palpate the bony prominences of the pelvis for tenderness or instability. Examine the perineum for laceration, hematoma, or active bleeding. If not checked earlier when placing a Foley catheter, examine the urethral meatus for blood. Blood loss from pelvic fractures can be critically significant and difficult to control, leading to a fatal hemorrhage. If there is major pelvic disruption, then the patient will need to be transferred to a trauma center. Prior to transfer, IV fluids and blood products are given. Bring the lower extremities together and apply an external pelvic sling made from a sheet or use the pneumatic antishock garment to reduce bleeding until the patient can get definitive care or embolization of major bleeding sites.

PERINEUM/RECTUM

The perineum, should be examined for contusions, hematomas, lacerations, and urethral bleeding. Perform a rectal examination prior to placing a urinary catheter. Determine sphincter muscle tone, rectal integrity, prostatic position, presence of a pelvic fracture, and the presence of blood in the stool. For the female patient, a vaginal examination should also be considered in the secondary survey.

EXTREMITY EXAMINATION

Look at all extremities looking for deformity, contusions, abrasions, intact sensation, penetrating injuries, pulses, and perfusion. The presence of a pulse does not exclude a proximal vascular injury or a compartment syndrome. Palpate long bones circumferentially assessing for tenderness, crepitation, or abnormal movement. Straighten severe angulations of the extremities if possible and apply splints and traction. Open fractures and wounds should be covered with sterile dressings. Inspect soft tissue injuries for foreign bodies, irrigate to minimize contamination, and debride devitalized tissues. Remember to check for fractures involving the bones of the hands, wrists, and feet since they are commonly missed until the patient regains consciousness.

BACK EXAMINATION

Examine the back, particularly in cases of penetrating trauma, looking for hematomas, exit or entry wounds, or spine tenderness. With the neck immobilized log roll the patient for examination.

SKIN

Examine for evidence of contusions, burns, penetration sites, petechiae, and signs of abuse.

NEUROLOGIC EXAMINATION

Obtain an additional Glasgow Coma Score and perform a more in-depth evaluation of motor, sensory, and cranial nerves. Check the fundi and look for rhinorrhea. Level of consciousness, pupillary examination, and sensorimotor examination, as quantified in the Glasgow Coma Scale, are invaluable in identifying a change in mental status. Presence of paresis or paralysis suggest a major neurologic injury. Conversely, lack of neurologic findings does not eliminate the possibility of a cervical cord injury, especially when the patient has a distracting injury and/or pain.

Any injured child is at risk for exposure to heat or cold. Because of their relatively larger body surface area, hypothermia can develop in the prehospital setting and/or in the ED. Hypothermia may impair circulatory dynamics and coagulation, worsen metabolic acidosis by increasing metabolic demand, and increase peripheral vascular resistance. The likelihood and risks of hypothermia can be minimized with the use of overhead warmers, warmed intravenous fluids, and warm blankets.

ADDITIONAL TREATMENT AND TESTS

Provide tetanus prophylaxis (toxoid and possibly tetanus immune globulin). This is also the time to make arrangements for other diagnostic tests. Consider the psychosocial aspects of traumatic injuries. Permit parents at the child's bedside as soon as the child's clinical status is stabilized.

BURNS

Burns are the second most common cause of accidental death among children <4 years of age and may often be a significant part of the problem in a multiply injured patient. For the principles and procedures of burn management (see Chapter 138).

IMAGING

A child with major blunt trauma needs three basic radiographs immediately, the AP chest, AP pelvis, and C-spine films. Chest films are more sensitive than clinical examination in smaller children for detecting hemothorax and pneumothorax. Check for widening of the mediastinum and fractured ribs. Pelvic fractures are important clinical indicators in that 80% of children with multiple fractures of the pelvis have concomitant abdominal or genitourinary injuries. Cervical spine films are obtained as appropriate. During the secondary survey, thoracolumbar and extremity films can be completed as indicated. Based on clinical findings in the primary and secondary surveys, further imaging studies may be needed.

CT Scan of Head

Indications for CT scanning of the brain include a Glasgow coma scale(GCS) <14, deteriorating neurologic examination, posttraumatic seizures, prolonged lethargy, prolonged vomiting, significant loss of consciousness, amnesia, and confounding medical problems, such as hemophilia (see Chapter 29).

CT Scan of Abdomen

Indications for abdominal CT scanning include a hemodynamically stable victim of blunt trauma with clinical signs of intraabdominal injury; hematuria >20 RBCs per high-powered field or even minimal hematuria with a history of deceleration injury; worrisome mechanism of trauma in the presence of neurologic compromise. Positive findings on abdominal CT scan are significantly increased if three of the following are present: Gross hematuria, lap belt injury, assault, or abuse as a mechanism of trauma, positive abdominal findings such as tenderness, trauma score <12, and significant neurologic compromise (GCS <10).

Some trauma centers use double-contrast CT scan for trauma patients. Diluted gastrograffin (20 mL/kg) is instilled

▶ **TABLE 28–14. DOSE OF CONTRAST MEDIA FOR RADIOGRAPHIC STUDIES**

Age (y)	Dose
Intravenous: 60% hypaque	
0 to 9	1 mL/0.45 kg bolus
10 or more	50 mL, followed by infusion of 50 to 100 mL during scan
Oral: 1.5% hypaque (20 mL to 1 L of fluid given po or NG)	
0–2	100 mL
3–5	150–200 mL
6–9	200–250 mL
>9	300–1000 mL
Adult	1000 mL
Oral: Gastrografin, 20 mL/kg via NG tube 20 min prior to scan	

via a nasogastric tube 20 minutes prior to CT scan and intravenous contrast after the initial survey is performed. During the CT scanning, the Foley catheter should be clamped to evaluate the bladder and the nasogastric tube should be pulled into the esophagus to avoid artifact (Table 28–14). Other centers use IV contrast only.

A limitation of CT scanning is the lack of sensitivity in diagnosing injuries to hollow viscous organs (bladder, intestinal perforations/rupture). If intraperitoneal fluid is found by CT scan with no apparent injury to the spleen or liver, consider injury to the bowel, bladder, or a vascular injury. Frequent reexaminations by the surgeon are needed or a DPL should be considered. CT scans will miss free intraperitoneal air in 75% of cases and lumbar spine injuries in 77% of cases. Therefore, if a patient is hemodynamically stable, consider obtaining thoracolumbar spine films (especially a lateral), an abdominal film looking for free air (e.g., left lateral decubitus film once C-spine injury is excluded), and a cystogram. If injury to bowel or bladder is confirmed, laparotomy is indicated.

Ultrasonography

Ultrasonography may be an alternative to CT scan in selected cases or when CT scan is not available. Ultrasound can diagnose injuries to the liver, spleen, and kidneys and can document intraperitoneal fluid. This modality is not a substitute for CT scan unless the examiner is very experienced in the use of ultrasound in traumatized children.[17,18]

Urologic Studies

If a patient has gross blood at the meatus, or the integrity of the urethra is in doubt because of the possible pelvic fracture, then a RUG should be performed. The study is performed by instilling contrast through a Foley catheter that has been inserted into the distal urethra and partially inflated (0.5–1.0 mL of saline in the balloon). If the urethra is found not to be damaged, the catheter can be advanced to perform a cystogram.

A "1-shot" intravenous pyelogram is a very useful and reasonable test to perform in the ED to evaluate renovascular status if the patient is too unstable for CT scan. A 2 to 4 mL/kg

▶ TABLE 28-15. **REVISED TRAUMA SCORE***

Revised Trauma Score	Glasgow Coma Score	Systolic Blood Pressure (mm Hg)	Respiratory Rate (breaths/min)
4	13–15	>89	10–20
3	9–12	76–89	>29
2	6–8	50–75	6–9
1	4–5	1–49	1–5
0	3	0	0

*A score of 0–4 is given for each variable then added (range, 0–12). A score ≥11 indicates potentially important trauma.

bolus of 50% diatrizoate sodium (Hypaque) is injected and a film of the abdomen is taken 5 minutes later. This will determine the absence or presence of blood supply to one or both kidneys and it may also show the function of the upper ureters. Knowledge of the status of the blood supply is very important because a renovascular intimal tear with occlusion or vascular disruption must be identified immediately. The warm ischemic time in which to diagnose, repair, and avoid irreparable damage to a devascularized kidney is only 6 hours.

▶ INJURY SEVERITY MEASURES

THE TRAUMA SCORES

The Revised Trauma Score (Table 28–15) was originally developed for rapid assessment, triage, measuring progression of injury, predicting outcome, and assisting in quality assessment. It is useful in the overall management of trauma patient but is less sensitive for severe injury to a single organ system. It is straightforward to calculate for all trauma patients. It allows for standardization of triage protocols and for scientific comparisons between groups of patients and institutions.[19, 20]

The pediatric trauma score (Table 28–16) was developed to reflect the unique injury pattern in children. It incorporates age into the score.

- Score >8: Associated with 100% survival
- Score <8: Should transfer patient to pediatric trauma center
- Score <0: 100% mortality

In a study by Nayduch et al.,[21] the Trauma Score had a better predictive value for overall outcome, whereas the pediatric trauma score was a better predictor for appropriate ED disposition. Unfortunately, no trauma score is totally reliable in predicting extent of either injuries or outcomes. For example, Jaimovich reviewed 305 pediatric trauma patients' functional long-term outcomes and found that the current trauma scoring systems fall short in identifying "nonsalvageable" survivors who make meaningful neurologic recovery.[22] In addition, study by Lieh-Lai et al.[23] demonstrated that a low GCS does not always predict the outcome of severe traumatic brain injury and in the absence of hypoxic insult—children with scores of 3 to 5 can recover independent function. Therefore, the trauma score or pediatric trauma score can be used to triage patients and predict outcome but exercise caution if used to predict functional outcome.

▶ DISPOSITION/TRANSFER

Facilities that receive trauma victims should have the appropriate personnel and patient care resources committed at all times. However, a majority of seriously injured children are not brought to comprehensive trauma centers. Children, therefore, can and should receive appropriate care at all hospitals where EMS policies have established that the facility is capable of receiving patients with life-threatening conditions. In a hospital without pediatric surgical consultants, early transfers to a pediatric trauma center, adult trauma center, or pediatric intensive care unit should be considered. Establish contingency plans for transfers, prearranged agreements between institutions prospectively (Table 28–5).

Children who appear to have clinical brain death should be considered for continued resuscitation since they may be candidates for organ donation and procurement. If heart, heart–lung, kidney, pancreas, and liver transplantation are considered, premortem management is essential to the viability of the organs. Considerations such as these are best handled in a facility that has the resources to do so. Sensitive parental consultation and support are paramount. Organ donation may provide traumatized families some consolation and strength in the face of such tremendous grief.

When dealing with a traumatized child, the physician must communicate openly and clearly with the family. Psychologic support is needed through the entire hospital course. Disposition and treatment decisions and progress reports need to be

▶ TABLE 28-16. **PEDIATRIC TRAUMA SCORE***

Variables	+2	+1	−1
Airway	Normal	Maintainable	Unmaintainable
CNS	Awake	Obtunded/LOC	Coma/Decerebrate
Body weight	>20 kg	10–20 kg	<10 kg
Systolic BP	>90 mm Hg	50–90 mm Hg	<50 mm Hg
Open wound	None	Minor	Major
Skeletal injury	None	Closed fracture	Open/multiple fractures
Cutaneous	None	Minor	

*A score of +2, +1, or −1 is given to each variable, and then added (range −6 to 12). A score ≥8 indicates potentially important trauma. LOC = loss of consciousness.

presented frequently, succinctly, and with sensitivity. Parents should be allowed to see the child and/or accompany him or her as soon as is practical.

REFERENCES

1. Arias E, MacDorman MF, Strobono DM, Guyer B. Annual summary of vital statistics. *Pediatrics.* 2003;112(6)(pt 1):1215–1230.
2. Danesco ER, Miller TR, Spicer RS. Incidence and costs of 1987–1994 childhood injuries: demographic breakdowns. *Pediatrics.* 2000;105(2):e27. Available at www.pediatrics.org/cgi/content/full/105/2/e27.
3. Miller TR, Romano EO, Spicer RS. The cost of childhood unintentional injuries and the value of prevention. *Future Child.* 2000;10(1):137–163.
4. Gausche-Hill M, Fuchs S, Yamamoto L, eds. *Advanced Pediatric Life Support: The Pediatric Emergency Medicine Resource.* Rev ed. Elk Grove Village, IL; Dallas, TX: American Academy of Pediatrics; American College of Emergency Physicians; 2007.
5. Legome EL. Trauma: general considerations. In: Harwood-Nuss AL, ed. *Clinical Practice of Emergency Medicine.* Philadelphia, PA: Lippincott; 2005:896.
6. Nathans AB, Jukovich GJ, Maier RV, et al. Relationship between trauma center volume and outcomes. *JAMA.* 2001;285:1164–1171.
7. Wright JL, Klein BL. Regionalized pediatric trauma systems. *Clin Pediatr Emerg Med.* 2001;2:3–12.
8. Fleisher G, Ludwig S, Henretig FM. *Textbook of Pediatric Emergency Medicine.* 5th ed. Baltimore, MD: Lippincott, Williams & Wilkins; 2006.
9. Tepas J III, Fallat ME, Moriarty T. Trauma. In: Gausche-Hill M, Fuchs S, Yamamoto L, eds. *Advanced Pediatric Life Support: The Pediatric Emergency Medicine Resource.* Rev ed. Elk Grove Village, IL; Dallas, TX: American Academy of Pediatrics; American College of Emergency Physicians; 2007:268–324.
10. ACS Committee on Trauma. *Advanced Trauma Life Support Manual.* Chicago, IL: American College of Surgeons; 2005:243–261.
11. Sadow KB, Teach SJ. Prehospital intravenous fluid therapy in the pediatric trauma patient. *Clin Pediatr Emerg Med.* 2001;2:23–27.
12. Bickell SP, O'Neill B, et al. Immediate versus delayed fluid resuscitation for hypotensive patients with penetrating torso injuries. *N Engl J Med.* 1994;331:1105–1109.
13. Teach SJ, Antosia RE, Lund DP, et al. Prehospital fluid therapy in pediatric trauma patients. *Pediatr Emerg Care.* 1995;11:5–8.
14. Waltzman ML, Mooney DP. Multiple trauma. In: Fleisher G, Ludwig S, Henretig FM, eds. *Textbook of Pediatric Emergency Medicine.* 5th ed. Baltimore, MD: Lippincott, Williams & Wilkins; 2006:1349–1360.
15. Sheik AA, Culbertson CB. Emergency department thoracotomy in children: Rationale for selective application. *J Trauma.* 1993;34:322.
16. Jaffe D, Weson D. Emergency management of blunt trauma in children. *N Engl J Med.* 1991;324:1477–1482.
17. Potoka DA, Saladino RA. Blunt abdominal trauma in the pediatric patient. *Clin Ped Emerg Med.* 2005;6(1):23–31.
18. Hegenbarth MA. Bedside ultrasound in the pediatric emergency department: basic skill or passing fancy? *Clin Ped Emerg Med.* 2004;5(4):201–216.
19. Tepas JJ III, Ramenofsky ML, Molitti DL, et al. The pediatric trauma score as a predictors of injury severity: an objective assessment. *J Trauma.* 1988;28:425–429.
20. Gaines BA. Pediatric trauma care: an ongoing evolution. *Clin Pediatr Emerg Med.* 2005;6:4–7.
21. Nayduch DA, Moylan J, et al. Comparison of the ability of adult and pediatric trauma scores to predict pediatric outcome following major trauma. *J Trauma.* 1991;31:452–457.
22. Jaimovich DG, Blostein PA, et al. Functional outcome of pediatric trauma patients identified as non-survivors. *J Trauma.* 1991;31:196–199.
23. Lieh-Lai MW, Theodorou AA, et al. Limitations of the Glasgow Coma Scale in predicting outcome in children with traumatic brain injury. *J Pediatr.* 1992;120:195–199.

CHAPTER 29

Head Trauma

Kimberly S. Quayle

▶ HIGH-YIELD FACTS

- The most common cause of head injury in children is falls. More severe injuries are likely caused by motor vehicle collisions, bicycle collisions, and assaults, including child abuse.
- Children with skull fractures are more likely to have an associated intracranial injury. However, intracranial injury may occur in the absence of skull fracture.
- Children with severe injuries, including those with altered mental status, focal neurologic deficits, or penetrating injuries, should undergo emergent computed tomography (CT) of the head and prompt neurosurgical consultation.
- Infants and children younger than 2 years may have subtle presentations despite clinically significant intracranial injury.
- Children with minor head injury and no loss of consciousness or brief loss of consciousness may be observed without CT of the head.
- Prevention of hypoxia, ischemia, and increased intracranial pressure is essential for children with severe head injuries.
- Although children have a greater likelihood of survival and recovery from brain injury than adults, they may be more vulnerable to long-term cognitive and behavioral dysfunction.

Traumatic brain injury is a significant cause of pediatric morbidity and mortality in the United States. More than 7000 children die each year as a result of traumatic brain injury, while another 60 000 are hospitalized, and an additional 500 000 seek care in emergency department.[1] Among children who die from trauma, 90% have an associated brain injury.[2] Pediatric brain injury leads to major morbidity from physical disability, seizures, and developmental delay. The most common cause of head injury in children is falls; however, severe injuries are more likely caused by motor vehicle collisions (with the child as occupant or pedestrian), bicycle collisions, and assaults, including child abuse particularly in the youngest children.[1,3] Boys are injured twice as commonly as girls.[2]

▶ PATHOPHYSIOLOGY

Primary brain injury occurs as a result of direct mechanical damage inflicted during the traumatic event. Secondary injuries occur from metabolic events such as hypoxia, ischemia, or increased intracranial pressure. The prognosis for recovery depends on the severity of the injuries. Anatomic features, specific injuries, and intracranial pressure physiology are important components in the pathophysiology of pediatric brain injury.

ANATOMY

The scalp is the outermost structure of the head and adjacent to the galea, which is a tendinous sheath connecting the frontalis and occipitalis muscles (Fig. 29–1). Beneath the galea is the subgaleal compartment where large hematomas may form in this space. The pericranium lies just below, tightly adhering to the skull. The outer and inner tables of the skull are separated by the diploic space. The thin, fibrous dura is next, and it contains few blood vessels compared to the underlying leptomeninges, the arachnoid, and pia. Small veins bridge the subdural space and drain into the dural sinuses. Dural attachments partially compartmentalize the brain. In the midline, the falx cerebri divides the right and left hemispheres of the brain. The tentorium divides the anterior and middle fossa from the posterior fossa, with an opening for the brain stem. Cerebrospinal fluid surrounds the brain within the subarachnoid space.

The outer structures protect the brain during everyday movements and minor trauma; however, these features can inflict damage when significant force is applied or sudden movement occurs. Movement of the brain within the vault along the uneven base of the skull may injure brain tissue. The unyielding, mature skull can contribute to brain injury when brain edema or an expanding hematoma develops. Subsequently, herniation across compartments can cause compression of vital structures, ischemia from vascular occlusion, and infarction.

In infants, the open sutures and thin calvarium produce a more flexible skull capable of absorbing greater impact. Incomplete myelinization contributes to greater plasticity of the brain as well. This flexibility permits more severe distortion between skull and dura, and cerebral vessels and brain, increasing susceptibility to hemorrhage. Finally, the disproportionately large size and weight of the head compared to the rest of the body of infants and young children contributes to an increased likelihood of head injury.

SPECIFIC INJURIES

The scalp is richly vascularized and, if injured, can bleed profusely. Scalp bleeding can lead to hemodynamically significant blood loss from relatively small lacerations, especially in infants and young children. Carefully explore open scalp wounds for skull integrity, depressions, or foreign bodies. The presenting sign of a subgaleal hematoma is an extensive soft tissue swelling that occurs several hours or days after the traumatic event and is commonly associated with a skull fracture. A subgaleal hematoma can persist for several days to weeks.

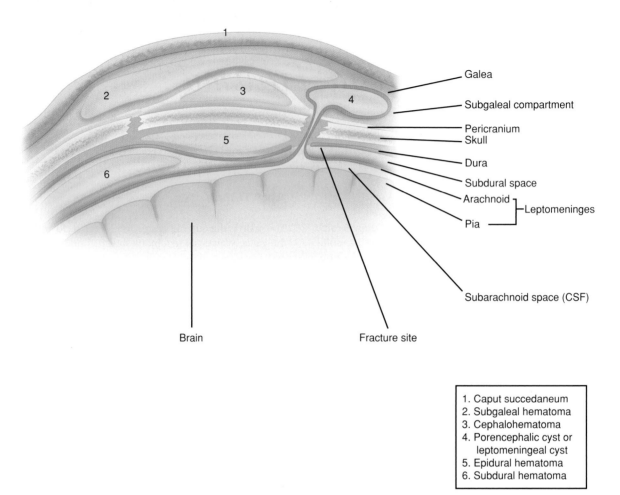

Figure 29–1. Traumatic head injuries.

Linear nondepressed skull fractures occur at the point of impact. The presence of a skull fracture indicates a significant blow to the head, and children with skull fractures are more likely to have an associated intracranial injury. However, the absence of a skull fracture does not exclude the presence of intracranial injury.[4] "Growing fractures" are unique to infants and young children. They may occur after a skull fracture in children younger than 2 years of age when associated with a dural tear. Rapid brain growth postinjury may be associated with the development of a leptomeningeal cyst, which is an extrusion of cerebrospinal fluid or brain tissue through the dural defect. Thus, children younger than 2 with a skull fracture require follow-up to detect a growing fracture.[2]

Basilar skull fractures typically occur at the petrous portion of the temporal bone, although they may occur anywhere along the base of the skull. Clinical signs suggesting a basilar skull fracture include hemotympanum, cerebrospinal fluid otorrhea, cerebrospinal fluid rhinorrhea, periorbital ecchymosis ("raccoon eyes"), or postauricular ecchymosis (Battle's sign). Radiologic diagnosis often requires detailed computed tomography (CT) imaging of the temporal bone, since plain skull radiographs or routine head CT scans may not be diagnostic.

Epidural hematomas occur more commonly in older children than infants and toddlers.[5] Most occur in combination with a temporal skull fracture and meningeal artery bleeding; the remainder are venous in origin. They may be life-threatening, but prompt diagnosis and surgical intervention make an excellent outcome possible. Signs and symptoms include headache, vomiting, and altered mental status, which may progress to signs and symptoms of uncal herniation with pupillary changes and hemiparesis. Patients classically present with an initial lucid period followed by a rapid deterioration in mental status, as the hemorrhage increases in size (Fig. 29–2).

Acute subdural hematomas occur more commonly than epidural hematomas in children.[2] Acute interhemispheric subdural hematomas, which occur more often in infants and young children, may be caused by shaking/impact injuries of abuse. Subdural hematomas usually result from tearing of the bridging veins and typically occur over the cerebral convexities. Subdural hematomas are often associated with more diffuse brain injury. They may progress more slowly than epidural bleeds, with symptoms commonly including irritability, vomiting, and alterations in mental status.

Parenchymal contusions are bruises or tears of brain tissue. Bony irregularities of the skull cause these cerebral contusions as the brain moves within the skull. A coup injury occurs at the site of impact, while a contrecoup injury occurs at a site remote from the impact. Intraparenchymal hemorrhages may

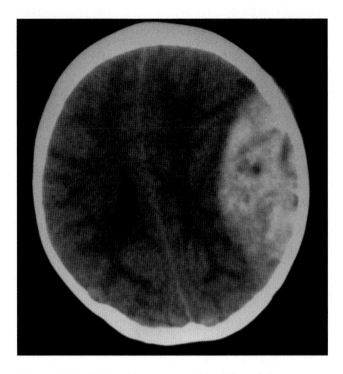

Figure 29–2. Epidural hematoma with midline shift.

also occur from shearing injury or penetrating wounds. They often occur in association with intracranial hematomas or skull fractures. Signs and symptoms may include decreased level of consciousness, focal neurologic findings, and seizures.

Penetrating injuries result from sharp-object penetration or gunshot wounds. Extensive brain injury is common and severity depends on the path of the object and location and degree of associated hemorrhage.

A concussion is defined as a "trauma-induced alteration in mental status that may or may not involve a loss of consciousness."[6] Additional symptoms may include vomiting, headache, dizziness, visual changes, as well as cognitive impairments and abnormal behavior. Most symptoms resolve after 48 hours; however, some symptoms may linger for weeks to months in a "postconcussive" syndrome.[7,8]

Diffuse brain swelling occurs more often in children than in adults.[9] The swelling usually results from a shearing or acceleration–deceleration injury. Prolonged coma or death may occur.

Nonaccidental trauma in infants and young children may result in the constellation of subdural hematoma, subarachnoid hemorrhage, and localized or diffuse brain edema (Fig. 29–3). Retinal hemorrhages, rib fractures, long bone fractures, and external signs of injury may also be present. Common symptoms of nonaccidental traumatic brain injury in infants may include lethargy, vomiting, irritability, seizures, and apnea. Many of these children may have severe alteration in consciousness.[10,11]

INTRACRANIAL PRESSURE AND HERNIATION SYNDROMES

The total volume of the intracranial vault is constant. Approximately 70% of this volume is brain, 20% is cerebrospinal and interstitial fluid, and 10% is blood. If any one of these three

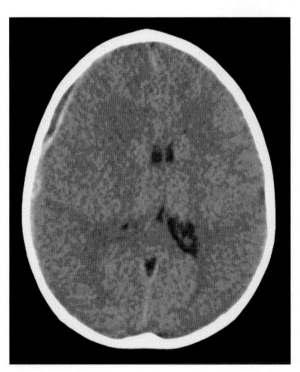

A

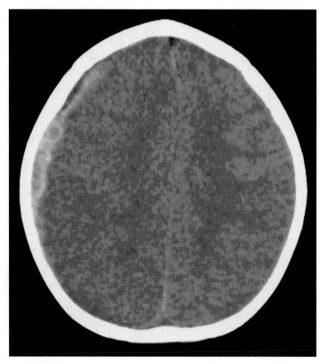

B

Figure 29–3. Right-sided subdural hematoma with associated midline shift and right hemispheric edema in an infant with nonaccidental head trauma.

components increases in volume, then the other two compartments must decrease or intracranial pressure rises. The main component of compensation is a displacement of cerebrospinal fluid into the spinal canal. Once this compensatory mechanism is maximized, any additional increases in volume cause elevation of intracranial pressure to abnormal levels (>15–20 mm Hg). Cerebral perfusion becomes impaired and irreversible ischemic damage to the brain ensues.

An intracranial mass or hematoma will occupy the fixed intracranial space, compress the normal brain tissue, and reduce blood flow. Cytotoxic cerebral edema occurs with fluid accumulation within damaged brain and glial cells. Interstitial cerebral edema results from decreased absorption of fluid following brain trauma. Vasogenic cerebral edema occurs as the endothelial cell barrier is compromised and leakage of fluid into the perivascular brain tissue occurs.

The volume of cerebrospinal fluid may also increase despite the compensatory redistribution of the fluid into the spinal canal. As brain and blood volumes increase, the ventricular spaces become compressed until redistribution is not possible. Additionally, if the cerebrospinal fluid pathways are compressed by edematous tissue, cerebrospinal fluid outflow ceases and ventricular dilation and hydrocephalus can occur.

Cerebral blood volume in head-injured children may be increased as a result of brain injury. The mechanisms of autoregulation of cerebral blood flow are complex; however, flow is often increased in head-injured children, possibly due to a loss of normal autoregulatory mechanisms leading to increased risk for brain swelling. Hypoxia and hypotension of the injured patient may also contribute to diffuse brain edema. Causes of diffuse brain swelling are likely multifactorial, including hyperemia, excitotoxic neurotransmitters, enhanced inflammatory response, and increased blood–brain permeability.

Diffusely or focally increased intracranial pressure may produce herniation. Cingulate herniation occurs as one cerebral hemisphere is displaced underneath the falx cerebri to the opposite side. A transtentorial or uncal herniation is of major clinical significance (Fig. 29–4). A mass lesion or hematoma

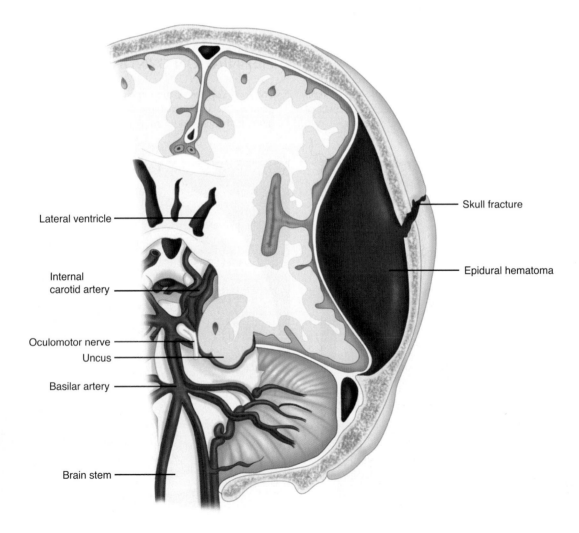

Lateral ventricle

Internal carotid artery

Oculomotor nerve

Uncus

Basilar artery

Brain stem

Skull fracture

Epidural hematoma

Figure 29–4. Anterior view of transtentorial uncal herniation caused by a large epidural hematoma. (With permission from American College of Emergency Physicians. *Emergency Medicine: A Comprehensive Study Guide.* 3rd ed. New York: McGraw-Hill; 1992.)

forces the ipsilateral uncus of the temporal lobe through the space between the cerebral peduncle and the tentorium. This causes ipsilateral compression of the oculomotor nerve and an ipsilateral dilated nonreactive pupil. The cerebral peduncle is compressed causing a contralateral hemiparesis. As the intracranial pressure increases and the brain stem is compressed, consciousness wanes. If herniation continues, ongoing brain stem deterioration occurs, progressing to apnea and death. Uncal herniation may be bilateral if there are bilateral lesions or diffuse edema. Herniation of the cerebellar tonsils downward through the foramen magnum occurs infrequently in children. Medullary compression from this herniation causes bradycardia, respiratory arrest, and death.

▶ ASSESSMENT

Assessment begins with a detailed history of the traumatic event, such as the mechanism of injury and the time and location of injury. Note the signs and symptoms occurring since the injury, including loss of consciousness, seizures, vomiting, headache, visual changes, altered mental status, weakness, and amnesia. Past medical history should include prior history of seizures, neurologic abnormalities, bleeding disorders, and immunization status. Child abuse should be suspected for a witnessed report of abuse, a history insufficient to explain the injuries present, a changing or inconsistent history, or a developmentally incompatible history.

Physical evaluation begins with the primary assessment. Airway obstruction by the tongue commonly occurs in unconscious children with serious head injury. Blood, vomitus, teeth, foreign bodies, or other debris may obstruct the airway as well. Establish an airway by positioning, suctioning, placing an oral airway, or intubation. Maintain cervical spine control in children with significant head injury until cervical spine injury is excluded. Manually stabilize the cervical spine during laryngoscopy.

Once the airway is established, assess ventilation by observing chest expansion, auscultate breath sounds, and assess for cyanosis or respiratory distress. Hypoventilation is treated with 100% oxygen, bag-valve-mask ventilation, and subsequent intubation of the trachea with consideration of rapid sequence technique.

Compared to awake intubation, the rapid sequence induction (RSI) technique produces an unconscious and paralyzed patient, creating an easier procedure for the physician and providing a better-tolerated procedure for the patient with less discomfort and less elevation of intracranial pressure. The RSI technique should also reduce the risk of aspiration in trauma patients, who should be presumed to have full stomach. The general procedure for RSI is discussed in Chapter 24; however, there are a few points of special note regarding the use of RSI in head trauma patients.

Ketamine is contraindicated in patients with head injury because it increases intracranial pressure, though this is being reevaluated. The use of succinylcholine is controversial in such patients because of concerns for possible increased intracranial pressure associated with its use. Rocuronium, a nondepolarizing muscle relaxant that does not increase intracranial pressure, is an alternative because its onset of action is similar to that of succinylcholine but its duration of action is significantly longer.

RSI for intubation is contraindicated in patients with major facial or laryngeal trauma or distorted facial and airway anatomy. These conditions may lead to a situation in which intubation or mask ventilation is unsuccessful.

Evaluate the circulation by checking heart rate, peripheral pulses, and perfusion. Control any life-threatening hemorrhage and maintain blood pressure so that there is adequate cerebral perfusion. Treat hypotension initially with isotonic fluid boluses. Hypovolemic shock is rare after an isolated head injury, although it does occur rarely in infants and young children. Other sources for hypovolemia must be identified.

After the rapid ABC (airway, breathing, circulation) assessment, a primary survey of neurologic disability follows. Ascertain the level of consciousness and categorize the patient as alert, responsive to verbal stimulus, responsive to painful stimulus, or unresponsive (AVPU). Evaluate the pupillary response. The remainder of the primary survey is completed prior to returning to a more detailed secondary neurologic examination. Examine the scalp and palpate for depressions. Evaluate the fontanel in the infant. Look for signs of basilar skull fracture. Evaluate extraocular movements, muscle tone, spontaneous movements, and posture. An older child should move the extremities in response to the examiner's request. Palpate the neck for tenderness or deformities. Note any stereotyped posturing. Decorticate posturing signifies damage to the cerebral cortex, white matter, or basal ganglia. Decerebrate posturing suggests damage to the midbrain.

In adults and older children, the Glasgow Coma Scale (GCS) is commonly used to assess and follow the level of consciousness in head-injured patients. The Glasgow Coma Scale evaluates for eye opening, best motor response, and best verbal response (Table 29–1). Use of this scale in infants and young children is limited due to this age group's underdeveloped verbal skills, so modifications have been made for the preverbal child (Table 29–2). Evaluation of young children and infants following head injury may be difficult, particularly the assessment of mental status and neurologic examination.

The neurologic status of a head-injured child must be reassessed regularly, particularly with regard to level of consciousness and vital signs. The frequency of reassessment should be dictated by the condition of the child.

▶ TABLE 29–1. GLASGOW COMA SCALE*

Eye opening (E)	Spontaneous	4
	To speech/voice	3
	To pain	2
	No response	1
Motor response (M)	Obeys commands	6
	Localizes pain	5
	Withdraws to pain	4
	Abnormal flexion-decorticate	3
	Abnormal extension-decerebrate	2
	No response	1
Verbal response (V)	Oriented	5
	Confused/disoriented	4
	Inappropriate words	3
	Incomprehensible sounds	2
	No response	1

*E + M + V = coma score (range: 3–15).

► TABLE 29-2. GLASGOW COMA SCALE*
MODIFIED FOR THE PREVERBAL CHILD

Eye opening (E)	Spontaneous	4
	To speech/voice	3
	To pain	2
	No response	1
Motor response (M)	Spontaneous movements	6
	Withdraws to touch	5
	Withdraws to pain	4
	Abnormal flexion	3
	Extensor response	2
	None	1
Verbal response (V)	Coos, babbles	5
	Irritable, cries	4
	Cries to pain	3
	Moans to pain	2
	None	1

*E + M + V = coma score (range: 3–15).
With permission from Reilly PL, Simpson DA, Sprod R, et al. Assessing the conscious level in infants and young children: a pediatric version of the Glasgow Coma Scale. *Childs Nerv Syst.* 1988;4:30.

► DIAGNOSTIC STUDIES

In children with serious injuries, complete blood count, type and cross-match, electrolytes, and coagulation studies should be done. Arterial blood gases, toxicology screens, and ethanol levels are obtained as indicated. Cervical spine films should be obtained in alert patients with neck pain or neurologic deficits and in all unconscious patients.

Computed tomography (CT) of the head is the diagnostic method of choice for identification of intracranial pathology in patients with acute head trauma. Skull radiographs are not routinely recommended. However, they may be useful in certain clinical situations, such as screening in young infants with scalp hematomas, in cases of suspected nonaccidental trauma, or when CT is not readily available. Children with severe injuries including those with altered mental status, focal neurologic deficits, or penetrating injuries should undergo emergent head CT and prompt neurosurgical consultation. Children with a known skull fracture or signs of a basilar or depressed skull fracture should also undergo head CT.

Consensus is lacking for the management of previously healthy children who are alert with normal, nonfocal neurologic examinations following minor head injury. The American Academy of Pediatrics has published recommendations for the evaluation of children 2 to 20 years of age with minor head injury, but not with multiple trauma, cervical spine injury, preexisting neurologic disorder, bleeding diathesis, suspected intentional head trauma, language barrier, or the presence of drugs or alcohol.[12] This practice parameter recommends observation by a reliable caretaker for neurologically normal children with no loss of consciousness or with brief loss of consciousness. Head CT scans may be obtained for children with brief loss of consciousness if desired by the physician and parents. Children without a history of loss of consciousness, but with a history of seizure, headache, vomiting, or amnesia, may be observed

without a head CT if they have an alert mental status and a normal neurologic examination.

Growing concerns regarding radiation exposure to the developing brain have prompted additional clinical studies to develop guidelines for the management of children with minor head injuries. Decision rules have been developed using the presence of skull fracture, mechanism of injury, and signs and symptoms to predict traumatic brain injury.[13,14] No single guideline has been widely adapted; however, a large multicenter study may produce such a guideline in the near future.

Infants and children younger than 2 years may have subtle presentations despite clinically significant intracranial injury. Published guidelines provide recommendations for the management of minor head injury in this age group as well.[15] Infants with high-risk findings, such as depressed mental status, focal neurologic deficit, signs of depressed or basilar skull fracture, seizure, irritability, acute skull fracture, bulging fontanel, vomiting five or more times or for more than 6 hours, or loss of consciousness for 1 minute or longer, should undergo prompt CT scanning. A head CT should be considered in infants at intermediate risk with vomiting three to four times, brief loss of consciousness or history of resolved lethargy or irritability. Head CT, skull radiographs or observation may be selected for infants with scalp hematomas, a higher-force mechanism of trauma, a fall onto a hard surface, or unwitnessed trauma. If skull radiographs are chosen based on lack of availability of CT or need for sedation, then the presence of a skull fracture should prompt transport to a facility capable of performing head CT. Infants at low risk who are asymptomatic and have a low-energy mechanism of trauma may be carefully observed by a reliable caretaker.

Patients who do not meet criteria for imaging may be observed at home by a reliable caretaker with careful instructions to return the child to medical attention if symptoms develop, worsen, or persist. Children who have normal head CT scans and normal mental status and neurologic examinations may also be observed at home, as the development of delayed intracranial injuries in these patients is rare. Children with isolated nondepressed skull fractures without intracranial injury may also be observed at home after discussion with the neurosurgeon.

► TREATMENT

The goal of management of head injury in children is to prevent secondary injury to the brain. Prevention of hypoxia, ischemia, and increased intracranial pressure is essential. Prompt neurosurgical intervention is necessary in the majority of seriously head-injured or multisystem-injured children.

As discussed earlier, endotracheal intubation and controlled ventilation are almost always required for patients with severe head injury. Intubate any child with a GCS of 8 or less. Hypoxemia may worsen the initial injury or cause secondary brain injury. Avoid hypercarbia as it can increase intracranial pressure. By following arterial blood gases and adjusting ventilator settings accordingly, it is possible to keep arterial P_{O_2} and P_{CO_2} near normal levels, unless the child has underlying pulmonary disease or injury. Modest hyperventilation (P_{CO_2} 35–40 Torr) is recommended for managing increased intracranial pressure.[16,17] In the emergency department setting, mild hyperventilation and correlation with end-tidal CO_2 may be used in unconscious patients, prior to insertion of an intracranial pressure monitor. More aggressive hyperventilation may be needed to treat acute deterioration, but other treatment may be more appropriate.

Hypotension has been associated with poor outcome in children with traumatic brain injury.[9] Brain perfusion must be preserved by maintaining normal intracranial pressure and normal mean arterial pressure. Cerebral perfusion pressure is equal to mean arterial pressure minus intracranial pressure. Hypotension should be treated with isotonic fluid boluses and inotropic medications as needed to maintain an adequate mean arterial blood pressure and cerebral perfusion pressure.

Mannitol is often used to maintain optimal intracranial pressure by reducing intravascular volume.[16] Fluid restriction may be used in conjunction; however, cerebral perfusion pressure must be maintained. Hypertonic saline (3%) has been studied in children with traumatic brain injury, but is not routinely used in the emergency setting. Syndromes of inappropriate antidiuretic hormone secretion or diabetes insipidus may occur in children with serious head injury; therefore, fluid balance and electrolyte status must be followed closely. Seizures may occur following brain injury. Most children with serious injuries are treated with fosphenytoin either to treat active seizures or for prophylaxis.[16]

Seriously brain-injured children must be monitored in an intensive care setting. Cardiopulmonary monitors, noninvasive blood pressure monitors or indwelling arterial catheters, and urinary catheters are commonly used. Intracranial pressure monitors may be used to detect acute changes in intracranial pressure, to limit indiscriminate therapies, to control intracranial pressure, and to reduce intracranial pressure directly by cerebrospinal fluid drainage. The patient should be positioned with a 30-degree elevation of the head. Corticosteroids and hypothermia are not routinely used to treat children with serious brain injury. Sedation and analgesia should be used as needed to limit wide fluctuations in intracranial pressure.[17] Coordination of the care for these children should involve neurosurgical, pediatric, and critical care physicians, most often in a tertiary care pediatric center.

The care for children with less serious injuries depends on the clinical situation. If children have persistent alteration in mental status despite a normal head CT, they should be admitted for observation with serial neurologic examinations. Children with protracted vomiting may need intravenous hydration and admission. Children with suspected child abuse should also be admitted for observation as well as evaluation of the social situation.

The majority of children who have minor head injuries can be observed safely at home by an adult caretaker with careful, detailed instructions to return if there is a change in condition. If a responsible caretaker cannot be identified, hospital admission for observation for the first 24 hours is warranted. Young athletes with concussions should delay return to play at least 1 week after the injury if the symptoms last longer than 15 minutes. With a history of any loss of consciousness, return to play should be 2 to 4 weeks after the injury.[6,7] Children with symptomatic head injury or isolated nondepressed skull fractures should be seen by their primary physician 24 hours after the emergency department visit.

▶ PROGNOSIS

Over the past 20 years, morbidity and mortality secondary to pediatric traumatic brain injury has dramatically declined.[18] Infants and children have long been thought to have better functional outcomes following a severe brain injury; however, new data suggests that children younger than 4 years of age have the poorest outcomes, compared to older children and adults. This may be related to the high incidence of nonaccidental trauma as cause for severe injury in this age group.[9] Early identification of neurobehavioral deficits is an important part of follow-up in children with significant head injury.

REFERENCES

1. Langlois JA, Rutland-Brown W, Thomas KE. *Traumatic Brain Injury in the United States.* Bethesda, MD: National Center for Injury Prevention and Control; 2006. http://www.cdc.gov/injury.
2. Atabaki SM. Pediatric head injury. *Pediat Rev.* 2007;28:215.
3. Keenan HT, Bratton SL. Epidemiology and outcomes of pediatric traumatic brain injury. *Dev Neurosci.* 2006;28:256.
4. Schnadower D, Vazquez H, Lee J, et al. Controversies in the evaluation and management of minor blunt head trauma in children. *Curr Opin Pediatr.* 2007;19:258.
5. Zuckerman GB, Conway EE. Accidental head injury. *Pediatr Ann.* 1997;26:621.
6. American Academy of Neurology. Practice parameter: the management of concussion in sports. *Neurology.* 1997;48:581.
7. Kirkwood MW, Yeates KO, Wilson PE. Pediatric sport-related concussion: a review of the clinical management of an oft-neglected population. *Pediatrics.* 2006;117:1359.
8. Ropper AH, Gorson KC. Concussion. *New Engl J Med.* 2007;356:166.
9. Kochanek PM. Pediatric traumatic brain injury: quo vadis? *Dev Neurosci.* 2006;28:244.
10. Duhaime AC, Christian CW, Rorke LB, et al. Nonaccidental head injury in infants—the shaken baby syndrome. *N Engl J Med.* 1998;338:1822.
11. Gerber P, Coffman K. Nonaccidental head trauma in infants. *Childs Nerv Syst.* 2007;23:499.
12. Committee on Quality Improvement, American Academy of Pediatrics. The management of minor closed head injury in children. *Pediatrics.* 1999;104:1407.
13. Palchak MJ, Holmes JF, Vance CW, et al. A decision rule for identifying children at low risk for brain injuries after blunt head trauma. *Ann Emerg Med.* 2003;42:492.
14. Dunning J, Daly JP, Lomas JP, et al. Derivation of the children's head injury algorithm for the prediction of important clinical events decision rule for head injury in children. *Arch Dis Child.* 2006;91:885.
15. Schutzman SA, Barnes P, Duhaime AC, et al. Evaluation and management of children younger than two years old with apparently minor head trauma: proposed guidelines. *Pediatrics.* 2001;107:983.
16. Adelson PD, Bratton SL, Carney NA, et al. Guidelines for the acute medical management of severe traumatic brain injury in infants, children, and adolescents. *Pediatr Crit Care Med.* 2003;4(suppl 3):S2.
17. Jankowitz BT, Adelson PD. Pediatric traumatic brain injury: past, present, and future. *Dev Neurosci.* 2006;28:264.
18. Mazzola CA, Adelson PD. Critical care management of head trauma in children. *Crit Care Med.* 2002;30(suppl):S393.

CHAPTER 30

Pediatric Cervical Spine Injury

Julie Leonard and Jeffrey Russell Leonard

▶ HIGH-YIELD FACTS

- Cervical spine injury should be suspected in any child who has suffered traumatic respiratory arrest and rapid sequence orotracheal intubation should be preformed with in-line cervical spine stabilization.
- Because of differences in anatomy and physiology, children sustain proportionally more upper cervical spine and spinal cord injury without radiographic abnormality (SCIWORA) injuries compared to adults.
- Standard radiographic screening for children consists of the AP, lateral, and open-mouth views; however, in younger or uncooperative children, the open-mouth view can be omitted. CT scan is more sensitive for bony injury and MRI for soft tissue injury.
- Although spine immobilization is indicated when cervical spine injury is suspected, there are documented complications and decisions to immobilize should be selective and target those at greatest risk for cervical spine injury.

Cervical spine injuries are serious, but rare events in children.[1,2] Emergency physicians are often the first to evaluate pediatric trauma patients with cervical spine injury and are required to quickly sort children with the potential for worsening neurological deficits from those with either no cervical spine injury or cervical sprain. Occasionally, these decisions are made in the absence of adequate cervical spine imaging when dealing with a child's unstable airway or other life-threatening injuries. These challenges raise some specific questions:

- Are there specific subsets of children who present to the emergency department and are at the highest risk for cervical spine injuries?
- Which children should be immobilized and how is this best achieved?
- How is the cervical spine "cleared"?
- If an artificial airway is needed, how should it be provided in children who may have cervical spine injuries?

▶ EPIDEMIOLOGY

Traumatic injury is the leading cause of morbidity and mortality in children, yet cervical spine injury represents a small subset of those injured. Cervical spine injury affects less than 1% of children undergoing emergency department trauma evaluation and only 1.5% of children enrolled in the National Pediatric Trauma Registry.[3,4] It is estimated that there is an overall 17% mortality associated with cervical spine injury in children; however, this rate may be as high as 60% in children ≤8 years.[4] This increased risk of mortality is likely associated with proportionately higher rate of upper cervical spine injury in young children.[4]

Within the pediatric population, motor vehicle collisions are the most common cause of cervical spine injuries.[5,6] However, the mechanisms vary by age. Neonates may suffer cervical spine injuries from birth trauma, particularly in the case of breech or forceps deliveries.[7,8] The incidence of nonaccidental trauma is likely underestimated in the pediatric population.[9] Sports-related injuries, pedestrians hit by motor vehicles, and falls are common mechanisms of cervical spine injury in older children and teenagers; while violent injuries, including assault and gunshot wounds, are causes of cervical spine injuries in the late teenage years.[5,6]

▶ ANATOMY AND PHYSIOLOGY

It is essential to understand the developmental anatomy of the pediatric spine. Although the development of the subaxial vertebrae is relatively consistent, the components of the craniocervical junction and upper cervical spine (occiput, atlas, and axis) have distinctive developmental patterns. Recognition of this is critical in differentiating fracture from normal developmental anatomy, as they may appear nearly identical radiographically.

The atlas (C1) has three primary ossification centers: one anterior arch and two neural arches. There are open cartilaginous synchondroses between the anterior arch and either neural arch as well as posteriorly between the two neural arches. By age 3, the neural arches are typically fused to form the solid posterior ring of C1. The neurocentral sychondrosis fuses by age 7.[10] Four identifiable ossification centers are present in the developing axis (C2).[10,11] The neural arches of C2 fuse posteriorly by age 3. The body of C2 fuses with the neural arches and the dens between ages 3 and 6. However, the subdental synchondrosis may be seen until ages 10 to 11. Any lucency at the base of the dens beyond this age is abnormal and should be considered a fracture.[12] Fortunately, each level of the subaxial cervical spine, including C3 to C7, follows the same developmental pattern. Three primary ossification centers occur at each level: a centrum for the body and two neural arches. In the subaxial spine, the neural arches fuse by age 3, whereas the body fuses with the neural arches by ages 3 to 6.[10] Secondary ossification centers in the transverse and spinous processes are present by puberty and fuse completely by the third decade.[10]

A relatively large head size in comparison with the remainder of the body, immature neck and paraspinal musculature, underdeveloped ligaments, incompletely ossified bone, anterior wedging of vertebral bodies, absent uncinate processes, and shallow, horizontally oriented facets all contribute to hypermobility in the pediatric cervical spine.[13–17] As a result, the fulcrum of motion in the pediatric cervical spine is at C2 to C3 rendering the upper cervical spine more prone to injury. With maturation of the spine and supporting soft tissues, the fulcrum migrates to C5 to C6 by age 14, making the biomechanics of the cervical spine and the injuries sustained similar to those observed in adults.[15,18]

► EVALUATION AND MANAGEMENT

All trauma evaluations begin with attention to the ABCs: airway, breathing, and circulation. Airway obstruction is common in the unconscious or severely injured trauma patients, and the mandibular block of tissue often obstructs the airway of the supine, unconscious child. Additionally, the child may be unable to cough or expectorate to clear mucus, vomitus, blood, or other debris. Lifting the mandible with a jaw-thrust maneuver often opens and improves the airway. The emergency practitioner must be cognizant of the potential for a cervical spine injury, which could be worsened by excessive motion of the spine (Fig. 30–1) and stabilize the cervical spine while performing the jaw-thrust maneuver.

The spine-injured patient may become hypopneic because of diminished diaphragmatic activity or intercostal muscle paralysis. Concomitant head or chest injuries and aspiration of gastric contents may further compromise ventilation. Therefore, supplemental humidified oxygen should routinely be provided and ventilation should be assisted whenever hypoventilation is suspected. Although the bag-mask technique will permit ventilation, its prolonged use increases the likelihood of aspiration of gastric contents. Therefore, the emergency practitioner may need to intubate the patient prior to completing full evaluation of the cervical spine. Cervical spine immobilization with an orthotic device was shown to make direct laryngoscopy three times more difficult compared to manual immobilization during intubation.[19] Manual in-line cervical stabilization, rapid sequence induction, and oral endotracheal intubation are the preferred techniques to achieve airway stabilization in children with suspected cervical spine injury (Fig. 30–2). In children, blind nasotracheal intubation is unreliable because it can be technically difficult. Emergency cricothyrotomy is relatively contraindicated in young children because of the small size of the cricothyroid membrane and the likelihood of causing permanent tracheal damage. The emergency physician must ensure an adequate airway for an injured child and protect the C-spine but not delay doing so while waiting for the cervical spine to be cleared.

Hypotension may be secondary to either hypovolemia or spinal shock. A clue to differentiating these is the pulse, which is slow in spinal shock and rapid in hypovolemic shock. Adequate fluid (crystalloid, colloid, and blood) is administered to combat hypovolemia. In the case of spinal shock, vaso-

pressors, such as dopamine, may be needed. The patient with spinal shock may be more sensitive to temperature variations than other patients and may require warming or cooling if subjected to extreme environmental temperatures either at the scene or during transport. Protect areas of the body that may have lost sensation from hard, protruding objects, as they may cause skin necrosis, especially on long transports.

Once the patient's cardiopulmonary status is stabilized, a thorough physical assessment and neurological examination is performed. Spinal cord injury should be suspected whenever there has been severe multiple trauma; significant trauma to the head, neck, or back; or any trauma associated with high-speed vehicular crashes and falls from heights. A useful diagnostic mnemonic is to evaluate the "six P's": Pain, Position, Paralysis, Paresthesia, Ptosis, and Priapism.

Conscious children old enough to talk may complain of pain localized to the involved vertebra. Head injury with diminished level of consciousness, intoxication, or significant injury of another part of the body may make the localization of pain unreliable. The patient's position may indicate a spine injury. A head tilt may be associated with a rotary subluxation of C1 on C2 or a high cervical injury. The prayer position (arms folded across the chest) may signify a fracture in the C4 to C6 area. Paresis or paralysis of the arms or legs should always suggest spine injury. Paresthesia, a "pins and needles" sensation or numbness or burning, may sometimes seem inconsequential, but these symptoms should always be taken as potential indicators of spine injury. Some patients complain of a transient shock-like or electrical sensation transmitted down the spine during neck flexion and/or rotation (Lhermitte's sign). Horner's syndrome (ptosis and a miotic pupil) suggests a cervical cord injury. Priapism is present only in approximately 3% to 5% of spine-injured patients, but indicates that the sympathetic nervous system is involved. Absence of the bulbocavernosus reflex in the presence of flaccid paralysis carries a grave prognosis. To elicit the bulbocavernosus reflex, a finger is inserted into the rectum, and then the glans of the penis or the head of the clitoris is squeezed. A normal response is a reflex contraction of the anal sphincter.

There are also characteristic cord syndromes (Table 30–1). In spinal shock, there is flaccid paralysis below the level of the lesion, absent reflexes, decreased sympathetic tone, and autonomic dysfunction. Sensation may be preserved, but if it is absent, the prognosis for recovery is poor. Central cord syndrome is often associated with extension injuries, which can cause circumferential pinching of the spinal cord by the ligamentum flavum. The anterior cord syndrome is associated with severe flexion injuries, especially teardrop fractures, in which a fragment of the fractured vertebral body is driven posteriorly into the anterior portion of the spinal cord.

Upper extremity position and function may provide clues not only to the presence of a cervical cord injury but also to the level of injury. With injuries at C5, patients can flex at the elbows, but are unable to extend them; with injuries at C6 to C7, they can flex and extend at the elbows; and injuries at the T1 level allow finger and wrist flexion.

During trauma evaluation, the emergency physician must determine whether or not a child is at risk for cervical spine injury and warrants cervical spine immobilization and radiographic evaluation. Clinical criteria for "clearing" the cervical spine have been established in adults. The National Emergency

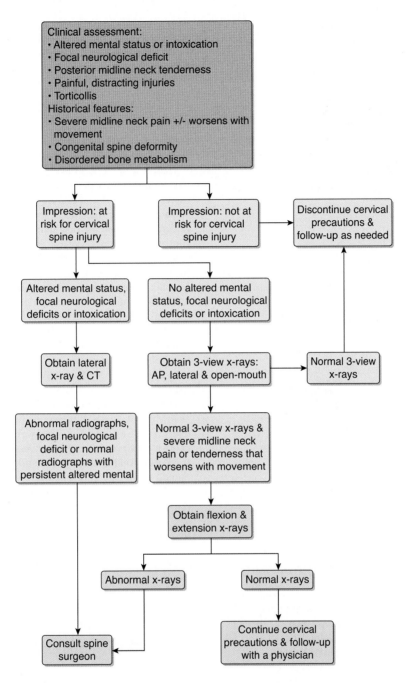

Figure 30–1. Algorithm for cervical spine clearance in blunt trauma injury.

X-ray Utilization Study (NEXUS) collaboration identified five clinical screening criteria (posterior midline cervical tenderness, altered alertness, distracting injury, intoxication, and focal neurological findings), which have nearly 100% sensitivity for cervical spine injury and had good interrater agreement among emergency physicians.[20–23] Alternatively, the Canadian C-spine Rule has been reported to have nearly 100% sensitivity for cervical spine injury in alert and stable adult trauma patients. The Canadian C-spine Rule was based on clinical, epidemiologic, and mechanism of injury variables.[24,25] Neither of these studies focused on children. Early attempts to define pediatric clinical screening criteria have tended to agree with the adult criteria, but are not generalizable because of small sample sizes that are not geographically, demographically, or clinically representative.[3,26–28] Furthermore, preverbal children who rarely experience cervical spine injury are particularly understudied and are potentially most at risk from inappropriate immobilization. Until further evidence for clinical risk stratification in pediatric cervical spine injury emerges, it is reasonable to rely on the NEXUS criteria coupled with the complaint of severe neck pain or the finding of severe craniofacial injuries to determine risk in children.

All trauma victims should be unstrapped and removed from the rigid long board, which is used for extrication and

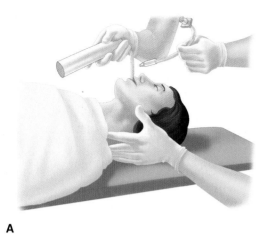

A

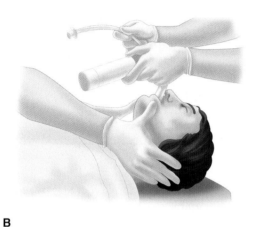

B

Figure 30–2. In-line stabilization for endotracheal intubation: (A) above and (B) below.

▶ **TABLE 30-1. SYNDROMES ASSOCIATED WITH SPINAL CORD INJURY**

Spinal shock	Brown-Séquard syndrome
• Flaccid below level of lesion	• Hemisection
• Absent reflexes	• Ipsilateral loss of
• Decreased sympathetic tone	○ Motor function
• Autonomic dysfunction (including hypotension)	○ Proprioception
• Sensation may not be preserved; if absent = total cord transection (poor prognosis)	• Contralateral loss of sensation:
	○ Pain
	○ Temperature
Central cord syndrome	Anterior cord syndrome
• Diminished or absent upper extremity function	• Complete motor paralysis
• Preserved lower extremity function	• Loss of pain and temperature sensation
• Associated with extension injuries	• Preservation of position and vibration sense
	• Associated with severe flexion injuries

patient transfers in the out-of-hospital setting. This aspect of "full spine immobilization" is known to be associated with adverse effects. Ventilation of trauma victims may be encumbered by full spinal immobilization. A study of healthy children who were fully immobilized demonstrated a mean reduction in FVC to 80% of their unrestrained supine FVC.[29] A similar significant decrease in mean FVC has been documented among adults.[30] Full spinal immobilization has been reported to cause substantial pain, which may last well beyond the immediate period of immobilization.[31–34] Furthermore, pain caused by spinal immobilization may be confused with pain caused by injury leading to unnecessary diagnostic evaluations. In spine-injured patients, prolonged immobilization on a rigid long board is associated with an increased risk of developing pressure sores during the immediate postinjury period.[35,36] The cervical collar can be discontinued once it has been determined either clinically or radiographically that the pediatric trauma victim is free of cervical spine injury.

If a child may be at risk for cervical spine injury, take steps to maintain neutral cervical spine positioning. In this position, the cervical spine is in lordosis and there is maximal spinal canal diameter. Achieving this position in children can be difficult. Studies evaluating spine positioning during immobilization indicate that patients, depending on habitus, are often immobilized in nonphysiologic positions. In children younger than 8 years, supine positioning without shoulder padding results in cervical kyphosis due to a relatively large head (Fig. 30–3).[37,38] In adults, however, supine positioning causes relative cervical lordosis.[39,40] The normal variation in the ratio of head to body among children results in a range of cervical spine positioning of up to 27-degree flexion or extension from neutral during immobilization for trauma transport.[41] Thus, as a child grows, padding may be required in either the shoulder or occipital regions to provide neutral positioning.

Children attended to in the prehospital setting often arrive at the emergency department with immobilization of the cervical spine. Rigid collars are available for infants and children; however, the availability of these devices is limited in

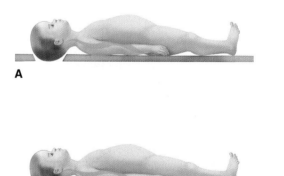

A

B

Figure 30–3. Backboard modifications for children. (A) Young child on a modified backboard that has a cutout to recess the occiput, obtaining a safe supine cervical positioning. (B) Young child on a modified backboard that has a double-mattress pad to raise the chest, obtaining a safe supine cervical positioning.

the prehospital setting. Cloth tape or straps across the fore-head and external orthoses, including a rigid backboard, are usually employed to complete the immobilization. When in the emergency department, extrication collars should be evaluated and replaced with an appropriately sized rigid cervical collar. The decision regarding the type of orthosis needed depends on the age of the patient, the affected levels, and the restriction of movement needed (flexion, extension, rotation, etc.). Studies have demonstrated that the commonly available rigid cervical collars, such as Aspen, Miami J, and Philadelphia, all provide significant restriction in neck movement but have subtle variations and the final choice of cervical collar is often based on availability and the recommendations of a spine surgeon.[42]

The evaluation of a child for potential cervical spine injury must be done carefully and requires some creativity. Sensation should be checked, both light touch and pressure. Evaluate for weakness by having the child handle an item or hold each extremity off of the stretcher for a count of 5 if the child is conscious and old enough to follow commands. More ingenuity is needed for the infant and toddler.

The results of the second National Acute Spinal Cord Injury Study were reported in May 1990.[43] The investigators reported that high-dose methylprednisolone (30 mg/kg) followed by 5.4 mg/kg/h for 23 hours, if given within 8 hours of acute spinal cord injury, improved the neurological recovery as compared to placebo or naloxone. Children younger than 13 years were excluded from the study. The putative mechanism of action is the ability of the steroid at these doses to inhibit oxygen free radical–induced lipid peroxidation. Lipid peroxidation is thought to mediate cell membrane degeneration and to explain other documented tissue-protective effects of steroids: support of energy metabolism, prevention of post-traumatic ischemia, reversal of intracellular calcium accumulation, prevention of neurofilament degradation, inhibition of vasoactive prostaglandin F_2 and thromboxane generation, and retardation of axonal degeneration. Still, there are no clinical trials confirming the efficacy of this regimen in children and it has become an acceptable option in neurosurgical practice to administer glucocorticoids to treat spinal cord injuries in children.[44]

► ANALYSIS OF RADIOGRAPHS

The standard screening series for adults consists of three views: cross-table lateral view (CTLV), anteroposterior view (AP), and open-mouth view (OM). The open-mouth view is used to visualize C1, C2, and the atlantoaxial and atlantooccipital articulations. Because the open-mouth view is difficult to obtain in younger children, the value of requiring the OM view in cervical spine screening has been questioned. The Waters view can be substituted to allow visualization of the odontoid projected through the foramen magnum. The steps in evaluating the CTLV are presented in Table 30–2. On the AP view, symmetry of longitudinal alignment of vertebral bodies, facets, pillars, and spinous processes is assessed. Evidence of linear or compression fractures as well as more subtle indicators such as stepoffs, subluxations, and malalignments are sought. On the OM view, the alignment of the atlantooccipital and atlantoaxial joints, alignment of the margins of the lateral arches of C1 with C2, and the position of the odontoid between the lateral arches

► **TABLE 30–2. CRITERIA FOR CLEARING THE LATERAL SPINE**

- All seven vertebral bodies are seen clearly, including the C7-T1 junction
- The posterior cervical line is properly aligned as are the four lordotic curves, which are the anterior longitudinal ligament line, the spinolaminal line, and the lips of the spinous processes
- The predental space is 4 to 5 mm
- All vertebrae are free of fractures and changes in density, which would suggest compression fractures or metastatic lesions
- The intervertebral and interspinous spaces are not more than 11 degrees at a single interspace.
- There is no fanning of spinous processes, which would suggest posterior ligament disruption
- The prevertebral soft tissue distance is less than 7 mm at C2 and less than 5 mm at C3–C4. Note that in children <2 y of age, the space may appear widened if it is not an inspiratory film
- No dislocation at the atlantooccipital region

of C1 are evaluated. These bony structures are also examined for fractures.

In a large multicentered prospective observational study, the sensitivity for cervical spine injury of a three-view standard plain radiograph series was 89.4% (95% CI, 86.9%–91.4%).[45] Within this cohort, the negative predictive value of normal screening films for any injury was 99.9% (95% CI, 99.9%–100.0%). The majority of missed patients had initial radiographs interpreted as nondiagnostic or inadequate (436 injuries in 237 patients) and further imaging was pursued. Retrospective series of spine-injured children suggest that the three-view series has comparable sensitivity in children.[27,46]

Other imaging modalities are available when the standard views fail to delineate the cervical anatomy adequately, which is frequently the case in the patient with altered mental status or when clinical suspicion of a cervical spine injury is high despite a negative screening series. These options include the swimmer's view to delineate the lower cervical spine, flexion and extension views, supine oblique views, thin-section tomography, computed tomography, and MRI. Some of these techniques, especially flexion and extension (stress) views, require positioning the head and neck out of neutral position and must be performed under careful medical supervision. One should not perform stress imaging of the cervical spine in patients who have altered mental status or who are otherwise incapable of clear communication about the effect of such manipulation. Flexion and extension views are indicated in neurologically intact children who have normal three-view screening films and complain of persistent midline, neck pain.[47] In a child with altered mental status, inadequate or abnormal plain three-view series, or focal neurological findings indicative of a cervical spine injury, thin-section CT scan is considered the diagnostic imaging of choice.[48] MRI is the modality of choice for assessing the supportive soft tissues of the spine and the spinal cord itself. Therefore, MRI can evaluate the extent of injury and offer prognostic information in situations in which cord damage is present, including SCIWORA. Additionally, MRI can be used to complete cervical spine injury clearance in the hemodynamically stable child with persistent altered mental status.[49,50]

► INJURY PATTERNS

ATLANTOOCCIPITAL DISLOCATION

Injuries involving the craniocervical junction are severe and frequently fatal (Figure 30–4).[51] High mortality rates associated with these injuries make estimation of true incidence difficult.[52] Children are at increased risk for craniocervical injury, particularly atlantooccipital dislocation (AOD), because of biomechanics of the pediatric cervical spine. Reported data suggest that the incidence of this injury is more than double of that observed in adults (15% vs. 6%).[53] Mechanisms which produce AOD include motor vehicle collisions or other high-impact trauma and results from excessive motion of the head relative to the upper cervical spine.[54]

ATLAS FRACTURES

Trauma with axial loading may result in a compressive force significant enough to cause a burst fracture of the atlas, oth-

erwise known as a Jefferson fracture (Fig. 30–5). Neurological injury is uncommon with Jefferson fractures because of the large canal diameter at this level and the propensity for burst fragments to project outward from the ring of C1.[55] True Jefferson fractures have four separate fracture lines involving both the anterior and posterior aspects of the C1 ring bilaterally. "Jefferson fracture" is also loosely applied to two- or three-point fractures of the atlas. Atlas fractures are stable unless there are severe compressive forces causing a combined C1 to C2 fracture complex or disruption of the transverse ligament with concomitant instability.[56] C1 injuries are initially evaluated with plain cervical spine x-rays. The Atlanto-dens interval (ADI) noted on lateral C-spine x-rays may be as much as 5 mm in pediatric patients.[57] ADI values in excess of 5 mm indicate transverse ligament disruption and resulting cervical instability (Fig. 30–6). The open-mouth view is useful for assessing transverse ligament stability. According to the Rule of Spence, a lateral mass overhang of C1 over C2 greater than 6.9 mm indicates transverse ligament disruption.[58]

ATLANTOAXIAL DISLOCATION

The atlantoaxial articulation provides significant rotation and to a lesser extent flexion–extension movement of the cervical spine.[59] Although the atlantoaxial articulation is effective in providing cervical rotatory motion, its structural design

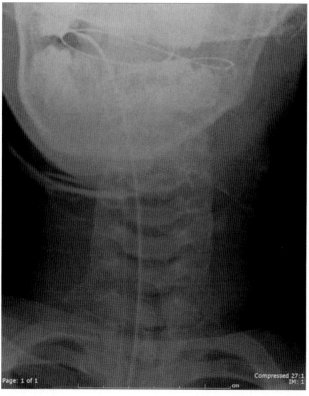

A

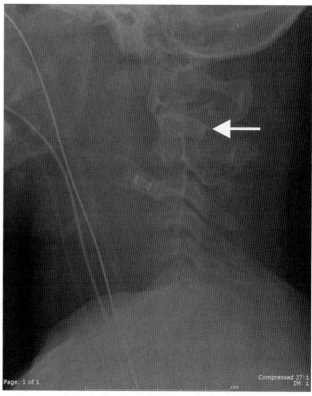

B

Figure 30–4. Ten-year-old unrestrained passenger in a high speed motor vehicle collision with respiratory arrest at scene. Atlantooccipital dislocation with longitudinal distraction and posterior dislocation.

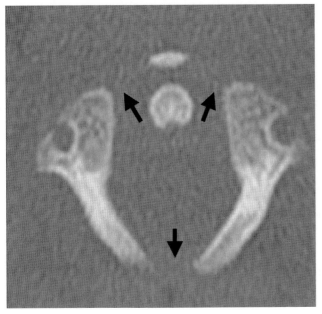 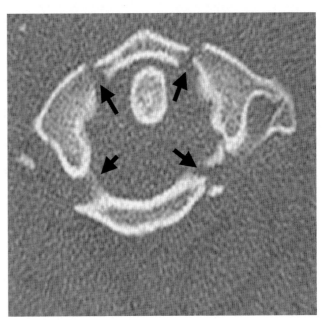

A   **B**

Figure 30–5. (A) Eleven-month-old infant (male) with an axial CT scan showing the normal anatomy of C1 with open synchondroses (three arrows) compared with (B) axial CT scan of C1 showing a Jefferson fracture in a 17-year-old suffered after landing on her head (four arrows).

predisposes it to a subset of traumatic injury patterns. High-energy injuries, such as motor vehicle–pedestrian collisions, may result in translational atlantoaxial subluxation (AAS).[60] Estimation of the true incidence of traumatic AAS is difficult because it carries a high mortality rate.[61] Some survivors will

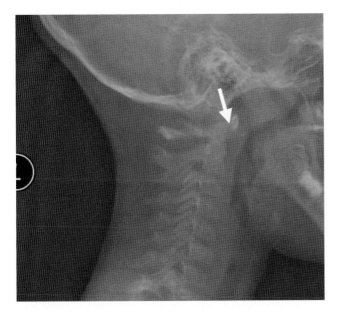

Figure 30–6. A normal atlantodental interval is defined as the distance between the dens and anterior arch of C1. A lateral x-ray taken of a 4-year-old after a fall shows a normal ADI (arrow).

present with severe head injury, while others present with the complaint of neck pain or subtle signs of myelopathy or C2 sensory changes.[60] Traumatic AAS is most commonly characterized by anterior translation of C1 on C2 and rupture of the transverse ligament of the atlas.[62] Severe hyperextension injuries with fracture of the anterior arch of C1 or the odontoid process define posterior AAS.

ATLANTOAXIAL ROTATORY INJURY

Atlantoaxial rotatory subluxation (AARS) can follow head and neck surgery. AARS also occurs in the setting of pharyngeal, upper respiratory tract or cervical infection (Grisel's syndrome), and after major and minor trauma.[63,64] On physical examination, patients have a painful "cock robin" torticollis characterized by chin rotation to the contralateral side and flexion of the neck. Patients with AARS are usually neurologically intact. Either C2 radiculopathy or myelopathy are only rarely present. Ligamentous laxity inherent in the pediatric spine predisposes children to rotatory subluxation of C1 on C2. In some cases, atlantoaxial rotatory fixation (AARF) can occur. In this situation, the neck remains locked in rotation. C1 to C2 facet dislocation and trapping of robust synovium in the articular surfaces may all contribute to AARF.[65] Severe neck pain may also prevent reduction of this position. Evaluation and diagnosis of AARS/AARF involve CT scan in addition to plain C-spine x-rays. Often, the anteroposterior (AP) x-ray is suggestive of the injury, which is then confirmed with CT. If the diagnosis is in question (physiologic C1 to C2 rotation is often present and is due to noncompliance of the pediatric patient with

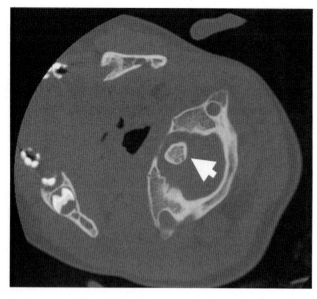
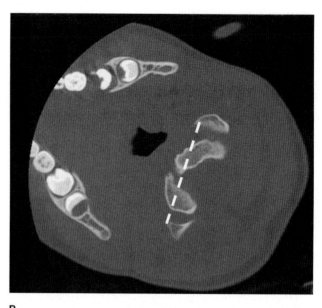

A   **B**

Figure 30–7. Seven-year-old presents after wrestling with no neurological deficits and a Cock-Robin deformity. Axial computed tomography (A and B) shows rotation of C1 about the dens (arrow A) with dislocation of the C1–2 joint resulting in anterior subluxation of C1 on C2 (dotted line).

positioning) or if AARF is suspected, dynamic CT scan may be performed (Fig. 30–7). With light sedation, the examiner can perform a CT scan in three positions: at rest, in neutral position, and rotated to the opposite side. This determines whether the AARS/AARF results from a true bony lock or from soft tissue blockage of rotation.[66]

AXIS FRACTURES

In children <7 years of age, the weakest point in the C2 body–dens complex is the cartilaginous subdental epiphysis ensuring that odontoid fractures nearly always involve this region.[67,68] While uncommon, significant displacement of the fractured dens can result in neurological deficit.[55,69] Without displacement of the fracture, it may be difficult to distinguish injury from normal anatomy; however, anterior angulation of the dens is common and may aid in identifying epiphysiolysis (Fig. 30–8).[68]

True fractures of the odontoid process are seen in older children and adolescents. The most common mechanism of injury is flexion with substantial force (e.g., motor vehicle collision). These fractures are classified by their location.[70] Type I odontoid fractures involve the superior portion of the dens and are caused by avulsion of the alar ligament. Type I fractures are rare, but are most often discovered in the setting of unstable craniocervical junction injuries.[71] Type II odontoid fractures involve the base of the neck of the dens and are considered unstable.[72,73] Type III odontoid fractures extend into the body of C2 such that the fracture fragment incorporates the entire odontoid process and a portion of the body of C2 (Fig. 30–9).[74] Bilateral pars interarticularis fractures of C2 or the "hangman's fracture" result from hyperextension with axial loading. The hangman's fracture may also result in

anterior subluxation of C2 on C3.[75] A critical distinction must be made between pathological C2 to C3 subluxation and C2 to C3 pseudosubluxation—a common physiologic finding on pediatric C-spine x-rays (Fig. 30–10).

Os odontoideum is a term used to describe a bony fragment with smooth cortical margins located cranially to the body of the axis, independent from a small or hypoplastic dens (Fig. 30–11).[76] It may appear to be an old, healed type I or type II dens fracture (Fig. 30–12). Historically thought to be a congenital anomaly related to nonunion of the dens to the C2 body, recent evidence favors fracture as the cause.[77–79] Congenital ligamentous or bony dysplasias (e.g., Morquio syndrome and Down's syndrome) and upper respiratory infections may also contribute to the development of os odontoideum.[80] Clinical significance of os odontoideum is determined by flexion-extension x-rays, which are used to evaluate the stability of the cruciate ligaments.

SUBAXIAL CERVICAL SPINE INJURIES

The biomechanics of the bony and ligamentous anatomy of levels of the subaxial cervical spine (C3–C7) are similar, allowing for grouping of injuries at these levels. Prior to 8 years of age, injury in the region is uncommon.[4] Mechanisms producing vertical axial loading (e.g., motor vehicle collisions, sports-related injuries, falls from height and diving into shallow water) cause compression or burst fractures of the vertebral body.[14,81] Compression fractures are generally considered stable and usually heal without surgical intervention. Burst fractures, however, can be unstable and involve retropulsion of bony fragments into the spinal canal (Fig. 30–13).

Flexion injury results in an avulsion fracture, which is identified by a small "teardrop" of bone observed at the

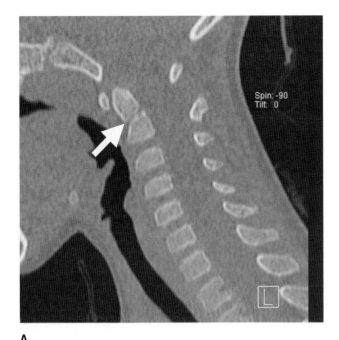

A

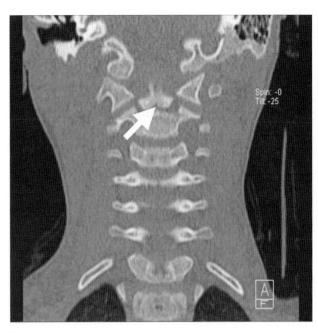

B

Figure 30–8. Sagittally (A) and coronally (B) reconstructed CT of the cervical spine from a 4-year-old after a fall showing a diastasis at the level of the synchondrosis of C2 (arrows).

anteroinferior margin of the vertebral body. A true teardrop fracture involves disruption of the facet joints, the anterior and posterior longitudinal ligaments, and the disk, and is thus considered unstable.[82] Flexion–extension x-rays and MRI may reveal subluxation or ligamentous damage, allowing the clinician to distinguish between a simple avulsion and a true unstable teardrop fracture. Hyperflexion with or without distraction may result in facet dislocation. Hyperflexion with rotation can cause unilateral facet dislocation, whereas hyperflexion alone may result in bilateral facet injuries. Various terms used to describe facet dislocation of varying degrees include perched, jumped, sprung, or locked (Fig. 30–14).

Flexion-distraction injuries can cause ligamentous disruption without fracture, potentially resulting in occult cervical

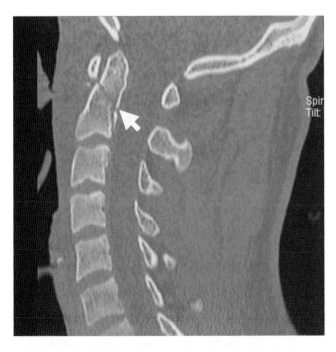

Figure 30–9. Sagittally reformatted CT scan of a 17-year-old presenting with a type III odontoid fracture through the body of C2 (arrow).

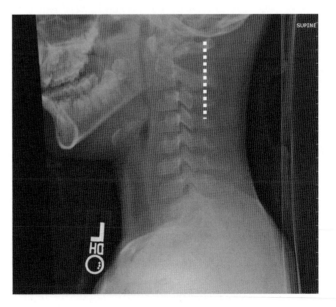

Figure 30–10. Eight-year-old presents status postmotor vehicle accident with the diagnosis of pseudosubluxation. There is mild subluxation of C2–3; however, the spinolaminar line is well aligned (dotted line).

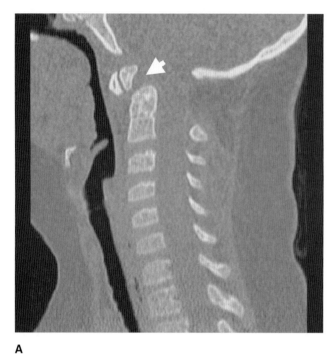

A

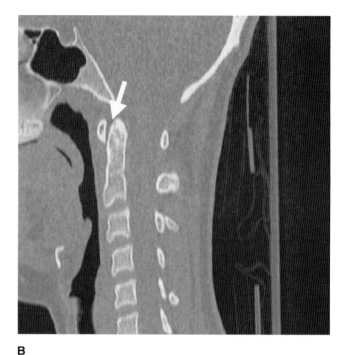

B

Figure 30–11. (A) A 17-year-old presents with progressive neck pain. Sagittally reformatted CT scan shows os odontoideum, which is subluxed with the arch of C1 relative to the body of C2 (arrow). (B) A 14-year-old presents status postmotor vehicle accident. This sagittally reformatted CT scan shows a normally aligned cervical spine with a normal atlantodental interval (arrow).

instability with normal plain radiographic findings. Subluxation may be apparent on neutral lateral cervical spine x-rays; however, flexion–extension views can reveal movement that would have otherwise been missed on neutral films. Posterior liga-

mentous disruption may present with increased interspinous distance on lateral x-ray or sagittal CT scan reconstructions. Hyperflexion or direct impact to the spinous process produces avulsion of a subaxial spinous process, often C7, and

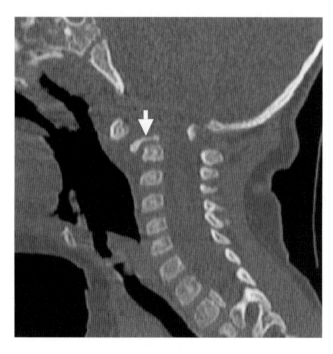

Figure 30–12. Sagittally reformatted CT scan of a 13-month-old presenting with a severely dysmorphic atlas. Bony corticated fragments anterior to C2 may represent old fracture of dens (arrow).

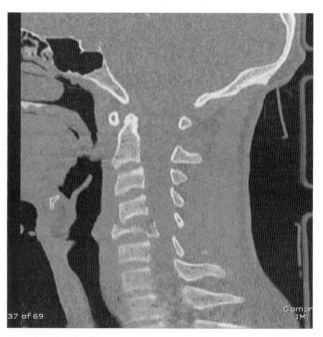

Figure 30–13. Sagittally reconstructed computed tomography of the cervical spine of a 15-year-old who suffered a C5 burst fracture while playing football. There is more than 50% loss of height and retropulsion of bony fragments into the spinal canal.

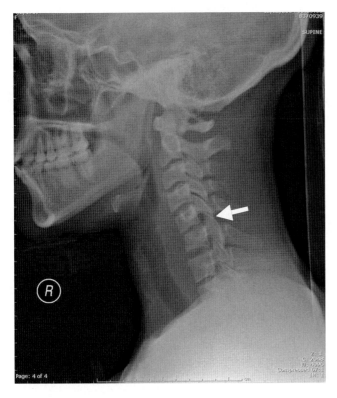

Figure 30–14. A 15-year-old restrained passenger who suffered subluxation at C5–6. Lateral plain x-rays show a unilateral perched facet (arrow).

is referred to as a "clay shoveler's fracture." Lateral mass, transverse process, or uncinate fractures occur with lateral hyperflexion. Alternatively, spinous process, laminar, and pedicle fractures are produced with hyperextension. Milder hyperextension followed by flexion is associated with classic "whiplash."

There is one more important type of fracture that is seen only in the pediatric population. Separation of the vertebral body from the end plate through the epiphysis is termed a physeal fracture.[83] Diagnosis is critical because certain subtypes of physeal fractures, specifically the Salter–Harris type I observed in young children, are unstable and require operative stabilization.[49]

SPINAL CORD INJURY WITHOUT RADIOGRAPHIC ABNORMALITY

SCIWORA was originally used to describe traumatic myelopathy in individuals with no radiographic evidence of vertebral injury on plain x-rays (including flexion–extension views), myelogram or CT scan. The reported incidence of SCIWORA ranges from 4% to 66% among all children with spinal cord injuries.[67] Most patients experience transient symptoms at the time of injury, ranging from Lhermitte's sign to paresthesias, weakness, or paralysis. Over time, the neurological course is variable.[67] Several studies suggest that the neurological examination on initial presentation is predictive of long-term outcome in SCIWORA. Children with mild deficits at presentation regain full function; however, the more severely injured chil-

dren tend to make a limited recovery.[22] SCIWORA occurs because the inherent hypermobility of the pediatric spine allows for transient deformation of the spinal column without fracture or ligamentous disruption at the expense of the spinal cord.[2] Bony and ligamentous structures strengthen as children get older and traumatic injury is more likely to cause a fracture.[31] SCIWORA remains a diagnosis of exclusion, and clinicians must be vigilant to rule out persistent ligamentous incompetence that may place the patient at risk for further injury. With more widespread use of MRI in traumatically injured patients, the definition and epidemiology of SCIWORA is continuing to evolve.

REFERENCES

1. U.S. Department of Health and Human Services. Healthy People 2010. http//www.healthypeople.gov. Accessed March 11, 2009.
2. Center for Disease Control and Prevention, National Center for Injury Prevention and Control. *Center for Disease Control Injury Research Agenda.* Atlanta, GA, 2002.
3. Viccellio P, Simon H, Pressman BD, et al. A prospective multicenter study of cervical spine injury in children. *Pediatrics.* 2001;108:e20.
4. Patel JC, Tepas DL III, Mollitt DL, et al. Pediatric cervical spine injuries: defining the disease. *J Pediatr Surg.* 2001;36:373.
5. Brown RL, Brunn MA, Garcia VF. Cervical spine injuries in children: a review of 103 patients treated consecutively at a level I pediatric trauma center. *J Pediatr Surg.* 2001;36:1107.
6. Cirak B, Ziegfeld S, Knight VM, et al. Spinal injuries in children. *J Pediatr Surg.* 2004;39:607.
7. Abroms IF, Bresnan MJ, Zuckerman JE, Fischer EG, Strand R. Cervical cord injuries secondary to hyperextension of the head in breech presentation. *Obstet Gynecol.* 1973;41:369.
8. Mills JF, Dargaville PA, Coleman LT, Rosenfeld JV, Ekert PG. Upper cervical spinal cord injury in neonates: the use of magnetic resonance imaging. *J Pediatr.* 2001;138:105.
9. Ghatan S, Ellenbogen RG. Pediatric spine and spinal cord injury after inflicted trauma. *Neurosurg Clin North Am.* 2002;13:227.
10. Pang D. Special problems of spinal stabilization in children. In: Cooper P, ed. *Management of Posttraumatic Spinal Instability.* Park Ridge, IL: American Association of Neurological Surgeons; 1990:181.
11. Ogden JA. Radiology of postnatal skeletal development-XI: the first cervical vertebra, XII: the second cervical vertebra. *Skeletal Radio.* 1984;12:12.
12. Harris JH Jr, Mirvis SE. The radiology of acute cervical spine trauma. In: Mitchell C, ed. *The Normal Cervical Spine.* 3rd ed. Baltimore, MD: Williams & Wilkins; 1996:1.
13. Koloska ER, Keller MS, Rallo MC, Weber TR. Characteristics of pediatric cervical spine injuries. *J Pediatr Surg.* 2001;36:100.
14. Roche C, Carty H. Spinal trauma in children. *Pediatr Radiol.* 2001;31:677.
15. McGrory BJ, Klassen RA, Chao EY, Staeheli JW, Weaver AL. Acute fractures and dislocations of the cervical spine in children and adolescents. *J Bone Joint Surg Am.* 1993;75:988.
16. Herman MJ, Pizzutillo PD. Cervical spine disorders in children. *Orthop Clin North Am.* 1999;30:457.
17. Pang D, Li V. Atlantoaxial rotatory fixation: 1. Biomechanics of normal rotation of the atlantoaxial joint in children. *Neurosurgery.* 2004;55:614.
18. Hadley MN, Bishop RC. Injuries of the craniocervical junction and upper cervical spine. In: Tindall GT, Cooper PR, Barrow

DL, eds. *The Practice of Neurosurgery.* Baltimore, MD: Williams & Wilkins; 1996:1687.

19. Heath KJ. The effect on laryngoscopy of different cervical spine immobilization techniques. *Anaesthesia.* 1994;49:843.

20. Hoffman JR, Schriger DL, Mower W, Luo JS, Zucker M. Low-risk criteria for cervical-spine radiography in blunt trauma: a prospective study. *Ann Emerg Med.* 1992;21:1454.

21. Hoffman JR, Mower WR, Wolfson AB, Todd KH, Zucker MI. Validity of a set of clinical criteria to rule out injury to the cervical spine in patients with blunt trauma. *NEJM.* 2000;343:94.

22. Touger M, Gennis P, Nathanson N, et al. Validity of a decision rule to reduce cervical spine radiography in elderly patients with blunt trauma. *Ann Emerg Med.* 2002;40(3):287.

23. Mahadevan S, Mower W, Hoffman JR, Peeples N, Goldberg W, Sonner R. Interrater reliability of cervical spine injury criteria in patients with blunt trauma. *Ann Emerg Med.* 1998;31(2):197.

24. Stiell IG, Wells GA, Vandemheen K, et al. The Canadian C-Spine Rule for radiography in alert and stable trauma patients. *J Am Med Assoc.* 2001;286:1841.

25. Stiell IG, Clement CM, McKnight RD, et al. The Canadian C-Spine Rule versus the NEXUS low-risk criteria in patients with trauma. *NEJM.* 2003;349:2510.

26. Rachesky I, Boyce WT, Duncan B, et al. Clinical prediction of cervical spine injuries in children. *Am J Dis Child.* 1987;141:199.

27. Jaffe DM, Binns H, Radkowski MA, et al. Developing a clinical algorithm for early management of cervical spine injuries in child trauma victims. *Ann Emerg Med.* 1987;16:270.

28. Binns H, Jaffe DM, Barthel MJ. An eight-variable model for prediction of cervical spine injury in children. *Am J Dis Child.* 1987;141:1249.

29. Schafermeyer RW, Ribbeck BM, Gaskins J, Thomason S, Harlan M, Attkisson A. Respiratory effects of spinal immobilization in children. *Ann Emerg Med.* 1991;20(9):1017.

30. Bauer D, Kowalski R. Effect of spinal immobilization devices on pulmonary function in the healthy nonsmoking man. *Ann Emerg Med.* 1988;17(9):915.

31. Lerner EB, Billittier AJ, Moscati R. Effects of neutral positioning with and without padding on spinal immobilization. *Prehosp Emerg Care.* 1998;2:112.

32. Chan D, Goldberg RM, Mason J, Chan L. Backboard versus mattress splint immobilization: a comparison of symptoms generated. *J Emerg Med.* 1996;14(3):293.

33. Chan D, Goldberg R, Tascone A, Harmon S, Chan L. The effect of spinal immobilization on healthy volunteers. *Emerg Med Serv.* 1994;23(1):48.

34. Cordell WH, Hollingsworth JC, Olinger ML, et al. Pain and tissue interface pressures during spine board immobilization. *Ann Emerg Med.* 1995;26:13.

35. Linares H, Mawson A, Suarez E, Biundo J. Association between pressure sores and immobilization in the immediate post-injury period. *Orthopedics.* 1987;10(4):571.

36. Mawson AR, Biundo JJ, Neville P, Linares HH, Winchester Y, Lopez A. Risk factors for early occurring pressure ulcers following spinal cord injury. *Am J Phys Med Rehabil.* 1988;67(3):123.

37. Herzenberg JE, Hensinger RN, Dedrick DK, Phillips WA. Emergency transport and positioning of young children who have an injury of the cervical spine. The standard backboard may be hazardous. *J Bone Joint Surg.* 1989;71 A(1):15.

38. Nypaver M, Treloar D. Neutral cervical spine positioning in children. *Ann Emerg Med.* 1994;23(2):208.

39. Schriger DL, Larmon B, LeGassick T, Blinman T. Spinal immobilization on a flat backboard: does it result in neutral position of the cervical spine? *Ann Emerg Med.* 1991;20(8):878.

40. DeLorenzo RA, Olson JE, Boska M, et al. Optimal positioning for cervical immobilization. *Ann Emerg Med.* 1996;28(3):301.

41. Curran C, Dietrich AM, Bowman MJ, Ginn-Pease ME, King DR, Kosnik E. Pediatric Cervical-Spine immobilization: achieving neutral position? *J Trauma.* 1995;39(4):729.

42. Tescher AN, Rindflesch AB, Youdas JW. Range-of-motion restriction and craniofacial tissue interface pressure from four cervical collars. *J Trauma.* 2007;63:1120.

43. Bracken MB, Shepard MJ, Collins WF, et al. A randomized, controlled trial of methylprednisolone or naloxone in the treatment of acute spinal-cord injury. *N Engl J Med.* 1990;322:1405.

44. Bracken MB, Shepard MJ, Holford TR, et al. Administration of methylprednisolone for 24 or 48 hours or tirilazad mesylate for 48 hours in the treatment of acute spinal cord injury. *JAMA.* 1997;277:1597.

45. Mower WR, Hoffman JR, Pollack CV, et al. Use of plain radiography to screen for cervical spine injuries. *Ann Emerg Med.* 2001;38(1):1.

46. Baker C, Kadish H, Schunk JE. Evaluation of pediatric spine injuries. *Am J Emerg Med.* 1999;17(3):230.

47. Pollack CV Jr, Hendey GW, Martin DR, Hoffman JR, Mower MR. Use of flexion-extension radiographs of the cervical spine in blunt trauma. *Ann Emerg Med.* 2001;38(1):8.

48. Rozycki GS, Tremblay L, Feliciano DV, et al. Prospective comparison of admission CT scan and plain film of the upper cervical spine in trauma patients with altered LOC. *J Trauma.* 2001;51(4):663.

49. Flynn JM, Closkey RF, Soroosh M, Dormans JP. Role of magnetic imaging in the assessment of pediatric cervical spine injuries. *J Pediatr Orthop.* 2002;22(5):573.

50. Frank JB, Lim CK, Flynn JM, Dormans JP. The efficacy of magnetic resonance imaging in pediatric cervical spine clearance. *Spine.* 2002;27(11):1176.

51. Montane I, Eismont FJ, Green BA. Traumatic occipitoatlantal dislocation. *Spine.* 1991;16:112.

52. Menezes A. Management of occipito-cervical instability. In: Cooper P, ed. *Management of Posttraumatic Spinal Instability.* Park Ridge, IL: American Association of Neurologic Surgeons; 1990:65.

53. Bucholz RW, Burkhead WZ. The pathological anatomy of fatal atlanto-occiptal dislocations. *J Bone Joint Surg Am.* 1979;61:248.

54. Bucholz RW, Burkhead WZ, Graham W, Petty C. Occult cervical spine injuries in fatal traffic accidents. *J Trauma.* 1979;19:768.

55. Ogden J. *Skeletal Injury in the Child.* Philadelphia, PA: W.B. Saunders; 1990.

56. Hadley MN, Dickman CA, Browner CM, Sonntag VKH. Acute traumatic atlas fractures: management and long-term outcome. *Neurosurgery.* 1988;23:31.

57. Locke GR, Gardner JI, Van Epps EF. Atlas-dens interval (ADI) in children: a survey based on 200 normal cervical spines. *Am J Roentgenol Radium Ther Nucl Med.* 1966;97:135.

58. Spence KF Jr, Decker S, Sell KW. Bursting atlantal fracture associated with rupture of the transverse ligament. *J Bone Joint Surg.* 1970;52:543.

59. Phillips WA, Hensinger RN. The management of rotatory atlanto-axial subluxation in children. *J Bone Joint Surg Am.* 1989;71:664.

60. DeBeer JD, Thomas M, Walters J, Anderson P. Traumatic atlantoaxial subluxation. *J Bone Joint Surg Br.* 1988;70:652.

61. Adams VI. Atlantoaxial dislocation-a pathological study of 14 traffic fatalities. *J Forensic Sci.* 1992;37:565.

62. Fielding JW, Cochran GB, Lawsing JF, Hohl M. Tears of the transverse ligament of the atlas. *J Bone Joint Surg Am.* 1974;56:1683.

63. Fielding JW, Hawkins RJ, Hensinger RN, Francis WR. Atlanto-axial rotatory deformities. *Orthop Clin North Am.* 1978;9A:955.

64. Grisel P. Enucleation des atlas et torticollis nasopharyngien. *Presse Med.* 1930;38:50.

65. Kawabe N, Hirotani H, Tanaka O. Pathomechanism of atlantoaxial rotatory fixation. *J Pediatr Orthop.* 1989;9:569.
66. Cowan IA, Inglis GS. Atlanto-axial rotatory fixation: improved demonstration using spiral CT. *Australas Radiol.* 1996;40:119.
67. Roche C, Carty H. Spinal trauma in children. *Pediatr Radiol.* 2001;31:677.
68. Lebwohl NH, Eismont FJ. Cervical spine injuries in children. In: Weinstein S, ed. *The Pediatric Spine: Principles and Practice.* 2nd ed. Philadelphia, PA: Lippincott Williams & Wilkins; 2001:553.
69. Sherk HH, Nicholson JT, Chung SMK. Fractures of the odontoid process in young children. *J Bone Joint Surg Am.* 1978;60:921.
70. Anderson LK, D'Alonzo RT. Fractures of the odontoid process of the axis. *J Bone Joint Surg Am.* 1974;56(8):1663.
71. Dickman CA, Hadley MN, Browner C, Sonntag VK. Neurosurgical management of acute atlas-axis combination fractures: a review of 25 cases. *J Neurosurg.* 1989;70:45.
72. Wang J, Vokshoor A, Kim S, Elton S, Kosnik E, Bartkowski H. Pediatric atlantoaxial instability: management with screw fixation. *Pediatr Neurosurg.* 1999;30:70.
73. Hadley MN, Browner CM, Liu SS, Sontag VK. New subtype of acute odontoid fractures (Type IIA). *Neurosurgery.* 1988;22:67.
74. Sonntag VK. Nonoperative management of cervical spine injuries. *Clin Neurosurg.* 1988;34:630.
75. Sumchai AP, Sternbach GL. Hangman's fracture in a 7-week-old infant. *Ann Emerg Med.* 1991;20(1):119.
76. Fielding JW, Hensinger RN, Hawkins RL. Os odontoideum. *J Bone Joint Surg Am.* 1980;62:376.
77. Wollin DG. The os odontoideum: separate odontoid process. *J Bone Joint Surg Am.* 1963;45:1459.
78. Dai L, Yuan W, Ni B, Jia L. Os odontoideum: etiology, diagnosis and management. *Surg Neurol.* 2000;53:106.
79. Ricciardi JEKH, Louis DS. Acquired os odontoideum following acute ligament injury. *J Bone Joint Surg Am.* 1976;58:410.
80. Menezes A. Os odontoideum: pathogenesis, dynamics and management. In: Marlin A, ed. *Concepts in Pediatric Neurosurgery.* Basel, Switzerlannd: Karger; 1988.
81. Osenbach RK, Menezes AH. Pediatric spinal cord and vertebral column injury. *Neurosurgery.* 1992;30:385.
82. Harris JH Jr, Edeiken-Monroe B, Kopanik DR. A practical classification of acute cervical spine injuries. *Orthop Clin North Am.* 1986;17:15.
83. Lawson JP, Ogden JA, Bucholz RW, Hughes SA. Physeal injuries of the cervical spine. *J Pediatr Orthop.* 1987;7:428.

CHAPTER 31

Thoracic Trauma

Karen O'Connell, Wendy Ann Lucid, and Todd Brian Taylor

▶ HIGH-YIELD FACTS

- Thoracic injuries occur less frequently in children than in adults, but remain a source of significant morbidity and mortality.
- Pediatric victims of thoracic trauma require rapid evaluation and management. Knowledge of pediatric-specific anatomy and injury patterns will help expedite the identification of injuries and allow for early surgical referral and treatment of potentially life-threatening chest injuries.
- Due to the increased compliance of the ribs and supporting structures, children are particularly susceptible to pulmonary contusion with little external signs of trauma.
- Treatment with needle and then chest tube thoracostomy should occur immediately in hemodynamically unstable or deteriorating victims of thoracic trauma. Uncertainty as to the side of a tension, pneumothorax should not prohibit initiation of this potentially life-saving procedure. Decompression of the alternate side should be done if immediate improvement is not seen with the initial thoracostomy.
- The most common site for aortic disruption in children is at the level of the ligamentum arteriosum, and it may be associated with aortic dissection. As in adults, morbidity and mortality is high with injuries to the great vessels.
- Gunshot wounds to the chest are associated with abdominal injuries in 30% to 40% of patients. Be aware of the possibility of concomitant injuries.

▶ EPIDEMIOLOGY AND SIGNIFICANCE

Traumatic injury is the most common cause of morbidity and mortality in children of age 1 to 14 years. While relatively rare in the pediatric trauma victim, it still accounts for approximately 5% to 10% of pediatric hospital admissions. Despite its low incidence, it remains a significant cause of death secondary to trauma. In isolation, thoracic trauma has a 5% mortality rate; however, when combined with head or abdominal trauma, the mortality rate increases dramatically. With multisystem injury, the risk of mortality may be as high as 40% to 50%.[1] The highest mortality rates involve injury to the heart and great vessels, hemothorax, and lung laceration.

The most common cause of thoracic injury is due to blunt trauma, with penetrating trauma accounting for only a small percentage of these injuries. Infants and toddlers are most often victims of passive injury such as motor vehicle crashes, falls, and nonaccidental trauma. School-age children and adolescents also have the risk of sports-related chest injuries. Adolescents are particularly at risk for high-energy injuries related to motor vehicle crashes, extreme sports, violence, and suicide. The most common injuries sustained include pulmonary contusion, pneumothorax, hemothorax, pneumohemothorax, and rib fractures.

When trauma is severe and results in cardiopulmonary arrest in the field, survival for both pediatric and adult victims is poor. Review of the trauma registry databases shows an overall mortality rate estimated at 95%, with victims of blunt traumatic arrest faring worse than those with a penetrating injury (97% vs. 89%, respectively).[2] A review of the National Pediatric Trauma Registry, however, estimates pediatric victims of traumatic arrest to fare better than their adult counterparts, with up to 25% of children surviving to hospital discharge.[3] For trauma patients suffering cardiac arrest, motor vehicle crashes, pedestrian accidents, and intentional injuries were the most common causes.

Over the past decade, designated pediatric trauma centers with improved prehospital pediatric care and rapid transport systems have improved the care of the injured child. Pediatric victims of trauma have improved survival when initial evaluation and resuscitation occur at designated pediatric trauma centers.[4] However, most injured children present to community hospital emergency departments or adult trauma centers. These patients must be managed in nonspecialty centers until arrangements for transport to an appropriate facility for definitive care is made. Improvements in the regionalization of pediatric trauma care have increased the likelihood that children sustaining even severe trauma may survive to arrival to an emergency department (ED). Because of anatomic reasons that will be discussed later in this chapter, even seemingly benign mechanisms of trauma have the potential of producing severe injuries in infants and young children. For these reasons, ED personnel need to be knowledgeable and well trained in the skills of pediatric trauma assessment and management.

▶ MECHANISM OF INJURY

BLUNT THORACIC TRAUMA

Blunt trauma accounts for the vast majority of serious chest injuries in children. Review of the National Pediatric Trauma Registry shows that approximately 80% to 90% of chest injuries in children are due to blunt forces compared to 10% to 20% from penetrating trauma. Of the blunt injuries, most are caused by motor vehicle crashes, falls, bicycle and pedestrian accidents. The mechanism of injury is important due to recognizable patterns of trauma associated with particular injuries. Thoracic trauma in children occurs relatively infrequently in isolation and is more often associated with multisystem injury. Due to its associated and concomitant injuries and high mortality rate, chest injury has become a marker of injury severity. Half of all serious blunt chest traumas result in rib fractures and pulmonary contusions, followed by pneumothorax and hemothorax at 20% and 10%, respectively.

PENETRATING THORACIC TRAUMA

Although penetrating mechanisms account for only about 15% of thoracic trauma in childhood, the incidence is increasing at an alarming rate, especially with respect to gunshot wounds. This increase is not only seen in the adolescent population at high risk for homicide, but also among younger children who are innocent victims of bystander violence. The overall mortality is about the same for blunt and penetrating trauma. Death from penetrating injury is more likely associated with the primary wound, whereas with blunt injury, mortality more often stems from associated injuries. Death associated with penetrating thoracic injury is often the result of massive hemorrhagic shock due to exsanguination or loss of cardiac filling potential associated with major vascular injuries, massive hemothorax, cardiac tamponade, and tension pneumothorax. In some cases, the use of autotransfusion has been beneficial to patients suffering massive hemorrhage. Because penetrating trauma is an independent predictor of mortality, there is an urgent need for immediate evaluation and treatment by the surgical trauma team.[5]

Concomitant abdominal injury should be suspected with penetrating trauma at or below the level of the sixth rib anteriorly, below the scapula posteriorly, or when stomach contents, chyme, or saliva are recovered from the chest tube. Gunshot wounds to the chest are associated with abdominal injuries in 30% to 40% of patients. Therefore, "isolated" thoracic trauma does not exclude abdominal injury, especially in the presence of abdominal tenderness or developing peritonitis.

▶ PATHOPHYSIOLOGY

There are critical differences in the pediatric anatomy that affect a child's risk of sustaining significant injuries from thoracic trauma (Table 31–1). The increased compliance of cartilaginous ribs allows for the dissipation of impact forces, protecting the ribs from fracture, but often leaving the underlying struc-

▶ **TABLE 31–1. PEDIATRIC ANATOMY AND PHYSIOLOGY**

Incomplete ossification of bony structures	Diminished functional residual capacity
Greater flexibility of thoracic cage	Greater mobility of mediastinal structures
More flexible ligamentous structures	Large cardiac reserve; delayed recognition of shock
Underdeveloped supporting musculature	Higher oxygen consumption per unit body mass
Narrow, short trachea	
More compressible trachea	

tures at increased risk for injury. Compliant ribs complicate thoracic trauma, allowing significant trauma to occur to intrathoracic structures (heart, lungs, airways, and vessels) with few or no apparent external signs of trauma. Even bruising, petechiae, and tenderness may be absent.

Children who sustain thoracic trauma have decreased respiratory compensation. They have higher oxygen consumption per unit body mass and a smaller lung functional residual capacity. Younger children are diaphragmatic breathers due to horizontally aligned ribs and immature intercostal musculature. Any intra-abdominal process that causes abdominal distension may hinder diaphragm excursion and lung expansion, decreasing total lung volume. Gastric distension is not uncommon in a child who is crying and tachypneic from pain or anxiety or when their breathing is assisted by bag-mask ventilation. When the natural movement of the diaphragm is impeded by a distended abdomen, accessory muscles are recruited to help with ventilation. When this type of abdominal breathing and respiratory distress is prolonged, fatigue leading to respiratory failure can occur.

The pediatric mediastinal structures have a higher percentage of elastin and are more mobile than an adult's. Thoracic injuries in children have a greater potential for interfering with the proper functioning of mediastinal structures. Interference with cardiac output has the potential to lead to rapid ventilatory and circulatory collapse, particularly in cases where preload volume is affected, as seen with tension pneumothorax.

▶ MANAGEMENT OF THORACIC INJURY

Priority for management lies in the recognition of injury and stabilization of the airway, breathing, and circulation. The unique pediatric anatomy places victims of thoracic trauma at an increased risk for airway and respiratory compromise and an increased risk for developing hypoxia. A variety of conditions can cause airway compromise, which should be considered potentially life-threatening. The narrow diameter of the pediatric trachea makes airway obstruction from foreign body, secretions, neck trauma, and the patients' own posterior pharyngeal structures more likely. The main objective is to obtain airway patency, while protecting and immobilizing the cervical spine. Use the jaw thrust maneuver, if needed, to open the airway. Avoid using a head-tilt, chin-lift mechanism when positioning the neck. Concentrate on adequate preoxygenation with 100% FiO_2, early rapid sequence intubation, and the maintenance of appropriate minute ventilation. (For discussion of rapid sequence see Chapter 23.

Physical signs of thoracic injury can be subtle in the child, even with severe injury. Respirations may appear shallow rather than labored, and central cyanosis can be absent in hemorrhagic shock due to a relative decrease in the amount of unsaturated hemoglobin. Therefore, absence of hypoxia detected by pulse oximetry does not exclude the presence of serious or life-threatening thoracic injuries. When shallow respirations are detected, end-tidal CO_2 monitoring may be employed to assess the adequacy of ventilation. In non-intubated patients, "side-stream" CO_2 monitoring by nasal prongs or cannula can help the provider monitor ventilatory function and detect early compromise. In patients who are intubated, "main-stream" or "in-line" end-tidal CO_2 monitoring should be performed.

Assess the circulatory status of a patient immediately. Children have a remarkable ability to compensate for significant hemorrhage. Cardiac output is determined by stroke volume (SV) and heart rate (HR) (CO = SV × HR). With volume loss, the pediatric patient may become profoundly tachycardic in order to maintain appropriate blood pressure and perfusion. Children may remain in a state of compensated hypovolemic shock until up to 40% of their blood volume is lost. For these reasons, a normal blood pressure in a patient who has suffered thoracic injury should be approached with caution. Hypotension is a late sign of shock in pediatric patients and should be avoided by early recognition and treatment and a high index of suspicion for blood loss. Initiate fluid resuscitation with two large-bore intravenous lines and the infusion of isotonic crystalloid solutions, such as normal saline or lactated ringers. If major vessel injury and hemorrhage shock are suspected, fluid resuscitation should continue with transfusion of donor blood products or by autotransfusion.

After the immediate life- and/or limb-threatening injuries are detected by the primary trauma survey and resuscitation initiated, a more comprehensive secondary survey will focus on the full evaluation of a trauma patient. During this secondary survey, more subtle findings of thoracic injury are often detected.

Diagnostic studies and treatment will vary depending on the clinical situation. With thoracic injury, a minimal workup includes supplemental oxygen, cardiac monitoring with continuous pulse oximetry, two large-bore intravenous lines, and

fluid resuscitation with crystalloid solutions or blood products. To access adequate oxygenation and ventilation, obtain an arterial blood gas. A baseline hemoglobin/hematocrit should be checked and a type and screen sent.

The chest radiograph is standard in the evaluation of chest trauma and is most likely to facilitate the diagnosis of a pneumothorax or hemothorax (Fig. 31–1). A portable chest radiograph is easily and rapidly obtained during trauma evaluations. There are clinical situations, however, that may dictate immediate treatment without a radiograph if the patient has clinical signs or symptoms of hypoxia and/or hypotension. In selected cases, where there is a high likelihood for thoracic injury, chest computed tomography (CT) may detect injuries not seen on routine chest radiograph and may lead to a change in patient management.

Concomitant abdominal and thoracic trauma requires a special approach. If surgical management of an abdominal injury is necessary, chest injuries requiring tube thoracostomy should be stabilized prior to being placed under general anesthesia. The abdominal injuries are repaired first if the clinical situation allows. After the abdomen is closed, a thoracotomy can be performed if necessary for other injuries and to irrigate the chest if it is contaminated with intestinal contents.

Thoracic injury in children is rare, but clinically important for the outcome and prognosis of pediatric victims of trauma. Studies by clinical researchers have helped guide best patient care practices. In the case of pediatric thoracic trauma, identification of predictors of thoracic injury may aid in early diagnosis and leads to improvements in the clinical and cost effectiveness of therapy. One group of researchers developed a model

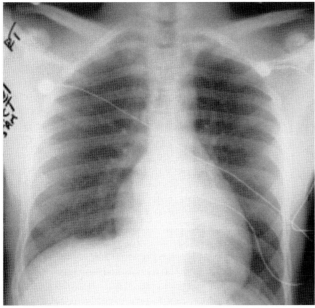

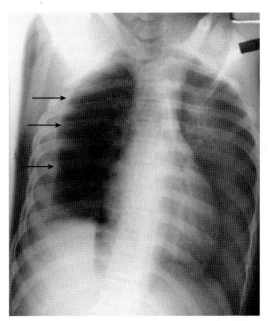

A   **B**

Figure 31–1. (A) An AP radiograph of a 14-year-old boy who was hit by a car. While there are no pathognomonic findings indicative of a hemothorax, in this clinical context the caretakers were concerned about the elevation of the right hemidiaphragm. In particular, the lateral position of the right hemidiaphragm apex makes the possibility of subpulmonic fluid even more likely. (B) The subsequent right lateral decubitus film, also done as a portable, demonstrates a significant hemothorax.

that maximizes sensitivity for identifying children with thoracic injuries, while also maximizing specificity.[6] The authors identified several independent predictors of thoracic injury, with the strength of association listed in decreasing order: abnormal chest auscultation findings; hypotension; abnormal external thoracic examination results; and elevated age-adjusted respiratory rate. Abnormal chest auscultation findings have the highest predictive value for thoracic injury. External evidence of thoracic trauma is uncommon in children. When abnormalities of the chest wall are found on examination, the likelihood of significant thoracic injury increases. Tachypnea, another important indicator, is often present in patients with pulmonary contusions. When this prediction model is utilized, patients without any of these findings are at very low risk for having clinically significant thoracic injuries.

▶ SPECIFIC INJURIES AND MANAGEMENT

PULMONARY CONTUSION, LACERATION, AND HEMATOMA

Pulmonary injuries are the most common type of thoracic trauma in children. Children are particularly susceptible to pulmonary contusion despite few external signs of trauma because of an increased compliance of the ribs and supporting structures. A search for other coexisting injuries is prudent in cases of pulmonary contusion because of their association with forceful mechanisms that often result in multisystem injuries.

Pulmonary contusion can be caused by blunt trauma to the chest wall or by high-speed penetrating trauma, such as a gunshot wound to the chest. Injured leaky capillary membranes allow bleeding or oozing of fluid into the interstitial and alveolar spaces leading to hypoxia and respiratory distress. The analogy of the "bruised lung" carries a more significant risk of hypoxia in the pediatric patient who has a decreased functional residual capacity and proportionally higher oxygen consumption. Pulmonary contusions manifest as areas of consolidation that interfere with gas exchange. Alveolar hemorrhage, edema, and consolidation lead to inadequate oxygenation, hypoventilation, and the development of a ventilation/perfusion mismatch. The majority of pulmonary contusions are detected on chest radiograph, but smaller areas of injury may only be diagnosed by chest CT scan.

Pulmonary lacerations are often associated with penetrating trauma, but may be the result of a rib fracture blunt trauma. Lacerations of lung parenchyma are diagnosed with the combination of mechanism of injury, clinical scenario of pulmonary compromise and hemorrhage, and thoracic imaging. Pulmonary lacerations have a cavitary appearance on chest radiograph, but the extent is more visible on the chest CT scan. Surgical repair is necessary when the laceration is associated with ongoing bleeding or air leakage. Pulmonary hematoma is uncommon, generally a self-limited injury, and rarely progresses to lung abscess

A high index of suspicion is necessary to identify early pulmonary contusion. Initial symptoms of parenchymal lung injury range from minimal-to-severe respiratory distress and/or hypoxia. Tachypnea is the chief physiologic response to hypoxia and should be noted early. Tachypnea and retractions may be severe due to limited pulmonary compliance because of the injury and greater chest wall compliance. Prolonged respiratory distress can lead to respiratory fatigue and failure. Knowledge of the mechanism of injury may be the only early clinical indicator of pulmonary contusion. The initial chest radiograph may not show the classic patchy infiltrate and physical examination may not reveal signs of pulmonary consolidation. In the early stages of injury, blood gas analysis may not be diagnostic if the alveolar–arterial gradient is still normal. However, as the injured lung parenchyma collapses and becomes congested, gas exchange is impaired, hypoxia ensues, and injury becomes more evident. Treatment is directed toward preventing hypoxia and respiratory failure. Most cases require only supplemental oxygen and close monitoring. Patients may need to be intubated and ventilated with higher positive end-expiratory pressures (PEEP) of greater than 5 cm H_2O, if the injuries have caused a decrease in lung compliance. Areas of contusion larger than 30% often require mechanical ventilation. Additional measures such as fluid restriction, early mobilization, and pain control should be taken to avoid worsening atelectasis. Early detection and treatment of secondary pneumonia may help prevent further complications. Spontaneous resolution of pulmonary contusions is the usual course unless the injury is complicated by a more diffuse reactive process, such as acute respiratory distress syndrome (ARDS). Excessive administration of crystalloid and aspiration of gastric contents are two factors that may precipitate the development of ARDS.

PNEUMOTHORAX

The clinician needs to appreciate the difference between spontaneous and traumatic pneumothorax. Spontaneous pneumothorax is caused by a ruptured bleb or small distal bronchiole that will easily seal itself and heal quickly. The air is reabsorbed over a few days often without intervention. A small spontaneous pneumothorax can be treated with close observation and followed with repeated chest radiographs to ensure resolution. At the most, they require a small chest tube.

In the setting of thoracic trauma, pneumothoraces occur in one-third of pediatric cases. The majority of these have associated injuries, while only one-third occur in isolation. Traumatic pneumothoraces have the potential to compromise patient stability. An uncomplicated pneumothorax is often asymptomatic. These may even be small enough to miss detection by chest radiograph (Figs. 31–2 and 31–3). However, all traumatic pneumothoraces have the potential to expand and are often associated with underlying pulmonary injury. Even a small pneumothorax can quickly develop into a more serious tension pneumothorax. A tension pneumothorax puts pressure on and often causes a shift in the mediastinal structures, which then affects cardiac filling and output (Fig. 31–4). An untreated tension pneumothorax may rapidly lead to cardiovascular collapse. For this reason, all traumatic pneumothoraces should be promptly drained with tube thoracostomy.

Treatment for small, isolated traumatic pneumothoraces include observation for at least 6 hours with a repeat chest radiograph. If there is no size increase, no underlying parenchymal injury, and the patient remains clinically stable, he or she may be discharged to return in 24 hours for

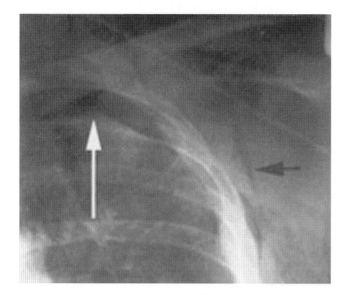

Figure 31–2. A CXR demonstrating a pneumothorax (white arrow) and overlying subcutaneous emphysema (black arrow), which can be seen tracking up to the neck. The lack of a tube thoracostomy indicates that the diagnosis of this pneumothorax was unfortunately made by this CXR instead of by the obvious physical exam findings.

a repeat evaluation. When a pneumothorax is large enough to cause a potential complication and warrants evacuation, a chest tube should be placed lateraly, or anteriorly. Treatment for larger traumatic pneumothoraces includes placing a large-caliber chest tube laterally and aimed posteriorly so that any underlying hemothorax may be drained as well. A large-bore chest tube will allow for the evacuation of air, blood, and thicker fluids. Under certain circumstances, stable patients with small, insignificant pneumothoraces should have chest tubes placed. This is particularly important when a patient with a

pneumothorax needs to undergo mechanical ventilation (for surgery or respiratory failure) or emergency transport, particularly by air, when changes in atmospheric pressure may cause an otherwise small pneumothorax to expand.

TENSION PNEUMOTHORAX

Tension pneumothorax occurs when the lung or airway develops a leak through a defect that acts like a one-way valve, allowing air to flow into the pleural cavity without a means of escape. As the amount of air increases, the pressure against the mediastinal structures shifts the mediastinum toward the opposite side and causing vascular compromise of the heart and great vessels. Cardiac decompensation ensues from mechanical impingement of blood flow and hypoxia from respiratory compromise. The clinician must do an immediate decompression with needle thoracostomy to relieve the tension and avoid imminent demise.

A tension pneumothorax may be caused by barotrauma from severe blunt compression of the chest cavity against a closed glottis or rib fractures that puncture the lung tissue. Penetrating injuries, such as stab wounds, can also cause a tension pneumothorax when the lung parenchyma is injured without a large enough chest wall defect to allow for spontaneous decompression. Many patients with tension pneumothorax present with severe respiratory distress, decreased breath sounds, and hyperresonance on the affected side. Subcutaneous emphysema may dissect superiorly into the neck or inferiorly into the abdomen and scrotal area. On physical examination, contralateral tracheal deviation, distended neck veins from compromised venous return, a narrow pulse pressure, and hypotension will alert the provider to the severe decrease in cardiac output. If the tension pneumothorax is not expeditiously decompressed, cardiovascular collapse will ensue.

The diagnosis of a suspected tension pneumothorax is made clinically. Treatment for a suspected tension pneumothorax should never be delayed to obtain a chest radiograph.

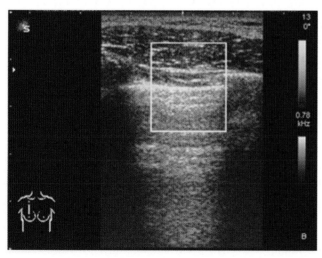

A

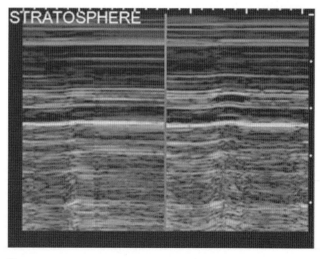

B

Figure 31–3. Ultrasound: Normal lung movement on Doppler (A) and M mode (B) demonstrating the absence of pneumothorax (the "seashore sign").

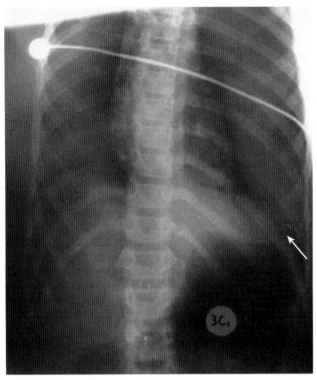

A

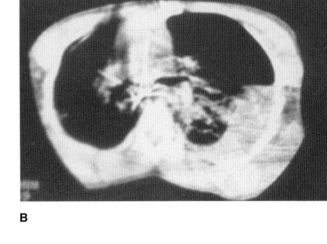

B

Figure 31–4. (A) A chest x-ray of a 12-year-old boy who was struck by a car. This hastily done, poor-quality film was taken when the child's mental status began to deteriorate. Note the left costophrenic angle, which is surprisingly deep. This is an example of a deep sulcus sign seen in an anterior pneumothorax. (B) The chest CT scan of the same patient clearly demonstrates the anterior pneumothorax.

Prehospital providers often perform this life-saving procedure in the field based on clinical suspicion alone. A tension pneumothorax is relieved by needle thoracostomy; for this procedure a needle catheter is attached to a valve or 3-way stop cock is inserted into the pleural cavity via the second intercostal space at the midclavicular line. Care must be taken to avoid the intercostal vessels by placing the needle just over the top of the third rib. Diagnosis of tension pneumothorax in children may be complicated by false transmission of breath sounds. This can confuse the clinical diagnosis; however, uncertainty as to the side of the tension pneumothorax should not prohibit initiation of empiric treatment if the patient is deteriorating. Decompression of the other side should be done if immediate improvement is not seen with the initial needle or tube thoracostomy. Definitive treatment is accomplished using a large-caliber (appropriate for age) thoracostomy tube placed laterally and directed posteriorly to allow drainage of a hemothorax that may often accompany tension pneumothorax in trauma patients. Table 31–2 outlines appropriate chest tube sizes for trauma patients.

▶ TABLE 31–2. **CHEST TUBE SIZES**

Weight (Kg)	Chest Tube Size (Fr)
<5	8–12
5–10	10–14
11–15	14–20
16–20	20–24
21–30	20–28
31–50	28–40
>50	32–40

HEMOTHORAX AND MASSIVE HEMOTHORAX

The mechanism for hemothorax is similar to that for pneumothorax. Blunt injuries and gunshot wounds typically cause bleeding from lung parenchyma and deep vascular structures. Stab wounds more often cause bleeding from injury to the intercostal vessels. Massive hemothorax is rare in children and when present, is usually a result of a forceful mechanisms, such as a high-speed motor vehicle crash, a fall from a great height, or a high-powered or close-range gunshot wound. Clinical findings vary in severity and involve both respiratory and circulatory systems. Auscultation of the chest often reveals decreased breath sounds and dullness to percussion on the affected side with or without obvious respiratory distress. Pneumothorax may coexist and compound the degree of respiratory distress seen on physical examination.

Rib fractures, penetrating trauma, chest compression, or shearing forces can cause major vascular injury. Injury to the intercostal or internal mammary vessels or lung parenchyma may result in significant bleeding, which is difficult to quantify on chest radiograph. A minimum of 10 mL/kg of blood is often necessary to be visualized. Any abnormal fluid collection in the traumatic setting is assumed to be blood. Removal of a hemothorax is necessary for both the evaluation of the quantity of blood loss and to prevent delayed complications due to fibrosis, empyema, and pneumonia. Collections of blood serve as culture media for bacteria and should be promptly drained to prevent the development of pneumonia and sepsis.

Large blood loss may occur in cases of massive hemothorax. Each hemothorax can hold 40% of a child's blood volume, enough blood loss to lead to decompensated hemorrhagic shock. Immediate drainage and observation for the volume and rate of ongoing blood loss is necessary. In cases where bleeding is uncontrolled or ongoing losses are significant, definitive surgical repair may be necessary. Fluid resuscitation should begin with crystalloid in the field. Preparation for transfusion should begin immediately and blood given as the clinical situation warrants. Critical patients may require immediate transfusion with O-negative blood, while more stable patients may be able to wait for type-specific or cross-matched blood. Both vital signs and the amount of output from the chest tube should be taken into account when deciding the need for immediate transfusion. Hemoglobin and hematocrit may not be useful initially because rapid blood loss does not allow for equilibration and these tests may not accurately reflect current blood volume.

Thoracostomy tubes should be placed as soon as the diagnosis of massive hemothorax is suspected. A large-caliber (approximately as wide as the intercostal space) tube should be used and inserted laterally and directed posteriorly to allow for drainage. Consider using an autotransfusion chest tube collection system, as this may be the most rapidly available source for blood transfusion. A chest radiograph should be taken soon after chest tube placement to confirm the position and to ensure reexpansion of the lung.

In certain circumstances, an emergency thoracotomy may be necessary to control massive hemorrhage. The decision to proceed with a thoracotomy will generally be made by the consulting surgeon. Guidelines include initial evacuated volume exceeding 10 to 15 mL/kg of blood or continued blood loss exceeding 2 to 4 mL/kg/h. Continued air leakage may be another reason to do so.

OPEN PNEUMOTHORAX

An open pneumothorax ("sucking" chest wound) is created when the chest wall is sufficiently injured to create bidirectional flow of air through the wound. This is most commonly associated with massive penetrating trauma, as seen with gunshot wounds. The normal expansion of the lung is impossible due to the loss of negative intrathoracic pressure and the normalization of pressures between the chest cavity and atmosphere. Inability to generate the negative pressure necessary to expand the lung compromises gas exchange and leads to hypoxia and hypercarbia. The compliant mediastinum allows for collapse of both lungs on inspiration, resulting in ineffective, paradoxical breathing.

Management of an open pneumothorax depends on the size of the chest wall defect and respiratory status. Small injuries, such as knife or gunshot wounds, can be treated by covering the chest wall defect with sterile petroleum dressing and placing a thoracostomy tube through a fresh incision. Size and location of the chest tube will depend on the extent of underlying injury. In general, a large-caliber tube placed laterally and directed posteriorly should be used, as an underlying hemothorax may be present. Small chest wall defects will seal and heal spontaneously and generally do not require surgical repair.

Prehospital treatment of a sucking chest wound may consist of placing a petroleum dressing with only three sides taped to create a flutter valve to allow for ongoing chest decompression while eliminating the sucking component of the chest wound. This should be converted to a sealed dressing with thoracostomy tube placed as soon as possible. Patients who are not spontaneously breathing or who have chest wall defects too large to adequately seal (such as in a blast injury) will require intubation and ventilatory support. Large wounds will often require urgent thoracotomy to repair the chest wall defect and underlying injuries.

TRAUMATIC TRACHEAL AND BRONCHIAL DISRUPTION

Traumatic tracheal and/or bronchial disruption is rare in children. Airway injury is more frequently seen in penetrating trauma, but high-speed, blunt injury may place significant shearing forces on the tracheal tree to generate a tear. In cases of crush injuries, severe compressive forces transmitted against a closed glottis may also disrupt the tracheobronchial tree. Although infrequent, these injuries carry a high mortality rate. A third to half of these patients die within the first hour after injury. Most injuries occur in the distal trachea or proximal bronchi. If the injury occurs low in the bronchial tree, air rupture into the pleural space may lead to tension pneumothorax. Symptoms range from mild respiratory distress to respiratory arrest.

Diagnosis of airway injury is made both clinically and radiographically (Fig. 31–5). Early bronchoscopy is diagnostic and should be considered in patients with these findings. Chest CT scan should also be utilized for better visualization and location of the injury. Treatment is variable and based on the specific lesion, stability of the patient, and other associated lesions.

In all cases where airway injury is suspected, endotracheal suctioning and other blind airway interventions should be avoided. Smaller, more distal injuries can be managed with a chest tube and observation. With more significant injuries, establishing an airway can be complicated, particularly when the trachea is disrupted or a peritracheal hematoma distorts the airway anatomy. When intubation is necessary, fiberoptic assistance will minimize further traumatic injury, especially in cases of incomplete tears. If a surgical airway becomes necessary, it should be placed below the level of the disruption by tracheostomy or cricothyrotomy. Inability to ventilate, once an airway has been established, requires emergency thoracotomy to repair or alleviate the disruption. Thoracotomy for definitive repair is also necessary in severe cases of uncontrolled bleeding.

TRAUMATIC ASPHYXIA

Traumatic asphyxia is an injury unique to children due to the increased compliance of the chest wall and absence of valves in the superior and inferior vena cava. Sudden, direct compression of the elastic pediatric thoracic cage against a closed glottis causes dramatic increases in intrathoracic pressure, temporary vena cava obstruction, and transmission of the pressure into the capillaries of the head and neck. This results in cyanosis, plethora, and petechiae of the head and neck regions, subconjunctival hemorrhages, face and neck edema, and rarely, intracranial hemorrhage. Clinical presentation varies depending

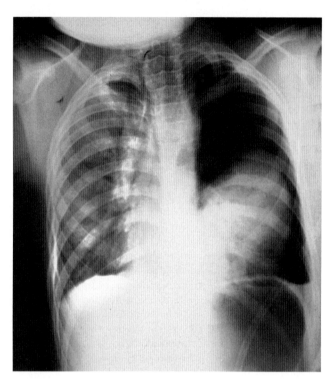

Figure 31–5. This 13-year-old child was hit by a car. The AP chest x-ray demonstrates an obvious left-sided pneumothorax, but the position of the left lung is peculiar. Rather than collapsing toward the hilum, the lung seems to have fallen to the dependent portion of the thorax. This is called the "fallen-lung sign." This is an extremely rare finding on x-ray, but when present, the abnormal position of the lung, together with the left-sided pneumothorax, are highly suggestive of rupture of the tracheobronchial tree. This was confirmed on a subsequent CT scan.

on the forces applied. More severe cases may present with respiratory distress, altered mental status, and seizures. Approximately one-third of these patients will experience a loss of consciousness. Transient and permanent visual disturbances can occur due to retinal hemorrhages and edema. The presence of traumatic asphyxia serves as a marker for associated head trauma, pulmonary contusions, and intra-abdominal injuries. Treatment involves removing the cause and tending to the resulting complications.

TRAUMATIC ESOPHAGEAL RUPTURE

Traumatic esophageal rupture is extremely rare in children. It occurs with severe blunt upper abdominal trauma in which stomach contents are forcefully injected into the esophagus against a closed cricopharyngeus muscle causing a rupture of the esophageal wall into the mediastinum. Clinical signs include pain and shock out of proportion to the apparent severity of injury. It may be associated with a pneumothorax that drains stomach contents or has signs of air leak equally and continuously throughout the respiratory cycle. Subcutaneous emphysema may dissect into the neck and be palpa-

▶ **TABLE 31–3. CHEST RADIOGRAPH FINDINGS IN AORTIC INJURY**

Widened mediastinum with obliteration of the aortic knob
Dilation of the ascending aorta
Deviation of the trachea (as evidenced by the endotracheal tube) to the right
Deviation of the esophagus (as evidenced by the nasogastric tube) to the right
Evidence of first and/or second rib fracture
Apical pleural cap (blood at the apex of the lung, seen more commonly on the left)

ble. Although rare in children, Hamman's sign (mediastinal crunch) may be appreciated as a crunching sound with heartbeats. Chest radiograph often reveals mediastinal emphysema and may be the only clue to the diagnosis. Fluoroscopy with water-soluble contrast or endoscopy can confirm the diagnosis. Urgent surgical repair with mediastinal drainage is required; occasionally delayed definitive repair may be necessary. With extensive esophageal damage, temporary esophageal diversion may be required. If unrecognized, this condition progresses rapidly to mediastinitis, sepsis, and death despite surgical intervention.

TRAUMATIC DIAPHRAGMATIC HERNIA

Traumatic diaphragmatic hernia in children is associated with both blunt and penetrating chest and/or abdominal trauma. It is more commonly associated with injuries involving forceful blunt trauma that cause a sudden increase in intra-abdominal pressure. One example is the "lap belt" complex, when children involved in motor vehicle crashes are improperly restrained with only lap belts. The small pelvis of a child allows for the displacement of the lab belt upward onto the abdomen. The acceleration/deceleration forces applied to the abdomen result in compressive forces that may injure the organs directly or cause intra-abdominal pressure significant enough to rupture the diaphragm. The left hemidiaphragm is involved in the majority of cases. Associated injuries involving the liver, spleen, and intestines are seen frequently. With penetrating trauma, diaphragmatic laceration is possible when the injury is sustained inferior to the nipple line.

Because of the few early symptoms, there is often a delay in the diagnosis of traumatic diaphragmatic hernia, with only 50% to 60% being diagnosed in the acute phase. Respiratory symptoms result not from the hernia itself, but from herniation of abdominal contents into the chest cavity. Lung function is compromised by the physical space constraint and compression of the lung parenchyma. Clinical findings may include contusions and abrasions of the upper abdomen and lower chest wall, but herniation can occur without external signs of trauma. Breath sounds may be decreased or bowel sounds heard on the affected side. Chest radiograph findings depend on the status of the abdominal contents and are outlined in Table 31–4. Knowledge of the forces and mechanism of injury and a high index of suspicion are necessary in the consideration of this diagnosis.

► **TABLE 31-4. CHEST RADIOGRAPH FINDINGS IN TRAUMATIC DIAPHRAGMATIC HERNIA**

Chest radiograph with acute herniation of abdominal
     contents
     Diagnostic with bowel or stomach presenting within the
          chest cavity
     Presence of the nasogastric tube in the chest

Chest radiograph with diaphragmatic tear but delayed
     herniation of abdominal contents
     Unexplained elevation of the hemidiaphragm
     Unrelieved acute gastric dilation
     Loculated subpulmonic hemopneumothorax
     Presence of the nasogastric tube in the chest

Acute traumatic diaphragmatic herniation requires surgical repair. However, initial management should concentrate on adequate oxygenation, ventilation, and stabilizing other injuries. A nasogastric tube should be placed to decompress the stomach and intubation with positive-pressure ventilation performed if respiratory status deteriorates. With delayed presentations, chest radiograph may demonstrate the pathology. Some cases may require confirmation by fluoroscopy or in rare cases by laparotomy.

RIB FRACTURES

Rib fractures are uncommon in children because of their compliant, cartilaginous thoracic cage. When rib fractures do occur, they are often the result of a direct blow to the chest or significant anterior–posterior forces seen with crush or squeezing mechanisms. The posterior–lateral aspect of the ribs is most susceptible to fracture from all causes. In isolation, rib fractures are rarely a source of mortality. However, because of the significant forces needed, such fractures serve as important markers for potentially serious underlying injuries. Evaluate the patient carefully for associated pulmonary contusions, pneumothorax, and hemothorax. When the first rib is involved, it is prudent to be suspicious for clavicular fractures, extremity trauma, head and neck injuries, central and peripheral nerve injuries, and major vascular trauma. Multiple rib fractures are often associated with multisystem organ involvement and carry a higher risk of morbidity and mortality. Lower rib fractures may be associated with abdominal injuries. Even when not associated with injuries to the abdominal organs, referred pain from rib fractures alone can confuse the diagnosis.

Without a clear history of trauma, and particularly if there are multiple fractures in various stages of healing, child abuse should be suspected. There are more than a million documented cases of child abuse each year in the United States, and up to 30% of these children will have sustained rib fractures. Children younger than one year of age are at the highest risk of abuse from shaking. These forces are frequently strong enough to cause rib fractures, significant intracranial hemorrhage, retinal hemorrhage, and metaphyseal fractures. This constellation of signs and symptoms is referred to as "shaken baby syndrome" or "shaken impact syndrome." When rib fractures are detected in infants and young children, an extensive workup is needed. (see Chapter 145). All cases of suspected child abuse should be immediately reported to child protective services and local law enforcement agencies.

Most rib fractures are diagnosed by screening chest radiograph. However, up to 50% of isolated rib fractures may not be diagnosed on the initial chest radiograph. Isolated rib fractures are self-limited in nature and often do not require any additional workup. In cases of multiple rib fractures or an isolated first rib fracture, further radiographic evaluation with rib series, chest CT scan, or angiography may be necessary to detect underlying injuries. Sternal fractures and costochondral separations are also not easily recognized on chest radiograph or rib series, but should be suspected if there is point tenderness, crepitus, or obvious deformity.

Simple rib fractures are well tolerated in children. Treatment involves optimizing the patient's respiratory effort with aggressive pain management and breathing therapy with incentive spirometry. In cases where pain is severe enough to cause splinting and atelectasis, intercostal nerve blocks may be necessary to facilitate the healing process. These efforts will help in the prevention of atelectasis and complicating pneumonias. Associated pneumothorax or hemothorax should be drained promptly to allow for better lung function.

FLAIL CHEST

Severe blunt trauma to the chest wall can cause more than two fractures to the same rib. When this occurs in more than two adjacent ribs, the structural integrity of the chest wall is compromised, causing a flail chest. This isolated segment of ribs moves paradoxically, making respirations ineffective. Children with large flail rib segments are at risk for respiratory failure.

Signs and symptoms include varying degrees of respiratory distress and hypoxia along with the classic paradoxical chest wall motion. Tenderness, bruising, and crepitus overlying the flail segments may also be present. Muscle spasm and respiratory splinting may obscure the clinical diagnosis by "stabilizing" and concealing the flail segments on physical examination.

Chest radiograph confirms the diagnosis (Fig. 31–6) and often reveals associated pulmonary contusion. Treatment is aimed at preventing hypoxia and respiratory failure. Treatment options are dependent on the extent of injury and the child's ability to compensate. Supplemental oxygen and close monitoring may be all that is required. The addition of intercostal or epidural nerve block for pain control is preferable to narcotic analgesia due to the potential for respiratory depression. Patients with paradoxical respirations from flail chest will need positive-pressure ventilation until rib fixation occurs. Few may need to be intubated and placed on PEEP for treatment. Large segments of flail ribs often require operative fixation.

SPINE INJURIES

Spine injuries are less frequent in children suffering thoracic trauma. Most injuries are sustained by motor vehicle crashes

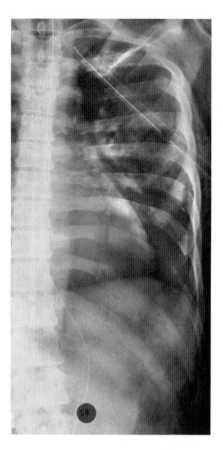

Figure 31–6. This is the x-ray of an adolescent who sustained significant blunt chest trauma. Note the fractures of ribs 4 through 10 seen medially that are indicative of posterior rib fractures, and the more peripheral fractures seen in ribs 4 through 8. This patient presented with paradoxical movement of the chest with breathing, crepitus of subcutaneous emphysema, and a pneumothorax that required placement of the chest tube (also seen on the x-ray).

and falls. Cervical and thoracic spine immobilization should be maintained until evaluation is complete and theses areas are cleared of injury. Potential spinal injuries include compression fractures from axial loading or falls; spinal cord and ligamentous injuries from spinal distraction due to hyperflexion and hyperextension mechanisms; and spinal cord contusions and hemorrhage from crush injuries.

Spine fractures may be detected on screening or detailed radiographs. If clinical suspicion remains high despite normal radiographs, CT scan can be helpful in detecting small fractures. When there is concern for spinal cord or ligamentous injury, magnetic resonance imaging (MRI) will be the most useful. If a child has suffered immediate or progressive neurologic deficits related to potential spinal cord injury, an MRI should be obtained immediately to evaluate for operative lesions such as expanding epidural hematomas causing cord compression. Remember that some patients have spinal cord injury without radiographic abnormality, which is discussed in Chapter 30.

CARDIOVASCULAR INJURIES

Cardiac and great vessel injuries are uncommon in children, but when they do occur, they increase the morbidity and mortality associated with thoracic trauma. Myocardial injury in children can occur in isolation or in association with multiple injuries. Myocardial contusion is the most common injury seen with blunt chest trauma. The most common injury seen with penetrating mechanisms is pericardial tamponade. Other more common injuries include ventricular rupture or laceration and valvular disruption. Rare complications of blunt thoracic trauma include great vessel injury, myocardial necrosis with subsequent aneurysm, traumatic aortic insufficiency, pericardial laceration, fatal cardiac herniation, coronary artery injury, and cardiac conduction system injury. Traumatic aortic rupture is the most common great vessel injured, but is still underreported since more than 50% of victims succumb to this injury before reaching the hospital. Injuries to other vessels are rare except in cases of penetrating trauma.

MYOCARDIAL CONTUSION

Cardiac contusion is the most common unsuspected and under diagnosed injury after blunt thoracic trauma. The National Pediatric Trauma Registry estimates that up to 5% of pediatric victims of blunt chest trauma suffer cardiac contusions. One study that looked at children who suffered blunt thoracic trauma severe enough to produce pulmonary contusion or rib fracture found that 43% of these patients had a significant cardiac contusion.[7] Cardiac injury is most often sustained as a result of motor vehicle crashes and pedestrian injuries. Pulmonary contusions are present in half and rib fractures present in a third of cases of cardiac contusion. Cardiac contusions tend to be more severe in cases of multisystem trauma.

Diagnosis should be made using a combination of clinical suspicion based on mechanism of injury, clinical examination findings, and cardiac-specific evaluation. Children may complain of significant tenderness in the anterior chest or poorly localized chest pain. However, up to half of patients with cardiac injury have no complaints of chest pain, and in most cases, there is no external evidence of trauma and the cardiac examination is normal. Tachycardia is the most sensitive and important indicator of myocardial injury and should be considered significant. Pain and anxiety only produce impressive tachycardia that can complicate the diagnostic process and mask concern for cardiac contusion. Children with more severely injured myocardium may present with dysrhythmias, hypotension, and signs of cardiac failure. ECG abnormalities are less common in children and a normal ECG may lead to a missed diagnosis if used as a defining tool alone. In a study where 43% of the cases of blunt chest trauma were diagnosed with a significant cardiac contusion, no patients had ECG abnormalities.[7] Diagnosis was made by abnormalities in cardiac function on echocardiography and radionuclide angiography/MUGA scan, and an elevation in cardiac enzymes. ECG abnormalities that are present in the ED serve as a better indicator for cardiac injury. Patients who present to the ED in a stable hemodynamic state and in normal sinus rhythm rarely develop serious cardiac sequelae. High-risk patients are evident on presentation to the ED. Elevation of cardiac-specific enzyme levels, specifically troponin I, is an important indicator of cardiac contusion.

Management of cardiac contusion is mostly supportive. Children with suspected cardiac injury should be admitted for observation with cardiac monitoring and serial measuring of cardiac enzymes. Cardiac-specific evaluation should focus on the assessment of function by echocardiography. Fluid management should be patient specific and adjusted accordingly.

CARDIAC TAMPONADE

Cardiac tamponade is a life-threatening condition that occurs when fluid (blood or serous fluid) fills the pericardial space to such an extent that venous return is compromised. Penetrating injuries, like stab and gunshot wounds, are the most common etiology. Gunshot wounds to this area typically cause sudden death. Blunt trauma is unlikely to cause this condition acutely. Even though the laceration of the pericardium may be quite small, life threatening hemorrhage may ensure. The coronary arteries and cardiac chambers are at or near arterial pressure, and therefore, the pericardial sac fills quickly with blood, causing normovolemic shock and death. This condition will rapidly progress from hypotension to pulseless electrical activity (PEA) unless prompt treatment is initiated.

Diagnosis of cardiac tamponade is made clinically, but confirmation is assisted with echocardiography. Clinical findings that are concerning for cardiac tamponade include the presence of a precordial wound, tachycardia, narrow pulse pressure, and pulsus paradoxus. Beck's triad with muffled or distant heart sounds, hypotension, and jugular venous distention may be present but may not be a reliable clinical indicator in the presence of hypovolemia.

Chest radiograph typically shows the classic "water bottle" cardiac silhouette. The ECG often shows tachycardia with extremely low voltage, or it may show evidence of acute myocardial infarction if a coronary artery has been lacerated.

Bedside echocardiography is diagnostic; however, treatment should not be delayed while waiting for the echocardiogram. Treatment should be based on clinical suspicion and a scenario of patient deterioration or arrest. Definitive treatment requires thoracotomy, pericardiotomy, and repair of the underlying injury. Although its role has become limited, in certain circumstances pericardiocentesis is both diagnostic and therapeutic. However, there is a high incidence of false-negative results, where a negative pericardiocentesis does not necessarily rule out a hemopericardium. With rapid bleeding into the pericardium, blood often clots, making it impossible to relieve the tamponade without a thoracotomy. Pericardiocentesis should only be performed by providers trained in emergency procedures because it carries significant risks, such as myocardial and coronary artery laceration, leading to hemopericardium, pneumothorax, and dysrhythmia. It should only be performed when the patient's condition is rapidly deteriorating and definitive thoracotomy is not readily available. Repeated aspirations may be necessary, so the needle or plastic angiocath is generally left in place until a thoracotomy can be done.

In certain circumstances, an emergency pericardial window may be necessary to open the pericardium to relieve the tamponade and control bleeding until definitive treatment can be performed. Bleeding may be controlled by directly clamping the injured area; however, the coronary arteries are particularly sensitive to pressure changes and compression and may easily be damaged. This procedure and chest thoracotomy should only be done by trained trauma or cardiovascular surgeons. Repeated pericardial aspiration and aggressive blood resuscitation are reasonable alternatives until a physician with expertise in emergency thoracotomy is available.

TRAUMATIC RUPTURE OF THE GREAT VESSELS

Rupture of the great vessels is extremely rare in children, in part due to the higher elastin content of their connective tissue. However, children and adults with Marfan's syndrome are more susceptible due to the intrinsic weakness of their uncrosslinked collagen. Aortic disruption at the level of the ligamentum arteriosum is the most common site in children and may be associated with aortic dissection. As in adults, morbidity and mortality are high with injuries to the great vessels. Paraplegia is the most significant complication suffered by survivors of thoracic aortic injury.

Blunt aortic injury is most commonly caused by rapid deceleration, as seen in high-speed automobile crashes and falls from great heights. More than 50% of these patients die at the scene. Many children will have significant associated injuries to the heart, lungs, abdomen, and central nervous system. Clinical signs include chest pain that may be localized to the anterior chest, back, or upper abdomen, and a murmur radiating to the back (rarely appreciated). It is not uncommon for there to be no external evidence of thoracic injury.

Making the diagnosis can be difficult, especially in children who are not prone to aortic injury. Chest radiograph findings (Table 31–4), although sometimes subtle, can increase suspicion for aortic injury. A widened mediastinum is the most common finding, but this alone does not confirm or necessarily warrant an angiogram. Chest CT scan will help better delineate the injuries, but may miss small tears. In cases where there is ongoing blood loss, diagnosis is confirmed by angiography.

Early surgical consultation with angiography is the diagnostic modality of choice in the appropriate clinical setting for suspected aortic rupture or dissection. Definitive treatment requires immediate surgical repair. Initial treatment should be directed toward the ABCs of trauma care and aggressive fluid resuscitation while the surgical team prepares for surgery. Hemopneumothorax should be treated with a thoracostomy tube unless an ED thoracotomy is indicated.

Penetrating trauma and impaled objects more often cause injury to the vena cava or pulmonary vessels than injury to the aorta. With isolated venous or pulmonary vessel injuries, patients often survive to surgery even with severe injuries. A vascular injury should be considered with any obvious wounds to the chest associated with hypotension. Hypovolemic shock is often present initially and may respond to fluid resuscitation only to recur as the slow venous bleeding progresses. Hemopneumothorax is universally associated with penetrating chest trauma and should be treated promptly and aggressively.

▶ PROCEDURES

These procedures should only be performed by physicians trained in the techniques and for the appropriate indication.

NEEDLE THORACOSTOMY

Needle thoracostomy is an emergent but temporary procedure used to relieve a pneumothorax, in particular a tension pneumothorax. This procedure can also be used in the diagnosis of a tension pneumothorax when an audible rush of air under pressure is heard upon decompression, and the patient's hemodynamic status improves when the excessive intrathoracic pressure is relieved. Uncertainty as to the side of the tension pneumothorax should not prohibit initiation of this potentially life-saving procedure. Decompression of the alternate side should be done if immediate improvement is not seen with the initial thoracostomy.

To perform this procedure, place the patient in a supine position and prepare the site in a sterile manner. An angiocath or butterfly needle attached to a syringe filled with 2 to 3 mL of saline is then inserted into the second or third intercostal space at the midclavicular line on the affected side while maintaining negative pressure on the syringe. The needle or catheter should be advanced over the superior aspect of the rib to avoid the intercostal neurovascular bundle. Decompression of a tension pneumothorax will occur spontaneously. Air return from a simple pneumothrorax will only be decompressed with aspiration, highlighting the importance of negative pressure on the syringe attached to the advancing needle. When air bubbles are visualized in the syringe or an audible rush of air is detected (in cases where a syringe is not attached), the pleural space has been entered. At this point a decrease in resistance should also be detectable. If a tension pneumothorax was relieved, the catheter should remain in place and air intermittently aspirated to prevent a reaccumulation of air under pressure. Place a large-bore chest tube (tube thoracostomy) as soon as possible and attach it to a drainage/suction device.

TUBE THORACOSTOMY

Performing tube thoracostomy (inserting a chest tube) (Fig. 31–7) is indicated for the drainage of air (pneumothorax), blood (hemothorax), or fluid (e.g., chylothorax) from the pleural space. The technique of insertion is similar to that of needle thoracostomy. The procedure, however, is more invasive and a sterile surgical field should be prepared. Select the appropriate size chest tube based on the patient's weight in kilograms (Table 31–2).

Tube thoracostomy is a painful procedure. Use local anesthetics at the insertion site and consider intravenous sedation and pain control in younger children who may have difficulty verbalizing pain. The trajectory of the tube should be planned; tubes intended to drain air should be directed anteriorly; tubes

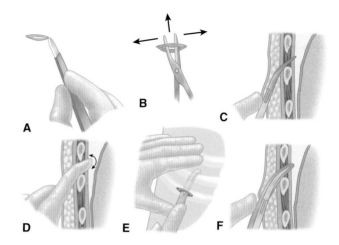

Figure 31–7. The tube thoracostomy. (A) The skin incision is made. (B) A tract is bluntly dissected in the subcutaneous tissues. (C) The Kelly clamp is forced into the pleural cavity. (D) A finger is inserted through the tract to feel for adhesions. (E) The chest tube is held in the Kelly clamp and inserted through the tract. (F) The chest tube is guided into the pleural cavity.

to drain fluid should be directed toward the patient's back. The most appropriate insertion sites are at the fourth or fifth intercostal space anterior to the midaxillary line. Insertion of the tube over the top of the rib, again to avoid the intercostal neurovascular bundle. To insert the tube, make a small skin incision parallel to the intercostal space approximately one or two intercostal spaces below the point of tube insertion into the pleural space. The incision should be large enough to allow for the passage of the chest tube, a hemostat attached to it, and the provider's finger. Using a blunt dissecting technique, a tunnel is made from the skin to the intercostal space. The blunt tip of the hemostats is then guided over the top of the rib and then pressure is applied to enter the pleural space. Once the tip is through, the hole is made larger by spreading the hemostats. The chest tube is then gripped by the hemostats and inserted using a finger as a guide. Once inserted, suture the chest tube in place and connect the tube to an underwater seal apparatus with or without suction. A postinsertion chest radiograph should be obtained to confirm proper placement of the tube and reexpansion of the lung.

Pericardiocentesis

Pericardiocentesis is performed when fluid aspiration from the pericardial space is necessary. The emergent removal of pericardial fluid can be lifesaving. The success rate of this procedure is variable, but the complication rate remains high. Complications include dysrhythmias, pneumothorax, hemopericardium, and ventricular puncture. For this reason, emergency pericardiocentesis should be performed for life-threatening cardiac tamponade by providers skilled in this technique.

Prior to this procedure, place the patient on a cardiac monitor, have airway patency secured, and IV access obtained. The patient should be placed in a slight reverse Trendelenburg position and a sterile field prepared. If ultrasonography is available, use it to visualize the pericardial fluid collection. Local anesthesia and sedation should be strongly considered in the awake patient undergoing this procedure. Special kits are available that include sterile drapes, large-bore angiocath needles, syringes, three-way stopcock, and an alligator clip with a wire for cardiac monitor guidance. For infants and young children, a 20-gauge spinal needle or a 1.5-inch, 18- to 20-gauge needle with a catheter may be used. For older children, an 18-gauge spinal needle or a 1.5-inch, 16-gauge needle with catheter may be used. An alligator clip is then attached to the hub of the appropriate-sized needle and connected to a precordial lead on an ECG monitor. This connection will detect any ventricular dysrhythmias that may be produced when the myocardium is irritated by the advancing needle. The insertion site for the needle is immediately inferior and 1 cm left of the xiphoid process. While applying negative pressure to the syringe, advance the needle at a 45-degree angle in the direction of the tip of the patient's left scapula until pericardial fluid or blood is obtained, or until ECG changes are noted. In adults or adolescents, a parasternal approach can be used. For this approach, the needle is inserted perpendicular to the skin surface at the left fifth intercostal space, just lateral to the sternum. For patients who may need ongoing drainage, place a pericardial catheter.

Emergency Department Thoracotomy

When cardiac arrest occurs following thoracic trauma, there are a few select injuries that may benefit from thoracotomy, including ventricular laceration, cardiac tamponade, thoracic arterial injuries, and intercostal arterial injuries. The decision to use ED thoracotomy is often based on the mechanism of injury and the presence of vital signs. All patients should have their vital signs assessed immediately upon arrival to the ED and should have a rapid assessment for the presence of penetrating trauma.

The role of ED thoracotomy in the resuscitation of victims of trauma has been a topic of continual debate. The indications for ED thoracotomy in the adult trauma patient are well established in the literature and have shown the procedure to be efficacious and cost-effective for selected patient populations. There is a consensus that ED thoracotomy is not indicated for adults suffering cardiac arrest in the field secondary to blunt thoracoabdominal trauma, whereas ED thoracotomy in cases of penetrating trauma has been shown to improve survival.[8,9] When a child arrives to an ED with no vital signs after a traumatic event, the ED physician will consider employing heroic ATLS (Advanced Traumatic Life Support) interventions when standard CPR fails to show improvement. There have been reports of various rates of success of ED thoracotomy in children, ranging from 0% to 26% for overall survival. Pediatric patients have a slightly better chance of survival from penetrating thoracic injuries (5%–36%) than from blunt thoracic trauma (0%–15%).[8] In most cases where patients arrive in the ED without vital signs and when cardiac arrest has occurred for more than 20 minutes, survival is unlikely. Extensive review of the literature has led to the following consensus on ED thoracotomy for pediatric patients: (1). Pediatric victims of blunt thoracoabdominal trauma who suffer cardiopulmonary arrest at the scene and do not have a return of cardiac function on arrival to the ED uniformly have a dismal chance of survival.

Even children suffering penetrating trauma who have lost vital signs in the field and have no return of cardiac function in the ED do not benefit from ED thoracotomy; (2). Children who have suffered penetrating or blunt thoracic trauma associated with detectable vital signs who deteriorate despite maximal conventional therapy have a better chance of survival from ED thoracotomy.[10]

▶ ORGAN DONATION

Victims of thoracic trauma and cardiopulmonary arrest who do not experience a return of spontaneous circulation may be eligible for organ donation. For this population, resuscitative efforts with external chest compressions, attempts at controlling hemorrhage, and restoration of blood volume may be continued until a decision regarding organ viability is made.

▶ LAW ENFORCEMENT

Most states require reporting of stab wounds, gunshot wounds, and assaults. Child abuse statutes also require reporting of suspected abuse. While treating pediatric trauma patients, one should also consider duty to report these injuries to local authorities and to child protective services.

▶ SUMMARY

Trauma is the number one cause of death and disability in children in the United States. Although uncommon in children, thoracic injuries are significant causes of childhood mortality secondary to trauma. For these reasons, the skillful management of thoracic injuries cannot be overemphasized. The approach to a child with thoracic trauma should follow guidelines set forth by the American Heart Association and the American College of Surgeons Committee on Trauma.[11] Isolated chest trauma is uncommon in children, making a complete and systematic approach necessary so as to not overlook frequently occurring concomitant injuries.

REFERENCES

1. Peclet MH, Newman KD, Eichelberger MR, et al. Thoracic trauma in children: an indicator of increased mortality. *J Pediatr Surg.* 1990;25(9):961–965.
2. Willis CD, Cameron PA, Bernard SA, Fitzgerald M. Cardiopulmonary resuscitation after traumatic cardiac arrest is not always futile. *Injury Int J Care Injured.* 2006;37:448–454.
3. Perron AD, Sing RF, Branas CC, Huynh T. Predicting survival in pediatric trauma patients receiving cardiopulmonary resuscitation in the prehospital setting. *Prehosp Emerg Care.* 2001;5(1):6–9.
4. Junkins EP, O'Connell KJ, Mann NC. Pediatric trauma systems in the United States: do they make a difference? *Clin Pediatr Emerg Med.* 2006;7:76–81.
5. Reinhorn M, Kaufman HL, Hirsch EF, Millham FH. Penetrating thoracic trauma in a pediatric population. *Ann Thorac Surg.* 1996;61(5):150–155.

6. Holmes JF, Brant WE, Bogren G, et al. Prevalence and importance of pneumothoraces visualized on abdominal computed tomographic scan in children with blunt trauma. *J Trauma.* 2001;50(3):516–520.

7. Ildstad ST, Tollerud DJ, Weiss RG, et al. Cardiac contusion in pediatric patients with blunt thoracic trauma. *J Pediatr Surg.* 1990;25(3):287–289.

8. Sheikh AA, Culbertson CB. Emergency department thoracotomy in children: rationale for selective application. *J Trauma.* 1993;34(3):323–328.

9. Branney SW, Moore EE, Feldhaus KM, Wolfe RE. Critical analysis of two decades of experience with postinjury emergency department thoracotomy in a regional trauma center. *J Trauma.* 1998;45(1):87–95.

10. Beaver BL, Colombani PM, Buck JR, et al. Efficacy of emergency thoracotomy in pediatric trauma. *J Pediatr Surg.* 1987; 22(1):19–23.

11. American College of Surgeons, Committee on Trauma; http:// www.facs.org/trauma/atls/index.html. Accessed January 26, 2009.

CHAPTER 32

Abdominal Trauma

Shireen M. Atabaki, Wendy Ann Lucid, and Todd Brian Taylor

▶ HIGH-YIELD FACTS

- Blunt abdominal trauma is proportionally more common in children and results in more injuries and deaths than penetrating trauma. However, penetrating trauma is far more lethal as a sole injury.
- Management of pediatric abdominal trauma requires a coordinated effort between the emergency physician, trauma surgeon, and pediatric referral center.
- The spleen and liver are the most commonly injured organs as a result of blunt abdominal trauma. Liver injuries constitute the most common cause of death.
- Care must be taken not to let the head and extremity components of Waddell's triad divert attention from the more subtle findings of intra-abdominal injury that may include life-threatening hemorrhage.
- Computed tomography (CT) scan has eliminated much of the difficulty surrounding the diagnosis of abdominal injuries and is the procedure of choice for stable pediatric trauma patients. However, CT scan is not without risk and must be used judiciously using the ALARA standard (as low as reasonably achievable).
- The focused abdominal sonography for trauma (FAST) ultrasound examination evaluates up to six areas of the abdomen with the principal objective of identifying hemoperitoneum. The FAST examination is less sensitive in children than adults.
- Perforations of the duodenum and proximal jejunum are the most common intestinal injuries and are usually associated with lap belt or bicycle handlebar injury.

Trauma is the most common cause of death in children. Abdominal trauma accounts for close to 200 000 visits to US emergency departments each year.[1] Serious abdominal injuries are relatively common in childhood and account for approximately 8% of admissions to pediatric trauma centers. Only 15% of these injuries require surgery and the majority of these are for penetrating wounds. Abdominal trauma is the third leading cause of traumatic death behind head and thoracic injuries, but it is the most common unrecognized cause of fatal injury in children.

Blunt abdominal trauma is proportionately more common in children and results in more injuries and deaths than penetrating trauma. Blunt trauma accounts for 85% of pediatric abdominal trauma (vs. 50% in adults) with 9% of these patients dying primarily from associated injuries. Yet penetrating trauma is far more lethal as the sole injury. Penetrating abdominal trauma accounts for only approximately 15% of the total cases, and of these 6% will die primarily from the penetrating wound. Children are susceptible to different injury patterns than adults. Blunt trauma from motor vehicle collisions causes more than half of the abdominal injuries seen in children and is the most lethal. Penetrating injuries in the pediatric population are increasing. Gunshot and stab wounds are particularly common in young adolescents and 75% are inflicted by an assailant as opposed to accidental shootings that occur most commonly from firearms discovered by children in the home. Accidental impalement occurs more often in children younger than 13 years and these injuries may involve such diverse items as scissors or picket fences.

Management of pediatric abdominal trauma requires a coordinated effort between the emergency physician, trauma surgeon, and pediatric referral center. Immediate stabilization and transfer of the most severely injured children to an appropriate trauma center when indicated will result in greatly improved outcomes.[2,3]

▶ PATTERNS OF INJURY

MOTOR VEHICLE COLLISIONS (TABLE 32–1)

Multisystem trauma, along with abdominal injury, is common when an automobile strikes a child. Waddell's triad (Fig. 32–1) demonstrates a pattern of injury for the pediatric pedestrian with impact first to the upper leg, then chest and abdomen, followed by head injury. Do not let the head and extremity components of Waddell's triad divert attention from the possibility of more serious intra-abdominal injury that may include life-threatening hemorrhage. The common belief that a unilateral femur fracture can result in hypovolemic shock in young children is questionable. Thus, in the hypotensive patient with blunt trauma, always complete a thorough investigation for potentially more serious abdominal injuries. In countries in which motorists drive on the right side of the road, the most common injuries are on the left side as children are often struck crossing the street, and such accidents frequently result in splenic injuries. With unrestrained occupants involved in motor vehicle collisions, head injuries are the most common and lethal injury, but abdominal injuries represent the most common cause of significant blood loss.

The *lap belt complex* in the restrained child (bursting injury of solid or hollow viscera, and rarely disruption of the diaphragm or lumbar spine) is characterized by ecchymosis, abrasion, or erythema in the pattern of a lap belt ("seat belt sign") across the abdomen (Figs. 32–2, 32–3) and flanks (Grey–Turner sign) and occurs in up to 10% of restrained children.

▶ TABLE 32–1. **PATTERNS OF INJURY BY MECHANISM**

Waddell's Triad	Lap Belt Complex	Fall from a Height
Pedestrian mechanism in child	Restrained occupant in MVC	
Midshaft femur fracture	Blowout diaphragm injury	Head injury
Abdominal injury	Duodenal injury	Multiple long bone fractures
Head injury	Solid organ injury; "Chance fracture" of lumbar spine occurs as a result of hyperflexion	Chest wall injury

The injury is thought to occur because of an improperly applied restraint that allows the lap belt to ride up and compress the abdomen as the child slides forward under the belt. Presence of the "seat belt sign" always warrants further evaluation and has been associated with increased risk of gastrointestinal injury.[4,5] The overall benefit of avoiding head injuries significantly outweighs any risk associated with seat belts, and proper fitting of restraints and use of booster seats should reduce this problem.

Injuries sustained in all-terrain vehicle crashes parallel motor vehicle collisions and have emerged as a frequent cause of abdominal trauma, accounting for a quarter of injuries and 19% of deaths.

BICYCLE CRASHES, SPORTS INJURIES, AND FALLS

Head trauma remains the predominant injury in bicycle crashes, although abdominal injury can occur if the child is impacted by the handlebars or falls to the ground. Handlebar injuries (Fig. 32–4) are particularly obscure, as most children show no serious sign of injury for hours to days after the impact. The mean elapsed time to onset of symptoms is almost 24 hours and as many as one-third are discharged home initially. The seriousness is illustrated by a mean length of stay exceeding 3 weeks for children requiring admission for a handlebar injury. Traumatic pancreatitis, often with pseudocyst formation, is the most common handlebar injury followed by injuries to the kidneys, spleen, and liver, duodenal hematoma, and bowel perforation. It is prudent to obtain an abdominal CT scan and observe children with a suspicion for this injury.

Sports-related trauma typically produces isolated organ injury because of a direct blow to the abdomen. The spleen, kidney, and gastrointestinal tract are particularly vulnerable. Falls rarely cause isolated serious abdominal injury unless there is a direct blow to the abdomen.

CHILD ABUSE

Significant abdominal injury occurs in only approximately 5% of child abuse cases, but it represents the second most common

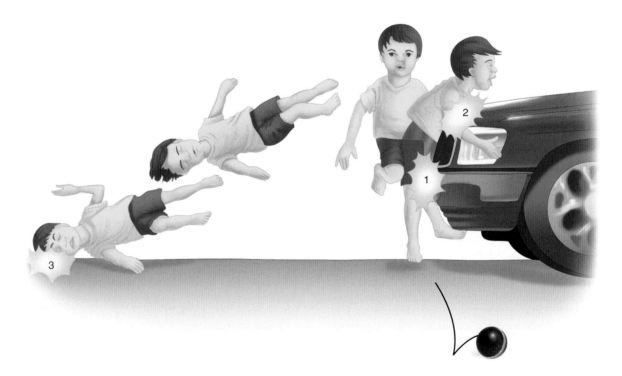

Figure 32–1. Waddel's triad. (With permission from: *Teaching Resource for Instructors of Prehospital Pediatrics—Advanced Life Support (TRIPP-ALS), Center for Pediatric Emergency Medicine.* New York, NY; 2002.)

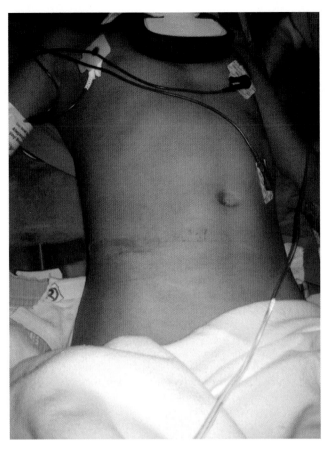

Figure 32-2. Seat belt sign. Ecchymosis, abrasion, and/or erythema across the anterior abdominal wall because of seat belt in a motor vehicle collision associated with intra-abdominal injury, disruption of the diaphragm, and Chance fracture of the lumbar spine.

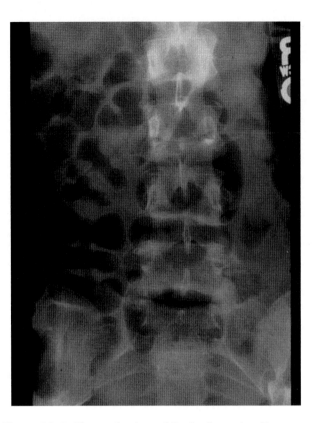

Figure 32-3. Chance fracture of the lumbar spine. Because of improperly applied lap belt which rides up and compresses the child's abdomen during a motor vehicle collision. (Courtesy of Dr. James F. Holmes, Department of Emergency Medicine, University of California, Davis Medical Center.)

cause of death after head injury. The diagnosis can be obscured by the inherent delay in seeking treatment, the surreptitious nature of the visit, and the lack of external signs of trauma in up to one-half of these patients. Common patterns of injury are to the liver and spleen with associated rib fractures.

▶ PATHOPHYSIOLOGY

Certain anatomic features predispose children to multiple rather than single injuries. Proportionally larger solid organs, poorly muscled protuberant abdomen, and flexible thin ribs contribute to the increased incidence of significant abdominal injury and potential for hemorrhage. The diagnosis of a major intra-abdominal hemorrhage may be delayed because children have the capacity to maintain normal blood pressure and pulse rate for age, even in the face of significant blood loss. External signs of injury, abdominal tenderness, and absence of bowel sounds seldom give clues to the ultimate need for surgery. Abdominal distention may be because of hemoperitoneum, peritonitis, or most commonly, gastric distention from crying, and air swallowing. This can confound the examination by masking or mimicking serious abdominal injury or bleeding. Severe dilation can result in respiratory compromise because of interference with diaphragm motion, gastric aspiration, or vagal

dampening of the normal tachycardic response. In children, the primary response to decreased cardiac output is increased heart rate; therefore vagal dampening can lead to precipitous circulatory collapse in the presence of hypovolemia.

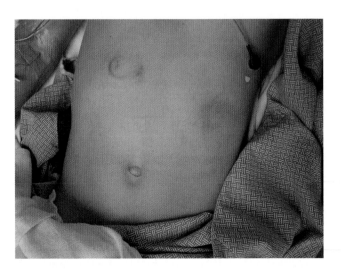

Figure 32-4. Bicycle handle bar injury associated with pancreatic trauma. (Courtesy of Dr. James F. Holmes, Department of Emergency Medicine, University of California, Davis Medical Center.)

► MANAGEMENT

GENERAL PRINCIPLES

A team approach in the evaluation and treatment of abdominal injuries, that includes the emergency physician, trauma surgeon, anesthesiologist, and surgical subspecialists, is ideal. In reality, many emergency physicians find themselves as the only physician initially and must approach the injured child in a systematic way, utilizing consultants appropriately and expeditiously. Blunt abdominal injuries rarely require surgical intervention, while penetrating trauma frequently does. Nevertheless, all unstable patients need immediate surgical consultation.

The basic principles of trauma evaluation and resuscitation should be followed in all cases of abdominal trauma. Evaluation of the abdomen is included in both the primary and secondary surveys. The following interventions are particularly important:

- Insert a nasogastric or orogastric tube to decompress the stomach and to check for blood or bile. Insert an orogastric tube if there is any suspicion of head trauma or basilar skull fracture.
- Place a urinary catheter to check for blood and urinary retention, if there is no gross blood at the meatus. Obtain a urinalysis.
- Complete a rectal examination to check for blood, prostate position in males, and rectal tone.
- Keep the child npo because of the possibility of surgery or development of paralytic ileus.
- Blood should be obtained for type and cros-match, electrolytes, CBC, serum amylase, and liver transaminases.

The mechanism of injury is important and guides the secondary survey and the ordering of specific tests or procedures. It is always important to log roll the patient to inspect the posterior torso for additional wounds. External injuries such as abrasions, lacerations, bruising, and characteristic markings such as tire tracks and seat belt marks should be noted.

Children respond differently to trauma and stress. A traumatized child may be more difficult to examine and may not show the familiar signs of impending demise as seen with adults. History may be limited and the child's reaction to pain may be difficult to assess. Designate a team member to take care of the child's emotional needs and to comfort them through the ordeal of trauma evaluation and treatment. Having the parent or caregiver at the bedside may assist greatly in consoling and evaluating the injured child. Over the past decade, many pediatric trauma centers have instituted policies on family member presence for trauma and pediatric resuscitation.[6-8] Family member presence has caused no delay in patient care.

PENETRATING ABDOMINAL TRAUMA

The diagnosis and treatment of penetrating abdominal injuries in children does not differ greatly from that for adults, and initial management is not dependent on identifying any specific injury. The hollow organs, because of their large volume, are most commonly injured, followed by the liver, kidney, spleen, and major vessels.

In children, the abdomen begins at the nipples, so penetrating wounds between the nipples and the groin potentially involve the peritoneal cavity and should be considered contaminated with a potential for infection. Surgical evaluation, wound debridement, and possible exploration, along with broad-spectrum intravenous antibiotics are necessary in all but the most minor of wounds. Location, size, and possible trajectory of entrance and exit wounds help to identify potential underlying injuries. At a minimum, the following should be performed when there has been significant penetrating abdominal trauma: placement of a nasogastric or orogastric tube; placement of a urinary catheter; upright posteroanterior chest radiograph with a lateral, if possible; supine, upright, and cross-table abdominal radiographs; obtain a CT scan of the abdomen with IV contrast for deep penetrating stab wounds and all gunshot wounds.

Gunshot wounds to the abdomen require immediate exploration. Most enter the peritoneal cavity and injure organs directly or indirectly through kinetic energy dissipation. The high morbidity and mortality associated with gunshot wounds is because of the destructive force of the missile and its fragments, rapid blood loss, complicated surgical repair, and postoperative complications.

Stab wounds pose the greatest threat to blood vessels. Commonly injured vessels include the aorta, inferior vena cava, the portal vein, and hepatic veins. However, stab wounds enter the peritoneal cavity only one-third of the time and only one-third of these require a visceral repair. Local exploration may be possible to rule out peritoneal penetration in minor stab wounds. Conservative management can be entertained if the patient meets the following criteria:

- No sign of shock or peritonitis with observation for 12 to 24 hours.
- No blood in the stomach, rectum, or urine.
- No evidence of free abdominal or retroperitoneal air on x-ray.
- No history or evidence of bowel or omental evisceration.
- Close observation with surgical consultation.

BLUNT ABDOMINAL TRAUMA

Both isolated abdominal and multisystem trauma present challenges in the pediatric patient because information is inherently difficult to obtain. Multiple other injuries may overshadow often subtle early abdominal findings and the physical examination may be only 55% to 65% accurate. For the emergency physician, the key to management is suspecting the diagnosis and obtaining appropriate studies and consultation. Minor mechanisms, such as falling 2 ft to the ground from a hammock, can result in significant splenic injury with minimal symptoms. Therefore observation, as well as repeat vital signs and serial abdominal examinations, may be warranted. Laboratory and radiologic studies may be necessary depending on clinical status, mechanism of injury, and suspicion for injury on physical examination.

Radiographs of the chest (supine or preferably upright posteroanterior plus a lateral) and supine abdomen and pelvis can give important clues to the diagnosis of abdominal injury (Table 32–2).

▶ TABLE 32–2. **RADIOGRAPHIC CLUES IN ABDOMINAL TRAUMA**

A ground glass appearance of the abdominal cavity may suggest intraperitoneal blood or urine

Medial displacement of the lateral border of the stomach, as evidenced by the nasogastric tube, suggests splenic laceration or hematoma as the enlarged spleen pushes the stomach aside

Obliteration of the psoas shadow or renal outline and fracture of the lower ribs suggest renal trauma

Bleeding from the short gastric vessels gives the fundal mucosa a "saw tooth" appearance

With nasogastric tube in place, the relative lack of gas in the distal small intestine suggests a duodenal or proximal jejunal hematoma

Air injected via the nasogastric tube may increase the chance of detecting a pneumoperitoneum indicative of perforated viscus

▶ TABLE 32–3. **CLINICAL FINDINGS PREDICTIVE OF INTRA-ABDOMINAL INJURY IN CHILDREN WITH BLUNT TRAUMA[9]**

ALT >125 or AST >200 (U/L)
Urinalysis >5 RBCs/hpf
Abdominal tenderness
Hematocrit <30%
Femur fracture

A persistently distended abdomen after nasogastric tube placement, hemodynamic instability not immediately responsive to fluid resuscitation, recurrent hypotension, or signs of peritoneal irritation warrant immediate surgical intervention by a surgeon experienced in pediatric abdominal injuries.

LABORATORY EVALUATION (DIAGNOSTIC STUDIES)

The child with blunt trauma is at high-risk for intra-abdominal injury if any of the laboratory or physical examination findings listed in Table 32–3 are present.[9]

Hemoglobin and hematocrit are seldom useful early in the evaluation, but may be valuable for comparison to baseline later in the management of the patient. However, if the initial hematocrit is <30% with other signs of impending shock, this suggests significant hemorrhage.[9] An initial hematocrit <24% is associated with high mortality, and transfusion should be initiated.

COMPUTED TOMOGRAPHY

CT scan has eliminated much of the difficulty surrounding the diagnosis of abdominal injuries and is the procedure of choice for stable trauma patients. Specialized studies should be ordered in consultation with the trauma surgeon to avoid unnecessary delay in definitive treatment. Indications for abdominal and pelvic CT scan are listed in Table 32–4. CT scan is useful for evaluation of the liver, kidney, spleen, retroperitoneum, and, to a lesser extent, gastrointestinal injuries. CT scan identification of pancreatic injury, diaphragm injury, and bowel perforation are much less sensitive and warrant a high index of suspicion with serial abdominal examinations to rule out occult injury.

Radiation exposure is the greatest risk associated with CT scan.[10] Abdominal CT scan carries a significantly high lifetime cancer mortality risk with radiation attributable risks from a single abdominal CT scan within the first and tenth years of

▶ TABLE 32–4. **COMPARISON OF TECHNIQUES FOR EVALUATION OF ABDOMINAL TRAUMA**

	Abdominal CT Scan	Abdominal Ultrasound
Indication	Relatively stable patient Multiple trauma or major thoracic, head, or orthopedic (pelvic) injury Physical findings or a mechanism suggesting possible abdominal injury Unexplained hypotension Hematuria (gross or microscopic >20 RBC/HPF), CNS injury, spinal injury, or mental status alteration precluding serial abdominal examination Declining hematocrit or unaccountable fluid and blood requirements	May be used as a triage tool and adjunct to the physical examination Evaluation of pancreatic injury and intra-abdominal fluid (presumably blood) May also be used to identify other intra-abdominal injuries when CT scan is not readily available.
Advantage	Relatively noninvasive High sensitivity and specificity Evaluates multiple organ systems simultaneously	Available at the bedside and more readily available than CT scan in some locales Can be used at the bedside for a FAST examination to evaluate for peritoneal fluid and blood
Disadvantage	Radiation risk 1/550 lifetime cancer mortality attributable to single CT scan of abdomen in first year of life Generally requires intravenous with or without oral contrast Time delay	Not as sensitive as CT scan

life estimated at 1/550 and 1/700 respectively.[11,12] Variation in practice with respect to CT scan of the child with blunt abdominal trauma persists. Clinical decision rules are necessary to reduce variability in medical management by providing evidence derived guidelines for clinical care; thereby, decreasing unnecessary radiation.[13,14]

Use of oral and intravenous contrast media has traditionally been thought to increase the sensitivity of abdominal CT scan. However, oral contrast is rarely used in the trauma setting because of the technical difficulty of administration and increased waiting time before scanning, risk of aspiration, and apparent limited value because of frequent lack of bowel opacification.[15]

DIAGNOSTIC PERITONEAL LAVAGE

Close observation, serial physical examinations, and particularly abdominal CT scan are utilized to the virtual exclusion of peritoneal lavage in pediatric patients. Diagnostic peritoneal lavage (DPL) may still be useful if these other modalities are unavailable or the child must undergo immediate general anesthesia for other injuries. Under these circumstances, DPL can often be performed in the operating suite. However, the usefulness of DPL remains questionable. It is neither organ-specific nor injury-specific, and cannot reliably assess retroperitoneal injury, and the decision to operate·for liver or splenic injuries is not based on the amount of intraperitoneal blood in children. In addition, the introduction of air and fluid into the abdomen and the resulting peritoneal irritation make subsequent radiographic and physical examinations more difficult.

The technique for DPL in children is similar to that for adults, although a small supraumbilical incision to avoid the bladder, in the young child, is preferred over the usual infraumbilical approach.

ABDOMINAL ULTRASOUND

Bedside ultrasound (US) is more readily available and has significantly reduced the need for DPL. It is particularly useful in the unstable patient as an immediate triage tool and adjunct to the physical examination. As such, it is best used for detecting intra-abdominal injuries that require immediate attention (such as in the setting of hypotension) rather than for a definitive diagnosis.[16–19] It is also useful when CT scan is not available and its greatest utility is in detecting intraperitoneal hemorrhage and pancreatic injuries. Overall, CT scan is more sensitive than US at detecting intra-abdominal injury in children.[20–22] In addition a highly experienced ultrasonographer is required to improve the sensitivity of the pediatric abdominal US. Abdominal US has 66% to 83% sensitivity for the detection of hemoperitoneum in the pediatric trauma patient and CT scan is recommended in the presence of a positive US.[23]

The use of bedside US has become part of the core emergency medicine curriculum and is often taught using the FAST method. The FAST examination evaluates up to six areas of the abdomen with the principal objective of identifying hemoperitoneum. Children who are hemodynamically unstable with abdominal trauma will require laparotomy regardless of the US and those that are stable are often managed nonsurgically even with abdominal organ injury. Therefore, the exact role of US in assessing pediatric abdominal trauma is still being evaluated.

▶ SPECIFIC INJURIES AND MANAGEMENT

SOLID ORGANS

Spleen

With blunt trauma, the spleen ranks first among the solid abdominal organs susceptible to major hemorrhage and second only to the liver in lethal injury. The typical blunt mechanism of injury is frequently from vehicular collisions. A right-sided blow to a pedestrian or fall can cause a contrecoup splenic injury. Penetrating injuries of all types can cause splenic injury and, as with liver stab wounds, it is often difficult to determine the extent of underlying injury based on the external signs of trauma. Mononucleosis, common in children, can result in splenic enlargement and predispose to splenic rupture with even mild impact. Patients with this condition should be warned about contact sports or any activity that could cause a blow to the abdomen until the spleen has returned to normal size, a minimum of 4 to 6 weeks.

Although diffuse abdominal pain may be the presenting complaint, typical findings with splenic injury are left upper quadrant abdominal pain, radiating to the left shoulder (Kehr's sign), associated with palpable tenderness on examination. Significant tenderness in the left upper abdomen and/or splenic enlargement should prompt surgical consultation and consideration of a CT scan. Frank splenic rupture may lead to shock and posttraumatic cardiac arrest. Persistent unexplained leukocytosis or hyperamylasemia also suggests splenic injury.

Abdominal CT scan is the study of choice to identify splenic injury. Abdominal radiographs may incidentally reveal a medially displaced gastric bubble secondary to the enlarged spleen. Once a splenic injury has been identified in the stable patient, management is focused on salvaging the spleen. The thick elastic splenic capsule in children and the usual transverse orientation of lacerations parallel to the vessels commonly results in spontaneous cessation of bleeding and allows nonsurgical management in 90% of cases.

Conservative management includes initial hospitalization for a few days of bed rest for grade 1 or 2 injuries and longer for higher-grade injuries, followed by a regimen of limited activity. Although spontaneous healing of splenic lacerations and subcapsular hematomas occurs in the overwhelming majority of cases, delayed spontaneous rupture can occur at any time and is most common on the third to fifth day. The commitment to conservative management includes close observation and frequent examination.

Children who develop hypotension not responsive to volume resuscitation obviously require surgery. When surgery is required for persistent bleeding, all efforts are made to salvage as much spleen as possible. The results of splenorrhaphy or partial splenectomy have been equally as good as nonsurgical management. There is a marked increase in infection and a 65-fold increase in lethal sepsis in children with splenectomy, particularly with encapsulated organisms (*Streptococcus pneumoniae, Haemophilus influenzae, Neisseria meningitidis, Staphylococcus aureus,* and *Escherichia coli).* The pneumococcal and *H. influenzae* (HIB) vaccines should be given to any patient undergoing partial or complete splenectomy, even though antibody response may be inconsistent and temporary.

Liver

The liver ranks second among solid abdominal organs for major hemorrhage and significant injury, but it is the most common source of *lethal* hemorrhage. Mortality from serious liver injuries may be as high as 10% to 20%. However, the majority of liver injuries in children are minor and remain undetected unless discovered incidentally by abnormal liver enzymes or imaging studies. Serum aspartate aminotransferase (AST) greater than 200U/L and alanine aminotranferase (ALT) greater than 125U/L have been associated with IAI (Table 32–3).[9] CT scan has revolutionized the diagnosis of liver injury and accounts for the increased recognition of this problem.

Mechanisms of injury are similar to those in splenic trauma. Symptoms depend largely on the extent of injury and range from nonspecific diffuse abdominal pain to posttraumatic cardiac arrest. Significant tenderness in the right upper abdomen and/or liver enlargement should prompt surgical consultation and CT scan evaluation.

Children with liver injuries who are not in shock or who respond to volume resuscitation rarely require surgery to control bleeding. However, nonsurgical management is not without complications. Those requiring late laparotomy have transfusion requirements greater than 50% of total blood volume (TBV) during the first 24 hours after injury and bleeding into the biliary tract (hematobilia) are not uncommon. Conservative management includes careful monitoring of vital signs, serial abdominal examinations, and serial hematocrit measurements.

Large stellate liver lacerations and subcapsular hematomas that have eroded through Glisson's capsule rarely stop bleeding without surgery. However, hepatic resection and biliary tree drains are rarely indicated, and direct suturing and drainage can manage most hepatic lacerations. In preparation for surgery, circulating blood volume should be restored since rapid hemorrhage can occur during surgery as blood clots are evacuated during repair.

Pancreas

The pancreas is rarely seriously injured in blunt pediatric trauma because of its deep position in the upper abdomen. However, it is in a fixed position anterior to the vertebral column and vulnerable to a direct blow to the upper central abdomen as seen with bicycle handlebar injury (Fig. 32–4). Pancreatic injuries are difficult to diagnose and signs such as elevated amylase and lipase may take up to 72 hours postinjury to present.

Traumatic pancreatitis without major pancreatic injury is most common, followed by pancreatic hematomas and, rarely, transection of the body or duct. Pancreatic transections often lead to pancreatic pseudocyst formation within 3 to 5 days and result in chronic intermittent attacks of abdominal pain, nausea, vomiting, and weight loss. Acutely, the leakage of pancreatic fluid into the lesser peritoneal sac causes a chemical peritonitis and pancreatic ascites. The classic triad of epigastric pain radiating to the back, a palpable abdominal mass with or without acute peritonitis or ascites, and hyperamylasemia are rarely detected in children.

CT scan may help identify severe pancreatic injury or evidence of pancreatic edema as an early indication of trauma, but is not as helpful in determining management. US may be more useful, but is also unlikely to change the early management. Elevated serum amylase may indicate pancreatic injury, but its absence does not preclude it.

Simple traumatic pancreatitis is treated similarly to other types of pancreatitis with bowel rest, nasogastric suction, intravenous fluids, and pain medication. Severe pancreatic injury will typically require surgical drainage with repair or partial resection of the pancreas. Pancreatic pseudocyst treatment involves 6 to 8 weeks of total parenteral nutrition followed by a surgical drainage procedure.

ABDOMINAL WALL

The muscles of the abdominal wall include the rectus abdominis anteriorly; the internal oblique, external oblique, and transversalis laterally; and posteriorly the erector spinae (sacrospinalis) muscle group, quadratus lumborum, latissimus dorsi, serratus posterioinferior, and the psoas (located deep and posterior). Hematomas of any of these muscles can occur, as well as concomitant injury to the spine and other skeletal structures. The psoas muscle is particularly susceptible to hematoma, even with minor trauma, in patients with a bleeding diathesis such as hemophilia, or those on warfarin.

Tenderness, bruising, swelling, or a mass of the abdominal wall may indicate a hematoma or simply a contusion. However, certain types of ecchymosis (such as the "seat belt sign") are indicative of intra-abdominal injury and the onset may occur several hours after the trauma. *Grey–Turner sign* is an ecchymosis in the abdominal or flank area and may represent a retroperitoneal hematoma. *Cullen's sign* is a bluish discoloration around the umbilicus and may represent an intraperitoneal hemorrhage. Abdominal wall injuries, other than large lacerations, are typically self-limited and consideration for other underlying injury is more important, as outlined in the previous sections. Differentiation between abdominal wall and deeper injury can be difficult, so a low threshold for abdominal CT scan is warranted.

Careful instructions should be given at discharge. Patients and caregivers are instructed to watch for vomiting, increasing pain, abdominal distention, hematuria, and fever. Assure close follow-up for reexamination within 24 hours for any significant abdominal wall injury.

HOLLOW ORGANS

Hollow visceral organs are injured in only 1% to 5% of children with blunt abdominal trauma. Of those requiring laparotomy up to 16% may have such injuries. Perforations of the duodenum and proximal jejunum are the most common and usually associated with a lap belt or bicycle handlebar injury. Penetrating trauma is more obvious and more likely to show early signs of injury, such as free air.

Without obvious evidence of free air on radiographs, the diagnosis of a perforated viscus in blunt trauma can be difficult. Tenderness may initially be localized and slowly worsen over 6 to 12 hours, accounting for the time necessary for peritonitis or obstruction to occur. Abdominal CT scan is not particularly sensitive for these injuries, and repeated physical examinations remain the most reliable indicator of enteric disruption. Surgical consultation should be obtained early in the management of these patients. Once the suspected diagnosis of perforated abdominal viscus has been made, treatment is straightforward with laparotomy to repair the injury. Most injuries can be repaired primarily; however, colon perforations often require a diverting colostomy.

Intramural hematomas of the duodenum or jejunum can cause symptoms of intestinal obstruction with pain, bilious vomiting, and gastric distention. The diagnosis can be made with US or upper GI series, which reveals the "coiled spring" sign. This problem rarely requires surgery. It may cause traumatic pancreatitis with involvement of the ampulla of Vater. Treatment is conservative and supportive including nasogastric suction and parenteral nutrition for up to 3 weeks.

When a large abdominal wall defect is present, as with a large stab wound or close-range shotgun wound, evisceration can occur. The bowel should be kept moist with saline-soaked gauze and not allowed to assume a dependent position that would increase edema of the bowel wall.

► SUMMARY

Evaluation and treatment of children with suspected abdominal trauma is challenging. Physiologic characteristics of children make vital signs and physical examination less predictive of serious injury than in adults. Therefore, other diagnostic clues such as mechanism of injury and maintaining a high suspicion for common injuries are paramount. An awareness of useful diagnostic tests such as abdominal CT scan and their limitations is also important. When treating the multisystem traumatized child, a systematic approach will lead to identification of less obvious injuries within the abdomen. Finally, it is wise to identify resources for treatment of pediatric trauma well in advance. The ability to provide definitive care in an efficient manner through trauma teams or expeditious transfer to a trauma center optimizes the chances of survival and limitation of morbidity.

REFERENCES

1. McCaig LF, Burt CW. National Hospital Ambulatory Medical Care Survey: 2003 emergency department summary. Advance data from vital and health statistics; no 358. Hyattsville, Maryland: National Center for Health Statistics; 2005.
2. Densmore JC, Im HJ, Oldham KT, Guise KS. American Academy of Pediatrics Policy statement on management of pediatric trauma. *Pediatrics*. 2008;121(4):849–854.
3. Densmore JC, Lim HJ, Oldham KT, Guise KS. Outcomes and delivery of care in pediatric injury. *J Pediatr Surg*. 2006;28(367):1–16.
4. Sokolove PE, Kuppermann N, Holmes JF. Association between the "seat belt sign" and intra-abdominal injury in children with blunt torso trauma. *Acad Emerg Med*. 2005;12(9):808–813.
5. Wotherspoon S, Chu K, Brown AF. Abdominal injury and the seat-belt sign. *Emerg Med*. 2001;13(1):61–65.
6. Sachetti A, Paston C, Carraccio C. Family members do not disrupt care when present during invasive procedures. *Acad Emerg Med*. 2005;12(5):477–479.
7. Robinson SM, Mackenzie-Ross S, Campbell-Hewson GL, et al. Psychological effect of witnessed resuscitation on bereaved relative. *Lancet*. 1998;352:614–617.
8. Helmer SD, Smith SR, Dort JM, et al. Family presence during trauma resuscitation: a survey of AAST and ENA members. *J Trauma*. 2000;48:1015–1024.
9. Holmes JF, Sokolove PE, Brant WE, et al. Identification of children with intra-abdominal injuries after blunt trauma. *Ann Emerg Med*. 2002;39:500–509.
10. Mettler FA Jr, Wiest PW, Locken JA, et al. CT scanning: patterns of use and dose. *J Radiol Prot*. 2000;20:353–359.
11. Brenner DJ, Elliston CD, Hall EJ, Berdon WE. Estimated risks of radiation-induced fatal cancer from pediatric CT. *AJR*. 2001;176:289–296.
12. Brenner DJ. Estimating cancer risks from pediatric CT: going from the qualitative to the quantitative. *Pediatr Radiol*. 2002;32:228–231.
13. Radiation risks and pediatric computed tomography (CT). A Guide for Health Care Providers. National Cancer Institute. http://www.cancer.gov/cancertopics/causes/radiation-risks-pediatric-CT. Updated December 22, 2008. Accessed January 10, 2008.
14. FDA Public Health Notification. Reducing radiation risk from computed tomography for pediatric and small adult patients. *Pediatr Radiol*. 2002;32:314–316.
15. Holmes JF, Offerman SR, Chang CH, et al. Performance of helical computed tomography without oral contrast for the detection of gastrointestinal injuries. *Ann Emerg Med*. 2004;43:120–128.
16. Holmes JF, Harris D, Battistella FD. Performance of abdominal ultrasonography in blunt trauma patients with out-of-hospital or emergency department hypotension. *Ann Emerg Med*. 2004;43:354–361.
17. Kaufmann RA, Towbin R, Babcock DS, et al. Upper abdominal trauma in children: imaging evaluation. *Am J Roentgenol*. 1984;142:449–460.
18. Rossi D, de Ville de Goyet J, Clement de Clety S, et al. Management of intra-abdominal organ injury following blunt abdominal trauma in children. *Intensive Care Med*. 1993;19:415–419.
19. Richardson MC, Hollman AS, Davis CF. Comparison of computed tomography and ultrasonographic imaging in the assessment of blunt abdominal trauma in children. *Br J Surg*. 1997;84:1144–1146.
20. Akgur FM, Aktug T, Olguner M, et al. Prospective study investigating routine usage of ultrasonography as the initial diagnostic modality for the evaluation of children sustaining blunt abdominal trauma. *J Trauma*. 1997;42(4):626–628.
21. Partrick DA, Bensard DD, Moore EE, et al. Ultrasound is an effective triage tool to evaluate blunt abdominal trauma in the pediatric population. *J Trauma*. 1998;45(1):57–63.
22. Richards JR, Knopf NA, Wang L, et al. Blunt abdominal trauma in children: evaluation with emergency US. *Radiology*. 2002;222:749–754.
23. Holmes JF, Gladman A, Chang CH. Performance of abdominal ultrasonography in pediatric blunt trauma patients: a meta-analysis. *J Ped Surg*. 2007;42:1588–1594.

CHAPTER 33

Genitourinary Trauma

Joyce C. Arpilleda

▶ HIGH-YIELD FACTS

- Perform a urinalysis on all major trauma patients as well as those suspected of having isolated genitourinary (GU) injury.
- Penetrating trauma between the nipples and perineum requires resuscitation efforts and careful evaluation for intra-abdominal and renal trauma.
- Renal trauma can lead to acute tubular necrosis with renal failure, delayed bleeding, infection, or abscess secondary to urinary extravasation.
- Consider bladder rupture in children who present with abdominal trauma with gross hematuria, blood at the urethral meatus, inability to void, or little urine upon urinary catheter placement.

▶ INTRODUCTION

Genitourinary tract injuries occur in 10% of abdominal trauma patients.[1–3] The kidney is the most commonly injured organ in the urinary tract, followed by the bladder, urethra, and ureter.[1,3] Renal injury occurs from trauma to the back, flank, lower thorax, or upper abdomen. Compared to adults, the pediatric kidney is more vulnerable to injury because there is less protection afforded by the pliable rib cage, weaker abdominal muscles, the relatively larger size of the kidneys in proportion to the rest of the child's body, less perirenal fat, and congenital abnormalities. Blunt trauma accounts for 80% to 95% of all renal injuries.[1,4–7] The most common cause of blunt trauma is motor vehicle collisions, that is, rapid deceleration.[8] Other common causes are sports activities. Penetrating trauma, for example, from gunshot wounds or stabbing injuries, accounts for approximately 10% of all renal injuries.[1,4]

Hemodynamically stable patients with hematuria and suspected urinary system injury are best evaluated by a contrast-enhanced CT scan. If CT scanning is not available, an intravenous pyelogram (IVP) is an alternative. Sexual and physical abuse should be considered in patients with perineal injuries, for example, burns, inconsistent mechanism of injury, previous injury, child's history, etc.

▶ INITIAL ASSESSMENT AND MANAGEMENT

As in all major traumas, management of genitourinary (GU) injuries begins with the basics of advanced trauma life support. After stabilizing the patient, specific organ systems are evaluated. The kidneys may be sources for major bleeding in patients with hypovolemic shock; however, shock due to an isolated renal fracture is uncommon since the kidneys are surrounded by a tight fascia which limits parenchymal bleeding to 25% or less of total blood volume. The vast majority of urologic injuries are not life-threatening; however, failure to diagnose them and any delay in treatment can lead to significant patient morbidity. Table 33–1 shows the initial assessment and management of GU injuries. A urine dipstick analysis is an initial screening test for hematuria; if positive for blood, perform a microscopic urinalysis. Hematuria may be absent in genitourinary injuries. Table 33–2 lists indications for further GU evaluation. Evaluation and testing for injury to the GU system and the abdomen is done simultaneously. The signs of GU trauma as seen in an anteroposterior pelvic plain film are as follows: (1) loss of the psoas shadow indicates retroperitoneal blood, (2) scoliosis with concavity to the side of injury, and (3) lower rib or transverse process fractures. Monitor urinary output (see Table 33–3).

▶ RENAL INJURIES

Blunt GU injuries occur most commonly with rapid deceleration. The kidneys are crushed against the ribs or vertebral column from their relatively fixed position within Gerota's fascia. This can result in contusion or parenchymal laceration. The vascular pedicle can be stretched, injuring the renal vein or artery and subsequent thrombosis.

Hematuria is present in more than 75% to 95% of cases of renal trauma.[5] However, ureteropelvic junction injuries, for example, renal pedicle injury, can occur without hematuria in 25% to 50% of patients.[9] In penetrating trauma, renal vessels or the ureter may be severed without hematuria.[10] Contusions, hematomas, or ecchymoses to the back or flank should lead one to suspect renal injury, requiring CT scan or IVP of the urinary tract. Hemodynamically unstable patients may require immediate surgery. Other indications for evaluating the urinary tract are gross or microscopic hematuria (>20 RBCs/hpf) with

1. penetrating abdominal trauma
2. hypotension with a systolic blood pressure less than 90 mm Hg
3. other intra-abdominal injuries from blunt trauma
4. rapid deceleration injury, for example, high-speed motor vehicle collisions, fall from a height.

CT scanning has become the gold standard and the best initial imaging study for patients suspected of having renal injury. It describes

▶ **TABLE 33–1. INITIAL ASSESSMENT AND MANAGEMENT OF GENITOURINARY INJURIES**

1. Inspect the back for signs of blunt and penetrating injuries and internal bleeding
2. Perineal assessment:
   a. Contusions and hematomas
   b. Lacerations
   c. Urethral bleeding
   d. Rectal examination is performed before placing a urinary catheter, i.e., a high-riding prostate is suspicious for a urethral disruption
3. Vaginal assessment:
   a. Blood in the vaginal vault
   b. Vaginal lacerations

1. the extent of damaged parenchymal tissue and perirenal hemorrhage or hematomas,
2. extravasation of urine,
3. renal pedicle or vascular injuries, and
4. injuries to other intra-abdominal structures.

The focused assessment sonography for trauma (FAST) scan has been popularized to evaluate blunt abdominal trauma. However, the FAST scan cannot differentiate between blood, extravasated urine, and other types of free fluid with regard to GU trauma. Thus, ultrasonography is less sensitive, compared to CT scan, for identifying renal injuries.[11,12]

Ninety-five percent of blunt renal injuries can be treated nonoperatively.[13] Most children who are initially hemodynamically unstable from blunt renal trauma do respond to rapid crystalloid fluid resuscitation. These children require admission to the intensive care unit for continuous monitoring. Major penetrating injuries to the kidneys with extravasation and hemodynamic instability usually require surgery. Upper tract injuries are rare and include thrombosis of the renal artery and disruption of the renal pedicle secondary to deceleration. They usually present with severe abdominal pain. Hematuria may be absent in these cases. IVP, CT scan, or renal arteriograms are the diagnostic studies of choice.

The classification of renal injuries is shown in Table 33–4. The grading system of the American Association for the Surgery of Trauma takes into account depth of injury, vascular involvement, and presence of urinary extravasation.[14,15] Grade I injuries are the most common type of renal trauma. They occur in approximately 80% of all renal injuries.[8] Subcapsular

▶ **TABLE 33–2. INDICATIONS FOR FURTHER GENITOURINARY EVALUATION**

1. Gross or microscopic hematuria >20 RBCs/hpf in children
2. Abdominal or flank pain. The flank is the area between the anterior and posterior axillary lines from the sixth intercostal space to the iliac crest
3. Hematoma
4. Mass
5. Flank ecchymosis (Gray Turner sign)
6. Periumbilical ecchymosis (Cullen sign)
7. Penetrating trauma that can injure the GU system

▶ **TABLE 33–3. URINARY OUTPUT BY AGE**

Age Group (y)	Urine Output (mL/kg/h)
Newborn and infant (0–1)	2
Toddler (1–3)	1.5
Older child through preadolescent (3–12)	1
Adolescent (>12)	0.5

hematoma is less common than perinephric hematoma in blunt trauma.[16] The hallmark of grade IV injuries is extravasation of opacified urine into the perirenal space on CT scan.[17] Urinary extravasation resolves spontaneously in approximately 80% of cases.[18] Grade IV segmental infarctions often resolve with conservative treatment.[8] In grade V injuries, the hallmark of complete avulsion of the ureteropelvic junction injury is noted by the absence of opacification of the distal ureter.

Renal pedicle injuries occur in up to 5% of all renal traumas.[19] Hematuria may be absent. The most common vascular pedicle injury from blunt trauma is renal artery occlusion. Traumatic renal infarction can occur at any time, even long after the initial renal trauma. Isolated renal vein injuries are the most infrequent type of renal vascular pedicle injury.[20] Renal vein thrombosis from trauma almost always occurs with an arterial or parenchymal injury.[21] A devascularized kidney will show no enhancement on CT scan.

Complications of renal trauma are urinary extravasation, urinoma, infected urinoma, secondary hemorrhage, perinephric abscess, pseudoaneurysm, hypertension, arteriovenous fistula, pulmonary complications, acute tubular necrosis with renal failure, chronic pyelonephritis, hydronephrosis, chronic calculi, and pseudocyst. These occur in 3% to 33% of patients with renal trauma.[8] Urinary extravasation is the most common complication.[22] This is present in grade IV parenchymal injury and grade V ureteropelvic junction avulsion. Urinoma is a urine collection that may occur in 1% to 7% of all renal trauma patients.[23] Intraperitoneal urine extravasation is usually due to a penetrating injury.[24] Secondary hemorrhage is common in grade V injuries and in penetrating trauma managed conservatively.[8] Secondary hemorrhage is often caused by a traumatic pseudoaneurysm or an arteriovenous fistula. Posttraumatic renovascular hypertension may occur weeks to decades later, with an average of 34 months after renal trauma.[14] Anomalous kidneys (hydronephrosis, tumor, horseshoe kidney, or polycystic kidney disease) are more easily injured with minor trauma and can present with hematuria of varying degrees.

▶ **URETERAL INJURIES**

Traumatic ureteral injuries are rare, occurring in less than 1% of all GU traumas.[25] The proximal ureter is protected by the psoas muscle and vertebrae; the distal ureter is protected by the bony pelvis. Penetrating trauma is the most common mechanism of injury. However, traumatic avulsion of the ureter occurs more commonly in children than adults and is usually due to blunt trauma. The pediatric spine is more mobile, allowing the renal pelvis and upper ureter to be compressed against

► TABLE 33–4. AMERICAN ASSOCIATION FOR THE SURGERY OF TRAUMA GRADING SYSTEM FOR RENAL INJURY

Grade*	Type of Injury	Description of Injury	Type of Injury	Description of Injury
I	Contusion	Microscopic or gross hematuria; urologic imaging studies normal	Hematoma	Subcapsular, nonexpanding without parenchymal laceration
II	Hematoma	Nonexpanding perirenal hematoma confined to retroperitoneum	Laceration	<1 cm parenchymal depth of renal cortex without urinary extravasation
III	Laceration	>1 cm parenchymal depth of renal cortex or medulla without collecting system rupture or urinary extravasation		
IV	Laceration	Parenchymal laceration extending through renal cortex, medulla, and collecting system	Vascular	Main renal artery or vein injury with contained hemorrhage. Segmental infarctions by thrombosis, dissection or laceration of segmental arteries.
V	Laceration	Completely shattered kidney. Uteropelvic junction avulsion.	Vascular	Avulsion or thrombosis of renal hilum main renal artery or vein which devascularizes kidney

*Advance one grade for bilateral injuries up to grade III.

the lower ribs or lumbar transverse processes. The ureter can be stretched by sudden extreme flexion of the trunk. Approximately 56% of patients with ureteral injuries are hypotensive.[25] Gross or microscopic hematuria is present in approximately 75% to 85% of these patients.[25,26] If there is complete ureteral transection or an adynamic segment of ureter, hematuria may not be present. CT scan with contrast is the best initial imaging study. CT scan with contrast is highly sensitive at detecting urine extravasation. It is important that, after initial scanning of the abdomen and pelvis, a second scan—approximately 10 minutes after contrast injection—is done to fully evaluate the collecting system and to assess urinary extravasation.[27] Ureteral transection is treated with ureteropyeostomy.

▶ BLADDER INJURIES

Bladder injuries are uncommon because of protection by the bony pelvis. However, approximately 10% of those with pelvic fractures have a concomitant bladder injury.[28] In the majority of children, the mechanism of injury for bladder injuries is due to motor vehicle collisions and can result in contusion or rupture. Bladder contusions, however, are self-limited. In young children, the bladder has an abdominal position and is more vulnerable to rupture when full. Bladder rupture requires surgical consultation for possible exploration, repair, debridement, and drainage. It is associated with a high mortality rate and that rate increases with delay in diagnosis. It should be considered in patients who have gross hematuria, blood at the urethral meatus, inability to void, or little to no urine flow on catheterization. These findings are indications for cystography.[29,30] Some of these patients have blood at the urethral meatus, the inability to urinate, or perineal ecchymosis and should have a retrograde urethrogram performed to evaluate the urethra before catheterization and cystography.

▶ URETHRAL INJURIES

Traumatic urethral injuries occur in approximately 10% of patients with pelvic fractures.[31] The mechanism of injury for urethral injuries is usually blunt trauma. These injuries are less common in children due to a more flexible pelvis. Urethral injuries are rare in females due to the hypermobility of the urethra and lack of bony attachments. Concomitant bladder injuries occur in 10% to 29% of patients with urethral injuries.[32] Examples of causes of urethral injuries are pelvic fracture, straddle injury, and urethral manipulation. Indications for a retrograde urethrogram before inserting a urinary catheter are as follows:

1. Gross hematuria.
2. Blood at the urethral meatus.
3. Inability to urinate.
4. Perineal or scrotal swelling and ecchymosis. A perineal "butterfly hematoma" is a classic finding.
5. An absent or high-riding, floating, or boggy prostrate on digital rectal examination.
6. Inability to insert a urethral catheter.
7. Unstable pelvic fracture.

Urethral disruptions may require insertion of a suprapubic catheter. The complications due to urethral injuries are

1. strictures,
2. incontinence,
3. impotence,
4. diverticulae,
5. fistulas, and
6. chordee.

A rectal examination can reveal a high-riding prostate indicating urethral disruption.

Anterior pelvic fractures usually accompany urethral injuries. Urethral disruptions are divided into those above (posterior) or below (anterior) the urogenital diaphragm. Posterior urethral injuries usually coincide with multisystem injuries and pelvic fractures. Penetrating anterior urethral and perineal injuries occur due to straddle injuries, for example, falls on a fence, and may be an isolated injury. Suspect a urethral tear when (1) there is blood at the urethral meatus or (2) ecchymoses or hematoma of the scrotum or perineum. Early urologic consultation is necessary.

▶ SCROTAL TRAUMA

Injuries to the external male genitalia result from the testis being forced against the pubic ramus. A common mechanism of injury is a straddle injury from a bicycle. Problems caused by scrotal trauma include testicular or appendage torsions, testicular dislocation, epididymitis, hematocele, hematoma, pyocele, hydrocele, and testicular rupture. Evaluate significant straddle injuries with a pelvic radiography to evaluate for fracture of the pubic ramus. Doppler ultrasound should be immediately available and can evaluate the testes for hematoma, rupture, dislocation, or blood flow and torsion. Delay of 4 to 6 hours may result in the loss of the testis, thus obtain urologic consultation early. If these conditions are ruled out, the patient may be discharged to home with urologic follow-up. Scrotal support and cold packs may help.

Testicular or epididymal rupture results from direct trauma when the testis is forced against the pubic ramus, which leads to tearing of the inelastic tunica albuginea with extrusion of the seminiferous tissue. This is rare in children. Suspect testicular or epididymal rupture when there is a recurrence of pain and delayed onset of scrotal swelling from hours to 3 days after the injury. Early surgical exploration is recommended. Complications include epididymoorchitis with localized redness, warmth, swelling, and fever.

Testicular dislocation occurs when the testis is forcibly displaced from the scrotum into the inguinal, acetabular, crural, perineal, penile, or abdominal region or extruded through a scrotal laceration. Testicular dislocations are rare. Consider this diagnosis when there is an empty hemiscrotum after trauma. Symptoms include scrotal pain, nausea, and vomiting. Obtain urologic consultation.

▶ PENILE INJURIES

The most common cause of penile injuries is from complications of circumcision. Other mechanisms of injury are direct blows from toilet seats, falls, and sports injuries; zipper entrapment of the foreskin; and tourniquet injuries. Most injuries are minor and can be treated conservatively. However, associated

GU injury may occur with major trauma. Urinalysis is recommended in significant penile injury. Retrograde urethrography is recommended as urethral injuries occur in up to 50% of patients with penile injury.[33,34] Superficial lacerations of the penis can be repaired as in any other laceration. Treatment of zipper injuries to the foreskin includes using bone cutters or similar device to cut the bridge of the sliding piece of the zipper. Scrotal exploration is recommended with the presence of a large hematocele or rupture of the tunica albuginea.[35]

Penile fracture, or corpus cavernosal rupture, from blunt trauma to an erect penis is uncommon. The most common mechanism of injury for a fractured penis is when an erect penis is forced against a solid object, for example, pubis, during sexual intercourse. The patient hears a "crack" or "pop" followed by pain, swelling, ecchymosis, deformity of the penis, and occasionally a palpated corporal defect. Urologic consultation is recommended. Consider a scrotal ultrasound or cavernosography as an adjunct to the physical examination in these cases.[36,37] Penile fractures can be treated conservatively except when penile deformity or urethral involvement are present. Urethral injuries occur in approximately one-third of patients with penile fractures.[38] Thus, indications for a retrograde urethrogram in patients with penile fractures are gross hematuria, blood at the meatus, and the inability to void.

Tourniquet injuries in an infant may present as balanitis, paraphimosis, or cellulitis of the penis. This may occur when hair surrounds the coronal groove and cuts into the shaft of the penis. Treatment usually involves removal of the band of hair and treating any infection. Follow up with a urologist if deeper injury is suspected.

▶ VULVAR AND VAGINAL INJURIES

Vaginal lacerations may occur from bony fragments from pelvic fracture(s) or from penetrating wounds. Confirm an intact urethra with a retrograde urethrogram before inserting a urinary catheter in cases such as gross hematuria; blood at the urethral meatus; inability to urinate; perineal or scrotal swelling and ecchymosis; an absent or high-riding, floating, or boggy prostrate on digital rectal examination; inability to insert a urethral catheter; and unstable pelvic fracture. A disrupted urethra may require a suprapubic tube placement. Perineal trauma in females often results from blunt trauma, for example, straddle injuries. Other mechanisms of injury include stretching of the perineum from the sudden abduction of the legs, for example, doing the splits causing tears; and penetrating injuries. Significant straddle injuries are screened with pelvic radiography to evaluate for a fracture of the ramus. Complications of perineal trauma are urinary retention, secondary infection, and urinary tract infection. Vulvar injuries are usually minor and can be treated with rest and cold packs. Large or expanding vulvar hematomas may require surgical drainage and are susceptible to secondary infection.

▶ PEDIATRIC SEXUAL ABUSE

Medical providers must evaluate the risk of child sexual abuse in all cases of genital trauma. The publication by the American Academy of Pediatrics (AAP) Committee on Child Abuse and Neglect includes a report on evaluation, reviews the definition and presentation, an outline for history taking, suggestions on performing the physical examination, discussion of indicated laboratory specimens, guidelines for reporting suspected cases, treatment, follow-up, and legal issues.[39] Child abuse should be considered when the history or reported mechanism does not match the injuries. All developmentally capable patients with suspected sexual abuse should be referred for formal forensic interview in a timely manner. Trained forensic interviewers can be from child advocacy centers, the police department, or child protective services (CPS). Children who are suspected to have been sexually abused warrant a screening examination.

Reasons for emergency examinations include, but are not limited to the following:

1. Complaints of pain in the genital area
2. Evidence or complaint of genital bleeding or injury
3. The alleged assault may have occurred within the previous 72 hours, depending on the state, and transfer of biologic material may have occurred for forensic analysis
4. Medical intervention is needed emergently for the health and safety of the child
5. Significant behavioral or emotional problems, for example, suicidal ideation/plan

The physical examination includes the following:

1. Placing the patient in a frog-leg position
2. Gentle labial traction on the labia majora, with the examiner tugging toward himself/herself with lateral traction, to visual the genitals, for example, labia minora, vestibule, hymen, and vaginal opening
3. Considering examination in the knee–chest position
4. Consulting a specialist if the examination is inadequate or if abnormalities are present
5. Avoiding a speculum examination in prepubertal children
6. Visual identification and/or photos of the genital anatomy before a speculum examination in adolescents

The majority of patients, who have disclosed sexual abuse or sexual assault, have normal examination results.[40] The absence of genital findings does not exclude sexual abuse. The Centers for Disease Control and Prevention (CDC) and the AAP have published guidelines for evaluating sexually transmitted infections in sexually abused children.[41,42] Each state has its own standards for forensic evidence collection. The AAP recommends that forensic evidence collection be considered when the victim presents within 72 hours of the assault.[43] Recommendations for interpretation of physical and laboratory findings are from the AAP Committee on Child Abuse and Neglect, the Ray E. Helfer Society (an honorary society for physician specialists in child abuse diagnosis and treatment), and Cornell University Special Interest Group in Child Abuse.[39,43] The CDC (www.cdc.gov) and AAP have published medication dosing guidelines for sexually transmitted disease prophylaxis.[41,42] A progestin-only regimen, that is, plan B (levonorgestrel), has been shown to be the most efficacious and least toxic of the postexposure prophylaxis to prevent pregnancy when started within 5 days of the sexual contact.[44] Patients with specific concern of sexual abuse based on

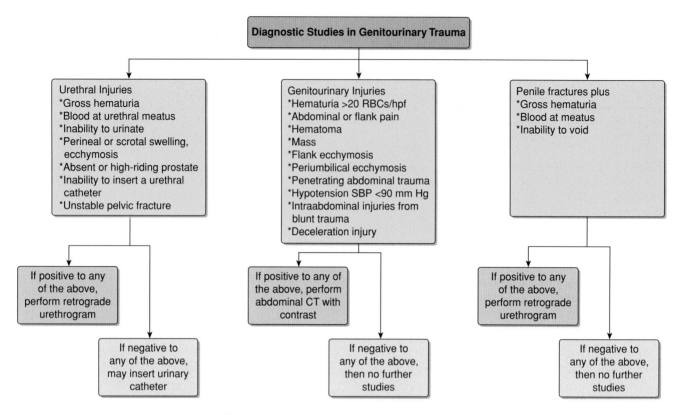

Figure 33–1. Diagnostic studies in GU trauma.

caretaker history or disclosure by the patient should have CPS involvement.

Accidental genital trauma may be confused with sexual abuse findings. Accidental genital trauma can present in the pediatric emergency department, most of which are due to straddle injuries.[45,46] Typical findings in straddle injuries are lysis of labial adhesions, lacerations in the gutter between the labia minora and the labia majora, labial contusions or hematomas, and injuries to the skin overlying the perineal body. Lysis of adhesions and small abrasions may also result from sexual abuse.[47] Injuries to the hymen or vagina are unusual.[48]

▶ SUMMARY

Approximately 3% to 10% of trauma patients have injury to the GU tract.[2,3] Figure 33–1 summarizes diagnostic studies in GU injuries. Hematuria is the hallmark of GU trauma. A urinalysis should be performed on all major trauma patients and those with minor GU injury (Fig. 33–1). Renal and urinary tract imaging is indicated in patients with penetrating trauma, gross hematuria, blunt trauma with shock or microscopic hematuria, clinical signs indicating abdominal organ injury, or significant deceleration injury. CT scan with contrast is the best initial imaging study to provide accurate American Association for the Surgery of Trauma grading by demonstrating the depth of injury and involvement of vessels or the collecting system. Delayed images are important in diagnosing urinary extravasation. Patients with pelvic injuries and gross hematuria should have a cystography. Consider urethral injuries in patients with pelvic

fractures. Those with blood at the urethral meatus, inability to urinate, perineal or scrotal ecchymosis, or an abnormal digital rectal examination should have a retrograde urethrography. Consider bladder rupture in those with abdominal trauma with gross hematuria, blood at the urethral meatus, inability to void, or little urine upon urinary catheterization. Ultrasound is recommended in scrotal trauma patients if the physical examination is inconclusive. Those with penetrating trauma to the external genitalia and those with blunt trauma to the penis with gross hematuria, blood at the meatus, or the inability to void require a retrograde urethrogram.

The GU tract has an amazing ability to heal itself. If the flow of urine can be maintained without obstruction, healing is likely to occur. The majority of renal injuries can be managed conservatively. Those with grade IV injuries, grade V injuries, or coexisting organ injuries more often require intervention or surgery.

Children with suspected sexual abuse often present to the emergency department. Most children who are sexually abused have normal genital examinations. Physicians should avoid interviewing the child, except to establish current symptoms that may impact examination or testing. Patients with sexual contact less than 72 hours before presentation may require forensic evidence collection.

▶ ACKNOWLEDGMENT

The author thanks Hannes Schweiger, PhD, for his assistance with the diagrams in the manuscript.

REFERENCES

1. Baverstock R, Simons R, McLoughlin M. Severe blunt renal trauma: a 7-year retrospective review from a provincial trauma centre. *Can J Urol.* 2001;8(5):1372–1376.

2. Carroll PR, McAninch JW. Staging of renal trauma. *Urol Clin North Am.* 1989;16:193–201.

3. Krieger JN, Algood CB, Mason JT, et al. Urological trauma in the Pacific Northwest: etiology, distribution, management and outcome. *J Urol.* 1984;132:70–73.

4. Miller KS, McAninch JW. Radiographic assessment of renal trauma: our 15-year experience. *J Urol.* 1995;154:352–355.

5. Sagalowsky AI, Peters PC. Genitourinary trauma. In: Walsh PC, Retik AB, Vaughan ED Jr, et al., eds. *Campbell's Urology.* Vol 3. 7th ed. Philadelphia, PA: WB Saunders; 1999:3085–3119.

6. Mee SL, McAninch JW, Robinson AL, et al. Radiographic assessment of renal trauma: a 10-year prospective study of patient selection. *J Urol.* 1989;141:1095–1098.

7. Nicolaisen GS, McAninch JW, Marshall GA, et al. Renal trauma: re-evaluation of the indications for radiographic assessment. *J Urol.* 1985;133:183–187.

8. Lee YJ, Oh SN, Rha SE, et al. Renal trauma. *Radiol Clin North Am.* 2007;45:581–592.

9. Kawashima A, Sandler CM, Corl FM, et al. Imaging of renal trauma: a comprehensive review. *Radiographics.* 2001;21(3):557–574.

10. Cass AS. Renovascular injuries from external trauma. Diagnosis, treatment, and outcome. *Urol Clin North Am.* 1989;16(2):213–220.

11. McGahan JP, Rose J, Coates TL, et al. Use of ultrasonography in the patient with acute abdominal trauma. *J Ultrasound Med.* 1997;16:653–662.

12. Perry MJ, Porte ME, Urwin GH. Limitations of ultrasound evaluation in acute closed renal trauma. *J R Coll Surg Edinb.* 1997;42:420–422.

13. American College of Surgeons Committee on Trauma. Abdominal trauma. In: *Advanced Trauma Life Support for Doctors, Student Course Manual.* 7th ed. Chicago, IL: American College of Surgeons; 2004:131–150.

14. Santucci RA, Wessells H, Bartsch G, et al. Evaluation and management of renal injuries: consensus statement of the renal trauma subcommittee. *BJU Int.* 2004;93(7):937–954.

15. Moore EE, Shackford SR, Pachter HL, et al. Organ injury scaling: spleen, liver, and kidney. *J Trauma.* 1989;29(12):1664–1666.

16. Smith JK, Kenney PJ. Imaging of renal trauma. *Radiol Clin North Am.* 2003;41(5):1019–1035.

17. Federle MP. Renal trauma. In: Pollack HM, McClennan BL, eds. *Clinical Urography.* Vol 2. 2nd ed. Philadelphia, PA: WB Saunders; 2000:1772–1784.

18. Heyns CF. Renal trauma: indications for imaging and surgical exploration. *BJU Int.* 2004;93(8):1165–1170.

19. Cass AS, Susset J, Khan A, et al. Renal pedicle injury in the multiple injured patient. *J Urol.* 1979;122(6):728–730.

20. Stables DP, Thatcher GN. Traumatic renal vein thrombosis associated with renal artery occlusion. *Br J Radiol.* 1973;46(541):64–66.

21. Kau E, Patel R, Fiske J, et al. Isolated renal vein thrombosis after blunt trauma. *Urology.* 2004;64(4):807–808.

22. Matthews LA, Smith EM, Spirnak JP. Nonoperative treatment of major blunt renal lacerations with urinary extravasation. *J Urol.* 1997;157(6):2056–2058.

23. Titton RL, Gervais DA, Hahn PF, et al. Urine leaks and urinomas: diagnosis and imaging-guided intervention. *Radiographics.* 2003;23(5):1133–1147.

24. Lang EK, Glorioso L III. Management of urinomas by percutaneous drainage procedures. *Radiol Clin North Am.* 1986;24(4):551–559.

25. Elliott SP, McAninch JW. Ureteral injuries from external violence: the 25-year experience at San Francisco General Hospital. *J Urol.* 2003;170:1213–1216.

26. Perez-Brayfeld MR, Keane TE, Krishnan A, et al. Gunshot wounds to the ureter: a 40-year experience at Grady Memorial Hospital. *J Urol.* 2001;166:119–121.

27. Brown SL, Elder JS, Spirnak JP. Are pediatric patients more susceptible to major renal injury from blunt trauma? A comparative study. *J Urol.* 1998;160:138–140.

28. Hochberg E, Stone NN. Bladder rupture associated with pelvic fracture due to blunt trauma. *Urology.* 1993;41:531–533.

29. Cass AS. The multiple injured patient with bladder trauma. *J Trauma.* 1984;24:731–734.

30. Carroll PR, McAninch JW. Major bladder trauma: mechanisms of injury and a unied method of diagnosis and repair. *J Urol.* 1984;132:254–257.

31. Glass RE, Flynn JT, King JB, et al. Urethral injury and fractured pelvis. *Br J Urol.* 1978;50:578–582.

32. Cass AS, Gleich P, Smith C. Simultaneous bladder and prostatomembranous urethral rupture from external trauma. *J Urol.* 1984;132:907–908.

33. Miles BJ, Poffenberger RJ, Farah RN, et al. Management of penile gunshot wounds. *Urology.* 1990;36:318–321.

34. Cline KJ, Mata JA, Venable DD, et al. Penetrating trauma to the male external genitalia. *J Trauma.* 1998;44:492–494.

35. Jankowski JT, Spirnak JP. Current recommendations for imaging in the management of urologic traumas. *Urol Clin North Am.* 2006;33:365–376.

36. Koga S, Saito Y, Arakaki Y, et al. Sonography in fracture of the penis. *Br J Urol.* 1993;72:228–229.

37. Karadeniz T, Topsakal M, Ariman A, et al. Penile fracture: differential diagnosis, management and outcome. *Br J Urol.* 1996;77:279–281.

38. Fergany AF, Angermeier KW, Montague DK. Review of Cleveland Clinic experience with penile fracture. *Urology.* 1999;54:352–355.

39. Kellogg NK; and the American Academy of Pediatrics Committee on Child Abuse and Neglect. Guidelines for the evaluation of sexual abuse in children. *Pediatrics.* 2005;116:506–512.

40. Heger A, Ticson L, Velasquez O. Children referred for possible sexual abuse: medical findings in 2384 children. *Child Abuse Negl.* 2002;26:RR-2645–RR-2659.

41. Centers for Disease Control and Prevention. Sexually transmitted diseases treatment guidelines 2002. *MMWR Recomm Rep.* 2002;51:69–73.

42. American Academy of Pediatrics. Sexually transmitted diseases. In: Pickering LK, ed. *Red book: 2003 Report of the Committee on Infectious Diseases.* 26th ed. Elk Grove Village, IL: American Academy of Pediatrics Publishing; 2003:159–167.

43. Adams JA, Kaplan RA, Starling SP, et al. Guidelines for medical care of children who may have been sexually abused. *J Pediatr Adolesc Gynecol.* 2007;20:163–172.

44. American Academy of Pediatrics Committee on Adolescence. Emergency contraception policy statement. *Pediatrics.* 2005;116:1026–1035.

45. Scheidler MG, Shultz BL, Schall L, et al. Mechanisms of blunt perineal injury in female pediatric patients. *J Pediatr Surg.* 2000;35:1317–1319.

46. Holland AJ, Cohen RC, McKertich KM, et al. Urethral trauma in children. *Pediatr Surg Int.* 2001;17:58–61.

47. Bernard D, Peters M, Makoroff K. The evaluation of suspected pediatric sexual abuse. *Clin Pediatr Emerg Med.* 2006;7:161–169.

48. Dowd MD, Fitzmaurice L, Knapp JF, et al. The interpretation of urogenital findings in children with straddle injuries. *J Pediatr Surg.* 1994;29:7–10.

CHAPTER 34

Maxillofacial Trauma

Joanna York and Stephen A. Colucciello

▶ HIGH-YIELD FACTS

- Maxillofacial trauma in children more often results in soft tissue injury than facial fractures.
- Up to 55% of seriously injured children with facial trauma also have intracranial injury, a much higher percentage than occurs with adults.
- The most urgent complication of facial trauma is airway compromise, which is most often associated with mid or lower face injury.
- The CT scan is the definitive diagnostic test for precise delineation of maxillofacial fractures.
- The mandible is the facial bone most frequently involved in posttraumatic developmental deformities.
- Timely referral of nasal fractures is of significant concern, as these injuries may have a profound effect on subsequent nasal and maxillofacial development.

Accurate bony alignment is important in the growing child, and missed fractures or inappropriate treatment may result in permanent facial deformity. A child with severe maxillofacial injury requires a team approach involving emergency physicians, pediatricians, general surgeons, maxillofacial specialists, and radiologists. Emergency specialists must recognize and prioritize injuries, manage the airway, stabilize the patient, read initial radiographs, and make appropriate consultations.

▶ INCIDENCE

Children have a lower incidence of facial fractures compared with adults. Facial fractures in the pediatric population comprise less than 15% of all facial fractures and they are especially rare below the age of 5. Their incidence peaks as children begin school and during puberty/adolescence with an increase in unsupervised sports, activities, and skeletal changes. Worldwide, the incidence of facial fractures is higher in boys than girls, attributed to more dangerous physical activities in boys.[1] This lower incidence of pediatric facial fractures is multifactorial and includes the protected environment of childhood as well as anatomic differences between children and adults. Great structural differences exist between birth and 10 years of age, with marked changes in bone composition and anatomy. Large fat pads in young children cushion impact and lessen forces transmitted to the facial bones that have flexible suture lines. Children have a high ratio of cancellous bone to cortical bone, which provides greater resilience and leads to a higher incidence of incomplete and greenstick fractures.[1–3] In addition, the presence of tooth buds within the jaws increases stability.[1] This contrasts with the comminuted fracture patterns seen in adults.

Fracture site distribution tends to shift from the upper aspect of the face in younger children to the lower face in older children. In early childhood, the skull is particularly prominent, whereas the face and mandible are small. This results in a high incidence of skull fractures in the younger age group. Development of paranasal sinuses weakens the anterior facial skeleton. LeForte fractures are uncommon in pediatrics and are almost never seen before age 2. For this reason, in children younger than 5 years, orbital and frontal skull fractures predominate, whereas in older children, maxillary and mandibular fractures become more prominent. The most frequently fractured bones are the nose (45%), mandible (32%), orbit (17%), and zygoma/maxilla (5%). The most common facial fractures in injured children requiring hospitalization are mandibular fractures. By the early teen years, the frequency and pattern of maxillofacial injury begins to mirror that found in adults.[1,3]

▶ ETIOLOGY

Motor vehicle crashes, including auto/pedestrian incidents, are the most frequent cause of facial injury, followed by falls, sporting injuries, and gunshot wounds. Altercations and sports-related injuries are significant causes of facial fractures in older children, accounting for up to 36% of injuries. Maxillofacial injuries due to child abuse have a high incidence of associated head and neck bruising and skull fractures are particularly common.

▶ ASSOCIATED INJURIES

Children with serious maxillofacial fractures often have associated injuries, in particular skull fractures and intracranial trauma. Up to 55% of seriously injured children with facial trauma may also have intracranial injury, a much higher percentage than occurs with adults.[4] This is due to the high energy necessary to disrupt the pediatric facial skeleton. Temporal bone fractures occur, often in conjunction with mandibular fractures, when force is transmitted along the mandible to the temporal bone. These temporal bone fractures are found most frequently in younger children. Periorbital fractures lead to intraocular injury in up to 10% of patients, mandating a careful ophthalmologic examination in these situations. Cervical spine fractures are rare in children younger than 8 years, but when present they have a high risk of morbidity and mortality. The upper three cervical vertebrae is the region most vulnerable to injury. In severe multiple trauma, the cervical spine should be evaluated initially with a three-view series or with CT scan, and a careful neurologic examination is paramount. Additional anteroposterior tomograms can be done to clarify findings on cervical spine radiographs. Helical CT scan has not proven superior to plain radiographs as a screening tool for cervical spine injury in children with blunt force trauma, as it results in increased radiation exposure and resourced without a reduction in sedation usage or time in the emergency department.[5] If an injury is suspected by radiography or clinical presentation, it is recommended that one obtain a CT scan. If the patient is unresponsive with a neurological deficit, magnetic resonance imaging (MRI) is the study of choice within 72 hours of admission and has been shown to be cost-effective.[6]

▶ EMERGENCY MANAGEMENT

The most urgent complication of facial trauma is airway compromise, which is most often associated with mid- and lower-face injury. Simple maneuvers, such as chin-lift jaw thrust, oropharyngeal suctioning, and oral or nasal airway, when appropriate provide immediate benefit.[4]

Infants younger than 3 months are obligate nose breathers, and nasal or midface trauma can lead to complete airway obstruction. Mandibular fractures can result in loss of support of the tongue and occlusion of the upper airway. These fractures may also produce hematomas of the floor of the mouth, which can displace tongue and obstruct the airway. In this situation, the physician should open the mouth and pull the tongue forward, either manually or with a large suture or towel clip. In children for whom cervical spine injury is not a consideration or has been ruled out, the child should be allowed to sit up and lean forward. If simple airway maneuvers do not suffice, orotracheal intubation with in-line immobilization is necessary. Nasotracheal intubation should be avoided with midface trauma to prevent passage of the tube into the cranial vault.[4] Nasotracheal intubation is also difficult in the young child, because of the presence of large adenoids. Uncontrolled bleeding into the pharynx may require intubation. If severe oropharyngeal bleeding persists, the pharynx may be packed with absorbent gauze to control bleeding and prevent aspiration when uncuffed endotracheal tubes are used.

If the child cannot be intubated, the physician must establish an airway surgically. Avoid emergency cricothyroidotomy in children younger than 12 years.[7] In children below this age, cricothyroidotomy causes numerous complications, including subglottic stenosis and tracheolaryngeal injury. Emergency tracheostomy results in fewer long-term complications, but is time consuming and requires great expertise. Percutaneous transtracheal jet ventilation is an excellent temporizing measure in these situations. Insert a needle into the cricothyroid membrane, and use oxygen at 50 psi (directly from the wall without a Christmas tree adaptor) with a 1:3 inspiration to expiration ratio (see Chapter 23).

Severe nasal hemorrhage may lead to aspiration and initially should be controlled by applying pressure to the external nares. If bleeding continues, consider nasopharyngeal packing. A Foley catheter is an effective emergency intervention. Insert the catheter along the floor of the nose, inflate the balloon in the nasopharynx, pull it anteriorly, and then place an anterior pack.[4]

▶ HISTORY

Obtain history regarding circumstances of injury from parents and prehospital care providers as well as from the child, if possible. Determine mechanism, time of injury and assess for loss of consciousness. Question the child about any visual problems, facial anesthesia, or pain with jaw movement.

▶ PHYSICAL EXAMINATION

Inspection of the face may reveal areas of swelling, ecchymosis, deformity, asymmetry, trismus, and malocclusion, all signs that suggest facial fractures. In addition to face-to-face inspection, a view from the child's head looking down or from the chin looking up may reveal otherwise unappreciated asymmetries. Posttraumatic Bell's palsy provides evidence of a temporal bone fracture. Carefully and systematically palpate the entire face starting with the skull and inferior to the mandible.[3]

EYES

The eyes must be evaluated for the presence of the pupillary light reflex. Hyphema, subconjunctival hemorrhage, and extraocular motions must be assessed. Subconjunctival hemorrhage is an important sign that often occurs in association with orbital, zygomatic, or maxillary fractures. Note the presence of proptosis or enophthalmos. Unequal pupil height may indicate orbital floor fracture. Lids must be retracted for adequate visualization of the globe, and visual acuity should be documented. Complete ocular examination is important in periorbital trauma because of the high incidence of globe injury (see Chapter 90).

Periorbital ecchymosis may occur in a wide variety of settings. Raccoon's eyes secondary to basal skull fracture usually occur 4 to 6 hours after a traumatic event, whereas direct trauma to the periorbital region may result in more immediate bruising. Bilateral periorbital ecchymosis also occurs in conjunction with LeFort II and III fractures.

Carefully palpate the *entire* orbital rim for tenderness or deformity. Many physicians neglect careful palpation of the superior orbital rim, concentrating instead on the inferior rim. Anesthesia above or below the eye may be secondary to supraorbital or infraorbital nerve injury and often occurs in conjunction with fractures.[4]

Telecanthus, an increased width between the medial canthi of the eyelids, with flattening of the medial canthus, is associated with nasal ethmoidal injury. In this situation, the medial canthal ligaments are torn or underlying bone is avulsed from the nasal orbital complex (Fig. 34–1). When present or there is tenderness over the medial orbital rim, a bimanual test for nasoethmoidal–orbital stability can help detect a fracture. Insert a clamp into the nose, and press the tip intranasally against the medial orbital rim opposite the canthal ligament. Apply

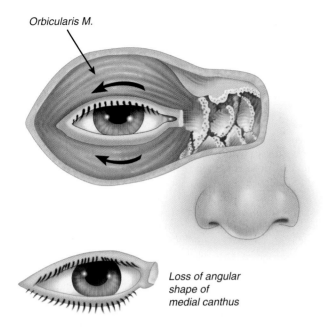

Figure 34–1. Telecanthus: Torn medial canthal ligament or bone avulsion causes flattening of the medial canthus.

counter pressure with a palpating finger against the external surface of the canthal ligament. A fractured medial orbital rim will move between the clamp and index finger. Topical intranasal anesthesia may be necessary to do this maneuver in the awake patient.[2] CT scanning of the face is a reasonable alternative to the bimanual test if telecanthus is present or there is tenderness over the medial canthus.

Subcutaneous emphysema about the eyes and maxillary area indicates a communication with a sinus or nasal antrum and may erupt when the child blows his or her nose.

EARS

Examine the pinna for presence of subperichondral hematoma. The ear canal must be examined for lacerations and cerebrospinal fluid (CSF) leak. Battle sign, ecchymosis over the mastoid area, appears several hours after injury resulting in basilar skull fracture. The presence of hemotympanum should also raise suspicion for this injury. Tympanic membrane rupture may occur with mandibular condyle fractures.

MIDFACE

Careful simultaneous palpation of the zygomatic arches is used to detect flattening of the arch. Intraoral palpation of the arch is also helpful in detecting minimally displaced fractures. LeFort III fractures produce elongation of the midface. LeFort fractures may also be identified by manipulation of the central maxillary arch. Grasp the central maxillary arch above the central incisors and attempt to mobilize the midface. LeFort classification is based upon which structures move anteriorly with traction. Specific LeFort fractures are outlined in detail later in the chapter.

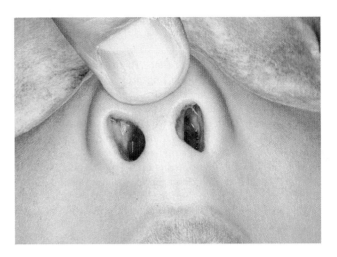

Figure 34–2. Photograph of nasal hematoma.

NOSE

The examining physician must carefully palpate the nose for crepitus and deformity, as edema may obscure bony anatomy. Examine the inside of the nose for septal hematoma, which may be recognized by a bluish, bulging mass on the septum, or by the subjective impression of an abnormally wide septum (Fig. 34–2). Pressure with a cotton swab will detect the presence of a soft, doughy swelling.[3]

With any significant facial trauma, it is important to assess for CSF rhinorrhea. The best test to distinguish CSF from nasal secretions, blood, or ear drainage is the β_2-transferrin assay. This is a protein produced by neuraminidase activity in the brain and is uniquely found in the CSF and perilymph. The detection of β_2-transferrin confirms a CSF fistula. The specificity nears 100% and the sensitivity is 91%.[8,9] In many hospitals, this is a send-out laboratory test. A simple test to order from the emergency department is the glucose concentration of the liquid in question. CSF will contain glucose while mucus will not.

INTRAORAL AND MANDIBULAR EXAMINATION

Injury of the inferior orbital nerve or inferior alveolar/mental nerve produces anesthesia of the upper or lower lip, respectively. Injury may be secondary to fracture of the bony canal or direct nerve contusion.

The emergency physician must observe movement of the patient's jaw through a full range of motion. Deviation to one side usually indicates ipsilateral subcondylar fracture, since dislocation of the jaw occurs infrequently in children. Difficulty in jaw movement may be secondary to mandibular fractures, injury to the temporomandibular joint (TMJ), or a depressed zygoma impinging upon the mandible or muscles of mastication. Trismus and malocclusion also occur with such injuries.[4]

It is important to palpate the condyles during jaw motion. This is easily done by placing the examining fingers in the external ear canal, and feeling the motion of the TMJ while the child opens and closes his or her mouth.[4]

Children, unlike adults, may suffer traumatic diastasis of the hard palate along the midline. To detect this injury, the physician must apply a distracting pressure upon the dental arches. Grasp and manipulate each tooth to assess for laxity and remove teeth that are in danger of falling into the airway. Permanent teeth may be saved in saline moistened gauze. Stress the mandible with lateral and medial pressures on the dental arches, and subsequently apply up and down manual pressure to test for bony disruption.[4] The cooperative child should be asked to bite down upon a tongue blade. Subsequent torque applied to the tongue blade will result in pain and reflex opening of the child's mouth in the presence of a mandibular fracture.

FACIAL LACERATIONS

Key to evaluating facial lacerations is an understanding of the relationship between the skin and the underlying vital structures. Injuries to the medial third of the upper or lower eyelids may result in lacrimal apparatus disruption. The course of the facial nerve and parotid duct must be kept in mind during examination (Fig. 34–3). Facial nerve injury will result in paralysis on the ipsilateral side. Suspect laceration of the parotid duct if saliva appears in the wound, or if blood is expressed at Stensen's duct. These signs may be elicited by massage of the parotid gland. Parotid duct injury is possible if a deep wound crosses a line drawn from the tragus to the midportion of the upper lip. The buccal branch of the facial nerve also parallels this line. Facial nerve injuries must be surgically repaired if they are posterior to a vertical line drawn through the lateral canthus. Injuries anterior to such a line are usually not repaired.

▶ IMAGING STUDIES

Obtaining imaging studies depends on the degree of injury and clinical stability of the child. Management of associated intracranial, thoracic, and abdominal injuries always takes precedence over imaging of the face.

The provider should have a low threshold for obtaining imaging studies in a seriously injured child, as the history and physical examination frequently are compromised. Modern CT scan images provide excellent detail of the midface structures, cranium, and mandibular condyle.[10] CT scans have dramatically increased the diagnostic accuracy of facial fractures in the pediatric patient and have become the standard of care for evaluating maxillofacial trauma victims. Although less expensive, plain radiographs are difficult to read in the pediatric patient due to tooth buds, poorly developed sinuses, and suture lines. Given the availability of high-resolution CT scanners, radiographs have fallen out of favor. CT scans provide consistently greater diagnostic accuracy of pediatric condylar fractures, sensitivity, and specificity than panoramic radiographs.[11] Specialized CT scan techniques, such as coronal views, thin slice scans (1.5–3 mm), and three-dimensional reconstructions, assist in surgical planning for these complex injuries. CT scan is particularly helpful in the presence of orbital fractures and evaluates the status of orbital contents. In children with neurologic findings, a facial and cervical spine scan may be performed after the head scan. Ultimately, MRI is often the study of choice for neuroimaging in a patient with a neurological injury but is usually obtained as an inpatient. It is a serious error to perform a CT scan of the face if it will delay the emergent care in a critically injured, unstable child. Treatment of serious, life-threatening injuries always takes precedence over facial imaging, and critical interventions must never be delayed for CT scans of the face. However, in many centers the addition

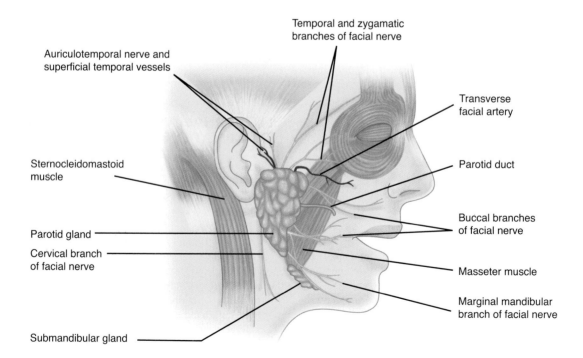

Temporal and zygamatic branches of facial nerve

Auriculotemporal nerve and superficial temporal vessels

Transverse facial artery

Parotid duct

Sternocleidomastoid muscle

Buccal branches of facial nerve

Parotid gland

Cervical branch of facial nerve

Masseter muscle

Marginal mandibular branch of facial nerve

Submandibular gland

Figure 34–3. Diagram of relationship of facial nerve and parotid duct.

of a facial CT scan (in conjunction with CT scan of the head, neck, abdomen, and pelvis) adds only seconds to the examination.

To obtain a high-quality scan, children may require sedation and, in some cases, paralysis and intubation. Agents useful in sedation include narcotics, such as fentanyl; benzodiazepines, such as midazolam; barbiturates; sedative hypnotics; and combination agents. Follow local guidelines for procedural sedation. Short-acting, intravenously administered, reversible agents are the safest choice.

▶ SPECIFIC INJURIES

NASAL FRACTURES

Nasal fractures are the most commonly encountered pediatric facial fracture, accounting for up to 50% of the total.[1] Initial control of hemorrhage is obtained with external digital pressure. If nasal packing is used, care must be taken to ensure that packing is not placed intracranially in the patient with midface trauma or signs of a basilar skull fracture. A particularly severe type of nasal fracture that occurs mostly in children is the "open book" type, where nasal bones separate in the midline along the suture.

Initially, nasal fractures may go undiagnosed secondary to edema and the difficulty in intranasal speculum examination.[1,2] For optimal repair of displaced nasal fractures, consultation should take place within 5 to 6 days postinjury, after which time fractures begin to unite and manipulation becomes increasingly difficult. Surgical reconstruction is generally contraindicated in the growing child and in the majority of nasal fractures anatomic realignment, hemostasis, and fixation are achieved by closed reduction with packing or splinting.[1] If the diagnosis is unclear, the child should be rechecked in 3 to 4 days after swelling has subsided to reassess for deformity or septal deviation.[3] The emergency specialist or the consultant may perform reexamination. Timely referral of nasal fractures is of significant medical and legal concern, as these injuries may have a profound effect on subsequent nasal and maxillofacial development.[2]

It is critical that emergency physicians recognize and treat septal hematomas. An untreated septal hematoma results in collapse of the septum and a "saddle" deformity of the nose due to septal cartilage necrosis. These hematomas may on rare occasion become infected and lead to septal perforation. Upon diagnosing a septal hematoma, the physician should anesthetize the area and then use a No. 11 blade to make an L-shaped incision through the mucoperiosteum along the floor of the nose and extend the incision vertically. The hematoma will then be evacuated through the flap (Fig. 34–4). Subsequent packing of the nasal antrum prevents reaccumulation, and the child must be referred to the appropriate specialist.

NASAL–ETHMOIDAL–ORBITAL FRACTURES

Nasal–ethmoidal–orbital (NEO) fractures occur when the bony structures of the nose are driven backward into the intraorbital

space. Fortunately, these injuries are rare in children. Telecanthus presents secondary to avulsion of one or both medial canthal ligaments. If this injury is suspected, perform the bimanual test for mobility as previously described or obtain a CT scan of the face to include coronal views. Associated injuries include orbital and optic nerve problems, as well as lacrimal system disruption.[12]

ORBITAL FRACTURES

The most common orbital fracture is the blowout fracture, which occurs when a blunt object, often a ball or fist, strikes the globe (Fig. 34–5). The intraorbital pressures increase suddenly and contents decompress through the orbit, most commonly the floor. Blowout fractures can also occur through the medial wall, the roof, and even the greater wing of the sphenoid bone. This may lead to entrapment of the inferior ocular muscles, with subsequent diplopia on upward gaze.[4] Urgent consultation is required in the presence of exophthalmus or extraocular muscle entrapment. If not treated early, ischemic muscle necrosis leads to muscle fibrosis, restriction of ocular motion, and persistent diplopia.[13] In these situations, orbital contents must be surgically released and the area of blowout covered with implants or bone grafts. Many cases of posttraumatic diplopia associated with blowout fractures may be due to muscle or nerve injury and not true mechanical entrapment. A CT scan can evaluate for entrapment.[4] Evaluation for associated ocular injury such as hyphema, retinal contusion, lens dislocation, and corneal lacerations must be performed and visual acuity documented. Facial CT scans provide accurate visualization of blowout fractures.

Patients with NEO or orbital fractures should be instructed not to blow their nose. Because patients with subcutaneous emphysema have a fracture into a sinus or the nasal antrum, many practitioners use antibiotics to cover common sinus pathogens. Such prophylaxis, however, has not been conclusively proved to reduce complications.[4] First-generation cephalosporins, trimethoprim/sulfamethoxazole, amoxicillin, or erythromycin are frequently used in outpatients.

FRONTAL SINUS AND SUPRAORBITAL FRACTURES

Supraorbital fractures involve the superior orbital rim or orbital roof. Exophthalmus and ptosis may be present with impairment of upward gaze. The *superior orbital fissure syndrome* results in paralysis of extraocular muscles, ptosis, and anesthesia in the ophthalmic division of the trigeminal nerve. The *orbital apex syndrome* is a combination of the superior orbital fissure syndrome plus optic nerve damage and results in blindness. These syndromes represent surgical emergencies and require immediate consultation and decompression.

Linear nondisplaced fractures of the anterior wall of the frontal sinus may be treated with observation and antibiotics in either an inpatient or an outpatient setting. If the posterior wall is involved, a CT scan will evaluate the possibility of depression and underlying brain injury. Posterior wall fractures should prompt neurosurgical as well as maxillofacial consultation.

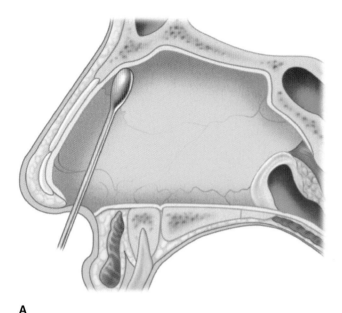

A

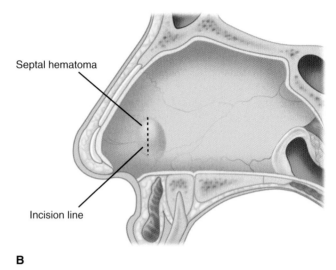

Septal hematoma

Incision line

B

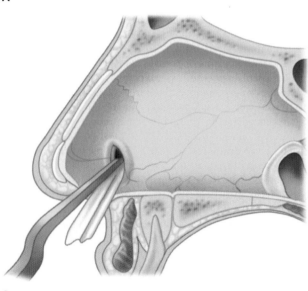

C

Figure 34–4. How to drain and pack a nasal hematoma.

MAXILLARY FRACTURES

Maxillary fractures are very uncommon in young children, but the incidence increases with age, as the paranasal sinuses develop. Because of the high degree of energy required to fracture the pediatric face, associated injuries, particularly intracranial, must be suspected.[3]

MALAR FRACTURES

The malar complex is often broken in a tripod fashion, with fractures at the infraorbital rim, across the zygomatic–frontal suture and along the zygomatic–temporal junction. Inward displacement of this fragment may result in impingement upon the mandible, giving rise to impaired mouth opening and tris-

mus. The zygomatic arch itself is frequently fractured in isolation. If a zygomatic complex fracture is without displacement, diplopia, or sensory deficits, it may be managed by observation. Open reduction and internal fixation is necessary for comminuted fractures.[1]

LEFORT FRACTURES

Fractures to the midface are classified according to the LeFort system, based on the horizontal level of the fracture. LeFort I is a transverse fracture that separates the hard palate from the lower portion of the pterygoid plate and nasal septum. Traction on the upper incisors produces movement of only the hard palate and dental arch. LeFort II or pyramidal fracture separates the central maxilla and palate from the rest of the craniofacial

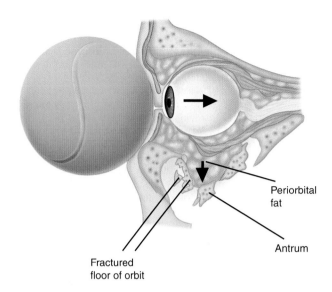

Figure 34–5. Orbital blowout fracture. Fracture of the orbital floor can lead to entrapment of fat and ocular muscles.

Periorbital fat

Antrum

Fractured floor of orbit

skeleton. Mobilization of the upper incisors will move the central pyramid of the face, including the nose. LeFort III, also known as craniofacial dysjunction, separates the facial skeleton from the rest of the cranium. The entire face, including inferior and lateral portions of the orbital rim, moves as a unit. "Pure" LeFort fractures are found more often in textbooks than in clinical practice. Fractures often do not fit the LeFort classification and demonstrate a mixed pattern—perhaps a LeFort II on one side and a LeFort III on the other. LeFort fractures may result in lengthening of the midface, occlusal abnormalities, orbital ecchymosis, and may be associated with basilar skull fractures.[3] CT scans are essential in their evaluation.

Children with LeFort fractures must be admitted and carefully assessed for associated injury. A maxillofacial specialist should be involved in their care.

MANDIBLE FRACTURES

Mandible fractures are the second most common facial fracture, following nasal bone injury. Because of its U-shaped structure, fractures of the mandible are often multiple. Blows or falls to the chin result in symphyseal or perisymphyseal injury, whereas lateral blows are more likely to produce body or angle fractures on the injured or contralateral side. The most frequently injured areas are the condyle (70%), followed by the body, angle, and symphysis.[4] Younger children suffer isolated condylar fractures and may present with deviation of the jaw to the affected side and trismus. Unlike the situation with adults, dislocation of the TMJ is very unusual in this age group. Physical examination is key in diagnosing these injuries, as radiographs may be nondiagnostic. Greenstick fractures, especially in the area of the condyles, are not well visualized on plain films. A recent study comparing the diagnostic accuracy of CT scan and panoramic radiographs in children 2 to 15 years old was 90% and 73%, respectively. Facial CT scan has become

the standard of care for suspected mandible fracture[11] in this age group. In teenagers 16 years and older, oral pan tomogram (Panorex) and posteroanterior mandible radiographs are appropriate initial tests.[14] Consultants may request a facial CT scan for follow-up care.

The mandible is the facial bone most frequently involved in posttraumatic developmental deformities. Crush injuries to the condyle prior to the age of 5 years have the greatest potential for developmental arrest, whereas condylar fractures in later childhood may be self-correcting. Arrested development results in severe facial deformity, micrognathia, and ankylosis of the TMJ. Raise the possibility of subsequent growth disturbances with the parents—the younger the child is, the more likely are the complications.[15]

Treatment of mandibular fractures is based on age, state of dentition, fracture location, bony integrity, and the presence of associated injuries. In general, mandibular fractures without displacement and malocclusion are managed by a liquid/soft diet, pain control, avoidance of physical activities, and close observation. Displaced mandibular fractures require reduction and immobilization.[1]

SOFT TISSUE INJURIES

Tissues that are clearly devitalized need *conservative* debridement. Emphasis must be placed on irrigation, foreign body removal, and cosmetic approximation of important landmarks such as the vermilion border of the lip and margins of the eyebrows. Eyebrows must not be shaved, as their regrowth is unpredictable. Hematomas of the pinna must be relieved: Otherwise a chronic deformity of cauliflower deformity of the ear may result. Drain hematomas of the external ear by either needle aspiration or formal incision, and then apply a pressure dressing to prevent reaccumulation.

Repair of lacerations to the salivary duct or to the lacrymal drainage system must be performed by a specialist. These repairs are achieved over a stent.

Despite the possibility of brisk bleeding, never blindly clamp inside a facial laceration due to the risk of injury to nerves or parotid duct. Direct pressure will control bleeding. Children may require sedation to ensure cooperation in the treatment of either complex or intraoral lacerations. Control of the tongue is necessary in glossal injury, and a large stitch placed in the tip of the tongue will retract it during suturing.

Penetrating wounds to the posterior pharynx occur when a child falls while carrying a pencil or foreign body in his or her mouth. Such wounds endanger carotid artery, jugular vein, and cranial nerves. Imaging studies, such as color flow Doppler, angiography, CT angiography, or MRI may be indicated.

▶ PAIN MANAGEMENT AND ANESTHESIA

Acute maxillofacial trauma produces injuries that are often extremely painful because of the presence of high numbers of nociceptive neurons in surrounding structures. Repair is frequently difficult in the uncooperative child and often requires the use of local and/or systemic analgesics, either alone or in combination.

Local anesthesia is the primary method of achieving immediate pain control. Nerve blocks rely on the deposition of anesthetic solutions in areas of nerve blocks and are an especially helpful technique. The most useful maxillofacial nerve blocks in acute injury are mental, inferior alveolar, infraorbital, and supraorbital. These procedures require patient cooperation, and in the uncooperative child local wound infiltration becomes the procedure of choice.[16] In the *very* uncooperative child, procedural sedation may be necessary.

Systemic analgesia, either enteral or parenteral, is often necessary for adequate pain control in the acute setting. Dose-appropriate use of nonsteroidal anti-inflammatory agents, opioids, or a combination of the two will be required for pain relief. In cases of lengthy repairs or uncooperative patients, implementation of procedural sedation may be necessary for adequate patient and physician comfort and safety. Both early and adequate analgesia will significantly aid the clinician in the immediate management of the suffering child.[16] Previously, some experts suggested that ketamine be avoided in patients with head injury as it was thought to increase intracranial pressure. However, a recent review of the literature found that ketamine does not increase intracranial pressure in neurological impaired patients during controlled ventilation and coadministration of a GABA receptor agonist. In fact, compared with other sedatives, level II and level III evidence indicate that hemodynamic stimulation induced by ketamine may improve cerebral perfusion.[17]

► CONCLUSIONS

Maxillofacial trauma in children more often results in soft tissue injury than facial fractures. When fractures do occur, associated injuries, particularly intracranial, may be present. Fractures heal rapidly over 2 to 3 weeks, and repair must be undertaken before bony union occurs. Conservative management is often the rule.

Late reduction of a fracture may result in unsatisfactory cosmesis secondary to arrested growth and distorted dentition. Aggressive airway management, assiduous search for associated injuries, and early consultation are the keys to successful emergency management of pediatric facial trauma.

REFERENCES

1. Zimmermann CE, Troulis MJ, Kaban LB. Pediatric facial fractures: recent advances in prevention, diagnosis, and management. *Int J Oral Maxillofac Surg.* 2005;35:2–13.
2. Schultz RC. Facial fractures in children and adolescents. In: Cohen M, ed. *Mastery of Plastic and Reconstructive Surgery.* Boston, MA: Little, Brown; 1995:1188–1198.
3. Koltai PJ, Rabkin D. Management of facial trauma in children. *Pediatr Clin North Am.* 1996;43:1253–1275.
4. Ellis E, Scott K. Assessment of patients with facial fractures. *Emerg Med Clin North Am.* 2000;18:411–448.
5. Adelgias KM, Grossman DC, Langer SG, et al. Use of helical computed tomography for imaging the pediatric cervical spine. *Acad Emer Med.* 2004;11:228–236.
6. Khanna G, El-Khoury GY. Imaging of cervical spine injuries of childhood. *Skeletal Radiol.* 2007;36:447–494.
7. Ceallaigh PO, Ekanaykaee K, Beirne CJ, et al. Diagnosis and management of common maxillofacial injuries in the emergency department. Part 1: Advanced trauma life support. *Emerg Med J.* 2006;23:796–797.
8. Nandapalan V, Watson I, Swift A. Beta-2-transferrin and cerebral spinal fluid rhinorrhea. *Clin Otolaryngol.* 1996;21(3):259–264.
9. Jones N, Becker D. Advances in the management of CSF leaks. *BMJ.* 2001;322(7279):122–123.
10. Hogg N, Horswell B. Hard tissue pediatric facial trauma: a review. *J Can Dental Assoc.* 2006;72(6):555–558.
11. Chacon G, Dawson K, Myall R. A comparative study of 2 imaging techniques for the diagnosis of condylar fractures in children. *J Oral Maxillofac Surg.* 2003;61:668–672.
12. Rhea JT, Rao PM, Novelline RA. Helical CT and three-dimensional CT of facial and orbital injury. *Radiol Clin North Am.* 1999;37:489–513.
13. Tse R, Allen L, Matic D. The white-eyed medial blowout fracture. *Plast Reconstr Surg.* 2007;119:277–286.
14. Ceallaigh PO, Ekanaykaee K, Beirne CJ, et al. Diagnosis and management of common maxillofacial injuries in the emergency department. Part 2: Mandibular fractures. *Emerg Med J.* 2006;23:927–928.
15. Dodson TB, Kaban LB. Special considerations for the pediatric emergency patient. *Emerg Med Clin North Am.* 2000;18:539–547.
16. Yagiela JA. Anesthesia and pain management. *Emerg Med Clin North Am.* 2000;18:449–470.
17. Himmelseher S, Durieux M. Revising a dogma: ketamine for patients with neurological Injury? *Anesth Analg.* 2005;101:524–534.

CHAPTER 35

Orthopedic Injuries

Greg Canty

▶ HIGH-YIELD FACTS

- Pediatric patients have unique patterns of injuries and fractures due to the immaturity of bone and the dynamic nature of skeletal growth. Fractures account for 10% to 15% of all childhood injuries.
- Fractures are more common than ligamentous injuries or sprains in children due to the relative weakness of the physis or growth plate.
- Injuries to the physis may lead to long-term growth abnormalities or growth arrest. Injuries to the physis occur in up to 18% of all pediatric fractures.
- Radiographs are more difficult to interpret and findings can be much more subtle in children than adults, as the physis is radiolucent and there are secondary ossification centers. Comparison views of the uninjured extremity can be helpful.
- The majority (75%) of physis fractures are Salter II fractures, and most of these are found after the age of 10 years.
- Up to 50% of fractures in children younger than 1 year are the result of nonaccidental trauma.

Orthopedic injuries are one of the most common reasons for pediatric visits to the emergency department (ED) with more than 40% of boys and 25% of girls experiencing a fracture before the age of 16. These injuries are often the result of either falls, recreation, sports, or motor vehicle accidents, but unfortunately situations like child abuse must also be considered with pediatric injuries.[1] Children with orthopedic injuries are often seen as diagnostic dilemmas because of the various injury patterns seen with growing bones and the challenges of interpreting pediatric x-rays. The better clinicians understand the growing skeleton, the more accurate the diagnosis and management of these injuries. Proper diagnosis allows for better outcomes and better anticipation of possible complications.

▶ THE IMMATURE SKELETON

The immature skeleton has unique characteristics to understand when comparing it to mature, adult bone. First, growing bone is much more porous and flexible leading to unique fracture patterns such as the greenstick, torus (buckle), and bowing (plastic deformation). Much of the immature skeleton consists of radiolucent cartilage that ossifies at different stages making some fractures difficult to visualize on radiographs. Growing bone is surrounded by a thick and active periosteum, which promotes faster healing and better remodeling than in adults. The most obvious characteristic on radiographs is the presence of the physis or "growth plate" at the end of growing bones. The radiolucent physis often leads to confusion and presents many challenges when interpreting radiographs.

The porous character and greater flexibility of the pediatric skeleton allows it to bend much further and absorb much more force before a fracture occurs. This "bending" characteristic is why incomplete fractures like the greenstick, torus, and bowing exist. These incomplete fractures occur when the bone "bends" without resulting in a complete, transverse fracture. The porous character is also why there is less comminution and less propagation seen with fractures of the immature skeleton.[2]

The largest obstacle to overcome when assessing pediatric orthopedic injuries is an understanding of the physis and the surrounding structures (Fig. 35–1). The growing bone begins at the joint surface with the epiphysis, and this area contains a large amount of radiolucent cartilage. The epiphysis is completely cartilaginous at birth (except for the distal femur) and begins to ossify at various stages during bone development, which starts to make it visible on radiographs. Portions of the cartilaginous epiphysis can fracture with very little, or no, radiographic evidence if ossification has not begun. When radiographs do reveal a fracture involving the epiphysis, it is important to remember that a much larger, radiolucent piece of cartilage is often attached. Clinicians should be suspicious of clicking and catching after pediatric injuries because it may be a sign that radiolucent, cartilaginous loose bodies have fractured into the joint. The most common sites for cartilaginous injuries are the distal femur, the patella, the distal humerus, and the radial head.

Next to the epiphysis sits the physis, or "the growth plate." The physis is a thin layer of radiolucent, growing cartilage that results in longitudinal growth of the bone. The physis is situated just between the epiphysis and the metaphysis. The physis is the weakest part of the bone and is often weaker then the surrounding ligamentous attachments. Because the physis is usually weaker than the surrounding ligaments, the same injury mechanism that results in adult sprains will often result in a physis fracture with children. Crossing over the physis, the next anatomic structure is the metaphysis. The metaphysis is the flare lying just between the growing physis and the long shaft of the bone known as the diaphysis.

The stronger and thicker periosteum that covers growing bones is less easily torn or stripped away when bones are fractured. As a result, this stronger periosteum helps to decrease the degree of displacement with fractures and aids as a hinge with reductions. The active periosteum is also the primary reason fractures remodel and heal so rapidly in children. It is very rare to see a nonunion in pediatric orthopedic injuries.

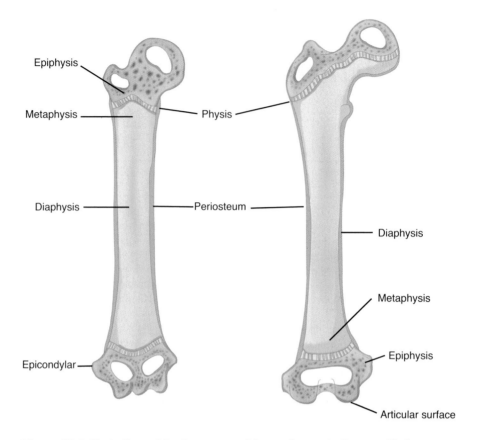

Figure 35–1. Illustrations of the humerus and femur demonstrating specific features of the immature skeleton.

► TERMINOLOGY

In order to communicate meaningfully with consultants and determine the best method of treatment, it is important to grasp the principles of fracture nomenclature and classification systems (Table 35–1). The precise anatomic location and morphology of a given fracture should be described using the "language of orthopedics." Like any language, "the language of orthopedics" requires knowledge, practice, and repetition. A good rule of thumb with any injury is to start with the age, gender, mechanism, location, and degree of soft tissue damage and finish with an excellent radiographic description of the injury. Any involvement of the physis requires further description using the Salter–Harris or Ogden classification systems described in Figure 35–2.[3]

► PHYSIS INJURIES

Just over 20% of all fractures in children involve the physis, or growth. When recognized and treated properly, most physis fractures heal well, but they do have an increased risk for complications such as growth arrest, overgrowth, and malunion. In order to better describe physis fractures and provide guidance for their management, Salter and Harris developed a practical classification system in 1963 that continues to be widely used today (Table 35–2 and Fig. 35–2). The Salter–Harris (SH)

classification depends upon the amount of radiographic involvement seen in the physis, epiphysis, and metaphysis. The SH classifications carry both prognostic and therapeutic implications. Other classification systems such as the Ogden (Table 35–2 and Fig. 35–2) have been developed, but none are as widely used due to the success of the Salter–Harris system.

Most physis fractures are either SH I or II, and these can be managed with closed reduction. Salter–Harris III and IV fractures involve both the physis and the articular surface, and these usually demand surgical fixation for the best prognosis. Type III and IV fractures also carry a worse prognosis for growth disturbance, but remember any physis fracture can result in growth deformities. Parents should be made aware of these risks whenever a physis injury is diagnosed. The SH V classification involves a crush injury to the physis and is difficult to appreciate on initial radiographs. The SH V fracture often goes unrecognized until growth arrest results, and then the diagnosis is made retrospectively. Any suspected physis fracture warrants close follow-up because of the increased risk of complications.[4]

► CLINICAL EVALUATION

The initial evaluation of all emergent patients begins with ensuring that the patient is stable of any life-threatening injuries. Many pediatric orthopedic injuries involve motor vehicle

▶ TABLE 35-1. **FRACTURE TERMINOLOGY**

Anatomic location
  Epiphysis: articular end of each long bone; completely cartilaginous at birth (except distal femur); secondary ossification centers develop and replace cartilage over time
  Physis (growth plate): cartilaginous structure between epiphysis and metaphysis responsible for longitudinal bone growth; injury may result in growth disturbance or arrest; weakest area of bone
  Metaphysis: flared end of diaphysis adjacent to the physis; represents new bone; structurally weak area
  Diaphysis: central shaft of long bone
  Apophysis: nonarticular bony prominence where muscles or tendons attach; not directly involved in longitudinal growth but contribute to bony contour; exposed to significant traction forces

Fracture patterns
  Avulsion: bony fragment pulled off by action of tendon or ligament
  Transverse: fracture line at right angle to long axis of bone
  Oblique: unstable fracture usually at about 30° to long axis of bone
  Spiral: rotational, oblique fracture (usually due to torsion)
  Comminuted: any fracture with more than two fracture fragments
  Bowing (plastic deformation): bending of bone without complete fracture; most often seen in ulna or fibula
  Torus (buckle fracture): compression of porous bone causes "buckle" near metaphysis
  Greenstick: incomplete fracture when energy starts a fracture but cannot complete it; tension side (convex) fractures after bone bends beyond limits, but compression side (concave) bows into plastic deformation; most common fracture pattern in children
  Pathologic: fracture through abnormal, weakened bone (i.e., tumors, osteomyelitis, cysts, inherited metabolic disorders)

Fracture descriptions
  Alignment: refers to longitudinal relationship of one fragment to another
  Displacement: deviation of fracture fragments from anatomic position; describe distal fragment in relation to proximal portion; varus displacement is toward midline of body; valgus displacement is away from midline of body
  Angulation: the apex of the angle formed by the two fracture fragments; direction will be opposite to the displacement of distal fragment
  Shortening: overlapping fracture fragments due to muscle contraction
  Malrotation: refers to the rotational alignment of one fragment to another
  Butterfly fragment: wedge-shaped fragment at apex of a fracture; caused by overload of both axial and angulation forces to the bone

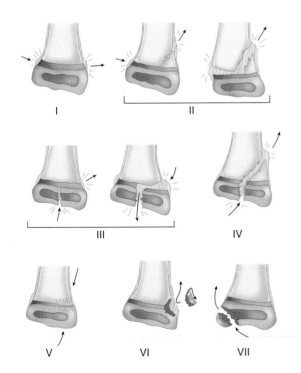

Figure 35–2. Examples of physis injuries classified by Salter–Harris (I–V) and Ogden (VI and VII).

accidents and multiple injuries, so life-threatening issues such as breathing, circulation, and internal injuries must be addressed first. The orthopedic evaluation in the pediatric patient can be complicated by pain, fear, and the developmental stage of the child. These issues are best overcome with proper pain control, reassurance, gaining the family's confidence, and understanding the patient's stage of development.

The history is the first and most underappreciated step in assessing orthopedic injuries. The history should be obtained from the patient with assistance from the family and any other witnesses. Any information about the timing of the event, surrounding circumstances, mechanism of injury, direction of force, and previous injuries is helpful. The time spent with the patient and family helps to build a relationship prior to the examination. Another important part of the history in pediatrics is to determine if the history seems plausible with the injury. Any incompatibility between the history and the injury should be a red flag for possible child abuse.

The physical examination begins with exposing the injured extremity and grossly assessing for any deformity or discoloration. Most experts then recommend examining the uninjured extremity to establish a baseline and reassure the patient. The injured extremity is examined closely for any swelling, deformity, or breaks in the skin suggestive of an open fracture. Joints above and below the injury are palpated for tenderness and taken through a range of motion. Any abnormalities should be noted and appropriate radiographs ordered. Distal

► TABLE 35–2. **CLASSIFICATION AND OVERVIEW OF PHYSIS INJURIES**

Type	Description
	Salter–Harris System
I	Fracture through the physis with complete separation of the epiphysis from the metaphysis; if periosteum remains intact, there may be little to no displacement; tenderness over growth plate/physis; diagnosis often on clinical suspicion alone because x-rays may be normal; good prognosis; usually results from shearing, torsion, or avulsion forces; immobilization and orthopedic referral recommended
II	Fracture along physis extending into metaphysis; triangular metaphysis fragment with variable displacement; most common physis injury; low risk of growth disturbance except in distal femur; closed reduction, immobilization, and orthopedic follow-up recommended
III	Fracture along physis extending into epiphysis and the articular surface; occurs in partially closed growth plates; usually requires surgical fixation to maintain articular surface; increased risk of growth disturbances, bony bridging, and posttraumatic arthritis
IV	Fracture line begins at articular surface and runs across the epiphysis, through the physis, and into the metaphysis; usually requires surgical fixation to maintain reduction and articular surface; significant risk of growth disturbance, bony bridging, and posttraumatic arthritis
V	Compression fracture of the physis not extending into the epiphysis or metaphysis; produced by axial compression; difficult or impossible diagnosis based on initial x-rays; diagnosed retrospectively based upon mechanism and growth arrest; high risk for growth disturbance
	Additional types from the Ogden system
VI	Peripheral shearing of the physis and surrounding structures; most commonly associated with lawn mower injuries, but may also be seen with sports, bicycle injuries, and deep infections; high risk for growth disturbance
VII	Fracture of the epiphysis; ligament pulls off portion of the epiphysis rather than tearing; results in fracture extending from the articular surface completely through the epiphysis without extending into the physis; very rare

neurologic and vascular assessments should be thorough and reassessed throughout the visit. Any suggestion of compartment syndrome or neurovascular compromise warrants emergent orthopedic consultation.

Appropriate radiographs begin with two views (AP and lateral) of the injury that are perpendicular to one another. Views of the joints proximal and distal to the injury are also helpful. Oblique radiographs of the injury may be helpful when suspicions persist, and comparison views of the uninjured extremity are another option to consider. More liberal use of radiographs is common in pediatrics because of the subtle x-ray findings and difficult examinations. Obtaining high-quality radiographs is the responsibility of the emergency physician, and inadequate views should never be accepted. The key to helpful radiographs is a good history and complete physical examination of the injured area prior to placing the request.[5]

► MANAGEMENT

Management of orthopedic injuries in the ED starts with pain control for patient comfort and optimal evaluation. Once pain control is established and the clinical evaluation is complete, management decisions center around whether operative or nonoperative care is necessary to stabilize the fracture (Fig. 35–3). Traditionally, most pediatric fractures have been managed by conservative, nonoperative means due to their tremendous ability to remodel and heal. Most are managed by closed reduction when necessary, and sent home with appropriate immobilization. Operative repair may be necessary, and consultation with an orthopedist is recommended for Salter–Harris III and IV fractures, most tibia fractures, all femur fractures, and any fracture with significant displacement. Emergent orthopedic consultation is required if there are any signs of neurovascular compromise, compartment syndrome, or the possibility of an open fracture. When present, compartment syndrome most often occurs in the forearm and lower leg. Early symptoms of compartment syndrome include pain out of proportion to the injury and extreme pain with passive range of motion. This is a limb-threatening complication, and one should not wait for late signs such as pallor, pulselessness, and paresthesias before consulting orthopedics. Open fractures need irrigation, antibiotics, and appropriate tetanus prophylaxis in the ED while awaiting orthopedic consultation.

The hallmarks of nonsurgical fracture care are closed reduction and immobilization. Closed reduction is necessary for significantly displaced or angulated fractures. Reduction is most often performed by orthopedists, but can also be performed by appropriately trained emergency physicians in many hospitals. The use of procedural sedation is strongly recommended for any attempts at fracture reduction.

Once a fracture has been reduced, or if it was initially nondisplaced, the focus becomes proper immobilization. Immobilization offers protection, decreases the risk for any further displacement, and improves patient comfort. The most common types of immobilization involve plaster or commercial splints. Casts are rarely applied in the ED because of the risks associated with progressive swelling in acute injuries. The types of splints differ in the degree of molding allowed, the ease of application, and the ability to properly immobilize

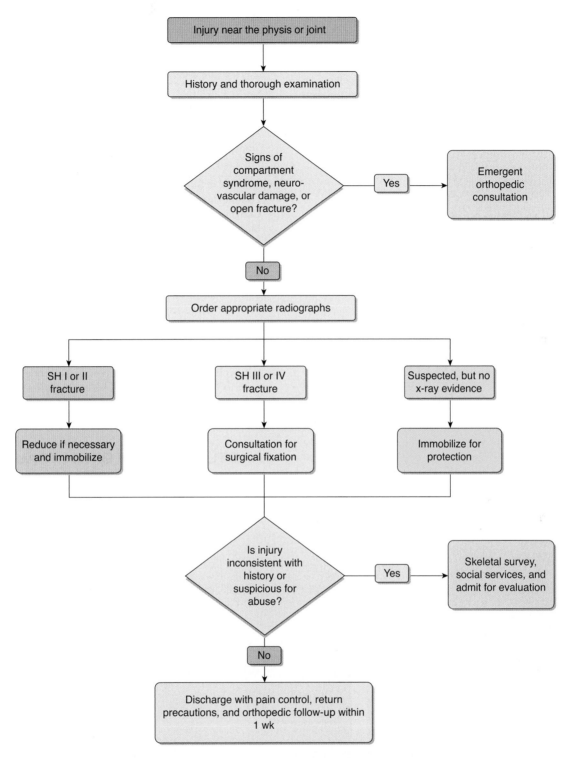

Figure 35–3. Algorithm for the management of physis injuries in children.

the injury. A sling and swathe provide immobilization for injuries of the clavicle, shoulder, and humerus. For supracondylar, elbow, forearm, and wrist injuries, a posterior long-arm splint with the elbow at 90 degrees and the hand in neutral works well. An ulnar gutter splint best immobilizes fractures of the fourth and fifth metacarpals. The scaphoid and thumb are immobilized with a thumb spica. Fractures to the distal fe-

mur, knee, and majority of the tibia require a long-leg posterior splint. Ankle and foot injuries can usually be immobilized in a posterior short-leg splint. When in doubt, always immobilize the joint proximal and distal to the injury.

The final step in caring for orthopedic injuries is to remember proper discharge instructions, and their importance cannot be overemphasized. Discharge instructions need to include information on splint/cast care, indications for returning to the ED, specific follow-up plans, and outpatient pain management. Elevation and ice are important to control pain and decrease swelling. Returning to the ED is emphasized for specific findings such as changes in extremity color, severe swelling, or a marked increase in pain. Follow-up plans should be clear and within 1 week due to the rapid rate of healing in children. Outpatient pain control is very important and should not be overlooked in children. Fractures and significant injuries need pain control to last until their orthopedic follow-up. Proper discharge instructions result in optimal patient care and fewer unnecessary returns to the ED.[6]

► SPECIAL CIRCUMSTANCES

FRACTURES OF CHILD ABUSE OR NONACCIDENTAL TRAUMA

Nonaccidental trauma is a major concern in pediatrics, and one that often presents with an orthopedic injury. Twenty-five to fifty percent of abused children will have a fracture and 10% of all injuries in children younger than 2 years are the result of nonaccidental trauma. The younger the patient with a fracture, the higher the suspicion should be for possible abuse (Table 35–3). Injuries such as "corner" femur fractures, transphyseal distal humerus fractures, spiral fractures, and "bucket-handle" fractures always raise concerns about nonaccidental trauma, but recent evidence shows the most common fracture with abuse is the routine transverse fracture (Fig. 35–4).[7] The biggest clue is not the fracture type, but the often underemphasized history. Any history that appears inconsistent with the type or degree of injury should raise concerns about possible abuse. The younger the child presenting with a fracture, the higher the

► **TABLE 35–3. RADIOGRAPHIC FINDINGS SUGGESTIVE OF NONACCIDENTAL TRAUMA**

Very High Index of Suspicion
   Any fracture with an inconsistent history or evasive explanation
   Metaphysis fractures (i.e., the "corner" or "bucket-handle" fracture)
   Rib or spinous process fractures
   Transphyseal distal humerus fractures
   Fractures at various stages of healing

High Index of Suspicion
   Lower extremity fractures in children less than 18 mo[9]
   Complex skull fractures
   Multiple fractures[10]
   Fractures of the hand or foot

Less Suspicion with plausible history
   Clavicle fracture
   Linear skull fracture
   Healing fracture following traumatic birth

likelihood the injury was nonaccidental. The law in all 50 states requires physicians to report any concerns about nonaccidental trauma to the proper authorities for further investigation. Any suspicion of nonaccidental trauma in young children requires a skeletal survey and hospital admission for further evaluation.[8]

FRACTURES FROM BIRTH TRAUMA

Fractures seen within the first few weeks of life may be due to birth trauma. Many of these fractures are found accidentally

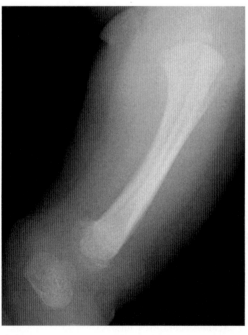

A

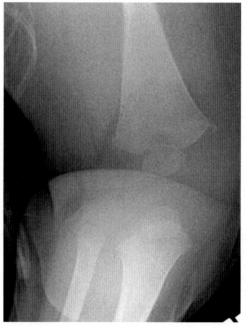

B

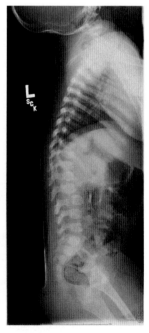

C

Figure 35–4. These are rare fractures which are often referred to as classics in nonaccidental trauma. (A) Illustrates a "bucket-handle" fracture of the distal tibia. (B) Illustrates a "corner" fracture of the distal femur. (C) Illustrates a lumbar fracture of L-2.

on chest x-rays, in evaluations for not moving an extremity, or on parental concerns about a "bump." The most common fracture from birth trauma involves the clavicle, but fractures of the femur and humerus are also not uncommon. Healing from birth injuries is rapid, and callus should be seen within 2 weeks of delivery. A lack of callus formation within this time-line or an absent history of traumatic delivery requires closer investigation for possible nonaccidental trauma.

▶ ACKNOWLEDGMENT

A special thanks to Valerie A. Dobiesz, MD, and Russell H. Greenfield, MD, who authored previous editions of this chapter.

REFERENCES

1. Landin LA. Epidemiology of children's fractures. *J Pediatr Orthop B.* 1997;6:79.
2. Xian CJ, Foster BK. The biologic aspects of children's fractures. In: Beaty JH, Kasser JR, eds. *Rockwood and Wilkins' Fractures in Children.* 6th ed. Philadelphia, PA: Lippincott Williams & Wilkins; 2006:21–50.
3. Wenger DR. Orthopedic literacy: fracture description and resource utilization. In: Wenger DR, Pring ME, eds. *Rang's Children's Fractures.* 3rd ed. Philadelphia, PA: Lippincott Williams & Wilkins; 2005:27–40.
4. Canale ST. Physis injuries. In: Green, NE, Swiontkowski MF, eds. *Skeletal Trauma in Children.* Philadelphia, PA: Saunders; 2003:17–56.
5. England SP, Sundberg S. Management of common pediatric fractures. *Pediatr Clin North Am.* 1996;43(5):991–1012.
6. Bachman D, Santora S. Orthopedic trauma. In: Fleisher GR, Ludwig S, Henretig FM, eds. *Textbook of Pediatric Emergency Medicine.* 5th ed. Philadelpia, PA: Lippincott Williams & Wilkins, 2006:1525–1569.
7. King J, Dietendorf D, Apthorp J, et al. Analysis of 429 fractures in 189 battered children. *J Pediatr Orthop.* 1988;8:585–589.
8. Campbell RM, Schrader T. Child abuse. In: Beaty JH, Kasser JR, eds. *Rockwood and Wilkins' Fractures in Children.* 6th ed. Philadelphia, PA: Lippincott Williams & Wilkins; 2006:223–253.
9. Coffey C, Haley K, Hayes J, et al. The risk of child abuse in infants and toddlers with lower extremity injuries. *J Pediatr Surg.* 2005;40:120–123.
10. Jenny C; for American Academy of Pediatrics Committee on Child Abuse and Neglect. Evaluating infants and young children with multiple fractures. *Pediatrics.* 2006;118:1299–1303.

CHAPTER 36

Pediatric Sports Injuries in the ED

Greg Canty

Over 30 million, or half of all children and adolescents, now participate in organized sports, and the number of children participating in nonorganized sports such as skateboarding, bicycling, and "extreme sports" is even harder to quantify. This boom in sporting activities has resulted in large numbers of patients presenting to the ED following sports-related injuries. Recent data indicate more than 20% of all pediatric injury-related visits involved a sports-related injury, and up to 10% of pediatric ED visits involve a sporting injury. The injuries include fractures, dislocations, contusions, sprains, strains, lacerations, and other injuries quite familiar to the ED physician. There are also a number of unique injuries and issues involving the pediatric athlete.[1–3] Injuries are not just musculoskeletal but also include neurologic injuries such as the challenging pediatric concussion and the "stinger" or brachioplexus injury. The challenge is recognizing the complexities of the growing skeleton and the developing nervous system. This chapter covers some of the unique injuries seen in the ED following sports injuries, and includes avulsion fractures, physeal fractures, overuse syndromes, pediatric concussions, and brachioplexus injuries. We also briefly discuss return-to-play recommendations because many of these patients are seeking definitive care for their injuries in the ED, and it is important to understand why the ED provider is not in a good position to answer all of these questions.

▶ FRACTURES

Fractures are very common in youth sports due to the weakness of the physis and the strength of the attached ligaments. Mechanisms that result in adult sprains frequently result in physeal fractures of the skeletally immature athlete due to the stronger ligaments pulling on the weaker bone. During adolescence, the skeleton starts to mature and both fractures and sprains become common. The most common injuries to the physis in athletes are the Salter–Harris (SH) I and II fractures. Once the physis begins to close during adolescence, unique fracture patterns like the SH III and IV also emerge. It is important to always keep in mind the stage of the growing skeleton when evaluating sports injuries, and remember "the younger the athlete, the more likely it's a fracture!"[4] (see Chapter 35).

▶ AVULSIONS

Avulsion injuries are usually fractures that occur when stronger tendons adhere to weaker areas of bone called secondary os-

sification centers or apophyses. These tendons attach to large muscle groups, and when a strong muscular contraction occurs, the tendon actually "pulls" the apophyses apart from the larger piece of bone. These injuries mostly appear in adolescent athletes as the muscle mass increases and the contraction forces become much greater. The most common site for avulsion fractures is the pelvis where the iliac crest, anterior inferior iliac spine (AIIS), anterior superior iliac spine (ASIS), or the ischium (Fig. 36–1) can have an avulsion injury. The tibial tubercle, greater and lesser trochanters, and phalanges are also frequent sites of avulsions. A unique avulsion of the knee is the tibial spine (eminence) avulsion which occurs following hyperextension. Management of avulsion fractures is usually nonoperative, but surgical repair may be necessary if there is a significant avulsion or intra-articular displacement. Most are managed with crutches and non–weight-bearing for 4 to 6 weeks.[5]

▶ DISLOCATIONS

Dislocations are rare until athletes reach adolescence. Once athletes start to mature, joint dislocations begin to appear, and seem to result from a combination of sporting activities and musculoskeletal forces. The most commonly dislocated joints are the proximal interphalangeal joint (PIP) of the hand, the patellofemoral joint of the knee, and the glenohumeral joint of the shoulder. Dislocations of the tibiotalar (ankle) joint or the hip are extremely rare during sporting activities.

Evaluation of suspected dislocations starts with pain control using narcotics or regional anesthesia. If time allows, prereduction radiographs can be taken in a timely manner. Reductions of larger joints, such as the glenohumeral or patellofemoral, are best achieved using some form of procedural sedation. Emergency medicine providers should be familiar with multiple techniques for reduction and should emphasize the gentlest methods possible to prevent further injury. Following reduction, all dislocations require careful neurovascular examination and postreduction radiographs to look for osteochondral injuries which frequently appear following dislocation and reduction. Common sites for these osteochondral injuries are the glenoid rim (Bankart), proximal humerus (Hill–Sachs), patella, and femoral condyle. Once radiographs confirm adequate reduction, all dislocations need immobilization with follow-up arranged for 3 to 5 days. Patients should be cautioned about the risk for recurrent dislocations, and recurrent dislocators need orthopedic referral.[5,6]

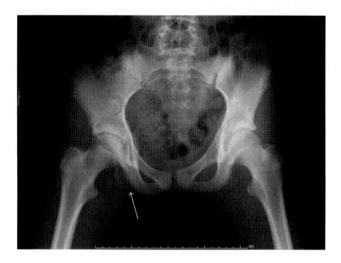

Figure 36–1. A 13-year-old girl who presented to the ED because of inability to bear weight after feeling a "pop" while doing the splits during gymnastics. Radiographs revealed an avulsion of her ischium.

▶ SPRAINS AND LIGAMENTOUS INJURIES

Much like dislocations, the incidence of sprains (ligamentous injuries) increases as athletes mature during adolescence. Beware of the preadolescent patient with a "sprain" because it is much more likely to be a physeal fracture. The sprained ankle is the most common sporting injury of adolescents, and 90% of these involve an inversion mechanism. Inversion of the ankle puts stress on the anterior talofibular ligament (ATFL) and the calcanofibular ligament (CF). It is important to palpate and stress each ligament as part of the ankle examination. The "high ankle sprain" or syndesmosis sprain has more anterior pain and often takes much longer to rehabilitate.[7]

Anterior cruciate ligament (ACL) injuries are increasing in young athletes due to the increased number of athletes in competitive sports, the increased number of female athletes, and better recognition of the injury. ACL injuries present to the ED as an acute traumatic knee effusion following a hyperextension mechanism. This mechanism should immediately alert the ED provider to the possibility of an ACL injury or a tibial spine avulsion depending upon the musculoskeletal age of the athlete. There is not an indication for routine MRI imaging of these injuries in the ED. Management is temporary protection with a knee extension immobilizer, compression bandage, and encouraging gentle range of motion.[8]

Ligamentous injuries, or sprains, are graded from I to III. (Table 36–1) Generalizations about management can be made based on the degree of severity. Most grade I and II sprains can be managed with protection and weight-bearing as tolerated. Grade III sprains require more stringent immobilization and non–weight-bearing. Follow-up, rehabilitation, and range-of-motion exercises should always be emphasized with discharge instructions.[9]

▶ TABLE 36–1. **GRADING OF LIGAMENTOUS INJURIES**

Grade I	Grade I sprains stretch the ligaments causing mild swelling and pain with stress testing, but no laxity.
Grade II	Grade II sprains partially tear the ligaments resulting in more moderate swelling and pain along with some laxity on stress testing. Despite the increased laxity, grade II sprains have a definitive end point with stress testing.
Grade III	Grade III sprains are complete tears of the ligaments with a tremendous amount of pain, swelling, and gross laxity on stress testing without any definitive end point.

▶ OVERUSE SYNDROMES

Overuse syndromes appear in the young athlete due to year-round training, repetitive activities, overtraining, and improper conditioning. ED physicians must be familiar with these syndromes because many of these patients will present to the ED with acute worsening of more chronic pain. One of the keys to diagnosis is inquiring about any chronic history of pain in the injured extremity, the type of sport(s) played, and the amount of practice and number of events. Stress fractures are an example of an overuse syndrome where acute worsening may lead to presentation in the ED. The most common stress fracture involves point tenderness along the proximal to middle third of the anterior tibia, but stress fractures also appear in the metatarsals, femur, and humerus. Spondylolysis usually appears in the lumbar spine, and it is a stress fracture of the pars interarticularis that worsens with back extension. Little League shoulder is a Salter–Harris I injury of the proximal humerus in repetitive overhead-throwing athletes like baseball pitchers, and the "Little League" elbow is a constellation of elbow pain, medial condyle tenderness, and a subtle flexion contracture from the repetitive stress of throwing. Other common overuse syndromes of the lower extremity include Osgood–Schlatter disease (tenderness over tibial tubercle), Sinding–Larsen–Johansson syndrome ("jumper's knee" with tenderness at the distal pole of the patella), and medial tibial stress syndrome ("shin splints" with diffuse tenderness over the middle to distal third of the medial tibia). Overuse syndromes are best managed by discontinuing the offending sports/activities and encouraging proper rehabilitation before resuming activities.[10,11]

▶ CONCUSSION AND BRACHIOPLEXUS INJURIES

Neurologic injuries are proof that sports injuries involve more than just musculoskeletal medicine. The growing knowledge base about concussions, or minor traumatic brain injuries (mTBI), has shown us that pediatric athletes recover much more slowly from concussions than the college or professional athlete, and must be managed more conservatively. The concussed athlete often presents to the ED with headaches, dizziness, posttraumatic amnesia, or confusion following a direct head blow. The physical and focal neurologic examination can be expected to be normal except for confused mental status (person, place, and time) or decreased cognitive function (immediate recall, delayed recall, and concentration). The majority of concussed patients do not need neuroimaging unless there are focal neurologic deficits, seizure activity, worsening headache, or a prolonged loss of consciousness (see Chapter 29). The severity of initial symptoms does not predict long-term outcomes nearly as well as following the continued duration of symptoms. As a result, much less emphasis is placed on initial grading of concussions, and much more emphasis is placed on close follow-up to monitor persistent symptoms.[12,13]

The brachioplexus injury is also called a "burner" or a "stinger," and occurs following injuries to the neck and shoulder region. These occur following traction on the plexus when the shoulder is depressed and the head is forced away from the injured side. The "burner" and "stinger" nicknames come from the sensation that extends down the injured extremity in a nondermatome pattern. These athletes can also have unilateral numbness, paresthesias, or weakness in the injured extremity, but beware of any bilateral symptoms or point tenderness of the cervical spine on examination. If there are any bilateral symptoms, radicular symptoms extending into the legs, or cervical spine tenderness to palpation, the patient should be immobilized until cervical injury can be excluded since these symptoms are much more suggestive of a spinal cord or cervical spine injury.[14]

▶ RETURN-TO-PLAY

Many athletes and their families are immediately interested in the ED about when an athlete can return to play following sports injuries. This is a conversation that cannot be properly answered in the department, and its implications should be understood. In order to return to play following a musculoskeletal injury, an athlete must be able to meet certain criteria for range of motion, functional ability, adequate strength, and minimal to no pain. In concussed athletes, we now know many of these young athletes continue to have prolonged symptoms that cannot be accurately predicted based on their ED presentation. Concussed athletes run the risk of increased disability with stacked concussions or even the risk of death due to second impact syndrome. Brachioplexus injuries must have resolution of their symptoms with a return to full strength and sensation before resuming activities. All of these criteria require following symptoms to resolution and cannot be accurately predicted by the ED physician. The issue of proper follow-up should be emphasized to the family during their ED visit, and explain why their return-to-play questions are best handled at follow-up.[15]

REFERENCES

1. Centers for Disease Control and Prevention (CDC). Non-fatal sports and recreational injuries treated in emergency departments-United States, July 2000–2001. *MMWR Morb Mortal Wkly Rep.* 2002;51(33):736–740.
2. Simon TD, Bublitz C, Hambidge SJ. Emergency department visits among pediatric patients for sports-related injury. *Pediatr Emerg Care.* 2006;2(5):309–315.
3. Burt CW, Overpeck MD. Emergency visits for sports-related injuries. *Ann Emerg Med.* 2001;37(3):301–308.
4. Wenger DR, Pring ME, eds. *Rang's Children's Fractures.* 3rd ed. Philadelphia, PA: Lippincott Williams & Wilkins; 2005:11–26.
5. LaBella CR. Common acute sports-related lower extremity injuries in children and adolescents. *Clin Pediatr Emerg Med* 2007;8:31–42.
6. Benjamin HJ, Hang BT. Common acute upper extremity injuries in sports. *Clin Pediatr Emerg Med* 2007;8:15–30.
7. Marsh JS, Daigneault JP. Ankle injuries in the pediatric population. *Curr Opin Pediatr* 2000;12:52–60.
8. Dorizas JA, Stanitski CL. Anterior cruciate ligament injury in the skeletally immature. *Orthop Clin North Am* 2003;34:355–363.
9. Chorley JN. Ankle sprain discharge instructions from the emergency department. *Pediatr Emerg Care* 2005;21:498–501.
10. Hogan KA, Gross RH. Overuse injuries in pediatric athletes. *Orthop Clin North Am.* 2003;34:405–415.
11. Lord J, Winell JJ. Overuse injuries in pediatric athletes. *Curr Opin Pediatr* 2004;16:47–50.
12. Buzzini SR, Guskiewicz KM. Sport-related concussion in the young athlete. *Curr Opin Pediatr* 2006;18(4):376–382.
13. Kirkwood MW, Yeates KO, Wilson PE. Pediatric sport-related concussion: a review of the clinical management of an oft-neglected population. *Pediatrics* 2006;117:1359–1371.
14. Bracker MD, ed. *The 5-Minute Sports Medicine Consult.* Philadelphia, PA: Lippincott Williams & Wilkins; 2001.
15. Gregory A. *Return to Play Issues.* Paper Presented at: American Academy of Pediatrics Sports Medicine Course; June 22, 2008; Vancouver, Canada.

CHAPTER 37

Injuries of the Upper Extremities

Jim R. Harley

▶ HIGH-YIELD FACTS

- The clavicle is the most common bone to be fractured in a shoulder injury.
- Small children with a clavicle fracture may present with refusal to move the arm after a fall.
- The proximal humerus epiphyseal plate is sometimes confused for a fracture.
- Children are more likely to suffer a Salter–Harris type II fracture separation of the proximal humerus than a true shoulder dislocation.
- Indirect radiographic evidence of elbow fracture includes the presence of a posterior fat pad, an exaggerated anterior fat pad, and an abnormal radiocapitellar or anterior humeral line. Further evidence may be obtained from normal comparison views and oblique views.
- Supracondylar fractures of the humerus can be associated with acute and delayed neurovascular compromise and require immediate orthopedic consultation.
- Nursemaid's elbow is the most common pediatric elbow injury. X-rays are not required if there is no elbow swelling.
- Fracture separation of the distal humeral physis may be the result of physical abuse.
- Fracture of the radius or ulna requires x-ray evaluation of the elbow and wrist to determine if a Monteggia or Galeazzi fracture is present.
- The normal cascade of the resting hand shows increasing flexion from the index to little fingers and from the distal interphalangeal (DIP) joints to the metacarpophalangeal (MCP) joints. Deviation from this normal cascade implies a tendon laceration.
- A Salter–Harris type I or II fracture of the distal phalanx may not be seen on x-ray because the epiphysis in young children may not be ossified. Look for a mallet deformity and inability to extend the DIP joint.
- Carpal fractures are rare in children due to the elasticity imparted by the cartilage surrounding the carpal bones. As in adults, scaphoid fractures are the most commonly encountered carpal fracture. A scaphoid view may improve fracture identification.

▶ INJURIES IN THE UPPER EXTREMITY

Children are prone to injuries of the upper extremity due to their natural curiosity, being active in sports, and due to risk-taking behaviors. Boys incur more injuries than girls. The high-est incidence of injuries occurs between 10 and 18 years of age. This chapter will review the diagnosis and management of injuries to the upper extremities and hands.

▶ THE CLAVICLE AND ACROMIOCLAVICULAR JOINT

The clavicle is the most commonly fractured bone during delivery and is the fourth most commonly fractured bone in older children. It is the most common bone fractured from a fall with a blow to the shoulder. The vast majority of injuries involve the area between the middle and distal third of the clavicle (>90%).[1] Young children sustain incomplete injuries (greenstick or bowing fractures), whereas older children and adolescents present more often with displaced fractures.

▶ MEDIAL CLAVICLE FRACTURES

Fractures of the medial clavicle are rare in children. The medial clavicular epiphysis is the last growth plate in the body to close, allowing physeal injuries to occur up to age 25. In contrast to adults, in whom sternoclavicular (SC) joint dislocations occur, children are most likely to experience Salter–Harris type I or II fracture, with or without epiphyseal separation. One must be careful in distinguishing a medial physeal injury from a posterior dislocation of the SC joint. Posterior dislocations of the SC joint, though rare, are important to diagnose as they are often associated with other complications such as brachial plexus injuries, pneumothorax, and vascular compromise. Accurate determination of medial clavicular fractures is often difficult. A CT scan is the best diagnostic procedure if the diagnosis is not clear after obtaining plain films.[2]

▶ DIAPHYSEAL CLAVICLE FRACTURES

The most common mechanism for a midshaft clavicle fracture is a fall on the shoulder. If the fall is unwitnessed, the only history may be refusal to move the arm. The patient presents with decreased or painful movement of the arm. The child may have point tenderness over the medial clavicle, localized swelling, crepitus, and tenting of the overlying skin. Radiographs will confirm the suspected injury (Fig. 37–1). Obtain two views, with one view directed 30 degrees cephalad. The physical examination, though, is very accurate in determining

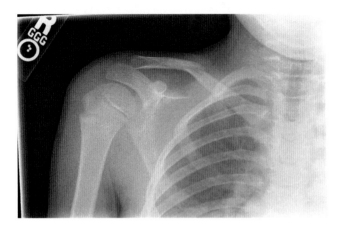

Figure 37–1. Midshaft clavicle fracture.

the presence of a midshaft fracture.[3] X-rays may not be necessary but parents or physician may be uncomfortable relying on physical examination alone.

A careful search for associated vascular injury is mandatory in the presence of a displaced clavicle fracture. Pulse changes and significant swelling may signal laceration or compression of the subclavian vessels, especially with posterior displacement of the fracture fragments, prompting emergent orthopedic, and vascular consultation. Auscultation of the lungs is important to assess for a possible pneumothorax and a chest radiograph is indicated if there is a high index of suspicion. Fortunately, associated injuries are extremely rare.

Shoulder compression during delivery often results in fracture of the clavicle. The clavicle is the most common bone to be fractured during delivery. The injury may be asymptomatic or present as pseudoparalysis (the infant will not move the arm but hand and forearm movement is normal).[4] Exuberant callus formation may call attention to the fracture a few weeks later. Initially, the deformity worries parents, but remodeling occurs and results in a normal appearance of the bone in 6 to 12 months.

Most clavicle fractures heal well without complication, and reduction is rarely necessary. Injuries due to birth trauma only require careful handling of the infant. Young children are placed in either a sling or a shoulder strap; older patients can be managed with a sling and swathe. Some children find the sling more comfortable than the shoulder strap or clavicle brace. Operative intervention is indicated in the presence of an open fracture or vascular complication. Adequate pain control is important but often given inadequately as these fractures can be very painful.[5] Parents should be told to expect a bump from callus formation to appear after about a month as the bone heals.

▶ LATERAL CLAVICLE INJURIES

Direct trauma to the lateral clavicle produces metaphyseal fractures in young children rather than true acromioclavicular joint separations, as seen in adolescents and adults. Avulsion of bone and periosteum occurs rather than ligamentous tearing. Weighted x-ray views are not recommended. The fracture heals well with the use of a sling and swathe, and surgery is only rarely indicated. Acromioclavicular separation is very rare before age 16. There will be tenderness over the acromioclavicular joint. Radiographs will show an increased distance between the coracoid process and the clavicle. Treatment is conservative with a sling or clavicle brace.

▶ SCAPULAR FRACTURES

Fractures of the scapula are very rare in children and occur infrequently in adolescents. They are often associated with high-energy injuries, so care must be taken to evaluate for more serious injuries. The fracture will be seen on plain radiographs. Special views may be necessary. The treatment of a scapular fracture is similar to a clavicle fracture.

▶ SHOULDER DISLOCATIONS

The same forces that result in shoulder dislocation in adults usually cause displaced Salter–Harris type II fracture separation of the proximal humerus in young children. Less than 2% of shoulder dislocations occur in patients younger than 10 years and 20% occur in patients aged 10 to 20 years. As with adults, when pediatric shoulder dislocations do occur, anterior dislocations are much more common than posterior or inferior dislocations.[2]

Inspection of the anteriorly dislocated shoulder reveals loss of the normally rounded contour, creating a squared-off appearance. The arm is held in slight abduction and external rotation, and the humeral head may be palpated anterior to the glenoid fossa. Radiographs should include an anteroposterior (AP) view of the shoulder and either a true scapular lateral or a transaxillary view. In general, adequate analgesia and relaxation should be provided before attempting reduction with either traction–countertraction, scapular manipulation, or external rotation techniques. Radiographs should be taken after reduction to look for occult fractures. After the reduction, the patient should be immobilized for 3 to 6 weeks then begin rehabilitation therapy. Posterior shoulder dislocations can occur following seizures or electrical injuries. The arm is held in adduction and internal rotation. The anterior shoulder appears abnormally flat, and the displaced humeral head may be palpable posteriorly. Orthopedic consultation is recommended in all cases of posterior shoulder dislocation.

Axillary nerve damage may accompany shoulder dislocation. Sensation over the deltoid muscle should be assessed before and after reduction. Other complications include greater tuberosity fractures, damage to the glenoid labrum, the Hill–Sachs deformity (a compression fracture of the posterolateral humeral head), rotator cuff injury, and recurrent dislocation. Younger patients with instability have a much higher rate of recurrence than older adults.

▶ HUMERUS FRACTURES

PROXIMAL HUMERUS FRACTURE

The proximal humerus epiphyseal ossification center appears at 6 months of age. The greater tuberosity ossification center appears at 3 years and the less tuberosity center at 5 years. The physis closes at age 14 to 17 years in girls, and 16 to 18 years

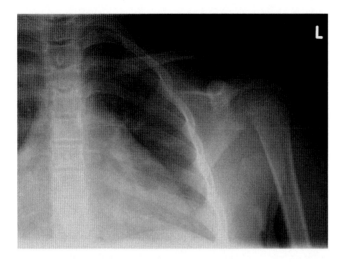

Figure 37–2. Normal proximal humerus epiphyseal plate.

in boys. Nearly 80% of the longitudinal growth of the humerus takes place at the proximal humeral epiphysis. Accordingly, the potential for remodeling is great.[6] The normal proximal humerus growth plate is often mistaken for a fracture (Fig. 37–2). A comparison view of the uninjured shoulder may be helpful.

Salter–Harris type I and type II fractures of the proximal humerus are frequently encountered. Type I fractures and proximal metaphyseal injuries, including greenstick and torus fractures, occur in youngsters aged 5 to 11 years. Children of age 11 to 15 years suffer the majority of proximal humerus fractures, usually type II injuries. Most proximal humerus fractures are nondisplaced due to the presence of a strong periosteal sleeve. Salter–Harris fracture types III, IV, and V are rare in this region.[2]

Patients with proximal humerus fractures will have point tenderness at the fracture site and swelling or an obvious deformity. Routine radiographic evaluation should include at least two views of the humerus at right angles to each other. Films should include the distal clavicle and acromion to look for an associated injury.

Most fractures of the proximal humerus heal well with only a sling and swathe. The decision for closed reduction attempt or operative treatment depends on the age of the patient, the degree of angulation and the amount of displacement. The younger the child, the more likely the fracture will heal without intervention.

HUMERUS SHAFT FRACTURES

Proximal and distal humerus fractures are much more common than diaphyseal injuries. Most humeral shaft fractures are the result of a direct blow to the area. The degree of displacement depends on the location of the fracture and the surrounding muscle attachments, which may pull the fragments out of alignment. A torsional force from a fall or severe twist may result in a spiral diaphyseal fracture. Nonaccidental trauma should be considered in children younger than 3 years with a spiral humerus fracture.

Midshaft fractures heal well even with angulation of up to 15 to 20 degrees and as much as 2 cm of overriding, due

to bony remodeling and longitudinal overgrowth that occurs in response to the fracture. A sling and swathe should be applied to young children. A sugar-tong splint can be used for adolescents.

Fractures involving the junction of the middle and distal thirds of the humerus may be associated with injury to the radial nerve. Motor and sensory functions should be assessed initially and following any manipulation. Acute radial nerve palsy has an excellent long-term prognosis, with reports of 80% to 100% recovery of function.[7]

▶ THE ELBOW

With injury in the area of the elbow, radiographic interpretation is complicated by the presence of numerous epiphyses and ossification centers that appear and fuse at different, but characteristic ages (Table 37–1). Matters are further complicated by the need for precise anatomic reduction of fracture fragments in order to avoid both early and late complications.

If the patient is in severe pain, analgesics should be given before x-rays. An adequate radiographic evaluation of the elbow consists of an AP view with the joint in extension and a true lateral view with the elbow flexed at a right angle. Frequently, adequate pain control is needed to flex the elbow fully for a true lateral radiograph. The anterior fat pad is located within the coronoid fossa and normally appears as a small lucency just anterior to the fossa on a true lateral x-ray of the elbow (Fig. 37–3). A joint space fluid collection may also cause the anterior fat pad to be pushed away from the joint and appear as a wind-blown sail—the "sail sign." The posterior fat pad sits deep down in the olecranon fossa and is not visible under normal circumstances. The presence of a posterior fat pad on a true lateral view of the elbow is always abnormal and suggests blood within the joint capsule. These abnormal fat pad signs are radiographic evidence of occult fracture of the distal humerus, proximal ulna, or radius (Fig. 37–4) and can only be detected with the elbow fully flexed at 90 degrees.

There are two reference lines that are useful in assessing elbow radiographs and helping to identify occult injury. The anterior humeral line, drawn along the anterior cortex of the distal humerus on a true lateral view of the elbow, should normally intersect the middle third of the capitellum distally. Posterior displacement of the capitellum may be consistent with an otherwise radiographically inapparent supracondylar fracture. The radiocapitellar line is drawn down the axis of the proximal radius on the true lateral view of the elbow and should bisect the capitellum regardless of the degree of flexion or extension

▶ TABLE 37–1. GROWTH CENTERS OF THE ELBOW: AVERAGE AGE OF OSSIFICATION ONSET

Capitellum	11 mo
Medial epicondyle	4–6 y
Radial head	5–6 y
Olecranon	6–8 y
Trochlea	9–10 y
Lateral epicondyle	10–12 y

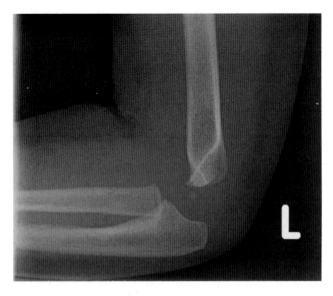

Figure 37–3. Normal elbow with thin anterior fat pad.

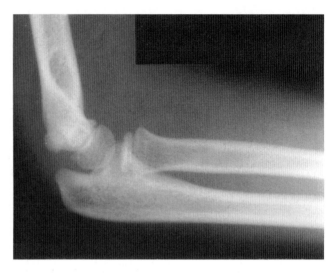

Figure 37–4. Note the posterior fat pad sign, signifying the presence of blood within the joint space.

present. Failure to do so suggests the presence of an occult radial neck fracture or radial head dislocation. Any question about the anatomic relationships can be further investigated using comparison views of the uninjured elbow.

► SUPRACONDYLAR HUMERUS FRACTURES

Supracondylar fractures account for 50% to 60% of all elbow fractures in children 3 to 10 years of age. A fall onto an outstretched hand causing violent hyperextension of the elbow is the usual mechanism of injury with supracondylar fractures of the distal humeral metaphysis. The olecranon process is forcibly thrust into the olecranon fossa, resulting in fracture

with posterior displacement of the distal fragment. On examination, there will be pain, swelling, deformity and functional impairment. A careful neurovascular examination is crucial to determine if there is an associated injury (Table 37–2). An AP and lateral radiograph should be obtained (Fig. 37–5). Oblique views may be useful to demonstrate occult fractures.[8]

Gartland distinguished three types of supracondylar fractures (Table 37–3).[9] Use of the anterior humeral line may be useful in determining whether the fracture is a type I or II (Fig. 37–5). Posterolateral type III fractures are more likely to damage the humeral artery or median nerve. Posteromedial type III fractures more commonly damage the radial nerve. Supracondylar humerus fractures are associated with a high incidence of early neurovascular complications (Fig. 37–6). Although puncture or actual laceration of the brachial artery

► TABLE 37–2. GUIDE TO UPPER EXTREMITY NEUROLOGIC EXAMINATION

Nerve	Muscle	Examination
Motor Function		
Radial	Extensor carpi radialis longus	Wrist extension
Ulnar	Flexor carpi ulnaris	Wrist flexion and adduction
Median	Interosseous	Finger spread
	Flexor carpi radialis	Wrist flexion and abduction
	Flexor digitorum profundus	Flexion of fingers at PIP
	Opponens pollicis	Opposition of thumb to little finger
Anterior inter-osseous	Flexor digitorum profundus	Flexion distal phalanx of index finger
Sensory		
Nerve	Sensory	
Radial	Dorsal web space between thumb and index finger	
Ulnar	Ulnar aspect palm and dorsum hand	
Median	Radial aspect palm and hand	
	Thumb, index, middle, radial aspect ring finger	

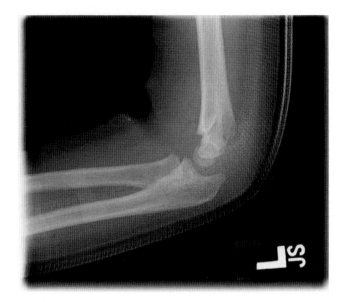

Figure 37–5. Type II supracondylar fracture. Notice the anterior humeral line that intersects the anterior portion of the capitellum.

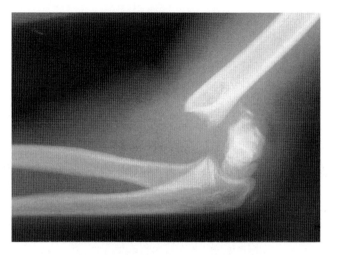

Figure 37–6. Comminuted supracondylar fracture with large joint effusion (Type III). The patient required fasciotomy and skin grafting due to neurovascular compromise.

are rare, the vessel may be compressed or contused or may undergo vasospasm at the fracture site. Signs of significant distal ischemia such as pallor and cyanosis of the fingers, prolonged capillary refill, or absence of the radial pulse indicate the need for prompt reduction of the fracture. If the vascular status is not improved, then surgical exploration is indicated. Patients are at risk of developing a forearm compartment syndrome. Unrecognized, this will lead to Volkmann's ischemic contracture and a nonfunctional hand and wrist. Forearm pain with passive flexion or extension of the fingers or distal parasthesias is an ominous early sign of compartment syndrome. Nerve impairment occurs in 10% to 20% of children with supracondylar fractures, yet the prognosis for return of function is good.[10] Radial, median, and ulnar nerve injuries, in descending order of frequency, have all been reported. A late complication of supracondylar humerus fractures is cubitus varus, a change in the carrying angle of the elbow.

The potential for significant complications with supracondylar humerus fractures mandates accurate diagnosis and urgent orthopedic consultation. Rotational and angular deformities must be meticulously reduced in order to preserve normal elbow function and prevent vascular compromise. Type I supracondylar fractures can be managed with casting but type II and III fractures require operative reduction and internal fixation. Most children are admitted for 24 to 48 hours of observation so that the neurovascular status of the extremity can

be reassessed frequently. Open reduction and internal fixation may be necessary.[11]

▶ THE MEDIAL AND LATERAL CONDYLES

Fractures involving the articular surface of the lateral condyle (capitellum) comprise 15% of all pediatric elbow fractures. The peak in incidence is at 6 years of age. The most likely mechanism of injury involves a fall on the outstretched arm with forearm supination or elbow flexion. Salter–Harris type IV fractures are common. The fracture fragment may become displaced and rotated, and the diagnosis is radiographically obvious if the ossified capitellum is notably displaced from the trochlea or radiocapitellar line. Clinically, swelling and tenderness are most pronounced at the lateral elbow. Although lateral condyle fractures are not usually associated with acute neurovascular injuries, they require aggressive intervention to prevent later complications such as nonunion, loss of elbow mobility, and growth arrest of the lateral condylar physis leading to eventual cubitus valgus and tardy ulnar palsy. Management is usually operative in all but nondisplaced fractures.

Fractures of the articular surface of the medial condyle, or trochlea, occur only rarely, but when present require precise anatomic reduction due to the intra-articular nature of the injury (Fig. 37–7). The most frequent complications associated with medial condylar fractures are nonunion and ulnar nerve neuropraxia.

▶ MEDIAL EPICONDYLAR FRACTURE

The epicondyles are located just proximal to the articulating surface of the distal humerus. The medial epicondyle is a traction apophysis to which the forearm flexors are attached. Fractures of the medial epicondyle are rarely encountered in children younger than 4 years, occurring most commonly in

▶ TABLE 37–3. SUPRACONDYLAR FRACTURE TYPES: DESCRIPTION

Type I	No displacement
Type II	Moderate displacement but contact between fragments remains
Type III	Complete displacement, fragments are not touching

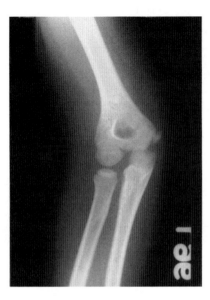

Figure 37–7. Nondisplaced fracture of the medial condyle in a 5-year-old.

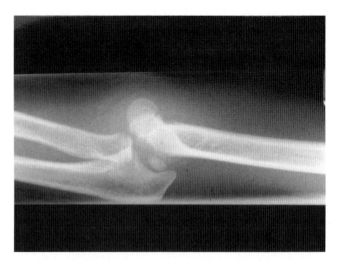

Figure 37–8. Posterior elbow dislocation with avulsion of the medial epicondyle.

children aged 7 to 15 years. These may occur as an avulsion injury due to a fall on the arm with forced hyperextension of the wrist and fingers. The vast majority of medial epicondylar fractures, however, are associated with elbow dislocations, occurring approximately 50% of the time (Fig. 37–7). The medial epicondyle may dislocate and then block reduction or become entrapped intra-articularly. The medial epicondyle *must* be identified as extra-articular after any elbow reduction. A more insidious injury to the medial epicondyle may occur with repetitive traction stress by the forearm flexors (Little Leaguer's elbow). Treatment is usually nonoperative, with severe displacement or ulnar nerve dysfunction considered relative indications for operative management.

► FRACTURE SEPARATION OF THE DISTAL HUMERAL PHYSIS

Although uncommon, this injury is important because of its association with nonaccidental trauma, such as with violent arm twisting. When present in children younger than 3 years, physical abuse should be suspected. The fracture can also occur following birth trauma. This injury is rare past age 3, after which supracondylar fractures predominate. Differentiation from elbow dislocation can be very difficult due to the lack of capitellar ossification. Orthopedic consultation is warranted, and closed reduction usually provides adequate healing.

► ELBOW DISLOCATIONS

Pediatric elbow dislocations occur infrequently, since most forces that would result in dislocations in adults usually cause fractures in children (Fig. 37–8). When elbow dislocations do occur, they are usually the result of a fall onto the slightly flexed, outstretched arm in an adolescent. As with adults, most dislocations are posterior.

Associated fractures are the rule and most commonly involve fracture of the medial epicondyle, coronoid process, radial head, or olecranon. Significant damage to the surrounding soft tissues also occurs, with damage to the neighboring nerves more common than brachial artery injury. Recovery of function of the ulnar nerve can be expected, but the prognosis is less optimistic with median nerve injury. Vascular compromise complicates up to 7% of pediatric elbow dislocations.[12]

Most dislocations can be reduced after providing adequate analgesia and muscle relaxation. The elbow should be flexed to 60 to 70 degrees and the forearm placed in supination. The proximal humerus is then stabilized by an assistant while longitudinal traction is applied at the wrist. Upon successful reduction, the elbow should be gently flexed and immobilized and the neurovascular status of the arm reappraised. A postreduction radiograph should be obtained with attention to verifying the location of the medial epicondyle as extra-articular.

► RADIAL HEAD SUBLUXATION

This most common pediatric elbow injury is called "nursemaid's elbow" or "pulled elbow." It occurs when abrupt axial traction is applied to the wrist or hand of the extended, pronated forearm of a child younger than 5 years, causing the annular ligament to slip free of the radial head and become entrapped between the radial head and capitellum. Left-sided injuries occur more commonly because of traction by predominantly right-handed adults walking at the child's side.[13]

A history of the patient being lifted by the arm may be obtained, but the precipitating event is often neither witnessed nor recognized. On presentation, the child appears comfortable yet refuses to reach for objects with the affected arm. On examination, the forearm is held in pronation with the elbow in slight flexion or fully extended. There is a remarkable lack of swelling and only mild tenderness over the radial head. The child resists all attempts at passive range of motion. Pain is worse with supination or pronation. Radiographic evaluation is not necessary in the presence of a clear history of precipitating arm traction. Figure 37–9 shows a useful algorithm for

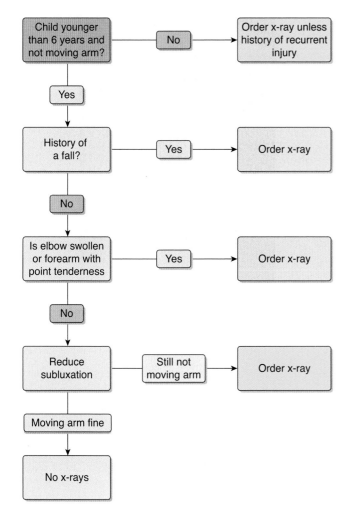

Figure 37–9. Algorithm for ordering radiographs in suspected radial head subluxation.

determining whether radiographs should be obtained prior to reduction. A key point is that if there is swelling present or a history of a fall, radiographs should be obtained. A nursemaid's elbow will not have appreciable swelling on examination.

There are two methods of reduction, supination and pronation. In the supination method, face the patient, place your thumb over the radial head, and place your opposite hand around the wrist. The forearm is supinated and flexed at the elbow. In the pronation method, the arm is extended at the elbow, a finger is placed over the radial head, and the forearm is pronated. A palpable or audible "pop" usually signals successful reduction. If the supination method does not work, one should try pronation. The pronation method may be less painful.[14] Typically, the patient again reaches for objects with the affected arm within 5 to 10 minutes of reduction. Offering a Popsicle may hasten recovery after successful reduction. No further treatment is necessary. If radiographs are obtained, the child often returns with normal arm movement after active positioning and inadvertent reduction by the technologist. The parents should be instructed not to lift their children by the wrists and informed about recurrence as it may be as high as 30%.

Several attempts at reduction may be necessary before the patient resumes normal use of the arm. Occasionally, radial traction prior to supination and flexion is necessary. If the subluxation occurred several hours earlier, it may be longer before normal function of the arm is observed. If normal use does not follow reduction attempts, alternative diagnoses should be considered. Immobilization with prompt orthopedic follow-up is indicated.

► FRACTURES OF THE RADIUS AND ULNA

The clavicle is the only bone broken more frequently than the radius and ulna during childhood. Three-quarters of all injuries involve the distal third of the forearm. Although an isolated fracture of one of the bones can occur, a high index of suspicion must be maintained for concomitant injury to the paired bone. The force precipitating a readily apparent injury may be transmitted to the paired bone and result in bowing, a greenstick fracture, or dislocation at a location distant from the obvious fracture site. For this reason, forearm x-rays should always include the wrist and elbow. Most fractures of the radius and ulna heal without significant complications.

► PROXIMAL RADIUS AND ULNA FRACTURES

A fall onto an extended, supinated arm with a valgus stress can result in fracture of the radial head or neck. Most proximal radius fractures in young children involve the narrow metaphyseal neck since the head is cartilaginous until ossification begins at age 5 years. Salter–Harris type I and type II radial neck fractures are most common. Salter–Harris type IV radial head fractures may be encountered in older children. Proximal radius fractures can occur in conjunction with elbow dislocations and are often associated with concomitant injury to the medial epicondyle, olecranon, and coronoid process.

An abnormal fat pad sign or abnormal radiocapitellar line on x-ray points to the presence of an occult radial head or radial neck fracture. Minimally, displaced or nondisplaced fractures can be treated in a posterior splint with the elbow flexed at 90 degrees. Complications include restriction of pronation and supination, as well as myositis ossificans.

Olecranon fractures occur commonly in combination with other elbow injuries, such as radial head dislocations, radial neck fractures, and fractures of the medial epicondyle. Isolated olecranon epiphyseal fractures are rare and are usually due to a direct blow to the posterior elbow. Nondisplaced injuries may be treated in a posterior splint. Healing usually takes place without complications, although nonunion and ulnar nerve neuropraxia do occur infrequently.

► DIAPHYSEAL RADIUS AND ULNA FRACTURES

Most forearm diaphyseal fractures are either greenstick or bowing injuries. Both bones may suffer greenstick or bowing injuries, or one bone may have a greenstick fracture while the

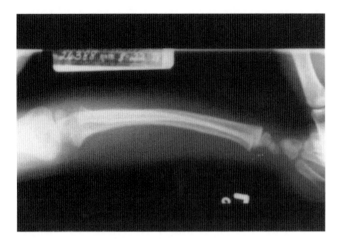

Figure 37–10. Radiographic appearance of midshaft bowing injury of both the radius and ulna.

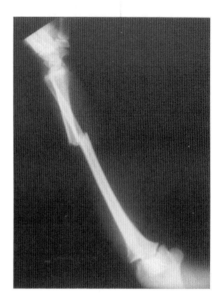

Figure 37–12. Galeazzi fracture in a 16-year-old.

paired bone is bowed (Fig. 37–10). The potential for remodeling of a bowing injury, or plastic deformation, is minimal in children older than 4 years. Bowing may restrict pronation and supination as well as result in permanent deformity of the extremity.

Overriding of fracture fragments in the presence of an isolated fracture of one of the forearm bones suggests either a Monteggia or Galeazzi fracture. An isolated fracture of the proximal ulna may be associated with concomitant dislocation of the radial head (Monteggia fracture). This combined injury may be inadvertently overlooked initially because attention is focused on the obvious ulnar fracture. An aberrant radiocapitellar line on plain x-ray is evidence of the accompanying radial head dislocation (Fig. 37–11). Closed reduction is usually successful. A fracture at the junction of the middle and distal thirds of the radius in association with distal radioul-

nar joint dislocation is called a Galeazzi fracture and is rare in children (Fig. 37–12).[15]

► DISTAL RADIUS AND ULNA FRACTURES

Fractures of the distal third of the radius and ulna are among the most common orthopedic injuries in children 6 to 12 years of age, often occurring after a fall onto an outstretched hand. There is a peak incidence in boys aged 12 to 14 years and girls aged 10 to 12 years. Torus fractures of the distal radius and ulna are frequently encountered and can be treated in a removable splint (Fig. 37–13).[16] These fractures can often be very subtle. One should have a high index of suspicion for a radius fracture when the patient has point tenderness over the distal radius.

The distal radial physis accounts for almost 80% of the longitudinal growth of the radius, but significant growth

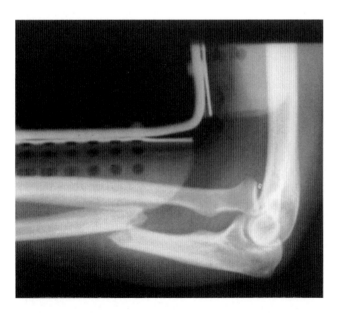

Figure 37–11. Fracture of the proximal ulna with radial head dislocation (Monteggia fracture). A line bisecting the proximal radius completely misses the capitellum.

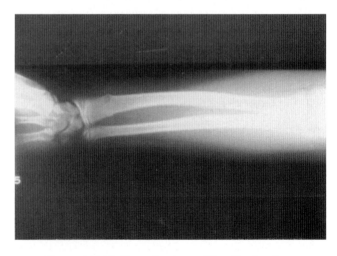

Figure 37–13. Torus fracture of the distal radius.

disturbance secondary to injury rarely occurs. Tenderness over the physis of the distal radius with a normal radiograph suggests nondisplaced Salter–Harris type I injury, and splinting with orthopedic follow-up is appropriate.

The capacity for angular remodeling after forearm fracture is great, but rotational remodeling does not occur and rotational abnormalities must be accurately corrected. The strong periosteal sleeve of the bones makes nonunion rare. Complications are uncommon, but vascular compromise or compartment syndrome can develop with any forearm fracture.[15]

HAND AND WRIST INJURIES

Pediatric hand injuries resulting in fractures occur less frequently in children than in adults. In younger children, the most common mechanism is to get the hand caught in a closing door resulting in a crush injury to the distal phalanxes. Approximately 25% of such injuries result in fractures. Amputations and tendon injuries are found occasionally. In the older age groups, injuries tend to occur as a result of athletic competition. Hand and wrist injuries occur in 3% to 9% of all sports injuries. Sprains are the most common, followed by contusions and fractures. Commonly encountered injuries include radius fractures, ligamentous injuries to the wrist and fingers, dislocations of the metacarpophalangeal (MCP), proxymal interphalangeal (PIP) and distal interphalangeal (DIP) joints.

Pediatric hand fractures represent 5% to 7% of all pediatric fractures. These injuries are sometimes difficult to diagnose and may be associated with long-term morbidity. This makes appropriate initial evaluation and treatment imperative. Fortunately, healing is rapid, tendon and joint complications are rare, and their ability to remodel is remarkable.

▶ PHYSICAL EXAMINATION

OBSERVATION

The physical examination of the hand begins with observation. One should look for lacerations, puncture wounds, soft-tissue swelling, deformity, and color. The resting hand should demonstrate increasing flexion from the index through little finger and increasing flexion of the joints, from the DIP through MCP joints. Disruption of this normal cascade implies a laceration to an extensor or flexor tendon. A complete flexor tendon laceration results in straightening of the finger due to the unopposed extensors. A complete extensor tendon laceration results in flexion of the finger due to the unopposed flexors.

Malrotation as a result of a phalangeal or metacarpal fracture will occasionally occur. Alignment may appear normal in extension but be grossly abnormal with the fingers flexed. Malrotation may lead to significant cosmetic and functional impairment, so the diagnosis should be made on initial presentation to avoid permanent disability. A useful method to test for malrotation is to have the patient alternately flex the fingers to the palm. Each finger converges to the same place on the palm, the tubercle of the scaphoid. Patients with significant malrotation will violate this pattern with the affected finger. Another method is to compare the planes of the fingernails with the fingers in flexion. The nail plates should be

approximately parallel and symmetric to the opposite hand. Any abnormal tilting is evidence of a rotational deformity.

PALPATION

Gently performed palpation of the injured hand can give significant information. This must be performed delicately since the pediatric patient is likely to be afraid and unwilling to allow examination freely. The examination should be performed with the patient's hand resting comfortably on a flat surface. One may use a fingertip or an object such as the eraser end of a pencil or the end of a cotton-tipped applicator to find the exact area of maximal tenderness. Maximal tenderness over the radial or ulnar aspect of an interphalangeal joint indicates a collateral ligament tear. Tenderness over the volar aspect of an interphalangeal joint indicates volar plate injury. Tenderness over the ulnar aspect of the thumb MCP joint indicates a gamekeeper's thumb (torn ulnar collateral ligament of the thumb). Pain elicited with palpation over the anatomic snuffbox is presumptive evidence for a scaphoid fracture.

CIRCULATION

Circulation is best assessed by observing color, testing for capillary refill, and determining skin temperature. A cyanotic, edematous hand indicates venous insufficiency. A pale cool hand or a finger with poor capillary filling indicates arterial insufficiency. Doppler ultrasound or an Allen test may determine adequacy or circulation. Brisk arterial bleeding can be managed by pressure. Blindly clamping arterial bleeders may cause further harm by damaging nerves, arteries, tendons, and muscle. Arterial bleeding from a volar laceration implies laceration of the digital nerve since these nerves are located superficial to the artery.

SENSATION

Sensation in the cooperative patient is best tested by two-point discrimination. Each digital nerve is alternately tested. This may be performed with a bent paper clip gently touching the tip of the finger along the longitudinal axis. The distance between the tips of the paper clip begins at 1 cm and is then made closer until the patient can no longer recognize one from two points. Normal two-point discrimination is 3 to 5 mm. In children too young or too afraid to cooperate, two other methods of sensory testing have been reported: loss of skin wrinkling and loss of sweating. After the hand is soaked in warm water for 30 minutes, the skin wrinkling usually seen is lost after digital nerve injury. Skin sweating is responsible for the "tackiness" of the fingertips and relies on intact sympathetic innervation. Following digital nerve injury, the ability to sweat is lost, and the skin takes on a smooth, silky texture. This may be tested by moving a smooth object, such as the barrel of a pen, over the fingertip. In the injured finger the barrel will move smoothly; in the normal finger there will be resistance. Even under the best of circumstances, such testing will be challenging in the emergency department. As always, a high index of suspicion is required for successful diagnosis.

MOTOR

The ulnar nerve is tested by having the patient abduct the index finger against resistance while palpating the first dorsal interosseus muscle. The median nerve is tested by having the patient palmar abduct the thumb against resistance while the examiner palpates the belly of the abductor pollicis brevis muscle, located on the radial aspect of the thenar eminence. The radial nerve is tested by having the patient extend the fingers and wrist against resistance. The anterior interosseous nerve (a branch of the median nerve) is evaluated by flexion of the distal phalanx of the index finger.

TENDON

Examination of the hand for tendon injury is particularly difficult in small children. The child's pain, anxiety, and unwillingness to cooperate, as well as partial tendon lacerations, all conspire to thwart the unwary examiner. The flexor digitorum profundus is tested by immobilizing the PIP and MCP joints and allowing the patient to flex the DIP joint against resistance. The flexor pollicis longus is tested by immobilizing the MCP joint of the thumb and allowing the patient to flex the interphalangeal (IP) joint. The flexor digitorum superficialis is tested by immobilizing the MCP joint and allowing the patient to flex the PIP joint against resistance. This test does not work for the index finger since the flexor digitorum profundus cannot be immobilized. To test the index finger, have the patient hyperextend the DIP joint with force against the thumb (thumb index pinch). If the patient is able to do this, the superficialis is intact. Patients with a superficialis laceration will not be able to hyperextend the DIP joint but will accomplish pinch by flexion of the DIP joint. The flexor carpi radialis is tested by flexion and radially deviation of the wrist against resistance. The flexor carpi ulnaris is tested by flexion and ulnar deviation of the wrist against resistance.

Since evaluating young patients is difficult, depending on age and willingness to cooperate, other tests may be required to determine tendon function. With the elbow resting on the table, allow the wrist to naturally fall into flexion. It is noted that the fingers fall into extension. When the wrist is relaxed in extension, the fingers fall into the normal cascade of flex-

▶ **TABLE 37–4. FLEXOR TENDONS OF THE HAND AND WRIST**

Tendon	Test of Function
Flexor digitorum superficialis	Hold MCP in neutral and flex PIP
Flexor digitorum profundus	Hold MCP and PIP in neutral and flex DIP
Flexor carpi radialis	Flex and radially deviate wrist
Flexor carpi ulnaris	Flex and ulnarly deviate wrist
Extensor digitorum communis	Extension of the fingers at the MCP joints
Flexor pollicis longus	Hold MCP straight, flex thumb across palm
Palmaris longus	No specific test

ion. This normal flexion and extension of the fingers relies on an intact tendon system. Another method to assess the flexor tendons is palpation of the forearm to create passive motion of the fingers. This is performed by pressing or squeezing the forearm at the junction of the middle and distal thirds on the ulnar–volar surface. This will cause flexion of the fingers, especially the three ulnar fingers. A similar test can be performed for the flexor pollicis longus by pressing on the distal forearm on the midvolar aspect. An intact flexor pollicis longus will result in flexion of the interphalangeal joint of the thumb. It is essential to know the normal muscle, tendon, and nerve anatomy to recognize injuries and arrange appropriate referrals. The flexor tendons and associated function are listed in Table 37–4. The extensor tendons are tested as described in Table 37–5. Note that the extensor tendons are divided into six different compartments.

RADIOGRAPHS

Oblique views of the fingers should be obtained along with the standard AP and lateral views of the hand. The epiphyses of the phalanxes and first metacarpal are located proximally. The epiphyses of the rest of the metacarpals are distal. Accessory bones should not be confused as fractures. In the lateral view,

▶ **TABLE 37–5. EXTENSOR TENDONS OF THE HAND**

Compartmend	Tendon	Test of Function
First	Abductor pollicis longus	Extension and abduction of the thumb
	Extensor pollicis brevis	Extension and abduction of the thumb
Second	Extensor carpi radialis longus and extensor carpi radialis brevis	Making fist while extending the wrist
Third	Extensor pollicis longus	Lifting the thumb off the surface of the table while the palm is flat on the table
Fourth	Extensor digitorum communis	Extension of the fingers at the MCP joints
	Extensor indicis proprius	Extension of the index finger at the MCP joint with the hand in a fist
Fifth	Extensor digiti minimi	Extension of the little finger while making a fist
Sixth	Extensor carpi ulnaris	Extension and ulnar deviation of the wrist

each finger should have more flexion than the next to avoid overlapping of finger images. A scaphoid or navicular view elongates the profile of the scaphoid and may improve fracture identification.

► FRACTURES OF THE PHALANGES

DISTAL PHALANX

Pediatric distal phalanx fractures are either a crush or hyperextension injuries. Crush injuries are quite common, usually resulting from entrapment in a closing door. In these injuries, the soft-tissue damage is more significant than the orthopedic injury. Wound care must be meticulous, the nail bed approximated with absorbable suture, and the finger splinted. Some authors recommend replacing the nail plate in the nail fold; however there is no evidence yet to suggest that this improves outcome. There is often an associated tuft fracture associated with nail bed injuries (Fig. 37–14). Some authors recommend prophylactic antibiotics when a tuft fracture is accompanied by a nail bed laceration but there is no evidence to suggest that there is a difference in outcome (see Chapter 39).

A hyperflexion force applied to the tip of the finger may result in one of two types of pediatric injuries (Fig. 37–15). In the preadolescent, a Salter–Harris type I or II fracture occurs with a mallet deformity. A mallet finger is the result of an avul-

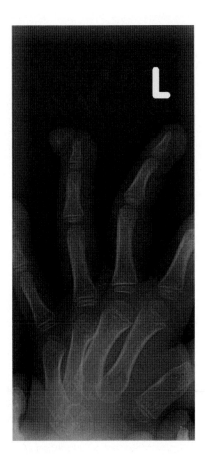

Figure 37–14. Partial finger tip amputation and tuft fracture.

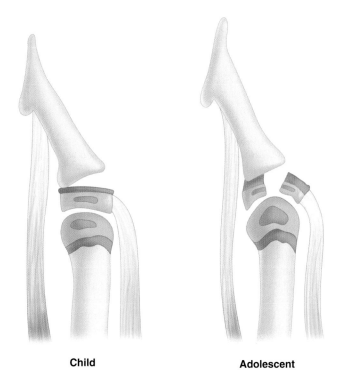

Child   **Adolescent**

Figure 37–15. Mallet injuries are caused by avulsion of the extensor tendon from the distal phalanx or from a fracture of the dorsal base of the distal phalanx. An extension lag at the DIP joint is present, and the patient is unable to actively extend the DIP joint. In children, a Salter–Harris type I or II fracture is seen. In the adolescent, a Salter–Harris type III fracture occurs. These fractures may be difficult to detect radiographically since the epiphysis is not fully ossified in children. Inability to actively extend the DIP joint and a mallet deformity reveal the extent of injury.

sion of the extensor tendon from the base of the distal phalanx. If a child has a mallet finger and inability to extend the distal phalanx, this injury should be assumed even if a fracture cannot be identified on radiographs. In the adolescent hyperflexion injury, a displaced Salter–Harris type III fracture occurs. These injuries are treated by wound care, closed reduction, and splinting in slight hyperextension. If adequate reduction is not obtained, then open reduction and Kirschner-wire fixation is performed. It is important to recognize the mallet deformity present in both of these injuries and treat and refer appropriately.[17]

MIDDLE AND PROXIMAL PHALANX

Middle and proximal phalangeal fractures commonly occur at the physis. These fractures are usually Salter–Harris type II fractures. They are reduced by flexion of the MCP joint and adduction of the finger. The wrist is placed in an ulnar gutter splint, and the patient is referred to an orthopedist. Salter–Harris type III fractures are ligament or tendon avulsion injuries. Displaced fractures usually require Kirschner-wire fixation. Fractures of the phalangeal shaft are not common in children. These fractures are usually minimally displaced. Splinting and referral is all that is necessary. Displaced fractures of the shaft or neck require splinting and acute referral.

▶ METACARPAL FRACTURES

Metacarpal fractures may occur in the epiphysis, physis, neck, shaft, or base. The neck is the most common area to be fractured. A displaced intra-articular fracture of the base of the thumb metacarpal, equivalent to the adult Bennett's fracture, is rare in children. These fractures are unstable Salter–Harris type III fractures and are treated by open reduction and Kirschner-wire fixation. Most other metacarpal fractures are undisplaced or minimally displaced and are treated initially by splint immobilization. Displaced fractures can generally be treated with closed reduction and splinting, but occasionally Kirschner-wire fixation is required.

The most common hand fracture is of the fifth metacarpal.[18] Typically, it results from an upset adolescent male striking someone or a solid object with a closed fist (Boxer's fracture). Closed reduction is indicated if there is more than 30 to 40 degrees of angulation. These fractures can be treated with an ulnar gutter splint with orthopedic referral.[17]

▶ CARPAL FRACTURES

Fractures of the carpal bones in children are exceedingly rare. The carpus is surrounded by cartilage that acts as a "shock absorber." Fractures are more likely to occur in the distal radius and ulna. Diagnosis of a carpal fractures can be difficult because of their rarity and obscurity with initial radiographs. Nafie found that 37% of carpal fractures were not seen on initial radiographs.[19] Scaphoid fractures are the most commonly encountered of the carpal bone fractures. The ossification center of the scaphoid appears by age 5 to 6 years. In the pediatric population, the peak age of scaphoid fractures is in early adolescence. The usual mechanism of injury is a fall on an outstretched hand. Physical examination may reveal limitation of range of motion from pain and swelling and tenderness in the "anatomic snuffbox." As in the adult, initial x-rays often appear normal. In a child with this presentation, application of a short-arm thumb spica splint with orthopedic referral is appropriate. Nonunion and avascular necrosis is rare in children because most injuries are avulsions or nondisplaced fractures through the distal third of the bone rather than fractures through the waist, as in adults. Other carpal bone fractures are very rare in children and are treated as in adults with splinting and orthopedic referral.[20]

▶ DISLOCATIONS

DISTAL INTERPHALANGEAL JOINT

DIP dislocations result from a hyperextension force. This dislocation generally displaces dorsally and is often open, due to the tight adherence of skin to bone in this area. Reduction is usually uncomplicated and consists of traction countertraction followed by flexion. Test active motion to ensure that the extensor and flexor tendons are functioning and that the volar plate is not interposed in the joint.

PROXIMAL INTERPHALANGEAL JOINT

PIP dislocations can occur in dorsal, volar, radial, or ulnar directions. Dorsal dislocations are the most common. These dislocations occur as a result of an axial load with concomitant hyperextension. Reduction is accomplished through slight hyperextension and longitudinal traction applied to the middle phalanx while correcting the ulnar or radial deformity. The finger is then gently flexed into position. Active range of motion is tested, and stress testing of the collateral ligaments and volar plate is performed. The finger is placed in a splint immobilizing the PIP (20–30 degrees of flexion) and MCP joints (60–70 degrees of flexion). Orthopedic referral is recommended. Volar dislocations are rare and may be irreducible due to entrapment of the proximal phalangeal condyle between the central tendon and lateral band. These dislocations may result in avulsion of the central slip of the extensor tendon leading to a late boutonnière deformity. Orthopedic referral is required.[17]

METACARPOPHALANGEAL JOINT

MCP joint dislocations sometimes occur in the pediatric age group. As in the adult, the thumb MCP dislocation is the most common (Fig. 37–16). It occurs as a result of a hyperextension

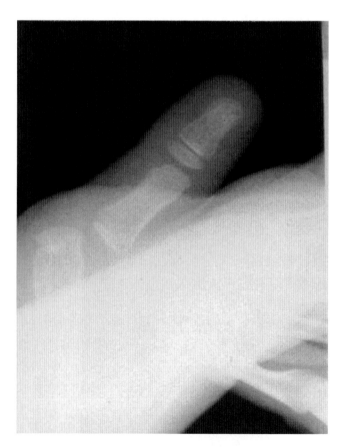

Figure 37–16. Carpometacarpal dislocation of the thumb.

force, usually from a fall on an outstretched hand. Dislocations may be simple reducible or complex irreducible. In the simple reducible dislocation, the proximal phalanx assumes a dorsal point at a 90-degree angle to the metacarpal. This dislocation can be reduced by gentle traction countertraction. Joint stability is assessed, the finger splinted, and the patient referred. The complex irreducible dislocation has the same mechanism of injury, but here, the proximal phalanx assumes a bayonet position parallel to the metacarpal. The volar plate is interposed in the joint, and the metacarpal head may also be trapped in the substance of the intrinsic muscles. Closed reduction is impossible. This dislocation can only be reduced by open reduction. Some authors recommend one attempt at gently performed closed reduction. Vigorous traction is to be avoided since this may convert a simple reducible dislocation to a complex irreducible one.

CARPOMETACARPAL JOINT

Carpometacarpal dislocations are rare in the pediatric age group. These injuries are generally a result of violent trauma that results in multiple dislocations or multiple fracture dislocations. These injuries require prompt orthopedic consultation for surgical intervention.

REFERENCES

1. Landin LA. Fracture patterns in children: analysis of 8682 fractures with special reference to incidence, etiology, and secular changes in Swedish urban populations. *Acta Orthop Scan.* 1982;54(suppl):1–109.
2. Bishop JY, Flatow EL. Pediatric shoulder trauma. *Clin Orthop.* 2005;432:41–48.
3. Shuster M, Agu-Laban RB, Boyd J, et al. Prospective evaluation of clinical assessment in the diagnosis and treatment of clavicle fracture: are radiographs really necessary? *Can J Emerg Med.* 2003;5:309–313.
4. Oppenheim WL, Davis A, Growden WA, et al. Clavicle fractures in the newborn. *Clin Orthop.* 1990;250:176–180.
5. Rogovik AL, Hussain S, Goldman RD. Physician pain reminder as an intervention to enhance analgesia for extremity and clavicle injury in pediatric emergency. *J Pain.* 2007;8:26–32.
6. Dameron TB Jr, Reibel DB. Fractures involving the proximal epiphyseal plate. *J Bone Joint Surg.* 1969;51:289–297.
7. Caviglia H, Garrido CP, Palazzi FF, et al. Pediatric fractures of the humerus. *Clin Orthop.* 2005;432:49–56.
8. Heras J, Duran D, de la Cerda J, et al. Supracondylar fractures of the humerus in children. *Clin Orthod Res.* 2005;432:57–64.
9. Gartland JJ. Management of supracondylar fractures in children. *Clin Orthod Res.* 1959;109:145–154.
10. Lyons ST, Quinn M, Stantski CL. Neurovascular injuries in type III humeral supracondylar fractures in children. *Clin Orthop.* 2000;376:62–67.
11. Shrader AW. Pediatric supracondylar fractures and pediatric physeal elbow fractures. *Orthop Clin North Am.* 2008;39:163–171.
12. Carson S, Woolridge DP, Colletti J, et al. Pediatric upper extremity injuries. *Pediatr Clin North Am.* 2006;53:41–67.
13. Schunk JE. Radial head subluxations: epidemiology and treatment of 87 episodes. *Ann Emerg Med.* 1990;19:1019.
14. Green DA, Linares MY, Garcia Pena MB, et al. Randomized comparison of pain perception during radial head subluxation reduction using supination-flexion or forced pronation. *Pediatr Emerg Care.* 2006;22:235–238.
15. Rodriguez-Merchan EC. Pediatric fractures of the forearm. *Clin Orthod Res.* 2005;432:65–72.
16. Plint AC, Perry JJ, Correll R, et al. A randomized trial of removable splinting versus casting for wrist buckle fractures in children. *Pediatrics.* 2006;117:691–697.
17. Valencia J, Leyva F, Gomez-Bajo GJ. Pediatric hand trauma. *Clin Orthop.* 2005;432:77–86.
18. Mahabir RC, Kazemi AR, Cannon WG, et al. Pediatric hand fractures: a review. *Pediatr Emerg Care.* 2001;17:153–156.
19. Nafie SA. Fractures of the carpal bone in children. *Injury.* 1987;18:117–119.
20. Goddard N. Carpal fractures in children. *Clin Orthop.* 2005;432:73–76.

CHAPTER 38

Injuries of the Pelvis and Lower Extremities

Greg Canty

▶ HIGH-YIELD FACTS

- Unstable pelvic fractures are present when there are multiple breaks in the pelvic ring. Suspect visceral injuries because of high-kinetic energy trauma.
- Reduction of a hip dislocation should take place prior to 12 hours after the injury. Complications include avascular necrosis (AVN) of the femoral head, degenerative arthritis, and sciatic nerve injury.
- Slipped capital femoral epiphysis (SCFE) is a disruption of the capital femoral physis that can occur over time. It is most common in overweight adolescent males and is diagnosed on the anteroposterior or frog-leg view of the pelvis.
- Legg-Calvé-Perthes disease is an idiopathic AVN of the femoral head that is most common in Caucasian children between 4 and 9 years of age. Radiographs demonstrate a small femoral head and epiphyseal collapse as a result of avascular necrosis.
- A spiral femur fracture in a nonambulatory infant or child suggests child abuse.
- Distal femoral epiphyseal fractures in children are significant because they can cause growth disturbances in the lower extremity.
- Ligamentous injuries of the knee are less likely to occur than are epiphyseal injuries. Proximal tibial epiphysis fractures can be significant because they can cause vascular compromise and growth disturbances.
- Spiral tibial shaft fractures are common in children because of twisting injuries and are termed toddler's fracture in those just learning to walk.
- Fibular head fractures can occur as a result of motor vehicle bumper injury in children. In order to exclude a significant peroneal nerve injury, make sure there is no foot drop of the affected extremity (loss of dorsiflexion).
- When examining the child with ankle pain, exclude injuries of the calcaneus, proximal fibula, and base of the fifth metatarsal.
- The most common fracture of the talus is in the neck, which occurs from forced dorsiflexion. This injury is often complicated by avascular necrosis.
- Midfoot fractures are rare because of the strong fibrous tissues that surround these bones, and are difficult to detect because of the irregularities of these bones. Lisfranc's fracture occurs at the base of the second metatarsal, where the stability of the midfoot is maintained.

- The Jones' fracture is a metatarsal neck fracture distal to the apophysis of the base of the fifth metatarsal. Although the apophysis of the fifth metatarsal runs parallel to the axis of the metatarsal shaft, fractures most often are perpendicular to the axis of the metatarsal shaft.

▶ PELVIC FRACTURES

Fractures of the pelvis are quite rare in children. In contrast to the brittle, adult pelvis, the young pelvis is protected by growing bone and a tremendous amount of cartilage. As a result of this pliability, the young pelvis can absorb tremendous amounts of energy before fracturing. Pelvic fractures in children usually result from high-energy trauma such as automobiles versus pedestrians, motor vehicle crashes, or significant falls. Pelvic fractures are classified depending on their involvement of the pelvic ring, the acetabulum, or one of the apophyses (avulsions). The violent forces necessary to cause pelvic fractures in children often result in multisystem trauma with a combination of head injuries, visceral organ damage, limb fractures, urogential injuries, vascular damage, and hematomas. Mortality and morbidity rates following pelvic fractures in children are much better than those seen in adults. Accompanying injuries usually pose the greatest risks to mortality and morbidity when dealing with pediatric pelvic fractures. The most pressing issue in the emergency department (ED) is to recognize and stabilize any accompanying injuries.[1]

Pelvic ring fractures are classified as either stable or unstable. Stable injuries include single breaks in the pelvic ring, diastasis of the pubic symphysis, and fractures of the iliac wings. Unstable injuries include those with two breaks inside the pelvic ring (Fig. 38–1) or those having a sacroiliac dislocation/fracture with an associated rami or pubic symphysis fracture. Stable fractures can be successfully managed nonoperatively. Unstable fractures always result from very high-energy trauma, and are usually accompanied by other severe injuries. Unstable fracture patterns may require external fixation or open reduction/internal fixation to stabilize the injury and allow better management of the accompanying injuries.

Fractures of the acetabulum are very rare in children, and almost all are associated with a hip dislocation. Dislocations of the hip may still be evident in the ED, or they may spontaneously reduce before presentation. The acetabulum will usually fracture where the triradiate cartilage meets the pelvis

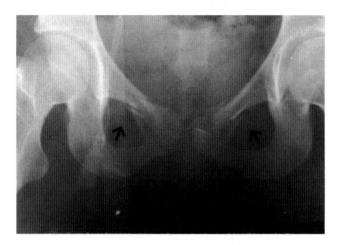

Figure 38–1. Bilateral pelvic rami fractures which are unstable and at high risk for accompanying visceral injuries.

(Fig. 38–2). Like pelvic ring fractures, these injuries are also associated with high-energy trauma. If the acetabular fracture is associated with a pelvic ring fracture, it is considered an unstable fracture like those discussed above.

Avulsion fractures of the pelvis are not associated with high-energy trauma, but are associated with adolescents playing sports (Fig. 38–3). These fractures occur when a muscle suddenly contracts against the resistance of a pelvic apophysis. Classic avulsion fractures and their associated attachments are the iliac crest (tensor fascia), anterior inferior iliac spine (rectus femoris), anterior superior iliac spine (sartorius), and the ischium (hamstrings). Avulsion fractures are not accompanied by multiple injuries and can usually be treated nonoperatively.

Evaluating any pelvic injury begins with identifying the mechanism (trauma, sports, etc.) followed by close inspection for any asymmetry, ecchymosis, or abrasions to the pelvis. Pain or crepitus elicited by compressing the iliac crests or by putting direct pressure on the pubic symphisis indicates a likely pelvic

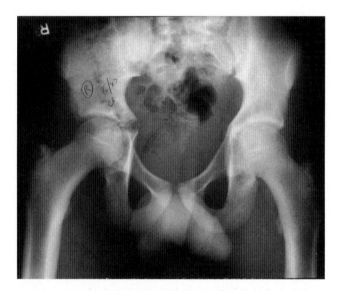

Figure 38–2. Fracture of the right acetabulum through the triradiate cartilage with a high risk for skeletal deformity. CT scans of the hip may be beneficial to assess joint stability.

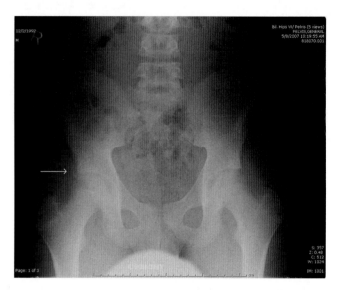

Figure 38–3. Right anterior inferior iliac spine (AIIS) avulsion fracture in a young track and field athlete. There also appears to be a previous injury to the ischial apophysis.

ring or acetabular fracture. Avulsions are point tender over the suspected apophysis, so the iliac crests, iliac spine, and ischium should be directly palpated. Because of the large number of multiple injuries with pelvic fractures, a thorough physical examination should follow with special attention to the abdomen, urogenitals, and rectum. AP radiographs of the pelvis are part of most trauma protocols, but many trauma patients are also getting abdominopelvic CT scans. The CT scan is more sensitive for detecting pelvic fractures, and the radiograph may be omitted when abdominopelvic scans are indicated.[2] Patients without CT scans who need better evaluation of possible ring fractures should get inlet/outlet views at 45 degrees. When a lateral view is desired, the cross-table lateral is preferred over the frog-leg because further displacement is a risk.

Pelvic fractures in children usually have good outcomes with conservative, nonsurgical management. Morbidity is closely related to the number and severity of accompanying injuries. Management in the ED focuses on stabilization of any associated injuries and controlling any signs of hemorrhage. Orthopedics should be consulted emergently if the fracture is open, unstable, or hemorrhaging is difficult to control. Orthopedics may elect to place an external fixator for temporary stabilization. Unstable fractures may be initially managed with bed rest in younger children, but most adolescents will need open reduction and internal fixation. Stable fractures of the pelvis can be treated with bed rest and non-weight-bearing for 4 to 6 weeks. Avulsion fractures heal well with protected weight bearing for 4 to 6 weeks, progressing from non-weight-bearing to partial-weight-bearing to gradual activities. Widely separated avulsions may need surgical fixation, but most can be successfully treated with conservative management.[3]

▶ HIP DISLOCATIONS

Dislocations of the hip are rare events in pediatrics and account for less than 5% of dislocations. Unlike in adults, the forces required for dislocation in young children are less violent because of their increased joint laxity and the shallow, nonossified acetabulum. The mechanism in younger children can be trivial falls or sporting injuries. Once the acetabulum deepens and ossifies during adolescence, much stronger forces are required to dislocate the hip. Most dislocations are posterior with the resulting leg shortened, flexed at the hip, and internally rotated. Anterior and obturator dislocations occur much less frequently. Dislocations may be complicated by fractures of the acetabulum or proximal femur.

Most hip dislocations present to the ED with severe discomfort, a shortened leg, a flexed hip, and internal rotation. Dislocations that spontaneously reduce before ED presentation are more challenging, but should be considered following any significant hip injury. After a thorough examination of the pulses and neurologic function in the lower extremity, an AP radiograph of the pelvis is needed to confirm hip dislocation. The radiograph must be reviewed closely for asymmetric joint spacing or associated acetabular and femoral neck fractures. Any suspicious radiographic findings require further radiographs or a CT scan to determine the extent of injury. Closed reduction with anesthesia and muscle relaxation is preferred unless an associated proximal femur or acetabular fracture is present. Dislocations with accompanying fractures require open reduction and fixation. Posterior dislocations are reduced by flexing the hip and knee to 90 degrees before applying axial traction to the thigh. A postreduction CT scan of the hip is necessary to look for any intra-articular fractures or fragments along with judging the adequacy of the reduction. Reductions should occur within 6 hours to decrease the risk of AVN and osteoarthritis. Delays in reduction make the procedure much more difficult. Bed rest and immobilization are recommended for 6 weeks once the dislocation is reduced.[3]

▶ PROXIMAL FEMUR FRACTURES

Proximal femur fractures are very rare in pediatrics and account for less than 1% of fractures around the hip. The proximal femur requires high-energy trauma for a fracture to occur. The fracture can occur at the physis, neck, or trochanteric region depending upon the forces involved. These fractures are complicated by the high risk of premature physeal closure and AVN of the femoral head. This risk is greatest with displaced transphyseal fractures. Transphyseal fractures and SCFE appear similar on x-rays, but their presentations are distinctly different. Transphyseal fractures occur in younger children following a significant trauma, and a SCFE is associated with obese teenagers lacking a major traumatic event. Any fracture of the proximal femur demands orthopedic consultation in the ED because the risk of complications is high and management is frequently surgical.

A few fractures of the proximal femur deserve separate mention because they are not a result of high-energy trauma like those mentioned above. The proximal femur has apophyses that can be avulsed by stronger adolescent muscles during sporting activities. A violent contraction of the iliopsoas can avulse the lesser trochanter, and the hip abductors may avulse the greater trochanter. Like avulsions of the pelvis, these fractures usually heal well with conservative management and progressive weight bearing over 4 weeks. In the rare instance, the avulsed fragment is significantly displaced, open reduction and fixation may be required.[4]

▶ FEMORAL SHAFT FRACTURES

Most fractures of the femur in children involve the femoral shaft. Femoral shaft fractures are classified and managed based upon the patient's age. The most common site of fracture is along the middle third of the shaft, but the proximal and distal third also occur regularly. Unlike adult femur fractures, the pediatric patient rarely experiences hypotension or shock because of an isolated femur fracture. If shocklike symptoms are present, look closely for accompanying injuries. In adolescents, where high-energy trauma is the mechanism, evaluate for injuries to the visceral organs.

When a femur fracture is suspected, the leg should be splinted following assessment of the distal pulses, testing of the distal nerves, and completion of needed resuscitation. Splinting and pain control should be achieved before radiographs are taken. Recheck the pulses and the neurovascular status after application of the splint. Suspected femur fractures need radiographs of the femoral shaft, hip, and knee to look for possible dislocations and accompanying injuries. Because of the intense amount of pain with femur fractures, patients may not localize pain as well as in other extremity fractures. Orthopedics should be involved in the management of all femoral shaft fractures. Hospital admission to orthopedics for pain control, observation, and definitive management is standard.

The nonambulatory infant or young toddler with a femur fracture should raise suspicions of child abuse. Spiral fractures from a twisting motion are classic for child abuse in this age group, but they are not pathognomonic. Nonambulatory patients with any type of femur fracture need a skeletal survey as part of their evaluation. The remarkable thing is the femur's ability to remodel and heal rapidly in these young patients. Most never need any surgical intervention and heal well with either a hip spica cast or a Pavlik harness.

The older toddler and young child often suffer femur fractures because of automobile versus pedestrian accidents. With the high-energy forces involved, these patients must be examined closely for concomitant, life-threatening injuries. Once they are stabilized in the ED, management is usually inpatient traction followed by closed reduction and spica casting.

Older children and adolescents typically present with femur fractures following high-energy trauma such as automobile accidents. The larger, stronger muscle groups in these patients increase the risk for limb shortening and malunion after reduction, so most of these injuries are managed with surgical placement of either an intramedullary rod or a flexible "Nancy" nail. These fractures used to be managed with prolonged traction until the callous was secure followed by a spica cast for many weeks. This prolonged traction/spica casting method has fallen out of favor for numerous reasons, and most in this age group are now managed surgically.[5]

▶ FRACTURES OF THE KNEE AND PATELLA

Injuries of the knee and patella are seen commonly in the ED. The most common mechanisms for these fractures are sports, falls, and autopedestrian accidents. Fractures around the knee are concerning because two-thirds of the lower extremity length comes from the physes of the distal femur and proximal tibia. There is a high risk of growth arrest or progressive deformity when either physis is fractured. Like all joints in pediatrics, the knee consists of strong ligaments attached to growing bone around the physis. The physis is the weakest part of the joint, so when a stronger ligament "pulls" upon a weaker physis, fractures often result. Ligamentous injuries are less common, but are becoming more recognized in adolescent sporting injuries.

The most common physeal fracture of the knee involves the distal femoral physis which accounts for 5% of all physeal fractures. Injuries to the distal femur physis usually result from high-energy trauma. If a nondisplaced Salter–Harris I (SH I) fracture occurs, the management is immobilization with a long-leg splint and no weight bearing. The most common pattern after a direct blow is a Salter–Harris II (SH II) fracture with a metaphyseal fragment. These require reduction and occasional pinning to ensure anatomic alignment. Even with proper management, a large number of these fractures will experience growth arrest. Salter–Harris III and IV (SH III and IV) fractures of the distal femoral physis require open reduction and fixation to properly align the joint surface and decrease the risk for subsequent arthritis.

The proximal tibial physis is much less commonly fractured because both the fibula and the insertion of the medial collateral ligament distal to the physis offer "protection." As a result of this protection, forces are transmitted away from the physis. The tibia does have its own challenges because, as adolescents mature, the tibia becomes the site for two unique types of avulsion fractures. The first unique avulsion fracture involves the tibial spine (tibial eminence or plateau). Avulsions of the tibial spine result from similar forces that would rupture the anterior cruciate ligament (ACL) in adults. In children, the mechanism is frequently hyperextension from falling off a bicycle or playing sports (Fig. 38–4). The second unique avulsion pattern involves the tibial tubercle. Forceful contractions of the strong quadriceps in adolescents can pull on the tibial tubercle enough to result in an avulsion. Depending upon their stage of skeletal maturity, this avulsion of the tubercle may extend up into the tibial physis or the articular surface of the knee (Fig. 38–5).

Fractures of the patella are less common in children than in adults. The growing patella is covered by a large amount of cartilaginous tissue that acts as padding against direct trauma. The most common patella fracture is transverse (Fig. 38–6) resulting from a direct blow. This should not be confused with the 5% of the population that have a non-pathologic bipartite patella in the superolateral corner of the patella. The history with a patellar fracture involves an acute injury incontrast to the bipartite patella where it is usually asymptomatic or associated with chronic symptoms. Adolescents may also present with a unique fracture of the patella called the "sleeve" fracture. The distal portion of the patella attaches to the tibia through the patella tendon. With a strong contraction of the quadriceps, the patella tendon may actually avulse a small "sleeve" of the inferior patella. Remember, the avulsed fragment also contains a larger piece of radiolucent cartilage and the "sleeve" fracture requires surgical repair.[6]

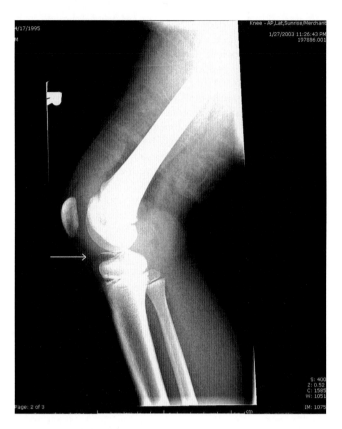

Figure 38–4. Tibial spine avulsion fracture after hyperextension in a young athlete.

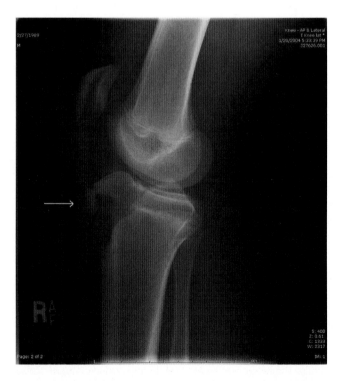

Figure 38–5. Tibial tubercle avulsion fracture in a basketball player requiring surgical fixation because of intra-articular extension.

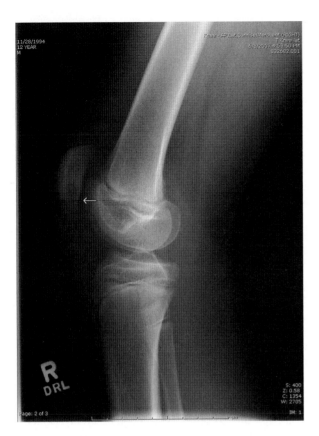

Figure 38–6. Transverse fracture of patella after a fall onto the knee.

Evaluating any knee injury begins with a good history looking for clues to the mechanism. The mechanism is particularly helpful in knee injuries to focus the examination and narrow the differential. Examination proceeds with the awareness that displaced physeal injuries can severe the popliteal artery, and assessment of the distal pulses is essential. The femur, tibia, patella, physes, and collateral ligaments should also be palpated to determine if point tenderness exists. When radiographs are indicated, a complete series includes an AP, lateral, and patella view.

Despite negative x-rays, any patient with significant tenderness of the physis or a traumatic effusion needs to be immobilized without weight bearing and closely followed-up by an orthopedist in 3 to 5 days. Acute traumatic effusions are always hemarthroses, and they indicate significant intra-articular pathology ranging from missed fractures to tears of the ligaments or menisci.[7]

▶ OSGOOD–SCHLATTER DISEASE

Osgood–Schlatter disease, also known as traumatic tibial apophysitis, causes inflammation and pain due to avulsion of the chondral portion of the tibial tuberosity. It is thought to be secondary to repeated forceful use of the quadriceps muscle and the knee's extensor mechanism. It is usually seen in physically active teenagers, especially boys between the ages of 14 and 16 years. It occurs bilaterally in up to 25% of patients. Patients often complain of pain below the knee exacerbated by physical activity and kneeling. The physical examination reveals tenderness and, possibly, swelling over the tibial tuberosity and knee radiographs may reveal irregularity or prominence of the tibial tuberosity. Management consists of temporary restriction of activity and relief of pain with nonsteroidal anti-inflammatory drugs (NSAIDs), realizing that this condition is usually self-limited.

▶ KNEE AND PATELLA DISLOCATIONS

Femur-on-tibia knee dislocations are extremely rare in children and result from motor vehicle accidents in most cases. They deserve consideration with any traumatic knee effusion because of the high risk of popliteal artery damage (40%) and peroneal nerve injury (33%) which can be limb-threatening. All knee dislocations need prompt reduction with sedation and analgesia followed by admission for frequent neurovascular checks.

Patellar dislocations appear regularly in adolescent athletes. Ninety percent of patella dislocations are lateral dislocations. Reduction may occur spontaneously when the patient extends the knee. If the patella remains displaced, then analgesia, sedation, and reduction should take place promptly. The diagnosis of a spontaneously reduced patellar dislocation can be achieved by performing the patellar apprehension test. This maneuver is positive when the knee is flexed 20 to 30 degrees and apprehension appears with attempts at lateral displacement of the patella. After reduction repeat radiographs are needed and the knee is immobilized in extension. Close follow-up is warranted because many will have osteochondral fragments from shearing of the patella or femoral condyle.[8]

▶ FRACTURES OF THE TIBIA AND FIBULA

Nonphyseal fractures of the tibia and fibula are the most common long bone fractures of the lower extremities in pediatric patients. Only forearm and supracondylar fractures are more common than tibial fractures. Fracturing both the tibia and the fibula is more common than an isolated tibia fracture, but both bone fractures require high energy. Isolated tibia fractures result from rotational and indirect forces. Fibula fractures are rarely seen in isolation, but plastic deformation may accompany with tibia fractures. Exercise caution with the "isolated" proximal fibula fracture because it is often in conjunction with a distal tibial physeal injury. Most fractures of the tibia and fibula require the involvement of an orthopedist but can be managed with closed reduction. Any displacement requires operative intervention, and the following patterns require special attention.

Fractures of the proximal tibial metaphysis (Fig. 38–7) require special attention because of their high risk for compartment syndrome and ischemia. Displacement of the proximal tibial metaphysis is worrisome because the tibial arteries run right along the surface of the tibia. If a tibial artery is damaged or severed, compartment syndrome or ischemia of the lower leg often results. Proximal tibia metaphyseal fractures require orthopedic involvement and frequent neurovascular checks.

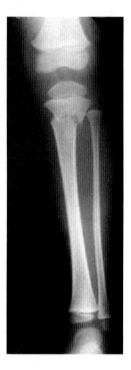

Figure 38–7. Fracture of the proximal tibial metaphysis after being stuck by a car. This injury is at high risk for compartment syndrome because of vascular damage of the tibial arteries. There is also a high risk of progressive valgus deformity.

The metaphyseal greenstick fracture has attracted plenty of attention by orthopedists because of its propensity to heal in a valgus deformity. Initial x-rays are often unimpressive, and the child may be immobilized without reduction. The difficulty is that many of these are actually in a slight valgus position which progresses with healing. As a result, greenstick fractures of the tibial metaphysis are best managed by completing the fracture and performing a reduction under anesthesia.

The toddler's fracture is an occult tibia fracture. The common scenario is a young child who presents to the ED with a limp or refusal to walk and an unimpressive examination. There may be history of a trivial injury, but most events are unwitnessed in younger children. The examination must include the entire extremity from the hip to the foot, but findings are usually absent or very subtle. The x-rays in the ED are frequently normal with the oblique views offering the most reward. These children are discharged with long-leg immobilization and orthopedic follow-up. Only in follow-up does a fracture appear as new callous bone formation becomes evident on x-ray. The presence of other symptoms at presentation such as fever, erythema, or other illnesses should prompt a different workup.[9]

▶ FRACTURES OF THE ANKLE AND FOOT

The pediatric ankle is frequently injured, and the forces generated are quite similar to those in adults. The big difference is the weaker physis and stronger ligaments make the likelihood of fracture much greater in pediatrics. The distal tibial and fibular physes are third to only the phalanges and dis-

tal radius in physeal fractures. The mechanisms resulting in adult ankle sprains result in childhood physeal fractures, and sports are the largest cause. Distinctive fracture patterns exist based upon the mechanism of injury and the stage of physeal closure. The foot must be examined closely with each ankle injury because concomitant fractures can occur.

Inversion and supination of the ankle often results in SH I and II physeal fractures of the distal fibular physis. The SH I is the most common ankle fracture. X-rays may be normal with the only findings being tenderness at the physis and mild swelling. Avulsions of the distal fibula can also be seen. Isolated fibular fractures can be managed with an ankle stirrup (sugar-tong) splint. Displaced fibular fractures are rare and always accompany SH III and IV fractures of the tibia. The displaced fibula fracture should reduce spontaneously when the tibia fracture is reduced, but if not, surgical fixation may be necessary.

The distal tibial physis most commonly fractures in a SH II pattern. The mechanism for this injury is eversion with plantar flexion, and it is often accompanied by a greenstick fracture of the fibula. The SH II fracture can be reduced in the ED using procedural sedation and a long-leg splint. The distal tibial physis closes in adolescents starting centrally to medially, but only later does the lateral portion close. This partial closure process in adolescence results in two distinctive fractures known as the SH III "Tillaux" fracture and the SH IV triplane fracture.[10] With an external rotation force of the ankle, the strong anterior tibiofibular ligament pulls off a portion of the lateral tibial physis resulting in the SH III Tillaux fracture (Fig. 38–8). The

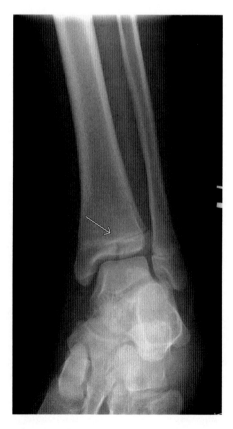

Figure 38–8. Mortise view of the ankle demonstrating a Salter–Harris III fracture of the tibia commonly referred to as a Tillaux fracture.

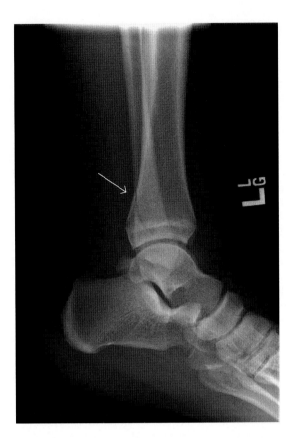

Figure 38–9. Lateral view of a Salter–Harris IV fracture of the tibia referred to as a triplane fracture. These fractures require a CT scan of the ankle to get a better understanding of fragment displacement and intra-articular damage.

Acute ankle injury*

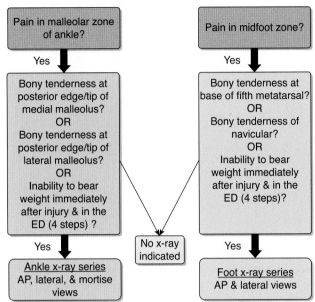

*Use with caution in children younger than 5 years

Figure 38–10. Ottawa ankle rules for use in adults and school-aged children.

SH IV triplane fracture results from a similar force but the fracture line extends into three planes crossing the epiphysis, physis, and metaphysis (Fig. 38–9). The Tillaux and triplane fractures are intra-articular and require surgical fixation to maintain the articular surface. CT scans are usually required in Tillaux and triplane fractures to reveal the amount of displacement and allow for better surgical planning. Physeal fractures of the tibia are complicated by the risk for growth arrest and intra-articular damage.[11]

Clinical decision rules for obtaining radiographs in the ED have been studied in adults and children because ankle injuries are so common. The popular Ottawa ankle rules (Fig. 38–10) have proven to be very sensitive in detecting pediatric ankle fractures and may be applied to school-aged children and adolescents. Exercise caution in patients younger than school age because physeal fractures are much more likely.[12] Radiographs of the ankle should include at least three views. In addition to the standard AP and lateral views, the mortise view gives an outline of the talus and surrounding spaces.

Nondisplaced fractures of the ankle are rare, but are immobilized in a stirrup splint with the added support of a posterior splint in many cases. Any significantly displaced fracture, intra-articular fracture, or open fracture needs orthopedic consultation in the ED for likely surgical fixation. Precise reduction is extremely important in ankle fractures because of the weight-bearing responsibilities and the risk of subsequent osteoarthritis.[13]

▶ FOOT FRACTURES

Fractures of the foot result from numerous mechanisms including inversions of the ankle, direct blows, twisting forces, falls, and axial loading. The vast majority of foot fractures involve the forefoot, which consists of the metatarsals and phalanges. Fractures of the forefoot are usually easy to recognize and managed without difficulty. However, rare injuries such as the Lisfranc or a hindfoot fracture can be diagnostic challenges with complications if they go unrecognized.

Phalangeal fractures are common, but rarely are they difficult to manage. They are easy to recognize by point tenderness and radiographic findings. Immobilization is with either a hard-sole shoe or a short-leg splint depending upon the family's preference. SH II fractures may require reduction following a digital block. Indications for surgical fixation are intra-articular fractures of the great toe with displacement at the proximal phalanx or any significant displacement that prevents remodeling.

Metatarsal fractures are the most common fractures of the foot, and they are often associated with an impressive amount of soft tissue swelling. Many of these are obvious after examination and standard radiographs, but complicated fractures require oblique views of the foot. Some lateral displacement can be accepted because of young children's tremendous ability to remodel, but remember this ability decreases as the patient nears skeletal maturity. The famous "Jones fracture" occurs in the proximal diaphyseal region of the fifth metatarsal, but it is very uncommon in children. Fractures are much more likely to be avulsions of the fifth metatarsal base (Fig. 38–11). It is important to understand the differences between avulsions that commonly occur with inversion injuries of the ankle, and the

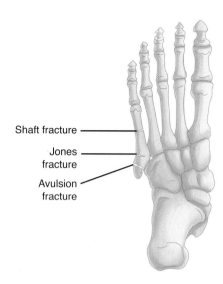

Figure 38–11. Fractures of the fifth metatarsal are much more likely to be avulsions or shaft fractures in pediatrics. The Jones fracture occurs at the metaphyseal–diaphyseal junction and is rare in children.

rare Jones fracture. Avulsions have a much better prognosis and heal rather quickly without surgical intervention. When complications do arise with metatarsal fractures, it is often because of compartment syndrome from severe swelling. Most metatarsal fractures can be effectively treated with a short-leg splint and closed reduction if displaced.

Midfoot fractures include the tarsal bones of the navicular, cuneiforms, and cuboid. These fractures result from direct trauma to the midfoot and may be difficult to detect. They can be managed with a non-weight-bearing posterior splint and follow-up unless significantly displaced. The rare tarsometatarsal fracture/dislocation (Lisfranc) involves the midfoot and is very rare in children (Fig. 38–12). The 'Lisfranc joint' is the entire tarsometatarsal junction where the second

metatarsal acts as a keystone with very strong ligamentous support. The Lisfranc presents as swelling in the midfoot with marked tenderness, and a fracture can be seen at the base of the second metatarsal with tarsometatarsal dislocation. It can be difficult to diagnose the Lisfranc injury on x-ray and oblique views of the midfoot are mandatory. The mechanism for the Lisfranc is usually a force of strong plantar flexion or abduction of the foot. Recognizing this injury is important because any dislocation or fracture displacement requires surgical fixation.

Hindfoot injuries include the talus and calcaneus which are rarely fractured in children. Calcaneal fractures result from significant falls and are associated with accompanying vertebral fractures, contralateral calcaneal fractures, and renal pedicle injuries in adults. These accompanying injuries occur in pediatrics but with much less frequency than in adults. Radiographs of the calcaneus are difficult to interpret and require AP, lateral, and axial views when a fracture is suspected. Some injuries may even require oblique views or a CT scan to make the diagnosis. Subtle compression fractures are detected in adolescents using Bohler's angle on lateral radiographs, but this measurement is much less reliable in younger children (Fig. 38–13). Any patient with a calcaneal fracture must also receive AP and lateral views of the thoracolumbar spine because of the risk of accompanying vertebral fractures. Pain and swelling is often marked with calcaneal injuries, and ED management consists of non-weight-bearing immobilization with a bulky posterior splint. Nonoperative management of pediatric calcaneal fractures is very successful unlike in adults.

Fractures of the talus typically involve the talar neck after a mechanism of forced dorsiflexion. Patients present with anterior ankle pain, swelling, and are unable to ambulate. Routine radiographs usually reveal the diagnosis, but occasionally a CT scan is indicated. Any signs of displacement require surgical repair, and all fractures of the talus must be followed closely because of their risk of osteonecrosis. A talar fracture seen in many parts of the country is the "snowboarder's fracture." This injury is a fracture of the lateral process of the talus because of dorsiflexion of the ankle and inversion of the hindfoot, which is common in snowboarding. Be suspicious of this

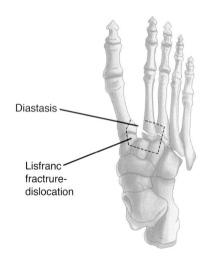

Figure 38–12. The rare Lisfranc injury consists of a tarsal–metatarsal dislocation. A fracture of the second metatarsal with dislocation is the most common pattern.

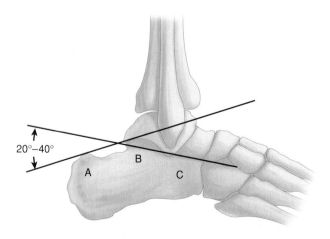

Figure 38–13. Bohler's angle to detect compression fractures of the calcaneus may be useful in adolescents, but it is unreliable in younger children.

fracture in any snowboarder who presents with anterolateral ankle pain. Unless displaced, fractures of the talus can be managed in the ED with non-weight-bearing immobilization in a posterior splint and close orthopedic follow-up.[14]

REFERENCES

1. Chia JP, Holland AJ, Little D, et al. Pelvic fractures and associated injuries in children. *J Trauma.* 2004;56:83–88.
2. Guillamondegul OD, Mahboubi S, Stafford PW, et al. The utility of the pelvic radiograph in the assessment of pediatric pelvic fractures. *J Trauma.* 2003;55:236–240.
3. Swiontkowski MF. Fractures and dislocations about the hips and pelvis. In: Green NE, Swiontkowski MF, eds. *Skeletal Trauma in Children.* 3rd ed. Philadelphia, PA: Saunders; 2003:371–406.
4. Blasier RD, Hughes LO. Fractures and traumatic dislocations of the hip in children. In: Beaty JH, Kasser JR, eds. *Rockwood and Wilkins' Fractures in Children.* 6th ed. Philadelphia, PA: Lippincott Williams & Wilkins; 2006:861–891.
5. Pring ME, Newton PO, Rang M. Femoral shaft. In: Wenger DR, Pring ME, eds. *Rang's Children's Fractures.* 3rd ed. Philadelphia, PA: Lippincott Williams & Wilkins; 2005:181–200.
6. Jones MH, Simon JE, Winell JJ. Pediatric knee fractures. *Curr Opin Pediatr.* 2005;17:43–47.
7. Luhman SJ. Acute traumatic knee effusions in children and adolescents. *J Pediatr Orthop.* 2003;23:199–202.
8. Fithian DC, Paxton EW, Stone ML, et al. Epidemiology and natural history of acute patellar dislocation. *Am J Sports Med.* 2004;32:1114–1121.
9. Lalonde FD, Wenger DR. Tibia. In: Wenger DR, Pring ME, eds. *Rang's Children's Fractures.* 3rd ed. Philadelphia, PA: Lippincott Williams & Wilkins; 2005:215–226.
10. Marsh JS, Daigneault JP. Ankle injuries in the pediatric population. *Curr Opin Pediatr.* 2000;12:52–60.
11. Koury SI, Stone CK, Harrell G, et al. Recognition and management of Tillaux fractures in adolescents. *Pediatr Emerg Care.* 1999;15:37–39.
12. Clarke KD, Tanner S. Evaluation of Ottawa ankle rules in children. *Pediatr Emerg Care.* 2003;19:73–78.
13. Cummings RJ. Distal tibial and fibular fractures. In: Beaty JH, Kasser JR, eds. *Rockwood and Wilkins' Fractures in Children.* 6th ed. Philadelphia, PA: Lippincott Williams & Wilkins; 2006:1077–1128.
14. Crawford AH, Al-Sayyad MJ. Fractures and dislocations of the foot and ankle. In: Green NE, Swiontkowski MF, eds. *Skeletal Trauma in Children.* Philadelphia, PA: Saunders; 2003:516–586.

CHAPTER 39

Soft Tissue Injury and Wound Repair

D. Matthew Sullivan

▶ HIGH-YIELD FACTS

- In assessing a child with a minor wound, exclude more serious, sometimes occult, injuries that take precedence in management.
- Physical examination of the wound must assess the length and depth of the injury, circulatory status, motor and sensory function, the presence of foreign bodies and contaminants, and the involvement of underlying structures.
- Topical anesthetics provide effective anesthesia and should be considered as a necessary adjuvant for pediatric lacerations.
- Irrigation with 5 to 8 psi is the appropriate method of choice for removing bacteria and debris from most wounds. Low-pressure irrigation does not adequately clean wounds.
- Many lacerations are suitable for closure using noninvasive methods of closure. With careful consideration, wounds closed in noninvasive fashion produce satisfying cosmetic results.
- Splint a wound overlying a joint in the position of function for 7 to 10 days.
- Antibiotics are indicated for patients who have significant host factors (immune-compromising disease), who present with a wound infection, who present for care late (12–24 hours), and in certain specific instances (intraoral lacerations, wounds of the hand, and cat bites).
- Outcome is dependent on wound care after discharge from the emergency department (ED). Patient and parents should be given thorough *after-care* instructions about care of the wound and what to expect.

Lacerations and soft tissue injuries are the most common reasons for children to present to the ED.[1] These encounters, if handled incorrectly, can be difficult for the child, parent, and physician. To maximize cosmetic and functional results, one should ensure meticulous wound care and repair. Many techniques exist to maximize the satisfaction and clinical results achieved in the ED and a solid understanding of the basic tenets of wound care is a necessary part of the emergency practitioner's arsenal.[2]

▶ SKIN AND SOFT TISSUE ANATOMY AND BIOMECHANICS

The skin is composed of the dermis, which provides most of the skin's tensile strength, and the epidermis, which protects the dermis from infection and desiccation. Dermal capillaries are fed by the nutrient vessels of the skin, and the epidermis,

which has no blood supply, is fed by diffusion of nutrients from the dermis. The subcutaneous tissue beneath the dermis is composed of loose connective and adipose tissue, large vessels, and nerves.[3]

The appearance and function of a healed wound is somewhat predicted by the magnitude of the tension on the surrounding skin, but there is great intra- and interindividual variability. The most cosmetically pleasing scar results when the long axis of the wound is in the direction of maximal static skin tension, along "Langer's lines" (Fig. 39–1). Examination of the wound in the ED is a reliable method to predict the appearance of the healed wound in the absence of confounding variables, such as the development of an infection or keloid. Dynamic skin tension (caused by joint movement and muscle contraction) also has an impact on the degree of scar formation and postrepair function. A wound intersecting the transverse axis of a joint may result in a significant contracture, since scars do not have the elasticity of uninjured tissue.

Unfortunately, soft tissue wounds are unplanned events and often have axes that are perpendicular to the direction of static skin tension or parallel to the dynamic skin tension. Therefore, it is always essential to warn the child and parent of possible adverse cosmetic outcomes.

▶ CLASSIFICATION OF MINOR INJURIES

LACERATIONS

Lacerations are cuts through the skin and, after contusions, are the most common type of soft tissue injury seen in the ED.[4,5] Lacerations that involve the dermal capillaries bleed and those through the subcutaneous fat often produce gaping wounds. The face, scalp, and hands are the most common sites of injury in the pediatric age group. Lacerations generally require more complicated treatment than other minor wounds. Much of this chapter deals with the assessment and treatment of lacerations. All lacerations can be associated with occult injuries and require thorough exploration to detect deeper injuries. The three main classes of lacerations are shear, tension, and compression.

Shear injuries are caused by sharp objects and generally cause little damage to adjacent tissues but can cause nerve, tendon, and vascular damage. Shears usually heal fastest and have the lowest incidence of wound infection.

Tension lacerations occur when stresses cause the skin to tear. There is often associated damage to the surrounding tissues, and these lacerations are irregularly shaped.

Compression lacerations occur during a crush injury and have irregular, often stellate, wound edges. They are often

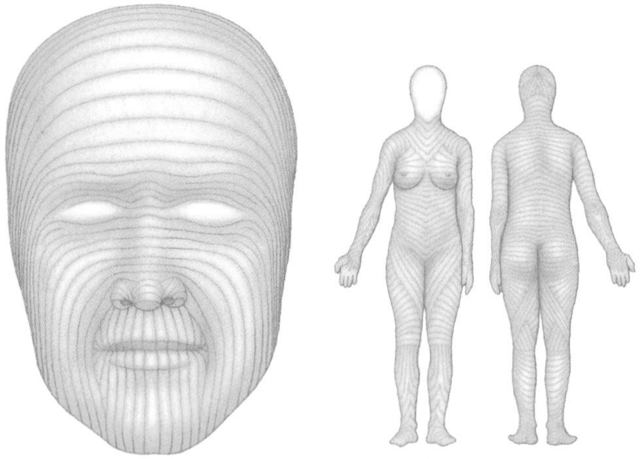

Figure 39–1. Lines of skin tension.

associated with a significant amount of injury to the adjacent skin, contusion to the underlying structures, and they have a higher incidence of wound infection than other types of lacerations.[6,7]

ABRASIONS

Abrasions are injuries in which layers of the skin are scraped or sheared away. In superficial abrasions, only the cornified epidermis is removed, there is minimal or no bleeding and healing is rapid. Deeper abrasions involving the dermis are prone to bleeding and are more susceptible to infection, pigment change, and prolonged healing.

CONTUSIONS AND HEMATOMAS

Contusions are the result of direct blows to the tissues and often injure underlying structures. Localized bleeding and edema can cause swelling and pain to the injured area, and on rare occasion, may result in secondary ischemic injuries. Management of all types of contusions involves elevation of the injured area, application of ice packs intermittently for the first 24 to 48 hours, and careful monitoring of circulation and neurologic function.

Hematomas are localized collections of extravasated blood that are relatively or completely confined within a space or potential space. Hematomas can be associated with most types of minor and major wounds; they must be observed closely for signs of infection and, in some instances, may benefit from drainage.

▶ PREHOSPITAL CARE

Prehospital care of minor wounds, includes control of bleeding and attention to the damage to underlying structures. Control of blood loss can almost always be accomplished by direct manual pressure or use of a pressure dressing. If bleeding is not controlled with these methods, inflation of a sphygmomanometer proximal to the bleeding site on an injured extremity can be safely employed even for prolonged (at least 2 hours) transport times. The attention to underlying structures and concomitant injuries includes careful assessment of neurovascular

status and may require prehospital attention (splinting, moist dressings) to maximize outcomes. Document what patients, parents, and providers have done in the prehospital setting.

▶ HISTORY AND PHYSICAL EXAMINATION

In assessing a child with a minor wound, first exclude more serious, sometimes occult injuries that will take precedence in management. Once more pressing injuries have been dealt with, the management of soft tissue injuries can be compartmentalized by addressing *host factors, wound factors,* and *after-care.*

The history of the injury should include the time and mechanism of the injury, the full extent of the injured areas, and whether there could be any possible contaminants or foreign bodies in the wound. For all wounds, obtain a detailed history of the patient's *host factors* with particular attention to the child's immunization status, whether the child has any medical problems or allergies, any medications that the child takes, and what prehospital wound care was performed prior to arrival in the ED. Always consider nonaccidental trauma, especially when the history and the injury pattern are inconsistent.

Addressing the *wound factors* involves a physical examination that must assess the length and depth of the injury, circulatory status, motor and sensory function, the presence of foreign bodies and contaminants, and the involvement of underlying structures (nerves, tendons, muscles, ligaments, vessels, bones, joints, and ducts). Whereas the sensory examination must precede the administration of anesthesia, the remainder of the examination should be performed with adequate anesthesia. To avoid fear in the child, anxiety in the parents, and frustration for everybody else, use a calm, unhurried, reassuring, and honest approach throughout the evaluation and management.

Test sensation by measuring two-point discrimination distal to an injury. For children younger than 3 years, use an appropriate stimulus to provide a sensory and a partial motor assessment. Since normal autonomic tone produces a degree of normal sweating, denervated fingers do not sweat, which may provide a clue to injury if this is not seen under magnification. Evaluate circulation by palpation of peripheral pulses and skin temperature, observation of skin color, and rapidity of capillary refill. Test tendons, muscles, and ligaments distal to an injury. With cooperative older children, it is possible to test these structures' functions individually. However, with younger, less cooperative children, one must rely on observation of symmetry, function, and exploration of the wound. Use a toy or light pen that requires manipulation by the child to help in evaluating motor function. Involve Child Life providers and observe the child at play to evaluate wounds that might involve underlying motor structures.[8]

▶ MANAGEMENT

INSTRUMENTS, SUTURES, STAPLES, TAPE, AND TISSUE ADHESIVES

The technical approach for wound closure depends on the *host* and *wound factors* of the laceration. Sutures, staples, surgical

▶ **TABLE 39–1. ADVANTAGES AND DISADVANTAGES OF COMMON WOUND CLOSURE TECHNIQUES**

Technique	Advantages	Disadvantages
Suture	Time honored Meticulous closure Greatest tensile strength Lowest dehiscence rate	Requires removal Requires anesthesia Greatest tissue reactivity Highest cost Slowest application Highest risk of needle stick
Staples	Rapid application Low tissue reactivity Low cost Low risk of needle stick	Less meticulous closure May interfere with imaging techniques
Tissue adhesive	Rapid application Patient comfort Resistant to bacterial growth No need for removal Low cost Low or no risk of needle stick	Lower tensile strength than sutures Dehiscence over high-tension areas Not useful on hands
Surgical tape	Least reactive Lowest infection rates Rapid application Patient comfort Low cost No risk of needle stick	Frequently falls off Lower tensile strength than sutures Highest rate of dehiscence Requires use of toxic adjuncts Cannot be used in areas with hair Cannot get wet

tape, closure devices, and tissue adhesives each have intrinsic pros and cons for their use (Table 39–1). Most wound repairs can be accomplished with basic instruments and supplies (Fig. 39–2):

- Gloves.[9,10]
- Needle driver.
- Forceps (noncrushing tips).
- No. 15 scalpel.
- Scissors.
- Sutures (Table 39–2), wound adhesive, closure devices, or staples.
- Sterile drape(s).

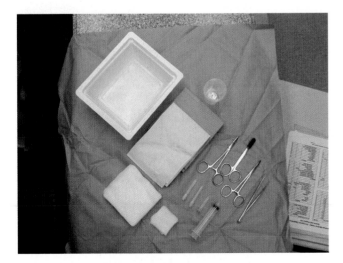

Figure 39–2. Standard laceration equipment.

- Anesthetic agent(s).
- Irrigation equipment.
- Sterile gauze.

A number of needle types are available for use, and manufacturers generally place a life-size and cross-sectional diagram of the needle on each suture package. The most common type of cross-sectional needle configuration used for wound repair is the cutting edge needle. Cutting edge needles come in many forms. Each cross-sectional type is designed for a specific purpose. Typical ED wound repair can be accomplished with reverse precision point cutting needles that are manufactured in various sizes, curvatures, and paired with differing thread types. Another type of common needle configuration is the tapered needle, which is not often used in the ED setting, as it is a bit more difficult to pass through the epidermis.

Suture choice is one of the most fundamental options in wound and laceration repair. Each suture type has inherent characteristics that are suited for specific uses. The most basic choice is absorbable versus nonabsorbable suture material. Historically, absorbable suture has been relegated to use as a deep (nonepidermal) closure, whereas nonabsorbable sutures were used externally (epidermal). Recently, strong consideration has been given toward the use of absorbable suture externally in order to eliminate the need for return visit for suture removal.[11] This diminishes both the stress of multiple encounters and the necessary operational resources. Because of the inflammatory response that absorbable sutures generate during the degradation process, the cosmetic outcome must be considered. Using absorbable sutures on noncosmetically important areas (extremities, trunk) has been studied and accepted[12]; the use of absorbable sutures on cosmetically critical regions (the face) has been studied with good outcomes

► TABLE 39–2. SUTURE TYPES AND CHARACTERISTICS

Type and Material	Properties
Nonabsorbable	
Silk	Easy to handle
	Lies flat when tied
	Forms secure knot because of presence of braid
	Induces more tissue reaction and has higher infection potential than other nonabsorbable
Nylon	Synthetic
	Less tissue reactivity and infection potential
	Does not tend to lie flat
	More difficult to handle than silk
	Decreased knot security because of lack of braid requires more throws per knot
Polypropylene	Similar to the properties of nylon sutures, although slightly easier to handle
Polyester	Infection potential greater than nylon and polypropylene, but less than silk and cotton
	Easier to handle and better knot security than nylon and polypropylene
Metal	Low tissue reactivity and infection potential
	Difficult to handle
	Uncomfortable for patient during healing
Polybutester	Equivalent to nylon and polypropylene in tensile strength and low infection potential
	Stretches easily, thus advantageous for wounds that tend to swell
Absorbable	
Plain gut	Phagocytosed by macrophages
	Maintains tensile strength for ~7 d
	High tissue reactivity and infection potential
Chromic gut	Similar to the properties of plain gut sutures, but maintains tensile strength for ~2–3 wk
Fast-absorbing	Similar to the properties of plain gut sutures, but breaks down gut within 5–7 d, thus does not require removal with scissors
Polyglycolic acid and polyglactin	Synthetic
	Cause less tissue reactivity and have lower infection potential than gut sutures
	Absorbed by enzymatic hydrolysis
	Braided, thus hold knots well, but have lots of drag through tissues if not coated with materials that reduce friction
	Gradually loses tensile strength over ~4 wk
Polydioxanone, polyglyconate, Poliglecaprone and glycoside	Synthetic monofilament (pass more smoothly through tissues)
	Cause less tissue reactivity than gut sutures
	Absorbed by enzymatic hydrolysis
Trimethylene carbonate	Retain ~60% of tensile strength at 28 d

compared with other standard methods.[13] Each wound requires a certain tensile strength for a certain amount of time and the characteristics of each suture type should be understood (Table 39–2).

Surgical staples are a useful alternative to suturing for selected wounds. Sharp lacerations of the scalp, trunk, and extremities are rapidly and effectively closed using staples. Staples induce a minimal inflammatory reaction and produce similar cosmetic results compared to suturing. Because of their site and mechanism, staples are often not well-suited for use in stellate or angulated wounds, hand wounds, or wounds which sit in recessed contours of the body. Recall that staples are hard and relatively nonmalleable when compared to sutures (Fig. 39–3). When stapling the scalp, ask the sleep position preference for patients or consider the position in which they will lay while hospitalized. Metallic staples are also radiopaque and give off a significant artifact when CT scan imaging is obtained. Magnetic resonance imaging (MRI) of metallic staples is safe as long as consideration is given to the heat that may be generated during the MRI. Absorbable intradermal staples

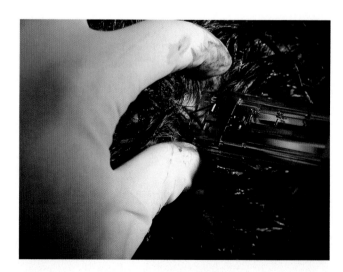

Figure 39–3. Scalp laceration.

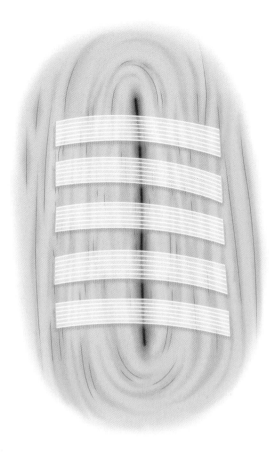

Figure 39–4. Skin-closure tapes should be applied perpendicular to the wound edges and spaced so that the edges do not gape.

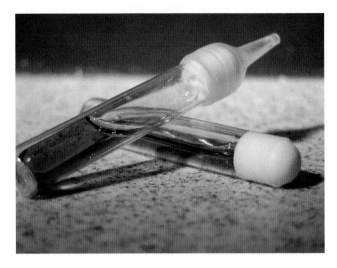

Figure 39–5. Tissue adhesive.

offer the advantage of rapid closure without the side effects of CT scan artifact or MRI heat development.

Steri-strips are an effective alternative for the closure of small linear lacerations that are under minimal tension (Fig. 39–4). Taped wounds offer an advantage over nonabsorbable sutured wounds in that they do not require return to the ED for removal. If applied with an adhesive such as tincture of benzoin, tape should remain in place for several days. Tape can also be used for skin closure of partial-thickness wounds and of wounds that are closed in a layered fashion with well-approximated wound edges. Tape closure is a reasonable alternative technique for the repair of multiple tangential skin flaps. Commercially available tape closure devices (Close-X) are well-suited for sharp, well demarcated lacerations but have not been vigorously studied in the pediatric population.[14]

Tissue adhesives have been used for many years and remain another option for rapid repair of pediatric lacerations (Fig. 39–5). Adhesives have slightly less tensile strength across wound edges and are therefore suited for use in low-tension wounds.[15,16] The failure of adhesives is typically because of the poor choice of wound type for adhesive use. Adhesives should not be used in wounds with high mobility (fingers, across joints). If you have concern that adhesives would not provide the strength, consider using deep absorbable sutures to provide that necessary strength, or avoid adhesives altogether. If tissue adhesives are to be used near the eye, use a ribbon of petroleum as a barrier to protect against inadvertent instillation of the adhesive into the eye. If the eye is accidentally glued shut, nail polish remover will free the eyelashes—DO NOT cut the lashes. While tissues adhesives provide their own waterproof and antimicrobial barrier, wound preparation remains at the same level of importance for wounds repaired with tissue adhesives as it does with any other wound closed by an invasive method. Care should be taken to ensure that adequate anesthesia, wound irrigation, and wound exploration occur regardless of the method of closure. With the right choice of wound, noninvasive repair can be faster, less painful, require no suture removal follow-up, and results in patient and parental satisfaction.[17]

ANALGESIA, LOCAL ANESTHESIA, NERVE BLOCKS, AND SEDATION

Analgesia, anesthesia, nerve blocks, and sedation are discussed in more detail in Chapter 23. Most wounds are adequately anesthetized using local infiltration of lidocaine, 1% to 2% with or without epinephrine, and this is still the standard approach. Lidocaine has a rapid onset of action and duration of action of approximately 1 to 2 hours. Commercial preparations/dilutions of epinephrine containing anesthetics are safer than older literature suggests and their use in regions supplied by end-arteries has been shown to be safe.[18] Consider the use of a longer-acting agent, such as bupivacaine, in order to spare patient repeated injections if wound repair may be interrupted. Bupivacaine's onset of action is moderate, and duration of action is approximately 2 to 6 hours.[19] For whatever local anesthetic agent is used, take care not to use more than the recommended dose per kilogram of the agent. For plain lidocaine and lidocaine with epinephrine, 4.5 mg/kg and 7 mg/kg are the recommended maximum doses, respectively.[20] Bicarbonate added to lidocaine, in a 1:10 dilution may also reduce the pain of injection.[21]

You should perform anesthetic infiltration prior to irrigation; however, for grossly contaminated wounds, it is occasionally necessary to irrigate gross contaminates prior to infiltration of anesthesia. Infiltration is achieved by means of a 25- to 27-gauge needle, injected slowly into the wound margins.[22]

The use of topical anesthetics on any wound prior to injectable anesthetics should be strongly considered as an adjuvant to care.[23] Topical lidocaine-adrenaline-tetracaine (LAT), as well as tetracaine-adrenaline-cocaine (TAC), has been shown to provide effective anesthesia for pediatric facial and scalp lacerations.[24,25] Use of LAT has compared favorably with TAC without the risks and administrative complications of cocaine.[26] The mixture can be applied to the wound by using saturated sponges, gauze pads, or cotton swabs held in place by a parent or caregiver wearing gloves. Transient anesthesia can also be obtained by applying a solution of 4% lidocaine to a wound prior to infiltration anesthesia or to an abrasion that requires mechanical scrubbing.

Use regional nerve blocks for large lacerations and for lacerations in areas where the anatomy will be distorted if local infiltration is performed. They are especially useful for anesthetizing digits, for facial lacerations, and wounds of the foot.

Moderate sedation is usually not required for the management of wounds in older children. However, for the child who is too uncooperative to permit adequate wound management, use chemical sedation with agents such as midazolam, fentanyl, nitrous oxide, or ketamine. Appropriate cardiac and respiratory monitoring should be performed during sedation, airway management equipment should be available at the bedside and reversal agents (naloxone and flumazenil) should be easily accessible. The patient should be discharged after the agents have worn off and the child has returned to an appropriate level of consciousness (see Chapter 19).

Some form of physical restraint during wound assessment and management may be necessary for children younger than 2 years and sometimes is required for children up to 5 or 6 years. You may immobilize a child using a folded sheet or a commercially available papoose board. Neither method provides adequate immobilization of the head. The perceived time benefit obtained through the use of physical restraints should be carefully balanced against the potential psychologic stressors that physical restraints might put on a child and/or the parents. Careful selection for cases for either chemical and/or physical restraint requires a thorough discussion of risk/benefit of each modality with the parents.

WOUND CLEANING AND PREPARATION

Controversy exists as to the proper physician attire during wound care. Some advocate routine donning of goggles, mask, gloves, cap, and gown. Certainly gloves, mask, and eye protection should always be worn, in keeping with universal precautions. As concern for skin infection rises (particularly methicillin-resistant *Staphylococcus aureus*), this topic may rise to a higher level of importance and scrutiny over time.

HEMOSTASIS

Hemostasis is necessary during all stages of wound management and usually is achieved by applying direct pressure for 10 to 20 minutes. Other methods that can be used for the control

of more brisk bleeding include elevation of the wound, infiltration of lidocaine with epinephrine, packing with absorbable gel foam, temporary instillation of hemostatic topical agents into the wound, or direct visualization and cautery or ligation of the offending vessel. Short-term (<30 minute) tourniquet use may be helpful for control of persistent, profound, or multiple sites of distal blood loss. Do not suture or clamp vessels blindly because of the risk of injuring adjacent structures.

ANTISEPSIS AND SCRUBBING

Clean the skin surrounding the wound prior to wound irrigation and repair. Various antiseptic skin cleansers can be used, including povidone–iodine and chlorhexidine gluconate. Non-ionic commercially available surfactants, such as Shur-Clens and Pharma Clens, mechanically lift bacteria from the skin, but possess no bactericidal activity.

Avoid mechanical scrubbing of the wound unless there is gross contamination. Although scrubbing can remove debris from the wound, it increases wound inflammation. If it is decided to perform scrubbing, use a fine-pore sponge (e.g., Optipore) to minimize tissue abrasion and a nonionic surfactant to minimize tissue toxicity and inflammation.

HAIR REMOVAL

Since infection rates are significantly greater in wounds that are shaved, remove hair by clipping if it interferes with the procedure. In almost all wounds, even those to the scalp, hair removal is not necessary. Moistening the hair in the area of the laceration with lubricating jelly usually keeps it out of the way. Never shave or clip the eyebrows. They serve as valuable landmarks for alignment during wound repair and, if removed, can take a long time to grow back.

IRRIGATION

Irrigation with between 5 and 8 psi of normal saline is the method of choice for removing bacteria and debris from most wounds.[27] Low-pressure irrigation with a bulb syringe does not adequately remove bacteria and debris from a wound.[28] The pressure delivered by a simple assembly consisting of an 18- to 20-gauge plastic catheter or needle attached to a 30-mL syringe is 6 to 8 psi.[29] Commercial systems to facilitate irrigation are available, including spring-loaded syringes with one-way valves connected to a standard intravenous (normal saline) setup, prepackaged irrigation fluids with irrigation nozzles, and cap devices that attach to standard fluid containers. Regardless of the system used, maintain the tip of the irrigation device between the wound and 5 cm above the intact skin. Use 200 to 300 mL of fluid for an average-sized low-risk wound and for increasing wound size or contamination, use more solution.

Normal saline remains the default irrigation fluid, and it is relatively inexpensive, decreases bacterial loads, and reduces wound infection rates. However, it is not bactericidal. Commercial strength povidone–iodine solution is tissue toxic and has no beneficial clinical effect on wound infection rates. When it is diluted to a 1% solution, however, it does not damage tissue and still retains its bactericidal properties but has no proven clinical benefit.[30] Tap water is cheaper than normal saline and is without tissue toxicity. Various method of tap water irrigation have been evaluated, and as long as irrigation pressures remain in the 5 to 8 psi range, tap water has been shown to be equivalent to normal saline.[31–33]

Antibiotic solutions have been studied for use in irrigation, but they cannot be routinely recommended for uncomplicated wounds. Nonionic surfactant agents (Shur-Clens, Pharma Clens) have been shown to remove bacteria and debris from wounds effectively. They are much more expensive than normal saline or 1% povidone–iodine solution and do not possess bactericidal activity or provide any additional benefit.[34] Hydrogen peroxide has no role in wound irrigation, as it impedes wound healing and has poor bactericidal activity. Benzalkonium chloride, although not as tissue toxic as hydrogen peroxide or 10% povidone–iodine, has a limited antimicrobial spectrum and has been associated with stock solution contamination by *Pseudomonas* organisms.

A consequence of irrigation is splatter, which can be minimized using one of many techniques.[35] Attaching a 4 × 4 inch gauze to the irrigation catheter or needle may provide minimal protection. Commercially available plastic shields (Zerowet) that attach directly to the irrigation syringe provide good protection against splatter while permitting visualization of the wound. An inexpensive version of these plastic shields is formed by puncturing the base of a sterile plastic medication cup with the irrigation needle. All the commercially available irrigation devices are prepackaged with some method of splatter control.

FOREIGN BODY EVALUATION

After anesthesia, perform wound exploration on all injuries to determine the extent of damage and to remove foreign material. The failure to diagnose foreign bodies in wounds is a frequent cause of litigation against emergency physicians.[36] Remove large debris from the wound with forceps. Inert foreign bodies such as glass or metal should be removed if possible (Fig. 39–6). Radiographs are occasionally required for precise localization of a foreign body, which can be aided by taping a radiopaque marker such as a paper clip to the skin overlying the suspected location. Other studies that can aid in the localization of foreign bodies include ultrasonography, CT scan, and MRI. If an inert foreign body is small and cannot easily be removed, it may be left in place and the patient or parent informed of its presence. Organic foreign bodies require urgent removal to prevent inflammatory reactions and potential infection. Consultation or urgent follow-up for surgical removal is warranted in cases where this type of material cannot be removed in the ED. Regardless of the findings on examination, or your ability to remove foreign bodies from the wound, parents and patients should be warned of potential residual contaminants in dirty wounds.

DEBRIDEMENT

Debridement is necessary in the management of contaminated wounds or wounds with nonviable tissue. Through removal

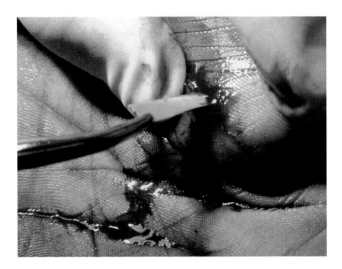

Figure 39–6. Foreign body in hand.

of contaminants and devitalized tissue from wounds, debridement increases a wound's ability to resist infection, shortens the period of inflammation, and creates a sharp, trimmed wound edge that is easier to repair and more cosmetically acceptable. If the devitalized edge of an irregular wound is debrided, the subcutaneous tissue of the wound can be undermined to avoid excess tension on the wound.

PRIMARY WOUND CLOSURE

Primary closure, using sutures, staples, tape, or tissue adhesive should be performed on lacerations that have been recently sustained (<24 hours on the face and <12 hours on other areas of the body), are relatively clean, and have minimal tissue devitalization. Prior to beginning closure, identify all the injured layers, such as fascia, subcutaneous tissue, muscle, tendon, and skin. During repair, always match each layer edge to its counterpart and ensure that when the sutures are placed, they enter and exit the appropriate layer at the same level so there is no overlapping of layers. A laceration that has been appropriately closed in layers usually does not need large or tight skin sutures to complete the closure. However, in hands and feet, placement of deep sutures increases the risk of infection, and they should be avoided in theses areas.

The size of suture to be used for wound closure depends on the tensile strength of the tissue in the wound. Use 3–0 suture for tissues with strong tension, such as fascia in an extremity, and 6–0 suture for tissues with light tension, such as the subcutaneous tissue of the face.

BURIED STITCH

Deep (buried) sutures serve four key functions and are required for many lacerations to ensure the best cosmetic result:

- They provide 2 to 3 weeks of additional support to the wound after the skin sutures are taken out or the tape is removed.

- They help to preserve the normal functioning of the underlying or involved muscles if the muscular fascia is sutured.
- They reduce the likelihood of the development of a hematoma or abscess by minimizing the dead space.
- They avoid the development of pitting in the injured region caused by inadequate healing of the deep tissues.

Unfortunately, deep sutures can result in damage to nerves, arteries, and tendons and can increase the risk of infection. Since suture material is a foreign body, even in clean or minimally contaminated wounds use as few deep sutures as necessary. The most common deep suture for laceration repair is the buried knot stitch, where one begins and ends at the base of the wound so as to bury the knot (Fig. 39–7).

The buried horizontal mattress stitch results in passage of suture material at the dermal–epidermal junction, with the knot placed subcuticularly below the dermis. The subcuticular stitch is a running buried suture at the dermal–epidermal junction that is actually used for skin closure (Fig. 39–8). Enter the skin initially approximately 3 mm to 2 cm from one end of the laceration, and allow the needle to emerge at the subcuticular plane at the wound apex. Pass the suture through the subcuticular tissue on alternate sides of the laceration. The point of entry of each stitch should be directly across from

or slightly behind the exit point of the previous stitch. At the other end of the laceration, burrow the needle again into the dermis to exit the skin 3 mm to 2 cm from the end. Ensure that there is no skin puckering, and then tape the free suture at both ends of the laceration in place. This stitch can be left in place if absorbable suture is used, or can be removed in 2 to 3 weeks if nonabsorbable suture is used. Use of the subcuticular stitch avoids skin suture marks but often requires more time to perform than other simpler methods for repair.

SKIN CLOSURE

If you choose to repair the epidermis and superficial layer of the dermis with sutures, place sutures such that the same depth and width is entered on both sides of the incision. A key to cosmetically acceptable closure is edge eversion, which is obtained by entering the skin at a 90-degree angle, and, in some cases, by using a skin hook. For wounds whose edges tend to invert despite proper technique, vertical mattress stitches can be used (Fig. 39–9). The number of sutures used to repair a laceration will vary with each case. For facial lacerations, sutures are generally placed 2 to 4 mm apart and 2 to 3 mm from the wound edge.

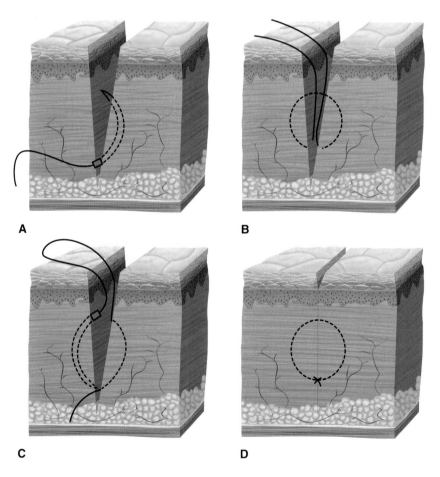

A

B

C

D

Figure 39–7. Buried subcutaneous stitch. This is particularly useful when approximating the subcutaneous tissue just beneath the skin edge, because it prevents irritation of the skin edge by the knot.

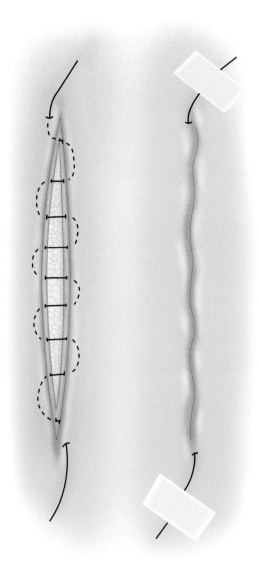

Figure 39–8. Subcuticular stitch. (See text for discussion.)

Simple Interrupted Stitch

The simple interrupted stitch is used most frequently for skin closure (Fig. 39–10). It involves placing separate loops of suture using proper eversion technique (i.e., entering skin at 90 degrees, including sufficient subcutaneous tissue), followed by tying and cutting each stitch. Although it is time consuming, if one stitch in the closure fails, the remaining stitches will hold the wound together. This technique is useful for stellate lacerations, wounds with multiple components, and lacerations that change direction. It is also helpful for approximation of landmarks on the skin, to achieve the best cosmetic result.

Running Stitch

The running or continuous stitch is well-suited for pediatric laceration repair for numerous reasons (Fig. 39–11): first, it is rapid; second, removal is easier; third, it provides more effective hemostasis; and finally, it distributes tension evenly along its length. The technique cannot be used over joints since, if one point were to break, the entire stitch would unravel.

To begin a simple running stitch, place an interrupted stitch at one end of the wound and cut only the free end of the suture. Continue suturing in a coil pattern, ensuring that the needle passes perpendicularly across the laceration with each pass. After each pass, tighten the loop slightly so that tension is equally distributed. To complete the stitch, place the final loop just beyond the end of the laceration and tie the suture with the last loop used as the tail. An interlocking continuous stitch can be used to reduce slippage of loops and for more irregular lacerations (Fig. 39–12). It is performed by pulling the needle through the previous loop each time it exits the skin. However, if the loops are tied too tightly, the resultant imprinting of the skin can increase the amount of tissue scarring.

Mattress Stitches

The horizontal mattress stitch can be used for single-layer closure of lacerations under tension (Fig. 39–13). It approximates skin edges closely, while providing some eversion, and decreases the time needed to suture because half the number of knots are tied. A running horizontal mattress suture can be used in areas of the body where loose skin could overlap or invert easily, such as the upper eyelids (Fig. 39–14).

The half-buried horizontal mattress stitch (corner stitch) is the suture of choice for closure of complex wounds with angulated (V-shaped) flaps (Fig. 39–15). Enter and exit the skin directly across from the flap and course the suture loop within the subcuticular tissue of the flap to maximize blood supply to the tip of the flap.

The vertical mattress stitch is helpful to evert skin edges (Fig. 39–9). It is useful in areas of the body with little subcutaneous tissue. The stitch begins in the same way as a simple interrupted stitch, but after the loop is made, reenter and reexit the skin approximately 1 to 2 mm from the wound edge and tie. A common technique is to alternate vertical mattress stitches with simple interrupted stitches to close a wound.

Knots

The knot used most commonly in the ED repair of lacerations is the surgeon's knot followed by one to four half-knots, usually formed as instrument ties. The single surgeon's knot allows for some give if any tissue edema develops.

Correction of Dog-Ears

When wound edges are not precisely aligned, an excess of skin on one or both ends ("dog-ears") result. A dog-ear can be corrected using the following technique (Fig. 39–16). First, elevate the excess skin with a skin hook and make an oblique incision from the apex of the wound toward the side of the dog-ear. Then undermine the flap and lay it flat, excise the excess triangle of skin, and complete the closure.

SECONDARY CLOSURE

Secondary closure is a technique that allows wounds to heal by granulation and reepithelialization. It is used to manage

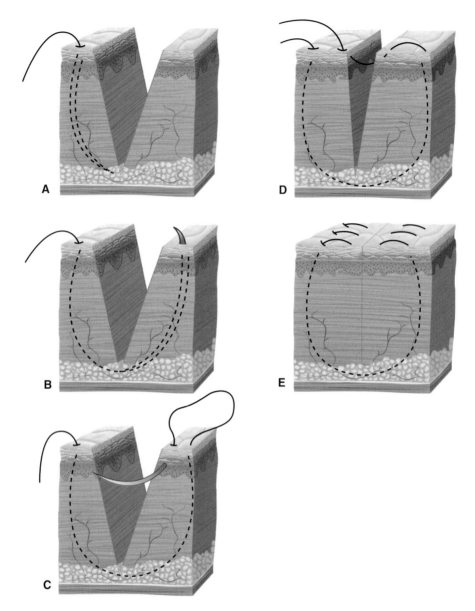

Figure 39–9. (A–E). Vertical mattress stitch. (See text for discussion.)

ulcerations, drained abscess cavities, deep puncture wounds, older or infected lacerations, and many animal bites. Daily packing is performed with saline-soaked gauze until granulation tissue closes the potential space.

DELAYED PRIMARY (TERTIARY) CLOSURE

Delayed primary closure with sutures is performed on wounds 3 to 5 days after they have been initially cleansed, debrided, and dressed appropriately.[37] Wounds amenable to this form of closure are those too contaminated for primary closure but not associated with significant tissue loss or devitalization. The utility of antibiotics during this "watch and wait" approach has not been closely studied.

WOUND DRESSING, DRAINS, AND IMMOBILIZATION

Sutured and stapled lacerations heal best in a moist environment. Thus, after laceration repair with sutures or staples, cleanse the skin of residual blood and povidone–iodine, and apply a light coat of antibiotic ointment. The use of topical antibiotic ointment for the prevention of infection has been shown to be clinically less effective after about 3 hours.[38] As such, if the antibiotic ointment is to be only used for purposes of maintaining a moist environment, a nonadherent dressing can be applied to the laceration instead (Adaptic, Telfa, Xeroform, or Vaseline gauze). Use a second layer of sterile gauze, or adhesive bandage (Band-Aid) to cover the ointment or nonadherent dressing. Alternatively, use an occlusive or semiocclusive dressing (Op-Site, Tegaderm, DuoDerm, or Biobrane).

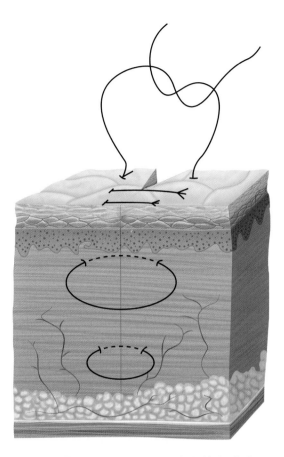

Figure 39–10. Simple interrupted stitch (with buried subcutaneous stitch). (See text for discussion.)

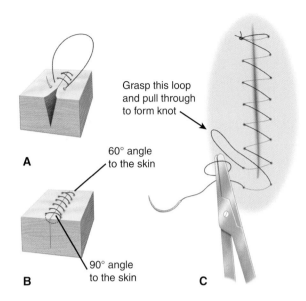

Figure 39–11. The simple continuous stitch. (A, B) This continuous suture is begun with a single suture that is tied to anchor the rest of the suture. The needle should be passed perpendicular to the skin edge and the suture threads should lie perpendicular to the wound margin, as with the simple interrupted suture. (C) To finish and tie off this continuous suture, grab the loop formed at the free end after insertion of the needle through the skin at its midpoint with the needle holder and pull on this loop. It will come together as if it were a single thread. Tie the needle end of the suture material and this "looped" free end as a simple interrupted suture would be tied. To complete the simple continuous stitch, a series of square knots is tied, with the loop as one of the ties.

If there is potential for the formation of a hematoma, apply a pressure dressing, taking care to avoid compression of arterial, venous, and lymphatic circulations.

Drains should rarely be used in sutured wounds. They act as foreign bodies and may promote rather than prevent infection. If a wound is considered a high risk for infection, attempt delayed primary closure rather than suturing and placing a drain in the wound. Drains should also not be used for hemostasis, which is better achieved by proper laceration repair, electrocauterization, and pressure dressings.

Splint a wound overlying a joint in the position of function for 7 to 10 days. For children, a bulky dressing may act as a splint and minimize motion at the wound, as well as prevent the child from tampering with the wound repair; it is especially helpful for hand and foot wounds.

ANTIBIOTIC USE AND TETANUS PROPHYLAXIS

More than 95% of wounds treated in the ED heal without complications if given appropriate wound care. Antibiotics should be considered in a few instances.[39] Antibiotics should be given to patients who present with a wound infection or with wounds that are more than 24-hours-old.[40] Other indications are for wounds heavily contaminated with feces or saliva, which may best be treated initially with secondary or delayed primary

closure. Intraoral lacerations appear to benefit from a short course (5 days) of penicillin.[41] Consider antibiotic use for any high-risk wounds in which there is involvement of cartilage, joint spaces, tendon, or bone, and despite literature that refutes the necessity, wounds of the hand are often covered with antibiotics.[42–45] Finally, consider antibiotics for high-risk wounds (contaminated or devitalized), especially in compromised hosts, such as children with sickle cell disease, diabetes, steroid use, or lymphoma.

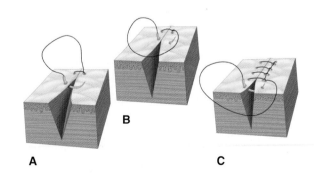

Figure 39–12. Continuous single lock stitch. (See text for discussion.)

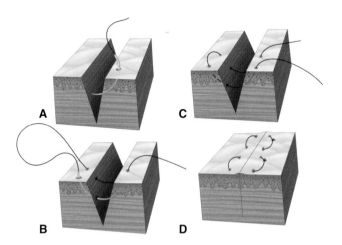

Figure 39–13. Horizontal mattress stitch. (A) The needle is passed 0.5–1 cm away from the wound edge deeply into the wound. (B) The needle is then passed through the opposite side and reenters the wound parallel to the initial suture. (C) One must enter the skin perpendicularly to provide some eversion of the wound edges and must enter and exit both the wound and skin at the same depth, otherwise "buckling" and irregularities occur in the wound margin. (D) The suture loop is then tied as shown.

When antibiotics are indicated, their effectiveness depends on early administration.[46] The first dose should therefore be given in the ED (preferably within 3 hours of the injury), regardless of the route of administration. The choice of antibiotics depends on the type of wound, although most infections are caused by sensitive staphylococci and streptococci that will respond to penicillin, first-generation cephalosporins or erythromycin for penicillin-allergic patients. Consideration of Methicillin-resistant *S. aureus* infection as a pathogen should be given, particularly to those patient who worsen or do not improve with standard therapy. Wounds contaminated with saliva generally respond to the same agents. Wounds contaminated with feces require coverage against facultative organ-

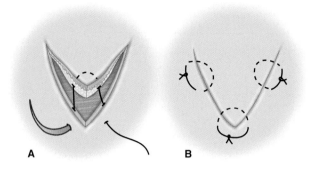

Figure 39–15. (A, B). Half-buried horizontal mattress stitch. This minimizes the vascular compromise at a corner flap. (See text for discussion.)

isms, coliforms, and obligate anaerobes. Reasonable choices would include second- and third-generation cephalosporins, or the combination of clindamycin and an aminoglycoside.

Mammalian bite wounds are a complex subject that merits more in-depth discussion. The cumulative research on the subject suggests that dog bites in normal hosts with low-risk wounds will do well with meticulous wound care, closure,[47] splinting, elevation, and close follow-up without antibiotics.[48] All noncanine bites merit a short course of antibiotics. Generally, 3 to 5 days of oral antibiotics are prescribed for these bite injuries, but no definitive studies have examined appropriate duration of therapy.

Tetanus prophylaxis begins with appropriate wound care. If the wound is tetanus prone, determine the child's immunization status (Fig. 39–17). If the child has a tetanus-prone wound and was not immunized or only partially immunized, or if their immunization status is unknown, treat the child as if they have no protection. Give human tetanus immune globulin (HTIG) 250 U IM and complete or initiate primary immunization. If a child has completed primary immunization and has received appropriate boosters, then HTIG is not required.[49]

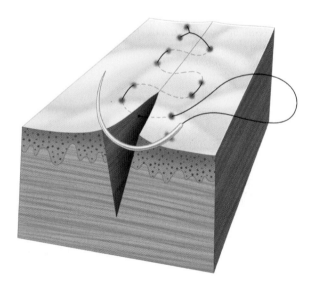

Figure 39–14. Continuous mattress stitch. (See text for discussion.)

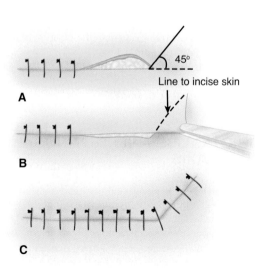

Figure 39–16. (A–C). The dog-ear. (See text for discussion.)

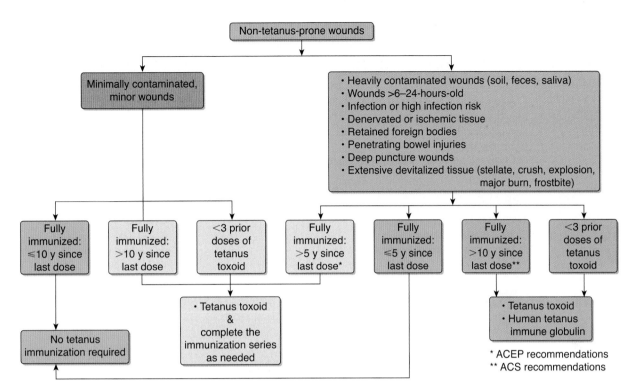

Figure 39–17. Tetanus immunization guidelines.

▶ POSTOPERATIVE WOUND CARE AND SUTURE REMOVAL

Successful outcome of wounds is partly dependent on wound care after discharge from the ED. Therefore, the patient and parents should be given thorough instructions about care of the wound and what to expect. Patients and families should be informed that all wounds of significance heal with scars, regardless of the quality of care. The final appearance of the scar cannot be predicted before 6 to 12 months after the repair. They should be informed about the possibility of infection and that there is always the possibility, despite appropriate management, of a residual foreign body in the wound.

Because lacerations are bridged by epithelial cells within 48 hours, the wound is less susceptible to the entry of bacteria after 2 days. Give instructions to keep the dressing in place and the wound clean for 24 to 48 hours. The dressing should be changed if it becomes soiled or soaked by exudate from the wound. The dressing may be removed to check for signs of infection, such as erythema, pain, warmth, purulent discharge, excessive edema, or red streaks suggestive of lymphangitis all of which mandate a reevaluation. If parental reliability is questionable, the patient should have the wound reexamined in the ED in 2 to 3 days. If there are no signs of infection, instruct the patient or parents to gently wash the wound daily with soap and water to remove dried blood and exudates.[50] Undiluted hydrogen peroxide should not be used, since it may destroy granulation tissue and newly formed epithelium. Generally, the wound should be protected with a dressing during the first week, with daily dressing changes. Once the dressing is removed, patients and parents should be instructed that sunscreen should be applied to the scar for at least 6 months to prevent hyperpigmentation of the scar.

Suture removal should be done at an appropriate time so as to prevent dehiscence of the wound seen with premature removal and to prevent suture track marks and stitch abscesses resulting from late removal (Table 39–3). Children both heal and form suture track marks faster than adults and thus need earlier suture removal. After appropriately timed suture removal, skin tape should be applied, since wound contraction and scar widening will continue to occur for several weeks after an injury.

Once the closure device, suture, or staples have been removed or the adhesive dissipates, wound healing continues and wound care remains important. Instruct your patients to avoid sun on the fresh scar and use sunscreen to avoid a hyperpigmented scar. Patients will often ask what can be done to prevent scar formation, and the literature suggests that the mechanical action of rubbing may be the common thread by which all the various commercially available topical products have positive effects.[51,52] Vitamin E preparations should be avoided because of potential local hypersensitivity reactions.[53]

▶ MANAGEMENT OF SELECTED INJURIES

ABRASIONS

It is generally sufficient to clean abrasions and dress them with a nonadherent dressing or antibiotic ointment that can be changed daily after cleaning. Deeper abrasions may be treated similar to skin graft donor sites with cleansing and a fine-mesh gauze dressing. It is important to remove any foreign bodies (e.g., gravel, dirt, or tar) to avoid infection or tattooing ("road rash") of the wound. Anesthesia for the cleansing of abrasions

▶ TABLE 39–3. **REPAIR OF SOFT TISSUE INJURIES BY BODY LOCATION**

Location	Type of Closure	Suture Removal
Scalp	Single tight layer with simple interrupted, vertical mattress, or horizontal mattress for hemostasis; galea requires close approximation, but preferably with single-layer closure	7–10 d
Pinna (ear)	Simple interrupted; stent dressing	4–6 d
Eyebrow	Layered closure	4–5 d
Eyelid	Horizontal mattress	3–5 d
Lip	Three layers (mucosa, muscle skin) if through and through, otherwise two layers	3–5 d
Oral cavity	Simple interrupted or horizontal mattress	7–8 days or allow to dissolve
Face	If full-thickness, layered closure	3–5 d
Neck	Two-layered closure	4–6 d
Trunk	Single or layered closure	7–12 d
Extremity	Single or layered; splint if over joint	10–14 d (joint) 7–10 d (other)
Hands and feet	Single-layer closure with simple interrupted or horizontal mattress; splint if over joint	10–14 d (joint) 7–10 d (other)
Nail beds		Allow to dissolve

can be difficult, and large abrasions may require general anesthesia or conscious sedation to permit adequate debridement. For smaller areas, topical anesthesia with 2% lidocaine or LAT solution, infiltration of local anesthetic, or nerve blocks can be used. Children with large or deep abrasions should have their wounds reexamined in 2 to 3 days for monitoring of healing.

SCALP LACERATIONS

There are five anatomic layers in the scalp: skin, superficial fascia, galea aponeurotica, subaponeurotic areolar connective tissue, and periosteum. The presence of a rich vascular supply and vessels that tend to remain patent when cut are responsible for the profuse bleeding associated with scalp injuries. Usually, the bleeding is halted by direct pressure, epinephrine infiltration, and rapid closure.

The subgaleal layer of connective tissue contains "emissary veins" that drain through vessels of the skull into the venous sinuses within the cranial vault. In scalp wounds that penetrate the galea, bacteria can be carried by these vessels, and while exceedingly rare, a wound infection can result in osteomyelitis, meningitis, or an intracranial abscess. Approximation of galeal lacerations will not only help to control bleeding, but may theoretically safeguard against the spread of infection.

Although most lacerations that involve multiple layers of tissue should be closed in layers, scalp wounds are best closed with a single layer of sutures that incorporates the skin, the subcutaneous fascia, and the galea. Some advocate separate closure of the galea with absorbable suture material, which allows its more careful approximation but introduces a foreign body into the wound, thus increasing chances of infection. In order to find the ends of the tied sutures these should be left longer than usual, and the use of blue nylon may also facilitate removal. Superficial scalp lacerations are also amenable to staple closure as was discussed earlier.

FOREHEAD LACERATIONS

Lacerations that are limited to the area above the supraorbital rim can be anesthetized with supraorbital and supratrochlear nerve blocks, thus avoiding tissue distortion associated with local infiltration. As for scalp lacerations, explore for skull fractures and foreign bodies. Close the forehead in layers, beginning with the approximation of the frontalis fascia. Continue the layered closure, taking care to align landmarks such as forehead furrows.

EYELID LACERATIONS

The thin, flexible skin of the eyelid is quite simple to suture (Fig. 39–18). However, it is essential that the emergency physician be aware of injuries that require consultation with

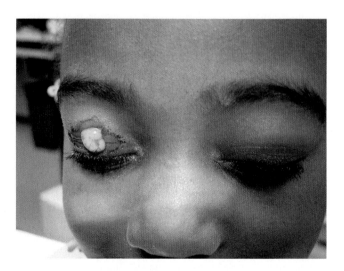

Figure 39–18. Eyelid laceration.

an ophthalmologist. A thorough eye examination needs to be performed whenever there is a laceration of the eyelid or periorbital region. Also, ensure that the levator palpebrae muscle and its tendinous attachment to the tarsal plate are intact, or ptosis may result. A laceration to the medial aspect of the lower lid often involves the lacrimal duct, which requires specialized repair by an ophthalmologist. If consultation is not required, close lid lacerations in a single layer with 6–0 suture, taking care to avoid skin inversion.

EAR LACERATIONS

Injuries to the ears require expedient cleansing, debridement of devitalized tissue, and coverage of exposed cartilage in order to avoid chondritis. Anesthesia of the external ear is simply accomplished with a field block of the auriculotemporal, greater auricular, and occipital nerves, performed by infiltration at the base of the auricle. Once cleansing and debridement of devitalized tissue is performed, approximate cartilage with 5–0 absorbable suture material placed through the posterior and anterior perichondrium. Keep tension to a minimum to prevent tearing of the cartilage. Finally, approximate the visible surface of the ear using 5–0 or 6–0 suture, ensuring approximation of landmarks such as folds. No cartilage should be left exposed. After repair, dress the ear with a compression dressing, including coverage of the anterior and posterior aspects of the auricle. This prevents accumulation of a perichondral hematoma, which can lead to necrosis of cartilage and subsequent deformity ("cauliflower ear").

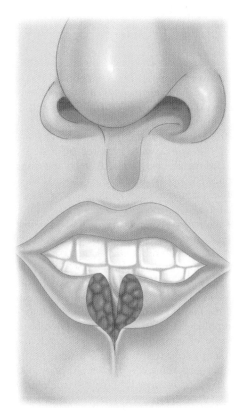

A

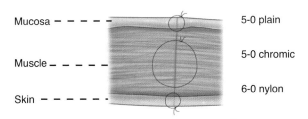

Mucosa — — — — —   5-0 plain

Muscle — — — —   5-0 chromic

Skin — — — — —   6-0 nylon

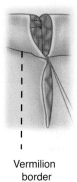

Muscle
approximation

Vermilion
border

Skin

B

Figure 39–19. Repair of through-and-through lip laceration.

LIP LACERATIONS

Lip lacerations are common in the pediatric age group and require careful attention to ensure a good cosmetic result (Fig. 39–19). Prior to beginning repair, inspect the oral mucosa and teeth for lacerations and trauma. Since local infiltration of anesthetic obscures the lip's landmarks, consider performing a mental nerve block for the repair of lower lip lacerations or an infraorbital nerve block for upper lip lacerations.

After anesthesia, cleanse and irrigate the wound in the usual manner, and then place the first stitch at the vermilion border. If deep sutures are required, leave the initial stitch untied and proceed with deep closure. Through-and-through lip lacerations require three-layer closure. Approximate the orbicularis oris muscle with 4–0 or 5–0 absorbable suture. Close the mucosa with 5–0 absorbable suture to obtain a tight seal. Finally, after irrigation of the outside surface, close the skin with 6–0 suture material (Fig. 39–20). Four-layer closure, including the subcutaneous layer, can be used to facilitate skin closure. Through-and-through lip lacerations are prone to infection, and prophylaxis with penicillin or erythromycin for 5 days has been shown to diminish infection rates.

FINGERTIP INJURIES

Young children often injure fingers in doors and windows. Distal fingertip injuries, even complete amputations, heal remarkably well in children. Therapy of distal fingertip amputations consists first of a digital block or local infiltration, followed by appropriate cleansing and dressing of the wound with antibiotic ointment or nonadherent gauze, and a splint or bulky dressing for protection while radiographs are obtained.

Prognosis of distal amputations depends on how much of the tip is lost. If the fingernail and nail bed are not involved, prognosis is excellent. If the bone is spared but there is involvement of the nail or nail bed, there may be shortening of the digit. Injuries involving the distal phalanx, especially those at the base of the nail, heal most poorly. More proximal amputations uniformly require consultation with a hand surgeon.

A paronychium is a cutaneous abscess at the lateral aspect of fingernails or toenails. Since the fingers and toes are

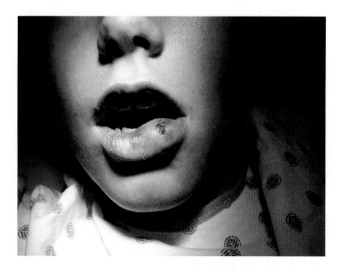

Figure 39–20. Lip laceration.

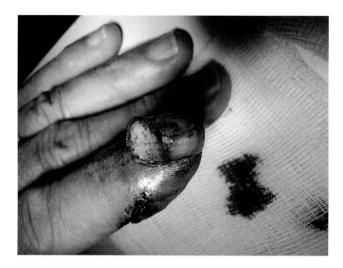

Figure 39–21. Nail/fingertip injury.

vulnerable to trauma during childhood, including nail biting and finger sucking, an acutely painful, swollen, erythematous, and tender paronychia is not an uncommon ED complaint. For fingers, an extensive procedure is rarely required for treatment of a paronychia. Most often, the cuticle (junction between the nail and the skin) can be elevated or incised with a No. 11 blade, and the abscess can be drained and irrigated. Systemic antibiotics are needed only when there is an accompanying cellulitis or lymphangitis. Paronychias of the toes are often caused by ingrown toenails. Thus, removal of the ingrown portion of the nail is required to avoid a recurrence. Since this is a more extensive and painful procedure, a digital nerve block in conjunction with moderate sedation should be considered.

A subungual hematoma is a collection of blood under a fingernail or toenail, usually sustained after a direct blow. If the nail is intact, pressure from the hematoma can cause substantial pain. If the hematoma involves less than 25% to 50% of the nail bed, trephinate the nail using one of a number of techniques. The use of electrocautery has most recently been advocated as the simplest, safest, and least painful method to drain a subungual hematoma. Prior to trephination, cleanse the nail and once blood escapes through the nail, remove the cautery to avoid nail bed damage. For subungual hematomas involving >50% of the nail bed, there is controversy as to what treatment is best. Nail removal used to be advocated, because of the perceived need to repair the underlying nail bed laceration. However, this practice has been questioned as long as the nail and surrounding nail fold are intact. Nail bed lacerations associated with disruption of the nail itself may be closed with 6–0 absorbable sutures (Fig. 39–21). Debridement should be kept to a minimum, and the paronychium and eponychium must be prevented from forming adhesions with the nail bed by packing the space with nonadherent gauze or using the nail itself as a stent after repair of the nail bed. If there is an underlying fracture of the distal phalanx, splint the finger and prescribe antibiotics appropriate for an open fracture.

PUNCTURE WOUNDS TO THE FOOT

Puncture wounds, most often to the foot, have a very low potential to result in significant morbidity.[54] While rare, cellulitis,

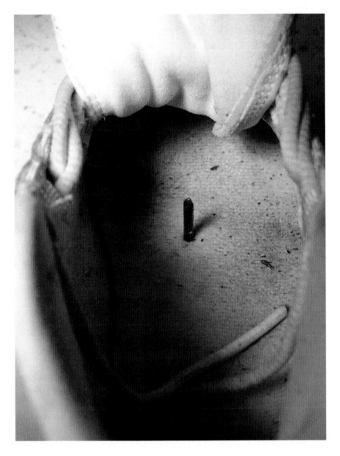

Figure 39–22. Puncture wound through tennis shoe.

plantar space infections, abscesses, retained foreign bodies, and osteomyelitis can result from a benign-appearing wound (Fig. 39–22). A reasonable approach to puncture wounds of the foot is to obtain a radiograph to ascertain bony involvement, air in the joint spaces, and radiopaque foreign bodies. Anesthetize the wound and then explore the puncture site, cleanse the wound, and remove any foreign bodies. The use of prophylactic antibiotics is controversial, and likely not warranted on a patient's initial accession to care. However, in the setting of infection at the time of presentation, debridement should be performed and broad-spectrum antibiotics should be given. For puncture wounds sustained through the sole of a tennis shoe, coverage was typically aimed at *Pseudomonas aeruginosa* as that pathogen has been associated with post-puncture osteomyelitis.[55] Patients who present quickly after puncture wounds, have normal host factors, and no evidence for retained foreign body may be discharged without antibiotics and reevaluated after 48 hours of elevation, non-weight-bearing, and meticulous wound care.[56]

► CONSULTATION GUIDELINES

Specialty consultation should be considered for the following:

- Complex or extensive wounds which exceed your resources or skill set.
- Wounds with large tissue defects not amenable to repair in the ED.

- Wounds in which there is tendon, nerve, joint, or critical vessel involvement.
- Lacerations involving the parotid or lacrimal ducts.
- Lacerations of the eyelid tarsal plates.
- Lacerations over fractures.
- Facial lacerations in which cosmetic results are a concern.
- Wounds about which there is physician uncertainty.

REFERENCES

1. Burt CW, McCaig LF. Trends in hospital emergency department utilization: United States, 1992–1999. *Vital Health Stat 13.* 2001:1–34, Data from the National Health Survey.
2. Hollander JE, Singer AJ. Laceration management [Review]. *Ann Emerg Med.* 1999; 34:356–367.
3. Singer AJ, Clark RA. Cutaneous wound healing [Review]. *N Engl J Med.* 1999;341:738–746.
4. Schappert SM. Ambulatory care visits to physician offices, hospital outpatient departments, and emergency departments: United States, 1997. *Vital Health Stat 13.* 2001:i–iv, Data from the National Health Survey, Review.
5. Slusarcick AL, McCaig LF. National Hospital Ambulatory Medical Care Survey: 1998 outpatient department summary. *Adv Data.* 2000:1–23.
6. Trott A. Mechanisms of surface soft tissue trauma [Review]. *Ann Emerg Med.* 1988;17:1279–1283.
7. Cardany CR, Rodeheaver G, Thacker J, Edgerton MT, Edlich RF. The crush injury: a high risk wound. *JACEP.* 1976;5:965–970.
8. Knapp JF. Updates in wound management for the pediatrician. *Pediatr Clinic North Am.* 1999;46:1202–1213.
9. Maitra AK, Adams JC, Maitra AK, Adams JC. Use of sterile gloves in the management of sutured hand wounds in the A&E department. *Injury.* 1986;17:193–195.
10. Perelman VS, Francis GJ, Rutledge T, Foote J, Martino F, Dranitsaris G. Sterile versus nonsterile gloves for repair of uncomplicated lacerations in the emergency department: a randomized controlled trial. *Ann Emerg Med.* 2004;43:362–370.
11. Karounis H, Gouin S, Eisman H, Chalut D, Pelletier H, Williams B. A randomized, controlled trial comparing long-term cosmetic outcomes of traumatic pediatric lacerations repaired with absorbable plain gut versus nonabsorbable nylon sutures. *Acad Emerg Med.* 2004;11:730–735.
12. Karounis H, Gouin S, Harley E, et al. Plain gut vs. non-absorbable nylon sutures in traumatic pediatric lacerations: long -term. *Acad Emerg Med.* 2002;9(5):448.
13. Holger JS, Wandersee SC, Hale DB, Holger JS, Wandersee SC, Hale DB. Cosmetic outcomes of facial lacerations repaired with tissue-adhesive, absorbable, and nonabsorbable sutures [see comment]. *Am J Emerg Med.* 2004;22:254–257.
14. Kuo F, Lee D, Rogers GS. Prospective, randomized, blinded study of a new wound closure film versus cutaneous suture for surgical wound closure. *Dermatol Surg.* 2006;32:676–681.
15. Singer AJ, Zimmerman T, Rooney J, Cameau P. Comparison of wound bursting strengths and surface characteristics of FDA approved tissue adhesives for skin closure. *J Adhes Sci Technol.* 2004;18:19–28.
16. Noordzij JP, Foresman PA, Rodeheaver GT, Quinn JV, Edlich RF. Tissue adhesive wound repair revisited. *J Emerg Med.* 1994;12:645–649.
17. Singer AJ, Hollander JE, Valentine SM, Turque TW, McCuskey CF, Quinn JV. Prospective, randomized, controlled trial of tissue adhesive (2-octylcyanoacrylate) vs. standard wound closure techniques for laceration repair. Stony Brook Octyl-cyanoacrylate Study Group. *Acad Emerg Med.* 1998;5:94–99.

18. Denkler K. A comprehensive review of epinephrine in the finger: to do or not to do [see comment] [Review]. *Plast Reconstr Surg.* 2001;108:114–124.

19. Spivey WH, McNamara RM, MacKenzie RS, Bhat S, Burdick WP. A clinical comparison of lidocaine and bupivacaine. *Ann Emerg Med.* 1987;16:752–757.

20. Scott DB. "Maximum recommended doses" of local anaesthetic drugs. *Br J Anaesth.* 1989;63:373–374.

21. Brogan GX Jr, Giarrusso E, Hollander JE, Cassara G, Maranga MC, Thode HC. Comparison of plain, warmed, and buffered lidocaine for anesthesia of traumatic wounds. *Ann Emerg Med.* 1995;26:121–125.

22. Bartfield JM, Sokaris SJ, Raccio-Robak N. Local anesthesia for lacerations: pain of infiltration inside vs. outside the wound. *Acad Emerg Med.* 1998;5:100–104.

23. Bartfield JM, Lee FS, Raccio-Robak N, Salluzzo RF, Asher SL. Topical tetracaine attenuates the pain of infiltration of buffered lidocaine. *Acad Emerg Med.* 1996;3:1001–1005.

24. Kennedy DW, Shaikh Z, Fardy MJ, Evans RJ, Crean SV. Topical adrenaline and cocaine gel for anaesthetising children's lacerations. An audit of acceptability and safety. *Emerg Med J.* 2004;21:194–196.

25. Schilling CG, Bank DE, Borchert BA, Klatzko MD, Uden DL. Tetracaine, epinephrine (adrenalin), and cocaine (TAC) versus lidocaine, epinephrine, and tetracaine (LET) for anesthesia of lacerations in children. *Ann Emerg Med.* 1995;25:203–208.

26. Schaffer DJ. Clinical comparison of TAC anesthetic solutions with and without cocaine. *Ann Emerg Med.* 1985;14:1077–1080.

27. Singer AJ, Hollander JE, Subramanian S, Malhotra AK, Villez PA. Pressure dynamics of various irrigation techniques commonly used in the emergency department [see comment]. *Ann Emerg Med.* 1994;24:36–40.

28. Stevenson TR, Thacker JG, Rodeheaver GT, Bacchetta C, Edgerton MT, Edlich RF. Cleansing the traumatic wound by high pressure syringe irrigation. *JACEP.* 1976;5:17–21.

29. Rodeheaver GT, Pettry D, Thacker JG, Edgerton MT, Edlich RF. Wound cleansing by high pressure irrigation. *Surg Gynecol Obstet.* 1975;141:357–362.

30. Lammers RL, Fourre M, Callaham ML, Boone T. Effect of povidone-iodine and saline soaking on bacterial counts in acute, traumatic, contaminated wounds. *Ann Emerg Med.* 1990;19:709–714.

31. Godinez FS, Grant-Levy TR, McGuirk TD, Letterle S, Eich M, O'Malley GF. Comparison of normal saline vs. tap water for irrigation of minor lacerations in the emergency department. *Acad Emerg Med.* 2002;9(5):396–397.

32. Valente JH, Forti RJ, Freundlich LF, Zandieh SO, Crain EF. Wound irrigation in children: saline solution or tap water? *Ann Emerg Med.* 2003;41:609–616.

33. Fernandez R, Griffiths R, Fernandez R, Griffiths R. Water for wound cleansing [Update of *Cochrane Database Syst Rev.* 2002;(4):CD003861; PMID: 12519612] [Review]. *Cochrane Database Syst Rev.* 2008:CD003861.

34. Dire DJ, Welsh AP. A comparison of wound irrigation solutions used in the emergency department. *Ann Emerg Med.* 1990;19:704–708.

35. Pigman EC, Karch DB, Scott JL. Splatter during jet irrigation cleansing of a wound model: a comparison of three inexpensive devices. *Ann Emerg Med.* 1993;22:1563–1567.

36. Sullivan DJ. Wound care: retained foreign bodies and missed tendon injuries. ED legal letter. 1998;9(5):45–56.

37. Dimick AR. Delayed wound closure: indications and techniques. *Ann Emerg Med.* 1988;17:1303–1304.

38. Dire DJ, Coppola M, Dwyer DA, Lorette JJ, Karr JL. Prospective evaluation of topical antibiotics for preventing infections in uncomplicated soft-tissue wounds repaired in the ED [see comment]. *Acad Emerg Med.* 1995;2:4–10.

39. Day TK. Controlled trial of prophylactic antibiotics in minor wounds requiring suture. *Lancet.* 1975;2:1174–1176.

40. Edlich RF, Rogers W, Kasper G, Kaufman D, Tsung MS, Wangensteen OH. Studies in the management of the contaminated wound. I. Optimal time for closure of contaminated open wounds. II. Comparison of resistance to infection of open and closed wounds during healing. *Am J Surg.* 1969;117:323–329.

41. Steele MT, Sainsbury CR, Robinson WA, Salomone JA III, Elenbaas RM. Prophylactic penicillin for intraoral wounds. *Ann Emerg Med.* 1989;18:847–852.

42. Grossman JA, Adams JP, Kunec J. Prophylactic antibiotics in simple hand lacerations. *JAMA.* 1981;245:1055–1056.

43. Haughey RE, Lammers RL, Wagner DK. Use of antibiotics in the initial management of soft tissue hand wounds. *Ann Emerg Med.* 1981;10:187–192.

44. Roberts AH, Teddy PJ. A prospective trial of prophylactic antibiotics in hand lacerations. *Br J Surg.* 1977;64:394–396.

45. Worlock P, Boland P, Darrell J, Hughes S. The role of prophylactic antibodies following hand injuries. *Br J Clin Pract.* 1980;34:290–292.

46. Morgan WJ, Hutchison D, Johnson HM, Morgan WJ, Hutchison D, Johnson HM. The delayed treatment of wounds of the hand and forearm under antibiotic cover. *Br J Surg.* 1980;67:140–141.

47. Maimaris C, Quinton DN. Dog-bite lacerations: a controlled trial of primary wound closure. *Arch Emerg Med.* 1988;5:156–161.

48. Garbutt F, Jenner R. Best evidence topic report. Wound closure in animal bites [Review]. *Emerg Med J.* 2004;21:589–590.

49. Thwaites CL, Farrar JJ. Preventing and treating tetanus. *BMJ.* 2003;326:117–118.

50. Noe JM, Keller M. Can stitches get wet? *Plast Reconstr Surg.* 1988;81:82–84.

51. Mustoe TA, Cooter RD, Gold MH, et al. International clinical recommendations on scar management [Review]. *Plast Reconstr Surg.* 2002;110:560–571.

52. Chung VQ, Kelley L, Marra D, et al. Onion extract gel versus petrolatum emollient on new surgical scars: prospective double-blinded study. *Dermatol Surg.* 2006;32:193–197.

53. Baumann LS, Spencer J. The effects of topical vitamin E on the cosmetic appearance of scars [see comment]. *Dermatol Surg.* 1999;25:311–315.

54. Weber EJ, Weber EJ. Plantar puncture wounds: a survey to determine the incidence of infection. *J Accid Emerg Med.* 1996;13:274–277.

55. Raz R, Miron D, Raz R, Miron D. Oral ciprofloxacin for treatment of infection following nail puncture wounds of the foot. *Clin Infect Dis.* 1995;21:194–195.

56. Schwab RA, Powers RD. Conservative therapy of plantar puncture wounds. *J Emerg Med.* 1995;13:291–295.

SECTION V

RESPIRATORY EMERGENCIES

CHAPTER 40

Upper Airway Emergencies

Richard M. Cantor and Linnea Wittick

▶ HIGH-YIELD FACTS

- Acute respiratory emergencies in the pediatric patient are common and may, if improperly treated, result in significant morbidity and mortality.
- The clinician must maintain an awareness of the unique anatomic and physiologic characteristics of the respiratory tract in the growing infant and child.
- Stridor may originate anywhere in the upper airway from the anterior nares to the subglottic region.
- The most common causes of acute upper airway obstruction are croup, epiglottitis, and foreign body obstruction. Additional processes include peritonsillar abscess, bacterial tracheitis, and retropharyngeal abscess.

Acute respiratory emergencies in the pediatric patient are common and may, if improperly treated, result in significant morbidity and mortality. Calm, decisive, and deliberate intervention is mandatory to ensure the most effective outcome. The clinician must maintain an awareness of the unique anatomic and physiologic characteristics of the respiratory tract in the growing infant and child. An expanded knowledge of the most frequent airway problems encountered in children will assist in arriving at the proper evaluation, treatment, and disposition of these patients. The ability to accurately assess the child in respiratory distress remains the most critical step in patient care.

▶ PATHOPHYSIOLOGY

UPPER AIRWAY CONSIDERATIONS

The small caliber of the upper airway in children makes it vulnerable to occlusion secondary to a variety of disease processes and also results in greater baseline airway resistance. Any process that further narrows the airway will cause an exponential rise in airway resistance and a secondary increase in the work of breathing. As the child perceives distress, an increase in respiratory effort will augment turbulence and increase resistance to a greater degree.

Since the young infant is primarily a nasal breather, any degree of obstruction of the nasopharynx may result in significant increase in work of breathing and present clinically as retractions. The large tongue of infants and small children can occlude the oropharynx. Any child who presents with altered mental status will be at risk for the development of upper airway obstruction secondary to a loss of muscle tone affecting the tongue. Occlusion of the oropharynx by this anatomic

structure is quite common in this setting. Interventions that can correct this anatomic blockage include either tilting of the head or lifting of the chin. Insertion of an orotracheal or a nasotracheal airway may also assist in alleviating respiratory distress.

Older children will frequently present with enlarged tonsillar and adenoidal tissues. Although they rarely cause an upper airway catastrophe, these structures are vulnerable to trauma and bleeding during clinical interventions such as insertion of an oral or nasal airway. The pediatric trachea is easily compressible because of incomplete closure of the cartilaginous rings. Any maneuver that overextends the neck will contribute to compression of this structure and secondary upper airway obstruction. The cricoid ring represents the narrowest portion of the upper airway and is often the site of occlusion in foreign body aspiration.

LOWER AIRWAY CONSIDERATIONS

The lower respiratory tract consists of all structures below the level of the midtrachea including the bronchi, bronchioles, and alveoli. Developmental immaturity of these structures is reflected by a decreased number of these subunits necessary for appropriate oxygenation and ventilation. In addition, the pediatric patient possesses a diminished pulmonary vascular bed. The relatively small caliber of the pediatric lower airway not only predisposes it to occlusion, but even partial obstruction will result in an augmented degree of airway resistance.

Immaturity of the musculoskeletal and central nervous systems can also contribute to the development of respiratory failure. In infancy, the diaphragm remains the primary muscle of respiration. Minor contributions are provided by the intercostal musculature. Any degree of abdominal distention will interfere with diaphragmatic function and cause secondary ventilatory insufficiency. The infant's diaphragm possesses muscle fibers that are more prone to fatigue compared with their adult counterparts. In addition, the chest wall of the pediatric patient is quite compliant, preventing adequate stabilization during periods of increased respiratory distress. Finally, infants are less sensitive to hypoxemia secondary to poor development of central respiratory control, which places this population at risk for insufficient respiratory response to disease states.

▶ SIGNS OF DISTRESS

Regardless of the specific disease process, abnormalities in respiratory function are eventually reflected in physical symptoms and signs ranging from subtle changes to obvious distress. Respiratory distress occurs when there is increased work of breathing or increased respiratory rate in order to maintain respiratory function necessary to meet the body's oxygen and ventilation requirements. Respiratory failure ensues when respiratory efforts cannot maintain adequate respiratory function, either oxygenation or ventilation.

Tachypnea (Table 28–3) represents the most common response of the child to augmented respiratory needs. Central stimulation by the medullary respiratory center is predominantly responsible for this physiologic response. Although most commonly caused by hypoxia and hypercarbia, tachypnea may also be a secondary response to metabolic acidosis, pain, or central nervous system insult. Tachycardia represents a protean sign of distress of any etiology in the pediatric patient. This would include the patient with respiratory compromise.

Infants and children readily use accessory muscles as a compensatory mechanism necessary to support the increased work of breathing. Intercostal, subcostal, sub- and supersternal, and supraclavicular retractions are commonly seen. In addition, the infant and child will demonstrate nasal flaring, if further compromised.

Pay specific attention to the child who generates a grunting sound at the end of expiration. This physiologic effort represents closure of the glottis at the end of expiration, which generates additional positive end-expiratory pressure, which in many disease states is necessary to prevent compromised alveoli from collapse. Grunting represents an ominous sign in the pediatric patient who presents with respiratory distress.

Many infants and children, especially children with upper airway compromise, will assume a "position of comfort," which represents the most adequate anatomic compensation they can generate relative to their disease state. Children with stridor will often assume an upright position, lean forward, and generate their own jaw thrust maneuver to facilitate opening of the upper airway. Patients with upper airway compromise may also prefer to breathe through an open mouth, which suggests dysphagia with inability to swallow secretions, or the general presence of air hunger. Patients with lower airway disease, specifically those with reactive airway components, will assume a "tripod position" consisting of upright posture, leaning forward, and support of the upper thorax by the use of extended arms. This position allows for full use of the thoracoabdominal axis for the work of breathing.

In situations in which significant excessive negative intrathoracic pressure is generated, venous return will increase to the heart, and left ventricular volume will be compromised. These intracardiac phenomena result in the generation of a pulsus paradoxus of greater than 20 mm Hg (normal, 0–10 mm Hg). The presence of an elevated pulsus paradoxus correlates well with severe respiratory distress.

The presence of cyanosis is an ominous sign in the pediatric patient. It represents inadequate oxygenation within the pulmonary bed or inadequate oxygen delivery by the cardiovascular system. Cyanosis of respiratory origin tends to be central rather than peripheral. A secondary effect of cyanosis may be the development of somnolence. The most common symptoms and signs of hypoxemia include agitation, irritability, and failure to maintain feeding efforts in the young infant. Clinically evident hypoxemia may not appear until P_{O_2} levels are dangerously low in the anemic child.

By far, the most reliable sign of respiratory failure remains the generation of an ineffective respiratory effort by the infant or child and an altered level of consciousness. Auscultation of the chest may reveal decreased air entry, poor breath sounds, and bradypnea as the child progresses toward respiratory failure. Concomitant with hypoxemia in infants is the development of bradycardia. Although bradycardia may also be due to excessive vagal stimulation, hypoxemia should be ruled out in all such cases of respiratory distress.

► GENERAL MANAGEMENT PRINCIPLES

Any child with respiratory distress requires supplemental oxygen. Humidified oxygen may be delivered in a variety of ways, including mask with or without rebreather apparatus, nasal prongs, face tent, or via an oxygen hood. Infants and children who feel threatened by the use of frightening equipment may be placed in the mother's arms and receive oxygen by tubing alone (at maximal flow) or by inserting the end of the tubing in a cup.

Specific diagnostic categories of respiratory distress offer the clinician various therapeutic modalities, which will improve the patient's status (see next section). General evaluative principles that should be applied to the infant or child in distress include the following. Use a standardized approach to the patient in mild-to-moderate distress by providing supplemental oxygen, allow the child to assume a position of comfort, and create a comfortable, nonthreatening environment for both parent and child. Avoid any noxious stimuli in the form of unnecessary procedures. Also maintain normothermia and hydration. Assess the degree of respiratory distress, at presentation and at appropriate intervals.

ARTERIAL BLOOD GASES

The arterial pH represents the balance between metabolic demand and respiratory expenditure. With metabolic acidosis, the respiratory system represents the primary compensatory mechanism for overall balance. In patients with excessive work of breathing, generation of lactate from respiratory musculature may remain uncompensated by hyperventilation, resulting in profound acidemia.

Measurement of $Paco_2$ provides the clinician with an estimate of alveolar ventilatory sufficiency. The absolute value must be interpreted in the face of the amount of respiratory effort the patient must generate to attain that particular $Paco_2$. Therefore, a $Paco_2$ of 40, although listed as within normal limits in most references, is less than acceptable when applied to an infant in distress with marked tachypnea. Any degree of fatigue in this patient will promote CO_2 retention and the rapid development of potentially irreversible respiratory failure. Tachypnea does not guarantee adequate ventilation, since many patients will fail to generate adequate tidal volumes and, in effect, be hypoventilating.

$Paco_2$ provides an estimate of alveolar gas exchange and a measure of the balance between tissue perfusion and metabolic demand. It is important to emphasize that the use of percutaneous oximetry only reflects oxygenation and may, in some circumstances, falsely represent the adequacy of ventilation. The use of oximetry should not replace the use of one's eyes and a stethoscope in evaluating the pediatric patient with respiratory distress.

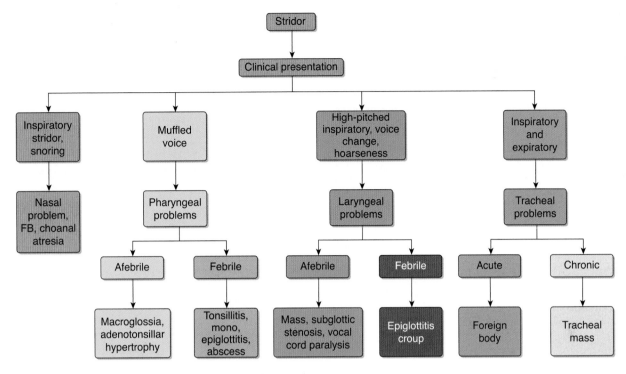

Figure 40-1. Algorithm for stridor.

RESPIRATORY FAILURE

Recognize the signs of respiratory failure. These include respiratory and central nervous system findings: decreased level of consciousness, progressive fatigue, increasing work of breathing, increasing respiratory rate, and poor color (cyanotic, ashen, or gray). Additional signs include diaphoresis, retractions, grunting, nasal flaring, decreased air movement on auscultation, and hypoventilation or apnea. This leads to acidosis, hypercapnea, and hypoxemia.

► ASSESSMENT AND MANAGEMENT OF SPECIFIC CLINICAL SCENARIOS (See Fig. 40-1)

Stridor, the hallmark of upper airway compromise, results from the generation of inspiratory turbulence transmitted against a narrowed lumen. Stridor may originate anywhere in the upper airway from the anterior nares to the subglottic region. In the young infant, stridor is most often the result of a congenital anomaly involving the tongue (macroglossia), larynx (laryngomalacia), and trachea (tracheomalacia). Congenital forms of stridor are often chronic in their presentation.

In the emergency department (ED), the most common causes of acute upper airway obstruction are croup, foreign body obstruction, and epiglottitis. Additional processes include bacterial tracheitis, peritonsillar abscess, and retropharyngeal abscess (Tables 40–1 and 40–2).

CROUP (VIRAL LARYNGOTRACHEOBRONCHITIS)

Laryngotracheobronchitis (croup) is a respiratory infection that diffusely affects the upper respiratory tract. This entity accounts for 90% of stridor with fever.[1-3] The subglottic region is most commonly affected, resulting in edematous and inflamed mucosa with a fibrinous exudate. Agents responsible

► TABLE 40-1. FEATURES OF UPPER AIRWAY DISORDERS

Disease Process	Age Group	Mode of Onset of Respiratory Distress
Severe tonsillitis	Late preschool or school age	Gradual
Peritonsillar abscess	Usually >8 y	Sudden increase in temperature, toxicity, and distress, with unilateral throat pain, "hot potato speech"
Retropharyngeal abscess	Infancy—3 y	Fever, toxicity, and distress after URI or pharyngitis
Epiglottitis	2–7 y	Acute onset of hyperpyrexia, with distress, dysphagia, and drooling
Croup	3 mo–3 y	Gradual onset of stridor and barking cough, after mild URI
Foreign body aspiration	Late infancy–4 y	Choking episode resulting in immediate or delayed respiratory distress
Bacterial Tracheitis	2–7 y	Acute onset of hyperpyrexia, distress, toxic appearance, pseudomembrane

▶ **TABLE 40–2. CLINICAL FEATURES OF ACUTE UPPER AIRWAY DISORDERS**

	Supraglottic Disorders (Epiglottitis/Bacterial Tracheitis)	Subglottic Disorders (Croup)
Stridor	Quiet	Wet and loud
Voice alteration	Muffled	Hoarse
Dysphagia	+	−
Postural preference	+	−
Barky cough	−	+
Fever	++	+
Toxicity	++	−
Trismus	+	−

▶ **TABLE 40–3. CLINICAL CROUP SCORE***

	Score
Inspiratory Breath Sounds	
Normal	0
Harsh with ronchi	1
Delayed	2
Stridor	
None	0
Inspiratory	1
Inspiratory and expiratory	2
Cough	
None	0
Hoarse cry	1
Bark	2
Retractions and Flaring	
None	0
Flaring, suprasternal retractions	1
As under 1, plus subcostal, and intercostal retractions	2
Cyanosis	
None	0
In air	1
In 40% O_2	2

*A score of 4 or more indicates moderately severe airway obstruction. A score of 7 or more, particularly when associated with $Paco_2 > 45$ and $Pao_2 < 70$ (in room air), indicates impending respiratory failure.

for croup are multiple, including parainfluenza types 1, 2, and 3, (most common); adenovirus; respiratory syncytial virus (RSV); and influenza. The seasonal predominance (winter) is related to the epidemiology of the most common causative agents.

Children from 1 to 3 years of age are usually affected. They often present, after several days of nonspecific upper respiratory infection (URI) symptoms, with a characteristic brassy or barking cough that is almost unique to croup. Inspiratory stridor eventually develops, ranging in severity from mild (only when crying or agitated) to severe (present at rest). Temperatures to 102°F are common in the course of the disease. Physical examination reveals a child with hoarse voice, coryza, and a slightly increased respiratory rate. Higher temperatures or the presence of a toxic appearance should alert the clinician to carefully consider other diagnoses (atypical epiglottitis or bacterial tracheitis). The usual evolution of symptoms is a worsening of symptoms for 3 to 5 days followed by resolution over a period of days. The vast majority of children tolerate this common disease without significant morbidity; however, a small percentage may develop complete upper airway obstruction.

A variety of croup scores have been developed that quantify and qualify a constellation of physical findings, assisting the clinician in estimating the severity of subglottic obstruction as mild, moderate, or severe (Table 40–3).[1,2]

The most common presentation will be the child with mild croup who may be treated as an outpatient if well hydrated and able to take oral liquids as long as the physician is comfortable with parental reliability. These patients will present with a history of a barky cough, mild respiratory distress, and stridor only with activity or agitation. As croup is a self-limited disease with treatment aimed solely at relieving symptoms, patients with a mild croup score can be discharged if the child improves with cool humidified oxygen therapy, the parents are reliable, and the child is older than 6 months. Cool mist therapy may be suggested.[4] The classic technique is to fill the bathroom with steam by running a hot shower. The parents can then sit with the child in this home version of a Turkish bath, for no more than 30 minutes at a time. A car ride in the cool night air with the windows slightly open may also diminish the child's symptoms. Follow-up within 24 hours should always be arranged

if the patient is discharged with instructions to return if symptoms worsen.

Patients with a moderate croup score (stridor at rest) require more aggressive treatment and longer observation. The use of oxygen, cool mist, and racemic epinephrine delivered by nebulizer will usually result in symptomatic improvement of the patient for up to 2 hours. The recommended dose for racemic epinephrine is 0.5 mL of a 0.25% solution dissolved in 2.5 mL of normal saline.[5–8] Peak effects have been demonstrated at 10 to 30 minutes, with duration of action lasting up to 2 hours. Racemic epinephrine does not shorten the duration of illness. It is important to remember that a child may experience a return to a pretreatment level of obstruction 1 to 2 hours after therapy as the effects of the medication wear off. The dose of racemic epinephrine may be repeated as needed until stridor at rest resolves. Although it is unproved, many believe that a child with severe croup may be successfully carried through the episode with racemic epinephrine therapy as often as every 20 minutes (as an inpatient), avoiding the need for intubation.

Corticosteroids are of benefit in preventing the progression of croup to complete obstruction by decreasing the amount of swelling of the laryngeal mucosa. Steroids have been shown to lessen the duration of illness, amount of time in the hospital, and the number of racemic epinephrine nebulizer treatments given.[4,8–11] If one plans to give corticosteroids (usually for the moderately or severely obstructed patient), they should be administered as soon as possible. Dexamethasone 0.6 mg/kg given one time orally or intramuscularly causes significant improvement in symptoms within 6 hours.

A child may be safely discharged to home after receiving both corticosteroids and racemic epinephrine treatments if, after 2 to 3 hours of ED observation, they demonstrate a normal respiratory effort, a normal level of consciousness, and no stridor at rest. Prompt follow-up should be arranged.

If a child has severe croup (score ≥ 7) or a decrease in oxygen saturations, it is prudent to admit that child to an intensive care setting. Treatment with oxygen, mist, racemic epinephrine, and corticosteroids should be initiated as soon as possible in the ED. Antibiotics may be needed if a bacterial etiology is suspected.

Children should be electively intubated for respiratory failure (lethargy, inability to maintain respiratory efforts, $Pao_2 < 70$ on 100% oxygen, or $Paco_2 > 60$), but this decision is best made in the intensive care setting. Children who develop severe upper airway obstruction from this disease do not do so suddenly but rather progress gradually over time. If intubation must be performed in the ED, an endotracheal (ET) tube 1 mm smaller than that calculated for age should be used to accommodate the subglottic edema and airway narrowing.

The following regimen is suggested for the patient with croup: avoid agitating the patient and provide humidified oxygen if indicated while allowing the patient to assume a position of comfort (usually in a parent's arms or lap). Initially, provide cool, moist air. If stridor at rest persists (or fatigue or distress is noted), administer aerosolized racemic epinephrine at a dose of 0.5 mL in 2.5 mL normal saline solution. Patients who receive this intervention are candidates for admission, or, at a minimum, observation within the ED for a period of 2 to 4 hours. Administer oral, intramuscular, or intravenous dexamethasone, 0.6 mg/kg. Intubate if clinically warranted.

Upright lateral neck radiographs, if desired, should be obtained for patients without suspicion of epiglottitis. Maintain close supervision of the patient while the films are obtained. The characteristic "steeple sign" with narrowing of the subglottic area may be noted but does not make the diagnosis of croup.

EPIGLOTTITIS (SUPRAGLOTTITIS)

Epiglottitis represents a true upper airway emergency with life-threatening complications if handled improperly. It may occur at any time of the year and in any age group. Traditionally, it most commonly involved children from 2 to 5 years of age. With the advent of the *Haemophilus influenzae* type B vaccine, the age range has shifted to more commonly involve older children and even adults.[12–16] Possible presentations include the following:

- The acute (over several hours) onset of fever, sore throat, and dysphagia with progression to signs of respiratory distress. The child will often assume a position of comfort consisting of voluntary upper airway posturing, that is, sitting upright, mouth open, with head, neck, and jaw extension. The voice will be muffled, and stridor, if present, may actually be quite minimal in intensity. The clinician will often note that these children appear "toxic." In severe cases, airway and swallowing mechanisms may be compromised to such a degree that profound drooling may ensue.

- Some children will be devoid of any respiratory symptoms. They will, however, complain of a severe sore throat and dysphagia. In the absence of signs of pharyngeal or tonsillar pathology, therefore, epiglottitis must be considered in this subgroup of patients. In addition, the presence of pharyngitis or uvulitis in no way excludes the possibility of epiglottitic involvement.

- Croup-like presentations in patients who fail to respond to traditional therapies should alert the clinician to the possibility of epiglottitis.

With the advent of the Hib vaccine, *H. influenzae* type b with accompanying bacteremia has become a less frequent cause of epiglottitis with *Streptococcus pneumoniae, Staphylococcus aureus,* and group A β-hemolytic streptococci becoming more common.[12–14] However, *H. influenzae* type B should not be discounted as it still causes disease in both unimmunized and immunized patients. Blood cultures will be positive in 80% to 90% of affected individuals. Other noninfectious etiologies of epiglottitis such as trauma, burns, leukemia, and angioneurotic edema have been reported as well.

The most important clinical consideration for patients with epiglottitis remains the fact that, if unrecognized, airway obstruction and respiratory arrest will most certainly occur. Factors contributing to airway and ventilatory deterioration include patient fatigue, aspiration of secretions, and sudden laryngospasm. All maneuvers that agitate the child should therefore be avoided, including separation from parents, alteration of optimal airway posture (lying down), fearful events (rectal temperatures, blood work, and radiographs), and gagging (forcible tongue blade examination of the oral cavity, suctioning).[17]

Radiographs, when obtained, should include anteroposterior and -lateral views of the soft tissues of the neck. Patients with suspected pneumonia should receive chest views as well. Under no circumstances should the child receive these evaluations if they promote agitation and subsequent worsening of stridor and airway compromise. The clinician must be prepared to emergently intubate and ventilate these patients at all times and in all places within the ED. In most cases, direct visualization and culture of the epiglottis itself will be performed in the operating suite prior to intubation (Fig. 40–2).

The following management guidelines should be followed to avoid undue morbidity and mortality.

Avoid agitating the child in any way. Provide supplemental oxygen in a nonthreatening manner and allow the patient to assume a position of comfort. Prepare equipment for bag-valve-mask (BVM) ventilation, ET intubation; needle cricothyrotomy, cricothyrotomy, and tracheostomy. Consult an expert in intubation and provision of a surgical airway and alert the operating room. Take the child to the operating room for direct visualization of the epiglottis and intubation.

If the child suffers a respiratory arrest, open the airway. Attempt BVM ventilation (usually effective).

If unable to ventilate, intubate. If unable to intubate, perform needle or surgical cricothyroidotomy.

Provide appropriate intravenous antibiotics (such as cefotaxime 50 mg/kg every 6 hours). Provide adequate sedation and restraint postintubation and transfer the patient to an intensive care unit for further treatment and monitoring.

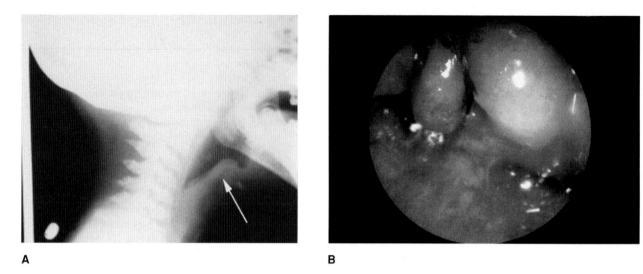

A **B**

Figure 40–2. Epiglottitis. (A) Lateral neck x-ray of a child with epiglottitis. (B) Endoscopic view of almost complete airway obstruction secondary to epiglottitis. Note the slit-like opening of the airway.

BACTERIAL TRACHEITIS

Bacterial tracheitis, also referred to as membranous tracheitis, represents a true upper airway emergency since, like supraglottitis, it may progress to full airway obstruction. Bacterial tracheitis is an infection of the subglottic region causing subglottic edema and pseudomembrane formation in the trachea and bronchi. With the decreasing incidence of *H. influenzae*, this uncommon upper airway infection has surpassed the incidence of epiglottitis, making it an important etiology of upper airway obstruction for the emergency physician to consider.[18,19] Bacterial tracheitis is polymicrobial, and culture most commonly grows out *S. aureus, S. pneumonii, H. influenzae, Pseudomonas,* and *Moraxella.* This entity occurs in the same age group as croup, with the average age at presentation being 3 years. Infections more commonly occur in boys than girls and usually occur during the fall and winter. Mortality lies between 18% and 40%, so prompt recognition and treatment is warranted. Significant morbidity such as ARDS, respiratory failure, cardiopulmonary arrest, shock, and multiorgan failure may occur. Symptoms are often very similar to both croup and epiglottitis making diagnosis difficult.

Symptoms begin with a prodrome of a mild upper respiratory tract infection lasting for 1 to 2 weeks. The patient then experiences a rapid deterioration with respiratory distress, increased work of breathing, high fevers, and a toxic appearance. These patients often appear anxious and lethargic. On physical examination, typical signs of upper airway obstruction such as stridor, tachypnea, retractions, and a barky cough are present. Occasionally, the infection extends into the lower airways and wheezing is present as well. If lateral neck radiographs are performed, subglottic and tracheal narrowing may be seen along with a ragged tracheal border secondary to the pseudomembrane. A chest radiograph may demonstrate a concomitant pneumonia in many children. Laboratory evaluation may demonstrate a leukocytosis with a left shift. Blood cultures are rarely useful. Tracheal cultures should be sent if the patient is intubated or bronchoscopy performed to help guide therapy.

Usually, patients with bacterial tracheitis experience such a rapid deterioration of their respiratory status and require mechanical ventilation. Definitive diagnosis occurs with visualization of a normal epiglottis and the presence of pus, inflammation, and in some cases a pseudomembrane in the subglottic region upon intubation. An endotrachial tube 1 mm smaller than normal should be used due to the tracheal wall edema. Meticulous ET tube suctioning in a pediatric intensive care unit (PICU) setting will usually maintain airway patency. Broad-spectrum antibiotic coverage that includes coverage for *S. aureus* is required. A third-generation cephalosporin, such as ceftriaxone, is a good initial choice, along with vancomycin until culture results are known. Toxic shock syndrome has been seen with staphylococcal tracheitis.

RETROPHARYNGEAL ABSCESS

Retropharyngeal abscesses are seen predominantly in children younger than 3 years secondary to suppurative cervical lymphadenopathy.[20] Older children may present with this entity, in many instances following penetrating trauma to the posterior oropharynx. Common organisms include group A β-hemolytic *Streptococcus* and *S. aureus.* Symptoms include high fever, muffled voice, difficulty swallowing, drooling, and, less frequently, inspiratory stridor. Dysphagia and drooling are more frequent findings than actual upper airway compromise. Cervical lymphadenitis and trismus also commonly present with retropharyngeal abscesses.

Children with retropharyngeal abscesses can present with a stiff neck or torticollis and often are initially diagnosed with meningitis. The presentation may also mimic supraglottitis if inspiratory stridor is present. Therefore, it is acceptable to make this diagnosis in the operating room on direct visualization.

A high index of suspicion must be maintained to accurately identify the child with a retropharyngeal abscess. Clinically noting a swelling of the wall of the posterior pharynx may make the diagnosis. Given the overlap in presentation with

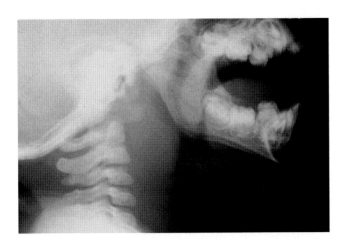

Figure 40–3. Retropharyngeal abscess lateral soft tissue neck x-ray demonstrating prevertebral soft tissue density consistent with retropharyngeal abscess.

supraglotittis, even if the diagnosis is suspected, it is prudent to first obtain a lateral neck film as a screening tool that may demonstrate prevertebral soft tissue swelling greater than 7 mm at the level of the second cervical vertebrae or greater than 14 mm at the level of the sixth cervical vertebrae and a normal epiglottis and aryepiglottic folds (Fig. 40–3). Attempting to visualize the oral cavity and posterior pharyngeal wall may be made in an older cooperative child as long as agitation does not ensue. In most suspected cases, a computed tomography (CT) scan of the neck will identify any soft tissue swelling, and in selected cases, the presence of free air would alert the specialist that surgical drainage may be necessary. An experienced radiologist may also be able to visualize an abscess by ultrasound.

All patients with a suspected retropharyngeal abscess should have an ENT consult. Children with cellulitis without a collection of pus are often treated with antibiotics. Airway management for severe or complete upper airway obstruction should include ET intubation under direct visualization to avoid rupture of the abscess. In children with partial airway obstruction, who do not demonstrate signs of respiratory failure, meticulous observation with all equipment and personnel on hand (a PICU setting) is acceptable. Antibiotics must cover the common organisms (*S. aureus*, *Streptococcus*, and anaerobes). Clindamycin is a good empiric choice and a third-generation cephalosporin. Management should be coordinated with an ENT consultant. Definitive therapy involves intraoperative drainage of the abscess after securing the airway by ET intubation.

PERITONSILLAR ABSCESS

Peritonsillar abscesses usually affect children older than 8 years. They are the most common deep infections of the head and neck, usually representing complications of recurrent bacterial tonsillitis, or in some cases, a superinfection of an existent Epstein–Barr infection.[21] Most are polymicrobial in origin, including group A *Streptococcus* (predominant), *Peptostreptococcus*, *Fusobacterium*, and other mouth flora, including anaerobes.

Historically, these patients present with increasing dysphagia and ipsilateral ear pain, with progression to trismus, dysarthria, and toxicity. Drooling is common. Patients will often have a "hot potato" phonation, representing splinting of the palatine muscles during normal speech.

The pharynx will be erythematous, with unilateral tonsillar swelling, which, in some cases, may displace the uvula toward the unaffected side. The soft palate may be displaced medially. Fluctuance may confirm the presence of underlying purulent fluid. Reactive cervical adenopathy is common. Severe, although uncommon, complications have been reported, including sternocleidomastoid spasm and torticollis, fasciitis, mediastinitis, and airway obstruction.

Often, the diagnosis may be made on examination alone.[22] The complete blood count will demonstrate an elevated white blood count count. Throat cultures (superficial) should be obtained in all cases. Serologic testing for Epstein–Barr virus infections should be performed as well. A CT scan of the neck with contrast should be done if any doubt exists as to the existence of a peritonsillar abscess after the examination. An experienced otolaryngologist should perform direct tonsillar needle aspiration, after adequate sedation/analgesia has been administered.[23] Selected individuals, after adequate drainage, may be considered for discharge from the ED after careful follow-up is arranged. Some patients require admission for drainage, intravenous hydration, and antibiotics (nafcillin or a third-generation cephalosporin).

▶ FOREIGN BODY OBSTRUCTION

Most foreign body aspirations occur in children younger than 5 years, with 65% of deaths affecting infants younger than 1 year.[24–26] Common offending agents are foods (e.g., peanuts, hard candies, frankfurters) and items commonly found in the home (e.g., disc batteries, coins, and marbles). Symptoms range from mild (cough only) to full-blown upper airway obstruction. It is imperative that the clinicians maintain a high index of suspicion relative to the possibility of foreign body aspiration, especially in the afebrile child with sudden onset of symptoms. In >50% of cases, there is no history of foreign body ingestion or a choking spell. Often, patients present multiple times for a respiratory illness that does not improve before the correct diagnosis is made. Some children may present with a recurring pneumonia or lung abscess in chronic foreign body aspiration.

Most patients will present with symptoms of partial obstruction. Evaluation should include anteroposterior and lateral views of the upper airway extending from the nasopharynx to the carina. More extensive radiographic investigations include inspiratory and expiratory chest radiographs, or, in younger, uncooperative patients, bilateral decubital views. These examinations are of great value in diagnosing foreign bodies that are radiolucent. The foreign body will act as a ball valve causing the affected lung to appear more inflated than usual. Atelectasis may also be seen in the affected lung. A high index of suspicion must be maintained in all suspected cases as the radiographs are not infrequently normal. Esophageal foreign bodies, if positioned at the thoracic inlet or carina, can compress the upper airway and cause symptoms and signs of airway obstruction.

Foreign body obstruction can cause complete or incomplete obstruction. It should be managed as follows:

- For acute complete obstruction:
  - Children younger than 1 year: give four back blows followed by chest thrusts.
  - Children older than 1 year: employ repetitive abdominal thrusts.
  - If unsuccessful, use Magill forceps under direct laryngoscopy to attempt removal of the foreign body.
  - If still unsuccessful, attempt vigorous BVM ventilation in preparation for brochoscopy.
- For incomplete obstruction (phonation, coughing present):
  - Provide supplemental oxygen.
  - Allow a position of comfort and avoid noxious stimuli.
  - Arrange for controlled airway evaluation in the operating room.
  - Aspirated foreign bodies must be removed by rigid bronchoscopy.

► SUMMARY

Competency in the management of the pediatric patient with respiratory distress is a necessary skill for the emergency physician. This chapter has provided an outlined overview of the most common upper airway disorders that one will encounter in general practice. Standardized therapeutic interventions will maximize overall clinical outcomes.

REFERENCES

1. Bjornson CL, Johnson DW. Croup-treatment update. *Pediatr Emerg Care.* 2005;21:863.
2. Malhotra A, Krilov LR. Viral croup. *Pediatr Rev.* 2001;22:5–12.
3. Rosekrans JA. Viral croup: current diagnosis and treatment. *Mayo Clin Proc.* 1998;73:1102–1106.
4. Neto G, Kentab B, Klassen T, et al. A randomized controlled trial of mist in the acute treatment of moderate croup. *Acad Emerg Med.* 2002;9:873–879.
5. Kelly PB, Simon JE. Racemic epinephrine use in croup and disposition. *Am J Emerg Med.* 1992;10:181.
6. Ledwith CA, Shea LM, Mauro RD. Safety and efficacy of nebulized racemic epinephrine in conjunction with oral dexamethasone and mist in the outpatient treatment of croup. *Ann Emerg Med.* 1995;25:331.
7. Prendergast M, Jones JS, Hartman D. Racemic epinephrine in the treatment of laryngotracheitis: can we identify children for outpatient therapy? *Am J Emerg Med.* 1994;12:613.
8. Rizos JD, DiGravio BE, Sehl MJ, et al. The disposition of children with croup treated with racemic epinephrine and dexamethasone in the emergency department. *J Emerg Med.* 1998;16:535.
9. Donaldson D, Poleski D, Knipple E, et al. Intramuscular versus oral dexamethasone for the treatment of moderate-to-severe croup: a randomized, double-blind trial. *Acad Emerg Med.* 2003;10:16–21.
10. Jonson DW, Jacobson S, Edney PC, et al. A comparison of nebulized budesonide, intramuscular dexamethasone, and placebo for moderately severe croup. *N Engl J Med.* 1998;339:498.
11. Rittichier KK, Ledwith CA. Outpatient treatment of moderate croup with dexamethasone: intravenous versus oral dosing. *Pediatrics.* 2000;106:1344–1348.
12. Hickerson SL, Kirby RS, Wheeler JG, et al. Epiglottis: a 9-year case review. *South Med J.* 1996;89:487.
13. Losek JD, Dewitz-Zink BA, Melzer-Lange M, et al. Epiglottitis: comparison of signs and symptoms in children less than 2 years old and older. *Ann Emerg Med.* 1990;19:55–58.
14. Mauro RD, Poole SR, Lockhart CH. Differentiation of epiglottitis from laryngotracheitis in the child with stridor. *Am J Dis Child.* 1988;142:679.
15. Shah RK, Roberson DW, Jones DT. Epiglottitis in the Hemophilus influenzae type B vaccine era; changing trends. *Laryngoscope.* 2004;114:557.
16. Kumar RK, Mashell K. Acute epiglottitis. *J Pediatr Child Health.* 1998;34:594.
17. Fulginiti VA. Acute supraglottitis (epiglottitis): to look or not? *Am J Dis Child.* 1988;142:597.
18. Hopkins A, Lahiri T, Salerno R, Heath B. Changing epidemiology of life-threatening upper airway infections: the reemergence of bacterial tracheitis. *Pediatrics.* 2006;188:1418–1421.
19. Bernstein T. Is bacterial tracheitis changing? A 14-month experience in a pediatric intensive care unit. *Clin Infect Dis.* 1998;27:458–462.
20. Craig FW, Schunk JE. Retropharyngeal abscess in children: clinical presentation, utility of imaging, and current management. *Pediatrics.* 2003;111:1394.
21. Hammerschlag PE, Hammerschlag MR. Peritonsillar, retropharyngeal, and parapharyngeal abscesses. In: Feigin RD, Cherry JD, eds. *Textbook of Pediatric Infectious Diseases.* Vol. 1. 5th ed. Philadelphia, PA: WB Saunders; 2004:172.
22. Herzon FS. Pediatric peritonsillar abscess: management guidelines. *Curr Probl Pediatr.* 1996;26:270–278.
23. Blotter JW. Otolaryngology consultation for peritonsillar abscess in the pediatric population. *Laryngoscope.* 2000;110:1698–1701.
24. Brownstein DR. Foreign bodies of the gastrointestinal tract and airway. In: Barkin RM, ed. *Pediatric Emergency Medicine Concepts and Clinical Practice.* 2nd ed. St. Louis, MO: Mosby-Year Book; 1997:371.
25. Chiu CY, Wong, KS, Lai SH. Factors predicting Early diagnosis of foreign body aspiration in children. *Pediatr Emerg Care.* 2005;21:161.
26. Rovin J, Rodgers BM. Pediatric foreign body aspiration. *Pediatr Rev.* 2000;21:86–89.

CHAPTER 41

Asthma

Kathleen M. Brown

▶ HIGH-YIELD FACTS

- Asthma is the most common chronic disease of childhood and is associated with significant morbidity and mortality.
- Inhaled albuterol remains the first line therapy for acute asthmatic exacerbations. Delivery of albuterol by metered dose inhaler has been shown to be superior to delivery by nebulization.
- Inhaled levoalbuterol has not been shown to have any significant benefit over racemic albuterol in acute asthma exacerbations.
- The addition of nebulized ipratroprium to the first 2 to 3 albuterol doses has been associated with a decreased need for hospitalization in pediatric patients with moderate-to-severe asthma exacerbations.
- Administration of oral corticosteroids in the emergency department has been shown to enhance recovery from an acute asthma exacerbation and decrease rates of hospitalization.
- Oral dexamethasone (one–two doses) has been shown to be as efficacious as a 5-day course of oral prednisone.
- Magnesium sulfate may be of benefit in patients with moderate-to-severe exacerbations who do not respond to initial bronchodilator therapy.
- Heliox has been suggested to be of benefit for patients with severe asthma exacerbations in small clinical trials, but convincing evidence of its benefit is not available.

Asthma is the most common chronic disease of childhood.[1] The current prevalence of asthma in the United States is estimated at 8.9%. It is the third most common reason for hospitalization of children in the United States, exceeded only by injuries and pneumonia. Acute exacerbations of asthma are often managed in emergency departments (EDs). In 2004, the number of children who sought care for an acute asthma exacerbation in a U.S. ED reached 754,000.[2]

Asthma is traditionally defined as intermittent, reversible obstructive airway disease. It is now known to be a chronic inflammatory disorder of the airways. The most recent National Heart Lung and Blood Institute (NHLBI) expert panel guidelines on the diagnosis and management of asthma define asthma as: a common chronic disorder of the airways that is complex and characterized by variable and recurring symptoms, airflow obstruction, bronchial hyperresponsiveness, and an underlying inflammation. The interaction of these features of asthma determines the clinical manifestations and severity of asthma and the response to treatment.[3]

▶ ETIOLOGY/PATHOPHYSIOLOGY

The major mechanisms thought to contribute to the pathophysiology of asthma are increased airway responsiveness, inflammation, mucus production, and submucosal edema. Airway responsiveness is defined as the ease with which airways narrow in response to various nonallergic stimuli. These stimuli include inhaled pharmacologic agents, such as histamine and methacholine, and physical stimuli, such as exercise. The level of airway responsiveness is reported to correlate with the severity of asthma symptoms and medication requirements. The critical role of airway inflammation in both the development of obstruction and the degree of hyperresponsiveness has been appreciated only recently. Pathologic specimens from patients demonstrate inflammation of the airways even in the mildest forms of the disease. Increased mucus production and submucosal edema add to the obstruction that occurs secondary to bronchospasm and inflammation.

These three components are synergistic and their relationship can be understood by dividing the mechanisms involved into stages. The early bronchospastic response is a classic antigen antibody reaction. When the patient is exposed to a specific antigen, mast cells are sensitized by reagin- or antigen-specific IgE antibody, which attaches to the cell wall. When this sensitized cell is reexposed to the specific antigen, mediators are released, including histamine, leukotrienes, and chemotactic factors that attract inflammatory cells to the area (Fig. 41–1). A predisposition to develop this response may be genetically based. In some patients, this initial inflammatory response is secondary to an infection. Whatever the cause of the inflammatory response, it is the convergence of these inflammatory cells that appears to correlate with the late asthmatic response. These inflammatory cells release a number of products that cause damage to the bronchial wall. Eosinophils play a large role in this process. They migrate to the bronchial wall in response to chemotactic substances released by macrophages, and are stimulated by mediators such as platelet activating factor (PAF) to release a number of substances which cause inflammation in the bronchial wall. Histamine is released from mast cells. It causes smooth muscle constriction and bronchospasm and plays a role in mucosal edema and mucus secretion. All inflammatory cells produce products which are the result of the action of phospholipase A2 on their membrane phospholipids. This leads to the formation of platelet activating factor (PAF) and arachidonic acid and its metabolites, including leukotrienes. These products cause smooth muscle contraction and mucosal edema. In addition to mucosal edema, hypersecretion, and bronchoconstriction, these cell products contribute to the sloughing of mucosal cells, which cause a

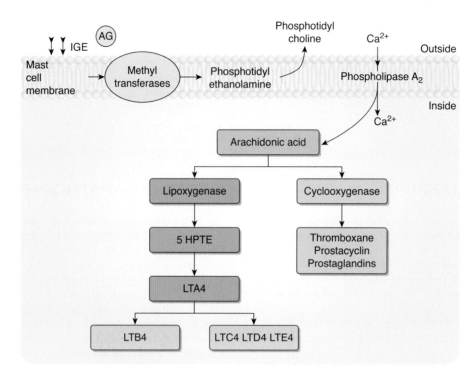

Figure 41-1. Pathophysiology of asthma.

loss of the protective effects of the epithelium and exposure of nerve fibers to irritants. Experimental models show that airway inflammation produces an alteration of the sensory nerve endings that may lead to bronchial hyperreactivity.

Once bronchial hyperactivity is present, nonspecific triggers may produce acute bronchospasm. The most common trigger is an upper respiratory infection. Other common triggers include inhaled allergens, exercise, and cold air. The level of airway responsiveness is not static. It may increase or decrease in response to various factors. Anxiety may potentiate bronchospasm through vagal efferentes. A vicious cycle can develop, in which continuous or repeated exposure to allergens, in sensitized persons, increases airway responsiveness. This is the chronic stage of asthma. Chronic asthma is not always reversible. During the immune response, proliferating fibroblasts deposit extensive networks of collagen that can lead to fibrosis, remodeling of the bronchioles, and irreversible airway disease.

All asthmatics have profound bronchoconstriction in response to cholinergic agonists, such as methacholine chloride suggesting that the parasympathetic nervous system is involved in the asthmatic response. The bulk of autonomic nerves in human airways are branches of the vagus nerve, whose efferent fibers enter the lung at the hilum and travel along the airways into the lungs. They are found throughout the length of the airways but predominately along the large- and medium-sized airways. Their postganglionic varicosities and terminals supply the smooth muscle and submucosal glands of the airways as well as vascular structures. Release of acetylcholine at these sites results in smooth muscle contraction and release of secretions from the submucosal glands. The level of parasympathetic activity can be augmented by neural reflexes that involve afferent and efferent vagal fibers. Stimuli that result in reflex bronchoconstriction include mechanical stimulation of

the airways, inhalation of certain particles, gases, aerosols, and cold and dry air. There is little direct sympathetic innervation of the bronchial tree. However, there are many β_2-adrenergic receptors in airway smooth muscle that are responsible for bronchoconstriction. The importance of the sympathetic nervous system is not in maintaining airway tone but in reversing bronchoconstriction.

There are several differences in the anatomy and physiology of a child compared to an adult who makes them more prone to obstruction and more vulnerable to respiratory failure. The peripheral airways are smaller and thus offer greater resistance to airflow. Infants do not possess collateral channels for ventilation that are present in older children and adults. In infancy, the diaphragm is the primary muscle of respiration. Any degree of abdominal distention will provide significant interference to diaphragmatic function and secondary ventilatory insufficiency. The infantile diaphragm possesses muscle fibers that are more prone to fatigue. The chest wall of the pediatric patient is more compliant preventing adequate stabilization during periods of increased respiratory distress. Viral infections, particularly respiratory syncytial virus (RSV), are the most common cause of acute wheezing illness in infants. The edematous inflammatory response in the airways leads to air trapping and hyperinflation, atelectasis, increased respiratory rate, and wheezing. This sequence of changes can rapidly progress to respiratory failure.

▶ CLINICAL PRESENTATION

Children with acute exacerbations of their asthma often seek care in an ED (Fig. 41-2). Asthma exacerbations are acute or subacute episodes of progressively worsening shortness of breath, increased cough, wheezing, and chest tightness—or

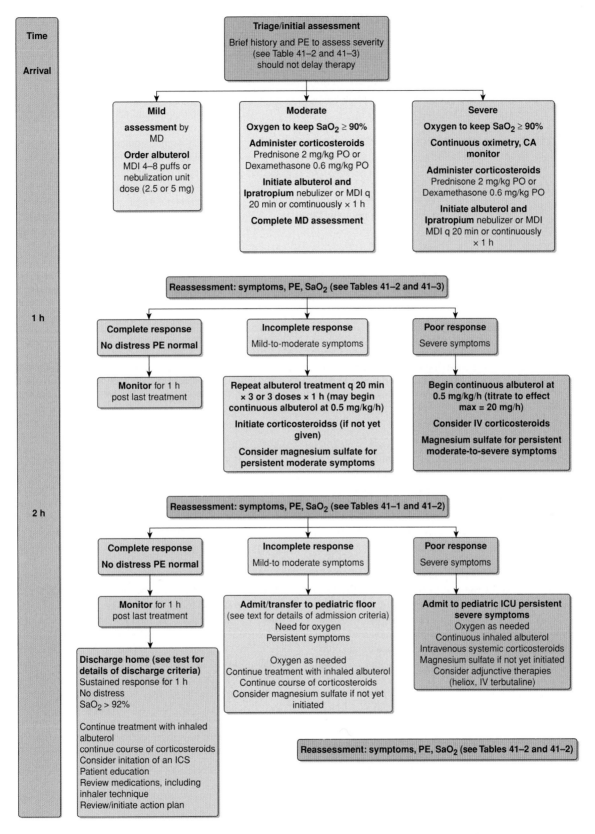

Figure 41–2. ED management of a child with an acute asthma exacerbation.

▶ **TABLE 41–1. CLASSIFYING SEVERITY OF ASTHMA EXACERBATIONS IN THE URGENT OR EMERGENCY CARE SETTING**

	Symptoms and Signs	Initial PEF (%) (or FEV₁)	Clinical Course
Mild	Dyspnea only with activity (assess tachypnea in young children)	PEF ≥70 predicted or personal best	• Usually cared for at home • Prompt relief with inhaled SABA • Possible short course of oral systemic corticosteroids
Moderate	Dyspnea interferes with or limits usual activity	PEF 40–69 predicted or personal best	• Usually requires office or ED visit • Relief from frequent inhaled SABA • Oral systemic corticosteroids; some symptoms last for 1–2 d after treatment is begun
Severe	Dyspnea at rest; interferes with conversation	PEF <40 predicted or personal best	• Usually requires ED visit and likely hospitalization • Partial relief from frequent inhaled SABA • Oral systemic corticosteroids; some symptoms last for >3 d after treatment is begun • Adjunctive therapies are helpful
Subset: Life threatening	Too dyspneic to speak; perspiring	PEF <25 predicted or personal best	• Requires ED/hospitalization; possible ICU • Minimal or no relief from frequent inhaled SABA • Intravenous corticosteroids • Adjunctive therapies are helpful

ED, emergency department; FEV₁, forced expiratory volume in 1 second; ICU, intensive care unit; PEF, peak expiratory flow; SABA, short-acting β₂-agonist.
Patients are instructed to use quick-relief medications if symptoms occur or if PEF drops below 80% predicted or personal best. If PEF is 50%–79%, the patient should monitor response to quick-relief medication carefully and consider contacting a clinician. If PEF is below 50%, immediate medical care is usually required. In the urgent or emergency care setting, the following parameters describe the severity and likely clinical course of an exacerbation.

some combination of these symptoms. Exacerbations are characterized by decreases in expiratory airflow that can be documented and quantified by simple measurement of lung function (spirometry). These objective measures more reliably indicate the severity of an exacerbation than does the severity of symptoms.[3] Unfortunately, spirometry is difficult to obtain in young children.[4] An initial history and physical examination should be obtained to help guide treatment. A more detailed history can be obtained while treatment is being initiated. Classification of the severity of the acute exacerbation is important as recommended therapy is often dependent on severity. Tables 41–1 and 41–2 illustrate the classification of asthma severity recommended by the National Heart Lung and Blood Institute (NHLBI) expert panel report.[3] Numeric asthma scores can also be used to classify severity and to measure effectiveness of treatment.[5–7]

The brief history should assess[3]:

• Time of onset and any potential causes of current exacerbation.
• Severity of symptoms, especially compared with previous exacerbations, and response to any treatment given before arrival to the ED.
• All current medications and time of last dose, especially of asthma medications.
• Estimate of number of previous unscheduled office visits, ED visits, and hospitalizations for asthma, particularly within the past year.
• Any prior episodes of respiratory insufficiency due to asthma.
• Other potentially complicating illness.

A family history of asthma, atopy, or allergic disease is common in patients with asthma. A recent history of an upper respiratory infection or exposure to a specific trigger is usually obtained. Other historical factors that should be elucidated include the patient's (or parents') perception of the severity of the attack, precipitating factors, history of past attacks, medications (last doses and recent changes), hydration status, and any other concurrent symptoms.

A rapid physical examination should be completed but should not delay initiation of therapy. The initial physical examination should focus on the severity of the exacerbation (see Table 41–2). Physical examination should start with a general assessment of the patient's degree of distress. Important clues are alertness, anxiety, fluid status, general health, positioning, ability to speak, and presence of cyanosis. The inability of the patient to lie down is significantly correlated with poor vital signs, arterial blood gases, and spirometry. Inability to speak was correlated in one study with hypoxia and a decreased peak flow rate. Vital signs may also have some prognostic value. Fever may point to a more complicated course and significant underlying disease. Increased pulse rate may be a sign of hypoxia. Pulsus paradoxus (a drop in systolic blood pressure of 10 mm Hg or more with inspiration) was believed to correlate with a worsening status but its usefulness has been questioned. Increased respiratory rates are usually seen in asthmatic exacerbations, but respiratory rate may decrease with fatigue in severe asthma. The lung examination may reveal a number of findings including diffuse wheezing. Wheezing results from turbulent airflow and occurs first on expiration alone, progressing to both inspiration and expiration. The wheezing may be localized and may shift in location with time as the relative

▶ TABLE 41-2. FORMAL EVALUATION OF ASTHMA EXACERBATION SEVERITY IN THE URGENT OR EMERGENCY CARE SETTING

	Mild	Moderate	Severe	Subset: Respiratory Arrest Imminent
Symptoms				
Breathlessness	While walking	While at rest (infant—softer, shorter cry, difficulty in feeding)	While at rest (infant—stops feeding)	
	Can lie down	Prefers sitting	Sits upright	
Talks in	Sentences	Phrases	Words	
Alertness	May be agitated	Usually agitated	Usually agitated	Drowsy or confused
Signs				
Respiratory rate	Increased	Increased	Often >30/min	
		Guide to rates of breathing in awake children:		
		Age	*Normal rate*	
		<2 mo	<60/min	
		2–12 mo	<50/min	
		1–5 y	<40/min	
		6–8 y	<30/min	
Use of accessory muscles; suprasternal retractions	Usually not	Commonly	Usually	Paradoxical thoracoabdominal movement
Wheeze	Moderate, often only end expiratory	Loud; throughout exhalation	Usually loud; throughout inhalation and exhalation	Absence of wheeze
Pulse/minute	<100	100–120	>120	Bradycardia
		Guide to normal pulse rates in children:		
		Age	*Normal rate*	
		2–12 mo	<160/min	
		1–2 y	<120/min	
		2–8 y	<110/min	
Pulsus paradoxus	Absent <10 mm Hg	May be present 10–25 mm Hg	Often present >25 mm Hg (adult) 20–40 mm Hg (child)	Absence suggests respiratory muscle fatigue
Functional Assessment				
PEF percentage predicted or percentage personal best	≥70%	Approx. 40%–69% or response lasts <2 h	<40 percentage	<25 percentage PEF testing may not be needed in very severe attacks
PaO₂ (on air)	Normal (test not usually necessary)	≥60 mm Hg (test not usually necessary)	<60 mm Hg: possible cyanosis	
and/or Pco₂	<42 mm Hg (test not usually necessary)	<42 mm Hg (test not usually necessary)	≥42 mm Hg: possible respiratory failure (see pages 393–394, 399)	
SaO₂ percentage (on air) at sea level	>95% (test not usually necessary)	90%–95% (test not usually necessary)	<90%	
		Hypercapnia (hypoventilation) develops more readily in young children than in adults and adolescents		

PaO_2, arterial oxygen pressure; Pco_2, partial pressure of carbon dioxide; PEF, peak expiratory flow; SaO_2, oxygen saturation.
The presence of several parameters, but not necessarily all, indicates the general classification of the exacerbation.
Many of these parameters have not been systematically studied, especially as they correlate with each other. Thus, they serve only as general guides.
The emotional impact of asthma symptoms on the patient and family is variable but must be recognized and addressed and can affect approaches to treatment and follow-up.

degree of obstruction may vary with location and time. If airway obstruction is severe, there will be little airflow and the chest may be quiet. Thus, wheezing is not a reliable indicator of the degree of obstruction. Lung examination may also reveal diffuse or localized rales, or a persistent cough with a clear lung examination. Air trapping due to occlusion of small airways leads to hyperinflation of the chest making it a less efficient muscle of inspiration and forcing the use of accessory muscles. The use of accessory muscles is a more reliable indicator of degree of obstruction. The presence of air leak is suggested by asymmetric breath sounds, tracheal deviation, or subcutaneous edema.

► LABORATORY AND RADIOGRAPHIC FINDINGS

Chest radiographs were shown to change the course of treatment in only 10% of asthmatics. Obtaining a chest x-ray is important for any child that presents with wheezing for the first time, as there are many illnesses that can present with wheezing. Thereafter, specific indications for a chest radiograph in a known asthmatic include clinical suspicion of consolidation, effusion, pneumothorax, or impending respiratory failure. Typical chest radiograph findings are hyperinflation, peribronchial cuffing, and areas of subsegmental atelectasis (Fig. 41–3). These findings are nonspecific and usually add little to the clinical assessment.

Spirometry can be used to assess a patient's degree of respiratory compromise. However, many children are not able to cooperate for spirometry. The simplest spirometry test, peak expiratory flow rate (PEFR), can usually be performed in children older than 5 years.[4] A PEFR of less than 30% to 50% of predicted or of the patient's personal best indicates severe airway obstruction.

Oximetry is another tool that may help assess severity. It correlates with ventilation perfusion mismatching and thus degree of obstruction. An initial pulse oximetry in infants and young children might be useful for assessing exacerbation severity but not for predicting the need for hospital admission.[8]

Blood gases may help assess the status of severe asthmatics but are not necessary for management of most acute asthma exacerbations. Hypoxia will be present early because of the ventilation perfusion mismatching. Pco_2 will be decreased early in the disease secondary to compensatory hyperventilation. As the obstruction progresses, the number of alveoli being adequately ventilated and perfused decreases and CO_2 retention occurs. Thus a "normal" or slightly elevated Pco_2 in a patient with an asthma exacerbation may be a sign of muscle fatigue and impending respiratory failure. Eventually, the hypoxia and hypercapnia lead to acidosis.

► DIFFERENTIAL DIAGNOSIS

The diagnosis of asthma is made by demonstrating episodic and reversible airway disease. This is most reliably accomplished by performing pulmonary function tests (PFTS). However, as discussed above, children younger than 6 years are generally unable to perform the tasks needed to get accurate PFTS. Therefore, the diagnosis in small children is usually made on a clinical basis. The diagnosis of asthma should be considered in all children with recurrent wheezing and symptom-free intervals, especially if there is a family history of asthma, atopy, or allergies. A personal history of atopy or allergies is also suggestive of the diagnosis of asthma in a wheezing child. Many children with asthma have their first asthmatic episode prior to 6 months of age. In infants, as in older children, viral infections are the most common trigger for asthma. Both infants who have asthma and those who do not may become infected with respiratory syncytial virus (RSV) or other viruses, and develop bronchiolitis as their first or only episode of wheezing. Therefore, in an infant with wheezing, it is often impossible to clinically differentiate between bronchiolitic wheezing and asthma. The most important clue to infantile asthma is a history of recurrent episodes of wheezing or persistent cough.

A list of other possible etiologies for wheezing in an infant or child is provided in Table 41–3. A history of prematurity or ventilatory support will help in identifying the infant with bronchopulmonary dysplasia (BPD). Cardiac examination may reveal other signs of cardiac failure in an infant with wheezing secondary to congenital heart disease. An association of signs and symptoms with feeding may suggest a tracheoesophageal fistula or recurrent aspiration. Clues to identifying the presence of a lower airway foreign body may come from the history (sudden onset and observed aspiration), chest examination (asymmetry), or radiographic studies (localized air trapping). A patient with cystic fibrosis may have clubbing of the digits, poor weight gain, or symptoms of malabsorption. It is often quoted that all that wheezes is not asthma. This is especially true in children and it is important to remember that even patients who come to the ED with a previous diagnosis of asthma and wheezing may have another etiology for their

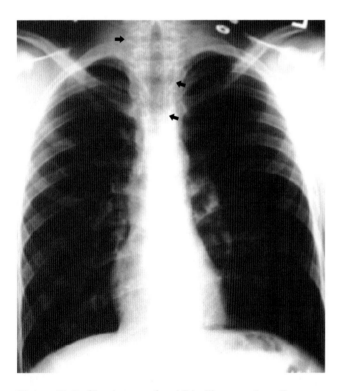

Figure 41–3. Chest x-ray of a child with an acute asthma exacerbation shows hyperinflation (abonormally lucent lungs). The diaphragm is flattened and relatively small and air is present within the mediastinum.

▶ **TABLE 41–3. DIFFERENTIAL DIAGNOSIS IN A WHEEZING INFANT**

Bronchiolitis
Foreign body aspiration
Immune deficiency
Immotile cilia
Bronchopulmonary dysplasia
Cystic fibrosis
Pneumonia
Anaphylaxis
Extrinsic airway compression
Vascular rings
Mediastinal masses
Aspiration
CHF

wheezing. Some patients with chronic cough, recurrent pneumonia, or chronic congestion may have a pathologic process similar to that of an asthmatic and benefit from the same modes of treatment.

▶ TREATMENT

Every patient with an acute asthma exacerbation needs rapid cardiopulmonary assessment. As noted above, a brief history and physical examination should be obtained but should not delay rapid initiation of therapy. The choice and intensity of therapy depends on the severity of the exacerbation and the patient's response to initial treatment. Recommended doses for asthma therapies are summarized in Table 41–4. Therapies that should be considered in all ED patients with an acute

exacerbation of their asthma include oxygen and fluids. Hypoxia can lead to hypoventilation and acidosis, which can cause pulmonary vasoconstriction, pulmonary hypertension, and right heart failure. Asthmatic patients are also often dehydrated due to decreased intake or vomiting and may require intravenous fluids. However, acute asthma is associated with increased secretion of antidiuretic hormone and with an increase in capillary permeability and interstitial fluid, thus overhydration may result in pulmonary edema. Antibiotics should be used in asthma only if evidence of concurrent infection exists. Chronic sinusitis, in particular, is thought to cause persistent asthmatic exacerbations.

β-ADRENERGIC AGONISTS

Adrenergic bronchodilators remain the first line of emergency treatment of asthma. Bronchodilation is produced by stimulation of β_2-adrenoreceptors, which mediate an increase in cyclic AMP via the enzyme adenyl cyclase. Cyclic AMP stimulates binding of calcium ions to the cell membrane, reducing the mycoplasmal calcium concentration with resultant bronchodilation (smooth muscle relaxation), and stabilization of mast cells (Fig. 41–4). Stabilization of mast cells retards the release of histamine and other inflammatory products. β-agonists also improve mucociliary clearance.

Albuterol is the most commonly used adrenergic agent in the United States because it combines a long duration of action with β_2 selectivity. Aerosol therapy is the most commonly used and recommended form of β-adrenergic agents. It has been shown to be as effective as IV or SC therapy and more effective than oral therapy. There are two main methods of delivering aerosolized medications. Numerous studies exist which suggest comparable efficacy of metered dose inhalers and jet

▶ **TABLE 41–4. MEDICATIONS FOR AN ACUTE ASTHMA EXACERBATION**

Medication	Route	Dose
β-adrenergic agents		
Albuterol solution for nebulization	Nebulizer	0.15 mg/kg (min. 2.5 mg, max. 5 mg) q 15–20 min. × 3
		May mix 3 doses with ipratropium in appropriate size holding chamber and run over 1 h
		Children <35 kg (7.5 mg albuterol and 500 μg ipratropium)
		Children >35 kg (15 mg albuterol and 1000 μg ipratropium)
	Continuous nebulization	0.3–0.6 mg/kg/h up to 20 mg/h
90 μg/puff	MDI	4–8 puffs q 20 min. × 3
Epinephrine (1:1000 solution)	SC	0.01 mg/kg (max. 0.3 mg)
Terbutaline (0.1%)	SC	0.01 mg/kg (max. 0.3 mg) q 20 min. × 3
	IV	Loading dose 10 μg/kg
		Infusion: 0.4 μg/kg/min. may titrate up to 6 μg/kg/min.
Corticosteroids		
Methylprednisolone	IV	2 mg/kg (max. 125 mg)
Prednisone/prednisolone	PO	2 mg/kg as loading dose in ED
		Discharge: 1–2 mg/kg/d (max. 60 mg) × 5 d
Dexamethasone phosphate	PO	0.6 mg/kg in ED (max. dose 16 mg)
Parenteral formulation)		Discharge: 0.6 mg/kg in 24 h
Anticholinergics		
Ipratropium bromide (500 μg/2 mL)	Nebulizer	250–500 μg q 20 min. × 2–3 doses (usually with albuterol)
18 μg/puff	MDI	4–8 puffs as needed
Magnesium sulfate	IV	50–75 mg/kg (max. 2.5 g) over 20 min.
Ketamine	IV	Induction: 1–2 mg/kg

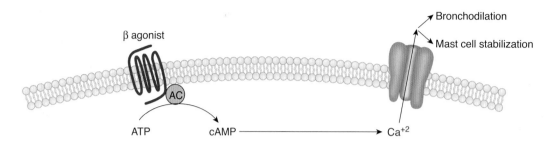

Figure 41–4. β-adrenergic agonist mechanism of action.

nebulization.[9,10] Metered dose inhalers (MDIs) are less expensive and more convenient, but require a cooperative (usually older) patient who understands the appropriate technique of administration. One method for enabling younger children to use an MDI more effectively is the use of an aero chamber or spacer, which provides a reservoir of particles for inspiration requiring less coordination of MDI activation with inhalation. Doses of 0.5 puffs/kg with a maximum of 6 to 8 puffs are recommended for treatment of an acute exacerbation. Particles generated by aerosolization vary in size. Only those in the 1 to 5 μm range are useful drug vehicles and are deposited in the lower airways. These represent only 10% of the output from an MDI, and 1% to 5% from jet nebulizer. The rest of the particles escape into the room, or are dissolved in mucus membranes and swallowed. Low flow rates and greater breath-holding periods optimize drug deposition in the lower airways. Oxygen flow rates of 6 to 7 L/min are recommended. Since so much of the drug escapes into the atmosphere, especially when being delivered to very young children, many physicians will administer "unit doses" (usually 2.5 or 5 mg albuterol/3 mL NS) for to all patients regardless of size. Larger nebulizer chambers allow for multiple unit doses to be placed in the chamber and run over a set period of time. This is less time-consuming for ED staff and avoids breaks in therapy in patients with moderate or severe exacerbations. Doses of 7.5 mg of albuterol mixed with 500 μg ipratropium for patients less than 35 kg and 15 mg albuterol with 1000 μg ipratropium in children greater than 35 kg can be mixed in the holding chamber and run over 1 hour. Continuous nebulization of albuterol at initial rates of greater than 3 mg/kg/h has also been shown to be safe and effective.[11] Continuous nebulization is usually started at approximately 0.5 mg/kg/h and titrated up or down as needed. The repeat assessments of the patient's clinical status should guide the frequency of aerosols or the rate of continuous nebulization.

Levalalbuterol (Xopenex) has been promoted as an alternative to racemic albuterol with the rationale that eliminating the isomer decreases side effects. However, no studies have demonstrated a benefit of this medication in the treatment of an acute asthma exacerbation.[12–14]

Other adrenergic medications are sometimes used in the treatment of acute asthmatic exacerbations. Inhaled epinephrine has not been shown to have any advantages over inhaled albuterol in acute asthma exacerbations.[15] Epinephrine is available as a subcutaneous (SC) injection. It is more toxic and no more effective than inhalation of a β_2 selective drug. Parenteral administration (0.01 mL/kg up to 0.3 mL of the 1:1000 solution SC) should be reserved for those patients who are unable to generate adequate tidal volume to deliver aerosolized drug to the bronchial tree. Subcutaneous terbutaline (0.01 mg/kg up to 0.25 mg), which is more β_2 specific, may be used as an alternative to subcutaneous epinephrine. It is preferred to SC epinephrine in the pregnant patient as SC epinephrine has been associated with fetal malformations from decreased uterine blood flow.

Intravenous (IV) terbutaline has been shown to be safe and effective in two small studies of pediatric patients with severe asthma exacerbations. Albuterol has been used as an IV medication in other countries. However, IV β-agonists have not been shown to have benefit over inhalational therapy. Isoproterenol was used as an IV preparation in the past in severe asthmatics. However, it can cause significant cardiac toxicity, especially in hypoxic patients. Therefore, isoproterenol is no longer recommended as a treatment for asthma.

Older inhaled β-adrenergic agents (isoetharine, metaproterenol) stimulate β_1 and β_2 receptors resulting, at least theoretically, in more undesirable side effects than albuterol. Inhaled epinephrine, which is available without a prescription, is much shorter acting than other inhaled β-agonists. Salmeterol is a longer-acting β_2-agonist that has a longer duration of action but slower onset than albuterol. It is not intended for frequent repetitive adminsistration.

Side effects associated with all β-adrenergic agonists are largely due to sympathomimetic effects and include tremors, anxiety, nausea, headache, vomiting, tachycardia, arrhythmia, hypertension, and hypotension. Nonsympathomimetic side effects include decreased oxygen saturation (secondary to altered V/Q matching), which is common, and paradoxical bronchospasm, which is rare. Metabolic side effects include hypokalemia, hypophosphotemia, hyperglycemia, and lactic acidosis. These side effects are often related to dose and route of administration and rarely require cessation of therapy. However, all patients receiving prolonged β-adrenergic therapy should have their oxygen saturation, heart rate, blood pressure, and serum electrolytes monitored closely.

ANTICHOLINERGICS

Atropine was the first drug used as a bronchodilator. It acts through interruption of parasympathetic transmission to the bronchial tree by decreasing the intracellular cyclic GMP (Fig. 41–5). This decreases the influence of cholinergic nerve endings on bronchial tone and dilates the airways. It fell into disfavor with discovery of epinephrine in the 1920s mainly because it produces anticholinergic side effects at doses only slightly above those required for bronchodilation. There has been a resurgence of interest in the use of anticholinergic agents in recent years due to our better understanding of the

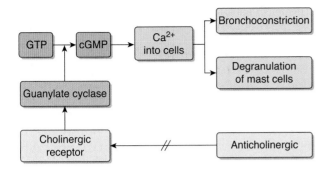

Figure 41–5. Anticholinergic agent mechanism of action.

cholinergic mechanisms that control airway caliber, and the development of synthetic analogues that are not appreciably absorbed across mucus membranes but retain their anticholinergic properties. Ipratropium bromide is a quaternary amine that fits into this category. There is evidence that its use in combination with β-agonists in pediatric patients with an acute exacerbation of their asthma is helpful in reducing rates of hospitalization.[16] It is most efficacious when given as two to three doses in combination with the initial two to three albuterol treatments in patients with moderate-to-severe exacerbations (see above for dosing). Reported side effects include dry mouth and a metallic taste.

CORTICOSTEROIDS

Multiple studies have demonstrated the effectiveness of corticosteroids in the treatment of asthma. The demonstrated benefits include rate of improvement measured by clinical scores and pulmonary function studies, increased rate of improvement, decreased duration of symptoms, decreased hospitalization rates, decreased relapse rates, and decreased need for β-agonists.[17,18] The use of steroids in the treatment of asthma has expanded greatly in the last few years. A clearer understanding of the inflammatory mechanisms involved in the pathogenesis of even mild asthma has led to a greater emphasis on the use of steroids. Corticosteroids are thought to have two mechanisms of action in improving asthmatic patients. It restores responsiveness to β adrenergics by increasing receptor numbers and lowering their threshold. Two mechanisms by which it reverses inflammation are inhibition of arachidonic acid metabolites via phospholipase and suppression of the PMN response to chemotactic stimuli. A number of studies have shown that corticosteroid benefit can occur promptly enough to affect the patient's disposition from the ED. Oral and parenteral corticosteroids are known to be equally efficacious.[19] Oral dosing is preferred in children when possible as it is less invasive. Intravenous dosing should be reserved for those patients who cannot tolerate oral medications, are requiring continuous β-agonist therapy, or have impending respiratory failure. Following a short course of corticosteroid therapy, adrenal suppression is minimal and clinically insignificant. Toxicity is chiefly related to duration of use and not to dose. Therefore, doses at the top of the dose response curve should be used and they should be stopped as soon as clinically allowable.

Early administration of corticosteroids has been shown to improve outcomes for patients who present to the ED with an acute asthma exacerbation.[20,21] Traditionally, 1 to 2 mg/kg of prednisone or an equivalent dose of another corticosteroid should be given as an initial bolus and then continued for another 4 days as a bid dose (total of 1–2 mg/kg for 5 days with a maximum single dose of 60 mg). One of the most common side effects or oral prednisolone (the liquid formulation of prednisone) is vomiting. This is especially problematic in children. Therefore, investigators have sought alternatives to this traditional therapy. Clinical trials have shown that 0.6 mg/kg of dexamethasone phosphate (maximum single dose of 16 mg) given at the time of ED evaluation and then 24 hours later resulted in similar clinical responses such as risk for hospitalization, return for additional care, or persistence of symptoms at 10 days, with a much lower (10 fold) rate of vomiting of the medication when compared to a 5-day course of 1 mg/kg/d of prednisolone (maximum daily dose of 60 mg).[22] Another trial demonstrated that a single dose of 0.6 mg/kg of dexamethasone phosphate (maximum dose 18 mg) given in the ED resulted in similar outcomes to a course of prednisolone 1 mg/kg/d bid for 5 days (maximum single dose 30 mg).[23] It is important to note that both of these trials used the parenteral form of dexamethasone phosphate administered orally and not a commercially available elixir of dexamethasone. The use of inhaled steroids in the acutely ill asthmatic patient has been investigated but a consistent significant benefit has not been reported.[24]

Inhaled corticosteroids should be considered for ongoing management of patients who have moderate or severe persistent asthma. They may be useful for children with mild persistent asthma if they seem to have increasing episodes of wheezing. There are many different inhaled steroids on the market. Most patients should start on the lowest effective dose. These do not have a role in the acute attack or for status asthmaticus.

MAGNESIUM

In patients who have not responded to therapy with β-agonists, ipratropium, and corticosteroids, additional therapies may be considered. Magnesium produces bronchodilation via counteraction of calcium-mediated smooth muscle constriction. There is conflicting literature on its benefits for pediatric patients with an acute asthma exacerbation.[25,26] However, a systematic review of the literature on IV magnesium for asthmatics of all ages did demonstrate a decrease in admission rate for those with severe acute asthma exacerbations.[27] Doses of 25 to 75 mg/kg IV over 20 minutes are recommended for patients with a moderate or severe acute asthma exacerbation who do not respond to initial therapy with albuterol and ipratropium.

HELIOX

Inhalation of a blend of helium and oxygen has also been suggested to be helpful for severe asthmatic patients unresponsive to other therapies. Because this mixture is less dense than air, there is less airway resistance and turbulence in the bronchi when it is inhaled. This may lead to decreased work of breathing and delay fatigue and respiratory failure until concurrent bronchodilator and anti-inflammatory therapy become effective. Current published literature on this subject is inconclusive as to its benefit and has not shown any significant complications with its use.[28,29] A recent systematic review of the role of heliox in acute asthma exacerbations concluded that the existing evidence does not provide support for the administration of helium–oxygen mixtures to all ED patients with acute asthma. At this time, heliox treatment does not have a role to play in the initial treatment of patients with acute asthma. Nevertheless, new evidence suggests certain beneficial effects in patients with more severe obstruction. Since these conclusions are based upon between-group comparisons and small studies, they should be interpreted with caution.[30]

INTUBATION/MECHANICAL VENTILATION

Indications for intubation of an asthmatic patient include decreased level of consciousness, apnea, exhaustion, rising $Paco_2$ after treatment, Pao_2 <60 mm Hg, and pH <7.2. An asthmatic may not immediately improve with intubation, since intubation does nothing to change lower airway obstruction. Intubation and mechanical ventilation may also put the patient at risk for serious complications. When intubating an asthmatic patient, the largest diameter tube appropriate for the patient's size is used to avoid increasing resistance even further. Although sedation is normally contraindicated in patients with asthma,[3] sedation and paralysis may be indicated to avoid barotrauma secondary to the child struggling during passage of the endotracheal (ET) tube. A modified rapid sequence induction should be used. The dissociative anesthetic ketamine is known to have bronchodilatory properties and therefore is a good choice for a sedative. Paralysis with succinylcholine may increase secretions but is not contraindicated. Pancuronium is thought to have bronchodilatory properties; however, its long duration of action outweighs this benefit. Vecuronium or rocuronium are recommended by most authors, when muscle paralysis is indicated in a pediatric patient with a severe asthmatic exacerbation. Once intubated, patients with asthma will require sedation and paralysis to maintain effective ventilation. They also require a long expiratory time to avoid air trapping due to airway obstruction. The ventilator may be providing a second inspired breath before the first breath has been fully expired (stacking breaths). Intrinsic PEEP may cause an increase in intrathoracic pressure that leads to decreased venous return to the heart and can cause hypotension. Air trapping also puts the patient at risk for the development of air leaks. Intubated asthmatic patients need to be watched carefully for the development of pneumothorax, or pneumomediastinum. Sudden changes in their respiratory or hemodynamic status may be due to a tension pneumothorax until proven otherwise. Ventilator settings should be adjusted to provide for adequate oxygenation with as low a peak pressure and PEEP as possible. The use of permissive hypercapnea (Pco_2) levels (as high as 70–90 mm Hg) has been associated with decreased morbidity and mortality rates in intubated asthmatic patients.

▶ DISPOSITION/OUTCOME

Despite appropriate therapy, approximately 10% to 25% of ED patients who have acute asthma will require hospitalization.[31] The decision to admit or discharge a patient from the ED af-

ter treatment for asthma can be difficult. There is a high relapse rate for patients discharged after treatment, and many patients return to the ED requiring further therapy or hospitalization. Numerous studies have been published attempting to establish objective criteria for admission. Clinical examination and scoring systems perform poorly in identifying patients requiring hospital admission.[7,32–35] However, these assessments may help to determine which patients should be admitted after an initial 1- to 2-hour period of treatment, leaving the ED resources for those who are more likely to go home after extended ED treatment and observation.[3] As noted above, an initial pulse oximetry in infants and young children might be useful for assessing exacerbation severity but not for predicting the need for hospital admission.[36] However, a repeat pulse oximetry of <92% to 94% at 1 hour was a better predictor of need for hospitalization, and it may be useful to move those infants and children into the hospital and out of the ED at that time.[35] Various spirometric parameters have also been proposed but have not proved to have adequate sensitivity and are often difficult to obtain in children.[4] To date, no objective criteria have been shown to be uniformly helpful in making this decision. The following risk factors have been identified as being associated with mortality: previous intubation (greatest predictor of subsequent death), two or more hospitalizations in the last year, three or more ED visits in the last year, use of systemic steroids, rapid progression of attacks, hypoxic seizures, severe nighttime wheezing, barotraumas, self-weaning from medications, lack of perception of the severity of the disease, poor medical management, poor access to medical care, and smoke exposure.

Patients discharged from the ED after an acute asthma exacerbation should be instructed to continue β-agonist use and be placed on a short course of corticosteroids. Steroid bursts for 5 days or less, if done no more than four times per year, do not require tapering. Immune suppression is clinically insignificant in patients with normal baseline immune function. Growth suppression does not occur, and the incidence of adverse psychiatric effects is low. One to two milligram per kilogram per day (maximum of 60 mg) prednisone for 5 days is the most commonly used regimen. However, as noted above, one or two doses of dexamethasone phosphate have been shown to have equivalent efficacy. Several other drugs are commonly used in the treatment of chronic asthma and should be considered as therapy for the patient being discharged from the ED. The use of inhaled steroids is encouraged for chronic treatment at home in moderately severe asthmatics. The addition of inhaled steroids to oral steroids in patients discharged from the ED can decrease the rate of relapse. The most recent National Heart Lung and Blood Institute (NHLBI) guidelines urge that those treating acute exacerbations of asthma work to prevent relapse of the exacerbation or recurrence of another exacerbation by providing: referral for follow-up asthma care within 1 to 4 weeks, an ED asthma discharge plan with instructions for medications prescribed at discharge and for increasing medications or seeking medical care if asthma worsens, review of inhaler technique whenever possible, and consideration of initiating inhaled corticosteroids.[3]

Despite the mortality and morbidity associated with this disease, the prognosis for most children with asthma is good. At least half of all children with asthma will be symptom free by adulthood.

REFERENCES

1. Eder W, Ege MJ, von Mutius E. The asthma epidemic. *N Engl J Med*. 2006;355:2226–2235.

2. Akinbami L. Asthma prevalence, health care use and mortality: United States, 2003–05, NCHS. www.cdc.gov/nchs/products/pubs/pubd/hestats/ashtma03–05/asthma03–05.htm. Accessed January 28, 2009.

3. EPR-3. *Expert Panel Report 3: Guidelines for the Diagnosis and Management of Asthma (EPR-3 2007)*. Bethesda, MD: U.S. Department of Healthand Human Services; National Institutes of Health; National Heart, Lung, and Blood Institute; National Asthma Education and Prevention Program, 2007. http://www.nhlbi.nih.gov/guidelines/asthma/asthgdln.htm. Accessed January 28, 2009.

4. Gorelick MH, Stevens MW, Schultz T, et al. Difficulty in obtaining peak expiratory flow measurements in children with acute asthma. *Pediatr Emerg Care*. 2004;20(1):22–26.

5. Ducharme FM, Chalut D, Plotnick L, et al. The pediatric respiratory assessment measure: a valid clinical score for assessing acute asthma severity from toddlers to teenagers. *J Pediatr*. 2008;152(4):476–480, 480.e1.

6. Carroll CL, Sekaran AK, Lerer T, et al. A modified pulmonary index score with predictive value for pediatric asthma exacerbations. *Ann Allergy Asthma Immunol*. 2005;94(3):355–359.

7. Gorelick MH, Stevens MW, Schultz TR, et al. Performance of a novel clinical score, the pediatric asthma severity score (PASS), in the evaluation of acute asthma. *Acad Emerg Med*. 2004;11(1):10–18.

8. Keahey L, Bulloch B, Becker AB, et al. Initial oxygen saturation as a predictor of admission in children presenting to the emergency department with acute asthma. *Ann Emerg Med*. 2002;40(3):300–307.

9. Cates CJ, Bestall JC, Adams NP. Holding chambers versus nebulisers for inhaled steroids in chronic asthma. *Cochrane Database Syst Rev*. 2006; (1). Art. No.: CD001491. DOI: 10.1002/14651858.CD001491.pub2.

10. Castro-Rodriguez JA, Rodrigo GJ. Beta-agonists through metered-dose inhaler with valved holding chamber versus nebulizer for acute exacerbation of wheezing or asthma in children under 5 years of age: a systematic review with meta-analysis. *J Pediatr*. 2005;145(2):172–177.

11. Camargo CA Jr, Spooner CH, Rowe BH. Continuous versus intermittent beta-agonists in the treatment of acute asthma. *Cochrane Database Syst Rev*. 2003;(4):CD001115.

12. Qureshi F, Zaritsky A, Welch C, et al. Clinical efficacy of racemic albuterol versus levalbuterol for the treatment of acute pediatric asthma. *Ann Emerg Med*. 2005;46(1):29–36.

13. Hardasmalani MD, DeBari V, Bithoney WG, Gold N. Levalbuterol vs. racemic albuterol in the treatment of acute exacerbation of asthma in children. *Ped Emerg Care*. 2005;21(7):415–419.

14. Ralston ME, Euwema MS, Knecht KR, et al. Comparison of levalbuterol and racemic albuterol combined with ipratropium bromide in acute pediatric asthma: a randomized controlled trial. *J Emerg Med*. 2005;29(1):29–35.

15. Plint AC, Osmond MH, Klassen TP. The efficacy of nebulized epinephrine in children with acute asthma: a randomized double blind trial. *Acad Emerg Med*. 2000;7:1097–1103.

16. Plotnick L, Ducharme F. Combined inhaled anticholinergics and beta2-agonists for initial treatment of acute asthma in children. *Cochrane Database Syst Rev*. 2000;(3). Art. No.: CD000060. DOI: 10.1002/14651858.CD000060.

17. Edmonds ML, Camargo CA Jr, Pollack CV Jr, et al. Early use of inhaled corticosteroids in the emergency department treatment of acute asthma. *Cochrane Database Syst Rev*. 2003;3: CD002308.

18. Rowe BH, Edmonds ML, Spooner CH, et al. Corticosteroid therapy for acute asthma. *Respir Med*. 2004;98(4):275–284.

19. Ratto D, Alfaro C, Sipsey J, et al. Are intravenous corticosteroids required in status asthmaticus? *JAMA*. 1988;260(4):527–529.

20. Rachelefsky G. Treating exacerbations of asthma in children: the role of systemic corticosteroids. *Pediatrics*. 2003;112(2):382–397.

21. Hendeles L. Selecting a systemic corticosteroid for acute asthma in young children. *J Pediatr*. 2003;142(2)(suppl):S40–S43.

22. Qureshi F, Zaritsky A, Poirier MP. Comparative efficacy of oral dexamethasone versus oral prednisone in acute pediatric asthma. *Pediatrics*. 2001;139:70–76.

23. Altamimi S, Robertson G, Jastaniah W, et al. Single-dose oral dexamethasone in the emergency management of children with exacerbations of mild to moderate asthma. *Pediatr Emerg Care*. 2006;22(12):786–793.

24. Rodrigues L, Coates AL, Schuh S, et al. High-dose inhaled fluticasone does not replace oral prednisolone in children with mild to moderate acute asthma. *Pediatrics*. 2006;118:644–650.

25. Ciarallo L, Brousseau D, Reinert S. Higher-dose intravenous magnesium therapy for children with moderate to severe acute asthma. *Arch Pediatr Adolesc Med*. 2000;154:97–99.

26. Scarfone RJ, Loiselle JM, Joffe MD, et al. A randomized trial of magnesium in the emergency department treatment of children with asthma. *Ann Emerg Med*. 2000;36:572–578.

27. Rowe BH, Bretzlaff JA, Bourdon C, et al. Intravenous magnesium sulfate treatment for acute asthma in the emergency department: a systematic review of the literature. *Ann Emerg Med*. 2000;36:181–190.

28. Martinon-Torres F, Rodriguez-Nunez A, Martinon-Sanchez JM. Heliox therapy in infants with acute bronchiolitis. *Pediatrics*. 2002;109:68–73.

29. Kim IK, Phrampus E, Venkataraman S, et al. Helium/oxygen-driven albuterol nebulization in the treatment of children with moderate to severe asthma exacerbations: a randomized, controlled trial. *Pediatrics*. 2005;116(5):1127–1133.

30. Rodrigo GJ, Pollack CV, Rodrigo C, Rowe BH. Heliox for nonintubated acute asthma patients. *Cochrane Database of Syst Rev*. 2006;(4). Art. No.: CD002884. DOI: 10.1002/14651858.CD002884.pub2.

31. Pollack CV Jr, Pollack ES, Baren JM, et al. Multicenter Airway Research Collaboration Investigators. A prospective multicenter study of patient factors associated with hospital admission from the emergency department among children with acute asthma. *Arch Pediatr Adolesc Med*. 2002;156(9):934–940.

32. Chey T, Jalaludin B, Hanson R, Leeder S. Validation of a predictive model for asthma admission in children: how accurate is it for predicting admissions? *J Clin Epidemiol*. 1999;52(12):1157–1163.

33. Keogh KA, Macarthur C, Parkin PC, et al. Predictors of hospitalization in children with acute asthma. *J Pediatr*. 2001;139(2):273–277.

34. Smith SR, Baty JD, Hodge D III, Validation of the pulmonary score: an asthma severity score for children. *Acad Emerg Med*. 2002;9(2):99–104.

35. Kelly AM, Kerr D, Powell C. Is severity assessment after one hour of treatment better for predicting the need for admission in acute asthma? *Respir Med*. 2004;98(8):777–781.

36. Sole D, Komatsu MK, Carvalho KV, et al. Pulse oximetry in the evaluation of the severity of acute asthma and/or wheezing in children. *J Asthma*. 1999;36(4):327–333.

CHAPTER 42

Bronchiolitis

Kathleen M. Brown

▶ HIGH-YIELD FACTS

- Bronchiolitis is a self-limited, virally mediated, acute inflammatory disease of the lower respiratory tract, resulting in obstruction of the small airways that occurs almost exclusively in infants.
- It is a clinical diagnosis characterized by rapid respiration, chest retractions and wheezing, and, frequently, hypoxia.
- Respiratory failure may occur secondary to respiratory muscle fatigue or apnea, especially in very young and premature infants.
- Treatment is largely supportive. Routine treatment with bronchodilators or corticosteroids has not been shown to be of benefit.
- Indications for hospital admission include need for supportive care (oxygen or IV fluids), persistent respiratory distress or respiratory failure, adjusted age <6 weeks, or significant underlying disease.

Bronchiolitis is a disease of the very young and occurs almost exclusively in children younger than 2 years. An attack rate of 11.4% in the first year of life and 6% in the second year of life was reported from one center. It is most common between the ages of 2 and 6 months. In the United States, it is the leading cause of hospitalization in infancy. It is the cause of more than 100 000 hospital admissions per year, which represents 17% of all hospitalizations of infants and an annual cost of more than $500 million.[1,2] It is more common in males than females and has a seasonal pattern, being most common in the winter and spring.[3]

Bronchiolitis is an acute inflammatory disease of the lower respiratory tract that is characterized by acute inflammation, edema and necrosis of epithelial cells lining small airways, increased mucus production, and bronchospasm.[4] The term is used to describe a clinical syndrome that occurs in infancy and is characterized by rapid respiration, chest retractions and wheezing, and, frequently, hypoxia.

▶ ETIOLOGY

The most common etiologic agent in bronchiolitis is respiratory syncytial virus (RSV). RSV is responsible for 70% of all bronchiolitis cases and for 80% to 100% of cases in winter months. Parainfluenza, adenovirus, and influenza account for most of the remaining cases.[5] Infection with RSV does not grant permanent or long-term immunity. Reinfections are common and

may be experienced throughout life.[6] Other viruses that are known to cause bronchiolitis are mumps, echovirus, and rhinovirus. *Mycoplasma pneumoniae* and *Chlamydia trachomatis* have also been associated with bronchiolitis. *Mycoplasma* has been shown to be the principal agent in school-age children with bronchiolitis. Adenovirus is associated with a particularly severe form of bronchiolitis that can lead to a chronic condition known as bronchiolitis obliterans.

▶ PATHOPHYSIOLOGY

Infection produces inflammation of the bronchiolar epithelium, which leads to necrosis, sloughing, and luminal obstruction. Ciliated epithelium that has sloughed is replaced by cuboidal cells without cilia. Increased mucus production and edema contribute further to airway obstruction. The absence of ciliated epithelium prevents adequate mobilization of secretions and debris. Histologic sections of the tracheobronchial tree of patients with bronchiolitis are very similar to those in asthmatics. The bronchioles and small bronchi are obstructed secondary to the submucosal edema, peribronchiolar cellular infiltrate, mucous plugging, and intraluminal debris. The obstruction is not uniform throughout the lungs. This leads to ventilation/perfusion mismatching and resultant hypoxia. The hypoxia leads to compensatory hyperventilation. If the obstruction is severe, hypercapnia may occur. Distal to the obstructed bronchiole, air trapping or atelectasis may occur. The epithelium usually regenerates from the basal layer within 3 to 4 days. However, functional regeneration of the ciliated epithelium usually requires approximately 2 weeks.

Adenovirus is associated with a particularly severe reaction termed bronchiolitis obliterans. In this disease, the destruction of the normal ciliated epithelium is extensive. The normal cells are replaced by stratified undifferentiated epithelium with an intense inflammatory response extending to the alveoli. During the reparative phase, extensive fibrosis and scarring leads to obliteration of the small airways.

▶ CLINICAL PRESENTATION

Typically, a child with bronchiolitis will have a prodrome of an upper respiratory tract infection. Parents will describe runny nose, low-grade fever, and decreased appetite for 1 to 2 days prior to the development of tachypnea and evidence of increased work of breathing. However, in some children lower-tract symptoms may develop over hours. Often, there will be

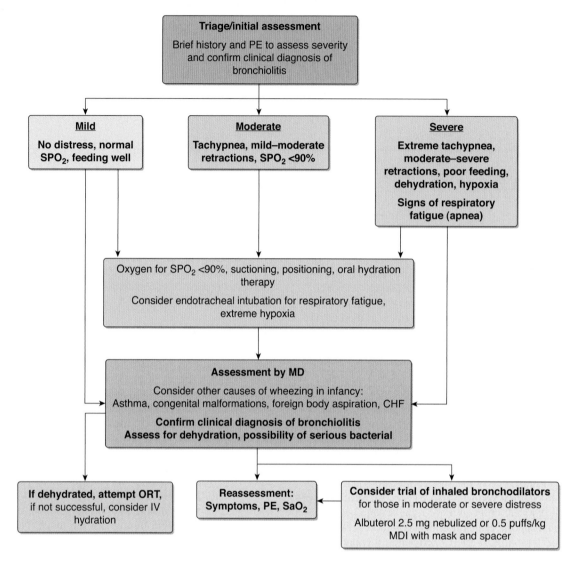

Figure 42–1. Management of a child with bronchiolitis.

a family or contact history of upper respiratory tract infection (Fig. 42–1).

Hyperventilation occurs as a compensatory response for hypoxia secondary to ventilation/perfusion mismatching. Respiratory rates of 70 to 90 per minute, or greater, are not uncommon. Flaring of the nasal alae and use of intercostal muscles may also be present. Respirations are shallow because of persistent distention of the lungs by the trapped air. Wheezing, prolonged expiration, and musical rales are common. The chest is often hyperexpanded and hyperresonant due to the air trapping. The liver and spleen may be displaced downward because of the hyperinflation and flattening of the diaphragm. Thoracoabdominal asynchrony may be present with breathing and correlates with the degree of obstruction. Fever is present in two-thirds of children with bronchiolitis. Despite these findings, the patient often has a nontoxic appearance.

Respiratory fatigue may occur since the broncholitic infant may increase his work of breathing up to sixfold. Apnea is not uncommon (18%–20% of those hospitalized with RSV bronchiolitis), especially in very young and premature infants. It generally occurs early in the illness often prior to the onset of other respiratory symptoms.

► LABORATORY AND RADIOGRAPHIC FINDINGS

A chest radiograph will reveal hyperinflation in the majority of patients with bronchiolitis. Peribronchial cuffing (thickening of the bronchiole walls) will be seen in approximately half. There may be areas of subsegmental atelectasis that can be difficult to differentiate from pneumonia. No study has convincingly demonstrated an association between radiographic findings and severity of disease.[7] A chest radiograph may be useful in ruling out the other disease processes in the differential diagnosis of bronchiolitis. However, there is controversy about whether all patients with a first-time episode of bronchiolitis should undergo a chest radiograph.[8] The American

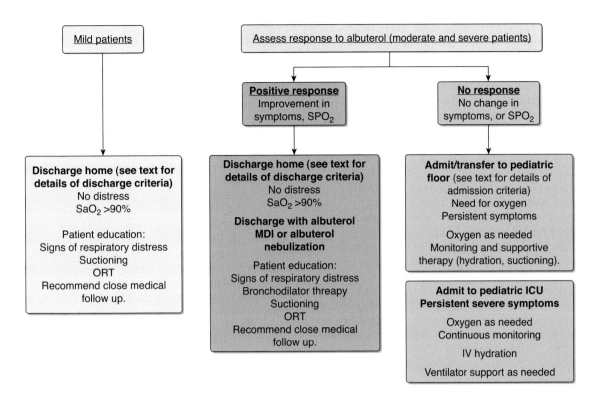

Figure 42–1. (*Continued*).

Academy of Pediatrics (AAP) practice guidelines for bronchiolitis state that the current evidence does not support routine radiography in children with bronchiolitis.[4] Laboratory studies are generally not helpful and not indicated in the acute management of bronchiolitis.[4,9] The use of complete blood counts has not been shown to be useful in either diagnosing bronchiolitis or guiding its therapy. Virologic tests for RSV, if obtained during peak RSV season, demonstrate a high predictive value. However, the knowledge gained from such testing rarely alters management decisions or outcomes for the vast majority of children with clinically diagnosed bronchiolitis.[10] Young febrile infants with clinical bronchiolitis are less likely to have SBI than febrile infants without bronchiolitis.[11]

Hypoxia is common and the patient should have oxygen saturations assessed with a pulse oximeter. Hypercarbia will be present in those with more severe obstruction. Respiratory rates greater than 60 breaths/min correlate well with carbon dioxide retention noted on blood gas analysis.

▶ DIFFERENTIAL DIAGNOSIS

The differential diagnosis for bronchiolitis is essentially the same as for asthma. Bronchiolitis may be very difficult to differentiate from infantile asthma. Response to bronchodilators does not exclude bronchiolitis, since some children with bronchiolitis may have some degree of bronchospasm. Since bronchiolitis most commonly occurs in infancy, pay particular attention to other processes that may mimic bronchiolitis and present in infancy. Congenital heart disease, cystic fibrosis, vascular rings, and other congenital anomalies may all mimic the findings of bronchiolitis. Infants and toddlers are particularly prone to foreign body aspiration, and this possibility must be considered.

▶ TREATMENT

Therapy is supportive. No medication has been shown to be beneficial in patients with bronchiolitis.[4,12–14] Since most children with bronchiolitis will have some degree of hypoxia, monitoring of oximetry and provision of oxygen, if needed, is important. The AAP practice guidelines on the diagnosis and management of bronchiolitis state that the supplemental oxygen is indicated if SpO_2 falls persistently below 90% in previously healthy infants. Oxygen may be discontinued if SpO_2 is at or above 90% and the infant is feeding well and has minimal respiratory distress.[4] Many children with bronchiolitis will have difficulty in drinking, secondary to their increased work of breathing. Intravenous hydration should be considered if the patient cannot take adequate oral fluids. As discussed above, a chest radiograph often reveals areas of opacity suggestive of pneumonia. However, no significant benefit has been demonstrated from routine antibiotic usage in patients with a clinical diagnosis of bronchiolitis.[4,15]

The association between bronchiolitis and the development of asthma, a disease in which steroids clearly are of benefit, has led some physicians to advocate their use in bronchiolitis. However, no study has convincingly documented their benefit and a meta-analysis of these studies also did not show a significant clinical benefit.[16,17] The majority of these studies were conducted on children hospitalized for bronchiolitis. A small, randomized-controlled study of the use of dexamethasone in infants with bronchiolitis presenting to an emergency department (ED) with bronchiolitis did show a reduction in rate of hospitalization.[18] However, a more recent, much larger, multicenter, and randomized-controlled trial of the use of dexamethasone in patients younger than 1 year presenting to an ED with a first episode consistent with brochiolitis (no previous history of wheezing) did not demonstrate a reduction in rate of hospitalization or any other clinical benefit. Even those children with a family history of asthma did not benefit from the administration of corticosteroid.[19] The use of inhaled steroids in children with bronchiolitis has also been studied. No study has shown a benefit of this therapy.

The use of oral bronchodilators (albuterol) has not been shown to be of benefit in these patients.[20–23] However, the use of inhaled bronchodilators in bronchiolitis remains controversial. Most clinicians believe that bronchodilators produce clinical improvement in some patients with bronchiolitis. However, systematic reviews looking at studies of the efficacy of β-agonists in bronchiolitis have not demonstrated a significant benefit of their routine use.[20–23] A systematic review, assessing the use of any bronchodilator therapy in bronchiolitis, demonstrated a modest improvement in clinical scores that was of questionable clinical significance. No difference was found in oxygenation or rates of hospitalization.[22] Despite the lack of proven benefit, most authors in this country recommend that patients with bronchiolitis, especially those with a past history of wheezing, should be given at least a trial of adrenergic bronchodilators. If there is no response to the trial dose, then therapy should be discontinued. The recent AAP practice guidelines on bronchiolitis state that a carefully monitored trial of α-adrenergic or β-adrenergic medication is an option. Inhaled bronchodilators should be continued only if there is a documented positive clinical response to the trial using an objective means of evaluation.[4] Some authors have suggested that the use of nebulized epinephrine therapy is superior to nebulized albuterol therapy in these patients. However, recent studies comparing racemic epinephrine to nebulized albuterol in patients with bronchiolitis have not shown that racemic epinephrine is more beneficial than nebulized albuterol therapy.[24,25]

The current AAP recommendations for ribavirin suggest that it should be used based on the particular clinical circumstances and physician's experience. This is a decision for the intensivist once the child is admitted.

Two to five percent of infants hospitalized for bronchiolitis will go on to develop respiratory failure and require mechanical support. There are no absolute criteria for endotracheal intubation. Suggested indications include P_{CO_2} greater than 60 to 65 mm Hg, recurrent apneic spells, decreasing mental status, and hypoxia despite oxygen therapy. Once intubated, these infants have many of the same problems that intubated asthmatics have and are at risk for air trapping and the development of air leaks. A mixture of helium and oxygen (heliox) has also been shown to be of benefit by some authors. However, no large-scale clinical trial of this therapy has been conducted.[26,27] Continuous positive airways pressure (CPAP) has also been used as an adjunctive therapy in patients with severe symptoms. One small clinical trial noted a decrease in the P_{CO_2} of patients who received CPAP versus those who received standard therapy.[28] There are also reports of successful management of severe bronchiolitis with extracorporeal membrane oxygenation (ECMO), in patients unresponsive to conventional therapy.

▶ DISPOSITION/OUTCOME

Bronchiolitis is a short-lived, self-limited disease lasting a few days. Most patients do not require admission. The disease is characterized by a high degree of variation. The clinical examination may vary depending on the infant's state of agitation, whether they have been recently suctioned and other factors. The decision as to which child requires admission sometimes can be difficult. One case–control study looked at whether oxygen saturation or clinical assessment could be used to predict patients who would return after discharge and require admission and found that they did not.[29] A recent multicenter trial attempted to identify factors associated with safe discharge from the ED. Of 1456 enrolled patients, 57% were discharged to home from the ED. The following factors predicted safe discharge to home: Age of ≥2 months, no history of intubation, history of eczema, age-specific respiratory rates (<45 breaths/min for 0–1.9 months, <43 breaths/min for 2–5.9 months, and <40 breaths/min for 6–23.9 months), no/mild retractions, initial oxygen saturation of ≥94%, fewer albuterol or epinephrine treatments in the first hour, and adequate oral intake. The importance of each factor varied slightly according to age.[30] Other suggested criteria for admission include age (adjusted for prematurity) less than 6 weeks, hypoxemia, and persistent respiratory distress. Children with a history of prematurity, congenital heart disease, bronchopulmonary dysplasia (BPD), underlying lung disease, and/or compromised immune function are at the highest risk for morbidity and mortality and admission should be considered. Follow-up within 24 hours is recommended for those who are discharged.

The overall mortality rate for infants with RSV bronchiolitis is 1% to 3%.[6] The mortality rate for infants within congenital heart disease and RSV bronchiolitis is 37%. It has been reported that 15% to 30% of infants who are hospitalized with bronchiolitis will require admission to an ICU or need ventilatory support. Up to 50% of infants with RSV bronchiolitis will go on to have recurrent wheezing. The only factor shown to increase the likelihood of subsequent wheezing is a family history of asthma, or atopy. Whether the initial infection causes changes that predispose to the development of asthma or patients with a genetic predisposition to reactive airway disease develop wheezing as a response to infection in infancy is controversial. Patients with bronchiolitis obliterans have a much poorer prognosis. They usually go on to have debilitating chronic lung disease.

REFERENCES

1. Shay DK, Holman RC, Newman RD, et al. Bronchiolitis-associated hospitalizations among US children, 1980–1996. *JAMA.* 1999;282(15):1440–1446.
2. Leader S, Kohlhase K. Respiratory syncytial virus-coded pediatric hospitalizations, 1997 to 1999. *Pediatr Infect Dis J.* 2002;21(7):629–632.
3. Mullins JA, Lamonte AC, Bresee JS, et al. Substantial variability in community respiratory syncytial virus season timing. *Pediatr Infect Dis J.* 2003;22:857–862.

4. American Academy of Pediatrics Subcommittee on Diagnosis and Management of Bronchiolitis. Diagnosis and management of bronchiolitis. *Pediatrics.* 2006;118(4):1774–1793.

5. Hall CB. Respiratory syncytial virus and parainfluenza virus. *N Engl J Med.* 2001;344:1917–1928.

6. Shay DK, Holman RC, Roosevelt GE, et al. Bronchiolitis-associated mortality and estimates of respiratory syncytial virus-associated deaths among US children, 1979–1997. *J Infect Dis.* 2001;183:16–22.

7. Dawson KP, Long A, Kennedy J, et al. The chest radiograph in acute bronchiolitis. *J Paediatr Child Health.* 1990;26:209–211.

8. Schuh S, Lalani A, Allen U, et al. Evaluation of the utility of radiography in acute bronchiolitis. *J Pediatr.* 2007;150(4):429–433.

9. Bordley WC, Viswanathan M, King VJ, et al. Diagnosis and testing in bronchiolitis: a systematic review. *Arch Pediatr Adolesc Med.* 2004;158(2):119–126.

10. Agency for Healthcare Research and Quality. *Management of Bronchiolitis in Infants and Children.* Evidence Report/Technology Assessment No. 69. Rockville, MD: Agency for Healthcare Research and Quality; 2003. AHRQ Publication No. 03-E009.

11. Bilavsky E, Shouval DS, Yarden-Bilavsky H, et al. A prospective study of the risk for serious bacterial infections in hospitalized febrile infants with or without bronchiolitis. *Pediatr Infect Dis J.* 2008;27(3):269–270.

12. King VJ, Viswanathan M, Bordley WC, et al. Pharmacologic treatment of bronchiolitis in infants and children: a systematic review. *Arch Pediatr Adolesc Med.* 2004;158(2):127–137.

13. Davison C, Ventre KM, Luchetti M, et al. Efficacy of interventions for bronchiolitis in critically ill infants: a systematic review and meta-analysis. *Pediatr Crit Care Med.* 2004;5(5):482–489.

14. Scarfone RJ. Controversies in the treatment of bronchiolitis. *Curr Opin Pediatr.* 2005;17(1):62–66.

15. Henderson M, Rubin E. Misuse of antimicrobials in children with asthma and bronchiolitis: a review. *Pediatr Infect Dis J.* 2001;20(2):214–215.

16. Patel H, Platt R, Lozano JM. Glucocorticoids for acute viral bronchiolitis in infants and young children. *Cochrane Database of Systematic Reviews* 2008, Issue 1. Art. No.: CD004878. DOI: 10.1002/14651858.CD004878.pub2.

17. Garrison MM, Christakis DA, Harvey E, et al. Systemic corticosteroids in infant bronchiolitis: a meta-analysis. *Pediatrics.* 2000;105(4):E44.

18. Schuh S, Coates AL, Binnie R, et al. Efficacy of oral dexamethasone in outpatients with acute bronchiolitis [see comment]. *J Pediatr.* 2002;140(1):27–32.

19. Corneli HM, Zorc JJ, Majahan P, et al; and Bronchiolitis Study Group of the Pediatric Emergency Care Applied Research Network (PECARN). A multicenter, randomized, controlled trial of dexamethasone for bronchiolitis. *N Engl J Med.* 2007;357(4):331–339.

20. Patel H, Gouin S, Platt RW. Randomized, double-blind, placebo-controlled trial of oral albuterol in infants with mild-to-moderate acute viral bronchiolitis. *J Peds.* 2003;14:509–514.

21. Everard ML et al. Anticholinergic drugs for wheeze in children under the age of 2 years. *Cochrane Database Syst Rev.* 3, 2005. ab001279.html.

22. Gadomski AM, Bhasale AL. Bronchodilators for bronchiolitis. *Cochrane Database of Systematic Reviews* 2006, Issue 3. Art. No.: CD001266. DOI: 10.1002/14651858.CD001266.pub.2.

23. Kellner JD, Ohlsson A, Gadomski AM, et al. Efficacy of bronchodilator therapy in bronchiolitis. A meta-analysis. *Arch Pediatr Adolesc Med.* 1996;150(11):1166–1172.

24. Wainwright C, Altamirano L, Cheney M, et al. A multicenter, randomized, double-blind, controlled trial of nebulized epinephrine in infants with acute bronchiolitis. *N Engl J Med.* 2003;349(1):27–35.

25. Mull CC, Scarfone RJ, Ferri L, et al. A randomized trial of nebulized epinephrine vs. albuterol in the emergency department treatment of bronchiolitis. *Arch Pediatr Adolesc Med.* 2004;158(2):113–118.

26. Martinon-Torres F et al. Heliox therapy in infants with acute bronchiolitis. *Pediatrics.* 2002;109:68–73.

27. Cambonie G, Milesi C, Fournier-Favre S, et al. Clinical effects of heliox administration for acute bronchiolitis in young infants. *Chest.* 2006;129(3):676–682.

28. Thia LP, McKenzie SA, Blyth TP, et al. Randomised controlled trial of nasal continuous positive airways pressure (CPAP) in bronchiolitis. *Arch Dis Child.* 2008;93(1):45–47.

29. Roback MG, Baskin MN. Failure of oxygen saturation and clinical assessment to predict which patients with bronchiolitis discharged from the emergency department will return requiring admission. *Pediatr Emerg Care.* 1997;13:9–11.

30. Mansbach JM, Clark S, Christopher NC, et al. Prospective multicenter study of bronchiolitis: predicting safe discharges from the emergency department. *Pediatrics.* 2008;121(4):680–688.

CHAPTER 43

Pneumonia

Sharon E. Mace

▶ HIGH-YIELD FACTS

- The incidence of pneumonia in children varies inversely with age.
- The primary predictor of the etiologic agent for infectious pneumonia is the patient's age.
- Pneumonia is usually part of a sepsis syndrome in the newborn, and, in an infant, presenting symptoms may be nonspecific.
- The most sensitive finding for diagnosing pneumonia in an infant is tachypnea.
- Most children with pneumonia can be managed as outpatients. Indications for admission include the following:
  - Hypoxia
  - Respiratory distress
  - Toxic appearance
  - Dehydration, age <3 months
  - Impaired immune function
  - Infections unresponsive to oral therapy
- The presence of underlying disease and the ability of the caregivers to provide care for the child should also be considered.
- Empiric antibiotic therapy should be based on the most likely etiologic organisms based on the child's age and clinical presentation.

Pneumonia, an inflammation of lung parenchyma, is most commonly due to an infectious etiology but may also have a noninfectious etiology from physical or chemical agents (Table 43–1). Various signs (such as rales) and symptoms (especially cough and fever) may lead to a presumptive "clinical" diagnosis of pneumonia, although in practice, pneumonia is determined by an abnormal chest radiograph showing pulmonary infiltrates. The clinical spectrum of pneumonia is highly variable whether in children, infants, or adults. It ranges from a mild illness to a life-threatening disease with significant morbidity and mortality. Considering the large numbers of microorganisms and other agents that can cause pneumonia, and the limitations of diagnostic testing, the exact cause is often difficult to determine. However, a constellation of clinical, radiologic, and ancillary/laboratory findings may suggest a likely pathogen, and therefore, appropriate therapy (Table 43–2).

▶ EPIDEMIOLOGY/OVERVIEW

Acute respiratory infections are among the most common infections encountered in pediatric patients. Acute upper respiratory tract infections are the number one diagnosis for all emergency department (ED) visits in children (age <15 years) in the United States.[1] According to some estimates, children may have up to 10 or more respiratory infections on an annual basis in early childhood.[2] Respiratory illnesses account for 20% of pediatric hospital admissions and nearly 10% of pediatric ED visits.[3] Pneumonia accounts for about 15% of all respiratory tract infections.[4]

In the United States, pneumonia is the leading cause of death from infectious disease in patients of all ages.[5] In adults, pneumonia is the sixth leading cause of death,[1,5] with one million hospitalizations[6] and 2 to 4 million cases of community-acquired pneumonia (CAP) annually.[5,6] In children (age <15 years) and excluding infants (age <1 year), pneumonia is the fourth leading cause of death (after trauma—both accidental and intentional, malignancy, and cardiovascular diseases) and the second most common hospital discharge diagnosis after injuries and poisoning.[1]

Pneumonia also has a significant morbidity with 200 000 hospital discharges annually (average length of stay of 3.2 days) for all infants and children (<18 years of age excluding newborns) in the United States.[1] CAP in children has a significant negative impact on patients and their families, with substantial financial and family care burden, which results in a decreased quality of life. On an annual basis, approximately 4% of children are diagnosed with pneumonia in the United States,[8] although the attack rate varies by age with the highest attack rate in the youngest patients. The attack rates are approximately 35 to 40 per 1000 infants (age <1 year), 30 to 35 per 1000 in the preschool age child (2–5 years), and 15 per 1000 school-age children (age 5–9 years) versus 6 to 12 per 1000 in children older than 9 years.[3]

The number of deaths from pneumonia in children in the United States has decreased by 97% from 1939 to 1996 due to several factors: the introduction of antibiotics, the widespread availability of vaccines, and improved access to medical care for poor children through the Medicaid program.[9] The fatality rate for pediatric pneumonia in the United States is <1%. Unfortunately, in spite of such progress, pediatric pneumonia remains a major cause of morbidity and mortality worldwide, especially in children younger than 5 years.[10] Worldwide, pneumonia is the number one killer of children and kills more children than AIDS, malaria, and measles combined.[10,11] Annually, the incidence of pneumonia in the developing countries is nearly 19 times that in the developed world.[10] The estimated annual new episodes of pneumonia are 150 million in developing countries alone and 2.1 million in developed countries according to the WHO,[12] resulting in 4 to 5 million pediatric deaths (20% of all pediatric deaths) worldwide yearly.[11,13] The

▶ TABLE 43–1. CAUSES OF PNEUMONIA*

Infectious	Noninfectious

Bacterial
 • Common
   ○ "Typical": streptococcus pneumonia ("pneumococcal pneumonia")
   ○ "Atypical": *M. pneumoniae*, chlamydophilia (formerly, chlamydia pneumoniae)
 • Less common
   ○ Typical: staphylococcus, group B streptococcus, *Listeria*, *Klebsiella*
   ○ Pseudomonas, *Hemophilus* (type B and nontype B), *M. catarrhalis*
   ○ Atypical: Legionella, *Bordetella pertussis*
 	
 Viral
 • Common
   ○ Respiratory syncytial virus
   ○ Human metapneumovirus
   ○ Parainfluenza
   ○ Influenza
 • Less Common
   ○ Coronavirus
   ○ Adenovirus
   ○ Rhinovirus
 • Other
   ○ Fungal
   ○ Rickettsial
   ○ Protozoal
	• Inflammation due to physical agents
	   ○ Inhalation (smoke/toxic inhalants) injury/pneumonia
	   ○ Lipoid pneumonia
	   ○ Kerosene pneumonia
	 • Inflammation due to chemical agents
	   ○ Drugs (chemotherapeutic agents: bleomycin, antibiotics: nitrofurantoin)
	   ○ Radiation pneumonitis
	 • Iatrogenic lung disease
	   ○ Graft versus host disease

*This is not an all-inclusive list but gives an overview of the various causes of pneumonia/pneumonitis.

WHO figures for clinical pneumonia include acute disease of the lower airway; for example, pneumonia, bronchiolitis, and reactive airway disease.[13]

▶ CLINICAL PRESENTATION

The clinical presentation in a child or infant with pneumonia is quite variable and is dependent on many factors including age, comorbidity, risk factors (Table 43–3), disease severity, and causative microorganism. The classic triad of fever, cough, and rales that is often present in adults or adolescents with pneumonia is rarely present in the young child or infant. Nonspecific signs and symptoms include lethargy, irritability, apnea, vomiting, poor feeding, isolated fever or hypothermia, and poor muscle tone are the rule in neonates. Pneumonia in newborns frequently occurs in the context of a sepsis syndrome.

Similarly, infants often lack the typical findings of pneumonia. They may present with nonspecific signs and symptoms. They may present with "a fever without source," sepsis, or vital sign abnormalities (fever, hypothermia, bradycardia, tachycardia, and tachypnea); gastrointestinal symptoms (poor feeding, vomiting, diarrhea, and abdominal pain); or grunting, lethargy, and shock. Infants with a bacterial pneumonia may be febrile with respiratory distress manifesting as tachypnea, retractions, and hypoxia, while infants with chlamydia

pneumonia may be afebrile and have a cough as their only symptom with a normal physical examination. The toddler with pneumonia frequently has a fever and a cough, although gastrointestinal complaints are common and may be the presenting symptom or chief complaint. The clinical presentation in older children and adolescents is similar to that in adults with cough, sometimes chest pain (which is usually pleuritic), and often generalized symptoms from abdominal pain to headache.

Although there is much overlap, two clinical presentations have been delineated: "typical" and "atypical" pneumonia. Typical pneumonia, presumed to be due to a bacterial microorganism, is characterized by sudden symptom onset with fever, chills, pleuritic chest pain, productive cough, a toxic appearance, and rales on lung examination. Atypical pneumonia is usually attributed to a viral etiology, mycoplasma, or chlamydia with a gradual onset of low-grade fever, nonproductive cough, malaise, headache, and physical examination findings that may include wheezing, a viral enanthem, an upper respiratory infection (URI) with pharyngitis, rhinitis, and conjunctivitis. However, determination of the etiologic agent based on clinical presentation alone may be unreliable.[14]

The clinical presentation usually indicates the severity of the pneumonia and the need for hospitalization or outpatient therapy. The lethargic infant who is not feeding or has respiratory distress likely has a more severe pneumonia needing

▶ **TABLE 43-2. PNEUMONIA SYNDROMES: PRESENTATION BASED ON ETIOLOGIC AGENT***

Signs and Symptoms	Bacterial	Viral	Chlamydia (Afebrile Pneumonia of Infancy)	Mycoplasma	Tuberculosis
Age	Any, especially neonates	Any, especially toddlers/preschoolers	1–4 mo (3–16 wk)	School-age adolescent	Any age >4 mo
Onset	Sudden (<50% occur after URI)	Gradual	Gradual	Gradual	Usually gradual may be acute
Cough	If age >10 y, ± sputum (if age <10 y, no sputum)	Dry cough	Dry cough can be only symptom	Usually dry cough	Cough often productive, sometimes hemoptysis
Other signs	Sometimes pleuritic chest pain	Sometimes coryza, sore throat, rash	Conjunctivitis in ~ 50% (may precede or occur with pneumonia)	Sometimes sore throat, rash, bullous otitis media, headache, myalgias	Weight loss, night sweats
Appearance	May be toxic	Nontoxic	Nontoxic	Nontoxic	Usually nontoxic
Fever	Usually high (>39°C)	Usually low grade	Usually afebrile	Usually low grade	Variable
Lung auscultation	Rales, decreased breath sounds	Rales, wheezing rhonchi	Rales, wheezing	Sometimes rales	Variable
White Blood Cell (WBC)	↑ WBC[†] ↑ neutrophils[†] ↑ bands	Normal or slightly ↑	Normal or slight ↑ WBC up to 15 000 range; may have eosinophia	↑ Lymphocytes, atypical lymphocytosis	Variable
Other laboratory tests	Obtain blood culture	Nasal washing for RSV may be helpful	Nasal washings may be helpful	Cold agglutinins often positive, bedside test	Sputum, gastric aspirates, skin testing (ppd)
Chest roentgenogram	Consolidation Pleural effusion Think *S. aureus* if pneumatoceles, pleural effusions, lung abscess	Hyperinflation Interstitial infiltrates	Hyperinflation Interstitial infiltrates	Variable patchy Interstitial infiltrates are most common	Variable: hilar adenopathy, infiltrates, cavitation, apical location

*The classic presentations for the various types of pneumonia are listed. However, a given patient may have all, some, or none of the given features even when the specific etiologic agent is known. There is overlap between the presentations. This is a general guide and not an absolute for any specific patient.
†Pertussis characteristically has an elevated WBC usually 15 000–40 000/mm³ with a marked lymphocytosis, although this may not be present in infants.

hospitalization than the playful nontoxic, well-appearing infant. Any infant or child with respiratory distress (e.g., hypoxia, cyanosis, grunting, flaring, retractions), or an altered mental status (whether lethargic or irritable, inconsolable, or unresponsive), undoubtedly has a severe pneumonia requiring hospital admission. Patients with any risk factors such as immunosuppression or chronic diseases (including chronic lung disease, congenital heart disease, and sickle cell disease) tend to have a more serious life-threatening pneumonia (Table 43–3). Immunosuppressed children or infants may have pneumonia from the "usual" organisms as well as from unusual pathogens.

Tachypnea may be an otherwise isolated finding in pediatric patients with pneumonia, especially in infants and young children. Although the absence of tachypnea has been purported to be the best finding for ruling out pneumonia,[15] contradictory results were noted in a study of patients with bacteremic pneumococcal pneumonia that found tachypnea in only 19% of patients.[16] Other findings in this study are as follows: 28% of patients had no respiratory symptoms, crackles (rales) occurred in only 14% of patients, 6% had only gastrointestinal symptoms, and 4% presented only with fever.[16]

A Canadian task force suggested evidenced-based guidelines for the diagnosis of pediatric pneumonia.[17] The absence of respiratory distress, tachypnea, crackles, and decreased breath sounds excluded pneumonia.[17] Unfortunately, when an attempt was made to validate these guidelines in pediatric patients in an urban ED, the results were dismal: only 45% sensitivity, 66% specificity, 25% positive predictive value, and 82% negative predictive value.[18] Another study that has not been validated also tried to determine predictive factors for pneumonia in a pediatric ED and had very poor specificity (5.7%–19.4%) but excellent sensitivity (93.1%–98%).[19] Tachypnea is a nonspecific sign and has many causes: fever, pain, anxiety, respiratory disease other than pneumonia, heart disease, and even metabolic disease. Thus, the results are not surprising.

▶ **TABLE 43-3. RISK FACTORS FOR PNEUMONIA***

- HOST:
- Prematurity
- Malnutrition
- Chronic disease
- HOST: pulmonary disease
- Acute
  - Upper respiratory infection (URI)†
  - Pneumonitis: chemical/physical agents
- Chronic
  - Cystic fibrosis
  - Bronchopulmonary dysplasia
  - Bronchiectasis
  - Pulmonary fibrosis
  - α 1-antitrypsin disease
  - Chronic obstructive lung disease
  - Pneumonitis
- HOST: neurologic diseases (may impair protective reflexes and swallowing, and increase aspiration risk)
- Muscular disorders (muscle weakness)
  - Cerebral palsy
  - Muscular dystrophy
  - Amyotrophic lateral sclerosis
- Central nervous system disease
  - Multiple sclerosis
  - Cerebrovascular accident (CVA)
- HOST: generalized immunosuppression
- Malignancy
- Human immunodeficiency virus (HIV)
- Iatrogenic
  - Medications: chemotherapeutic drugs, corticosteroids, others
  - Radiation therapy
- HOST: primary immunologic diseases
- Defects of white blood cells (neutrophils, lymphocytes): in number and/or of function
- Chronic granulomatous disease
- Neutropenia
- Leukopenia
- Lymphopenia
- Chediak–Higashi syndrome
- HOST: systemic disease
- Congenital heart disease (CHD) (not all CHD, but mainly those that may affect pulmonary blood flow or cause congestive heart failure)
- Congestive heart failure
- Pulmonary edema
- Host bronchial obstruction
- Foreign body
- Pulmonary neoplasm: primary or metastic
- Host: aspiration
- Gastroesophageal reflux
- Neuromuscular/neurologic disorders
- Tracheoesophageal fistula
- HOST: anatomic abnormalities
- Cleft palate, tracheosphageal fistula, pulmonary sequestration
- HOST: iatrogenic
- Direct access to respiratory tract (bypass of upper airway defense mechanisms)
  - Intubation
  - Tracheostomy
  - Surgery, invasive pulmonary procedures
- Impaired Reflexes
  - Medications: narcotics, sedatives, paralytics
  - Anesthesia
- Environmental
- Cigarette smoking: secondhand smoke in household
- Day care
- Crowded living conditions
- Low socioeconomic status
- Inhaled pollutants: household: wood burning stoves, poor air quality (smog), polluted environments
- Microorganism: virulence factors

---

*An overview of risk factors that predispose an individual to pneumonia is given. This is not intended to be an all-inclusive list.
†Preceding URI destroys normal epithelial cell barrier, impairs mucociliary system, alters normal native bacterial flora in upper respiratory tract, and inhibits cellular defense mechanisms.

Although rales, decreased breath sounds, and wheezing may be heard in pediatric patients with pneumonia, such findings may be absent with "normal" auscultation of the lungs. Rales may not be heard in infants or young children because of poor inspiration, poor ventilation of affected areas, transmission of sounds throughout the chest, which precludes localization, and noisy upper airway sounds. Respiratory distress and signs of increased work of breathing, retractions, grunting, flaring, head bobbing, or paradoxical (seesaw) breathing may occur in children with pneumonia. Abdominal pain and/or distention from swallowed air, an ileus, or diaphragmatic irritation from lower lobe pneumonia may occur. Meningismus, without meningeal infections, can occur with upper lobe pneumonia.

Other physical examination findings may be useful in detecting the source of the pneumonia as with contiguous or hematogenous spread from other sites, and in diagnos-

ing comorbidity (e.g., immunosuppression, chronic diseases), extrapulmonary findings suggesting specific etiologic agents may occur: such as conjunctivitis with chlamydia, pharyngitis with streptococcal or mycoplasma, a preceding or co-existent URI, and skin exanthems with bacterial or viral pathogens. The physical examination may reveal complications of pneumonia, such as dehydration, pleural effusion, respiratory failure, or even sepsis.

▶ **RISK FACTORS FOR PNEUMONIA**

There are numerous factors that increase an individual's susceptibility to pneumonia. Any process that negatively impacts host defense mechanisms predisposes to pneumonia. Such factors that impair host defenses may be congenital (such as a tracheoesophageal fistula) or acquired (e.g., human immunodeficiency virus [HIV]): a primary pulmonary disorder, (e.g., bronchopulmonary dysplasia, chronic obstructive pulmonary lung disease, cystic fibrosis), versus a "nonpulmonary" disease (e.g., muscular dystrophy, cerebral palsy, or congestive heart failure), or a "systemic" disease (e.g., malignancy) and even iatrogenic (anesthesia/sedation/medications or invasive procedures to the upper airway or lungs and chest) (Table 43–3). Environmental factors are also associated with both an increased incidence and a severity of respiratory infections.[2]

In pediatric patients, perhaps, the most common condition that predisposes to pneumonia is a preceding viral URI. Such viral URIs suppress the host's normal respiratory anatomic and physiologic mechanisms by destroying the normal respiratory epithelium that acts as a cellular barrier, altering the native bacterial flora in the upper respiratory tract, impairing the mucociliary system, and even inhibiting phagocytosis.

▶ PATHOPHYSIOLOGY

Numerous host defense mechanisms are employed by the body to keep the lower respiratory tract (below the vocal cords) sterile. Microbes most commonly reach the lung parenchyma after infective particles are aspirated from the upper respiratory tract. Less frequently, hematogenous spread occurs during bacteremia or from a distant focal infection. Contiguous spread and iatrogenic spread postoperatively following thoracic surgery or after invasive chest or upper airway procedures can also occur, but are less common.

The respiratory epithelium serves as a mucosal barrier. The mucociliary apparatus works to clear foreign materials including microorganisms from the airway. Coughing is a physiologic reflex, which also acts to clear foreign material from the respiratory tract. If microorganisms are able to reach the lung parenchyma, the lymphatic channels that drain to regional lymph nodes, and macrophages in the alveoli and terminal bronchioles work to clear microorganisms.

A series of steps needs to occur for any microbe to be cleared from the lower respiratory tract. First, the microorganism must be detected by the host cells, which involves pattern-recognition receptors. Once the antigens of the infecting microbe are identified by the cells of the host, various cytokines from tumor necrosis factor (TNF) to the interleukins (e.g., interleukin-1, interleukin-8) are secreted that mediate the host's inflammatory response. Sentinel cells in the lungs (e.g., alveolar macrophages and dendritic cells) alert other cells in the body (such as neutrophils), which are then recruited to kill the invading microbes and to direct the body's immune responses. With bacterial infections, neutrophils migrate into the lung, while viruses and intracellular pathogens (such as Mycobacterium) are attacked by the host's cell-mediated immunity. Various chemokines secreted by lung cells affect such processes as chemotaxis, the production and release of cells/cellular products, and cellular activation. Small lymphocytes and opsonins enhance the phagocytosis and killing of microorganisms. Secretory immunoglobulins, particularly IgA, augment bacterial lysis as well as neutralizing various toxins and certain viruses. The transudation of plasma fluids enables substances from complement to immunoglobulins M and G (IgM, IgG), necessary for bacterial opsonization to reach the sites of microbial infection in the lungs. However, the accumulation of inflammatory cells and fluids produces the clinical manifestations and radiologic findings of pneumonia.

When a pulmonary infection occurs, neutrophils travel from pulmonary capillaries into the lung's air spaces. Neutrophils kill microorganisms by two mechanisms: phagocytosis or by neutrophil extracellular trap (NET).[20] After ingestion of the microbes (e.g., phagocytosis), the neutrophil uses reactive oxygen species (such as hypochlorite), antimicrobial proteins (e.g., lactoferrin), and/or degradative enzymes (e.g., elastase) to kill the ingested microorganism. Neutrophils also extrude NET. NET is a meshwork of chromatin that contains antimicrobial proteins. The NET traps and then kills the extracellular microbe, a process that can be likened to a spider ensnaring a victim in its web.

Pathogenic organisms have evolved ways to escape the body's defense mechanism. For example, pneumococci are adept at avoiding recognition by the lung epithelial cells, perhaps by misleading or avoiding the pattern recognition receptors on lung cells. Pneumococcus has the ability to prevent the release of chemokines (such as tumor necrosis factor α [TNF alpha], or interleukin-1) by the lung's sentinel cells. A DNase virulence factor that cleaves NETs and releases bacteria has also been identified. *Streptococcus pneumoniae* also contains the virulence factor, pneumolysin, which is a pore-forming protein that allows the microbe to kill the host cell. All of these properties of the invading microorganisms may, at least partly, explain why neutrophils can fail to contain and kill pneumococci. These various processes, in turn, activate the complement system, which leads to an inflammatory response.

Unfortunately, although inflammation is essential for host defense mechanisms, it may also result in injury to the lungs. The substances produced by neutrophils, including degredative enzymes (e.g., proteases) and reactive oxygen species, can also kill lung cells and destroy host tissues. The host's inflammatory response causes cellular migration and the secretion of fluids which results in an excess of extravascular plasma fluids that can interfere with the exchange of gases across the alveolar capillary membrane and cause noncardiogenic pulmonary edema, cause respiratory distress/failure, and precipitate the acute respiratory distress syndrome (ARDS). When respiratory epithelium is infected, host cells may be killed, protective ciliary activity is destroyed, and the dead cells may slough into the airway. The net result is an accumulation of cellular debris and mucus stasis. This narrows the airway causing hyperinflation and air trapping as well as increased dead space ventilation. Destroyed alveolar cells can no longer produce surfactant. The inflammatory response along with the destroyed epithelial cells may lead to atelectasis with increased intrapulmonary shunting, hyaline membrane formation, and noncardiogenic pulmonary edema.

▶ ETIOLOGY

Unfortunately, the exact causative microorganism is usually unknown to the clinician, at least initially. The specific etiologic agent of pneumonia is determined, at best, only about one-third of the time,[21,22] although this percentage may improve in the future with better diagnostic testing. Recent studies, using extensive state-of-the-art diagnostic tests, identified a respiratory pathogen in 79% to 85% of pediatric patients with a lower respiratory tract infection.[23,24] However, this was in hospitalized patients after an "expanded diagnostic armamentarium", which included the following: bacterial cultures, viral cultures, direct fluorescent antibody (DFA) test, PCR test, and serology; done on nasopharyngeal swabs and blood, as well as on tracheal aspirate and/or pleural fluid.[23,24]

Although rapid antigen testing for specific microorganisms, especially the viruses, is becoming more widespread, it is not always available in all places at all hours 24/7, and there are technological limitations with many of the methods. Furthermore, an increased battery of diagnostic tests involves additional samples from the patient, time for the tests to be run, and costs.

Two important caveats need to be remembered: detection of a pathogen does not necessarily mean that organism is the cause of the current infection. An elevated acute serology sample may denote a prior infection, thus the need for paired serology samples. The organisms detected may or may not be the offending etiologic agent. Nasal carriage of some organisms does occur and they may not be the etiologic agent of the pneumonia. The yield for even "good" sputum and blood cultures may be low, especially for fastidious, difficult-to-grow organisms. Some organisms need special culture material and handling, and may take days or weeks to grow. Second, coexistence of pathogens is quite common with concomitant viral and bacterial infections occurring in children from 20% to 53% of the time.[23–31] So the presence of a given virus does not necessarily rule out a bacterial etiology or vice versa. The isolated virus or bacteria may be part of a coexistent infection or a "bystander" and not a cause of the pneumonia.[31]

▶ ATYPICAL PNEUMONIA

The term atypical pneumonia arose at the onset of the antibiotic era, in the 1940s when the sulfonamides and penicillins were introduced and referred to those cases of pneumonia that did not respond to these two antibiotics and using the available testing (bacterial Gram stain and culture) no organism could be identified. Thus, primary atypical pneumonia (PAP) meant that no causative microorganism could be identified. Over the years, with the new field of virology and other improved diagnostic techniques, many organisms that cause atypical pneumonia have been identified. These include viruses, *Mycoplasma pneumoniae*, Chlamydophilia (previously known as Chlamydia pneumoniae), Legionella, and Pneumocystis, to name a few. Currently, atypical pneumonias are characterized by: failure to identify an etiologic agent on routine Gram stain or sputum culture, and chest radiograph appearance showing a nonlobar, patchy, or interstitial pattern.

▶ PEDIATRIC PNEUMONIA: MOST COMMON ORGANISMS

The prevailing pathogens responsible for pneumonia in pediatric patients are dependent on the patient's age, comorbid-

ity, immunizations, day care attendance, and epidemiologic factors including seasonal variations/recent local outbreaks. There is a seasonal variation with the incidence of pneumonia peaking in the winter.[32] Most types of pneumonia including bacterial pneumonia and RSV pneumonia occur more frequently during the fall/winter when indoor crowding promotes aerosolized transmission of microorganisms, although they can occur year-round. If the causative organism cannot be determined, age is the best predictor of the pathogen (Table 43–4). In pediatric patients of all ages, *S. pneumoniae* is the most common bacteria causing pneumonia, while RSV is the most frequent viral cause of pneumonia and *M. pneumoniae* is the most common cause of "atypical" pneumonia with Chlamydophilia (chlamydia) pneumoniae second.[21,23–26,28–32] Overall, the most common organisms identified in ambulatory children with CAP regardless of age according to several studies were *S. pneumoniae* (17.5%–30%), viruses (20%–39%), *M. pneumoniae* (7%–29.5%), and Chlamydophilia (Chlamydia) pneumoniae (6%–15%),[21,28,30,32] with RSV being the most common virus (21%–28%).[28,30,33] The findings were similar in hospitalized children with CAP.[31] A bacteria was detected in 31% to 60% of patients with *S. pneumoniae* being the most frequent bacterial etiologic agent (9%–44% of patients), while viruses were noted in 45% to 66% of patients with RSV being the most common virus occurring in 42% to 59% of patients, and mycoplasma was detected in 7% to 22% of patients.[24–26,30]

In all age groups excluding neonates, the most common pathogens causing severe pneumonia necessitating an intensive care unit admission are *S. pneumoniae*, *Staphylococcus aureus*, group A streptococcus, *Haemophilus influenzae* type B, adenovirus, and *M. pneumoniae*.[19,20,22,35] Coinfections of *S. pneumoniae* with other organisms were common: bacterial–viral (with RSV) or bacterial–bacterial (with *M. pneumoniae* or *C. pneumoniae*).[24–27]

Human metapneumovirus has recently been identified as a leading cause of respiratory tract infection in the first few years of life.[34] It has a clinical spectrum similar to RSV: with bronchiolitis occurring in 59%, croup in 18%, asthma exacerbation in 14%, and pneumonia in 8%.[34] It occurs most frequently during the winter months. The mean age of infected children is 11.6 months.[34]

It is likely that the recent introduction of the pneumococcal vaccine will alter the relative frequency of the various pathogens,[35] as occurred after the introduction of and widespread immunization with the Hib vaccine. Prior to the Hib vaccine, *H. influenzae* type B pneumonia was a frequent cause of pneumonia in children. After widespread immunization with Hib, other pathogens emerged with increasing frequency and *H. influenzae* type B infections had a precipitous decline.[35]

▶ PNEUMONIA BASED ON PEDIATRIC AGE GROUP

NEONATE

Neonatal (birth to 1 month) pneumonia is usually due to aspiration of maternal genital organisms acquired during labor and delivery. The predominant organism is group B Streptococcus followed by enteric gram-negative bacilli, generally

▶ TABLE 43-4. **COMMON PATHOGENS BASED ON AGE***

Age (Pediatric)	Most Common Etiologic Group	Specific Microorganism
Neonate (≤30 d)	1. Bacteria 2. Viruses	Bacteria: Common: Group B *Streptococcus*, gram-negative enteric bacteria (*E. coli*, *Klebsiella*), *L. monocytogenes* Less common: staphylococci, *H. influenza* (type B)† Viruses: Herpes simplex, cytomegalovirus, rubella
Infant (1–3 mo)	1. "Atypical" bacteria 2. Viruses 3. Bacteria	Atypical bacteria: Common: "Afebrile Pneumonia" (*C. trachomatis*) Viruses: Common: Respiratory syncytial virus (RSV) Less common: Parainfluenza, influenza, adenovirus Bacteria: *S. pneumonia*, *H. influenzae* (nontype B), *H. influenzae* type B† plus same bacteria as for neonates
Infant/very young child (3–24 mo)	1. Viruses 2. Bacteria	Viruses: Common: RSV, human metapneumovirus, parainfluenza Less common: adenovirus, rhinovirus, others Bacteria: Common: *S. pneumoniae*, *H. influenzae* (nontype B) Less common: *M. catarrhalis*, *M. pneumoniae*, group A streptococci, *S. aureus*, *H. influenzae* type B†
Toddler (Preschooler) (2–5 y)	1. Viruses 2. Bacteria 3. Atypical	Viruses: Common: RSV, parainfluenza, influenza, adenovirus Bacteria: Common: *S. pneumoniae*, *H. influenzae* (nontype B) Less common: *H. influenzae* (type B)†, *S. aureus*, Group A *Streptococcus*, *M. catarrhalis* Atypical: Common: *M. pneumoniae* Less common: Chlamydophilia (Chlamydia) pneumoniae
School Age and Adolescents (5–18 y)	1. Atypical 2. Bacteria 3. Viruses	Atypical: Common: *M. pneumoniae* Less common: Chlamydophilia (Chlamydia) pneumoniae Bacteria: Common: *S. pneumoniae* Less common: *H. influenzae* (nontype B) Viruses: Common: influenza, adenovirus Less common: rhinovirus, parainfluenza

*The most likely organisms (but not all possibilities) are listed. Assumes immunocompetent patient.
†Marked ↓ since widespread Hib immunization.

Escherichia coli and *Klebsiella pneumoniae*. Other less common etiologic agents include *Listeria monocytogenes*, other streptococci (group A and B-hemolytic species), *S. aureus*, *B. pertussis*, anaerobic bacteria, and viruses (most often, herpes simplex, cytomegalovirus, and then rubella).

INFANTS: 1 TO 3 MONTHS

Infants aged 4 to 8 weeks may still have pneumonia caused by organisms predominantly found in neonates; specifically, Group B streptococci, gram-negative enteric bacteria, and

L. monocytogenes. In addition, viruses (especially RSV and parainfluenza), chlamydia ("afebrile pneumonia of infancy"), and staphylococci may be a cause of pneumonia in infants 1 to 3 months of age. The predominant organisms causing pneumonia differ between early infancy (aged 4–12 weeks) versus older infants. In infants aged 4 to 12 weeks, the prevailing pathogens are (in order of prevalence) *Chlamydia trachomatis*, viruses (RSV and parainfluenza), *S. pneumoniae*, and *B. pertussis*.[36]

"Afebrile pneumonia of infancy" or "afebrile pneumonitis" or atypical pneumonia typically occurs in infants from 3–4 weeks to 16 weeks old. The classic presentation is that of an afebrile infant 1 to 4 months of age with a prominent dry cough who looks well. There is a gradual symptom onset beginning with nasal congestion followed by a dry cough. Conjunctivitis either preceding or concurrent with the respiratory symptoms is found in approximately half of the infants. The infant usually appears nontoxic without positive physical examination findings including clear lungs on auscultation except for conjunctivitis and a cough that may be paroxysmal like pertussis. The chest radiograph usually demonstrates an interstitial pneumonia while the total WBC count is normal but eosinophilia is present. The etiologic agent is *C. trachomatis*, although *Ureaplasma urealyticum*, *Mycoplasma hominis*, *Pneumocystis carinii*, and *B. pertussis* have also been associated with this afebrile pneumonia of infancy (but are not proven etiologic agents). Generally, "chlamydia pneumonia" is a mild disease but the cough may interfere with usual activities (e.g., feeding, sleeping) and significant respiratory distress with tachypnea, retractions, and hypoxia can occur. Apnea is also a major concern with chlamydia pneumonia as well as with other causes of respiratory infections (such as RSV or pertussis) in young infants which explains why admission, whether as an inpatient or to an observation unit, is often considered in infants younger than 6 months with lower respiratory tract infections (LRTI). A macrolide erythromycin, azithromycin, or clarithromycin, is the drug of choice for chlamydia pneumonia. Azithromycin may be better-tolerated (e.g., less gastrointestinal side effects) than erythromycin or clarithromycin.[37,38]

INFANTS: 3 TO 24 MONTHS

In older infants (3–12 months) and very young children (12–24 months), viruses are the most common etiologic agent causing pneumonia. The viruses implicated in the majority of lower respiratory tract infections (LRTI) including pneumonia in this age group are RSV, human metapneumovirus, parainfluenza, less frequently, adenovirus and rhinovirus, and numerous other viral agents.[34] The most common pathogens responsible for bacterial pneumonia in the 3- to 24-month age group are *S. pneumoniae*, *H. influenzae* (non-B-type), *Moraxella catarrhalis*, *M. pneumoniae*, group A streptococci, and *S. aureus*. There has been a precipitous decline in *H. influenzae* type B invasive disease, including pneumonia, after the Hib vaccine was included in the vaccination program.[35]

TODDLER/PRESCHOOLER

Viruses remain the most common cause of pneumonia in this developmental age group, although the relative frequency of bacterial etiologic agents increases. The most frequent viral pathogens are RSV, parainfluenza, adenovirus, and influenza and less frequently, adenovirus and rhinovirus; while the bacterial pathogens are *S. pneumoniae*, *H. influenzae*, (non-B-type), followed by the "atypicals" *M. pneumoniae* and Chlamydophilia (Chlamydia) pneumoniae, and less frequently *S. aureus*, group A streptococcus, and *M. catarrhalis*.[31] The Hib vaccine does not confer immunity against nontype B *H. influenzae*, which has increased in frequency as an etiologic agent of bacterial pneumonia and other infections.

SCHOOL AGE AND ADOLESCENTS

The "atypical" bacterial organisms, *M. pneumoniae* and less commonly Chlamydophilia (chlamydia) pneumoniae, are the predominant pathogens causing pneumonia in this age group followed by *S. pneumoniae* and viruses (RSV, parainfluenza, influenza, adenovirus, and rhinovirus). Mycoplasma accounts for approximately one-fifth of all cases of pneumonia in the general population. The incidence of *M. pneumoniae* increases from school age (9%–16%), adolescents (16%–21%), and up to 30% to 50% in college students and military recruits.

SEVERE, LIFE-THREATENING PNEUMONIA

In pediatric patients excluding newborns, the most common organisms that can lead to severe, life-threatening pneumonia needing an intensive care unit admission are *S. pneumoniae*, *S. aureus*, group A streptococcus, *H. influenzae* b, adenovirus, and *M. pneumoniae*.[31-39]

▶ SPECIFIC PATHOGENS

STREPTOCOCCUS PNEUMONIAE

The most common cause of bacterial pneumonia in all ages of pediatric patients excluding neonates has been *S. pneumoniae*. The classic presentation of pneumococcal pneumonia is the sudden onset of fever, chills, cough (a productive cough with blood-tinged sputum or hemoptysis may occur in adolescents and adults), pleuritic chest pain, and dyspnea. Patients with functional (e.g., sickle cell disease) or anatomic asplenia are at increased risk for pneumococcal disease. Routine immunization with pneumococcal conjugate vaccine PCV7 (Prevnar) and also PPV23 (Pneumovax) in high-risk children is recommended.[35] The incidence of all invasive pneumococcal infections has decreased by 80% for children <2 years of age and approximately 90% for vaccine/vaccine-related serotypes and has also decreased in older children and adults since the recommendation in 2000 for the routine use of PCV7 in infants.[35] Whether serotype replacement is occurring remains to be determined.

STAPHYLOCOCCUS AUREUS

S. aureus is an uncommon but rapidly progressive fulminant illness. *S. aureus* pneumonia may be primary with no extrapulmonary site of infection or secondary with ≥1 nonpulmonary site of infection. Blood cultures are positive in 20% to 30% of patients with primary *S. aureus* pneumonia. Pleural effusions and pneumatoceles (noted in 45%–60% of patients) are not uncommon.

HAEMOPHILUS INFLUENZAE

H. influenzae infections including pneumonia are most prevalent in young children. Extrapulmonary infections (such as otitis media, meningitis, pericarditis, and epiglottitis) are common in patients with *H. influenzae* type B pneumonia. There has been a marked decline in infections due to *H. influenzae* type B since the Hib vaccine administered. However, *H. influenzae* type B remains a significant life-threatening pathogen and *H. influenzae* nontype B pneumonia also occurs.

MYCOPLASMA PNEUMONIAE

Generally, *M. pneumoniae* is characterized by a low-grade fever and nonproductive cough. Other symptoms that may occur include headache, myalgias, abdominal pain, and vomiting. The pulmonary examination may reveal rales or decreased breath sounds, or may be normal. Typical laboratory studies include normal WBC, elevated transaminases, and positive cold agglutinins. Neurologic complications including meningoencephalitis, transverse myelitis, Guillain–Barre syndrome, and cerebellar ataxia occur in approximately 7% of patients with mycoplasma pneumonia.

RESPIRATORY SYNCYTIAL VIRUS

RSV is the most common pediatric viral pneumonia particularly in infancy.[31] Although the most common presentation of RSV infection is bronchiolitis, RSV pneumonia can also occur and both can coexist (up to one-third of infants with RSV bronchiolitis will also have pneumonia). The typical findings with an RSV infection include a low-grade fever; signs of URI, cough, wheezing, and/or rales; WBC normal or mildly increased with a lymphocytosis; and variable chest radiographic findings with air bronchograms, atelectasis, and/or hyperinflation.

OTHER SPECIFIC PATHOGENS AND UNUSUAL CAUSES OF PNEUMONIA

Gram-negative bacilli including pseudomonas should be considered in neonates and in patients who have been recently hospitalized. Group A streptococcus can cause invasive disease ranging from pneumonia and empyema to necrotizing fasciitis. Pneumonia secondary to anaerobes can occur with any condition (such as neurologic disorders or congenital anomalies) that predispose to aspiration (Table 43–4). Mycobacterial infection should always be in the differential diagnosis of pneumonia. Tuberculosis is a particular concern in patients with HIV/AIDS and in immigrants.

Other unusual etiologic agents causing pneumonia are associated with a specific location, animal exposure, or hobbies. Recent travel to or residence in an endemic region may suggest pneumonia secondary to coccidiomycosis (southwestern United States), histoplasmosis (Mississippi/Ohio river valley), or hantavirus (southwestern United States). Exposure to/contact with an infected individual(s) and travel or residence in an endemic area may be a clue to severe acute respiratory syndrome (SARS) or tuberculosis (TB). Occupational or avocational exposure and exposure to pets or other animals also can be associated with certain pneumonias (Table 43–5).

▶ **TABLE 43–5. VARIABLES ASSOCIATED WITH UNUSUAL CAUSES OF PNEUMONIA**

Endemic region and/or exposure to infected individuals
   Severe acute respiratory syndrome exposure to infected individual and/or in endemic area
   Tuberculosis exposure to infected individual and/or in endemic area

Location
   Cocidiomycosis: location/recent travel to southwestern United States (San Joaquin Valley, S. California, New Mexico, Southern Arizona, and Southwest Texas)
   Histoplasmosis: Mississippi/Ohio River Valley
   Hantavirus: southwestern United States (4 corners area of Arizona, New Mexico, Nevada, and Utah)
   Meliodosis: south/central America, W. Indies, Australia, Southeast Asia, Guam

Contaminated environment
   Legionnaires' disease: contaminated water supply, air coolers, (open water source)

Animal exposure
   Psitticosis exotic birds (parrots, cockatoos, etc.), turkeys, pigeons
   Anthrax cattle, horses, swine, animal hides

Brucellosis: unpasteurized dairy products, cattle, goats, pigs
Bubonic plague lagomorphs (squirrels, rabbits, chipmunks, etc.), rats
Hantavirus: rodent excretions, urine, saliva, droppings

Histoplasmosis: soil with bird or bat droppings
Leptospirosis: water contaminated with animal urine, wild dogs, cats, rodents, cattle, horses, pigs
Pasteurella: multocida-infected dogs, cats
Q fever: secretions of infected animals or contact with the animals (cattle, sheep, goats, and other domestic animals)
Tularemia: hunting, trapping, skinning of infected animals

▶ LABORATORY STUDIES

Laboratory studies may not be necessary in every patient with suspected pneumonia, such as the well-appearing afebrile pediatric patient presenting with a cough that has a good oral intake and is in no distress. However, in some patients laboratory studies may be useful in identifying the underlying disease and potential complications. The WBC is usually normal or mildly elevated with a viral pneumonia.[40] With *M. pneumoniae* or *C. pneumoniae*, a normal WBC is characteristic. Lymphocytosis is typically present with a viral, Chlamydia or pertussis pneumonia. A markedly elevated total WBC and lymphocytosis is characteristic of pertussis (see Chapter 44). Eosinophilia often occurs with *C. pneumoniae* or a parasitic infection. Leukopenia may portend a poor prognosis. Leukocytosis ($>15\,000$ cells/mm^3)[41–44] with bandemia is generally present with a bacterial pneumonia.[41–44] A markedly increased WBC ($>25\,000$ mm^3) is highly suggestive of a bacterial etiologic agent, frequently with bacteremia and a greater complication rate.[44] Although there is a conflicting report indicating that, an elevated WBC >15 000 did not differentiate between viral or bacterial pneumonia.[23] Whether coinfections were present, the range of diagnostic testing used to detect the various etiologic agents, and which specific bacteria or virus was present (e.g., some bacteria and viruses are more virulent than others), the time of presentation, the treatment given, and other variables could all affect the results of these various studies and explain the different findings. In a study of febrile children presenting to an ED, 26% of febrile pediatric ED patients with a WBC >20 000/mm[3] had an occult pneumonia on the chest radiograph.[45]

Positive blood cultures in the 16% to 30% range have been reported for adults with pneumococcal pneumonia in previous reports,[40,45–48] while more recent studies in children and adults with community-acquired pneumonia found a 1% to 16% yield with *S. pneumoniae* being the most common bacteria isolated.[21] There is probably a higher yield for blood cultures in hospitalized (10%–15%)[21] versus ambulatory patients, which reflects a higher incidence of bacterial pneumonia (such as *S. pneumoniae*) in hospitalized patients compared with a greater incidence of viral and atypical pneumonia in outpatients.[40] Although the yield from blood cultures is low and their use has been questioned by some,[49] most recommendations include obtaining blood cultures in febrile toxic or ill-appearing hospitalized patients[50] with the understanding that mandating blood cultures in all hospitalized patients (versus targeting more critically ill patients) is probably neither necessary nor cost effective.[51]

In children, sputum cultures have limited utility since children younger than 10 years rarely produce sputum and obtaining a high-quality sputum uncontaminated by mouth/pharyngeal flora is difficult. However, sputum samples may be useful in selected cases and to confirm TB. Nasopharyngeal and throat cultures for bacteria are not useful and may be misleading because of contamination with oral flora. Conversely, nasopharyngeal and/or throat cultures for viruses, pertussis, and the atypicals (e.g., mycoplasma and chlamydia) may help reveal the pathogen causing the pneumonia.

Rapid viral antigen testing (such as for RSV, influenza, and parainfluenza) and fluorescent antibody testing for *B. pertussis* and *C. trachomatis* are available and have the advantage of yielding results more quickly than a culture. Bacterial antigen testing for pneumonia, however, has limited utility because of poor sensitivity and specificity. Serologic testing, which usually involves acute and convalescent sera may be helpful in selected patients in whom the diagnosis is uncertain or the pneumonia persistent and unresponsive to therapy.

Positive cold agglutinins occur in 70% to 90% of patients with *M. pneumoniae* but may be negative in young children and may also be positive with viral infections. The bedside cold agglutinin test is confirmed by putting several drops of blood in a blue coagulation tube then placing the tube in ice water for 15 to 30 seconds. Course floccular agglutination that disappears with rewarming is a positive test. Currently, with Legionella pneumonia, the diagnostic test of choice is Legionella urinary antigen which remains positive weeks after the infection but it only detects Legionella pneumophila and not other Legionella species. Tuberculosis skin testing may be indicated with apical and/or cavitary pneumonia.

Invasive diagnostic testing including transtracheal aspiration, bronchoalveolar lavage, percutaneous, or open-lung biopsy is generally reserved for patients with severe disease unresponsive to therapy, especially if they are immunocompromised.

▶ RADIOGRAPHIC EVALUATION

The chest roentgenogram may help in making the diagnosis by eliminating many possible infectious and noninfectious causes for the patient's symptoms (Table 43–6). The chest roentgenogram is essential in confirming the diagnosis of pneumonia, may indicate the likely pathogen, and is valuable in detecting complications such as a pleural effusion, abscess, or pneumatoceles. An abnormal chest roentgenogram characteristic of a specific pneumonia may identify those patients who will (or will not) benefit from specific therapy including antimicrobials. Although the need for a chest radiograph in a well-appearing low-risk child/infant with clinically mild pneumonia who has close follow-up and reliable caregiver has been questioned,[15] the chest radiograph is noninvasive, painless, easily obtained, readily available, fairly inexpensive, has a low risk of radiation (although it is not zero), reliable, can yield valuable information, and is indicated in most patients with a clinical suspicion of pneumonia.[47]

There are three major categories of pneumonia: lobar (alveolar), bronchopneumonia (lobular), and interstitial (Fig. 43–1).[42,52] Bacterial infections, specifically *S. pneumoniae* and *Klebsiella*, tend to have a lobar (originating in the airspace) or segmental consolidation,[23,42,52] while bronchopneumonia (lobular) pneumonia has small fluffy infiltrates and peribronchial markings (a patchy or stringy consolidation) and is commonly due to mycoplasma and bacteria, particularly *S. aureus* and many gram-negative bacteria. Initially, lobular pneumonia may be segmental since it originates in the airways rather than the airspaces but commonly spreads to other areas and may be bilateral. Acute interstitial pneumonia is characterized by hyperinflation, peribronchial cuffing (thickening), and increased bronchovascular markings, and may have a nodular appearance. Viral pneumonia usually has an interstitial pattern; however, lobar or segmental consolidation can also occur.[40] Of the three radiologic categories of pneumonia, lobar (alveolar) is fairly specific (but not sensitive) for bacterial pneumonia,[40,42]

▶ TABLE 43–6. VARIABLES THAT MAY SIMULATE "PNEUMONIA" ON A CHEST RADIOGRAPH

- Thymus (in an infant)
- Breast shadow
- Soft-tissue shadow
- Poor inspiration
- Underpenetrated film
- Uneven grid on film
- When in doubt, consider repeating the chest radiograph to obtain better quality films
- If pleural effusion is a possibility, consider lateral decubitus films
- Obtain apical lordotic views for disease in the upper lobes
- Consider inspiratory/expiratory films if a foreign body is present which may demonstrate unequal aeration bilaterally and "air-trapping"

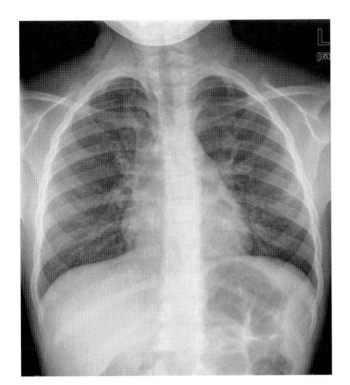

A

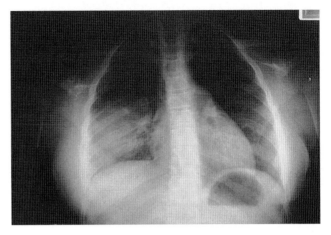

B

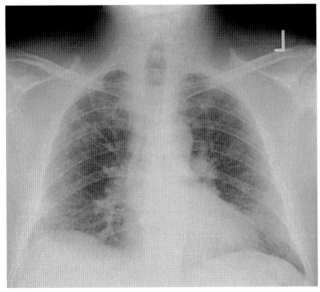

C

Figure 43-1. There are three main categories of pneumonia: (A) lobar (alveolar) bilateral patchy infiltrates. (B) Bronchopneumonia (lobular)—note consolidation in the superior segment of the right lower lobe. (C) Interstitial—note reticular nodular opacities bilaterally with small lung volumes consistent with usual interstitial pneumonitis (UIP) on pathology.

while viral pneumonia tends to have an interstitial or bilateral bronchoalveolar or peribronchial infiltrates.[21]

A "round" pneumonia is a large solitary consolidated spherical-shaped ("round") lesion, which is typically due to *S. pneumoniae*. The presence of pneumatoceles, pleural effusion, and/or empyema suggests *S. aureus*. Pneumonia due to *C. trachomatis* generally appears as diffuse alveolar or perihilar interstitial infiltrates with hyperexpansion. Classically, *M. pneumoniae* appear as lower lobe streaky or patchy infiltrates, although 10% to 25% of the time, different patterns occur including lobar infiltrates.

Studies have documented that interobserver agreement among radiologists' readings of chest radiographs regarding pneumonia is poor.[53,54] Moreover, radiologists' readings of chest radiographs in febrile 3- to 24-month-old children are biased by information from the treating physician.[55] Overall, using a chest radiograph to differentiate viral from bacterial pneumonia has widely varying results with sensitivities of 42% to 80% and specificities of 42% to 100%.[15] In summary, although the radiographic patterns may be suggestive of a specific etiologic agent (bacterial vs. viral, or even a specific microorganism such as *S. aureus*), overlap occurs and it is not possible to make the diagnosis of bacterial versus viral pneumonia on a chest roentgenogram. However, the chest radiograph can add valuable information which along with other data may lead to the likely pathogen.

Occasionally, a patient with clinical signs and symptoms of pneumonia may have a negative chest radiograph and later after treatment, a repeat roentgenogram may become positive for pneumonia.[41] Similarly, a patient may have recovered from pneumonia and have clear lungs on auscultation yet the radiograph may still demonstrate pneumonia.[41] There may be a temporal disconnect between the clinical findings and the radiograph, which may take 6 to 8 weeks for the radiographic findings to resolve. The converse is also true. A patient, especially a young infant, may have a significant pattern of pneumonia on the chest roentgenogram yet lack clinical signs of pneumonia, such as rales.[41]

Some have questioned whether infants with just a fever but no clinical findings of pulmonary disease (e.g. rales, rhonchi, wheezing, tachypnea, grunting, flaring, cough coryza) warrant a chest radiograph. The absence of these respiratory findings predicts a normal chest radiograph about 99% of the time. Unfortunately, although this may have negative predictive value, it may overlook many cases of pneumonia. A small study with only 16 patients with documented radiographic findings of pneumonia that recommended using similar clinical criteria to determine the need for chest roentgenograms[56] has been criticized for methodologic flaws.[57] In one study, 28% of patients with bacteremic pneumococcal pneumonia documented by positive blood cultures had no respiratory symptoms whatsoever.[16] Similarly, the absence of tachypnea has been cited as the best physical examination (PE) finding for ruling out pneumonia.[15] Yet in the study of bacteremic pneumococcal pneumonia patients, 81% of patients did *not* have tachypnea. The "best" PE finding was positive only 19% of the time, and would miss 81% of the bacteremic pneumonia patients.[16] It has also been documented that young infants with a high fever and leukocytosis may have an occult pneumonia (in 26%), so a chest radiograph may be warranted in these patients.[45,58]

In selected patients with equivocal chest radiographs, other plain films may be helpful. Computed tomography (CT) scan is rarely needed but may be useful in complicated patients or those in whom the diagnosis is uncertain.

▶ DIFFERENTIAL DIAGNOSIS

The differential diagnosis of pneumonia is extensive and includes both infectious and noninfectious etiologies. (Table 43–7). The history and physical examination and the chest radiograph along with ancillary studies in some patients (Table 43–2) are the key to establishing the etiology and initiating appropriate therapy (Tables 43–8 and 43–9).

▶ MANAGEMENT

Management of pneumonia centers on supportive care, appropriate use of antimicrobials, and in some patients' hospitalization. Evaluation begins with a determination of severity and of the need for hospital admission (Table 43–10). Any patient with altered mental status, hypoxia, respiratory distress, or respira-

▶ **TABLE 43–7. DIFFERENTIAL DIAGNOSIS OF PNEUMONIA NONINFECTIOUS CONDITIONS***

Pulmonary
- Congenital anatomic abnormalities
  - Congenital lobar emphysema
  - Vascular rings
  - Pulmonary sequestration
  - Cystic malformation
  - Bronchogenic cyst
- Rheumatologic/inflammatory disorders affecting the lungs
  - Collagen vascular diseases: systemic lupus erythematous ("lupus pneumonia"), juvenile rheumatoid arthritis
- Sarcoidosis
- Hematologic/oncologic disorders
  - Sickle cell vaso-occlusive crisis
  - Histiocytosis
  - Neoplasm: primary, metastatic
- Vascular
  - Pulmonary emboli
  - Pulmonary infarction
  - Fat emboli
- Aspiration
  - Foreign body
  - Chemical
- Recurrent aspiration
  - Neuromuscular disorders
  - Gastroesophageal reflux
  - Tracheoesophageal fistula
- Cardiovascular
  - Congestive heart failure
  - Congenital heart disease
- Chronic pulmonary disease
  - Cystic fibrosis
  - Asthma
  - Pulmonary fibrosis
  - Bronchiectasis
  - Bronchopulmonary dysplasia (BPD) (Chronic lung disease of infancy = CLD)
  - α1-antitrypsin disease
- Other pulmonary disorders
  - Pleural effusion
  - Empyema
  - Acute respiratory distress syndrome (ARDS)

* Included are some disorders that may present clinically like pneumonia and/or may have a radiographic appearance like that of pneumonia.

tory failure has severe pneumonia, which warrants admission. Indicators of respiratory distress include cyanosis, hypoxemia, retractions, grunting, flaring, abdominal (seesaw) respirations, head bobbing, altered mental status, restlessness (secondary to hypoxia), somnolence (possibly due to hypercarbia), and nonspecific vital sign abnormalities such as tachycardia, tachypnea, bradycardia, bradypnea, and apnea. Pulse oximetry should be determined in all pneumonia patients and those patients with low oxygen saturation should receive supplemental oxygen. There is almost universal agreement that a previously healthy child with pneumonia with a pulse oximetry <90% should be admitted, and a majority of physicians would also admit children with a pulse oximetry level <93%.[59]

▶ TABLE 43-8. COMMON BACTERIAL CAUSES OF PNEUMONIA AND EMPIRIC THERAPY*

Age (Pediatric)	Common Bacterial Pathogens	Empiric Therapy (Parenteral)	Empiric Therapy (Oral)
Neonate (≤30 d)	Group B *Streptococcus* Gram-negative enteric bacteria (*E. coli, Klebsiella*) *L. monocytogenes*	Ampicillin plus Third-generation† cephalosporin (cefotaxime) or Gentamycin	Inpatient‡
Infant (1–3 mo)	Febrile pneumonia: (*S. pneumoniae*) *H. influenza* (nontype B) *H. influenza* (type B) Afebrile pneumonitis: (*C. trachomatis*)	Third-generation Cephalosporin (cefuroxime) Macrolides: azithromycin clarithromycin erythromycin	Inpatient‡ Macrolides: azithromycin clarithromycin erythromycin
Infant/Young Child/Toddler/Preschool (3 mo –5 y)	*S. pneumoniae* *H. influenzae* (nontype B) Group A *Streptococcus* *C. trachomatis* (infant) *M. pneumoniae* (toddler)	Third-generation Cephalosporin (cefuroxime) Macrolides: azithromycin clarithromycin erythromycin	Augmentin
School Age/Adolescent (>5–18 y)	*S. pneumoniae* *M. pneumoniae*	Third-generation Cephalosporin plus Macrolide	Macrolide
Any Age Critically Ill/ICU Patient	Staphylococci Any of the above	Vancomycin or clindamycin§ Third-generation Cephalosporin plus Macrolide plus Vancomycin (or clindamycin)	Inpatient‡ Inpatient‡

*This table is one possible option for empiric therapy which may change based on future resistance patterns and epidemiologic factors. If other specific pathogens are suspected, such as a gram-negative bacteria, other antibiotics (such as piperacillin tazobactam) may be indicated.
†Avoid ceftriaxone in neonates because of concern over possible hyperbilirubinemia.
‡Hospital admission recommended in neonates, infants 1–3 mo of age, if staphylococcal pneumonia, or critically ill patients.
§If vancomycin or clindamycin can not be given due to resistance or allergies, the "antistaphylococcal cillins" (nafcillin, oxacillin, and methacillin) can be considered.

Supportive care not only includes respiratory care but also includes control of fever, maintaining of hydration (may need intravenous fluids), and treatment of complications. Respiratory care may involve supplemental oxygen, suctioning, cardiorespiratory monitoring, bronchodilators for wheezing, humidification, and, in a few cases, intubation and mechanical ventilation. Apnea and/or respiratory failure may occur precipitously in infants younger than 6 months, so monitoring and inpatient observation may be indicated.

Complications of pneumonia range from dehydration, apnea, pleural effusions, empyema, pneumatoceles, shock, pneumothorax, bacteremia, sepsis, shock, to bronchiolitis obliterans. Additional foci of infection may be present such as meningitis, epiglottitis, septic arthritis, pericarditis, soft tissue/skin infections, and otitis media. Thoracentesis of a pleural effusion or empyema may be diagnostic and therapeutic.[60] Selected pleural effusions (e.g., a large effusion that is interfering with respiration) and any empyema generally require drainage with a chest tube.

Most patients with bacterial pneumonia improve rapidly (with defervescence and symptom improvement within 1–2 days) once therapy including appropriate antibiotics is begun unless complications occur, although resolution of chest radiographic abnormalities may take ≥6 to 8 weeks. Failure to improve or worsening symptoms suggests possible complications or a misdiagnosis such as another infection (including TB, fungal, or parasitic infection), foreign body, other pulmonary disease, and underlying systemic conditions (e.g., malignancy, HIV, autoimmune disorder, immunologic disorder) as the cause for the nonresolving or recurrent pneumonia. Many patients with pneumonia, including most atypical pneumonias (e.g., viral, mycoplasma, *C. pneumoniae*), and some bacterial pneumonias in nonimmunosuppressed older-age children may be treated as an outpatient. All pediatric patients discharged from the ED with pneumonia should have close follow-up in 1 to 2 days with their primary care provider. Another option to inpatient hospitalization is admission to an ED observation unit, especially if it is early in the clinical course or difficult

► **TABLE 43-9. DRUG DOSAGE PARENTERAL (IV/IM)**

Aminopenicillin
- Ampicillin
  ○ 25–50 mg/kg q 6 h (if severe/critical 50–100 mg/kg q 6 h)
  ○ Neonate: 25–50 mg/kg q dose given q 6, 8, or 12 h depending on postnatal age and weight
  ○ Adult: 1–2 g q 4–6 h
  ○ Maximum: 12 g q day

Aminoglycoside
- Gentamycin
  ○ 2.5 mg/kg q 8 h
  ○ Neonate: 2.5 mg/kg q dose given q 8, 12, or 24 h depending on postnatal age and weight
  ○ Adult: 3–5 mg/kg/d

Third-generation cephalosporin
- Cefotaxime
  ○ 50 mg/kg q 6 h
  ○ Neonate: 50 mg/kg q dose given 6, 8, or 12 h depending on postnatal age and weight
  ○ Maximum: 2 g q dose (age > 1 mo)
- Ceftriaxone
  ○ 50 mg/kg q 12 h
  ○ Neonate: Use other third-generation cephalosporin due to concern for hyperbilirubinemia
  ○ Adult: 1–2 g q 12 or 24 h
  ○ Maximum: 4 g q dose

Macrolide
- Erythromycin
  ○ 10 mg/kg q 6 h, (oral therapy preferred, should replace IV as soon as possible, avoid IM)

- Neonate: 10 mg/kg q dose given q 8 or 12 h depending on postnatal age and weight, po
- Adult: 1 g q 6 h
- Maximum: 500 mg q dose or 2 g/d
- Azithromycin
  ○ 10 mg/kg IV first day (first dose), then 5 mg/kg
  ○ Adult: 500 mg
  ○ Maximum: 500 mg
- Vancomycin
  ○ 10 mg/kg q 6 h
  ○ Neonate: 15 mg/kg q dose given q 6, 8, 12, or 24 h depending on postnatal age and weight
  ○ Adult: 1 g q dose
  ○ Maximum: 1 g q dose, 4 g/d
- Clindamycin
  ○ 10 mg/kg q 6 h
  ○ Neonate: 5 mg/kg/dose given q 6, 8, or 12 h depending on age and weight
  ○ Adult: 1.2 g q dose q 6 h
  ○ Maximum: 1.2 g q dose, 4.8 g q dose

Drug Dosage ORAL
Aminopenicillin with β-lactamase inhibition
- Amoxicillin-clavulanic Acid
  ○ 40 mg/kg q 12 h (age ≥3 mo)
  ○ Adult: 875 mg q 12 h

Macrolides
- Erythromycin (same as parenteral)
- Azithromycin (same as parenteral)
- Clarithromycin
  ○ Child 7.5 mg/kg/dose q 12 h
  ○ Adult: 500 mg q 12 h
  ○ Maximum: 500 mg q dose

The first dose which should be given in the ED in hospitalized patients is listed. Dosages assume normal renal and hepatic function. Dosages may be adjusted depending on the clinical condition. The dose for the child or infant is listed first then the neonate dose and adult dose.
Outpatient therapy is usually for 7–10 d (except for azithromycin which is given for 5 d) for community-acquired pneumonia
Of the macrolides, azithromycin may be better tolerated (e.g., less GI side effects), although erythromycin is less expensive.
Azithromycin and clarithromycin are not approved for neonates but have been used in infants to treat infections such as pertussis (see Chapter 44). Avoid IM erythromycin. Oral erythromycin preferred, switch from IV to oral as soon as possible.

► **TABLE 43-10. INDICATIONS FOR HOSPITAL ADMISSION—PNEUMONIA**

- Neonate (≤30 d)
- Young infant (≤3–6 mo)
- Inability to tolerate fluids or medications
- Lack of response to outpatient therapy
- Psychosocial issues (compliance with therapy, follow-up)
- Comorbidity (bronchopulmonary dysplasia, sickle cell disease, etc.)
- Respiratory distress
- Hypoxemia
- Complications of pneumonia (lung abscess, empyema, fistula, etc.)
- Bacteremia
- Sepsis
- Dehydration
- Suspicion of specific virulent pathogens (e.g., *P. carinii*, *S. aureus*)

to assess the severity of the pneumonia or there are any other concerns.[61]

► **EMPIRIC THERAPY**

Since the specific etiologic agent is likely unknown, empiric therapy is the rule and is determined by the likely pathogen(s) based on the patient's age, need for hospitalization/illness severity, and epidemiologic factors (Table 43–8). In patients needing hospital admission, the first dose of antibiotic(s) should be administered in the ED. Newborns should be hospitalized and double antibiotic coverage begun with ampicillin for *Listeria* and enterococci and either a third-generation cephalosporin (e.g., cefotaxime) or an aminoglycoside (e.g., gentamycin). Ceftriaxone is not usually given to neonates because of a concern that it could lead to an increased bilirubin. Similarly, hospitalization is generally recommended for young infants (aged 1–3 months) because of immunologic immunity, pneumonia is often part of a sepsis syndrome, signs/symptoms of sepsis are subtle and nonspecific, and complications such as apnea and/or respiratory failure can occur. For the 1- to 3-month old, a third-generation cephalosporin (e.g., cefuroxime) is one option and, if an afebrile pneumonitis or pertussis is suspected, a macrolide or a sulfonamide should be administered.

For the older infant and preschool child (3 months up to 5 years), a third-generation cephalosporin and a macrolide for inpatients are one antibiotic regimen which should provide empiric coverage for the atypicals (macrolide for mycoplasma and chlamydia) and ceftriaxone for other bacterial organisms, while amoxicillin-clavulanate is an option in the outpatients. For school-age children and adolescents (age >5 years up to age 18 years), inpatient therapy could be ceftriaxone and a macrolide while outpatient therapy could be with a macrolide alone (Table 43–8).

In any age patient, if there is any concern for a staphylococcal pneumonia, especially if the patient is seriously ill, then antistaphylococcal therapy with vancomycin or clindamycin, or even nafcillin/oxacillin/methicillin (depending on resistance patterns) should be added. Vancomycin is a reasonable choice if methicillin resistant *S. aureus* is a possibility and clindamycin or one of the "antistaphylococcal cillins" (e.g., oxacillin, methicillin, or nafcillin) is an appropriate antibiotic for vancomycin resistant enterococci until sensitivities are known.[62] Fulminant viral pneumonia can occur, particularly in immunocompromised patients, and empiric viral therapy may be needed: such as acyclovir (for varicella pneumonia), ribivirin for high-risk patients with RSV pneumonia, gancyclovir for cytomegalovirus pneumonia, amantadine for influenza, or prednisone and zidovudine for HIV patients with lymphocytic interstitial pneumonia.

▶ SUMMARY

Pneumonia is one of the most common illnesses encountered in pediatric patients. The clinical spectrum ranges from mild to severe life-threatening disease with management ranging from outpatient therapy, use of an ED observation unit to inpatient hospitalization, and even intensive care unit admission. Since there is a vast number of microorganisms that can cause pneumonia and since diagnostic testing has limitations, the specific etiologic agent is generally not known in the ED. Management includes supportive therapy and often empiric therapy, which is based on many variables: patient age, comorbidity, clinical picture, ancillary (radiology and laboratory) studies, and epidemiology.

REFERENCES

1. *US Census Bureau Statistical Abstract of the United States: 2008.* 127th ed. Washington, DC: United States Government Printing Office; 2007. Tables 110–115.
2. Chase PS, Hilton NS. Pneumonia. In: Reisdorff EJ, Roberts MR, Wiegenstein JG, eds. *Pediatric Emergency Medicine.* Philadelphia, PA: WB Saunders; 2003:280–290.
3. Lichenstein R, Suggs AH, Campbell J. Pediatric pneumonia. *Emerg Med Clin North Am.* 2003;21:437–451.
4. Campbell PW, Stokes DC. Pneumonia. In: Loughlin GM, Eigen H, eds. *Respiratory Diseases in Children Diagnosis and Management.* Baltimore, MD: Williams and Wilkins; 1994:351–372.
5. Moran GJ, Talan DA. Pneumonia. In: Marx JA, Hockberger RS, Walls RM, et al., eds. *Rosen's Emergency Medicine: Concepts and Clinical Practice.* 6th ed. Philadelphia, PA: Mosby Elsevier; 2006:1128–1142.
6. Mandell LA, Bartlett JG, Dowell SF, et al. Update of practice guidelines for the management of community-acquired pneumonia in immunocompetent adults. *Clin Infect Dis.* 2003;37:1405–1433.
7. Shoham Y, Dagan R, Givon-Lair N, et al. Community-acquired pneumonia in children: quantifying the burden on patients and their families including decrease in quality of life. *Pediatrics.* 2005;115(5):1213–1219.
8. Rafei K, Lichenstein R. Airway infectious disease emergencies. *Pediatr Clin North Am.* 2006;53:215–242.
9. Dowell SF, Kuproni BA, Zell ER, et al. Mortality from pneumonia in children in the United States, 1939 through 1996. *N Engl J Med.* 2000;342:1399–1407.
10. Wardlaw T, Salama P, White Johansson E. Pneumonia: the leading killer of children. *Lancet.* 2006;368:1048–1050.
11. Mulholland K. Childhood pneumonia mortality—a permanent global emergency. *Lancet.* 2007;307:285–289.
12. Rudan I, Tomaskovic L, Boschi-Pinto C, et al. WHO Child Health Epidemiology Reference Group. Global estimate of the incidence of clinical pneumonia among children under five years of age. *Bull World Health Organ.* 2004;82:895–903.
13. Sectish TC, Prober CG. Pneumonia. In: Kliegman RM, Behrman RF, Jensen HB, Stanton BF, eds. *Nelson Textbook of Pediatrics.* Philadelphia, PA: WB Saunders Elsevier; 2007:1795–1806.
14. Fang GD, Fine M, Orloff J, et al. New and emerging etiologies for community-acquired pneumonia with implications for therapy. *Medicine (Baltimore).* 1990;69:307–316.
15. Margolis P, Gadomoski A. Does this infant have pneumonia? *JAMA.* 1998;279:308–313.
16. Toikka P, Virkki R, Mertsola J, et al. Bacteremic pneumococcal pneumonia in children. *Clin Infect Dis.* 1999;29(3):568–572.
17. Jadavji T, Law B, Level MH, et al. A practical guide for the diagnosis and treatment of pediatric pneumonia. *CMAJ.* 1997;165(5):S703-S711.
18. Rothrock SG, Green SM, Fanelli JM, et al. Do published guidelines predict pneumonia in children presenting to an urban ED? *Pediatr Emerg Care.* 2001;17:240–243.
19. Lynch T, Platt R, Gouin S, et al. Can we predict which children with clinically suspected pneumonia will have the presence of focal infiltrates on chest radiographs? *Pediatrics.* 2004;113(3):e186–e189. http://www.pediatrics.org/cgi/content/full/113/3/e186. Accessed May 17, 2008.
20. Mizgend JP. Acute lower respiratory tract infection. *N Engl J Med.* 2008;358:716–727.
21. McCracken GH Jr. Diagnosis and management of pneumonia in children. *Pediatr Infect Dis.* 2000;19:924–928.
22. Ruuskanen O, Mertsola J. Childhood community-acquired pneumonia. *Semin Respir Infect.* 1999;14(2):163–172.
23. Virkki R, Juven T, Rikalainen H, et al. Differentiation of bacterial and viral pneumonia in children. *Thorax.* 2002;57:438–441.
24. Michelow IC, Olsen K, Lozano J, et al. Epidemiology and clinical characteristics of community-acquired pneumonia in hospitalized children. *Pediatrics.* 2004;113(4):701–707.
25. Nohynek H, Eskola J, Laine E, et al. The causes of hospital-treated acute lower respiratory tract infection in children. *AJDC.* 1991;145:618–622.
26. Paisley JW, Lauer BA, McIntosh K, et al. Pathogens associated with acute lower respiratory tract infection in young children. *Pediatr Infect Dis J.* 1984;3(1):14–19.

27. Hietala J, Uhari M, Tuokko H, et al. Mixed bacterial and viral infections are common in children. *Pediatr Infect Dis J.* 1989;8(10):683–686.

28. Turner RB, Lande AE, Chase P, et al. Pneumonia in pediatric outpatients: cause and clinical manifestations. *J Pediatr.* 1987;111:194–200.

29. Juven T, Mertsola J, Waris M, et al. Etiology and treatment of community-acquired pneumonia in ambulatory children. *Pediatr Infect Dis J.* 2000;19:293–298.

30. Heiskanen-Kosma T, Korppi M, Jokinen C, et al. Etiology of childhood pneumonia: serologic results of a prospective population-based study. *Pediatr Infect Dis J.* 1998;18:98–101.

31. McIntosh K. Community-acquired pneumonia in children. *N Engl J Med.* 2002;346:429–437.

32. Van den Bruel A, Bartholomeusen S, Aertgeerts B, et al. Serious infections in children: an incidence study in family practice. *BMC Fam Pract.* 2006;7:23–32.

33. Wubbel L, Muniz L, Ahmed A, et al. Etiology and treatment of community-acquired pneumonia. *Pediatr Infect Dis J.* 1999;18:98–104.

34. Williams JV, Harris PA, Tollefson SJ, et al. Human metapneumovirus and lower respiratory tract disease in otherwise healthy infants and children. *N Engl J Med.* 2004;350:443–450.

35. Pickering LK, ed. *Streptococcus Pneumoniae, Pneumococcal Infections Red Book 2006 Report of the Committee on Infectious Diseases.* 27th ed. Evanston, IL. American Academy of Pediatrics; 2006.

36. Davies HD, Matlow A, Petric M, et al. Prospective comparative study of viral, bacterial, and atypical organisms identified in pneumonia and bronchiolitis in hospitalized Canadian infants. *Pediatr Infect Dis J.* 1996;15(4):371–375.

37. Harris JA, Kolokathis A, Campbell M, et al. Safety and efficacy of azithromycin in the treatment of community-acquired pneumonia in children. *Pediatr Infect Dis J.* 1998;17:865–871.

38. Block S, Hedrick J, Hammerschlag M, et al. Mycoplasma pneumoniae and chlamydia pneumoniae in pediatric community-acquired pneumonia: comparative efficacy and safety of clarithromycin vs. erythromycin ethylsuccinate. *Pediatr Infect Dis J.* 1995;14:471–477.

39. Stein RT, Marostica PJC. Community-acquired bacterial pneumonia. In: Chernick V, Boat TF, Wilmott RW, Bush A, eds. *Kendig's Disorders of the Respiratory Tract in Children.* 7th ed. Philadelphia, PA: Saunders Elsevier; 2006:441–452.

40. Cohen GJ. Management of infections of the lower respiratory tract in children. *Pediatr Infect Dis J.* 1987;6(3):317–323.

41. Klein JO. Bacterial pneumonia. In: Feigin RD, Cherry JD, Demmber GJ, Kaplan SL, eds. *Textbook of Pediatric Infectious Diseases.* 5th ed. Philadelphia, PA: Saunders; 2004:299–310.

42. Korppi M, Kroger L, Laitinen M. White blood cell and differential counts in acute respiratory viral and bacterial infections in children. *Scand J Infect Dis.* 1993;25(4):435–440.

43. Toikka P, Virkki R, Mertsola J, et al. Bacteremic pneumococcal pneumonia in children. *Clin Infect Dis.* 1999;29(3):568–577.

44. Mazur LJ, Kline MW, Lorin MI. Extreme leukocytosis in patients presenting to a pediatric emergency department. *Pediatr Emerg Care.* 1991;7(4):215–218.

45. Bachur R, Perry H, Harper MB. Occult pneumonias: empiric chest radiographs in febrile children with leukocytosis. *Ann Emerg Med.* 1999;33(2):166–173.

46. Austrian R, Gold J. Pneumococcal bacteremia with special references to bacteremic pneumococcal pneumonia. *Ann Intern Med.* 1964;60:759–776.

47. Donowitz GR, Mandell GL. Acute pneumonia. In: Mandell GL, Bennett JE, Dolin R, ed. *Mandell, Douglas, and Bennett's Principles and Practice of Infectious Diseases.* Philadelphia, PA: Elsevier Churchill Livingstone; 2005:819–844.

48. Bohte R, vanFurth R, van den Broek PJ. Aetiology of community-acquired pneumonia. A prospective study among adults requiring admission to hospital. *Thorax.* 1995;50:543–547.

49. Kennedy M, Bates DW, Wright SB, et al. Do emergency department blood cultures change practice in patients with pneumonia. *Ann Emerg Med.* 2005;46(5):393–400.

50. Kumar P, McKean MC. Evidence based paediatrics: review of BTS guidelines for the management of community acquired pneumonia in children. *J Infection.* 2004;48:134–138.

51. Moran GJ, Abrahamian FM. Blood cultures for community-acquired pneumonia: can we hit the target without a shotgun? *Ann Emerg Med.* 2005;46(5):407–408.

52. Adler BH, Effmann EL. Pneumonia and Pulmonary Infection. In: Slovia TL, ed. *Caffey's Pediatric Diagnostic Imaging.* Vol 2. 11th ed. Philadelphia, PA: Mosby Elsevier; 2008:1184–1228.

53. Albaum MN, Hill LC, Murphy M, et al. Interobserver reliability of the chest radiograph in community acquired pneumonia. *Chest.* 1996;110(2):343–350.

54. Davies HD, Wang EEL, Manson D, et al. Reliability of the chest radiograph in the diagnosis of lower respiratory tract infections in young children. *J Pediatr.* 1997;130(1):159–160.

55. Kramer MS, Roberts-Brauer R, Williams RL. Bias and overcall in interpreting chest radiographs in young febrile children. *Pediatrics.* 1992;90(1)(Pt 1):11–13.

56. Losek JD, Kishaba RG, Berens RJ, et al. Indications for chest roentgenogram in the febrile young infant. *Pediatr Emerg Care.* 1989;5(3):149–152.

57. Lewis RJ. Letter to the editor. *Pediatr Emerg Care.* 1990;6(1):78.

58. Kirelik S, Alverson B. Pediatric respiratory emergencies: disease of the lungs. In: Marx JA, Hockberger RS, Walls RM, et al., eds. *Rosen's Emergency Medicine Concepts and Clinical Practice.* 6th ed. Philadelphia, PA: Mosby Elsevier; 2006:2554–2567.

59. Brown L, Dannenburg B. Pulse oximetry in discharge decision-making: a survey of emergency physicians. *CJEM.* 2002;4:388–393.

60. Anderson E, Mace SE. Lung abscess and empyema. In: Tintinalli JE, Cline D, Cydulka RK, et al., eds. *Tintinalli's Emergency Medicine.* New York, NY: McGraw-Hill; 2008:chap 5.

61. Mace SE. Pediatric observation medicine. *Emerg Med Clin North Am.* 2001;19(1):239–254.

62. Staphylococcal Infections. In: Pickering LK, Baker CJ, Long SS, et al., eds. *Red Book 2006 Report of the Committee of Infectious Diseases.* 27th ed. Elk Grove Village, IL: American Academy of Pediatrics; 2006:598–610.

CHAPTER 44

Pertussis

Sharon E. Mace

▶ HIGH-YIELD FACTS

- Pertussis occurs most commonly in infants younger than 6 months but can occur in any age group.
- The initial or catarrhal stage is characterized by upper respiratory tract symptoms and lasts 7 to 10 days. This is followed by a paroxysmal phase characterized by episodic bouts of staccato cough lasting 2 to 4 weeks.
- Diagnosis is usually based on history and physical examination. Fluorescent antibody testing is currently the most utilized confirmatory test, but it has a low sensitivity and poor predictive value. The polymerase chain reaction test has a much higher sensitivity.
- The mainstay of treatment is supportive therapy including oxygen for hypoxia and intravenous fluids for dehydration. Erythromycin is an effective therapy only if given prior to the paroxysmal stage.
- Prophylactic therapy should be given to close contacts.
- Indications for hospital admission include young age (younger than 1 year), hypoxia, and dehydration.

▶ INTRODUCTION

Pertussis is an acute, bacterial, highly contagious, respiratory infection with a significant associated morbidity and mortality, especially in infants. In spite of widespread vaccination, the incidence of pertussis has been increasing, especially in adolescents and young adults.[1-3] Pertussis or "whooping cough" is characterized by severe episodes of coughing followed by a forceful inspiration against a partially closed glottis, which causes the "classic whooping sound."

In the prevaccine era, pertussis was the number one cause of death in children (age ≤ 13 years old) from a communicable disease in the United States. Pertussis accounted for more infant deaths than diphtheria, poliomyelitis, measles, and scarlet fever combined.[4] Worldwide, on an annual basis, there are 60 million cases of pertussis with more than half a million deaths. In developing countries and in countries where vaccination rates are low, a high incidence of pertussis continues.[4]

After the introduction of a vaccine in the United States in 1940s, the incidence of pertussis declined precipitously, from approximately 250 000 cases yearly in the 1930s to just more than 1000 cases in 1976.[5,6] Since then, the incidence has been rising worldwide, including in the United States with 25 827 cases in 2004.[6] The actual incidence of pertussis is much greater since pertussis is significantly underreported.[7] The rates of reported pertussis are estimated to be 40- to 160-fold less than actual rates, with asymptomatic infections 4 to 22 times more common than symptomatic infection.[8] The rising incidence is due to multiple factors: waning immunity after childhood immunization, better diagnostic tests, greater health care provider awareness, improved reporting techniques, and decreased pertussis immunization in certain patient populations such as immigrants and those unimmunized for religious or other reasons.[9]

▶ MICROBIOLOGY

Pertussis is caused by *Bordetella pertussis*. *B. pertussis* belongs to the Bordetella genus of bacteria, which are small gram-negative fastidious pleomorphic coccobacilli that are very difficult to grow. They require special media for culture, which makes a definitive diagnosis by culture challenging. Other Bordetella species can also cause disease. *B. parapertussis* causes a milder pertussis-like respiratory illness. *B. bronchiseptica*, known to cause respiratory illness in animals ("kennel cough"), can also cause respiratory illness in humans, generally occurring in immunocompromised patients.

▶ PATHOPHYSIOLOGY

B. pertussis infection is transmitted in aerosolized droplets during coughing. The bacteria are inhaled and adhere to the nasopharyngeal ciliated epithelium, where they proliferate and disseminate throughout the ciliated lower respiratory airway. Occasionally, the bacteria will also invade the pulmonary alveoli thus causing primary pertussis pneumonia, although secondary pneumonia from other bacterial or viral pathogens can also occur. The spread of *B. pertussis* is limited to the respiratory epithelium. Therefore, it is almost never recovered from the bloodstream. Bacteremia is not a feature of the disease and blood cultures are not helpful in making the diagnosis.

B. pertussis produces various substances and toxins, which increase its virulence by promoting cellular attachment or hampering host defenses, and these are responsible for various manifestations of the disease. For example, the pertussis toxin, thought to promote its virulence, is responsible for the lymphocytosis and increased insulin secretion (which occasionally causes hypoglycemia) that occur with the disease. An inactivated form of pertussis toxin is a component of the acellular pertussis vaccine.

▶ EPIDEMIOLOGY

Pertussis is a highly contagious disease. Humans are the only reservoir for *B. pertussis* and it does not survive for prolonged periods in the environment.[10] Attack rates in individuals exposed to aerosol droplets at close proximity (distance ≤ 5 ft) are as high as 100%.[10] Secondary attack rates in susceptible household contacts are 50% to 100%, while an outbreak on a college campus had a conservatively estimated attack rate of 13%. Even in those individuals who are fully immunized or are naturally immune, the subclinical infection rate after household exposure is up to 80%.[4]

The case fatality rate is greatest in children especially in infants, with 84% of fatalities occurring in infants younger than 6 months.[11] Other studies and reports state that the morbidity is highest in infants (24%) versus older children (5%) or adolescents (16%),[12] although a relatively high morbidity (28%) has been reported in adults.[13,14] Similarly, hospitalization rates are greatest for infants younger than 6 months (up to 80%), followed by infants aged 6 to 11 months (30%), and are lowest for adolescents (<10%).[10,15,16] According to data from 1990 to 1996,[17] the overwhelming majority of hospital admissions (83%), deaths (91%), and complications (66% of pneumonia, 59% of seizures, 71% of encephalopathy) occurred in infants.

Pertussis is endemic with epidemic cycles occurring every 3 to 4 years after accretion of a susceptible cohort. Vaccination or natural disease does not confer lifelong or complete immunity against the disease or reinfection. Approximately 3 to 5 years postimmunization, protection against pertussis begins to decline and there is none after 12 years.[2,5] Thus, in the United States, adults lack adequate antibody to pertussis.[18] This explains why pertussis outbreaks increased in frequency in the elderly, in residential facilities, in nursing homes, and in health care facilities—because of waning levels of antibody and thus, protective immunity over time.[19] The primary reservoir for pertussis are adults and adolescents suffering from cough, who are often not identified as having pertussis.[18]

► CLINICAL PRESENTATION

The clinical case definition for pertussis (endemic or sporadic) by the World Health Organization and the CDC is an acute cough illness ≥ 14 days, without other apparent cause, plus any one of the following: paroxysms of coughing, inspiratory whoop, or post-tussive emesis. The classic presentation of pertussis occurs in three phases (catarrhal, paroxysmal, and convalescent stages) over 6 weeks following a 3- to 12-day incubation period. Nondescript signs and symptoms, such as congestion, rhinorrhea, sneezing, low-grade fever, lacrimation, and conjunctival suffusion, are characteristic of the catarrhal stages (Table 44–1). As these symptoms wane, coughing heralds the onset of the paroxysmal stage. A dry, irritant, intermittent hacking cough progresses into paroxysms of coughing, often with the characteristic "whoop"—a forceful inspiratory gasp—which

► TABLE 44–1. THREE STAGES OF THE DISEASE

- Initial or catarrhal stage is characterized by upper respiratory tract symptoms and lasts for 7 to 10 days.
- Paroxysmal phase characterized by episodic bouts of staccato cough lasting 2 to 4 weeks.
- Convalescent stage where the symptoms gradually wane.

gives pertussis the designation "whooping cough." Classically, whooping cough presents in well-appearing, even playful, toddlers who, without any real provocation, suddenly appear anxious and may reach for their parents just prior to the onslaught of a rapid-fire series of uninterrupted coughs, during which the toddlers' chin and chest are held forward, their tongue protrudes, and their face turns a purple color. The coughing stops abruptly, and then a loud whoop occurs (caused by movement of inspired air over a partially closed glottis), followed by post-tussive emesis and post-tussive exhaustion. Post-tussive vomiting occurs in patients of all ages and is so characteristic that its presence should suggest the diagnosis in patients of any age.

The paroxysmal stage evolves into the convalescent stage. The coughing episodes during the convalescent phase decrease in terms of severity, duration, and number of episodes except in infants. Conversely, in infants during the convalescent stage, the cough becomes more prominent and the whoop louder. Many patients lack the classic signs and symptoms and/or have an atypical presentation.

Very young infants (≤3 months of age) often do not have the classic three-stage presentation of pertussis. The catarrhal stage may be unrecognized or shortened to only a few days. The cough (expiratory grunt) and the whoop (forceful inspiratory gasp) may not be a significant feature. A well-appearing infant, after minimal stimulation (such as sucking or stretching or from a sound or light), will start to choke, gasp, and turn red in the face. Paradoxically, the coughing or "whooping" may worsen during the convalescent phase instead of gradually getting better. Infants may have a prolonged convalescent stage with episodic paroxysmal coughing spells continuing during their first year of life with paroxysmal spells triggered by other (non-pertussis) respiratory illnesses.

Another presentation of this disease in infants younger than 6 months is silent paroxysms. The infant appears to be coughing or not breathing and there are no audible sounds. If the paroxysm lasts long enough, the child may become unresponsive. Between bouts of paroxysmal coughing, the physical examination is usually normal. Physical examination findings are minimal except for the cough and frequently, petechiae on the upper body and conjunctival hemorrhages from the severe coughing. Patients generally do not have any lung findings on examination, such as rales or wheezing, unless they also have a complication, for example, pneumonia.

► DIAGNOSTIC EVALUATION

Consider pertussis in any patient with a chief complaint of cough, particularly if associated signs and symptoms, such as rales, wheezing, sore throat, myalgias, malaise, fever, exanthemas, exanthemas, are absent. One out of five college students with no known contact with pertussis, who had a coughing illness lasting more than 1 week, had pertussis as confirmed by laboratory studies. According to Senzilet et al., in the United States, 21% of adolescents and adults with a prolonged cough (>1 week) have pertussis.[20] Infants younger than 3 months presenting with cyanosis or apnea should have pertussis considered in their differential diagnosis.

In the catarrhal stage, leukocytosis from 15 000 to 40 000 cells/mm[3] is generally present, but may reach 100 000 mm[3].

This is secondary to an absolute lymphocytosis[21] of normal small size lymphocytes of both T- and B-cell origin. This is unlike the large atypical lymphocytes found with viral illnesses such as mononucleosis, which may serve as a clue to the diagnosis. Polymorphonuclear leukocytosis implies a secondary bacterial infection or another disease. Extreme leukocytosis (median 94 000 cells/L) and/or thrombocytosis (median 82 × 109 cells/L) is associated with increased disease severity and death.[22]

Mild abnormalities (such as a perihilar infiltrate, edema, or alelectasis) are noted on the chest roentgenogram in most hospitalized infants. Parenchymal consolidation indicates a secondary bacterial infection. The forceful coughing may lead to radiographic findings of pneumothorax, pneumomediastinum, or soft tissue emphysema. Another abnormality may be hypoglycemia, which occurs infrequently.

LABORATORY DIAGNOSIS

B. pertussis is a fastidious organism that is difficult to grow, taking 3 to 7 days to appear on the culture media. It must be cultured on a specific medium (Regan Lowe/Bordet/Gengou medium permeated with antibiotics in order to decrease the growth of competing bacteria).[23] The pertussis organism is more difficult to grow if the patient has already received antibiotics or if the patient is in the paroxysmal phase. The sensitivity of pertussis cultures is only 15% to 45% even when patients have been coughing for more than 21 days.[24] Culture of pertussis does yield definitive diagnosis and is the gold standard. It has a high specificity (>95%) and allows for antibiotic susceptibility testing and DNA fingerprinting.[23,24] Unfortunately, it takes several days, needs specific culture media not always readily available, and needs meticulous specimen collection, transport, and isolation techniques. Specimens for testing are obtained by placing a flexible dacron or calcium alginate swab for 15 to 30 seconds in the posterior nasopharynx or until the patient coughs. Specific transport medium may be needed depending on the length of time the specimen is being "transported" prior to incubation of the specimen on the culture medium.

Direct fluorescent antibody (DFA) testing of nasopharyngeal secretions, using specific antibody for B. pertussis and B. parapertussis gives results within several hours but has low sensitivity and specificity and may have cross-reactivity with normal nasopharyngeal flora. It has been replaced by PCR testing. PCR testing has a higher sensitivity than culture, a high specificity (>95%), and quick results (usually <48 hours). However, false positives secondary to contamination can occur, the methods are not universally standardized or validated, and laboratories require adequately trained personnel with appropriate quality improvement measures. Some experts recommend doing a culture and PCR during the infectious period, which is 3 weeks from onset of cough or 4 weeks from symptom onset.[24]

Serology using IgG/IgA ELISA testing is specific but requires blood samples, has a low sensitivity depending on the disease duration, and is a delayed diagnosis, which limits its clinical usefulness. Acute and convalescent serology samples are the most sensitive tests in immunized individuals and for epidemiologic studies.

DIFFERENTIAL DIAGNOSIS

The differential diagnosis includes other infectious respiratory pathogens as well as noninfectious etiologies from reactive airway disease or asthma to gastroesophageal reflux and foreign body aspiration, all of which can cause paroxysmal and/or intractable coughing. Infectious agents considered in the differential include other Bordetella species (e.g., B. parapertussis and B. bronchiseptica), viruses such as parainfluenza, influenza A and B, and respiratory syncytial virus, bacteria such as Mycoplasma pneumoniae and Chlamydia. Coinfections can occur such that a patient with documented pertussis may also be symptomatic from another viral, bacterial, or fungal respiratory pathogen, and the documented presence of another pathogen does not rule out pertussis. According to a recent study, one-third of hospitalized infants with pertussis (documented by positive B. pertussis cultures) also had a concurrent respiratory syncytial viral infection.[25]

► COMPLICATIONS

Complications occur most frequently in the youngest infants. The overall complication rate in a large multicenter European study was 6%, but jumped to 24% in infants younger than 6 months.[14] Apnea, pneumonia, respiratory failure, and dehydration/weight loss from the vomiting and trouble feeding are the most common complications of an acute pertussis infection. Seizures and death are infrequent complications of pertussis. Apnea is a complication occurring almost entirely in infants, particularly those younger than 6 months. One Canadian study found that nearly one-third (31%) of children younger than 2 years had apnea,[26] while another study found a 16% incidence of apnea or cyanosis in infants younger than 6 months.[14] Although apnea is generally linked with paroxysmal coughing, it may occur spontaneously and is thought to be secondary to parasympathetic (vagal) stimulation.

Pneumonia may occur from a secondary bacterial infection or a primary infection from the pertussis. Pneumonia was found to be the most frequent complication in one German study and was also found to be responsible for almost one-third (29%) of complications.[14] According to one Canadian study, pneumonia was generally noted in school-age children (age 4–9 years), although 9% of hospitalized pediatric patients with pertussis younger than 2 years old had pneumonia.[26] The CDC reported similar results in children younger than 6 months with a 12% to 13% incidence of pneumonia documented by chest radiograph.[27,28]

Vomiting is extremely common with a cited incidence of 50% in several studies.[14,26] Indeed, the diagnosis of pertussis should be considered in anyone with post-tussive emesis. Neurologic complications of pertussis, fortunately, are rare with new-onset seizures reported in 1% to 2% of children (age < 2 years old) and encephalopathy in <1% (probably due to hypoxia).[27,28]

The mortality from pertussis is <1% with the overwhelming majority of deaths occurring in the youngest patients especially those younger than 6 months of age. Factors associated with an increased risk of death (other than young age) are intubation for pneumonia, leukocytosis, and pneumonia at initial

▶ TABLE 44–2. ORAL DOSAGES RECOMMENDED

	Infant	Children >1 month	Adult
Azithromycin	10 mg/kg/d for 5 days	10 mg/kg, day 1; 5 mg/kg, days 2–5 Maximum 500 mg/d	500 mg, day 1; 250 mg, days 2–5
Erythromycin	10 mg/kg/dose qid for 14 days	10–12.5 mg/kg Maximum 2 g/d	500 mg qid, 14 days
Clarithromycin	Do not use	7.5 mg/kg bid, 7 days	500 mg bid, 7 days

presentation.[29] Pertussis is considered an infrequent cause of sudden infant death due to fatal apnea in infants with pertussis. It has been suggested that SIDS infants be considered for examination of pertussis, especially if there is a history of cough in the infant and/or family member(s).

▶ TREATMENT

The management of pertussis focuses on supportive care ranging from avoidance of triggers for paroxysmal coughing, such as cold ambient temperatures or strenuous activity, to hospitalization for careful monitoring of respiratory and fluid, electrolyte and nutritional status. In a Canadian study, intensive care unit admission occurred in 16% and mechanical ventilation in 5% of admitted patients (age < 2 years).[26]

Reasons for hospitalization include complications, whether respiratory, including apnea, cyanosis, pneumonia, or respiratory distress; or neurologic, including seizures or encephalopathy; or dehydration/weight loss from the vomiting and inability to feed. Place the patient in isolation and monitor respiratory rate, heart rate, and oxygen saturation. Some patients may need intravenous hydration and/or nasogastric feedings.

Antimicrobial therapy is recommended in any patient considered to have clinical pertussis or a laboratory verified diagnosis of pertussis, even if asymptomatic, irrespective of age. Antibiotic therapy may shorten the duration and severity of symptoms and decreases the transmission to others. The variable results of treatment, in many of the studies, are likely due to the time when treatment was started and the stage of the illness. Antibiotic therapy also eliminates nasopharyngeal carriage, which prevents transmission. Antibiotic therapy is very important in infants younger than 6 months. If untreated, they have a greater risk of complications and remain carriers much longer than older children and adults.

The antibiotics of choice are the macrolide class. All three macrolides, that is, erythromycin, clarithromycin, and azithromycin are effective, although erythromycin may not be well tolerated due to the gastrointestinal side effects.[30] Trimethoprim-sulfamethoxazole (TMP-SMX) is an alternative antibiotic in patients in whom a macrolide is contraindicated or not tolerated due to side effects.[30] TMP-SMX is contraindicated in late trimester of pregnancy because of the potential for bilirubin displacement and risk of kernicterus in the fetus and infant. Other antibiotics are not recommended because of inconsistent bactericidal activity against *B. pertussis* (as with the β-lactam antibiotics, for example, cephalosporins, ampicillin, amoxicillin), failure to eradicate nasopharyngeal carriage (e.g., ampicillin, amoxicillin), or possible adverse effects in children (doxycycline, fluorooquinolones).

One should treat infants older than 1 month and younger than 6 months with a macrolide antibiotic according to both the Red Book (American Academy of Pediatric Committee on Infectious Diseases) and the CDC; even though azithromycin and clarithromycin are not approved by the United States Food and Drug Administration for use in infants younger than 6 months.[30] The newer macrolides appear to be better tolerated and have a more convenient dosing schedule than erythromycin, although erythromycin is less expensive. For neonates (age < 1 month), both the Red Book and the CDC recommend azithromycin (fewer side effects) with erythromycin as an alternative but do not recommend clarithromycin[30] due to association of hypertrophic pyloric stenosis (Table 44–2 for dosages).

▶ HYPERTROPHIC PYLORIC STENOSIS

An association between hypertrophic pyloric stenosis and the use of erythromycin or azithromycin has been reported.[31] This led to the recommendation that hypertrophic pyloric stenosis be considered in any young infant who develops vomiting within 1 month of macrolide therapy given as a neonate.

▶ PREVENTION

POSTEXPOSURE PROPHYLAXIS

Antimicrobial prophylaxis is given at the same dosage as for treatment, which is unlike most prophylaxis regimens. Prophylaxis can prevent the development of symptoms when given to asymptomatic contacts within 21 days of the onset of cough in the index case, although efficacy after 21 days is not established. Antimicrobial prophylaxis is recommended for all close contacts (irrespective of immunization status), although widespread prophylaxis for an entire classroom/school is not recommended.[30] Close contacts include household members and childcare workers. In the health care setting, close contacts are individuals who have had direct contact with secretions (nasal, oral, or respiratory) from a symptomatic patient or who had a face-to-face exposure within 3 ft of a symptomatic patient, or shared the same confined space in close proximity with a symptomatic patient for ≥1 hour. Nosocomial outbreaks are aborted by antimicrobial prophylaxis of exposed health care workers (HCWs) and patients.

Antibiotic prophylaxis is also recommended for exposed individuals at high risk for severe or complicated pertussis.

High-risk patients include young age (<1 year especially <4 months), immunodeficient patients, and/or those with significant comorbidity (e.g., chronic lung disease, respiratory insufficiency). Women in the third trimester of pregnancy should also be given postexposure prophylaxis because of the high risk to young infants.

VACCINATION

Vaccination is very effective, conferring 95% protection against severe disease and 64% protection against mild disease. There are two types of pertussis vaccine: killed whole-cell vaccine and acellular vaccine. The acellular vaccine has fewer reactions, is more expensive, and is the vaccine used in the United States. The whole-cell vaccine has more side effects but is widely used in the developing world. The Red Book and the CDC recommend routine vaccination of children and adolescents with five doses of diphtheria, tetanus toxoid, and acellular pertussis (DTaP) at 2, 4, 6, 15, to 18 months and 4 to 6 years of age.[30]

With the resurgence of pertussis in recent years, a booster vaccination (Tdap) in adolescents and adults is recommended, either adacell (for ages 11–64 years) or boostrix (for age 10–18 years). The booster immunizations (Tdap) for previously immunized individuals differ from DTaP used for primary immunizations in that it contains lower quantities of the diphtheria and pertussis toxoids than the equivalent pediatric DTaP (daptacel or infantrix). It has comparable side effects, of which the most frequent are injection site pain and febrile reactions, and has documented safety and immunogenicity.

Nosocomial outbreaks of pertussis have been reported and infected HCWs can expose at-risk infants, children, and adults. To control such outbreaks, vaccination of HCWs with a single Tdap vaccination has been recommended by the Advisory Committee on Immunization Practices and the Healthcare Infection Control Practices Advisory Committee.

OTHER PREVENTION MEASURES

Isolation using standard precautions and droplet precautions (mask within 3 ft) are recommended for hospitalized pertussis patients until 5 days after effective therapy has ended or 3 weeks after symptom onset in untreated patients. Exposed individuals should have close observation for signs/symptoms of pertussis for 20 days postcontact, particularly if their vaccination history is unknown or incomplete. Postexposure immunization (active with pertussis vaccine or passive with immunoglobulin) does not prevent infection. Patients with pertussis should not return to work in health care facilities, day care, or schools until after antibiotic therapy for 5 days, and should stay away from infants/young children, especially if they have not been immunized.

▶ SUMMARY

Pertussis ("whooping cough"), an acute, highly communicable respiratory disease caused by *B. pertussis*, is the only vaccine-preventable disease on the increase in the United States. It was considered a disease of childhood, however, there is an increasing incidence in adolescents and adults secondary to waning immunity and they serve as a reservoir for disease transmission. The classic presentation of pertussis involves severe coughing spells ending with a "whooping sound." Asymptomatic patients with atypical presentations can occur. The disease can be mild or asymptomatic in older children, adolescents, and adults. In young children, especially infants, pertussis can be a life-threatening illness. There are several new recommendations for pertussis vaccination in adolescents, adults, and for health care personnel. Definitive laboratory diagnostic testing for pertussis can be difficult and clinical suspicion remains the cornerstone for diagnosis.

REFERENCES

1. Schafer S, Gillette H, Hedberg K, et al. A community-wide pertussis outbreak. *Arch Intern Med.* 2006;166:1317–1321.
2. Galanis E, King AS, Halperin SA. Changing epidemiology and emerging risk groups for pertussis. *CMAJ.* 2006;174(4):451–452.
3. Hewlett EL, Edwards KM. Clinical practice: pertussis-not just for kids. *N Eng J Med.* 2005;352:1215–1222.
4. Long SS. Pertussis (Bordetella pertussis and B. parapertussis). In: Kliegman RM, Behrman RF, Jensen JB, et al. eds. *Nelson Textbook of Pediatrics.* Philadelphia, PA: WB Saunders Elsevier; 2007.
5. Edwards K, Freeman DM. Adolescent and adult pertussis: disease burden and prevention. *Curr Opin Pediatr.* 2006;18(1):77–80.
6. Centers for Disease Control and Prevention. Historical summaries of notifiable diseases in the United States. *MMWR Morb Mortal Wkly Rep.* 2005;52(54):1–85.
7. Crowcroft NS, Andrews N, Rooney C, et al. Deaths from pertussis are underestimated in England. *Arch Dis Child.* 2002;86:336–338.
8. Cherry JD. Epidemiology of pertussis. *Pediatr Infect Dis J.* 2006;25(4):361–362.
9. Munoz FM. Pertussis in infants, children, and adolescents: diagnosis, treatment, and prevention. *Semin Pediatr Infect Dis.* 2006;17:14–19.
10. Hewlett EL. Bordetella species. In: Mandell GL, Bennett JE, Dolin R, eds. *Principles and Practice of Infectious Diseases.* 6th ed. New York, NY: Elsevier Churchill Livingston; 2005:2701–2708.
11. Centers for Disease Control and Prevention. Summary of notifiable diseases, United States, 1998. *MMWR Morb Mortal Wkly Rep.* 1999;47(53):53.
12. Raguckus SE, Vanden Bussche HL, Jacobs C, et al. Pertussis resurgence: diagnosis, treatment, prevention, and beyond. *Pharmacotherapy.* 2007;27(1):41–52.
13. DeSerres G, Shadmani R, Duval B, et al. Morbidity of pertussis in adolescents and adults. *J Infect Dis.* 2000;182:174–179.
14. Heininger U, Klich K, Stehr K, et al. Clinical findings in Bordetella pertussis infections: results of a prospective multicenter surveillance study. *Pediatrics.* 1997;100:e10. www.pediatrics.org/cgi/content/full/100/6/e10. Accessed May 21, 2008.
15. Greenberg DP, Wirsing von Konig CH, Heininger U. Health burden of pertussis in infants and children. *Pediatr Infect Dis J.* 2005;24:S39–S43.
16. Rothstein E, Edwards K. Health burden of pertussis in adolescents and adults. *Pediatr Infect Dis J.* 2005;24:S44–S47.
17. Guris D, Strebel PM, Bardenheier B, et al. Changing epidemiology of pertussis in the United States: increased reported

incidence among adolescents and adults, 1990–1996. *Clin Infect Dis.* 1999;28:1230–1237.

18. Ward JI, Cherry JD, Change SJ, et al. Bordetella pertussis infections in vaccinated and unvaccinated adolescents and adults, as assessed in a national prospective randomized acellular pertussis vaccine trial (APERT). *Clin Infect Dis.* 2006;43:151–157.

19. Halperin SA. The control of pertussis—2007 and beyond. *N Engl J Med.* 2007;356(2):110–113.

20. Senzilet LD, Halperin SA, Spika JS, et al. Pertussis is a frequent cause of prolonged cough illness in adults and adolescents. *Clin Infect Dis.* 2001;32:1691.

21. Guinto-Ocampo H, Bennett JE, Attia MW. Predicting pertussis in infants. *Pediatr Emerg Care.* 2008;24(1):16–20.

22. Postels-Multani S, Schmitt HJ, et al. Symptoms and complications of pertussis in adults. *Infection.* 1995;23:139.

23. Singh M, Lingappan K. Whooping cough the current scene. *Chest.* 2006;130(5):1547–1553.

24. Crowcroft NS, Pebody RG. Recent developments in pertussis. *Lancet.* 2006;367:1926–1936.

25. Crowcroft NS, Booy R, Harrison T, et al. Severe and unrecognized: pertussis in UK infants. *Arch Dis Child.* 2003;88:802.

26. Halperin SA, Wang EE, Law B, et al. Epidemiological features of pertussis in hospitalized patients in Canada, 1991–1997: report of the Immunization Monitoring Program Active (IMPACT). *Clin Infect Dis.* 1999;28:1238.

27. Guris D, Strebel PM, Bardenheier B, et al. Pertussis—United States, 1997–2000. *MMWR Morb Mortal Wkly Rep.* 2002;51:73–76.

28. Pertussis—United States, 2001–2003. *MMWR Morb Mortal Wkly Rep.* 2005;54:1283–1286.

29. Mikelova LK, Halperin SA, Scheifele D, et al. Predictors of death in infants hospitalized with pertussis: a case-controlled study of 16 pertussis deaths in Canada. *J Pediatr.* 2003;143:576.

30. Committee on Infectious Diseases. American Academy of Pediatrics Pertussis (whooping cough). In: Pickering LK, Baker CJ, Long SS, et al. eds. *Red Book: 2006 Report of the Committee on Infectious Diseases.* 27th ed. Elk Grove Village, IL: American Academy of Pediatrics; 2006:498–520.

31. Mahon BE, Rosenman MB, Kleinman MB. Maternal and infant use of erythromycin and other macrolide antibiotics as risk factors for infantile hypertrophic pyloric stenosis. *J Pediatr.* 2001;139:380.

CHAPTER 45

Bronchopulmonary Dysplasia

Madeline Matar Joseph

▶ HIGH-YIELD FACTS

- Bronchopulmonary dysplasia (BPD) is a chronic lung disease of infancy that follows neonatal lung disease. Oxygen requirement at 36 weeks corrected postgestational age predicts the development of BPD.
- Infants with BPD, ranging from mild asymptomatic disease to crippling cardiopulmonary dysfunction, may present to the ED with an exacerbation of their chronic lung disease. Exacerbations are most often secondary to viral upper respiratory infections.
- The treatment of an exacerbation in a patient with BPD is mainly supportive. Oxygen, ventilatory support, and fluids are provided, if indicated.
- Bronchodilators and corticosteroids are often effective in these patients and are used in a similar fashion to the way they are used for asthma. Diuretics have been shown to improve lung function and survival in some patients.
- Indications for admission include respiratory distress, need for ventilatory support, new infiltrates, infection with respiratory syncytial virus (RSV), inability of family to manage exacerbation at home.

▶ BACKGROUND

Despite advances in the prevention and management of neonatal acute respiratory illness, BPD persists as one of the major complications in surviving very-low-birth weight infants.[1] BPD is a form of chronic lung disease of infancy that follows preterm neonatal lung disease treated with oxygen and positive-pressure ventilation (PPV). The original insult may be hyaline membrane disease, apnea, persistent fetal circulation, complex congenital heart disease, or any illness requiring prolonged mechanical ventilation as a neonate.

The overall rate of BPD is approximately 15% for premature infants requiring mechanical ventilation. The incidence of BPD, defined as oxygen dependency at 36 weeks postmenstrual age (PMA), in infants with birth weights between 500 and 1500 g, ranges between 3% and 43% in different centers.[1] The use of antenatal steroids, surfactant and improved respiratory care has increased survival of immature infants, those at higher risk for developing BPD.

The definition of BPD has evolved over the last four decades. Previous definitions of BPD were based on the presence of a supplemental oxygen requirement at 4 weeks of age. However, this is not predictive of the development of BPD in infants born at less than 30 weeks' gestation. A June 2000 National Institute of Child Health and Human Development/National Heart, Lung, and Blood Institute Workshop proposed a severity-based definition of BPD for infants younger than 32 weeks' gestational age (GA). (Table 45–1) Oxygen requirement at 36 weeks corrected for postgestational age has been shown to be an excellent predictor of the development of BPD in this group of infants.[2]

▶ ETIOLOGY/PATHOPHYSIOLOGY

The pathogenesis of BPD remains complex and not fully understood. BPD results from a variety of toxic factors that can injure small airways and that can interfere with alveolarization (septation), leading to reduction in the overall surface area for gas exchange and clinically significant pulmonary dysfunction. The developing pulmonary microvasculature can also be injured.

An increased incidence of reactive airway disease is found in the families of infants who develop BPD. This suggests that some infants may be genetically predisposed to the development of BPD. The major host susceptibility factor associated with BPD is immature lungs secondary to prematurity (22–32 weeks' gestational age) followed by the presence of symptomatic patent ductus arteriosus (PDA). The left-to-right shunting through the PDA produces an increase in pulmonary blood flow and in lung fluid, negatively affecting lung function and gas exchange leading to increased risk of BPD.[3] In addition, male infants with BPD tend to have more severe disease and worse neurodevelopmental outcome. The primary lung injury often leads to increased permeability of the lungs and the presence of neutrophils and macrophages. These cells produce proteases and other cytotoxic products including oxygen radicals capable of producing pulmonary membrane damage. Factors involved in secondary injury include mechanical ventilation, oxygen toxicity, infection and inflammatory mediators.[4]

MECHANICAL VENTILATION

The treatment necessary to recruit alveoli and prevent atelectasis in the immature lung such as surfactant replacement with oxygen supplementation, continuous positive airway pressure (CPAP), and mechanical ventilation may cause lung injury and activate the inflammatory cascade. Trauma secondary to PPV is generally referred to as barotrauma. Volutrauma suggests the occurrence of lung injury secondary to excessive tidal volume from PPV. Many modes of ventilation and many ventilator strategies have been studied to potentially reduce lung

▶ TABLE 45–1. **SEVERITY OF BPD**

Severity of BPD	O₂ Supplement >28 Weeks PMA	O₂ Supplement >36 Weeks PMA
Mild	Yes	None
Moderate	Yes	Yes, <30% O₂
Severe	Yes	Yes, >30% O₂ and/or PP

PMA, postmenstrual age; PP, positive pressure.

injury. In 1996, Bernstein et al. compared synchronized intermittent mechanical ventilation (SIMV) with intermittent mechanical ventilation in preterm infants with RDS. Infants weighing <1000 g who received SIMV had less BPD than did other infants.[5]

Other researchers used high-frequency jet ventilation (HFJV) or high-frequency oscillatory ventilation (HFOV) to prevent barotrauma or to rescue infants when conventional ventilation failed. Results have been mixed. Several investigators comparing primary HFOV or HFJV with conventional ventilation suggested that high-volume strategies that effectively recruit alveoli may prevent BPD. In the Provo multicenter HFOV trial, surfactant was administered, and infants were randomly assigned to receive conventional ventilation or HFOV with a lung-recruitment strategy. Patients given HFOV had minimal BPD at the age of 30 days and needed less oxygen than the others did at discharge.[6] PPV with various forms of nasal CPAP has been reported to decrease injury to the developing lung, and it may reduce the development of BPD. Van Marter and colleagues described BPD rates in different centers using various ventilation strategies.[7] Centers that used more CPAP and less intubation, surfactant, and indomethacin had the lowest rates of BPD.

OXYGEN THERAPY

The major antioxidant enzymes in humans are superoxide dismutase, glutathione peroxidase, and catalase. Activity of antioxidant enzymes tend to increase during the last trimester of pregnancy, similar to surfactant production, alveolarization, and development of the pulmonary vasculature preparing the fetus for transition from a relatively hypoxic intrauterine environment to a relatively hyperoxic extrauterine environment. Therefore, preterm birth exposes the neonate to high oxygen concentrations without having the antioxidant enzymes leading to an increase in the risk of injury due to oxygen free radicals. In 2003, Davis and others reported that supplementation with superoxide dismutase, in ventilated preterm infants with RDS, substantially improved their clinical pulmonary status and markedly reduced readmissions among treated subjects compared with placebo-treated control group.[8] Further trials are currently underway to examine the effects of supplementation with superoxide dismutase in preterm infants at high risk for BPD.

Ideal oxygen saturation for term or preterm neonates of various gestational ages has not been definitively determined. In practice, many clinicians have adopted conservative oxygen saturation parameters (i.e., 88%–92%). A delicate balance exists to optimally promote neonatal pulmonary (alveolar and vascular) and retinal vascular homeostasis.

INFLAMMATION

Elevated levels of interleukin-6 and placental growth factor in the umbilical venous blood of preterm neonates are associated with increased incidence of BPD. This inflammation likely affects alveolarization and vascularization of the pulmonary system of the second-trimester fetus. Activation of leukocytes after cell injury caused by oxygen free radicals, barotrauma, infection, and other stimuli may begin the process of destruction and abnormal lung repair that results in acute lung injury then BPD. Metabolites of arachidonic acid, lysoplatelet factor, prostaglandin, and prostacyclin may cause vasodilation, increase capillary permeability with subsequent albumin leakage, and inhibit surfactant function. These effects increase oxygenation and ventilation requirements and potentially increase rates of BPD. Activation of transcription factors, such as nuclear factor-kappa B in early postnatal life, is associated with death or BPD. α1-proteinase inhibitor mitigates the action of elastases and is activated by oxygen free radicals. Increased activity and decreased function of α1-proteinase inhibitor may worsen lung injury in neonates. A decrease in BPD and in the need for continued ventilator support is found in neonates given supplemental α1-proteinase inhibitor.[9]

INFECTION

Schelonka and colleagues summarized findings from 23 studies of *U. urealyticum* and concluded that infection with this organism is associated with increased rates of BPD.[10] Infection—either antenatal chorioamnionitis and funisitis or postnatal infection—may activate the inflammatory cascade and damage the preterm lung, resulting in BPD. In fact, any clinically significant episode of sepsis in the vulnerable preterm neonate greatly increases the risk of BPD, especially if the infection increases the baby's requirement for oxygen and mechanical ventilation.

MALNUTRITION

Malnutrition is frequently seen in sick neonates. It may have profound effects on lung defenses and repair capabilities. Vitamins A and E are nutritional antioxidants that may help prevent lipid peroxidation and maintain cell integrity. However, supplementation of vitamin E in preterm neonates does not prevent BPD. Data from meta-analyses reported in a Cochrane Database review of vitamin A supplementation suggest that vitamin A supplementation reduces the risk of BPD in neonates born prematurely and death at 36 weeks.[11]

The way neonates react to lung injury also plays a role in the development of BPD. The principal histologic finding in the lungs of neonates with BPD is an extensive fibroproliferative response far in excess of the needs to repair the damage that occurred. This may be due to neonates having an increased number of pulmonary neuroendocrine cells (PNEC). These are among the first cells to differentiate in regenerating endothelium and demonstrate a proliferative response to lung injury. The multifactorial nature of the pathogenesis of this disease accounts for the great variability in severity of the clinical presentation of these patients.

▶ CLINICAL PRESENTATION

BPD causes not only significant complications in the newborn period, but is associated with continuing mortality, cardiopulmonary dysfunction, rehospitalization, growth failure, and poor neurodevelopmental outcome after hospital discharge. The clinical spectrum of infants with chronic lung disease ranges from mild symptomatic disease to crippling cardiopulmonary dysfunction. Follow-up of pediatric patients with BPD to adulthood demonstrated that patients had airway hyperreactivity, abnormal pulmonary function, and hyperinflation, as noted on chest radiography.[12,13] Blayney et al. found persistence of respiratory symptoms and abnormal pulmonary function in children aged 7 and 10 years.[14]

Patients who are likely to present to the ED are those who have been discharged home from the neonatal intensive care unit, typically at about 3 to 6 months of age. These children are often on home oxygen, bronchodilators, apnea monitors, and other medications. They will present to the ED with an exacerbation of their chronic lung disease most often secondary to a viral upper respiratory infection. Parents may describe increased respiratory distress, poor feeding, lethargy or irritability, and an increased oxygen requirement.

On physical examination, infants with chronic lung disease will usually be small for age and have hyperinflated chests (increased anteroposterior diameter). They will have tachypnea, rales, wheezes, or areas of decreased breath sounds. They may also have signs of an upper respiratory infection, including fever.

▶ LABORATORY AND RADIOGRAPHIC FINDINGS

A chest radiograph will reveal variable degrees of hyperinflation with areas of "scarring" (cystic or fibrotic areas). Comparison with old films is required to differentiate these areas from acute processes.

Oximetry should be checked on all patients with BPD. The results should be interpreted in light of the baseline level of hypoxia and usual need for oxygen therapy. Blood gas results can be helpful in assessing the more severely symptomatic patient. The results will also need to be compared with previous results, as these children will often have hypercarbia and hypoxia at baseline.

▶ DIFFERENTIAL DIAGNOSIS

In most cases, the diagnosis of BPD will be evident from the history. As many BPD exacerbations are triggered by upper respiratory infections, and often involve reactive airways as part of the pathology, the signs and symptoms of an exacerbation may overlap considerably with that of pneumonia, asthma, or bronchiolitis. Often these problems are coexistent and are the cause of the exacerbation. A chest radiograph can be helpful in identifying pneumonia if the radiograph can be compared to previous films. Testing for RSV will help identify those patients who may need hospitalization.

▶ TREATMENT

The treatment of an exacerbation in a patient with BPD is mainly supportive. The most effective treatments for ameliorating symptoms or preventing exacerbation in established BPD patients include oxygen therapy, inhaled glucocorticoid therapy, and vaccination against respiratory pathogens. Many other strategies for the prevention or treatment of BPD have been proposed, but have weaker or conflicting evidence of effectiveness. Oxygen is provided, if indicated. The patient's fluid status is assessed and intravenous fluids provided, if indicated. Mechanical ventilation may be necessary for recurrent apnea spells (most commonly with RSV infections), worsening hypercarbia, or refractory hypoxemia.

Bronchodilators are often effective in these patients and should be used as they are for asthma. Systemic corticosteroids are thought to be effective in acute exacerbations, but their chronic use is associated with many side effects, most notably the recently recognized adverse effects on neurodevelopment, which precludes their routine use for the prevention or treatment of BPD.[15] Inhaled steroids have been shown to increase the ability to extubate children who are chronically ventilated but its efficacy in nonventilated patients has not been demonstrated. A review by Shah et al. found no evidence that early-inhaled steroids confer important advantages over systemic steroids in the management of ventilator-dependent preterm infants. Neither inhaled steroids nor systemic steroids can be recommended as a part of standard practice for ventilated preterm infants. Because they might have fewer adverse effects than systemic steroids, further randomized controlled trials of inhaled steroids are needed, which address risk/benefit ratio of different delivery techniques, dosing schedules, and long-term effects, with particular attention to neurodevelopmental outcome.[16]

Parenteral diuretics have been shown to improve lung function and survival in some patients. Studies have looked at the effectiveness of aerosolized furosemide for patients with BPD, but no conclusive benefit has been demonstrated.[17]

▶ DISPOSITION

Some patients who present to the ED with exacerbation caused by an upper respiratory infection can be managed at home. However, children with BPD often have a very fragile respiratory status and can become very sick with relatively minor insults. Indications for inpatient management include increased respiratory distress, increasing hypoxia or hypercarbia, new pulmonary infiltrates or inability to keep up with appropriate fluid intake. Patients with BPD and RSV infections are at high risk for complications of RSV and need to be hospitalized. Prematurely born infants, who had a symptomatic RSV lower respiratory tract infection and/or respiratory morbidity at follow-up, had worse lung function prior to neonatal unit discharge.[18] In 1998, the Food and Drug Administration approved palivizumab (Synagis) for the prevention of severe lower respiratory tract infection secondary to RSV in pediatric patients at high risk for developing disease that required hospitalization. Four years of retrospective and prospective data on the use of palivizumab in clinical practice has accumulated a wealth of "real life" information on the clinical effectiveness of RSV immunoprophylaxis in a large cohort of high-risk infants.[19]

It is important to remember that the home care of these children requires a tremendous amount of work on the part of the parents or other caretakers even when the child is not acutely ill. Parents may have difficulty coping with an exacerbation. This factor should be considered when making a decision to discharge a patient for home care.

REFERENCES

1. Lemons JA, Bauer CR, Oh W, et al. Very low birth weight outcomes of the national institute of child health and human development neonatal research network, January 1995 through December 1996. *Pediatrics.* 2001;107:1–8.
2. Ehrenkranz RA, Walsh MC, Vohr BR, et al. Validation of the national institutes of health consensus definition of bronchopulmonary dysplasia. *Pediatrics.* 2005;116(6):1353–1360.
3. Del Moral T, Claure N, Van Buskirk S, et al. Duration of patent ductus arteriosus as a risk factor for bronchopulmonary dysplasia. *Pediatr Res.* 2001;49:282A.
4. Davis Jonathan W, Sweet David G. Pathophysiology and prevention of bronchopulmonary dysplasia. *Curr Pediatr Rev.* 2008;4(1):2–14.
5. Bernstein G, Mannino FL, Heldt GP, et al. Randomized multicenter trial comparing synchronized and conventional intermittent mandatory ventilation in neonates. *J Pediatr.* 1996;128(4):453–463.
6. Gerstmann DR, Minton SD, Stoddard RA, et al. The Provo multicenter early high-frequency oscillatory ventilation trial: improved pulmonary and clinical outcome in respiratory distress syndrome. *Pediatrics.* 1996;98(6, pt 1):1044–1057.
7. Van Marter LJ, Allred EN, Pagano M, et al. Do clinical markers of barotraumas and oxygen toxicity explain interhospital variation in rates of chronic lung disease?. The Neonatology Committee for the Development Network. *Pediatrics.* 2000;105(6):1194–1201.
8. Davis JM, Richter SE, Biswas S, et al. Long-term follow up of premature infants treated with prophylactic, intratracheal recombinant human CuZn superoxide dismutase. *J Perinatol.* 2000;20(4):213–216.
9. Stiskal JA, Dunn MS, Shennan AT, et al. Alpha 1-proteinase inhibitor therapy for the prevention of chronic lung disease of prematurity: a randomized, controlled trial. *Pediatrics.* 1998;101(1, pt 1):89–94.
10. Schelonka RL, Katz B, Waites KB, et al. Critical appraisal of the role of ureaplasma in the development of brochopulmonary dysplasia with meta-analytic techniques. *Pediatr Infect Dis J.* 2005;24(12):1033–1039.
11. Darlow BA, Graham PJ. Vitamin A supplementation to prevent mortality and short and long-term morbidity in very low birth weight infants. *Cochrane Database Syst Rev.* 2007;(4):CD000501.
12. Bhandari A, Bhandari V. Pathogenesis, pathology and pathophysiology of pulmonary sequelae of bronchopulmonary dysplasia in premature infants. *Front Biosci.* 2003;8:e370–e380.
13. Northway WH Jr. Bronchopulmonary dysplasia: twenty-five years later. *Pediatrics.* 1992;89(5, pt1):969–973.
14. Blayney M, Kaerem E, Whyte H, et al. Bronchopulmonary dysplasia: improvement in lung function between 7 and 10 years of age. *J Pediatr.* 1991;118(2)201–206.
15. D'Angio CT, Maniscalco WM. Bronchopulmonary dysplasia in preterm infants: pathophysiology and management strategies. *Paediatr Drugs.* 2004;6(5):303–330.
16. Shah SS, Ohlsson A, Halliday H, Shah VS. Inhaled versus systemic corticosteroids for preventing chronic lung disease in ventilated very low birth weight preterm neonates. *Cochrane Database Syst Rev.* 2003;(1):CD002058.
17. Brion LP, Primhak RA, Yong W. Aerosolized diuretics for preterm infants with chronic lung disease. *Cochrane Database Syst Rev.* 2006;(3):CD001694.
18. Broughton S, Bhat R, Roberts A, et al. Diminished lung function, RSV infection, and respiratory morbidity in prematurely born infants. *Arch Dis Child.* 2006;91(1):26–30.
19. Romero JR. Palivizumab prophylaxis of respiratory syncytial virus disease from 1998 to 2002: results from four years of palivizumab usage. *Pediatr Infect Dis J.* 2003;22(2 suppl):S46–S54.

CHAPTER 46

Cystic Fibrosis

Sabah F. Iqbal, Kathleen M. Brown, and Bruce L. Klein

▶ HIGH-YIELD FACTS

- Cystic fibrosis (CF) is a generalized defect in all of the exocrine gland secretions.
- Patients not yet diagnosed with CF may present to the emergency department (ED) with a history of failure to thrive chronic or recurrent pulmonary infections or gastrointestinal problems.
- Patients with known CF may present with a pulmonary exacerbation, pneumothorax, hemoptysis, or cor pulmonale. Nonpulmonary acute complications include meconium ileus equivalent, rectal prolapse, and electrolyte abnormalities.
- Bronchodilators and antibiotics are first-line therapies for a pulmonary exacerbation. Other possible therapies include anti-inflammatory medications, mucolytic agents, and chest physiotherapy.

Cystic fibrosis (CF) is the most common, life-limiting, autosomal recessive disease among Caucasians in the United States.[1,2] It occurs in approximately 1 in 3500 white births and is being diagnosed increasingly in non-Caucasians as well[1] (Fig. 46–1).

Most patients with CF have the classic triad of manifestations:

- Chronic pulmonary disease
- Malabsorption due to pancreatic insufficiency
- Elevated concentrations of sweat sodium and chloride.[2]

However, there is considerable individual variation in the clinical manifestations, severity, and course of the disease.

▶ ETIOLOGY/PATHOPHYSIOLOGY

CF is caused by mutations in the gene that encodes the cystic fibrosis transmembrane conductance regulator (CFTR) protein.[1,3–5] This protein, which is located in the epithelial cell membrane, functions normally as a cAMP-activated chloride channel, transporting chloride (and passively water) out of the cell into the adjacent lumen.[1,4,5] CFTR also plays a role in bicarbonate transport from the cell into the lumen.[1,4,5] In addition, for airway epithelial cells at least, CFTR is involved in regulating sodium channels, helping to limit sodium (and water) reabsorption from the lumen to the cells.[1,4,5] In sweat gland ductal cells, CFTR transports chloride in the opposite direction, i.e., from the lumen into the cell.[1]

The CFTR gene is located on the long arm of chromosome 7.[4] The most common mutation that causes CF (F508del)—

and more than 1500 less-common mutations—have been identified.[1,4] At least four categories of mutations have been identified: (1) defective CFTR production; (2) defective CFTR processing; (3) defective regulation; and (4) defective conduction.[1,3,4] Organs that express the CFTR gene (particularly the sinuses, lungs, pancreas, liver, gastrointestinal (GI) tract, and reproductive system) are the ones affected by the mutations.[4] The relationship between genotype and clinical manifestations is not always straightforward, however.[1,4]

The most important pathophysiologic consequence of these CFTR "defects" is diminished water in mucous and most exocrine secretions (along with associated electrolyte and other abnormalities).[1,2,4] Mucous and exocrine secretions are more viscid, and they are difficult to clear, causing airway and ductal obstruction.[1,2–4,6] In the airways, these mucous (and possibly other) abnormalities also predispose to chronic infection with a characteristic group of bacterial organisms and inflammation.[1–6] Exactly why this predisposition to specific infections occurs has yet to be fully elucidated. Various hypotheses have been proposed (Table 46–1), which are discussed in some detail in the references.[1–5]

Pancreatic exocrine insufficiency (which results in GI malabsorption and malnutrition) follows from the low volume of pancreatic secretions reaching the GI tract as well as their abnormal bicarbonate-, enzyme-, and water-deficient content.[1,2,4] Pancreatic endocrine insufficiency (resulting in diabetes mellitus)—or even acute pancreatitis—may ensue eventually, due to pancreatic autodigestion by stagnant activated enzymes.[1–4,6] Abnormal intestinal mucous and biliary secretions also play roles in the malabsorptive and various GI and hepatobiliary obstructive sequelae found in CF.[2] CF patients have elevated sweat chloride (and sodium) concentrations because of defective chloride transport out of the primary sweat by the sweat gland duct cells.[1]

▶ CLINICAL PRESENTATION

Patients who have not yet been diagnosed with CF, and are untreated, may present to the ED for a variety of complaints. Failure to thrive with a history of chronic GI and/or respiratory problems is a typical presentation.[2] CF should be considered in any patient with chronic diarrhea, recurrent respiratory infections (especially with bronchiectasis or clubbing), or atypical asthma.[2] Hypoproteinemia and edema may develop in those with prominent malabsorption.[2] Malabsorption may also lead to vitamin deficiencies, especially of fat-soluble vitamins.[1,2] Hemorrhage due to vitamin K deficiency and neurologic abnormalities and hemolytic anemia from vitamin E deficiency

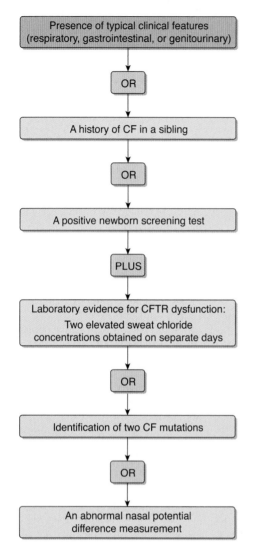

Figure 46–1. Algorithm for diagnosis of CF.[1]

have been described.[1,2] Refer patients with clinical findings suggestive of CF for diagnostic evaluation.

Known CF patients can present to the ED with various acute complications and the most common is a pulmonary exacerbation, manifested by an increase of respiratory symptoms.

▶ **TABLE 46–1. FACTORS HYPOTHESIZED TO PREDISPOSE TO AIRWAY INFECTION WITH CHARACTERISTIC ORGANISMS IN CF PATIENTS**

Anaerobic/microaerophilic growth conditions leading to bacterial mucoid transformation and resistance
Decreased mucociliary clearance of bacteria
Inability of epithelial cell membrane F508del CFTR to bind *P. aeruginosa*
Inactivation of "defensins" by elevated luminal chloride concentrations
Increased epithelial cell membrane asialoGM1 receptors, resulting in increased binding of *P. aeruginosa* and *S. aureus*
Low concentrations of cytokine interleukin-10
Low concentrations of lipoxins, which suppress neutrophilic inflammation

Pulmonary exacerbations are thought to be due to more active airway infection. The youngest CF patients have infections caused by *Staphylococcus aureus* or *Hemophilus influenzae*. Eventually, however, *Pseudomonas aeruginosa* becomes the most prevalent organism.[4,5,7,8] In chronically infected CF patients, *P. aeruginosa* tends to mutate, becoming more mucoid, less motile, and very difficult to eradicate with antibiotics.[4,7,8] *Burkholderia* (formerly *Pseudomonas*) *cepacia* is a particularly virulent organism in CF patients.[1,5] Nontuberculous mycobacterial infections can occur and are difficult to eradicate.[1]

Chronic airway infection and inflammation, along with repeated exacerbations, result in destruction of the airway.[1,4,5,9] Bronchiolitis develops initially, accompanied by bronchitis later.[1] With prolonged disease, bronchiolar obliteration, bronchiolectasis, and bronchiectasis ensue.[1,5] Mucous plugging and airway obstruction are prominent features of CF, leading to atelectasis, enlarged air spaces, and ventilation–perfusion mismatching.[1,5]

Pneumothorax (sometimes a tension pneumothorax) results from the rupture of an emphysematous bulla or bleb and must be excluded in any CF patient who deteriorates suddenly.[1,2] It is not unusual in older teenagers and adults, or in patients with significant impairment in lung function. It can often recur.[2,10] Pneumothorax is a poor prognostic indicator and is associated with a subsequent increase in hospitalizations, hospital days, and 2-year mortality.[10]

CF patients frequently have hemoptysis, especially during exacerbations.[1] Bleeding is usually minor and not dangerous. Massive hemoptysis—acute bleeding >240 mL/d or >100 mL/d over several days—is not rare and can cause life-threatening asphyxia or hypotension.[11] It is thought to result from persistent airway inflammation and erosion into markedly enlarged bronchial arteries (which contain systemic pressures).[11] Like pneumothorax, massive hemoptysis is more prevalent in older patients and in those with more severe pulmonary impairment.[11] *S. aureus* in sputum cultures is also associated with an increased risk.[11] Massive hemoptysis is a poor prognostic indicator, similar to pneumothorax.[11]

Hematemesis occurs less often but must be distinguished from hemoptysis.[2] It is due to bleeding esophageal varices secondary to portal hypertension from advanced cirrhosis.[2]

Patients with progressively worsening lung disease eventually develop pulmonary hypertension and right ventricular hypertrophy (cor pulmonale).[2] A respiratory exacerbation may precipitate congestive heart failure.[2] In time, most CF patients die of respiratory failure complicated by cor pulmonale.

Acute GI complications of CF include meconium ileus, meconium ileus equivalent, and rectal prolapse.[1,2] Newborns with meconium ileus present with symptoms and signs of intestinal obstruction (Fig. 46–2). They usually have passed no stool or only a small amount since birth.[1,2] Intestinal obstruction can also occur in older children with CF who have difficulty passing the dry, putty-like stool from the terminal ileum into the cecum, and is called meconium ileus equivalent.[1,2] Intestinal perforation (which sometimes occurs prenatally in meconium ileus), intussusception, and volvulus are other potential related consequences.[1,2] Similarly, constipation and crampy abdominal pain are common in CF patients. Rectal prolapse is associated with CF and is most commonly seen in children younger than 3 years old.[1,2]

CF patients have elevated sweat chloride and sodium concentrations, giving them their characteristically salty taste.[1,2,4]

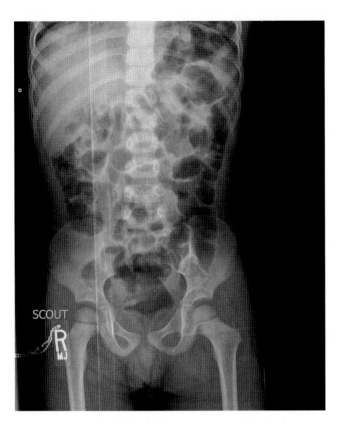

Figure 46–2. Intestinal obstruction.

Sweat salt and water losses, with associated renal compensation, can lead to acute or chronic electrolyte depletion and dehydration.[2] These occur most commonly in infants with gastroenteritis and poor oral intake, or during the hot summer months, especially in arid climates.[1,2]

As patients approach adulthood, they may develop additional complications, such as diabetes mellitus (20% of young adults), obstructive biliary tract disease (up to 30% of adults), and obstructive azospermia (95% of postpubertal males).[1]

▶ LABORATORY AND RADIOGRAPHIC FINDINGS

Many states now test for CF in newborn screens, leading to earlier detection in most cases and, possibly, improved survival.[4,12] A referral for evaluation should be made for any patient in whom the diagnosis is suspected.[2] Recommended criteria and testing for diagnosing CF are identified in Figure 46–1.[1] DNA mutation analysis is available for detection of patients and carriers.[1] Traditionally, a pilocarpine iontophoresis sweat test has been a part of the diagnostic evaluation in any patient with suspected CF.[1,12] This test measures the chloride concentration in sweat. Values >60 mEq/L are considered positive; however, this cutoff is not 100% sensitive for diagnosing CF.[1,4] Of note, sweat testing can be difficult to perform accurately, is time consuming, and is usually not available in the ED.[1]

During pulmonary exacerbations, oxygen saturation should be measured via pulse oximetry initially. Blood gas determinations may be useful in managing patients with respiratory failure, particularly those who have had good lung

▶ TABLE 46–2. SOME NON-CF CAUSES OF PROTRACTED OR RECURRENT PULMONARY SYMPTOMS

Asthma
Bronchopulmonary dysplasia
Congenital bronchial or pulmonary abnormalities
Foreign body
Immotile cilia syndrome
Immunodeficiency disorders
Intrathoracic neoplasms

functions and suffer acute decompensations likely to respond to therapy.[2] The evaluation should include sputum or, if unobtainable, lower pharyngeal or throat culture, in order to guide antibiotic therapy.[1,8]

Compare the chest x-ray during an exacerbation with the most recent previous ones.[2] Common chest x-ray findings include hyperinflation, diffuse peribronchial thickening, and areas of atelectasis and fluffy infiltrates.[1,2] Patients with cor pulmonale have comparatively larger hearts—as opposed to the narrow hearts usually seen in CF patients—and prominent pulmonary vasculature.[2] Any patient with a sudden deterioration in pulmonary status must have a pneumothorax excluded by chest x-ray. Patients with meconium ileus or meconium ileus equivalent have dilated loops of bowel on abdominal films. A bubbly granular density in the lower abdomen, representing the meconium or fecal mass, may also be seen.[2]

In patients with significant hemoptysis or hematemesis, blood should be sent for complete blood count, type and cross-match, and prothrombin time. Hyponatremic, hypokalemic, hypochloremic alkalosis is the classic electrolyte abnormality, and can be a diagnostic clue, particularly when seen in a patient with other findings suggestive of CF.[1,2]

▶ DIFFERENTIAL DIAGNOSIS

CF may be confused with a variety of different disorders. Table 46–2 lists some non-CF causes of protracted or recurrent pulmonary symptoms. Table 46–3 lists other causes of exocrine

▶ TABLE 46–3. NON-CF CAUSES OF EXOCRINE PANCREATIC INSUFFICIENCY (ALL RARE IN CHILDREN)[1]

Alagille syndrome
Autoimmune polyendocrinopathy-candidiasis-ectodermal dystrophy
Chronic pancreatitis
Congenital pancreatic hypoplasia
Congenital rubella
Duodenal atresia and stenosis
Enterokinase deficiency
Isolated pancreatic enzyme deficiency (amylase, lipase, colipase, lipase-colipase, trypsinogen)
Johanson-Blizzard syndrome
Nesidioblastosis, following pancreatectomy
Pearson syndrome
Protein-calorie malnutrition
Shwachman syndrome

▶ **TABLE 46–4. NON-CF CONDITIONS ASSOCIATED WITH ELEVATED SWEAT ELECTROLYTE CONCENTRATIONS[1]**

Adrenal insufficiency	Hypoparathyroidism
Autonomic dysfunction	Hypothyroidism
Ectodermal dysplasia	Malnutrition
Familial cholestasis	Mauriac syndrome
Fucosidosis	Mucopolysaccharidoses
Glucose-6-phosphatase deficiency	Nephrosis with edema
Hereditary nephrogenic diabetes insipidus	Pancreatitis
HIV	Pseudohypoaldosteronism

pancreatic insufficiency.[1] Table 46–4 lists other conditions that are associated with elevated sweat electrolyte concentrations.[1]

▶ TREATMENT

Much of the decision making in CF involves issues of chronic care. However, sometimes the ED physician must begin treating one of the acute complications of the disease, most commonly a pulmonary exacerbation (Fig. 46–3). Therapy for the latter is aimed at relieving airway obstruction and treating infection.[1] Oxygen should be administered if indicated by pulse oximetry or arterial blood gas.[2] Airway obstruction in CF tends to be only partially reversible, because of the inflammation as well as any preexisting structural damage. Inhaled β₂-adrenergic bronchodilators are often effective in the short term and should be used in those who respond clinically.[1,2] Methylxanthines are rarely prescribed nowadays.

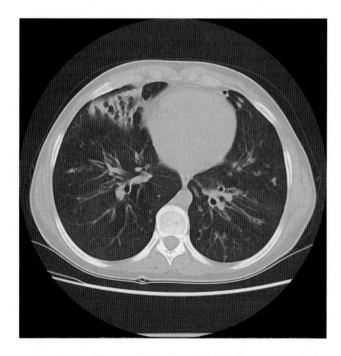

Figure 46–3. CT scan of the lung.

Antimicrobial therapy during an exacerbation results in a decreased bacterial load and improved pulmonary function.[7] Until current sputum culture results are known, prior results can help guide antibiotic selection.[1,2,5,8] If recent results are unavailable, empiric therapy should be aimed at the most common organisms seen in CF patients: *S. aureus* and *H. influenzae* in infants and young children, and *P. aeruginosa*, which is often present by the end of the first decade of life.[4,5,7,8] CF patients with exacerbations due to *P. aeruginosa* should be treated with combination antibiotics, because treatment with a single antibiotic has been associated with rapid pseudomonal resistance.[1,8] Inhaled antibiotics, particularly tobramycin, was noted to be safe and effective for patients colonized with Pseudomonas and can be used in an acute exacerbation. For patients with massive hemoptysis, anti-staphylococcal therapy should be considered.[11] Decisions regarding specific antibiotics must be individualized and should be made in consultation with the patient's CF specialist.

Pulmozyme (recombinant human deoxyribonuclease) is a "mucolytic" medication, which is administered via nebulization. It reduces sputum viscosity by enzymatically degrading the excessive DNA from dead neutrophils and other cells in airway mucous.[4,5] Pulmozyme has been shown to improve pulmonary function and decrease the number of exacerbations when used for long term in selected CF patients.[1] Although it is generally employed for chronic management, it can be continued during an acute exacerbation as well. Nebulized hypertonic saline has been proposed as an alternative method of clearing secretions.[1,4,5] Chest physiotherapy and postural drainage techniques are well accepted (although not as well proven) for clearing secretions in CF patients.[1,4,5]

Although still under study, anti-inflammatory medications may be beneficial in the long-term—and, possibly, acute—care of certain CF patients. Macrolides (e.g., azithromycin), which possess anti-inflammatory in addition to antibacterial properties, and high-dose ibuprofen seem promising.[1,4,5,13–17] Inhaled steroids are commonly used for long-term care, but this is controversial.[1,4,5,13] Some CF centers administer intravenous steroids for acute exacerbations. However, chronic administration of oral steroids is not recommended for most patients.[1,4,5,13]

Pneumothoraces greater than 10% of the hemithorax on AP chest x-ray should be evacuated by tube thoracostomy (via a chest tube or pleural drain), at least initially.[2] A tension pneumothorax should be aspirated first (through a large-bore IV catheter), followed by tube thoracostomy.[2]

Significant hemoptysis (>30–60 mL) is an indication for inpatient observation.[1,2] Vitamin K should be administered if the prothrombin time is prolonged.[1,2] Guidelines for replacement with packed red blood cells, fresh frozen plasma, etc., are the same as for bleeding from other sources.[2] For massive hemoptysis, ligation or embolization of the bleeding vessel may be necessary.[1,2]

Cor pulmonale may require treatment with oxygen and diuretics, in addition to treatment for the underlying lung disease. Before deciding to intubate and mechanically ventilate a CF patient in respiratory failure, the ED physician must consider the baseline pulmonary function, disease course, and patient and parental expectations.[2] In general, a patient is a candidate for ventilation if the pulmonary function has been good and this bout of respiratory failure was precipitated by an acute insult, such as asthma or pneumonia.[1,2] Ventilation may not be warranted; however, if the pulmonary function has been very poor and had been steadily declining despite aggressive medical therapy.[2] This is a terribly difficult decision, of course, and should be made in conjunction with the patient, parents, and chronic care provider.[2] Recently, a number of patients with CF have undergone double lung (or heart-lung) transplants, although further study is required to determine whether these truly lengthen survival.[1,2,4,18]

For meconium ileus or meconium ileus equivalent, a diatrizoate (Gastrografin) enema should be administered to relieve the obstruction.[1,2] Laparotomy is indicated for bowel perforation or volvulus, or if the enema is unsuccessful in relieving the obstruction or reducing an intussusception.[1,2]

Infants with significant dehydration and electrolyte losses should receive a 20 mL/kg normal saline bolus initially.[2] More than one bolus may be necessary. Once urine output is established (and after the bolus(es)), potassium chloride should be added to the fluids.[2] Serum electrolytes should be monitored frequently to help guide fluid therapy.[2]

▶ OUTCOME

Many more CF patients now survive to adulthood, with their median cumulative survival exceeding 35 years of age.[1] Factors contributing to this improved survival include earlier diagnosis, better nutrition, aggressive treatment of pulmonary infections, and prompt recognition and treatment of the numerous life-limiting and life-threatening complications of CF.

REFERENCES

1. Boat TF, Acton JD. Cystic fibrosis. In: Behrman RE, Kliegman RM, Jenson HB, Stanton BF, eds. *Nelson Textbook of Pediatrics*. Philadelphia, PA: Elsevier Science; 2007:1803–1817.
2. Scanlin TF. Cystic fibrosis. In: Fleisher GR, Ludwig S, Henretig FM, eds. *Textbook of Pediatric Emergency Medicine*. Philadelphia, PA: Lippincott Williams & Wilkins; 2006:1161–1166.
3. Katkin JP. Genetics and pathogenesis of cystic fibrosis. In: Rose BD, ed. *UpToDate*. Waltham, MA: UpToDate; 2008.
4. Ratjen F, Doring G. Cystic fibrosis. *Lancet*. 2003;361:681–689.
5. Rowe SM, Clancy JP. Advances in cystic fibrosis therapies. *Curr Opin Pediatr*. 2006;18:604–613.
6. Katkin JP. Clinical manifestations of pulmonary disease in cystic fibrosis. In: Rose BD, ed. *UpToDate*. Waltham, MA: UpToDate; 2008.
7. Goss CH, Burns JL. Exacerbations in cystic fibrosis 1: epidemiology and pathogenesis. *Thorax*. 2007;62:360–367.
8. Lahiri T. Approaches to treatment of initial pseudomonas aeruginosa infection in children who have cystic fibrosis. *Clin Chest Med*. 2007;28:307–318.
9. Hilliard TN, Regamey N, Shute JK, et al. Airway remodelling in children with cystic fibrosis. *Thorax*. 2007;62:1074–1080.
10. Flume PA, Strange C, Ye X, et al. Pneumothorax in cystic fibrosis. *Chest*. 2005;128:720–728.
11. Flume PA, Yankaskas JR, Ebeling M, et al. Massive hemoptysis in cystic fibrosis. *Chest*. 2005;128:729–738.
12. Rock MJ. Newborn screening for cystic fibrosis. *Clin Chest Med*. 2007;28:297–305.
13. Bush A, Davies J. Non-steroidal anti-inflammatory therapy for inflammatory lung disease in cystic fibrosis (at least at the moment). *J Pediatr*. 2007;151:228–230.
14. Rabin HR, Butler SM, Wohl MEB, et al. Pulmonary exacerbations in cystic fibrosis. *Pediatr Pulmonol*. 2004;37:400–406.
15. Clement A, Tamalet A, Leroux E, et al. Long term effects of azithromycin in patients with cystic fibrosis: a double blind, placebo controlled trial. *Thorax*. 2006;61:895–902.
16. Shinkai M, Rubin BK. Macrolides and airway inflammation in children. *Paediatr Respir Rev*. 2005;6:227–235.
17. Lands LC, Milner R, Cantin AM, et al. High-dose ibuprofen in cystic fibrosis: Canadian safety and effectiveness trial. *J Pediatr*. 2007;151:249–254.
18. Liou TG, Adler FR, Cox DR, et al. Lung transplantation and survival in children with cystic fibrosis. *N Engl J Med*. 2007;357:2143–2152.

SECTION VI

CARDIOVASCULAR EMERGENCIES

CHAPTER 47

Congenital Heart Disease

Timothy Horeczko and Kelly D. Young

▶ HIGH-YIELD FACTS

- Ductal-dependent lesions typically present with sudden-onset cardiogenic shock at 1 to 2 weeks of life and require immediate prostaglandin E_1 infusion.
- Congestive heart failure typically presents in the first 6 months of infancy in children with left-to-right shunting lesions and requires immediate stabilization and medical management.
- Aortic coarctation may present with hypertension and the complications of hypertension. The median age of presentation is 5 years. Blood pressure will be higher in the upper extremities compared with the lower extremities.
- The number of survivors of cardiac surgery for congenital heart lesions is rapidly increasing, and emergency physicians should be aware of common complications, such as arrhythmias, residual or recurrent lesions, and endocarditis.
- Children commonly have benign cardiac murmurs, which are usually softer, lower pitched, and early to midsystolic compared with pathologic murmurs.

The term "congenital heart disease" encompasses a wide variety of lesions. The emergency physician must not only recognize and manage previously undiagnosed congenital heart disease but also anticipate complications in a rapidly growing population of survivors of congenital heart surgery. This chapter reviews the common presentations and management of cyanotic and acyanotic congenital heart lesions and also discusses complications seen in postoperative congenital cardiac patients.

▶ EPIDEMIOLOGY

Congenital heart lesions occur in approximately 8 in 1000 live births in the United States, which includes lesions ranging from mild to severe but does not include common lesions such as bicuspid aortic valve (1%–2% of the population) or mitral valve prolapse. Significant congenital heart lesions can go undetected by prenatal ultrasound and may not present immediately after birth.[1] Overall, neither gender is predominant, but individual lesions may be more common in either males or females. The vast majority of patients will have isolated congenital heart lesions, which are multifactorial in origin. Approximately 10% of cases can be attributed to genetic causes. Many genetic syndromes (e.g., the trisomies, connective tissue disorders) and teratogens (e.g., congenital rubella infec-

tion) are associated with a higher risk of specific congenital heart lesions (Table 47–1). Most patients present during infancy (Fig. 47–1).

▶ PHYSIOLOGY

FETAL CIRCULATION

Oxygenated blood from the placenta enters the fetus through the single umbilical vein (Fig. 47–2). Approximately half of this blood bypasses the liver via the *ductus venosus*, flowing directly into the inferior vena cava (IVC). The majority is then directed from the IVC across the *foramen ovale* into the left atrium, bypassing the right heart and pulmonary circulation. This highly oxygenated blood in the left atrium mixes with pulmonary venous return, enters the left ventricle and the ascending aorta, and perfuses the cerebral circulation. Deoxygenated blood from the cerebral circulation drains into the superior vena cava, entering the right atrium, right ventricle, and pulmonary artery. Since pulmonary vascular resistance is high in the fetus, most of this blood bypasses the pulmonary circulation by way of the *ductus arteriosus* and enters the descending aorta. Two-thirds of this descending aorta outflow returns to the placenta via the umbilical arteries, and one-third perfuses the lower part of the fetus.

NEONATAL CIRCULATION

In the first hours of life, the newborn's pulmonary arterioles dilate and pulmonary vascular resistance begins to fall, resulting in increased pulmonary blood flow. Separation from the low-resistance placental circuit results in increased systemic blood pressure, which also reduces blood flow through the ductus arteriosus. The smooth muscle of the ductus arteriosus constricts in response to increased blood P_{O_2}; it is functionally closed by 15 hours of life. In the normal infant, the ductus arteriosus becomes the ligamentum arteriosum by 2 to 3 weeks of age. The foramen ovale closes by 3 months of age.

The neonatal myocardium is inefficient in extracting oxygen at the cellular level; its baseline oxygen requirement is high and it is unable to increase its contractility in response to demand. When increased cardiac output is needed, the neonate responds with an increasing heart rate. Thus, the physiology in the young infant is one of rate-dependent cardiac output, increased oxygen consumption, and a lower systolic reserve. These factors predispose children with congenital heart disease to congestive heart failure (CHF). In addition, neonates and

▶ **TABLE 47–1. SELECTED SYNDROMES ASSOCIATED WITH CONGENITAL HEART DISEASE[2,3]**

Syndrome	Incidence	Common Features	Congenital Heart Lesions
Down syndrome (trisomy 21)	1 in 1000	Decreased tone, epicanthal folds, hypothyroidism, esophageal, and duodenal atresia	Atrial septal defect, ventricular septal defect
Klinefelter syndrome (47 XXY)	Boys only 1 in 1000	Gynecomastia, hypogonadism	Mitral valve prolapse, left ventricular dysfunction
Noonan syndrome (AD or new mutation)	1:1000 to 1:2500	Webbed neck, wide-set eyes, epicanthal folds, short stature, lymphedema, blood dyscrasias	Pulmonic valve abnormalities, pulmonic stenosis, hypertrophic cardiomyopathy
Turner syndrome (XO syndrome)	Girls only 1:2000	Web neck, lymphedema, lack of secondary sexual characteristics, musculoskeletal and renal defects	Coarctation of the aorta, bicuspid aortic valve, secondary hypertension
DiGeorge syndrome (deletions, mutations)	1:3000	Hypocalcemia, immunodeficiency, hypoparathyroidism, thymic aplasia	Conotruncal anomalies, interrupted aortic arch, tetralogy of Fallot, truncus arteriosus, ventricular septal defect
Edwards syndrome (trisomy 18)	Girls >> Boys 1 in 3000	Coloboma, pectus carinatum, clenched hands/crossed legs, renal disease	Atrial septal defect, ventricular septal defect, patent ductus arteriosus
Marfan syndrome (fibrillin mutation)	1:5000 30% FamHx	Arched palate, scoliosis, ectopia lentis, thoracic cage defects; tall; thin, long fingers, arms, legs	Aortic aneurysm, mitral valve prolapse, risk of endocarditis
Patau syndrome (trisomy 13)	1 in 10 000	Cleft palate, close-set eyes, polydactyly, omphalocoele, seizures, apnea	Dextrocardia, atrial septal defect, ventricular septal defect, patent ductus arteriosus
Williams syndrome (elastin deletions)	1:20 000	Hearing/visual problems, hypercalcemia, cystic kidneys, diverticula, sudden death	Supravalvular aortic stenosis, pulmonic stenosis, ventricular hypertrophy
Holt–Oram syndrome (heart–hand syndrome)	1:100 000	Upper limb bone aplasia or hypoplasia, heart block	Atrial septal defect, ventricular septal defect
Fetal alcohol syndrome	0.2 in 1000 to 1.5 in 1000	Microcephaly, smooth philtrum, short stature, developmental delay, risk of neonatal withdrawal	Valvular defects (various), cardiomyopathies
Lithium exposure	1:10 during treatment	Hypertonicity, hypothyroidism	Ebstein's anomaly, atrial septal defect
Rubella, congenital	Mostly during outbreaks	Deafness, ophthalmic defects, "Blueberry muffin baby," sepsis	Atrial septal defect, ventricular septal defect, pulmonic stenosis, patent ductus arteriosus

young infants may be slow to change their in utero physiology and may still shunt blood via the foramen ovale or a patent ductus arteriosus (PDA). This may present as high pulmonary vascular resistance, which is responsive to oxygen (oxygen decreases resistance) and a prominent right ventricle (seen as right-axis deviation [RAD] on electrocardiogram).

▶ EVALUATION

HISTORY

General health, including growth, development, and susceptibility to respiratory illnesses should be assessed. Pregnancy, birth, and family history may provide valuable clues to specific genetic or teratogenic etiologies. Symptoms of CHF should be sought: poor feeding, longer feeding times than the average infant, poor growth or failure to thrive, sweating with feeding, irritability or lethargy, weak cry, increased respiratory effort, dyspnea, tachypnea, and coughing. Ask about cyanosis or cyanotic episodes, which may be more noticeable during crying or exercise.

PHYSICAL EXAMINATION

As with any patient encounter, evaluation begins with a first impression of the patient's overall well-being. The pediatric assessment triangle (PAT) is used to assess rapidly a child's severity of illness and to determine urgency for life support. Its three components—appearance, work of breathing, and circulation to skin—give powerful information across the room using only visual and auditory clues.[4] This rapid global assessment is especially useful in the undifferentiated patient

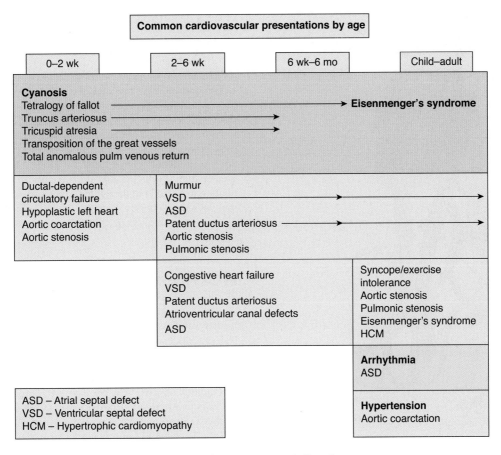

Common cardiovascular presentations by age

0–2 wk	2–6 wk	6 wk–6 mo	Child–adult

Cyanosis
Tetralogy of fallot ———————————————→ **Eisenmenger's syndrome**
Truncus arteriosus —————————————→
Tricuspid atresia ——————————————→
Transposition of the great vessels
Total anomalous pulm venous return

Ductal-dependent
circulatory failure
Hypoplastic left heart
Aortic coarctation
Aortic stenosis

Murmur
VSD ————————————————————————→
ASD
Patent ductus arteriosus ——————————→
Aortic stenosis
Pulmonic stenosis

Congestive heart failure
VSD
Patent ductus arteriosus
Atrioventricular canal defects
ASD

Syncope/exercise
intolerance
Aortic stenosis
Pulmonic stenosis
Eisenmenger's syndrome
HCM

Arrhythmia
ASD

ASD – Atrial septal defect
VSD – Ventricular septal defect
HCM – Hypertrophic cardiomyopathy

Hypertension
Aortic coarctation

Figure 47–1. Common presentations by age.

who may be suffering from sequelae of congenital heart disease.

Check vital signs, including four-extremity blood pressures and pulse quality, in the upper and lower extremities in the sick infant. Color and general appearance may be significant clues for classifying the lesion into one of three categories:

- Pink: congestive heart failure, L → R shunt
- Blue: cyanotic heart disease, R → L shunt
- Gray: outflow obstruction, hypoperfusion, and shock.

For cyanosis to be clinically apparent, 3 to 5 g of deoxygenated hemoglobin must be present (correlating to an oxygen saturation of 80%–85%). Therefore, if the child is anemic, cyanosis may be less easily recognized. Peripheral cyanosis, acrocyanosis, and mottling may be seen in normal newborns. Nail beds (look also for clubbing) and mucous membranes are the best locations to assess for central cyanosis. Auscultate for murmurs, S1 and S2, and extra sounds. If the child is quiet and comfortable when you first enter the room, take advantage of the situation to auscultate the heart and lungs before upsetting the child with other elements of the physical examination. Murmurs are commonly heard in normal children (Table 47–2). Generally speaking, normal murmurs are never diastolic, late systolic, or pansystolic. Examine the abdomen for hepatomegaly. A normal infant's liver is palpable 1 to 3 cm below the right subcostal margin. Examine the child for dysmorphic features suggestive of a genetic or teratogenic syndrome.

HYPEROXIA TEST

The single most sensitive and specific test in the initial evaluation of a neonate with suspected congenital heart disease (in the absence of readily available echocardiography) is the *hyperoxia test*. An arterial blood gas is sampled with the patient on room air (if tolerated), and repeated after a few minutes of high-flow oxygen. When a child breathes high-flow oxygen ("100%" O_2), an arterial P_{O_2} of greater than 250 torr virtually excludes hypoxia due to congenital heart disease ("passed" hyperoxia test)[1]. An arterial P_{O_2} of less than 100 torr in a patient without obvious lung disease is indicative of a right-to-left shunt and extremely predictive of cyanotic congenital heart disease ("failed" hyperoxia test). A value of 100 to 250 torr may indicate structural heart disease with complete intracardiac mixing. Ideally, blood is sampled from both preductal (right upper extremity) and postductal sites (any other extremity) and carefully labeled as to site and F_{IO_2}. When done in both sites, valuable information about the possible lesion may be obtained, such as differential cyanosis. For example, a markedly higher oxygen level in the right upper extremity versus the lower extremities may indicate aortic arch obstruction.

Regardless of site used, the hyperoxia test should be conducted on all neonates with suspected congenital heart disease, not just those who appear cyanotic. Pulse oximetry is not an appropriate substitute for an arterial blood gas; it is not sensitive enough to determine "pass or fail" of the test, since a

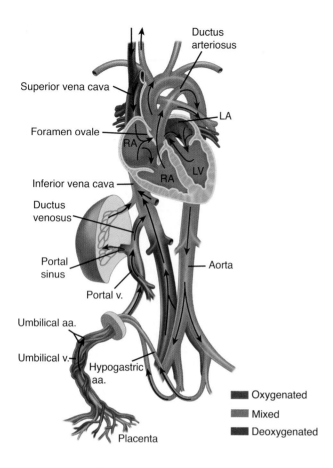

Figure 47-2. Fetal circulation.

child breathing high-flow O_2 and registering 100% on pulse oximetry may actually have an arterial Po_2 of anywhere from 80 torr to 680 torr. *Most importantly, a neonate who fails the hyperoxia test should be presumed to have critical congenital heart disease and should receive prostaglandin E_1 immediately until a definitive anatomic diagnosis is made.*

OTHER ANCILLARY TESTS

Chronically cyanotic children usually compensate with polycythemia. A cyanotic child's oxygen-carrying capacity will be further compromised by anemia, and a "normal" hematocrit by usual standards may be inadequate for the cyanotic child. Obtain a chest radiograph (CXR) to evaluate cardiomegaly, chamber enlargement, and pulmonary vascularity. Evaluate an electrocardiogram (ECG) for conduction and rhythm disturbances, chamber forces, and rare ischemic changes. Consult a pediatric handbook as ECG normals vary greatly by age. Age and chamber force differences may seem intimidating to the clinician, but a few basic principles may provide a guide (see also Tables 47–3 and 47–4). For example, one striking difference between adult and pediatric ECGs is the inclusion of additional leads such as the right ventricular leads V3R or V4R (and less frequently the posterior left ventricular lead V7). Neonates and young children have a natural right-axis deviation, which may obscure the typical findings of right-sided disease; the addition

of leads V3R or V4R increases the yield in detecting right atrial or ventricular hypertrophy when congenital heart disease is suspected[5] (Fig. 47–3).

There are other features that are important to interpreting the pediatric ECG. Sinus bradycardia must be recognized in the sick infant. Intervals are analyzed for drug effects and for long Q–T syndrome. Neonatal right-sided forces such as RAD and right ventricular hypertrophy will transition gradually to adult form by age 3 to 4 years. Right bundle-branch block is common, and left bundle-branch block is rare. Ischemic changes are rare and differ from those in adults. However, Q waves greater than 35 ms, ST elevation greater than 2 mm, or ventricular arrhythmia in the setting of a worrisome clinical setting may indicate ischemia. T-wave changes, especially T-wave inversions are common in children and are rarely ischemic (juvenile T waves).

▶ CLASSIFICATION

Lesions are usually classified as **cyanotic** or **acyanotic** and further subclassified according to whether or not the lesion is ductal-dependent; that is, whether the lesion depends on a patent ductus arteriosus to deliver partially oxygenated blood to the systemic circulation.

Cyanotic lesions: "The Six Terrible (Turqouise) Ts" include Truncus Arteriosus, Transposition of the Great Arteries, Total Anomalous Pulmonary Venous Return, Tetralogy of Fallot*, Tricuspid Abnormalities* (Tricuspid Atresia, Ebstein's Anomaly), "Tons" of Others* ("*Tiny Heart*"—Hypoplastic Left Heart Syndrome, "*Terminated Aorta*"—Interrupted Aortic Arch) (**Ductal-dependent lesions*).

Acyanotic lesions: "**PiCk A Very Powerful Approach to Acyanosis**" include **P**ulmonic Stenosis*, **C**oarctation of the Aorta*, **A**trioseptal Defect, **V**entriculoseptal Defect, **P**atent Ductus Arteriosus, **A**ortic Stenosis, **A**trioventriculoseptal defects (**Ductal-dependent lesions*).

▶ BRIEF SURVEY OF INDIVIDUAL LESIONS

Truncus arteriosus involves a single arterial trunk supplying both the pulmonary and systemic circulations (Fig. 47–4). A ventricular septal defect (VSD) is usually present. Initially cyanosis may be mild or absent. A murmur is detected in the first few days, pulses are bounding, and there is a single S2. The patient may have symptoms of CHF and recurrent pulmonary infections. CXR shows cardiomegaly and increased pulmonary blood flow (PBF). ECG shows left ventricular hypertrophy (LVH), right ventricular hypertrophy (RVH), or both.

Transposition of the great arteries (TGA) is the most common cyanotic lesion to present in the first week of life. The right ventricle feeds the aorta, whereas the left ventricle feeds the pulmonary artery (Fig. 47–5). Mixing occurs via an atrial septal defect (ASD) or patent foramen ovale, ventricular septal defect, or patent ductus arteriosus (PDA) to sustain life, as the pulmonary and systemic circulations are in parallel. Symptoms include cyanosis and tachypnea in the first days of life; often

▶ **TABLE 47-2. NORMAL BENIGN CARDIAC MURMURS**

Murmur	Age	Character	Positioning	Etiology	Differential Diagnosis
Still's vibratory	Most common benign in children 2–6 y old, can occur infant to adolescent	I–III/VI early systolic ejection murmur, left lower sternal border to apex, twanging musical quality	Louder when patient supine	Postulated to be from ventricular false tendons	VSD murmur is harsher
Pulmonary flow murmur	Child to young adult	II–III/VI crescendo–decrescendo, early-to-midsystolic, left upper sternal border, second intercostal space	Louder when patient supine, increased on full expiration	Flow in the pulmonary outflow tract	ASD has fixed split S2; pulmonic stenosis has higher pitched, longer murmur, ejection click
Peripheral pulmonic stenosis	Newborn to 1-y-old	I–II/VI low-pitched, early-to-midsystolic ejection murmur in the pulmonic area and radiating to axillae and back	Increased with viral respiratory infections, lower heart rate, decreased with tachycardia	Turbulence at the peripheral pulmonary artery branches due to narrow angles in infants	Significant branch pulmonary artery stenosis in Williams syndrome; congenital rubella has higher-pitched murmur, extends beyond S2; older child
Supraclavicular or brachio-cephalic	Child to young adult	Crescendo–decrescendo, systolic, low-pitched, above the clavicles, radiating to neck, abrupt onset and brief	Decreases with rapid hyperextension of the shoulders	Flow through the major brachiocephalic vessels arising from the aorta	Idiopathic hypertrophic subaortic stenosis: louder with valsalva and softer with rapid squatting. Aortic stenosis: higher-pitched, ejection click
Venous hum	Child	Faint to grade VI, continuous, humming, low ant. neck to lateral sternocleidomastoid muscle to ant. chest infraclavicular	Louder when sitting, looking away from murmur; softer when lying, with compressed jugular vein or head turned toward murmur	Turbulence from the internal jugular and subclavian veins entering the superior vena cava	Patent ductus arteriosus has machinery murmur, not compressible, bounding pulses
Mammary souffle	Pregnant, lactating, rarely adolescent	High-pitched, systole into diastole, ant. chest over breast, varies day to day		Plethora of vessels over chest wall	Patent ductus arteriosus has machinery murmur, does not vary day to day

▶ **TABLE 47-4. AGE-SPECIFIC QRS AXIS**

Age	Range	Mean
1–7 d	80–160	125
1–4 wk	60–160	110
1–3 mo	40–120	80
3–6 mo	20–80	65
6–12 mo	0–100	65
1–3 y	20–100	55

Source: With permission from Hakim SN, Toepper WC. Cardiac disease in children. In: Rosen P, Barkin RM, eds. *Emergency Medicine: Concepts and Clinical Practice II.* St. Louis, MO: Mosby-Year Book; 1992:546.

▶ **TABLE 47-3. DURATION OF ECG INTERVALS (VALUES IN SECONDS)**

Age	P-R Limits	QRS Limits	QTc Limits
0–7 d	0.08–0.12	0.04–0.10	0.34–0.54
7–30 d	0.08–0.12	0.04–0.07	0.30–0.50
1–3 mo	0.08–0.16	0.05–0.08	0.46–0.47
3–6 mo	0.08–0.12	0.05–0.08	0.35–0.46
6–12 mo	0.08–0.14	0.04–0.08	0.31–0.49
1–3 y	0.08–0.16	0.04–0.08	0.34–0.43

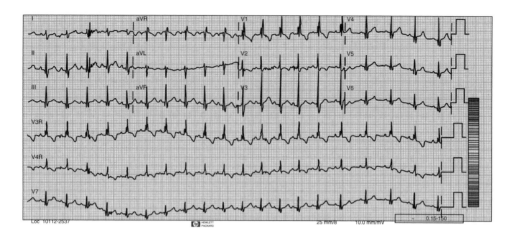

Figure 47–3. Pediatric ECG with right ventricular hypertrophy in a patient with ASD.

there is no murmur. CXR may be normal or may have an "egg on a string" appearance. ECG shows RAD and RVH but may be normal in the first days of life. If the mixing lesion is small, the patient presents early with cyanosis. If there is a large VSD, the infant may present with CHF and cyanosis at 2 to 6 weeks of age.

Total anomalous pulmonary venous return (TAPVR) has many variations depending on whether it is total or partial (from one to four veins connecting anomalously to a location other than the left atrium, usually to the right atrium) and where the veins terminate (Fig. 47–6). Cyanosis is mild to moderate, depending on the degree of mixing of the right and left circulations. There is often little murmur, but the S2 is widely split. CXR may show a "snowman" appearance, and ECG may show RVH, RAD, and right atrial enlargement (RAE).

Tetralogy of Fallot (TOF) is the most common cyanotic congenital heart disease seen in children older than 4 years. It consists of right ventricular (RV) outflow obstruction with resultant right ventricular hypertrophy (RVH), a large VSD, and an overriding aorta (Fig. 47–7). Patients have a loud, harsh, pansystolic murmur in the left sternal border, and often a single S2. CXR shows a boot-shaped heart (*coeur en sabot*), a decreased PBF, and in 25%, a right-sided aortic arch. ECG shows RAD and RVH. Severity ranges widely, and depends on the degree of RV outflow obstruction.

Tricuspid atresia must be accompanied by an intra-atrial right-to-left shunt (ASD or patent foramen ovale) (Fig. 47–8). Tricuspid atresia is rare and findings depend on the presence or absence of a VSD and presence or hypoplasia of the right ventricle. *Ebstein's anomaly* is a displacement of the tricuspid valve into the RV. Severity varies widely depending on the degree of displacement.

Hypoplastic left heart syndrome (HLHS) is a rare anomaly in which the right ventricle perfuses both circulations via the pulmonary artery (Fig. 47–9). The systemic circulation is perfused through a PDA. Management spans the entire range of no treatment, palliative surgery, and cardiac transplantation, depending on the parents' choice and resources available.

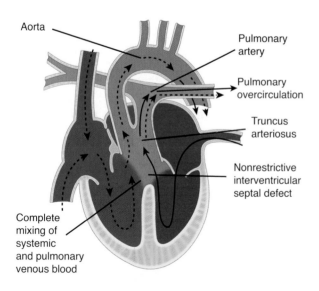

Figure 47–4. Truncus arteriosus.

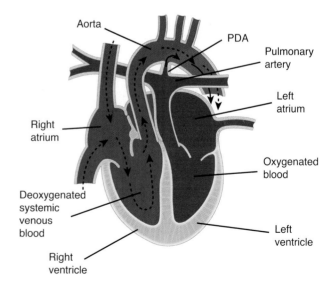

Figure 47–5. Transposition of the great arteries.

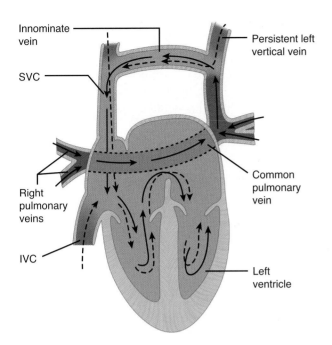

Figure 47–6. Total anomalous pulmonary venous connection.

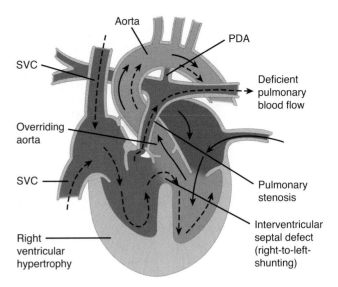

Figure 47–7. Tetralogy of Fallot.

Pulmonic stenosis (PS) often produces no symptoms and may be recognized when a murmur is noted during routine physical examination (Fig. 47–10). Once pulmonic stenosis is moderate to severe, there may be cyanosis on exertion, syncope, RV failure, and even sudden death. An ejection click is typically heard before the systolic ejection murmur in the left second to third intercostal space. CXR shows a prominent main pulmonary artery and normal to decreased PBF. ECG may be normal or show RVH.

Aortic coarctation accounts for 10% of congenital heart lesions. The narrowing most commonly occurs just distal to the left subclavian artery branch. Symptoms range from CHF in in-

fancy to hypertension in childhood or adulthood (Fig. 47–11). The median age at referral is 5 to 8 years. Blood pressure is elevated in the upper compared with the lower extremities, and femoral pulses are weak or absent. Children may complain of pain in the legs after exercise. A systolic ejection murmur at the apex radiates to the interscapular back. There may be a diastolic murmur of aortic regurgitation as well. In some patients a thrill is felt in the suprasternal notch. CXR is normal initially, but may show notching of ribs 3 through 8 posteriorly as collateral circulation develops. ECG shows LVH in the severely affected infant. Children may present with complications of hypertension, including intracranial hemorrhage.

Atrial septal defect (ASD) accounts for 12% of congenital heart lesions. Many patients are asymptomatic and undiagnosed until childhood or even adulthood. A soft systolic

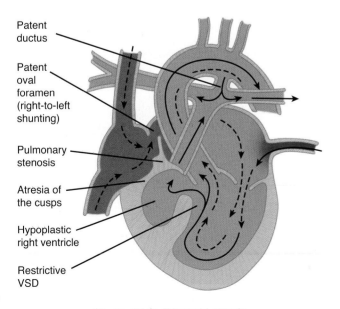

Figure 47–8. Tricuspid atresia.

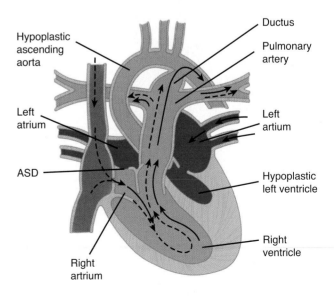

Figure 47–9. Hypoplastic left heart syndrome.

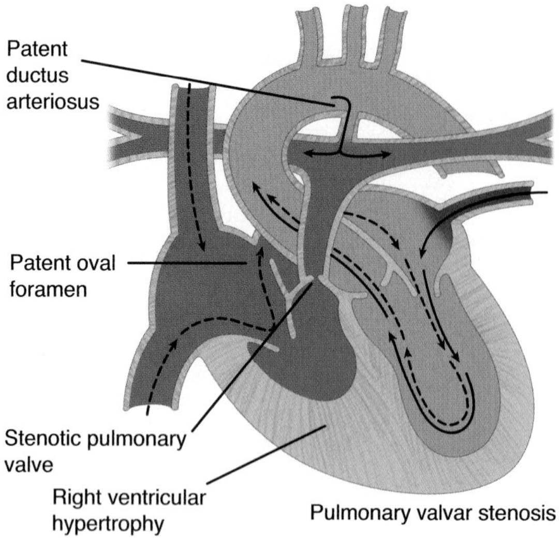

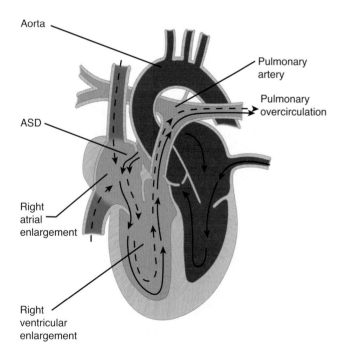

Figure 47–10. Pulmonary stenosis.

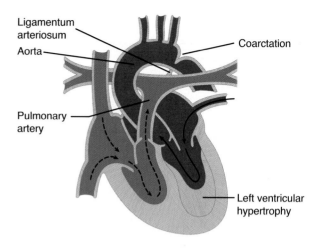

Figure 47–11. Coarctation of the aorta.

ejection murmur of increased pulmonic flow is heard in the left upper sternal border, and S2 is widely split and fixed (does not close with respiration) (Fig. 47–12). CXR shows right-sided chamber enlargement and increased PBF, and ECG shows an RSR' in lead V1, often right bundle-branch block, and an increased PR interval.

Ventricular septal defect (VSD) is the most common congenital heart lesion. Small VSDs have a high rate of spontaneous closure. A harsh pansystolic murmur is heard in the left lower sternal border. If the defect is large, respiratory symptoms and CHF develop in the first 3 months of life. As pulmonary vascular resistance decreases, left-to-right shunting via the VSD increases (Fig. 47–13). CXR may be normal or show

signs of CHF. ECG may show LVH, RVH, and left atrial enlargement (LAE) if the defect is large.

Patent ductus arteriosus (PDA) occurs in 8:1000 premature infants and 2:1000 full-term infants. A continuous machinery-like murmur is heard in the left second intercostal space, first appearing at 2 to 5 days of age. Prior to this, the pulmonary vascular resistance is high enough that there is no significant left-to-right shunting through the ductus. The diastolic runoff into the PDA generates bounding pulses. Infants may develop CHF, or may compensate with myocardial hypertrophy and present later with exercise intolerance. CXR shows increased PBF and possible cardiomegaly (Fig. 47–14). ECG is normal or shows LVH. Premature infants often respond to indomethacin with closure of the PDA.

Aortic stenosis (AS), often associated with a bicuspid aortic valve, may be asymptomatic; however, severe aortic stenosis can present as shock in an infant (Fig. 47–15). Once symptomatic, patients complain of dyspnea on exertion, fatigue, abdominal pain, increased sweating, and exertional syncope

Figure 47–12. Atrial septal defect.

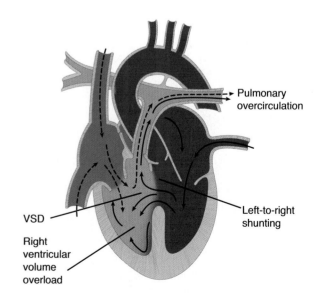

Figure 47–13. Ventricular septal defect.

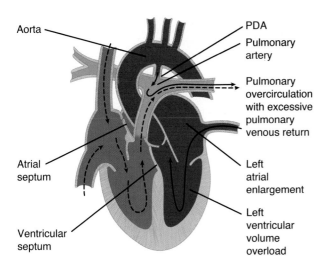

Figure 47–14. Patent ductus arteriosus.

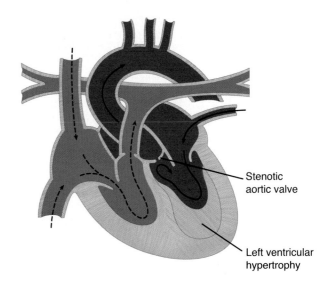

Figure 47–15. Aortic stenosis.

(indicative of critical aortic stenosis). An ejection click is heard before the systolic ejection murmur in the right upper sternal border, radiating into the neck. There may be a left ventricular thrill or heave. CXR may be normal and ECG reflects LVH.

Atrioventricular septal defect or AV canal is associated with Down syndrome (Fig. 47–16). Symptoms include those of CHF, poor growth, and frequent respiratory infections. CXR shows increased PBF and cardiomegaly. ECG shows an increased PR interval, RAE and/or LAE, and RVH. The axis is often superior (extreme left-axis deviation).

▶ COMMON PRESENTATIONS

Rather than memorizing a multitude of individual lesions, the emergency physician should concentrate on a few scenarios of presentations: the undifferentiated sick infant,

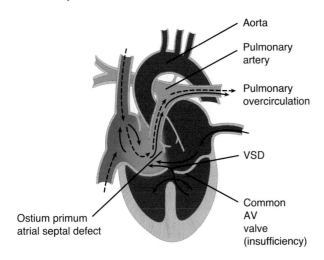

Complete AV-canel
(artrial and ventricular level left-to-right shunting

Figure 47–16. AV septal defect.

ductal-dependent lesions, CHF, hypoxemic "Tet" spells, and presentations seen in older children. These scenarios require rapid emergency management to prevent further decompensation and cardiac arrest. Knowledge of the exact lesion is often not necessary to provide the critical management needed in these cases.

UNDIFFERENTIATED SICK INFANT

In emergency medicine, patients present in two main categories: the "H&P patient" and the "ABC patient". The "H&P patient" is typically stable, with a chronic or subacute presentation; the emergency physician has some time to examine, run tests, observe, and come to a diagnosis. The "ABC patient" presents acutely in distress or in extremis and the emergency physician must be ready to diagnose and treat simultaneously.

The sick infant is the prototype of the "ABC" patient; often with little information available and the need to intervene is palpable. Since there is significant similarity in presentation between congenital heart disease and other similarly life-threatening disorders, a systematic approach is needed for the wide differential diagnosis (Fig. 47–17). The mnemonic "THE MISFITS" outlines the broad and varied causes of acute illness in very young children.[6]

T—Trauma (accidental and nonaccidental)

H—Heart disease and hypovolemia

E—Endocrine (congenital adrenal hyperplasia and thyrotoxicosis)

M—Metabolic (electrolyte abnormalities)

I—Inborn errors of metabolism

S—Sepsis (meningitis, pneumonia, and pyelonephritis)

F—Formula problems (over- or underdilution)

I—Intestinal disasters (intussusception, necrotizing enterocolitis, and volvulus)

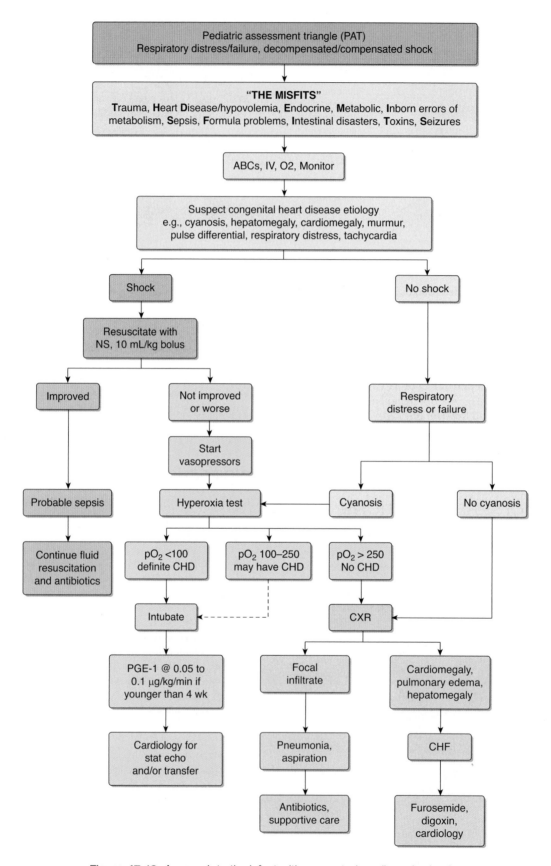

Figure 47–16. Approach to the infant with suspected cardiogenic shock.

T—Toxins

S—Seizures

As with any sick infant, assessment and intervention in airway, breathing, and circulation is critical, with close attention to vital signs, such as tachycardia and tachypnea. Always check blood glucose and keep the infant warm during the course of evaluation and treatment. Even with a detailed differential diagnosis, final diagnosis may not be possible until much later in the child's management because conditions such as sepsis and congenital heart disease have significant overlap. For example, concomitant treatment with fluids, antibiotics, and possibly prostaglandin E_1 (PGE_1) is appropriate in these circumstances.

The most important mantra in the care for the sick newborn is that neonates who present in shock in the first few weeks of life are presumed to have ductal-dependent systemic flow until proven otherwise. Resuscitation depends on opening the ductus arteriosus with PGE_1. It is appropriate to start PGE_1 before a definitive anatomic diagnosis is made.[1]

This dictum should be balanced with an even more basic tenet of emergency medicine: perform an intervention and carefully evaluate its effect. This is true for any patient, but essential in treating critically ill newborns. An algorithmic approach reminds the emergency physician of possible pathways, not to usurp clinical judgment. For example, some children with congenital heart disease may worsen with supplemental oxygen; at baseline, an infant with congenital heart disease may have preexisting pulmonary hypertension that shunts blood to the systemic circulation, maintaining adequate blood pressure. Overoxygenation can dilate the pulmonary vasculature to the point where it shunts blood away from the systemic circulation, causing sustained hypotension and either no improvement or worsening of the patient's condition with oxygen therapy.[7] Oxygen is a cornerstone of therapy in sick infants and the physician should not hesitate to begin treatment with oxygen. However, this rare adverse effect serves to illustrate the importance of assessment, intervention, and reassessment.

DUCTAL-DEPENDENT LESIONS AND CARDIOGENIC SHOCK

Lesions which are completely dependent on a patent ductus arteriosus for systemic or pulmonary blood flow present with acute onset circulatory failure and shock when the ductus closes, typically within the first week of life. Such lesions include hypoplastic left heart syndrome (HLHS), severe aortic coarctation, interrupted aortic arch, and lesions such as pulmonary atresia or transposition of the great arteries (TGA) without a mixing lesion, such as a VSD. No symptoms or signs of congenital heart disease may have been noted prior to presentation, in the newborn nursery or at home. Ductal-dependent cardiac failure should be suspected in any infant in the first week of life with sudden-onset circulatory collapse leading to hypoperfusion, hypotension, severe acidosis, and cyanosis. Infants may present in the second week of life, but rarely present beyond 4 weeks of age.

As noted above, the mainstay of therapy for suspected ductal-dependent cardiac shock is PGE_1 infusion. PGE_1 main-

tains the patency of the ductus arteriosus. It is infused initially at 0.05 to 0.1 µg/kg/min and advanced to 0.2 µg/kg/min if necessary.[8] When an increase in PaO_2 is noted, titrate down to the lowest effective dose; the usual dosage range is 0.01 to 0.4 µg/kg/min. Adverse effects include hyperthermia, apnea, hypotension, rash, tremors, focal seizures, and bradycardia. Nevertheless, PGE_1 is critical for infants in ductal-dependent cardiac shock and should be initiated in the emergency department. Be prepared to provide definitive airway management in the case of apnea, and to add inotropic medications as needed for circulatory support. Other etiologies for shock must be entertained and treated as well, such as sepsis. A pediatric cardiologist must be consulted immediately and the patient admitted to the pediatric or neonatal intensive care unit.

CONGESTIVE HEART FAILURE

Children differ from adults both in the causes and in the presentation of CHF. A common scenario is that of an infant 2- to 6-months old with a left-to-right shunting lesion (VSD, PDA, AV canal defect, or less commonly, an ASD alone) resulting in volume overload and CHF (Fig. 47–18). Excessive pressure load from left-sided obstruction (e.g., aortic coarctation, aortic stenosis) may also result in CHF. Causes other than congenital heart lesions include myocardial dysfunction (e.g., cardiomyopathies) and dysrhythmias.

Symptoms are gradual in onset and may be subtle. They include poor feeding (increased time to feed) or sweating while feeding; poor growth; irritability, lethargy, or a weak cry; increased respiratory effort, dyspnea, tachypnea, chronic cough, or wheezing; and increased frequency of respiratory infections.

Physical examination may reveal the following: tachypnea, retractions, nasal flaring, grunting, wheezing, or rales (although less commonly than in adults). One may also find tachycardia, a gallop rhythm, hyperactive precordium, murmur, poor peripheral pulses with delayed capillary refill, and

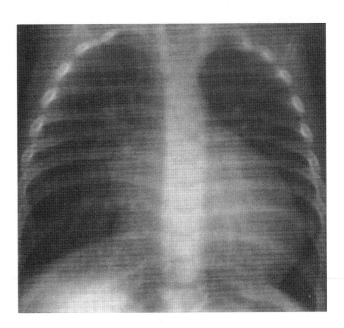

Figure 47–17. Congestive heart failure.

▶ **TABLE 47–5. MEAN BNP VALUES IN CHILDREN[10]**

Study	No. of Patients	Age Range	Kit Used	Mean BNP Level (pg/mL)
Koch and Singer	12	Day 0–1	Biosite	231.6 SD 197.5
Koch and Singer	14	Day 4–6	Biosite	48.4 SD 49.1
Kunii et al.	11	Day 1	Shiono RIA	118.8 SD 83.2
Kunii et al.	11	Day 7	Shiono RIA	15.3 SD 7.8
Soldin et al.	50	<31 d	Biosite	97.5th percentile: 1585

Biosite, San Diego, CA; Shiono RIA, Shionogi, Osaka, Japan.

hepatomegaly (a cardinal sign of CHF in infants). Jugular venous distension and peripheral edema, often seen in adults with CHF, are rarely seen in young children. If present, edema is best appreciated in the eyelids, sacrum, and legs. More commonly, children will present with hepatic congestion or hepatomegaly, as the relatively pliable liver becomes congested with venous blood. CXR shows cardiomegaly (cardiothoracic ratio >0.55 in infants, >0.50 for children older than 1 year) and increased pulmonary vascularity. When evaluating for cardiomegaly, remember that infants often have a prominent thymus shadow overlying the heart; the thymus gives an appearance of an enlarged mediastinum and will be apparent as anterior to the heart on the lateral film. ECG findings depend on the specific lesion.

Treatment includes oxygen to keep saturations about 95%. Overoxygenating the patient may lead to pulmonary vascular dilation and worsened failure. Keep the infant in a semireclining position (such as when in an infant car seat) if possible. Fluid and sodium restriction is necessary, and furosemide should be given at 1 mg/kg intravenously. Nitrates are not first-line emergent therapy in children. In consultation with a pediatric cardiologist, the patient should be started on digoxin. Consult a pediatric drug handbook for digitalization doses. Patients may require sedation, but closely monitor their airway and ventilatory efforts. Make preparations for endotracheal intubation and ventilatory support in the event that they are needed. If a patient's respiratory status allows, a trial of continuous positive airway pressure (CPAP) may be applied nasally in an attempt to avoid the need for intubation. If the patient is in shock, fluids must be used cautiously (boluses of only 5 mL/kg, if at all), and inotropic support with dopamine or dobutamine may be more appropriate. Complete blood count, chemistry panel, calcium level, rapid bedside glucose test, and arterial blood gas should be assessed. Monitor vital signs, including blood pressure, cardiac rhythm, and oxygen saturation, continuously.

B-TYPE NATRIURETIC PEPTIDE ASSAY

The role of B-type natriuretic peptide (BNP) is well described in specific congenital heart lesions in children. It may be used judiciously in the emergency department as an ancillary screening tool in the evaluation of the dyspneic young child. BNP levels spike at birth with the physiologic transition from fetal to neonatal circulation, reaching a plateau at day 3 to 4; BNP levels subsequently fall to a constant level during infancy.[9] As natriuretic peptides do not cross the placenta, BNP measurements will reflect the neonate's own production and clearance.

The interpretation of normal BNP ranges is currently under continued investigation, with variability due to age of patient, kits used, and specific cardiac lesions. Nonetheless, multiple studies have resulted in an attempt to provide normal mean BNP values in children (Table 47–5). There are as of yet no established BNP "cutoff" values in children to support definitively or to rule out CHF. Currently, BNP values can be interpreted as either consistent with the normal mean value or not. The standard deviations are reported as a reference, and not as a diagnostic tool. As always, the physician should note the normal laboratory values used at each institution.

In the case of CHF in children, just as in adults, the patient's clinical presentation will often provide an adequate basis to make the diagnosis. No single laboratory test should replace or supercede a clinician's judgment. However, in the undifferentiated dyspneic child, a BNP level may help to exclude the diagnosis if very low and support the diagnosis if markedly high.

HYPOXEMIC "TET" SPELLS

Sudden-onset spells of increased cyanosis may occur in young children with tetralogy of Fallot and less commonly in other complex lesions with decreased PBF, such as tricuspid atresia. Various theories exist regarding the initiation of a spell. The classic teaching is a sudden "clamping down" of the pulmonary infundibular right ventricular outflow tract, leading to increased right-to-left shunting; although not a complete explanation, this provides a useful model to understand spell physiology. The increased right-to-left shunting leads to hypoxemia, cyanosis, and acidosis. Attempts at compensation occur via hyperventilation and decreased systemic vascular resistance (SVR) to increase cardiac output. Decreased SVR and increased venous return result in further shunting, perpetuating a cycle of ongoing shunting, and hypoxemia.

Spells are most common in children younger than 2 years and often occur when SVR is naturally decreased: in the morning after awakening, after a feed, after defecation, and after a bout of crying. Symptoms include restlessness, irritability, or lethargy. Signs include a sudden increase in cyanosis and occasional syncope. Hyperpnea is a cardinal sign of hypoxemic spells. Previously appreciated murmurs of left-to-right shunting may disappear during a spell. The "tet spell" may occur in a previously acyanotic patient and may be the first presentation of a child with previously unrecognized congenital heart disease. Spells must be differentiated from seizures, CHF, and

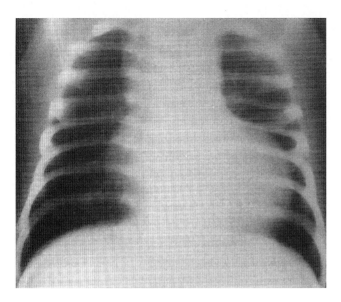

Figure 47–18. Tetralogy of Fallot.

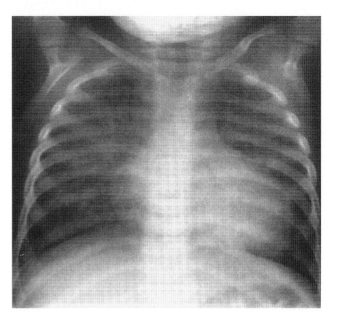

Figure 47–19. Coarctation of the aorta.

respiratory disease. Differentiating factors include history of congenital heart disease, profound cyanosis unresponsive to oxygen, and presence of features consistent with tetralogy of Fallot (Fig. 47–19).

Keep the child as calm as possible, in a position of comfort with a parent present. Avoid unnecessary painful or stressful procedures. Provide oxygen, although it will have little effect in shunt-induced hypoxemia. Place the child in a knee-chest position (to simulate squatting) to increase SVR. Older children may even have a history of squatting on their own to abort spells. Morphine, 0.05 to 0.2 mg/kg intravenous or intramuscular is the traditional first-line medical therapy, although the exact mechanism by which it "breaks" the spell is unknown. Administer a fluid bolus of 10 mL/kg normal saline intravenously to counteract the vasodilatory effects of morphine and to ensure adequate preload, on which pulmonary flow is dependent.

Successful therapy will be evidenced by improved pulse oximetry, decreased cyanosis, decreased hyperpnea, and a calmer child. If the above therapies are unsuccessful, propranolol 0.1 to 0.25 mg/kg (mechanism of action unclear) by a slow intravenous route may be given and repeated once after 15 minutes. Phenylephrine 5 to 20 μg/kg/dose (agonist resulting in increased SVR) intravenously may be used and repeated every 10 to 15 minutes as necessary. Propranolol and phenylephrine are customarily given in consultation with a cardiologist. If these interventions fail, general anesthesia may be necessary.

PRESENTATIONS IN OLDER CHILDREN AND ADULTS

Clinically, unapparent lesions are frequently discovered by recognition of a murmur during routine physical examination. Common lesions include ASD, small VSD, PDA, PS, AS, and aortic coarctation. Patients with an ASD will also be noted to have a fixed, split S2. Adult patients with unrepaired ASD may present with atrial arrhythmias, often in the fourth decade of life. Patients with PDA and AS may present with dyspnea on exertion and fatigue. Patients with critical AS may present with syncope. Patients with critical PS may present with cyanosis on exertion, right-sided heart failure, or syncope. Patients with aortic coarctation (Fig. 47–20) are often diagnosed during evaluation for hypertension. They may present with symptoms resulting from the hypertension such as headache, intracranial hemorrhage, dizziness, palpitations, or epistaxis. Occasionally, they may complain of claudication due to decreased perfusion of the lower extremities.

HYPERTROPHIC CARDIOMYOPATHY

Hypertrophic cardiomyopathy is a genetic disorder of sarcomeric proteins that results in varying degrees of left ventricular hypertrophy, found in 1:500 of the general population.[11] It is a primary myopathy, not secondary to hypertension or aortic stenosis. The term hypertrophic cardiomyopathy (HCM) includes both hypertrophic obstructive cardiomyopathy (HOCM) and idiopathic hypertrophic subaortic stenosis (IHSS). The distinction is made depending on the degree of outflow obstruction and/or asymmetric hypertrophy found in each case. The shared feature is diastolic dysfunction, with resultant impaired cardiac output on exertion.

Approximately half of patients with hypertrophic cardiomyopathy have a family history. Young children may be asymptomatic, and the first clinical manifestation may be sudden death. Children and young adults may complain of dyspnea, angina, fatigue, or syncope, especially after strenuous exercise. Patients often have a harsh systolic murmur increasing after the first heart sound ("diamond-shaped") best heard at the lower left sternal border or apex; this may be accompanied by an S4. The murmur may be more prominent with tachycardia or Valsalva maneuver, which both reduce ventricular volume, mimicking the conditions of exercise in these patients. Conversely, the murmur may decrease with squatting, hand grip, or leg raise, which augment venous return and increase ventricular volume. Patients may also demonstrate a prominent apical impulse and rapidly rising carotid impulse on physical examination.

ECG may show LVH and/or wide Q waves. Chest radiograph may be normal or reflect a mild-to-moderate increase in the size of the cardiac silhouette. Echocardiography is the mainstay of diagnosis. Treatment options span from medication such as β-blockers or calcium-channel blockers to septal myomectomy to placement of an automated implantable cardioverter-defibrillator. Any child with a history consistent with arrhythmia or syncope warrants inpatient investigation, including urgent echocardiography and possibly electrophysiology studies. If the clinician has high suspicion of HCM in a currently asymptomatic child without high-risk historical features such as arrhythmia or syncope, nonemergent referral to a cardiologist is recommended.[12] The child should avoid dehydration and refrain from strenuous activity until a definitive diagnosis is obtained.

ISOLATED CORONARY ARTERY ANOMALIES

Congenital lesions of the coronary arteries are uncommon, occurring in less than 1% of the population.[13] During fetal development, abnormalities may form affecting the number (duplication of artery), site of origin (e.g., from pulmonary trunk), anatomic course (e.g., between the aorta and pulmonary trunk), anomalous termination (e.g., fistula formation), or structure (stenosis and atresia) of the coronary arteries and virtually any coronary artery may be affected. These lesions may be isolated to a single coronary artery or associated with other congenital heart defects.

Depending on the lesion, patients may present from infancy to young adulthood. Neonates with an isolated coronary artery anomaly (ICAA) may demonstrate anginal symptoms with irritability, episodic diaphoresis and/or color change when symptomatic. Older infants may have poor feeding, dyspnea, failure to thrive, or unexplained episodes of pallor. Diaphoresis during feeding is an ominous sign, reflecting both a decreased "exercise tolerance" and a splanchnic steal syndrome. Older children and young adults typically present with more familiar ischemic symptoms such as angina and dyspnea. Unfortunately, a child's first presentation may be sudden death.

A rare but serious lesion primarily affects neonates—anomalous origin of the left coronary artery arising from the pulmonary artery (ALCAPA), also called Bland–White–Garland syndrome.[14,15] Most children present within the first few months of life, often with nonspecific complaints such as irritability; they are often misdiagnosed with colic. Signs and symptoms of CHF, such as tachypnea, tachycardia, poor feeding, and weight gain may ensue. On physical examination, the baby may be completely normal or show signs of CHF. ECG may show an anterolateral infarct pattern with deep and wide Q waves laterally and absent Q waves inferiorly. Chest x-ray may be consistent with CHF. Echocardiography with Doppler

flow is often diagnostic, especially if retrograde flow from the left coronary artery to the pulmonary trunk is shown.

Surgical correction is necessary to restore blood flow. Emergency department care is supportive, with great attention paid to volume status and very careful use of diuretics and nitrates if needed. Titrate oxygen to effect; 100% oxygen may dilate pulmonary vasculature and create a steal syndrome from the right coronary artery to the pulmonary arteries in this lesion. Although isolated coronary artery anomalies are rare, they should be considered in the child with unexplained age-specific anginal symptoms.

EISENMENGER SYNDROME

Patients with a large left-to-right shunt left unrepaired, either by choice or because the lesion was never recognized, gradually develop pulmonary vascular disease due to the increased volume overload. When pulmonary hypertension becomes severe enough, the direction of shunting will reverse to right to left, and cyanosis ensues. Typically, this occurs in adolescence to early adulthood. Patients may complain of decreased exercise tolerance, dyspnea on exertion, hemoptysis, palpitations due to atrial arrhythmias, and symptoms of hyperviscosity due to chronic polycythemia (vision disturbances, fatigue, headache, dizziness, paresthesias, and even cerebrovascular accident). Brain abscesses can occur with right-to-left passage of an infected embolus. On examination, the murmur may no longer be present with the disappearance of left-to-right shunting, and S2 is loud due to the pulmonary hypertension. CXR shows decreased vasculature (pruned pattern), and ECG shows RVH. Although no definitive therapy exists, other than heart–lung transplant, patients should avoid dehydration, heavy exertion, altitude, vasodilators, and pregnancy, which is associated with a high-mortality rate. Symptoms of hyperviscosity may be treated with phlebotomy and isovolemic replacement. Patients should be medically managed by a cardiologist to optimize cardiac function as long as possible.

▶ CARE OF THE POSTCARDIAC SURGERY CONGENITAL HEART PATIENT

CATEGORIES OF REPAIR

Patients with true complete repairs generally lead a normal life after repair. True complete repairs are typically performed successfully for ASD, VSD, PDA, aortic coarctation, and TGA (switch procedure). Repairs of tetralogy of Fallot, AV canal, and valve obstructions typically result in anatomic repairs with residual lesions, and late complications may occur (Table 47–6). Repairs requiring prosthetic materials such as pulmonary atresia, truncus arteriosus, and prosthetic valve replacements will require replacement of the prosthetic material due to growth of the child or degeneration of the material. Physiologic repairs improve the patient's blood flow physiology but do not result in normal cardiac anatomy. These palliative repairs, which include the Fontan operation for lesions resulting in a functionally single ventricle and the Mustard

▶ **TABLE 47–6. SELECTED CARDIAC PROCEDURES AND COMPLICATIONS[16,17]**

Procedure	Lesions Addressed	Complications
Atrial septostomy (i.e., Rashkind procedure) Surgical defect created to mix blood between atria	Hypoplastic left heart TGA Tricuspid atresia	Arrhythmias
Blalock-Taussig shunt, modified Palliative systemic-to-pulmonary shunt; uses systemic arterial flow to increase PBF	Hypoplastic left heart Pulmonic stenosis Tetralogy of Fallot Tricuspid atresia	Infective endocarditis Paradoxical embolism Shunt thrombosis Excessive PBF with mild CHF
Fontan, modified Fontan Anastamosis of SVC to right pulmonary artery (Glenn procedure) followed by anastamosis of right atrium to IVC. Separates systemic, pulmonary circuits	Hypoplastic left heart Tricuspid atresia	Atrial arrhythmias Intracardiac thrombosis Thromboembolism in either arterial or venous circulation Protein-losing enteropathy
Glenn, modified Glenn SVC to right pulmonary artery shunts. Step toward Fontan procedure; palliative	Hypoplastic left heart Tricuspid atresia	Same as Fontan
Orthotopic heart transplant Donor heart is grafted onto recipient's intact chambers and/or great vessels	Hypoplastic left heart Pulmonary atresia	Viral, bacterial, or protozoal infections, especially CMV, PCP; acute, subacute, or chronic rejection
Norwood Complete restructuring of flow, including Aortic arch reconstruction, modified Blalock-Taussig, creation of surgical VSD; multiple stages	Hypoplastic left heart	Excessive PBF with low systemic cardiac output
Rastelli operation for TOF VSD patch closure, reconstruction of right ventricular outflow with homograft or prosthetic valve	Tetralogy of Fallot	Arrhythmias Infective endocarditis
Ross Pulmonary root autograft to replace aortic root and replacement of the pulmonic valve	Aortic stenosis	Arrhythmias Left ventricular hypertrophy
Repair of ASD, VSD Various patches using autologous and synthetic materials	ASD VSD	Arrhythmias (more common in ASD than VSD repair)
TGA repair Various: Arterial switch of Jatene, Mustard, Rastelli for TGA, Senning procedures	TGA	Supraventricular tachycardia Sick sinus syndrome Tricuspid regurgitation
Valvotomy Opening of stenotic aortic or pulmonary valves either via balloon or open procedure	Aortic stenosis Pulmonic stenosis	Arrhythmia Infective endocarditis

CMV, cytomegalovirus; PCP, pneumocystis carinii, i.e., pneumocystis jirovecii.

operation and Arterial Switch of Jatene for TGA, invariably produce late complications

There exists a myriad of variations of congenital heart disease and procedures for repair (Table 47–6). The key concept for care of these children is a careful examination and consideration of complications such as arrhythmias, infective endocarditis (IE), and thromboembolism. Consultation with the child's cardiologist or primary care physician may be helpful in the management and disposition of postoperative patients.

POSTOPERATIVE COMPLICATIONS

Arrhythmias are the most common problem and may present with symptoms of palpitations, decreased appetite, emesis, and decreased exercise tolerance.[18,19] Arrhythmias may be a result of the surgical repair, the underlying lesion (e.g., Ebstein's anomaly), or medical therapy (e.g., digoxin toxicity). Supraventricular tachycardia (SVT) is the most common clinically significant arrhythmia and is seen in lesions repaired with atriotomy (Senning, Mustard, Fontan, ASD repair, and

TAPVR repair). Bradycardia due to sinoatrial nodal disease is seen in 20% of patients status post-Fontan repair, and first-degree block may occur after AV canal repair. Ventricular arrhythmias occur uncommonly after VSD or TOF repair and are decreasing further due to increased use of transatrial approaches to repair. Right bundle-branch block is common after VSD, TOF, and AV canal repairs. Premature ventricular contractions are benign if isolated and unifocal (order a 24-hour Holter monitor test); consult a cardiologist if they are frequent, coupled, or multifocal. Isolated, infrequent premature atrial contractions are common in normal and postcardiac surgery patients.

Residual or recurrent lesions occur as a complication of repair, due to incomplete success of the repair, outgrowing prosthetic materials, or from conduit stenosis. Coarctation recurs in 10% of repaired patients. Recurrent stenosis after PS or AS repair is common, as is aortic insufficiency after AS repair. Recurrent stenosis may be recognized by a new murmur or a change in exercise tolerance. A residual small VSD around the borders of the patch is present in 15% to 25% of patients after VSD or TOF repair; most close spontaneously within 6 to 12 months.

Endocarditis is a significant complication seen in congenital heart patients before and after surgical repair (Table 47–7). The rate in patients with uncorrected congenital heart disease is 0.1% to 0.2% per patient-year; this decreases to 0.02% after correction for many lesions. Unrepaired complex congenital heart disease carries the highest risk, at 1.5% per patient-year. ASDs of the ostium secundum type are the lowest risk lesions and do not require prophylaxis for procedures, even if unrepaired. Patients with repaired ASD, VSD, PDA, aortic coarctation, and PS (no mechanical valve) without residual lesions, and patients' status post–heart transplantation or pacemaker insertion also carry a low risk and do not require prophylaxis. Patients' status post-AS or -TOF repair and those with prosthetic valves remain at high risk. Antibiotic prophylaxis should be given to patients at high risk prior to invasive procedures likely to produce bac-

> ▶ **TABLE 47–7. CARDIAC CONDITIONS ASSOCIATED WITH THE HIGHEST RISK OF ADVERSE OUTCOME FROM ENDOCARDITIS[21]**

- Prosthetic cardiac valve or prosthetic material used for cardiac valve repair
- Previous infective endocarditis
- Congenital heart disease*:
  ○ Unrepaired cyanotic CHD, including palliative shunts and conduits
  ○ Completely repaired congenital heart defect with prosthetic material or device, whether placed by surgery or by catheter intervention, during the first 6 mo after the procedure[†]
  ○ Repaired CHD with residual defects at the site or adjacent to the site of a prosthetic patch or prosthetic device (which inhibit endotheliazation)
- Cardiac transplantation recipients who develop cardiac valvulopathy

*Except for the conditions listed above, antibiotic prophylaxis is no longer recommended for any other form of CHD.
[†]Prophylaxis is reasonable because endotheliazation of prosthetic material occurs within 6 mo after the procedure.

> ▶ **TABLE 47–8. PROCEDURES FOR WHICH PROPHYLAXIS IS RECOMMENDED[21]**

All dental procedures that involve manipulation of gingival tissue or the periapical region of teeth or perforation of the oral mucosa*
Consider prophylaxis for incisional procedures on the respiratory tract, infected skin, or musculoskeletal tissue only for high-risk patients.

*The following procedures do not need prophylaxis: routine anesthetic injections through noninfected tissue, taking dental radiographs, placement of removable prosthodontic or orthodontic appliances, adjustment of orthodontic appliances, placement of orthodontic brackets, shedding of deciduous teeth, and bleeding from trauma to the lips or oral mucosa.

teremia, such as dental procedures. See Tables 47–8 and 47–9 for procedures requiring prophylaxis and antibiotic regimens used.

Other complications common in patients with congenital heart disease include poor growth, electrolyte disturbances due to medications, cerebral embolus in patients with right-to-left shunts (health care workers should be particularly careful to avoid air embolus during intravenous line placement), and increased susceptibility to respiratory illnesses. Cardiac patients may have a particularly difficult time with respiratory syncytial virus infections.

CARDIAC TRANSPLANT PATIENTS

Patients who are status post heart transplant are at risk for acute or chronic rejection, post-transplant lymphoproliferative disorder (PTLD), and infectious complications associated with their immunosuppressive or immunomodulating medication regimen.[20] In contrast to other types of transplantation, acute and chronic cardiac rejection is not defined by the timing after the operation; rather it is the clinical presentation that delineates them. Acute rejection is defined as a distinct episode that prompts intensification of immunosuppressive therapy, either based on cardiac dysfunction or based on histologic diagnosis. Symptoms of acute rejection vary widely, and may include fever, myalgias, vomiting, and shock. Less commonly, children may experience chest pain and/or have ECG changes, such as decreased R-wave amplitude. Laboratory studies, such as cardiac markers, are often nondiagnostic. An echocardiogram may show diastolic dysfunction, but early in the course it may not be present.

Whereas acute cardiac rejection is a fulminant presentation, chronic rejection is an ongoing process that mostly involves development of atherosclerotic disease. Ischemic symptoms such as decreased exercise tolerance, fatigue, and chest pain may be present. Syncope or sudden death may result from an arrhythmia. As in acute rejection, the diagnosis is clinical.

Post-transplant lymphoproliferative disorder (PTLD) is associated with the Epstein–Barr virus and occurs most often within a year of transplant, but may develop many years later. PTLD is a B-cell lymphoma resulting in masses throughout the body, most notably in the abdomen, chest, head and neck. Symptoms include a mononucleosis-like syndrome of fever,

▶ TABLE 47-9. REGIMENS FOR PROPHYLAXIS FOR INFECTIVE
ENDOCARDITIS[21]

Situation	Agent	Single Dose 30–60 Min Before Procedure	
		Adults	Children
Oral	Amoxicillin	2 g po	50 mg/kg po
Unable to take oral medications	Cefazolin or Ceftriaxone	1 g IM or IV	50 mg/kg IM or IV
Allergic to penicillin or ampicillin—Oral	Cephalexin OR	2 g po	50 mg/kg po
	Clindamycin OR	600 mg po	20 mg/kg po
	Azithromycin or Clarithromycin	500 mg po	15 mg/kg po
Allergic to penicillin or ampicillin—Unable to take oral medications	Cefazolin or Ceftriaxone OR	1 g IM or IV	50 mg/kg IM or IV
	Clindamycin	600 mg IM or IV	20 mg/kg IM or IV

lymphadenopathy, and abdominal pain. The diagnosis is based on clinical suspicion from history and physical examination with radiologic findings consistent with scattered lymphoid masses.

PREVENTION OF INFECTIVE ENDOCARDITIS

In 2007, the American Heart Association (AHA) in conjunction with the American Academy of Pediatrics (AAP) and the Infectious Diseases Society of America (IDSA) published revised guidelines for the prevention of infective endocarditis (IE).[21,22] The changes simplify and greatly narrow the recommendations to provide prophylaxis for only the higher risk patients and procedures. Antibiotic prophylaxis solely to prevent IE is no longer indicated for gastrointestinal and genitourinary procedures. The committee found that it is still reasonable to give prophylaxis for procedures on the respiratory tract, infected skin, or musculoskeletal tissue only for high-risk patients (see Tables 47–7 to 47–9).

OUTPATIENT REFERRAL

Children with complications associated with congenital heart disease and those with a new diagnosis in the emergency department are invariably admitted for stabilization and/or investigation of the lesion. A currently asymptomatic child may have high-risk historical features, including symptoms associated with exertion, recurrent episodes, symptoms while recumbent, associated chest pain or palpitations, and family history of sudden death or childhood cardiac disease; children with one or more of these features should also be admitted in consultation with a pediatric cardiologist.[23]

An otherwise well child with no high-risk historical features and a normal ECG may present to the ED with signs and symptoms necessitating an expedited outpatient workup. Any well child with only unexplained poor feeding may be referred to his primary care physician. Appropriate outpatient cardiology referrals from the emergency department include otherwise well children with diaphoresis with eating, unexplained significant murmur, or exercise intolerance. Parent education is crucial in understanding both the importance of primary care and (if needed) subspecialty follow-up, as well as return precautions to the ED.

▶ SUMMARY

Emergency physicians should concentrate on recognition and management of a few common presentations seen in congenital heart disease patients, especially ductal-dependent circulatory failure and CHF. Physicians are unlikely to determine the specific lesion in the emergency department without an echocardiogram, and knowledge of the exact lesion is often unnecessary for appropriate therapy. The number of adolescent and adult survivors of congenital heart disease repair is rapidly increasing, and these patients are subject to certain complications that emergency physicians must be prepared to recognize and manage.

REFERENCES

1. Cloherty JP, Eichenwald EC, Stark AR. *Manual of Neonatal Care.* 5th ed. Philadelphia, PA: Lipincott Williams & Wilkins; 2004:407–453.
2. Bernstein D. Congenital heart disease. In: Behrman RE, Kliegman RM, Jenson HB, eds. *Nelson Textbook of Pediatrics.* 17th ed. Philadelphia, PA: Saunders; 2004: chap 417.
3. Seidman J, et al. Genetic factors in myocardial disease. In: Libby P, Bonow RO, Mann DL, Zipes DP, eds. *Braunwald's Heart Disease: A Textbook of Cardiovascular Medicine.* 8th ed. Philadelphia, PA: Saunders; 2007: chap 10.
4. Dieckman RA. Pediatric assessment. In: Gausche-Hill M, Fuchs S, Yamamoto L, eds. *APLS: The Pediatric Emergency Medicine Resource.* 4th ed. Sudbury, MA: Jones and Bartlett Publishers; 2004:21–48.
5. Sharieff G, Rao S. The pediatric ECG. *Emerg Med Clin North Am.* 2006;24:195–208.

6. Brousseau T, Sharieff G. Newborn emergencies: the first 30 days of life. *Pediatr Clin North Am*. 2006;53:69–84.

7. Sacchetti A, Wernovsky G, Paston C, et al. Hypoventilation and hypoxia in reversal of cardiogenic shock in and infant with congenital heart disease. *Emerg Med J*. 2004;21:636–638.

8. Lee C, Robertson J, Shilkovski N. *The Harriet Lane Handbook*. 17th ed. Philadelphia, PA: Mosby; 2005:704.

9. Silberbach M, Hannon D. Presentation of congenital heart disease in the neonate and young infant. *Pediatr Rev*. 2007;28:123–131.

10. El-Khuffash A, Molloy EJ. Are B-type natriuretic peptide (BNP) and N-terminal-pro-BNP useful in neonates? *Arch Dis Child Fetal Neonatal Ed*. 2007;92:F320–F324.

11. Wynne J, Braunwald E. Cardiomyopathy and myocarditis. In: Kasper DL, Braunwald E, Hauser SL, Longo DL, Jameson JL, Fauci AS, eds. *Harrison's Principles of Internal Medicine*. 16th ed. New York, NY: McGraw-Hill; 2005:1410–1412.

12. Niemann JT. The cardiomyopathies, myocarditis, and pericardial disease. In: Tintinalli J, Kelen G, Stapczynski J, eds. *Emergency Medicine: A Comprehensive Study Guide*. 6th ed. New York, NY: McGraw-Hill; 2004:379–380.

13. Shirani J. Isolated coronary artery anomalies, in cardiology: coronary artery disease. *eMedicine*. http://www.emedicine.com. Updated March 13, 2008. Accessed March 18, 2008.

14. Pelech A. Coronary artery anomalies, in pediatrics: cardiac disease and critical care medicine. *eMedicine*. http://www.emedicine.com. Updated August 18, 2006. Accessed March 18, 2008.

15. Mancini M. Anomalous left coronary artery from the pulmonary artery, in pediatrics: cardiac disease and critical care medicine. *eMedicine*. http://www.emedicine.com. Updated July 27, 2006. Accessed March 18, 2008.

16. Artman M, Mahony L, Teitel D. *Neonatal Cardiology*. New York, NY: McGraw-Hill; 2002:64–135.

17. Reitz B, Yuh DD. *Congenital Cardiac Surgery*. New York, NY: McGraw-Hill; 2002:30–160.

18. Artman M, Mahony L, Teitel D. *Neonatal Cardiology*. New York, NY: McGraw-Hill; 2002:64–135.

19. Rosenkranz ER. Pediatric surgery for the primary care pediatrician, part I: caring for the former pediatric cardiac surgery patient. *Pediatr Clin North Am*. 1998;45:907.

20. Woods WA, et al. Care of the acute ill pediatric heart transplant recipient. *Ped Emerg Care*. 2007;23(10):721–724.

21. American Heart Association. Prevention of infective endocarditis: guidelines from the American Heart Association. *Circulation*. 2007;116:1736–1754.

22. Baltimore R. New recommendations for the prevention of infective endocarditis. *Curr Opin Pediatr*. 2008;20:85–89.

23. Hauda W, Mayer T. Syncope and sudden death. In: Tintinalli J, Kelen G, Stapczynski J, eds. *Emergency Medicine: A Comprehensive Study Guide*. 6th ed. New York, NY: McGraw-Hill; 2004:838–842.

CHAPTER 48

Congestive Heart Failure

Donna M. Moro-Sutherland, William C. Toepper, and Joilo Barbosa

▶ HIGH-YIELD FACTS

- Congestive heart failure (CHF) is a clinical syndrome and a directed history and physical examination can provide valuable clues to the presence and possible etiologies of heart failure.
- Abnormal vital signs such as unexplained tachycardia or tachypnea with normal temperature may suggest cardiac disease.
- Tachycardia of heart failure is often "monotonous" or incessant, and does not typically respond to treatment (i.e., volume, antipyretics, pain medications, etc.)
- Tachypnea, failure to thrive, or diaphoresis with feeding, accompanied by an abnormal lung examination, tachycardia, hyperactive precordium, gallop, and hepatomegaly suggest CHF in an infant.
- New-onset heart failure may be less overtly symptomatic in older children. Malaise, decrease in the level of daily activity, and weight loss may be the only complaint. Symptoms of abdominal pain and nausea and anorexia can be present, sometimes diverting attention from the real cause.
- New biomarker, B-type natriuretic peptide (BNP) may help with the diagnosis of suspected CHF in some cases.
- Management is directed at the cause. Medications to consider include diuretics, vasodilators, inotropes, and neurohumoral modulators.

▶ INTRODUCTION

Heart failure is a "clinical syndrome in which heart disease reduces cardiac output, increases venous pressures, and is accompanied by molecular abnormalities that cause progressive deterioration of the failing heart and premature myocardial cell death."[1] It is a failure of the cardiovascular system to meet metabolic demands. Heart failure results from the interplay of hemodynamic, neurohumoral, cellular, and developmental factors. Function is no longer dependent on supply and demand of the heart but on improving hemodynamics, improving symptoms, and providing myocardial preservation, and remodeling at the same time. CHF has many etiologies (Table 48–1). In the younger infant, CHF is most likely related to structural heart disease yet respiratory illnesses, anemia, and infection must be considered and appropriately managed. In an older child, the etiology may have a structural, metabolic, and/or environmental origin.[2–4]

▶ PATHOPHYSIOLOGY

Cardiac output is determined by four factors: preload, afterload, contractility, and rate. Preload, or filling volume, is increased in left-to-right shunts. *Afterload*, or the resistance the ventricles face upon ejection of blood, is important in outlet obstruction or systemic hypertension. *Contractility* is altered in cardiomyopathy. *Rate* can either be too slow, resulting in inadequate output, or too fast, decreasing diastolic filling.[2]

In acute CHF, end-organ hypoperfusion explains most clinical features. Decreased flow to the kidney results in renin/angiotensin-based salt and water retention, and an increased circulating volume. In addition, angiotensin II, a potent vasoconstrictor, increases vascular resistance resulting in a rise in blood pressure. Sympathetic discharge, as a result of decreased oxygen delivery, results in improved contractility. Redistribution of blood from skin and skeletal muscle to heart, brain, and kidney improves vital function. As the disease process worsens, physiologic mechanisms are unable to keep up. Overcompensation results in symptoms. Salt and water retention produces edema. Increased adrenergic response and tachycardia cause inadequate diastolic filling. Diaphoresis during feeding is secondary to catecholamine release. Decreased skin perfusion results in mottling and pallor. Increased systemic vascular resistance increases myocardial demand, causing hypertrophy or dilation. Valve insufficiency or myocardial ischemia can cause further decrease in cardiac output.[3–5]

In chronic CHF, myocardial cells die from energy starvation, from cytotoxic mechanisms leading to necrosis, or from the acceleration of apoptosis. This loss of myocytes leads to cardiac dilation, increased afterload, wall tension, and further systolic dysfunction.[3,5,6]

▶ HISTORY AND PHYSICAL EXAMINATION

Signs of CHF vary with the age of the child. When evaluating an infant with suspected CHF, questions related to feeding and nutritional status are extremely important (Table 48–2). Poor weight gain, cachexia, and malnutrition may be a sign of a flailing heart in an infant. As CHF worsens, failure to thrive may be the key to uncompensated CHF.

In an older child, questions regarding exercise ability, fatigability, shortness of breath, weight gain, or weight loss are important when considering heart failure. Fatigue and/or report of a lower than normal energy level may be the chief complaint in an adolescent. As failure worsens, complaints of cool

▶ **TABLE 48-1. ETIOLOGIC BASIS OF CHF**

Preload (Volume Overload)	Contractility
Left-to-right shunt: VSD, PDA, AV fistula, atrioventricular canal defects, Epstein's anomaly	Inflammatory: infectious (myocarditis), cardiomyopathy
Anemia: iron deficiency, sickle cell, thalassemia	Rheumatic: rheumatic fever, early Kawasaki, SLE
Iatrogenic	Toxin: digoxin, Ca^{2+} channel/β-blocker, cocaine and other stimulants
Afterload (increased SVR)	Traumatic: cardiac tamponade, myocardial contusion
Congenital: coarctation of the aorta, aortic stenosis, pulmonary stenosis	Metabolic: electrolyte abnormality, hypothyroidism
Systemic hypertension	Other: Asphyxia, hypoglycemia, hypocalcemia, sepsis

VSD, ventricular septal defect; PDA, patent ductus arteriosus; AV, arteriovenous; SLE, systemic lupus erythematosus.

extremities, exercise intolerance, dizziness, or syncope may be elicited.[4,6,7]

New-onset heart failure may be less overtly symptomatic in older children. Malaise, decrease in the level of daily activity, and weight loss may be the only complaint. Symptoms of abdominal pain and nausea and anorexia can be present and sometimes divert attention from the real cause.

The first manifestation of CHF is usually "tachycardia." This is especially important in the infant with suspected heart failure. An infant's myocardium is "stiffer" and less distensible, and hence the infant is unable to increase the stroke volume as an older child does. An infant compensates primarily by raising heart rate. Abnormal vital signs such as unexplained tachycardia or tachypnea with normal temperature may suggest cardiac disease. Tachycardia of heart failure is often "monotonous" or incessant, and does not respond to treatment (i.e., volume, antipyretics, and pain medications). Left-sided heart failure is associated with pulmonary venous congestion, whereas right-sided heart failure is associated with signs of systemic venous congestion[4,6] Table 48-3.

Physical examination should evaluate for resting tachycardia, tachypnea, hepatomegaly, ascites, edema, and diminished perfusion. Facial edema and anasarca are late signs. Pedal edema and neck vein distention are rare. Cardiac examination should focus on heart rate, presence of gallops, new murmurs, displaced PMI, an RV impulse, and perfusion deficits. A pathologic murmur or gallop rhythm is characteristic for CHF.[4]

▶ **TABLE 48-2. KEY QUESTIONS ON HISTORY WITH SUSPECTED CHF**

Infant	Older Child
Feeding: tachypnea with feeds, gagging, diaphoresis, time to complete feeding	Exercise capacity; exercise intolerance
Weight: weight gain; poor weight gain, cachexia, malnutrition, and failure to thrive	Easy fatigability; lower than usual energy levels, malaise
	Dizziness
	Syncope
	Orthopnea
	Paroxysmal nocturnal dyspnea
	Weight gain
	Weight loss

▶ LABORATORY EVALUATION

Laboratory testing includes arterial blood gas, complete blood cell count with hemoglobin concentration, electrolytes, calcium, BUN, creatinine, lactic acid, liver function tests, and urinalysis. A metabolic and respiratory acidemia is generally present due to pulmonary congestion and poor tissue perfusion; hyponatremia and hypochloremia secondary to free water retention, and elevated creatinine levels due to poor renal perfusion and compromised renal function also occur. Elevated lactic acid is present with significant tissue hypoxia. The hemoglobin and hematocrit should be checked since severe anemia can precipitate high-output cardiac failure and accentuate heart failure.[4] In infants, knowing the calcium level is critical. The infant relies on the circulating calcium and, if low, will add to the difficulty in managing these infants. Cortisol level may be drawn and if low, corticosteroids may be considered in the management of heart failure.

Newer laboratory tests assessing neurohormonal markers in heart failure have evolved. Elevated norepinephrine, aldosterone, angiotensin II, and vasopressin levels have all been linked to worse outcomes in patient with chronic CHF. One laboratory test in particular, such as β-type natriuretic peptide (BNP), is being used to diagnosis CHF in numerous clinical scenarios. The measurement of serum BNP is useful in differentiating a pulmonary cause of dyspnea from a cardiac cause of dyspnea.[4,7,8]

In children, an elevated BNP level correlates positively with heart failure and negatively with ejection fraction. An elevated BNP in the setting of heart failure is related to an increased morbidity and mortality. A BNP >100 pg/mL is considered abnormal; between 100 and 500, the test is inconclusive; and a level >500 pg/mL is indicative for heart failure in children (see chapter 46).[8]

▶ DIAGNOSTIC STUDIES

Ancillary tests include a chest radiograph, electrocardiogram, and echocardiogram.

CHEST RADIOGRAPH

The chest radiograph (CXR) helps to assess heart size and pulmonary congestion. The chest radiograph is a reliable tool for measuring volume overload. A cardiothoracic ratio of greater

▶ TABLE 48-3. **SIGNS AND SYMPTOMS OF CHF IN CHILDREN**

Pulmonary Venous Congestion (L → R Shunt, Pulmonary Edema, Poor Oxygenation)	Systemic Venous Congestion (Increased Right-Sided Filling Pressure)	Impaired Cardiac Output (Decreased Contractility and Perfusion)
Tachypnea	Hepatomegaly	Decreased pulses
Wheezing (cardiac asthma)	Ascites	Delayed capillary refill (cool extremities)
Rales	Pleural effusion	Fatigue
Nasal flaring or grunting	Peripheral edema	Pallor
Retractions	Weight gain	Sweating
Cough or chest congestion	JVD (rare in children)	Poor weight gain (failure to thrive)
Poor feeding		Dizziness
Irritability		Altered consciousness
		Syncope

JVD, jugular venous distension.

than 0.55 in infants and greater than 0.5 in children is the standard for cardiomegaly. CXR typically demonstrates cardiomegaly with prominent pulmonary vascular markings of pulmonary edema. But, remember a normal CXR does not rule out heart failure[4] (Figs. 48–1 and 48–2).

ELECTROCARDIOGRAM

The electrocardiogram (EKG) may give information regarding atrial enlargement, ventricular hypertrophy, strain, and changes in ST segment or T-wave morphology. These findings are generally nonspecific. Frequently, the EKG shows sinus tachycardia with low-voltage QRS complexes with or without low-voltage or inverted T waves. With worsening failure, the evidence and care of brady (atrioventricular block) and tachyarrthymias (ventricular tachycardia, supraventricular tachycardia, atrial fibrillation) may be necessary. Wide Q waves and ST-segment changes indicting myocardial infarction can be seen[4] (Fig. 48–3).

ECHOCARDIOGRAPHY

The quickest way to assess cardiac function in the emergency department is with two-dimensional echocardiography (ECHO). It is utilized to assess cardiac anatomy in congenital heart disease, but also in estimating gradients, shunting, and cardiac output. Assessment of right ventricular function has always been challenging due to the geometric limitations.

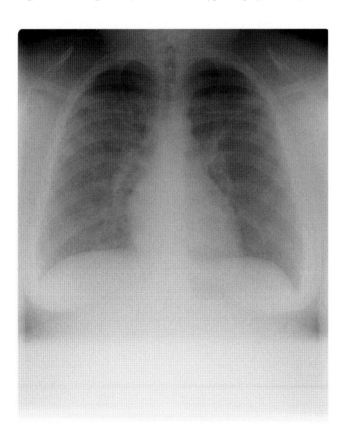
Figure 48–1. Normal CXR.

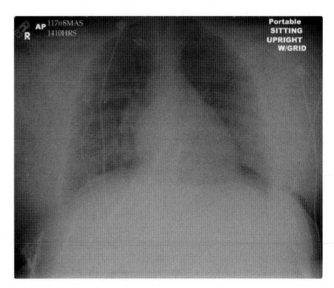
Figure 48–2. Pulmonary edema.

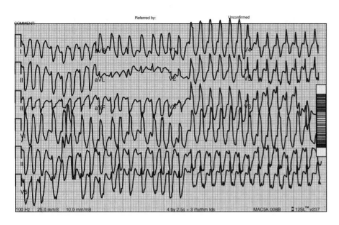

Figure 48–3. EKG: Patient with CHF with tachyarrhythmia.

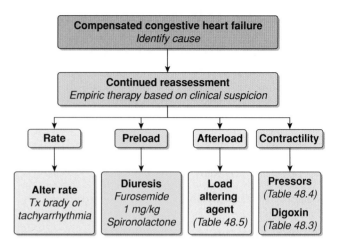

Figure 48–4. Management of compensated (chronic) CHF in children.

Newer echocardiographic techniques are providing information regarding diastolic dysfunction, which may be as important as systolic dysfunction in pediatric heart failure. ECHO gives information regarding the myocardial disease, such as hypertrophic cardiomyopathy, restrictive cardiomyopathy, and dilated cardiomyopathy, all of which can present as heart failure. ECHO typically reveals a dilated, dysfunctional left ventricle consistent with dilated cardiomegaly. A pericardial effusion is frequently present.[4]

▶ TREATMENT

Management of heart failure is multidimensional and requires a stepwise approach. A pediatric cardiologist should be involved early on in the child's care. In an emergency department, setting the goal is to recognize the child in acute CHF and begin management, remembering always the ABCs.

The management of acute CHF is difficult and can be dangerous without knowledge of the underlying cause. Therapy is directed toward the cause. The goal is to reduce cardiac contractility, reduce afterload, improve oxygenation, and enhance nutrition. Medications to consider include diuretics, vasodilators, inotropes, and neurohumoral modulators.[3,7,9–13] Current therapy for acute heart failure focuses on improving myocardial performance with inotropic agents, adjustments to afterload and preload, and on correcting the underlying cause. When the cause is known, correctable tasks must be undertaken. Examples include interventional techniques for obstructive lesions, exchange transfusion for profound anemia, or pericardiocentesis for cardiac tamponade. When the cause is unknown, empiric therapy is initiated based on the need to control rate, decrease preload, and improve afterload and/or contractility (Fig. 48–4). Diuretics help with increased work of breathing, peripheral edema, and ascites.

TREATMENT OF CHF

Pharmacologic therapy is directed at the specific cause when dealing with known cardiac disease with CHF. Empiric therapy is based on clinical suspicion. Treatment involves the use of diuretics, angiotensin-converting enzyme (ACE) inhibitors, digoxin, and β-blockade.[7,9–13]

Fluid overload is treated with furosemide (Lasix) 1 mg/kg/dose intravenously. Digoxin improves contractility by both blocking the sodium–potassium pump and increasing intracellular calcium, making actin–myosin bridging more forceful. Digoxin also slows heart rate and relieves diaphoresis through adrenergic withdrawal. It is useful in the stable, well-known patient, but is contraindicated in CHF associated with acute myocarditis because of its arrhythmogenic effects on the irritable myocardium.[7,9] Dosing is outlined in Table 48–4.

Afterload reduction is obtained orally by ACE inhibitors or intravenously by other agents such as hydralazine, nitroprusside, and alprostadil. In the setting of low output with increased systemic resistance, such as in hypertensive cardiomyopathy, afterload reduction with ACE inhibitors may be helpful. Contraindications include patients with renal insufficiency and those with right-to-left shunts. In right-to-left shunt, the systemic circulation may improve at the expense of the pulmonary circulation.[7,9]

Contractility can be supported with intravenous agents (dopamine) or mixed agents (dobutamine, inamrinone, milrinone). Milrinone, a phosphodiesterase inhibitor has gained popularity in many institutions as a first-line agent. Milrinone is shown to increase cardiac muscle contractility, vascular smooth muscle relaxation, and cardiac output without increasing myocardial oxygen consumption or ventricular afterload.[13] Inamrinone is a positive inotrope with the additional benefit of

▶ TABLE 48–4. ORAL DOSING GUIDELINES FOR DIGOXIN*

Age and Weight	Acute Digitalization (μg/kg)†	Maintenance
Premature infant	20	5 μg/kg/d
Full-term infant	30	4–5 μg/kg q12h
2–24 mo	40–50	5–10 μg/kg q12h
>24 mo	30–40	4–5 μg/kg q12h

*IV dose is 75% of po dose.
†Daily dose = 1/2 given initially, then 1/4 given at 8 h, and 1/4 given at 16 h.

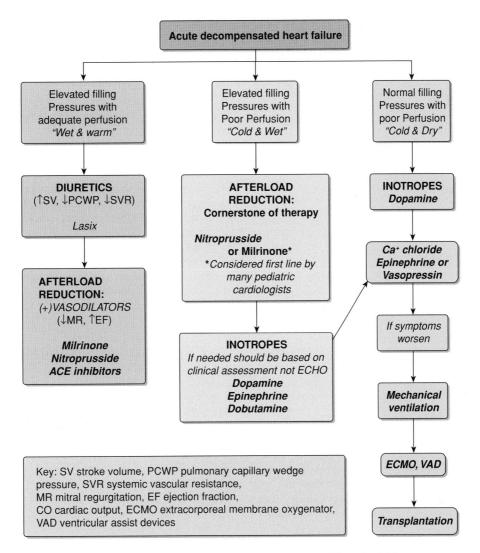

Figure 48–5. Management of acute decompensated heart failure in children.

decreasing pulmonary vascular resistance. It may be beneficial in digoxin-refractory patients. Its potent vasodilatory effects may cause hypotension. Dobutamine has fallen out of favor because of increased mortality in adult heart failure patients.

β-Blockers may have a role in chronic CHF. They "upregulate" cell wall receptors, increasing contractility.[7,9] The decision to begin long-term agents, digoxin, inamrinone, or β-blockers, is best made in consultation with a pediatric cardiologist or intensivist. An algorithmic approach to CHF is presented in Figures 48–4 and 48–5.

The child in moderate-to-severe CHF will require the intensive care unit or transfer to a tertiary care facility. Intubation may be necessary to improve oxygenation and provide positive end-expiratory pressure (PEEP), useful in pulmonary edema. Inotropic support includes dopamine to increase contractility and blood pressure, dobutamine for its more pronounced effect on contractility, and epinephrine to improve blood pressure[13] (Table 48–5).

In severe cases, such as myocarditis with cardiogenic shock, the weakened myocardium ineffectively pumps against increased afterload. Vasodilators such as sodium nitroprusside may be helpful. It has venodilator and arteriolar dilator effects and is easily titratable[7,13] (Table 48–6).

► FUTURE MODALITIES IN THE TREATMENT OF PEDIATRIC CHF

β_2-Blockers are being used more frequently in the pediatric patient. Carvedilol, a β-adrenergic blocker with vasodilating action appears to be beneficial in chronic CHF in adults. In adult clinical trials, Carvedilol has been shown to improve survival, decrease symptoms, improve ventricular function, decrease hospitalizations, enhance ventricular remodeling, decrease free radicals and adverse neurohumoral factors, decrease arrhythmias, and slow progression of heart failure. In recent multicenter pediatric clinical trial, Carvedilol as an adjunct to standard therapy for pediatric heart failure improved symptoms and left ventricular function. Because of its potential side effects of hypotension and its negative inotropic action, Carvedilol should be started at a low dose and only

▶ TABLE 48-5. **INOTROPIC AGENTS: DOSAGE AND PHARMACOLOGIC EFFECTS**

Drug	Dose (μg/kg/min)	Comments
Dopamine	1–5	Stimulates dopamine receptors in renal, cerebral, mesenteric, and pulmonary vasculature
	6–20	↑ HR, ↑ contractility, and ↑ afterload
		Side effects: tachycardia, dysrhythmias, increased myocardial oxygen consumption
Dobutamine	2–10	↑ HR, ↑ contractility, and vasodilation
		Side effects: tachycardia, dysrhythmias
		Fallen out of favor
Epinephrine	0.05–1	↑ HR, ↑ contractility, ↑ afterload, and vasodilation
		Dose-dependent actions: tachycardia, proarrhythmia effects, increased myocardial oxygen consumption
Norepinephrine	0.1	↑ HR, ↑ contractility, ↑ afterload
		Side effects: bradycardia, arrhythmias
Inamrinone	5–10	↑ HR, ↑ contractility, ↑ afterload
	Load: 1 mg/kg IV over 2–3 min	Side effects: hypotension, tachycardia, myocardial ischemia
Milrinone	0.25–1	↑ HR, ↑ contractility, ↑ afterload
	Load: 50 μg/kg IV slowly over 15 min	Side effects: hypotension, dysrhythmias, renal toxic in adults

after the patient has been stabilized on digoxin, diuretics, and ACE inhibitors. Carvedilol most likely will be beneficial in children with CHF, due to dilated cardiomyopathy, who have been stabilized on more traditional therapy but remain symptomatic.[3,7,13,14]

Nesiritide (β-type natriuretic peptide) is one of the newest therapies in the treatment of decompensated CHF in adults. It possesses vasodilatory, natriuretic, diuretic, and neurohormonal effects. It has been shown to rapidly improve hemodynamics and induce diuresis in adult patients with moderate-to-severe CHF. It does not appear to have proarrhythmic effects. Pediatric cardiologists have been reporting on small numbers of pediatric patients in the last 5 years with similar results. The pediatric patients generally diuresed and had symptomatic improvement in response to an infusion of Nesiritide with only dose-related hypotension and asymptomatic hyponatremia as recognized side effects. Nesiritide infusion, alone or in combination, is felt to be an alternative for decompensated heart failure in children. It is associated with decreased thirst and improved urine output and functional status, and it may be efficacious in the treatment of pediatric heart failure.[13,15–18]

Spironolactone (Aldactone) has become increasingly important in the management of chronic heart failure in adults. Spironolactone has an effect on cardiac function in addition to its weak diuretic effect. The RALES (Randomized Aldactone Evaluation Study) demonstrated a significant decrease in morbidity and mortality when incorporated into the treatment regimen of adults with significant symptomatic CHF. It is not known if these benefits apply to children but is being used more often by pediatric cardiologists in the management of CHF in children.[13]

Levosimendan, a calcium sensitizer, is a promising new agent in a new class of medications. Levosimendan increases both inotropic and vasodilation without increasing calcium levels or myocardial oxygen demand.[13,19]

Other options are extracorporeal membrane oxygenation (ECMO) and ventricular assist devices (VAD), which are being utilized in children with CHF who are not responding to medical management. The hope is to extend the child's life while awaiting cardiac transplantation or recovery from the infection.[7,13,20]

▶ SUMMARY

In all age groups, a directed history and physical examination can provide valuable clues to the presence and possible etiologies of impending decompensated heart failure. Remember

▶ TABLE 48-6. **LOAD-ALTERING AGENTS**

Drug	Dose	Comments
Nitroprusside	0.5–10 μg/kg/min IV	Cyanide toxicity
Captopril	Infants: 0.1–0.5 mg/kg/d po q8–12h	Neutropenia, cough, proteinuria
Nitroglycerin	2–10 μg/kg/min IV	Use not well established in children
Inamrinone	0.5–2 mg/kg, then 5–10 μm/kg/min IV	Hypotension, thrombocytopenia, hepatic dysfunction
Enalapril	0.1 mg/kg/d po div qd/bid, not to exceed 0.5 mg/kg/d	
Alprostadil (PGE1)	0.05–0.1 μg/kg/min IV	For ductal-dependent lesions

that early on tachycardia is generally the only sign and reassessments are key. Abdominal pain has been found to be the key presenting symptom for a great number of patients with heart failure. The goal is to reduce cardiac contractility, reduce afterload, improve oxygenation, and enhance nutrition. Medications to consider include diuretics, vasodilators, inotropes, and neurohumoral modulators. Current therapy for acute heart failure focuses on improving myocardial performance with inotropic agents, adjustments to afterload and preload, and on correcting the underlying cause. Digoxin is falling out of favor and newer agents are now being used to manage pediatric heart failure.

REFERENCES

1. Katz AM. Overview, definition, historical aspects. In: Katz AM, ed. *Heart Failure: Pathophysiology, Molecular Biology and Clinical Management*. Philadelphia, PA: Lippincott Williams & Wilkins; 2000:3.
2. O'Laughlin MP. Congestive heart failure in children. *Pediatr Clin North Am*. 1999;46:263–273.
3. Balaguru D, Artman M, Auslender M. Management of heart failure in children. *Curr Probl Pediatr*. 2000;30:5–30.
4. Kim JJ, Rossano JW, Nelson DP, et al. Heart failure in infants and children: etiology, pathophysiology, and diagnosis of heart failure (chapter 66a). *Roger's Textbook of Pediatric Intensive Care*. 4th ed. Philadelphia, PA: Lippincott Williams & Wilkins; 2008:1064–1074.
5. Fenton M, Burch M. Understanding chronic heart failure. *Arch Dis Child*. 2007;92(9):812–816.
6. Satou GM, Herzberg G, Erickson LC. Heart failure, congestive. http://www.emedicine.com/PED/topic2636.htm. Updated June 26, 2006. Accessed September 12, 2008.
7. Balfour I. Management of chronic congestive heart failure in children. *Curr Treat Options Cardiovas Med*. 2004;6:407–416.
8. Koulouri S, Acherman RJ, Wong PC, et al. Utility of B-type natriuretic peptide in differentiating congestive heart failure from lung disease in pediatric patients with respiratory distress. *Pediatr Cardiol*. 2004;25(4):341–346.
9. Auslender M, Artman M. Overview of the management of pediatric heart failure. *Prog Pediatr Cardiol*. 2000(11):231–241.
10. Shaddy RE. Optimizing treatment for chronic congestive heart failure in children. *Crit Care Med*. 2001;29(10):S237–S213.
11. Ross RD. Medical management of chronic heart failure in children. *Am J Cardiovasc Drugs*. 2001;1(1):37–44.
12. Sarma M, Nair MNG, Jatana SK, et al. Congestive heart failure in infants and children. *MJAFI*. 2003;59:228–233.
13. Rossano JW, Price JF, Nelson DP. Treatment of heart failure in infants and children: medical management (chapter 67A). *Roger's Textbook of Pediatric Intensive Care*. 4th ed. Philadelphia, PA: Lippincott Williams & Wilkins; 2008:1093–1108.
14. Bruns LA, Kichuk M, Lamour JM, et al. Carvediol as therapy in pediatric heart failure: an initial multicenter experience. *J Pediatr*. 2001;138(4):505–511.
15. Feingold B, Law YM. Nesiritide use in pediatric patients with congestive heart failure. *J Heart Transplant*. 2004;23(12):1455–1459.
16. Mahle WT, Cuadrado AR, Kirshbom PM, et al. Nesiritide in infants and children with congestive heart failure. *Pediatr Crit Care Med*. 2005;6(5):543–546.
17. Jefferies JL, Denfield SW, Price JF, et al. A prospective evaluation of nesiritide in the treatment of pediatric heart failure. *Pediatr Cardiol*. 2006;27(4):402–407.
18. Jefferies JL, Price JF, Denfield SW, et al. Safety and efficacy of nesiritide in pediatric heart failure. *J Card Fail*. 2007;13(7):541–548.
19. Auslender M. New drugs in the treatment of heart failure. *Prog Pediatric Cardiol* 2000(12):119–124.
20. Rosenthal D, Chrisant MRK, Edens E, et al. International society for heart and lung transplantation: practice guidelines for management of heart failure in children. *J Heart Lung Transplant*. 2004;23(12):1313–1333.

CHAPTER 49

Inflammatory and Infectious Heart Disease

William T. Tsai

▶ HIGH-YIELD FACTS

- Pericarditis presents with chest pain in the older child. Pleuritic or positional chest pain, fever, tachycardia, friction rub, and electrocardiographic changes may help narrow the differential.
- Myocarditis has protean manifestations with symptom complexes that range from sudden death to signs attributable to congestive heart failure and cardiogenic shock.
- Children with acute myocarditis should be admitted to a pediatric intensive care unit for careful monitoring and aggressive supportive management.
- Echocardiography should be performed in patients with suspected myocarditis.
- The at-risk patient with endocarditis presents with unexplained fever, myalgia, new murmur, and elevated acute-phase reactants.

▶ INTRODUCTION

Inflammatory diseases of the heart may affect the pericardium, myocardium, or endocardium. Pancarditis describes inflammation involving all layers of the heart. Such inflammatory cardiac disorders may be infectious, noninfectious, or rheumatologic and enter into the differential diagnosis in children presenting with complaints that range from chest pain, to acute gastrointestinal symptoms, to symptoms of cardiovascular collapse.

This chapter will discuss the presentation, diagnosis, and management of pericarditis, myocarditis, and endocarditis in children presenting to the emergency department.

▶ PERICARDITIS

Pericarditis usually follows a benign clinical course. Presenting symptoms include pleuritic or positional chest pain, fever, dyspnea, or abdominal pain. Causes overlap with those of myocarditis (Table 49–1).

Signs include a pericardial friction rub and tachycardia. If there is a pericardial effusion, one may not hear a friction rub because the visceral and parietal pleura are not apposed. As effusions increase in volume, dyspnea or shock may develop. In the presence of pericardial tamponade, distended jugular veins and hepatomegaly may become noticeable. As cardiac output decreases because of decreased cardiac stroke volume, delayed capillary refill, decreased urine output, and hypotension develop. Pulsus paradoxus, an exaggerated decrease in systolic blood pressure during inspiration, may be appreciated.[1]

Cardiomegaly occurs on chest radiography when moderate or large pleural effusions are present (Fig. 49–1). In patients with little or no effusion, the chest radiograph is normal. The electrocardiogram may be diagnostic with diffuse ST-T wave changes. PR depression may occur. A decreased QRS amplitude or electrical alternans may be seen with large effusions. Echocardiography will rapidly demonstrate the presence, size, and location of a pericardial effusion and can rapidly identify cardiac tamponade using 2D and Doppler techniques. It is important in guiding pericardiocentesis if drainage is necessary (Fig. 49–2).

Management depends on the presence and extent of pericardial effusion. Treatment is generally supportive and includes treatment with NSAIDs and cardiology consultation. Consider hospitalization in children with effusion. Obtain urgent cardiology and critical care consultation in children with large effusions and hemodynamic instability.

Children with pericarditis and pericardial effusion, who exhibit signs of hemodynamic instability secondary to cardiac tamponade, should have emergent pericardiocentesis. While pericardiocentesis can be lifesaving in cases of tamponade, the possibility of severe complications and the high overall rate of complications mandates that this procedure be performed by clinicians with considerable experience and expertise.[2]

▶ MYOCARDITIS

Acute myocarditis is a serious, but relatively uncommon diagnosis in the emergency department. Symptoms can progress from those of a nonspecific respiratory illness to those of cardiovascular collapse and death in a short period of time. The clinical course varies from those with subclinical disease to those with fulminant disease which is associated with cardiogenic shock and is often fatal. Others have an indolent course that progresses over time to dilated cardiomyopathy with chronic congestive heart failure. Signs and symptoms may point to an obvious cardiac etiology, but subtler and misleading presentations require the clinician to have a high index of suspicion.

The incidence of myocarditis in the United States is not known because of patients with subclinical infection and

▶ **TABLE 49–1.** **ETIOLOGY OF PERICARDITIS**

Infectious:
    Viral: coxsackievirus, enterovirus, adenovirus, hepatitis B
       virus, human immunodeficiency virus, Epstein–Barr
       virus, cytomegalovirus
    Bacterial: *Streptococcus pneumoniae*, *Staphylococcus*
       aureus, *Haemophilus pneumoniae*, *Neisseria*
       meningitidis
    Fungal: histoplasmosis, coccidioidomycosis, *Candida*
    Other: Lyme disease, mycobacteria

Noninfectious
    Rheumatic fever
    Autoimmune: juvenile rheumatoid arthritis, systemic lupus
       erythematosus, acute rheumatic fever
    Uremia
    Radiation
    Hypersensitivity to drugs
    Postpericardiotomy syndrome

Idiopathic

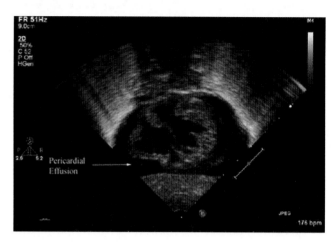

Figure 49–2. Subcostal view echocardiogram of a patient. A large pericardial effusion is seen surrounding the right and left ventricle.

difficulties in precise diagnosis. Myocarditis was found at autopsy in between 3% and 40% of infants and children with sudden death.[3–5] Frequently, a diagnosis of myocarditis is suspected but never confirmed. More recently, a survey of the incidence of pediatric cardiomyopathy in two regions of the United States, the incidence of myocarditis as a cause of dilated cardiomyopathy was approximately 0.2 per 100 000 children.[6]

ETIOLOGY

In cases of suspected myocarditis, an etiologic agent is identified in less than one-third of the time.[7] Laboratory techniques include observing acute and convalescent titer for specific viruses, viral cultures from fluid or tissue, and PCR amplification of viral genome. Viral etiologies predominate, however bacteria, rickettsia, fungi, and parasites are known agents (Table 49–1).

CLINICAL PRESENTATION

Myocarditis is difficult to diagnose because signs and symptoms may mimic other very common disorders. Frequently, it is not until later in the clinical course that these symptoms are noted to be of cardiac origin. The clinical presentation can be divided into specific symptom complexes based on presentation (Table 49–2). In general, the pathophysiology of the

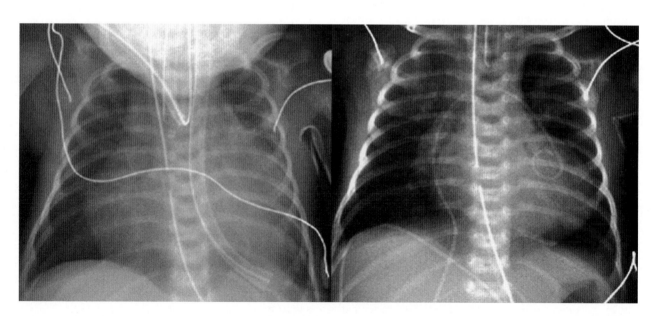

Figure 49–1. Left. Chest radiograph of an infant with cardiomegaly secondary to a large pericardial effusion. Right, same infant after placement of a pericardiocentesis catheter.

▶ **TABLE 49–2. MYOCARDITIS PRESENTING SYMPTOM COMPLEXES**

Respiratory	Difficulty breathing, retractions, wheezing
Gastrointestinal	Vomiting, diarrhea, abdominal pain
Cardiac	Chest pain, palpitations, congestive heart failure
Hypoperfusion	Lethargy, syncope, shock

symptom complexes follows the gradual onset of congestive heart failure to frank cardiogenic shock.

Complaints include cough, wheeze, congestion, fever, or tachypnea. Bronchospasm responding poorly to conventional therapy may suggest early myocarditis. Red flags include the child who is tachypneic, but lack symptoms of wheezing or supporting evidence for the diagnosis of pneumonia. Other signs and symptoms include those associated with congestive heart failure, poor feeding, cyanosis, and grunting. Murmur, gallop rhythm, rales, or organomegaly may confirm the diagnosis (Table 49–3). Myocarditis should be considered in any child who deteriorates despite aggressive treatment for bronchospasm or reactive airway disease.[8]

The onset of metabolic acidosis secondary to severe hypoperfusion (cardiogenic shock) accounts for some of the symptoms seen. Metabolic acidosis can cause tachypnea, retractions, and grunting.[9,10] Gastrointestinal symptoms arise because of viral syndromes but also because of gastrointestinal hypoperfusion. Severe acidosis may also affect mental status causing lethargy and coma.

DIAGNOSIS

Diagnosis requires a high index of suspicion. Unfortunately, standard laboratory, radiographic, and electrocardiographic testing is nonspecific. Chest radiograph is positive in only 42% to 75% of cases (Fig. 49–3).[8,9,10]

Elevations in CPK, LDH, troponin,[11] and BNP lack specificity.[7] Indicators of inflammation such as ESR and CRP are nonspecific. Electrocardiographic changes include nonspecific ST-T wave and axis changes. Rarely, heart block of infarct patterns may emerge.

Patients, who may have myocarditis, should receive echocardiography. Findings include increased end-diastolic

▶ **TABLE 49–3. PHYSICAL FINDINGS**

	n (%)
Respiratory distress, tachypnea	21 (68)
Tachycardia	18 (58)
Lethargy	12 (39)
Hepatomegaly	11 (36)
Abnormal heart sounds	10 (32)
Fever	9 (30)
Hypotension	7 (23)
Pallor	6 (19)
Peripheral edema, cyanosis	5 (16)
Cyanosis, hypoxia	3 (10)

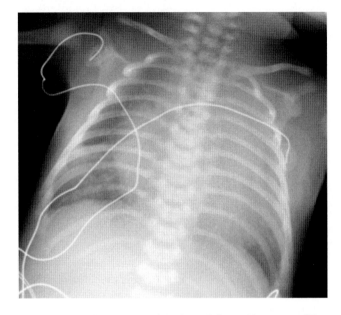

Figure 49–3. Chest radiograph in an infant with myocarditis. Note cardiomegaly and increased vascular congestion consistent with pulmonary edema.

chamber dimensions, reduced shortening fraction, atrioventricular valve regurgitation, and regional wall abnormalities (Fig. 49–4).

TREATMENT

Children with acute myocarditis should be admitted to a pediatric intensive care unit (PICU) for continuous monitoring because of the risks of ventricular ectopy and cardiogenic shock. Preferably, the PICU should have the ability to provide aggressive mechanical cardiac support, if needed. Initial management includes the treatment of congestive heart failure or cardiogenic shock. Consider use of invasive monitoring. Ionotropic support with dopamine, dobutamine, epinephrine,

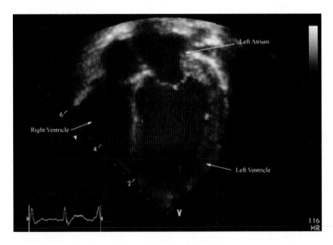

Figure 49–4. Apical 4 chamber echocardiogram from infant in Figure 49-3, showing left ventricular dilation. Ejection fraction 28%.

or milrinone may be necessary. An aggressive approach to dysrhythmias may prevent sudden death. Heart block is an indication for transvenous pacing. Meticulous supportive care of acid–base derangements, metabolic abnormalities, and fluid status is mandatory. The use of corticosteroids and other immunosuppressants is not well supported by current studies.[12] The use of intravenous immunoglobulin remains controversial.[13] Patients with fulminant myocarditis should receive aggressive mechanical support of the circulation because of the excellent long-term prognosis if these patients can survive the initial period of cardiogenic shock.[14] Ultimately, transplantation may be required for end-stage cardiomyopathy because of myocarditis.

▶ ENDOCARDITIS

Bacterial endocarditis occurs in children with congenital heart disease or central venous catheters or in adolescents, who use intravenous drugs. Seeding can occur via dental caries, skin infections, and manipulation of the airway, gastrointestinal tract, or genitourinary tract. Staphylococcal and streptococcal species predominate, with HACEK organisms (*Hemophilus, Actinobacillus, Cardiobacterium, Eikenella, Kingella*) and *Candida* as occasional offenders. Diagnosis is suspected in the at-risk patient in the presence of unexplained fever, weakness, myalgia, and arthralgia. A new murmur is present in fewer than 50% of cases. Other findings may include congestive heart failure secondary to valvular insufficiency, petechiae, or new neurologic findings. Adult cutaneous hallmarks such as Janeway lesions or Osler nodes are rare. Blood culture will identify the organism in 90% of cases. Other supportive data include elevated acute-phase reactants such as white blood cell count or erythrocyte sedimentation rate, anemia, hematuria, or embolic infiltrates. The echocardiogram has a 70% to 80% detection rate, with failure occurring in children who have complex congenital heart disease.

Identification of the causative organism allows more specific antibiotic therapy. However, in the sickest patients, start appropriate broad-spectrum coverage in consultation with a consultant. Bacteremia will persist in some patients despite antibiotics. Removal of vegetation or valve replacement may be indicated. Other sequelae, such as threatened or recurrent embolization, severe valve failure, recalcitrant arrhythmia secondary to vegetation, or myocardial abscess may require. Pulmonary or neurologic emboli are dependent on the location of the vegetations and presence of intracardiac shunting. Overall, endocarditis carries a mortality rate of 6% to 14%.

Because of the high mortality rate, prevention of endocarditis is important. The emergency physician plays an important role in endocarditis prophylaxis. Indications are dynamic. American Heart Association guidelines for at-risk patients are summarized in Table 49–4.

▶ ACUTE RHEUMATIC FEVER

Valvular involvement characterizes the carditis of acute rheumatic fever. The acute phase begins 2 to 3 weeks after a group A streptococcal illness. Jones criteria are outlined in Table 32–7. Typically, carditis follows arthritis and can involve

▶ **TABLE 49–4. ENDOCARDITIS PROPHYLAXIS IN CARDIAC CONDITIONS**[15]

Endocarditis Prophylaxis Recommended

High risk
  Prosthetic valves
  Previous bacterial endocarditis
  Complex cyanotic malformations
  Surgical systemopulmonary shunts
Moderate risk
  Rheumatic or acquired valvular dysfunction
  Hypertrophic cardiomyopathy
  MVP with regurgitation or thickened leaflets
  Most other complex cardiac malformations

Endocarditis Prophylaxis Not Recommended
Isolated secundum ASD
Repaired secundum ASD, VSD, PDA, without residua after 6 mo
Innocent murmurs
Previous Kawasaki syndrome without valvular dysfunction
Previous rheumatic fever without valvular dysfunction
Cardiac pacemakers and implanted defibrillators

ASD, atrial septal defect; VSD, ventriculoseptal defect; PDA, patent ductus arteriosus; MVP, mitral valve prolapse.
Source: Adapted from Dajani AS, Taubert KA, Gerber MA, et al[15]. Prevention of bacterial endocarditis: recommendations by the American Heart Association. JAMA. 1997;277:1794.

the three layers of the heart. A benign acute phase can be followed years later with valvular insufficiency. Mitral insufficiency is most common and is characterized by a holosystolic, high-pitched, blowing apical murmur radiating to the axilla. Regurgitant aortic murmurs are middiastolic, high-pitched, and blowing, located at the base, radiating into the neck. Other cardiac findings include tachycardia, gallop rhythm, pericardial rub, or congestive heart failure. The ECG may demonstrate PR prolongation, conduction delays, left ventricular hypertrophy, or dysrhythmia. Echocardiography is helpful in the follow-up of patients with rheumatic heart disease and may have a role in the evaluation of patients without murmur or with subclinical heart involvement.[16]

Treatment during the acute phase includes hospitalization and bed rest and cardiac rehabilitation follows. High-dose aspirin is started upon confirmation of the diagnosis. Penicillin or erythromycin is given to eradicate residual streptococci. Corticosteroids are controversial and may have a role in the treatment of carditis or chorea. Long-term follow-up of patients with acute rheumatic fever includes surveillance for recurrence, endocarditis prophylaxis, and treatment of chronic failure. Patients without early cardiac involvement are unlikely to develop delayed valvular disease.

REFERENCES

1. Deshpande JK, Tobias JD, Johns JA. Inflammatory heart disease. In: Nichols DG, Cameron DE, Greeley WJ, et al, eds. *Critical Heart Disease In Infants And Children.* St. Louis, MO: Mosby; 1995:937–960.

2. Reeves SD. Pericardiocentesis. In: King C, Henretig FM, eds. *Textbook Of Pediatric Emergency Procedures.* Phildelphia, PA: Lippincott Williams & Wilkins; 2008:709–714.

3. Forcada P, Beigelman R, Milei J. Inapparent myocarditis and sudden death in pediatrics. Diagnosis by immunohistochimical staining. *Int J Cardiol.* 1996;56:93.

4. Neuspiel DR, Kuller LH. Sudden and unexpected natural death in childhood and adolescence. *JAMA.* 1985;254:1321.

5. Topaz O, Edwards JE. Pathologic features of sudden death in children, adolescents, and young adults. *Chest.* 1985;87: 476.

6. Lipshultz SE, Sleeper LA, Towbin JA, et al. The incidence of pediatric cardiomyopathy in two regions of the United States. *N Engl J Med.* 2003;348:1647–1655.

7. Feldman AM, McNamara D. Medical progress: myocarditis. *N Engl J Med.* 2000;343:1388–1398.

8. Freedman SB, Haladyn JK, Floh A, et al. Pediatric myocarditis: emergency department clinical findings and diagnostic evaluation. *Pediatrics.* 2007;120:1278–1285.

9. Bonadio WA, Losek JD. Infants with myocarditis presenting with severe respiratory distress and shock. *Pediatr Emerg Care.* 1987;3:110.

10. Press S, Lipkind RS. Acute myocarditis in infants. Initial presentation. *Clin Pediatr.* 1990;29:73.

11. Soongswang J, Durongpisitkul K, Nona A, et al. Cardiac troponin T: a marker in the diagnosis of acute myocarditis in children. *Pediatr Cardiol.* 2005;26:45–49.

12. Mason JW, O'Connell JB, Herskowitz A, et al. A clinical trial of immunosuppressive therapy for myocarditis. The myocarditis treatment trial investigators. *N Engl J Med.* 1995;333: 269.

13. Drucker NA, Colan SD, Lewis AB, et al. Gamma-globulin treatment of acute myocarditis in the pediatric population. *Circulation.* 1994;89:252.

14. McCarthy RE, Boehmer JP, Hruban R, et al. Long-term outcome of fulminant myocarditis as compared with acute (nonfulminant) myocarditis. *N Engl J Med.* 2000;342:690–695.

15. Dajani AS, Taubert KA, Gerber MA, et al. Prevention of bacterial endocarditis: recommendations by the American Heart Association. *JAMA.* 1997;277:1794.

16. Committee on Rheumatic Fever, Endocarditis, and Kawasaki disease; and American Heart Association. Guidelines for the diagnosis of rheumatic fever. *JAMA.* 1992;268:2069.

CHAPTER 50

Dysrhythmias in Children

Ghazala Q. Sharieff and Stephanie Donige

▶ HIGH-YIELD FACTS

- Dysrhythmias in children are classified according to rate, QRS width, and clinical stability.
- Sinus bradycardia in the neonate always requires aggressive investigation and prompt resuscitation.
- Infants with paroxysmal supraventricular tachycardia (PSVT) may present in a low output state with irritability, poor feeding, tachypnea, and diaphoresis.
- Vagal maneuvers and adenosine convert most episodes of PSVT. Verapamil is contraindicated in children <2 years of age.
- Accessory pathway is the most common mechanism for PSVT in the child, but is difficult to appreciate during PSVT. Digoxin may precipitate ventricular tachycardia (VT) and is only used under the supervision of a pediatric cardiologist.
- Atrial fibrillation or flutter associated with accessory pathway disease or hypertrophic cardiomyopathy puts a child at high risk for 1:1 conduction, ventricular tachycardia, and sudden death.
- The electrocardiogram (ECG) is important in the evaluation of the syncopal patient, looking for wide complex tachycardia, long QT syndrome (QTc > 0.46s), or hypertrophic myocardopathy (LVH).

Disorders of rate and rhythm are fortunately rare in the pediatric population. Supraventricular tachycardias (SVTs) have predictable etiologies based on age. Rhythm disturbances, such as sinus bradycardia, can be life-threatening in the neonate.

Dysrhythmias in children are usually the result of cardiac lesions with a poorer prognosis than patients with structurally normal heart. Noncardiac causes, such as hypoxia, electrolyte imbalance, toxins, and inflammatory disease, must be considered in the child, as should cardioactive drugs, such as digoxin or over-the-counter cold remedies. Initial evaluation of the child with idiopathic or unexplained dysrhythmia includes an echocardiogram.

Age is an important consideration in the child with dysrhythmia. Some ventricular dysrhythmias disappear with age. Other conditions associated with an escape pacemaker worsen with age. The ventricular rate in third-degree heart block may be adequate for the 2-month-old child but will not provide an adequate cardiac output for the child at age 12. Age is also a factor in the clinical presentation of the dysrhythmia. The infant may present with poor feeding, tachypnea, irritability, or signs of a low output state. Caregivers often note that their baby is "not acting right." The older child presents with specific symptoms, such as syncope from decreased cerebral blood flow, chest pain from decreased coronary blood flow, or palpitations. Adolescents involved in competitive athletics with syncope, palpitations, or worrisome chest pain should be investigated promptly. Normal ranges for heart rate and blood pressure are listed in Tables 50–1 and 50–2.

The initial emergency management of dysrhythmias is dependent on three factors: rate, QRS width, and clinical stability. Decisions should be based on 12-lead ECG interpretation as single-lead monitor strips can be misleading. Rapid rates may appear supraventricular in origin in the child with sinus tachycardia. Children tolerate most rhythm disturbances well, providing ample time for precise interpretation. A brief review of the natural history and management of pediatric rhythm disturbances follows.

▶ SLOW RATES

SINUS BRADYCARDIA

Sinus bradycardia may be a manifestation of serious underlying disease or a normal physiologic variant; therefore, each child must be approached individually. Athletes commonly will be bradycardic and the approach to these patients differs significantly from newborns and younger children with bradycardia. Serious causes of bradycardia include hypoxia, hypothyroidism, hypoglycemia, hypo- or hyperkalemia, tension pneumothorax, cardiac tamponade, toxins, coronary or pulmonary thrombosis, or increased intracranial pressure. Sinus bradycardia can be a manifestation of calcium channel blocker, β-blocker, or digoxin toxicity. Treating the underlying condition corrects the rate. If the cause is unclear and oxygenation and ventilation are adequate, an unstable patient is given epinephrine 1:10 000, at 0.01 mg/kg IV/IO or 1:1000, at 0.1 mg/kg via the endotracheal tube (0.1 mL/kg of either solution). High-dose epinephrine via the intravenous route is no longer recommended unless there is concern for β-blocker overdose.[1] Atropine, 0.02 mg/kg (minimum dose 0.1 mg), is reserved for patients with either vagally mediated bradycardia or first- and second-degree heart blocks. The maximum dose for children is 0.5 mg and 1.0 mg for adolescents.[2–4]

ATRIOVENTRICULAR BLOCKS

Complete atrioventricular (AV) block may be congenital or acquired. Congenital blocks associated with structural disease, such as an AV canal, have a poor prognosis than blocks associated with maternal collagen vascular disease. Maternal

▶ **TABLE 50-1. EXPECTED HEART RATES ACCORDING TO AGE²**

Age	Rate (Mean)
0–3 mo	80–205 (140)
3 mo–2 y	75–190 (130)
2–10 y	60–140 (80)
> 10 y	50–100 (75)

antibodies cause fibrosis and destruction of the conduction system. Complete AV block is suspected in utero in the setting of sustained fetal bradycardia, polyhydramnios, and congestive heart failure (CHF). Rates of 50 to 80 beats per minute (bpm) are typical in complete AV block. Symptoms are rate dependent and most patients with rates >50 bpm are rarely symptomatic. An alternative explanation for instability must be pursued in patients with heart rates approaching 80 bpm. Treatment of neonatal symptomatic bradycardia due to AV block includes control of CHF, isoproterenol, and temporary transcutaneous, transthoracic, or umbilical transvenous pacing.

Acquired third-degree block is associated with myocarditis, endocarditis, rheumatic fever, cardiomyopathy, Lyme disease, or tumor. Postoperative blocks are less common today because of advances in intraoperative mapping. Postoperative blocks may last for years or occur years after surgery. Unlike congenital third-degree block, QRS complexes are usually wide. Treatment is similar, except patients with syncope must be paced immediately.

PACEMAKERS IN CHILDREN

The indications for pediatric pacemakers differ from indications in adults. The most common is symptomatic bradycardia. Occasionally, an asymptomatic child with an extremely low heart rate needs pacing. Postoperative or acquired AV blocks require permanent pacing beyond 10 to 14 days. Other indications include the long QT syndrome and cardioinhibitory syncope lasting >10 seconds.

Advances in adult pacemakers have improved the management of children with dysrhythmia. Most permanent pedi-

▶ **TABLE 50-2. EXPECTED SYSTOLIC AND DIASTOLIC BLOOD PRESSURES ACCORDING TO AGE**

Age	Systolic BP (mm Hg)	Diastolic BP (mm Hg)
0 d	60–76	30–45
1–4 d	67–84	35–53
1 mo	73–94	36–56
3 mo	78–103	44–65
6 mo	82–105	46–68
1 y	67–104	20–60
2 y	70–106	25–65
7 y	79–115	38–78
15 y	93–131	45–85

atric pacemakers are transvenous. Epicardial units are reserved for premature infants and those with right-to-left shunts. Choice of mode depends on disease. For example, children with sinus disease require atrial pacing. Ventricular pacing is unnecessary because AV conduction is normal. Children with congenital or acquired AV block require dual chamber pacing. Isolated ventricular pacing is employed in the very young. Most units can be programmed to sense, demand, or inhibit at the atrial or ventricular level, depending on the needs of the child. Also, they may be programmed to sense motion or breathing.

Syncope or palpitations in a child with a pacemaker suggests malfunction. Chest radiography may reveal wire fracture or lead displacement. Most malfunctions are not mechanical and require external reprogramming. Uncaptured paced beats outside the refractory period require investigation. If the problem is not easily resolved, the patient should be admitted.

Temporary transvenous pacemakers are rarely necessary in children. Most temporary pacing is transcutaneous. Transthoracic pacing via pericardiocentesis catheter should be considered in the very unstable infant.

▶ FAST RATES

PAROXYSMAL SUPRAVENTRICULAR TACHYCARDIA

The most common dysrhythmia in the child is paroxysmal supraventricular tachycardia (PSVT). PSVT is differentiated from sinus tachycardia by its abrupt onset, rates > 220 bpm, the absence of normal P waves (Fig. 50–1), or by little rate variation during stressful activities, such as phlebotomy. Symptoms of PSVT in infants include poor feeding, tachypnea, and irritability. They may appear ill or septic. Infants tolerate PSVT well but usually present within 24 hours of onset. Occasionally, it is associated with fever, infection, drug exposure, or congenital heart disease, but it is usually caused by one of the two following mechanisms: AV reciprocating tachycardia or AV nodal reentry. Younger children are more likely to have accessory pathway tachycardia, which is very important in choosing treatment.

AV reciprocating tachycardia or accessory pathway tachycardia is most common in children. Conduction during PSVT is usually orthodromic, with antegrade AV conduction and retrograde accessory pathway conduction (Fig. 50–2). Conduction during sinus rhythm can be via the accessory pathway, resulting in a short PR interval and appearance of a delta wave. This characterizes the Wolff–Parkinson–White (WPW) syndrome. Some accessory pathways only conduct retrograde during bouts of PSVT and are termed "concealed" because they are not apparent on surface ECG.

The other mechanism, AV nodal reentry, is more common in adults, but may be responsible for one-third of cases of PSVT in adolescents. Within the AV node, fast pathways with long refractory periods are blocked during a PAC, allowing for antegrade conduction down the slow tract. The impulse then propagates up the fast tract, initiating reentry. Distinguishing nodal from accessory pathway PSVT is difficult during episodes of PSVT. Negative P waves in II, III, and avF may indicate retrograde conduction through the accessory pathway but they are

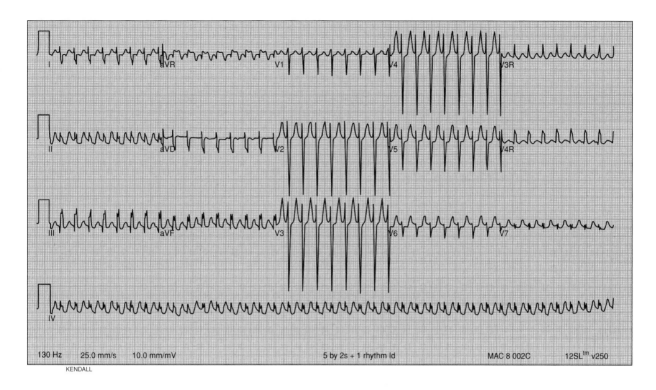

Figure 50–1. SVT, with concomitant right ventricular hypertrophy. This 4-year-old male was postoperative from repair of congenital heart disease (Fontan repair). He was eventually converted to normal sinus rhythm after multiple doses of adenosine.

usually buried in the QRS complex. Pointed or peaked T waves suggest retrograde P waves. P waves are almost never seen in AV nodal reentry. Lack of delta wave during sinus rhythm does not rule out concealed accessory tracts. Information from parents may be helpful, but first episodes of PSVT or unstudied children make diagnosis in the ED difficult.

Unstable PSVT is treated with synchronized cardioversion, 0.5 J/kg, increasing to 2 J/kg as needed. Vagal maneuvers may convert stable patients. A bag containing ice and some water is placed over the nose and forehead for intervals of 15 to 20 seconds. Another technique is to have the child blow into an occluded straw. Ocular pressure or nasogastric stimulation is discouraged. If vagal maneuvers fail, adenosine, 0.1 mg/kg followed by 0.2 mg/kg, is recommended. Adenosine terminates nodal and accessory pathway tachycardia by blocking adenosine receptors in the AV node and slowing conduction. Transient side effects include headache, flushing, and chest pain. Rhythm disturbances, such as atrial fibrillation, accelerated ventricular rhythm, and wide-complex tachycardia, may require resuscitation. Other side effects include bronchospasm, apnea, and asystole. Adenosine can be used in hypotension but should be avoided in the patient on theophylline.

Digitalis is commonly used to prolong AV nodal conduction and refractoriness of fast and slow tracts. A pediatric cardiologist should be consulted prior to administration as it can promote accessory pathway conduction and ventricular tachycardia; therefore, it is best used in the well-known, stable patient with AV nodal reentry. It may take hours to work and if cardioversion is necessary, there is a risk of ventricular fibrillation.

Verapamil is not routinely used and is reserved for children >2 to 3 years of age. Hypotension, cardiovascular collapse, and death have occurred in infants. Older children with stable but recalcitrant PSVT may respond to IV verapamil, 0.1 mg/kg slowly. Calcium chloride, 10 mg/kg, and IV saline should be available to treat hypotension.

β-Blockers such as propanolol or esmolol may be used with caution, as propanolol may cause hypotension, tachycardia, or ventricular fibrillation. If the above measures fail or PSVT resumes, procainamide may be useful. Procainamide is preferred in narrow complex tachycardia thought to be ventricular. A 5- to 15-mg/kg bolus is given over 20 to 30 minutes, watching for hypotension or prolongation of the QRS complex. Amiodarone, 5 mg/kg administered over 20 to 60 minutes, is another option. However, it should not be given in conjunction with procainamide because of the risk of refractory hypotension or increased prolongation of the QRS interval. Propranolol, 0.1 mg/kg IV, is useful in WPW or other accessory pathway diseases. Esmolol dosage is 0.1 to 0.5 mg/kg IV over 1 minute, then 0.05 mg/kg/min, titrated as noted in PALS protocols. β-Blockers, calcium channel blockers, and digoxin should be avoided in SVT or atrial fibrillation/flutter with a wide complex (i.e., WPW) as these agents can increase the transmission through the bypass tract and induce ventricular fibrillation.

Any infant with new onset PSVT should be hospitalized and structural heart disease must be ruled out. Infants are likely to have accessory pathway disease and require further therapy. A child with immediate recurrence is at higher risk for repeat episodes or recalcitrant PSVT and may require surgical ablation.

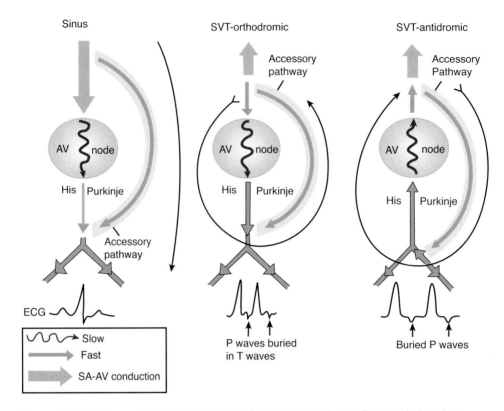

Figure 50–2. Diagrammatic representation of accessory pathway disease during sinus rhythm and PSVT. Sinus—short PR, delta wave, characteristic of WPW; Orthodromic—fast retrograde conduction through accessory pathway leads to reentry. His–Purkinje conduction is normal, complexes are narrow. Retrograde P waves are abnormally directed and buried in T wave; Antidromic (rare)—fast antegrade conduction through accessory pathway leads to abnormal His–Purkinje conduction and wide complexes. Retrograde P waves are abnormally directed and buried in T waves.

► ATRIAL FLUTTER AND FIBRILLATION

Atrial flutter and fibrillation in children are rare. Children with congenital heart disease, rheumatic fever, or dilated cardiomyopathy are at highest risk. Patients with atrial flutter or fibrillation, in combination with an accessory pathway or hypertrophic cardiomyopathy, are at high risk for sudden death. Unstable patients are cardioverted with 0.5 J/kg. Overdrive pacing 10 to 20 bpm faster than the flutter rate may also be effective. Cardioversion may be the only option. Patients with long-standing atrial disease associated with a diseased sinus node are at risk for bradycardia or asystole on termination. Pacing must be available. Consultation with a pediatric cardiologist is helpful if one chooses drug therapy as the choices vary based on left ventricular function and whether WPW is suspected or known. The long-term prognosis of children with congenital heart disease and atrial fibrillation or flutter may depend on the elimination of all flutter activity.

PREMATURE VENTRICULAR CONTRACTIONS

Premature ventricular contractions (PVCs) in the infant and young child are rare. Unifocal PVCs begin appearing in healthy children during adolescence. The patient is usually asymptomatic and has a normal physical examination, chest x-ray, and ECG. Unusual morphology, such as multifocal PVCs, coupling, or the "R on T" phenomenon, are rarely cause for emergency intervention in the asymptomatic child with normal QT interval. Continuous ECG monitor may define and quantify the PVCs. PVCs that diminish during exercise or stress are benign and require no therapy. Patients with myocarditis, cardiomyopathy, congenital heart disease, or who are postoperative from cardiac surgery, are at greater risk and may require treatment. Syncope or exercise-induced PVCs may also require therapy. Lidocaine, procainamide, or amiodarone may be useful using guidelines similar for ventricular tachycardia (see "Ventricular Tachycardia").

ACCELERATED IDIOVENTRICULAR RHYTHM

Accelerated idioventricular rhythm (AIVR) is a benign pediatric dysrhythmia that has the appearance of ventricular tachycardia. Rates are rarely faster than 150 bpm. AIVR begins gradually with fusion beats and is a monomorphic, wide-complex rhythm that originates from an accelerated ventricular focus. Diagnosis can be difficult in the new patient. Patients with AIVR are stable. Unstable wide-complex tachycardia is not AIVR and should be converted immediately. AIVR rarely responds to medication but can be a warning of a residual hemodynamic abnormality associated with corrected congenital heart disease.

VENTRICULAR TACHYCARDIA

Ventricular tachycardia (VT) is rare in children and can be confused with other forms of tachycardia. It is distinguished from PSVT by wide QRS complexes, >0.08 to 0.09 seconds, depending on age. Complexes as narrow as 0.06 seconds have been noted in infantile VT (Fig. 50–3). Wide complexes can be seen in PSVT but this is rare. Antegrade accessory pathway conduction can result in wide and bizarre-looking QRS complexes that simulate VT. Rates averaging 250 bpm are rarely helpful in differentiating PSVT from VT but may be helpful in distinguishing VT from AIVR, with average rates of 150. AV dissociation with P wave and QRS independence can also help distinguish VT from PSVT.

Idiopathic ventricular tachycardia is occasionally encountered in a child who is completely asymptomatic and has a normal heart. It is usually not treated. Serious causes, such as electrolyte disturbance, toxins, or myocarditis, should be considered. Structural heart disease, tumor, cardiomyopathy, or long QT syndrome may be the cause. VT in the setting of a diseased heart or congenital lesion is much more ominous than with normal anatomy. It usually requires aggressive evaluation and treatment. Recurrent exercise-induced syncope is often because of VT. The initial workup may be negative. A search for a small myocardial tumor, early cardiomyopathy, or occult myocarditis may be necessary. EPS or biopsy may be necessary to guide treatment.

Regardless of etiology, unstable wide-complex tachycardia should be synchronously cardioverted with 0.5 to 1 J/kg. After conversion, lidocaine may be given, 1 mg/kg bolus, followed by 15 to 50 μg/kg/min infusion. Amiodarone, 5 mg/kg over 1 hour, may be given for patients with stable ventricular tachycardia. In addition, procainamide may be useful for wide-complex tachycardia of uncertain origin because of its effect both above and below the AV node. An initial dose of 10 to 15 mg/kg over 30 to 45 minutes is followed by 20 to 80 μg/kg/min drip. Adenosine is safe and may be useful in the rare case of PSVT with aberrancy. It should be used only in stable situations when other traditional therapies have failed.

VENTRICULAR FIBRILLATION

Ventricular fibrillation is an uncommon rhythm in the pediatric population, but is certainly life-threatening. Causes include postoperative complications from congenital heart disease repair, severe hypoxemia, hyperkalemia, medications (digitalis, quinidine, catecholamines, and anesthesia), myocarditis, and myocardial infarction. The hallmark of ventricular fibrillation is chaotic irregular ventricular contractions without circulation to the body the rhythm. The electrocardiogram reveals a rapid rate, with bizarre QRS complexes with varying sizes and configurations.

In patients with unwitnessed arrests, CPR is beneficial immediately prior to defibrillation. It has been shown that giving

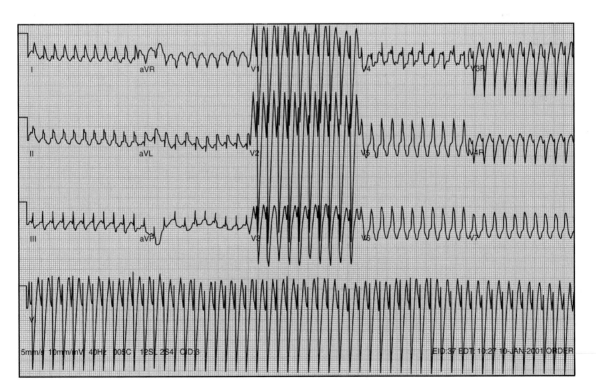

Figure 50–3. Ventricular tachycardia. This is an example, of an extraordinarily fast ventricular tachycardia with a heart rate of almost 300 BPM. (Courtesy of CDR Jonathan T. Fleenor, MD, Naval Medical Center, San Diego.)

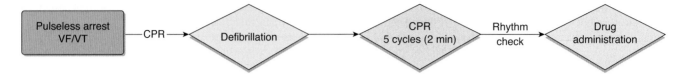

Figure 50–4. Sequence of resuscitation, in pulseless arrest with ventricular fibrillation (VF) and ventricular tachycardia (VT).

CPR prior to defibrillation increased survival rates from 4% to 22%.[5] The dosages of defibrillation are now 2 J/kg followed by 4 J/kg for subsequent dosages, regardless of the type of defibrillator. It is important to note that stacked shocks are no longer recommended. A single shock is recommended fol-lowed by CPR largely because of the prolonged period of time to administer three shocks. Do not interrupt CPR until 5 cy-cles or 2 minutes for a pulse/rhythm check (Fig. 50–4). More specifically, the treatment of each rhythm disturbance can be classified according to the tachycardia algorithm (Fig. 50–5).

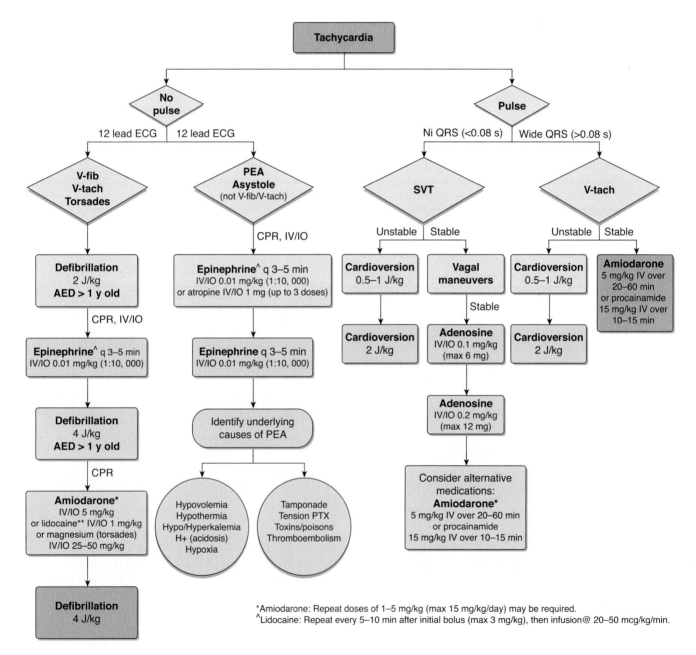

Figure 50–5. Tachycardia algorithm. (With permission from Ralston M, Hazinski M, Zaritsky A, Schexnayder S, Kleinman M. Pediatric assessment. *Pediatric Advanced Life Support, Provider Manual.* American Heart Association; 2006:1–32.)

The presence or absence of a pulse determines which arm of the algorithm to initiate.

For the most part, the algorithm drug dosages remain the same in the updated 2005 AHA recommendations. Drug delivery should not interrupt CPR. The timing of drug delivery is less important than minimizing interruption of chest compressions. Amiodarone is the preferred drug for treatment for pulseless arrest, since it is more effective. Lidocaine is only recommended when amiodarone is unavailable.[6] It is important to note that amiodarone and procainamide should not be administered together as they can lead to severe hypotension and prolongation of the QT interval. High-dose epinephrine (1:1000 concentration via IV) is not recommended in any age group, and is actually associated with a worse outcome, especially in cases of asphyxia.[2–4] Therefore, the standard recommended dose is (0.01 mg/kg IV/IO) for all doses, which correlates to 0.1 mL/kg. Although the preferred routes of administration are intravenous or intraosseous, it may be given via the endotracheal tube when such access is unable to be obtained (0.1 mg/kg ETT). In exceptional cases, such as β-blocker overdose, high-dose epinephrine may be considered. Magnesium sulphate at a dose of 25 to 50 mg/kg (maximum 2 g) should be given for torsades de pointes.

In the community, AEDs have been shown to increase survival rates. There has been sufficient evidence to show that AEDs can safely be used for those older than 1 year. In a sudden witnessed collapse, the AED should be used as soon as it becomes available. However, if the collapse is unwitnessed, CPR should be performed for 5 cycles or 2 minutes, prior to the use of the AED. Pediatric AED pads and energy levels should be used in those 1 to 8 years of age.[2] If the pediatric dose is unavailable, the adult dose is a reasonable alternative.

▶ OTHER CARDIAC CONDITIONS ASSOCIATED WITH DYSRHYTHMIAS

LONG QT SYNDROME

LQTS should be considered and an ECG be obtained on any patient presenting with a suggestive history, including First-degree relatives of known LQTS carrier, family history of syncope, seizures, or sudden death, a sibling with sudden infant death syndrome, seizure of unknown etiology, unexplained near-drowning. Other risk factors include congenital deafness and bradycardia in infants. Jervell and Lange-Nielsen first described the association of syncope, sudden death, deafness, and long QT interval in 1957. In 1963, Romano described the syndrome in normal-hearing patients. Congenital LQTS is an inherited syndrome characterized by paroxysmal ventricular tachycardia and torsades de pointes. It can be emotionally induced or stress related and can progress to ventricular fibrillation and sudden death. Acquired QT prolongation associated with drugs (Table 50–3), anorexia nervosa, bulimia, and electrolyte derangements can also predispose to dysrhythmia. The congenital form is the most common form affecting the child.

The QT interval should be manually measured, with Lead II generally accepted as being the most accurate. In order to account for the normal physiologic shortening of the QT interval that occurs with increasing heart rate, the corrected QT inter-

▶ **TABLE 50–3. DRUGS THAT PROLONG THE QT INTERVAL**

Antiarrhythmics (class 1 A and 3)
Antiemetic (droperidol)
Antifungals (ketoconazole)
Antihistamines (astemizole, terfenadine)
Antimicrobials (erythromycin, trimethoprim-sulfamethoxazole)
Antipsychotics (haloperidol, risperidone)
Organophosphate insecticides
Phenothiazines (thioridazine)
Promotility agents (cisapride)
Tricyclic antidepressants (amitryptyline)

val (QT_c) is calculated using the Bazett formula: $QT_c = QT/\sqrt{RR}$. For greatest accuracy, the QT and preceding RR intervals should be measured for three consecutive beats and averaged. The current practice identifies a $QT_c \geq 460$ ms as prolonged. A QT_c value between 420 and 460 ms is borderline and warrants additional assessment.[7] Although ECGs automatically calculate the QT and QT_c, in those patients with suggestive history an ECG with manual calculation of the QT_c should be performed, as the computer calculation often is inaccurate. If the diagnosis of LQTS is suspected but the screening ECG is not diagnostic, increasing sympathetic activity such as with vagal maneuvers may trigger abnormalities on electrocardiogram. These abnormalities include QT interval prolongation, prominent U waves, T-wave alternans, and ventricular dysrhythmias (Fig. 50–6).

Patients presenting with LQTS may require emergency intervention. Patients presenting with an episode of polymorphic ventricular tachycardia or torsades de pointes of unknown etiology should receive IV magnesium sulfate (25–50 mg/kg maximum 2 g). Serum electrolytes and a toxicology screen should be obtained. β-Blockers may be useful in suppressing catecholamine surges and further dysrhythmic activity. In those patients with torsades owing to prolonged QT, they may worsen acutely, while those with normal QT improve. Patients with recurrent ventricular tachycardia may require temporary transcutaneous ventricular pacing.

Any patient with a compatible history, borderline prolongation of the QT interval with symptoms, or identified prolonged QT syndrome should be referred to a cardiologist for further management. Admission is limited to those who are symptomatic or have cardiovascular compromise. Holter monitoring may be helpful in capturing a prolonged QT interval not apparent on a resting ECG. Therapy is aimed at reducing sympathetic activity of the heart, either pharmacologically or surgically. β-Blockers are generally recommended as the initial therapy of choice. β-Blockers have been shown to effectively eradicate dysrhythmias in 60% of patients, and to decrease mortality from 71% in untreated patient, to 6% in those who are treated.[8] The most commonly used are propanolol (2–4 mg/kg/d, maximum 60 mg/d) and nadolol (0.5–1 mg/kg/d, maximum 2.5 mg/kg/d). Patients with severe asthma in whom β-blockers are contraindicated may be candidates for pacer therapy. Approximately 20% of patients remain refractory to treatment with β-blockers, and continue to experience recurrent syncope. Alternative therapies include left-sided cervicothoracic sympathetic ganglionectomy, and implantation of automatic implantable cardiac defibrillators.

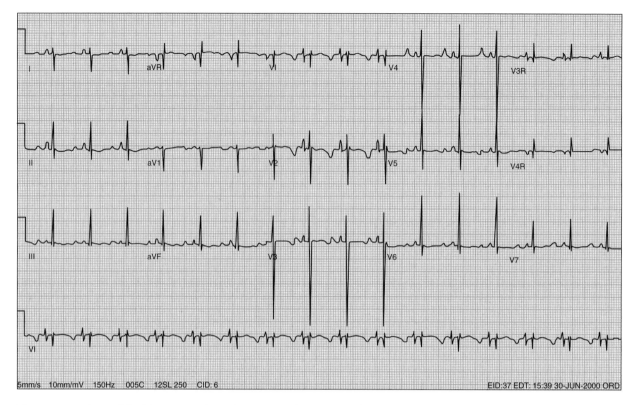

Figure 50–6. Long QT without associated heart block. Markedly prolonged QT interval calculated with the Bazett formula [6]: QTc = QT/(square root of the preceding RR interval); QTc = 0.452/(square root of 0.612); QTc = 578 ms; Of note, for improved accuracy average three consecutive R-R intervals and QT intervals, where each small box = 0.04 ms. (Courtesy of CDR Jonathan T. Fleenor, MD, Naval Medical Center, San Diego.)

Once a patient is diagnosed with LQTS, and ECG should be performed on all other family members. All affected individuals, regardless of age, should be restricted from competitive sports, but not necessarily recreational sports. Patients should be educated to avoid triggering factors, such as certain medications, loud noises, emotionally stressful situations, and dehydration. Because of the high risk of unexpected cardiac events, family members and close friends should be instructed in CPR and even consider purchasing a home AED.

HYPERTROPHIC CARDIOMYOPATHY

Hypertrophic cardiomyopathy (HC) is characterized by a hypertrophied, nondilated left ventricle. Symptoms include chest pain, dyspnea, syncope, or sudden death. Clinical presentation varies. Some patients are asymptomatic. The majority of symptomatic adults suffer from CHF secondary to insufficient diastolic filling. Dysrhythmias include atrial fibrillation and ventricular tachyarrhythmia, the leading causes of sudden death. Outflow obstruction is rare. Mortality rates of 3% are probably overestimated due to sampling bias and may lead to an overly aggressive approach to therapy. This is especially true of the asymptomatic individual. However, pediatric HC tends to be more serious, with mortality rates in infants approaching 6%. Other risk factors include advanced symptoms at diagnosis, LV dysfunction, and a family history of sudden death. Atrial fibrillation is especially dangerous in the HC patient. The ECG may provide a clue to the diagnosis. Look for narrow Q waves in leads 1 and avL combined with increased voltage in V2 and V5.

Signs of HC include late systolic murmur and paradoxical splitting of S_2. LV or septal hypertrophy on ECG is a poor prognostic sign. Echocardiogram is diagnostic. Therapy depends on the clinical manifestation. β-Blockers are the mainstay of therapy for CHF, effective in relieving dyspnea and chest pain. β-Blockers have no effect on rates of sudden death. Atrial fibrillation should be controlled because of its association with rapid ventricular rate and decreased outflow. Amiodarone may be effective, but has also been associated with sudden death in some symptomatic patients. Implantable defibrillators may be preferred. Dual chamber pacing and surgical myectomy may be necessary for significant outflow obstruction.

► SUMMARY

Children, fortunately, rarely have dysrythmias, and can remain stable for longer periods of time. The clinician needs to assess the patient for stability, for type of rhythm disturbance, and for the appropriate therapy.

REFERENCES

1. Perondi M, Reis A, Paiva E, Nadkarni V, Berg R. A comparison of high-dose and standard-dose epinephrine in children with cardiac arrest. *N Engl J Med*. 2004;350(17):1708–1709.

2. Ralston M, Hazinski M, Zaritsky A, Schexnayder S, Kleinman M. Pediatric assessment. *Pediatric Advanced Life Support, Provider Manual.* American Heart Association; 2006:1–32.
3. ECC Committee. 2005 American Heart Association guidelines for cardiopulmonary resuscitation and emergency cardiovascular care: Part 13: Neonatal resuscitation guidelines. *Circulation.* 2005;112:188–195.
4. ECC Committee. Highlights of the 2005 American Heart Association guidelines for cardiopulmonary resuscitation and emergency cardiovascular care. *Currents.* 2006;15(4):23–27.
5. Wik L, Kramer-Johansen J, Myklebust H, et al. Quality of cardiopulmonary resuscitation during out-of-hospital cardiac arrest. *JAMA.* 2005;293:299–304.
6. Dorian P, Cass D, Schwartz B, Cooper R, Gelaznikas R, Barr A. Amiodarone as compared with lidocaine for shock-resistant ventricular fibrillation. *N Engl J Med.* 2002;346:884–890.
7. Ackerman MJ. The long QT syndrome: ion channel diseases of the heart. *Mayo Clin Proc.* 1998;73:250–269.
8. Schwartz PJ. Idiopathic long QT syndrome: progress and questions. *Am Heart J.* 1985;399–411.

CHAPTER 51

Pediatric Hypertension

Emily C. MacNeill

▶ HIGH-YIELD FACTS

- Hypertension is defined as blood pressures ≥ 90th percentile for age and height matched normal values. Stage 2 hypertension (≥ 99th percentile) requires urgent evaluation and treatment.
- The differential diagnosis of hypertension changes with the age of the patient.
- Evaluation of the hypertensive patient should focus on the cause of hypertension, and evaluate the patient for signs of end-organ damage.
- Initiation of oral antihypertensive agents should be done in conjunction with the physician who will be following up with the patients.
- Patients with a hypertensive emergency should be aggressively treated and admitted to a pediatric nephrologist or other hypertension specialist.

Hypertension is an unusual finding in pediatric patients; however, when present, it must be quickly recognized and treated to avoid damage to the renal, cardiovascular, and neurologic systems. It has become a common practice to not routinely take blood pressures of children younger than 3 years in the emergency department (ED) setting. The onus is on the practitioner to keep a watchful eye out for young patients who have risk factors for hypertension. Blood pressures must be measured accurately and abnormal values confirmed before initiating an evaluation. The normal ranges for blood pressure change with age and height and not all elevated pressures require immediate treatment. An understanding of the etiologies of high blood pressures in the pediatric patient and a stepwise approach to hypertensive children ensures that patients will receive appropriate management.

▶ MEASURING BLOOD PRESSURE

Management of hypertension in children requires an accurate measurement of blood pressure. This can be difficult with the pediatric patient, as accuracy requires a seated and relaxed patient as well as selection of the appropriate size cuff. Cuffs that are too large will yield an erroneously low blood pressure and conversely, cuffs that are too small will yield a high reading. The bladder width should be approximately 40% of the circumference of the width of the arm at mid point between the acromion and the olecranon process. The length of the bladder should reach around 80% to 100% of the circumference of the arm.[1]

Many EDs utilize automated oscillometric devices that can be very accurate at all age ranges as long as they are calibrated regularly. It is important, however, that any abnormal reading be repeated by manual sphyngomanometry. In addition, abnormally high readings should be correlated with blood pressure measurements obtained from both upper extremities as well as at least one lower extremity.

▶ DEFINING HYPERTENSION

Although there has been some debate over the years as to defining pediatric hypertension, the National High Blood Pressure Education Program (NHBPEP) put forth the following definitions of hypertension in the *Fourth Report on the Diagnosis, Evaluation, and Treatment of High Blood Pressure in Children and Adolescents*: hypertension is either a systolic (sBP) or diastolic pressure (dBP) ≥95th percentile of age and height matched normal values and prehypertension is between the 90th and 95th percentile (Fig. 51–1). Hypertension is then further broken down into two stages: stage 1 hypertension is defined as sBP or dBP between the 95th and 99th percentile and stage 2 hypertension is ≥99th percentile. While all stages of hypertension require some further evaluation, many patients with stage 1 hypertension can be safely discharged from the ED with close follow-up. Stage 2 hypertensive patients require more urgent evaluation and treatment. This terminology differs from the vague concept of hypertensive urgency versus emergency. Hypertensive urgency describes a state of elevated pressures with potential to cause end-organ damage without any evidence of damage. Hypertensive emergency, on the other hand, is used to describe a state where end-organ damage is apparent.

Primary or essential hypertension is the most common cause of elevated blood pressure in adult populations, as secondary hypertension is a rare entity; this is not so in children. Emergency physicians must look for disease processes that can cause secondary hypertension in pediatric patients. This is especially true for very young children, children with stage 2 hypertension, and children with signs or symptoms of concurrent illnesses. There is some debate regarding a rise in essential hypertension in adolescents and school-age children and its link to increased obesity.[1,2] It is important for the emergency physician to know that patients with essential hypertension often present differently than those with secondary disease. Patients with primary hypertension usually present with mild stage 1 hypertension with few, if any, symptoms. These children usually have a family history of hypertension or cardiovascular disease and often have an elevated body mass index.[1] These

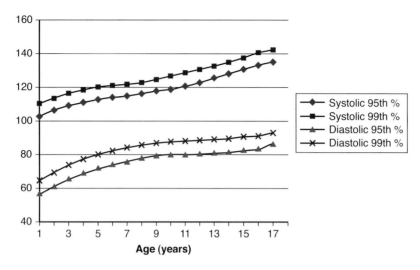

Figure 51–1. Hypertensive values according to age. From the Fourth Report on the Diagnosis, Evaluation, and Treatment of High Blood Pressure in Children and Adolescents from 2004. Data points are taken from males at the 50th percentile for height. Females and smaller children will have slightly lower blood pressure thresholds.

are the patients who are more likely to be discharged from the ED without initiation of pharmacologic intervention. Patients with secondary hypertension often present with stage 2 hypertension and can have more overt signs of end-organ damage: encephalopathy, seizure, congestive heart failure, chest pain, hematuria, or edema to name a few.

▶ DIFFERENTIAL DIAGNOSIS

The differential diagnosis for the etiology of secondary hypertension in the pediatric patient is broad (Table 51–1). As with many pediatric diseases, the differential diagnosis for hypertension is dependent on the age of the patient. Table 51–2 demonstrates the most prominent causes of hypertension among patients of different ages. In the neonatal popula-

tion, the most common causes are renal vessel thromboses/stenoses, coarctation of the aorta and congenital renal anomalies. Renal parenchymal abnormalities are uncommon in early infancy and then become the most common cause of hypertension in the school-age child. Essential hypertension is becoming more prevalent in school-age children and is becoming predominant in the adolescent patient.

The emergency physician should be aware that there are numerous, less common causes, of hypertension in children. Endocrine abnormalities, such as hyperthyroidism, and hypercortisol states (from endogenous production or exogenous exposure) can be imminently dangerous. Heavy metal poisoning is also associated with hypertension and exposure to substances such as lead should be ascertained.

▶ ASSESSMENT

HISTORY

The history should focus on elucidating the cause and effect (if any) of hypertension in the child. First and foremost, a history

▶ TABLE 51–1. ETIOLOGY OF SECONDARY HYPERTENSION IN CHILDREN

Renal
  Glomerulonephritis
  Obstructive uropathy
  Hemolytic uremic syndrome
  Renal tumors
  Pyelonephritis
  Acute renal failure
  Congenital malformation
  Renovascular

Cardiovascular
  Coarctation of aorta
  Aortic insufficiency
  Vasculitis

Neurologic
  Trauma
  Increased intracranial pressure
  Guillain–Barre syndrome

Endocrine
  Hypercortisol states
  Adrenal dysfunction
  Hyperparathyroidism
  Hyperthyroidism

Toxicologic
  Oral contraceptives
  Steroids (corticosteroids and anabolic)
  Stimulants (amphetamines, ephedrine)
  Heavy metal exposures
  Cyclosporine

▶ TABLE 51–2. COMMON ETIOLOGY OF HYPERTENSION IN CHILDREN ACCORDING TO AGE

Age	Etiology
Infancy	Congenital renal disease, aortic coarctation, renal artery/vein thrombosis
Early childhood	Renal parenchymal disease, aortic coarctation, renal vessel disease
School age	Renal parenchymal disease, essential hypertension, renal vessel disease
Adolescent	Essential hypertension, renal parenchymal disease

of hypertension and medication use for this problem should be ascertained because sudden withdrawal of medication can lead to pathologic increase in blood pressures. A full medication history of both prescription and recreational drugs is important; oral contraceptives and steroids as well as cocaine and amphetamines can cause elevated pressures. Birth history indicating problems such as umbilical artery catheterization as well as premature infant with chronic lung disease is a risk factor for high blood pressure. Renal disease can both cause and be an effect of elevated pressures. Thus, inquiry into the symptoms of renal disease is vital for children with hypertension, specifically gross hematuria, edema, generalized fatigue, and recent infections. Endocrine problems can cause symptoms in addition to hypertension such as flushing and tachycardia and weight changes. It is especially important in the obese patient to inquire about sleep disturbance, as sleep-disordered breathing is associated with hypertension.

The effects of elevated blood pressures on the pediatric patient can be quite vague. As stated above, the kidneys can be profoundly affected by prolonged high pressures with few signs. Symptoms are more often recognized in the cardiovascular and neurologic systems. Chest pain, exertional dyspnea, and palpitations can occur. It is important to ask about headaches, visual disturbances, and in more severe cases, altered mental status and convulsions.

PHYSICAL EXAMINATION

Again, the role of the emergency physician in the evaluation of the hypertensive child is to look carefully for clues to the etiology and the effects of high blood pressure. As with any physical examination, pay attention to the vital signs. Blood pressure measurements should be performed in both upper extremities and at least in one lower extremity. Leg pressures should measure at least 10 to 20 mm Hg higher than arm pressures and, if not, could signify coarctation of the aorta. Tachycardia can point toward an endocrine etiology, whereas bradycardia can signify increased intracranial pressure and impending herniation. After vital signs, the most important part of the physical examination is the neurologic examination, especially in the younger child, as altered mental status can be a cause or a result of pathologically elevated pressures. Fundoscopic examination should be attempted to look for elevated intracranial pressure as well as signs of long-term hypertension. Examination of the cardiovascular system includes checking pulses in all four extremities, evaluation for murmurs and gallops, as well as location of the cardiac apex.

Other physical findings can provide important clues. Adenotonsillar hypertrophy cause sleep disturbance that can lead to hypertension. Signs of heart failure should be noted, such as pulmonary edema or hepatomegaly. Edema in the lower extremities or periorbitally can indicate renal disease. Evaluate the skin for striae, flushing, acne, hirsutism, and acanthosis nigricans, all of which are signs of endocrine abnormalities. Young children should also undergo a urogenital examination to evaluate for ambiguous genitalia.

TESTING

Two things must be accomplished in the ED: initiate testing for the etiology and for end-organ damage and decide whether the child requires admission or can be safely discharged with follow-up (Fig. 51–2). The results of initial screening examinations can help with this decision. An electrocardiogram, a CBC, and a basic metabolic panel as well as urinalysis and urine culture should be done on every patient with blood pressures > 95th percentile prior to deciding disposition from the ED. Electrocardiogram can show left ventricular hypertrophy in the cases of prolonged or severe hypertension and can be a useful tool for deciding whether a child requires more urgent reduction in blood pressure. Electrolytes can evaluate for mineralocorticoid function and an elevated glucose, in the setting of obesity, can point toward a diabetic with primary hypertension. BUN and creatinine are vital, as acute renal failure and numerous parenchymal and glomerular kidney disorders can cause hypertension. A CBC should be performed to look for signs of infection and anemia.

If a child is to be admitted with hypertensive urgency or emergency, it is helpful to obtain other tests that the child will require for the workup. These tests include rennin levels, plasma and urine steroids, plasma and urine catecholamines, drug screening, and heavy metal levels, if deemed appropriate. Clearly, if the child shows signs of neurologic dysfunction, a head CT scan is mandatory. Patients with severe hypertension will need an echocardiogram, but if the child is not in extremis and has neither critical valvular disease nor aortic coarctation, this can be completed as part of the inpatient evaluation.

▶ TREATMENT

GOALS

It is crucial for the ED physician to be comfortable using parenteral antihypertensive medications in the setting of hypertensive emergency. The medications used are similar to those used in adults; however, side effects and indications can be different in the pediatric patient. Thus, it is important to know not the medications, but to be aware of doses and side effects for each drug (Table 51–3). ED physicians should also have some degree of familiarity with oral agents, as many patients will present on these medications or they may require initiation of therapy by the ED physician in conjunction with a specialist (Table 51–4).

According to the *Fourth Report on the Diagnosis, Evaluation, and Treatment of High Blood Pressure in Children and Adolescents*, parenteral medications should be reserved for patients with hypertensive emergencies. The goal of treatment should be a relatively slow reduction of pressure so as not to underperfuse vital organs. The blood pressure should decrease by 25% over the first 8 hours; medications can then be titrated to normalization of blood pressure over the next 26 to 48 hours. Children with stage 2 hypertension who have no evidence of end-organ damage can be started on oral antihypertensive agents.[1]

▶ INDIVIDUAL AGENTS

SODIUM NITROPRUSSIDE

Sodium nitroprusside lowers blood pressure by dilating both the arterial and venous side of the circulation, dramatically

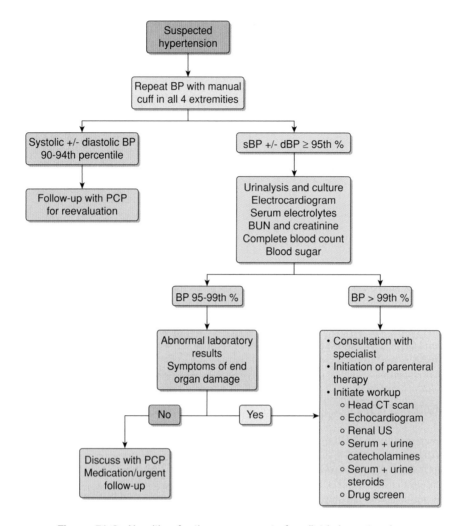

Figure 51–2. Algorithm for the assessment of pediatric hypertension.

increasing the size of the capillary beds. Its quick onset of action makes it a very useful drug for hypertensive emergencies. The short half-life of the drug allows for easy titration and in fact, blood pressures will return to baseline within minutes of turning off a sodium nitroprusside drip. The starting dose of nitroprusside is 0.3 to 0.5 μg/kg/min with a maximum of 8 μg/kg/min.[3]

Side effects for nitroprusside include an increase in intracranial pressure, so it should be used with caution in the setting of head injury or hypertensive encephalopathy. Also, nitroprusside is metabolized into cyanide by the red blood cells, which is then metabolized into thiocyanate by the liver and then excreted by the kidneys. Prolonged use, and/or higher doses in small children can lead to cyanide poisoning.

▶ TABLE 51–3. **MEDICATIONS USEFUL IN HYPERTENSIVE EMERGENCY**

Route	Drug	Dose	Onset of Action	Comments
Continuous IV drip	Nitroprusside	0.3–8 μg/kg/min	Seconds	May cause increased ICP
	Labetolol	0.5–3.0 mg/kg/h*	2–10 min	Contraindicated with asthma; avoid use with congenital heart disease/heart failure
	Esmolol	50–300 μg/kg/min†	Seconds	Avoid with asthma
	Nicardipine	0.5–3.0 μg/kg/min	2–5 min	Caution with increased ICP
IV bolus	Hydralazine	0.1–0.5 mg/kg/dose (max. 20 mg/dose)	5–30 min	May cause reflex tachycardia
	Enalopril	5–10 μg/kg/dose	15–60 min	Do not use with bilateral renal artery stenosis

*An initial bolus of 0.2–1 mg/kg can be given followed by 0.25–1.5 mg/kg/h drip. Labetolol can also be given at 0.2–1 mg/kg in single doses (with a maximum of 20 mg/dose).
†A loading dose of 100–500 μg/kg is used to start this medication.

▶ **TABLE 51–4. ORAL AGENTS FOR THE MANAGEMENT OF PEDIATRIC HYPERTENSION**

Agent	Initial Dose (mg/kg/dose)	Maximum Dose Per Day, (mg/kg)/ max mg	Frequency
ACE Inhibitors			
Captopril	0.3–0.5	6	tid
Lisinopril	0.07	0.6/40	qid
Angiotensin-receptor blocker			
Losartan	0.7	1.4/100	qid
Diuretics			
Furosemide	0.5	6	qid–bid
Hydrochlorothiazide	1	3/50	qid
Spironolactone	1	3.3/100	qid–bid
Calcium channel blocker			
Nifedipine	0.25–0.5/d	3/120	qid–bid
β-blocker			
Atenolol	0.5–1	2/100	qid–bid
Propranolol	1–2	4/640	bid–tid

Thiocyanate levels need to be followed in prolonged administration and the drug should be discontinued after approximately 48 hours. Because of its metabolic pathway, it should be used with caution in children with renal insufficiency or liver impairment.[4]

α OR β BLOCKADE

Labetolol has been used for many years in both adult and pediatric hypertensive crises. It acts as both an α- and a β-blocker; smooth muscle relaxation peripherally allows a decrease in blood pressure. Despite its efficacy, there are a few drawbacks to this drug. Its half-life is quite a bit longer than that of nitroprusside, approximately 3 to 5 hours. Thus, overshooting the desired blood pressure decrease cannot be easily reversed. Because of its β blockade, it is contraindicated in children who suffer from asthma or chronic lung disease. It also is a negative inotrope and should probably not be used with children with congenital heart disease.[3]

Esmolol is a selective β-blocker that appears to be more cardioselective and some people recommend its use in children with hypertensive crisis in the setting of congenital heart disease.

There are drugs such as prazosin and clonidine that are selective α inhibitors that have the benefit of not worsening bronchospasm. The main drawback with clonidine is its oral administration and a severe rebound hypertension once the drug is withdrawn.

CALCIUM CHANNEL BLOCKADE

There are two drugs in the calcium channel blocker class that can be used to treat hypertension in children: nicardipine and nifedipine. Nicardipine is administered intravenously and can be titrated carefully with its rapid onset of action and short half-

life. There is not much published data on the use of this drug in children but case reports have been published for its use in pediatric patients, especially those in whom other agents are contraindicated. Nifedipine is an oral agent available in liquid-filled capsules and is not used often in acute settings. The capsule can be opened and administered sublingually as a last resort for children with hypertensive emergency, when IV access is an issue. This agent should be used with great caution as it can be difficult to dose and can cause excessive drop in blood pressure.[5] Also, it has a short half-life with potential for rebound hypertension.[3] Its use is better restricted to long-term management of hypertension in its extended release form.

ACE INHIBITORS

This class of drugs inhibits angiotensin converting enzyme (ACE) that converts renin to angiotensin. Angiotensin is a potent vasoconstrictor, so the result of inhibiting ACE is vascular relaxation and decrease in blood pressure. There are many oral forms that have been studied and are both efficacious and safe in pediatric populations such as lisinopril. There is also an intravenous version of enalopril called enaloprilat that can theoretically be used for pediatric hypertensive emergency, although it is found to be most effective with children who have high renin states.[4]

HYDRALAZINE

Hydralazine is a drug that has, in the past, been given for rapid lowering of blood pressure; this is accomplished by pure arteriolar dilatation. It has not been shown to be more effective than sodium nitroprusside, can have a less predictable effect on blood pressure, and can also cause significant tachycardia.[4] At this time, there are numerous superior choices to hydralazine for blood pressure lowering.

DIURETICS

Diuretics work by decreasing intra- and extravascular volumes. Unfortunately, the body becomes accustomed to this effect, leading to medication resistance. The most commonly used agents are loop diuretics, thiazides, and potassium-sparing diuretics, and all are safe to use initially. Side effects of these medications are mainly electrolyte imbalances that should be evaluated in patients who take them for prolonged periods of time. Both loop diuretics and thiazides can cause hypokalemia and hyperlipidemia; loop diuretics also cause hypercalcemia and thiazides can cause calciuria.[4]

▶ SUMMARY

As the incidence of hypertension in the pediatric population is increasing, it is vital that the emergency physicians recognize and treat pathologically elevated pressures in their patients. This requires knowledge of the normal blood pressures in children and the differential diagnosis of hypertension appropriate for that patient's age group. While definitive diagnosis and treatment of hypertension does not often occur in the ED, the responsibility of initial screening for both life-threatening causes (such as aortic coarctation) and end-organ damage lies with the emergency physician. Patients can then be routed to the appropriate specialist as an inpatient or with an outpatient referral for long-term management. The physician should also have familiarity and comfort with the treatment of hypertensive emergency; this includes knowledge of a few pressure-lowering agents, their dosing administration, as well as their side effects and contraindications. An understanding of blood pressure management is crucial to prevent long-term morbidity in the hypertensive pediatric patient.

REFERENCES

1. National High Blood Pressure Education Working Group on High Blood Pressure in Children and Adolescents. The Fourth Report on the Diagnosis, Evaluation, and Treatment of High Blood Pressure in Children and Adolescents. *Pediatrics.* 2004;114:555–576.
2. Chiolero A, Bovet P, Paradis G, et al. Has blood pressure increased in children in response to the obesity epidemic. *Pediatrics.* 2007;119(3):544–553.
3. Constantine E, Linakis J. The assessment and management of hypertensive emergencies and urgencies in children. *Pediatr Emerg Care.* 2005;21(6):391–396.
4. Temple ME, Nahate MC. Treatment of pediatric hypertension. *Pharmacotherapy.* 2000;20(2):140–150.
5. Adelman RD, Coppo R, Dillon MJ. The emergency management of severe hypertension. *Pediatr Nephrol.* 2000;14:422–427.

CHAPTER 52

Thromboembolic Disease

Lee S. Benjamin

▶ HIGH-YIELD FACTS

- The single greatest risk factor for thromboembolic disease in children is an indwelling central venous catheter.
- Disease patterns for pulmonary embolism in children and adolescents are similar to those in adults, yet diagnosis and management is often delayed or inappropriate.
- Arterial thromboembolism is more common in neonates and children with cardiac disorders, likely due to the use of umbilical artery catheters, cardiac catheters, ECMO circuits, and valvular disease.
- Advanced imaging studies have historically been the mainstay of diagnosis for pulmonary embolism as well, as most chest radiographs in children are normal.
- Anticoagulation is achieved acutely with unfractionated heparin or low-molecular-weight heparin (LMWH), followed by long-term anticoagulation with either LMWH or warfarin.

▶ THROMBOEMBOLIC DISEASE

Although rare, thromboembolic events (TEs) increasingly occur in children, with a current rate of 5 episodes per 100 000 pediatric hospitalizations.[1] Deep vein thrombosis (DVT) is the most common TE in children with pulmonary embolism (PE) relatively rare at 8% of venous thrombotic events (VTE).[2] Arterial thromboembolism (ATE) is more common in neonates and children with cardiac disorders, likely due to the use of umbilical artery catheters, cardiac catheters, ECMO circuits, and valvular disease.[3] After briefly discussing ATE, this chapter will focus on the risk factors, clinical presentation, diagnosis, and management of venous thromboembolism (VTE), with stroke discussed further in Chapter 59.

▶ ARTERIAL THROMBOEMBOLISM

ATE leads to higher morbidity and mortality than VTE.[4,5] Previously healthy children with no underlying risk factors rarely present with ATE, although 22% of pediatric patients developing ischemic stroke have no identifiable underlying risk factors.[6] Among critically ill children, 96% of ATE are catheter related, either secondary to peripheral catheter use or cardiac catheterization.[7] Non–catheter-related ATE occur in patients with underlying hematologic risk factors similar to those correlated with VTE, yet also include organ transplantation and vasculitides such as Kawasaki disease and Takayasu arteritis.[8,9] Complications of ATE include stroke, limb loss, and dysfunction of the involved distal organs.

▶ RISK FACTORS FOR THROMBOEMBOLISM

Risk factors for developing VTE assume two primary forms: inherited and acquired. Inherited thrombophilias such as protein C[10] and S deficiencies,[11] antithrombin deficiency,[12] and the presence of lupus anticoagulant[13] are considered high-risk states, with factor V Leiden disease, prothrombin mutation, elevated factor VIII, hyperhomocysteinemia, elevated lipoprotein (a), dysfibrinogenemia, and hypo/dysplasminogenemia considered lower risk.[14,15] Healthy children with a single thrombophilic trait rarely present with TE, but the risk increases with multiple thrombophilic traits or with the addition of acquired risk factors.[16,17]

Acquired risk factors are numerous. The most consistent risk factor for development of VTE is central venous catheter placement. In neonatal TE, 65% to 90% are catheter related, and 64% of non-neonate TE is associated with central venous lines.[3,18] Commonly cited acquired risk factors are listed in Table 52–1. Among medical conditions, one of the most concerning risk factors for TE is cancer. Both acute leukemia and sarcoma carry high risk of VTE.[3,19] Contrary to the high adult VTE rate in brain cancer,[20] children with brain tumors have an incidence of clinically apparent TE in only 0.64% of patients.[21] Trauma has anecdotally been considered a risk factor for TE. However, when specifically studied, VTE appears quite rare in pediatric trauma. Incidence rate for all children younger than 17 years admitted to a trauma center after injury was only 0.06%.[22] Other studies concur with this very low rate of VTE. The highest traumatic risk factors for VTE include spinal cord injury, major vascular injury, older age, central line placement, and operative interventions.[23,24]

▶ DIAGNOSIS OF VENOUS THROMBOEMBOLISM

CLINICAL PRESENTATION

The first challenge of diagnosing VTE is clinically suspecting it. In many children, VTE is unsuspected, but found on routine management of common conditions, as in radiographic monitoring of osteomyelitis.[25] Furthermore, it is impossible to know if a patient has underlying inherited risk factors for VTE if they have not had a previous event and prothrombotic evaluation. Therefore, if a patient presents with signs or symptoms of VTE, a thorough search for predisposing conditions is warranted, including obtaining a family history specifically aimed at identifying VTE.

▶ **TABLE 52–1. FREQUENTLY CITED ACQUIRED RISK FACTORS FOR THROMBOEMBOLISM**

Indwelling catheters	Dehydration
Malignancy*	Vasculitis
Surgery	Immunosuppression
Pregnancy	Obesity
Infection	Stem cell/bone marrow transplant
Oral contraceptive use diabetes mellitus	Liver failure
	Dehydration
Nephrotic syndrome	Hyperlipidemia
Congenital heart disease	Sickle cell anemia
Congestive heart failure	Immobility
Vascular malformations	Burns
Trauma*	

*see text.

Clinically, DVT presents as pain, swelling, and erythema of the involved extremity. The differential diagnosis includes musculoskeletal injury, tumor, infection, arteriovenous malformation, and cystic lesions including Baker's cyst in the lower extremity.[26–29] In contrast to adults, DVTs in children commonly occur in the upper venous system correlating strongly with the common locations of central venous catheters.[3]

PE provides an even more complicated scenario. Even when well studied in adults, a significant proportion of patients lack some of the characteristic clinical findings of pleuritic chest pain, shortness of breath, tachycardia, tachypnea, hypoxia, and signs or symptoms of DVT.[30,31] Multiple templates provide a diagnostic guideline for adults.[32–34] However, none have been validated in children.

LABORATORY TESTING

Baseline PT, PTT, TT, ABG, and type and screen should be considered for a patient with suspected VTE requiring treatment. Factor Xa is used to monitor anticoagulation with low-molecular-weight heparin (LMWH), but is not helpful in the initial evaluation. The serum D-dimer test is an assay assessing for fibrin breakdown products, and is commonly used to rule out adult VTE in combination with a low-pretest probability.[32,35] It is not well studied in children and should not be relied on as a screening test as up to 40% of pediatric patients with proven VTE have negative assays.[36] Once VTE is established, persistently elevated D-dimer levels do predict risk of further events or complications.[37,38]

IMAGING

DVT diagnosis is historically based on imaging with either ultrasound (US) or venogram, yet pitfalls remain. US is the most commonly accepted initial imaging modality, based on technical ease and noninvasive nature of the test. Sensitivity in the lower extremities is high, and US is the standard diagnostic tool. If inconclusive and clinical suspicion is high, venography, CT venogram, or MR venogram may be useful. US is also

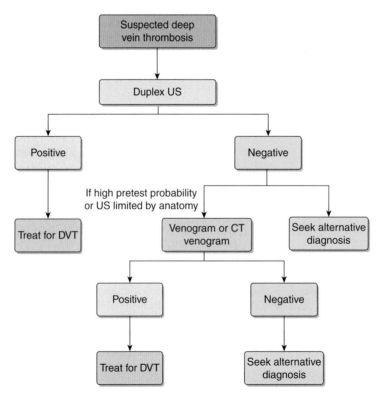

Figure 52–1. Diagnostic algorithm for deep vein thrombosis. DVT, deep vein thrombosis; US, ultrasound; CT, computed tomography.

effective in the neck and upper extremities themselves; however, sensitivity drops as low as 37% in upper extremity DVT due to poor visualization of the subclavian vein, brachiocephalic vein, and superior vena cava due to skeletal structures. Other studies for upper extremity DVT include venography, CT venogram, MR venogram, and echocardiogram, and should be considered if US is unable to visualize the potential thrombosis[39,40] (Fig. 52–1).

Advanced imaging studies have historically been the mainstay of diagnosis for PE as well, since most chest radiographs in children are normal.[41] Use of both perfusion lung scans (V/Q) and CT imaging may lead to the diagnosis. No studies document the efficacy of these tests in children; however, V/Q scans with perfusion defects should be assumed to be PE as most pediatric patients lack chronic pulmonary diseases.[42] If a chest radiograph is void of significant disease, and the patient is able to comply, it is the author's opinion that V/Q be the imaging study of choice for PE. If the study is nondiagnostic, further imaging with CT should be obtained, which may provide other useful information.[43] Pulmonary angiography, the previous standard diagnostic tool, remains an option as well[41] (Fig. 52–2). MRI has also been used to evalu-

ate PE; however, it has poor sensitivity in children, limiting its usefulness.[44,45]

Other VTE that may be encountered include renal vein, inferior vena cava (IVC), and right atrium thrombosis. The prior presents with flank mass, pain, hematuria, thrombocytopenia, and hypertension. IVC thrombosis may present with bilateral lower extremity swelling, pallor, cyanosis, or pain, and is associated with significant long-term disease. Cardiac thrombus is associated with catheter malfunction and congestive heart failure. All of these processes are most common in ill neonates and infants who had indwelling catheters, with few outliers.[46,47] US remains the standard imaging modality for evaluating these pathological processes.

TREATMENT

The mainstay of treatment in thromboembolic disease is anticoagulation to prevent further clot formation, and should be done in conjunction with a pediatric hematologist, when possible. Anticoagulation is achieved acutely with unfractionated heparin (UH) or LMWH, followed by long-term anticoagulation

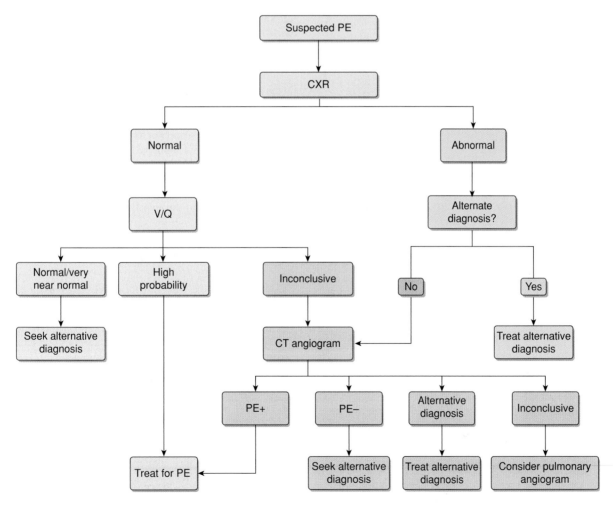

Figure 52–2. Diagnostic algorithm for pulmonary embolism. PE, pulmonary embolism; CXR, chest radiograph; V/Q, ventilation-perfusion scan; CT, computed tomography.

▶ **TABLE 52-2. ANTICOAGULANT AND THROMBOLYTIC DOSING GUIDELINES FOR ACUTE THROMBOEMBOLISM**

Anticoagulants

Heparin

  Unfractionated heparin[50]

  Loading dose: 75 U/kg IV over 10 min

  Maintenance dose for infants <1 y: 28 U/kg/h

  Maintenance dose for children >1 y: 20 U/kg/h

Obtain aPTT 4 h after loading dose, and 4 h after each adjustment

Adjustment to maintain aPTT 60 to 85 s:

aPTT: < 50, bolus 50 U/kg IV with 10% increase in rate

  50–59, 10% increase in rate

  60–85, maintain rate

  86–95, 10% decrease in rate

  96–120, stop drip for 30 min, resume with 10% decrease in rate

  >120, stop drip for 60 min, resume with 15% decrease in rate

Once therapeutic, check daily ABC, aPTT

Low-molecular-weight heparin (LMWH)

  Enoxaparin[52,53]

    Age <2 mo Term: 1.7 mg/kg q 12 h; preterm: 2 mg/kg q 12 h

    Age >2 mo 1.0 mg/kg q 12 h

  Dalteparin[54]

    All ages 129 ± 43 U/kg q 24 h

Thrombolytic agents

Tissue plasminogen activator (tPA)[57,58]

  Neonate 0.06 mg/kg/h

  Non-neonate 0.01 mg/kg/h

with either LMWH or warfarin. LMWH has the advantages of predictable pharmacokinetics, minimizing the frequency of monitoring, and subcutaneous dosing, limiting the need for intravenous access. Its activity is not affected by other medications or diet, as with warfarin, and may be used for long-term anticoagulation.[48] Heparin dosing in children is not well studied; however, infants appear to require higher doses per unit body weight than do older children due to physiologically low levels of antithrombin.[49] Older children who have acquired antithrombin deficiency usually require higher doses of heparin as well. See Table 52–2 for dosing recommendations for UH and LMWH.[50–54]

Thrombolytics are effective in the pediatric population, but not without risk at higher doses. Tissue plasminogen activator (tPA), the most studied thrombolytic for children, can be given continuously for the treatment of arterial thrombosis, extensive DVT, or massive PE.[51,55] Major complications associated with tPA therapy occur in 40% of patients receiving the medication at higher rates of 0.1 to 0.5 mg/kg/h, requiring transfusion with packed red blood cells. Predictors of major complications include higher dose, significantly longer duration of tPA therapy, and a greater decline in post-tPA therapy fibrinogen levels.[56] Low-dose continuous infusions (0.03–0.06 mg/kg/h) are effective in treating acute thrombosis in children with only

minor bleeding common at this rate, but life-threatening hemorrhage is rare (Table 52–2). The coadministration of heparin is necessary when using tPA, as tPA does not inhibit clot propagation or alter hypercoagulability.[57,58] Contraindications for thrombolytics exist in adults; however, no absolute contraindications exist for children.[51]

Surgical thrombectomy is another uncommonly used treatment modality for TE. Authors report both open thrombectomy and catheter aspiration thrombectomy in the pediatric literature.[59,60]

COMPLICATIONS

Complications of thromboembolism are common. Mortality directly attributable to VTE has been reported as 2% to 9%, with 14% of total deaths in one cohort attributed to central venous line associated thrombosis. Eight to 18.5% have recurrent thrombosis, and 12% to 21% develop postphlebitic syndrome, clinically described by extremity swelling and pain due to venous insufficiency.[2,18] High levels of D-dimer may indicate that a child is at increased risk of thrombus persistence or recurrence or onset of the postphlebitic syndrome.[37] Thrombolysis may significantly decrease the development of postphlebitic syndrome.[61] The complication of heparin-induced thrombocytopenia (HIT) is reported primarily in children undergoing anticoagulation with UH,[62] yet there are case reports of children developing HIT while using LMWH as well.[63]

In summary, TE is becoming more commonly recognized in the pediatric population. Those at high risk for TE commonly have indwelling central catheters, as well as other predisposing diseases, either inherited or acquired. The clinician must have high index of suspicion for this diagnosis, must be familiar with limitations of imaging techniques, and must be able to initiate appropriate therapy. Future directions in pediatric VTE undoubtedly include developing validated protocols for diagnosing DVT and PE, as well as further evaluating the use of anticoagulants and thrombolytics.

REFERENCES

1. Stein PD, Kayali F, Olson RE. Incidence of venous thromboembolism in infants and children: data from the National Hospital Discharge Survey. *J Pediatr.* 2004;145(4):563–565.
2. Andrew M, David M, Adams M, et al. Venous thromboembolic complications (VTE) in children: first analyses of the Canadian Registry of VTE. *Blood.* 1994;83(5):1251–1257.
3. Kuhle S, Massicotte P, Chan A, et al. Systemic thromboembolism in children. Data from the 1–800-NO-CLOTS Consultation Service. *Thromb Haemost.* 2004;92(4):722–728.
4. Bonduel M, Sciuccati G, Hepner M, et al. Arterial ischemic stroke and cerebral venous thrombosis in children: a 12-year Argentinean registry. *Acta Haematol.* 2006;115(3–4):180–185.
5. Monagle P, Newall F, Barnes C, et al. Arterial thromboembolic disease: a single-centre case series study. *J Paediatr Child Health.* 2008;44(1–2):28–32.
6. Bowen MD, Burak CR, Barron TF. Childhood ischemic stroke in a nonurban population. *J Child Neurol.* 2005;20(3):194–197.

7. Albisetti M, Schmugge M, Haas R, et al. Arterial thromboembolic complications in critically ill children. *J Crit Care.* 2005;20(3):296–300.

8. Suzuki A, Kamiya T, Kuwahara N, et al. Coronary arterial lesions of Kawasaki disease: cardiac catheterization findings of 1100 cases. *Pediatr Cardiol.* 1986;7(1):3–9.

9. Zheng D, Fan D, Liu L. Takayasu arteritis in China: a report of 530 cases. *Heart Vessels Suppl.* 1992;7:32–36.

10. Griffin JH, Evatt B, Zimmerman TS, et al. Deficiency of protein C in congenital thrombotic disease. *J Clin Invest.* 1981;68(5):1370–1373.

11. Schwarz HP, Fischer M, Hopmeier P, et al. Plasma protein S deficiency in familial thrombotic disease. *Blood.* 1984;64(6):1297–1300.

12. Egeberg O. An inherited hemorrhagic trait with characteristics resembling both mild hemophilia of type A and Von Willebrand's disease. *Scand J Clin Lab Invest.* 1965;17(suppl 84):25–32.

13. Manco-Johnson MJ, Nuss R. Lupus anticoagulant in children with thrombosis. *Am J Hematol.* 1995;48(4):240–243.

14. Nowak-Gottl U, Dubbers A, Kececioglu D, et al. Factor V Leiden, protein C, and lipoprotein (a) in catheter-related thrombosis in childhood: a prospective study. *J Pediatr.* 1997;131(4):608–612.

15. Koster T, Blann AD, Briet E, et al. Role of clotting factor VIII in effect of von Willebrand factor on occurrence of deep-vein thrombosis. *Lancet.* 1995;345(8943):152–155.

16. Kosch A, Junker R, Kurnik K, et al. Prothrombotic risk factors in children with spontaneous venous thrombosis and their asymptomatic parents: a family study. *Thromb Res.* 2000;99(6):531–537.

17. Tormene D, Simioni P, Prandoni P, et al. The incidence of venous thromboembolism in thrombophilic children: a prospective cohort study. *Blood.* 2002;100(7):2403–2405.

18. Monagle P, Adams M, Mahoney M, et al. Outcome of pediatric thromboembolic disease: a report from the Canadian Childhood Thrombophilia Registry. *Pediatr Res.* 2000;47(6):763–766.

19. Paz-Priel I, Long L, Helman LJ, et al. Thromboembolic events in children and young adults with pediatric sarcoma. *J Clin Oncol.* 2007;25(12):1519–1524.

20. Marras LC, Geerts WH, Perry JR. The risk of venous thromboembolism is increased throughout the course of malignant glioma: an evidence-based review. *Cancer.* 2000;89(3):640–646.

21. Tabori U, Beni-Adani L, Dvir R, et al. Risk of venous thromboembolism in pediatric patients with brain tumors. *Pediatr Blood Cancer.* 2004;43(6):633–636.

22. Azu MC, McCormack JE, Scriven RJ, et al. Venous thromboembolic events in pediatric trauma patients: is prophylaxis necessary? *J Trauma.* 2005;59(6):1345–1349.

23. David M, Andrew M. Venous thromboembolic complications in children. *J Pediatr.* 1993;123(3):337–346.

24. Vavilala MS, Nathens AB, Jurkovich GJ, et al. Risk factors for venous thromboembolism in pediatric trauma. *J Trauma.* 2002;52(5):922–927.

25. Crary SE, Buchanan GR, Drake CE, et al. Venous thrombosis and thromboembolism in children with osteomyelitis. *J Pediatr.* 2006;149(4):537–541.

26. Balint PV, Sturrock RD. Inflamed retrocalcaneal bursa and Achilles tendonitis in psoriatic arthritis demonstrated by ultrasonography. *Ann Rheum Dis.* 2000;59(12):931–933.

27. Christenson JT. Popliteal venous aneurysm: a report on three cases presenting with chronic venous insufficiency without embolic events. *Phlebology.* 2007;22(2):56–59.

28. Langsfeld M, Matteson B, Johnson W, et al. Baker's cysts mimicking the symptoms of deep vein thrombosis: diagnosis with venous duplex scanning. *J Vasc Surg.* 1997;25(4):658–662.

29. Kane D, Balint PV, Gibney R, et al. Differential diagnosis of calf pain with musculoskeletal ultrasound imaging. *Ann Rheum Dis.* 2004;63(1):11–14.

30. Stein PD, Goldhaber SZ, Henry JW. Alveolar-arterial oxygen gradient in the assessment of acute pulmonary embolism. *Chest.* 1995;107(1):139–143.

31. Stein PD, Henry JW. Clinical characteristics of patients with acute pulmonary embolism stratified according to their presenting syndromes. *Chest.* 1997;112(4):974–979.

32. Wells PS, Anderson DR, Rodger M, et al. Derivation of a simple clinical model to categorize patients probability of pulmonary embolism: increasing the models utility with the SimpliRED D-dimer. *Thromb Haemost.* 2000;83(3):416–420.

33. Kline JA, Nelson RD, Jackson RE, et al. Criteria for the safe use of D-dimer testing in emergency department patients with suspected pulmonary embolism: a multicenter US study. *Ann Emerg Med.* 2002;39(2):144–152.

34. Wicki J, Perneger TV, Junod AF, et al. Assessing clinical probability of pulmonary embolism in the emergency ward: a simple score. *Arch Intern Med.* 2001;161(1):92–97.

35. Wells PS, Anderson DR, Rodger M, et al. Evaluation of D-dimer in the diagnosis of suspected deep-vein thrombosis. *N Engl J Med.* 2003;349(13):1227–1235.

36. Rajpurkar M, Warrier I, Chitlur M, et al. Pulmonary embolism-experience at a single children's hospital. *Thromb Res.* 2007;119(6):699–703.

37. Goldenberg NA, Knapp-Clevenger R, Manco-Johnson MJ. Elevated plasma factor VIII and D-dimer levels as predictors of poor outcomes of thrombosis in children. *N Engl J Med.* 2004;351(11):1081–1088.

38. Palareti G, Legnani C, Cosmi B, et al. Predictive value of D-dimer test for recurrent venous thromboembolism after anticoagulation withdrawal in subjects with a previous idiopathic event and in carriers of congenital thrombophilia. *Circulation.* 2003;108(3):313–318.

39. Male C, Chait P, Ginsberg JS, et al. Comparison of venography and ultrasound for the diagnosis of asymptomatic deep vein thrombosis in the upper body in children: results of the PARKAA study. Prophylactic Antithrombin Replacement in Kids with ALL treated with Asparaginase. *Thromb Haemost.* 2002;87(4):593–598.

40. Qanadli SD, El Hajjam M, Bruckert F, et al. Helical CT phlebography of the superior vena cava: diagnosis and evaluation of venous obstruction. *AJR Am J Roentgenol.* 1999;172(5):1327–1333.

41. Uderzo C, Faccini P, Rovelli A, et al. Pulmonary thromboembolism in childhood leukemia: 8-years' experience in a pediatric hematology center. *J Clin Oncol.* 1995;13(11):2805–2812.

42. Babyn PS, Gahunia HK, Massicotte P. Pulmonary thromboembolism in children. *Pediatr Radiol.* 2005;35(3):258–274.

43. Tsai KL, Gupta E, Haramati LB. Pulmonary atelectasis: a frequent alternative diagnosis in patients undergoing CT-PA for suspected pulmonary embolism. *Emerg Radiol.* 2004;10(5):282–286.

44. Oudkerk M, van Beek EJ, Wielopolski P, et al. Comparison of contrast-enhanced magnetic resonance angiography and conventional pulmonary angiography for the diagnosis of pulmonary embolism: a prospective study. *Lancet.* 2002;359(9318):1643–1647.

45. Pleszewski B, Chartrand-Lefebvre C, Qanadli SD, et al. Gadolinium-enhanced pulmonary magnetic resonance angiography in the diagnosis of acute pulmonary embolism: a prospective study on 48 patients. *Clin Imaging.* 2006;30(3):166–172.

46. Zigman A, Yazbeck S, Emil S, et al. Renal vein thrombosis: a 10-year review. *J Pediatr Surg.* 2000;35(11):1540–1542.
47. Hausler M, Hubner D, Delhaas T, et al. Long term complications of inferior vena cava thrombosis. *Arch Dis Child.* 2001;85(3):228–233.
48. Parasuraman S, Goldhaber SZ. Venous thromboembolism in children. *Circulation.* 2006;113(2):e12–e16.
49. McDonald MM, Hathaway WE, Reeve EB, et al. Biochemical and functional study of antithrombin III in newborn infants. *Thromb Haemost.* 1982;47(1):56–58.
50. Michelson AD, Bovill E, Andrew M. Antithrombotic therapy in children. *Chest.* 1995;108(4 suppl):506S–522S.
51. Monagle P, Chan A, Massicotte P, et al. Antithrombotic therapy in children: the Seventh ACCP Conference on Antithrombotic and Thrombolytic Therapy. *Chest.* 2004;126(3 suppl):645S–687S.
52. Massicotte P, Adams M, Marzinotto V, et al. Low-molecular-weight heparin in pediatric patients with thrombotic disease: a dose finding study. *J Pediatr.* 1996;128(3):313–318.
53. Malowany JI, Monagle P, Knoppert DC, et al. Enoxaparin for neonatal thrombosis: a call for a higher dose for neonates. *Thromb Res.* 2008; January 17:18207492.
54. Nohe N, Flemmer A, Rumler R, et al. The low molecular weight heparin dalteparin for prophylaxis and therapy of thrombosis in childhood: a report on 48 cases. *Eur J Pediatr.* 1999;158(suppl 3):S134–S139.
55. Monagle P, Michelson AD, Bovill E, et al. Antithrombotic therapy in children. *Chest.* 2001;119(1 suppl):344S–370S.
56. Gupta AA, Leaker M, Andrew M, et al. Safety and outcomes of thrombolysis with tissue plasminogen activator for treatment of intravascular thrombosis in children. *J Pediatr.* 2001;139(5):682–688.
57. Wang M, Hays T, Balasa V, et al. Low-dose tissue plasminogen activator thrombolysis in children. *J Pediatr Hematol Oncol.* 2003;25(5):379–386.
58. Manco-Johnson MJ, Grabowski EF, Hellgreen M, et al. Recommendations for tPA thrombolysis in children. On behalf of the Scientific Subcommittee on Perinatal and Pediatric Thrombosis of the Scientific and Standardization Committee of the International Society of Thrombosis and Haemostasis. *Thromb Haemost.* 2002;88(1):157–158.
59. Dittrich S, Schlensak C, Kececioglu D. Successful thrombectomy of the superior vena cava thrombosis in a newborn after cardiopulmonary bypass surgery. *Interact Cardiovasc Thorac Surg.* 2003;2(4):692–693.
60. Sur JP, Garg RK, Jolly N. Rheolytic percutaneous thrombectomy for acute pulmonary embolism in a pediatric patient. *Catheter Cardiovasc Interv.* 2007;70(3):450–453.
61. Goldenberg NA, Durham JD, Knapp-Clevenger R, et al. A thrombolytic regimen for high-risk deep venous thrombosis may substantially reduce the risk of post thrombotic syndrome in children. *Blood.* 2007;110(1):45–53.
62. Klenner AF, Lubenow N, Raschke R, et al. Heparin-induced thrombocytopenia in children: 12 new cases and review of the literature. *Thromb Haemost.* 2004;91(4):719–724.
63. Dager WE, White RH. Low-molecular-weight heparin-induced thrombocytopenia in a child. *Ann Pharmacother.* 2004;38(2):247–250.

SECTION VII

NEUROLOGIC EMERGENCIES

CHAPTER 53

Syncope

Susan Fuchs

▶ HIGH-YIELD FACTS

- Most syncope in children is neurocardiogenic/vasovagal.
- Situational events that cause a Valsalvalike maneuver can cause syncope.
- Prolonged QT syndrome is an uncommon but important cause of syncope in children.
- A head upright tilt-table test may diagnose neurocardiogenic syncope in selected cases.

Syncope refers to a sudden and transient loss of consciousness and postural tone. Although in the pediatric age group it accounts for less than 1% of emergency department visits, 15% to 50% of children will have experienced a syncopal episode by age 18.[1] Syncope can be a manifestation of serious underlying pathology and always warrants careful evaluation. Unlike the adult population, in which syncope often results from malignant cardiac arrhythmias, in the pediatric population it is more often secondary to neurally mediated causes and is therefore discussed in the section on neurologic emergencies.[1]

▶ PATHOPHYSIOLOGY

The pathophysiology of syncope varies with etiology (Table 53–1), but it always results from momentarily inadequate delivery of oxygen and glucose to the brain. Syncope can result from inadequate cardiac output, which can be secondary to obstruction of blood flow, or to an arrhythmia. It can also result from inappropriate autonomic compensation for the normal fall in blood pressure that occurs on rising from a sitting or supine position. Respiratory disturbances, especially hyperventilation that results in hypocapnia and cerebral vasoconstriction, can also cause syncope.[1]

▶ HISTORY

The first component in the evaluation of a patient with syncope is to determine that momentary loss of consciousness actually occurred. It is common for patients to confuse acute dizziness or vertigo with loss of consciousness. For patients who did indeed lose consciousness, the events antecedent to the syncopal episode are elicited. A prodrome of light-headedness, nausea, dizziness or vision changes, a sudden change in posture, emotional excitement, respiratory difficulty, palpitations, exercise, and any history of trauma are essential information. Past history of syncope is sought, as is any history of medica-

tion or drug ingestion that would explain a precipitous fall in blood pressure. Patients are queried carefully about any history of congenital heart disease, any family history of heart disease, or family history of sudden death in children or young adults.[2,3]

An important consideration in any patient with a history of loss of consciousness is the possibility that the patient may have suffered a seizure. In contrast to syncope, seizures are usually accompanied by some form of muscle twitching or convulsions, and are usually followed by a postictal phase, during which the patient has confusion, disorientation, or other mental status changes, usually lasting more than 5 minutes.[4] Convulsions are unusual during syncopal episodes except during very severe events, or with reflex anoxic seizures, and patients generally have normal mental status upon recovery from the episode.[2,5]

▶ PHYSICAL EXAMINATION

The physical examination focuses upon establishing the hemodynamic stability of the patient. Particular attention is paid to vital signs, especially to pulse and orthostatic blood pressure. A positive test is a decrease in systolic blood pressure by 20 mm Hg or an increase in heart rate (20 beats per minute), on going from lying to sitting, or sitting to standing. However, if the patient has recurrent symptoms, the test is considered positive.[6] The patient's mental status is carefully evaluated, and a full neurologic examination is performed.

For all patients, a careful cardiac examination is indicated. The regularity of the pulse is noted, as is the quality of the peripheral pulses. The heart is auscultated carefully to detect the presence of a murmur that may indicate congenital heart disease, especially aortic stenosis (systolic ejection murmur and ejection click). The presence of gallops, rubs, thrills, or carotid bruits is noted. The quality and presence of all peripheral pulses are evaluated. Diminished pulses should prompt blood pressure measurements in all extremities to check for coarctation of the aorta.[6]

▶ LABORATORY STUDIES
(Fig. 53–1)

The selection of laboratory studies of use in the evaluation of the syncope patient is largely guided by the history and physical examination. For a patient with a history of fasting or diabetes, blood glucose is indicated. In the presence of pallor or a history of blood loss, hemoglobin measurement is obtained.

▶ **TABLE 53–1. CAUSES OF SYNCOPE**

Neurocardiogenic/vasodepressor/vasovagal
  Orthostatic hypotension
  Environmental triggers
  Sympathetic withdrawal
  Situational syncope
  Reflex syncope (pallid breath-holding spells)

Cardiac mediated syncope
  Arrhythmias
    Supraventricular tachycardias
    Atrial flutter
    Wolfe–Parkinson–White syndrome
    Ventricular tachycardia
    Ventricular fibrillation
    Conduction disturbances
    Atrioventricular block
    Prolonged QTc
    Short QTc
    Brugada syndrome
    Sick sinus syndrome
    Arrhythmogenic right ventricular dysplasia (ARVD)
  Obstructive lesions
    Aortic stenosis
    Pulmonic stenosis
    Idiopathic hypertrophic subaortic stenosis
    Hypertrophic cardiomyopathy
    Mitral stenosis
    Coarctation of the aorta
    Tetralogy of Fallot
    Anomalous origin of the left coronary artery
    Tumors
  Other
    Myocarditis
    Pericarditis
    Cardiac tamponade
    Cardiomyopathy
    Pulmonary hypertension

Noncardiac
  Metabolic
    Hypoglycemia
    Hypocalcemia
    Hypomagnesemia
  Toxic
  Seizures
  Psychogenic
    Hyperventilation
    Hysteria

With permission from Chaves-Carbello E. Syncope and paroxysmal disorders other than epilepsy. In: Swaiman KF, Ashwal S, Ferriero DM, eds. *Pediatric Neurology, Principles and Practice.* 4th ed. Philadelphia, PA: Mosby/Elsevier; 2006:1209–1223.
With permission from Coleman B, Salerno JC. Causes of syncope in children and adolescents. In: Rose BD, ed. *UpToDate.* Waltham, MA: UpToDate; 2007.
With permission from Strieper MG. Distinguishing benign syncope from life-threatening cardiac causes of syncope. *Semin Pediatr Neurol.* 2005;12:32–38.

Electrolyte abnormalities are uncommon, but if an arrhythmia is suspected, then serum potassium, calcium, and magnesium are measured. Other studies including arterial blood gas, toxicology screening, and pregnancy testing may be indicated in certain clinical scenarios.[6]

For all patients with a history of syncope, a 12-lead electrocardiogram (ECG) is indicated. This provides information concerning potential conduction defects or arrhythmias. Special attention is paid to determination of the corrected QT interval (QTc), since prolonged QT syndrome, as well as a short QTc are causes of syncope in children. Other abnormalities to note include bradyarrhythmias, AV block, delta waves (preexcitation/WPW), epsilon waves (ARVD), and ST segment elevation in V_1–V_3 (Brugada syndrome), and left ventricular hypertrophy or strain patterns (hypertrophic cardiomyopathy). If abnormalities are seen, or if a cardiac abnormality is strongly suspected, further evaluation will include a 24-hour ambulatory (Holter) monitor or continuous loop event monitoring and cardiology consultation.[4,6]

Other studies are dependent upon the suspected etiology. If the event is thought to be a seizure, (rather than syncope), an EEG is appropriate. The head upright tilt-table test helps confirm the diagnosis of neurocardiogenic syncope, but is often reserved for those with recurrent unexplained syncope or presyncope, syncope resulting in injury, or exercise-induced syncope.[3]

▶ SPECIFIC ETIOLOGIES OF SYNCOPE

NEUROCARDIOGENIC (AUTONOMIC, VASODEPRESSOR, VASOVAGAL) SYNCOPE

The most common syncope in children is neurocardiogenic (vasodepressor or vasovagal) syncope. There is a sudden, brief loss of consciousness because of vasodilatation and decreased peripheral resistance, resulting in decreased arterial pressure, hypotension, bradycardia, and then decreased cerebral blood flow (Bezold–Jarisch reflex). Current theories suggest that the systemic vasodilation and the changes in heart rate and blood pressure are caused by sympathetic withdrawal, rather than increased parasympathetic (vagal) activity.[1] Orthostatic hypotension may be a result of volume depletion, anemia, or drugs, but it can also be because of a paradoxic response to the vasodepressor reaction.[4,6] A tilt-table test can be performed by a cardiologist to diagnose true neurocardiogenic syncope. A positive head upright tilt-table test response, consisting of an initial increase in heart rate followed by bradycardia and syncope, may warrant drug therapy if frequent episodes occur.[1]

Environmental factors, such as prolonged standing, heat, fatigue, crowding, or hunger, can trigger syncope. Emotional stress or a recent illness can also play a role. Patients may have symptoms beforehand such as blurred vision, dizziness, nausea, or pallor. This is what is commonly referred to as a "simple faint." Placing the person in a supine position with the head down usually results in improvement, although the patient may still complain of dizziness.[6]

The term situational syncope can be used for those patients that have syncope triggered by specific events. The

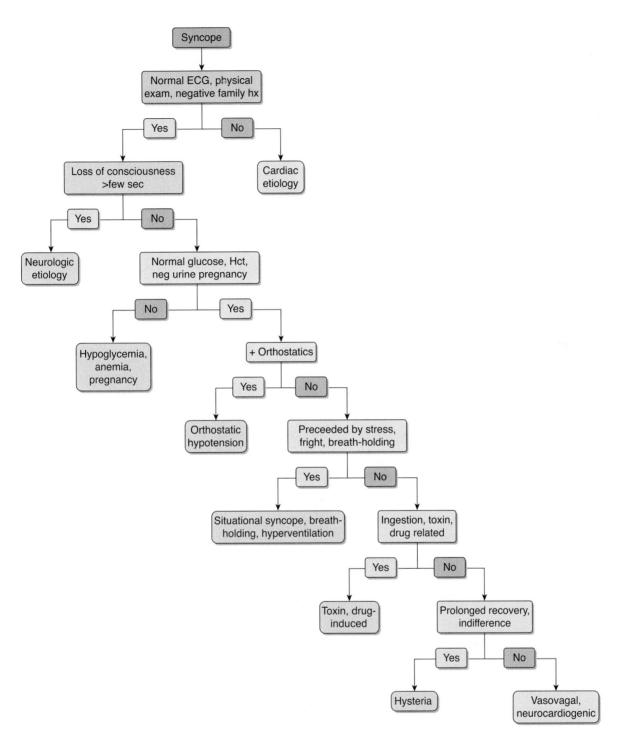

Figure 53–1. Diagnostic approach to the patient with syncope.

common denominator is that these actions are accompanied by a Valsalva-like maneuver. This includes coughing, micturition, hairgrooming, diving, weight lifting, and sneezing. Another form is carotid sinus syncope, which occurs with head rotation or pressure on the carotid sinus. This can occur with shaving or tight collars.[1]

Breath-holding spells are another example of reflex syncope. The age of onset of breath-holding spells is 6 to 18

months.[5] The two types of breath-holding spells are classified based on the color change:

- The pallid breath-holding spell is a form of reflex syncope. Pallid breath-holding spells are usually provoked by some mild antecedent trauma (usually to the head), pain, or fright. The child may gasp and cry, then become quiet, lose postural tone and consciousness, and become pale. The child may have clonic movements and incontinence in more severe episodes. The child regains consciousness in less than 1 minute, but may be tired after the episode for several hours.[5]

- A cyanotic breath-holding spell is often precipitated by anger or frustration. The child cries, becomes quiet, and holds the breath in expiration. This apnea is associated with cyanosis and there may be a loss of consciousness, limpness, or opisthotonic posturing, with recovery usually within 1 minute.[5]

CARDIAC SYNCOPE

Cardiac syncope is important to exclude, as this is the type that is truly life-threatening. The differential in this subgroup includes arrhythmia, obstruction, cyanosis, and other cardiac etiologies. Arrhythmias that result in a heart rate that is too fast or too slow can cause a decrease in cardiac output and lead to decreased cerebral perfusion. Included in this group are supraventricular tachycardia (SVT), atrial tachycardia, Wolff–Parkinson–White syndrome, atrial flutter, ventricular tachycardia, and ventricular fibrillation. Conduction abnormalities such as AV block, sick sinus syndrome (may occur after cardiac surgery), long QT syndrome, congenital short QT, or Brugada syndrome may be present.

Long QT Syndrome (Fig. 53–2)

Long QT syndrome is a disorder of myocardial repolarization that can lead to polymorphic ventricular tachycardia (torsades

de pointes). There are congenital forms; Romano–Ward syndrome (autosomal dominant), and Jervell and Lange–Nielsen syndrome (autosomal recessive). The latter form is associated with sensioneural deafness. There are also acquired forms usually the result of the metabolic disorders such as hypokalemia and hypomagnesemia, some medications (quinidine, procainamide), or a combination of medications (erythromycin or ketoconazole and terfenadine).[6] Although prolongation of the corrected QTc is the main requirement, this value changes with the patient's age, and sex. (QTc is >450 ms in males and >460 in females).[7] To calculate the QTc, use Bazett's formula $QTc = QT/\sqrt{RR}$.[2] After evaluation by a cardiologist, treatments include β-blockers, implantable defibrillators, and avoidance of medication that prolong the QT interval.[8]

Congenital Short QT Syndrome

This syndrome has led to sudden cardiac death, syncope, and atrial fibrillation. The QTC is ≤0.30 ms.[2]

Brugada Syndrome

Patients with this inherited autosomal dominant disorder have a characteristic ECG pattern: ST segment elevation (≥2 mm) in leads V_1–V_3. There is an increased risk of sudden cardiac death resulting from polymorphic ventricular tachyarrhythmias.[9] Although it is more likely to occur in young males, with a reported mean age of sudden death at 40 years, children have been detected with this disorder during family screening, and there was no male predominance, and febrile illness was the most important precipitating event.[9]

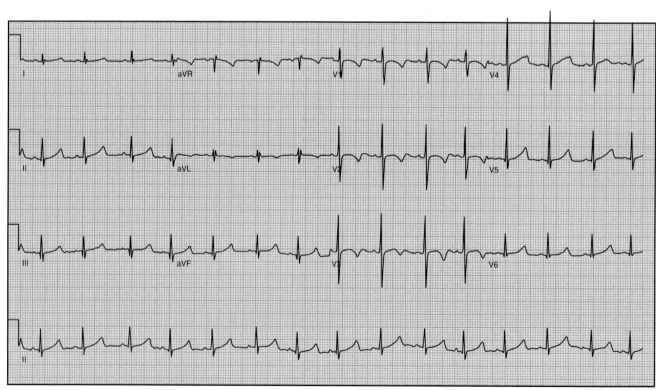

5mm/s 10mm/mV 40Hz MUSE 7.0.0 12SL 235 CID: 76 EID:4 EDT: 11:43 18-JUL-2003 ORDER:

Figure 53–2. Long QT syndrome.

Arrhythmogenic Right Ventricular Dysplasia/Cardiomyopathy

Arrhythmogenic right ventricular dysplasia/cardiomyopathy (ARVD) is characterized by ventricular tachycardia and abnormalities of the right ventricle, caused by myocyte replacement by fibrosis or adipose tissue. Although sudden cardiac death may be the presenting feature (mean age of 30 years), PVCs, syncope, and ventricular tachycardia with left bundle branch block may be forewarning findings. Diagnosis is based on ECG findings (epsilon waves after the QRS) as well as structural, and functional criteria.[2,6,8]

All these problems should be excluded by evaluation of a 12-lead electrocardiogram and rhythm strip. If the problem is intermittent, 24-hour Holter monitoring and referral to a cardiologist should be included in the evaluation.

Obstructive lesions can impair cardiac output and cerebral blood flow, leading to syncope. These include congenital lesions such as aortic stenosis, pulmonic stenosis, idiopathic hypertrophic subaortic stenosis (IHSS), hypertrophic cardiomyopathy, mitral stenosis, coarctation of the aorta, tetralogy of Fallot, anomalous origin of the left coronary artery, and transposition of the great vessels. Children who have undergone surgical correction of tetraology, transposition, and aortic stenosis are at greater risk of arrhythmias.[2] The presence of chest pain and syncope with exercise, as well as a murmur on physical examination, can suggest left ventricular outflow obstruction because of IHSS or aortic stenosis. Cyanosis with or without syncope can result from increased resistance to pulmonary blood flow, causing an increase in the right-to-left shunting of blood. These spells can occur in children with tetralogy of Fallot, tricuspid atresia, and Eisenmenger's syndrome.

Evaluation for these disorders includes an ECG, chest radiograph, echocardiogram, and cardiology consultation.[2]

Hypertrophic Cardiomyopathy

This autosomal dominant disorder is characterized by asymmetric hypertrophy of the left ventricle, without dilatation. It is a common cause of sudden death associated with exercise in young patients. Syncope is a major risk factor for sudden death. The mechanisms that cause syncope and sudden death include bradyarrhythmias, ventricular arrhythmias, severe outflow tract obstruction, and decreased blood pressure in response to exercise.[2,8] Implantable defibrillators have been used to treat this disorder with some success.[8]

Acquired lesions include cardiac tumors and conditions secondary to myocarditis, pericarditis, cardiac tamponade, cardiomyopathy, and pulmonary hypertension. Primary pulmonary hypertension can cause dyspnea on exertion but can also cause syncope from inadequate cardiac output. Evaluation includes a 12-lead ECG, chest radiograph, and prompt cardiology referral.[2]

NONCARDIAC SYNCOPE

Noncardiac causes of syncope include neurologic, metabolic, psychologic, and toxicologic problems. Seizures should be considered whenever there is a loss of consciousness, especially if accompanied by increased muscle tone or tonic-clonic movements. If syncope occurs while the child is in a recumbent position, a seizure is a likely diagnosis. The diagnostic workup should proceed based on the most likely etiology and type of seizure.[2]

Hypoglycemia is the main metabolic disorder that can cause syncope. Prior to a loss of consciousness there is often a period of confusion and weakness. Hypocalcemia and hypomagnesemia can also cause syncope, but this is secondary to the arrhythmias generated by these disorders.

Psychologic causes of syncope include hyperventilation and hysteria. Hyperventilation results in hypocapnia, which causes cerebral vasoconstriction and decreased cerebral blood flow. The patient may complain of shortness of breath, chest tightness, numb fingers before syncope ensues.[1] Hysteric syncope occurs when the patient mimics a loss of consciousness and falls to the ground without injury. No abnormalities of heart rate, blood pressure, or skin color are detected, and clues regarding surrounding events may point to the correct diagnosis, such as prolonged recovery after the event, and indifference to syncope.[2,3]

Drug-induced syncope can be caused by prescription drugs, over-the-counter medications, or drugs of abuse. Drugs of abuse such as cocaine are well known to result in syncope as well as more serious cardiac arrhythmias. Marijuana, alcohol, and opiates can all cause a loss of consciousness.[1,2] Inhalant use can result in ventricular tachycardia and death. Antihypertensive agents, phenothiazines, calcium channel blockers, nitrates, and barbiturates can block the increased blood pressure response, and β-blockers and digitalis will block the tachycardia needed to respond to decreased systemic vascular resistance prior to syncope. Some of the newer antihistamines can cause prolonged QT and even torsades de pointes, if given with macrolides or ketoconazole.[1]

▶ TREATMENT

Although most children will not require specific therapy, treatment should be based on the etiology and frequency of syncopal episodes. A child with hypoglycemia requires glucose, and one with anemia or hypotension may benefit from intravenous fluids while a workup for the etiology is ongoing. If a cardiac etiology is suspected, depending on the urgency of the situation, further studies could be performed on an inpatient or outpatient basis, but activity restrictions may be needed while awaiting evaluation. Treatment of a child with orthostatic syncope with β-blockers or mineralocorticoids should await formal head upright tilt-table testing. If a neurologic etiology is suspected, treatment with anticonvulsive medications should be based on neurologic consultation. If the emergency department evaluation and workup is negative, with the likely etiology being neurocardiogenic, or a simple faint, reassurance may be all that is needed. Avoidance of specific triggers or environmental factors can prevent most attacks. Those with a prodromal phase can be taught to sit or lie down before the loss of tone and consciousness occurs.

DISPOSITION

Most patients with syncope can be discharged from the emergency department with appropriate follow-up. Those who require admission have conditions with a cardiac origin that require urgent evaluation: arrhythmias (SVT, atrial flutter, ventricular tachycardia, or fibrillation), conduction abnormalities (third-degree AV block, sick sinus syndrome), or newly diagnosed or worsening of obstructive lesions (aortic stenosis, pulmonic stenosis, IHSS).[6] Patients with arrhythmias precipitated by drugs require inpatient monitoring, for at least the half-life of the offending agent. Patients with cyanosis with syncope, those with abnormal neurologic examinations, and those with orthostatic syncope who do not resolve with fluids, and have no other etiology should also be admitted.[6]

REFERENCES

1. Chaves-Carbello E. Syncope and paroxysmal disorders other than epilepsy. In: Swaiman KF, Ashwal S, Ferriero DM, eds. *Pediatric Neurology, Principles and Practice.* 4th ed. Philadelphia, PA: Mosby/Elsevier; 2006:1209–1223.
2. Coleman B, Salerno JC. Causes of syncope in children and adolescents. In: Rose BD, ed. *UpToDate.* Waltham, MA: UpToDate; 2007.
3. Strieper MG. Distinguishing benign syncope from life-threatening cardiac causes of syncope. *Semin Pediatr Neurol.* 2005;12:32–38.
4. Kapoor WN. Syncope. *N Engl J Med.* 2000;343:1856.
5. Roddy SM. Breath-holding spells and reflex anoxic seizures. In: Swaiman KF, Ashwal S, Ferriero DM, ed. *Pediatric Neurology, Principles and Practice.* 4th ed. Philadelphia, PA: Mosby/Elsevier; 2006:53;1203–1208.
6. Coleman B, Salerno JC. Emergent evaluation of syncope in children and adolescents. In: Rose BD, ed. *UpToDate.* Waltham, MA: UpToDate; 2007.
7. Schwartz PJ, Moss AJ, Vincent GM, et al. Diagnostic criteria for the long QT syndrome; an update. *Circulation.* 1993;88:782.
8. Strickberger SA, Benson DW, Biaggioni I, et al. AHA/ACCF Scientific statement on the evlautaion of syncope. *Circulation.* 2006;113:316–327.
9. Probst V, Denjoy I, Meregalli PG, et al. Clinical aspects and prognosis of Brugada syndrome in children. *Circulation.* 2007;115:2042–2048.

CHAPTER 54

Ataxia

Susan Fuchs

▶ HIGH-YIELD FACTS

- Ataxia can result from a variety of lesions, including damage to the peripheral nerves, spinal cord, cerebellum, and cerebral hemispheres. One of the most common etiologies is drug intoxication, especially with alcohol, benzodiazepines, or phenytoin.
- Findings of cerebellar dysfunction include nystagmus, staggering, wide-based gait, and titubation. In addition, a sensory examination for light touch and pinprick, position, and vibration sense should be performed because lower extremity sensory impairment can cause ataxia.
- In a patient with acute ataxia, the history and physical examination focus on excluding acute infectious etiologies, such as meningitis or encephalitis, lesions that result in increased intracranial pressure, such as hemorrhage and tumors, and toxic ingestions.
- A common cause of ataxia in children younger than 5 years is acute cerebellar ataxia, a postinfectious phenomenon that often occurs about 2 weeks after a viral illness. The onset of ataxia is insidious and predominantly affects the gait, although dysmetria, nystagmus, and dysarthria can occur.
- In children, the most common cause of intermittent ataxia is a migraine headache that involves the basilar artery. Besides ataxia, associated symptoms include blurred vision, visual field deficits, vertigo, and headache.
- Chronic progressive ataxia has an insidious onset and progresses slowly over weeks to months. The differential diagnosis consists of brain tumors, hydrocephalus, and neurodegenerative disorders.
- The combination of ataxia, headache, irritability, and vomiting in a child younger than 6 years is characteristic of a medulloblastoma.
- Hereditary causes of ataxia include spinocerebellar ataxias, of which there are 28 types. Friedrich's ataxia is common autosomal recessive ataxia, which usually manifests before 10 years of age. It is characterized by ataxia, nystagmus, kyphoscoliosis, cardiomyopathy, and distal muscle wasting.
- Patients with progressive ataxia require an aggressive evaluation in the emergency department. All patients are examined for signs of increased intracranial pressure, which in some cases can be severe enough to result in the threat of uncal herniation.
- The emergency department evaluation of chronic nonprogressive ataxia consists of ensuring, by a careful history and physical examination, that the problem is indeed stable.

Ataxia is a disorder of intentional movement, characterized by impaired balance and coordination. It can variably affect the trunk or extremities. Severe truncal ataxia is sometimes referred to as titubation. Ataxia of the extremities can result in a wide-based gait or can cause dysmetria, which is the tendency of the limbs to overshoot a target, with subsequent movements attempting to correct the overshoot.[1,2]

Ataxia can be congenital/genetic or acquired. Acquired ataxia is often classified as acute, episodic/intermittent, or chronic.[1]

▶ PATHOPHYSIOLOGY

Ataxia can result from a variety of lesions, including damage to the peripheral nerves, spinal cord, cerebellum, and cerebral hemispheres. Lesions of the cerebellum can be further categorized as affecting the hemispheres, which results in ipsilateral limb hypotonia, tremor, and dysmetria, but spare speech. With walking, these patients tend to veer to the side of the lesion. Lesions of the midline vermis cause truncal ataxia or titubation, dysarthria, and gait abnormalities.[1] Damage to the spinal cord can cause ataxia when the patient stands with the eyes closed, which is referred to as a positive Romberg's sign. Patients with cerebellar ataxia have findings whether their eyes are open or closed.

Metabolic and systemic disorders can also cause ataxia. One of the most common etiologies is drug intoxication, especially with alcohol, benzodiazepines, or phenytoin.[2,3]

▶ EVALUATION

True ataxia must be distinguished from problems with similar neurologic manifestations. Vestibular disorders can cause vertigo, a sensation of abnormal movement or spinning that can cause a severe gait disturbance, nausea, and vomiting. Vertigo is often accompanied by nystagmus. Myopathies can be confused with ataxia, as can peripheral neuropathies. On physical examination, myopathies are characterized by muscle weakness, whereas peripheral neuropathies are accompanied by decreased reflexes. Chorea is a disorder characterized by involuntary movements and incoordination. It is distinguished from ataxia in that it occurs at rest, whereas ataxia is manifested during intentional movement.

PHYSICAL EXAMINATION

Vital signs and a thorough physical examination should be performed. Findings of cerebellar dysfunction include nystagmus, staggering, wide-based gait, titubation, and speech abnormalities. Specific neurologic tests include the following:

- Finger to nose with eyes closed (to look for intention tremor)
- Finger to nose to (examiner's) finger; dysmetria is poor coordination of voluntary movements, and results in under- or overshooting the target (tests cerebellar integrity when limb strength and sensation is intact)
- Heel-to-shin maneuvers (test cerebellar integrity when limb strength and sensation are intact)
- Rapid alternating hand movements—difficulty is termed dysdiadochokinesia (tests cerebellar function)
- Heel and toe walking (with hemispheric lesions there is a tendency to veer in one direction)
- Tandem gait (with hemispheric lesions there is a tendency to veer in one direction)
- Walking in a circle (with hemispheric lesions there is a tendency to veer in one direction) [1,2]

In addition, a sensory examination for light touch and pinprick, position, and vibration sense should be performed because lower extremity sensory impairment can cause ataxia.

For diagnostic purposes, it is useful to categorize ataxia as acute, intermittent, or chronic. Chronic ataxia is further categorized as progressive or nonprogressive (Table 54–1).

▶ ACUTE ATAXIA

Acute ataxia generally has an onset of <24 hours. Drug toxicity and infections are the most common etiologies. Acute metabolic processes, such as hypoglycemia, are also implicated, although they are usually accompanied by multiple systemic manifestations.

In a patient with acute ataxia, the history and physical examination focus on excluding acute infectious etiologies, such as meningitis or encephalitis, recent infections, or immunizations; lesions that result in increased intracranial pressure, such as trauma, hemorrhage, and tumors; and toxic ingestions. Central nervous system infections are usually characterized by fever and headache, and often by mental status changes. The physical examination may reveal neck stiffness. Lesions that cause increased intracranial pressure are associated with headache and vomiting, and the physical examination may reveal papilledema.[2,4] In the case of a cerebellar hemorrhage, the onset of ataxia is extremely sudden, whereas with posterior fossa tumors, the history will usually reveal a more protracted process.[2] Toxic ingestions are likely in patients on anticonvulsants and are especially common in toddlers. Acute ataxia can also occur after head trauma, in which it can result from a cerebellar hemorrhage or basilar skull fracture.

Any ataxic patient in whom an acute infectious process is considered requires a lumbar puncture. It is imperative that, prior to lumbar puncture, increased intracranial pressure be excluded by computed tomography (CT) scan of the brain.[1,2,4] In any case in which ingestion of a toxic substance is suspected, a toxicology screen is indicated. Specific toxins to assess include anticonvulsants, benzodiazepines, tricyclic antidepressants, sedative/hypnotics, and alcohol.

Certain causes of acute ataxia are almost unique to the pediatric population and deserve special mention. Guillain–

▶ TABLE 54–1. CAUSES OF ATAXIA

Acute
  Postinfectious/immune mediated
    Acute cerebellar
    Polymyoclonus/opsoclonus
    Guillain–Barré/Miller–Fisher syndromes
    Tick paralysis
    Acute demyelinating encephalomyelitis (ADEM)
  Posttraumatic
    Hematoma
    Mass
    Vertebrobasilar dissection
  Infection
    Meningitis
    Encephalitis
  Polyneuritis
  Posterior fossa tumors
  Intoxications
    Alcohol
    Anticonvulsants
    Benzodiazepines
    Cyclic antidepressants
    Sedative-hypnotics
    Inhalants
    Carbon monoxide
    Lead

Intermittent
  Migraine & migraine variants
  Seizures
  Multiple sclerosis
  Metabolic/Inborn errors
  Urea cycle defects
  Amino acid disorders
  Organic acid disorders
  Recurrent genetic ataxias

Chronic
  Progressive
    Tumor
    Abscess
    Hydrocephalus
    Degenerative
  Nonprogressive
    Cerebral palsy
    Sequelae of
      Head trauma
      Lead poisoning
      Cerebellar malformations: Dandy–Walker cysts,
        Agenesis, Hypoplasia

Barré syndrome can present with ataxia, although the associated findings of areflexia and, in the Miller–Fisher variant, ophthalmoplegia distinguish it from acute cerebellar ataxia. Many childhood illnesses and immunizations have been postulated as inciting an autoimmune phenomenon, which can result in acute cerebellar ataxia, acute demyelinating encephalomyelitis (ADEM), or brain stem encephalitis.[1]

ACUTE CEREBELLAR ATAXIA

A common cause of ataxia in children younger than 5 years is acute cerebellar ataxia. The onset of ataxia is insidious and predominantly affects the gait, although dysmetria, nystagmus, and dysarthria can occur. The affected child is afebrile, and has a normal level of consciousness. Acute cerebellar ataxia is thought to be a postinfectious phenomenon and often occurs 2 weeks after a viral illness. Ataxia has been reported after infection with varicella, influenza, mumps, Epstein–Barr virus, echovirus 6, coxsackie B virus, and other viruses. The gait abnormalities come on abruptly, and are maximum at onset, with the trunk affected more than the extremities.[1] It is a self-limiting illness with an excellent prognosis. Although therapies such as steroids and intravenous immune globulin have been used, there is really no specific therapy.[5] Acute cerebellar ataxia is a diagnosis of exclusion.

MYOCLONIC ENCEPHALOPATHY OF INFANCY (OPSOCLONUS/MYOCLONUS)

Myoclonic encephalopathy of infancy (polymyoclonus/ opsoclonus) is another cause of acute ataxia. This syndrome occurs in children from 6 months to 3 years of age, in association with occult neuroblastoma, viral disease, aseptic meningitis (especially mumps), and unknown or miscellaneous causes. It is differentiated from acute cerebellar ataxia by its association with opsoclonus (rapid, chaotic conjugate eye movements), which occur in association with polymyoclonus (severe myoclonic jerks of the limbs and trunk or head).[1] Irritability and vomiting can also occur. Diagnostic tests that should be initiated in the emergency department (ED) include chest and abdominal CT, urine vanillylmandelic acid (VMA), and lumbar puncture to exclude aseptic meningitis.[1] Treatment for the parainfectious form includes ACTH and oral glucocorticoids. Treatment for those with a neuroblastoma should be in consultation with a pediatric oncologist. Unfortunately, for those without an underlying cause, intellectual impairment is often associated with this movement disorder.[1]

ACUTE POSTINFECTIOUS DEMYELINATING ENCEPHALOMYELITIS

This is a multifocal immune-mediated encephalopathy characterized by ataxia, alteration in level of consciousness, and neurological deficits. Seizures, cranial neuropathies, hemiparesis and transverse myelitis are common. The patient may have fever, headache, and meningismus. It develops during the recovery from a viral illness, or after vaccination. Repeated episodes of this should prompt a workup for multiple sclerosis.[1]

TUMORS

Up to 60% of childhood brain tumors occur in the brain stem or cerebellum. Those that arise in the posterior fossa often have a slow onset of symptoms including ataxia, headache, and vomiting. However, hydrocephalus from obstruction or a bleed into the tumor can cause abrupt symptoms and decompensation.[1]

GUILLAIN–BARRÉ SYNDROME/ MILLER–FISHER SYNDROME

This is an acute demyelinating polyradiculoneuropathy that occurs after an infection or immunization. Although it predominantly affects the motor nerves resulting in weakness, 15% of patients develop a loss of sensory input to the cerebellum resulting in a sensory ataxia. The ataxia and weakness is progressive over several days. The Miller–Fisher syndrome is a form of GBS that results in ataxia, areflexia, and ophthalmoplegia. It occurs 5 to 10 days after an infectious illness, especially *Campylobacter gastroenteritis*.[1,2] Diagnostic tests include lumbar puncture looking for cytoalbuminologic dissociation and anti-GQ1b antibody for the Miller–Fisher variant. Patients suspected of these syndromes should be admitted to the hospital for further testing and monitoring as disease progression is variable. Electromyography is helpful to diagnose both GBS where specific abnormalities are seen. It is less helpful in diagnosing the Miller–Fisher syndrome, but may demonstrate abnormalities.[1]

INTERMITTENT/EPISODIC ATAXIA

Intermittent or episodic ataxia occurs as acute episodes that are similar in nature. In children, the most common cause of intermittent ataxia is a migraine headache that involves the basilar artery. Besides ataxia, associated symptoms include blurred vision, visual field deficits, vertigo, and headache. In a child experiencing the first basilar migraine, it is essential to exclude an acute infectious process, toxic ingestion, or mass lesion.[1]

Partial complex seizures can also cause intermittent ataxia but are often associated with alteration of consciousness and possibly characteristic motor manifestations.

Rarely, inborn errors of metabolism result in intermittent ataxia. These include maple syrup urine disease, Hartnup's disease, urea cycle defects (citrullinemia, ornithine transcarbamylase deficiency, and arginosuccinic aciduria), multiple carboxylase deficiencies (biotinidase deficiency and isovaleric academia), pyruvate decarboxylase and pyruvate dehydrogenase deficiencies, and ataxia with vitamin E deficiency.[1,6]

Patients with intermittent ataxia may not require radiographic or laboratory evaluation in the ED if they present with a known diagnosis. Patients suspected of having seizures are referred for an electroencephalogram (EEG). The rare patient suspected of having an undiagnosed inborn error of metabolism is referred to a pediatric geneticist or endocrinologist.

► CHRONIC PROGRESSIVE ATAXIA

Chronic progressive ataxia has an insidious onset and progresses slowly over weeks to months. The differential diagnosis consists of brain tumors, hydrocephalus, and neurodegenerative disorders.

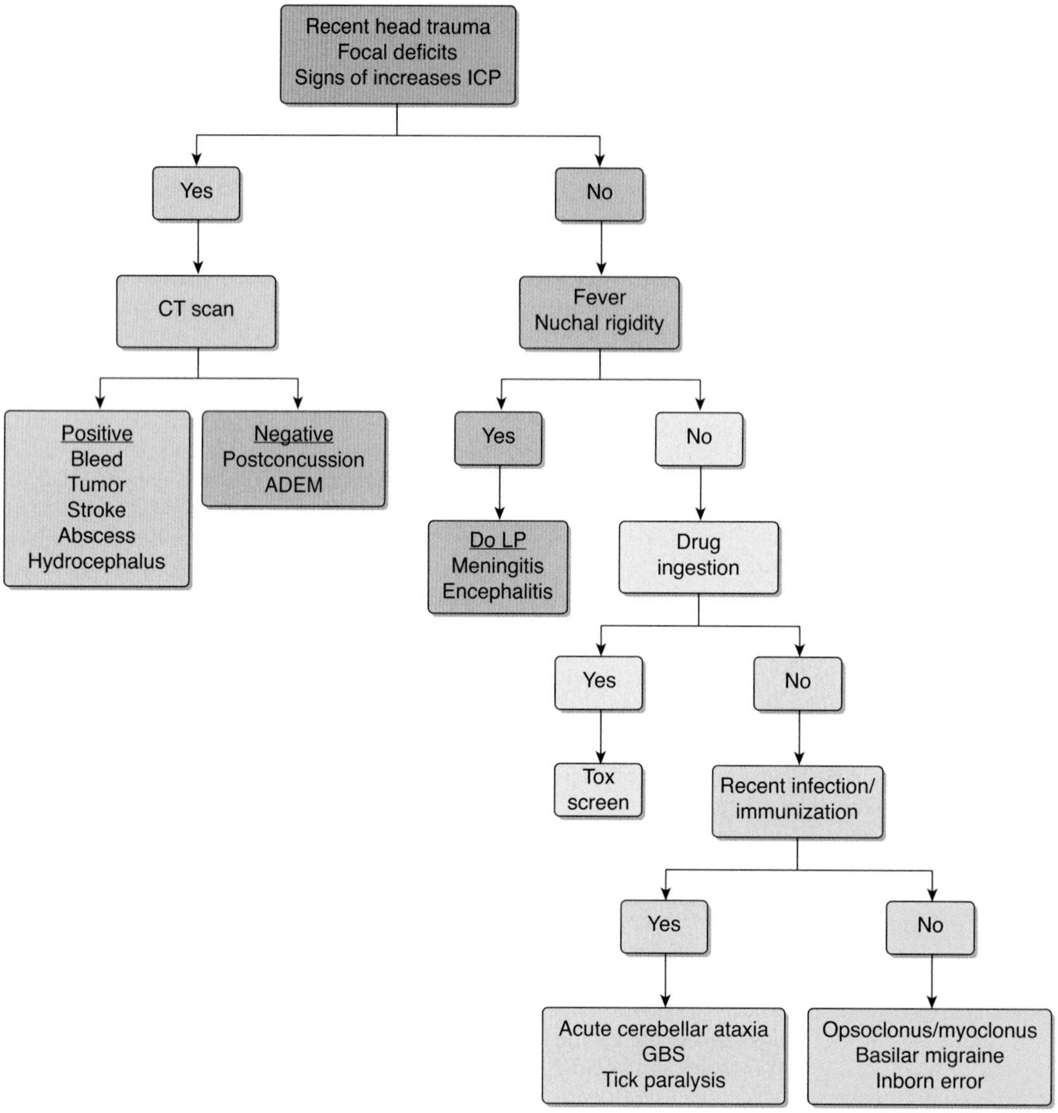

Figure 54–1. ED evaluation of acute ataxia.

The combination of ataxia, headache, irritability, and vomiting in a child younger than 9 years is characteristic of a cerebellar tumor, most commonly a medulloblastoma.[7] Cerebellar astrocytomas are located in the cerebellar hemispheres and cause ipsilateral limb ataxia, headache, and double vision. They occur most commonly in school-age children. Brain stem gliomas present with ataxia and are often accompanied by cranial nerve palsies or spasticity. In some cases, posterior fossa tumors have a relatively acute presentation.

Hydrocephalus, whether congenital or acquired, can cause ataxia. It is often accompanied by headache and vomiting and, when the patient presents late in the course of illness, can be associated with critically increased intracranial pressure.

Neurodegenerative diseases are a group of inherited disorders that can cause spinocerebellar degeneration and progressive ataxia. These include Refsum's disease and Bassen–Kornzweig syndrome (abetalipoproteinemia with hypovitaminosis A), which are treatable by diet (dietary restriction of phytanic acid and the addition of vitamin E, respectively).[6] Leigh syndrome (subacute necrotizing encephaolmyelopathy)

consists of developmental delay or psychomotor regression with ataxia, dystonia, seizures, and lactic acidosis. It is thought to be due to a mitochondrial disorder.[6]

Other hereditary causes of ataxia include spinocerebellar ataxias, of which there are 28 types.[8] Friedrich's ataxia is the most common autosomal recessive ataxia, which usually manifests before 10 years of age. It is characterized by ataxia, nystagmus, kyphoscoliosis, cardiomyopathy, and distal muscle wasting.[5] Patients with ataxia–telangiectasia present with ataxia before the onset of the ocular and facial telangiectasias.[9] Patients with progressive ataxia require an aggressive evaluation in the ED. All patients are examined for signs of increased intracranial pressure, which in some cases can be severe enough to result in the threat of uncal herniation. A CT scan of the brain is indicated in any patient with signs of a mass lesion or hydrocephalus. Many of these patients are candidates for an emergency placement of a ventricular shunt. Patients with suspected neurodegenerative diseases are referred to a pediatric neurologist for further evaluation and specific diagnosis.

▶ CHRONIC NONPROGRESSIVE ATAXIA

Chronic nonprogressive ataxia may be a sequela of head trauma, meningitis, or lead poisoning. It can also result from congenital malformations, such as cerebellar agenesis or hypoplasia or the Chiari type I malformation (herniation of the cerebellar tonsils into the foramen magnum).[2]

The ED evaluation of chronic nonprogressive ataxia consists of ensuring, by a careful history and physical examination, that the problem is indeed stable. Patients with an unknown diagnosis may benefit from CT or magnetic resonance imaging of the brain (see Figure 54–1).

REFERENCES

1. Ryan MM, Engle EC. Acute ataxia in childhood. *J Child Neurol.* 2003;18:309–316.
2. Agrawal D. Approach to the child with acute ataxia. In: Rose BD, ed. *UpToDate.* Waltham, MA: UpToDate; 2007.
3. Maricich SM, Zoghbi HY. The cerebellum and the hereditary ataxias. In: Swaiman KF, Ashwal S, Ferriero DM, eds. *Pediatric Neurology: Principles and Practice.* 4th ed. Philadelphia, PA: Mosby/Elsevier; 2006:1241–1247.
4. Friday JH. Ataxia. In: Fleisher GR, Ludwig S, Henretig FM, eds. *Textbook of Pediatric Emergency Medicine.* 5th ed. Philadelphia, PA: Lippincott, Williams & Wilkins; 2006:189–192.
5. Sanger TD, Mink JW. Movement disorders. In: Swaiman KF, Ashwal S, Ferriero DM, eds. *Pediatric Neurology: Principles and Practice.* 4th ed. Philadelphia, PA: Mosby/Elsevier; 2006:1295–1297.
6. Opal P, Zoghbi HY. Overview of the hereditary ataxias. In: Rose BD, ed. *UpToDate.* Waltham, MA: UpToDate; 2007.
7. Pomeroy SL. Pathogensesis and clinical features of medulloblastoma. In: Rose BD, ed. *UpToDate.* Waltham, MA: UpToDate; 2007.
8. Opal P, Zoghbi HY. The spinocereballar ataxias. In: Rose BD, ed. *UpToDate.* Waltham, MA: UpToDate; 2007.
9. Opal P, Bonilla FA, Lederman HM. Ataxia-telangiectasia. In: Rose BD, ed. *UpToDate.* Waltham, MA: UpToDate; 2007.

CHAPTER 55

Weakness

Susan Fuchs

► HIGH-YIELD FACTS

- Upper motor neuron diseases usually present with asymmetrical weakness contralateral to the lesion. Lower motor neuron diseases present with symmetrical weakness that can be isolated to specific muscle groups.
- Involvement of bulbar muscles is manifested by cranial nerve findings, facial muscle weakness, and chewing or swallowing difficulties. Bulbar involvement can occur in both upper and lower motor neuron disorders.
- Neuropathies are disorders of nerves and tend to cause distal muscle weakness, hypesthesias or paresthesias, and decreased reflexes, especially early in the disease.
- Myopathies are disorders of muscle and can be inflammatory or congenital. Inflammatory myopathies usually involve proximal muscles and are associated with muscle pain or tenderness.
- Guillain–Barré syndrome often starts with nonspecific muscular pain, most often in the thighs. The pain is followed by weakness, which is most often symmetrical and distal, progresses upward, and, in some cases, results in total paralysis within 24 hours.
- Transverse myelitis is a syndrome characterized by acute dysfunction at a level of the spinal cord. A mass lesion must be emergently excluded.
- Tick paralysis is caused by a neurotoxin from the Rocky Mountain wood tick or the Eastern dog tick.
- Food-borne botulism results from ingestion of toxins contained in improperly canned foods. Diarrhea and vomiting are followed by neurologic symptoms, such as blurred vision, dysarthria, and diplopia, followed by weakness of the extremities.
- Infantile botulism is caused by colonization of the intestinal tract by spores of *Clostridium botulinum*. Many cases are linked to nearby construction projects, as soil harbors the spores. A prominent early manifestation is constipation.

The term "weakness" can refer to a general phenomenon that affects all or most of the body or may refer to a specific area, such as an extremity. The complaint can imply generalized fatigue, refusal to walk, increased clumsiness, loss of bowel or bladder function, or focal motor weakness. In infants, weakness can imply lethargy, poor feeding, or poor head control. Slowly progressive forms of weakness may be due to congenital disorders. The child may present at a time when the weakness is mild, yet progressive. Others may have paralysis at the time of presentation. The primary focus in this chapter is on weakness arising from neuromuscular disorders.

► PATHOPHYSIOLOGY

The pathophysiology of weakness varies with the etiology and the specific area affected. Terms that are applied to neuromuscular disorders include the following:

- Paresis implies a complete or partial weakness.
- Paraparesis is weakness of the lower half of the body.
- Quadraparesis is weakness involving all limbs.
- Hemiparesis is weakness of one side.[1]
- Quadriplegia is paralysis of all limbs; it usually results from a spinal cord lesion.
- Hemiplegia, involving one side of the body, generally results from a lesion in the brain.

Abnormalities of the neuromuscular system are further classified as arising from an upper or lower motor neuron unit. The upper motor neuron unit arises in the motor strip of cerebral cortex, traverses the corticospinal tract, and ends in the spinal cord adjacent to the anterior horn cell.[2,3] Upper motor neuron diseases involving the cerebral cortex or spinal cord usually present with asymmetrical weakness that is contralateral to the lesion, and are associated with hyperreflexia, increased muscle tone, and the absence of atrophy or fasciculations I.[3,4] The lower motor neuron unit includes the anterior horn cells, peripheral nerve, neuromuscular junction, and muscle fibers. Lower motor neuron diseases present with symmetrical weakness that can be isolated to specific muscle groups, and are associated with decreased muscle tone and depressed reflexes. Depending on whether the disorder is acute or chronic, atrophy and fasciculations may be present (Table 55–1).[2,3,5]

Involvement of bulbar muscles is manifested by cranial nerve findings, facial muscle weakness, and chewing or swallowing difficulties. Bulbar involvement can occur in both upper and lower motor neuron disorders.[1]

In the patient presenting with weakness, it is important to distinguish between a neuropathy and myopathy. Neuropathies are disorders of nerves, and tend to produce distal muscle weakness, hypesthesias or paresthesias, and decreased reflexes, especially early in the disease. The progression of weakness and sensory loss is in a stocking and glove distribution.[6] Myopathies are disorders of muscle, and can be inflammatory, infectious, congenital, or metabolic. Inflammatory myopathies usually involve proximal muscles and are often associated with muscle pain or tenderness. Reflexes become decreased late in the disease. Congenital myopathies tend to involve specific muscle groups, and can present at birth with hypotonia and weakness, or in older children with a more insidious progression.[3,7]

▶ TABLE 55–1. **UPPER VERSUS LOWER MOTOR NEURON FINDINGS**

Upper motor neuron lesions
   1. Asymmetric weakness
   2. Increased muscle tone
   3. No atrophy/fasciculations
   4. Hyperreflexia/clonus

Lower motor neuron lesions
   1. Symmetrical weakness
   2. Decreased muscle tone
   3. Atrophy/fasciculations
   4. Diminished reflexes

▶ DIAGNOSIS

HISTORY

It is vital to distinguish between acute and chronic disorders, since this information will direct the remainder of the workup. The location of the initial weakness is elicited, and weakness is established as focal or general. Focal weakness is further characterized as predominantly proximal or distal. The rate of progression of symptoms is characterized as acute, which implies minutes to hours; subacute, meaning hours to days; and slowly progressive, which involves a prolonged period. Acute onset or rapid progression implies spinal cord compression or a vascular event involving the spinal cord or brain. Subacute progression can be due to infection, inflammation, toxin, or tumor. Slowly progressive symptoms imply a chronic or congenital disorder.[3] Defining the progression of symptoms is facilitated by asking the parents questions regarding progressive difficulty in walking, recent difficulty climbing up or down stairs, or inability to go from a sitting to standing position unaided. The loss of developmental milestones implies a degenerative disorder.

The patient and parents are questioned regarding symptoms preceding the onset of weakness, such as recent illness, fever, headache, neck or back pain, and loss of bowel or bladder function. A history of recent trauma to the head or neck and the presence of underlying medical problems is elicited. Prior episodes of weakness may suggest an intermittent metabolic problem. A family history of weakness suggests a congenital disorder. A history of exposure to drugs or heavy metals suggests poisoning. A pertinent travel history is indicated, since weakness can be a manifestation of entities such as tick paralysis, or from ciguatera poisoning. A careful antenatal history is indicated to rule out a perinatal insult, as is an immunization history to evaluate the possibility of a vaccine-related complication.

PHYSICAL EXAMINATION

The physical examination begins with observation of mental status, posture, gait, and the ability of the child to get on the examining table or to sit unaided. The vital signs are assessed, with particular attention to respiratory rate and effort since many neuromuscular disorders are associated with a risk of respiratory failure. Blood pressure and pulse are carefully mon-

▶ TABLE 55–2. **EVALUATING MUSCLE STRENGTH**

0: Total lack of contraction
1: Muscle twitch/trace contraction
2: Movement/weak contraction without gravity
3: Movement/weak contraction against gravity
4: Movement against some but not full resistance
5: Normal motor strength against full resistance

itored, since some neuromuscular disorders, such as Guillain–Barré syndrome, are associated with autonomic instability.

The patient's general appearance is noted, with attention given to general muscular development and the presence of kyphosis, scoliosis, or lordosis, which can all suggest a congenital disorder. The patient's facial expression is noted. Lack of facial expression, snarl, or slack jaw suggests myasthenia gravis. Ptosis can be due to myasthenia or myotonic dystrophy. Gross inspection of the muscles is performed, noting the presence of wasting, fasciculation, or hypertrophy.

The neurologic examination includes an evaluation of pupillary size and reactivity and the remainder of the cranial nerves. If possible, the fundus is examined and the visual fields are assessed. One way to test facial strength is to have children blow out their cheeks and resist compression.[6] For patients old enough to cooperate, motor strength in the extremities is evaluated and rated on a scale of 0 to 5 (Table 55–2). For infants who cannot cooperate with the examination, it is possible to perform a general assessment of muscle tone and integrity by holding the baby under the arms and placing the feet on the bed. Infants with normal tone will not slide through an examiner's hands and will actively kick both legs against the resistance of the bed. In an outstretched prone position, infants supported on the trunk should hold their head up, flex the limbs, and keep their back straight.[2] Older children can be asked to walk on their toes and heels. The ability to walk on the heels but not the toes suggests intraspinal pathology, although toe walking can occur with upper motor neuron disorders that cause spasticity.[6]

Deep tendon reflexes at the knees, ankles, elbows, and wrists are elicited (Table 55–3).[1] Hyperreflexia or sustained clonus indicates an upper motor neuron lesion, whereas absent or decreased reflexes imply a problem in a lower motor distribution.[2] Other reflexes to be noted include the anal wink, the plantar response, and abdominal and cremasteric responses.

Sensory evaluation includes touch, pain, position, vibration, and temperature. Touch and pain are evaluated by assessing soft versus sharp stimulation and two-point discrimination. Position sense is assessed by asking the child to indicate the direction in which an examiner moves a finger or toe.

▶ TABLE 55–3. **EVALUATING DEEP TENDON REFLEXES**

0: Absent
1: Reduced
2: Normal
3: Increased
4: Clonus

Temperature sensation can be assessed by the use of a cold stethoscope or by touching the child with cold or warm water. Vibration can be tested using a tuning fork on both thumbs (interphalangeal joint) and big toes.[1]

The sensations of touch and position-vibration do not cross in the spinal cord on their way to the brain, whereas those of pain and temperature do. An abnormality of touch and position on one side and pain and temperature on the other suggests a cord lesion. The unilateral loss of all sensations suggests a brain lesion. A stocking and glove distribution of sensory loss suggests a peripheral neuropathy.

LABORATORY EVALUATION

The laboratory evaluation is based on the provisional diagnosis. Generally, complete blood counts and serum electrolytes are indicated. Elevated serum creatine kinase is nonspecific but is found in children with active inflammatory myopathies and is elevated in congenital myopathies. Urine is assessed for the presence of myoglobin and, in selected cases, is used for toxicology screening.

For patients with a suspected spinal cord lesion, radiographs are indicated. Even if they are negative, any patient suspected of having a developing lesion of the spinal cord requires evaluation by magnetic resonance imaging (MRI). If this is unavailable, computed tomography (CT) of the spine may be helpful.

For patients with suspected central nervous system lesions, a CT scan of the brain is indicated. Some patients may require a lumbar puncture.[3]

Electromyography and nerve conduction studies are indicated if lower motor neuron disease is suspected, and to distinguish neurogenic from myopathic etiologies.[2,6] Muscle biopsies are also of value to diagnose specific neuromuscular diseases.[2]

▶ SPECIFIC CAUSES OF WEAKNESS

Weakness due to certain causes is common enough in the pediatric ED population to justify specific discussion.

GUILLAIN–BARRÉ SYNDROME

Also known as acute inflammatory demyelinating polyradiculoneuropathy (AIDP), Guillain–Barré syndrome occurs in both children and adults. It is more common in the adult patient population. The pathogenesis is unknown, but it is thought to result from an immune response to an antecedent viral infection that triggers demyelination of nerve roots and peripheral nerves. Campylobacter infection is the most common preceding illness, occurring in 30% of cases. Other infections include cytomegalovirus, EBV, herpes simplex, *Hemophilus influenzae, Mycoplasma pneumoniae*, hepatitis A and B, enterovirus, and *Chlamydophila pneumoniae*.[8] The form of GBS associated with campylobacter also results in acute axonal degeneration.[8] The syndrome often starts with paresthesias in the toes and fingers, and nonspecific muscular pain, most often in the thighs. The pain is followed by weakness, which is most often symmetric and distal, and results in trouble walking.[8] Weakness progresses upward and, in some cases, results in total paralysis within 24 hours. Cranial nerve involvement is common, with bilateral facial weakness. Deep tendon reflexes are usually absent, but plantar responses remain downgoing. Autonomic involvement can produce labile changes in blood pressure and bowel and bladder incontinence. The degree of weakness and the rate of progression of disease vary considerably. Laboratory findings are generally not helpful, although spinal fluid analysis may reveal a high protein (>45 mg/dL) and usually has fewer than 10 white blood cells.[8]

Diagnostic criteria exist which combine clinical, laboratory, and electrophysiologic features. Electrophysiologic studies demonstrate motor conduction bock, and slowed nerve conduction velocities.[9]

The basic treatment for Guillain–Barré syndrome is supportive care. Patients with vital capacity ½ normal for age usually require ventilatory support. Approximately 20% of patients require mechanical ventilation, which is associated with a poorer prognosis.[10] Attention is given to fluid and electrolyte balance, heart rate, cardiac rhythm, blood pressure, and nutritional needs. Steroids and other immunosuppressive agents are of no value. Intravenous immunoglobulin (IVIG) has been shown to shorten the course, as have limited studies on plasmsapheresis.[10] The American Academy of Neurology states that IVIG or plasmapheresis are treatment options for children with severe GBS.[10,11]

There are several variants of GBS/AIDP in children, including Miller–Fisher syndrome, which is characterized by ophthalmoplegia, hyporeflexia, and ataxia. Acute motor and sensory axonal neuropathy (ASMAN) and acute motor axonal neuropathy (AMAN) occur mainly in China, and are associated with a preceeding campylobacter infection.[8] The latter two forms consist of acute ascending weakness, hyporelexia, and elevated CSF protein, with ASMAN having a more prolonged course and limited recovery.[8,9]

TRANSVERSE MYELITIS

Transverse myelitis is a syndrome characterized by acute dysfunction at a level of the spinal cord. It can occur as an isolated phenomenon or as part of another illness, such as multiple sclerosis. As such, it represents a syndrome rather than a distinct entity. The onset can be insidious, but is usually over 24 to 48 hours. Patients may initially complain of paresthesias and weakness of the lower extremities. Those with the rapid form often complain of back pain. Progressive weakness, paraplegia, and urinary retention usually result, and a sensory level may develop, most commonly in the thoracic area. Flaccid paralysis and decreased reflexes are characteristic early in the process but are later followed by increased muscle tone.[12]

For a patient with signs of a rapidly advancing spinal cord lesion, it is imperative to exclude a treatable mass lesion that could be compressing the cord, such as an epidural abscess or hemorrhage. This is usually done by MRI, which shows a gladolinium signal abnormality over the spinal cord, and may show swelling on weighted T2 images. Most patients with transverse myelitis recover some function. Corticosteroids may benefit some patients.[12]

Tick Paralysis

Tick paralysis is caused by a neurotoxin from the Rocky Mountain wood tick (*Dermacentor andersoni*) or the Eastern dog tick (*Dermacentor variabilis*). The tick produces a neurotoxin that prevents liberation of acetylcholine at neuromuscular junctions. Several days after the tick attaches, the patient begins to experience paresthesias, fatigue, and weakness, which progresses to ataxia and difficulty walking. Deep tendon reflexes are absent. In some cases, there can be facial and bulbar muscle involvement, or unilateral paralysis. If the tick is not removed, flaccid paralysis and death can result. Removal of the tick is generally curative within a few hours.[6,13]

BOTULISM

Infection with *C. botulinum* can produce three neurologic diseases. Ultimately, symptoms result from a toxin generated from spores of the bacteria that inhibits calcium-dependent release of acetylcholine at the prejunction of terminal nerve fibers.[14]

Food-borne botulism results from ingestion of food containing the toxin. Diarrhea and vomiting are followed by neurologic symptoms, often secondary to cranial nerve dysfunction. Blurred vision, dysarthria, and diplopia can occur and can be followed by weakness of the extremities. Mucous membranes of the mouth and pharynx may be dry. Deep tendon reflexes may be weak or absent. Antitoxin may be effective in food-borne botulism.[14]

Wound botulism results from infection of a contaminated wound, 4 to 14 days after the wound is infected. Clinically, it is usually indistinguishable from food-borne botulism. Treatment includes wound debridement and antibiotic therapy. Antitoxin may also be useful.[14]

Infantile botulism is caused by colonization of the intestinal tract by spores of *C. botulinum*, which releases toxin that is systemically absorbed. It has been related to the ingestion of contaminated honey, but many cases are linked to nearby construction projects, as soil harbors the spores. The affected age group is 6 weeks to 9 months. A prominent manifestation is constipation. The infant develops a descending paralysis, with ptosis, difficulty in sucking and swallowing, and reduced facial expression and can become hypotonic. Symmetrical paralysis can develop with occasional respiratory involvement.[14]

Diagnosis is by isolating the toxin in the infant's stool. Electromyography is also useful. The management of infant botulism is supportive and may require mechanical ventilation. Treatment with antitoxin and antibiotics does not seem to be of benefit.

MYASTHENIA GRAVIS

The term myasthenia gravis comprises a group of autoimmune diseases characterized by easy fatigability. It is associated with anti-acetylcholine receptor antibodies resulting in decreased transmission of nerve impulses across the neuromuscular junction. It is the most common disorder of the myoneural junction in children.[14] In children, the striated muscles innervated by the cranial nerves are particularly affected. The diagnosis is usually established by demonstrating improvement in muscle strength after administration of the anticholinesterase edrophonium (Tensilon). The two basic categories of myasthenia gravis in the pediatric population are as follows:

- Neonatal transient myasthenia
- Juvenile myasthenia gravis

Neonatal transient myasthenia gravis occurs in infants born to mothers with the disease, and is caused by maternal anti-acetylcholine receptor antibodies that cross the placenta. It affects 10% to 15% of infants whose mothers have myasthenia gravis. The infant may have a weak cry or suck, ptosis, generalized weakness, hypotonia, and respiratory distress. It presents in the first few hours of life, but may be delayed up to 3 days. Treatment is with neostigmine or pyridostigmine. The disease usually improves in 4 to 6 weeks, but may last for months.[14]

Juvenile myasthenia gravis is similar to that seen in adults. It commonly has its onset at around 10 years of age, and is more common in females. Ptosis, ophthalmoplegia, and weakness of other facial muscles are commonly present. This results in difficulty in chewing, dysarthria, and dysphagia. Bulbar weakness develops in 75% of patients.[14] Symmetrical limb weakness is usually present, and affects the proximal muscles more than the distal muscles. The disease tends to become worse throughout the day, but can also worsen with stress or exertion. Symptoms and signs can be scored on a validated myasthenia scoring system and activities of daily living scale. Both remissions and exacerbations are common. To diagnose myasthenia gravis, the edrophomium (tensilon) test is helpful, but electrophysiologic testing and the presence of serum anti-acetylcholine receptor antibodies are more specific.[14] The primary treatment is with anticholinesterase agents. In refractory or severe cases, immunosuppressive agents, corticosteroids, IVIG, plasmapheresis, or thymectomy may be necessary. Erythromycin, tetracycline, aminoglycoside antibiotics, anesthetic drugs, neuromuscular blockers, and muscle relaxants therapy can exacerbate symptoms and should be avoided.[14,15]

Myasthenic Crisis

Occasionally, exacerbations of symptoms can occur that result in profound weakness, difficulty in swallowing secretions, and respiratory insufficiency. It is often precipitated by infection, surgery, or decreasing immunosuppressive drugs. It can also be exacerbated by the use of antibiotic therapy, especially aminoglycosides as well as antiarrhythmics, and ophthalmologic medications.[15] If a myasthenic crisis is suspected, the patient is admitted to an intensive care unit where respiratory status can be monitored, and elective intubation can occur if needed.

Cholinergic Crisis

Patients with myasthenia gravis can also suffer from overdose of anticholinesterase medications, which can provoke a cholinergic crisis. Unfortunately, the symptoms of cholinergic excess are similar to those of a myasthenic crisis. In both, increasing weakness is the predominant finding.[16] Patients suffering a cholinergic crisis may also have associated vomiting, diarrhea, and hypersalivation. In patients with obvious severe cholinergic excess, atropine or glycopyrrolate may be useful in drying airway secretions.[16] However, in most cases, it will be difficult to distinguish between a cholinergic crisis and an exacerbation of myasthenia, and hospital admission and close observation are indicated.

BELL'S PALSY

Bell's palsy is a condition that results in unilateral facial weakness. In severe cases, there can be total paralysis of the facial muscles. It is thought to result from swelling and edema of cranial nerve VII, the facial nerve, as it traverses the facial canal within the temporal bone. As such, it is a peripheral neuropathy, and the distribution of the weakness reflects the territory innervated by the facial nerve. The nerve has motor, sensory, and autonomic functions and, in addition to supplying the muscles of the face, it innervates the lacrimal and salivary glands, and the anterior two-thirds of the tongue. In most cases, Bell's palsy is idiopathic. Certain conditions are associated with unilateral facial weakness, including viral infections, otitis media, Lyme disease, and temporal bone trauma.[17]

Symptoms may begin with ear pain, which is followed by the development of facial weakness, characterized by a drooping mouth and inability to close the eye on the affected side. In some cases, lacrimation and taste are impaired. Inability to close the mouth can make eating and drinking difficult.[17]

The lesion is identified as a peripheral neuropathy, as opposed to a lesion of the central nervous system, by the fact that Bell's palsy affects the muscles of the forehead on the side of the lesion. In a lesion of the central nervous system, the forehead is spared, because it receives innervation from both sides of the brain. A lesion in a cerebral hemisphere will cause weakness confined to the lower part of the face.[17]

Laboratory studies are not necessary in uncomplicated cases. If the child has been in a Lyme disease endemic region, testing may be useful. If mastoiditis is suspected, a CT scan is helpful.[17]

The prognosis of Bell's palsy is generally good, with recovery usually beginning in 2 to 4 weeks, but may take 6 to 14 weeks to resolve fully. Steroid therapy may be beneficial if started early in the course of illness, and is given for 1 week. Treatment includes lubricating solutions for the eye on the affected side to maintain moisture of the cornea.[17] Patients with inability to close the eye may require patching. In young children, ophthalmologic consultation may be advisable.

MYOPATHIES

Myopathies are diseases that affect skeletal muscle. They are relatively uncommon in children, and, in most cases, a child affected with a myopathy will present to the ED with a known diagnosis. Many myopathies are congenital.

Muscular Dystrophies

Muscular dystrophies are disorders associated with progressive degeneration of muscle. The many different varieties of muscular dystrophy vary in their mode of inheritance, age of onset, muscles involved, progression of disease, and ultimate outcome. The most common is Duchenne muscular dystrophy,

usually an X-linked recessive disorder resulting in the absence of the protein dystrophin.[7] Clinical manifestations usually become apparent before age 4, when patients begin to develop weakness of the hip girdle and shoulder muscles. Patients may have difficulty standing and characteristically rise from all fours by placing their hands on the thighs and pushing up (Gower's sign). There is hypertrophy of the calf muscles. The disease is characterized by a progressive loss of muscle strength. Lordosis and kyphoscoliosis develop as the disease progresses. Pulmonary involvement due to weakness of the diaphragmatic and intercostal muscles results in impaired lung function. While the use of mechanical ventilators has increased survival, pulmonary infections and respiratory insufficiency are the main causes of mortality.[7] Cardiac insufficiency and cardiomyopathy of varying degrees occur in the majority of children. In adolescence, cardiac fibrosis can lead to left ventricular dysfunction, arrhythmias, heart failure, and sudden death.[7] The use of daily prednisone is the only treatment. It has been shown to improve ambulation, reduce contractures, and preserve respiratory function.[7]

Periodic Paralysis

Periodic paralysis is an example of metabolic myopathies that result in muscle weakness. The disorders are usually inherited, but can also be acquired. The inherited forms are autosomal dominant. There are several varieties, which include the channelopathies affecting the potassium, sodium, and calcium channels in skeletal muscle.[18]

Hypokalemic periodic paralysis is actually one of five channelopathies that is due to a disorder in the skeletal muscle sodium, calcium, or potassium channel gene, or is associated with thyroid disease, or cardiac dysrhythmias (Anderson syndrome).[18] Most episodes of hypokalemic periodic paralysis have their onset during the first or second decade of life. They are often precipitated by excitement, cold, rest after exercise, or ingestion of high-carbohydrate meals, but can also be associated with hyperthyroidism, excessive insulin, renal tubular acidosis, or laxative abuse. Paralysis usually begins proximally and spreads distally. The patient may be areflexic. The episode can last for 6 to 12 hours.[6,18] Attacks tend to decrease with age. Serum potassium during an attack is usually decreased compared with a baseline value. Treatment with oral potassium during an attack may be helpful; intravenous potassium may be needed for severe attacks. Long-term therapy with a low-sodium and low-carbohydrate diet, avoidance of exposure to cold, and potassium supplement can be beneficial. Acetazolamide taken daily may reduce the number of attacks.[18]

The three forms of hyperkalemic periodic paralysis are also autosomal dominant conditions associated with intermittent attacks beginning in the first decade of life. Attacks can be provoked by cold exposure, periods of rest following heavy exertion, and oral potassium loads. Weakness can develop rapidly, and lasts a shorter period of time than that of hypokalemic periodic paralysis.[6,18] Myalgia develops at the outset, and is followed by proximal then distal muscle weakness. Some patients develop myotonia during attacks.[18] The serum potassium is elevated above baseline values, although the degree of hyperkalemia varies. Treatment with oral glucose may speed recovery. Most attacks respond to treatment with glucose and insulin. In severe cases, intravenous calcium gluconate is necessary. In such cases, nebulized albuterol is also helpful.[18] Preventive treatment includes avoidance of exposure to cold and avoidance of fasting. Eating frequent high-carbohydrate meals may be helpful, as is treatment with hydrochlorothiazide or acetazolamide.[18]

Viral Myositis

Viral myositis is a common cause of weakness in children. It may follow influenza or other viral illnesses. Fever and other constitutional symptoms are accompanied by myalgias. Affected muscles are tender to touch, and may be boggy. The creatine kinase is often elevated. The urine should be examined for myoglobinuria, as this may indicate rhabdomyolysis, a serious complication. Most cases are self-limited, and are treated with bed rest, hydration, and NSAIDs or acetaminophen.[3,19,20]

Trichinosis

This is caused by ingestion of inadequately cooked meat (usually pork) containing the parasitic nematode *Trichinella spiralis*. While most infections are asymptomatic, invasion of the muscles results in an acute systemic infection characterized by fever, headache, generalized myalgias, abdominal pain, and weakness 2 to 12 days after ingestion of the meat. Myalgias and weakness are more profound in the third week of infection. Other complications include myocarditis and CNS infection. Diagnosis is by serum antibody levels, which peak 3 to 4 weeks after infection. Many patients also have elevated creatine kinase and eosinophilic leuckocytosis. Treatment includes thiabendazole and prednisone, to prevent a Herxheimer-like reaction after degeneration of the larvae.[19]

Pyomyositis

This is an abscess or multifocal abscesses within the muscle. While it is more likely to occur in an immunocompromised host, it has been occurring more frequently with the emergence of methicillin resistant *Staphylococcus aureus* (MRSA). Other bacterial causes include streptococci, *Escherichia coli*, *Yersinia*, and Legionella.[3,19] The child presents with fever, muscle pain, and tenderness. The abscess can be seen on ultrasound, CT scan, or MRI. Treatment involves appropriate intravenous antibiotics.[3,19]

Poliomyelitis

Although polio is rare, there are still sporadic cases. The virus attacks the anterior horn cells, resulting in asymmetrical weakness. The child may develop nuchal rigidity, muscle tightness, and fever. In infants younger than 1 year, spasm of the back muscles is also prominent. Bulbar involvement results in respiratory compromise, circulatory and autonomic instability, and mandates ventilatory support. The cerebrospinal fluid has pleocytosis with mononuclear cells, and a normal or slightly elevated protein.[5]

West Nile Virus

This RNA virus has rapidly become endemic in the United States, due to its vector of the *Culex* mosquito. Although most infections are asymptomatic, those that are symptomatic are more severe in the elderly; there have been cases in children as well. Symptoms include fever, headache, nausea, vomiting, and meningoencephalitis. Weakness may develop, and may be asymmetric or involve the face. Diagnosis is by demonstrating a rising IgM titer, or by reverse transcriptase PCR.[5]

▶ DISPOSITION

The disposition of a patient with weakness depends on the degree of disability and the nature of the underlying problem. In any patient in whom the development of respiratory compromise is a possibility, hospital admission and close observation is recommended.

REFERENCES

1. Gelb D. The detailed neurologic examination in adults. In: Rose BD, ed. *UpToDate*. Waltham, MA: UpToDate; 2007.
2. Swaiman KF. Muscular tone and gait disturbances. In: Swaiman KF, Ashwal S, Ferriero DM, eds. *Pediatric Neurology, Principles & Practice*. 4th ed. Philadelphia, PA: Mosby/Elsevier; 2006: 65–76.
3. Tsarouhas N, Decker JM. Weakness. In: Fleisher GR, Ludwig S, Henretig FM, eds. *Textbook of Pediatric Emergency Medicine*. 5th ed. Philadelphia, PA: Lippincott Williams & Wilkins; 2006:691–699.
4. Miller ML. Approach to the patient with muscle weakness. In: Rose BD, ed. *UpToDate*. Waltham, MA: UpToDate; 2006.
5. Connolly AM, Iannaccone ST. Anterior horn cell and cranial motor neuron disease. In: Swaiman KF, Ashwal S, Ferriero DM, eds. *Pediatric Neurology, Principles & Practice*. 4th ed. Philadelphia, PA: Mosby/Elsevier; 2006:1859–1885.
6. Fenichel GM. Flaccid limb weakness in childhood. In: Fenichel GM, ed. *Clinical Pediatric Neurology, A Signs and Symptoms Approach*. 5th ed. Philadelphia, PA: Elsevier/Saunders; 2005:171–197.
7. Escolar DM, Leshner RT. Muscular dystrophies. In: Swaiman KF, Ashwal S, Ferriero DM, eds. *Pediatric Neurology, Principles & Practice*. 4th ed. Philadelphia, PA: Mosby/Elsevier; 2006:1969–2014.
8. Cruse RP. Overview of Guillain-Barre syndrome in children. In: Rose BD, ed. *UpToDate*. Waltham, MA: UpToDate; 2007.
9. Sladky JT, Ashwal S. Inflammatory neuropathies. In: Swaiman KF, Ashwal S, Ferriero DM, eds. *Pediatric Neurology, Principles & Practice*. 4th ed. Philadelphia, PA: Mosby/Elsevier; 2006:1919–1939.
10. Cruse RP. Treatment of Guillain-Barre syndrome in children. In: Rose BD, ed. *UpToDate*. Waltham, MA: UpToDate; 2005.
11. Hughes RAC, Wijdicks EFM, Barohn R, et al. Practice parameter: Immunotherapy for Guillain-Barre syndrome. *Neurology*. 2003;61:736–740.
12. Lotze TE. differential diagnosis of acute central nervous system demyelination. In: Rose BD, ed. *UpToDate*. Waltham, MA: UpToDate; 2007.
13. Sexton DJ. Tick paralysis. In: Rose BD, ed. *UpToDate*. Waltham, MA: UpToDate; 2006.
14. Wolfe GI, Barohn RJ. Diseases of the neuromuscular junction. In: Swaiman KF, Ashwal S, Ferriero DM, eds. *Pediatric Neurology, Principles & Practice*. 4th ed. Philadelphia, PA: Mosby/Elsevier; 2006:1941–1968.
15. Bird SJ. Myasthenic crisis. In: Rose BD, ed. *UpToDate*. Waltham, MA: UpToDate; 2007.

16. Bird SJ. Treatment of myasthenia gravis. In: Rose BD, ed. *UpToDate*. Waltham, MA: UpToDate; 2007.

17. Smith SA, Ouvier: peripheral neuropathies. In: Swaiman KF, Ashwal S, Ferriero DM, eds. *Pediatric Neurology, Principles & Practice*. 4th ed. Philadelphia, PA: Mosby/Elsevier; 2006:1887–1895.

18. Moxley RT, Tawil R. Channelopathies: myotonic disorders and periodic paralysis. In: Swaiman KF, Ashwal S, Ferriero DM, eds. *Pediatric Neurology, Principles & Practice*. 4th ed. Philadelphia, PA: Mosby/Elsevier; 2006:2093–2109.

19. Amato AA, Kissel JT. Inflammatory myopathies. In: Swaiman KF, Ashwal S, Ferriero DM, eds. *Pediatric Neurology, Principles & Practice*. 4th ed. Philadelphia, PA: Mosby/Elsevier; 2006:2075–2084.

20. Miller ML. Viral myositis. In: Rose BD, ed. *UpToDate*. Waltham, MA: UpToDate. 2007.

CHAPTER 56

Headache

Susan Fuchs

▶ HIGH-YIELD FACTS

- Most headaches in children are benign.
- Headaches can be classified as primary or secondary
- Brain tumor headaches in children are associated with neurologic findings such as papilledema, ataxia, and weakness in 85% of cases within 8 weeks of onset, and in virtually all cases by 24 weeks
- Pseudotumor cerebri causes headache in the absence of a mass lesion.

Headaches are common in childhood. As many as 82% of children experience a headache by the age of 15 years.[1,2] Although they usually do not result from serious disease, headaches are sometimes the manifestation of life-threatening illness. It is incumbent on the emergency physician to distinguish those headaches that result from benign, self-limited processes from those that can result in serious morbidity or mortality.

Headaches can be classified as primary or secondary. Primary headaches include migraine, tension-type, and cluster headaches, and are based on criteria defined by the International Headache Society and the International Classification of Headache Disorders.[3] Secondary headaches have identifiable etiologies based on history and physical examination. These include headaches attributed to head or neck trauma, infection, a vascular disorder such as bleed or stroke, a nonvascular intracranial disorder such as elevated intracranial pressure or a neoplasm, or a toxic substance such as carbon monoxide. Facial pain, sinus, and dental problems can also cause headaches. Some patients with psychiatric disorders will complain of headache.[3] The brain itself is not sensitive to pain, but there are pain-sensitive structures in the skin, the muscles, the vascular sinuses, the intracranial blood vessels, and the meninges at the base of the brain. Inflammation, dilation, irritation, and displacement of the pain-sensitive areas can result in a headache.

▶ EVALUATION

The evaluation of a child for a headache includes information on the headache history. Based on this information, the headache can be classified as acute (sudden, first), acute and recurrent (episodic), chronic and progressive (steadily worsening), or chronic and nonprogressive.[1,4] One way to help determine headache etiology is demonstrated in Table 56–1.

The following information should be obtained: age at onset, frequency and duration (minutes, days), time of onset (day, night, schooldays only), location (frontal, temporal, occipital), quality of pain (stabbing, pressure, pounding), associated symptoms (nausea/vomiting, photophobia), warning signs or aura (blurred vision, vertigo, nausea, weakness), precipitating factors (stress, coughing, certain foods), relieving factors (sleep), recent trauma, change in school or home environment, response to treatment at home, and family history of migraines.[1,4]

The physical evaluation includes general appearance, blood pressure and temperature, height, weight, and head circumference. The eyes are assessed for extraocular nerve palsies or nystagmus. A fundascopic examination evaluates the possibility of papilledema. Examination of the head assesses the temporomandibular joints and sinuses. The neck is ausculted for bruits that would indicate an arteriovenous malformation, and assessed for the presence of meningismus or rigidity. The skin is examined for café-au-lait spots, neurofibromas, and ash leaf spots. The neurologic examination includes strength testing, deep tendon reflexes, Romberg test, gait testing, cerebellar tests, Brudzinskis and Kernig's sign.[1,4,5]

The main concern for a physician is whether intracranial pathology exists. One study identified seven predictors for space-occupying lesions. These included sleep-related headache, absence of family history of migraine, vomiting, absence of visual symptoms, headache less than 6 months, confusion and an abnormal neurologic examination.[6] Brain tumor headaches in children are associated with neurologic findings including papilledema, ataxia, weakness in 85% of cases within 8 weeks of onset, and in virtually all cases by 24 weeks.[4,7] Although many brain tumors in children have a midline cerebellar origin (primary neuroectodermal tumor, medulloblastoma, cerebellar astrocytoma, ependymoma), signs and symptoms will still occur. Look for non-lateralizing signs such as morning or evening occurrence, vomiting, head tilt, double vision, declining school performance, a change in personality and gait changes.[8] Other life-threatening causes of headache that should not be missed include bacterial meningitis, orbital or cerebral abscess, viral encephalitis, hydrocephalus, intracranial hemorrhage, hypertensive encephalopathy, and carbon monoxide poisoning.

In a study of acute headaches in children presenting to an emergency department (ED), 55% had a URI with fever, 18% had a primary headache (migraine, tension), 7% had viral meningitis, 2% were postictal, 2% were postconcussive, 2.5% had a tumor, 2% had shunt malfunction, 1.5% suffered a hemorrhage, and 7% were of undetermined etiology.[9]

▶ **TABLE 56–1.** **HEADACHE ETIOLOGY**

Acute, Localized	Acute, Generalized	Acute, Recurrent	Chronic, Progressive	Chronic, Nonprogressive
Sinusitis, otitis, viral infection: flu	Systemic infection: flu, meningitis	Migraine	Idiopathic intracranial hypertension	Tension-type
Posttrauma	Hypertension		Space occupying lesion (tumor, abscess, hemorrhage, hydrocephalus)	Psychiatric (depression, school phobia)
Dental abscess, TMJ	Hemorrhage			
First migraine	Exertional, first migraine			

▶ LABORATORY STUDIES

Laboratory studies should be performed based upon the suspected etiology of the headache. If the blood pressure is elevated, electrolytes, BUN, creatinine, and urinalysis are appropriate. For a child with a fever, CBC, blood cultures, and cerebrospinal fluid (CSF) studies, if a lumbar puncture is performed, are appropriate.

▶ NEUROIMAGING

Neuroimaging should be performed for a child with signs of increased intracranial pressure, focal symptoms, an abnormal neurologic examination, skin lesions suggestive of a neurocutaneous syndrome, recent head trauma, and a progressive neurologic disorder[6] (Fig. 56–1). While a computed tomography (CT) scan is usually adequate to see a space-occupying

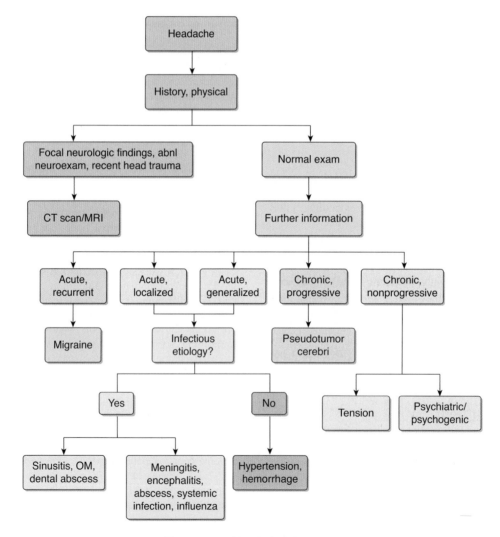

Figure 56–1. Headache algorithm.

► **TABLE 56–2. PRIMARY HEADACHE CHARACTERISTICS**

Symptom	Migraine	Tension	Cluster
Location	Unilateral 60%–70%, bilateral 30%	Bilateral	Always unilateral, begins around eye, temple
Characteristics	Gradual onset, crescendo, pulsating, mod-severe,	Pressure, tightness, waxes, and wanes	Begins quickly, crescendo, deep, continuous, excruciating pain
Patient appearance	Prefers rest in dark, quiet room	May remain active, or may rest	Remains active
Duration	4–72 h	Variable	30 min–3 h
Associated symptoms	Nausea, vomiting, photophobia, phonophobia, ± aura	None	Ipsilateral eye lacrimation, redness, rhinorrhea, sweating, Horner syndrome

lesion, bleed, hydrocephalus, and abscess, a magnetic resonance imaging (MRI) may be needed to demonstrate sellar lesions, some small posterior fossa lesions, white matter abnormalities, and congenital anomalies. However, MRI may not be immediately available, and frequently requires the child be sedated for the procedure.[1,5]

The main issue in many cases of pediatric headache is that the examination is normal or that this is a recurrent headache, so do these children really require neuroimaging? A decision analysis for diagnostic strategies of children suspected of having brain tumor headaches developed some neuroimaging strategies. A child with a low risk of a brain tumor (0.01% = 1 in 10,000) has a nonmigraine headache for more than 6 months and a normal neurologic examination. In such cases, no neuroimaging is indicated, but there should be close clinical follow-up. An intermediate risk group (0.4% = 4 in 1000) is the child with migraine symptoms and a normal neurologic examination; a CT scan followed by an MRI was an effective plan. High-risk children (4% = 4 in 100) were those with a headache less than 6 months, sleep-related headache, vomiting confusion, no visual symptoms, no family history of migraine, and an abnormal neurologic examination; they should undergo MRI.[6]

The American Academy of Neurology and the Child Neurology Society developed a practice parameter for the evaluation of children and adolescents with recurrent headaches. They stated that routine neuroimaging is not recommended in children with recurrent headaches and a normal neurologic examination. Neuroimaging should be considered in the child with headache who has an abnormal neurologic examination consisting of focal findings, signs of increased intracranial pressure, altered level of consciousness, or coexistent seizures or both. Neuroimaging should be considered in children with historical features to suggest recent onset of severe headache, change in the type of headache, or features that suggest neurologic dysfunction.[2]

► LUMBAR PUNCTURE

A child suspected of having meningitis/encephalitis requires a lumbar puncture (LP). If there is concern for a subarachnoid hemorrhage, an LP can be diagnostic if the CT was inconclusive. In addition, if idiopathic intracranial hypertension (pseudotumor cerebri) is being considered, and LP with an opening pressure is required (>25 cm H_2O, with normal CSF findings is diagnostic).

► PRIMARY HEADACHES

The characteristics of primary headaches are described in Table 56–2.

MIGRAINE HEADACHES

Migraine headaches are an example of recurrent headaches. The mean age of onset is 7.2 years for males and 10.9 years for females, but the prevalence increases from 3% in children aged 3 to 7 years to 8% to 23% for children aged 11 to 15 years.[10] In the younger age group, males are more affected than females, but this reverses by the older age group.[11] The headache tends to be unilateral, throbbing or pulsating, lasts 1 to 48 hours, is often associated with nausea and vomiting, and is relieved with sleep.[11,12] There is a genetic predisposition to migraines, with a positive family history in most cases.[12]

The classification of migraines includes migraine with aura (classic), migraine without aura (common), and childhood periodic syndromes that are commonly precursors of migraine (abdominal migraines, benign paroxysmal vertigo of childhood, and cyclic vomiting).[11,13] The IHS classification of pediatric migraine without aura, which accounts for 60% to 85% of cases, includes the following:

(A) At least five attacks fulfilling criteria B to D.
(B) Headache attacks lasting 1 to 72 hours.
(C) Headache has at least two of the following: either bilateral or unilateral location (frontal/temporal, but not occipital), pulsating quality, moderate-to-severe intensity aggravated by routine physical activities such as walking.
(D) At least one of the following during the headache: nausea and/or vomiting, photophobia, and phonophobia (may be inferred from behavior).[10,11]

Pediatric migraine with aura occurs in 15% to 30% of patients and the diagnostic criteria includes the following:

(A) At least two attacks fulfilling criteria B to D,
(B) An aura consisting of at least one of the following: (1) fully reversible visual symptoms such as flickering lights or spots, (2) fully reversible sensory symptoms such as pins and needles or numbness, or (3) fully reversible dysphasic speech disturbances. Motor weakness is not a criteria

(C) At least two of the following: (1) homonymous visual symptoms or unilateral sensory symptoms, (2) at least one aura symptom develops gradually over ≥5 minutes or different aura symptoms occur in succession ≥5 minutes, (3) each symptom lasts ≥5 minutes and ≤60 minutes,

(D) Symptoms are not attributable to another disorder.[11]

Several theories exist as to the pathophysiology of migraines. It is a primary neuronal process associated with intracranial and extracranial changes that have a genetic predisposition.[11,12] Antidromic stimulation of the trigeminal nerve releases substance P, calcitonin generated peptide, and other vasoactive polypeptides that cause pain and vasodilatation (neurogenic inflammation). There is also a cortical spreading depression of Leao, which is neuronal and glial hyperpolarization followed by depolarization that causes the aura of migraine, activates trigeminal afferents, and alters blood–brain barrier permeability, resulting in the headache.[11,12]

A variant of a migraine with aura that occurs in 3% to 19% of childhood migraines is the basilar artery migraine, which results in ataxia and vertigo, at times accompanied by visual disturbances. The headache is usually occipital in location. Familial hemiplegic migraine is a migraine with aura that includes motor weakness, and even some degree of hemiparesis. It has an autosomal dominant pattern of inheritance, and is due to a mutation in the calcium channel gene CACNA1 A.[11,13]

Benign paroxysmal vertigo is a migraine precursor. This occurs in children aged 2 to 6 years and consists of sudden, brief episodes when the child cannot stand upright without support. There is no loss of consciousness, but nystagmus is often seen. The episode lasts for several minutes, and then the child recovers completely.[11,13,14]

Cyclic vomiting syndrome is recurrent episodes of severe vomiting that last for a few hours to days, separated by symptom-free periods. Treatment includes IV fluids with glucose, antiemetic medication, and sometimes sedation.[11,13]

Abdominal migraine is recurrent episodes of abdominal pain lasting 1 to 72 hours, usually vague, and midline or periumbilical in location. It may be accompanied by nausea, vomiting, anorexia, or pallor.[11,13]

TREATMENT

Reassurance and patient, and parental education are the first steps. Patients should keep a headache diary in order to see if there are any precipitating factors. These include emotional stress, anxiety, menstruation, missing a meal, lack of sleep, and environmental factors such as bright lights, loud noises, and perfumes. Certain foods such as those that contain tyramine (aged cheese), sodium nitrite (hot dogs, smoked meats), or monosodium glutamate (Chinese food) can precipitate migraines, as can caffeine-containing beverages, chocolate, red wine, and certain drugs (such as oral contraceptives, antihypertensive medications, cimetidine, and H_2 blockers).[8,14]

ED treatment of migraines consists of providing analgesia and treating associated symptoms such as nausea during the acute attack. Analgesics such as acetaminophen or ibuprofen are often effective.[10] If the child is unable to tolerate oral NSAIDs, intravenous ketorolac can be used.[15]

Sumatriptan is a selective 5-HT agonist that can be given subcutaneously (6 mg) (although not FDA approved for children < 16 years) or as a nasal spray for children older than 12 years.[10,15] There are no data regarding oral use of sumatriptan, and other triptans are not approved for children.[10,15]

For children older than 10 years who present to the ED with a migraine headache, dihydroergotamine mesylate (DHE) 0.25 to 1.0 mg over 3 minutes intravenously may be beneficial, especially if given with metoclopramide. For nausea, antiemetics such as ondansetron, promethazine, metoclopramide, or prochlorperazine have been used.[15]

Preventive treatments include cyprohepatdine, β-blockers, antidepressants, anticonvulsants, and calcium channel blockers, but conclusive data are lacking regarding their use in children and adolescents.[10,15] Methods such as relaxation therapy and biofeedback may be beneficial. Those children who have frequent headaches and those with headaches that are unresponsive to abortive measures should be placed on prophylactic medications after consultation with a neurologist.

TENSION-TYPE HEADACHES

Tension-type headaches or muscle contraction or stress headaches tend to be chronic and nonprogressive in nature, with the pain described as band-like, bilateral, or generalized. There is no accompanying aura, and nausea is rare. The headache can last for 30 minutes to days and can be accompanied by photophobia or phonophobia but is not aggravated by physical activity.[16] There are three subtypes of tension-type headache: infrequent, occurring less than 1 day a month; frequent episodic, occurring 1 to 14 days a month; and chronic, occurring 15 or more days a month.[3,16]

The pathophysiology of tension-type headache is unknown but includes the trigeminal neurovascular system, unstable serotonergic neurotransmission, and muscle contraction producing vasoconstriction and ischemia.[16]

The diagnosis of tension-type headache is usually based upon clinical criteria, but the differential diagnosis includes infection, increased intracranial pressure, Chiari I malformation, and chronic sinus infection.[16] Of note, the physical and neurologic examination of a child with tension-type headaches is normal.

Tension-type headaches are generally managed with emotional support, and mild analgesics, such as acetaminophen and ibuprofen. Reassuring the family that the problem is not organic and advising the patient to avoid precipitating factors, such as stress, is an important part of therapy. Behavioral techniques, such as biofeedback, and relaxation exercises may be useful. In cases of frequent of chronic headaches, treatment with an antidepressant such as amitriptyline may be of benefit.[16]

CLUSTER HEADACHES

Cluster headaches are uncommon in children younger than 10 years of age. The headache is unilateral, occurs in the frontal or periorbital region, and is often described as ice-pick like. The headache lasts 15 minutes to 3 hours, and is associated with ipsilateral lacrimation, redness of the eye, and ipsilateral nasal congestion; the cheek may become flushed and warm. The patient may develop Horner syndrome—miosis, ptosis, and, facial anhidrosis—on the side of the headache.[1,17] The headache tends to occur at the same time each day during a cluster. Patients are unable to lie down or rest because of the pain.[17] Abortive treatment consists of 100% oxygen given for 20 minutes; sumatriptan and octreotride have been used in adults.[17]

► SECONDARY HEADACHES

BRAIN TUMORS AND HYDROCEPHALUS

The presence of a headache that is made worse by lying down, or that comes on with coughing, sneezing, or straining at stool and then disappears, suggests increased intracranial pressure. Headaches associated with disorders related to increased intracranial pressure are of a progressive nature. Papilledema is often found on funduscopic examination. A complete neurologic examination may disclose other abnormalities, such as ataxia with a cerebellar tumor, or cranial nerve findings with hydrocephalus. Differentiation of these disorders is by CT scan or MRI with appropriate consultation if hydrocephalus or a tumor is found.

IDIOPATHIC INTRACRANIAL HYPERTENSION (PSEUDOTUMOR CEREBRI)

Idiopathic intracranial hypertension or pseudotumor cerebri is a condition associated with increased intracranial pressure in the absence of a mass lesion or other obvious etiology. It results from impaired reabsorption of CSF. While many cases are idiopathic, it is associated with obesity, pregnancy, high doses of vitamin A, birth control pills, retinoic acid, tetracycline, infections including mastoiditis and otitis media, endocrinopathies, systemic lupus erythematosus, and steroid withdrawal.[8,14,18] Patients may have papilledema on examination. The CT scan in such patients often reveals small ventricles and an enlarged cisterna magna. Lumbar puncture will reveal an opening pressure > 25 cm H_2O, with normal protein, glucose, and cell count. Therapy includes treating the underlying cause, serial lumbar punctures to relieve acute symptoms, and acetazolamide 25 mg/kg to reduce the formation of CSF.[4]

HYPERTENSIVE ENCEPHALOPATHY

Severe elevation in blood pressure can cause headache and if untreated can result in the development of encephalopathy and seizures. This should be suspected in a patient with a severe headache whose diastolic blood pressure is greater than the 95th percentile for age. In young children, the development of hypertension is often secondary to an acute illness, such as fulminant glomerulonephritis. It can also be secondary to acute exacerbations in patients with known hypertension. In severe cases, hypertension can result in cardiac as well as neurologic dysfunction. Since other causes of increased intracranial pressure can also occasionally result in hypertension, it is essential that they be excluded. This includes coarctation of the aorta, so blood pressure should be checked in all extremities.

Acute therapy in the ED is individualized, based on complete physical examination findings, degree of hypertension, and past history of hypertension. Patients with encephalopathy and seizures require rapid reduction of blood pressure with an agent such as nitroprusside. The patient is admitted for blood pressure control and complete evaluation.

ACUTE HEMORRHAGE

The child presenting with a severe headache of sudden onset, with or without neck or back pain, may have suffered an intracranial hemorrhage. The patient's mental status can range from normal to coma. Focal findings and seizures may or may not be present. Spontaneous intracranial hemorrhage usually results from either a ruptured aneurysm or arteriovenous malformation. It can also occur in association with coagulopathies. The diagnosis and management are further discussed in the section on cerebrovascular syndromes.

MENINGITIS/ENCEPHALITIS/BRAIN ABSCESS

The association of headache with a fever and stiff neck implies an infectious etiology, such as bacterial meningitis, encephalitis, or brain abscess. A brain abscess can result from orbital cellulitis, extension from sinusitis, or in children with congenital heart disease caused by right-to-left intracardiac shunt.[5] Viral encephalitis can present with mild neck stiffness along with a change in behavior, fever, and headache. Specific etiologies to consider include herpes simplex and West Nile virus.[5] If there are no focal findings or signs of increased intracranial pressure on physical examination, a lumbar puncture is performed and will provide the diagnosis. CSF is sent for culture, cell count, protein, and glucose, with bacterial and viral cultures. If there are focal neurologic abnormalities or signs of increased intracranial pressure, a brain abscess is possible and a CT scan or MRI of the brain with and without contrast is performed prior to a lumbar puncture to avoid the potential for herniation. Hospital admission is required for children with these problems; the neurologic examination, serum electrolytes, and fluid status need to be monitored closely. Antibiotics are required for bacterial meningitis and brain abscess; acyclovir is the treatment for herpes simplex virus infection.

► OTHER ETIOLOGIES OF HEADACHE

Included in this group are problems that originate outside the calvarium but that can result in headache, either directly or through referred pain. They include sinusitis, otitis media, dental caries or abscess, pharyngitis, temporomandibular joint abnormalities, postconcussion or posttraumatic syndrome, and ophthalmologic problems, such as refractive errors or astigmatism. It can also include systemic infections, such as influenza, or strep throat. Toxic exposures, especially to carbon monoxide, can also cause headache.

► PSYCHIATRIC/PSYCHOGENIC HEADACHES

Psychiatric-related or psychogenic headaches tend to be chronic and nonprogressive and are characterized by vague complaints and nonspecific symptoms. They may result from stress, adjustment reactions, conversion reactions, depression, and malingering. In the ED, they are a diagnosis of exclusion.

REFERENCES

1. Brazis PW, Lee AG. Approach to the child with headache. In: Rose BD, ed. *UpToDate*. Waltham, MA: UpToDate; 2008.
2. Lewis DW, Ashwal S, Dahl G, et al. Practice parameter: evaluation of children and adolescents with recurrent headaches: report of the quality standards subcommittee of the American Academy of Neurology and the practice committee of the child neurology society. *Neurology*. 2002;59:490–498.
3. Headache Classification Committee of the International Headache Society. *The International Classification of Headache Disorders*. 2nd ed. *Cephalagia*. 2004;24(suppl 1):1–160. Available at: http://www.i-h-s.org and http://www.ihs-classification.org. Accessed Feb 22, 2008.
4. Lewis D. Headache treatment. When, how, what can I do?. Presented at: American Academy of Pediatrics, National Conference and Exhibition; October 2007; San Francisco, CA.
5. King C. Emergency evaluation of headache in children. In: Rose BD, *UpToDate*. Waltham, MA: UpToDate; 2008.
6. Medina LS, Kuntz KM, Pomeroy SL. Children with headache suspected of having a brain tumor: a cost-effectiveness analysis of diagnostic studies. *Pediatrics*. 2001;108:255–263.
7. Honig PJ, Charney EB. Children with brain tumor headaches: distinguishing features. *Am J Dis Child*. 1982;136:121–124.
8. Melvin J, Lewis D. Headache in the pediatric ED. Presented at: American Academy of Pediatrics, National Conference and Exhibition. Section on Emergency Medicine meeting; October 2007; San Francisco, CA.
9. Lewis DW, Qureshi F. Acute headache in children and adolescents presenting to the emergency department. *Headache*. 2000;40:200–203.
10. Lewis D, Ashwal S, Hershey A, et al. Practice parameter: pharmacological treatment of migraine headaches in children and adolescents: report of the American Academy of Neurology quality standards subcommittee and the practice committee of the child neurology society. *Neurology*. 2004;63:2215–2224.
11. Lewis DW. Pediatric migraine. *Pediatr Rev*. 2007;28:43–53.
12. Cruse RP. Pathophysiology, clinical features, and diagnosis of migraine in children. In: Rose BD, ed. *UpToDate*. Waltham, MA: UpToDate; 2007.
13. Cruse RP. Classification of migraine in children. In: Rose BD, ed. *UpToDate*. Waltham, MA: UpToDate; 2007.
14. Fisher PG. Headaches: When do I worry?. Who do I scan?. Presented at: American Academy of Pediatrics, National Conference and Exhibition; October 2007; San Francisco, CA.
15. Cruse RP. Management of migraine in children. In: Rose BD, ed. *UpToDate*. Waltham, MA: UpToDate; 2007.
16. Cruse RP. Tension headache in children. In: Rose BD, ed. *UpToDate*. Waltham, MA: UpToDate; 2007.
17. Bajwa ZH, Sabahat AS. Approach to patient with headache syndromes other than migraine. In: Rose BD, ed. *UpToDate*. Waltham, MA: UpToDate; 2008.
18. Gorelick MH, Blackwell CD. Neurologic emergencies. In: Fleisher GR, Ludwig S, Henretig FM, eds. *Textbook of Pediatric Emergency Medicine*. 5th ed. Philadelphia, PA: Lippincott Williams & Wilkins; 2006:759–781.

CHAPTER 57

Hydrocephalus

Susan Fuchs

▶ HIGH-YIELD FACTS

- Hydrocephalus refers to the excess accumulation of cerebrospinal fluid (CSF). Most cases result from congenital or acquired obstructions to the flow of CSF from the brain to the spinal canal.
- Infants with hydrocephalus are often diagnosed on routine examination by finding head circumference disproportionately large for age or splitting of the cranial sutures.
- Older children with hydrocephalus will usually complain of headache, which is often progressive in nature, worse in the morning, awakens the patient from sleep, and is exacerbated by lying down or straining.
- It is imperative to begin treatment in the unstable patient before herniation occurs. Patients who are lethargic on presentation, those with a Glasgow Coma Scale <8, or those who deteriorate in the emergency department are intubated following rapid sequence induction procedures and ventilated to maintain P_{CO_2} at 35 torr. If there are signs of herniation such as unequal pupils, fixed and dilated pupils, or posturing, mild hyperventilation can be helpful on a short-term basis.
- Patients who do not respond with an improved mental status after intubation and controlled ventilation may benefit from diuretic therapy with mannitol or furosemide.
- After the patient is stabilized, a computed tomography scan or magnetic resonance image of the brain is performed to define the lesion and plan definitive treatment.

Hydrocephalus refers to the excess accumulation of CSF. This can occur because of obstruction of CSF flow, reduced absorption, or excess production. Most (70%) of CSF is produced by the choroid plexus and absorbed by the arachnoid villi and granulations. Flow direction is from the lateral to third ventricle via the foramen of Monro. It then flows through the aqueduct of Sylvius to the fourth ventricles and exits via the foramina of Luschka (2) and Magendie to the basal cisterns.[1,2] It then divides between the spinal subarachnoid space and the subarachnoid cisterns. CSF is absorbed through arachnoid villi covering the brain and leptomeninges, across the ependymal lining of the ventricles, and the spinal subarachnoid space.[1,2] Although there are several ways to categorize hydrocephalus based on the site of excess fluid collection, the primary concern in the emergency department is determining the etiology of the problem and instituting appropriate treatment.

Most cases of hydrocephalus result from congenital or acquired obstructions to the flow of CSF from the brain to the spinal canal. Congenital malformations include the Arnold–Chiari malformation, which is elongation and downward displacement of the brain stem into the fourth ventricle, and the Dandy–Walker malformation, which is a posterior fossa cyst that causes obstruction at the outlet of the fourth ventricle at the foramen of Luschka and Magendie.[2] Intrauterine infections such as toxoplasmosis, rubella, cytomegalovirus, herpes, and syphilis can lead to hydrocephalus through inflammation of the ependymal lining of the ventricular system and lead to CSF flow obstruction.[1] Intraventricular hemorrhage in preterm newborns can also lead to hydrocephalus. Beyond the neonatal period, the most common causes of acquired hydrocephalus are mass lesions, which include tumors, cysts, and abscesses. Other acquired causes of hydrocephalus are meningitis, encephalitis, posthemorrhagic adhesions, and vascular malformations.[1,2]

▶ CLINICAL PRESENTATION

The clinical presentation of hydrocephalus depends on the age of the patient and the rate at which it develops.

Infants with hydrocephalus are often diagnosed on routine examination by finding head circumference disproportionately large for age or splitting of the cranial sutures. The unfused sutures of the infant allow the calvarium to expand and function as a pressure relief phenomenon. When the limitations of suture expansion are reached, intracranial pressure begins to rise precipitously, and the infant may experience irritability, poor feeding, or other behavioral changes. When intracranial pressure becomes severely elevated, the infant develops vomiting and lethargy, which can signal impending herniation. In addition to split sutures, the physical examination may reveal a bulging anterior fontanel and engorged scalp veins. Dysfunction of cranial nerve III may result in loss of upward gaze, or the "sundown or setting-sun" sign. Bobble-head doll movements may also occur, especially with aqueductal stenosis or a third ventricle cyst.[1]

Older children with hydrocephalus will usually complain of headache, which is often progressive in nature, worse in the morning, awakens the patient from sleep, and is exacerbated by lying down or straining. The child may suffer visual symptoms that are difficult to specify, but may result in the patient being perceived as unusually clumsy. Gait disturbances can occur, especially ataxia, which is characteristic of children with posterior fossa tumors. As with infants, older children develop vomiting as intracranial pressure begins to become severely elevated. Papilledema is a late finding in children and is rarely found in infants, but it implies a severe increase in intracranial pressure.

► MANAGEMENT

In the emergency department, the primary goal of management of the child with hydrocephalus is the assessment and control of elevated intracranial pressure. Patients may be quite stable or in imminent danger of herniation. Cushing's triad of hypertension, bradycardia, and abnormal respiratory patterns is a late sign of elevated intracranial pressure. Specific signs of herniation depend on the part of the brain involved. In uncal herniation, there is compression of the third cranial nerve with dilation of the ipsilateral pupil and contralateral hemiparesis. Herniation of the cerebellar tonsils through the foramen magnum is preceded by headache and stiff neck and characterized by fixed, dilated pupils. The loss of leg function on one side suggests herniation under the falx. Central herniation occurs when both cerebral hemispheres compress the midbrain and results in decreased level of consciousness, constricted pupils, and Cheyne–Stokes respirations.

It is imperative to begin treatment in the unstable patient before herniation occurs. Patients who are lethargic on presentation, those with a Glasgow Coma Scale <8, or those who deteriorate in the emergency department are intubated following rapid sequence induction procedures. Prior to intubation, ventilation with a bag-valve-mask device to attain a Pco_2 of 35 torr may provide sufficient cerebral vasoconstriction to re-

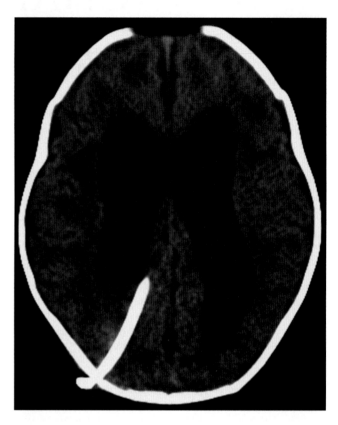

Figure 57–2. Hydrocephalus after ventriculoperitoneal shunt placement.

duce intracranial pressure enough to avert herniation. If there are signs of herniation such as unequal pupils, fixed and dilated pupils, or posturing, mild hyperventilation can be helpful on a short-term basis.[3,4] Ventilation is continued after intubation, keeping oxygenation and blood pressure within normal values. Patients who do not respond with an improved mental status to intubation and ventilation may benefit from diuretic therapy with mannitol (0.25–1 g/kg) or furosemide (1 mg/kg). It is appropriate to elevate the head of the bed 15 to 30 degrees.[4]

After the patient is stabilized, a computed tomography scan or magnetic resonance image of the brain is performed to define the lesion and plan definitive treatment. For those children with hydrocephalus because of an obstruction in CSF flow, management includes insertion of a catheter from the ventricle to a distal site by a neurosurgeon. The most common site is the peritoneal cavity (VP), although the right atrium (VA) and pleura are also used (VP) (Figs. 57–1 and 57–2). If the cause of the increased intracranial pressure is due to trauma resulting in bleeding or cerebral edema, therapy usually includes placement of an intracranial pressure monitoring device by a neurosurgeon. In dire circumstances, a percutaneous ventricular tap may be performed.

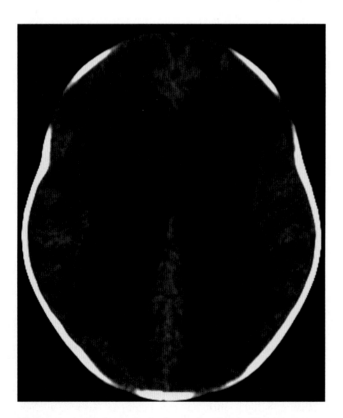

Figure 57–1. Hydrocephalus because of aqueductal stenosis.

REFERENCES

1. Gleeson JG, Dobyns WB, Plawner L, Ashwal S. Congenital structural defects. In: Swaiman KF, Ashwal S, Ferriero DM, eds.

Pediatric Neurology: Principles and Practice. 4th ed. Philadelphia, PA: Mosby/Elsevier; 2006:425–433.

2. Fishman M. Hydrocephalus. In: Rose BD, ed. *UpToDate.* Waltham, MA: UpToDate; 2006.

3. 2005 American Heart Association Guidelines for cardiopulmonary resucitation and emergency cardiovascular care. Part 12: pediatric advanced life support. *Circulation.* 2005;112(suppl 4):IV181.

4. Tepas JJ, Fallat ME, Moriarty, TM. Trauma. In: Gausche-Hill M, Fuchs S, Yamamoto L, eds. *APLS The Pediatric Emergency Medicine Resource.* 4th ed. Sudbury, MA: Jones and Bartlett Publishers; 2004:295–298.

CHAPTER 58

Cerebral Palsy

Susan Fuchs

▶ HIGH-YIELD FACTS

- Cerebral palsy (CP) is a common condition associated with "special needs" children who require care in emergency departments.
- The major abnormality in all forms of CP is abnormal muscle tone.
- Breakthrough seizures are common.
- Respiratory problems, often resulting from chronic aspiration, commonly result in emergency department visits in CP victims.
- Severely impaired patients may require a multidisciplinary approach in the emergency department.

Cerebral palsy (CP) is a nonprogressive motor disorder reported to occur in 1.2 to 2.5 per 1000 children. It is usually evident within the first 3 to 4 years of life.[1] The injury that results in CP can occur during the antepartum, peripartum, or postnatal period. Prematurity remains the most important risk factor, but there is also a higher risk of CP with multiple births, even those not born prematurely.[1] The Task Force on Neonatal Encephalopathy has developed four essential criteria for asphyxial CP. Evidence of metabolic acidosis (umbilical artery pH < 7 and base deficit ≥ 12 mmol/L at delivery), early onset of severe or moderate neonatal encephalopathy in infants older than 34 weeks gestation, CP of the spastic quadriplegia or dyskinetic type, and exclusion of other identifiable etiologies.[2] They have also developed a list of peripartum events that may be related to the development of CP, but are not specifically asphyxial in nature: a sentinel hypoxic event occurring immediately before or after delivery, a sudden and sustained fetal bradycardia or absence of fetal heart rate variability, Apgar score of 0 to 5 at 5 minutes, onset of multisystem involvement within 72 hours, early imaging studies showing evidence of an acute nonfocal cerebral abnormality.[2] Other etiologies include congenital abnormalities, brain malformations, stroke in the perinatal period, intracranial hemorrhage, intrauterine infection, premature birth, genetic abnormalities, metabolic abnormalities, and kernicterus.[1,3]

Although the disorder is not in itself an emergency department diagnosis, children with CP have associated problems that often result in emergency department visits. The emergency department physician must realize that each child with CP has different abilities and problems and that each family has different parent–child relationships and coping mechanisms.

▶ CLINICAL PRESENTATION

There are several forms of CP, with the classification systems based on the extremities involved, tone, and the ability to perform normal activity. The major disorder is of muscle tone, but there can also be neurologic disorders such as seizures, vision disturbances, and impaired intelligence.

Spastic CP includes several variants: spastic quadriplegia, spastic diplegia, and spastic hemiplegia. Spastic CP is the most common variant, with 70% to 80% of children with CP in one of these groups.

Spastic quadriplegia is characterized by a generalized increase in muscle tone, deep tendon reflexes, and rigidity of the limbs on both flexion and extension. Although the lower extremities are generally more severely affected, in severe forms the child is stiff and assumes a posture of decerebrate rigidity. Many children have pseudobulbar involvement, resulting in swallowing difficulties and recurrent aspiration. Intellectual impairment is severe, and half have a tonic–clonic seizure disorder.[1,4]

Spastic diplegia is characterized by bilateral spasticity, with greater involvement of the lower extremities than the upper. It is the most common form of CP diagnosed in preterm infants. Early in life, when rigidity predominates, the legs are held in extension and in a scissored pattern because of adductor spasm. As spasticity progresses, flexion of the hips and knees develops, ultimately leading to contractures.[1] In those less severely affected, dorsiflexion of the feet with increased ankle tone results in toe-walking. Other manifestations include convergent strabismus, delayed speech development, and seizure disorders. Intellectual impairment parallels the motor deficit.

Spastic hemiplegia (hemiparesis) is a unilateral paresis that usually affects the upper extremity more than the lower. Some degree of spasticity and flexion contracture usually results. One of the initial symptoms is fisting, which is an exaggerated palmar grasp reflex. The gait may be circumductive, with swinging of the affected leg like an arc. The extent of functional impairment varies, with fine movements of the hand affected most. Sensory impairment, growth disturbance, and involuntary movements of the affected limbs can occur. In addition, facial weakness, visual disturbances, and seizures can occur.[1]

Another classification of CP is extrapyramidal or dyskinetic, which accounts for 10% to 15% of cases. Dyskinesia is difficulty performing voluntary movements. The variants are based on the types of movement and defects in posture more than the tone, with all four extremities involved to varying degrees. Athetoid CP involves slow, continuous writhing motions and usually involves the distal limbs. Ballismus is characterized by violent, jerky motions of the arms and legs. Choreic CP movements, which are rapid and irregular muscle contractions, result from disorganized tone and can involve the limbs, face, or trunk. Those with tremulous CP have involuntary, rhythmic contractions of opposing muscles. Dystonic CP results in repetitive twisting movements of the limbs and trunk, although the head and neck can also be involved.[1,4]

The remaining forms of CP are less common and include rigid (5%), atonic (hypotonic), and ataxic (1%). Ataxic CP presents with a wide-based gait and truncal ataxia. There are many children (10%–15%) who have a mixed form of CP, with two or more types of the above-mentioned forms. This group can be difficult to diagnose, as the expression of CP may change during their early years.

▶ COMPLICATIONS

Many complications can occur in the patient with CP, with the type depending on the degree of the patient's impairment. The most common problem in CP patients presenting to the emergency department is breakthrough seizures. The management of seizures is discussed in Chapter 38.

Respiratory difficulties also commonly present to the emergency department. Chronic aspiration can result in reactive airway disease and, for some patients, chronic hypoxia and hypercarbia. Acute pneumonia is common after aspiration and is often difficult to diagnose in patients whose baseline chest radiographs are abnormal. Poor coughing mechanisms contribute to pulmonary pathology. In CP patients with evidence of pneumonia, aggressive antibiotic therapy is indicated. Admission to the hospital may be necessary if the child is unable to take oral antibiotics or needs chest physiotherapy or supplemental oxygen. In many cases, functional lung impairment mandates a low threshold for hospital admission. The management of patients with bronchospasm includes aggressive therapy with bronchodilators.

Many children with CP have significant feeding difficulties that require placement of a gastrostomy tube or button, with or without a fundoplication, (often used when aspiration is a risk).[5] In some patients, a gastrojejunal feeding tube is inserted. Malfunction of either tube can result in vomiting, especially for patients without a fundoplication. Feeding tube malfunction can also result in the inability to deliver feedings and medications, which predisposes to dehydration and subtherapeutic levels of anticonvulsants. When the tube needs to be replaced, correct positioning can be confirmed by an abdominal radiograph, accompanied by the injection of radiopaque contrast.

Many patients with CP who are significantly impaired are not toilet trained and are vulnerable to urinary tract infections and perineal skin breakdown that can result in infection. In addition to a chest radiograph to rule out pneumonia, all febrile CP patients require a urinalysis and urine culture.

Although there is no cure for CP, an important goal of emergency department management is ensuring that the child is receiving adequate overall therapy through a multidisciplinary approach and that the family is comfortable with the child's management.

REFERENCES

1. Swaiman KF, Wu Y. Cerebral palsy. In: Swaiman KF, Ashwal S, Ferriero DM, eds. *Pediatric Neurology: Principles & Practice.* 4th ed. Philadelphia, PA: Mosby/Elsevier; 2006:491–504.
2. American College of Obstetrics and Gynecologists; and American Academy of Pediatrics. Neonatal encephalopathy and cerebral palsy: executive summary. *Obstet Gynecol.* 2004;103:780–781.
3. Miller G. Epidemiology and etiology of cerebral palsy. In: Rose BD, ed. *UpToDate.* Waltham, MA: UpToDate; 2007.
4. Miller G. Clinical features and diagnosis of cerebral palsy. In: Rose BD, ed. *UpToDate.* Waltham, MA: UpToDate; 2007.
5. Miller G. Management and prognosis of cerebral palsy. In: Rose BD, ed. *UpToDate.* Waltham, MA: UpToDate; 2007.

CHAPTER 59

Cerebrovascular Syndromes

Susan Fuchs

► HIGH-YIELD FACTS

- In U.S. children, hemorrhagic strokes are more common than ischemic strokes, with a hemorrhagic incidence of 7.8/100 000 per year versus 2.9/100 000 per year for ischemic strokes.
- Ischemic strokes are caused by vascular occlusion of an artery, usually because of thromboembolism (arterial ischemic stroke) or occlusion of venous sinuses or cerebral veins (sinovenous thrombosis).
- A history of complex congenital heart disease, prosthetic heart valve, recent cardiac surgery, or ECMO should raise suspicion of an embolic phenomenon. Twenty-five percent of patients with sickle cell disease will develop cerebrovascular problems.
- Magnetic resonance imaging (MRI) is more sensitive in detecting small infarcts, infarcts of the brain stem and cerebellum, and hemorrhagic conversion of infarcts than a CT scan.
- A computed tomography (CT) scan will show a tumor and abscess, and may show loss of gray/white differentiation and dense triangle sign (hyperdense thrombus in posterior part of superior sagittal sinus), but may not detect an acute hemorrhage.
- Magnetic resonance angiography can be done at the time of the MRI to visualize the flow through the cerebral arteries. MRI can also be used with magnetic resonance venography (MRV) to diagnose sinovenous thrombosis.
- For patients in whom a hemorrhagic stroke is suspected and in whom the CT scan is negative, a lumbar puncture is indicated. Particularly with a small subarachnoid hemorrhage, the CT scan may not reveal blood.
- The key function of the emergency department is stabilization of the patient's respiratory and cardiovascular status, especially the blood pressure. In the event of an ischemic infarct, a precipitous decline in blood pressure is avoided, since it can worsen cerebral ischemia, but if hypotension is present, careful fluid resuscitation and inotropic support may be needed.
- Serum glucose should be monitored closely as hypoglycemia can worsen the effect of the stroke, and hyperglycemia can increase infarct size.
- Specific therapy is directed at the etiology of the stroke, such as correction of clotting abnormalities, antibiotics for infections, antiepileptic medication for seizures, and surgery for evacuation of a hematoma. For patients with sickle cell disease, exchange transfusion is indicated for ischemic stroke.

Although they are uncommon in children when compared to adults, both ischemic and hemorrhagic strokes occur. In U.S. children, hemorrhagic strokes are more common than ischemic strokes, with an incidence of 7.8/100 000 per year for hemorrhagic events versus 2.9/100 000 per year for ischemic events.[1] Ischemic strokes can be categorized as arterial ischemic strokes (AIS) and cerebral sinovenous thrombosis (CSVT). In the pediatric population, arterial ischemic stroke usually results from a thromboembolism. Occlusion of venous sinuses or cerebral veins can result in cerebral sinovenous thrombosis. The peak age of AIS is neonatal and childhood[2], whereas the peak age of CSVT is neonatal and adolescence.[3] This chapter will focus on the older age group.

The signs of AIS vary with age and the area of the brain affected by ischemia; they include focal neurologic findings such as hemiparesis, cranial nerve palsies, visual field deficits, and aphasia. Seizures may or may not occur.[1,2] Cerebral sinovenous thrombosis (CSVT) may present with diffuse neurologic signs and seizures, but symptoms vary with age and etiology. Infants present with seizures, jitteriness, or lethargy, while older children have headaches, vomiting, possible seizures, fever, and focal neurologic deficits.[1,4] Strokes that can result from vascular rupture are classified as hemorrhagic. The two main types are intracerberal and subarachnoid hemorrhage. Signs of hemorrhagic stroke include severe headache, decreased level of consciousness, focal neurologic signs, and seizures.[1]

The arterial circulation to the brain is via the anterior carotids and the posterior vertebral and basilar arteries, which link via communicating arteries to form the circle of Willis. Cerebral arteries can thrombose due to damage to the arterial wall, emboli, or prothrombotic conditions. Infarction occurs when loss of blood supply to cerebral tissue results in ischemia, hypoxia, and depletion of energy and carbohydrate stores. The extent of neuronal damage depends on the severity and length of time of ischemia, the availability of collateral circulation, and the metabolic needs of the brain.[1]

In children, risk factors associated with AIS include cardiac disease, coagulation and hematologic disorders, infection, vasculitis, cancer, metabolic disorders, moyamoya, sickle cell anemia, and perinatal complications. In some cases, no risk factor is defined, whereas in others there may actually be multiple risk factors. This is in stark contrast to adults, in whom arteriosclerosis is the leading risk factor for AIS, along with hypertension, smoking, diabetes, and hypercholesterolemia.[1,2,5]

Sinovenous thrombosis can occur due to thrombophlebitis, hemoconcentration, or coagulation abnormalities. Occlusion of the sinuses or other cerebral vessels results in increased venous pressure and blood–brain barrier disruption,

▶ **TABLE 59-1. PREDISPOSING CONDITIONS FOR ISCHEMIC STROKE**

Cardiac
  Congenital heart disease (s/p Fontan, ECMO)
  Rheumatic heart disease
  Bacterial endocarditis
  Arrhythmias
  Cardiomyopathy
  Prosthetic heart valves
  Ventriculoseptal defect/atrial septal defect
  Patent foramen ovale

Infection
  Meningitis
  Encephalitis

Vasculopathy
  Moyamoya disease
  Postvaricella angiopathy
  Postradiation vasculopathy
  Transient cerebral arteriopathy

Systemic disorders
  Systemic lupus erythematosus
  Polyarteritis nodosa
  Nephrotic syndrome
  Inflammatory bowel disease
  Takayasu's arteritis
  Dermatomyositis
  Rheumatoid arthritis
  Diabetes mellitus

Hematologic disorders
  Sickle cell disease
  Leukemia
  Iron deficiency anemia
  Polycythemia
  Thrombocytosis
  Thrombotic thrombocytopenic purpura
  Idiopathic thrombocytopenic purpura

Acquired prothrombotic states
  Lupus anticoagulant
  Anticardiolipin antibodies
  Protein S deficiency
  Protein C deficiency

Antithrombin III deficiency
Plasminogen deficiency
Pregnancy

Congenital prothrombotic disorders
  Factor V Leiden gene defect
  Prothrombin gene G20 210A mutation
  Methyltetrahydrofolate reductase
  Antithrombin III deficiency

Trauma
  Head injury
  Neck injury
  Intraoral trauma
  Child abuse

Drugs
  Cocaine
  Oral contraceptives
  Antineoplastic agents (e.g., L-asparaginase)
  Steroids
  LSD
  Amphetamines

Metabolic disorders
  Hyperhomocystinuria
  Mitochondrial encephalomyopathy (MELAS)
  Hyperlipidemia
  Cerebral autosomal dominant arteriopathy with subcortical
    infarct and leukoencephalopathy (CADASIL)

Neurocutaneous syndromes
  Neurofibromatosis
  Sturge–Weber syndrome
  Tuberous sclerosis

Hereditary disorders
  Ehlers–Danlos syndrome
  Fabry's disease

Vasospastic disorders
  Migraine

With permission from DeVeber Ga. Cerebrovascular disease. In: Swaiman KF, Ashwal S, Ferriero DM, eds. *Pediatric Neurology: Principles and Practice.* 4th ed. Philadelphia, PA: Mosby/Elsevier; 2006:1759–1801.
With permission from Bernard TJ, Goldenberg NA. Pediatric arterial ischemic stroke. *Pediatr Clin North Am.* 2008;55:323–338.
With permission from Smith SE. Ischemic stroke in children and young adults: etiology and clinical features. In: Rose BD, ed. *UpToDate.* Waltham, MA: UpToDate; 2008.

which leads to vasogenic edema. As pressure continues to increase, cerebral edema and decreased cerebral perfusion result. In some cases, the vessels leak and the infarcts become hemorrhagic. In addition, there is a risk of developing communicating hydrocephalus after sinovenous thrombosis of the sagittal sinus or with sinus hypertension, because the arachnoid granulations, which absorb CSF, become nonfunctional.[1]

Risk factors associated with CSVT are prothrombotic disorders, dehydration, systemic infection, otitis media, mastoiditis, sinusitis, hematologic disorders, drugs, cardiac disease, cancer, and perinatal complications.[1,3,4] The underlying diseases that cause AIS and CSVT are listed in Tables 59–1 and 59–2, respectively.

Hemorrhagic strokes involve the rupture of cerebral blood vessels with leakage of blood into the brain parenchyma, subarachnoid space, or ventricular system. The location of the hemorrhage defines the two major types of stroke as intracerebral/intraparenchymal or subarachnoid, and determines the pathophysiology, risk factors, and clinical findings.[1]

Intracerebral hemorrhage occurs when arteries or veins rupture into intracerebral areas or brain parenchyma. Damage occurs to the blood–brain barrier, resulting in cerebral edema;

▶ TABLE 59-2. **RISK FACTORS FOR CSVT**

Septic
  Otitis media
  Mastoiditis
  Sinusitis
Indwelling central lines
Prothrombotic
  Protein S deficiency
  Protein C deficiency
  Antiphospholipid antibodies
  Antithrombin III deficiency
  Factor V Leiden gene defect
  Prothrombin G20 210A mutation
  Hyperhomocysteinemia
Dehydration
Systemic infection
  Systemic lupus erythematosus
  Nephrotic syndrome
Hematologic disorders
  Polycythemia
Malignancy
  L-asparaginase treatment
Cardiac disease
Oral contraceptives
Head injury
Pregnancy

With permission from DeVeber Ga. Cerebrovascular disease. In: Swaiman KF, Ashwal S, Ferriero DM, eds. *Pediatric Neurology: Principles and Practice*. 4th ed. Philadelphia, PA: Mosby/Elsevier; 2006:1759–1801.
With permission from Ferro JM, Canhao P. Etiology, clinical features, and diagnosis of cerebral venous thrombosis. In: Rose BD, ed. *UpToDate*. Waltham, MA: UpToDate; 2008.
With permission from Goldenberg NA, Bernard TJ. Venous thromboembolism in children. *Pediatr Clin North Am*. 2008;55:305–322.

▶ TABLE 59-3. **CONDITIONS PREDISPOSING TO HEMORRHAGIC STROKE**

Vascular malformations
  Aneurysms
  Arteriovenous malformations
  Cavernous malformation

Coagulation defects
  Hemophilia
  Disseminated intravascular coagulation
  Idiopathic thrombocytopenia purpura
  Vitamin K deficiency
  Anticoagulation treatment
  Leukemia
  Aplastic anemia
  Factor deficiencies

Systemic disorders
  Hypertension
  Sickle cell disease

Drug
  Amphetamines
  Phenylpropanolamine
  Cocaine

Head trauma
  Child abuse

Brain tumors

Infection
  Herpes simplex
  Varicella

Congenital syndromes
  Ehlers–Danlos Syndrome
  Neurofibromatosis
  Tuberous sclerosis

With permission from DeVeber Ga. Cerebrovascular disease. In: Swaiman KF, Ashwal S, Ferriero DM, eds. *Pediatric Neurology: Principles and Practice*. 4th ed. Philadelphia, PA: Mosby/Elsevier; 2006:1759–1801.

when large, the hematoma can cause a mass effect. In children the greatest risk factor is head trauma, followed by aneurysms and vascular malformations.

Subarachnoid hemorrhage results from rupture of an aneurysm (usually proximal arteries at the circle of Willis) or an arteriovenous malformation (AVM). Secondary effects include ischemic infarction due to blood in the subarachnoid space that causes vasospasm of the cerebral arteries and hydrocephalus. Risk factors include disorders associated with vascular malformations, aneurysms, sickle cell disease, and hypertension. However, hemorrhagic strokes are occasionally associated with systemic diseases and coagulopathies.[1] These conditions are summarized in Table 59–3.

▶ DIAGNOSIS

HISTORY

The presenting signs and symptoms of a stroke depend somewhat on the type of stroke and the age of the patient. Arterial ischemic strokes usually have a rapid onset, so there may be little in the history to warn of the impending event. Patients often suffer sudden seizures, or focal neurologic findings, especially hemiplegia. A history of recurrent headaches, transient ischemic attacks, or focal seizures may be obtained, but these do not provide a specific diagnosis, and often confuse the issue.[1] An AIS involving a large vessel may present with loss of consciousness and multiple focal neurologic deficits.[2] A stroke due to a metabolic disorder may have a progressive course. A prenatal AIS often does not present until age 4 to 8 months as an evolving hemiparesis.[2]

An older child with a CSVT may present with slowly progressive signs, such as fever, vomiting, or headache. A young infant may have dilated scalp veins, eyelid swelling, and a large anterior fontanelle.[1]

An older child with a hemorrhagic stroke may have a history of severe headache or, especially in the case of subarachnoid hemorrhage, neck pain. A large bleed will usually result in a sudden alteration in consciousness and perhaps seizures, but a small bleed may result in subtle focal neurologic signs, including cranial nerve palsies.[1]

A history of cardiac disorders, especially complex congenital heart disease, prosthetic heart valve, or recent cardiac surgery should raise suspicion of an embolic phenomenon. The presence of fever and headache should raise concern about meningitis. However, systemic infections, such as mycoplasma, Rocky Mountain spotted fever, and others, have been associated with cerebral infarction due to thrombophlebitis of cerebral vessels.[1] A recent infection with varicella is of concern, because postvaricella angiopathy can include basal ganglia infarction and stenosis of large arteries. Inherited coagulation disorders such as deficiency of protein C, protein S, antithrombin III, and plasminogen, or the presence of factor V Leiden, anticardiolipin antibody, or lupus anticoagulant can all lead to thromboembolism.[1,3,4]

A history of sickle cell disease is extremely important to elicit, because 25% of patients will develop cerebrovascular problems.[1] The presence of systemic lupus erythematosus and other forms of vasculitis such as polyarteritis nodosa, mixed connective tissue disease, or Takayasu's arteritis have all been associated with arterial ischemic and sinovenous thrombosis.

Metabolic disorders, such as homozygous homocystinuria (hyperhomocysteinemia), which have a thrombotic effect, can cause arterial and venous thrombosis. Fabry's disease (deficiency of α-galactosidase A) can lead to lacunar infarcts, and hyperlipidemia has also been associated with childhood strokes. The MELAS syndrome (mitochondrial myopathy, encephalopathy, lactic acidosis, and stroke-like episodes) is characterized by episodes of nausea, vomiting, headaches, seizures, and hemiparesis, which initially resolve, but ultimately lead to persistent deficits and cortical blindness.[1,2] Neurocutaneous disorders such as neurofibromatosis, Sturge–Weber syndrome, and tuberous sclerosis are all associated with both ischemic and hemorrhagic strokes.

Any history of trauma is significant and suggests a hemorrhagic lesion. Intraoral trauma can cause dissection of the carotid artery, and injury to the vertebral arteries can occur after neck trauma.

Children who have had radiation for optic gliomas or pituitary or suprasellar tumors can develop postradiation vasculitis.

Adolescents in particular are questioned regarding illicit drug ingestion, particularly cocaine. Additional questions are directed toward detecting one of the underlying etiologies noted in Tables 59–1, 59–2, and 59–3.

PHYSICAL EXAMINATION

Stabilization of the patient is the first priority, since seizures may occur in younger children at the time of or shortly after the stroke. Complete vital signs include temperature and blood pressure. If trauma is suspected, the head and neck are immobilized. A thorough examination includes auscultation over the head, eyes, and carotid arteries listening for bruits, as well as a careful auscultation of the heart for murmurs, clicks suggestive of valvular disease, arrhythmias, or indications of prior cardiac surgery. The eyes are examined for extraocular movements, pupillary responses, and the visual fields. The eyes will look toward the lesion if the cerebral hemisphere is involved, but away with brain stem involvement. The skin is examined for petechiae, café au lait spots, neurofibromas, or telangiectasias.

Neurologic assessment includes determination of degree of weakness, cranial nerve dysfunction, and the side and extent

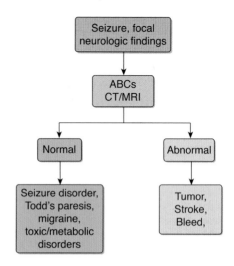

Figure 59–1. Differential diagnosis for stroke.

to which the extremities are involved. If the facial muscles and tongue are involved, there is dysarthria, but involvement of the basal ganglia, thalamus, or cerebral hemispheres can result in aphasia. It may be difficult to assess sensory impairment due to aphasia.

Some disorders that can be confused with a stroke include complicated migraines, partial seizures, Todd's paralysis, brain tumors, brain abscesses, and subdural hematoma. Most will be diagnosed during the workup of the suspected stroke (Fig. 59–1).

DIAGNOSTIC EVALUATION

Baseline laboratory studies include a complete blood count with differential and platelet count and coagulation studies. If sickle cell disease is a possibility, a sickle cell preparation and hemoglobin electrophoresis are performed. Further coagulation studies are indicated if hemophilia or other coagulopathies, such as protein S or C or antithrombin III deficiencies, are suspected. Other studies should include electrolytes, BUN, creatinine, glucose, sedimentation rate, and CRP, as well as a urinalysis looking for red cells or protein, and a urine pregnancy test in females.[1,2,5] Studies evaluating a hypercoagulable/prothrombotic state include antinuclear antibodies, protein S, protein C, factor V Leiden mutation, prothrombin 20210A, antithrombin III activity, homocysteine concentration, and anticardiolipin levels.[1–4,6] If a fever is present, blood culture, urine culture, and CSF studies are indicated. Blood and CSF viral titers of varicella zoster, herpes zoster, EBV enterovirus, and parvovirus may be helpful.[2] If a metabolic disorder is suspected, blood lactate, pyruvate, carnitine, and serum amino acids are ordered, and urine is sent for organic acids.[2] An electrocardiogram and an echocardiogram should be performed on all children in whom underlying heart disease is suspected.[6]

Imaging studies provide information that will help differentiate an ischemic from a hemorrhagic stroke. Magnetic resonance imaging (MRI) is more sensitive than a computed tomography (CT) scan in detecting small infarcts, infarcts of the brain stem and cerebellum, and infarcts that become hemorrhagic.[1,2] A CT scan will show a tumor or abscess, and may show loss of gray/white differentiation and the dense triangle sign

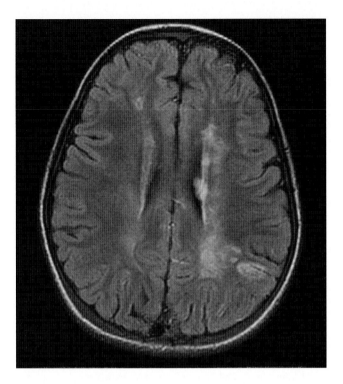

Figure 59-2. MRI—T2 hyperintensity representing recent infarct in left parietal lobe.

(hyperdense thrombus in posterior part of superior sagittal sinus). However, a CT scan may not detect a small acute hemorrhage.[1,2,4] CT scan is also normal in up to 30% of CSVT, so MRI is the preferred study in these cases.[4] Magnetic resonance angiography (MRA) correlates well with angiography, and can be done at the time of the MRI to visualize the flow through the cerebral arteries.[1] MRI can also be used with magnetic resonance venography (MRV) to diagnose CSVT.[3] The visualization of a thrombus and the absence of a flow-related signal provide the diagnosis (Fig. 59–2).

The gold standard to visualize intracranial and extracranial vessels is cerebral angiography. Other modalities that may prove useful include single-photon emission CT (SPECT), Doppler imaging of the carotid arteries, transcranial Doppler, and transcranial ultrasound.[1,7]

For patients in whom a hemorrhagic stroke is suspected, in whom the CT scan is negative, and who have no signs of increased intracranial pressure, a lumbar puncture is indicated. Particularly in a small subarachnoid hemorrhage, the CT scan may not reveal blood. The CSF is evaluated for the presence of red blood cells, which, in the absence of a traumatic lumbar puncture, indicates hemorrhage, especially if the blood does not clear during CSF collection. In some cases, the CSF may appear xanthrochromic, which is also consistent with hemorrhage.[1]

▶ TREATMENT

The key function of the ED is stabilization of the patient's respiratory and cardiovascular status, especially the blood pressure. In the event of an ischemic infarct, a precipitous decline in blood pressure is avoided, since it can worsen cerebral ischemia.[1,2] If hypotension is present, careful fluid resuscitation and inotropic support may be needed. If there are signs of impending herniation, mannitol (0.25 to 1 g/kg intravenously over 20 minutes) and controlled ventilation may be required. Serum glucose should be monitored closely because hypoglycemia can worsen the effect of the stroke, and hyperglycemia can increase the infarct size. Maintenance of normal body temperature is also important, since hyperthermia can worsen ischemic brain damage. The patient should be kept with the bed at 0 to 15 degree of head elevation for AIS.[5] Specific therapy is directed at the etiology of the stroke, such as correction of clotting abnormalities, antibiotics for infections, antiepileptic medication for seizures, and surgery for evacuation of a hematoma. In patients with sickle cell disease, hydration and exchange transfusion to reduce hemoglobin S to <30% is indicated[2,6,7] (see Chapter 2). Depending on the etiology of the stroke in children, there is some use for antithrombotic agents, but dosing and efficacy still need to be determined for some therapies.[1-3] The American College of Chest Physicians (ACCP) recommends treatment of children with non–sickle cell AIS with unfractionated heparin (UFH) or low-molecular-weight heparin (LMWH) for 5 to 7 days, while the Royal College of Physicians recommends initial treatment with aspirin.[2,6]

Treatment of CSVT includes hydration, antibiotics for cases due to infection, control of seizures and elevated intracranial pressure, and treatment with UFH or LMWH initially.[1,3,8] The use of steroids is indicated only if there is proven vasculitis with progression of stenosis, but they are rarely indicated in the ED.

▶ DISPOSITION

Children who have suffered strokes are admitted to an intensive care setting for close monitoring of blood pressure, fluid status, temperature, glucose, neurologic function, and antithrombotic therapy.

▶ OUTCOME/DISABILITY

For children with AIS, a middle cerebral artery territory stroke volume >10% of intracranial volume and initial presentation with altered level of consciousness are predictors of poor outcome.[6] The risk of recurrence ranges from 6% to 40%; the presence of vasculopathy appears to be an important risk factor, since children with evidence of abnormal vessels had a stroke recurrence rate of 66%, while those with normal vascular imaging had no recurrence.[2,6]

For CSVT, outcome depends on etiology, but mortality ranges from 4% to 20%, with a recurrence rate of 17%.[3] For children with sickle cell disease, effective prevention or recurrent stroke includes chronic transfusion therapy, and hydroxyurea.[7]

▶ SPECIFIC CONDITIONS

MOYAMOYA

Moyamoya is characterized by an abnormal network of small collateral vessels, which develop due to idiopathic stenosis and occlusion of large cerebral arteries involving the circle of Willis.

The "puff of smoke" appearance on angiogram is due to the collateral vessels.[1,9] The etiology is unknown, but there is a relatively high incidence in Asian and Japanese populations, with a family history in 10% of patients.[9] In children, the presentation is more often with ischemic events such as TIA or stroke, rather than a hemorrhagic stroke and seizures, which occur more in adults.[9] The prognosis in children is worse in children <3 years of age compared to patients between 3 and 6 years; both age groups have a worse prognosis than adults.[10] Moyamoya syndrome includes the typical angiographic pattern, but is secondary to an etiology such as trisomy 21, sickle cell disease, and cranial radiation.[2,5]

► POSTVARICELLA ANGIOPATHY AND TRANSIENT CEREBRAL ARTERIOPATHY

In children with AIS, varicella-associated angiopathy accounts for one-third of cases.[1] The mechanism is thought to be a transient acute vasculitis. Characteristic findings include basal ganglia infarction and intracranial narrowing of the distal internal carotid or proximal anterior, middle, or posterior cerebral arteries.[1,2]

Transient cerebral angiopathy is characterized by unilateral focal or segmental stenosis of the distal carotid arteries and vessels in the proximal circle of Willis vessels. These lesions may resolve or stabilize within 6 months.[2,5] This results in infarction in the internal capsule or basal ganglia. The average age of onset is 5 years, and etiology is thought to be viral, and when preceded by varicella within 12 months is termed postvaricella angiopathy.[1]

REFERENCES

1. DeVeber GA. Cerebrovascular disease. In: Swaiman KF, Ashwal S, Ferriero DM, eds. *Pediatric Neurology: Principles and Practice.*4th ed. Philadelphia, PA: Mosby/Elsevier; 2006:1759–1801.
2. Bernard TJ, Goldenberg NA. Pediatric arterial ischemic stroke. *Pediatr Clin North Am.* 2008;55:323–338.
3. Goldenberg NA, Bernard TJ. Venous thromboembolism in children. *Pediatr Clin North Am.* 2008;55:305–322.
4. Ferro JM, Canhao P. Etiology, clinical features, and diagnosis of cerebral venous thrombosis. In: Rose BD, ed. *UpToDate.* Waltham, MA: UpToDate; 2008.
5. Smith SE. Ischemic stroke in children and young adults: etiology and clinical features. In: Rose BD, ed. *UpToDate.* Waltham, MA: UpToDate; 2008.
6. Smith SE. Ischemic stroke in children and young adults: evaluation, initial management, and prognosis. In: Rose BD, ed. *UpToDate.* Waltham, MA: UpToDate; 2008.
7. Dreyer Z. Cerebrovascular disease in sickle cell disease. In: Rose BD, ed. *UpToDate.* Waltham, MA: UpToDate; 2008.
8. Sebire G, Tabarki B, Saunders DE, et al. Cerebral venous sinus thrombosis in children: risk factors, presentation, diagnosis, and outcome. *Brain.* 2005;128:477–489.
9. Suwanwela NC. Moyamoya disease. In: Rose BD, ed. *UpToDate.* Waltham, MA: UpToDate; 2007.
10. Kim S-K, Seol HJ, Cho B-K, et al. Moyamoya disease among young patients: its aggressive clinical course and the role of active surgical treatment. *Neurosurgery.* 2004;54:840–846.

SECTION VIII

INFECTIOUS EMERGENCIES

CHAPTER 60

Influenza

Karen C. Hayani and Arthur L. Frank

▶ HIGH-YIELD FACTS

- Influenza is an enveloped single-stranded RNA virus found in animals and humans, which is one of the most important causes of respiratory illness throughout the world.
- Influenza usually causes yearly winter epidemics in temperate climates, but new strains that have the potential to cause infrequent but severe worldwide pandemics can arise.
- Although there are only three main serotypes, new strains of influenza are regularly formed by mutations and genetic reassortment, which change the viral surface antigens, thereby facilitating spread in populations that do not have antibody.
- Influenza is transmitted by inhalation of infected droplets and aerosols (from persons with coughing or sneezing) or by direct contact with contaminated animals or objects.
- The incubation period is 1 to 4 days (average of 2 days).
- Viral shedding of influenza begins 24 hours before the onset of clinical illness and can last for 1 to 2 weeks.
- The most common symptoms in teenagers and adults include fever, cough, headache, sore throat, and malaise. Children may present with atypical symptoms that include lower respiratory tract symptoms. Infants may present with fever and "rule out sepsis" or with apnea.
- In patients with lower respiratory symptoms, it may be difficult to distinguish primary influenza pneumonia from secondary bacterial pneumonia (both clinically and radiographically).
- Routine laboratories, such as CBC, are usually less helpful than culture or PCR of nasopharyngeal secretions for influenza and other respiratory viruses.
- Most influenza infections are self-limited and require only supportive care; however, antiviral medications can be considered for the following:
  ○ Children who are at risk for severe or complicated infection (such as immunocompromised children and children with underlying cardiopulmonary disease)
  ○ Healthy children with severe symptoms
  ○ Children with special environmental circumstances (such as immunocompromised family members)
- If antiviral medications are started, they should be started within the first 24 to 48 hours of symptoms and given for 5 days. They shorten the duration of symptoms, but prevention of serious complications, such as viral or secondary bacterial pneumonia, is less well documented.
- In the clinic or emergency department, droplet precautions as well as standard precautions should be used, with close attention paid to good hand-washing.

- The Web site of the Centers for Disease Control (CDC), www.cdc.gov, is regularly updated, and provides the following:
  ○ Helpful information sheets that are easily downloaded for parents and patients
  ○ Current recommendations for physicians, including immunization and antiviral medication information
- Information regarding local epidemiology and outbreaks can be obtained from local health departments.

Symptomatic influenza infection is commonly called "flu." Flu can affect individuals of any age. The name influenza originated in the 15th century from the Italian word *influenza*, meaning influence. It was thought that the disease was due to adverse astrological influences. It was first used in English in the 1700s.

The virus is a member of the Orthomyxoviridae family, typically spheroid or ovoid in shape, and approximately 80 to 120 nm in diameter (Figs. 60–1 and 60–2). It has multiple segments of single-stranded, negative-sense RNA. Influenza A and B have eight gene segments, while influenza C has seven gene segments. The genome is surrounded by an envelope, made of a lipid bilayer, within which are embedded matrix proteins M1 and M2. The M1 proteins are located on the interior surface of the envelope and provide stablility to the virus, while the M2 proteins serve as ion channels that facilitate uncoating of the virus in the host lysosome. The envelope is studded with glycoproteins, approximately 80% of which are hemagglutinin (HA) and approximately 20% are neuraminidase (NA). HA is the viral molecule that binds to the host sialic acid sugar, enabling attachment of the virus to the host epithelial cell. Once attachment has taken place, the process of endocytosis allows for entry of the virus into the cell. HA is the major stimulus for the host immune response. NA is involved in release of newly formed virions from the host cell and it prevents reduced infectivity from aggregation of virions. The HA and NA glycoproteins determine the strain of the virus. Minor changes in these antigens are called **antigenic drift**, which usually occurs on a yearly basis. A major change in these glycoproteins is called **antigenic shift**, and this can cause worldwide pandemics. Antigenic drift and shift are important in the spread of influenza because new strains are able to evade the host immune system, which may not recognize the virus even after previous exposure to different influenza strains (Table 60–1 and Fig. 60–3).[1]

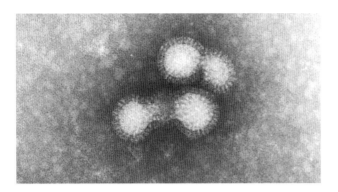

Figure 60–1. Electron microscopic photograph of influenza virus. (With permission from Fauci et al. *Harrison's Principles of Internal Medicine.* 17th ed. McGraw-Hill; 2008.)

► EPIDEMIOLOGY AND TRANSMISSION

Influenza is perhaps the most familiar respiratory infection besides the common cold. The influenza virus is found worldwide, but the origins of many human strains can be traced to Asia. Person-to-person transmission, close contact, air travel, and migratory birds all play a role in the global spread of the virus. Each year in the United States, approximately 25 to 50 million people become symptomatically infected with one of the influenza strains despite massive immunization campaigns. In temperate areas, increased incidence of influenza is seen during winter months not because of cold climate but because of increased crowding indoors and easier transmission from person to person. The virus usually spreads through inhalation of infected droplets or aerosols from a cough or a sneeze but can also spread by direct contact with infected animals or fomites. Once infected, a person usually sheds the virus for 7 days, starting 24 hours prior to the onset of symptoms. Shedding can be prolonged in young children and immunocompromised patients.[2] Since 1977, annual epidemics have often been due to two predominant strains that circulate simultaneously. Over the last several years, influenza A strains with the H1N1 and H3N2 serotypes have been present, with either type being predominant during any 1 year.[3] In addition, both influenza A and B viruses can cocirculate and other viruses, such as RSV or parainfluenza, may circulate simultaneously with influenza during any single season. When there

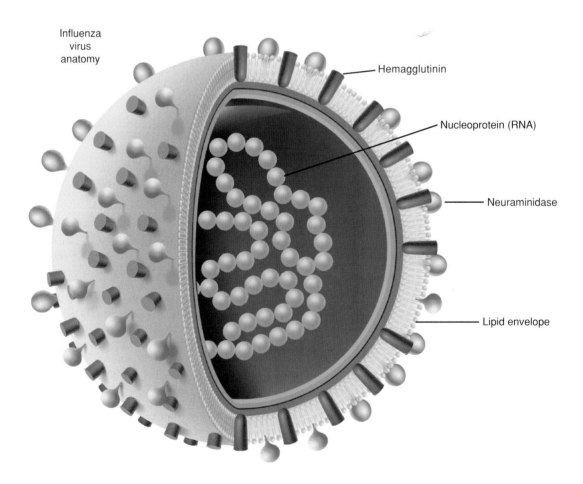

Figure 60–2. Diagram of influenza virus with key features shown. (With permission from Brooks GF, Butel JS, Morse SA. *Jawetz, Melnick, & Adelberg's Medical Microbiology.* 24th ed. McGraw-Hill; 2007.)

▶ TABLE 60-1. **TERMS ASSOCIATED WITH INFLUENZA**

Term	Commentary
Influenza	Orthomyxoviridae family of viruses Single-stranded, enveloped, RNA virus (negative sense) Segmented genome (7 or 8 segments)
Major types	A, B, and C
Serotypes	Determined by hemagglutinin (HA) and neuraminidase (NA) surface glycoproteins

Strains (strain variants)	Identified by World Health Organization (WHO) naming system
	  Major type (A, B, or C)
	  Geographic area of origin
	  Isolate number
	  Year of isolation
	  HA and NA serotype (if influenza A)
	Examples:
	  Influenza A/New Caledonia/20/99 (H1N1)
	  Influenza A /Texas/1/77 (H3N2)
	  Influenza B/Hong Kong/20/2003

Hemagglutinin (HA)	Surface glycoprotein Important for attachment to the sialic acid receptor on the host epithelial cell Neutralizing response of host is mostly determined by ability to recognize HA Influenza A has 16 different HA (designated as H1 to H16)
Neuraminidase (NA)	Surface glycoprotein Cleaves host cell membrane sialic acid, enabling release of virions Prevents viral aggregation, thus promoting infectivity and free release of virions Target of host immune response Influenza A has 9 different NA (designated as N1–N9) NA inhibitors include oseltamivir and zanamivir
Matrix protein 1 (M1)	Protein located on the inner surface on the viral envelope Provides stability to virus
Matrix protein 2 (M2)	Protein located within the envelope of influenza A only Forms an ion channel Facilitates uncoating of the virus M2 inhibitors include amantadine and rimantadine (active against influenza A only)
Antigenic drift	Minor changes in HA and NA Due to random, frequent genetic mutations Occurs in both influenza A and influenza B Leads to seasonal, yearly epidemics Drift is anticipated in yearly vaccine formulation Example: drift within H1N1 or within H3N2
Antigenic shift	Major changes in HA and NA Due to rare genetic events: when an animal strain mutates and is able to infect human hosts, or when a human strain takes on the genes from an animal strain (reassortment) Occurs only in influenza A Leads to large, worldwide pandemics, many years apart Pandemics occur because human populations lack immunity Example: shift from H1N1 to H2N2, and then to H3N2, etc.
Epidemic	Occurs annually Due to antigenic drift Seasonal (November to March in temperate climates) Caused by one or two predominant serotypes
Pandemic	Occurs rarely, only at infrequent intervals (many years) Due to antigenic shift

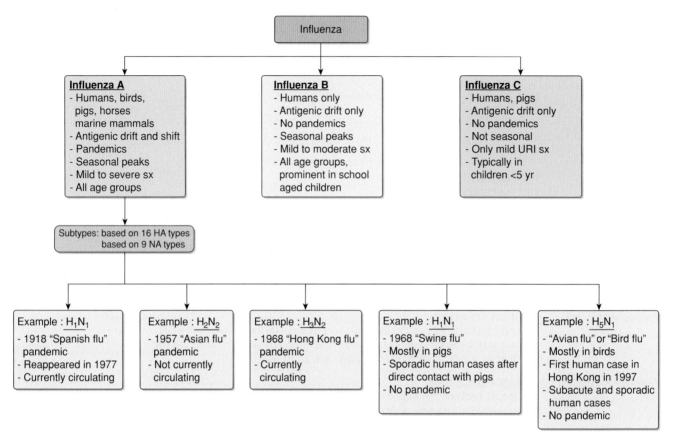

Figure 60–3. Classification of influenza viruses.

► **TABLE 60–2. RESPIRATORY VIRUSES TO CONSIDER IN THE DIFFERENTIAL DIAGNOSIS OF INFLUENZA (WITH ACCOMPANYING CLINICAL TIPS)**

Influenza A—"Common flu" (example: H1N1 or H3N2)
  Wide variety of symptoms with potentially severe systemic disease

Influenza A—"Avian flu" (example: H5N1)
  Usually bird exposure history, but risk of future pandemic with human–human spread

Influenza A—"Swine flu"
  Specific pig exposure history

Influenza B
  School-age children predominant
  Rarely can cause myositis

Influenza C
  Rare and clinically insignificant

Parainfluenza 1, 2, and 3
  Season is different than influenza (spring and fall in temperate climates)
  Nonspecific febrile illness with hospital admission in young infants (para 3)
  Croup (para 1 and 2)

Respiratory syncytial virus (RSV)
  Seasonal overlap with influenza (winter in temperate climates)

Large number of hospital admissions in infants with bronchiolitis
Premature infants may have received preventative monthly monoclonal anti-RSV antibody
Transmission especially by contaminated fomites

Human Metapneumovirus (hMPV)
  Clinically and epidemiologically similar to RSV, but smaller number of cases

Adenovirus
  Wide range of clinical severity (common cold to fatal disseminated infection)
  Acute pneumonia can be the initial clinical presentation

Coronaviruses (Co-V)
  Severe acute respiratory syndrome (SARS-CoV)
    Severe life-threatening disease is likely
    History of travel to an area where SARS is occurring
  Non-SARS Co-V
    Generally mild upper respiratory infections

Bocaviruses
  Recently discovered by molecular testing
  Full clinical spectrum unclear, but likely mild respiratory disease

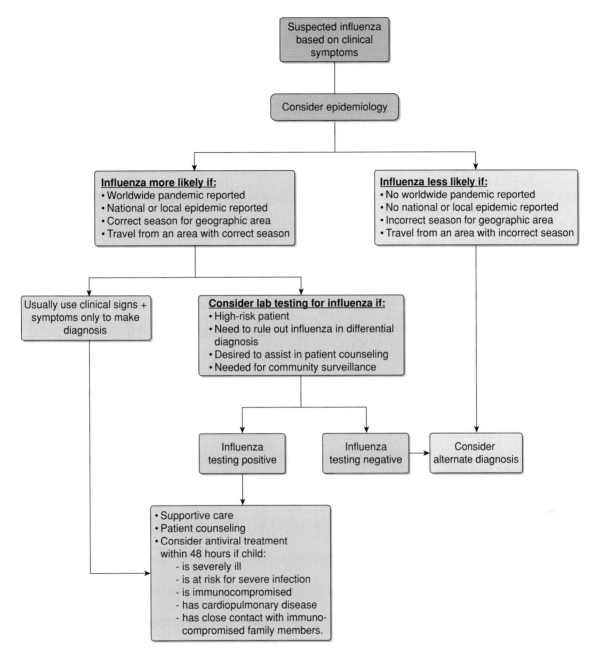

Figure 60–4. Management of suspected influenza in children.

is coinfection with human and animal influenza viruses, the segmented nature of the genome allows for reassortment between the viruses and the emergence of new serotypes with new HA or NA glycoproteins. Since populations lack immunity, worldwide pandemics can result.

▶ PATHOPHYSIOLOGY

When the influenza virus is inhaled, it enters the respiratory epithelium and causes loss of ciliary function, decreased mucus production, and desquamation. This damaged lining of the respiratory tract is a potential portal of entry for secondary bacterial infections. The infection can spread to lower airways by inhalation into the alveoli or by contiguous spread. Systemic

infection can occur causing a variety of clinical complications. The host responds with a humoral IgG as well as a mucosal IgA antibody response to the viral HA and NA antigens. Cytotoxic T lymphocytes also play a role.[4] The host defenses include production of interleukin-6 and interferon-α, which result in many of the systemic clinical symptoms of influenza.[3]

▶ CLINICAL PRESENTATION

The incubation period of influenza is 2 to 4 days and varies with viral strain and host factors, such as age and underlying conditions. Classically, the onset of symptoms is acute and in children and adults usually includes fever, chills, headache, sore throat, dry cough, and myalgias. Otitis media and conjunctivitis can also occur. Any part of the respiratory tract can be affected, and although upper respiratory tract symptoms are most common, croup, bronchitis, and pneumonia can also develop. Pneumonia can be either due to the virus itself or due to a secondary bacterial infection and the two are difficult to distinguish. The development of thick productive cough and lobar consolidation on chest radiograph are suggestive of the latter. In older children, acute calf pain and refusal to walk may indicate myositis, which is seen more often following influenza B than influenza A. Young children may present with fever alone ("rule out sepsis") or may have GI symptoms such as vomiting, abdominal pain, and diarrhea. Infants may present with apnea. Rarely, influenza can cause myocarditis, seizures, encephalopathy, encephalitis, transverse myelitis, or Guillain–Barré syndrome. In Japan, a severe, acute necrotizing encephalopathy due to influenza has been reported in young children. It is associated with rapid progression to seizures and coma.[5] Reye syndrome can develop when aspirin is used during influenza infection and the incidence of this syndrome has decreased greatly with the widespread use of acetaminophen or ibuprofen for fever in children. Deaths usually occur due to complications, including secondary bacterial infections. In December 2006 and January 2007, for example, the CDC reported an increased number of deaths in children coinfected with influenza and community acquired–methicillin-resistant *Staphylococcus aureus* (CA-MRSA) pneumonia and an advisory was issued alerting health care professionals to this trend.[6]

▶ DIFFERENTIAL DIAGNOSIS AND CLINICAL MANAGEMENT

The clinical presentation of influenza overlaps with other respiratory viruses, especially RSV and human metapneumovirus, which often circulate in the community during the same season. Table 60–2 outlines some features of various respiratory viruses that are a part of the differential diagnosis of influenza. Figure 60–4 summarizes an approach to the management of infants and children who may present to the clinic or emergency department with influenza.

▶ LABORATORY AND RADIOGRAPHIC FINDINGS

During winter months in temperate climates, many children seen in the clinic or emergency department are diagnosed with "viral syndrome" depending on history and physical examination. In many cases, symptoms are mild, supportive care alone is appropriate, and no diagnostic testing is necessary. Making a specific diagnosis with respect to influenza or other respiratory viruses may be helpful and appropriate, however, when patients are infants, have underlying diseases, or have severe symptoms. Specific identification may also be helpful in determining the epidemiology of influenza and other viruses in a community during a certain season. Table 60–3 outlines the features of the laboratory tests most commonly available. In general, rapid tests, such as PCR, done on nasopharyngeal specimens are the most sensitive and specific and identify the major type but not the strain of influenza. They are often part

▶ **TABLE 60–3. LABORATORY TESTING IN INFLUENZA VIRUS INFECTION**

Polymerase chain reaction (PCR) testing for influenza A and B:
  Done on nasopharyngeal specimens
  Often part of a PCR panel that may include parainfluenza, respiratory syncycial virus (RSV), and human metapneumovirus (hMPV)
  High sensitivity and specificity
  Rapid results

Direct fluorescent antigen (DFA) and indirect fluorescent: antigen (IFA) testing
  Done on nasopharyngeal specimens
  Rapid results

Viral culture:
  Done on nasopharyngeal specimens
  Viral isolation within 2–6 d

Complete blood count (CBC) with differential:
  Usually not helpful, nonspecific
  If done for other reasons, it may show mild WBC elevation with predominance of lymphocytes

Serology
  Usually not helpful in acute infection:
  Can be helpful in making the diagnosis retrospectively, but only if acute and convalescent sera (obtained 1–2 wk apart) are available

of an extended panel and results are obtained more quickly than by viral culture. Routine laboratory tests, such as CBC, are often not needed, but may be helpful in patients with lower respiratory tract symptoms. WBC counts of <5000/mm^3 are often seen with influenza and other viruses and elevated WBC counts with predominantly polymorphonuclear cells suggest secondary bacterial infection. Serology is not useful acutely, but may be helpful if a diagnosis needs to be made in retrospect. Chest radiographs are not routinely indicated, but if done due to suspected lower respiratory tract disease may help distinguish viral from secondary bacterial pneumonia.

▶ TREATMENT

Most influenza infections require only supportive therapy. This includes fluids, rest, and ibuprofen or acetaminophen for fever. Aspirin (salicylates) should never be given to children with respiratory viral infections, because of the risk of Reye syndrome. If children are already taking aspirin (for Kawasaki disease, e.g.), it should be stopped immediately. Over-the-counter decongestants are not recommended, especially in children younger than 2 years because these might be harmful. Several antiviral medications are approved for use in children (Table 60–4).[7,8] These antiviral medications should not be given routinely, but can be considered in children who are at risk for severe or complicated infection, for example, immunocompromised children or children with underlying cardiopulmonary disease, healthy children with severe symptoms, or children with special environmental circumstances (for example,

▶ TABLE 60–4. ANTIVIRAL MEDICATIONS USED FOR INFLUENZA PROPHYLAXIS AND TREATMENT*

Generic Name	Brand Name (in the United States)	Class of Drug	Active Against Influenza Types	Route of Administration	Approved for Treatment	Approved for Prophylaxis	Side Effects or Precautions
Amantidine	Symmetrel	Adamantane (inhibits M2 protein)	A only	Oral	≥1 y of age but not currently recommended in the United States due to resistance	≥1 y of age but not currently recommended in the United States due to resistance	Hypotension, edema Dizziness, headache Confusion Livedeo reticularis Nausea, vomiting Urinary retention
Rimantidine	Flumadine	Adamantane (inhibits M2 protein)	A only	Oral	≥13 y of age but not currently recommended in the United States due to resistance	≥1 y of age but not currently recommended in the United States due to resistance	Hypotension Dizziness, headache Confusion CNS effects less than with amantidine Nausea, vomiting Urinary retention
Oseltamivir	Tamiflu	Neuraminidase (NA) inhibitor	A and B	Oral	≥1 y of age	≥1 y of age	Unstable angina Arrhythmia Dizziness, headache Rash Worsening of diabetes Nausea, vomiting Anemia Hepatitis Conjunctivitis Neuropsychiatric effects†
Zanamivir	Relenza	Neuraminidase (NA) inhibitor	A and B	Inhaled	≥7 y of age	>5 y of age	Bronchospasm Allergic reactions

*Ribavirin has been studied for use in influenza infections for many years, but despite positive results initially, there has been no consistent documentation of significant clinical benefit in practice. Ribavirin is currently not recommended for either prophylaxis or treatment of the influenza viruses.
†As of November 2007, the precautions for oseltamivir include neuropsychiatric effects. This is based on rare postmarketing reports (mostly from Japan) of delirium and abnormal behavior leading to injury and, in some cases, resulting in fatal outcomes. These events were reported primarily in pediatric patients and often had an abrupt onset and rapid resolution.

▶ TABLE 60-5. INFLUENZA VACCINES*

Vaccine	Brand Names	Route Given	Approved for Age Groups	Dose (mL)	Number of Doses	Contraindications
Trivalent inactivated influenza vaccine (TIV)	Fluzone	IM	6–35 mo	0.25 mL	1 or 2[†]	Children <6 mo of age Persons with history of hypersensitivity including anaphylactic reaction to chicken or egg proteins or other TIV vaccine components
	Fluvirin	IM	≥36 mo	0.5 mL	1 or 2[†]	Persons with moderate or severe acute illness
	Fluarix	IM	≥4 y	0.5 mL	1 or 2[†]	
	FluLaval	IM	≥18 y	0.5 mL	1	
		IM	≥18 y	0.5 mL	1	
Live attenuated influenza vaccine (LAIV)	Flumist	Nasal spray	2–49 y of age if healthy and nonpregnant	0.2 mL (spray ½ dose into each nostril)	1 or 2[‡]	Persons <2 y of age or >50 y of age Persons considered to be at high risk for severe influenza (including those with asthma) Persons with history of hypersensitivity including anaphylactic reaction to egg proteins or other LAIV vaccine components Children or adolescents receiving aspirin Known or suspected immunodeficiency History of Guillain–Barré syndrome Pregnant women

*With permission from www. cdc.gov/flu. 2007–2008 Influenza Prevention and Control Recommendations. Recommendations of the Advisory Committee on Immunization Practices (ACIP).

[†]For children aged 6 mo to 8 y who are receiving TIV for the first time, two doses administered at least 1 mo apart are recommended. For those who received only one dose in their first year of vaccination, two doses should be given the following year.

[‡]For children aged 5 to 8 y who are receiving LAIV for the first time, two doses administered at least 6 wk apart are recommended. For those who received only one dose in their first year of vaccination, two doses should be given the following year.

close contact with immunocompromised family members).[2] Adamantanes (amantidine and rimantidine) and neuaminidase inhibitors (oseltamivir and zanamavir) can shorten the duration of symptoms if started within 24 to 48 hours of the onset of symptoms, but prevention of complications of influenza is less well documented. If treatment is indicated, the level of antiviral resistance in a community is important in determining which medication to prescribe. This information can be obtained from the CDC or local health department. In January 2006, for example, the CDC recommended that neither amantidine nor rimantidine be used for treatment or prophylaxis, because of a global spread of adamantine resistance.[2] Oseltamavir has become the drug of choice; however, as of February 2008, 8% of U.S. influenza A (H1N1) isolates were oseltamivir resistant.[9] Thus, in cases of life-threatening influenza illness, use of two antiviral medications (one from each class of drug) should be considered. In addition, if secondary bacterial pneumonia is suspected, physicians should be aware of the prevalence of CA-MRSA in their communities when choosing empiric antibiotics.[6]

▶ PREVENTION: IMMUNIZATION AND PROPHYLAXIS

Influenza vaccines are newly formulated every year in the summer depending on predictions of the three most likely strains to circulate the following winter. Each year the trivalent inactivated (TIV) and the live attenuated (LAIV) influenza vac-

cines are based on the same strains and this usually includes two influenza A strains and one influenza B strain. Usually, one of the strains is new and two are strains that were in the formulation of the vaccine from the previous year. For example, the new strain in the 2007 to 2008 influenza vaccine was A/Solomon Islands/3/2006(H1N1-) like and the strains being repeated were A/Wisconsin/67/2005(H3N2-) like and B/Malaysia/2506/2004-like viruses.[10] The features of the two types of influenza vaccines (TIV and LAIV) are outlined in Table 60–5. Prevention against influenza can also include prophylaxis with antiviral medications in certain circumstances.[11] The medications approved for prophylaxis in various age groups are outlined in Table 60–4. Since the CDC recommendations for vaccination and prophylaxis change frequently depending in part on epidemiological conditions, the CDC Web site should be consulted. Additional helpful Web sites for up-to-date information on influenza are listed in Table 60–6.

▶ TABLE 60–6. HELPFUL WEB SITES

Centers for Disease Control and Prevention (CDC)
including the Advisory Committee on Immunization Practices (ACIP)—www. cdc.gov
American Academy of Pediatrics (AAP) including the Red Book Committee (Committee on Infectious Diseases)—www.aap.org
World Health Organization (WHO)—www.who.org
Infectious Diseases Society of America (IDSA)—www.idsociety.org
Pediatric Infectious Diseases Society (PIDS)—www.pids.org
American Academy of Emergency Medicine (AAEM)—www.aaem.org
National Network for Immunization Information (NNII)—www.immunizationinfo.org
These Web sites are regularly updated and can provide:
handouts for patients and parents (easily downloaded)
educational materials (posters, pamphlets) for health care professionals and staff
recommendations for immunizations and antiviral medications
recent trends in influenza epidemiology, antiviral drug resistance patterns, etc.
upcoming meetings, lectures, and seminars for health care professionals
contact phone numbers and e-mail addresses

REFERENCES

1. Treanor JJ. Influenza viruses. In: Mandell GL, Bennett JE, Dolin R, eds. *Principles and Practice of Infectious Diseases.* 6th ed. Philadelphia, PA: Elsevier Churchill Livingstone; 2005:2060–2085.
2. American Academy of Pediatrics. Influenza. In: Pickering LK, Baker CJ, Long SS, McMillan JA, eds. *Red Book: 2006 Report of the Committee on Infectious Diseases.* 27th ed. Elk Grove Village, IL: American Academy of Pediatrics; 2006:401–411.
3. Subbarao K. Influenza viruses. In: Long SS, Picering LK, Prober CG, eds. *Principles and Practice of Pediatric Infectious Diseases.* 3rd ed. Philadelphia, PA: Elsevier Churchill Livingstone; 2008:1130–1138.
4. Glezen WP. Orthomyxoviridae. In: Feigin RD, Cherry JD, Demmler GJ, Kaplan SL, eds. *Textbook of Pediatric Infectious Diseases.* 5th ed. Philadelphia, PA: Saunders; 2004:2252–2269.
5. Grose C. The puzzling picture of acute necrotizing encedphalopathy after influenza A and B virus infection in young children. *Pediatr Infect Dis J.* 2004;23:253–254.
6. Severe methicillin-resistant staphylococcus aureus community-acquired pneumonia associated with influenza—Louisiana and Georgia, December 2006–January 2007. *MMWR Morb Mortal Wkly Rep.* 2007;56(14):325–329.
7. Taketomo CK, Hodding JH, Kraus DM, eds. *Pediatric Dosage Handbook.* 11th ed. Hudson, OH: Lexi-Comp. Inc; 2004:78–79, 881–882, 1041–1042.
8. *Physician's Desk Reference.* 62nd ed. Montvale, NJ: Thompson Healthcare Inc; 2008:1552–1555.
9. CDC. Update: influenza activity—United States, September 30, 2007–February 9, 2008. *MMWR Morb Mortal Wkly Rep.* 2008;57:1–5.
10. Centers for Disease Control and Prevention. *2007–2008 Influenza Prevention and Control Recommendations.* Atlanta, GA: Centers for Disease Control and Prevention. http://www.cdc.gov/flu/professionals/acip/primarychanges.htm. April 1, 2008.
11. Committee on Infectious Diseases, American Academy of Pediatrics. Antiviral therapy and prophylaxis for influenza in children: clinical report. *Pediatrics.* 2007;119(4):8523–8860.

CHAPTER 61

Meningitis

Steven Lelyveld and Gary R. Strange

▶ HIGH-YIELD FACTS

- Early meningitis is not easy to diagnose. Especially in young infants, signs and symptoms are notoriously nonspecific.
- Organisms enter the cerebrospinal fluid by hematogenous spread or by direct extension from the nasopharynx or other adjacent structures. Many of the pathologic changes are not primarily due to infection but result from the response of the human immune system to the infection.
- An increasing majority of all cases of meningitis are aseptic and most of these cases have a benign outcome.
- For children younger than 1 month, the predominant organisms are group B *Streptococcus, Escherichia coli,* and *Listeria monocytogenes.*
- The incidence of *Haemophilus influenzae* type b, which was the most common etiologic agent of childhood bacterial meningitis, has dropped dramatically since the introduction of the conjugate vaccine against this organism. *Streptococcus pneumoniae* is now the major cause of infant bacterial meningitis in the United States and *Neisseria meningitidis* is the most common cause in the 2- to 18-year age group.
- Neonatal cerebrospinal fluid contains more cells and protein and less glucose than that of older children.
- Newborns are generally treated with an initial dose of ampicillin, 100 mg/kg, and an aminoglycoside, such as gentamicin, 2.5 mg/kg. Depending on local sensitivities, a cephalosporin active against gram-negative bacilli, such as cefotaxime, 50 mg/kg, may be substituted for the aminoglycoside.
- Vancomycin is the only antibiotic to which all strains of pneumococci are susceptible and it is therefore added to a broad-spectrum cephalosporin for comprehensive therapy (vancomycin, 15 mg/kg/dose bid, and cefotaxime, 50 mg/kg/dose tid) for infants and small children.
- In the unstable child, lumbar puncture should be withheld until after stabilization and antibiotic administration.
- Steroids may be beneficial in reducing the sequelae of bacterial meningitis. Major sequelae include hearing loss, seizures, and decreased mental ability.

Over the past 20 years, there has been a significant change in the epidemiology of bacterial meningitis, which is now predominantly a disease of adults. The most important contributor to this change has been the >99% decrease in frequency of *H. influenzae* type B (Hib), which was the most common etiologic agent of childhood bacterial meningitis, since the introduction of the conjugate Hib vaccine in the late 1980s.[1,2] In 2006, there were only 29 cases of invasive *H. influenzae* type B reported in children younger than 5 years.[3] *S. pneumoniae* was the major cause of bacterial meningitis in infants 1 month to 2 years of age in the United States until the heptavalent pneumococcal conjugate vaccine (PCV7) that covers 80% of invasive serotypes was introduced in 2000. In 2005, there were 13 000 fewer cases of *S. pneumoniae* meningitis and bacteremia annually in children <5 years of age compared to 1998 to 1999, just prior to the introduction of the vaccine. The overall incidence of pneumococcal disease in this age group declined from 98.7 to 23.4 cases per 100 000.[4] A 23-valent pneumococcal vaccine is also available for older children and adults with underlying diseases. *N. meningitidis* is now the most common cause of meningitis in infants and children, with a peak caused by serogroup B below age 2 and second peak at 18-year age. There is no vaccine for serogroup B. A tetravalent vaccine (A, C, Y, or W-135) is effective against 75% of cases older than 2 years.[5,6] For children younger than 1 month, the predominant organisms are group B *Streptococcus, E. coli,* and *L. monocytogenes* (Fig. 61–1).

Since the introduction of the Hib and PCV7 vaccines, an increasing majority of all cases of meningitis are aseptic. Most of these cases have a benign outcome. Of the viral causes of meningitis, over 80% are seasonal enteroviruses, predominantly echovirus and coxsackievirus. Mumps, herpes simplex, varicella, measles, and arboviruses have all been described as central nervous system pathogens.

▶ PATHOPHYSIOLOGY

Most pathogens enter the subarachnoid space by hematogenous spread. In addition, they may enter through a mechanical disruption, as in a fracture of the base of the skull, or by direct extension from an infection in the ear, mastoid air cells, sinuses, orbit, or other adjacent structure. Under normal circumstances, the blood–brain barrier provides an adequate defense against invasive disease. However, once it is breached, natural defense mechanisms are unable to stop the multiplication of organisms. An alteration in the cerebral capillary endothelial cells ensues, with weakening of the blood–brain barrier.

Many of the pathologic changes of meningitis are not primarily because of infection, but result from the response of the human immune system to the infection. A complicated series of interactions among immune, vascular, and central nervous system cells; cytokines and chemokines; matrix metalloproteinases; and free radical molecules is ultimately responsible for many of the changes that occur in bacterial meningitis, including neuronal death. Cytotoxic and vasogenic cerebral edema cause an increase in intracranial pressure, which in

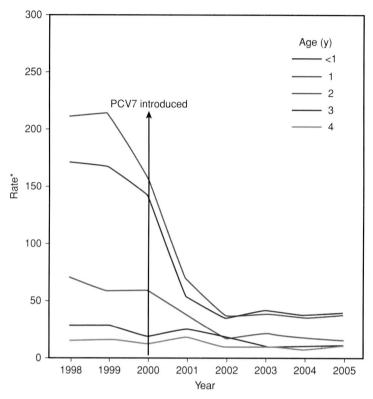

*Per 100 000 population.
†California (one county); the state of Connecticut; Georgia (20 counties);
Maryland (six counties); Minnesota (seven counties); New York (seven
counties); Oregon (three counties); and Tennessee (four counties).

Figure 61–1. Changes in the incidence rate before and after
introduction of 7-valent pneumococcal conjugate vaccine (PCV7) by
age and year. (Reprinted with permission from CDC. Invasive
pneumococcal disease in children 5 years after conjugate vaccine
introduction—Eight States, 1998–2005. *MMWR.* 2008;57(06):144–148.)

turn leads to decreased cerebral perfusion pressure, decreased
blood flow, regional hypoxia, and focal ischemia of the brain.[7]

▶ PRESENTATION

The "classic" signs and symptoms of meningitis include
headache, photophobia, stiff neck, change in mental status, bulging fontanelle, nausea, and vomiting (Table 61–1).
The Brudzinski sign occurs when the irritated meninges are
stretched, with neck flexion causing the hips and knees to flex
involuntarily (Fig. 61–2). The Kernig sign of nerve root irritation is present when the hip is flexed to 90 degrees and the
examiner is unable to passively extend the leg fully (Fig. 61–3).
Children with meningeal irritation often resist walking or being carried, preferring to remain recumbent, often in a fetal
position. These signs and symptoms, related to meningeal irritation, are reasonably reliable in older infants and children,
but their absence does not rule out intracranial infection.[8,9]

The younger the child, the less obvious the signs and
symptoms until late in the course of the disease. Neonates and
young infants are likely to present with poor feeding, irritability, inconsolability, or listlessness. Nuchal rigidity, the resistance to flexion of the neck in the anteroposterior plane only,

has been considered one of the most specific signs of meningitis. However, nuchal rigidity is seen in <15% of children
with meningitis younger than 18 months and, in one study,
was found to be present in 21% of children being evaluated
for meningitis who were subsequently found to have normal
cerebrospinal fluid (CSF).

▶ TABLE 61–1. SIGNS AND SYMPTOMS OF MENINGITIS AT PRESENTATION

Manifestation	% of Cases
History of fever	>95
Lethargy	87–95
Vomiting	54–71
Upper respiratory infection symptoms	46–55
Seizures	22–23
Temperature >38.3°C	59–77
Altered mental status	53–78
ENT infection	22–42
Nuchal rigidity	54–59
Brudzinski sign	10–13
Kernig sign	9–11
Focal neurologic defect	5–6

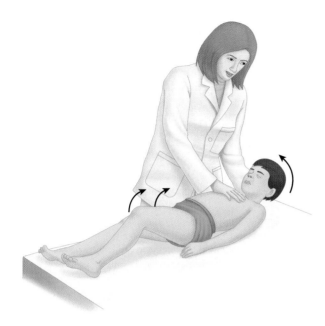

Figure 61–2. Brudsinski sign. With the patient supine and the examiner's hand on the patient's chest, passive neck flexion (arrow at right) results in flexion at the hips (arrows at left), which is often asymmetric. The sign is present with meningeal irritation and inflammation such as that seen in meningitis, but also in subarachnoid hemorrhage.

Meningitis may take either an insidious (90%) or fulminant (10%) course. If the course is insidious, the patient has a high likelihood of presenting to a physician days before diagnosis with a nonspecific illness. This is especially true when the pathogen is *Pneumococcus*. The duration of illness before diagnosis can be up to 2 weeks, with a median of 36 to 72 hours. Many of these children would have been treated with oral antibiotics before the diagnosis of meningitis is considered. Partial treatment may complicate the diagnostic process, but antibiotic treatment prior to diagnosis of central nervous system infec-

Sensitivity-5%
Specificity-95%

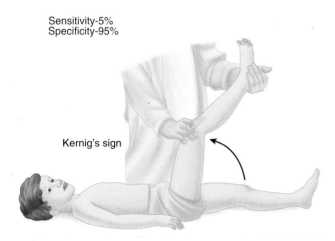

Kernig's sign

Figure 61–3. Kernig sign. With the patient supine and the examiner's hand on the patient's chest, the hip is flexed to 90 degrees and the examiner attempts to passively extend the leg fully. Inability to passively extend the leg to its full extent is a positive Kernig sign.

tion may also be associated with reduction in disease-related sequelae.[10]

The more fulminant the course, the worse the prognosis. Typically, meningococcal disease presents with a more fulminant course. Concomitant meningococcal bacteremia rapidly progresses to petechiae, purpura fulminans, and cardiovascular collapse. As other causes of pediatric meningitis have been contained, meningococcal disease has become a leading infectious cause of death.[6,11]

The management of any of the bacterial meningitides may be complicated by hemorrhage into the adrenal cortex, the Friderichsen–Waterhouse syndrome.

▶ DIFFERENTIAL DIAGNOSIS

In the early phases, meningitis may be confused with gastroenteritis, upper respiratory infection, pneumonia, otitis media, or minor viral syndromes. As the alteration of mental status becomes more severe, the diagnoses of encephalitis, subarachnoid or subdural hemorrhage with or without direct trauma or abuse, cerebral abscess, and Reye's syndrome must be considered. Toxic ingestions, seizure disorders, diabetic ketoacidosis, hypothyroidism, and other altered metabolic states may initially be confused with meningitis but do not have the same prodrome or fever. A young child with intussusception may present with vomiting, altered mental status, and cardiovascular collapse. Many of these children are evaluated for meningitis before their diagnosis is clear.[12]

▶ MANAGEMENT

UNSTABLE PATIENTS

Whenever meningitis is suspected, the diagnostic test of choice is the lumbar puncture with cerebrospinal fluid (CSF) analysis. However, it is imperative not to neglect the ABCs while performing diagnostic procedures. Care must be taken to ensure proper oxygenation and cardiovascular stabilization. In the unstable child, lumbar puncture should be withheld until after stabilization and antibiotic administration.[13] Although the early administration of antibiotics may prevent recovery of the organism on culture of CSF,[14] early appropriate antibiotic therapy should be the goal. However, studies have not definitively shown a correlation between early treatment and clinical outcome.[7,10] Drawing of specimens for blood cultures prior to administration of antibiotics provides another avenue for identification of specific pathogens and usually can be accomplished without delaying antibiotic administration.[15]

The unstable patient with meningitis may have respiratory compromise, shock, increased intracranial pressure, seizures, or hypoglycemia. The first priority is to ensure an open airway and adequate ventilation. Supplemental oxygen is always administered. Inadequate ventilation or oxygenation, based on clinical assessment or blood gas results, requires assistance with the bag-valve-mask technique, followed by endotracheal intubation.[15]

Patients with evidence of shock are treated with rapid intravenous or intraosseous infusion of crystalloid solution in 20 mL/kg aliquots. However, careful assessment of the need for continuing fluid resuscitation should be made because fluid

▶ **TABLE 61–2. NORMAL CEREBROSPINAL FLUID (CSF) VALUES**

Parameter	Preterm Infant	Term Infant	Child
Cell count	9 (0–25) WBC/mm^3	8 (0–22) WBC/mm^3	0–7
WBC/mm^3	57% PMNs	61% PMNs	0% PMNs
Glucose	24–63 mg/dL (mean 52)	34–119 mg/dL (mean 52)	40–80 mg/dL
CSF/blood glucose ratio	55%–105%	44%–128%	50%
Protein	65–150 mg/dL (mean 115)	20–170 mg/dL (mean 90)	5–40 mg/dL

overload can lead to worsening of cerebral edema. Fluid restriction is not routinely indicated and therefore once the patient is stabilized, fluid should be given at the usual maintenance rate.[15]

If signs of increased intracranial pressure (worsening mental status, papilledema, full fontanelle, and widening of sutures) develop, elevate the head at 30 degrees and initiate controlled ventilation to keep the Paco$_2$ between 30 and 35 mm Hg. Patients who do not respond to controlled ventilation may benefit from the use of diuretic therapy with mannitol (0.25–1 g/kg) or furosemide (1 mg/kg).[15]

Seizures are controlled with rapid-acting benzodiazepines followed by phenytoin (see Chapter 7).[15]

The blood glucose level should be rapidly assessed. If the blood glucose is <40 mg/dL, administer an infusion of glucose (250 to 500 mg/kg) as 10% dextrose for neonates, 25% dextrose for infants younger than 2 years, and 50% dextrose for older infants and children.

STABLE PATIENTS

In stable patients with manifestations suggestive of meningitis, phlebotomy for diagnostic studies is followed promptly by lumbar puncture. The threshold for clinical suspicion of meningitis should be particularly low for certain patients:

- Neonates
- Immunocompromised children
- Children who have been in close contact with cases of meningitis
- Children with documented bacteremia

The initial workup includes a complete blood count (CBC),[16] electrolytes, glucose, renal functions, and blood culture. Specific tests may be performed to detect bacterial capsular antigens but are not often helpful in the acute situation.[15]

Once it is safe to do so, a lumbar puncture is performed. The expected laboratory parameters for CSF analysis are age-related (Table 61–2). A low white blood cell count, with predominantly mononuclear cells, and normal glucose and protein are more consistent with a viral etiology. High protein, low sugar, and elevated polymorphonuclear leukocytes (PMNs) suggest bacterial etiology.[17]

ANTIBIOTIC TREATMENT

Antibiotic treatment is directed by the specific organisms, if known, or by the predominant organisms depending on age of the patient, if the specific agent is not known.

Newborns are generally treated with an initial dose of ampicillin, 100 mg/kg, and an aminoglycoside, such as gentamicin, 2.5 mg/kg. Depending on local sensitivities, a cephalosporin active against gram-negative bacilli, such as cefotaxime, 50 mg/kg, may be substituted for the aminoglycoside.[18]

Infants and children are generally treated with a cephalosporin (ceftriaxone 100 mg/kg/dose qd or cefotaxime 50 mg/kg/dose tid). In areas where cephalosporins are of limited availability, the combination of ampicillin, 100 mg/kg/dose qid, and chloramphenicol, 25 mg/kg/dose bid, is an option. If the organism is known to be *S. pneumoniae* or if gram-positive cocci are seen on Gram stain of the CSF, penicillin and cephalosporin resistance is possible. Vancomycin is the only antibiotic to which all strains of pneumococci are susceptible, and it is therefore added to a broad-spectrum cephalosporin for comprehensive therapy (vancomycin, 15 mg/kg/dose bid, and cefotaxime, 50 mg/kg/dose tid).[13,19,20]

CORTICOSTEROID TREATMENT

The role of steroids in the management of meningitis is controversial. When given prior to the antibiotic, the anti-inflammatory effect of dexamethasone (0.15 mg/kg intravenously) decreases intracranial pressure, cerebral edema, and CSF lactate concentrations. Dexamethasone significantly decreases hearing loss and other neurologic sequelae in meningitis caused by *H. influenzae* type B. Clinical trials and meta-analyses suggest that dexamethasone therapy improves the outcome for patients with bacterial meningitis caused by other agents, but the evidence is not yet conclusive. For *S. pneumoniae*, dexamethasone should be considered, after weighing the potential benefits and risks. In addition, some authorities argue that steroids may strengthen the blood–brain barrier and limit the penetration of intravenously administered antibiotics into the CSF. However, this does not appear to be a significant consideration with commonly used antibiotics such as vancomycin, ceftriaxone, and cefotaxime. Currently, there is no clear consensus on the empiric use of steroids for meningitis when the bacterial agent is unknown.[13,21]

▶ SEQUELAE

The vast majority of children with aseptic meningitis have a self-limited illness without subsequent problems. In spite of modern antibiotic treatment, the mortality of *H. influenzae* type B meningitis is 5% to 10%, and for *S. pneumoniae* meningitis, it is 20% to 40%. Up to 20% of survivors will have some long-term sequelae. These include mild learning defects, sensorineural hearing loss, afebrile seizures, and multiple neurologic defects, including retardation and blindness. Other neurologic defects, such as hemiparesis, ataxia, cranial nerve palsy, and abnormal extensor reflexes, may be present initially but may resolve in a few months.[22-24]

REFERENCES

1. Schuchat A, Rosentein Messonnier N. From pandemic suspect to the postvaccine era: the haemophilus influenzae story. *Clin Infect Dis.* 2007;44:817–819.
2. Short WR, Tunkel AR. Changing epidemiology of bacterial meningitis in the United States. *Curr Infect Dis Rep.* 2000;2:327–331.
3. CDC. Summary of notifiable diseases—United States, 2006. *MMWR.* 2008;55(53):1–94.
4. CDC. Invasive pneumococcal disease in children 5 years after conjugate vaccine introduction—Eight States, 1998–2005. *MMWR.* 2008;57(06):144–148.
5. CDC. Prevention and control of meningococcal disease: recommendations of the advisory committee on immunization practices (ACIP). *MMWR.* 2005;54(RR-7):1–21.
6. Rosenstein NE, Perkins BA, Stephens DS, et al. Medical progress: meningococcal disease. *N Engl J Med.* 2001;344:1378–1388.
7. Aronin SI. Bacterial meningitis: principles and practical aspects of therapy. *Curr Infect Dis Rep.* 2000;2:337–344.
8. Van de Beek D, De Gans J, Spanjaard L, et al. Clinical features and prognostic factors in adults with bacterial meningitis. *N Engl J Med.* 2004;351:1849–1859.
9. Oosterbrink R, Moons K, Theunissen C, et al. Signs of meningeal irritation at the emergency department: how often bacterial meningitis? *Pediatr Emerg Care.* 2001;17:161–164.
10. Bonsu B, Harper M. Fever interval before diagnosis, prior antibiotic treatment and clinical outcome for young children with bacterial meningitis. *Clin Infect Dis.* 2001;32:566–572.
11. Thompson MJ, Ninis N, Perera R, et al. Clinical recognition of meningococcal disease in children and adolescents. *Lancet.* 2006;367(9508):397–403.
12. Levy M, Wong E, Fried D. Diseases that mimic meningitis. *Clin Pediatr.* 1990;29:254–260.
13. Quagliarello VJ, Scheld WM. Treatment of bacterial meningitis. *N Engl J Med.* 1997;336:708–716.
14. Kanegaye JT, Soliemanzadeh P, Bradley JS. Lumbar puncture in pediatric bacterial meningitis: defining the time interval for recovery of cerebral spinal fluid pathogens after parenteral antibiotic treatment. *Pediatrics.* 2001;108:1169–1174.
15. Strange GR, Ahrens WR. Meningitis: evidence to guide an evolving standard of care. *Pediatr Emerg Med Pract.* 2005;2(4):1–24.
16. Bonsu B, Harper MB. Utility of the peripheral blood count white cell count for identifying sick young infants who need lumbar puncture. *Ann Emerg Med.* 2003;41:206–214.
17. Negrini B, Kelleher KM, Wald ER. Cerebrospinal fluid abnormalities in aseptic versus bacterial meningitis. *Pediatrics.* 2000;105:316–319.
18. Committee on Infectious Diseases. *Red Book: 2006 Report of the Committee on Infectious Diseases.* 27th ed. Elk Grove Village, IL: American Academy of Pediatrics; 2006.
19. Buckingham SC, McCullers JA, et al. Early vancomycin therapy and adverse outcomes in children with pneumococcal meningitis. *Pediatrics.* 2006;117(5):1688–1694.
20. Wang VJ, Malley R, Fleisher GR, et al. Antibiotic treatment of children with unsuspected meningococcal disease. *Arch Pediatr Adolesc Med.* 2000;154:556–560.
21. Greenwood BM. Corticosteroids for acute bacterial meningitis. *N Engl J Med.* 2007;357:2507–2509.
22. Baraff LJ, Lee SI, Schriger DL. Outcomes of bacterial meningitis in children: a meta-analysis. *Pediatr Infect Dis.* 1993;12:389–395.
23. Wellman MB, Sommer DD, McKenna J. Sensorineural hearing loss in postmeningitic children. *Otol Neurotol.* 2003;24:907–912.
24. Carter JA, Neville BG, Newton CR. Neuro-cognitive impairment following acquired central nervous system infections in childhood: a systematic review. *Brain Res Rev.* 2003;43:57–69.

CHAPTER 62

Toxic Shock Syndrome

Shabnam Jain and Anthony Cooley

► HIGH-YIELD FACTS

- Toxic shock syndrome (TSS) is an acute, toxin-mediated illness characterized by fever, erythematous rash, hypotension, multiorgan involvement, and desquamation.
- Most cases of TSS have been associated with *Staphylococcus aureus*. However, group A Streptococcus (GAS) can cause a similar disease known as streptococcal TSS (STSS).
- Menstrual and nonmenstrual cases of TSS are now reported with almost equal frequency. Predisposing factors for nonmenstrual TSS are surgical and nonsurgical trauma, burns, and postpartum conditions. Predisposing factors for STSS are varicella, NSAID use, and deep-seated GAS infections.
- TSS is a rare disease and is less common in children than adults. However, it is serious and can be life-threatening unless diagnosed rapidly and managed aggressively.
- STSS patients may have severe pain and hyperesthesia out of proportion to the degree of skin involvement.
- Abnormal laboratory values reflect the multisystem involvement in TSS.
- Management depends on prompt recognition, identification, and removal of the infectious focus. In addition, antibiotics and hemodynamic support are essential.
- Clindamycin has been recommended as the antibiotic of choice for both TSS and STSS (along with penicillin G for GAS).
- The most important initial therapy is aggressive volume replacement. Crystalloids or fresh frozen plasma may be used for the management of hypotension, with pressors added if fluids alone are not sufficient.
- TSS can mimic many common diseases and should be considered in any patient who has unexplained fever, rash, and a toxic condition out of proportion to local findings. Early recognition is critical because the clinical course can be fulminant.

Toxic shock syndrome (TSS) is a rare acute febrile disease characterized by fever, diffuse erythroderma (that later desquamates), vomiting, abdominal pain, diarrhea, myalgia, and nonspecific neurologic abnormalities.[1] It can progress rapidly to hypotension, multiorgan failure, and death.[2]

TSS was first described in 1978 in seven children with *Staphylococcus aureus* infections. In 1980, TSS was noted in menstruating women. An epidemic developed associated with continuous tampon use by women who had vaginal colonization with toxin-producing strains of *S. aureus*. With the withdrawal of superabsorbent tampons from the market, menstrual

TSS is now rare. However, nonmenstrual TSS continues to occur in children and adults; it is most commonly associated with cutaneous infections. Menstrual and nonmenstrual TSS are now reported in almost equal frequency.[1] TSS is more common in adults than children.

Since the late 1980s, with the resurgence of highly invasive streptococcal infections, a toxic shocklike syndrome has been reported. Most authors accept the abbreviation "sTSS" to distinguish streptococcal from staphylococcal TSS.[3]

Because TSS and sTSS are syndromes, the diagnosis is made when several clinical signs are found together. The Centers for Disease Control and Prevention (CDC) have formulated case definitions for both TSS and sTSS (Tables 62–1 and 62–2).[4,5]

► ETIOLOGY AND PATHOGENESIS

The pathogenesis of TSS is thought to be related to production of a toxin, currently referred to as toxic shock syndrome toxin-1 (TSST-1). It is likely that more than one toxin may be involved. These toxins are thought to be superantigens, which are a group of proteins that can overactivate the immune system, bypassing certain steps in the usual antigen-mediated immune response sequence.[6] This causes massive T-cell stimulation and an overwhelming immune cascade that is destructive to all end organs. This is why such a global response to these toxins is exhibited, with every major organ affected in full-blown disease.

The majority of cases TSS are caused by coagulase-positive *S. aureus*, although recently, coagulase-negative strains have been isolated. It often develops from a site of colonization rather than infection.[1]

STSS is caused by invasive group A streptococci (GAS) which are thought to produce the streptococcal enterotoxin. It occurs most commonly following varicella in previously healthy children and/or during the use of NSAIDs. Sites of infection in sTSS are much deeper than in staphylococcal TSS, such as infection following blunt trauma.[1]

When superantigens come in contact with cells, they react, with various consequences depending on the cell type. Activation of blood vessel muscle cells leads to vasodilation and hypotension, activation of skin cells leads to rash, activation of gut cells leads to diarrhea, and activation of muscle cells leads to pain and cramps.[3]

The most impressive aspect of the pathophysiology of TSS is the massive vasodilatation and rapid movement of serum proteins and fluid from the intravascular to the extravascular

▶ TABLE 62–1. **TOXIC SHOCK SYNDROME: CENTERS FOR DISEASE CONTROL CASE DEFINITION**

Fever	Temperature $\geq$ 38.9°C
Rash	Diffuse macular erythroderma.
Desquamation	1–2 wk after onset of illness, particularly on palms and soles
Hypotension	Systolic blood pressure $\leq$ 90 mm Hg for adults and systolic blood pressure <fifth percentile for age in children younger than 16 y; orthostatic hypotension, syncope, or dizziness.
Involvement of $\geq$3 of the following organ systems clinically or by abnormal laboratory tests:	
Gastrointestinal	Vomiting or diarrhea at onset of illness
Muscular	Severe myalgia or CPK > twice normal
Mucous membranes	Vaginal, conjunctival, or oropharyngeal hyperemia
Renal	BUN or serum creatinine > twice normal or pyuria ($\geq$5 leucocytes per hpf) in the absence of a urinary tract infection
Hematologic	Platelet count < 100 000/mm^3
Hepatic	Total bilirubin, ALT or AST > twice normal
Central nervous system	Disorientation or altered consciousness without focal neurologic signs when fever and hypotension are absent
Negative results on the following tests, if obtained:	
Negative	Blood, throat, or CSF culture
Negative	Serologic tests for Rocky Mountain spotted fever, leptospirosis, or measles

space. This results in oliguria, hypotension, edema, and low central venous pressure. The multisystem collapse seen in TSS may be either a reflection of the rapid onset of shock or may be from direct effects of toxin(s) on the parenchymal cells of the involved organs.

▶ EPIDEMIOLOGY

The CDC have reported a decrease in the annual incidence of TSS, presumably from the increased awareness of risk associated with tampon use. Today, only half of the cases are associated with tampon use, whereas the other half occur in children, men, and nonmenstruating women. Nonmenstrual cases occur in a variety of clinical settings, but are chiefly associated with postpartum or cutaneous/subcutaneous *S. aureus* infections. Predisposing factors include burns, abrasions, abscesses, and nasal packing.

In the United Kingdom, it was estimated that 3% to 13% of children admitted to a burn unit developed TSS.[7] TSS is more common in children with burns of relatively low body surface area. Although children have a higher incidence of minor *S. aureus* infection than adults, the incidence and mortality of TSS in children are lower. The location of infection probably plays a role in the elaboration of toxin. The immunologic status of the individual may also play a role. Studies have shown that patients with TSS do not develop a significant antibody response to TSST-1. Therefore, there is a significant recurrence rate for TSS (30%). Secondary cases are milder and occur within 3 months of the original episode; the overall mortality rate is 5%.[4]

The incidence of sTSS corresponds to the incidence of invasive GAS disease, which varies according to geographic location and occurs in clusters. Varicella is an important risk factor for invasive GAS infections in previously healthy children. An association between NSAID use and the development of sTSS has been reported.[1]

▶ TABLE 62–2. **STREPTOCOCCAL TOXIC SHOCK SYNDROME: CENTERS FOR DISEASE CONTROL CASE DEFINITION**

An illness with the following clinical manifestations occurring within the first 48 h of illness or hospitalization:	
Hypotension	Systolic BP $\leq$90 for adults or < fifth percentile for children younger than 16 y
Involvement of two or more of the following:	
Renal	Creatinine $\geq$2 mg/dL for adults or $\geq$ twice upper limit for age, or greater than twofold increase over baseline
Coagulopathy	Platelet count $\leq$100 000/mm^3 or DIC, low fibrinogen level, and fibrin degradation products present
Liver	Total bilirubin, ALT, or AST $\geq$ twice normal or greater than twofold increase over baseline
Acute respiratory distress syndrome	Acute onset diffuse pulmonary infiltrates and hypoxemia without cardiac failure, diffuse capillary leak (edema, effusions, hypoalbuminemia)
Rash	Generalized erythroderma, desquamation
Soft tissue necrosis	Necrotizing fasciitis, myositis, gangrene
Laboratory findings	Isolation of group A *Streptococcus*

► TABLE 62–3. ABBREVIATED CRITERIA FOR DIAGNOSIS OF TSS IN CHILDREN

Fever ≥39°C
Rash
Diarrhea ± vomiting
Irritability
Lymphopenia

► CLINICAL MANIFESTATIONS

TSS (caused by staphylococcus or streptococcus) is characterized by an acute illness with fever, hypotension, and multisystem organ involvement (including renal failure). Because this can be difficult to distinguish from other childhood illnesses in their early stages, the CDC has established clinical criteria for diagnosis. CDC criteria for TSS and sTSS may not be applicable to children. So, in 1990, abbreviated diagnostic criteria were proposed for use in children (Table 62–3).[8]

TSS should be considered in any patient who has unexplained fever, rash, and a toxic appearance. Patients with menstrual TSS usually present between the third and fifth day of menses. A typical presentation in a child could be a toddler with a small, 2-day-old burn and a sudden deterioration in clinical condition.[6] The symptoms, signs, and laboratory abnormalities reflect multiple organ involvement. There is sudden onset of high fever, over 38.9°C (with chills), vomiting, diarrhea, myalgia, dizziness, and diffuse rash. Additional symptoms include headache, arthralgia, sore throat, abdominal pain, and stiff neck. There may be orthostatic dizziness or syncope. Diarrhea (which may be profuse and watery) and vomiting occur in about half of the cases.[6]

Patients with TSS appear acutely ill. Physical examination may reveal hypotension or orthostatic blood pressure changes. In the acute stage, which lasts 24 to 48 hours, the patient may be agitated, disoriented, or obtunded. Hyperemia of the conjunctiva and vagina is seen (Fig. 62–1). Tender edematous external genitalia, vaginal mucosal erythema, scant purulent cer-

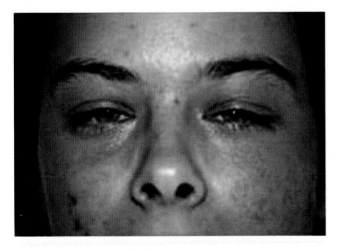

Figure 62–1. Erythema of the bulbar conjunctivae associated with facial erythema and edema in a female with menstrual toxic shock syndrome (TSS).

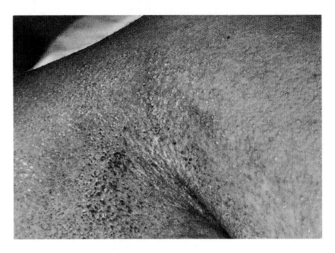

Figure 62–2. Blanching, nonpruritic erythroderma with a "rough" texture in a patient with toxic shock syndrome.

vical discharge, and bilateral–adnexal tenderness are seen in menstruation-related TSS.

Skin findings can be dramatic and present as a severe erythroderma and erythema of mucus membranes (Fig. 62–2).

Between the fifth and tenth hospital day, a generalized pruritic maculopapular rash develops in about 25% of patients. The skin rash is diffuse and blanches. It fades within 3 days of its appearance and is followed by a fine generalized desquamation of the skin, with peeling over the soles, fingers, toes, and palms.

Abnormal laboratory values reflect the multisystem involvement in TSS. No specific laboratory test can make the diagnosis, but there are several frequently found abnormalities. Leucocytosis, with an increase in immature forms, is frequently seen. Lymphopenia has been reported as a useful way to confirm diagnosis. Platelet count may be low. Azotemia and abnormal urinary sediment are seen with the development of acute renal failure. Liver function tests frequently show some elevation of liver enzymes and bilirubin. Electrolyte abnormalities vary and may include hyponatremia. With severe hypotension, the patient may be acidotic. Clotting studies are normal or mildly abnormal; untreated patients may show clinical evidence of coagulopathy. Cultures of blood, throat, and cerebrospinal fluid may be useful. However, only 5% of blood cultures are positive.[9] Vaginal culture should be done, as well as culture from any identifiable focus of infection. *Staphylococcus* will be cultured from the cervix or vagina of more than 85% of patients with menstrual TSS. The majority of the above tests return to normal by 7 to 10 days after onset of illness.

Mild episodes of TSS are more difficult to diagnose. The presence of any combination of fever, headache, sore throat, diarrhea, vomiting, orthostatic dizziness, syncope, or myalgias in a menstruating woman should raise the possibility of TSS. There is no diagnostic laboratory test; the presence of *S. aureus* on culture is not diagnostic because non-TSST-1–producing *S. aureus* may be cultured from the cervix or vagina of up to 10% of well women. However, the presence of desquamation during a febrile illness should prompt the clinician to obtain cultures for *S. aureus*. Other laboratory data do not reflect multisystem involvement in mild cases. Thus, strong support for the fact that the signs and symptoms did represent mild TSS will depend on the development of the typical desquamation of palms, soles, toes, and fingers.

STSS presents as sudden onset of shock and organ failure in the presence of any streptococcal infection. Tender erythroderma is the most suggestive symptom of sTSS. It appears abruptly and the hyperesthesia may seem out of proportion to the degree of skin involvement. These patients should be evaluated for GAS necrotizing fasciitis.[2]

Because the initial presentation of sTSS may not be obvious, clinicians should maintain a high index of suspicion. Those most suspect include children with varicella, skin injury, well-localized or unusually severe tenderness, and infection at sites of blunt trauma.

▶ DIFFERENTIAL DIAGNOSIS

Several other systemic illnesses with fever, rash, diarrhea, myalgias, and multisystem involvement resemble TSS. Kawasaki disease also is characterized by fever, conjunctival hyperemia, and erythema of mucus membranes with desquamation. Although it is clinically similar, it lacks many of the features of TSS, including diffuse myalgia, vomiting, abdominal pain, diarrhea, azotemia, thrombocytopenia, and shock. Kawasaki disease occurs typically in children younger than 5 years.

The clinical picture of staphylococcal scarlet fever is also very similar to TSS. They are both illnesses caused by toxin-producing staphylococci. Pathology specimens or serologic evidence of the exfoliation toxin differentiates the two entities. Streptococcal scarlet fever is rare after the age of 10. The "sandpaper" rash of scarlet fever is distinct from the macular rash of TSS. Rather than the tender erythroderma seen with sTSS, scarlet fever causes a nontender erythematous sandpaperlike rash.

Sepsis syndrome, once called septic shock, must always be considered in the differential diagnosis of TSS. In sepsis syndrome, multiplying bacteria cause inflammation to develop rapidly because of the body's own immune response, but without the development of superantigens.[3] Hypotension is common to both sepsis and TSS; therefore, initial management is always the same. However, the appearance of a rash and the laboratory abnormalities associated with TSS will aid in distinguishing these two entities.

Other conditions, such as Rocky Mountain spotted fever, leptospirosis, meningococcemia, Stevens–Johnson syndrome, and staphylococcal scalded skin syndrome, may resemble TSS.

▶ MANAGEMENT

The cause of TSS is bacteria and their toxins, which produce inflammatory changes that compromise many organ systems.[3] Therefore, management is aimed at blocking the effects of the toxin and removing bacteria that might synthesize more toxin and supporting the major organ systems, especially the cardiovascular, renal and respiratory systems.

Management depends on prompt recognition. Some authors recommend that all patients with fever and erythroderma be hospitalized for at least 24 hours of close monitoring.[10] Early identification of the infectious focus is critical. The focus must be drained and foreign material (such as nasal

packing or a retained tampon) promptly removed. Cultures should be obtained. Antibiotic therapy is essential for recovery from the acute episode, but is also important for eradication of the organism to reduce the recurrence rate. Traditionally, β-lactamase–resistant antistaphylococcal antibiotics, such as oxacillin or nafcillin, had been the recommended treatment. However, because of the recent emergence of community-associated methicillin-resistant *Staphylococcus aureus*, clindamycin or vancomycin is now recommended.[1] Although of unproven efficacy, elimination of nasal carriage of bacteria with mupirocin or rifampin may be considered.[11] For sTSS, combination therapy with intravenous penicillin G and clindamycin is recommended.[1] Penicillin acts against replicating bacteria and clindamycin may reduce toxin production.

Initial parenteral antibiotic coverage for both GAS and *S. aureus* infection should be instituted because of the similarity in the clinical appearance of TSS and sTSS. Therefore, clindamycin usually is the antibiotic of choice for both TSS and sTSS (in addition to penicillin G for GAS).

Adjunctive therapy to neutralize toxins includes intravenous immunoglobulins or fresh frozen plasma. Either provides passive immunity with antibodies that bind to superantigens to stop them from activating cells and preventing further damage.[3]

The remainder of therapy depends on the severity and extent of symptoms. The most important initial therapy is aggressive management of hypovolemic shock with large volumes of crystalloids or fresh frozen plasma; pressors may be added if fluids alone are not sufficient.

Continuous monitoring of heart rate, blood pressure, respiratory rate, urinary output, central venous pressure, and pulmonary wedge pressure is required. As volume resuscitation progresses, chest radiographs, blood gases, and electrolytes need to be followed. Thrombocytopenia may require platelet transfusions. If ARDS occurs, mechanical ventilation will become necessary.

Corticosteroids, aimed at reducing the host response contribution to the inflammatory cascade, have not been shown conclusively to affect outcome. The majority of patients become afebrile and normotensive within 48 hours of hospitalization. The erythema disappears within a few days and the muscle pain and weakness resolve in 7 to 10 days.

▶ RECURRENCES

More than half of the patients not treated with a β-lactamase–resistant antibiotic have recurrences. Most recurrent episodes occur by the second month following the initial episode, on the same day of menses as the prior attack. In the majority of patients, the initial episode is the most severe.

▶ THE FUTURE

Toxoid vaccines against superantigens and monoclonal antibody against TSST-1 are being studied.[1] It remains unexplained why some people develop TSS while others do not.

TSS is the best example of superantigen-mediated disease. Early recognition and aggressive management are the keys to reducing morbidity and mortality from this treatable condition.

REFERENCES

1. Chuang YY, Huang YC, Lin TY. Toxic shock syndrome in children: epidemiology, pathogenesis, and management. *Padiatr Drugs.* 2005;7(1):11–25.
2. Martin JM, Green M. Group A streptococcus. *Semin Pediatr Infect Dis.* 2006;17(3):140–148.
3. Lillitos P, Harford D, Michie C. Toxic shock syndrome. *Emerg Nurse.* 2007;15(6):28–33.
4. Centers of Disease Control And Prevention. *Toxic Shock Syndrome.* 1997; http://www.cdc.gov/ncphi/disss/nndss/print/toxic_shock_syndrome_current.htm. Accessed March 24, 2008.
5. Centers for Disease Control and Prevention. *Streptococcal Toxic Shock Syndrome.* 1996. http://www.cdc.gov/ncphi/disss/nndss/print/streptococcalcurrent.htm. Accessed March 24, 2008.
6. Young AE, Thornton KL. Toxic shock syndrome in burns: diagnosis and management. *Arch Dis Child Educ Pract Ed.* 2007;92(4):e97–e100.
7. Edwards-Jones V, Dawson MM, Childs C. A survey into toxic shock syndrome (TSS) in UK burns units. *Burns.* 2000;26(4):323–333.
8. Cole RP, Shakespeare PG. Toxic shock syndrome in scalded children. *Burns.* 1990;16(3):221–224.
9. American Academy of Pediatrics. In: LK P et al., eds. *Red Book: 2006 Report of the Committee on Infectious Diseases.* Elk Grove Village, IL: American Academy of Pediatrics; 2006:660–665.
10. Byer RL, Bachur RG. Clinical deterioration among patients with fever and erythroderma. *Pediatrics.* 2006;118(6):2450–2460.
11. Wu CC. Possible therapies of septic shock: based on animal studies and clinical trials. *Curr Pharm Des.* 2006;12(27):3535–3541.

CHAPTER 63

Kawasaki Disease

Anthony Cooley and Shabnam Jain

▶ HIGH-YIELD FACTS

- The principal pathologic feature of Kawasaki disease (KD) is an acute vasculitis that affects the microvessels (arterioles, venules, and capillaries) anywhere in the body.
- Since there are no pathognomonic laboratory findings, the diagnosis is established clinically by the presence of fever and at least four of five clinical features (conjunctival injection, oropharynx erythema, cervical adenopathy, hand and foot erythema/swelling, and rash).
- As many as 20% of children will have incomplete KD, with only two of conventional diagnostic criteria. Elevated C-reactive protein or erythrocyte sedimentation rate should raise suspicion in these children and consultation with a local expert is advised.
- Caution should be used when trying to exclude the diagnosis of KD based on a positive screen for an infectious etiology. Positive screening tests for infection may identify a concomitant infection, carrier state, or viral shedding.
- All patients diagnosed with Kawasaki syndrome should be hospitalized immediately for administration of intravenous gamma globulin, aspirin therapy, and cardiac evaluation.
- The overall mortality rate of Kawasaki syndrome in American children ranges from 0.1% to 0.2%, with infants younger than 1 year at greatest risk. Mortality peaks 15 to 45 days after the onset of fever. Patients receiving treatment within the first 8 to 10 days of the onset of fever have the best prognosis.

Kawasaki disease (KD), or mucocutaneous lymph node syndrome, is an acute, self-limited, multisystem vasculitis of unclear etiology. KD is the leading cause of acquired heart disease in children in the United States and Japan. The diagnosis is based entirely on fulfilling a defined set of clinical criteria; there are no pathognomonic laboratory findings.

Cases usually occur in clusters throughout the year, particularly during winter and spring. The peak incidence is in children 18 to 24 months of age, with 80% to 85% of cases occurring in children younger than 5 years. It is most common in children of Asian and Pacific Island descent and more common in males than females (1.5:1).[1,2]

▶ ETIOLOGY AND PATHOGENESIS

The etiology is unknown. Given its clinical presentation and epidemiology, an infectious agent or immune response to an infectious agent could be argued. It has been hypothesized that this syndrome may be a unique response of genetically predisposed individuals to some unidentified microbial agent. Alternatively, KD may be an unexplained immunologic response to known microbial agents. Environmental toxins have been suggested but never proven as having a role.[1]

The principal pathologic feature of this syndrome is an acute, nonspecific vasculitis that affects the microvessels (arterioles, venules, and capillaries). Nearly every organ system is involved. In the heart, the vasculitis results in aneurysm formation in 20% to 25% of untreated patients.

▶ CLINICAL FINDINGS

Without pathognomonic laboratory or clinical findings, the diagnosis is established using clinical criteria. Classically, KD is diagnosed by the presence of fever for 5 days and four of five other physical findings (Table 63–1):

- Conjunctival injection without discharge.
- Lip and pharyngeal erythema without exudate.
- Cervical adenopathy.
- Hand and foot swelling and erythema.
- Skin rash (Figs. 63–1 and 63–2).

All symptoms do not need to be present simultaneously to make the diagnosis. When at least four criteria are present, most experts will make the diagnosis of KD on the fourth day of fever.[1,3]

▶ TABLE 63–1. DIAGNOSTIC CRITERIA FOR KAWASAKI SYNDROME

Fever persisting for ≥5 d
And at least four of the following findings:
   Bilateral, painless bulbar conjunctival injection without exudate
   Mucous membrane changes of the oropharynx including injected, dry, cracked lips, and oral mucosal; pharyngeal injection; "strawberry tongue"
   Peripheral extremity changes including erythema and edema of hands and feet in the acute phase; periungual and generalized desquamation in the convalescent phase
   Polymorphous truncal exanthema usually erythematous but may be pustular
   Acute, nonpurulent cervical lymphadenopathy usually >1.5 cm
Findings cannot be explained by some other known disease process

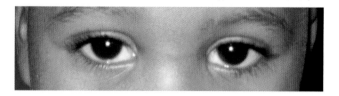

Figure 63–1. Conjunctival injection of Kawasaki disease.

The failure to recognize and treat KD has become a growing concern, particularly in infants. Cases of incomplete KD are being diagnosed with increasing frequency. Up to 20% of children with coronary artery aneurysms fail to meet the classical definition of KD.[3] Therefore, incomplete KD should be considered in children with 5 days of fever and at least two of the classic criteria. Then, a stepwise approach is taken to make the diagnosis (Fig. 63–3). First, acute-phase reactant (C-reactive protein or erythrocyte sedimentation rate) elevation

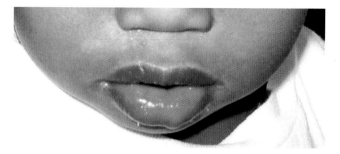

Figure 63–2. Lip findings in Kawasaki disease.

is considered. If present, then supplemental laboratory criteria and echocardiogram findings suggest presence of disease and the need for treatment (Fig. 63–3). Infants younger than 6 months with fever lasting for more than 7 days should be included in this algorithm, even without any physical findings.[1]

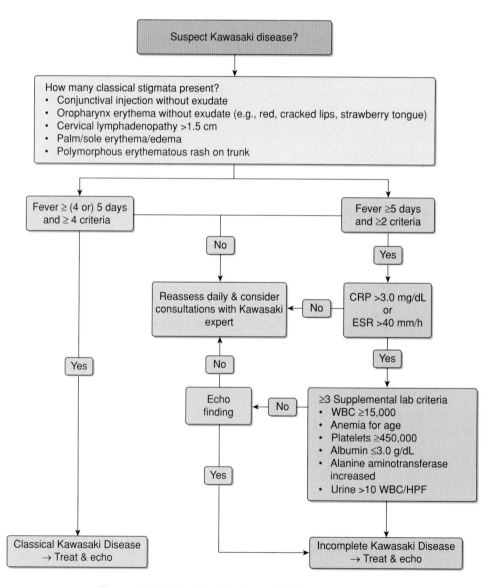

Figure 63–3. Algorithm for diagnosing Kawasaki disease.

▶ PHASES OF KD

ACUTE OR FEBRILE PHASE

The acute phase lasts 7 to 15 days and is the period when most diagnostic clinical features occur. Fever defines this phase. Lasting 7 to 15 days (mean 12 days), the fever typically is unremitting, even with antipyretics. It often is high and associated with irritability.

All physical findings are a consequence of the vasculitis. Bulbar conjunctivitis is bilateral, nonexudative, and spares the limbus. It may persist for several weeks. Mucocutaneous changes may include bright red erythema of the lips with cracking, a strawberry tongue, and hyperemia of the oral mucous membranes. The pharynx may be erythematous, but exudate is not present.

Cervical adenopathy is an early feature. Nodes may not be prominent but they should be at least 1.5 cm in diameter to be considered part of disease. Involvement of the anterior cervical chain is most common and may be unilateral. The lymphadenopathy is nonsuppurative and may disappear rapidly.

Skin changes usually accompany the fever throughout the acute phase and then gradually fade. These rashes are red, polymorphous, and develop in most children. It may be morbilliform, maculopapular, scarlatiniform, or pustular, but vesiculation does not occur.[4,5] The rash may actually vary in character from place to place in a single child. It is mostly seen on the trunk and may be prominent in the diaper area.

Changes in the peripheral extremities occur within a few days after onset. Any part of the hands and feet may be edematous. The palms and soles may be erythematous.

There are many other ancillary features and alternate presentations of KD. In fact, involvement of almost any system can occur (see "Other Complications"). Arthralgia and arthritis, urethritis, gastrointestinal complaints, uveitis, and meningitis are the most common. Although they are not considered diagnostic criteria, these other findings are helpful in supporting the diagnosis.

SUBACUTE PHASE

The subacute phase lasts for approximately 2 to 4 weeks and begins with resolution of fever and elevation of platelet count. It ends with the return of platelet counts to near normal levels.

The subacute phase is dominated by desquamation that may begin before the resolution of fever. Desquamation is a common feature of KD. It is noted first in the periungual region, with peeling underneath the fingernails and toenails. It may also be prominent in the diaper area.

Thrombocytosis is another constant feature of the subacute phase, with platelet counts in the range of 500 000 to 3 000 000/mm^3. Thrombocytosis is rare in the first week of the illness, appears in the second week, peaks in the third week, and returns gradually to normal about a month after onset in uncomplicated illness.

It is during the subacute phase that complications such as coronary artery aneurysms and hydrops of the gall bladder develop (although coronary artery aneurysms may develop during the acute phase as well).

RECOVERY OR CONVALESCENT PHASE

The recovery phase may last months to years. Some coronary artery disease is first recognized during this phase. Resolution of coronary artery disease hopefully occurs during this phase.

▶ ANCILLARY DATA

Laboratory findings are nonspecific in KD. The complete blood count often shows an elevated white blood cell count with a left shift. A mild hemolytic anemia may be present. Elevated platelet counts occur in the subacute phase but are usually normal in the acute phase. Acute-phase reactants (CRP, ESR) are markedly elevated. Urinalysis demonstrates moderate pyuria from urethritis. Bilirubinuria may occur as an early sign of hydrops of the gall bladder.

Chest radiographs may show evidence of pulmonary infiltrates or cardiomegaly. The electrocardiogram may show dysrhythmias, prolonged PR or QT intervals (QTc), and nonspecific ST-T wave changes. Two-dimensional echocardiography may demonstrate coronary artery dilation or aneurysms, pericardial effusion, or decreased contractility.

▶ DIFFERENTIAL DIAGNOSIS

The differential diagnosis is extensive because of the nonspecific nature of the clinical features (Table 63–2). Most viral exanthems can be eliminated based on the clinical course or by epidemiology, the absence of expected findings, or immunization status. Group A β-hemolytic streptococcal or staphylococcal infection usually can be excluded by failure to isolate the

▶ TABLE 63–2. DIFFERENTIAL DIAGNOSIS FOR KAWASAKI SYNDROME

Viral Illnesses
  Rubeola (measles)
  Rubella
  Epstein–Barr virus infection
  Adenovirus infection
  Enterovirus infection
Bacterial Infections
  Toxic shock syndrome
  Scarlet fever
Rickettsial Diseases
  Rocky Mountain spotted fever
  Leptospirosis
Rheumatologic Disease
  Juvenile rheumatoid arthritis
  Systemic lupus erythematosus
  Acute rheumatic fever
Drug/Toxin Reactions
  Serum sickness
  Stevens–Johnson syndrome
  Mercury hypersensitivity (acrodynia)

specific organisms but caution should be used when trying to exclude the diagnosis of KD based on a positive screen for an infectious etiology. Positive screening tests for infection may identify a concomitant infection, carrier-state, or viral shedding. Toxic shock syndrome and rickettsial diseases usually present with thrombocytopenia rather than thrombocytosis.

► COMPLICATIONS

CARDIOVASCULAR

The most serious manifestation of KD is cardiac involvement. In fact, cardiac disease accounts for the vast majority of long-term morbidity and mortality. Furthermore, KD has surpassed rheumatic fever as the leading cause of acquired heart disease in American children. Patients with KD have a 20% to 25% risk of developing coronary aneurysms without treatment. With treatment, this risk drops to 5%. With coronary aneurysms, sudden cardiac death or myocardial infarction may occur. Mortality peaks 15 to 45 days after the first day of fever.[1]

The generalized vasculitis of KD affects coronary arteries as it does all vessels. Initially, there is an influx of neutrophils which are quickly replaced by mononuclear cells, lymphocytes, and plasma cells. Affected vessels suffer dissociation of smooth muscle cells and destruction of the elastic lamina. All of this leads to aneurysm formation. Coronary artery aneurysms typically occur after the first week but before the fourth week of illness. It is uncommon for them to develop after the sixth week.[1]

Auscultation of the heart often reveals a hyperdynamic precordium, tachycardia, gallop rhythm, and flow murmur (associated with anemia). Electrocardiographic changes can be seen and include low voltage and ST depression in the first week of illness, as well as PR prolongation, QT interval prolongation, and ST elevation in the second and third weeks.

Echocardiography is the most sensitive technique for delineating coronary aneurysms. It should be performed as soon as the diagnosis is made, but treatment should not be delayed waiting for echocardiography. Myocarditis is universal and patients may have decreased left ventricular function. Patients at higher risk for development of coronary artery involvement can be determined based on clinical symptoms and signs (Table 63–3).

The most common cause of early death in Kawasaki syndrome is from cardiac sequelae, with a peak occurrence

► TABLE 63–3. RISK FACTORS FOR THE DEVELOPMENT OF CARDIAC SEQUELAE IN KAWASAKI SYNDROME

Male sex
Age <1 y or >8 y
Prolonged fever (>10 d)
Peripheral white blood cell bandemia
Hemoglobin <10 g/dL
Platelets <350 000/µL
Erythrocyte sedimentation rate >101 mm/h
Electrocardiographic abnormality

between 15 and 45 days after the onset of fever. Extremely elevated platelet counts and hypercoagulability place these children with coronary vasculitis at risk for coronary thromboses and myocardial infarction. Aneurysmal rupture is also a risk. Late death may occur from coronary occlusive disease, rupture of an aneurysm several years after onset, or small blood vessel disease of the heart.

OTHER COMPLICATIONS

Urethritis is common, affecting 70% of patients. A sterile pyuria is characterized by white blood cells on microscopy but absence of leukocyte esterase on urinalysis. The latter test is negative because the urethritis is caused by monocytic and lymphocytic infiltration.

Gallbladder hydrops (acute acalculous distention of gallbladder) occurs in 15% of patients. A tender right upper quadrant mass may be palpated. Serum bilirubin will be elevated and the diagnosis can be confirmed by ultrasonography. Even without gall bladder involvement, children may have abdominal pain, vomiting, or diarrhea because of gut vasculitis.

Uveitis occurs in 25% to 50% of patients. Between 10% and 20% develop arthralgia or arthritis. Hearing loss may occur. Aseptic meningitis is also possible.

► MANAGEMENT

All patients diagnosed with KD should be hospitalized immediately for

- administration of intravenous gamma globulin (IVIG).
- aspirin therapy.
- cardiac evaluation.

Routine testing includes complete blood count, erythrocyte sedimentation rate, C-reactive protein, liver profile, bag urinalysis, and echocardiogram.

IVIG has been shown to decrease the incidence of coronary artery aneurysm from 25% to 5%, when given during the acute phase of disease. The dose of IVGG is 2 g/kg infused over 8 to 12 hours as a single dose. IVIG given before the eighth day of fever reduces the risk of cardiac sequelae. However, IVIG should be given to any child who presents later with KD with continuing fever or aneurysm with persistent signs of inflammation.

Aspirin has two roles in the treatment of KD. High-dose aspirin (100 mg/kg/d divided into four doses) is used for its anti-inflammatory effect. Duration of high-dose treatment varies from 48 hours after defervescence to the 14th day of the illness, depending on the center. This is followed by low-dose aspirin (3–5 mg/kg/d as a single-day dose) for its antiplatelet effects; this is continued for at least 6 to 8 weeks and until resolution of coronary abnormalities.

Ten percent of children will have refractory disease, with persistence of fever 36 hours after completion of IVIG. The majority will respond to a second dose of IVIG. For those refractory to this second dose of IVIG, there is limited data about how best to treat them. A third dose of IVIG, high-dose corticosteroids, and tumor necrosis factor inhibitors have been used by experts in some centers.

▶ PROGNOSIS

The prognosis for patients receiving treatment within the first 8 to 10 days of the illness is excellent.

Most aneurysms resolve within the first year with no apparent sequelae. Of the 5% with coronary aneurysms after treatment, 1% persists as giant aneurysms and the remainder regress. Even in patients with regression, there is debate about cardiac risk later in life. Patients may be at greater risk for atherosclerosis.[6] Additionally, it is possible that some patients will have persistently poorly compliant fibrotic vessel walls. All patients with a history of KD should be followed by a cardiologist at regular intervals.

The overall mortality rate of Kawasaki syndrome in American children is between 1 and 2 per 1000.[1] It is higher in infants younger than 1 year.

REFERENCES

1. American Academy of Pediatrics. Diagnosis, treatment, and long-tern management of Kawasaki disease: a statement for health professionals from the committee on rheumatic fever, endocarditis, and Kawasaki disease, councli on cardiovascular disease in the young; and American Heart Association. http://www.pediatrics.org/cgi/full/114/6/1708.
2. Belay ED, Maddox RA, Holman RC, et al. Kawasaki syndrome and risk factors for coronary artery abnormalities: United States, 1994–2003. *Pediatr Infect Dis J.* 2006;25(30):245–249.
3. Witt MT, Minich LL, Bohnsack JF, et al. Kawasaki disease: more patients are being diagnosed who do not meet American Heart Association criteria. *Pediatrics.* 1999;104; e10.
4. Ulloa-Gutierrez R, Acón-Rojas F, Camacho-Badilla K, et al. Pustular rash in Kawasaki syndrome. *Pediatr Infect Dis J.* 2007;26(12):1163–1165.
5. Kwan Y, Leung C. Pustulo-vesicular skin eruption in a child with probably Kawasaki disease. *Eur J Pediatr.* 2005;164(12):770–771.
6. McCrindle BW, McIntyre S, Kim C, et al. Are patients after Kawasaki disease at increased risk for accelerated athersclerosis? *J Pediatr.* 2007;151(3):244–248.

CHAPTER 64

The Pediatric HIV Patient in the ED

John F. Marcinak

▶ HIGH-YIELD FACTS

- Use of highly active antiretroviral therapy (HAART) in children and adolescents has improved survival, decreased hospitalization rates, and transformed HIV infection from a uniformly fatal to a chronic disease.
- The epidemic of HIV in pediatrics has changed from a predominance of infection in infants with perinatal HIV infection to adolescents between 13 and 24 years of age infected through sexual transmission, either heterosexual or men who have sex with men.
- The Centers for Disease Control and Prevention has recommended routine HIV testing for all patients 13 to 64 years of age in health care settings, including the emergency department (ED).
- Rapid HIV tests with high sensitivity and specificity, using blood or oral fluid specimens, are available for diagnostic testing for HIV in the ED.
- Acute HIV infection presents most often as an infectious mononucleosis-like illness and is best diagnosed through use of nucleic acid amplification tests, such as the HIV-1 RNA PCR which measures the viral load in a patient's blood.
- Use of standard precautions, knowledge of the pediatric HIV patient's CD4 count and percentage, as well as communication with the patient's HIV provider are important principles to guide management in the ED.
- Acute HIV infection should be considered in the adolescent who presents to the ED with fever, pharyngitis, oral ulcers, lymphadenopathy, gastrointestinal symptoms, and a maculopapular or papulovesicular rash.
- Infections most likely to be seen in the pediatric or adolescent HIV patient with a CD4 percentage < 25 include herpes zoster and oral candidiasis.
- An important life-threatening complication of antiretroviral therapy to recognize in the pediatric or adolescent patient seen in the ED is lactic acidosis.
- The issue of postexposure prophylaxis for children and adolescents for nonoccupational exposure to HIV is likely to be encountered in the ED setting. Guidelines have been established to aid in the decision-making process for the appropriate use of antiretroviral medications for nonoccupational postexposure prophylaxis (nPEP).

Since human immunodeficiency virus (HIV) infection was first identified in 1981, the epidemic of HIV in the pediatric age group has affected a disproportionate number of infants born to mothers with HIV infection. These infants with perinatal HIV infection were born with what was considered a fatal infection but has now been transformed into a chronic disease.

Many of these infants with perinatal HIV infection have now reached adolescence. Decreased rates of hospitalization[1] and mortality[1-3] have recently been found in children and adolescents with perinatal HIV-1 infection. The most likely reason for improved survival of children with HIV infection has been the introduction of highly active antiretroviral therapy (HAART), which was first begun in 1996 and by 1999 was being received by almost three-quarters of children and adolescents with HIV infection.[1] Decreased rates of hospitalization have also corresponded to an expanded use of HAART. Many children with perinatal HIV infection are diagnosed during infancy or early childhood, but it is possible for the diagnosis to be made later in school age or early adolescence. Up to 25% of perinatally infected children develop severe immunosuppression in the first year of life, but the majority of children have a slower progression to AIDS with a mean time period of 6 to 9 years.[4] With the advent of HAART therapy, the natural history of HIV-1 infection in children has been altered. However, there are children treated with HAART who have not been able to achieve or sustain viral suppression over time. These children have a poorer prognosis than children who achieve complete viral suppression and are at risk for complications of AIDS. The natural history of HIV infection in adolescents with horizontally acquired HIV infection is similar to that of adults. In the absence of antiretroviral (ARV) therapy, a 13-year-old adolescent would be expected to develop AIDS 10 to 12 years after primary infection with HIV.[4]

▶ EPIDEMIOLOGY

In the United States, HIV infection affects a disproportionate number of nonhispanic black and hispanic children and adolescents. Nonhispanic black and hispanic women are also overrepresented in the HIV epidemic. This has important implications for the racial distribution of infants with perinatal infection. There has been a significant decline in mother-to-child transmission (MTCT) of HIV since 1994. This has been attributed to U.S. Public Health Service Guidelines regarding use of zidovudine (ZDV) to reduce MTCT of HIV (1994) and universal HIV counseling and voluntary HIV testing of pregnant women (1995). Cases of MTCT have declined from an estimated 1650 HIV-infected infants born each year during the mid-1990s to 144 to 236 in 2002.[5]

As previously noted, there are a growing number of HIV perinatally infected children who are surviving into the age of adolescence. Compared to adolescents with newly acquired HIV infection, these adolescents are more likely to have received HAART that is prolonging the life of the adolescents

▶ **TABLE 64–1. DISTRIBUTION OF HIV INFECTION AND AIDS CASES REPORTED AMONG 13- TO 19-YEAR-OLD ADOLESCENTS (BY SEX) IN 2005**

Sex	HIV Infection (%)*	AIDS (%)†
Female	36	43
Male	64	57

*Data from 33 states with confidential name-based HIV infection reporting since 2001.
†Reported in 2005—United States and dependent areas.
Source: US Centers for Disease Control.

with perinatal HIV infection. Newly acquired HIV in adolescents is still a significant public health problem. Half of new HIV infections in the United States are occurring in youths aged 13 to 24 years and 75% of infected youths are in racial or ethnic minority groups.[6] Adolescent females are also at a significant risk for HIV infection and development of AIDS. In 2005, adolescent females aged 13 to 19 years accounted for over one-third of the cases of HIV infection reported to the Centers for Disease Control and Prevention (CDC). These cases came from 33 states that have used confidential name-based HIV infection surveillance since 2001 and also over 40% of AIDS case reports from the District of Columbia, the 50 states, and U.S. territories (Table 64–1). In addition, approximately 25% of sexually transmitted infections (STIs) reported in the United States are among adolescents. This is of significance since the risk of HIV transmission increases if either partner is infected with an STI. In addition, female adolescents have unique risk factors of biological vulnerability, which increase susceptibility to HIV acquisition. These include the physical development of the cervix during puberty; the cervix is composed of single-layer columnar epithelial cells, which are more susceptible to infection. In addition, STIs are often asymptomatic in women and transmission of HIV from male to female is more efficient than from female to male.[6]

▶ DIAGNOSIS

The diagnosis of HIV infection in the pediatric and adolescent age group depends upon a number of factors, most important of which include age, clinical presentation, and the diagnostic test employed. Two important examples regarding the use of HIV antibody testing by enzyme immunoassay (EIA) is that the HIV EIA should not be used for diagnosis of HIV in infants younger than 18 months or for diagnosis of acute HIV infection in an older pediatric or adolescent patient. In September 2006, CDC proposed revised recommendations for HIV testing in health care settings, which includes hospital EDs.[7] The rationale for routine HIV testing includes the quality of the screening tests available as well as the need to know the diagnosis, which is strongly related to prevention and care. Routine testing for HIV infection is recommended for all patients aged 13 to 64 years (not risk based). Screening should be voluntary with the patient's knowledge and understanding, and consent for testing is included in the consent for care with testing performed unless the patient declines (referred to as "opt-out" screening). A patient with a positive HIV test must

be linked to care and have access to prevention counseling. However, prevention counseling is not required as part of the HIV screening program.

The use of rapid HIV testing in the ED as a strategy to identify persons with previously undiagnosed HIV infection has received considerable attention over the past few years. As of February 2008, there are currently six rapid HIV tests approved by the U.S. Food and Drug Administration using blood (either whole blood, serum, or plasma) and/or oral fluid (one only). Four of these tests are easy to perform with negligible chance for error and therefore CLIA (Clinical Laboratory Improvements Amendments) waived. These rapid HIV tests have shown a very high sensitivity and specificity (both > 99%) for diagnosing HIV infection.[8] Use of rapid HIV testing has been shown to be feasible and acceptable for patients as part of routine health care services in three EDs (Los Angeles, New York, and Oakland) using an opt-in (patients offered testing and testing performed if agreed and written consent provided) method for consent for HIV testing.[9] Overall, 1.0% of patients tested were HIV positive and 12.4% of the HIV-positive groups were in the age range of 12 to 24 years. However, only Oakland tested patients who were ≥ 12 years old while the other 2 sites enrolled patients ≥ 18 years. A recent study of routine HIV screening using the OraQuick Rapid HIV (1/2 antibody test with an oral fluid specimen) in adolescents and adults aged 13 to 64 years seen in urban EDs found opt-out HIV testing to be feasible with 60% of the patients who were offered HIV screening accepting the test.[10] In this study, 26 (1.1% of all patients tested) had a positive rapid HIV test, but only 13 (50%) could be reached for follow-up. Of the 13 who could be reached for follow-up, there were 4 false-positive test results, but in this setting the specificity of the rapid HIV test was still 99.8%. Of the 9 with confirmatory HIV testing, 8 (89%) were successfully linked to care. In another cross-sectional survey study of the acceptance of opt-out routine rapid HIV testing in adults ≥ 18 years seen in an urban ED, 81% of those surveyed indicated that they would agree to have an HIV test using an opt-out strategy.[11] However, 11% indicated a need for an explanation of opt-out screening. There is currently no information available regarding the acceptance of opt-out HIV testing of adolescents in an ED setting.

With the long incubation period from acquisition of HIV infection to development of AIDS, an adolescent infected with HIV may not be diagnosed until the early thirties. However, another opportunity to make the diagnosis of HIV infection early in the course of the infection is to recognize acute HIV infection. Acute infection with HIV is usually associated with a self-limited infectious mononucleosis-like illness. A study performed on stored serum samples that were initially collected for Epstein–Barr virus heterophil antibody testing and were negative revealed that 7 of 563 (1.2%) were consistent with acute HIV-1 infection.[12] The specimens from these seven patients had very high quantitative HIV-1 RNA (viral load) levels and four of the seven had negative HIV ELISA results. The appearance of HIV-1 markers in plasma donors with primary HIV infection has established a pattern of detection of various diagnostic tests.[13] Currently, there are also third-generation HIV EIAs that, in addition to detecting IgG, also detect IgM antibodies, which develop earlier after infection.[14] The viral load, as measured by quantitative RNA PCR, is the test with the shortest time from infection to development of a positive test

▶ **TABLE 64-2. TIME OF HIV INFECTION FOR VARIOUS DIAGNOSTIC HIV-1 MARKERS**

Marker	Time at Which HIV Can First Be Detected
Antibody*	22 d
p 24 antigen	16 d
RNA by PCR	9 d

*Third-generation, IgM sensitive EIA (enzyme immunoassay).
Data from Fiebig EW, Wright DJ, Rawal BD, et al. Dynamics of HIV viremia and antibody seroconversion in plasma donors: implications for diagnosis and staging of primary HIV infection. *AIDS*. 2003;17:1871.
Data from Branson BM. State of the art for diagnosis of HIV infection. *Clin Infect Dis*. 2007;45:S221.

(Table 64–2). Testing for both HIV-1 RNA and HIV antibody should be performed when acute HIV infection is being considered.

▶ CLINICAL PRESENTATIONS

The pediatric and adolescent patient with perinatal HIV infection will have occasion to be seen in the ED setting. There are a few important principles that guide ED management of the child or adolescent known to have HIV infection. These include understanding of appropriate infection-control procedures, noting the patient's CD4 count/percentage, and consultation with the patient's primary HIV care provider.[15] First, standard precautions should be followed by all health care personnel who care for HIV-infected patients in the ED. Second, knowledge of the patient's CD4 count and percentage reflects the risk of a patient for developing an opportunistic infection and disease progression. In pediatric patients < 13 years of age, a CD4 percentage ≥ 25% indicates no immune suppression, while a CD4 percentage of 15 to 24 indicates moderate immune suppression and < 15% represents severe immune suppression.[16] Finally, close communication with the patient's primary HIV provider will be of great assistance in appropriate management and follow-up of the pediatric or adolescent patient with HIV seen in the ED.

Although the number of new perinatal HIV infections in the United States has significantly declined, it is important to consider HIV infection in an infant who presents to the ED with significant respiratory distress, including cough, tachypnea, and hypoxia and in whom maternal HIV positive status has not been recognized during pregnancy. These infants are most likely to present at 3 to 6 months of age with diffuse interstitial infiltrates on chest x-ray, which results in respiratory failure. The diagnosis of pneumocystis pneumonia (PCP) caused by *Pneumocystis jiroveci* can be best confirmed by direct fluorescent antibody (DFA) staining of a specimen obtained by bronchoalveolar lavage (BAL). Although opportunistic infections such as PCP would certainly raise the suspicion of HIV infection, other common serious bacterial infections such as pneumonia, recurrent otitis media and sinusitis, meningitis, and sepsis can be the first manifestations of disease in children with HIV infection. In a series of 172 children with perinatal HIV infection diagnosed between 1981 and 1987, prior

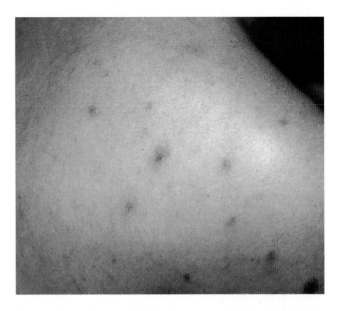

Figure 64–1. Primary HIV infection. A maculopapular rash is seen in more than half of persons with symptomatic acute HIV infection. This less typical papular/vesicular rash was present in a patient with primary HIV infection. (Courtesy of Gregory K. Robbins, MD, MPH.)

to advent of the use of ARV therapy in children, most children became symptomatic before 1 year of age, although close to one-quarter presented with symptomatic disease after the age of 2 years.[17] Failure to thrive and developmental delay can also be the presenting clinical findings in children with HIV infection.

An adolescent with acute HIV infection will often present with fever, pharyngitis, oral ulcers, lymphadenopathy, and gastrointestinal symptoms.[18] A maculopapular rash is seen in more than 50% of cases reported in most series but a papulovesicular rash can also be seen (Fig. 64–1). Other common clinical manifestations of acute HIV infection include arthralgias, myalgias, genital ulcers, aseptic meningitis, encephalopathy, and peripheral neuropathy. More unusual manifestations of acute HIV infection have included clinical hepatitis, acute pneumonitis, aplastic anemia, vasculitis, rhabdomyolysis Guillain–Barré syndrome, and facial nerve palsy.[19] The most common laboratory abnormalities found in acute HIV infection include leukopenia, lymphopenia, and thrombocytopenia.

▶ COMPLICATIONS IN HIV-INFECTED PATIENTS

There are many complications that can occur with HIV-infected pediatric and adolescent patients, both infectious and noninfectious. In the ED, most pediatric and adolescent patients with HIV infection will be prescribed HAART therapy. It is important to be aware of what opportunistic illnesses and infections are likely to still occur in the HAART era. A large multicenter cohort study designed to examine long-term outcomes in HIV-infected children currently provides the best data to answer this question. The incidence of opportunistic and other infections was determined in 2767 HIV-infected infants, children, and

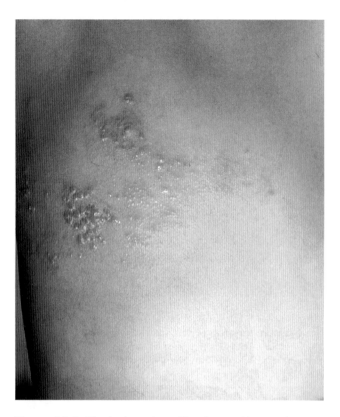

Figure 64–2. Single dermatomal involvement in a patient with herpes zoster infection in a thoracic distribution.

adolescents for a 4-year period between 2001 and 2004.[20] In this study, the percentage of children receiving HAART remained stable from 69% to 71% over the 4 years. The four most common first-time infections found were bacterial pneumonia, herpes zoster (Fig. 64–2), oral candidiasis, and dermatophyte infections with incidence rates (IR) per 100 person-years of 2.15, 1.11, 0.93, and 0.88, respectively. At the time of first infection, one-half of all children had a CD4 percentage of at least 25%. Of the four most common infections, the two more likely to occur in children with a CD4 percentage < 25 were herpes zoster (60%) and oral candidiasis (73%). Less commonly reported opportunistic infections, such as PCP and disseminated *Mycobacterium avium* complex, occurred in children with CD4 percentage < 25. In a 2004 study of 811 perinatally HIV-infected children, substantial herpes zoster was still found to be occurring (IR of 5.9 per 100 person-years). CD4 percentage < 15 was a significant risk factor.[21] In another related study in the same setting, 1927 children with perinatal HIV infection who were receiving HAART were followed from 2000 to 2003 and occurrence of opportunistic illnesses determined.[22] Overall, 12.7% developed opportunistic illnesses during follow-up and opportunistic illness was strongly associated with a CD4 percentage < 15. This data emphasizes the importance of knowing the most recent CD4 count and percentage in the child or adolescent with HIV infection who presents to the ED.

Children and adolescents with HIV infection can have significant oral and dental lesions. These include dental caries, gingivitis, aphthous ulcers, herpes stomatitis, oral candidiasis, and tongue lesions, such as depapillated tongue and median

rhomboid glossitis. A recent study in HIV perinatally infected children receiving HAART found that the two most common conditions seen were dental caries and gingivitis in 20% each.[23] Overall, oral lesions were most common in children with severe immunosuppression (CD4 percentage < 15). Bilateral cervical lymph node, as well as parotid gland, enlargement can also occur and is more common with severe immunosuppression. Patients with generalized cervical, axillary, and inguinal lymphadenopathy are also more likely to have uncontrolled viral replication with elevated viral loads as measured by RNA PCR. If an HIV-infected child or adolescent presents with asymmetric lymphadenopathy that has persisted for weeks in spite of antibiotic therapy, a malignancy such as lymphoma (most commonly non-Hodgkin lymphoma) and Hodgkin disease[24] should be strongly considered.

The HIV-infected child or adolescent may present to the ED with a chief complaint of pain. Pain in children and adolescents with HIV/AIDS is multifactorial and has been associated with increased mortality.[25] In a study of 985 HIV-infected children followed between 1995 and 1999, the prevalence of pain remained relatively constant during each year of observation, averaging 20%. Reporting of pain was significantly associated with female gender and lower CD4 percentage and there was also a significant association between report of pain and mortality. Some of the diagnoses observed to have painful manifestations, which occurred in at least one-third, include peripheral neuropathy (53%), aphthous ulcers (40%), urinary tract infection (40%), candidiasis (36%), colitis (35%), and cellulitis (33%).

Pediatric and adolescent patients with HIV infection may also develop central nervous system infections, such as acute bacterial meningitis or encephalitis caused by HIV or other opportunistic infections. A number of neurologic complications associated with HIV infection can also occur. These can involve the peripheral nervous system, such as peripheral neuropathy, or the central nervous system, manifesting as HIV-associated neurocognitive disorder (HAND). In addition, the incidence of psychiatric hospitalizations among HIV-infected children and adolescents younger than 15 years have been reported to be significantly higher than the same age group in the general pediatric population.[26] The most common reasons for hospitalization were depression, behavioral disorders, and suicidal ideation/attempts.

ARV therapy in children and adolescents can be associated with a number of adverse effects. Although the benefits of ARV therapy include decreased HIV progression and improved survival, there are potential downsides of therapy. These include the development of drug resistance and adverse effects, including toxicity and long-term complications.[27] Regarding adverse effects, the organs most involved include the gastrointestinal tract, liver, pancreas, skin, bone marrow, bone, and nervous system. The experience with the use of combination ARV therapy has led to the recognition of several distinct adverse drug effects. These include mitochondrial dysfunction (including lactic acidosis and hepatic toxicity), metabolic abnormalities (such as fat maldistribution, body habitus changes, hyperlipidemia, hyperglycemia and insulin resistance, osteopenia, osteoporosis, and osteonecrosis), hematologic complications, and allergic reactions.[28] Currently, the four main classes of ARV drugs available for pediatric patients include the nucleoside/nucleotide analogue reverse transcriptase inhibitors

► TABLE 64–3. DISTINCT ADVERSE DRUG EVENTS WITH INDIVIDUAL OR CLASSES OF ANTIRETROVIRAL (ARV) THERAPY

Adverse Event	Class of ARV	Associated Individual ARVs
Lactic acidosis	NRTIs	Didanosine, Stavudine, Zidovudine Lamivudine
Hepatic toxicity	All NRTIs, NNRTIs, PIs	Common to all the classes
	Fusion inhibitor	Enfuvurtide
Hyperglycemia	PIs	Common to the entire class
Hematologic (anemia and neutropenia)	NRTIs	Zidovudine, Didanosine, Stavudine
Skin rash (maculopapular)	NNRTIs	Common to the entire class
	PIs	Amprenavir, Fosamprenavir, Atazanavir, Darunavir, Tipranavir
	NRTIs	Abacavir
Hypersensitivity reaction	NRTIs	Abacavir
	NRTIs	Nevirapine
	Fusion inhibitor	Enfuvurtide
Stevens-Johnson syndrome	NNRTIs	Nevirapine, Efavirenz, Delaviridine

NRTIs, nucleoside analogue reverse transcriptase inhibitors; NNRTIs, nonnucleoside analogue reverse transcriptase inhibitors; PIs, protease inhibitors.

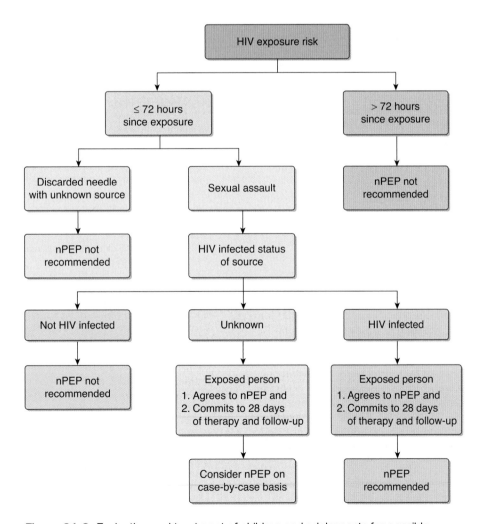

Figure 64–3. Evaluation and treatment of children and adolescents for possible nonoccupational exposure to HIV from a discarded needle or sexual assault.

(NRTIs/NtRTIs), non-nucleoside analogue reverse transcriptase inhibitors (NNRTIs), protease inhibitors (PIs), and fusion inhibitors. It is important to determine the complete list of the ARV medications the pediatric or adolescent patient is receiving because significant adverse events are associated with specific individual or groups of ARV medications (Table 64–3). Life-threatening and fatal cases of lactic acidosis have been reported in HIV-infected children.[29,30] The onset can be acute or subacute and initial symptoms are nonspecific with generalized fatigue, weakness, and myalgias. Gastrointestinal (nausea, vomiting, diarrhea, abdominal pain, and anorexia), respiratory (tachypnea and dyspnea), or neurologic symptoms (motor weakness) can occur. Diagnostic evaluation should include serum lactate, serum bicarbonate, hepatic transaminases, serum albumin, amylase, lipase, and arterial blood gases. Imaging studies, such as abdominal ultrasound or CT scan, should be considered to evaluate for hepatic steatosis or pancreatitis. All ARV drugs should be discontinued during the evaluation for lactic acidosis in HIV-infected children.

▶ POSTEXPOSURE PROPHYLAXIS

In the pediatric ED, the issue of HIV postexposure prophylaxis in children and adolescents is particularly relevant as it relates to nonoccupational exposure. The two areas where the decision to offer nonoccupational postexposure prophylaxis (nPEP) is most likely to arise is in the setting of a needlestick injury and sexual assault. Both the American Academy of Pediatrics[31] and the CDC[32] have issued nPEP guidelines. There have been no confirmed reports of HIV transmission from percutaneous injury by a needle found in the community. Victims of sexual assault are at much higher risk for HIV transmission. This would include a child who is a victim of sexual abuse as well as an adolescent who is a victim of sexual assault or reports unprotected sex with a partner who is known to have HIV. Use of nPEP should be considered only if the exposure has occurred within 72 hours, the exposed patient voluntarily accepts nPEP and agrees to 28 days of ARV medications for prophylaxis and appropriate follow-up (Fig. 64–3). The preferred ARV medications recommended by the CDC are three drug HAART regimens that are either NNRTI- or PI-based.[32] Completion of a 28-day course of ARV medications and close follow-up may be difficult in adolescents who are victims of sexual assault.[33,34] In a recent prospective study of nPEP for HIV in adolescents who presented to a pediatric ED within 72 hours of sexual assault, only 27% completed the entire recommended course of a two-medication ARV regimen for nPEP and about half experienced adverse events associated with the medications.[34] In adolescent victims of sexual assault in whom nPEP is recommended or considered, a 3- to 5-day starter pack of ARV medications should be offered if nPEP is accepted by the adolescent. Contact and follow-up with a pediatric and adolescent HIV provider should be strongly encouraged.

REFERENCES

1. Gortmaker SL, Hughs M, Cervia J, et al. Effect of combination therapy including protease inhibitors on mortality among children and adolescents infected with HIV-1. *N Engl J Med.* 2001;345:1522.

2. Selik RM, Lindegren ML. Changes in deaths reported with human immunodeficiency virus infection among United States children less than thirteen years old, 1987–1999. *Pediatr Infect Dis J.* 2003;22:635.

3. Viani RM, Araneta MRG, Deville JG, et al. Decrease in hospitalization and mortality rates among children with perinatally acquired HIV type 1 infection receiving highly active antiretroviral therapy. *Clin Infect Dis.* 2004;39:725.

4. Aldrovandi GM. The natural history of pediatric HIV disease. In: Zeichner S, Read J, eds. *Textbook of Pediatric HIV Care.* New York: Cambridge University Press; 2005:68–83.

5. Centers for Disease Control and Prevention. Reduction in perinatal transmission of HIV infection—United States, 1982–2005. *MMWR Morb Mortal Wkly Rep.* 2006;55(21):592.

6. Futterman D. Perspective-HIV in adolescents and young adults: Half of all new infections in the United States. *Topics HIV Med.* 2005;13:101.

7. Centers for Disease Control and Prevention. Revised recommendations for HIV testing of adults, adolescents, and pregnant women in health-care settings. *MMWR Morb Mortal Wkly Rep.* 2006;55(RR-14):1.

8. Greenwald JL, Burstein GR, Pincus J, et al. A rapid review of rapid HIV antibody tests. *Curr Infect Dis Rep.* 2006;8:125.

9. Centers for Disease Control and Prevention. Rapid HIV testing in emergency departments-three U. S. sites, January 2005-March 2006. *MMWR Morb Mortal Wkly Rep.* 2007;56(24):597.

10. Brown J, Shesser R, Simon G, et al. Routine HIV screening in the emergency department using the new US Centers for Disease Control and Prevention guidelines: results from a high-prevalence area. *J Acquir Immune Defic Syndr.* 2007;46:395.

11. Haukoos J, Hopkins E, Byyny RL. Patient acceptance of rapid HIV testing practices in an urban emergency department: assessment of the 2006 CDC recommendations for HIV screening in health care settings. *Ann Emerg Med.* 2008;51:303.

12. Rosenberg ES, Caliendo AM, Walker BD. Acute HIV infection among patients tested for mononucleosis. *N Engl J Med.* 1999;340:969.

13. Fiebig EW, Wright DJ, Rawal BD, et al. Dynamics of HIV viremia and antibody seroconversion in plasma donors: implications for diagnosis and staging of primary HIV infection. *AIDS.* 2003;17:1871.

14. Branson BM. State of the art for diagnosis of HIV infection. *Clin Infect Dis.* 2007;45:S221.

15. Church JA. Pediatric HIV in the emergency department. *Clin Pediatr Emerg Med.* 2007;8:117.

16. Centers for Disease Control and Prevention. 1994 revised classification system for human immunodeficiency virus infection in children less than 13 years of age. *MMWR Morb Mortal Wkly Rep.* 1994;43(RR-12):1.

17. Scott GB, Hutto C, Makuch RW, et al. Survival in children with perinatally acquired human immunodeficiency virus type 1 infection. *N Engl J Med.* 1989;321:1791.

18. Aggarwal M, Rein J. Acute human immunodeficiency syndrome in and adolescent. *Pediatrics.* 2003;112:e323.

19. Russel ND, Sepkowitz KA. Primary HIV infection: clinical, immunologic, and virologic predictors of progression. *AIDS Reader.* 1998;8:164.

20. Gona P, Van Dyke RB, Williams PL, et al. Incidence of opportunistic and other infections in HIV-infected children in the HAART era. *JAMA.* 2006;296:292.

21. Anderson J, Levin M, Williams P, et al. Incidence and predictors of herpes zoster in pediatric HIV in the HAART era. http://www.retroconference.org/2006/Denver, CO 2006. Accessed March 15, 2008.

22. Ylitalo N, Brogly S, Hughes MD, et al. Risk factors for opportunistic illnesses in children with human immunodeficiency virus in the era of highly active antiretroviral therapy. *Arch Pediatr Adolesc Med.* 2006;160:778.

23. Okunseri C, Badner V, Wiznia A, et al. Prevalence of oral lesions and percent CD4+ T-lymphocytes in HIV-infected children on antiretroviral therapy. *AIDS Patient Care.* 2003;17:5.

24. Kest H, Brogly S, McSherry G, et al. Malignancy in perinatally human immunodeficiency virus-infected children in the United States. *Pediatr Infect Dis J.* 2005;24:237.

25. Gaughan DM, Hughes MD, Seage GR III, et al. The prevalence of pain in pediatric human immunodeficiency virus/acquired immunodeficiency syndrome as reported by participants in the pediatric late outcomes study(PACTG 219). *Pediatrics.* 2002;109:1144.

26. Gaughan DM, Hughes MD, Oleske JM, et al. Psychiatric hospitalizations among children and youths with human immunodefiency virus infection. *Pediatrics.* 2004;113:e544.

27. Yogev R. Balancing the upside and downside of antiretroviral therapy in children. *JAMA.* 2005;293:2272.

28. The National Institutes of Health. Guidelines for the use of antiretroviral agents in pediatric HIV infection. *Supplement III: Adverse Drug Effects.* Bethesda, MD; 2008. http://AIDSinfo.nih.gov/. Accessed March 15, 2008.

29. Carter RW, Singh J, Archambault C, et al. Severe lactic acidosis in association with reverse transcriptase inhibitors with potential response to L-carnitine in a pediatric HIV-positive patient. *AIDS Patient Care STDs.* 2004;18:131.

30. Rey C, Prieto S, Medina A, et al. Fatal lactic acidosis during antiretroviral therapy. *Pediatr Crit Care Med.* 2003;4:485.

31. Havens PL; and Committee on Pediatric AIDS. Postexposure prophylaxis in children and adolescents for nonoccupational exposure to human immunodeficiency virus. *Pediatrics.* 2003;111:1475.

32. Centers for Disease Control and Prevention. Antiretroviral postexposure prophylaxis after sexual, injection-drug use, or other nonoccupational exposure to HIV in the United States; Recommendations from the US Department of Health and Human Services. *MMWP Morb Mortal Wkly Rep.* 2005; 54(RR-2):1.

33. Olshen E, Hsu K, Woods ER, et al. Use of hunan immunodeficiency virus postexposure prophylaxis in adolescent sexual assault victims. *Arch Pediatr Adolesc Med.* 2006;160: 674.

34. Neu N, Hefferan-Vacca S, Millery M, et al. Postexposure prophylaxis for HIV in children and adolescents after sexual assault: a prospective observational study in an urban medical center. *Sex Transm Dis.* 2007;34:65.

CHAPTER 65

Tick-Borne Infections

Scott A. Heinrich, Marcie Stoshak-Chavez, and Kemedy K. McQuillen

▶ HIGH-YIELD FACTS

- The best ways to prevent tick-borne diseases are to avoid tick exposure and ensure prompt tick removal if bites do occur. Children that are going to be in rural, wooded areas in endemic regions should wear long-sleeved shirts buttoned at the cuff and long pants tucked into their socks. Clothing may be sprayed with 0.5% permethrin and diethyltoluamide (DEET) can also be used at concentrations of 20% to 30%.
- Attached ticks should be removed as soon as possible to lessen the risk of infection. Viscous lidocaine may be applied to kill the tick and anesthetize the site, followed by gentle, continuous traction with a pair of fine forceps to the tick's head, ensuring that the tick is not crushed.
- *Borrelia burgdorferi*, the most common cause of Lyme disease in the United States, is a gram-negative organism that is transmitted by ticks of the *Ixodes ricinus* complex.
- The most common manifestation of early-localized Lyme disease is erythema migrans, the "bull's eye" rash, which usually begins within 7 to 10 days of tick infection.
- Antibiotics recommended for children with erythema migrans are
  - amoxicillin (50 mg/kg/d in three divided doses, maximum of 500 mg/dose)
  - cefuroxime axetil (30 mg/kg/d in two divided doses, maximum of 500 mg/dose)
  - doxycycline (4 mg/kg/d in two divided doses, maximum of 100 mg/dose)
    – if the child is ≥ 8 years old
- Rocky Mountain spotted fever (RMSF) is the most common tick-borne rickettsial disease in the United States and is one of the most virulent human infections identified.
- The American dog tick (*Dermacentor variabilis*) is the primary vector of *R. rickettsii* in most of the United States, while the Rocky Mountain wood tick (*D. andersoni*) is a major culprit in the mountain states and Canada.
- Symptoms of RMSF usually appear approximately 7 days after tick exposure, although a history of tick bite is only elicited in 50% to 60% of patients. The initial phase of RMSF infection is characterized by sudden onset of fever, malaise, and severe headache, with accompanying nonspecific symptoms such as myalgias, nausea and vomiting, abdominal pain, anorexia, and photophobia.
- The rash of RMSF usually begins as blanching, erythematous macules on the wrists and ankles, and spreads centripetally to the arms, legs, and trunks within hours. The palms and soles are also involved.
- Because RMSF has a 20% mortality rate if untreated and up to a 5% rate if treated, and rapid confirmatory diagnosis is not easily achieved, antibiotic therapy should be started when the disease is suspected. Doxycycline is the drug of choice for treating RMSF regardless of the child's age.

Ticks are capable of transmitting numerous diseases to children including bacterial, viral, and parasitic pathogens. Many of the tick-borne diseases have higher incidences in children than in the general population, thus clinicians who treat the pediatric population must be especially aware of them. As most patients do not recall a tick bite, tick-borne illnesses should be included in the differential diagnosis of nonspecific febrile illnesses, especially in the presence of an associated rash (Fig. 65–1).

The best ways to prevent tick-borne diseases are to avoid tick exposure and ensure prompt tick removal if bites do occur. Children that are going to be in rural, wooded areas in endemic regions should wear long-sleeved shirts buttoned at the cuff and long pants tucked into their socks. Clothing may be sprayed with 0.5% permethrin. DEET, a commercially available insect repellant, can also be used at concentrations of 20% to 30%. Attached ticks should be removed as soon as possible to lessen the risk of infection. First, viscous lidocaine may be applied to kill the tick and anesthetize the site. Next, gentle, continuous traction is applied with a pair of fine forceps to the tick's head, ensuring that the tick is not crushed. Lastly, ensure that all parts of the tick have been removed.[1]

▶ LYME DISEASE

Lyme disease is currently the most common vector-borne illness in both the United States and Europe, with more than 20 000 new cases reported each year in the United States.[1,2] Ninety-three percent of the reported cases in the United States occur in the 10 reference states where Lyme disease is endemic: Connecticut, Delaware, Maryland, Massachusetts, Minnesota, New Jersey, New York, Pennsylvania, Rhode Island, and Wisconsin.[3] Figure 65–2 shows the endemic distribution of cases throughout the United States. Lyme disease occurs most commonly in children, with 61% of cases occurring in children aged 5 to 14 years, although there is a median age of 41 years and a bimodal distribution.[2] There is a slight male predominance. The vast majority (74%) of patients have illness onset between the warmer months of May and August.[2]

Lyme borreliosis is caused by infection with a spirochete of the group *B. burgdorferi* sensu lato.[4] In Europe, most of

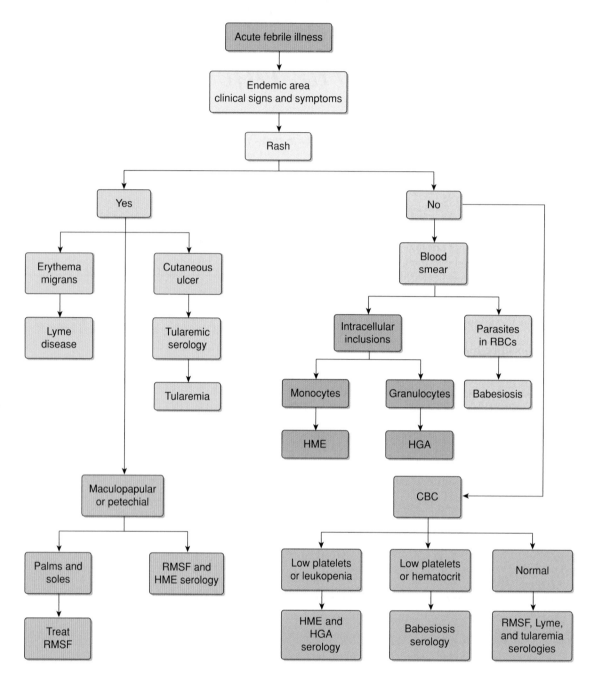

Figure 65–1. Algorithm for differentiating between tick-borne illnesses. This algorithm should be used as a general guide based on common clinical signs and symptoms and should not be used for final diagnosis.

the illness is caused by *B. afzeli* and *B. garinii*, while in the United States only *B. burgdorferi* is pathogenic in humans.[5] *B. burgdorferi* is a gram-negative organism that is maintained and transmitted by ticks of the *I. ricinus* complex.[6] *I. scapularis* (also called *I. dammini*) predominates in the northeast and northcentral regions of the United States (Figs. 65–3 and 65–4), while *I. pacificus* is present on the West Coast and *I. ricinus* in Europe. Many animals may serve as reservoirs for *Borrelia* including birds, mice, deer, voles, dormice, and some lizards.[4]

Lyme disease is spread when an infected tick feeds on an individual, transmitting the *Borrelia* spirochete. There are var-

ious factors that affect the likelihood of *B. burgdorferi* spread. The percentage of ticks infected in a given geographic area is first and probably most important. In the northeast and Midwest United States, 30% to 40% of adult *I. scapularis* and 10% to 20% of nymphal stage ticks are infected with *B. burgdorferi*, while in Europe, the number is nearer to 20%. However, only about 1% to 3% of *I. pacificus* ticks on the West Coast of the United States are infected with *B. burgdorferi*.[4] A second factor that determines the spread of disease is the duration of tick attachment and feeding. For a substantial rate of transmission to occur, the tick has to be attached for more than 48 hours.[6]

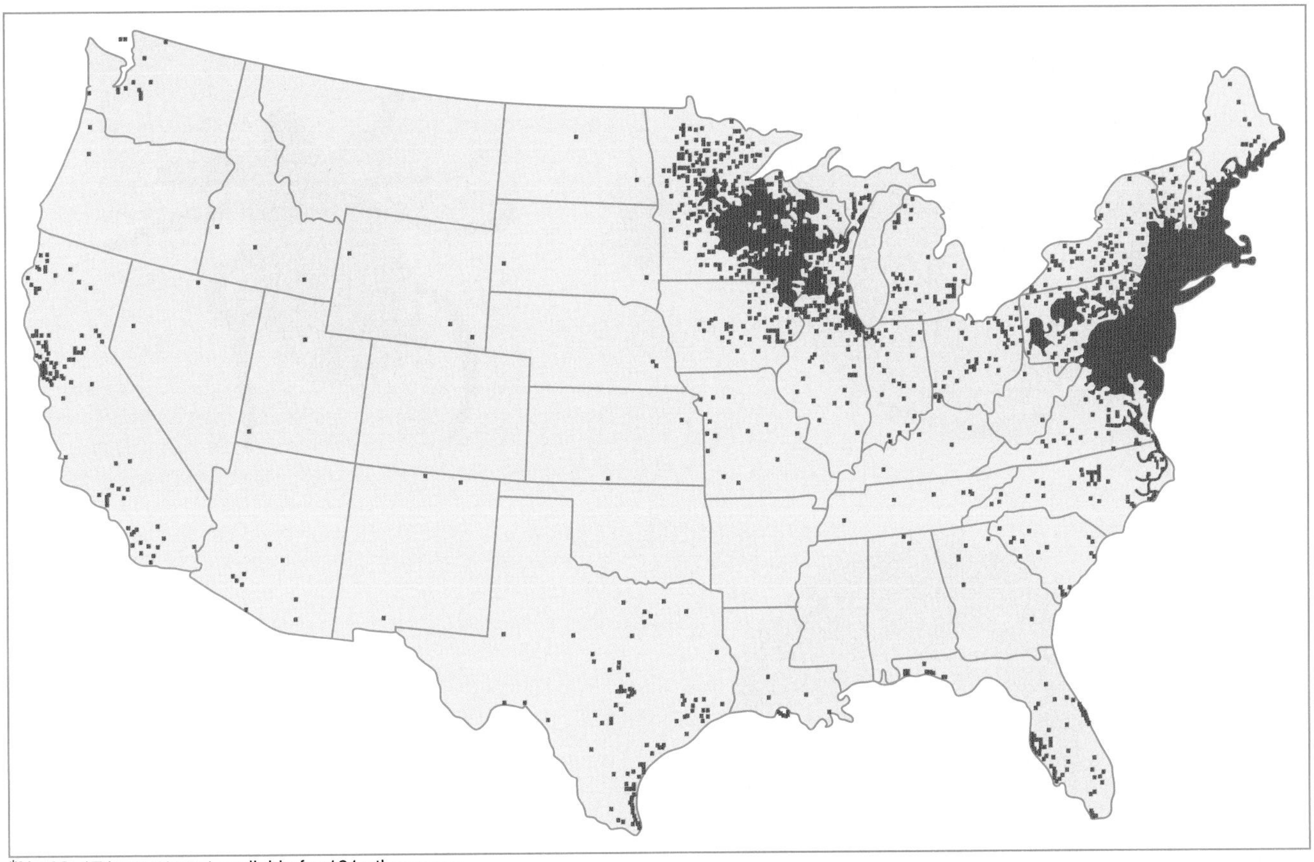

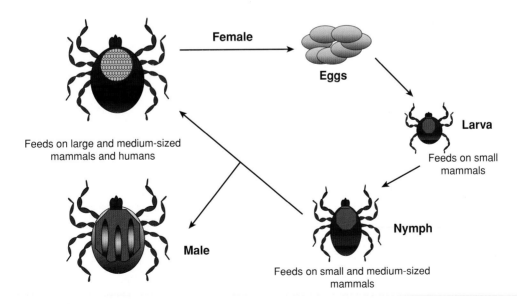

*N =23, 174; county not available for 131 other cases.
†One dot was placed randomly within the county of patient residence for each reported case.

Figure 65–2. Number of newly reported Lyme disease cases by county in the United States, 2005. (Photo courtesy of CDC.)

Female

Eggs

Larva

Feeds on small
mammals

Feeds on large and medium-sized
mammals and humans

Male

Nymph

Feeds on small and medium-sized
mammals

Figure 65–3. Life cycle of *Ixodes scapularis*. The larva does not transmit Lyme disease and can be differentiated from other life stages by the presence of six legs. (Image courtesy of Centers for Disease Control and Prevention, part of the United States Department of Health and Human Services.)

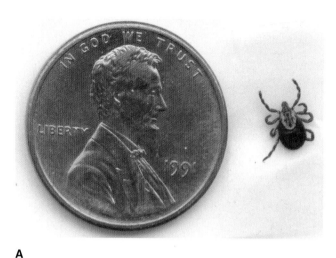

A

B

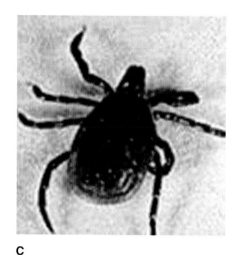

C

Figure 65–4. **(A).** Adult female dog tick on the left. Dog ticks do not transmit Lyme disease, but are an important vector of RMSF and human monocyte erlichiosis. **(B)** Adult female deer tick. **(C)** Engorged adult female deer tick on the right. (Photos courtesy of Scott Bauer at Wikimedia Commons. http://commons.wikimedia.org.   Accessed March 30, 2008.)

Clinical Lyme borreliosis infection is typically divided into three stages:

- Early localized disease
- Early disseminated disease
- Late Lyme disease

The most common manifestation of early localized disease is erythema migrans, or the bull's eye rash (Fig. 65–5). Erythema migrans usually begins within 7 to 10 days of tick infection, although it may present as early as one day and as late as 30 days.[4,7] The rash is seen in up to 85% of infected patients and is classically described as an erythematous macular or papular rash that spreads centrifugally to form an erythematous annular plaque. An influenza-like illness characterized by fever, regional lymphadenopathy, and nonspecific constitutional syndrome often accompanies erythema migrans.

The second stage of Lyme infection, early disseminated disease, is characterized by multiorgan disease resulting from the hematogenous spread of *B. burgdorferi*. This stage can include episodes of arthralgias or myalgias lasting hours to days, severe headaches, conjunctivitis, cranial nerve palsies (especially facial nerve palsy), meningitis, and multiple annular skin

lesions.[8] Carditis, presenting as atrioventricular block, can be seen but is rare in children.

The third stage, late Lyme disease, involves recurring large joint arthritis and neuroborreliosis that manifests as peripheral neuropathy, paresthesias, radicular pain, or encephalopathy. The majority of patients with erythema migrans who are not treated will go on to have complications of late-stage Lyme disease—60% will develop monoarticular or oligoarticular arthritis, 10% will have neurologic manifestations (facial nerve palsy being most common), and approximately 5% will have cardiac complications (varying degrees of AV block, pericarditis, myocarditis, tachyarrythmias, congestive heart failure, junctional rhythms, and prolonged QT intervals).[9] The arthritis of Lyme disease most commonly affects large joints, especially the knee, although virtually any joint can be involved. Joint swelling is usually out of proportion to the discomfort experienced by the patient. The arthritis usually occurs months after the initial inoculation, lasts for 1 to 2 weeks and may recur. The differential diagnosis of Lyme arthritis includes septic joint, acute rheumatic fever, juvenile rheumatoid arthritis, and postinfectious reactive arthritis.

The diagnosis of erythema migrans in endemic areas is purely clinical, and is the only manifestation of Lyme disease

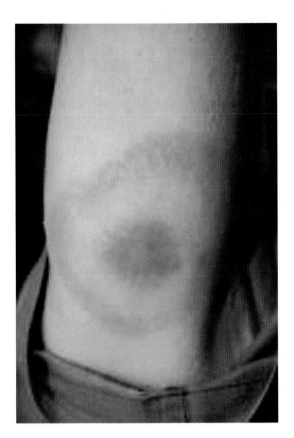

Figure 65-5. Erythema migrans. A single erythematous rash in the pattern of a bulls-eye. This rash is pathognomonic for Lyme disease. (Photo courtesy of CDC/James Gathany.)

that is sufficient to make the diagnosis without laboratory data.[2] If there is uncertainty about diagnosis, serum samples from the acute phase and subsequent convalescent phase should be tested using the recommended two-tier testing. Two-tier testing involves serology followed by confirmatory Western blot tests. Most patients with early neurologic Lyme disease are seropositive; although those with a negative two-tier test, may have a

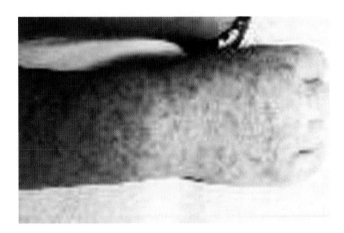

Figure 65-6. Rocky Mountain spotted fever. A child's hand and wrist displaying the characteristic spotted rash of RMSF. (Photo courtesy of CDC.)

convalescent-phase sample sent approximately 2 weeks after the acute-phase sample. Lyme carditis, although a rare pediatric manifestation, will usually (up to 85% of cases) occur concomitantly with erythema migrans and thus can be diagnosed clinically. However, in the absence of erythema migrans, the diagnosis of Lyme carditis requires the presence of antibodies directed against *B. burgdorferi* in either acute- or convalescent-phase serum samples. Lyme arthritis, and late-neurologic Lyme disease, such as peripheral neuropathy, encephalomyelitis, and encephalopathy, should be confirmed with two-tier testing that includes an ELISA and IgG immunoblot. Synovial fluid PCR and CSF serologies may help to confirm Lyme arthritis and encephalomyelitis, respectively.

The Infectious Diseases Society of America published evidence-based guidelines for the management of patients with Lyme disease in 2006 (Table 65-1).[1] Antibiotics recommended for children with erythema migrans are

- amoxicillin (50 mg/kg/d in three divided doses, maximum of 500 mg/dose)
- cefuroxime axetil (30 mg/kg/d in two divided doses, maximum of 500 mg/dose)
- doxycycline (4 mg/kg/d in two divided doses, maximum of 100 mg/dose)
  - If the child is ≥ 8 years old

The recommended treatment duration is for 14 to 21 days. Although macrolides have been found to be less effective, they may be prescribed for patients that are intolerant of the above medications.

Children with Lyme meningitis and other early neurologic manifestations of Lyme disease should receive ceftriaxone (50–75 mg/kg/d, maximum 2 g/d) in a daily intravenous dose. An alternative is cefotaxime (150–200 mg/kg/d in three or four divided doses, maximum 6 g/d) or penicillin G (200 000–400 000 U/kg/d every 4 hours, maximum 18–24 million units/d). For patients that are β-lactam intolerant, children ≥8 years old have been successfully treated with oral doxycycline at the same dosages mentioned above. Treatment should be continued for 14 days. Children with late-neurologic sequella should also receive the above antibiotics but for 2 to 4 weeks.

Children with Lyme carditis should be given a parental antibiotic similar to those with early neurologic Lyme disease. Therapy can be completed with the same oral antibiotic regimen as for children with erythema migrans for a total of 14 days. Treatment for Lyme arthritis is the same as that for erythema migrans; although with persistent or recurrent joint swelling after a course of oral antibiotic therapy, re-treatment with a 4-week course of oral antibiotics or a 2- to 4-week course of ceftriaxone is recommended.

▶ ROCKY MOUNTAIN SPOTTED FEVER

RMSF is the most common tick-borne rickettsial disease in the United States and is one of the most virulent human infections identified.[10] RMSF is found only in North and South America, and in the United States is found in all 48 contiguous states, except Vermont and Maine. Most of the cases are reported in the south Atlantic region, the Pacific region, and the west south-central region, with more than half of reported cases

▶ TABLE 65–1. PREVENTION AND TREATMENT OF LYME DISEASE

	Drug	Dose	Duration (Range)
I. scapularis bite*	Doxycycline[†]	4 mg/kg/d (maximum dose: 200 mg)	1 dose
Erythema migrans	Doxycycline[†]	4 mg/kg/d bid (maximum dose: 100 mg)	14 d (10–21 d)
	Amoxicillin	50 mg/kg/d tid (maximum dose: 500 mg)	14 d (14–21 d)
	Cefuroxime axetil	30 mg/kg/d bid (maximum dose: 500 mg)	14 d (14–21 d)
Erythema migrans with heart block ± myopericarditis[‡]	Doxycycline[†]	4 mg/kg/d bid (maximum dose: 100 mg)	14 d (10–21 d)
	Amoxicillin	50 mg/kg/d tid (maximum dose: 500 mg)	14 d (14–21 d)
	Cefuroxime axetil	30 mg/kg/d bid (maximum dose: 500 mg)	14 d (14–21 d)
	Ceftriaxone (IV or IM)	50–75 mg/kg once daily (maximum dose: 2000 mg)	14 d (14–21 d)
	Cefotaxime (IV)	150–200 mg/kg/d tid (maximum dose: 2000 mg)	14 d (14–21 d)
Erythema migrans with uncomplicated facial nerve palsy	Doxycycline[†]	4 mg/kg/d bid (maximum dose: 100 mg)	14 d (14–21 d)
	Amoxicillin	50 mg/kg/d tid (maximum dose: 500 mg)	14 d (14–21 d)
	Cefuroxime axetil	30 mg/kg/d bid (maximum dose: 500 mg)	14 d (14–21 d)
Erythema migrans with meningitis or radiculopathy	Ceftriaxone (IV or IM)	50–75 mg/kg once daily (maximum dose: 2000 mg)	14 d (10–28 d)
	Cefotaxime (IV)	150–200 mg/kg/d tid (maximum dose: 2000 mg)	14 d (10–28 d)
Lyme arthritis	Doxycycline[†]	4 mg/kg/d bid (maximum dose: 100 mg)	28 d
	Amoxicillin	50 mg/kg/d tid (maximum dose: 500 mg)	28 d
	Cefuroxime axetil	30 mg/kg/d bid (maximum dose: 500 mg)	28 d
Late CNS Lyme	Ceftriaxone (IV or IM)	50–75 mg/kg once daily (maximum dose: 2000 mg)	2–4 wk
	Cefotaxime (IV)	150–200 mg/kg/d tid (maximum dose: 2000 mg)	2–4 wk

*Only if tick is adult or nymphal & has been attached for ≥36 h, prophylaxis can be started within 72 h of tick removal, the local tick infection rate with *B. burgdorferi* is ≥ 20%, & doxycycline treatment is not contraindicated [18].
[†]Doxycycline is contraindicated in children younger than 8 years and pregnant/lactating women.
[‡]Hospitalized patients should receive parenteral therapy initially.

from just five states (North Carolina, Tennessee, Oklahoma, South Carolina, and Arkansas).[11] Contrary to its name, only 2% of cases are reported in the Mountain States. The highest incidence of infection has been reported in children less than 10 years old and adults aged 40 to 64 years, with males making up the majority of patients. Ninety to ninety-three percent of cases of RMSF in the United States occur in the warmer months between April and September.

RMSF is caused by *Rickettsia rickettsii*, an obligate intracellular gram-negative coccobacillus that typically infects the host's vascular endothelial cells. *R. rickettsii* is transmitted by the bite of an infected tick, usually a hard tick of the family Ixodidae, which serves as both a vector and reservoir for the bacterium. The American dog tick (*D. variabilis*) is the primary vector of *R. rickettsii* in most of the United States (Fig. 65–4A), while the Rocky Mountain wood tick (*D. andersoni*) is a major culprit in the Mountain States and Canada. Transmission requires a minimum period of tick attachment of 4 to 6 hours, although the requirement may be as long as 24 hours. *R. rickettsii* infection can also occur with exposure to crushed tick tissues, fluids, feces or through blood transfusions.[10]

Symptoms of RMSF usually appear approximately 7 days after tick exposure, although a history of tick bite is only elicited in 50% to 60% of patients. The initial phase of RMSF infection is characterized by sudden onset of fever, malaise, and severe headache, with accompanying nonspecific symptoms such as myalgias, nausea and vomiting, abdominal pain, anorexia, and photophobia (Fig. 65–1). Not surprisingly, RMSF may be misdiagnosed as a viral syndrome during this phase. The classic triad of RMSF (fever, rash, headache) is only seen

in 3% of patients in the first 3 days, although it is usually seen in the majority of patients within the first 2 weeks.[10] A rash usually appears between 2 and 5 days, although up to 10% of children may not develop a rash. The rash of RMSF usually begins as blanching, erythematous macules on the wrists and ankles, and spreads centripetally to the arms, legs, and trunks within hours (Fig. 65–6). Palms and soles are also involved. By the end of the first week, the characteristic petechial rash will develop in 35% to 60% of patients. Some patients may develop neurologic symptoms such as meningismus, altered mental status, amnesia, coma, seizures, cranial nerve palsies, central deafness, and cortical blindness. Other manifestations are less commonly reported but include conjunctivitis, periorbital and peripheral edema, congestive heart failure, arrhythmias, myocarditis, shock, hepatomegaly, and jaundice.

Diagnosing RMSF can be difficult because the early signs and symptoms are often nonspecific and may be mistaken for other tick-borne diseases, viral infections, or bacterial infections, including meningococcemia. Although there are serologic studies available, there currently is no rapid confirmatory test for RMSF. The reference standard for RMSF is generally considered the immunofluorescence assay (IFA). IgG antibodies generally do not form until 7 to 10 days after the onset of illness, thus acute and convalescent titers (≥3 weeks apart) may be required for a positive test. Laboratory findings that may be helpful include hyponatremia (20% of patients) and thrombocytopenia (33% of patients).

Because RMSF has a 20% mortality rate if untreated and up to a 5% rate if treated, and rapid confirmatory diagnosis is not easily achieved, antibiotic therapy should be started when the disease is suspected. Doxycycline is the drug of choice for treating RMSF regardless of the child's age. The recommended dosage is 2.2 mg/kg twice daily for children ≤45 kg and 100 mg twice daily for children >45 kg. The optimal duration of treatment has not yet been established, but the current recommendations are to treat for 3 days after the fever subsides and until there is evidence of clinical improvement. This usually results in duration of treatment of 7 to 10 days. In children with life-threatening illness, it may be reasonable to add an antibiotic (e.g., cefotaxime, ceftriaxone) active against *Neisseria meningitidis* as this condition may be difficult to distinguish from RMSF.

▶ TULAREMIA

Tularemia is caused by infection with the gram-negative coccobacillus, *Francisella tularensis*. *F. tularensis* is found worldwide and has been reported in every US state except Hawaii.[12] Ticks of the *Dermacentor* spp. and *Amblyomma* spp. are the vectors for *F. tularensis* in the United States, while rabbits, hares, and deer serve as the principal vectors.[13] Most patients in the United States acquire tularemia infection from tick bites or from contact with infected mammals, usually rabbits.[12] More than half of all reported tularemia cases are from just four states: Arkansas, Missouri, South Dakota, and Oklahoma, in descending order. The annual incidence shows a bimodal distribution with children aged 5 to 9 years and adults ≥75 years having the highest incidence. More than two-third of cases are reported during the summer months of May to August, although cases are reported year round.

Tularemia infection is commonly classified into six categories: ulceroglandular, glandular, oculoglandular, oropharyngeal, pneumonic, and typhoidal. The ulceroglandular form is the most common, while the latter four are less common in children. Clinical manifestations of tularemia infection depend on the method of inoculation, with the organism gaining access to the host via the skin, mucosa, ingestion, or inhalation. Tularemia infection presents as an acute febrile illness with an incubation period averaging 3 to 5 days (range 1–21 days), and disease severity ranges from mild to severe (Fig. 65–1).[8] Children present with abrupt-onset fever, myalgia, chills, vomiting, fatigue, and headache. Ulceroglandular tularemia presents with an ulcerating eschar at the inoculation site with painful regional lymphadenopathy, whereas the glandular form lacks the inoculation eschar.

Laboratory findings of tularemia are nonspecific but may include a normal or elevated WBC count, pyuria, and hepatic function abnormalities. *F. tularensis* is difficult to isolate in blood or tissue cultures but can be isolated using special media. It is very important to notify laboratory personnel when tularemia is suspected to prevent airborne spread of the organism. Tularemia is usually diagnosed by serologic testing. A ≥4-fold increase in titers between the acute and convalescent stages confirms the diagnosis, whereas a single titer of 1:160 or more is consistent with recent or past tularemia infection.[8] Aminoglycosides are currently first-line therapy for tularemia. Gentamicin can be given at 2.5 mg/kg IV/IM three times daily for 10 days. Doxycycline and chloramphenicol are alternative choices, although they are bacteriostatic and are associated

with increased relapses. Fluoroquinolones have been effective in treating tularemia, but their efficacy is not yet proven.

▶ BABESIOSIS

Babesiosis, a malaria-like disease, is caused by intraerythrocytic protozoa *Babesia microti* and *B. equi*. Domesticated mammals, rodents, and deer serve as the major zoonotic reservoirs, while *Ixodes* ticks are the principal vectors. Because Lyme disease is also transmitted by *Ixodes* ticks, coinfection with babesiosis may occur. Babesiosis may also be spread by blood transfusions and transplacental or perinatal transmission.

Most cases of babesiosis in North America are asymptomatic, especially in endemic areas. Children usually have a milder clinical course than adults. Symptom onset is usually gradual and begins between 1 and 4 weeks after the bite of an infected tick. The initial disease is marked by nonspecific symptoms such as fevers, chills, diaphoresis, fatigue, myalgia, malaise, headaches, nausea, and abdominal pain (Fig. 65–1). Babesiosis infection can be prolonged, lasting weeks to months. On physical examination, hepatomegaly and splenomegaly may be present. Laboratory findings may reveal thrombocytopenia, anemia, liver dysfunction, renal dysfunction, and evidence of hemolysis.

Babesiosis may be treated with either atovaquone (20 mg/kg orally every 12 hours, maximum 750 mg/dose) and azithromycin (10 mg/kg orally once on day 1 then 5 mg/kg daily thereafter) or clindamycin (7–10 mg/kg orally or intravenously every 6–8 hours, maximum 600 mg/dose) and quinine (8 mg/kg orally every 8 hours, maximum 650 mg/dose). Children should be treated for 7 to 10 days. More serious infections should be treated with clindamycin and quinine. RBC exchange transfusion may be necessary for children with severe babesiosis as evidenced by high-grade parasitemia (≥10%), significant hemolysis, or pulmonary, renal, or hepatic compromise.[2]

▶ HUMAN MONOCYTE EHRLICHIOSIS

Human monocyte ehrlichiosis (HME) is caused in the United States by *Ehrlichia chaffeensis*, a small, intracellular, gram-negative coccobacillus that infects circulating leukocytes. The principal tick vectors for HME are *D. variabilis* and *A. americanum,* and the main reservoirs of disease are deer, dogs, and other large mammals.[14] Similar to RMSF, the incidence of HME is highest in the south and southeastern regions of the United States. Unlike RMSF and Lyme disease, most of the reported cases of HME occur in adults rather than children.

HME causes a clinical syndrome in children very similar to RMSF. A tick-bite history is obtained in up to 90% of children within the preceding 3 weeks of illness onset.[13] Almost all children present with fever and headache; myalgia, anorexia, nausea, abdominal pain, and vomiting are frequently seen (Fig. 65–1). Although only one-third of adults have a rash, two-third of children will have a rash that commonly affects the trunk, extremities, or both. The rash appears for a median of 5 days after illness onset and can be macular, maculopapular, or petechial. Less commonly, children may have diarrhea, lymphadenopathy, or changes in mental status.[8] Rarely, the disease may lead to pneumonitis, respiratory failure, encephalitis, meningitis, shock, or disseminated intravascular coagulation. Laboratory testing characteristically shows signs of hepatic injury and myelosuppression, such as increased transaminases, thrombocytopenia, leukopenia, and anemia. Hyponatremia may also be seen.

HME diagnosis is usually confirmed by serology studies showing a ≥4-fold change in antibody titer by indirect IFA between acute- and convalescent-phase samples. A single IFA titer >64 in conjunction with identifying intracytoplasmic inclusions of replicating organisms in monocytes or detecting ehrlichial DNA by PCR in clinical specimens may also confirm the diagnosis.[8] The treatment of choice for children with HME is doxycycline at previously mentioned doses for 3 days after defervescence or for a minimum of 5 to 10 days. An alternative for children who cannot tolerate doxycycline is rifampin.

▶ HUMAN GRANULOCYTIC ANAPLASMOSIS

Human granulocytic anaplasmosis (HGA), formerly human granulocytic ehrlichiosis, is caused by infection with the gram-negative, intracellular coccobacillus, *Anaplasma phagocytophila*. The disease shares a geographic distribution with Lyme disease as well as a tick vector, *Ixodes*. Unlike Lyme disease, HGA is currently very rare in children. Clinical manifestations of HGA, similar to HME, are usually nonspecific and include fever, chills, headache, and myalgias (Fig. 65–1). Rash is rare in HGA. The disease is usually mild and self-limited with symptoms resolving within 30 days in most patients, regardless of antibiotic treatment.[2] However, serious manifestations can occur, especially in patients with conditions that suppress the immune system.

Diagnosis of HGA is most sensitively accomplished by serologic testing using IFA of acute- and convalescent-phase samples. *A. phagocytophilia* can also be detected in blood using PCR, smear examination, or culture.[2] The current IDSA recommendations for treatment are summarized here. Children ≥8 years old may be treated with doxycycline for 10 days, severely ill children <8 years old without concomitant Lyme disease may receive doxycycline for 4 to 5 days, and those with concomitant Lyme disease should receive amoxicillin or cefuroxime axetil at the conclusion of doxycycline therapy for a total of 14 days of antibiotic therapy. Children with mild disease with a drug allergy or <8 years old can receive rifampin for 7 to 10 days at 10 mg/kg twice daily (maximum 300 mg/dose).

▶ COLORADO TICK FEVER

Colorado tick fever occurs when an RNA virus is transmitted by the bite of the wood tick *D. andersoni*. The disease is endemic to the western mountainous regions of the United States and Canada, and its zoonotic reservoirs are deer, marmots, and porcupine.[13] The disease usually presents as an acute, self-limited, febrile illness with headaches, chills, myalgias, and photophobia (Fig. 65–1). Symptoms begin 3 to 7 days after a tick bite and may be accompanied by a macular or petechial rash. Treatment for the disease is supportive.

REFERENCES

1. Wormser GP, Dattwyler RJ, Shapiro ED, et al. The clinical assessment, treatment, and prevention of Lyme disease, human granulocytic anaplasmosis and babesiosis: clinical practice guidelines by the Infectious Disease Society of America. *Clin Infect Dis.* 2006;43:1089–1134.
2. Centers for Disease Control and Prevention. Lyme disease—United States, 2003–2005. *MMWR Morb Mortal Wkly Rep.* 2007; 56:573–576.
3. US Department of Health and Human Services. *Healthy people 2010* (conference ed., in 2 Vols.). Washington, DC: US Department of Health and Human Services; 2000. http://www.health.gov/healthypeople.
4. Hengge UR, Tannapfel A, Tyring SK, et al. Lyme borrelosis. *Lancet Infect Dis.* 2003;3:489–500.
5. Parola P, Raoult D. Ticks and tickborne bacterial diseases in humans: an emerging infectious threat. *Clin Infect Dis.* 2001;32:897–928.
6. Piesman J. Dynamics of *Borrelia burgdorferi* transmission by nymphal *Ixodes dammini* ticks. *J Infect Dis.* 1993;167:1082–1085.
7. Depietropaolo DL, Powers JH, Gill JM. Diagnosis of Lyme disease. *Am Fam Physician.* 2005;72:297–304.
8. Buckingham SC. Tick-borne infections in children: epidemiology, clinical manifestations, and optimal management strategies. *Pediatr Drugs.* 2005;7:163–176.
9. Wormser GP. Early Lyme disease. *N Engl J Med.* 2006;354:2794.
10. Dantas-Torres F. Rocky Mountain spotted fever. *Lancet Infect Dis.* 2007;7:724–732.
11. Razzaq S, Schutze GE. Rocky Mountain spotted fever: a physician's challenge. *Pediatr Rev.* 2005;26:125–130.
12. Centers for Disease Control and Prevention. *Tularemia—United States,* 1990–2000. *MMWR Morb Mortal Wkly Rep.* 2002;51:182–184.
13. Meredith JT. Zoonotic infections. In: Tintinalli JA, Kelen GD, Stapczynski JS, eds. *Emergency Medicine: A Comprehensive Study Guide.* 6th ed. New York, NY: McGraw-Hill; 2004:970–973.
14. Bryant KA, Marshall GS. Clinical manifestations of tick-borne infections in children. *Clin Diagn Lab Immunol.* 2000;7:523–527.

CHAPTER 66

Common Parasitic Infestations

Steven Lelyveld and Gary R. Strange

► HIGH-YIELD FACTS

- Three major groups of parasites cause human disease:
  ○ Protozoa
  ○ Helminths
    – Nematodes (roundworms)
    – Cestodes (flatworms)
    – Trematodes (flukes)
  ○ Arthropods
- Virtually all organ systems are at risk for parasitic infestation, with symptoms depending on the system(s) involved. Arthropods are predominantly surface dwellers and cause pruritus and rash. Nematodes and cestodes infest the gut, producing diarrhea, abdominal pain, and nutritional derangement, but, along with trematodes, they may migrate to the lungs and solid organs.
- *Ascaris lumbricoides* is the largest and most prevalent human nematode, with an estimated one billion cases worldwide. Albendazole (400 mg orally as a single dose) or ivermectin (150–200 µg/kg orally as a single dose) is curative.
- *Enterobius vermicularis* (pinworm) is present in all parts of the United States and affects individuals of all ages and socioeconomic levels, with the most common presentation being that of a toddler or small child with anal itch. Scotch tape, placed sticky side to perianal skin when the child first awakens and then viewed under low power, is usually diagnostic, but repeated examination may be necessary to find the eggs.
- *Trichuris trichiura* (whipworm) lives predominantly in the cecum and can cause malabsorptive symptoms, pain, bloody diarrhea, and fever but is usually asymptomatic. A heavy worm burden may cause a colitislike picture and rectal prolapse and can be associated with anemia and developmental and cognitive deficits.
- The hookworms, *Necator americanus* and *Ancylostoma duodenale*, are found between 36-degrees north and 30-degrees south latitude and are one of the most prevalent infectious diseases of humans, with an estimated one billion individuals affected. Although a broad spectrum of symptoms is possible, the hallmark of hookworm infestation is the microcytic, hypochromic anemia of iron deficiency.
- Symptoms of schistosome infestation appear only in those with heavy infestation and are commonly frequency, dysuria, and hematuria with *Schistosoma haematobium* and colicky abdominal pain and bloody diarrhea with the other agents. None of these flukes are endemic in the continental United States.
- The avian schistosome *Trichobilharzia ocellata* is spread by migratory birds to the freshwater lakes of the northern United States. The cercariae cause dermatitis, known as swimmer's itch.
- Most patients with amoebic infestation carry amebas asymptomatically in the cecum and large intestine. Heavy infestations of *Entamoeba histolytica* produce a colitislike picture ("gay bowel syndrome") with nausea, vomiting, bloating, pain, bloody diarrhea, and leukocytosis without eosinophilia.
- Infection with chloroquine resistant malaria should be high in the differential diagnosis of febrile children returning from international travel.
- Resistance of head lice to permethrin is now common, with reported insecticidal activity down to 28% in one study. The combination of 1% permethrin with trimethoprim/sulfamethoxazole has been reported to be 95% effective, compared with 80% for permethrin alone.

Parasitic diseases are ubiquitous. In spite of advances in sanitation throughout the world, new medications, and the heightened awareness of health care providers, between one-fourth and one-half of the world's population has a parasitic infestation at any given time. An increasingly mobile society has made disease containment nearly impossible. Travel (for business and pleasure), immigration, and the importation of vectors as a consequence of international trade have all led to an increase in disease. The increased number of immunocompromised hosts has also led to an increased expression of these infestations. This chapter reviews the major parasitic infestations causing human disease in the United States.

The oral exploratory behavior of the child, coupled with a poor capacity to avoid arthropods, places the child at particular risk for acquiring parasites. Important factors in the history are included in Table 66–1.

Three major groups of parasites cause human disease: protozoa, helminths, and arthropods. Further, there are three important subgroups of helminths that cause human disease: nematodes (roundworms), cestodes (flatworms), and trematodes (flukes).

Virtually all organ systems are at risk for infestation, with symptoms depending on the system(s) involved. Arthropods are predominantly surface dwellers. They cause pruritus and rash. Nematodes and cestodes infest the gut, producing diarrhea, abdominal pain, and nutritional derangement. Along with trematodes, the other helminths may migrate to the lungs and

TABLE 66-1. IMPORTANT ASPECTS OF THE HISTORY IN THE CHILD OR ADOLESCENT WITH POSSIBLE PARASITIC INFESTATION

Camping trips
Travel to regions with questionable sanitation and water purification practices or a warm climate
Method of food acquisition and preparation
Exposure to pets and other animals, both domestic and wild
Participation in day care
Living in confined situations
Mental retardation
Adolescent drug abuse
Homosexual contacts
Sexual abuse
Blood transfusions

solid organs and are associated with malnutrition and inhibited growth and development. Protozoa may live in the gut for generations, shedding cysts in the stool. Like helminths, they can also, under proper circumstances, travel throughout the body. Some parasites only begin to produce symptoms months to years after the first exposure. In addition, the symptoms produced depend on the stage of the parasitic life cycle.

The varied and nonspecific symptoms produced place parasitic infestation on the expanded differential diagnosis of most patients presenting to the emergency department.

The challenge to the pediatric emergency physician is, therefore, to be aware of the patterns of worldwide distribution of these organisms and the symptoms they produce. It is important not to overlook the possibility of parasitic infestation when treating large numbers of patients with common complaints. A list of common emergency department complaints and the major human parasites that produce them is given in Table 66–2.

▶ NEMATODES (ROUNDWORMS)

ASCARIASIS

A. lumbricoides is the largest and most prevalent human nematode, with an estimated one billion cases worldwide. Although it is most commonly found in tropical and subtropical climates, it is present throughout the United States. Ascariasis is most common in preschool and early school age children.

From an egg measuring 65 by 45 μm, this nematode can grow to a length of 30 cm. After being deposited in the stool, the egg matures over 3 weeks. Upon ingestion, the egg hatches in the small intestine (Fig. 66–1). The larvae burrow through the gut mucosa, enter the bloodstream, and migrate to the lungs. They cause shortness of breath, hemoptysis, eosinophilia, fever, and Loffler's pneumonia as they break through the alveoli, migrate up the bronchial tree, and are swallowed. Maturing to the adult form, *A. lumbricoides* can live freely in the

▶ **TABLE 66-2. SYMPTOMS OF PARASITIC DISEASE**

Symptom	Possible Cause
Abdominal pain	*Ascaris, Clonorchis, Diphyllobothrium, Entamoeba, Fasciola, Giardia.* hookworm, *Hymenolepsis, Schistosoma, Taenia, Trichuris*
Anemia	*Babesia, Diphyllobothrium,* hookworm, *Leishmania donovani, Plasmodium* species, *Trichuris*
Asthma	*Ascaris, Strongyloides, Toxocara*
Conjunctivitis and keratitis	Filariae (*Onchocerca volvulus*), *Taenia, Trichinella, Trypanosoma*
Diarrhea	*Dientamoeba, Entamoeba, Fasciola, Fasciolopsis, Giardia,* hookworm, *Hymenolepsis, L. donovani, Palantidium, Schistosoma, Strongyloides, Taenia, Trichinella, Trichuris*
Edema	*Fasciolopsis,* Filariae (*Wuchereria bancrofti*), *Trichinella, Trypanosoma*
Eosinophilia	*Ascaris, Dracunculus, Fasciola,* Filariae (*W. bancrofti, Brugia malayi*) fluke (*Paragonimus westermani, Chlonorchis sinensis, Fasciolopsisbuski*), *Hymnenolepsis,* hookworm, *Schistosoma, Strongyloides, Taenia, Toxocara, Trichinella, Trichuris*
Fever	*Ascaris, Babesia, Entamoeba, Fasciola,* Filariae (*W. bancrofti*), fluke (*C. sinensis*), *Giardia, L. donovani, Plasmodium* species, *Toxocara, T. trichiura, Trypanosoma*
Hemoptysis	*Ascaris, Echinococcus, Paragonimus*
Hepatomegaly	Fluke (*C. sinensis, Opisthorchis viverrini, Fasciola*), *L. donovani, Plasmodium* species, tapeworm (*Echinococcus*), *Schistosoma, Toxocara, Trypanosoma*
Intestinal obstruction	*Ascaris, Diphyllobothrium,* fluke (*Fasciolopsis buski*), *Strongyloides, Taenia*
Jaundice	Fluke (*C. sinensis, O. viverrini*), *Plasmodium* species
Meningitis	*Acanthamoeba,* malaria (*Plasmodium falciparum*), *Naegleria,* primary amebic meningoencephalitis, *Toxocara, Trichinella, Trypanosoma*
Myocardial disease	*Taenia, Trichinella, Trypanosoma (T. cruzi)*
Nausea and vomiting	*Ascaris, Entamoeba, Giardia, Leishmania, Taenia, Trichinella, Trichuris*
Pneumonia	*Ascaris,* Filariae (*W. bancrofti, B. malayi*), fluke (*P. westermani*), *Strongyloides, Trichinella*
Pruritus	*Dientamoeba, Enterobius,* Filariae (*O. volvulus*), *Trichuris*
Seizures	*Hymenolepsis, Trichinella, Paragonimus,* tapeworm (*Echinococcus, Cysticercus*)
Skin ulcers	*Dracunculus,* hookworm, *L. donovani, Trypanosoma*
Splenomegaly	*Babesia, Toxoplasma, Plasmodium*
Urticaria	*Ascaris, Dracunculus, Fasciola, Strongyloides, Trichinella*

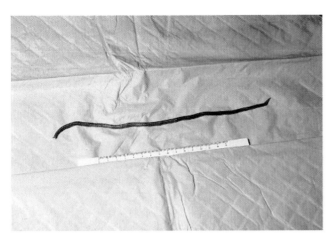

Figure 66–1. *Ascaris lumbricoides* after passage from the anus.

small intestine for up to a year, shedding eggs in the stool. At this stage, it usually remains asymptomatic but can cause gastrointestinal symptoms, including pain, protein mal-absorption, biliary duct or bowel obstruction, and appendicitis.

Although stool testing for ova is diagnostic, serologic hemagglutination and flocculation tests are available.

Albendazole (400 mg orally as a single dose) or ivermectin (150–200 μ/kg orally as a single dose) is curative. Piperazine salts (50–75 mg/kg for 2 days) are recommended for ascaria-

sis complicated by intestinal or biliary obstruction, since they cause relatively rapid expulsion of the worms.[1–4] If multiple infestations are present, it is recommended that *Ascaris* be treated first, as treatment of other parasites may stimulate a large worm burden to migrate simultaneously, causing obstruction.

There is controversy in regard to the clinical significance of *Ascaris* infestation. However, approximately 20 000 deaths annually are attributed to *Ascaris*, mostly because of intestinal obstruction. Preventive therapy in endemic regions may be considered.

ENTEROBIASIS

E. vermicularis (pinworm) is present in all parts of the United States and affects individuals of all ages and socioeconomic levels. The most common presentation is that of a toddler or small child with anal itch. The egg is oval, approximately 50 by 25 μm in size. It is inhaled or ingested and hatches between the ileum and ascending colon, growing to an adult length of 3 to 10 mm. The adult may live and copulate in the colon for 1 to 2 months. The gravid female migrates to the anus, where it deposits embryonated eggs, usually during early morning hours (Fig. 66–2A). When the host stirs, the adult will migrate back into the body, causing symptoms of pruritus ani, dysuria, enuresis, and vaginitis. Scratching and hand–mouth behavior reinoculates the host, and the cycle repeats. Granulomas of the pelvic peritoneum and female genital tract may occur. Scotch

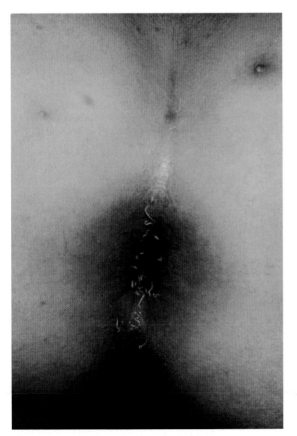

A

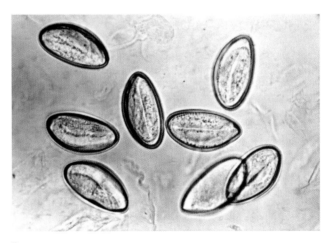

B

Figure 66–2. **(A)** Pinworms. Multiple tiny pearly white worms are seen at the anus. **(B)** This photomicrograph depicts the eggs of the nematode, or round worm, *Enterobius vermicularis*, mounted on cellulose tape. (Courtesy of the Centers for Disease Control Public Health Image Library.)

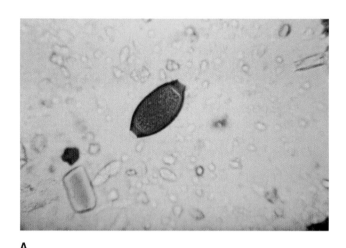

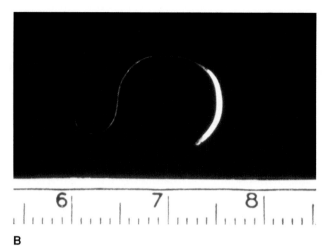

A **B**

Figure 66–3. **(A)** This micrograph depicts an egg from the "human whipworm," Trichuris trichiura, the causal agent of "Trichuriasis." **(B)** This micrograph of an adult Trichuris female human whipworm, reveals that its size in centimeters is approximately 4 cm (A and B.) (Courtesy of the Centers for Disease Control Public Health Image Library.)

tape, placed sticky side to perianal skin when the child first awakens and then viewed under low power (Fig. 66–2B), is usually diagnostic; but repeated examination may be necessary to find the eggs. Treatment is with albendazole, 400 mg orally. Pyrantel pamoate (11 mg/kg) or mebendazole (100 mg) may also be used.[1,3–5] Each drug is given as a single dose, with a repeat given 2 weeks later to remove secondary hatchings.

TRICHURIS TRICHIURA

T. trichiura (whipworm) is found in southern Appalachia, southwest Louisiana, and other warm rural areas. The life cycle mimics that of *E. vermicularis*. The eggs are of similar size and configuration, with the addition of a rounded cap at each pole (Fig. 66–3A). The adult resembles *E. vermicularis*, with a long whiplike projection at one end (Fig. 66–3B). It lives predominantly in the cecum and can cause malabsorptive symptoms, pain, bloody diarrhea, and fever but is usually asymptomatic. A heavy worm burden may cause a colitislike picture and rectal prolapse and can be associated with anemia and developmental and cognitive deficits.[6] Treatment is with albendazole (400 mg daily for 3 days) or mebendazole (100 mg bid for 3 days). Community control should be considered in heavily endemic areas.[1,3,4]

TRICHINOSIS

Trichinella spiralis is found throughout the United States, with increasing prevalence in the Northeast and Mid-Atlantic states. Although <100 cases of clinical disease are reported annually, cysts are found at autopsy in the diaphragms of 4% of patients. Current control efforts include laws governing the feeding of swine destined for sale to the public, specifically the heat treatment of garbage used as feed and recommendations for the preparation of meat in the home.[4]

Digestive enzymes liberate the encysted larvae, which lodge in the duodenum and jejunum, grow, and, within 2 days,

mature and copulate. The females give birth to living larvae that bore through the mucosa, become blood-borne, and migrate to striated muscle, heart, lung, and brain. Host defenses produce inflammation at each site. Although a classic triad of fever, myalgia, and periorbital edema has been described, symptoms of gastroenteritis, pneumonia, myocarditis, meningitis, and seizures can occur.

Although most cases are mild and self-limited, the history and physical examination, along with elevation of muscle enzymes and eosinophilia, may suggest the need for further investigation. Serologic tests are available from the Centers for Disease Control and Prevention. Muscle biopsy is confirmative.

Treatment, with aspirin and steroids, is initially aimed at reducing the inflammatory symptoms. Mebendazole (200–400 mg tid for 3 days and then 400 mg tid for 10 days) or albendazole (400 mg bid for 8–14 days) is indicated for severe disease but may not be effective after encystment.[1,3]

HOOKWORMS

The hookworms, *N. americanus* and *A. duodenale*, are found between 36-degree north and 30-degree south latitude and are one of the most prevalent infectious diseases of humans, with an estimated one billion individuals affected.[7] The eggs hatch in the soil, releasing rhabditiform larvae 275 μm long that feed on bacteria and organic debris (Fig. 66–4). They double in length, molt, and may survive as filariform larvae for several weeks. Upon contact, they burrow through the skin, causing pruritus (ground itch), enter the blood, travel to the lung, and are ingested, like *A. lumbricoides*. Although a broad spectrum of symptoms is possible, the hallmark of hookworm infestation is the microcytic, hypochromic anemia of iron deficiency. Each adult hookworm may ingest up to 0.05 mL of blood a day. Children with chronic hookworm disease may develop a characteristic yellow–green pallor called chlorosis. Although more commonly seen with the dog and cat hookworms (*Ancylostoma braziliense*), these hookworms can also cause

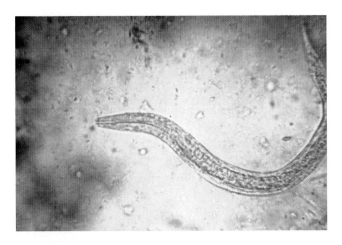

Figure 66–4. This micrograph depicts a hookworm rhabditiform larva, which represents its early, noninfectious immature stage. (Courtesy of the Centers for Disease Control Public Health Image Library.)

the serpentine track of cutaneous larva migrans. Finding the ova in stool is diagnostic. Albendazole (400 mg qid for 2–3 days), mebendazole (100 mg bid for 3 days), or pyrantel pamoate (11 mg/kg–maximum 1 g qid for 3 days) is recommended. Cutaneous larva migrans is usually self-limited, but topical application of 10% thiabendzole, ivermectin (150–200 μg orally), or albendazole (400 mg qid for 3 days) may hasten resolution.[1,3,8]

STRONGYLOIDIASIS

Strongyloides stercoralis (threadworm) is found in southern Appalachia, Kentucky, and Tennessee.[4] Like the hookworms, it penetrates the skin, producing pruritus and cutaneous larva migrans. Pulmonary and gastrointestinal symptoms occur as the larvae migrate. The human is a definitive host. Ongoing autoinfection is slowed by the host's immune response, but immunocompromised patients and the elderly may suffer fatal infestation. The rise in the acquired immunodeficiency syndrome (AIDS) has been mirrored by a rise in reported cases of *Strongyloides* infestation. Infestation is extremely common in institutionalized mentally disabled children.[7] A definitive diagnosis is made by recovering *Strongyloides* in stool, sputum, or duodenal aspirate. Ivermectin (200 μg qid for 2 days) is recommended. Albendazole (400 mg bid for 7 days) or thiabendazole (50 mg/kg/d divided bid, maximum 3 g/d for 2 days) may also be used. In disseminated strongyloidiasis, treatment may need to continue for up to 2 weeks.[1,3]

FILARIAL NEMATODES

The filarial nematodes *Wuchereria bancrofti* (elephantiasis), *Onchocerca volvulus* and *Loa loa* (river blindness), and *Dracunculus medinensis* (Guinea worms) cause significant worldwide morbidity. They are rarely encountered in the United States; when they are, it is usually in immigrants from parts of the world where they are endemic.

▶ TREMATODES (FLUKES)

Flukes are oval, flat worms with a ventral sucker for nutrition and attachment. Eggs are shed in the stool of definitive hosts, hatch into miracidia, and enter an intermediate host such as a snail or other crustacean, fish, or bird. They develop into cercariae, which leave the intermediate host to become free living prior to infesting the definitive host on contact with contaminated water. The intermediate host may also be ingested, releasing this infective form of the parasite. Symptoms are produced as the fluke reaches its destination. *Fasciolopsis buski* infests the gut; *Fasciola hepatica, Opisthorchis* (formerly *Clonorchis) sinensis*, and *Schistosoma mansoni* the liver; *S. haematobium* the bladder; and *Paragonimus westermani* the lung. Acute schistosomiasis is an immune complex, febrile disease associated with early infection. Symptoms appear only in those with heavy infestation and are commonly frequency, dysuria, and hematuria with *S. haematobium* and colicky abdominal pain and bloody diarrhea with the other agents. None of these flukes are endemic in the contiguous United States. Praziquantel (40 mg/kg/d divided into 2 doses for 1 or 2 days) is recommended for *S. haematobium, S. mansoni*, and *S. intercalatum*. A higher dose, 60 mg/kg/d divided into 3 doses for 1 day, is recommended for *S. japonica* and *S. mekongi*.[1,3]

Of particular interest to the pediatric emergency physician is the avian schistosome, *Trichobilharzia ocellata*. Spread by migratory birds to the freshwater lakes of the northern United States, the cercariae cause dermatitis, known as swimmer's itch. The intense reaction produced by host defenses is treated with heat and antipruritics. Severe cases are treated with thiabendazole cream.

▶ CESTODES (FLATWORMS AND TAPEWORMS)

Cestodes attach to the gut of the definitive host with hooks or suckers at the head (scolex), from which grow segmented proglottids. Each proglottid is equipped to produce large volumes of eggs. These eggs, along with terminal proglottids, pass in the stool and are ingested by the intermediate host. The eggs hatch into a larval stage, either cysticercus (larva with a single scolex in a fluid-filled cyst), cysticercoid (larva with the single scolex filling the cyst), coenurus (a cyst with grapelike daughter cysts internally containing protoscolices), or hydatid cysts (mature cyst filled with numerous immature cysts), depending on the species. Symptoms are produced as these larvae act as space-occupying lesions or cause inflammation. When the intermediate host is ingested by the definitive host, the larvae attach to the intestine and the cycle repeats.

Four cestodes produce most clinical disease seen in the United States: *Taenia solium, Taenia saginatum, Diphyllobothrium latum* and *Echinococcus granulosus. T. solium* (pork tapeworm), and *Taenia saginatum* (beef tapeworm) infestations are generally asymptomatic and are diagnosed when a parent brings a proglottid to the emergency department for identification (Fig. 66–5). A history of raw meat consumption may be elicited. Patients occasionally will have gastrointestinal complaints. When *T. solium* enters the cysticercus phase, it may migrate to the heart, brain, breast, eye, skin, or other solid organ. Subcutaneous nodules, visual field defects, focal

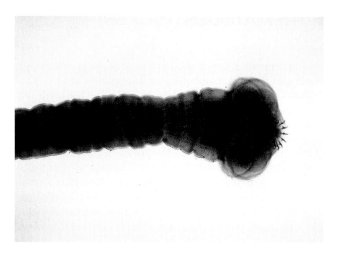

Figure 66–5. Scolex of *Taenia solium*. (Courtesy of the Centers for Disease Control Public Health Image Library.)

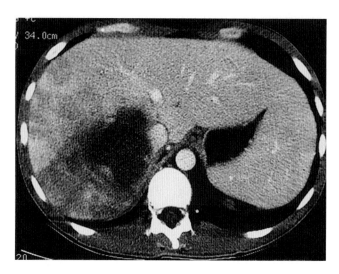

Figure 66–7. Abdominal CT scan of a large amebic abscess of the right lobe of the liver.

neurologic findings, acute psychosis, and obstructive hydrocephalus may develop years after infestation. Calcified cysts may be found on plain radiographs, and cysts may be seen as a ring of calcification on computed tomography.

D. latum (fish tapeworm) is becoming more prevalent with the increased popularity of raw fish. Because *D. latum* absorbs >50 times more vitamin B_{12} than *Taenia*, it causes pernicious anemia.

Echinococcus granulosus (sheep tapeworm) is found in agricultural countries. Most reported cases are from the southeastern United States. Symptomatology is secondary to hydatid cyst formation with mass effect (Fig. 66–6).

Most tapeworms are treated with praziquantel (5–25 mg/kg once). *Echinococcus* infection and cysticercosis respond best to albendazole (15 mg/kg/d divided tid for 28 days).[1,3]

▶ PROTOZOA

E. HISTOLYTICA

E. histolytica is a water-borne single-cell organism. It is found in epidemic proportion after heavy rain in areas of subop-

timal sanitation and among closely confined populations. In addition to ingestion of contaminated water, it may be spread by direct human contact, both sexually and in breast milk.[4] Most patients carry amebas asymptomatically in the cecum and large intestine. Heavy infestations of *E. histolytica* produce a colitislike picture ("gay bowel"). These patients may present with nausea, vomiting, bloating, pain, bloody diarrhea, and leukocytosis without eosinophilia. The amebas live at the base of large flask-shaped ulcers. When the infection is severe, direct inspection will reveal pseudopolyps of normal tissue on a base of ulcerative disease. *E. histolytica* has the capacity to invade the blood, causing abscess formation in the liver (Fig. 66–7), lung, brain, and breast.[9] Diagnosis is confirmed with stool specimen or colonoscopic aspiration. Metronidazole (35–50 mg/kg/d divided tid for 10 days) followed by iodoquinol (40 mg/kg/d divided tid for 20 days) is recommended to eradicate this infestation.[1,3]

DIENTAMOEBA FRAGILIS

Dientamoeba fragilis is a flagellate that lives in the cecum and proximal large bowel and has worldwide distribution. It is generally not invasive, does not form cysts, and closely resembles *Trichomonas*, except for the lack of a flagellum. It may be found in children in day care, causing the local mucosal irritative symptoms of abdominal pain, decreased appetite, diarrhea, and eosinophilia. It is diagnosed when trophozoites are found in the stool after the use of permanent stains.[4,10] The treatment is iodoquinol (40 mg/kg/d divided tid for 20 days).[1,3]

GIARDIA LAMBLIA

This flagellate thrives in the relatively alkaline pH of the duodenum and proximal small bowel (Fig. 66–8). Infestation occurs after ingestion of contaminated water or other fecal–oral behavior. It is commonly found in day care centers; among travelers, immunocompromised children, and patients with

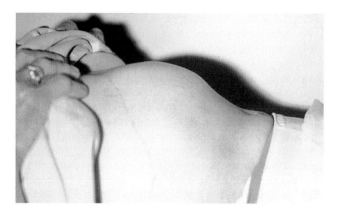

Figure 66–6. Abdominal bulge from intraperitoneal cyst of echinococcosis.

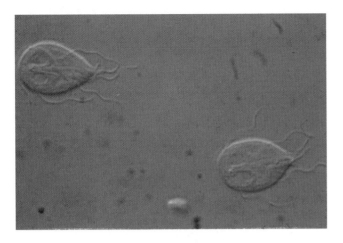

Figure 66–8. Flagellated, binucleate Giardia trophozoite.

cystic fibrosis; and in association with hepatic or pancreatic disease. Flatulence, nonbloody diarrhea or constipation, abdominal distention, and pain are common symptoms. Fever, weight loss, and fat, carbohydrate, and vitamin malabsorption can occur. Although cysts may appear in the stool, it is often necessary to perform duodenal aspiration to confirm the diagnosis. Metronidazole (15 mg/kg/d divided tid for 5 days) is recommended.

TRYPANOSOMES

The vectors that transmit *Trypanosoma gambiense, Trypanosoma rhodesiense* (African sleeping sickness), and *Trypanosoma cruzi* (Chagas' disease) are not endemic to the United States. However, they may be passed on through blood transfusions and breast feeding from infected adults. Although infestation initially mimics a viral illness, patients will later develop alterations in mental status, myocarditis, megacolon, and megaesophagus. If a history of travel to an endemic area by the parent or child is elicited, serologic tests and biopsy of affected organs are indicated. When the diagnosis has been confirmed, treatment is with nifurtimox, suramin, or melarsoprol.[1,3]

MALARIA

In 2006, 1474 cases of malaria were reported to the Centers for Disease Control and Prevention.[11] Over the past 10 years, the number of cases has remained stable at approximately 1000 a year. Of the cases reported in the United States between 2000 and 2005, 695 were US residents aged younger than 18 years. Most cases are because of either *Plasmodium falciparum* or *Plasmodium vivax*. Less common causative agents are *Plasmodium ovale, Plasmodium malariae,* and *P. knowlesi*. *P. knowlesi* is a primate malaria parasite, similar to *P. malariae,* that is commonly found in Southeast Asia. *P. knowlesi* causes malaria in long-tailed macaques but may also infect humans.[12] Two-thirds of all cases of malaria are imported from sub-Saharan Africa. For further discussion of the diagnosis and treatment of malaria, see Chapter 67.

BABESIOSIS

Babesia microti has an erythrocytic phase similar to that of malaria. It is transmitted by the deer tick *Ixodes dammini* from a rodent reservoir and is therefore found in the same geographic distribution as Lyme disease (northeastern states, Wisconsin, and Minnesota). When symptomatic, patients present with fever, malaise, hemolytic anemia, jaundice, and renal failure. Upon blood smear inspection, it may be difficult to distinguish *B. microti* from the ring form of *P. falciparum*. Treatment is with clindamycin (20–40 mg/kg/d divided tid) and quinine (25 mg/kg/d divided tid) for 7 to 10 days. Alternatively, a 7-to 10-day regimen of atovaquone (20 mg/kg q12 h) and azithromycin (12 mg/kg daily) has been shown to be effective and to have fewer adverse reactions.[1,3,13]

PNEUMOCYSTIS

Pneumocystis jiroveci (formerly *carinii*) has a low virulence and is found in the latent phase in a large percentage of the American population. When the host is immunocompromised, trophozoites replicate in alveolar spaces and spread through the vascular and lymphatic beds. The patient experiences respiratory distress, fever, and nonproductive cough with limited auscultatory findings. The radiograph may be normal or symmetric interstitial ground glass infiltrates in the middle and lower lung fields may be seen.[4]

Pneumocystis reactivation occurs in debilitated patients and those with suppressed immune responses. It is found in more than 60% of patients with HIV infection. The overall mortality rate in children is 40%, rising to 100% once radiographic changes occur in untreated non-AIDS patients.

Given the high incidence of asymptomatic carriers, the diagnostic method of choice is silver nitrate methenamine stain of a lung biopsy specimen in the proper clinical setting. Treatment is with trimethoprim (15–20 mg/kg/d) and sulfamethoxazole (75–100 mg/kg/d) in 3 or 4 divided doses orally or pentamidine (3–4 mg/kg/d) intravenously for 2 to 3 weeks.[1,3]

COCCIDIA

Cryptosporidium, Isospora belli, and *Toxoplasma gondii* belong to the protozoan subclass *Coccidia*, which also includes *Plasmodium*. Modes of transmission include direct human contact and ingestion of fecally contaminated food and water. *Toxoplasma* is also transmitted transplacentally, with blood transfusion and organ transplantation. Intermediate hosts include farm animals *(Cryptosporidium)*, cats *(Toxoplasma)*, and other mammals.[4]

Although some children harbor *Cryptosporidium* and *Isospora* asymptomatically, both organisms can cause a secretory, choleralike diarrhea after a 2-week incubation. Large volumes of watery, nonbloody, leukocyte-free stool may produce significant dehydration. Fever, headache, and anorexia are followed by malabsorption of lactose and fat. These symptoms are self-limited and last for up to 3 weeks. The oocysts may be shed for an additional month. Immunocompromised children may manifest infective symptoms of the liver, gallbladder, appendix, and lung as well as a reactive arthritis. No toxins have been demonstrated, and the pathogenic mechanism of this spectrum of symptoms is not known. Direct examination of stool with a modified Ziehl–Neelsen stain is the diagnostic method of choice. There is no proven antiparasitic cure. Octreotide (300–500 μg tid subcutaneously) may control the diarrhea of patients with HIV.

The trophozoites of *T. gondii* have a predilection for the brain, heart, and bone, although they can invade any nucleated cell. Approximately 2500 infants are born annually in the United States with congenital disease, 10% of whom have the *Toxoplasma* triad of hydrocephalus, chorioretinitis, and intracranial calcification. The long-term prognosis for these children is poor.

Acquired toxoplasmosis in the immune-competent host is asymptomatic but may produce a subclinical reaction in the reticuloendothelial system. For patients with AIDS and other types of immunocompromise, reactivation produces severe CNS involvement and dissemination to the heart and lungs. Between 30% and 40% of AIDS patients will develop *Toxoplasma* encephalitis or mass lesions of the brain and cranial nerves. The diagnosis is made by antigen detection or by seeing a ring formation on computed tomography with contrast (Fig. 66–9). Prompt treatment with pryimethamine (2 mg/kg/d for 3 days and then 1 mg/kg/d for 4 weeks–maximum 25 mg/d) and sul-

fadiazine (100–200 mg/kg/d for 4 weeks) is recommended.[1,3] However, there is a high fatality rate once *Toxoplasma* becomes reactivated.

► ARTHROPODS

PEDICULOSIS

The parasites *Pediculus humanus capitis* (head louse) (Fig. 66–10), *Pediculus humanus corporis* (body louse) (Fig. 66–11), and *Phthirus pubis* (pubic or crab louse) (Fig. 66–12) are 1 to 2 mm long. They attach 0.8 mm long eggs (nits) firmly to hair shafts, close to the skin (Fig. 66–13). Lice are transmitted by direct human contact or the sharing of clothing or other personal articles. They are not transmitted to or from domestic animals and are found on children with proper hygiene. They require a hair-bearing surface, with the adult viable for only 2 days and the nit for 10 days off the host. The most common complaint is itching. *P. pubis* may produce blue-colored macules (maculae ceruleae).[4]

A 10-minute rinse with 1% permethrin (Nix) has been reported to kill adult lice and 90% of nits.[1,3] It may, however, exacerbate the pruritus and erythema. It is too toxic to use near the eyes, where petrolatum is recommended to suffocate the lice. Eyelid lice in prepubescent children should alert the physician to the possibility of sexual abuse. Care must be taken to delouse other family members and the child's environment.

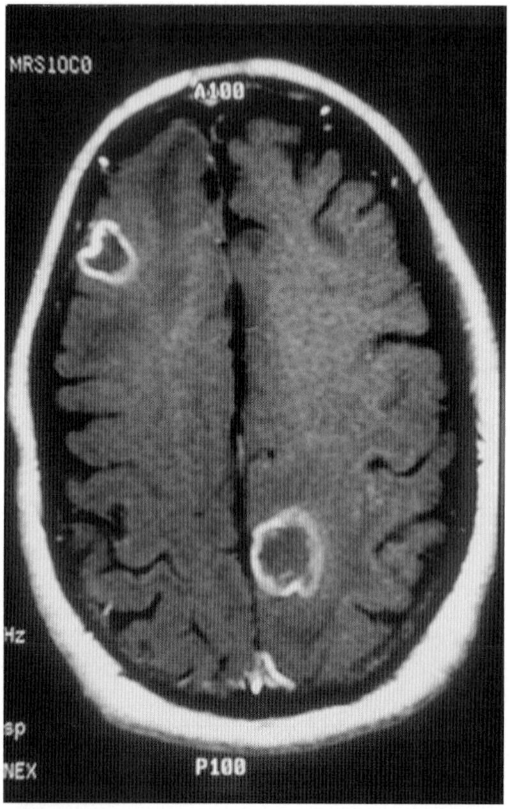

Figure 66–9. Contrast head CT scan showing typical multiple ring-enhancing lesions seen in *T. gondii* CNS infection.

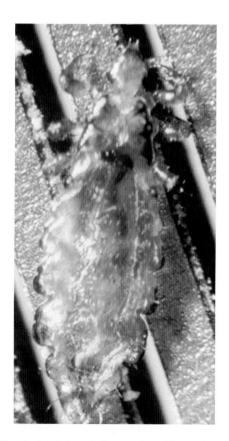

Figure 66–10. Adult female human head louse (Pediculus capitis) on a nit (louse-egg) comb.

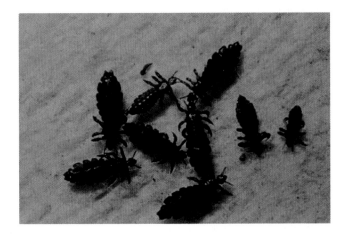

Figure 66–11. Pediculosis humanus corporis, the body louse.

A spray of permethrin and piperonyl butoxide should be employed on furniture and bedding used in the previous 2 days. Alternatively, objects can be sealed in plastic bags for 2 weeks until all adults and nits are no longer viable. Dead nits can be removed from hair shafts with a fine-toothed comb.

Resistance to permethrin is now common, with reported insecticidal activity down to 28% in one study. The combination of 1% permethrin with trimethoprim/sulfamethoxazole has been reported to be 95% effective, compared with 80% for permethrin alone.[14]

SCABIES

Sarcoptes scabiei (scabies) are transmitted by direct close and prolonged human contact. Scabies will not flourish on other animals. Following a 3- to 6-week incubation, the 200 to 400 μ-long scabies mite burrows between the fingers and toes as well as in the groin, external genitalia, and axillae, depositing eggs in the tunnel as she goes. The itch is worse at night, with infants sleeping poorly and rubbing their hands and feet together. Small red, raised, papules are formed, which may progress to vesicles and pustules. Secondary excoriations are also present. The diagnosis is made clinically. However, one

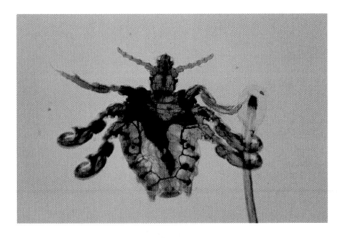

Figure 66–12. Pediculosis *Phthirus pubis*, the crab louse.

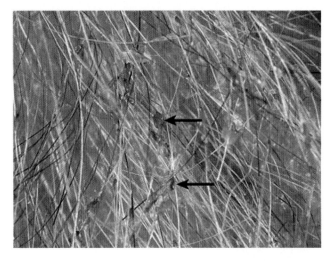

Figure 66–13. Pediculosis capitis: multiple nits on scalp hair. Myriads of nits (oval, grayish-white egg capsules) are firmly attached to the hair shafts, visualized with a lens. On close examination, these have a bottle shape.

may scrape burrows or papules overlaid with mineral oil and inspect the scrapings for adults, eggs, and excreta for confirmation (Fig. 66–14). A single application of 5% permethrin cream is curative for children older than 2 months. Younger children may be treated with sulfur precipitated in petrolatum.[1,3] The long incubation period makes treating the entire family advisable. As the parasite lives less than 24 hours off the host, environmental decontamination may not be necessary.

MYIASIS

Myiasis occurs when fly larvae invade the human body. Under normal circumstances, these larvae live off decaying organic matter. In very unusual circumstances, particularly with debilitated and malnourished children, maggots may be found in

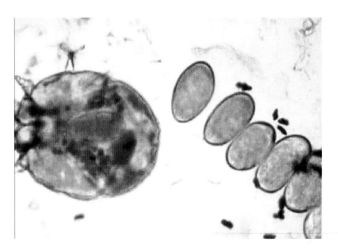

Figure 66–14. Scabies. Microscopic examination of a mineral oil preparation after scraping a burrow reveals a gravid female mite with oval, gray eggs and fecal pellets.

the nasal mucosa, eye, diaper area, or skin. Surgical excision is required and is curative.

REFERENCES

1. Drugs for parasitic infections. *Med Lett Drugs Ther.* 2007 (suppl):1–15.
2. Georgiev VS. Pharmacotherapy of ascarisis. *Expert Opin Pharmacother.* 2001;2:223–239.
3. Liu LX, Weller PF. Antiparasitic drugs. *N Engl J Med.* 1996; 334(18):1178–1184.
4. Recommendations of the International Task Force for Disease Eradication. *MMWR Recomm Rep.* 1993;42(RR-16):1–25.
5. Georgiev VS. Chemotherapy of enterobiasis (oxyuriasis). *Expert Opin Pharmacother.* 2001;2:267–275.
6. Stephenson LS, Holland CV, Cooper ES. The public health significance of trichuris trichiura. *Parasitiology.* 2000; 121(suppl):S72–S95.
7. Nair D. Screening for strongyloides infection among the institutionalized mentally disabled. *J Am Board Fam Pract.* 2001; 14:51–53.
8. Georgiev VS. Necatoriasis: treatment and developmental therapeutics. *Expert Opin Pharmacother.* 2000;9:1065–1078.
9. Stanley SL. Pathophysiology of amoebiasis. *Trends Parasitol.* 2001;17:280–285.
10. Windsor JJ, Johnson EH. Dientamoeba fragilis: the unflagellated human flagellate. *Br J Biomed Sci.* 1999;56:293–306.
11. Centers for Disease Control and Prevention. Summary of notifiable diseases—United States, 2006. *MMWR Morb Mortal Wkly Rep.* 2008;55(53):1–100.
12. Cox-Singh J, Davis TME, Lee K-S, Shamsul SSG, et al. Plasmodium knowlesi malaria in humans is widely distributed and potentially life threatening. *Clin Infect Dis.* 2008;46:165–171.
13. Krause PJ, Lepore T, Sikand VK, et al. Atovaquone and azithromycin for the treatment of babesiosis. *N Engl J Med.* 2000;343:1454–1458.
14. Hipolito RB, Mallorca FG, Zuniga-Macaraig ZO, et al. Head lice infestation: single drug versus combination therapy with one percent permethrin and trimethoprim/sulfamethoxazole. *Pediatrics.* 201;107:E30.
15. Thank HD, Elsas RM, Veenstra J. Airport malaria: report of a case and a brief overview of the literature. *Neth J Med.* 2002; 60(11):441–443.
16. Suh KN, Kain KC, Keystone JS. Malaria. *CMAJ.* 2004;170(11): 1693–1702.
17. Svenson JE, MacLean JD, Gyorkos TJ, et al. Imported malaria: clinical presentation and examination of symptomatic travelers. *Arch Intern Med.* 1995;155:861.

CHAPTER 67

Imported Diseases/Diseases in the Traveling Child

Thomas L. Hurt

▶ HIGH-YIELD FACTS

- Nonspecific viral illness is the most common final diagnosis in pediatric patients admitted to the hospital with febrile illnesses after traveling.
- Blood cultures and thin and thick smears for malaria are important initial tests for all travelers returning from an area endemic for malaria. If the first smears are negative and the diagnosis is not established, repeat smears should be obtained every 8 to 24 hours until it is certain that malaria is not the cause of the fever.
- Anemia is common in many diseases but hemoconcentration, especially in combination with thrombocytopenia, may indicate dengue fever.
- Eosinophilia is defined as a peripheral eosinophil count of > 400 to 500 cells/mm^3. In the returning traveler, especially if fever is noted, helminth infection is suggested.
- Malaria most commonly presents as a nonspecific influenza-like syndrome with high fever, chills, rigors, sweats, and headache and is frequently misdiagnosed as a viral syndrome. These symptoms are unreliable in clinical practice and no combination of fever pattern, duration of symptoms, or physical findings can reliably rule out malaria.
- The laboratory diagnosis of malaria has not changed markedly over the past century. The use of thick and thin peripheral blood smears using Giemsa stain remains the "accepted diagnostic technique for malaria."
- The most practical approach in the emergency department is to assume that all malaria is chloroquine resistant.
- Falciparum malaria can progress rapidly to become a medical emergency. If falciparum malaria is diagnosed or reasonably suspected, the patient should be admitted to the hospital and treatment started.
- In a critically ill child with malaria, *falciparum* should be presumed until proven otherwise and parenteral treatment with quinine or quinidine should be started. These medications require cardiac monitoring with particular attention to the QT interval and to hypotension.
- If neither quinidine nor quinine is available, clindamycin can be used as a temporizing medication.
- Classic dengue fever is an acute onset febrile illness with a variety of nonspecific symptoms. In addition to fever, the most commonly reported symptoms in older children and adolescents include rash, headache, retro-orbital pain, myalgias, and arthralgias. The arthralgias and myalgias can be so severe that dengue fever has been given the nickname "breakbone fever."
- The etiology of traveler's diarrhea (TD) has been somewhat elusive as medical workups infrequently yield a bacteria, virus, or parasite. However, the fact that prophylactic antimicrobial agents markedly reduce the attack rate suggests that an infectious bacterial process is often responsible.
- The most important intervention for diarrhea is replacement of fluid and electrolyte losses.
- There is theoretical concern that antimotility agents may prolong the course of disease caused by invasive enteropathogens. Use in children remains controversial because of concerns that it might aggravate disease caused by invasive enteric pathogens.
- Typhoid fever (TF) continues to be a global health problem, but in the developed world it is now thought of primarily as a travel-related disease.

Emergency department physicians face the challenging task of evaluating patients who have returned with illnesses acquired while abroad. Nearly two million children travel internationally every year.[1] International adoptees and immigrants make up another group of children who bring "imported" diseases home with them.

Fortunately, emergency physicians encounter these "imported" diseases only infrequently. It is this same infrequency, though, that can result in missed diagnoses and incorrect treatment. The evaluation and treatment of the ill-child traveler is aided by an awareness of possible pathogens, knowledge of the geographic distribution and incubation periods of specific pathogens, knowledge of the patient's immunization and chemoprophylaxis status, recognition of signs and symptoms of specific illnesses, and application of a systematic approach to diagnosis and treatment of these unfamiliar diseases.

Nonspecific viral illness is the most common final diagnosis in pediatric patients admitted to the hospital with febrile illnesses after traveling. Malaria is a less frequent but potentially more life-threatening diagnosis. Malaria is the diagnosis in up to 41% of returning pediatric travelers admitted to hospitals in the United Kingdom. Diarrhea illnesses are the cause of fever in 27% of hospitalized pediatric travelers.[2–4] The list of all possible tropical diseases in children is extremely lengthy, but those diseases that are likely to be diagnosed in the emergency department make up a much shorter list. Some diseases

▶ **TABLE 67–1. IMPORTED DISEASES**

Disease	Organism Vector	Clinical Manifestation	Treatment
Plasmodium protozoa	Malaria (mosquito)	Fever, hepatosplenomegaly	Antimalarials: quinine, quinidine, doxycycline, clindamycin
Spotted fevers	Rickettsiae (tick)	Fever, headache, malaise, rash	Doxycycline
Yellow fever	Group B arbovirus (mosquito)	Fever, headache, vomiting, jaundice	Supportive
Dengue shock syndrome	Arbovirus (mosquito)	Fever, severe body aches, purpura	Supportive
Enteric fever	*S. typhi* or *paratyphi* (fecal)	Fever, abdominal pain, rash	Ceftriaxone or fluoroquinolones
Hemorrhagic fevers (Ebola, Marburg)	Filoviruses, ebola, and Marburg (direct contact with infected host)	Fever, DIC, shock	Supportive
Leptospirosis	Leptospiro interrogans (contaminated freshwater)	Fever, ictohemorrhagic "Weil's disease"	Cephalosporins, penicillins, doxycycline
Rabies	Rabies virus (animal bite)	Fever, pain, paresthesias, encephalitis, death	Postexposure vaccine, supportive care
Leishmaniasis	Parasite from sand flea bite	Cutaneous sores, abdominal visceral swelling and pain	Antimonials
Strongyloides	Helminthic parasite – cutaneous entry	Rapidly spreading serpiginous rash—larva currens	Ivermectin, thiabendazole
Schistosomiasis	Intestinal and urinary freshwater flatworms	Fever, back pain, paresthesias	Praziquantel
Cysticercosis	Pork tapeworm Taenia solium	Seizures	Praziquantel
Amebiasis	*E. histolytica*	Abdominal pain, bloody diarrhea	Mebendazole, iodoquinol
Roundworm (ascariasis)	Ascaria lumbrigoides	Abdominal pain, Loeffler syndrome	Mebendazole Pyrantel pamoate

are especially important to bear in mind because they have the potential of rapidly becoming life-threatening. The physician should focus on those illnesses that carry the greatest risk of morbidity and mortality. Illnesses which have specific public health concerns (e.g., viral hemorrhagic fevers, tuberculosis) must also be kept in mind. Table 67–1 provides a partial list of imported diseases.

▶ IMMUNIZATIONS AND CHEMOPROPHYLAXIS

Information about the patient's immunization and chemoprophylaxis status may help narrow the possible causes of a febrile illness. Proper scheduling of some vaccines provides immunity, which is nearly 100% effective. Immunizations against yellow fever, hepatitis A, and hepatitis B are in this category.[5] Other vaccines are less effective and significant illness can occur in spite of immunizations. Typhoid vaccines offer 70% to 80% protection.[6] The most important immunizations a child should receive prior to travel are the "routine" immunizations. Children residing in developed countries who are not vaccinated against the "routine" infections have the benefit of relative protection through local herd immunity. Diseases such as diphtheria, measles, and polio occur in periodic outbreaks in many countries and for traveling children, "routine" vaccines against polio, diphtheria, tetanus, and measles may not provide adequate immunity if a booster is not given before the travel.[7] Arriving adoptees from developing countries comprise

a patient population that is unique since they often are only partially immunized or have received no immunizations at all. Immunization records for these patients may not be accurate.[8]

Detailed information for schedules of routine immunizations can be found in the current edition of the Report of the Committee on Infectious Diseases (*Red Book*).[9] Table 67–2 lists some of the recommended travel vaccines.

▶ TRAVEL LOCATIONS

Disease exposure differs according to the region of the world. Knowledge of the distribution of various diseases can help include or exclude the likelihood of a specific disease in a returning traveler. As an example, yellow fever is not found in Southeast Asia but travel to parts of Africa or South America may expose the patient to this disease. Table 67–3 provides a list of infections found in specific locations.

▶ INCUBATION PERIODS

Knowledge of incubation periods can help exclude some diseases entirely. For example, a patient who develops a fever 3 days after returning from a 7-day trip to Tanzania (incubation period less than 10 days) may have a rickettsial infection, dengue fever, or viral hemorrhagic fever such as yellow fever because these diseases typically have incubation periods of less than 2 weeks. Hepatitis A would be very unlikely because

▶ **TABLE 67-2. RECOMMENDED TRAVEL VACCINES**

Vaccines	Comments
Hepatitis A	Efficacy 94%–100%
Rabies	Antibodies exist for at least 2 y after the primary series.
Preexposure vaccines	
Human diploid cell vaccine (HDCV)	
Rabies vaccine adsorbed (RVA)	
Purified chick embryo cell vaccine (PCEC)	
Postexposure treatment	
Passive and active immunization	
Meningococcus	Antibody concentrations decrease rapidly over 2–3 y.
Vaccine available for children >2 y	
Typhoid	Approximately 70%–80% effective
Oral vaccine and parenteral vaccine are available in the United States	
Yellow fever	Provides at least 10 y protection
Available at approved state health department centers	

it has a mean incubation period of 4 weeks. Knowledge of the incubation periods can serve as guidelines, but not hard and fast rules. Table 67–4 lists the incubation periods for a variety of illnesses that may be contracted abroad.

▶ SOURCES OF INFORMATION FOR INTERNATIONAL TRAVEL-RELATED DISEASES

A variety of sources can provide region-specific and disease-specific information. The *Red Book* provides general information on worldwide exposure risk.[9] The CDC Division of Quarantine publishes a biweekly summary of Health Information for International Travel (the *Blue Sheet*), which shows where cholera and yellow fever are currently being reported. The Parasitology Division of the National Institute of Health offers special expertise in the evaluation of eosinophilia. A partial list of Web sites providing information on international travel-related infections is provided in Table 67–5.

▶ **TABLE 67-3. INFECTIONS AND GEOGRAPHIC LOCATIONS***

Caribbean: malaria (Haiti), dengue fever, leishmaniasis

South and Central America: malaria, dengue fever, hepatitis A, cholera, leishmaniasis, yellow fever, amebiasis, viral encephalitis, schistosomiasis

Pacific Islands: malaria, dengue fever, hepatitis A, Japanese encephalitis

Southeast Asia, Far East, South Asia (India, Pakistan, Bangladesh, Nepal, and Sri Lanka): malaria, dengue fever, hepatitis A, Japanese encephalitis, cholera, rickettsial diseases, leishmaniasis

Middle East and North Africa: malaria, hepatitis A, leishmaniasis, tick typhus, schistosomiasis, brucellosis

Subsaharan Africa: malaria, hepatitis A, cholera, yellow fever, amebiasis, typhus, schistosomiasis

Europe and former Soviet Union: hepatitis, tick typhus, Lyme disease, leishmaniasis, diphtheria, polio, brucellosis, tick-borne encephalitis

Australia/New Zealand/North America: rocky mountain spotted fever, Lyme disease, viral encephalitis

*Dysentery, typhoid and tuberculosis are worldwide in distribution.

▶ **TABLE 67-4. INCUBATION PERIODS FOR TRAVEL-RELATED INFECTIOUS DISEASES**

Incubation Period	Infectious Disease
Short (<2 wk)	Malaria (especially *P. falciparum*)
	Viral hemorrhagic fevers—including dengue fever
	Rickettsioses: louse, flea-born, typhus
	Enteric fever
	Influenza
	Plague
	Anthrax
	Rabies
Mid (2–6 wk)	Malaria (especially *P. falciparum*)
	Rickettsioses: spotted fever group
	Enteric fever
	Leptospirosis
	Brucellosis
	Viral hepatitis
	Strongyloides
	Rabies
Long (>6 wk)	Malaria
	Tuberculosis
	Viral hepatitis
	Enteric protozoal infections and helminthes infections
	Schistosomiasis
	Amebic liver abscess
	Leishmaniasis
	Rabies

▶ TABLE 67–5. **INTERNET REFERENCES FOR TRAVEL-RELATED ILLNESSES**

1. CDC "Health Information for International Traveler" (Yellow Book)
   General travelers' health information, region- and destination-specific recommendations, including vaccinations and malaria prophylaxis — http://www.cdc.gov/travel/yellowbook.pdf

2. Centers for Disease Control and Prevention: Travelers' Health Information
   Recommendations for specific travel destinations, links to other sites, travel advisories, and outbreak notices — http://www.cdc.gov/travel/

3. World Health Organization (WHO) Yellow Book, "International Travel and Health"
   General travelers' health recommendations; with country-specific malarial risks. Very useful for current outbreaks. — http://www.who.int/ith/

4. Morbidity and Mortality Weekly Report, International bulletins
   Surveillance summaries & outbreak investigations. — http://www.cdc.gov/mmwr

5. American Society of Tropical Medicine and Hygiene (ASTMH)
   Current information on tropical disease prevention and control and worldwide outbreaks. — http://www.astmh.org

6. World Health Organization (WHO) Infectious Disease Health Topics
   Maps of travel-related diseases & general information. — http://www.who.int//health-topics/

▶ RISK FACTORS

It is important to ask about activity-based risk factors. Was there contact with others who were ill? Epidemics of meningococcal disease have occurred in travelers to Mecca and Nepal.[10] Did the patient swim or raft in any freshwater? Leptospirosis is transmitted by exposure to nonchlorinated freshwater. Was there a history of insect or animal bite? Children have the highest incidence of rabies worldwide.[11] Obtain the sexual history in anyone old enough to be involved in any sexual activity.

▶ PHYSICAL EXAMINATION

The physical examination can provide clues to the diagnosis. The presence of jaundice may suggest hepatitis, dengue fever, liver flukes, or liver abscesses. A rash may suggest any number of possibilities, but petechiae and/or purpura suggest bacterial sepsis, dengue fever, viral hemorrhagic fevers, or rickettsial diseases. Respiratory symptoms may suggest influenza, pneumonia, tuberculosis, or Loeffler syndrome. Table 67–6 provides a limited differential diagnosis for some travel-related diseases based on physical findings.

▶ DIAGNOSTIC STUDIES/LABORATORY INVESTIGATIONS

Blood cultures and thin and thick smears for malaria are important initial tests for all travelers returning from an area endemic for malaria. If the first smears are negative and the diagnosis is not established, repeat smears should be obtained every 8 to 24 hours until it is certain that malaria is not the cause of the fever.[12]

In addition to malaria smears and blood cultures, recommended basic laboratory tests include a complete blood count (CBC) with differential, chemistry panel that includes liver function tests, urinalysis, urine culture, and stool studies. It is very practical to obtain a tube of serum that can be stored

▶ TABLE 67–6. **PHYSICAL FINDINGS FOR SOME IMPORTED DISEASES**

Physical Finding	Jaundice	Petechiae/ Ecchymosis	Hepatomegaly	Splenomegaly	Wheezing	Neurologic Complaints
Disease	Hepatitis	Meningococcus	Malaria	Malaria	Loeffler syndrome	Rabies
	Malaria	Dengue fever	Hepatitis	Typhoid	Tropical pulmonary eosinophilia	Neurocysti- cercosis
	Relapsing fevers	Yellow fever	Typhoid	Dengue fever	Tuberculosis	Neuroschisto- somiasis
	Leptospirosis	Rickettsial diseases	Leishmaniasis	Leishmaniasis		
	Dengue fever	Viral hemorrhagic fevers	Leptospirosis	Brucellosis		
	Liver abscess		Amebic liver abscess	Typhus		

for future paired (acute and convalescent) serologic tests.[12] Storing this tube of serum when the patient is first evaluated may provide the diagnosis when a sample obtained at a later date is compared to the first.

Specific laboratory findings may provide clues to the diagnosis. Anemia is common in many diseases but hemoconcentration, especially in combination with thrombocytopenia, may indicate dengue fever.[13] Thrombocytopenia is common in dengue fever and also in malaria. A low or normal white blood count is most typically found with malaria.[14] A low white blood count with a bandemia can be consistent with *Shigella* infection whereas a low white blood count with a lymphocytosis is more typical of a viral illness or a rickettsial infection.[15] The presence of atypical lymphocytes suggests acute mononucleosis. A leukocytosis with a predominance of neutrophils suggests a bacterial infection but can also occur with a spirochetal disease such as leptospirosis or *Borrelia* (relapsing fever). Mild-to-moderate elevation of liver enzymes can be seen in many diseases, including acute mononucleosis, enteroviral infections, typhoid fever, dengue fever, typhus, viral hemorrhagic fevers, leptospirosis, shigellosis, and viral hepatitis. Markedly elevated transaminases are consistent with viral hepatitides. Elevated levels of lactate dehydrogenase and bilirubin in connection with mild-to-moderate elevation of transaminases are frequently found in patients with malaria.[14] Hypoglycemia should raise suspicion for the possibility of malaria as well.[12]

SIGNIFICANCE OF EOSINOPHILIA

Eosinophilia is defined as a peripheral eosinophil count of >400 to 500 cells/mm^3.[16,17] It develops as an immune response to a variety of processes such as allergic disorders, drug-related hypersensitivity reactions, collagen vascular disease, and malignancies. In the returning traveler, especially if fever is noted, helminth infection is suggested. Eosinophilia is seen especially during the early acute tissue invasive phase of infestation as compared to the later chronic phase of illness.[18] Diagnoses to be considered in febrile travelers with eosinophilia include ascariasis, strongyloides, acute schistosomiasis, toxocariasis, trichinosis, lymphatic filariasis, coccidiomycosis, echinococcus, tapeworm (cestode infestation), and lung and liver flukes. The more common intestinal protozoa, *Giardia lamblia* and *Entamoeba histolytica*, do not cause eosinophilia.

The initial evaluation of returning travelers with eosinophilia should include an examination of the stool for ova and parasites. Depending on the geographical areas of travel and the clinical findings, the evaluating physician may consider imaging studies such as chest x-rays (coccidiomycosis), CT scans of the head (cysticercosis), or ultrasound of the liver (amebic abscesses or echinococcal cysts).

Helminth infections often occur without eosinophilia. Conversely, when blood eosinophilia is noted, it has only limited predictive value for the presence of travel-related infections. In a Swiss study of returning travelers, the positive predictive value of eosinophilia for helminth infection was only 18.9%. However, if eosinophilia was extreme (≥16% of the total WBC count), the probability of finding a definite diagnosis reached >60% and the positive predictive value for a helminth infection was 46.6%.[16]

See Figure 67–1 for a systematic approach to evaluating the returning child traveler.

▶ SPECIFIC DISEASES OF IMPORTANCE

MALARIA

Malaria is endemic to the tropics and is responsible for 2.7 million deaths per year. The great majority of these deaths are in children. Approximately 1200 cases a year are reported in the United States and almost all of these are acquired abroad. Malaria is a treatable disease with significant potential for mortality. It should be at the top of the physician's differential when evaluating a returning febrile traveler.[19] Malaria should also be suspected in febrile neonates born to mothers who have lived in a malaria area (transplacental transmission) and in febrile adoptees from endemic areas. Even those travelers who spent "no" time in an endemic area can contract malaria from mosquito bites during brief transfer stops or layovers in airports (so-called "runway" or "airport malaria").[20]

Malaria is transmitted by the night-biting *Anopheles* mosquito. It is a protozoal infection caused by any of four species (*vivax*, *ovale*, *malariae*, and *falciparum*) of the genus *Plasmodium*. Close to 90% of the global cases of malaria are caused by *Plasmodium falciparum*.

Malaria most commonly presents as a nonspecific influenza-like syndrome with high fever, chills, rigors, sweats, and headache and is frequently misdiagnosed as a viral syndrome. Other manifestations include nausea, vomiting, diarrhea, abdominal pain, cough, arthralgias, and back pain. These symptoms are unreliable in clinical practice and no combination of fever pattern, duration of symptoms, or physical findings can reliably rule out malaria.[21] Malaria can present with prominent gastrointestinal symptoms and can be misdiagnosed as acute gastroenteritis. Physicians are taught that a 48- or 72-hour periodic fever, which reflects the reproductive cycle of the *Plasmodium* organism, is the hallmark of infection and can distinguish malaria from other causes of fever, but many patients do not have cyclical fevers and only about half of the patients have fever at the time of presentation.[22] Daily fever is the most common complaint in pediatric patients but only about a third have a history of paroxysmal fevers. Hepatomegaly is commonly noted and splenomegaly is reported in up to 68% of patients.[19] Potentially fatal complications of *P. falciparum* include cerebral malaria, severe hemolytic anemia (blackwater fever), hypoglycemia, noncardiogenic pulmonary edema, respiratory failure, renal failure, metabolic acidosis, shock, and vascular collapse.

Laboratory studies may show anemia, thrombocytopenia, and moderately elevated liver function tests with hyperbilirubinemia. Leukocytosis is unusual with normal white blood counts or leukopenia being more common. Hypoglycemia is frequently noted.

The laboratory diagnosis of malaria has not changed markedly over the past century. The use of thick and thin peripheral blood smears using Giemsa stain remains the "accepted diagnostic technique for malaria."[23] These "malaria smears" are the most widely available diagnostic tests in the United States, since most hospital laboratories are able to

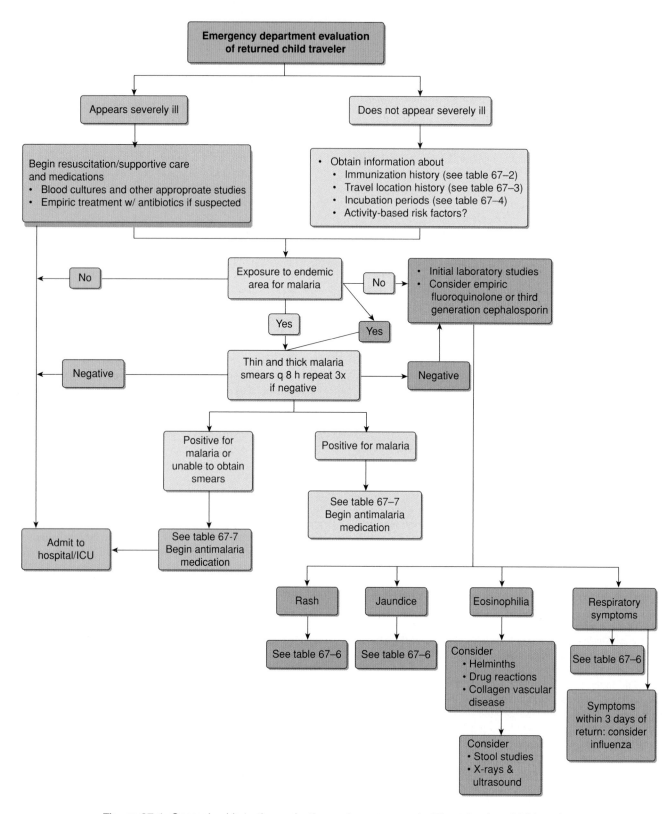

Figure 67–1. General guide to the evaluation and management of the returning child traveler.

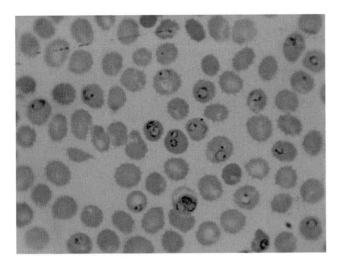

Figure 67-2. Thin smear showing parasites within red blood cells. The thin smear is helpful for species identification. (Courtesy of Angkor Hospital for Children, Siem Reap, Cambodia.)

perform Giemsa stains on peripheral blood.[24] Both thick and thin smears should be examined. Thick smears give a higher sensitivity than thin smears by a factor of 10 since a larger volume of blood is examined (Fig. 67–2). Thin smears are used primarily for speciation and determination of the degree of parasitemia (Fig. 67–3). The sensitivity of these tests is limited by the experience of the microscopist. Since malaria is not endemic to the United States, many US hospitals have few microscopists skilled at reading these smears. One set of negative films is not enough to rule out disease and it is recommended that smears be repeated every 8 to 24 hours for at least three negative sets before malaria is ruled out.[25]

A study from Toronto demonstrated that in nonendemic centers there is an average 7.6-day delay in the onset of treat-

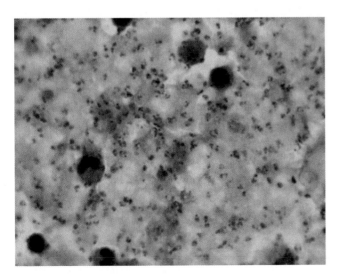

Figure 67-3. The thick smear is most helpful for discovery of intracellular parasites. (Courtesy of Angkor Hospital for Children, Siem Reap, Cambodia.)

ment of *P. falciparum* due to a combination of factors: failure of physicians to consider malaria, slow and inaccurate laboratory diagnosis, and failure to initiate prompt and appropriate therapy.[25] In many hospital laboratories, malaria smears may be read only once a day or may be considered a "send-out." If unable to arrange for reliable and quick reading of these smears, one should consider admitting even relatively well-appearing febrile children with a history of travel to malaria-endemic areas for observation and diagnosis. This recommendation holds particularly true for patients at risk for *P. falciparum*, which can be rapidly fatal.

Alternative diagnostic techniques exist but are not readily available in all hospital laboratories. Fluorescent microscopy is at least as sensitive as thick smears but is relatively expensive. It is often not able to distinguish species.[23] Rapid antigen detection tests have the advantages of a quick turn around time and low technical requirements, but are mostly available only outside the United States. They have poor capability for speciation and the sensitivity of the tests varies with the degree of parasitemia and therefore cannot exclude disease.[26] PCR techniques are sensitive (>90%) and almost 100% specific[23] but in the United States, these tests are only available on a limited basis in certain government-sponsored laboratories.

Treatment options for malaria depend upon the severity of the illness, the species and whether or not it is resistant to chloroquine. The most practical approach in the emergency department is to assume that all malaria is chloroquine resistant. Falciparum malaria can progress rapidly to become a medical emergency. If falciparum malaria is diagnosed or reasonably suspected, the patient should be admitted to the hospital and treatment started.[27] Any febrile child traveler who presents with altered mental status, respiratory distress, signs of shock, or severe laboratory abnormalities should be admitted to the intensive care unit (ICU). Malaria should be high on the differential. In a critically ill child with malaria, *falciparum* should be presumed until proven otherwise and parenteral treatment with quinine or quinidine should be started. These medications require cardiac monitoring with particular attention to the QT interval and to hypotension. Both quinidine and quinine, as well as malaria itself, can cause hypoglycemia and frequent serum glucose checks should be made. If neither quinidine nor quinine is available, clindamycin can be used as a temporizing medication. Because chloroquine-resistant species are now found throughout the world, combination oral therapy with quinine/quinidine and sulfadoxine-pyrimethamine or clindamycin (if <7 years old) or doxycycline (if >7 years old) is recommended as first-line treatment for children with malaria, even in those who are well appearing. Other agents include atovaquone-proguanil in children weighing >5 kg, mefloquine, lumefantrine, halofantrine, and artemisinin derivatives. Information pertaining to diagnosis, regional resistance, and treatment guidelines is available on the CDC Web site: www.cdc.gov. Recommendations for the initial treatment of malaria are found in Table 67–7.

DENGUE FEVER

Dengue fever is the most significant arboviral infection of humans. This flavivirus is endemic to most tropical parts of the world and infects an estimated 100 million people annually. It

▶ TABLE 67–7. **TREATMENT OF MALARIA**

Medication	Dose	
Patients with malaria who are seriously ill or cannot take oral medications (all species of plasmodium)		
IV quinidine gluconate	10 mg/kg IV load in NS over 1–2 h, then infuse 0.02 mg/kg/min with cardiac monitoring	
Patients with uncomplicated chloroquine-resistant _P. falciparum_ or _Plasmodium vivax_ (90% of patients)		
Oral quinine sulfate Plus	25 mg/kg/d (max. 650 mg/dose) ÷ tid × 3–7 d	
Doxycycline Or	2 mg/kg/d (max. 100 mg) × 7 d	
Pyrimethamine sulfadoxine	<1 y, ¼ tablet 1–3 y, ½ tablet 4–8 y, 1 tablet 9–14 y, 2 tablets >14 y, 3 tablets	Note 1. Single oral dose 2. Sulfa allergy risk
Or		
Clindamycin (if _P. falciparum_)	20–40 mg/kg/d ÷ tid × 5 d (max 900 mg/dose)	
Suspected or proven malaria from areas without _P. falciparum_ or _P. vivax_		
Chloroquine phosphate	10 mg/kg of base (max. 600 mg), then 5 mg/kg of base at 6, 24, and 48 h	
Plus		
Doxycycline Or	3 mg/kg (max. 200 mg) once daily × 3 d	
Pyrimethamine sulfadoxine	<1 y, ¼ tablet 1–3 y, ½ tablet 4–8 y, 1 tablet 9–14 y, 2 tablets >14 y, 3 tablets	Note 1. Single oral dose 2. Sulfa allergy risk

is most commonly transmitted via the day-biting female _Aedes aegypti_ and _Aedes albopictus_ mosquitoes. Dengue virus causes a range of illness from benign minor fever to hemorrhagic phenomena that may lead to circulatory collapse (dengue shock syndrome [DSS]) and death. DSS is responsible for about 15,000 deaths annually.[13]

Classic dengue fever is an acute onset febrile illness with a variety of nonspecific symptoms. It may be difficult to distinguish dengue fever from more familiar viral diseases such as influenza. Infants and younger children most commonly present with fever and vomiting and are likely to develop hepatomegaly. In addition to fever, the most commonly reported symptoms in older children and adolescents include rash, headache, retro-orbital pain, myalgias, and arthralgias.[28] The arthralgias and myalgias can be so severe that dengue fever has been given the nickname "breakbone fever." In the majority of individuals, dengue fever is very uncomfortable, but self-limiting and benign.

The primary concern is the potential for progression of the disease to the hemorrhagic form that can lead to systemic shock. Clinical manifestations in dengue hemorrhagic fever (DHF) include high fever, hepatomegaly, bleeding (from the mucosa, GI tract, or injection sites), and skin findings such as petechiae, purpura, and easy bruising. Circulatory failure is seen as the disease progresses to DSS.

A CBC should be obtained to check the hematocrit and platelets. Thrombocytopenia (≤100,000 cells/mm³) and hemo-

concentration (a rise in the hematocrit of >20% of baseline for age) are indicators of worsening disease. The WHO considers fever combined with hemoconcentration or any hemorrhagic manifestation including easy bruising and thrombocytopenia sufficient to establish a provisional diagnosis of DHF.[29] Increased vascular permeability and abnormal hemostasis may cause coagulopathy and DIC. Other abnormal laboratory findings include elevated liver transaminases and albuminuria. Hepatic dysfunction seems to be more common in infants.

Treatment is primarily symptomatic and supportive. Acetaminophen is recommended for pain and fever. NSAIDs and aspirin should not be used because they affect platelet-clotting function. Patients with suspected DHF/DSS should be admitted and managed supportively with fluid resuscitation, supplemental oxygen, and blood products as needed.

Definitive diagnosis of dengue fever cannot be established in the emergency department, but blood should be drawn for attempted virus isolation if the patient presents within the first 5 days of illness. Acute and convalescent serologies can help identify dengue viral infection.

Currently, there is no vaccine for dengue fever. Dengue virus has four distinct serotypes and exposure to one serotype does not establish cross-immunity to the remaining three. Exposure to a second infection (i.e., second serotype) increases the risk for progression to DHF and DSS, especially in children.[30] Exposure to a third infection makes DHF or DSS very likely. An effective vaccine will have to offer 100%

protection against all serotypes. It is estimated that a vaccine for dengue fever will be available in the near future.[31]

DIARRHEA: FOOD- AND WATERBORNE INFECTIONS

Travelers' diarrhea (TD) affects millions of international travelers of all ages every year. Some report the risk of TD to be as high as 50%.[32,33] Infectious causes usually occur due to ingestion of fecally contaminated food and water.

The most important risk factor is the destination of travel. North Africa has the highest incidence rate for TD (66%) followed by India (61.3%), East Africa (30.6%), Southeast Asia (29.8%), and Latin America (27.2%).[34] For all destinations, the highest attack rates and the most severe diarrhea diseases occur in children younger than 2 years (60%) followed by adolescents (39%). On average, TD starts on the eighth day of travel but can occur any time during or after travel. The majority of TD cases occur between 5 and 15 days after arrival with a reported range from 3 to 31 days.

In addition to diarrhea, the most common signs and symptoms of TD in children include abdominal cramping (67%), nausea and vomiting (18%), fever (14%), and mucous (5%) or blood (2%) in stools.[34] Tenesmus and fecal urgency can also occur.

The etiology of TD has been somewhat elusive as medical workups infrequently yield a bacteria, virus, or parasite. However, the fact that prophylactic antimicrobial agents markedly reduce the attack rate suggests that an infectious bacterial process is often responsible.[35] In one study, the most common microorganisms found in all children with TD included *Rotavirus* (24%), *Cryptosporidium* (15%), *Salmonella* (12%), *Campylobacter* (8%), *Shigella* (2%), enteropathogenic *Escherichia coli* (4%), enterotoxigenic *E. coli* (2%), and enterohemorrhagic *E. coli* (2%).[36]

The need for laboratory testing varies based on the duration of symptoms and severity of illness. Laboratory testing is indicated for those with more significant disease (severe diarrhea and dehydration, severe abdominal pain, and bloody stools) and persistent symptoms. The disease agents of persistent and chronic diarrhea are different from those of acute TD. Evaluation in chronic diarrhea should include a search for bacteria, parasites, overgrowth syndromes, and lactase deficiency.

The most important intervention for diarrhea is replacement of fluid and electrolyte losses. It is also important to consider the differences between the traveler with diarrhea and the nontraveler with diarrhea. In the nontraveler child in a developed country, antibiotics have no significant role in empiric treatment of acute diarrhea. Since viruses predominate as the cause in most of these cases of diarrhea, overuse of antibiotics may lead to both antibiotic resistance and risk for potential adverse reactions. Treatment focus in these children is prevention and replacement of fluid losses.

Current evidence suggests that TD in children is predominately bacterial. The adult literature has clearly shown that treatment with antibiotics decreases both the severity and duration of TD.[37,38] There is evidence that oral rehydration in conjunction with antibiotic treatment decreases pediatric diarrhea duration in developing countries.[39]

The traditional empiric antibiotic treatment of choice for TD in children has been a 3- to 5-day course of trimethoprim-sulfamethoxizole (TMP-SMX). Because of emerging TMP-SMX resistance, other agents are now recommended including macrolides and quinolones. Azithromycin should be considered in areas where *Campylobacter* is common. It has also been shown to be effective against *Shigella* and in one study was felt to be comparable to levofloxacin.[40] It is well tolerated by children and has an advantage of once-a-day dosing. Fluoroquinolones are the drugs of choice in adults with TD and may soon be approved for use in children. Fluoroquinolones have been avoided in children younger than 12 years due to potential issues with bone growth and arthropathies. Multiple studies using fluoroquinolones, (primarily ciprofloxacin), in children with chronic conditions such as cystic fibrosis have shown no increase in adverse events as compared to placebo or other antibiotics.[41-43] Some travel medicine specialists advocate ciprofloxacin as the drug of choice for TD treatment in all ages, including infants and children.[44] Cefixime is an alternative treatment for TD in children. Cefixime has been shown to be effective against *Shigella*, *E. coli*, and *Salmonella* in regions where TMP-SMX resistance is substantial.[45]

There is theoretical concern that antimotility agents may prolong the course of disease caused by invasive enteropathogens.[46] Loperamide is the antimotility agent of choice for treatment of adult TD and when used alone has been shown to reduce the frequency of diarrhea and the duration of illness.[47] The combination of an antimicrobial and loperamide appears to yield even better results than either treatment alone.[48] Although loperamide is approved for use in children older than 2 years, some authorities do not recommend antimotility agents in young children or feel that there is insufficient data to support their use.[46] Others consider loperamide to be safe in children older than 2 years but hesitate to recommend it if there is indication of an invasive organism.[44] Use in children remains controversial due to concerns that it might aggravate disease caused by invasive enteric pathogens. Recent studies involving children with gastroenteritis have documented statistically significant beneficial effects of loperamide with a minimum of side effects.[49] Despite this, the American Academy of Pediatrics still recommends against the use of loperamide in the management of acute diarrhea in children, whether travel-related or not.[34] Many sources also recommend against bismuth subsalicylate (BSS) use in children. It has been shown to decrease unformed stools in adults by 50%, but concern exists due to the potential risk of salicylate toxicity and Reyes syndrome in children. A group in Santiago, Chile, recently evaluated BSS as an adjunct to rehydration therapy in a double-blind, placebo-controlled study in children hospitalized for acute diarrhea and noted shortened disease length and hospital stay.[50] Another group of infants studied in Peru also had a significant reduction in stool output and hospital stays.[51] Both studies reported no adverse side effects or salicylate toxicity.

TYPHOID AND PARATYPHOID ENTERIC FEVERS

Typhoid fever (TF) is caused by *Salmonella enterica*, serotype *typhi*. *Salmonella paratyphi* causes an identical clinical syndrome. The term enteric fever is sometimes used in place of typhoid fever to describe either syndrome. There is no animal reservoir. Disease occurs only in humans and is transmitted via the fecal-oral route due to contaminated food and water. Asymptomatic intestinal carriers of *S. typhi* in disease-endemic areas unknowingly contribute as sources of infection.

TF continues to be a global health problem, but in the developed world, it is now thought of primarily as a travel-related disease. The incidence of TF in the United States steadily declined in the first half of the twentieth century and since the late 1970s has remained at around 500 cases per year. Between 1994 and 1999, the CDC reported that 74% of U.S. TF patients had recently traveled. The risk for travelers varies by the geographic region visited. In the CDC reports, 76% of TF cases were associated with travel to only six countries—India (30%), Pakistan (13%), Mexico (12%), Bangladesh (8%), the Philippines (8%), and Haiti (5%).[52] Reports indicate that the Indian subcontinent has an overall higher risk for acquiring TF than travel to any other region.[53] Travelers who acquire TF are rarely immunized against it, indicating that failure to vaccinate, not vaccine failure, is the primary problem.

In indigenous populations, TF affects infants less than older children and adolescents. The incidence of TF peaks between the ages of 5 and 12 years. A 5-year review of US cases of TF (1994–1999) showed that only 7% were in children <2 years of age and 41% were in the 2- to 17-year age group.[54]

The typical incubation period is 5 to 21 days but the range is broad—from 3 to 60 days. Presenting symptoms include fever, chills, frontal headache, anorexia, nausea, and malaise. Hepatomegaly and splenomegaly may occur. Infants and young children with TF frequently present with a different syndrome of symptoms when compared to older children and adults. While constipation is a feature of TF in adults and older children, diarrhea is a more common GI symptom in younger children.

Symptoms progress during the first week and rash may occur. Erythematous blanching maculopapular "rose spots" are reported in 5% to 30% of cases. They usually erupt on the trunk rather than the extremities. Rose spots are easier to see on light-skinned individuals and can be missed in dark-skinned patients.

TF is notable for prolonged high fevers, often continuing for 10 to 14 days. Relative bradycardia in response to fever is common in TF, although it is not specific for it. If untreated, the disease course is prolonged for more than 1 month.

Laboratory data commonly show a leukopenia, anemia, and thrombocytopenia. Liver function tests, both bilirubin and transaminases, may be moderately elevated (two–three times the normal rate). These laboratory findings are similar to those seen in both dengue fever and malaria.

Diagnosis of TF is based on identifying *S. typhi* in blood or stool cultures. Blood cultures are most likely to be positive during the acute febrile phase in the first 2 weeks of illness. Stool and urine cultures have only a 10% to 15% yield during the first week with higher yields in weeks 3 and 4 (75%).

The inexpensive Widal test quantitatively measures antibodies against antigens of *Salmonella*. It is commonly used in developing countries but numerous studies have shown it to be limited by poor sensitivity and specificity. A newer enzyme-linked immunosorbent assay (ELISA) detects antilipopolysaccharide and antiflagellin antibodies against *S. typhi* proteins and has a reported sensitivity of 94% and specificity of 97%.[55]

While not all patients with TF have fluid losses from diarrhea, they are bacteremic and can be septic. Early recognition and treatment is essential. Antibiotics should be started empirically after cultures are drawn and fluids should be replaced as needed. Historically, TF was treated with chloramphenicol. Because of bacterial resistance, ampicillin and cotrimoxazole were then used. Multidrug resistance has developed worldwide. Third-generation cephalosporins and fluoroquinolones are now considered the best choice for empiric treatment.

Use of ciprofloxacin for TF in children has increased in Southern Asia due to resistance to other drugs. A study by Doherty et al. showed no adverse effects on bone growth when ciprofloxacin was used to treat TF.[56] Third-generation cephalosporins are effective against *S. typhi* when administered for 5 to 7 days. Ceftriaxone can be given daily and can be given to those who are vomiting. Cefixime has been shown to be a safe and effective option for treatment of multidrug resistant enteric fever.[57] It is simpler and more cost-effective since it is an oral option in the third-generation cephalosporin class.

Azithromycin is a once-a-day oral approach that has a shorter duration of therapy that may improve compliance. A recent study of children aged 3 to 17 years showed a 94% cure of TF with a 5-day azithromycin course.[58] See Table 67–8 for a guide to antibiotic therapy for TD and enteric fever.

▶ TABLE 67–8. ANTIBIOTIC THERAPY FOR TRAVELERS DIARRHEA AND ENTERIC FEVER

Antibiotic	Dose	Advantages	Effectiveness in Children
Ciprofloxacin	30 mg/kg/D IV or po ÷ bid	Oral or parenteral	Use is controversial in children younger than 12 y
Ceftriaxone	50–75 mg/kg/d maximum 2.5 g/d	Parenteral Once a day dosing	Highly effective
Cefixime	10–15 mg/kg/d ÷ bid	Oral dosing	Highly effective
Azithromycin	12 mg/kg/d on day 1 (max. 1g) followed by 6 mg/kg/d	Oral dosing	Highly effective
Trimethoprim/ sulfamethoxazole (TMP/SMX)	8 mg/kg/dose (TMP) ÷ bid	Oral dosing	Significant resistance worldwide

REFERENCES

1. Maloney SA. *Semin Pediatr Infect Dis*. 2004;15(3):137–149.

2. Klein JL, Millman GC. Prospective, hospital based study of fever in children in the United Kingdom who had recently spent time in the tropics. *BMJ*. 1998;316:1425–1426.

3. Riordan FA, Tarlow MJ. Imported Infections in East Birmingham children. *Postgrad Med J*. 1998;74:36–37.

4. West NS, Riordan FAI. Fever in returned travelers: a prospective review of hospital admissions for a 2½ year period. *Arch Dis Child*. 2003;88:432–434.

5. Strickland GT. Fever in the returned traveler. *Med Clin North Am*. 1992;76:1375–1392.

6. Engels EA, Falagas ME, Lau J, et al. Typhoid fever vaccines: a meta-analysis of studies on efficacy and toxicity. *BMJ*. 1998;316(7125):110–116.

7. Wilson ME. Travel-related vaccines. *Infect Dis Clin North Am*. 2001;15(1):231–251.

8. Centers for Disease Control. Update: measles among children adopted from China. *MMWR Morb Mortal Wkly Rep*. 2004; 53(21):459.

9. Pickering LK, ed. *2006 Red Book: Report of the Committee on Infectious Diseases*. 27th ed. Elk Grove Village, IL: American Academy of Pediatrics; 2006.

10. Mayer LW, Reeves MW, Al-Hamdan N, et al. Outbreak of W135 meningococcal disease in 2000: not emergence of a new W135 strain but a clonal expansion within the electrophoretic type-37 complex. *J Infect Dis*. 2002;185(11):1596–1605.

11. Rotivel Y, Goudal M, Wirth S, et al. Rabies is a risk for traveling children. *Arch Pediatr*. 1998:561–567.

12. Suh KN, Kozarsky PE, Keystone JS. Evaluation of fever in the returned traveler. *Med Clin North Am*. 1999;83:997–1017.

13. Jelinek T. Dengue fever in international travelers. *Clin Infect Dis*. 2000;31(1):144–147.

14. Murphy GS, Oldfield EC III. Falciparum malaria. *Infect Dis Clin North Am*. 1996;10:747.

15. Edleston M, Pierini S. Fevers/systemic signs. In: *Oxford Handbook of Tropical Medicine*. New York, NY: Oxford University Press; 1999:192–245.

16. Schulte C, Krebs B, Jelinek T, et al. Diagnostic significance of blood eosinophilia in returning travelers. *Clin Infect Dis*. 2002;34:407–411.

17. Ryan ET, Wilson ME, Kain KC. Illness after international travel. *N Engl J Med*. 2002;347:505–516.

18. Wolfe MS. Eosinophilia in the returning traveler. *Med Clin North Am*. 1999;83(4):1019–1032.

19. Suh KN, Kain KC, Keystone JS. Malaria. *CMAJ*. 2004; 170(11):1693–1702.

20. Thang HD, Elsas RM, Veenstra J. Airport malaria: report of a case and a brief overview of the literature. *Neth J Med*. 2002; 60(11):441–443.

21. Svenson JE, Gyorkos TW, MacLean JD. Diagnosis of malaria in the febrile traveler. *Am J Trop Med Hyg*. 1995;53(5):518–521.

22. Svenson JE, MacLean JD, Gyorkos TJ, et al. Imported malaria: clinical presentation and examination of symptomatic travelers. *Arch Intern Med*. 1995;155:861.

23. Makler MT, Palmer CJ, Ager AL. A review of practical techniques for the diagnosis of malaria. *Ann Trop Med Parasitol*. 1998;92(4):419–433.

24. Thellier M, Datry A, Alfa Cisse O, et al. Diagnosis of malaria using thick bloodsmears: definition and evaluation of a faster protocol with improved readability. *Ann Trop Med Parasitol*. 2002;96(2):115–124.

25. Kain KC, Harrington MA, Tennyson S, et al. Imported malaria: prospective analysis of problems in diagnosis and management. *Clin Infect Dis*. 1998;27(1):142–149.

26. *Malaria Diagnosis—New Perspectives*. Report of a Joint WHO/USAID Informal Consultation October 25–27, 1999.

27. McLellan SL. Evaluation of fever in the returned traveler. *Prim Care*. 2002;29(4):947–969.

28. Nunes-Araujo FR, Ferreira MS, Nishioka SD. Dengue fever in Brazilian adults and children:assessment of clinical findings and their validity for diagnosis. *Ann Trop Med Parasitol*. 2003;97(4):415–419.

29. *Fact Sheet: Dengue and Dengue Haemorrhagic Fever*. Geneva, Switzerland: World Health Organization. Fact Sheet No. 117.

30. Wichmann O, Hongsiriwon S, Bowonwatanuwong C, et al. Risk factors and clinical features associated with severe dengue infection in adults and children during the 2001 epidemic in Chonburi, Thailand. *Trop Med Int Health*. 2004;9(9):1022–1029.

31. World Health Organization publication. *Dengue Haemorrhagic Fever: Diagnosis, Treatment, Prevention and Control*. 2nd ed. Geneva, Switzerland: World Health Organization; 1997.

32. *Travelers' Health. The Yellow Book Health Information for International Travel, 2001–2002*. Centers for Disease Control Webpage. http://www.cdc.gov/travel/diarrhea.htm.

33. Dallimore J, Cooke J, Forbes K. Morbidity on youth expeditions to developing countries. *Wilderness Environ Med*. 2002;13:1–4.

34. Pitzinger B, Steffen R, Tschopp A. Incidence and clinical features of travelers' diarrhea in infants and children. *Pediatr Infect Dis J*. 1991;10(10):719–723.

35. Ramaswamy K, Jacobson K. Infectious diarrhea in children. *Gastroenterol Clin*. 2001;30(3):611–624.

36. Staat MA. Travelers diarrhea. *Pediatri Infect Dis J*. 1999;18:373–374.

37. Ansdell VE, Ericsson CD. Prevention and empiric treatment of travelers' diarrhea. *Med Clin North Am*. 1999;83:945–973.

38. DuPont HL. What's new in enteric infectious diseases at home and abroad. *Curr Opin in Infect Dis*. 2005;18:407–412.

39. DuPont HL, Jiangh ZD, Okhysen PC, et al. A randomized, double-blind, placebo-controlled trial of rifaximin to prevent traveler's diarrhea. *NEJM*. 2005;142:805–812.

40. Adachi JA, Ericsson CD, Jiang ZD, et al. Azithromycin found to be comparable to levofloxacin for the treatment of US travelers with acute diarrhea acquired in Mexico. *Clin Infect Dis*. 2003;37:1165–1171.

41. Kubin R. Safety and efficacy of ciprofloxacin in pediatric patients. *Infection*. 1993;21:413–421.

42. Heggers JP, Villarreal C, Edgar P, et al. Ciprofloxacin as a therapeutic modality in pediatric burn wound infections: efficacious or contraindicated? *Arch Surg*. 1998;133:1247–1250.

43. Singh UK, Sinha RK, Prasad B, et al. Ciprofloxacin in children: is arthropathy a limitation? *India J Pediatr*. 2000;67:386–387.

44. Rose SR, Keystone J. *International Travel Health Guide*. 13th ed. Northampton, MA: Travel Medicine; 2006:71.

45. Martin JM, Pitetti R, Maffei F, et al. Treatment of shigellosis with cefixime: two days versus five days. *Pediatri Infect Dis*. 2000;19:522–526.

46. Motala C, Hill ID, Mann MD, et al. Effect of loperamide on stool output and duration of acute infectious diarrhea in infants. *J Pediatr*. 1990;177:467–471.

47. Johnson PC, Ericsson CD, DuPont HL, et al. Comparison of loperamide with bismuth subsalicylate for the treatment of acute travelers' diarrhea. *JAMA*. 1986;255:757–760.

48. Ericsson CD, DuPont HF, Matthewson JS. Single dose of ofloxacin plus loperamide compared with a single dose or three days of oflaxacin in treatment of travelers' diarrhea. *J Travel Med*. 1997;4:3–7.

49. Kaplan MA, Prior MJ, McKonly KI, et al. A multi-center randomized controlled trial of liquid loperamide product versus placebo in the treatment of acute diarrhea in children. *Clin Pediatr*. 1999;38:579–591.

50. Soriano-Brucher H, Avendano P, O'Ryan M, et al. Bismuth

subsalicylate in the treatment of acute diarrhea in children: a clinical study. *Pediatrics.* 1991;87(1):18–22.

51. Figueroa-Quintanilla D, Salazar-Lindo E, Sack RB, et al. A controlled trial of bismuth subsalicylate in infants with acute watery diarrheal disease. *N Engl J Med.* 1993;328(23):1653–1658.

52. Steinberg EB, Bishop R, Haber P, et al. Typhoid fever in travelers: who should be targeted for prevention? *Clin Infect Dis.* 2004;39:186–191.

53. Connor BA, Schwartz E. Typhoid and paratyphoid fever in travelers. *Lancet Infect Dis.* 2005;5:623–628.

54. Mahle WT, Levine MM. Salmonella typhi infection in children younger than five years of age. *Pediatr Infect Dis J.* 1993;12: 627–631.

55. Jesudason MV. Diagnosis of typhoid fever by the detection of anti-LPS and anti-flagellin antibiodies by ELISA. *Indian J Med Res.* 1998;107:204–207.

56. Doherty CP, Saha SK, Cutting WA. Typhoid fever, ciprofloxacin and growth in young children. *Ann Trop Paediatr.* 2000;20: 297–303.

57. Memon IA, Billoo AG, Memon HI. Cefixime: an oral option for the treatment of multidrug-resistant enteric fever in children. *South Med J.* 1997;12:1204.

58. Frenck RW, Mansour A, Nakhia I, et al. Short-course azithromycin for the treatment of uncomplicated typhoid fever in children and adolescents. *Clin Infect Dis.* 2004;38:951–957.

CHAPTER 68

Bioterrorism: A Pediatric Perspective

Janet Lin and Timothy B. Erickson

▶ HIGH-YIELD FACTS

- Children are more likely than adults to have severe illness following a biological exposure.
- Vulnerabilities, such as a lack of pediatric expertise, equipment, or facilities within disaster planning and EMS systems, could be exacerbated by a terrorist attack involving children.
- Antibiotics that are infrequently used in children, such as tetracyclines and fluoroquinolones, may be the drugs of choice for children in the setting of bioterrorism.
- Infection control practices should be employed since secondary transmission is likely with biological agents such as plague, smallpox, and hemorrhagic fevers.

▶ BIOLOGICAL AGENTS

Pediatric needs in the planning, preparation, and response to biological disasters or acts of terrorism is essential.[1] Nearly all child health professionals can benefit from bioterrorism disaster training and education.[2] Children remain potential victims of biological terrorism. In recent years, children have been specific targets of terrorists' acts.[3] Consequently, it is necessary to address the needs of pediatric patients after a potential terrorist or disaster incident.

Specific to bioterrorism, more fulminant infectious diseases are possible in children because of immunologic immaturity and a more permeable blood–brain barrier. Furthermore, many drugs used to treat illness from bioagents were historically avoided during childhood because of potential developmental toxicity. Finally, it is anticipated that specific vulnerabilities such as lack of pediatric expertise, equipment, or facilities within disaster planning and EMS systems might be exacerbated by a terrorist attack involving children.[4]

In contrast to a chemical attack, a covert biological attack will simulate a natural outbreak, with an incubation period rather than producing immediate mass casualties.[5] The Centers for Disease Control and Prevention (CDC) has developed a list of "critical agents for health preparedness" that encompasses organisms with the most potentially devastating consequences that would require the most critical medical responses if released by a bioterrorist.[6] According to this classification scheme, the highest overall public health impact and requirement for intensive preparedness as well as intervention would stem from an aerosolized release of:

- Variola virus (smallpox).
- *Bacillus anthracis* (anthrax).
- *Yersinia pestis* (plague*)*.
- *Clostridia botulinum* (botulism).
- *Francisella tularensis* (tularemia).
- Filoviridae/Arenaviridae, such as Ebola, Marburg, or Lassa fever viruses that produce hemorrhagic fevers.

Each of these identified agents will be discussed in the following paragraphs. The remaining agents are identified in Table 68–1.

Although any of the highest risk biological agents listed above can be seen in the pediatric patient, several agents might closely resemble some of the more common childhood illnesses, particularly in their initial stages. The awareness of these similarities and, more importantly, their differences, are critical for all health care professionals.[7]

ANTHRAX

Anthrax occurs in nature following contact with infected animals or animal products. Ninety-five percent of naturally occurring anthrax is cutaneous disease. It is associated with less than 1% mortality if treated, but approximately 20% mortality if untreated. The risk is mostly occupational in nature from close contact with herbivores such as sheep, goats, and cattle. Naturally occurring inhalational anthrax accounts for less than 5% of reported cases. The historical mortality rate of inhalational anthrax is approximately 90%. The mortality from the US mail associated outbreak in 2001 was 45%. The decrease in mortality is most likely because of improved supportive care and the improved antibiotic treatment available today. Naturally occurring gastrointestinal (GI) anthrax accounts for less than 5% of reported cases. It is very difficult to diagnose and is frequently fatal.[4,8]

Figure 68–1 demonstrates the pathophysiology of disease development. The site of entry into the body is typically the skin, lungs, or GI tract. Low level germination at those sites occur leading to localized edema and necrosis. The agent is taken up by the macrophage where further germination occurs. The macrophage may carry the germinating bacteria to regional lymph nodes. The release of exotoxins, such as edema toxin and lethal toxin, can lead to cell death and necrosis in the affected areas (e.g., hemorrhagic adenitis). The resultant release of tumor necrosis factor (TNF) and other cytokines can affect other homeostatic mechanisms and contribute to shock and death. Once the local necrosis occurs, there can be a large release of anthrax bacilli into the blood stream causing septicemia and the seeding of other organs such as the meninges and lungs.

The hallmark of cutaneous disease is a single or few lesions that are painless throughout all stages, starting with

▶ **TABLE 68–1. CRITICAL BIOLOGICAL AGENT CATEGORIES FOR PUBLIC HEALTH PREPAREDNESS**

Biological Agent	Disease
Category A	
Bacillus anthracis	Anthrax
Yersenia pestis	Plague
Variola major	Smallpox
Clostridium botulinum (botulinum toxins)	Botulism
Francisella tularensis	Tularemia
Filoviruses and arenaviruses (e.g., *Ebola virus, Lassa virus*)	Viral hemorrhagic fevers
Category B	
Coxiella burnetii	Q fever
Brucella spp.	Brucellosis
Burkholderia mallei	Glanders
Burkholderia pseudomallei	Melioidosis
Alphaviruses (Venezuelan equine, eastern equine, western equine encephalomyelitis viruses)	Encephalitis
Rickettsia prowazekii	Typhus fever
Toxins (e.g., ricin, staphylococcal enterotoxin B)	Toxic syndromes
Chlamydia psittaci	Psittacosis
Food safety threats (e.g., *Salmonella spp., Escherichia coli* O157:H7)	
Water safety threats (e.g., *Vibrio cholerae, Cryhptosporidium parvum*)	
Category C	
Emerging threat agents (e.g., *Nipah virus, hantavirus*)	

With permission from Centers for Disease Control and Prevention (CDC). Bioterrorism website. www.bt.gov/bioterrorism/factsheets. 2008. Bethesda, MD.

a papule or macule that may be pruritic. Over the next 1 to 2 days, single or multiple vesicles or large bullae appear with clear or serosanguineous fluid. This dries into an ulcer with surrounding gelatinous, often extensive, nonpitting edema. If the edema involves the head or the neck, airway compromise can occur. Several days later, this progresses to a black depressed eschar at the base of the ulcer (Fig. 68–2). Purulence or significant erythema and evidence of inflammation should raise the suspicion of secondary bacterial infection such as cellulitis.

B. anthracis spores are highly stable and highly infectious upon inhalation and it is this form that has been manufactured for use in biological warfare. Illness resulting from an aerosolized release of anthrax spores is likely associated with an incubation period of 1 to 60 days, followed by fever, myalgias, cough, and chest pain.

Children, particularly infants and toddlers, present with nonspecific symptom complexes primarily limited to fever, vomiting, cough, and dyspnea.[9] Children with anthrax present with a wide range of clinical signs and symptoms, which differ somewhat from the presenting features of adults with anthrax. Like adults, children with GI anthrax have two distinct clinical presentations: upper tract disease characterized by dysphagia and oropharyngeal findings and lower tract disease characterized by fever, abdominal pain, and nausea and vomiting. Additionally, children with inhalational disease may have "atypical" presentations including primary meningoencephalitis. Children with inhalational anthrax have abnormal chest roentgenograms; however, children with other forms of anthrax usually have normal roentgenograms.[10]

With inhalational anthrax, transient clinical improvement might occur, but is followed by the abrupt onset of sepsis,

hypotension, and death within 24 to 36 hours. Hemorrhagic meningitis is expected in 50% of cases, as would a very high overall case fatality rate. Hallmarks of the illness include gram-positive bacilli on tissue biopsy, blood smear, or spinal fluid microscopy, and chest radiograph findings of mediastinal widening from lymphadenitis. Pulmonary infiltrates or effusions may also be seen.

There are no clinical trials assessing the treatment of inhalational anthrax in humans. Early antibiotic administration is likely to be the most important determinant of outcome in the setting of anthrax infection. Cutaneous anthrax without systemic sequelae can be adequately treated with oral doxycycline or ciprofloxacin. Any other form or anthrax should be admitted and treated with intravenous antibiotics. Those patients potentially exposed to anthrax spores should receive antibiotic prophylaxis for 60 days. Treatment and prophylaxis recommendations are summarized in Table 68–2.[4,8] Unlike plague, secondary transmission of inhalational anthrax does not occur, although it has been described with cutaneous anthrax. Standard blood and bodily fluid precautions are indicated.

PLAGUE

Y. pestis, the bacteria that causes plague, classically spreads in nature from infected fleas to humans. Historically, plague is most well known as the cause of Justinian's plague and the black death (during the middle 6th and 14th centuries, respectively), which were two devastating epidemics that killed millions of people. A third epidemic began in China and eventually spread to all continents. Between 1896 and 1930,

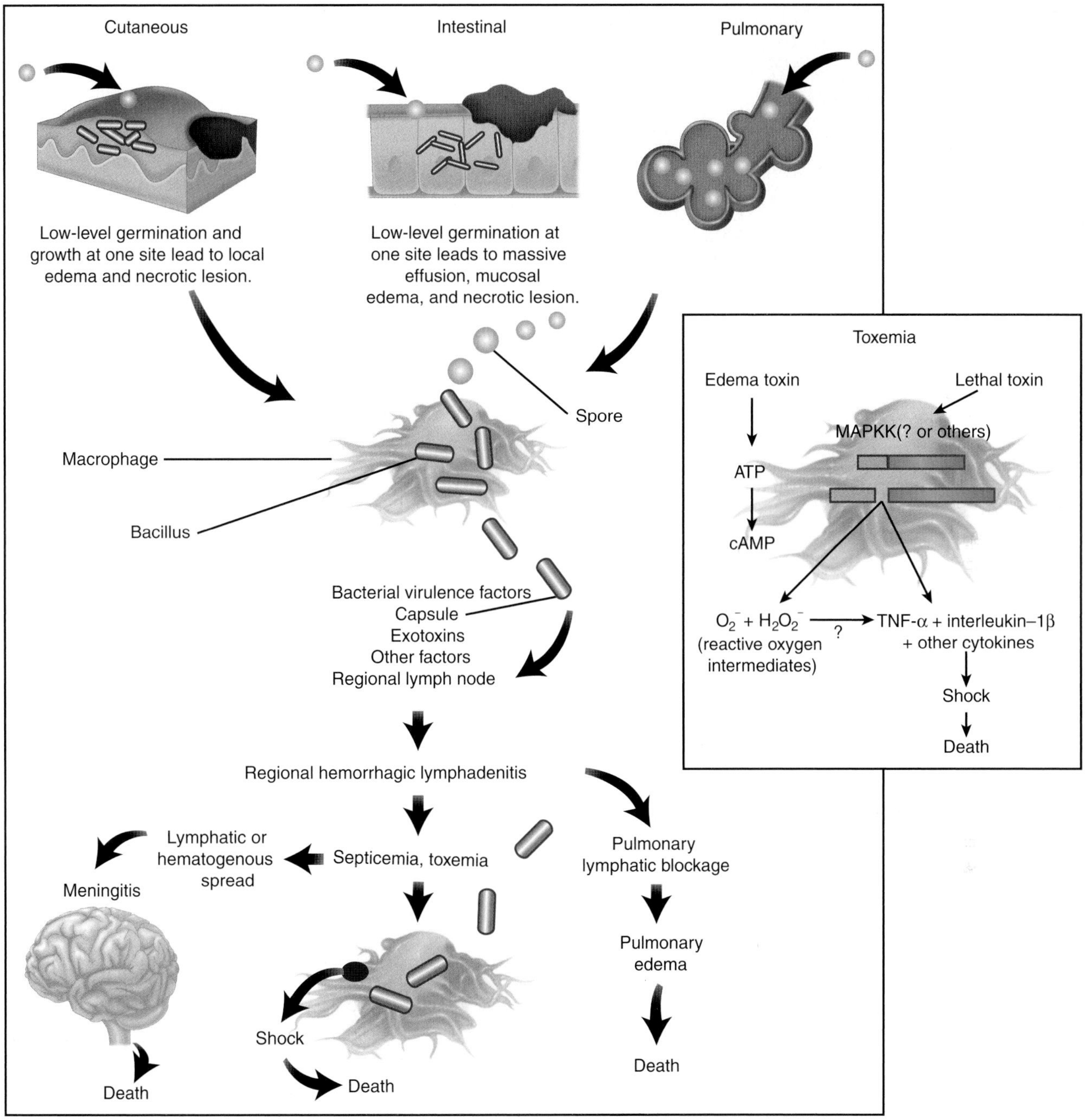

Figure 68–1. The pathophysiology of disease development in anthrax. (With permission from Dixon TC, Meselson M, Guillemin J, Hanna PC. Anthrax. *N Engl J Med*. 1999;341(11):815–826.)

more than 12 million deaths and almost 30 million cases were documented. Research during the last pandemic led to the discovery of *Y. pestis* as the causative agent. Transmission of bubonic plague occurs through a flea bite, bite or scratch of an infected animal, or direct contact from an infected carcass. Pneumonic plague occurs via inhalation of respiratory droplets from an infected animal or person-to-person spread. Pneumonic plague can be primary inhalational or secondary resulting from spread via the bloodstream in bubonic or septicemic cases.[11] Naturally occurring plague most often is asso-

ciated with the bubonic type, occurs in the southwest United States primarily during the months of April to October or during hunting season. Oftentimes, there is an associated rodent die off that precedes the presentation of the disease in humans. An aerosol-mediated bioterrorist attack would be associated with pneumonic plague and would not present with the same epidemiologic factors mentioned above.

Clinical manifestations include tender lymphadenopathy, if associated with bubonic plague, and multiorgan failure, if associated with septicemic plague. It often presents with

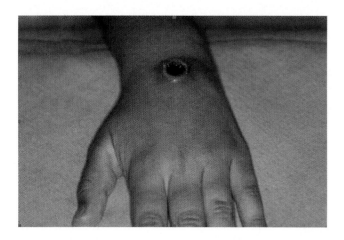

Figure 68–2. Cutaneous anthrax. webs.wichita.edu/.../ lecture20/anthrax`hand.jpg. (With permission from CDC public domain images)

nonspecific respiratory signs and symptoms beginning from 1 to 6 days after exposure. An intense cough with thin bloody sputum is a characteristic finding. GI signs and symptoms can be very prominent, and at times may mimic an acute abdomen. Petechiae, purpura, and an overwhelming picture of DIC may occur. Rapid progression to death occurs in those not treated with antibiotics within 24 hours of symptom onset. A clue to the diagnosis of *Y. pestis* is a classic bipolar, "safety pin"-staining bacilli on Gram's staining of the sputum or lymph node aspirate.

Treatment consists of antibiotic treatment with streptomycin, gentamicin, doxycycline, ciprofloxacin, or chloramphenicol. Doxycycline or ciprofloxacin are the antibiotic choices for postexposure prophylaxis. Because secondary transmission of pneumonic plague occurs, standard blood and bodily fluid, as well as droplet precautions are necessary as is postexposure prophylaxis for those exposed to pneumonic

▶ **TABLE 68–2. INITIAL ANTIBIOTIC THERAPY FOR SELECTED BACTERIAL AGENTS OF BIOTERRORISM IN CHILDREN**

Agent	Antibiotics	Dose and Route
Inhalational Anthrax*	Ciprofloxacin	10–15 mg/kg IV q 12 h (max 400 mg/dose) or
	Doxycycline	2.2 mg/kg IV (max 100 mg) q 12 h and
	Clindamycin	10–15 mg/kg IV q 8 h and
	Penicillin G	400–600K u/kg/d IV divided q 4 h
Cutaneous Anthrax*	Ciprofloxacin	10–15 mg/kg po q 12 h (max 1 gm/d) or
	Doxycycline	2.2 mg/kg po (max 100 mg) q 12 h
Plague	Streptomycin	15 mg/kg IM q 12 h (max 2 g/d) or
	Gentamicin	2.5 mg/kg IM or IV q 8 h (q 12 h in neonates younger than 1 wk) or
	Doxycycline	2.2 mg/kg IV q 12 h (max 200 mg/d)
	(Ciprofloxacin 15 mg/kg IV q12 h or chloramphenicol 25 mg/kg IV q 6 h (max 4 gm/d) might also be considered; especially chloramphenicol for plague meningitis)	
Tularemia	Streptomycin	15 mg/kg IM q 12 h (max 2 g/d) or
	Gentamicin	2.5 mg/kg IM or IV q 8 h (q 12 h in neonates younger than 1 wk) or
	Doxycycline	2.2 mg/kg IV q 12 h (max 200 mg/d)
	(Chloramphenicol or ciprofloxacin may also be considered)	
Mass Casualty Setting or Prophylaxis		
Inhalational Anthrax*	Ciprofloxacin	10–15 mg/kg po q 12 h (max 1 g/d) × 60 d or
	Doxycycline	2.2 mg/kg (max 100 mg) po q 12 h × 60 d
Plague	Doxycycline	2.2 mg/kg po q 12 h (max 200 mg/d) or
	Ciprofloxacin	20 mg/kg po q 12 h (max 1 g/d)
Tularemia	Doxycycline	2.2 mg/kg po q 12 h (max 200 mg/d) or
	Ciprofloxacin	15 mg/kg po q 12 h (max 1 g/d)

*Amoxicillin could be substituted after 14 d of ciprofloxacin or doxycycline if strain susceptible at 40–80 mg/kg/d divided q 8 h to complete a 60-day course of therapy.

plague victims.[12] Treatment and prophylaxis recommendations are summarized in Table 68–2.

SMALLPOX

A global campaign, begun in 1967 under the guidance of the World Health Organization (WHO), succeeded in eradicating smallpox in 1977. The last documented case worldwide was reported in Somalia. The last documented case of smallpox reported in the United States was in 1949. Routine smallpox vaccination in the United States was discontinued in 1972. Therefore, the majority of US citizens are susceptible to an outbreak. Samples of the virus have been stored in laboratory research freezers. If a terrorist had access to stored smallpox virus, a release could produce a chaotic situation.[13]

Smallpox is caused by a member of the Orthopoxvirus group. Smallpox afflicts only humans, as there are no known animal hosts. The diagnosis of smallpox is made clinically, with laboratory confirmation through the CDC.

Smallpox has an incubation period of 7 to 17 days. Clinical illness is characterized by a severe prodrome of high fever, rigors, vomiting, headache, and backache. The classic exanthem begins 2 to 4 days later, on the face (Fig. 68–3) and distal portions of the extremities (Fig. 68–4), with macules progressing to papules, umbilicated pustules, and then scabs. The centrifugal onset and synchronous nature of the rash helps to distinguish it from chickenpox (Fig. 68–5).

If used as a biological weapon, smallpox represents a serious threat to the general population because it carries a high case-fatality rate of 30% or more among unvaccinated persons and there is no specific therapy. Although smallpox has long been feared as the most devastating of all infectious diseases, its potential for devastation today is far greater than at any previous time. In a now highly susceptible, mobile population, smallpox would be able to spread widely and rapidly throughout this country and the world.

Smallpox also has a high potential for secondary spread from person-to-person. Transmission occurs primarily through close face-to-face contact via droplet nuclei. However, smallpox can also be transmitted via an airborne route in the setting of an infected patient with a severe cough, and from direct

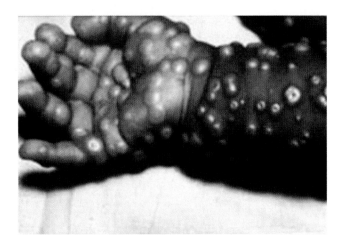

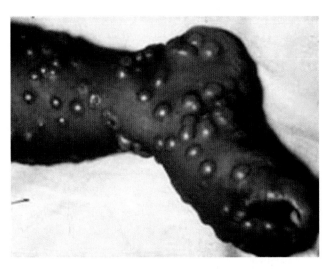

Figure 68–4. Smallpox on hands and feet of a child. chsweb.lr.k12.nj.us/psidelsky/smallpox.htm. (With permission from CDC public domain images)

aerosol inhalation. One of the most concerning things about smallpox is the potential for the disease to spread exponentially. The secondary attack rate is estimated to be 25% to 40% in unvaccinated contacts, meaning that at least one of every three or four persons exposed to smallpox would develop disease. Historically, three to four contacts were infected per index case. However, it is expected that up to 10 to 20 contacts in a mostly nonimmune population would be infected.[4] There is also very high potential for nosocomial spread.

Vaccination with the smallpox vaccine within 3 to 4 days of exposure may prevent disease or lessen the severity of the disease.[14] Historically, the vaccine was given to children. Currently, it is not being offered to children for preevent prophylaxis and it is not recommended for postexposure use in children younger than 1 year. In the United States, virtually all children, and adults younger than 35 years, are unvaccinated, and have no immunity to smallpox. Thus, their potential susceptibility to fulminant disease might actually be greater than in those older Americans who were immunized before 1972. The only currently available vaccine has been tested on adults, not children.[13] A "ring vaccination strategy" is now being recommended by the CDC. With this plan, cases of smallpox are rapidly identified, infected individuals are isolated, and

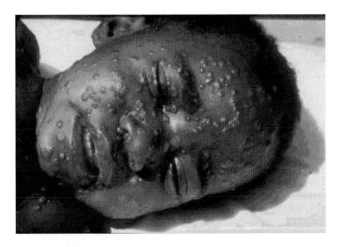

Figure 68–3. Facial smallpox. cache.view/images.com. (With permission from CDC public domain images)

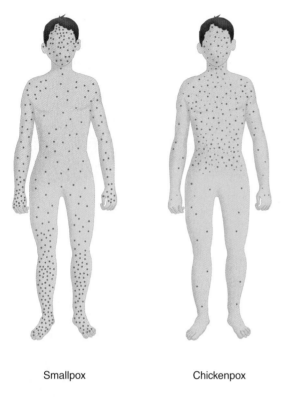

Smallpox   Chickenpox

Figure 68–5. Smallpox versus chickenpox distribution. www.bt.cdc.gov/agent/smallpox/images/smpxman1.gif. (With permission from CDC public domain images)

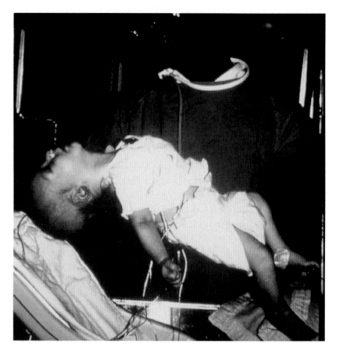

Figure 68–6. Infantile botulism. www.rnceus.com/biot/botul.html. (With permission from CDC public domain images)

contacts of the infected individuals as well as their contacts are immunized immediately.[15]

As mentioned, there is no specific treatment for smallpox. The mainstay of treatment is supportive therapy plus antibiotics as indicated for treatment of any secondary bacterial infections. No antiviral substances have yet proven effective for the treatment of smallpox. Airborne, droplet, and standard blood and bodily fluid precautions are indicated when caring for victims until all their scabs separate. Universal fluid precautions are also recommended for close contacts of victims until 17 days from their last exposure.

BOTULISM

Botulism is found throughout the world. Three forms of naturally occurring human botulism exist: foodborne, wound, and infantile (Fig. 68–6). Fewer than 200 cases of all forms of botulism are reported annually in the United States.[16]

Botulism is an obligate anaerobe, spore-forming, grampositive rod. The bacteria produces its effect through botulinum toxin. All forms of botulism result from absorption of botulinum toxin into the circulation from either a mucosal surface (gut, lung) or a wound. Botulinum toxin does not penetrate intact skin. The toxin is taken up by skeletal muscle motor neurons where it irreversibly inhibits the release of acetylcholine, resulting in postsynaptic muscle paralysis. The paralysis persists until axonal branches regenerate. Wound botulism and intestinal botulism are infectious diseases that result from production of botulinum toxin by *C. botulinum* either in devi-

talized (i.e., anaerobic) tissue or in the intestinal lumen, respectively. Neither would result from bioterrorist use of botulinum toxin.

A fourth, man-made form, results from aerosolized and purified botulinum toxin and is called inhalational botulism. This mode of transmission has been demonstrated experimentally in primates, has been attempted by bioterrorists, and has been the intended outcome of at least one country's specially designed missiles and artillery shells. Inhalational botulism has occurred accidentally in humans. A brief report from West Germany in 1962 described three veterinary personnel who were exposed to aerosolized botulinum toxin while disposing of rabbits and guinea pigs whose fur was coated with aerosolized type A botulinum toxin.

Patients with botulism typically present acutely with an afebrile, symmetric, descending flaccid paralysis that always begins in bulbar musculature. It always presents with multiple cranial nerve palsies. Patients may complain of difficulty seeing, speaking, and/or swallowing. Prominent neurologic findings include ptosis, diplopia, blurred vision, often enlarged or sluggishly reactive pupils, dysarthria, dysphonia, dysphagia, and descending paralysis. The mouth may appear dry because of peripheral parasympathetic nervous system cholinergic blockade. The incubation period lasts anywhere from 2 hours to 8 days.

Because botulism is toxin mediated there is no transmission from person-to person. Respiratory isolation is not needed. The mainstays of treatment are supportive and passive immunization with one of two antitoxins. The trivalent botulinum antitoxin is available through the CDC and may be used to treat children of any age with subtypes A, B, or E. The heptavalent antitoxin (subtypes A, B, C, D, E, F, G) is available through US army. In 2006, the Department of Health and Human Services approved the delivery of the heptavalent antitoxin into the Strategic National Stockpile in 2007. Botulism immune globulin (BIG) is used to treat infant botulism.[16]

TULAREMIA

Tularemia is a zoonotic illness that most commonly manifests in an ulceroglandular form after exposure to diseased animal fluids or bites from infected deerflies, mosquitoes, or ticks. The classic animal reservoir is the lagomorphs (rabbits). While not highly fatal, its extremely high infectivity and its ability to escape laboratory detection make it an agent of potential use for bioterrorism.[17] Typical symptoms occur following a 2- to 10-day incubation period. These include sudden fever, chills, diarrhea, dry cough, muscle aches, joint pain, and progressive weakness or prostration. The presentation of other symptoms such as ulcers on the skin or mouth, swollen and painful lymph nodes, and sore throat vary depending on how a patient is exposed to the bacteria. An aerosolized release (as would be implicated in a bioterrorist attack) would likely result in clinical findings similar to community-acquired pneumonia, often developing chest pain and difficulty breathing. Patchy infiltrates and hilar adenopathy might be seen on a chest radiograph.

Tularemia can be treated with several antibiotics. Currently, the treatment of choice is streptomycin administered by intramuscular injection. Alternatively, gentamicin, a more widely available aminoglycoside, can be given intravenously. Other antibiotics that are used include tetracyclines and chloramphenicol but they tend to have a higher primary failure and relapse rate. Mass casualty prophylaxis can be achieved with doxycycline or ciprofloxacin. Person-to-person transmission does not occur, and respiratory isolation is not required. Treatment and prophylaxis recommendations are summarized in Table 68–2.[4,8]

VIRAL HEMORRHAGIC FEVERS

Several families of viruses that share similar and defining features cause viral hemorrhagic fevers. The two most noteworthy families are the Filoviridae and the Arenaviridae because they are both highly contagious and are associated with a high mortality rate. Filoviruses cause Ebola and Marburg hemorrhagic fevers and an arenavirus causes Lassa fever. These RNA viruses are dependent on a natural animal or arthropod reservoir. Rodents, ticks, and mosquitoes are common vectors; however, the vector for Marburg and Ebola viruses are unknown. Humans become infected by a bite or when they come into contact with an infected host vector. However, documented cases of human-to-human transmission occur with Ebola, Marburg, and Lassa hemorrhagic fever viruses. Symptoms most often include fever, dizziness, fatigue, exhaustion, and muscle aches. While not all hemorrhagic fevers cause bleeding, severe forms of the disease may present with bleeding under the skin, internal organ bleeding, and bleeding from body orifices. Fulminant illnesses will present with shock and, oftentimes, multiorgan system failure. Supportive care and blood product replacement are the mainstays of therapy. Ribavirin (an antiviral medication) is possibly effective in treating some patients with an arenavirus illness (Lassa fever). Secondary transmission is likely with Ebola, Marburg, and Lassa fever, necessitating airborne isolation with standard blood and bodily fluid precautions.[18]

A unique feature of previous Ebola outbreaks has been the relative sparing of children. In an African study from Uganda, analysis revealed that 90 out of the 218 national laboratory confirmed Ebola cases were children and adolescents with a case fatality rate of 40%. The mean age was 8 years, with the youngest child being 3 day old. Children younger than 5 years contributed to the highest admission rate (35%) and case fatality among children and adolescents. All (100%) of Ebola positive children and adolescents were febrile while only 16% had hemorrhagic manifestations. Strategies to shield children from exposure to dying and sick Ebola relatives are recommended in the event of future Ebola outbreaks. Health education to children and adolescents to avoid contact with sick and their body fluids should be emphasized.[19]

▶ PEDIATRIC BIOLOGICAL AGENT EXPOSURE MANAGEMENT

In addition to the unique pediatric issues involved in general emergency preparedness, terrorism preparedness must consider several additional issues. These include the unique vulnerabilities of children to various agents as well as limited availability of age- and weight-appropriate antibiotics and antidotes. Although children may respond more readily to therapeutic intervention, they are at the same time more susceptible to various agents and conditions and more likely to deteriorate if they are not monitored carefully.[20]

Recent consensus recommendations for the antibiotic treatment and prophylaxis of anthrax, plague, and tularemia, in children, are based on clinical and evidence-based criteria and do not necessarily correspond to the Federal and Drug Administration (FDA) approved indications or labeling of these drugs. Foremost, as detailed in Table 68–2, many of the highest threat bioterrorist agents are appropriately treated in adults with ciprofloxacin or doxycycline.[4,8] The fluoroquinolone and tetracycline classes of antibiotics have each been considered as relatively contraindicated in young children. The fluoroquinolone concern has primarily stemmed from arthropathy and growth abnormality noted in animal studies. The tetracyclines are known to stain children's teeth, particularly in those children younger than 8 years taking prolonged or repeated courses.

The past decade has seen a great deal of clinical use of ciprofloxacin in young children with cancer, cystic fibrosis, shigellosis, typhoid fever, and neonatal sepsis. There is no evidence of arthropathy or slower rates of bone growth in these children. In fact, in 2001, the FDA approved ciprofloxacin for use in bioterrorist-related anthrax exposures for children as well as for adults.

Among the tetracyclines, doxycycline is least likely to cause dental staining. It is now recognized as the drug of choice for treatment in children with life-threatening, rickettsial infections, such as Rocky Mountain spotted fever and erlichiosis. In this setting, has been used without evidence of dental staining. This reevaluation has mitigated much of the previous concern regarding fluoroquinolone and doxycycline use in children.

Finally, the pediatric health care professional must be in contact with their local, state, and federal public health infrastructure as soon as a potential biological agent is perceived clinically. Most states are now setting up contingency plans and means to address these issues in a systematic way. This involves the local health departments, regional poison control centers, police departments, fire departments, National Guard units, and federal agencies such as the CDC and the FBI. The key component however, is actually identifying a biological agent in the community and then moving quickly to isolate those that may be at risk of spreading the infection.[21]

REFERENCES

1. Markenson D, Redlener I. Pediatric terrorism preparedness national guidelines and recommendations. *Biosecur Bioterror.* 2004;2(4):301–319.
2. Hu Y, Adams R, Boscarino J, et al. Training needs of pediatricians facing the environmental health and bioterroism consequences after September 11th. *Mt Sinai J Med.* 2006;73(8):1156–1164.
3. Michael WS, Julia AM; and Committee on Environmental Health; Committee on Infectious Disease. Chemical-biological terrorism and its impact on children. *Pediatrics.* 2006;118(3):1267–1278.
4. White S, Walters F. Weapons of mass destruction. In: Erickson TB, Ahrens WR, Aks S, Baum C, eds. *Pediatric Toxicology: Diagnosis and Management of the Poisoned Child.* New York, NY: McGraw-Hill; 2005.
5. Centers for Disease Control and Prevention (CDC). Bioterrorism website. http//www.bt.cdc.gov/bioterrorism/factsheets.asp. 2008. Bethesda, MD. Accessed January 2, 2008.
6. Henretig FM, Ciesklak TJ, Eitzen EM. Biological and chemical terrorism. *J Pediatr.* 2002;141(3):311.
7. Stocker JT. Clincial and pathological differential diagnosis of selected potential bioterrorism agents of interest to pediatric health care providers. *Clin Lab Med.* 2006;26(2):329–344.
8. Walter FG. Bioterrorism Agents. In: Walter FG, ed. *Advanced Hazmat Life Support (AHLS) for Toxic Terrorism.* Tucson, AZ: Arizona Board of Regents; 2003. www.http//aemrc.Arizona.edu.
9. Place R, Hanfling D, Howell J, et al. Bioterrorism-related inhalational anthrax: can extrapolated adult guidelines be applied to a pediatric population? *Biosecur Bioterror.* 2007;5(1):35–42.
10. Bravata DM, Wang E, Holty JE, et al. Pediatric anthrax: implications for bioterrorism preparedness. *Evid Rep Technol Assess.* 2006;(141):1–48.
11. Dennis DT, Chow CC. Plague. *Pediatr Infect Dis J.* 2004;23(1):69–71.
12. Koirala J. Plague: disease, management, and recognition of act of terrorism. *Infect Dis Clin North Am.* 2006;20(2):273–287.
13. Baltimore R, Jenson H. Should smallpox vaccine be tested in children? *Curr Opin Infect Dis.* 2003;1693):237–239.
14. Waecker NJ, Hale BR. Smallpox vaccination: what the pediatrician needs to know. *Pediatr Ann.* 2003;32(3):178.
15. American Academy of Pediatrics; Committee on Infectious Disease. Small pox vaccine. *Pediatrics.* 2002;110(4):841–845.
16. Villar RG, Elliott SP, Davenport KM. Botulism: the many faces of botulinum toxin and its potential for bioterrorism. *Infect Dis Clin North Am.* 2006;20(2):313–327.
17. Dennis D, Inglesby T, Henderson D, et al. Tulermia as a biological weapon: medical and public health management. *JAMA.* 2001;285(21):2763–2773.
18. Peters CJ. Marburg and ebola—arming ourselves against the deadly filoviruses. *N Engl J Med.* 2005;352(25):2571–2573.
19. Mupere E, Kaducu OF, Yoti Z. Ebola haemorrhagic fever among hospitalised children and adolescents in northern Uganda: epidemiologic and clinical observations. *Afr Health Sci.* 2001;1(2):60–65.
20. Markenson D, Reynolds S; and American Academy of Pediatrics; Committee on Pediatric Emergency Medicine; Task Force on Terrorism. The pediatrician and disaster preparedness. *Pediatrics.* 2006;117(2):e340–e362.
21. Cross JT, Altemeier W. A pediatrician's view. skin manifestations of bioterrorism. *Pediatr Ann.* 2000;29(1):7–9.

SECTION IX

IMMUNOLOGIC EMERGENCIES

CHAPTER 69

Common Allergic Presentations: Allergic Conjunctivitis/Rhinitis

William R. Ahrens

▶ HIGH-YIELD FACTS

- Allergic conjunctivitis/rhinitis are associated with considerable morbidity when undertreated.
- The diagnosis of allergic conjunctivitis/rhinitis is often missed or delayed.
- Complications of allergic conjunctivitis/rhinitis include exacerbation of asthma, sinusitis, middle ear infections and effusions, and sleep disturbances.
- There are multiple medical modalities for the treatment of allergic conjunctivitis/rhinitis.

▶ INTRODUCTION

Patients with symptoms related to common allergies are frequently treated in emergency departments. Often, the specific diagnosis of an allergic reaction is missed. This is especially true in the pediatric patient, in whom upper respiratory infections, which have clinical manifestations similar to allergic presentations, are extremely common. Recognizing and either initiating treatment or referring pediatric patients with allergic diseases for further follow-up is important because undertreatment of these illnesses can result in long-term morbidity. It is becoming increasingly well studied and appreciated that the symptoms of uncontrolled allergic symptoms have significant negative impact on the quality of patients' lives. Common allergic presentations in the emergency department include asthma, eczema, allergic conjunctivitis, and allergic rhinitis. Current literature emphasizes the interrelationship and overlap between these illnesses, especially allergic conjunctivitis and rhinitis: the two diseases are often discussed together as allergic rhinoconjunctivis.[1–5] Asthma and eczema are discussed in detail in other chapters; this chapter will focus on allergic conjunctivitis and allergic rhinitis.

▶ PATHOPHYSIOLOGY

Allergic illnesses are most commonly seen in patients with a history of atopy, which is defined as a genetically determined hypersensitivity to environmental antigens.[6] The most common form of hypersensitivity, type 1, is associated with IgE antibody and is the cause of most of the allergic presentations seen in the emergency department. Contact of IgE antibody with mast cells triggers mast cell degranulation, which results in the release of multiple inflammatory mediators; early-phase reactants include leukotriene C_4 and prostaglandin D_2. The late-phase response involves the recruitment of neutrophils, eosinophils, and macrophages. Histamine released on mast cell activation can cause pruritis, bronchospasm, increased vascular permeability, and vasodilation.[6] Asthma, hay fever, allergic conjunctivitis, and allergic rhinitis can all be triggered by type 1 responses to environmental antigens. The most severe manifestation of a type 1 reaction is anaphylaxis, which can be fatal. Anaphylaxis is discussed in a separate chapter. Common indoor allergens include house dust mites, cockroaches, and pet allergens; these often cause persistent, perennial symptoms. Outdoor allergens include pollen from grass and trees—these tend to cause seasonal symptoms.[1–5]

▶ CLINICAL PRESENTATION

ALLERGIC CONJUNCTIVITIS

The conjunctiva in a mucosa is similar to the nasal mucosa and possesses a relatively large surface area that reacts to the same allergens. The conjunctiva is connected to the nose via the lacrimal ducts; in this sense, it is part of the airway. The association of allergic conjunctivitis with allergic rhinitis is such that some authors group the two together under the heading "allergic rhinoconjunctivitis." There are several specific classifications of allergic conjunctivitis.[7]

Seasonal allergic conjunctivitis (SAC) implies that patients have symptoms for a defined period of time. Patients with perennial conjunctivitis (PAC) have symptoms year round. Together, SAC and PAC account for approximately 98% of allergic eye disease in patients.[8] Patients with SAC and PAC usually have atopic symptoms and a family history of atopy. A fairly high percentage complains specifically of concomitant nasal symptoms. Itching of the eyes is an important symptom; without itching the diagnosis of allergic conjunctivitis is unlikely. Physical findings include injection of the conjunctival vessels, chemosis, and eyelid edema (Fig. 69–1). Increased vascular permeability can result in conjunctival edema. Corneal involvement is uncommon and vision is rarely affected.

Vernal keratoconjunctivitis (VKC) is a chronic bilateral inflammation of the conjunctiva that predominantly occurs in

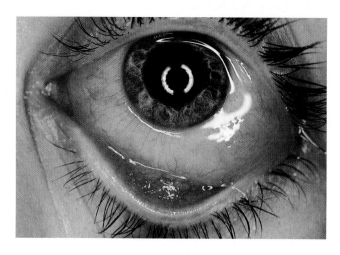
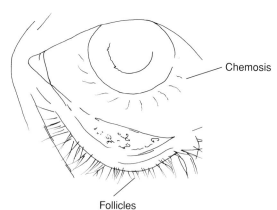

Figure 69–1. Allergic conjunctivitis conjunctival injection, chemosis, and a follicular response in the inferior palpebral conjunctiva in this patient with allergic conjunctivitis secondary to cat fur.

children (Fig. 69–2). It is most common in hot dry environments and typically occurs during spring months. Affected individual also has a family history of atopy. VKC has a male predominance. As with SAC and PAC, itching is an important symptom; photophobia and a foreign body sensation can be present. The eyelid skin is usually not involved. Eye discharge tends to be thick and mucoid. There are two types of VPC. In the palpebral variety, giant papillae are commonly found on the superior tarsal conjunctiva; the inferior tarsal conjunctiva is generally unaffected. The limbal variety of VKC is more common in dark-skinned individuals; papillae occur at the limbus. VKC can be complicated by punctuate epithelial kertopathy, which can lead to a corneal shield ulcer, especially in very young patients.[7–9]

Atopic keratoconjunctivitis (AKC) is a bilateral inflammation of the conjunctiva and eyelids and is strongly associated with dermatitis. It most commonly occurs in adults. Symptoms tend to be perennial. Cornea and lens may also be involved. Itching of the eyelids is a common symptom, but redness, photophobia, and pain can occur. Eye discharge tends to be clear and watery. Colonization of the eyelid margins with staphylococcus is common and can result in blepharitis. Corneal involvement ranges from punctuate epithelial kertopathy to corneal neovascularization and scarring. Keratoconus can result from chronic eye rubbing. It is most common in older patients.[7–9]

Giant papillary conjunctivitis (GPC) is an immune-mediated inflammatory disorder of the superior tarsal conjunctiva; it is characterized by the presence of "giant" papillae, characteristically greater than 0.3 mm in diameter. GPC may be a reaction to ocular irritants: contact lenses are associated with this disorder. Ocular itching is associated with a mucoid or watery discharge.[7]

▶ DIFFERENTIAL DIAGNOSIS

The differential diagnosis of conjunctivitis includes acute bacterial or viral infection and allergic disorders. Bacterial conjunctivitis is usually an acute illness associated with a purulent discharge. Viral conjunctivitis is also usually an acute process; while the discharge tends to be more watery than in bacterial conjunctivitis, the two can be difficult to differentiate. Both bacterial and viral conjunctivitis are often associated with upper respiratory infection. A careful history can help distinguish infectious from allergic conjunctivitis, since patients with the allergic conjunctivitis usually have a personal or family history of atopic illnesses, and allergic symptoms are often seasonal. Allergists and opthalmologist can perform complex chemical analysis of inflammatory mediators present in tears or ocular discharge that are characteristic of allergic disease; these tests are impractical in the emergency department.[7,8]

TREATMENT

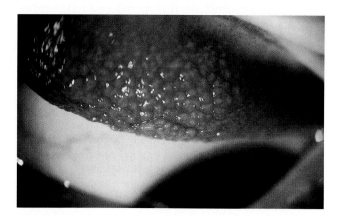

Figure 69–2. Vernal conjunctivitis—the tarsal conjunctiva demonstrates giant papillae and a cobblestone appearance pathognomonic for vernal conjunctivitis.

The treatment of each type of ocular allergy begins with trying to avoid the allergic stimulus or stimuli that trigger the illness. Artificial tears can provide some relief. There are multiple medical treatments for each type of ocular allergy, including systemic and topical (ophthalmic) antihistamines, topical mast cell stabilizers, topical nonsteroidal anti-inflammatory agents, and topical steroids. The treatment of patients suspected of having VKC, AKC, and GPC is best initiated and followed by an opthalmologist and/or allergist. Treatment for SAC and PAC can be initiated in the emergency department with a topical antihistamine alone or in combination with a mast cell stabilizer (cromolyn sodium). Antihistamines have the advantage of providing relatively rapid relief; mast cell stabilizers have a delayed effect. Treating ocular symptoms may decrease nasal symptoms. Topical steroids are reserved for patients of allergic conjunctivitis not responding to other therapy, since they can cause complications such as glaucoma and cataracts. Research is ongoing in an attempt to find treatments directed at more specific immunologic triggers of allergic conjunctivitis.[7–12]

► ALLERGIC RHINITIS OR ALLERGIC RHINOCONJUNCTIVITIS

The prevalence of allergic rhinoconjunctivitis has doubled in the past 20 years.[1] The diagnosis is often missed, which is not surprising given the prevalence of rhinorrhea in the pediatric population. More than 1.5 million children were brought to emergency departments in 2004 with complaints related to rhinorrhea.[13] The most common cause of rhinorrhea in children is acute upper respiratory infection. It is important to diagnose those patients who have allergic rhinoconjunctivitis from those with self-limited infections because appropriate treatment can decrease morbidity. Untreated or undertreated, allergic rhinoconjunctivitis is associated with sleep disturbances and impairment of daily activities and school performance. Generalized fatigue and malaise is common. Allergic rhinitis is the second most common predisposing factor for sinusitis after upper respiratory infection.[13,14] Postnasal drip can cause chronic cough and exacerbate the symptoms of asthma.[1,13]

The same allergens responsible for the ASC and PAC cause allergic rhinitis; however, not all children with ocular and nasal symptoms are sensitized to an identifiable antigen. Affected children often have a history of asthma, eczema, chronic sinusitis, and otitis media with effusion. Thus, patients with these conditions should be questioned regarding symptoms such as persistent nasal discharge or sneezing. Children with prolonged nasal symptoms or those who "always have a cold" are likely to be suffering from allergic rhinitis. Allergic rhinitis is characterized as intermittent or persistent; it is further characterized as mild or moderate/severe (Table 69–1).

The symptoms of allergic rhinitis are largely the result of histamine released from mast cells. They include nasal congestion, itching, sneezing, and discharge. Complaints of itchy and watery eyes are common; fever is not. Symptoms can be seasonal or perennial. Classic physical findings associated with allergic rhinitis include "allergic shiners," darkening of the lower eyelids due to suborbital edema; the "allergic salute," upward rubbing of the nose with the hand to relieve nasal itching; and the "allergic crease" (a transverse line across the nasal bridge due to the "nasal salute"). Nasal discharge from

► **TABLE 69-1. CLASSIFICATION OF ALLERGIC RHINOCONJUNCTIVITIS IN CHILDREN**

Intermittent: symptoms less than 4 d/wk and present less than 4 wk
Persistent: symptoms more than 4 d and present for more than 4 wk
Mild severity: no sleep disturbance, impairment of school or daily activities, symptoms well tolerated
Moderate to severe: sleep is disturbed, school and daily activities are disturbed, symptoms are well-tolerated

With permission from de Groot H, Brand PL, Wytske FF, et al. Allergic rhinoconjunctivitis in children. *BMJ.* 2007;335:985.

AR tends to be more watery and clear than in patients with acute upper respiratory infection. The oropharyngeal cavity is inspected for signs of postnasal drip, and sinuses are assessed for tenderness. Physical examination may reveal conjunctival injection and watery eye discharge from concomitant allergic conjunctivitis.[1–3,13]

There is no test available in the emergency department to confirm the diagnosis of allergic rhinitis. Assessment depends on history and physical examination, of which the most important components are the presence of other manifestations of atopy. An abbreviated list of the differential diagnosis of rhinitis is given in Table 69–2.

TREATMENT

Treatment of allergic rhinitis can begin in the emergency department, or patients can be referred to their primary care physician or an allergist for definitive management (Fig. 69–3). The most effective medications for allergic rhinitis are intranasal glucocortocoids; they reduce symptoms and improve quality of life. Second-generation antihistamines such as cetirizine and loratadine are also effective in children. Disodium cromoglycate is less effective than glucocortocoids or antihistamines. Intranasal decongestants can improve symptoms in the short term, but rebound mucosal swelling can occur with prolonged use. Children with nonremitting symptoms or those in whom allergic disease is negatively impacting quality of life should be referred to an allergist.

► **TABLE 69-2. PARTIAL LIST OF THE DIFFERENTIAL DIAGNOSIS OF RHINORRHEA**

Viral upper respiratory infections
Sinusitis
Allergic rhinitis
Vasomotor rhinitis
Nasal foreign bodies
Nasal polyps
Nasal septum deviation
Immunologic or inflammatory disorders

With permission from Ferdman RM, Linzer JF. The runny nose in the emergency department. *Clin Pediatr Emerg Med.* 2007;8:123.

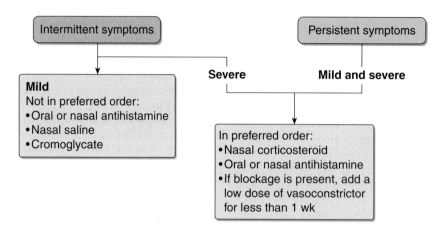

Figure 69–3. Algorithm for the management of allergic rhinoconjunctivitis in children.

REFERENCES

1. De Groot H, Brand PL, Fokkens WF, et al. Allergic rhinoconjunctivitis in children. *BMJ.* 2007;335:985.
2. Magnan A, Meunier JP, Saugnac C, et al. Frequency and impact of allergic rhinitis in asthma patients in everyday general medical practice: a French observational cross-sectional study. *Allergy.* 2008;63:292.
3. Global Initiative for Asthma. Global strategy for asthma prevention and management. 2007; 71. www.gina.asthma.org.
4. Blais MS. Allergic rhinoconjunctivitis: burden of disease. *Allergy Asthma Proc.* 2007;28:393.
5. Lack G. Pediatric allergic rhinitis and comorbid disorders. *J Allergy Clin Immunol.* 2001;108:S9.
6. Stedmans Medical Dictionary. 27th ed. Lippincott Williams & Wilkins; 2008. www.stedmans.com/section.cfm/45
7. Majudar PA. Conjunctivitis, allergic. *Emedicine.* 2008, www.emedicine.com/oph/topic85.htm. Accessed April 2008.
8. Ono SJ, Abelson MB. Allergic conjunctivitis: update on pathophysiology and prospects for future treatment. *J Allergy Clin Immunol.* 2005;115:118.
9. Jun J, Bielory L, Raizman MB. Vernal conjunctivitis. *Immunol Allergy Clin North Am.* 2008;28:59.
10. Bielory L, Katelaris CH, Lightman S, et al. Treating the ocular component of allergic rhinoconjunctivitis related eye disorders. *MedGenMed.* 2007;9:35.
11. Bielory L, Lien KW, Bigelsen S. Efficacy and tolerability of newer antihistamines in the treatment of allergic conjunctivitis. *Drugs.* 2005;65:215.
12. Bielory L. Ocular symptom reduction in patients with seasonal allergic rhinitis treated with the intranasal corticosteroid monetasone fluorate. *Ann Aller Asthma Immunol.* 2008;100:272.
13. Ferdman RM, Linzer JF. The runny nose in the emergency department: rhinitis and sinusitis. *Clin Pediatr Emerg Med.* 2007;8:123.
14. Ramadan H. Pediatric sinusitis, medical treatment. *Emedicine.* 2006, http://www.emedicine.com/Ent/topic612.html. Accessed April 2008.

CHAPTER 70

Anaphylaxis

E. Bradshaw Bunney

► HIGH-YIELD FACTS

- More than 50% of anaphylaxis cases are idiopathic; therefore, a high index of suspicion is needed to make the diagnosis in children.
- Airway compromise can occur rapidly.
- Epinephrine is the first-line medication for the treatment of moderate-to-severe anaphylaxis.
- In severe anaphylaxis if 2 to 3 fluid boluses (20 cc/kg) are given, as well as epinephrine; if hypotension persists, an epinephrine drip is indicated.

Anaphylaxis is a severe, potentially life-threatening hypersensitivity reaction characterized by skin or mucosal manifestations that include a pruritic rash, urticaria, or angioedema, respiratory compromise associated with airway edema and bronchospasm, and/or cardiovascular compromise that can result in distributive shock. It occurs within minutes to hours after exposure to an offending allergen. The estimated risk of anaphylaxis per person in the United States is 1% to 3%; this may be an underestimate of the true severity of the problem.[1] Food allergy is the most common cause of anaphylaxis, and leads to approximately 150 fatalities in the United States each year.[1] Since in over 50% of episodes of anaphylaxis cases no precipitating cause is identified, the emergency physician must have a high level of suspicion for the disorder in order to recognize the symptoms and initiate proper treatment.[2]

► PATHOPHYSIOLOGY

Anaphylaxis is an immunologic reaction. An initial exposure to an allergen results in the development of a specific IgE antibody to the antigen. The IgE antibody resides on the cell membrane of basophil and mast cells. When a subsequent exposure to the allergen occurs, the allergen binds to the IgE on the basophil and mast cells, and stimulates the release of multiple mediators, including histamine, leukotriene C4, prostaglandin D2, and tryptase. These mediators lead to increased production and release of respiratory secretions, increased bronchial smooth muscle tone, decreased vascular smooth muscle tone, and increased capillary permeability. An anaphylactoid reaction involves the release of similar mediators without involvement of the immune system. Intravenous (IV) contrast allergy is an example of an anaphylactoid reaction.

► ALLERGENS

Food is the number one cause of anaphylaxis; More than 90% of food-related anaphylaxis is caused by exposure to nuts and shellfish.[3,4] In infants, cow's milk and eggs are the most common causes of anaphylaxis.[5] Once the food that caused the anaphylaxis is identified, thorough education of the parents and child is necessary to avoid reexposure.

Insect stings are a common cause of a localized allergic reaction and can also cause anaphylaxis. There is a fatality rate of fewer than 100 deaths per year in the United States.[4]

Drug-related allergies are quite common, but fortunately anaphylaxis from medications is relatively rare. The most common medications causing anaphylaxis are aspirin, NSAIDs, and β-lactam antibiotics. IV administration of medication has a higher incidence of anaphylaxis and more rapid onset of the anaphylactic symptoms.

Latex allergy is becoming an increasingly common cause of allergic reaction in children; it can occur following exposure to gloves, or tourniquets, or a Foley catheter. Chui found that in pediatric patients, risk factors for developing a latex allergy included spina bifida, surgery in the first year of life, multiple surgeries, urogenital malformations, and atopy. Atopy is the genetic predisposition to produce IgE to common proteins, and can lead to hay fever, allergies to dust and grass pollen, and asthma.

Parents often worry about the risk of childhood immunizations causing an allergic reaction or anaphylaxis: Bohlke recently published that the risk of anaphylaxis is approximately 0.65 per million doses of vaccine.[6]

► PRESENTATION

In general, anaphylaxis is categorized as mild, moderate, and severe. Mild anaphylaxis consists primarily of skin and mucosal manifestations. These include redness, flushing, urticaria (hives), itching, and angioedema. In addition, mild anaphylaxis can produce some wheezing or throat irritation and mild tachycardia, without respiratory or cardiovascular compromise. Moderate anaphylaxis has the same cutaneous manifestations, with the addition of difficulty breathing, barky cough, stridor, light-headedness, and tachycardia. Severe anaphylaxis can cause severe respiratory distress and cardiovascular manifestations that range from hypotension and tachycardia to fulminant shock. Gastrointestinal symptoms such as vomiting, diarrhea, and crampy abdominal pain frequently accompany moderate-to-severe anaphylaxis.

In an anaphylactic reaction, the onset of symptoms ranges from minutes to a few hours after contact with an allergen, thus a history of such exposure is helpful in those patients with known severe allergies. However, since 50% of anaphylactic reactions are idiopathic, the diagnosis often needs to be made based on the constellation of symptoms at presentation, and not on information about an allergen exposure. Therefore, it is critical that the clinician considers anaphylaxis in a hypotensive child with respiratory distress.

The diagnosis is made easier when the characteristic urticarial rash is present. However, if the clinician fails to look at the skin because he or she is focusing on the critical nature of the patient the rash can be missed. In addition, up to 10% of children with anaphylaxis will present without a rash.[1,2,4]

Although most patients with anaphylaxis who are hypotensive will be tachycardic, insect stings have been associated with hypotension and a relative bradycardia. The cause of the bradycardia is unknown.[7]

▶ ANCILLARY TESTS

In general, laboratory tests or radiographic tests will not help to diagnose anaphylaxis. Some advocate the use of serial measurement of tryptase when the diagnosis is uncertain.[8]

▶ TREATMENT

As with all critically ill children, treatment begins with establishing an airway. The airway may be difficult to secure in the child with severe mucosal edema. Immediate endotracheal intubation is done in any child at risk of respiratory arrest. The clinician must always consider rescue airway techniques they may need to employ, such as cricothyrotomy and jet insufflation, should endotracheal intubation not be possible. Oxygen (100%) is indicated in all anaphylactic children with respiratory symptoms who are hypoxic. The medications used to treat anaphylaxis are listed in Table 70–1.

Epinephrine is the primary drug of choice for treating moderate-to-severe forms of anaphylaxis. The dose is 0.01 mL/kg of 1:1000 IM or SC every 15 minutes, or 0.01 mL/kg of 1:10 000 IV. Recent studies have shown that IM is preferred over SC because of more efficient absorption.[9] Inhaled epinephrine has been shown not to achieve the serum epinephrine levels needed to treat anaphylaxis and should not be used either in the emergency department or in the prehospital setting.[10] It is important to remember in children with moderate-to-severe anaphylaxis that there is no contraindication to the use of epinephrine.[3,4] In a recent review of the emergency department management of anaphylaxis, only 24% of

children in moderate-to-severe anaphylaxis got epinephrine.[11] Bronchospasm may respond to inhaled β-agonists.

IV fluids are the second mainstay of treating anaphylaxis in patients who are hypotensive. The relaxation of the vascular smooth muscle combined with the increased capillary permeability leads to considerable third-space accumulation of fluids, which can result in distributive shock. IV crystalloids are given as a 20 cc/kg bolus over 10 to 20 minutes; multiple boluses may be necessary. If hypotension persists, then an epinephrine or dopamine drip should be considered.[3,4]

H-1 antihistamines such as diphenhydramine are often used in treating anaphylaxis, particularly the histamine-related rash and pruritus, but do replace epinephrine as the first-line agent in moderate-to-severe anaphylaxis. Some authors have advocated not using diphenhydramine except in truly mild cases because of the sedative effect and possible decrease in respiratory drive.[3]

H-2 antihistamines such as cimetidine have been used in the treatment of anaphylaxis based on theoretical efficacy, but have not been proven to be of benefit.

Steroids, such as methylprednisolone, have been used to prevent recurrence of symptoms or a delayed reaction, based on their anti-inflammatory properties; the evidence for this is weak, and they are not a first-line medications in the treatment of anaphylaxis.[3,4] On rare occasions, methylprednisolone has been shown to actually cause anaphylaxis.[12]

Removal of the allergen, if possible, is always done. The child should remain lying or in Trendelenburg position until symptoms have completely resolved. There is evidence that abrupt changes in position, from lying to sitting or standing, has been associated with fatalities in pediatric, anaphylactic patients.[11]

▶ SPECIAL CONDITIONS

Exercise-induced anaphylaxis is initially characterized by mild fleeting, pinpoint wheals that are brought on by an increase in body temperature; symptoms can then progress toward respiratory and vascular compromise. Food-dependent exercise-induced anaphylaxis (FDEIA) is characterized by anaphylaxis during or soon after exercise which was preceded by the ingestion of a causal food. Neither the exercise alone nor the food will trigger the allergic response. The exercise can consist of mild or aggressive aerobic activity. Five to fifteen percent of exercise-related anaphylaxis can be caused by FDEIA. The most common food associated with FDEIA is wheat.[13]

On rare occasion, anaphylaxis has been associated with the use of anesthetic agents. In one study, the most frequent cause of anesthetic-induced anaphylaxis was from the paralytic agents, succinylcholine, and rocuronium.[14]

▶ TABLE 70–1. MEDICATIONS USED FOR THE TREATMENT OF ANAPHYLAXIS

Epinephrine	0.01 mL/kg 1:1000	IM or SC	Every 15 min
	0.01 mL/kg 1:10 000	IV	Every 15 min
Albuterol	0.03–0.05 mL/kg 0.5% solution	Nebulized	Every 15 min
Diphenhydramine	1–2 mg/kg	PO or IV or IM	Every 4–6 h
Cimetidine	5–10 mg/kg	PO or IV or IM	Every 6 h
Methylprednisolone	1–2 mg/kg	IV or IM	Every 6 h

▶ DISPOSITION

In general, any child with severe anaphylaxis involving vascular collapse should be admitted to the ICU. Any child with respiratory symptoms that have completely resolved should be observed for 6 to 8 hours before discharge to ensure that a delayed phase reaction does not occur.[3] Patients being discharged are given strict instructions to return if symptoms recur. Patients with first time anaphylaxis are referred to an allergist.

Autoinjectable epinephrine is used by patients for immediate treatment of anaphylaxis symptoms outside the hospital. They are single use and come in two doses, 0.3 mg and 0.15 mg. Many have advocated that additional, smaller doses, be produced in order to better serve the pediatric population. A general guideline proposed by Sicherer is that the 0.15 mg dose is used in children weighing 10 to 25 kg, and the 0.3 mg dose be used in children weighing 25 kg and over. Although the 0.3 mg dose in a 25 kg child is 1.2 times the recommended dose, some authors recommend this dose because the benefit of aggressively treating anaphylaxis outweighs the small potential risk of overdosing with epinephrine in otherwise healthy children.[15,16] Those that should go home with an autoinjectable epinephrine are those with cardiovascular or respiratory reaction, exercise-induced anaphylaxis, idiopathic anaphylaxis, and persistent asthma with a food allergy.[3]

REFERENCES

1. Chiu AM, Kelly KJ. Anaphylaxis: drug allergy, insect stings, and latex. *Immunol Allergy Clin North Am.* 2005;5:389.
2. Webb LM, Lieberman P. Anaphylaxis: a review of 601 cases. *Ann Allergy Asthma Immunol.* 2006;97:39.
3. Muraro A, Roberts G, Clark A, et al. The management of anaphylaxis in childhood: position paper of the European academy of allergology and clinical immunology. *Allergy.* 2007;62: 857.
4. National Guidelines Clearinghouse. http://www.guidelines. gov/summary/summary.aspx?doc'id=6887&nbr=004211& string=anaphylaxis 2005. Accessed March 5, 2008.
5. Simons FE. Anaphylaxis in infants: can recognition and management be improved? *J Allergy Clin Immunol.* 2007;120:537.
6. Bohlke K, Davis RL, Marcy SM, et al. Risk of anaphylaxis after vaccination of children and adolescents. *Pediatrics.* 2003; 112:815.
7. Brown SG. Cardiovascular aspects of anaphylaxis: implications for treatment and diagnosis. *Curr Opin Allergy Clin Immunol.* 2005;5:359.
8. Tewari A, Du TG, Lack G. The difficulties of diagnosing food-dependent exercise-induced anaphylaxis in childhood—a case study and review. *Pediatr Allergy Immunol.* 2006;17:157.
9. Sicherer SH. Advances in anaphylaxis and hypersensitivity reactions to foods, drugs, and insect venom. *J Allergy Clin Immunol.* 2003;111(3 suppl):S829.
10. Simons FE, Gu X, Johnston LM, et al. Can epinephrine inhalations be substituted for epinephrine injection in children at risk for systemic anaphylaxis? *Pediatrics.* 2000;106:1040.
11. Stone KD. Advances in pediatric allergy. *Curr Opin Pediatr.* 2004;16:571.
12. Schonwald S. Methylprednisolone anaphylaxis. *Am J Emerg Med.* 1999;17:583.
13. Du TG. Food-dependent exercise-induced anaphylaxis in childhood. *Pediatr Allergy Immunol.* 2007;18:455.
14. Laxenaire MC, Mertes PM. Anaphylaxis during anaesthesia. Results of a two-year survey in France. *Br J Anaesth.* 2001;87:549.
15. Sicherer SH, Simons FE. Self-injectable epinephrine for first-aid management of anaphylaxis. *Pediatrics.* 2007;119:638.
16. Simons FE, Gu X, Silver NA, Simons KJ. EpiPen Jr versus EpiPen in young children weighing 15 to 30 kg at risk for anaphylaxis. *J Allergy Clin Immunol.* 2002;109:171.

SECTION X

GASTROINTESTINAL EMERGENCIES

CHAPTER 71

Abdominal Pain

Philip H. Ewing

▶ HIGH-YIELD FACTS

- A surgical emergency should always be ruled out when evaluating a patient with abdominal pain.
- If a patient complains of abdominal pain, an examination of the external genitalia and a digital rectal examination should be a part of a routine examination.
- Ovarian and testicular torsions are important causes of abdominal pain that should not be overlooked.
- Ionizing radiation exposure should be considered when ordering CT for determination of the cause of abdominal pain.
- Intussusception should always be considered in infants/children with intermittent abdominal pain associated with vomiting.
- If an organic cause of abdominal pain has been ruled out, the patient and family need to be reassured and given appropriate, close follow-up through a primary care physician.

The chief complaint of abdominal pain elicits a broad differential in the mind of the practitioner. The most common discharge diagnoses in pediatric patients with abdominal pain are conditions such as acute gastroenteritis, constipation, and "viral syndrome." However, serious clinical problems that require medical or surgical intervention may present with the same symptoms as disease processes that are benign and self-limited. No differential for abdominal pain is complete without abuse or nonaccidental trauma, especially in the younger, more vulnerable patient. Traumatic abdominal pain, as well as pain related to tumors, will be addressed in Chapters 32 and 103, respectively. The most frequently encountered surgical and medical causes of abdominal pain are addressed in this chapter including causes of abdominal pain that are unique to the female and male reproductive tracts.

▶ THE HISTORY AND EXAMINATION FOR ABDOMINAL PAIN

Abdominal pain can be either visceral or somatic in nature. Visceral pain is poorly localized and may be difficult to describe, even in older children. Somatic pain is an intense and readily localized sensation that indicates the presence of inflammation. The brain modulates the perception of pain; patients with comparable pathologies may range from stoic to incapacitated depending on the influence of the environment upon their perception of pain. Referred pain syndromes manifested as abdominal pain may be characteristic of a variety of clinical problems.

The history and physical examination of a pediatric patient with abdominal pain can be complex due to the frightening and unfamiliar environment of the emergency department (ED). Communication is enhanced when the provider can establish an effective relationship with the patient and the caregiver. Infants and toddlers may not provide useful or relevant information, so the physician must rely on the caregivers for historical data. Careful observation may provide abundant information about a child's diagnosis. With older patients, the presence of a parent or caregiver may influence the effectiveness of an interview. This is certainly true for adolescents where an accurate sexual history may be impossible to obtain with a parent at the bedside. Creating an opportunity for the patient to be examined in private without presence of the caregiver can be an effective way of establishing a trusting relationship that may yield important historical information. Finally, the physician should attempt to formulate questions that are appropriate for the child's level of development, regardless of the patient's age. Open-ended questions are preferable and should be used in place of "yes or no" questions that may exceed the child's level of comprehension. A detailed surgical history should be obtained. Intra-abdominal adhesions may be causing an obstruction at a previous surgical site. An age-appropriate differential diagnosis may be altered if there is history of surgery that alters the normal anatomy of the GI tract, such as a Nissen fundoplasty or a Ladd's procedure.

The history should help to create a preliminary differential diagnosis, and it should include abdominal conditions, systemic illnesses, and referred pain syndromes. Afferent nerves from distant organs can share central pathways that allow pain from one organ to be interpreted as if the stimulus is affecting another organ. A classic example is a right lower-lobe pneumonia that refers pain to the abdomen mimicking appendicitis. Conversely, some conditions that are intra-abdominal in origin may produce pain syndromes that are manifested in other locations. Examples are shoulder pain due to hepatic irritation (right), or splenic rupture (left), and groin pain from renal stone disease. Characteristic referred pain syndromes should alert the practitioner to include an abdominal process in the differential diagnosis. Table 71–1 lists extra-abdominal and systemic conditions that may present as abdominal pain.[1]

A traditional bedside examination may not be possible in frightened infants and small children. The examination may actually begin by observing the patient walking to an examination room. Approach the child with caution in a nonthreatening way. The patient should be allowed to sit with the parent as long as a complete examination may be obtained. While the child is in the parent's lap, the physician may carefully observe, auscultate, palpate, and percuss the abdomen. A complete

▶ **TABLE 71–1. EXTRABDOMINAL AND SYSTEMIC CAUSES OF ABDOMINAL PAIN**

▶ **TABLE 71–1. EXTRABDOMINAL AND SYSTEMIC CAUSES OF ABDOMINAL PAIN**

- Asthma
- Pneumonia
- Heart disease
- Toxin exposure, ingestion, or overdose
- Collagen vascular disease
- Diabetic ketoacidosis
- Black widow spider bite
- Hemolytic–uremic syndrome
- Inborn error of metabolism
- Sepsis
- Abdominal epilepsy/migraine
- Henoch–Schönlein purpura
- Mononeucloisis
- Pharyngitis

examination includes the genitalia and perineum, in addition to a rectal examination when appropriate. It is important not to miss diagnoses such as an incarcerated inguinal hernia presenting with refusal to feed or a testicular torsion in an embarrassed male presenting with abdominal pain.

▶ DIAGNOSTIC TESTS FOR ABDOMINAL PAIN

Diagnostic testing may assist decision making in the ED and is often a useful screening tool for patients with a concerning history but an equivocal examination or vice versa. Laboratory testing and diagnostic imaging should be focused to confirm clinical suspicion. For instance, a patient with a brief history of abdominal pain and vomiting need not have testing for electrolytes, blood urea nitrogen, or creatinine since they are unlikely to have a significant metabolic derangement. A patient with panhypopituitarism, who presents with the same history, may require those tests regardless of the duration of vomiting. Table 71–2 reviews ancillary laboratory test that may be helpful in sorting out the cause of abdominal pain.

Ultrasonography, plain radiography, and computed tomography (CT) represent the most common imaging per-

▶ **TABLE 71–2. LABORATORY TESTS FOR ABDOMINAL PAIN**

- Hematologic/infectious/inflammatory conditions—complete blood count with differential, erythrocyte sedimentation rate, blood culture
- Pancreatiitis—amylase, lipase
- Specific bile duct enzymes—γ-glutyl transferase
- Liver injury—alanine transaminase, aspartate transaminase
- Liver function tests—protein fractions, prothrombin time, partial thromboplastin time, alkaline phosphatase, bilirubin, ammonia, glucose
- Renal—electrolytes, blood urea nitrogen, urinalysis, urine culture

▶ **TABLE 71–3. IONIZING RADIATION FROM COMMON RADIOLOGICAL IMAGING**

• Two-view chest radiography	• 0.16 mSv
• Adult abdominal CT	• 10 mSv
• Neonatal abdominal CT	• 20 mSv
• Barium enema	• 15 mSv

The estimated lifetime attributable risk of death from any cancer after an abdominal CT in a pediatric patient ranges from 0.06% to 0.14%. Six to fourteen patients in 10 000 are likely to develop fatal cancer after a single exposure.
With permission from Brenner DJ, Hall EJ. Computed tomography—an increasing source of radiation exposure. *N Engl J Med.* 2007;357:2277–2284.

formed for assessment of abdominal pain. Attention should be paid to the potential effects of ionizing radiation. Young infants and children are particularly vulnerable to the long-term effects of ionizing radiation, and the widespread use of CT for diagnostic imaging may increase the risk of cancer in the future. Table 71–3 compares the radiation exposure from various imaging.[2] This somewhat hypothetical data should not limit the clinician from obtaining important tests, but protocols and algorithms that achieve timely diagnosis with a minimum amount of radiation should be developed and adopted. Plain films are often the primary step during a sequence of imaging modalities. It is imperative to obtain images that compare the patient in prone or decubitus and upright positions to identify presence of bowel gas throughout the intestines and rule out obstruction. Appropriate images should be able to demonstrate the presence of extraluminal air or a mass effect that may direct further imaging. Contrasted CT scans are an important tool that should be used judiciously due to the risk of contrast-induced nephropathy. A detailed past medical history can be helpful in discovering patients who are at risk, but a serum creatinine level is a quick screening tool.

Ultrasound is emerging as a diagnostic adjunct for many conditions that are addressed in the ED. The main advantage of diagnostic ultrasound is that it does not expose the patient to ionizing radiation like other radiological modalities. The portability of the ultrasound apparatus allows the machine can be moved to the patient's bedside for a rapid examination in an unstable child. Ultrasound allows for rapid diagnosis in the hands of an experienced practitioner, and rarely requires sedation. Table 71–4 lists conditions that ultrasonography may serve as an aid to diagnosis. See Chapter 20 for more details on imaging modalities.

▶ **TABLE 71–4. ULTRASOUND AS FIRST IMAGING OF CHOICE**

- Appendicitis
- Choledocholithiasis
- Intussusception
- Pregnancy and ectopic pregnancy
- Renal stones
- Ovarian/testicular torsion
- Abdominal trauma

IS A SURGEON NEEDED?

In the assessment of an infant or child with abdominal pain, one of the most important issues to determine early is if the pain is due to a surgically correctable cause. While not all of the following conditions require immediate surgical correction, it is prudent to have early surgical involvement to ensure that prompt intervention can be made should the patient's condition deteriorate.[3]

▶ OBSTRUCTION

Abdominal obstruction will present with colicky, cramping abdominal pain usually associated with vomiting, often bilious in nature. In young infants, irritability and inconsolable crying must alert the examining physician to consider obstruction. Bilious emesis in a newborn infant must be considered malrotation with midgut volvulus until proven otherwise. This can progress to an abdominal catastrophe if not recognized early. However, bilious emesis does not occur in all patients with malrotation, so the diagnosis should also be considered in infants with poor feeding, recurrent emesis, abdominal distention, or failure to thrive. Malrotation occurs in utero when the midgut fails to rotate counterclockwise, preventing the normal abdominal orientation of the intestine where there cecum rotates into the right lower quadrant. A nasogastric tube should be placed prior to upper gastrointestinal fluoroscopy with radio-opaque oral contrast, which is the study of choice. A diagnostic study shows that the duodenum does not cross the midline, assuming a corkscrew-like appearance.[4]

Early diagnosis of intussusception is particularly important because when delayed, bowel ischemia can produce disastrous results. Intussusception occurs when a portion of bowel prolapses into another section of bowel, most often in children, infants, and toddlers. A strong visual comparison is that of the antique collapsing telescope where the smaller sections fit into the larger section. As the bowel prolapses, the associated mesentery is pulled along and blood flow to the bowel is compromised. Classically, the resultant ischemia can be recognized as intermittent colicky pain that may be associated with lethargy or somnolence. Some patients will draw their legs up toward the abdomen when experiencing episodes of pain. Vomiting is common and occasionally may be bilious. An abdominal mass, usually right sided, may be present. A late sign is the currant jelly stool that indicates extensive bowel ischemia proceeding to sloughing of the intestinal mucosa. Radiographs may demonstrate a right-sided abdominal mass or target lesion; however, a negative examination does not rule out intussusception. Even when negative or equivocal, plain film of the abdomen can identify the presence of extraluminal free air, which can complicate reduction when performed with an enema. Air contrast enemas are emerging as the therapy of choice in appropriate patients. Advantages include less radiation than barium enemas and reduced complications should there be a bowel perforation. Ultrasound-guided enemas are also used, achieving the lowest possible radiation exposure. Surgical intervention is mandatory for patients whose intussusceptions cannot be reduced with an enema. Special consideration should be given to older patients who develop intussus-

ception. Patients at and beyond the age of 2 to 5 years have an increased incidence of a pathologic lead point as the cause of prolapse. Pathologic lead points could include soft tissue masses, polyps, Henoch–Schöenlein purpura, and Meckel's diverticula (see Chapter 9).

An incarcerated hernia can be a difficult diagnosis to make since an infant may not present with abdominal pain, but rather irritability and the refusal to feed. Careful examination must include an evaluation of the genitalia because prompt diagnosis and reduction may obviate the need for emergent surgical intervention. Incarcerated hernias most often occur when bowel prolapses through a patent inguinal canal. Hernias that are not reducible through traditional means (cold packs, Trendelenburg positioning, or massage) require surgical attention because of the risk of bowel ischemia and perforation. Patients with hernias that are successfully reduced in the ED do not require immediate surgical consultation; however, the child should be able to feed normally prior to discharge and the caregivers should be given detailed discharge instructions. Referral for elective surgical closure is appropriate.

▶ PERITONEAL IRRITATION, INFLAMMATION

Intra-abdominal sepsis with abdominal pain from peritoneal irritation may have many causes, of which appendicitis is one of the most frequent. Other entities are less common and occur within groups with specific risk factors. Acute appendicitis classically produces abdominal pain that is initially vague and periumbilical and within hours of onset localizes to the right lower quadrant. Vomiting, anorrhexia, and low-grade fever are usually present. Table 71–5 reviews helpful clinical signs of appendicitis and peritoneal irritation. If the diagnosis is not made in 24 to 48 hours, appendicitis can progress to perforation with intra-abdominal abscess formation and sepsis. The concern for complications is what drives the conservative approach diagnosis and early surgical consultation in the ED. Early recognition of appendicitis before perforation occurs can be a clinical challenge in infants and young children complicated by the frequency of abdominal pain and a child's inability to describe or localize pain. It is also common for the clinical condition of the patient to improve, and abdominal pain temporarily resolve when an appendix perforates. Data demonstrates a 90% perforation rate by the time diagnosis is made in children younger than 5 years. Because of its high incidence, many authors have approached the diagnosis of appendicitis to identify the most important diagnostic studies to support early recognition.[5,6] The diagnosis may be made clinically on the basis of right lower quadrant pain on examination, but the white blood count and a urinalysis may assist in decision making. Imaging studies can include plain films, CT scans, and abdominal ultrasounds. Ultrasound is very "user-dependent" but is quite accurate in thin children and may be particularly useful for females with right-sided pain where ovarian torsion is in the differential. Figure 71–1 provides a diagnostic algorithm for appendicitis. Once the diagnosis is confirmed, the surgical approach to appendectomy can be either open or laparoscopic[3] (see Chapter 9).

- McBurney's sign: rebound RLQ pain
- Rosving's sign: rebound tenderness referred from LLQ to RLQ
- Psoas sign: pain with passive extension of the thigh while the knee is extended
- Obturator sign: right knee pulled laterally while hip flexed 90 degrees

Spontaneous or primary peritonitis is a condition that is often associated with disease processes such as nephrotic syndrome, which may result from ascites in the face of a relative immunodeficiency. Antibiotic therapy should be directed at the typical causative organisms including *Streptococcus* species and gram-negative rods, but other organisms should be considered especially if the patient has an indwelling catheter for peritoneal dialysis.

Necrotizing enterocolitis (NEC) is often thought to be a condition that is restricted to premature infants. While it is primarily diagnosed in the neonatal intensive care unit (NICU), NEC can be seen in neonates after being discharged to home. Risk factors include prematurity and difficulty in transitioning at birth, identified by a complicated resuscitation. Infants may present with irritability due to abdominal pain, poor feeding, and bloody stools. Directed resuscitation in the ED is mandatory and conservative treatment involves admission for bowel rest, parenteral antibiotics, and early surgical consultation. Some infants will require surgical resection of the involved areas that typically include those in watershed areas of the small intestine. As with patients in the NICU, there is a risk of losing the involved portions of the bowel and the patients with extensive losses may develop short gut syndrome.

Even though there may be a significant warning sign in abnormal stooling from birth, the recognition of Hirschsprung's disease may be delayed and patients can present with significant disease, including toxic megacolon. The disease is characterized by the lack of parasympathetic ganglia to the affected portion of the colon making peristaltic efforts of the bowel ineffective at moving stool through the colon. When the distal rectum is involved, digital rectal examination may be diagnostic since the lack of rectal tone gives the sensation of inserting one's finger into a glove when there is loss of the dilated rectal vault. Antibiotics and decompression of the bowel may be indicated to stabilize the patient before a diagnostic workup. This may include a barium enema demonstrating a "transition zone," rectal manometry, or a suction biopsy of the rectum and colon.

NONSURGICAL CAUSES OF ABDOMINAL PAIN

Acute Gastroenteritis

Vomiting and diarrhea frequently accompany the chief complaint of abdominal pain, and commonly present together. The temptation to automatically diagnose such a patient with acute gastroenteritis can be dangerous as the symptoms are very nonspecific. Be particularly concerned with the patient who presents with vomiting and abdominal pain without diarrhea. Surgically correctable disease must be ruled out.

Urinary Tract Infections

A common source of abdominal discomfort in children is both upper and lower urinary tract infections (UTI). Patients may have fever, nausea, emesis, abdominal pain, and urinary

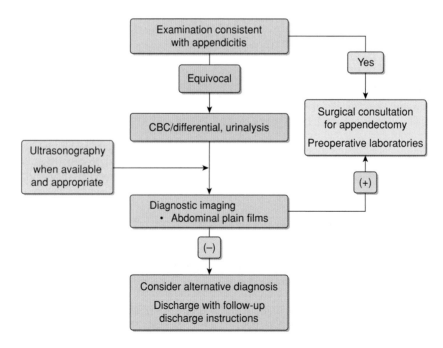

Figure 71–1. Algorithm for the diagnosis of appendicitis.

symptoms such as frequency, urgency, and dysuria. Screening urinalysis, culture, and Gram stain can identify affected patients. An oral course of antibiotics will suffice for treatment of patients who appear nontoxic. Inpatient, parenteral antibiotics required for infants younger than 2 to 6 months and ill patients where the risk of pyelonephritis, bacteremia, and urosepsis is greater (see Chapter 84).

Constipation

One of the most common causes of colicky, cramping abdominal pain in children is constipation. The pain may limit their everyday function and progress to cause nausea and vomiting. Some patients will present with recurrent UTIs secondary to obstruction. Often the patient will have encoparesis, loose, or liquid stools resulting from leakage around impacted stool in the distal colon and rectum. The etiology of the symptoms often has significant behavioral overlay.

Colic

Although not likely an abdominal condition, colic often presents when parents interpret prolonged periods of crying as abdominal pain. Some parents describe an infant who strains to pass a stool. First, it is important to rule out pathologic causes for the infant's irritable behavior. Efforts should be directed to supporting the parents and empowering them with knowledge about the benign nature of the symptoms and giving them ample resources for stress relief. The parents can be exasperated and this puts the infant at risk for abuse because it stresses the parent–child dyad. An emergency provider must help them partner with their primary care physician to ensure that the family has ample follow-up after discharge.

Bleeding and Pain

Abdominal pain associated with bleeding from the gastrointestinal tract has many causes and is discussed in detail in Chapter 72. The history should attempt to quantify the amount of blood lost as well as its quality: bright red blood, dark blood, clots, or coffee ground emesis. Patients with a recent history of facial trauma and developing nausea and abdominal pain may have epistaxis when blood from the nose has been swallowed. Others who have had protracted emesis may develop Mallory–Weiss tears with subsequent bloody emesis. A nasogastric lavage with isotonic saline may be necessary to quantify the amount of bleeding and whether the bleeding is controlled.

Infants and toddlers may present with stool that are hard and covered or streaked with blood. The act of passing hard stools is painful and may cause anal fissures. A close examination of the anal opening with ample retraction of the skin of the perineum may be needed to discover the fissure. A more serious disease process is hemolytic uremic syndrome (HUS) that presents with anemia, thrombocytopenia, and renal failure. Abdominal pain with bloody diarrhea can be part of the prodrome; the causative agent is often *Escherichia coli* O157:H7. Patients with HUS require aggressive fluid resuscitation and treatment of hemolutic anemia and coagulation dis-

orders. The characteristic rash of Henoch–Schöenlein purpura can also present with pain in the abdomen, arthralgias, and blood in the stool. The blood may be only occult in nature, and the physician should remember to obtain a urinalysis looking for proteinuria and hematuria with RBC casts, which can identify whether the patient will develop renal complications.

Liver/Pancreatic Pain

Gallbladder disease, including gallstone complications, is not common in the pediatric population but there are groups who are at risk, including patients with ongoing hemolytic disease such as sickle cell anemia. Patients with enteric infections and Kawasaki disease may also manifest biliary tract problems with pain. Patients may present with recurrent postprandial colicky epigastric or right upper quadrant abdominal pain. Upon diagnosis, the patient should be made NPO, given pain control, and started on antibiotics. Symptoms of gallstone movement through the bile duct should prompt appropriate diagnostic imaging and surgical or gastroenterology consultation.

Pancreatitis is another uncommon disease in the pediatric population. Obesity appears to be increasing the incidence of pancreatitis in children and adolescents. Patients may present with abdominal pain radiating to the back after high-fat meals in conjunction with pale stools. Some children will develop the disease as a result of an infection or exposure, while others will develop pancreatitis as a manifestation of a systemic or genetic disorder such as cystic fibrosis of hereditary pancreatitis. Lipase and amylase will be elevated. Care is mainly supportive, emphasizing pain control and bowel rest. They will often require hospitalization, fluids, and continuous nasogastric drainage till pain is resolved.

Jaundice and abdominal pain may be the first manifestations of hepatitis. The etiology of hepatitis can be related to infection, drug exposure (especially acetaminophen), systemic disease, or diseases inherent to the liver and biliary tree. The diagnostic pathway should include laboratory studies to assess damage to the liver, hepatic function, investigations into possible etiologies, and imaging of the biliary tract. In complicated patients, early consultation with gastroenterology is essential to ensure that the patient is followed to identify possible progression to liver failure. See Chapter 75 for a detailed discussion of hepatitis.

Inflammatory Bowel Disease

Inflammatory bowel disease (IBD) is another uncommon cause of abdominal pain in children; however, the undiagnosed patient may present repeatedly to the ED for complaints of abdominal pain. This can be frustrating for the patient, family, and the provider. The pain may be vague in nature, but it may be associated with melena or frankly bloody stool. The subset of patients with Crohn's disease may have early manifestations of the disease in the perianal area, including fistulae and skin tags. Patients with significant bowel involvement may progress to obstruction, perforation, or sepsis. At a minimum, the patient should have a CBC, liver function tests, and assessment of inflammatory markers. Patients with IBD will require gastroenterology consultation for long-term management, but a strong relationship with the primary care provider will reduce unnecessary ED visits and improve care.

GYNECOLOGIC CAUSES OF ABDOMINAL PAIN

The complexity of decision making about the causes of abdominal pain is increased when considering the adolescent female. Pubescent females may have abdominal pain that can cause significant morbidity if left untreated. Ovarian cysts and tumors may cause pain but may also lead to ovarian torsion, so it is imperative to consider this diagnosis even in young girls. Additional complexities are introduced when puberty begins and with the onset of sexual activity. Dysmenorrhea and endometriosis should be considered in young women with recurrent abdominal pain. Pelvic inflammatory disease is possible when an adolescent has lower abdominal pain, cervical motion tenderness, and fever. Pregnancy and ectopic pregnancy should also be a consideration in any adolescent with abdominal pain.

GENITAL PROBLEMS IN MALES WITH ABDOMINAL PAIN

A diagnostic examination for abdominal pain must include careful evaluation of both the genitalia and rectum. Acute scrotal or testicular pain often presents as abdominal pain. Testicular torsion, torsion of the appendix testes, orchitis, and epididymitis can be reviewed in Chapter 82.

REFERENCES

1. McCollough M, Sharieff GQ. Abdominal pain in children. *Ped Clin North Am.* 2006;53(1):107–137.
2. Brenner DJ, Hall EJ. Computed tomography—an increasing source of radiation exposure. *N Engl J Med.* 2007;357:2277–2284.
3. Mattei P. Minimally invasive surgery in the diagnosis and treatment of abdominal pain in children. *Curr Opin Pediatr.* 2007; 19:338–343.
4. McCollough M, Sharieff GQ. Abdominal surgical emergencies in infants and young children. *Emerg Med Clin North Am.* 2003;21:909–935.
5. Bundy DG, Byerly JS, Liles EA, et al. Does this child have appendicitis? *JAMA.* 2007;298:438–451.
6. Hagendorf BA, Clarke JR, Burd RS. The optimal initial management of children with suspected appendicitis: a decision analysis. *J Pediatr Surg.* 2004;39:880–885.

SUGGESTED READINGS

Bachur RG. Abdominal emergencies. In: Fleisher GR, Ludwig S, Henretig FM, et al., eds. *Textbook of Pediatric Emergency Medicine.* Philadelphia, PA: Lippincott, Williams & Wilkins; 2006:1605–1630.

Durbin DR, Liacouras CA. Gastrointestinal emergencies. In: Fleisher GR, Ludwig S, Henretig FM, et al., eds. *Textbook of Pediatric Emergency Medicine.* Philadelphia, PA: Lippincott, Williams & Wilkins; 2006:1087–1112.

Ruddy RM. Pain—abdomen. In: Fleisher GR, Ludwig S, Henretig FM, et al., eds. *Textbook of Pediatric Emergency Medicine.* Philadelphia, PA: Lippincott, Williams & Wilkins; 2006:469–476.

CHAPTER 72

Gastrointestinal Bleeding

Rebecca L. Partridge

▶ HIGH-YIELD FACTS

- Pulse rate and quality can help determine the presence of a significant gastrointestinal (GI) bleed.
- Examination of the posterior pharynx in patients with hematemesis may reveal a posterior nosebleed as the cause.
- Cefdinir and Rifampin can cause red stools and be mistaken for a GI bleed.
- The Apt-Downey test can differentiate swallowed maternal blood from neonatal GI bleeding.
- Vascular malformations are a rare but serious cause of both upper and lower GI bleeding.
- The ligament of Treitz is the anatomic separation between upper and lower GI bleeding.
- Melena indicates proximal bleeding, while hematochezia is seen with bleeding from the distal colon and rectum.

▶ A GENERAL APPROACH TO GASTROINTESTINAL BLEEDING

Gastrointestinal (GI) bleeding is a common and anxiety-provoking experience for both parents and children. Although the exact incidence of gastrointestinal bleeding in children is unknown, hematemesis and hematochezia are common emergency department complaints. In healthy children, most gastrointestinal bleeding is minor and self-limited, but occasionally the bleeding can be severe and even life-threatening.

As with any chief complaint, initial assessment must focus on rapid assessment and stabilization. Although most children with gastrointestinal bleeding will be clinically stable, rarely a child with a massive gastrointestinal bleed may present critically ill. A child's airway can be jeopardized by profuse bleeding with aspiration of blood, or decreased mental status from blood loss. If the airway is compromised or the child is at risk for aspiration, endotracheal intubation should be quickly performed. A nasogastric tube may be required to keep the stomach decompressed and to minimize vomiting. Assessment of a child's circulation is critical, and if there is any concern about excessive or continued blood loss, two large-bore IVs should be immediately placed. Pulse rate and quality and capillary refill time and blood pressure should be rapidly assessed to determine the need for fluid resuscitation. Fluids should be given as crystalloid boluses, but if blood loss is severe, repletion with blood products including packed red blood cells and fresh frozen plasma may be required.

Once stability of a child's airway, breathing, and circulation has been confirmed, further history and physical examination can be obtained. Asking about the color, timing, and volume of bleeding is essential, although it is often difficult for parents and children to accurately assess the volume of blood loss. Associated symptoms such as abdominal pain, preceding vomiting, fever, and stool patterns are also helpful. Some patients have a history of conditions such as coagulopathy, liver, or bowel disease known to put them at risk for gastrointestinal bleeding. In addition, medications such as NSAIDs, corticosteroids, or anticoagulants are known to increase the risk for bleeding

Although the source of gastrointestinal bleeding is often difficult to visualize, certain physical examination findings can assist in the diagnosis. Vital signs, particularly pulse rate and quality, are essential in determining if a patient has experienced a hemodynamically significant bleed, and other assessments of circulation such as capillary refill and skin color are also helpful adjuncts. Examination of the nose and pharynx may reveal a bleeding source. Signs of liver disease, such as jaundice, hepatosplenomegaly, or ascites, may be evident, and a careful abdominal examination is essential. In patients with a lower gastrointestinal bleed, a careful rectal and anal examination may reveal a benign diagnosis such as anal fissure or hemorrhoids.

In patients with small or resolved gastrointestinal bleeding, minimal diagnostic testing may be required. If there is any question about the presence of blood in vomit or stool, a guaiac test may be performed. Patients with any significant bleed may require a measurement of hematocrit to assess for anemia, keeping in mind this may not reflect anemia if blood loss is acute, and serial measurements may be required. A platelet count should also be performed. Assessment of liver and kidney function may be required in some patients as well as tests of coagulation such as prothrombin time and partial thromboplastin time. Performing a type and screen is also essential if there is excessive or continued blood loss.

Patients presenting with hematemesis may require gastric lavage. Although ineffective for hemostasis, placement of a nasogastric tube with instillation of room temperature saline and suctioning of gastric secretions may be helpful in assessing if bleeding is continuing. Gastric lavage can be helpful in determining if blood is upper gastrointestinal in origin, but cannot rule out continued bleeding, particularly if bleeding is duodenal in origin. Placement of a nasogastric tube may also help decompress the stomach and reduce further vomiting.

Patients with recurrent, continued, or massive gastrointestinal bleeding may require endoscopy. Both upper and lower endoscopies can identify the source of bleeding and may be therapeutic as well. Thermal coagulation, sclerotherapy, banding, and excision may all be performed through the endoscope.

It is important to also keep in mind that although gastrointestinal bleeding is extremely anxiety-provoking, all that is red is not necessarily a gastrointestinal bleed. Ingestion of red food dyes, medications such as cefdinir or rifampin, and foods such as beets or blueberries can all color the vomitus and stool. Bismuth salicylate, iron, and spinach can also turn stools very dark and be mistaken for melena. False positive guaiac tests may be seen if patients have ingested red meat or peroxidase-containing fruits and vegetables such as cauliflower, broccoli, turnips, or radishes.[1] Newborns may present with either hematemesis or melena secondary to ingested maternal blood, and the source of the bleeding can be distinguished with the Apt–Downey test in which adult hemoglobin turns brown in an alkaline environment. In addition, sources outside the gastrointestinal tract such as epistaxis, hemoptysis, hematuria, or menstrual blood commonly result in the appearance of an upper or lower gastrointestinal bleed.

▶ UPPER GASTROINTESTINAL BLEEDING

Upper gastrointestinal bleeding is classically defined as occurring proximal to the ligament of Treitz, and causes vary by age (Table 72–1). Although hematemesis is always upper gastrointestinal in origin, up to 75% of lower gastrointestinal bleeding is actually upper in origin, presenting as melena or even bright red rectal bleeding if bleeding is brisk and transit time is rapid. Upper gastrointestinal bleeding also carries a higher mortality rate compared to lower gastrointestinal bleeding.[2] Upper gastrointestinal bleeding can originate in the esophagus, stomach, or duodenum.

ESOPHAGUS

Inflammatory disorders of the esophagus can result in irritation of the mucosa and subsequent bleeding. Gastroesophageal re-

flux is the most common cause of esophageal inflammation and may present with regurgitation, abdominal or chest pain, cough, and food refusal.[3] (See Chapter 73 for a detailed review of gastroesophageal reflux.) Esophageal infections from *Candida*, cytomegalovirus, and herpes also occur, more commonly in immunocompromised children, although they can occur in otherwise healthy children as well. These patients typically present with severe chest or abdominal pain, fever, dysphagia, and odynophagia, and if bleeding occurs, it is typically small in volume. Many patients with reflux esophagitis can be treated empirically with acid suppression, but children with infections of the esophagus often require further evaluation and possibly inpatient treatment depending on the severity of their symptoms. Patients with severe or persistent symptoms may require endoscopy.

Lacerations of esophageal mucosa (Mallory Weiss tears) can occur in patients with repeated retching, vomiting, or paroxysmal cough.[4] These lesions typically occur at the gastroesophageal junction or in the cardia of the stomach. Abdominal pain is typically minimal.[5] Most bleeding from Mallory Weiss tears is self-limited and relatively small in volume,[6] and most patients can be successfully treated with anti-emetics and acid suppression.[7]

Children with known liver disease or portal hypertension are at risk for esophageal varices, coagulopathy, and subsequent significant gastrointestinal bleeding (Fig. 72–1). Even otherwise healthy children can have undiagnosed extrahepatic portal hypertension and develop bleeding varices. Variceal bleeding can present with bleeding ranging from minimal to life-threatening and carries with it a mortality rate of up to 8%.[8] These patients may require red cell or platelet transfusions and correction of coagulation defects with fresh frozen plasma or vitamin K. Fortunately, variceal bleeding is self-limited in up to 50% of patients.[4] Endoscopy is particularly important in

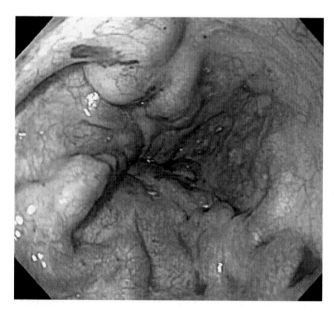

Figure 72–1. Multiple oozing esophageal varices seen, extending to gastroesophageal junction in a child with portal hypertension. (Photo courtesy of Dr. Brian Riedel, Pediatric Gastroenterology, Vanderbilt University Medical Center.)

▶ **TABLE 72–1. CAUSES OF UPPER GASTROINTESTINAL BLEEDING (BY AGE)**

Age	Small Volume	Large Volume
Newborn	Gastritis Stress ulcers Esophagitis	Ingested maternal blood Vitamin K deficiency A-V malformation Bleeding disorders/DIC
Infant	Gastritis Esophagitis Mallory–Weiss tear	Peptic ulcer disease A-V malformation
Child	Gastritis Esophagitis Foreign body Mallory–Weiss tear	Esophageal varices Peptic ulcer disease A-V malformation

patients with variceal bleeding as it offers not only a diagnosis but also allows therapeutic sclerotherapy or banding. If endoscopy is not feasible, medical therapy with intravenous vasopressin or somatostatin can be effective in controlling variceal bleeding.[7,8]

STOMACH/DUODENUM

Gastritis and peptic ulcer disease are common etiologies for upper gastrointestinal bleeding (Fig. 72–2). Medications such as NSAIDs, corticosteroids, and iron are known to increase the risk for gastric and duodenal inflammation. Infection with *Helicobacter pylori* is a common cause of gastric and duodenal ulcers in healthy children.[9] Critically ill children are particularly at risk for development of "stress gastritis," and prophylaxis with acid-suppressing drugs is essential. Patients with gastritis or ulcers often present with epigastric or left upper quadrant abdominal pain, which is relieved by eating. Hematemesis can occur and is usually self-limited,[7] although it can be massive and even life-threatening, particularly if ulceration and perforation occur. Although the gold standard for the diagnosis of *H. pylori* infection is endoscopy with biopsy, noninvasive testing for *H. pylori* fecal antigen testing is a reliable, highly sensitive test and may be feasible in the emergency department.[10] Gastritis and peptic ulcers can be treated with acid suppression and close follow-up provided the bleeding is minimal and has stopped.[11] Antimicrobial therapy should be included if infection with *H. pylori* is a factor. Endoscopy may be required for severe or persistent symptoms.

Vascular malformations are a rare but important cause of gastrointestinal bleeding and can be present anywhere along the gastrointestinal tract. They typically present with painless, massive, and recurrent hemorrhage in the absence of other symptoms. Endoscopy is valuable for lesions in the upper gastrointestinal tract or colon and allows for therapeutic interventions. Some vascular lesions are visible on CT scan or MRI.[12] For persistent bleeding (at least 0.1 mL/min), a radioisotope-labeled red cell scan may be diagnostic. Although difficult to perform in children, angiography may assist the diagnosis if bleeding is brisk (1–2 mL/min),[5] and treatment may be possible by embolization. An important lesion occurring in the upper gastrointestinal tract is the Dieulafoy malformation. These bleeding submucosal vessels occur in the stomach without overlying ulceration. They can result in massive bleeding and may retract, making them difficult to identify on endoscopy.[2]

Although ingestion of foreign bodies is a common event in pediatrics, rarely this can result in upper gastrointestinal bleeding. Young children in particular may not provide a history of ingestion; thus, a high level of suspicion is required in patients with a history of choking, unexplained coughing, dysphagia, or food refusal. Some objects may be visible on plain film, but most patients with suspected ingested foreign body and gastrointestinal bleeding will require further investigations including CT scan or endoscopy for diagnosis. (See Chapter 74 for a detailed discussion of gastrointestinal foreign bodies.)

► LOWER GASTROINTESTINAL BLEEDING

Lower gastrointestinal bleeding can occur anywhere from the ligament of Treitz to the anus and varies by age (Table 72–2). Although lower gastrointestinal bleeding is a common complaint, encompassing 0.3% of pediatric emergency department visits, most causes are relatively benign and self-limited.[1] The actual bleeding source, however, can occasionally be difficult to identify. Lower gastrointestinal bleeding can present as melena or hematochezia. Melena typically indicates a more proximal source and occurs when blood has been present in the gastrointestinal tract for a prolonged period of time, resulting in breakdown of hemoglobin.[13] Small volume hematochezia

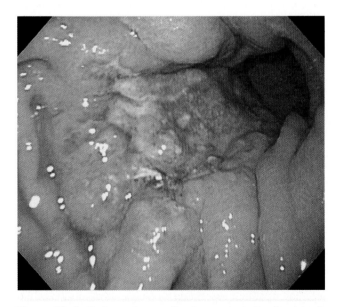

Figure 72–2. Deep crater peptic ulcer seen in the fundus of the stomach on endoscopy. (Photo courtesy of Dr. Brian Riedel, Pediatric Gastroenterology, Vanderbilt University Medical Center.)

► TABLE 72–2. CAUSES OF LOWER GASTROINTESTINAL BLEEDING (BY AGE)

Age	Small Volume	Large Volume
Newborn	NEC Anal fissure Volvulus Duplication	Ingested maternal blood DIC AVM
Infant	Allergic colitis Enterocolitis Nodular lymphoid hyperplasia Duplication Intussusception Anal fissure Rectal prolapse	Meckel's diverticulum AVM
Child	IBD Hemorrhoid HSP Toxic megacolon Enterocolitis	Juvenile polyp Meckel's diverticulum AVM

is typically from the distal colon or anus, although large volume rectal bleeding can result from lesions any place along the gastrointestinal tract if bleeding is brisk. Lower gastrointestinal bleeding can occur in the small intestine, colon, rectum, or anus.

INTESTINE

A common cause of lower gastrointestinal bleeding is infectious enterocolitis. Enterocolitis occurs among children of all ages and can result in abdominal pain, fever, and bloody stools. Common pathogens implicated in bloody diarrhea include *Salmonella, Shigella, Campylobacter jejuni, Yersinia enterocolitica, Escherichia coli, Clostridium difficile,* and *Entamoeba histolytica.*[1] Although most enterocolitis is self-limited, rare complications such as hemolytic uremic syndrome can occur; thus, children with infectious enterocolitis and bloody diarrhea may require additional testing and close follow-up. Diagnosis is commonly made by stool culture or antigen testing. Many infections in otherwise healthy children do not require treatment, and in some cases, treatment with antimicrobials may worsen the clinical course. Treatment with appropriate antimicrobials is recommended, however, for patients with documented *Shigella, Campylobacter, C. difficile,* and *E. histolytica.*[14] Antimotility agents should generally be avoided.

Necrotizing enterocolitis (NEC) is a rare but serious cause of lower gastrointestinal bleeding in young infants. Although most often seen in the newborn intensive care unit, occasionally neonates may present to the emergency department. These infants often have a history of prematurity, significant anoxic stress at birth, or cyanotic congenital heart disease.[15,16] Infants with NEC typically appear ill, with lethargy, abdominal distension, vomiting, and bloody stools. Abdominal radiographs reveal distended loops of bowel and pneumatosis intestinalis. Treatment involves appropriate resuscitation, bowel rest, broad-spectrum antimicrobials, and early surgical consultation.[15]

Children with Hirschprung's disease can develop toxic megacolon and present acutely ill with abdominal distension, fever, explosive diarrhea, hematochezia, and abdominal pain. Toxic megacolon can be the presentation of Hirschprung's disease, but can also occur after surgical resection of the aganglionic segment, particularly in children with longer segment disease or Down syndrome.[17] Intestinal dilatation with air–fluid levels is often seen on plain abdominal x-ray, often with an intestinal cutoff sign (abrupt cutoff of intestinal distension at the pelvic brim, Fig. 72–3).[18] Treatment involves bowel decompression, hydration, and broad-spectrum antibiotics.[17]

Obstructive disorders of the intestine can also lead to lower gastrointestinal bleeding. Although typically small in volume, the bleeding associated with obstruction is typically secondary to tissue ischemia. The most common cause of bleeding from obstruction is intussusception. Intussusception most commonly occurs in children younger than 2 years. These children typically present with intermittent colicky abdominal pain and vomiting, although some children present with only generalized illness and malaise. Intussusception can occur anywhere within the bowel, but most commonly at the ileocecal junction. A sausage-shaped abdominal mass may be palpated in

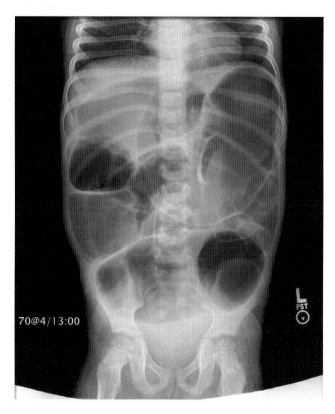

Figure 72–3. Intestinal cutoff sign seen in a child with toxic megacolon. This child had previously undergone resection of his aganglionic colon segment. Note the massive intestinal distension. (Photo courtesy of Dr. Thomas J. Abramo, Pediatric Emergency Medicine, Vanderbilt University Medical Center.)

the right lower quadrant or anywhere along the ascending or transverse colon, depending on the extent of bowel telescoping. Bleeding from an intussusception is described as "currant-jelly," and occurs late in the course, after bowel ischemia has occurred.[1] Abdominal radiographs may show a "target sign" or paucity of bowel gas in the right lower quadrant, but may also be normal.[15] Ultrasound is a common modality to diagnose intussusception. Air-contrast enema can be both diagnostic and therapeutic for intussusception, but complications such as failure to reduce the intussusception or bowel perforation can occur, and surgical consultation may be warranted.

Volvulus can also present with rectal bleeding from bowel ischemia. It is most common in neonates and typically presents with bilious vomiting, abdominal distension, and feeding problems. Abdominal radiographs may reveal a paucity of gas in the abdomen with a "double bubble sign," with foci of gas seen in the stomach and duodenum. An upper gastrointestinal contrast study is the diagnostic study of choice. Appropriate resuscitation, antimicrobials, and emergent surgical reduction of the volvulus are critical to preserve bowel viability. Duplication of the bowel can also result in bowel ischemia and bleeding from intussusception, volvulus, or expansion of the duplication.[1]

Otherwise asymptomatic bleeding of the small intestine can be due to lesions such as a Meckel's diverticulum or juvenile polyp. Meckel's diverticulum occurs when the

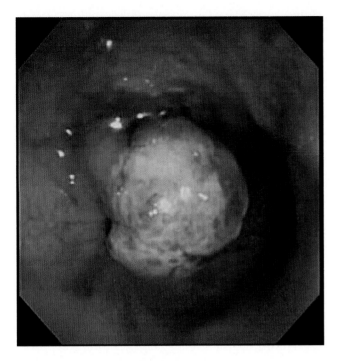

Figure 72–4. A 0.7-cm pedunculated polyp was identified in the sigmoid colon of a child presenting with painless rectal bleeding. (Photo courtesy of Dr. Brian Riedel, Pediatric Gastroenterology, Vanderbilt University Medical Center.)

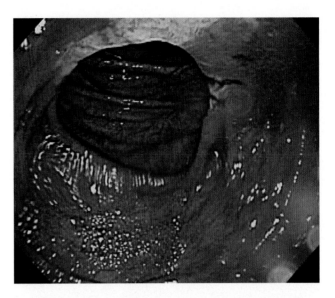

Figure 72–5. Edema, friability, and ulceration of colon seen on endoscopy in a child with ulcerative colitis. (Photo courtesy of Dr. Brian Riedel, Pediatric Gastroenterology, Vanderbilt University Medical Center.)

omphalomesenteric duct is incompletely obliterated early in fetal life. Two percent of the population has this 2-in long diverticulum within 2 ft. of the ileocecum.[1,19] If the diverticulum contains ectopic gastric mucosa, ulceration and massive bleeding can occur. Patients typically present before age 2 and are well-appearing with painless rectal bleeding. A radionuclide scan with technetium-99 m pertechnate is diagnostic.[1] This radioisotope binds preferentially to gastric mucosa. Treatment involves surgical consultation and resection. Meckel's diverticulum can also act as a lead point for intussusception.[19] Duplications of the small intestine can also contain ectopic gastric mucosa. Juvenile polyps are a common cause of gastrointestinal bleeding outside the neonatal period. Bleeding is typically painless, recurrent, and small in amount. Most polyps in children are solitary, benign, and occur within the left colon, often in the rectosigmoid region.[13] Diagnosis is typically made on endoscopy, which may also allow for excision if the polyp is small (Fig. 72–4).

Inflammatory disorders of the intestine are also a common cause of lower gastrointestinal bleeding. Infants most commonly have milk protein allergic colitis. These infants are well-appearing, but present with a history of bloody stools and occasionally vomiting or failure to thrive. Cow milk and soy milk are the most commonly implicated allergens, although in a significant number of infants the allergen is unknown.[20] Diagnostic testing is difficult, and most infants are diagnosed clinically and treated empirically by exclusion of any known allergens from the infant's or breast-feeding mother's diet.[20] Even with dietary modification, however, bloody stools can persist for weeks.[19]

Inflammatory bowel disease including ulcerative colitis and Crohn's disease commonly results in rectal bleeding (Fig. 72–5). Most common in adolescents, inflammatory bowel disease often mimics other causes of colitis, causing crampy abdominal pain, frequent bloody stools, tenesmus, and weight loss. While ulcerative colitis typically only involves the colon, Crohn's disease can involve any portion of the gastrointestinal tract. Laboratory evaluation may reveal anemia, thrombocytosis, and elevated ESR. Colonoscopy with biopsy is required for diagnosis in most cases.[22] Therapy involves anti-inflammatory and immunosuppressive medication and occasionally surgical intervention.

Henoch–Schönlein Purpura (HSP) is a common immune-mediated vasculitis, which can involve the entire gastrointestinal tract. Children with HSP often have gastrointestinal manifestations including abdominal pain, vomiting, and bloody stools or melena. Most commonly, bleeding is due to mucosal hemorrhage, but intussusception is also common among children with HSP. Diagnosis of HSP is made clinically, which can offer a challenge as gastrointestinal manifestations can precede the pathognomonic purpuric skin changes. Although there is no current consensus on treatment, administration of corticosteroids may ameliorate some gastrointestinal symptoms in HSP.[23]

Colonic lymphonodular hyperplasia from protein allergy or infection can result in asymptomatic, small volume bleeding. More common in infants and young children, these inflammatory patches may result in flecks or small amounts of blood mixed in the stool of otherwise asymptomatic children. Lymphonodular hyperplasia is typically diagnosed on colonoscopy and does not require any specific treatment[24] (Fig. 72–6).

RECTUM/ANUS

Benign lesions of the rectum and anus can also cause apparent lower gastrointestinal bleeding. The most common cause of rectal bleeding in infants is an anal fissure. These infants

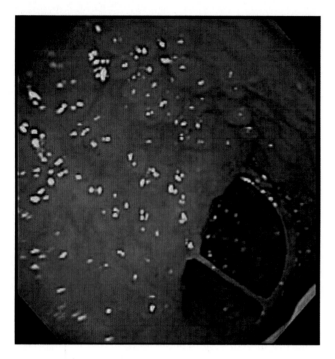

Figure 72–6. Diffuse lymphnodular hyperplasia is seen in this child undergoing colonoscopy for rectal bleeding. (Photo courtesy of Dr. Brian Riedel, Pediatric Gastroenterology, Vanderbilt University Medical Center.)

typically pass a painful, hard stool with bright red blood seen on the surface of the stool. Hemorrhoids are uncommon in young children but can occur in constipated adolescents. They result in painful defecation, often with the blood on the outside of the stool. Diagnosis is made on physical examination, and treatment involves dietary modifications or medications to soften the stool. Young children with constipation are also predisposed to rectal prolapse, which may result in scant rec-

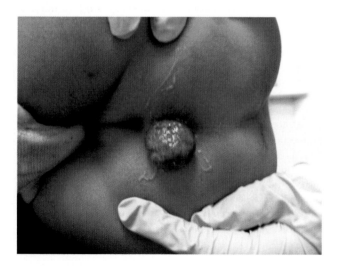

Figure 72–7. Rectal prolapse was seen on examination of this child presenting with rectal pain and bleeding. (Photo courtesy of Dr. Thomas J. Abramo, Pediatric Emergency Medicine, Vanderbilt University Medical Center.)

tal bleeding (Fig. 72–7). The prolapsed segment often self-reduces, and the diagnosis is made on history and physical examination alone. If a child presents with rectal prolapse, firm constant pressure will typically result in reduction, otherwise surgical consultation is necessary. Softening the stool will minimize recurrence. Trauma from sexual abuse may also present as rectal bleeding (see Chapter 145 for more details) (Fig. 72–7).

► CONCLUSIONS

Gastrointestinal bleeding is a common complaint in the pediatric emergency department and may result in considerable anxiety for families but is only rarely associated with significant morbidity or mortality. Although the etiology can sometimes be challenging to identify, close attention to the volume, timing, and color of the bleeding as well as other associated signs and symptoms will often point to a diagnosis.

REFERENCES

1. Leung AK, Wong AL. Lower gastrointestinal bleeding in children. *Pediatr Emerg Care.* 2002;18:319.
2. Burke SJ, Golzarian J, Weldon D, et al. Nonvariceal upper gastrointestinal bleeding. *Eur Radiol.* 2007;17:1714.
3. Gupta SK, Hassall E, Chiu YL, et al. Presenting symptoms of nonerosive and erosive esophagitis in pediatric patients. *Dig Dis Sci.* 2006;51:858.
4. Chawla S, Seth D, Mahajan P, et al. Upper gastrointestinal bleeding in children. *Clin Pediatr (Phila).* 2007;46:16.
5. Boyle JT. Gastrointestinal bleeding in infants and children. *Pediatr Rev.* 2008;29:39.
6. Esrailian E, Gralnek IM. Nonvariceal upper gastrointestinal bleeding: epidemiology and diagnosis. *Gastroenterol Clin North Am.* 2005;35:589.
7. Rodgers BM. Upper gastrointestinal hemorrhage. *Pediatr Rev.* 1999;20:171.
8. Molleston JP. Variceal bleeding in children. *J Pediatr Gastroenterol Nutr.* 2003;37:538.
9. Blecker U, Gold BD. Gastritis and peptic ulcer disease in childhood. *Eur J Pediatr.* 1999;158:541.
10. Sabbi T, De Angelis P, Colistro F, et al. Efficacy of noninvasive tests in the diagnosis of *Helicobacter pylori* infection in pediatric patients. *Arch Pediatr Adolesc Med.* 2005;159:238.
11. Olson AD, Fendrick AM, Deutsch D, et al. Evaluation of initial noninvasive therapy in pediatric patients presenting with suspected ulcer disease. *Gastrointest Endosc.* 1996;44:554.
12. Dubois J, Rypens F, Garel L, et al. Pediatric gastrointestinal vascular anomalies: imaging and therapeutic issues. *Pediatr Radiol.* 2007;37:566.
13. Lawrence WW, Wright JL. Causes of rectal bleeding in children. *Pediatr Rev.* 2001;22:394.
14. Pickering LK, Baker CJ, Long SS, et al. *Red Book: 2006 Report of the Committee on Infectious Diseases.* 27th ed. Elk Grove Village, IL: American Academy of Pediatrics; 2006.
15. McCollough M, Sharieff GQ. Abdominal surgical emergencies in infants and young children. *Emerg Med Clin North Am.* 2003;21:909.
16. Hostetler MA, Schulman M. Necrotizing enterocolitis presenting in the emergency department: case report and review of differential considerations for vomiting in the neonate. *J Emerg Med.* 2001;21:165.

17. Dasgupta R, Langer J. Evaluation and management of persistent problems after surgery for Hirschprung disease in a child. *J Pediatr Gastroenterol Nutr.* 2008;46:13.

18. Elhalaby EA, Coran AG, Blane CE, et al. Enterocolitis associated with Hirschprung's disease: a clinical-radiological characterization based on 168 patients. *J Pediatr Surg.* 1995;30:76.

19. Rodrigues F, Brandao N, Duque V, et al. Herpes simplex virus esophagitis in immunocompetent children. *J Pediatr Gastroenterol Nutr.* 2004;39:560.

20. Aryola T, Ruuska T, Keranen J, et al. Rectal bleeding in infancy: clinical, allergological, and microbiological examination. *Pediatrics.* 2006;117:e760.

21. Xanthakos SA, Schwimmer JB, Melin-Aldana H, et al. Prevalence and outcome of allergic colitis in healthy infants with rectal bleeding: a prospective cohort study. *J Pediatr Gastroenterol Nutr.* 2005;41:16.

22. Beattie RM, Croft NM, Fell JM, et al. Inflammatory bowel disease. *Arch Dis Child.* 2006;91:426.

23. Weiss PF, Feinstein JA, Luan X, et al. Effects of corticosteroid on Henoch-Schoenlein purpura: a systematic review. *Pediatrics.* 2007;120:1079.

24. Berezin S, Newman LJ. Lower gastrointestinal bleeding in infants owing to lymphonodular hyperplasia of the colon. *Pediatr Emerg Care.* 1987;3:164.

CHAPTER 73

Gastroesophageal Reflux

Jamie N. Deis and Thomas J. Abramo

▶ HIGH-YIELD FACTS

- Gastroesophageal reflux (GER) occurs in two thirds of normal infants for the first year of life.
- Symptomatic GER (GERD) in infants includes excessive crying, irritability, arching of back during feeds, sleep disturbance, and poor weight gain.
- Severe GERD may include aspiration pneumonia, and acute life-threatening events.
- Treatment for mild GERD includes smaller, more frequent feedings, thickened formula with cereal, and elevating the head of the crib; for severe cases, H2 receptor antagonists or proton pump inhibitors may be considered.
- Esophageal pH probe, intraluminal impedance monitoring, upper GI imaging, and endoscopy may be helpful in selected cases of GERD for defining cause and recognizing complications.
- Complications are most common in children with neurologic impairment and swallowing dysfunction.

Gastroesophageal reflux (GER) is the most common esophageal disorder in children of all ages[1] and a frequent reason for visits to the pediatric emergency department. It occurs when gastric contents pass into the esophagus through transient relaxations in the lower esophageal sphincter. While the pathophysiology of GER in infants, children, and adults is similar, the symptoms and clinical presentation can be quite different (Table 73–1).

▶ GASTROESOPHAGEAL REFLUX IN INFANTS

GER is nearly universal in infants, occurring in up to 67% of healthy, thriving infants by 4 to 5 months of age.[2] There are multiple factors that predispose infants to GER including immaturity of the esophagus and lower esophageal sphincter, incomplete propagation of esophageal contractions, short length of the abdominal esophagus, and liquid diet.[3,4]

CLINICAL PRESENTATION OF GER IN INFANTS

The great majority of infants with physiologic reflux are "happy spitters." These infants typically regurgitate small volumes of breast milk or formula after feedings but are relatively unaffected by it. They gain weight appropriately and typically "out-

grow" their symptoms by 12 months of age as esophageal and gastric motility mature.[2]

A small number of infants will develop complications of reflux, referred to as gastroesophageal reflux disease (GERD). Infants with GERD may present with excessive crying, irritability, arching, sleep disturbance, feeding aversion, and poor weight gain.[5,6] Excessive crying and arching typically occur during or shortly after feeds when gastric acid enters the esophagus and causes discomfort. These stereotypic stretching and arching movements can be mistaken for seizures in a condition known as Sandifer syndrome. Over time, infants with severe symptoms may develop an aversion to feeding and failure to thrive.

GER may induce respiratory symptoms in infants including chronic cough, stridor, and wheezing. In severe cases, aspiration pneumonia may occur. Reflux in infants may also manifest as an acute life-threatening event (ALTE) with cyanosis and respiratory distress. This occurs when reflux causes laryngospasm and bronchospasm.

DIFFERENTIAL DIAGNOSIS OF GER IN INFANTS

The main challenge in evaluating infants with symptoms of reflux is distinguishing reflux from true vomiting. Reflux typically occurs when infants "burp" during or shortly after feeds and does not involve forceful muscle contraction. Vomiting occurs when stomach contents are forcefully expelled into the esophagus and out of the mouth by contractions of the abdominal and chest wall muscles. While this distinction can be difficult in infants, vomiting should prompt consideration of other diagnoses including milk protein allergy, food allergy, esophageal web, hiatal hernia, pyloric stenosis (Fig. 73–1), intestinal

▶ TABLE 73–1. **COMMON SYMPTOMS OF GASTROESOPHAGEAL REFLUX**

Infants	Older Children and Adolescents
Regurgitation	Abdominal pain
Feeding aversion	Heartburn
Excessive crying	Chest pain
Irritability	Dysphagia
Arching	Chronic cough
Sleep disturbance	Wheezing
Cough, wheezing, stridor	Sinusitis
Apnea or ALTE	

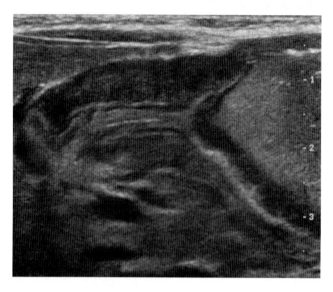

Figure 73–1. Abdominal ultrasound image in a 2-month old infant with vomiting shows thickened pyloric muscle consistent with pyloric stenosis. (Courtesy of Herman Kan, MD.)

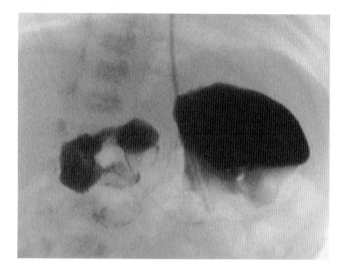

Figure 73–2. Upper gastrointestinal series in an infant with vomiting shows characteristic "corkscrew sign" indicating malrotation with midgut volvulus. (Courtesy of Herman Kan, MD.)

obstruction, infection, inborn errors of metabolism, and increased intracranial pressure (Table 73–2).

EVALUATION OF GER IN INFANTS

The majority of cases of infantile GER can be diagnosed by history and physical examination alone. Extensive workup in the emergency department is not generally indicated unless an anatomic or metabolic abnormality is suspected. The upper gastrointestinal series (UGI) is nonspecific for GER but can identify anatomic abnormalities including vascular rings, esophageal and intestinal webs, strictures, hiatal hernia, pyloric stenosis, and malrotation (Fig. 73–2). If indicated, esophageal pH probe monitoring and upper endoscopy can be performed in the outpatient setting.

▶ **TABLE 73–2. DIFFERENTIAL DIAGNOSIS OF VOMITING IN INFANTS**

Obstruction	Neurologic
Pyloric stenosis	Hydrocephalus
Esophageal web	Subdural hematoma
Duodenal web/atresia	
Malrotation	
Intussusception	
Infection	Allergic
Sepsis	Milk protein allergy
Urinary tract infection	Food allergy
Meningitis	
Otitis media	
Toxic/metabolic	Other
Inborn errors of metabolism	Overfeeding
Urea cycle defects	Post-tussive emesis
Lead poisoning	

TREATMENT OF GER IN INFANTS

Conservative Therapy

Conservative therapy is the treatment of choice for mild infantile reflux. Simple alterations in the feeding routine such as smaller volume feeds, frequent burping, and prone positioning at 45 to 60 degrees after feeds may reduce the frequency of reflux. Thickening feeds with cereal may also reduce the number of reflux events and increase the infant's relative sleep time.[7]

Acid Suppression

If symptoms persist despite these measures, a trial of acid suppression with an H2 receptor antagonist may be warranted. H2 receptor antagonists, such as famotidine and ranitidine, are recommended as first-line pharmacologic therapy for infants because of their excellent safety profile.[1] Proton pump inhibitors (PPIs) are highly effective antireflux medications that decrease gastric acid secretion by inhibiting the H^+K^+-ATPase pump. Because of their superior efficacy, PPIs are now the mainstay of treatment in GER in older children and adults.[8] While PPIs have been used to treat refractory GER in infants, there are limited studies in this patient population. None of the PPIs are currently FDA approved for use in children younger than 1 year.[9]

Prokinetic Agents

Prokinetic agents such as domperidone and metoclopramide have been used to treat infantile GER, but use of prokinetic agents has declined in recent years. This class of medications is associated with an increased risk of side effects including dystonic reactions, and there is no convincing evidence that prokinetic agents have any clinical benefit in the treatment of childhood GERD.[10–12]

► GER IN CHILDREN AND ADOLESCENTS

CLINICAL PRESENTATION

The prevalence of GER in children aged 3 to 18 years ranges from 1.8% to 22%.[13] In older children, GER may present with epigastric abdominal pain, heartburn, noncardiac chest pain, dysphagia, and vomiting. Older children may also have extraesophageal symptoms including chronic cough, recurrent otitis media, sinusitis, laryngitis, and stridor.[8,14] In children with asthma, GER may precipitate bronchospasm and wheezing.

DIFFERENTIAL DIAGNOSIS OF GER IN CHILDREN AND ADOLESCENTS

Diagnoses to consider in the older child with chronic vomiting include increased intracranial pressure, rumination, bulimia, and intestinal obstruction. The differential for children with epigastric pain and dysphagia should also include peptic ulcer disease, achalasia, infectious esophagitis, pill esophagitis, and eosinophilic esophagitis (EE).

Eosinophilic Esophagitis

EE is now increasingly recognized as a common cause of dysphagia, abdominal pain, and vomiting in children and adolescents. Children with EE have high levels of eosinophils in their esophagus as part of an allergic response to food antigens.[15] Many of the symptoms of EE mimic those of GER. However, the common medications used to treat reflux are generally not effective against EE. While many patients with EE will have a strong medical history of allergic symptoms, the diagnosis can only be made by endoscopy with biopsy.[15]

EVALUATION OF GER IN CHILDREN AND ADOLESCENTS

As with infants, the majority of cases of GER in older children can be diagnosed by history and physical examination alone. In typical GER, an empiric trial of acid suppression may be the most simple and definitive test. GER symptoms usually respond to treatment with proton pump inhibitors within 1 to 2 weeks.[8] When anatomic abnormalities are suspected, an upper gastrointestinal series (UGI) may be helpful. Additional testing, including esophageal pH monitoring and upper endoscopy, can usually be performed on an outpatient basis.

Esophageal pH probe monitoring measures the duration and frequency of acid reflux episodes, but the results are subject to a number of technical factors including the type and number of probes used, the position of the probe in the esophagus, and the duration of the study.[16,17] Patient variables such as diet, activity level, and position can also affect the

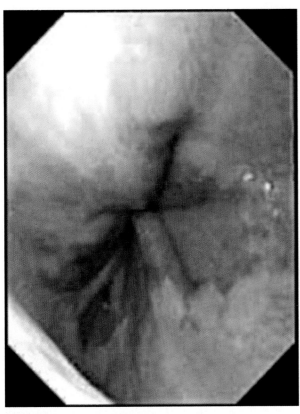

A

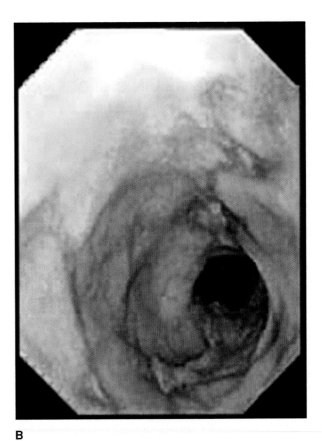

B

Figure 73–3. Endoscopic appearance of reflux esophagitis. (**A**) Esophageal erythema and erosions. (**B**) Severe erosive disease. Source: McPhee SJ, Papadakis MA, Tierney Jr, LM: *Current Medical Diagnosis & Treatment* 2008, 47th Edition: http://www.accessmedicine.com.

▶ **TABLE 73–3. COMPLICATIONS OF GASTROESOPHAGEAL REFLUX**

Esophageal Complications	Pulmonary Complications	ENT Complications
Erosive esophagitis	Apnea or ALTE	Sinusitis
Esophageal stricture	Chronic cough	Otitis media
Barrett's esophagus	Asthma	Laryngitis
Adenocarcinoma	Aspiration pneumonia	Dental erosions

results.[16,17] Intraluminal impedance monitoring, which is based on the concept that passage of a bolus changes impedance between esophageal segments, may complement esophageal pH monitoring by measuring nonacid reflux episodes. To date, however, there is an absence of literature demonstrating improved clinical outcome with the use of impedance tracing.[18] Upper endoscopy is the test of choice to document evidence of mucosal injury and esophagitis (Fig. 73–3). Endoscopy can also help identify complications of longstanding reflux including esophageal strictures and Barrett's esophagus (premalignant metaplasia).

COMPLICATIONS OF GERD

Children with reflux may develop both esophageal and extraesophageal complications of GERD (Table 73–3). Complications are most common in children with neurologic impairment and swallowing dysfunction. Additional risk factors include prematurity, history of esophageal atresia, obesity, and strong family history of severe reflux.[14]

TREATMENT OF GER IN CHILDREN AND ADOLESCENTS

The goals of treatment in pediatric GER are elimination of symptoms, mucosal healing, prevention of complications, and maintenance of remission.[1,8] Treatment options include conservative therapy with lifestyle modifications, pharmacologic therapy with acid suppression, and surgical management.

Conservative Therapy

Dietary and lifestyle modifications may help reduce the symptoms of GER in older children and adolescents. Weight loss along with simple dietary changes, such as avoidance of chocolate, fatty foods, and citrus fruits may reduce the frequency of reflux. Nocturnal symptoms of reflux may be reduced by elevating of the head of the bed or sleeping in the left lateral decubitus position.[19]

Pharmacologic Therapy

In children with mild or infrequent symptoms of GER, antacids and H2 receptor antagonists may be sufficient for treating symptoms. H2 receptor antagonists are considered first-line therapy for young children with GER due to their excellent safety profile, but PPIs are quickly becoming the mainstay of pharmacologic management of GER in older children and adolescents. The PPIs are highly effective antireflux medica-

tions that decrease gastric acid secretion by inhibiting the H^+K^+-ATPase pump. Numerous randomized control trials have shown that PPIs are superior to H2 receptor antagonists in healing esophagitis and maintaining remission in adults.[20,21] Although no placebo-controlled studies have been performed in children, multiple case series have shown symptomatic and endoscopic improvement with PPIs in children.[22–24] Only two PPIs are currently approved for use in children, omeprazole and lansoprazole.[25]

Surgical Therapy

Antireflux surgery may be required in children with severe GERD who fail medical management and develop complications of reflux including severe esophagitis, strictures, and recurrent aspiration pneumonia. The most common antireflux surgical procedure is the fundoplication in which the fundus of the stomach is either partially or completely wrapped around the esophagus just above the gastroesophageal junction. Complications can occur after antireflux surgery. If the wrap is too loose, symptoms may persist. If the wrap is too tight, new symptoms such as excessive gas and abdominal bloating may occur.

▶ SUMMARY

Gastroesophageal reflux is common in children of all ages. Most infants with physiologic reflux can be successfully managed with conservative measures alone, and the majority will have resolution of symptoms by 12 months of age. Further evaluation is indicated when the diagnosis is uncertain and when reflux-related complications occur. In older children with reflux, specific diagnostic tests are selected based on the clinical concern in each child. Current treatment options include conservative therapy with lifestyle modifications, medical therapy with acid-suppressing medications, and antireflux surgery. Children with severe, chronic reflux may develop both esophageal and extraesophageal complications.

REFERENCES

1. Chawla S, Seth D, Mahajan P, et al. Gastroesophageal reflux disorder: a review for primary care providers. *Clin Pediatr.* 2006;45:7–13.
2. Nelson SP, Chen EH, Syniar GM, et al. Prevalence of symptoms of gastroesophageal reflux during infancy: a pediatric practice-based survey: Pediatric Practice Research Group. *Arch Pediatr Adolesc Med.* 1997;151:569–572.
3. Vandenplas Y, Hassall E. Mechanisms of gastroesophageal reflux and gastroesophageal reflux disease. *J Pediatr Gastroenterol Nutr.* 2002;35(2):119–136.

4. Omari TI, Miki K, Fraser R, et al. Esophageal body and lower esophageal sphincter function in healthy premature infants. *Gastroenterology.* 1995;109(6):1757–1764.

5. Feranchak AP, Orenstein SR, Cohn JF. Behaviors associated with onset of gastroesophageal reflux episodes in infants. Prospective study using splitscreen video and pH probe. *Clin Pediatr.* 1994;33(11):654–662.

6. Hart JJ. Pediatric gastroesophageal reflux. *Am Fam Physician.* 1996;54(8):2463–2472.

7. Orenstein SR, Magill HL, Brooks P. Thickening of infant feedings for therapy of gastroesophageal reflux. *J Pediatr.* 1987;110(2):181–186.

8. Richter JE. The many manifestations of gastroesophageal reflux disease: presentation, evaluation, and treatment. *Gastroenterol Clin North Am.* 2007;36:577–599.

9. Barron JJ. Proton pump inhibitor utilization patterns in infants. *J Pediatr Gastroenterol Nutr.* 2007;45(4):421–427.

10. Di Lorenzo C. Gastroesophageal reflux: not a time to "relax." *J Pediatr.* 2006;149(4):436–438.

11. Rudolph CD, Mazur LJ, Liptak GS, et al. Guidelines for evaluation and treatment of gastroesophageal reflux in infants and children: recommendations of the North American Society for Pediatric Gastroenterology and Nutrition. *J Pediatr Gastroenterol Nutr.* 2001;32(suppl 2):S1–S31.

12. Hibbs AM, Lorch SA. Metoclopramide for the treatment of gastroesophageal reflux disease in infants: a systematic review. *Pediatrics.* 2006;118(2):746–752.

13. Nelson SP, Chen EH, Syniar GM, et al. Prevalence of symptoms of gastroesophageal reflux during childhood: a pediatric practice-based survey. *Arch Pediatr Adolesc Med.* 2000;54:150–154.

14. Michail S. Gastroesophageal reflux. *Pediatr Rev.* 2007;28:101–110.

15. Liacouras CA, Ruchelli E. Eosinophilic esophagitis. *Curr Opin Pediatr.* 2004;16:560–566.

16. Vandenplas Y, Franckx-Goossens A, Pipeleers-Marichal M, et al. Area under pH 4: advantages of a new parameter in the interpretation of esophageal pH monitoring data in infants. *J Pediatr Gastroenterol Nutr.* 1989;9(1):34–39.

17. Friesen CA, Hayes R, Hodge C, et al. Comparison of methods of assessing 24-hour intraesophageal pH recordings in children. *J Pediatr Gastroenterol Nutr.* 1992;14:252–255.

18. Vandenplas Y, Salvatore S, Vieira MC, et al. Will esophageal impedance replace pH monitoring? *Pediatrics.* 2007;119(1):118–122.

19. Kaltenbach T, Crockett S, Gerson LB. Are lifestyle measures effective in patients with gastroesophageal reflux disease? An evidence-based approach. *Arch Intern Med.* 2006;166:965–971.

20. Van Pinxteren B, Numans ME, Bonis PA, et al. Short term treatment with proton pump inhibitors, H2RAs and prokinetics for gastro-oesophageal reflux disease-like symptoms and endoscopy negative reflux disease. *Cochrane Database Syst Rev.* 2004;3:CD002095.

21. Donnellan C, Sharma N, Preston C, et al. Medical treatments for the maintenance therapy of reflux oesophagitis and endoscopic negative reflux disease. *Cochrane Database Syst Rev.* 2004;3:CD003245.

22. Gunasekaran S, Hassall E. Efficacy and safety of omeprazole for severe gastroesophageal reflux in children. *J Pediatr.* 1993;123:148–154.

23. Israel DM, Hassall E. Omeprazole and other proton pump inhibitors: pharmacology, efficacy and safety, with special reference to use in children. *J Pediatr Gastroenterol Nutr.* 1998;27:568–579.

24. Hassall E, Israel DM, Shepherd R; and the International Pediatric Omeprazole Study Group. Omeprazole for treatment of chronic erosive esophagitis in children: a multicenter study of efficacy, safety, tolerability and dose requirements. *J Pediatr.* 2000;137:800–807.

25. Hassall E. Decisions in diagnosing and managing chronic gastroesophageal reflux disease in children. *J Pediatr.* 2005;146:S3–S12.

CHAPTER 74

Gastrointestinal Foreign Bodies

Philip H. Ewing

► HIGH-YIELD FACTS

- Handheld metal detectors may allow rapid localization of metallic foreign bodies without further imaging.
- A coin that has passed the thoracic inlet of the esophagus can be observed and will usually pass through the gastrointestinal (GI) tract without problems.
- Sharp objects that pass the pylorus should be treated conservatively, but carefully observed for signs of obstruction.
- Lead containing objects must get past the acid medium of the stomach to avoid leaching of lead and absorption.
- Multiple ingested magnets must be retrieved.
- Watchful waiting is acceptable in most cases of foreign body ingestion.

Foreign bodies are a common cause of pediatric emergency department (ED) visits. Objects lodged in the upper esophagus can be a threat to airway patency and require prompt removal under controlled conditions, whenever possible. Many, if not most, objects do not cause symptoms and pass uneventfully through the GI tract. Some foreign bodies become impacted, typically in anatomical sites that are narrow or tortuous. Some of these impaction sites are amenable to procedural removal, while others may require surgical intervention.

► ETIOLOGY

Exploration of the environment is the hallmark of early childhood development. Learning about the environment involves cataloging objects by their sight, smell, sound, touch, and taste. From nearly the moment that infants begin to grasp objects, they are at risk of ingesting a foreign body. Small colorful objects can be particularly problematic, so we are alerted to the choking hazards of toys and products that have small parts. Developmentally inappropriate foods can also cause problems. A hot dog or nuts offered to a child who does not have molars to grind and process the food can cause choking and aspiration. Older children develop more complex behaviors and will hide objects within close reach. Foreign bodies that are squirreled away in the mouth can be swallowed nonintentionally when a child is distracted or startled. Toddlers may insert an object into other body orifices during the process of body exploration.

According to the American Association of Poison Control Centers Toxic Exposure Surveillance System, in excess of 92 000 pediatric foreign body ingestions occurred in 2003.[1] A number of ingestions will go unnoticed and many will not be reported to poison control, so it is difficult to translate this statistic into a number of ED visits. Nevertheless, it is clear that the health care burden for managing ingested foreign bodies is high. Fortunately, morbidity and mortality are the exception, especially when objects threatening the airway are excluded. Most objects will travel through the GI tract without incident. Those that cause symptoms are likely to do so because of the location in which they are impacted.

ANATOMIC SITES FOR OBSTRUCTION

Three frequent sites of impaction are in the esophagus. The first major site is at the thoracic inlet, which is the first narrowing of the GI tract. In general, symptoms may include a vague discomfort of the throat and chest, drooling, and coughing with gagging. When pulmonary complaints are associated with foreign body ingestion, it is important to consider both aspiration and tracheal obstruction from impingement on the trachea by esophageal foreign bodies. Figure 74–1 demonstrates an example of how an esophageal foreign body can cause airway obstruction requiring emergent removal in the ED. The next anatomical esophageal narrowing occurs at the area where the aorta traverses the esophagus. Secondary pulmonary symptoms in this region are much less likely. Objects impacted at the last esophageal narrowing, the gastroesophageal junction, are likely to complain of chest and abdominal discomfort.

Objects that have passed into the stomach are likely to pass through the rest of the GI tract without incident. An exception is gastric bezoars that are composed of conglomerations of substances that are difficult for the stomach to digest, for example, milk, hair, and pill fragments (iron, aspirin). The pylorus and the tortuous curves of the duodenum are another sites of impaction, especially for longer or sharp objects. Impaction is likely to cause localized pain. Once a foreign body has passed into the duodenum, it is probably not accessible by procedural methods, e.g., endoscopy, and surgical intervention becomes the only option for symptomatic foreign bodies until they pass through the ileocecal junction. The ileocecal junction is the last narrowing of the small intestine and is a common place for impaction of difficult to digest foods, such as seeds and nuts. The large diameter of the colon allows for rapid passage of foreign bodies, although turns at the hepatic flexure, splenic flexure, and rectocolonic juncture can cause problems. The last obstacle is the anal sphincter (Table 74–1).

The history surrounding the ingestion is important for defining the risk and designing a plan of care. The most important aspects of the ingestion are the child's symptoms, the

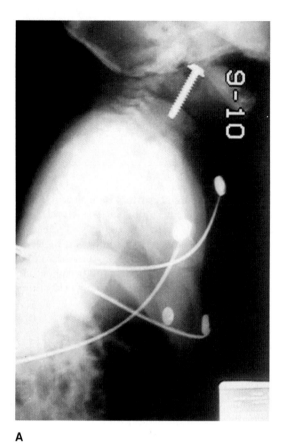

A

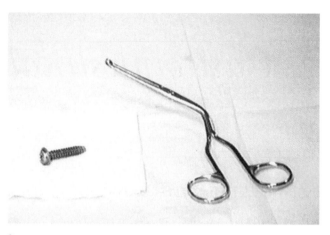

B

Figure 74–1. (**A**) Ingested screw trapped at the thoracic inlet, causing airway obstruction. (**B**) Screw removed with McGill forceps.

nature of the object, the time of ingestion, and the child's past medical history. First, ensure that the child's airway is not in danger of obstruction. Presenting symptoms can be helpful in estimating the location of the object. The nature of the object itself is important to determine the likelihood of passage, the risk of toxicity to the tissues, and the likelihood of tissue reaction to the object. In general, objects that are smaller than 5 cm are likely to navigate the GI tract without obstruction.[2] This includes a swallowed coin, the most common ingested foreign body. If a coin requires endoscopic removal, it will usually be trapped at the thoracic inlet (Fig. 74–2). This rule of thumb may not hold true for multiple ingested items, which have an increased propensity for impaction. The procedures to remove the objects become more difficult technically when there is more than one object present.[3]

Multiple magnets are particularly problematic. Magnets in different parts of the bowel may attract one another and trap

▶ **TABLE 74–1. CONDITIONS INCREASING THE RISK OF ESOPHAGEAL OBSTRUCTION**

Esophageal atresia/tracheoesophageal fistula

Esophageal stricture
  Congenital esophageal stenosis
  Esophageal web
  Previous esophageal injury—button battery erosion, caustic ingestion

Cancer requiring radiation therapy to the head and neck

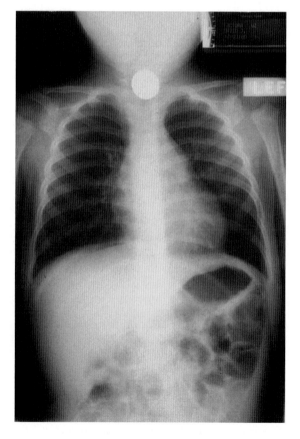

Figure 74–2. Coin at thoracic inlet.

► **TABLE 74-2. ESOPHAGEAL COINS**

Segment	Pulmonary Symptoms	GI Symptoms	Likelihood of Initial Location (%)	Likelihood of Passage (%)
Proximal	±	+	60–80	14
Middle	–	+	5–20	43
Distal	–	+	10–20	67

The esophageal segment refers to coins lodged above the thoracic inlet (proximal), above the aortic arch (middle), and above the gastroesophageal sphincter (distal). Pulmonary symptoms: respiratory distress, stridor, and cough. GI symptoms: drooling, pain, and dysphagia.[2,9]

the tissues from the bowel wall in between, causing irritation, ischemia, and erosion through the bowel wall.[4] This could lead to peritonitis, sepsis, or obstruction. Another consideration is whether a foreign body will cause a reaction with the tissues in the GI tract. As an example, button batteries have been shown to cause erosion through the esophageal wall if they become lodged in one location resulting in tissue erosion, perforation, and mediastinitis. These effects are not seen if the battery travels through the GI tract unimpeded. As a rule, button batteries that are lodged in any one location of the GI tract should be referred for prompt endoscopic removal. Table 74-1 reviews conditions increasing the risk of esophageal abnormality.[2,5]

► DIAGNOSIS

Radiographic imaging, ultrasonography, and metal detectors can be useful in determining the location of an object. Unfortunately, not all objects are amenable to these techniques; radiolucent and nonmetallic foreign bodies can be very difficult to localize. A metal detector may be useful to pinpoint the location of ingested metallic foreign bodies and can track their movement through the GI tract.[6] Usually metal detectors are used as a screening tool to identify the child that may require diagnostic imaging. Studies have proven that this technique is a viable and effective method for the use in the ED and may reduce the need for further imaging.

Symptoms should drive the requests for imaging. Patients with esophageal pain and secondary airway symptoms require imaging of the soft tissues of the neck and chest. A chest radiograph to include the upper abdomen may suffice for a child with only throat or epigastric discomfort. Occasionally, a barium swallow may be helpful to help locate a nonradiopaque object that is causing chest or epigastric discomfort. Poorly imaged by radiographs, cartilaginous fishbones that are lodged in the esophagus may be easier to visualize as a filling defect on a barium swallow. The most common place for small fishbones to lodge is in the friable tonsillar tissues. As a child swallows fish with small bones, the tonsils act as a sieve trapping the bones. Using a tongue blade and forceps the caregiver can remove these bones and resolve symptoms.

► THERAPEUTIC OPTIONS

The management of swallowed foreign bodies that pass the thoracic inlet is conservative for the vast majority of patients.

Table 74-2 reviews the natural history of foreign bodies lodged in the esophagus, the most common sites of obstruction, and the likelihood of spontaneous passage.[2,7] Coins lodged at the thoracic inlet should be retrieved. Coins at the middle or distal esophagus can be observed at home, 24 hours for spontaneous passage. An asymptomatic object should be left to pass through the GI tract at its own pace. This "watchful waiting" approach has been documented to be safe, although it is important to provide the caregivers with detailed discharge instructions describing signs and symptoms of intestinal obstruction. Sharp objects should always be retrieved if they are trapped in the esophagus (Fig. 74–3) or stomach. If a sharp object passes through the pylorus, it will probably continue through the GI tract without incident. Very close monitoring for symptoms should be arranged. Objects can be expected to pass in the stool in days to weeks.

Essentially, there is no human data to support the use of medical adjuncts to aid the passage of foreign body through the gastrointestinal tract. Only procedural approaches have demonstrated utility. Glucagon has been shown to decrease

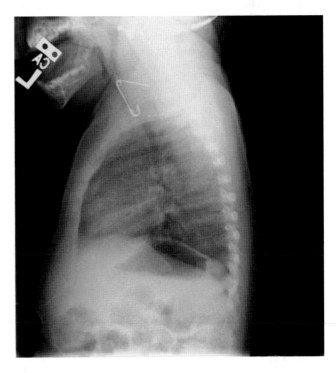

Figure 74–3. Open safety pin caught in upper esophagus.

esophageal smooth muscle tone. In theory, decreased tone would prevent an object from becoming impacted and would allow for more effective peristalsis. However, data has demonstrated that glucagon decreased passage of coins when compared to placebo.[8] 5-HT agonists have been proposed as well; their effects are increased peristalsis and decreased gastric emptying. Human studies of the 5-HT agonists used in the presence of an esophageal coin have not been performed. Some physicians have advocated the use of cathartics to promote clearance of a foreign body that has reached the stomach. No data demonstrate the efficacy of this approach. Furthermore, it can be argued that the side effects produced by cathartics and stool softeners may mimic the symptoms of intestinal obstruction. This intervention may complicate the watchful waiting approach that is effective in the vast majority of cases of the swallowed foreign body. For the rare occurrence of lead foreign bodies trapped in the stomach, protein pump inhibitors may be considered to reduce acid while arranging endoscopic removal.

► PROCEDURAL/SURGICAL APPROACHES

Procedural removal of an esophageal or gastric foreign body usually requires admission and a trip to the operating room for endoscopy. A number of procedures for the removal of ingested objects trapped in the esophagus have been described. Blind procedures using a foley catheter to retrieve objects at the thoracic inlet, or bougienage to advance a foreign body in the middle or lower esophagus have been described. However, these options do not allow direct or indirect visualization of the object and may increase risk of mechanical injury to the esophagus and its complications. Fluoroscopy allows the practitioner the luxury of visualization of radiopaque foreign bodies during the procedure. One technique employing fluoroscopy and endoscopic forceps has demonstrated effectiveness in a small study where the mean subject age was 34 months.[9] None of these approaches are easily performed in a child who cannot cooperate with the provider. As a result, many younger patients should be referred to a specialist capable of endoscopy for removal under sedation or anesthesia.

► SMALL BOWEL

Foreign bodies that are lodged in the small bowel are uncommon. While asymptomatic radiopaque objects may be located using metal detectors or radiographs, those patients that are significantly symptomatic should have foreign bodies removed by a surgeon. Another class of small intestinal foreign bodies that deserves discussion is the drug packet that has been either "stuffed" in an attempt to hide evidence from law enforcement or "packed" during an attempt to smuggle a drug across borders. Interestingly, the "stuffed" drug packet is the most likely to leak or rupture, as it was not intended to protect the contents

during passage through the gut; however, the ingested amount is usually small—not as likely to be toxic. The same cannot be said for packers who may be carrying a lethal amount of drug in very secure packaging. Whole bowel irrigation and activated charcoal should be considered for both subsets of patients to ensure that the ingested drugs are not absorbed.[10] Further therapy should be directed at the symptoms that develop should a package rupture.

► COLONIC/RECTAL FOREIGN BODIES

In the pediatric population, lower gastrointestinal foreign bodies are significantly less common than foreign bodies in any other part of the intestine. Nevertheless, the rectal foreign body may occur, as there is no limit to where a child may place a foreign object. An object that can be visualized can be removed with gentle traction. A surgeon should remove impacted objects that do not release with traction or those that cannot be visualized.

REFERENCES

1. Watson WA, Litovitz TL, Klein-Schwartz W, et al. 2003 Annual report of the American Association of Poison Control Centers Toxic Exposure Surveillance System. *Am J Emerg Med.* 2004;22:335–404.
2. Schunk JE. Foreign body—ingestion/aspiration. In: Fleisher GR, Ludwig S, Henretig FM, et al. *Textbook of Pediatric Emergency Medicine.* Philadelphia, PA: Lippincott Williams & Wilkins; 2006:307–314.
3. Jona JZ, Glicklich M, Cohen RD. The contraindications for blind esophageal bougienage for coin ingestion in children. *J Pediatr Surg.* 1988;23:328–330.
4. Centers for Disease Control and Prevention. Gastrointestinal Injuries from Magnet Ingestion in Children—United States, 2003–2006. http://www. cdc.gov/mmwr/preview/mmwrhtml/mm5548a3.htm Bethesda, MD: Centers for Disease Control and Prevention; 2007.
5. Cox JA, Rudolph CD. Anatomic disorders of the esophagus. In: Rudolph CD, Rudolph AM, Hostetter, et al. *Rudolph's Pediatrics.* New York, NY: McGraw-Hill; 2003:1385–1387.
6. Lee JB, Ahmad S, Gale CP. Detection of coins ingested by children using a handheld metal detector: a systematic review. *Emerg Med J.* 2005;22:838–854.
7. Mehta D, Attia M Quintana E, et al. Glucagon use for esophageal coin dislodgement in children: a prospective, double-blind, placebo controlled trial. *Acad Emerg Med.* 2001;8:200–203.
8. Gauderer MW, DeCou JM, Abrams RS, et al. The 'penny pincher': a new technique for fast and safe removal of esophageal coins. *J Pediatr Surg.* 2000;35:276–278.
9. Waltzman ML. Management of esophageal coins. *Pediatr Emerg Care.* 2006;22:367–371.
10. Osterhoudt KC, Burns EM, Shannon M, et al. Toxicologic emergencies. In: Fleisher GR, Ludwig S, Henretig FM, et al. *Textbook of Pediatric Emergency Medicine.* Philadelphia, PA: Lippincott Williams & Wilkins; 2006:951–1007.

CHAPTER 75

Liver and Gallbladder

Ashley Kumar and Susan M. Scott

▶ HIGH-YIELD FACTS

- Jaundice within the first 24 hours of life is NEVER normal.
- Urinary tract infections can be associated with the onset of unconjugated hyperbilirubinemia after a week of age.
- Conjugated hyperbilirubinemia is never normal at any age and mandates consultation with a pediatric gastroenterologist.
- The treatment of breast milk jaundice is not the cessation of breast-feeding.
- Consider exchange transfusion if levels >20 mg/dL.
- Consider hemolytic disease with unconjugated hyperbilirubinemia beyond the neonatal period.
- Postexposure prophylaxis is available for some types of hepatitis.
- RUQ pain can be an important clue to the recognition and diagnosis of hepatic dysfunction.
- Normal serum liver transaminases do not rule out liver failure.
- Always think of biliary atresia in an infant younger than 2 months with direct hyperbilirubinemia.
- Acute cholangitis should be suspected in any patient with fever and jaundice who has had surgical correction of biliary atresia.
- Think of choledochal cyst when presented with a patient with history of recurrent jaundice.
- Cholesterol stones account for up to 90% of gallstones in adolescents.
- Gallbladder hydrops does not occur in isolation; look for the underlying cause.

▶ HYPERBILIRUBINEMIA

Hemoglobin is released from red blood cells, broken down into heme, and ultimately reduced to unconjugated bilirubin, which is then bound to serum albumin. Unconjugated (indirect) bilirubin is converted into conjugated (direct) bilirubin in the liver and stored in the gallbladder. Bile is released into the intestines to assist in digestion and cholesterol metabolism as well as absorption of lipids and fat-soluble vitamins. Hyperbilirubinemia indicates either increased production of or impaired excretion of bilirubin and is the result of numerous etiologies, some pathologic and some physiologic. Increased red blood cell destruction may lead to unconjugated hyperbilirubinemia. Impairment of bile secretion from the liver or excretion from the gallbladder may lead to conjugated hyperbilirubinemia.

The patient's age and the type of hyperbilirubinemia, whether direct or indirect, are important factors in determining the cause and treatment. Hyperbilirubinemia within the first day of life is never normal and can be concerning within the first week of life. Multiple etiologies, including serious bacterial infection, must be considered with prompt diagnosis and treatment imperative for the prevention of serious side effects. Hyperbilirubinemia in older children and adolescents is concerning for hemolysis, extrahepatic obstruction, or hepatocellular injury.

NEONATAL HYPERBILIRUBINEMIA, UNCONJUGATED

The most common causes of indirect hyperbilirubinemia in the first week of life are physiologic jaundice, breast milk jaundice, and hemolysis. Associated conditions increasing the risk for development of hyperbilirubinemia include infection, prematurity, maternal diabetes, breast-feeding, infant hypothyroidism, and poor feeding leading to delayed intestinal transit. Physiologic jaundice is self-limited with bilirubin levels peaking by the third day of life and returning to normal over the next 2 weeks. These infants are well with no risk factors or associated conditions. Breast milk jaundice is thought to be caused by decreased hepatic excretion and intestinal resorption of unconjugated bilirubin. Bilirubin levels are initially normal and increase to a peak at 2 to 3 weeks of life. With breast milk jaundice, bilirubin levels may remain elevated for 3 weeks to 2 months, and then resolve. Birth trauma resulting in cephalohematomas, hemorrhage, and/or bruising can lead to excessive red cell breakdown and jaundice. Maternal–fetal blood group incompatibility, primarily ABO incompatibility, can also result in hyperbilirubinemia and is associated with a higher risk of kernicterus, thus making prompt recognition and treatment imperative[1,2] (Fig. 75–1).

Recognition

A careful history should be performed including prenatal and perinatal history with identification of maternal blood type, if possible. Family history should be directed to the identification of childhood liver disease, metabolic abnormalities, or hemolytic anemias. The presence of jaundice with fever, lethargy, and poor feeding should alert the physician to the possibility of infection. Urinary tract infections are associated with the onset of unconjugated hyperbilirubinemia after a week of age. In addition to jaundice, scleral icterus or hepatomegaly may be present on physical examination.

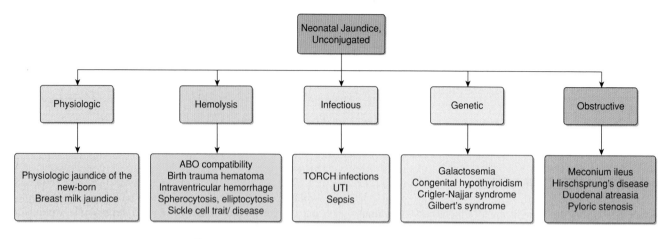

Figure 75–1. Neonatal unconjugated hyperbilirubinemia.

Ancillary Studies

Initial studies include total and direct bilirubin to confirm the diagnosis. If the infant is admitted a, CBC with reticulocyte count, direct antibody test, blood type, serum albumin, and urine for reducing substances should be obtained. Testing for G6PD should be considered if suggested by ethnic or geographic origin. If serious bacterial infection is suspected, a full sepsis workup should be performed with prompt administration of antibiotics.

Management/Complications

Bilirubin level, chronologic age, gestational age, and clinical status of the patient are all considerations in the initiation of phototherapy. The American Academy of Pediatrics guideline for the initiation of phototherapy in infants of 35 or more weeks' gestation is available on their website.[3] Ensure that the patient is appropriately hydrated while providing phototherapy. It is important to remember that premature infants and those with significant comorbidity require treatment at lower bilirubin levels.

Breast milk jaundice should not be treated by withholding breast milk, if at all possible. Supplementation may be appropriate with expressed breast milk or formula if the infant is dehydrated or intake is inadequate.

Bilirubin level >20 mg/dL can be associated with neurotoxicity, encephalopathy, and kernicterus. Kernicterus is the result of deposition of bilirubin in the brain, most importantly in the basal ganglia. Initial symptoms of kernicterus include poor feeding and lethargy, with ensuing opisthotonos, seizures, and death. Kernicterus is associated with long-term impairment of coordination, hearing, and learning abilities. Exchange transfusion must be considered in infants with bilirubin levels approaching 20 to 25 mg/dL and in consultation with a neonatologist.[3]

NEONATAL HYPERBILIRUBINEMIA, CONJUGATED

Direct hyperbilirubinemia is defined as a direct bilirubin concentration > 2 mg/dL, or if the direct concentration is greater than 20% total bilirubin. Neonatal direct hyperbililrubinemia is never normal and indicates hepatobiliary dysfunction. The most common causes of conjugated hyperbilirubinemia infants are biliary atresia, extrahepatic biliary obstruction, neonatal hepatitis, and α_1-antitrypsin (α_1-AT) deficiency.[4] Biliary disorders will be discussed later in this chapter.

Neonatal hepatitis has multiple etiologies including viral, bacterial, idiopathic, and in association with total parenteral nutrition. TORCH infections (toxoplasmosis, rubella cytomegalovirus, hepatitis B, or HIV) are the most common infectious causes. Neonatal hepatitis presents with prolonged jaundice, vomiting, and poor feeding. Symptoms usually appear in the first few weeks of life but may appear as late as 2 to 3 months. Physical examination may reveal, in addition to jaundice, hepatomegaly, altered mental status, or signs of a bleeding diathesis.[5] α_1-AT is a protease inhibitor produced in the endoplasmic reticulum (ER) within hepatocytes. The majority of α_1-AT is made in the liver. Lack of α_1-AT results in an abnormally folded protein, and because this protein cannot be degraded, it is retained within the ER. Only patients homozygous for disease will have clinical expression. In children, it is the most common deficiency hereditary cause of both acute and chronic liver disease, as well as the most common inherited disorder leading to liver transplantation.[4] Patient presentation is highly variable from neonatal hepatitis to portal hypertension in the older child. In the neonatal period, these patients are indistinguishable from those with idiopathic neonatal hepatitis. Diagnosis is based on α_1-AT (Pi) phenotype, and liver biopsy demonstrating deposits within a dilated rough ER demonstrating PAS-positive, diastase resistant granules.[4,5]

Diagnosis/Recognition

The patient's medical history should include prenatal and perinatal information as well as a detailed family history of childhood liver disease, metabolic abnormalities, or hemolytic anemias. Parents should be questioned about the presence of pale stools, which raises the suspicion for cholestasis. Jaundice, scleral icterus, hepatomegaly, and splenomegaly may be present on physical examination (Fig. 75–2).

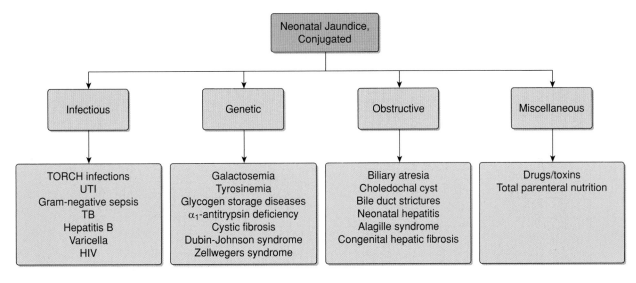

Figure 75–2. Neonatal conjugated hyperbilirubinemia.

Ancillary Studies

Diagnosis and identification of pathologic causes is the key. Initial studies include total and direct bilirubin levels to confirm the diagnosis. Further workup is urgent and diagnostic studies to be considered include CBC and reticulocyte count, blood type of infant and mother, direct antibody test, liver function tests, urine for reducing substances, thyroid function tests, TORCH titers, α_1-AT, and sweat test for cystic fibrosis.

Management/Complications

Any infant with direct hyperbilirubinemia requires a consult with a pediatric gastroenterologist and possible hospital admission. Patients should be monitored closely for potential complications of cholestasis, particulary coagulopathy and fat malabsorption with poor weight gain. Enhancing nutrition and fat-soluble vitamin supplementation is essential.

HYPERBILIRUBINEMIA BEYOND THE NEONATAL PERIOD

In children and adolescents, unconjugated hyperbilirubinemia is most commonly caused by hemolytic processes resulting in the overproduction of bilirubin. Included in the differential are sickle cell disease, hereditary spherocytosis, and G6PD deficiency. If hemolysis is not evident, primary liver dysfunction must be considered. Causes of hepatocellular injury include viral and drug-related hepatitis and can lead to significant injury and resulting jaundice. Although autoimmune hepatitis and Wilson's disease are less common causes of hyperbilirubinemia, these diagnoses must be considered.

Conjugated hyperbilirubinemia beyond the neonatal period is caused by biliary obstruction or hepatocellular injury. The most common causes of obstruction are cholelithiasis, tumor, or choledochal cyst.[4]

Ancillary Studies

In addition to bilirubin levels, consider CBC with smear and liver function tests. If unconjugated hyperbilirubinemia is present, an ultrasound is the appropriate imaging study.

▶ HEPATITIS

Although most children with viral hepatitis have minimal and nonspecific symptoms, it is important to establish a diagnosis and etiology as postexposure prophylaxis is available for some variants. The hepatitis A and B vaccines have significantly decreased the incidence of hepatitis in children.[6,7]

Diagnosis

In children, hepatitis presents with a prodrome of nonspecific symptoms including malaise, anorexia, nausea, vomiting, fever, and abdominal pain followed by the onset of scleral icterus and jaundice. A high index of suspicion must be maintained by the clinician as these patients are often diagnosed with viral gastroenteritis.

Ancillary Studies

Elevated levels of AST/ALT are diagnostic of hepatocellular injury. Indicators of hepatic function may be abnormal including ammonia, prothrombin time, and glucose. Serodiagnostic testing should be obtained for hepatitis A, B, C, CMV, and EBV with further testing as indicated. Table 75–1 reviews the symptoms, spread, risks, and management of the various types of viral hepatitis.

Management

Management is supportive care. The majority of patients can be managed at home, but children with poor intake may need hospitalization for intravenous fluids.

▶ TABLE 75–1. CHARACTERISTICS AND MANAGEMENT OF VIRAL HEPATITIS

Hepatitis	Spread	Symptoms	Labs	Vaccine Available	Chronic Hepatitis	Risk Factors	Treatment	Postexposure Prophylaxis
A	Fecal–oral	Flu-like, fever, jaundice, malaise, self-limiting	HAV total antibody, anti-HAV IgM; IgM present at onset	Yes	No	Close personal contact with an infected person, household or personal contact with a child care center, international travel, a recognized outbreak, homosexual activity, IV drug use	Supportive, no therapy for acute infection	IM immune globulin given within 2 wk postexposure
B	Blood, body fluids, sexual, IV drug use	Subacute illness with nonspecific symptoms, clinical hepatitis with jaundice, fulminant fatal hepatitis	HBsAg, HBeAg, HBV DNA	Yes	Yes	Unknown maternal HBsAg status at birth, needle sharing, perinatal exposure, multiple sexual partners, occupational exposure to blood, incarceration	Supportive, no therapy for acute infection	Infants, Hep B immune globulin; otherwise Hep B vaccine + Hep B Ig or Hep B vaccine alone
C	Exposure to blood of HCV infected patients such as IV drug use, tattoos, piercings, or multiple sexual partners	Similar to Hep A and B, with mild onset, asymptomatic, 20% patients with jaundice	Anti-HCV IgG, HCV DNA	No	Yes	Current/former IV drug users, blood/blood product recipient prior to 1992, inmates, long-term hemodialysis patients	Supportive, no therapy for acute infection	None
D	Only if acute or chronic HBV coinfection present; blood, sexual contact, IV drug use	Causes patient with mild HBV symptoms to progress to severe disease	IgM anti-HDV	No	No	HBV coinfection	Supportive, no therapy for acute infection	HBV vaccine
E	Fecal–oral, commonly found in wild/domestic animals	Jaundice, fever, abdominal pain, arthralgia	Anti-HEV IgG, anti-HEV IgM	No	No	Travel to endemic country	Supportive, no therapy for acute infection	None

FULMINANT HEPATIC FAILURE

Fulminant hepatic failure is an acute or chronically progressive event with the loss of vital hepatic functions resulting in hyperbilirubinemia, hypoglycemia, coagulopathy, hypoproteinemia, and altered mental status from encephalopathy. Acute fulminant liver failure has a mortality approaching 60% to 80% without liver transplant. The causes of fulminant hepatic failure include infection, metabolic derangements, and toxin exposure. In neonates, it is thought to have an infectious (such as HSV) or metabolic (such as Wilson's disease) source. In children, fulminant hepatic failure is most commonly a complication of viral hepatitis or toxin induced (mushrooms) or pharmacologic exposure (acetaminophen, anticonvulsants).

An uncommon but severe cause of liver failure is *Reye's syndrome*. Reye's syndrome occurs following a viral illness (most commonly influenza B) with vomiting and rapid onset of hepatic dysfunction, encephalopathy, and cerebral edema. Antecedent treatment with aspirin has been associated with Reye's syndrome. The liver can recover from this injury and prognosis is dependent on extent of cerebral edema.[3]

Diagnosis/Recognition

By history, most patients have an unremarkable medical history with no preexisting liver disease. The majority of patients have nonspecific complaints including nausea, vomiting, anorexia, and abdominal pain, particularly right upper quadrant. As failure progresses, jaundice develops and is often the symptom prompting medical attention. With the onset of coagulopathy, bruising and bleeding may occur. Hemorrhage can be significant, especially if occurs from gastric and esophageal varices resulting from portal hypertension. Patients may also have a characteristic breath odor, "fetor hepaticus." Encephalopathy correlates with the severity of liver dysfunction and can progress from simple fatigue and drowsiness to unresponsiveness secondary to cerebral edema and elevated intracranial pressure.

Ancillary Studies

Liver enzymes and bilirubin levels may be elevated but can return to normal as the number of viable hepatocytes decreases. Markers of synthetic function, that is albumin, clotting studies, and ammonia, are abnormal and are useful indicators of function. Hypoglycemia is a common complication and serum glucose must be monitored closely. As hepatorenal syndrome occurs in well more than half of the cases of fulminant hepatic failure, monitoring of renal function and urine function is necessary. Liver biopsy shows patchy or confluent necrosis of hepatocytes, without evidence of hepatic regeneration.

Management/Complications

Treatment is supportive with close monitoring often in an intensive care unit. Consistent monitoring of the following is imperative: serum glucose, electrolytes, calcium, phosphorous, magnesium, clotting studies, and ammonia. Intravenous glucose may be necessary for the treatment of persistent hypoglycemia. If indicated, the patient with encephalopathy may need airway control and treatment of cerebral edema. Accompanying coagulopathy is managed with the administration of vitamin K.[8]

Prognosis is based on the underlying cause of liver failure and stage of hepatic encephalopathy. Poor prognosis is associated with

1. jaundice >7 days prior to onset of encephalopathy.
2. PT >50 seconds.
3. serum bilirubin >17.5 mg/dL.

Although the liver is capable of regeneration, in fulminant hepatic failure, the injury/insult may be so significant and widespread that regeneration does not occur.

▶ BILIARY TRACT DISEASE

Biliary tract abnormalities seen in infancy include biliary atresia, choledochal cyst, and the potentially life-threatening disorder associated with both, that is *acute cholangitis*. Acute biliary tract disease in childhood includes cholelithiasis, cholecystitis, and hydrops of the gallbladder.

BILIARY ATRESIA

Biliary atresia is a cause of neonatal conjugated hyperbilirubinemia and may be surgically correctable. Biliary atresia occurs in 1:10 000 to 1:18 000 births in European Americans, with a higher incidence in Asian Americans, especially Asian American females. The most common form of biliary atresia is extrahepatic with the absence of all extrahepatic biliary structures.[9]

Diagnosis

Hyperbilirubinemia as a result of biliary atresia usually occurs within 2 to 3 weeks of age. Parents will report stools that are light yellow, gray, or acholic. Hepatomegaly is also present. If the diagnosis is delayed beyond 2 months of age, the patient may also demonstrate poor weight gain, ascites, and splenomegaly.

Ancillary Studies

Initial laboratory studies will reveal conjugated hyperbilirubinemia. If the diagnosis is delayed, other serologic abnormalities occur resulting from hepatic damage and poor nutrition. Visualization of the biliary tree, by either ultrasound or nuclear medicine hepatobiliary studies (DISIDA) scan, can determine presence of obstruction and define abnormalities. Liver biopsy is a conclusive diagnostic test in greater than 90% of cases, but laparotomy and operative cholangiography are definitive.[10]

Management

Treatment is both supportive care and surgical correction. The definitive treatment is hepatoportoenterostomy (Kasai procedure). Early surgical correction is vital as the success rate of the procedure declines if performed after 3 months of age. Two-thirds of patients with biliary atresia will advance to liver failure and need liver transplantation. Supportive treatment includes caloric and nutritional supplementation with fat-soluble vitamins (A, D, E, K), and ursodeoxycholic acid.

Acute cholangitis is a complication associated with surgical correction of biliary atresia or removal of a choledochal cyst. It is the result of an ascending biliary infection or obstruction and patients present with fever, worsening jaundice, and elevated serum transaminases. Prompt recognition and institution of broad-spectrum antibiotics is imperative, as the morbidity and mortality associated with this disorder is significant.

CHOLEDOCHAL CYST

Choledochal cysts are congenital anomalies of the biliary tract and an extrahepatic cause of conjugated hyperbilirubinemia from cholestasis. Incidence is four times higher in females and higher in Asian Americans.[11]

Diagnosis

The patients present with recurrent episodes of jaundice, pancreatitis, and abdominal pain. A right-sided abdominal mass may be palpated. In infancy, it can be clinically impossible to separate choledochal cysts from biliary atresia.[11]

Ancillary Studies

In addition to liver function tests, an ultrasound of the abdomen is indicated.

Management

Referral to a pediatric gastroenterologist and pediatric surgeon is indicated. The urgency of these consultations is dependent on the clinical status of the patient.

CHOLELITHIASIS AND CHOLECYSTITIS

Acute cholecystitis is a relatively uncommon entity in children and indicates gallbladder inflammation in the presence of gallstones. Gallstones occur more commonly in females than males, especially adolescent females. Gallstones develop as a result of abdominal surgery, sepsis, necrotizing enterocolitis, parenteral nutrition, hemolysis, or disorders with enhanced biliary enterohepatic circulation such as cystic fibrosis or Crohn's disease.[12] Adolescents have cholesterol stones secondary to obesity, pregnancy, and/or the use of oral contraceptives. Acalculous cholecystitis or inflammation of the gallbladder in the absence of stones is more common than cholelithiasis and can be caused by bacterial infections (e.g., Streptococcus, Salmonella, Klebsiella), viral infections, and parasitic infestations (e.g., Giardia, ascarus).[13]

Diagnosis

The patients present with biliary colic, which is acute in onset and colicky in nature. The pain is usually right upper quadrant or epigastric, increases in intensity over 15 to 20 minutes and lasts up to 4 hours. The pain may radiate to the back or shoulder and is often associated with meals. Systemic symptoms include fever, jaundice, and vomiting. The classic triad is right upper quadrant pain, fever, and leukocytosis.

Ancillary Studies

Typically, there are abnormalities of liver function and a leukocytosis. The gallbladder can be visualized via ultrasound, but the gold standard for imaging is hepatobiliary scintigraphy. As the patient may be vomiting, it is important to monitor the fluid/electrolyte status.

Management

Treatment should include IV hydration and pain control. Febrile patients may need admission and IV antibiotics, usually ampicillin and gentamicin, plus clindamycin or metronidazole. Patients with adequate pain control with oral medications can be managed as an outpatient with surgical follow-up. Complications of cholecystitis include gallbladder perforation, bile peritonitis, pancreatitis, sepsis, and abscess/fistula formation.[13]

► HYDROPS OF THE GALLBLADDER

Gallbladder hydrops is an acute noninfectious process leading to an enlarged gallbladder without gallstones. It occasionally occurs as a complication of viral gastroenteritis, Kawasaki disease, streptococcal pharyngitis, mesenteric adenitis, or nephrotic syndrome. These patients will present with abdominal pain, elevation in liver enzymes, and possibly hepatomegaly. Ultrasound is diagnostic. This condition resolves when the underlying infection is treated. NSAIDs can be given for pain control.[11,13]

REFERENCES

1. Hostetler MA. Neonatal jaundice. In: Marx JA, Hockberger RS, Walls RM, Adams JG, eds. *Rosen's Emergency Medicine: Concepts and Clinical Practice.* 6th ed. Philadelphia, PA: Mosby; 2006;2601–2605.
2. Moyer V, Freese DK, Whitington PF, et al. Guideline for the Evaluation of Cholestatic Jaundice on Infants: Recommendations of the North American Society for Pediatric Gastroenterology, Hepatology and Nutrition. *J Pediatr Gastroenterol Nutr.* 2004;39:115–128.
3. American Academy of Pediatrics: Subcommittee on Hyperbilirubinemia. Management of Hyperbilirubinemia in the Newborn Infant 35 or More Weeks of Gestation. *Pediatrics.* 2004;114:297–316.
4. Harb R, Thomas DW. Conjugated hyperbilirubinemia: screening and treatment in older infants and children. *Pediatr Rev.* 2007;28:83–90.
5. Rudolph JA, Balistrer WF. Metabolic diseases of the liver. In: Behrman RE, Kliegman RM, Jenson HB, eds. *Nelson Textbook of Pediatrics.* 17th ed. Philadelphia, PA: Saunders; 2004;1319–1324.
6. American Academy of Pediatrics. Hepatitis A. In: Pickering LK, Baker CJ, Long SS, McMillan JA, eds. *Red Book: 2006 Report of the Committee on Infectious Diseases.* 27th ed. Elk

Grove Village, IL: American Academy of Pediatrics; 2006:326–334.

7. American Academy of Pediatrics. Hepatitis B. In: Pickering LK, Baker CJ, Long SS, McMillan JA, eds. *Red Book: 2006 Report of the Committee on Infectious Diseases*. 27th ed. Elk Grove Village, IL: American Academy of Pediatrics; 2006:335–354.

8. Suchy F. Drug- and toxin-induced liver injury. In: Behrman RE, Kliegman RM, Jenson HB, eds. *Nelson Textbook of Pediatrics*. 17th ed. Philadelphia, PA: Saunders; 2004:1339–1340.

9. Rosenthal P. Disorders of the biliary tract: other disorders. In: Walker WA, Kleinman RE, Sherman PM, Shneider BL, Sanderson IR, eds. *Pediatric Gastrointestinal Disease: Pathophysiology, Diagnosis, and Management*. 4th ed. Lewiston, NY: BC Decker Inc; 2004:1139–1141.

10. Zalen GS et al. Biliary Atresia. *Pediatr Rev.* 2006;27:243–248.

11. Sokol RJ, Narkewicz MR. Liver and pancreas. In: Hay WW Jr, Levin MJ, Sondheimer JM, Deterding RR, eds. *Current Diagnosis and Treatment in Pediatrics*. 18th ed. Chicago, IL: McGraw-Hill; 2007:638–673.

12. Broderick A, Sweeney BT. Gallbladder disease. In: Walker WA, Kleinman RE, Sherman PM, Shneider BL, Sanderson IR, eds. *Pediatric Gastrointestinal Disease: Pathophysiology, Diagnosis, and Management*. 4th ed. Lewiston, NY: BC Decker Inc; 2004:1551–1562.

13. Hostetler MA. Neonatal jaundice. In: Marx JA, Hockberger RS, Walls RM, Adams JG, eds. *Rosen's Emergency Medicine: Concepts and Clinical Practice*. 6th ed. Philadelphia, PA: Mosby; 2006:220–2621.

SECTION XI

ENDOCRINE EMERGENCIES

CHAPTER 76

Disorders of Glucose Metabolism

Nicholas Furtado

▶ HIGH-YIELD FACTS

- Diabetic ketoacidosis (DKA) is a complex endocrine condition caused by an absolute or relative lack of insulin. It is characterized by hyperglycemia, dehydration, ketosis, and metabolic acidosis.
- DKA is often insidious in onset with slow progression of the illness.
- Definition of DKA by biochemical criteria includes the following:
  - Hyperglycemia: Blood glucose > 200 mg/dL
  - Venous pH < 7.3 or bicarbonate < 15 mmol/L
  - Ketonemia and ketonuria
- In type 2 diabetes mellitus, hyperglycemic hyperosmolar state (HHS) can occur and is defined by the following:
  - Plasma glucose concentration > 600 mg/dL
  - Arterial pH > 7.30
  - Serum bicarbonate > 15 mmol/L
  - Small ketonuria and absent or mild ketonemia
  - Serum osmolarity ≥ 320 mOsm/kg
  - Stupor or coma

Treatment of diabetic ketoacidosis (DKA) consists of rapid assessment, replacement of the patient's fluid and electrolyte deficit, and reversal of the central pathophysiologic process by the administration of insulin.

The initial fluid resuscitation is with normal saline at a dose of 10 to 20 mL/kg over 1 to 2 hours. After the initial bolus, the patient's cardiovascular status is reevaluated and a second bolus may be administered.

An initial bolus of insulin is unnecessary and can increase the risk for cerebral edema. The insulin infusion starting dose is 0.1 U/kg/h and this should continue till resolution of DKA (pH > 7.3, bicarbonate > 15 mmol/L).

Potassium replacement therapy is started once normal or low serum potassium is ensured and urine output is established. The usual dose of potassium is twice-daily maintenance or 3 to 4 mEq/kg per 24 hours provided as 40 mEq/L in the IV fluids, with half as potassium chloride and half as potassium phosphate.

Cerebral edema occurs in 0.5% to 0.9% of DKA patients and the mortality rate is 21% to 24%. The predisposing factors are younger age, new onset diabetes, and longer duration of symptoms.

Newborns and young infants with hypoglycemia may be asymptomatic or may manifest nonspecific symptoms. Older children exhibit more classic symptoms of hypoglycemia, including sweating, tachycardia, tremor, anxiety, tachypnea, and weakness.

Treatment of hypoglycemia

- In newborns, give 10% dextrose 2 mL/kg (0.2 g/kg) as a bolus, followed by infusion at 6 to 9 mg/kg/min
- In children, give 10% dextrose at 5 mL/kg (0.5 g/kg) as a bolus, followed by continuous infusion at 6 to 9 mg/kg/min
- If an IV line is not possible, then give glucagon 0.03 mg/kg (maximum dose 1 mg) subcutaneously

Admission of the hypoglycemic patient is indicated when there is no obvious cause, toxic ingestion as with oral hypoglycemic agents is suspected, administration of long-acting insulin was the cause, and if there are persistent neurological deficits.

▶ DIABETIC KETOACIDOSIS

DKA is a complex endocrine condition caused by an absolute or relative lack of insulin. It is characterized by hyperglycemia, dehydration, ketosis, and metabolic acidosis.

EPIDEMIOLOGY

The annual incidence of DKA in the United States ranges from 4.6 to 8 episodes per 1000 patients with diabetes. Diabetes is one of the most common diseases occurring in teenagers. DKA is seen as the initial presentation of diabetes in approximately 25% of young children.[1] The risk of DKA in children and adolescents with type 1 diabetes is 1 to 10 per 100 person per year.[2-5] In young patients, DKA accounts for 70% of diabetes-related deaths.

PATHOPHYSIOLOGY

In DKA, a lack of insulin and stress lead to increase in the levels of counterregulatory hormones—glucagon, epinephrine, cortisol, and growth hormone (Fig. 76–1). Gluconeogenesis and glycogenolysis occur in the liver and proteolysis occurs in peripheral tissues. Lipolysis occurs in fatty tissues, forming the ketoacids, β-hydroxybutyrate, and acetoacetic acid. The combination of hyperglycemia and ketoacidosis causes a hyperosmolar diuresis that results in loss of fluids and electrolytes. The combination of ketonemia and hypoperfusion then results in high anion gap metabolic acidosis.

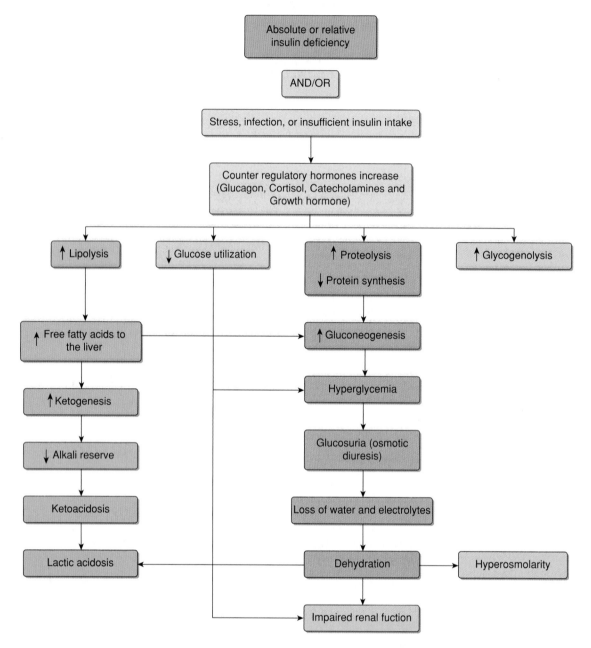

Figure 76–1. Pathophysiology of DKA. (With permission from Wolfsdorf J, Glaser N, Sperling MA. Diabetic ketoacidosis in infants, children, and adolescents: a consensus statement from the American Diabetes Association. *Diabetes Care.* 2006;29(5):1150–1159.)

PRECIPITATING FACTORS

DkA is precipitated by a variety of causes. DKA at diagnosis is more common in younger children <5 years and families with poor access to health care.[2] In adolescents, noncompliance with insulin is a main cause of DKA. The risk of DKA is increased in peripubertal and adolescent girls, children with clinical depression or eating disorders, and those on insulin pump therapy (due to use of short-acting insulin).[2,5,6] In the Diabetes Control and Complications Trial (DCCT), the incidence of DKA in patients on insulin pumps was double than that in the multiple-injection group.[7]

CLINICAL MANIFESTATIONS

History

- DKA is often insidious in onset with slow progression of the illness
- Fatigue and malaise
- Nausea/vomiting
- Abdominal pain
- Polydipsia
- Polyuria
- Polyphagia

- Significant weight loss
- Fever

Physical Findings

- Altered mental status characterized by drowsiness, progressive obtundation, and loss of consiousness without evidence of head trauma
- Tachycardia
- Acidosis: tachypnea or hyperventilation or deep, rapid, sighing respirations called Kussmaul respirations
- Normal or low blood pressure
- Dehydration: poor peripheral perfusion and delayed capillary refill
- Poor perfusion
- Lethargy and weakness
- Fever if infection precipitated the episode
- Acetone odor of the breath reflecting metabolic acidosis
- Nonspecific elevation of serum amylase

Laboratory Studies

Initial laboratory studies include a complete blood count, serum electrolytes, glucose, calcium, phosphorus, and serum acetone. An arterial blood gas and bedside tests for blood sugar and urine ketones can be done for rapid diagnosis of DKA. An initial electrocardiogram can be performed to assess for T-wave changes.

Definition of DKA (biochemical criteria)[8]

- Hyperglycemia: blood glucose > 200 mg/dL
- Venous pH < 7.3 or bicarbonate < 15 mmol/L
- Ketonemia and ketonuria

DKA can be classified by the degree of acidosis into mild, moderate, and severe.[9]

- Mild: Venous pH < 7.3 or bicarbonate < 15 mmol/L
- Moderate: pH < 7.2, bicarbonate < 10 mmol/L
- Severe: pH < 7.1, bicarbonate < 5 mmol/L

In type 2 diabetes mellitus, hyperglycemic hyperosmolar state (HHS) can occur.[10] This is defined by the following:

- Plasma glucose concentration > 600 mg/dL
- Arterial pH > 7.30
- Serum bicarbonate > 15 mmol/L
- Small ketonuria and absent or mild ketonemia
- Serum osmolarity ≥ 320 mOsm/kg
- Stupor or coma

MANAGEMENT

Treatment of DKA consists of rapid assessment, replacement of the patient's fluid and electrolyte deficit, and reversal of the central pathophysiologic process by the administration of insulin.

Assessment

- Perform a quick clinical assessment and bedside tests to confirm the diagnosis.

- Weigh the patient and use weight for calculation of fluid and electrolyte therapy
- Assess the level of dehydration
- Assess the level of consciousness using the Glasgow Coma Scale
- Obtain blood samples and start peripheral IV line
- Perform an ECG

Supportive Measures

- Airway management for obtunded or comatose patients
- Oxygen at 100% concentration is to be administered to patients in respiratory or circulatory failure and shock
- Maintain good peripheral or central IV access
- Continuous cardiac monitoring is to be used for assessment of T-wave changes[11]
- After obtaining samples for cultures, intravenous antibiotics are to be started as soon as possible for patients with DKA precipitated by febrile illness
- As soon as hemodynamic stability is achieved, child should be transferred to a intensive care unit to be managed by a pediatric intensive care specialist with consultation from a pediatric endocrinologist

FLUID RESUSCITATION

Children with DKA are at least 5% to 10% dehydrated.[12,13] Because clinical estimates are usually inaccurate,[14] it is practical to estimate for moderate DKA, 5% to 7% dehydration, and for severe DKA, 7% to 10% dehydration.[1] The initial fluid resuscitation is with normal saline at a dose of 10 to 20 mL/kg over 1 to 2 hours. After the initial bolus, the patient's cardiovascular status is reevaluated and a second bolus may be administered. The association between rate of fluid resuscitation and development of cerebral edema is not convincing.[15]

After the initial fluid resuscitation, rehydration is continued with 0.9% normal saline or Ringer's lactate for 4 to 6 hours depending on state of hydration, serum sodium, and hemodynamic status of the patient.[16] Subsequently, the remaining fluid deficit should be replaced slowly over 48 hours with a solution of tonicity greater or equal to 0.45% saline with added potassium chloride, potassium phosphate or potassium acetate.[16–18]

In addition to assessment of dehydration, calculation of effective osmolarity can guide fluid and electrolyte therapy. In patients with extreme hyperosmolarity, some recommend continuing therapy with isotonic fluids until serum osmolarity decreases below 320 mOsm/L. The formula for serum osmolality is as follows (blood urea is not included because of low osmolality):

$$\text{Serum osmolality (mOsm/L)} = 2[\text{serum Na (mEq/L)}] + \text{blood glucose (mg/dL)}/18$$

INSULIN THERAPY

The absolute or relative lack of insulin and increase in counterregulatory hormones causes hyperglycemia and DKA (Fig. 76–1). With initial fluid resuscitation, there is some decrease in blood glucose[20,21]; however, normalization of blood glucose and suppression of lipolysis requires low-dose, continuous, intravenous insulin infusion.[22] This provides slow, reliable, and

▶ **TABLE 76-1. LOSS OF FLUIDS AND ELECTROLYTES IN DKA AND MAINTAINANCE REQUIREMENTS IN NORMAL CHILDREN**

	Average Loss (kg)	24-h Maintenance Requirements (kg)
Water	70 mL (30–100)	<10 kg: 100 mL/kg/24 h 11–20 kg: 1000 mL + 50 mL/kg/24 h for each kg over 10 >20 kg: 1500 mL + 20 mL/kg/24 h for each kg over 20[19] For children over 10 kg: body surface area can be used ($1500\ mL/m^2/24\ h$)
Sodium	6 mEq (5–13)	2–4 mEq
Potassium	5 mEq (3–6)	2–3 mEq
Chloride	4 mEq (3–9)	2–3 mEq
Phosphate	1.5–7.5 mEq	3–6 mEq

titratable systemic absorption of insulin. An initial bolus of insulin is unnecessary and can increase the risk for cerebral edema.[23,24] The starting dose is 0.1 U/kg/h and this should continue till resolution of DKA (pH > 7.3, bicarbonate > 15 mmol/L). On occasion, the infusion may have to be decreased to 0.05 unit/kg/h when there is marked sensitivity to insulin or conversely it may need to be increased to 0.15 to 0.2 U/kg/h to lower the serum glucose and reverse the ketosis if the patient's serum glucose is unresponsive to the initial starting dose of 0.1 U/kg/h. The goal of therapy is to decrease the serum glucose by 75 to 100 mg/L/h. When the serum glucose reaches 250 mg/dL, 5% glucose is added to the infusing fluid. If the serum glucose is dropping precipitously, a glucose solution of ≥ 10% may need to be administered. It is dangerous to discontinue the insulin infusion completely if the patient has moderate-to-large serum ketones, since this can worsen the ketoacidosis.

During the initial resuscitation phase, the patient should be given nothing by mouth. As the patient improves, oral intake of water or ice may be provided and advanced to clear liquids as tolerated. When the serum glucose normalizes, metabolic acidosis improves and serum ketones decrease to trace, the insulin infusion is discontinued and switched to subcutaneous insulin and oral intake of liquids or solids. Subcutaneous insulin is administered 30 minutes prior to discontinuing the insulin infusion to allow for absorption of the subcutaneous insulin dose and hence prevent rebound hyperglycemia and ketoacidosis.

If low-dose IV insulin cannot be administered because of the circumstances, then subcutaneous (SC) or intramuscular intermittent doses of short- or rapid-acting insulin analog may be used.[25] The initial dose is 0.3 unit/kg followed in 1 h by SC insulin lispro or aspart at 0.1 unit/kg every hour or 0.15 to 20 units/kg every 2 hours. If blood sugar falls to below 250 mg/dL before resolution of DKA, then start 5% glucose IV and continue as before. When DKA resolves and blood sugar is < 250 mg/dL, reduce insulin to 0.05 unit/kg to keep blood sugar at about 200 mg/dL.

POTASSIUM

Children with DKA are potassium-depleted with a deficit of 3 to 6 mEq/L/kg.[13] This loss is primarily intracellular potassium, which is drawn out of the cells by hypertonicity and in exchange for hydrogen ions and also by efflux during glycogenolysis and proteolysis. Potassium is also lost by vomiting and osmotic diuresis.[26] Although there is total body depletion of potassium, the initial serum potassium can be normal, increased, or decreased.[27] When the insulin infusion is started, potassium is driven back into the cells with decrease in serum levels.[28] Hypokalemia is most common after several hours of rehydration. Both severe hypo- and hyperkalemia can cause life-threatening cardiac arrhythmias; therefore, it is essential that the patient's serum potassium be determined as soon as possible. Alternatively, an ECG can be used to determine if the child has evidence of hyper- or hypokalemia.[11] Serum potassium levels should be checked every 2 to 4 hours. Replacement therapy is started once normal or low serum potassium is ensured and urine output is established. The usual dose of potassium is twice-daily maintenance (Table 76–1) or 3 to 4 mEq/kg per 24 hours provided as 40 mEq/L in the IV fluids, with half as potassium chloride and half as potassium phosphate. The maximum recommended rate of IV potassium is usually 0.5 mEq/kg/h.

SODIUM

The osmotic diuresis usually induces sodium depletion in patients with DKA. In DKA, both the hyperglycemia and hyperlipidemia cause pseudohyponatremia. In addition, the osmotic movement of water into the extracellular space causes dilutional hyponatremia.[29,30] Therefore, corrected serum sodium should be used for monitoring changes during therapy. The formula for corrected serum sodium is as follows:

$$\text{Corrected serum sodium (mEq/L)} = \text{Measured Na} + 0.016 \times (\text{Serum glucose} - 100)$$

The corrected serum sodium should not be allowed to drop faster than 10 to 12 mEq/L per 24 hours. If significant hyponatremia is present, the first 6 to 8 hours of correction should occur with 0.9% NS. During the continuing resuscitation, sodium levels are monitored every 4 hours and as the glucose falls, the reported level of serum sodium should increase. A fall in serum sodium during continued fluid resuscitation may indicate excess accumulation of free water and may be a risk factor for the development of cerebral edema. If this happens, the sodium content of the fluid may need to be increased.[31,32]

PHOSPHATE

Depletion of phosphate during DKA occurs as a result of osmotic diuresis.[12,13] Clinically significant hypophosphatemia can cause impaired cardiac function and insulin resistance. Usually after starting insulin, serum phosphate decreases and clinically significant hypophosphatemia can occur if food is not started after 24 hours of fluid therapy.[12,13] Prospective studies have not shown clinical benefit from phosphate replacement.[33,34] Supplementation is indicated if the serum level is < 2 mEq/L and can be administered with potassium replacement as potassium phosphate alone or with potassium chloride. During phosphate replacement, monitor serum calcium for development of hypocalcemia.[35,36]

ACIDOSIS

The acidosis that is fundamental to DKA is usually reversible with fluid resuscitation and insulin therapy. Controlled trials have shown no clinical benefit from bicarbonate administration.[37,38] Bicarbonate causes paradoxical CNS acidosis, rapid onset hypokalemia, and increase in serum osmolality.[39,40] Despite these adverse effects and lack of clinical benefit, its cautious use may be considered in patients with severe acidosis (pH < 6.9 or serum bicarbonate < 5 mEq/L) and hyperkalemia, which are associated with insulin resistance and cardiac arrhythmias. If bicarbonate is considered necessary, administer 1 to 2 mEq/kg over 60 minutes.[26]

COMPLICATIONS

Complications of DKA therapy include the following:

- Inadequate rehydration
- Hypoglycemia
- Hypokalemia
- Hyperchloremic acidosis
- Cerebral edema

Hypoglycemia is common, especially in young diabetics, who tend to be extremely sensitive to insulin and labile. Adjusting the insulin infusion and providing supplemental intravenous and oral glucose according to the principles outlined above will successfully correct this.

Hypokalemia occurs within several hours of initiation of therapy and can lead to arrhythmias. Therefore, cardiac monitoring is essential during therapy for DKA. Treatment is with potassium replacement, as discussed above.

Cerebral edema occurs in 0.5% to 0.9% of DKA patients and the mortality rate is 21% to 24%.[41,42] The predisposing factors are younger age, new onset diabetes and longer duration of symptoms.[43,44] Other risk factors that may be identified at diagnosis or during therapy include administration of insulin in the first hour of fluid replacement, high fluid volume replacement within the first 4 hours,[24] severe acidosis and hypocapnia at presentation after adjusting for acidosis,[42] high serum urea nitrogen, attenuated rise of corrected serum sodium during treatment,[31] and the use of bicarbonate.[42]

The warning signs of cerebral edema are as follows:

- Headache and slowing of the heart rate
- Change in neurological status (restlessness, irritability, increased drowsiness, and incontinence)
- Focal neurological signs (cranial nerve palsy)
- Rising blood pressure
- Decrease in O_2 saturation

Diagnostic criteria for use in the bedside evaluation of neurological state for the early diagnosis of cerebral edema include the following:[45]

- Abnormal motor or verbal response to pain
- Decorticate or decelerate posture
- Cranial nerve palsy (III, IV, and VI)
- Abnormal respiratory pattern (grunting, tachypnea, Cheyne-Stokes breathing, and apnea)

Major criteria

- Atered mentation or fluctuating level of consciousness
- Sustained deceleration of the heart rate
- Age inappropriate incontinence

Minor criteria

- Vomiting
- Headache
- Lethargy (not easily arousable)
- Diastolic BP > 90 mm Hg
- Age < 5 y

One diagnostic criterion and two major criteria or one major and two minor criteria have a sensitivity of 92% for the diagnosis of cerebral edema in DKA.

TREATMENT OF CEREBRAL EDEMA

- IV mannitol 0.5 to 1 g/kg over 20 minutes to be repeated if there is no response in 30 minutes[46,47]
- Fluid restriction by one-third
- Hypertonic saline 3%, 5 to 10 mL/kg over 30 minutes[48]
- Elevate the head of the bed
- Hyperventilation to maintain a P_{CO_2} < 22 mm Hg, although aggressive hyperventilation may be associated with poor outcome[49]
- After treatment of cerebral edema, a CT scan should be performed to rule out other causes of neurological deterioration such as thrombosis or hemorrhage

DISPOSITION

All patients presenting with DKA as the initial presentation of diabetes are hospitalized at a center where a physician trained in management of pediatric DKA and/or a pediatric endocrinologist are available for consultation. Patients with severe acidosis are best treated in a pediatric intensive care unit for reasons of close monitoring and need for repeated blood sampling.

Children with prolonged illness, decreased level of consciousness, and those at increased risk for cerebral edema at presentation must be admitted to a pediatric intensive care unit

► TABLE 76-2. **DEFINITION OF HYPOGLYCEMIA**

Age	Plasma Glucose* (mg/dL)
3–24 h	<40
Over 24 h	<45
Infants (1 mo to 1 y) and children (>1 y)	<50

*Whole blood glucose values are 10%–15% higher.

for management.[8,50] Occasionally, children with recurrent and mild DKA, with good family support, may be treated in the emergency department and discharged and followed up as an outpatient in consultation with their endocrinologist.[8]

► HYPOGLYCEMIA

Hypoglycemia is most common in early neonatal life and may reflect a normal adaptive processes to extrauterine life.[51] In contrast to adults, infants and children are more prone to early development hypoglycemia when fasting because of higher metabolic rate and lower stores of glycogen.[52,53] Hypoglycemia is pathological when low blood glucose levels are recurrent and persistent leading to acute systemic effects and long-term neurological sequelae.[54,55] In childhood and adolescence, hypoglycemia usually presents as a complication of aggressive treatment for insulin-dependent diabetes mellitus [56,57] (Table 76–2).

The plasma glucose level at which obvious signs and symptoms of hypoglycemia are manifest is variable and depends on the age and clinical characteristics of the patient.

PATHOPHYSIOLOGY

The homeostasis of glucose is maintained by a complex balance between the exogenous supply of food and the body's regulatory hormones. Insulin and its counterregulatory hormones (glucagon, epinephrine, cortisol, and growth hormone) and their interaction on the liver, muscle, and adipose tissue control glucose levels in the blood. When adequate levels are not maintained, hypoglycemia occurs (Fig. 76–2). Glucose is the main energy substrate for the central nervous system and most other organs in the body. Hence hypoglycemia results in the acute increase in counterregulatory hormones causing autonomic symptoms and central nervous system (CNS) dysfunction and sequelae.

SIGNS AND SYMPTOMS

Newborns and young infants may be asymptomatic or may manifest nonspecific symptoms (Tables 76–3 and 76–4). Older children exhibit more classic symptoms of hypoglycemia, including sweating, tachycardia, tremor, anxiety, tachypnea, and weakness. Neuroglycopenia, which is a condition of prolonged and severe hypoglycemia manifested on the CNS, can result in permanent neurologic sequelae.

DIAGNOSTIC EVALUATION

Evaluation of an infant or child with hypoglycemia should include a detailed history of the past including perinatal history, acute or recurrent symptoms, and physical examination.[58]

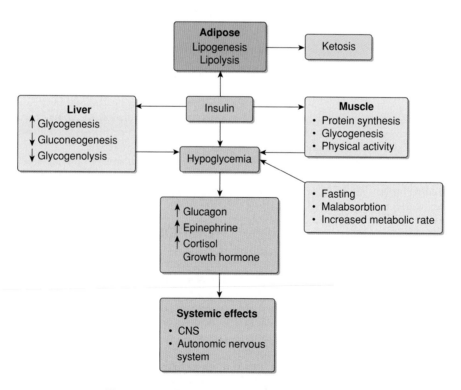

Figure 76–2. Pathophysiology of hypoglycemia.

▶ **TABLE 76-3. SYMPTOMS OF HYPOGLYCEMIA**

Symptoms of Hypoglycemia		
In Children		
Autonomic Nervous System (Acute)	Central Nervous System (Prolonged)	In Infancy
Sweating	Headache	Cyanotic episodes
Jitteriness, tremor	Visual disturbances	Apnea
Tachycardia	Lethargy	Refusal to feed
Anxiety	Restlessness/irritability	Jitteryness
Weakness	Mental confusion	Myoclonic jerks
Nausea, vomiting	Difficulty with speech/thought	Hypothermia
	Convulsions	Sweating
	Personality changes	Somnolence
	Permanent neurological sequelae	

History

- Perinatal history: birth weight, maternal diabetes
- Dietary relationship to acute symptoms: time after food or association with starvation
- Past history and family history: symptoms, mortality
- Toxic ingestion
- Growth and development
- Signs and symptoms of the current episode

Physical Examination

- Anthropmetrics: short stature, macrosomia
- Macroglossia, hepatomegaly, jaundice

- Midline defects: single central incisor, cleft lip/palate, microphallus, undescended testis
- Skin pigmentation due to adrenal insufficiency
- Hyperventilation (acidosis)

Laboratory Tests

- A rapid screen for the plasma glucose level at the bed-side
- A critical sample which includes repeat blood glucose and other important studies such as insulin, C-peptide, growth hormone, cortisol, and glucagon levels
- A bedside urine test for ketones

▶ **TABLE 76-4. ETIOLOGY OF HYPOGLYCEMIA IN INFANTS AND CHILDREN**

Etiology of Hypoglycemia		
Ketone Negative	Ketone Positive	Other Causes
Hyperinsulinemic states	Hormone deficiency	Amino acid and organic acid disorders
K ATP channel mutations	Panhypopituitarism	Maple syrup urine disease
Glutamate dehydrogenase gene mutation	Isolated growth hormone deficiency	Propionic acidemia
Glucokinase gene mutation	ACTH deficiency	Methyl malonic acidemia
B cell adenoma	Adrenal insufficiency	Tyrosinosis
Beckwith–Wiedemann syndrome	Glucagon deficiency	Glutaric aciduria
Insulin administration (Munchausens by proxy)	Epinephrine deficiency	3-methyl-glutaric aciduria
Disorders of fatty acid oxidation	Lack of substrate	Drugs toxicity
Primary carnitine deficiency	Ketotic hypoglycemia	Salicylates
Carnitine transporter defect	Glycogen storage disease	Alcohol
Carnitine palmitoyl transferase deficiency	Glucose-6 phosphatase deficiency	Oral hypoglycemic agents
Long-, medium-, short-chain fatty acid acyl CoA dehydrogenase deficiency	Amylo-1,6 glucosidase deficiency	Insulin
	Liver phosphorylase deficiency	β-blockers
	Glycogen synthetase deficiency	Systemic disease
	Disorders of Gluconeogenesis	Sepsis
	Fructose-1, 6 diphosphatase deficiency	Malabsorbtion
	Phosphoenol pyruvate carboxy kinase deficiency	Malnutrition
	Other enzyme defects	Polycythemia
	Galacosemia	
	Fructose intolerance	

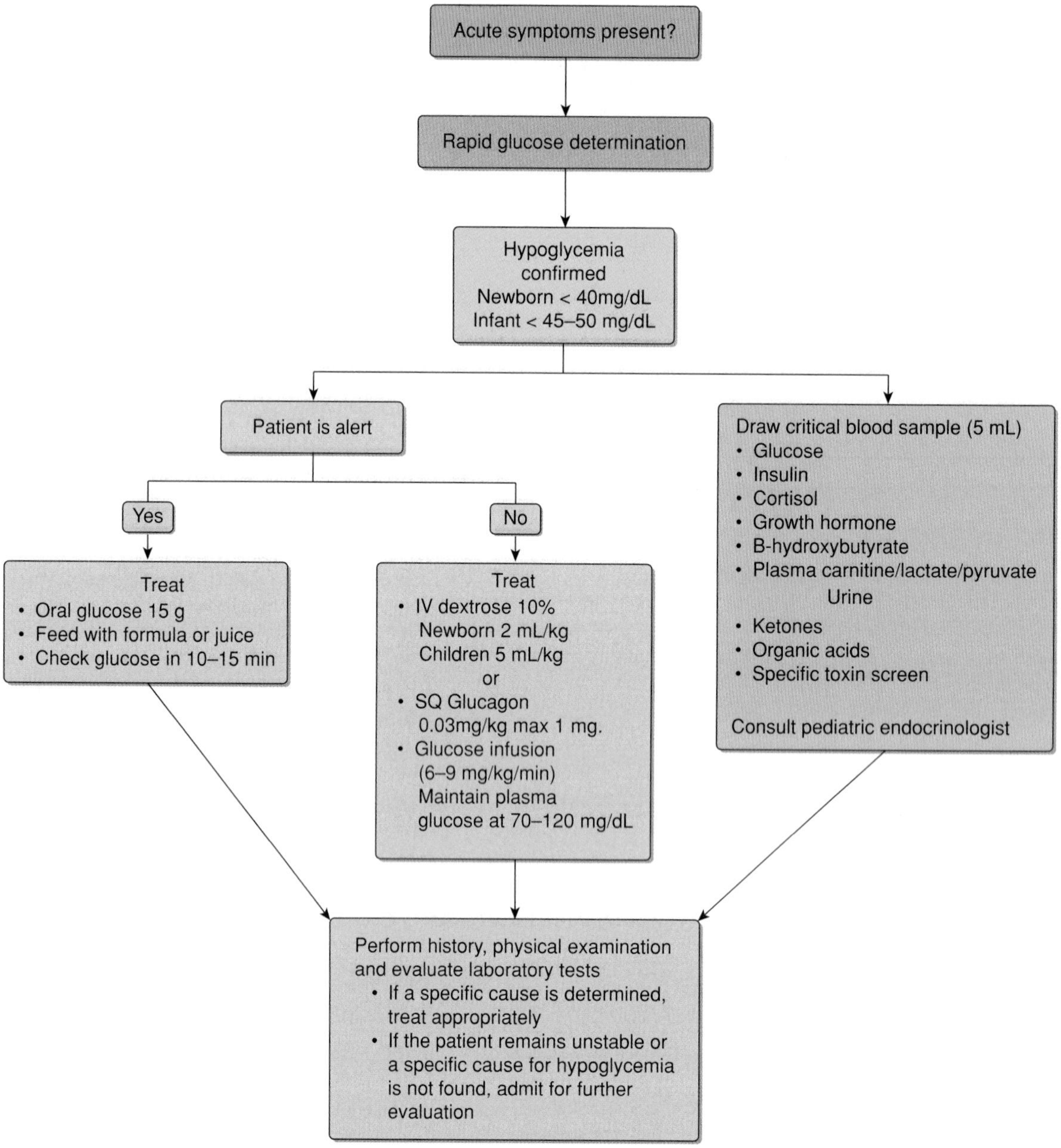

Figure 76–3. Acute management of hypoglycemia in infants and children.

MANAGEMENT

Maintenance of normal plasma glucose levels (70–120 mg/dL) is a must for preserving CNS function (Fig. 76–3).

PROVIDE ADEQUATE SUBSTRATE

- If the patient is alert, oral glucose 15 g, formula feeds, or juice can be given
- If the patient is not alert, start an IV and take the critical blood sample simultaneously
  - In newborns, give 10% dextrose 2 mL/kg (0.2g/kg) as a bolus, followed by infusion at 6 to 9 mg/kg/min

- In children, give 10% dextrose at 5 mL/kg (0.5 g/kg) as a bolus, followed by continuous infusion at 6 to 9 mg/kg/min
- If an IV line is not possible, then give glucagon 0.03 mg/kg (maximum dose 1 mg) subcutaneously
- If the history, physical examination, and laboratory tests suggest a specific cause for hypoglycemia, then the following drugs may be given as appropriate:
  - Growth hormone 0.1 mg/kg/dose
  - Hydrocortisone 5 mg/kg/dose po
  - Diazoxide 10 to 20 mg/kg/day po
  - Somatostatin (Octreotide) 2 to 4 μg/kg/d divided into 2 to 4 doses SQ/IV
  - Carnitine 100 mg/kg/d

DISPOSITION

Admission of the patient is indicated when there is no obvious cause, toxic ingestion as with oral hypoglycemic agents is suspected, administration of long-acting insulin was the cause, and if there are persistent neurological deficits. Discharge may be considered after a high carbohydrate meal if an obvious cause is found and treated with rapid reversal of symptoms. For all insulin-dependent diabetics with hypoglycemia, discharge should be coordinated with a pediatric endocrinologist and the child's family after appropriate adjustment of insulin dose.

REFERENCES

1. Wolfsdorf J, Glaser N, Sperling MA. Diabetic ketoacidosis in infants, children, and adolescents: a consensus statement from the American Diabetes Association. *Diabetes Care.* 2006;29(5):1150–1159.
2. Rewers A, Chase HP, Mackenzie T, et al. Predictors of acute complications in children with type 1 diabetes. *JAMA.* 2002;287(19):2511–2518.
3. Rosilio M, Cotton JB, Wieliczko MC, et al. Factors associated with glycemic control. A cross-sectional nationwide study in 2,579 French children with type 1 diabetes. The French Pediatric Diabetes Group. *Diabetes Care.* 1998;21(7):1146–1153.
4. Smith CP, Firth D, Bennett S, Howard C, Chisholm P. Ketoacidosis occurring in newly diagnosed and established diabetic children. *Acta Paediatr.* 1998;87(5):537–541.
5. Hanas R, Lindgren F, Lindblad B. Diabetic ketoacidosis and cerebral oedema in Sweden—a 2-year paediatric population study. *Diabet Med.* 2007;24(10):1080–1085.
6. Hanas R, Ludvigsson J. Hypoglycemia and ketoacidosis with insulin pump therapy in children and adolescents. *Pediatr Diabetes.* 2006;7(suppl 4):32–38.
7. Keen H. The diabetes control and complications trial (DCCT). *Health Trends.* 1994;26(2):41–43.
8. Dunger DB, Sperling MA, Acerini CL, et al. European Society for Paediatric Endocrinology/Lawson Wilkins Pediatric Endocrine Society consensus statement on diabetic ketoacidosis in children and adolescents. *Pediatrics.* 2004;113(2): e133–e140.
9. Chase HP, Garg SK, Jelley DH. Diabetic ketoacidosis in children and the role of outpatient management. *Pediatr Rev.* 1990;11(10):297–304.
10. Kitabchi AE, Umpierrez GE, Murphy MB, et al. Management of hyperglycemic crises in patients with diabetes. *Diabetes Care.* 2001;24(1):131–153.
11. Malone JI, Brodsky SJ. The value of electrocardiogram monitoring in diabetic ketoacidosis. *Diabetes Care.* 1980;3(4):543–547.
12. Atchley DW, Loeb RF, Richards DW, Benedict EM, Driscoll ME. On diabetic acidosis: a detailed study of electrolyte balances following the withdrawal and reestablishment of insulin therapy. *J Clin Invest.* 1933;12(2):297–326.
13. Nabarro JD, Spencer AG, Stowers JM. Metabolic studies in severe diabetic ketosis. *Q J Med.* 1952;21(82):225–248.
14. Koves IH, Neutze J, Donath S, et al. The accuracy of clinical assessment of dehydration during diabetic ketoacidosis in childhood. *Diabetes Care.* 2004;27(10):2485–2487.
15. Brown TB. Cerebral oedema in childhood diabetic ketoacidosis: is treatment a factor? *Emerg Med J.* 2004;21(2):141–144.
16. Harris GD, Fiordalisi I. Physiologic management of DKA. *Arch Dis Child.* 2002;87(5):451–452.
17. Hale PM, Rezvani I, Braunstein AW, Lipman TH, Martinez N, Garibaldi L. Factors predicting cerebral edema in young children with diabetic ketoacidosis and new onset type I diabetes. *Acta Paediatr.* 1997;86(6):626–631.
18. Rother KI, Schwenk WF. Effect of rehydration fluid with 75 mmol/L of sodium on serum sodium concentration and serum osmolality in young patients with diabetic ketoacidosis. *Mayo Clin Proc.* 1994;69(12):1149–1153.
19. Friedman AL. Pediatric hydration therapy: historical review and a new approach. *Kidney Int.* 2005;67(1):380–388.
20. Waldhausl W, Kleinberger G, Korn A, Dudczak R, Bratusch-Marrain P, Nowotny P. Severe hyperglycemia: effects of rehydration on endocrine derangements and blood glucose concentration. *Diabetes.* 1979;28(6):577–584.
21. Owen OE, Licht JH, Sapir DG. Renal function and effects of partial rehydration during diabetic ketoacidosis. *Diabetes.* 1981;30(6):510–518.
22. Kitabchi AE. Low-dose insulin therapy in diabetic ketoacidosis: fact or fiction? *Diabetes Metab Rev.* 1989;5(4):337–363.
23. Dunger DB, Edge JA. Predicting cerebral edema during diabetic ketoacidosis. *N Engl J Med.* 2001;344(4):302–303.
24. Edge JA, Jakes RW, Roy Y, et al. The UK case-control study of cerebral oedema complicating diabetic ketoacidosis in children. *Diabetologia.* 2006;49(9):2002–2009.
25. Fisher JN, Shahshahani MN, Kitabchi AE. Diabetic ketoacidosis: low-dose insulin therapy by various routes. *N Engl J Med.* 1977;297(5):238–241.
26. Wolfsdorf J, Craig ME, Daneman D, et al. Diabetic ketoacidosis. *Pediatr Diabetes.* 2007;8(1):28–43.
27. Adrogue HJ, Lederer ED, Suki WN, Eknoyan G. Determinants of plasma potassium levels in diabetic ketoacidosis. *Medicine (Baltimore).* 1986;65(3):163–172.
28. DeFronzo RA, Felig P, Ferrannini E, Wahren J. Effect of graded doses of insulin on splanchnic and peripheral potassium metabolism in man. *Am J Physiol.* 1980;238(5):E421–E427.
29. Katz MA. Hyperglycemia-induced hyponatremia—calculation of expected serum sodium depression. *N Engl J Med.* 1973; 289(16):843–844.
30. Hillier TA, Abbott RD, Barrett EJ. Hyponatremia: evaluating the correction factor for hyperglycemia. *Am J Med.* 1999;106(4): 399–403.
31. Harris GD, Fiordalisi I, Harris WL, Mosovich LL, Finberg L. Minimizing the risk of brain herniation during treatment of diabetic ketoacidemia: a retrospective and prospective study. *J Pediatr.* 1990;117(1)(Pt 1):22–31.
32. Duck SC, Wyatt DT. Factors associated with brain herniation in the treatment of diabetic ketoacidosis. *J Pediatr.* 1988;113(1) (Pt 1):10–14.
33. Gibby OM, Veale KE, Hayes TM, Jones JG, Wardrop CA. Oxygen availability from the blood and the effect of phosphate replacement on erythrocyte 2,3-diphosphoglycerate and haemoglobin-oxygen affinity in diabetic ketoacidosis. *Diabetologia.* 1978;15(5):381–385.
34. Wilson HK, Keuer SP, Lea AS, Boyd AE III, Eknoyan G. Phosphate therapy in diabetic ketoacidosis. *Arch Intern Med.* 1982;142(3):517–520.
35. Zipf WB, Bacon GE, Spencer ML, Kelch RP, Hopwood NJ, Hawker CD. Hypocalcemia, hypomagnesemia, and transient hypoparathyroidism during therapy with potassium phosphate in diabetic ketoacidosis. *Diabetes Care.* 1979;2(3):265–268.
36. Winter RJ, Harris CJ, Phillips LS, Green OC. Diabetic ketoacidosis. Induction of hypocalcemia and hypomagnesemia by phosphate therapy. *Am J Med.* 1979;67(5):897–900.
37. Hale PJ, Crase J, Nattrass M. Metabolic effects of bicarbonate in the treatment of diabetic ketoacidosis. *Br Med J (Clin Res Ed).* 1984;289(6451):1035–1038.

38. Green SM, Rothrock SG, Ho JD, et al. Failure of adjunctive bicarbonate to improve outcome in severe pediatric diabetic ketoacidosis. *Ann Emerg Med.* 1998;31(1):41–48.

39. Assal JP, Aoki TT, Manzano FM, Kozak GP. Metabolic effects of sodium bicarbonate in management of diabetic ketoacidosis. *Diabetes.* 1974;23(5):405–411.

40. Soler NG, Bennett MA, Dixon K, FitzGerald MG, Malins JM. Potassium balance during treatment of diabetic ketoacidosis with special reference to the use of bicarbonate. *Lancet.* 1972;2(7779):665–667.

41. Edge JA, Hawkins MM, Winter DL, Dunger DB. The risk and outcome of cerebral oedema developing during diabetic ketoacidosis. *Arch Dis Child.* 2001;85(1):16–22.

42. Glaser N, Barnett P, McCaslin I, et al. Risk factors for cerebral edema in children with diabetic ketoacidosis. The Pediatric Emergency Medicine Collaborative Research Committee of the American Academy of Pediatrics. *N Engl J Med.* 2001;344(4):264–269.

43. Rosenbloom AL. Intracerebral crises during treatment of diabetic ketoacidosis. *Diabetes Care.* 1990;13(1):22–33.

44. Bello FA, Sotos JF. Cerebral oedema in diabetic ketoacidosis in children. *Lancet.* 1990;336(8706):64.

45. Muir AB, Quisling RG, Yang MC, Rosenbloom AL. Cerebral edema in childhood diabetic ketoacidosis: natural history, radiographic findings, and early identification. *Diabetes Care.* 2004;27(7):1541–1546.

46. Franklin B, Liu J, Ginsberg-Fellner F. Cerebral edema and ophthalmoplegia reversed by mannitol in a new case of insulin-dependent diabetes mellitus. *Pediatrics.* 1982;69(1):87–90.

47. Shabbir N, Oberfield SE, Corrales R, Kairam R, Levine LS. Recovery from symptomatic brain swelling in diabetic ketoacidosis. *Clin Pediatr (Phila).* 1992;31(9):570–573.

48. Curtis JR, Bohn D, Daneman D. Use of hypertonic saline in the treatment of cerebral edema in diabetic ketoacidosis (DKA). *Pediatr Diabetes.* 2001;2(4):191–194.

49. Marcin JP, Glaser N, Barnett P, et al. Factors associated with adverse outcomes in children with diabetic ketoacidosis-related cerebral edema. *J Pediatr.* 2002;141(6):793–797.

50. Monroe KW, King W, Atchison JA. Use of PRISM scores in triage of pediatric patients with diabetic ketoacidosis. *Am J Manag Care.* 1997;3(2):253–258.

51. Cornblath M. Neonatal hypoglycemia 30 years later: does it injure the brain? Historical summary and present challenges. *Acta Paediatr Jpn.* 1997;39(suppl 1):S7-S11.

52. Haymond MW, Karl IE, Clarke WL, Pagliara AS, Santiago JV. Differences in circulating gluconeogenic substrates during short-term fasting in men, women, and children. *Metabolism.* 1982;31(1):33–42.

53. Chaussain JL, Georges P, Calzada L, Job JC. Glycemic response to 24-hour fast in normal children: III. Influence of age. *J Pediatr.* 1977;91(5):711–714.

54. Pildes RS, Cornblath M, Warren I, et al. A prospective controlled study of neonatal hypoglycemia. *Pediatrics.* 1974;54(1):5–14.

55. Anderson JM, Milner RD, Strich SJ. Effects of neonatal hypoglycaemia on the nervous system: a pathological study. *J Neurol Neurosurg Psychiatry.* 1967;30(4):295–310.

56. Becker DJ, Ryan CM. Hypoglycemia: a complication of diabetes therapy in children. *Trends Endocrinol Metab.* 2000;11(5):198–202.

57. Ryan C, Gurtunca N, Becker D. Hypoglycemia: a complication of diabetes therapy in children. *Pediatr Clin North Am.* 2005;52(6):1705–1733.

58. Haymond MW. Hypoglycemia in infants and children. *Endocrinol Metab Clin North Am.* 1989;18(1):211–252.

CHAPTER 77

Adrenal Insufficiency

Nicholas Furtado

▶ HIGH-YIELD FACTS

- Adrenal insufficiency (AI) results from deficiency of glucocorticoid (cortisol) and mineralocorticoid (aldosterone) secreted by the adrenal cortex.
- Glucocorticoid deficiency impairs gluconeogenesis and glycogenolysis, resulting in fasting hypoglycemia.
- Aldosterone deficiency results in decreased sodium retention by the kidney and distal renal tubular exchange of potassium and hydrogen ions for sodium, resulting in osmotic diuresis, hyponatremia, hypovolemia, hyperkalemia, acidosis, and prerenal azotemia.
- AI is classified into primary (adrenocortical failure itself), secondary (pituitary), or tertiary (hypothalamic) types. AI, because of withdrawal from exogenous steroid administration, is the most common cause of adrenal crisis.
- Symptoms of AI are usually nonspecific such as fatigue, anorexia, abdominal pain, nausea, or diarrhea but it can present as cardiovascular collapse or shock and hence a high index of suspicion is required.
- The most common cause of primary AI in infants is congenital adrenal hyperplasia (CAH).
- Acquired causes of primary AI in children are less common than congenital disorders.
- Acquired AI results from autoimmune, infectious, infiltrative, hemorrhagic, or toxic causes.
- Acute management consists of rapid fluid resuscitation, correction of hypoglycemia, hyperkalemia, and acidosis and stress doses of hydrocortisone (50–75 mg/m^2 IV).

The adrenal cortex produces two main hormones: glucocortcoid (cortisol) and mineralocorticoid (aldosterone). AI is a clinical state that results from the inability of the adrenal cortex to produce these hormones in response to stress.

▶ PATHOPHYSIOLOGY

Primary AI results from congenital or acquired adrenal gland dysfunction. Secondary and tertiary AI result from pituitary or hypothalamic underfunction, respectively. Glucocorticoid deficiency impairs gluconeogenesis and glycogenolysis, and decreases the sensitivity of the vascular system to angiotensin II and norepinephrine, resulting in hypoglycemia, tachycardia, and mild hypotension. Aldosterone deficiency causes decreased sodium retention by the kidney, osmotic diuresis, hyponatremia, hypovolemia, and dehydration. In addition, it causes a decreased distal renal tubular exchange of potassium and hydrogen ions for sodium ions, leading to hyperkalemia and acidosis. Androgen deficiency in primary AI leads to ambiguous genitalia and underdeveloped secondary sexual characteristics in prepubertal children. In addition, in primary AI, the lack of negative feedback from cortisol on the anterior pituitary causes oversecretion of ACTH and propiomelanocortin that in turn stimulate skin hyperpigmentation (Fig. 77–1).

▶ ETIOLOGY AND EPIDEMIOLOGY

The commonest cause of AI in North America is the abrupt withdrawal of glucocorticoids while on chronic treatment.[1] Children who have been on glucocorticoid therapy for 2 to 4 weeks tend to have prolonged suppression of the hypothalamopituitary axis leading to secondary AI after treatment is stopped.[2] The most common cause of primary AI in children is CAH, with an incidence of 1 in 10 000 to 18 000 live births.[3] In long-term studies of children with AI, most have primary AI and, of these, approximately 72% are found to have CAH.[4,5]

CAH results from a deficiency in the enzymatic activity of one of the enzymes in the cortisol biosynthetic pathway, the commonest being 21-hydroxylase deficiency. Mortality for CAH is five times that of the general population but this has improved with the present recommendation for universal screening of newborns.[6,7] Other rarer forms of congenital primary AI are congenital adrenal hypoplasia, adrenal aplasia or hemorrhage associated with a traumatic delivery,[8] familial isolated glucocorticoid deficiency, the "triple A syndrome," consisting of AI, alacrima, and achalasia of the esophagus, and adrenoleukodystrophy (ALD) (Table 77–1).

Acquired causes of primary AI in children are less common than congenital disorders and result from autoimmune, infectious, infiltrative, hemorrhagic, or ablative disorders of the adrenal cortex. Granulomatous, degenerative, or storage diseases that involve the adrenal gland, such as tuberculosis, histoplasmosis, or lysosomal acid lipase deficiency (Wolman's disease), also cause acquired primary AI. The most common cause of this is autoimmune adrenalitis, which accounts for 80% of all cases. Acute AI in fulminating sepsis or

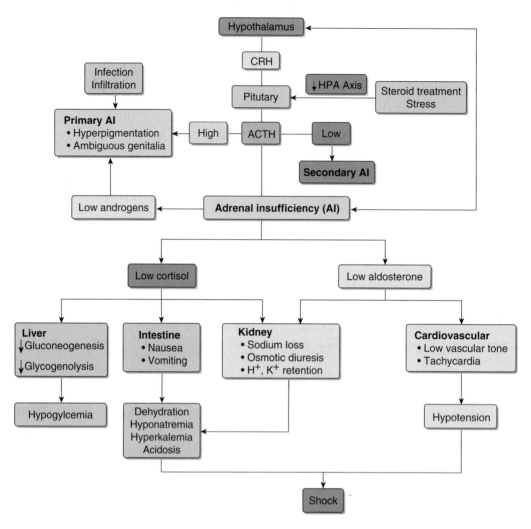

Figure 77-1. Pathophysiology of adrenal insufficiency.

meningococcemia may be indicated by catecholamine resistant shock and low plasma cortisol levels.[9–11]

Secondary AI that is not because of pharmacologic glucocorticoid withdrawal can result from any process that interferes with the pituitary's ability to secrete ACTH, such as tumors, craniopharyngioma, infections, infiltrative diseases of the pituitary, lymphocytic hypophysitis, head trauma, and intracranial aneurysms (Table 77–1). Most of these coexist with other pituitary hormone deficiencies and there is history of pituitary insult or abnormality of the hypothalamopituitary axis on MRI.[12]

▶ CLINICAL PRESENTATION

AI can present with vague and nonspecific symptoms (Table 77–2) and diagnosis is delayed in many cases.[5] Acute insufficiency or Addison's crisis is typically encountered in a previously undiagnosed child who has been subjected to the stress of an acute illness, inadequate administration of stress steroid dosing in known cases, or abrupt withdrawal in the context of prolonged steroid therapy. In all these clinical situations, the presentation is characterized by dehydration, hypotension, hypoglycemia, or altered sensorium. Hypoglycemia occurs most commonly in young children.

Physical clues to AI include hyperpigmentation of the face, neck, hands, areas subject to friction such as elbows, knees, and knuckles, the buccal mucosa, areolae, scars, and moles (Fig. 77–2).[13] Other skin findings are vitiligo, secondary to autoimmune melanocyte destruction, and chronic mucocutaneous candidiasis, as part of autoimmune polyendocrinopathy type 1. In the absence of history of steroid withdrawal, secondary AI is usually associated with signs of other pituitary hormone deficiencies such as growth failure, delayed puberty, secondary hypothyroidism, and diabetes insipidus.[13]

▶ TABLE 77-1. ETIOLOGY OF ADRENAL INSUFFICIENCY IN CHILDREN

Primary	Secondary
Congenital	Hypothalamus Congenital
Congenital–adrenal hyperplasia	Septooptic dysplasia
Congenital–adrenal hypoplasia	CRH deficiency
Triple A	Maternal hypocortisolemia acquired
ACTH resistance	Steroid withdrawal after chronic use
Glucocorticoid resistance	Inflammatory disorders
Metabolic diseases	Trauma
Adrenoleukodystrophy	Cranial radiation therapy
Zellweger	Surgery
Smith-Lemli-Opitz	Tumors
Wolman	Infiltrative disease
Mitochondrial disease	Pituitary Congenital
Kearnes–Sayre syndrome	Aplasia/hypoplasia
Acquired	Multiple anterior pituitary hormone deficiency
Autoimmune adrenalitis	Isolated ACTH deficiency acquired
Isolated	Steroid withdrawal
Autoimmune polyendocrinopathy I and II	Trauma
Hemorrhage/infarction	Craniopharyngioma
Trauma	Radiation therapy
Waterhouse Frederichsen syndrome	Lymphocytic hypophysitis
Anticoagulation	
Drugs	
Etomidate, ketoconazole, rifampin, phenytoin,	
medroxyprogesterone, barbiturates	
Infections	
HIV, CMV, tuberculosis, blastomycosis,	
coccidiomycosis, histoplasmosis.	
Infiltrative	
Hemocromatosis, sarcoidosis, histiocytosis,	
amyloidosis, neoplasm	

▶ TABLE 77-2. SIGNS AND SYMPTOMS OF ADRENAL INSUFFICIENCY

Cortisol Deficiency (Serum Level < 10 μg/dL)	Aldosterone Deficiency
Weakness and fatigability	Hyponatremia
Weight loss	Hyperkalemia
Hypotension	Dehydration
Shock	Prerenal azotemia
Gastroentestinal problems (nausea, vomiting, diarrhea, abdominal pain)	Acidosis
	Androgen excess in CAH
	Virilization
Hyperpigmentation	Ambiguous genitalia (clitoromegaly, fused labia majora)
Hypoglycemia	
Anemia	Cryptorchidism
Eosiniphilia	
Mild hyponatremia	
High ACTH levels (>100 pg/mL)	

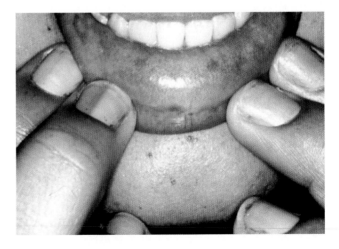

Figure 77-2. Skin, nail, and mucosal changes in primary adrenal insufficiency.

In the rare case of missed neonatal screening for CAH, ambiguous genitalia may be present (Fig. 77–3).

▶ LABORATORY FINDINGS

Laboratory findings and common abnormalities of AI are based on the pathophysiology (Fig. 77–1) and summarized in Table 77–2 above. The diagnosis of primary AI is confirmed by the documentation of an elevated plasma ACTH level (>100 picogram/mL) and a low serum cortisol level (<10μg/dL).[13] Mineralocorticoid deficiency is confirmed by documentation of low aldosterone levels associated with hyperemia with or without hyperkalemia and hyponatremia.[13] Secondary AI is diagnosed by documenting simultaneously low blood ACTH and cortisol levels.

▶ DIFFERENTIAL DIAGNOSIS

The differential diagnosis of acute AI must include all causes of hyponatremia, hyperkalemia, ketotic hypoglycemia, and shock in children and is summarized in Table 77–3.

▶ MANAGEMENT

Recognizing adrenal crisis immediately requires a high index of suspicion and is warranted in children presenting with unexplained shock and hypoglycemia. The patient's airway should be stabilized, the child placed on continuous cardiac monitoring, and rapid fluid resuscitation is started with 5% dextrose and normal saline. If sepsis is suspected, appropriate culture samples should be taken and antibiotics administered. If there is no previous history of AI, prior to specific treatment, a critical blood sample must be collected for ACTH, cortisol, aldosterone, and plasma renin activity. If CAH is suspected, 17-hydroxyprogesterone and androgen levels should also be requested. Correction of specific disturbances such as hypoglycemia, hypokalemia, and the administration of stress doses of hydrocortisone are outlined in the clinical pathway in Figure 77–4.

▶ DISPOSITION

All patients presenting to an emergency department in acute adrenal crisis must be admitted to the pediatric intensive care unit for continued parenteral fluid replacement and steroid maintenance therapy. A pediatric endocrinologist must be consulted for further inpatient evaluation, management, and continuity of care. Children with known AI and mild symptoms may be managed as an outpatient with consultation and close follow-up with their pediatric endocrinologist.

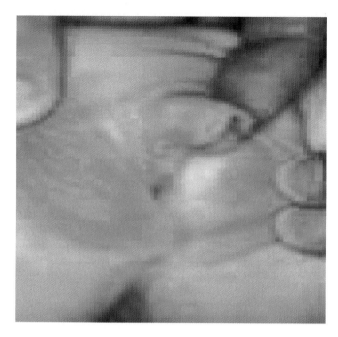

Figure 77–3. Clitoromegaly in a neonate with congenital adrenal hyperplasia.

▶ TABLE 77–3. DIFFERENTIAL DIAGNOSIS OF ACUTE ADRENAL INSUFFICIENCY

Hyponatremia	Hypoglycemia
Excessive intake of free water	Growth hormone deficiency
Psychogenic polydipsia	Ketotic hypoglycemia
Water enemas	Inborn errors of carbohydrate metabolism
Overhydration	Liver disease
Decreased water output	
Cardiac failure	
Renal failure	
Liver failure	
SIADH	
Sodium deficiency states	
GI losses	
Cerebral salt wasting	
Decreased intake	
Third spacing	
Burns	
Trauma	
Malnutrition	
Hyperkalemia	Shock
Renal disease	Sepsis
Trauma	Hypovolemic shock, dehydration
Burns	Cardiogenic shock
Iatrogenic	

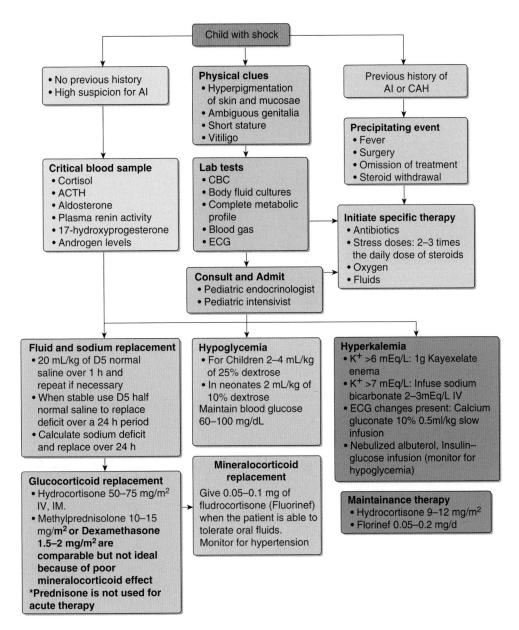

Figure 77–4. Clinical pathway for management of acute adrenal insufficiency.

REFERENCES

1. Arlt W, Allolio B. Adrenal insufficiency. *Lancet.* 2003; 361(9372):1881–1893.
2. Root A, Shulman DI. Clinical adrenal disorders. In: Pescovitz OEE, ed. *Pediatric Endocrinology, Mechanisms, Manifestations, and Management.* Philadelphia, PA: Lippincott Williams & Wilkins; 2004;568–600.
3. Kovacs J, Votava F, Heinze G, et al. Lessons from 30 years of clinical diagnosis and treatment of congenital adrenal hyperplasia in five middle European countries. *J Clin Endocrinol Metab.* 2001;86(7):2958–2964.
4. Perry R, Kecha O, Paquette J, Huot C, Van Vliet G, Deal C. Primary adrenal insufficiency in children: twenty years experience at the sainte-justine hospital, montreal. *J Clin Endocrinol Metab.* 2005;90(6):3243–3250.
5. Simm PJ, McDonnell CM, Zacharin MR. Primary adrenal insufficiency in childhood and adolescence: advances in diagnosis and management. *J Paediatr Child Health.* 2004;40(11):596–599.
6. Swerdlow AJ, Higgins CD, Brook CG, et al. Mortality in patients with congenital adrenal hyperplasia: a cohort study. *J Pediatr.* 1998;133(4):516–520.
7. White PC, Speiser PW. Congenital adrenal hyperplasia due to 21-hydroxylase deficiency. *Endocrine Rev.* 2000;21(3):245–291.
8. Velaphi SC, Perlman JM. Neonatal adrenal hemorrhage: clinical and abdominal sonographic findings. *Clin Pediatr (Phila).* 2001;40(10):545–548.

9. Riordan FA, Thomson AP, Ratcliffe JM, Sills JA, Diver MJ, Hart CA. Admission cortisol and adrenocorticotrophic hormone levels in children with meningococcal disease: evidence of adrenal insufficiency? *Crit Care Med.* 1999;27(10):2257–2261.

10. Pizarro CF, Troster EJ, Damiani D, Carcillo JA. Absolute and relative adrenal insufficiency in children with septic shock. *Crit Care Med.* 2005;33(4):855–859.

11. Pizarro CF, Troster EJ. Adrenal function in sepsis and septic shock. *J Pediatr (Rio J).* 2007;83(5 suppl):S155–S162.

12. Walvoord EC, Rosenman MB, Eugster EA. Prevalence of adrenocorticotropin deficiency in children with idiopathic growth hormone deficiency. *J Clin Endocrinol Metab.* 2004;89(10):5030–5034.

13. Shulman DI, Palmert MR, Kemp SF. Adrenal insufficiency: still a cause of morbidity and death in childhood. *Pediatrics.* 2007;119(2):e484–e494.

14. Castillo L, Chernow B. Endocrine disorders. In: Holbrook P, ed. *Textbook of Pediatric Critical care.* Philadelphia, PA: W. B. Saunders; 1993.

CHAPTER 78

Hyperthyroidism

Nicholas Furtado

▶ HIGH-YIELD FACTS

- Thyrotoxicosis is a hypermetabolic clinical state of thyroid hormone excess either caused by overproduction of thyroid hormone by the thyroid gland or by administration of exogenous synthetic hormone.
- The most common disorder causing thyrotoxicosis in children is Graves' disease.
- Thyroid hormones upregulate β-adrenergic receptors causing symptoms of sympathetic nervous system overactivity.
- Signs of sympathetic hyperactivity include tremor, brisk deep tendon reflexes, tachycardia, supraventricular tachycardia, flow murmur, overactive precordium, and a widened pulse pressure. Other cardiac disturbances such as atrial fibrillation and congestive heart failure (CHF) may also occur.
- Precipitating factors for thyroid storm in a patient with hyperthyroidism are thyroid surgery, withdrawal of antithyroid medications, radioiodine therapy, palpation of a goiter, iodinated contrast dyes, and stress.
- Physical findings in Graves' disease, such as eye signs, are usually subtle in children.
- Thyroid storm is suggested by severe hyperpyrexia, atrial dysrhythmia, CHF, delirium or psychosis, severe gastrointestinal hyperactivity, and hepatic dysfunction with jaundice.
- Treatment consists of antithyroid drugs propylthiouracil (PTU) at a dosage of 175 mg/m^2/d or 4 to 6 mg/kg/d at 6- or 8-hour intervals, iodine therapy started 1 hour after antithyroid medication is initiated, β-adrenergic blockade with propranolol, 10 to 20 mg every 12 to 8 hours, and supportive management.

Hyperthyroidism is a state of increased production and secretion of thyroid hormones resulting in the hypermetabolic clinical syndrome of thyrotoxicosis. The term thyroid storm refers to an extreme state of decompensated thyrotoxicosis and is a thyroid emergency that can be potentially fatal.

▶ EPIDEMIOLOGY

The most common cause of hyperthyroidism in children is Graves' disease. This disease occurs in 1 in 5000 children with a peak incidence between 11 and 15 years of age. The male to female ratio is 1:5.[1] Although the true incidence of childhood thyrotoxicosis is unknown, 5% of all thyrotoxicosis occurs in childhood[2] and 0.6% to 10% of neonates born to mothers with Graves' disease will show signs of thyrotoxicosis.[3] The reported mortality in neonatal thyrotoxicosis is as high as 20%.[4]

Because childhood hyperthyroidism occurs mostly in adolescents, thyroid storm also occurs more frequently in this group.[2] (Figure 78–1).

▶ PATHOPHYSIOLOGY

Thyrotoxicosis results from thyroid hormone excess either caused by overproduction of thyroid hormone by the thyroid gland or by administration of synthetic hormone. Increased concentration of serum free thyroid hormone is almost always found in thyrotoxicosis. In Graves' disease, activated B-lymphocytes produce antibodies against antigen shared by the thyroid gland and eye muscle.[1,5] Thyrotropin receptor-stimulating antibodies (TRSAb) bind to TSH receptors to increase thyroid hormone production. In congenital hyperthyroidism, transplacental transfer of TRSAb from the mother with Graves' disease stimulates the thyroid gland to cause hyperthyroidism or thyrotoxicoxis.[1,3,4]

The actions of thyroid hormone at the cellular level include calorigenesis, acceleration of substrate turnover, amino acid, and lipid metabolism and stimulation of water and ion transport. Thyroid hormones also activate the adrenergic system by upregulation of β-adrenergic receptors causing symptoms of sympathetic nervous system overactivity, including hyperthermia. Why some individuals with hyperthyroidism have few symptoms and others develop the most extreme clinical manifestation of thyroid hormone excess, thyroid storm, is still poorly understood. In thyroid storm, the clinical manifestations of thyroid hormone excess are thought to be because of an uncoupling of oxidative phosphorylation secondary to the illness, resulting in an enhanced rate of lipolysis, with fatty acid oxidation, increased oxygen consumption, calorigenisis, and hyperthermia. Specific conditions such as thyroid surgery, withdrawal of antithyroid medications, radioiodine therapy, palpation of a generous goiter, and iodinated contrast dyes are known to precipitate thyroid storm in a patient with hyperthyroidism.

▶ ETIOLOGY

The causes of thyrotoxicosis may be divided into conditions in which the source of excess thyroid hormone is endogenous or exogenous (Table 78–1). The most common disorder causing thyrotoxicosis in children, as in adults, is the autoimmune disorder, Graves' disease.[2,6,7] In 5% to 10% of thyrotoxicosis, the cause is autoimmune thyroiditis or hashitoxicosis. In an even smaller percentage of patients, subacute thyroiditis

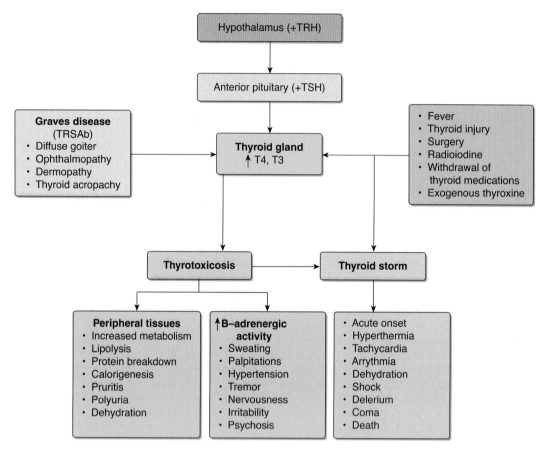

Figure 78–1. Etiology and pathophysiology of thyrotoxicosis and thyroid storm.

▶ **TABLE 78–1. ETIOLOGY OF HYPERTHYROIDISM**

Increased Endogenous Thyroid Hormone	Increase in Exogenous Thyroid Hormone
Autoimmune thyroid disease	Exogenous thyroid hormone intake
Graves' disease (commonest cause)	Excessive replacement therapy
Hashitoxicosis	Intentional suppressive therapy with thyroxine
Neonatal or congenital hyperthyroidism	Factitious hyperthyroidism (Munchausen's
Autonomous thyroid tissue	syndrome)
Toxic adenoma	
Toxic multinodular goiter	
McCune–Albright syndrome	
TSH-mediated hyperthyroidism	
TSH-producing pituitary adenoma	
Human chorionic gonadotropin-mediated	
hyperthyroidism	
hydatidiform mole	
Hyperthyroidism because of subacute thyroiditis	
Subacute lymphocytic thyroiditis	
Amiodarone (iodine-induced hyperthyroidism)	
Radiation thyroiditis	
Palpation thyroiditis	

can cause thyrotoxicosis because of destruction of thyroid tissue. This process is usually because of viral or granulomatous diseases, classically presents with a painful thyroid gland and is self-limiting. Autonomously functioning thyroid nodules (toxic adenoma) are sometimes encountered in children.[1] Multinodular goiters with thyrotoxicosis are unusual in childhood. Rarely, hyperthyroidism is secondary to TSH over-secretion from a pituitary tumor or because of isolated pituitary resistance to negative feedback control by thyroid hormones on a genetic basis. The possibility of a molar pregnancy, which produces a thyroid stimulating hormone, must be considered in adolescent females with thyrotoxicosis.[8] Administration of iodine-containing medications, such as dyes, to patients with a nodular goiter may rarely induce hyperthyroidism in Hashimoto's thyroiditis, endemic goiter, multinodular goiter, and nontoxic diffuse goiter. Finally, thyrotoxicosis can occur as the result of intentional excess thyroxine or triiodothyronine intake or it can be because of overtreatment.

▶ CLINICAL PRESENTATION

Children who present with thyrotoxicosis have symptoms of nervousness, palpitations, weight loss, muscle weakness, and fatigue. A history of developmental delay and declining school performance may be found.[9] Other symptoms include tremulousness, anxiety, excessive sweating, temperature intolerance, and emotional lability. Gastrointestinal overactivity with symptoms of frequent stools is common. An increased appetite is classically present. However, an apathetic state, including decreased appetite, occasionally occurs.

The signs of Graves' disease are similar to those seen in adults but the ophthalmologic signs are usually milder in children.[10,11] Signs of sympathetic and cardiac overactivity are common. These include tremor, brisk deep tendon reflexes, tachycardia, supraventricular tachycardia, flow murmur, overactive precordium, and a widened pulse pressure. Other cardiac atrioventricular conduction disturbances may occur, such as atrial fibrillation, atrioventricular block, or sinoatrial block. CHF may develop because of the inability of cardiac function to meet metabolic demands and papillary muscle dysfunction, causing mitral valve prolapse, may occur.[12,13] Except in neonates and children with underlying cardiac disease, CHF is uncommon in childhood thyrotoxicosis. In thyroid storm, severe hyperpyrexia, atrial dysrhythmia and CHF, delirium or psychosis, severe gastrointestinal hyperactivity, and hepatic dysfunction with jaundice are present.[14]. A history of a precipitating event, illness, or major stress, should be identified.

▶ DIFFERENTIAL DIAGNOSIS

Conditions that cause tachydysrhythmias (atrial flutter, atrial fibrillation, and ventricular tachycardia) must be differentiated from hyperthyroidism.[15] These include electrolyte disturbances and cardiac disease. The murmur of mitral valve prolapse in association with tachycardia may lead to a mistaken diagnosis of CHF and cardiac valvular disease. The patient who is febrile and appears "toxic" may have sepsis alone or as a precipitating factor in thyroid storm. Intoxication with adrenergic and anticholinergic drugs may also mimic the hypermetabolic

▶ **TABLE 78–2. DIFFERENTIAL DIAGNOSES FOR THYROTOXICOSIS AND THYROID STORM**

Neuropsychiatric	Others
Meningitis	Malignant hyperthermia
Encephalopathy	Septic shock
Psychosis	Toxicity
Anxiety disorder, panic	Adrenergic drug intoxication
disorder	Anticholinergic drug
Cardiovascular	intoxication
Hypertension	
Tachyarrhythmia (Atrial	
fibrillation, SVT)	
Valvular heart disease	
Congestive cardiac	
failure	
Gastrointestinal	
Liver failure	
Severe gastroenteritis	
and dehydration	

state seen in thyrotoxicosis. Gastrointestinal hyperactivity may imitate an acute abdomen in thyroid storm (Table 78–2).

▶ MANAGEMENT

Treatment of severe thyrotoxicosis or thyroid storm is directed at preventing further thyroid hormone synthesis and secretion, alleviating the acute peripheral effects of excess thyroid hormone, and supportive measures.[2–4,6,7,14,16]

Initial laboratory tests should include the measurement of total and free T_4, T_3, and TSH levels, along with a complete metabolic profile.

Blockade of thyroid hormone synthesis should be initiated and continued until the crisis resolves:

- PTU at a dosage of 175 mg/m^2/d or 4 to 6 mg/kg/d divided and given at 6- or 8-hour intervals or 200 mg every 4 hours.
- Methimazole 30 mg every 6 hours.

Blockade of release of thyroid hormone:

- Start 1 to 3 hours after antithyroid medication is initiated.
- Sodium Iodide 0.05 mg IV every 12 hours.
- Lugol's solution (5% iodine) 3 to 5 drops orally every 8 hours.
- Lithium 600 mg oral loading dose followed by 300 mg every 6 hours (do not use with CHF, renal failure, arrythmia).

Inhibition of peripheral T_4 and T_3 conversion:

- Dexamethasone 2 mg IV followed by 2 mg orally every 6 hours.

β-adrenergic antagonists:

- Propranolol 10 to 20 mg orally every 8 hours in children and adolescents.

Hyperthermia:

- Acetaminophen.

- Cooling blankets, ice packs.
- Salicylates must be avoided because they can displace thyroid hormone from binding sites, potentially worsening the hypermetabolic state.

Fluid resuscitation:

- Normal saline, 20 mL/kg, is administered; then the fluid deficit is calculated and replaced in the form of half normal saline with 5% dextrose over the next 24 to 48 hours.

Cardiovascular complications:

- Arrythmias and CHF are treated with antiarrhythmics, digoxin, and diuretics.
- In all cases the precipitating event causing severe thyrotoxicosis must be sought and treated.

▶ TREATMENT OF NEONATAL THYROTOXICOSIS

Neonatal hyperthyroidism, characterized by growth failure, microcephaly, wide-eyed stare and symptoms of tachycardia, and irritability is usually seen a few days after birth; Occasionally, the onset can be delayed by weeks. Neonatal thyrotoxicosis is usually seen in newborns whose mothers are on antithyroid drugs[1]

Antithyroid treatment:

- PTU 5 to 10 mg every 8 hours.
- Iodide drops (sodium or potassium salt) 1 drop every 8 hours orally.
- β-adrenergic blockade.
- Propranolol 2 mg/kg/d every 12 hours.

Supportive measures:

- Treatment of CHF, arrhythmia, airway management, fluid, and caloric replacement.

▶ DISPOSITION

Treatment and disposition of children with thyrotoxicosis should always be undertaken in the consultation with a pedi-atric endocrinologist. Children with severe thyrotoxicosis, thyroid storm, and those with cardiovascular complications, such as arrhythmia, CHF, and shock, should be admitted to a pediatric intensive care unit for further management.

REFERENCES

1. LaFranchi S. Hyperthyroidism. In: Behrman R, Kliegman R, Jenson H, eds. *Nelson Textbook of Pediatrics*. Philadelphia, PA: Saunders; 2004:1884–1887.
2. Madhusmita M. Thyroid Storm. http://www.emedicine.com. 2006;8–22.
3. Zimmerman D. Fetal and neonatal hyperthyroidism. *Thyroid*. 1999;9(7):727–733.
4. Ogilvy-Stuart AL. Neonatal thyroid disorders. *Arch Dis Child Fetal Neonatal Ed*. 2002;87(3):F165–F171.
5. Weetman AP. Graves' disease. *N Engl J Med*. 2000;343(17):1236–1248.
6. LaFranchi S, Hanna CE, Mandel SH. Constitutional delay of growth: expected versus final adult height. *Pediatrics*. 1991;87(1):82–87.
7. Kwon KT, Tsai VW. Metabolic emergencies. *Emerg Med Clin North Am*. 2007;25(4):1041–1060, vi.
8. Misra M, Levitsky LL, Lee MM. Transient hyperthyroidism in an adolescent with hydatidiform mole. *J Pediatr*. 2002;140(3):362–366.
9. Segni M, Leonardi E, Mazzoncini B, Pucarelli I, Pasquino AM. Special features of Graves' disease in early childhood. *Thyroid*. 1999;9(9):871–877.
10. Chan W, Wong GW, Fan DS, Cheng AC, Lam DS, Ng JS. Ophthalmopathy in childhood Graves' disease. *Br J Ophthalmol*. 2002;86(7):740–742.
11. Nordyke RA, Gilbert FI Jr, Harada AS. Graves' disease. Influence of age on clinical findings. *Arch Intern Med*. 1988;148(3):626–631.
12. Klein I. Thyroid hormone and the cardiovascular system. *Am J Med*. 1990;88(6):631–637.
13. Klein I, Danzi S. Thyroid disease and the heart. *Circulation*. 2007;116(15):1725–1735.
14. Burch HB, Wartofsky L. Life-threatening thyrotoxicosis. Thyroid storm. *Endocrinol Metab Clin North Am*. 1993;22(2):263–277.
15. Doniger SJ, Sharieff GQ. Pediatric dysrhythmias. *Pediatr Clin North Am*. 2006;53(1):85–105, vi.
16. Zimmerman D, Gan-Gaisano M. Hyperthyroidism in children and adolescents. *Pediatr Clin North Am*. 1990;37(6):1273–1295.

CHAPTER 79

Rickets

Carla Minutti

▶ HIGH-YIELD FACTS

- Vitamin D deficiency is the major cause of rickets around the world.
- Nutritional rickets continues to be reported in the United States and in other developed nations, especially in minority ethnic groups and immigrants.
- Vitamin D deficiency in childhood and rickets continue to be public health problems in the Middle East, North Africa, and some parts of Asia.
- The recommended adequate intake of vitamin D by the National Academy of Sciences to prevent vitamin D deficiency in normal infants, children, and adolescents is 200 IU/d.
- It is recommended that all infants (breast-fed or not) who are ingesting less than 500 mL/d of vitamin D-fortified formula or milk have a minimum intake of 200 IU of vitamin D per day beginning during the first 2 months of life.
- Other organizations and individuals recommend a daily intake of 400 to 2000 IU of vitamin D daily as a preventive dose, for infants through 18 years of age.
- Vitamin D supplementation is critically important for breast-fed infants and for infants and children living in an inner-city area and those with increased skin pigmentation.

Rickets is defined as the failure of osteoid to calcify in a growing person. Osteomalacia is the failure of osteoid to calcify in the adult.[1] Osteoid is the collagen-containing organic matrix of the bones. Rickets results from vitamin D deficiency or the abnormal metabolism of vitamin D. Vitamin D deficiency is the major cause of rickets around the world.[2,3] Less commonly, deficiency of calcium or phosphorus may produce rickets. In this chapter, we will focus on vitamin D-deficient (nutritional) rickets and will mention some important characteristics of other causes of rickets.

Vitamin D (cholecalciferol or vitamin D_3) is formed in the skin under the stimulus of ultraviolet (UV) light. UV light was the only significant source of vitamin D until ergosterol (vitamin D_2), contained in fish liver oil, was introduced as a dietary supplement in 1918.[4]

Rickets became a public health problem when the factories of the industrial revolution triggered a massive migration to overcrowded cities and produced so much contamination that UV light rays were blocked. Rickets was probably the first childhood disease caused by environmental pollution. Early in the 20th century, vitamin D was named as the factor responsible for causing rickets. Fish liver oil and exposure to sunlight were recognized to have a role in the prevention and treatment of rickets.[5]

After vitamin D was discovered, many public health initiatives were implemented. Education of the population on the importance of sunlight exposure and fortification of dairy and other food products with vitamin D resulted in the eradication of rickets from North America.[4] In the last two or three decades, we have seen a resurgence of rickets, with vitamin D deficiency and several other factors contributing to the resurgence. Nutritional rickets continues to be reported in the United States and other developed nations, especially in minority ethnic groups and immigrants.[2,3,6,7] The exact prevalence in the United States is unknown.[8] The majority of the reported cases occurred in individuals with dark skin and breast-fed infants who did not receive vitamin D supplementation.[8] Vitamin D deficiency in childhood and rickets continue to be public health problems in the Middle East, North Africa, and some parts of Asia.[2,3,6] Vitamin D deficiency is currently a highly prevalent condition among infants, children, and adolescents in the United States and around the world.[8] Relatively high rates of subclinical vitamin D deficiency in infants, children, and adolescents have also been reported in several states in North America.[8]

▶ ETIOLOGY

The causes of rickets are summarized in Table 79–1.

VITAMIN D DEFICIENCY

Studies suggest that vitamin D intake in adults is inadequate to prevent a state of deficiency. Deficiency in adults is defined by most experts as a level less than 20 ng/mL. Insufficiency is defined as levels of 21 to 29 ng/mL and sufficiency as levels of 30 ng/mL or greater.[9,10] Among infants and young children, the Institute of Medicine and the American Academy of Pediatrics have defined vitamin D deficiency as a level below 11 ng/mL. However, children with skeletal abnormalities characteristic of vitamin D-deficient rickets have been found to have levels between 11 and 15 ng/mL. The definition for adult vitamin D deficiency (<20 ng/mL) is being increasingly applied for children (Table 79–2).[6] By the above definition, it has been estimated that one billion people worldwide have vitamin D deficiency or insufficiency.[11]

Recent studies have shown that, among pregnant women, vitamin D deficiency and insufficiency are highly prevalent, even when prenatal vitamins are being administered.[11,12] When the mother has a low vitamin D level, the infant can be born with a relative vitamin D deficiency resulting from decreased maternal transfer. Deficiencies of vitamin D and calcium in

▶ TABLE 79–1. **ETIOLOGY OF RICKETS**

Vitamin D Deficiency
  Dietary deficiency
  Maternal vitamin D deficiency (congenital rickets)
  Breast-fed infants
  Infants and children who are fed macrobiotic diets
Deficient Endogenous Synthesis
  Deficient exposure to UV light
    Sunscreen use
    Skin pigment
    Pollution
    Season/latitude
Decreased Bioavailability
  Gastrointestinal tract disorders
    Severe intestinal malabsorption
  Obesity (sequestration of vitamin D in body fat)
Disorders of Vitamin D Metabolism
  Decreased synthesis of calcidiol
    Hepatobiliary disease
  Accelerated catabolism of calcidiol
    Use of anticonvulsants: phenobarbital and phenytoin
  Hereditary
    Vitamin D-resistant (absent or abnormal receptors)
    Vitamin D-dependent (defect in 1α-hydroxylase)
  Aquired
    Chronic renal disease
    Decreased synthesis of calcitriol
Calcium Deficiency
  Nutritional deprivation
  Hypercalciuria
Phosphate Deficiency
  Nutritional deprivation or use of antacids
  Hereditary
    X-linked hypophosphatemic rickets
    Hypophosphatemic rickets with hypercalciuria
  Acquired
    Sporadic hypophosphatemic osteomalacia
    Oncogenic osteomalacia
    Neurofibromatosis and fibrous dysplasia
Other Rare Causes
  Primary mineralization defects
  Defective osteoid
  Toxicities, such as aluminum (8, 9)

▶ TABLE 79–2. **VITAMIN D LEVELS IN ADULTS***

	25-Hydroxyvitamin D (calcidiol)	
	ng/mL	nmol/L
Deficiency	<20	50
Insufficiency	21–29	—
Sufficiency	>30	75

*Among infants and young children, the Institute of Medicine and the AAP have defined vitamin D deficiency as a level below 11 ng/mL (27.5 mol/L); however, the definitions described above are increasingly being applied to children.

utero may prevent the maximum deposition of calcium in the bones. There is also a positive correlation between maternal vitamin D levels during pregnancy and lactation and the development of rickets in infancy and childhood.[13]

DECREASED SUNLIGHT EXPOSURE

In comparison to sunlight, diet provides on average less than 10% of the body's vitamin D requirements. A lightly pigmented adult, with 10 to 15 minutes of full body sunlight exposure during summer, will generate between 10 000 to 20 000 IU of vitamin D in a day.[14] It is very difficult to determine what is adequate sunlight exposure for a given infant or child.

The Centers for Disease Control and Prevention and many other organizations in recent years have launched a major public health campaign to decrease the incidence of skin cancer and photoaging by recommending the limitation of exposure to UV light. Epidemiologic evidence suggests that the age at which direct sunlight exposure is initiated is more important than the total sunlight exposure over a lifetime in determining the risk of skin cancer. Guidelines for decreasing sun exposure, including keeping young children out of direct sunlight, the use of protective clothing, as well as sunscreens, have been implemented.[15] Many factors limit the amount of sunlight exposure for a given individual. These include season of the year, latitude, pollution, lifestyle or cultural practices, and skin pigment.[6,16] This results in increased dependence on dietary vitamin D to maintain vitamin D sufficiency.

BREAST-FEEDING AND FORMULA FEEDING

All infant formulas, evaporated milks and almost all whole milk sold in the United States contain 400 IU of vitamin D per liter, while breast milk contains only 12 to 60 IU/L.[20] Thus, the recommended adequate intake of vitamin D of 200 IU cannot be met with human milk as the sole source of vitamin D for the breast-fed infant. In addition, the breast milk of a mother with vitamin D deficiency will contain less vitamin D than normal, adding to the risk of developing rickets.[17] This has led to the advice to supplement the breast-fed infant with 200 IU of vitamin D per day. Supplementation should begin within the first 2 months of life.[15] Some infants receive both breast milk and formula. If an infant is ingesting at least 500 mL/d of formula, he or she will receive the recommended vitamin D intake of 200 IU/d.[15]

POLLUTION

Living in an inner-city area also is a risk factor for rickets because of the presence of smog, which reduces the amount of UV radiation that reaches the residents.

RICKETS OF PREMATURITY

Preterm infants, especially the ones with very low-birth-weight (VLBW), are at a relatively high risk of developing rickets. In the third trimester of gestation, bone mineral density shows the highest rate of increase. In this stage, the requirement for calcium and phosphorus is at its maximum level. It is of the utmost importance that nutrition be especially adapted in infants with birth weights of less than 1500 grams. In utero, the fetus receives approximately 120 to 140 mg/kg of calcium and 70 to 80 mg/kg of phosphorus, but breast milk contains only 60 mg/kg of calcium and 30 mg/kg of phosphorus. It is easy to see that these levels are inadequate and that infants with VLBW need special supplementation if breast milk is their primary dietary source to gain bone mass. Recommended daily intake for premature infants is 100 to 160 mg/kg/d of highly bioavailable calcium salts, 60 to 90 mg/kg/d of phosphorus, and 800 to 1000 IU of vitamin D.[18]

► PATHOPHYSIOLOGY

Understanding of the pathophysiology of vitamin D-deficient rickets requires knowledge of the biochemistry of vitamin D. Vitamin D is a prohormone. In the human body, vitamin D can be either exogenous or endogenous.

Exogenous vitamin D_2 (ergosterol) can be acquired through a healthy diet and/or vitamin supplements. Dietary sources of vitamin D include fatty fish and fortified food products, including dairy, infant formula, juice, and cereals.[19]

Endogenous vitamin D_3 (cholecalciferol) is synthesized in the dermis and epidermis from 7-dehydrocholesterol by exposure to the UV light fraction of sunlight (Fig. 79–1). UV rays convert 7-dehydrocholesterol to precholecalciferol.

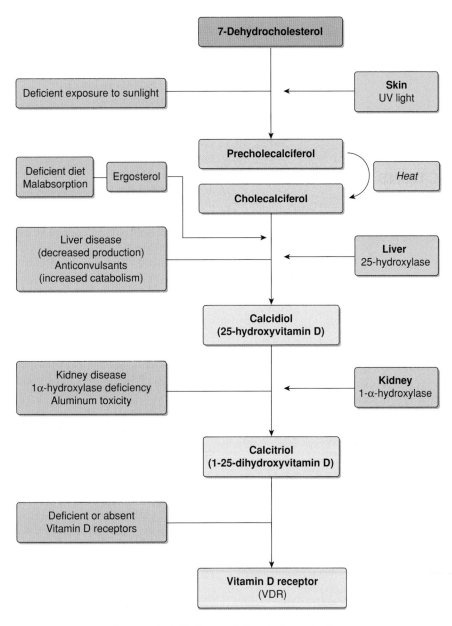

Figure 79–1. Pathway of vitamin D production.

Precholecalciferol is then, through thermal isomerization, converted to cholecalciferol.[6,20] Excessive exposure to sunlight degrades any excess precholecalciferol or cholecalciferol preventing any intoxication with vitamin D. Vitamin D (either D_2 or D_3) can be deposited in and then released from fat cells.

Both vitamin D_2 or D_3 are activated by hydroxylation at two different sites. The first hydroxylation occurs mainly in the liver (although this process may also occur in the kidneys and intestine), by vitamin D-25 hydroxylase, producing calcidiol (25-hydroxyvitamin D or 25-hydroxycholecalciferol). This step is substrate-dependent and measuring this metabolite is used to measure vitamin D status.[6,20] This step in the vitamin D activation path is a self-limiting feedback system, which is needed because 25-hydroxyvitamin D persists only for several days in the human body, while vitamin D can be stored for months.

The second hydroxylation occurs primarily, but not exclusively, in the kidney, where 25-hydroxyvitamin D is converted to the active metabolite calcitriol (1,25-dihydroxycholecalciferol or 1,25-dihydroxyvitamin D), a hormone, by the enzyme 1α-hydroxylase. Activity of 1α-hydroxylase is stimulated by parathyroid hormone (PTH). Hypocalcemia and hypophosphatemia also stimulate 1α-hydroxylase.

Inhibitors of 1α-hydroxylase are calcium, phosphate, and calcitriol.

Deficient or underactive 1α-hydroxylase is the cause for vitamin D-dependent rickets.[6,20]

CALCITRIOL ACTIONS

The actions of calcitriol are mediated primarily through interaction with the intracellular vitamin D receptor (VDR). The vitamin D receptor (VDR) may be absent or abnormal and this is the cause for vitamin D-resistant rickets.

Calcitriol increases intestinal calcium absorption from 10%–15% to 30%–40% and phosphorus absorption from 60% to 80% (Table 79–3).[11] Calcitriol also stimulates an increase in vitamin D-24 hydroxylase activity (that catalyzes conversion of 1,25-hydroxyvitamin D into the biologically inert calcitriol acid). The enzyme vitamin D-24-hydroxylase is found in a wide range of normal tissues and is believed to be important in the removal of vitamin D metabolites.[11] Calcitriol suppresses synthesis and secretion of PTH and inhibits 1α-hydroxylase activity. At high levels, it may induce increased osteoclastic activity. All these actions increase the concentrations of calcium and phosphorus in extracellular fluid. The increase of calcium and phosphorus in extracellular fluid leads to the calcification of osteoid.

If vitamin D levels are low, calcium absorption from the intestines is inadequate and serum calcium concentrations begin to decrease. Hypocalcemia stimulates PTH secretion. PTH increases the activity of enzyme 1α-hydroxylase and thus increases levels of calcitriol, and it also enhances the tubular reabsorption of calcium, restoring calcium levels. Elevated PTH produces renal phosphate loss and serum phosphorus levels decline, further reducing calcification potential. Hypocalcemia usually precedes a decrease in serum phosphorus.

Calcitriol increases mobilization of calcium from the bone matrix, by stimulation of transformation of preosteoclasts into mature osteoclasts. Mature osteoclasts remove calcium and

▶ **TABLE 79–3. ACTIONS OF CALCITRIOL**

Bone	Small Intestines
Increased mineralization (through calcium and phosphorus absorption)	Increased absorption of calcium
Increased osteoclastic activity (to release calcium and phosphorus)	Increased absorption of phosphorus
	Decreased absorption of magnesium

Parathyroid Glands	Kidney
Decreased PTH synthesis and secretion	Autoregulation of calcitriol production
	Enhanced tubular reabsorption of calcium
	Decreased excretion of phosphorus

Other
Decreases production of type 1 collagen
Stimulates 24-hydroxylation of 25-hydroxyvitamin D

phosphorus from the bone to maintain normal levels in the blood.

As vitamin D deficiency progresses, serum calcium continues to decrease. PTH continues to increase to counteract the decline in serum calcium, calcium is mobilized from the bone and bone matrix breakdown occurs. At some point, mineral absorption becomes inadequate to maintain normal serum calcium despite elevated PTH.

Prolonged vitamin D deficiency eventually is associated with both hypocalcemia and hypophosphatemia. Bone does not calcify normally in the absence of calcium and phosphorus. In several weeks to months, rachitic bone changes become apparent. The result is a frayed zone of nonrigid tissue (unmineralized osteoid) at the metaphysis level. Mobilization of calcium and bone matrix breakdown are associated with an increase level of alkaline phosphatase. Alkaline phosphatase is produced by very active osteoblast cells.

▶ CLINICAL MANIFESTATIONS

SIGNS AND SYMPTOMS

Figure 79–2 provides an algorithm to guide the diagnosis of vitamin D-deficiency rickets.

Patients with rickets may present with hypocalcemic signs and symptoms. Signs and symptoms of hypocalcemia relate more to the velocity of the fall in calcium levels than on the actual serum concentration. The more acute the drop in calcium, the more likely clinical symptoms will be expressed. Usually, signs of hypocalcemia are always present when the ionized calcium concentration falls below 2.5mg/dL.[21]

Symptoms of hypocalcemia result from enhanced neuronal excitability, which causes tetany—spontaneous,

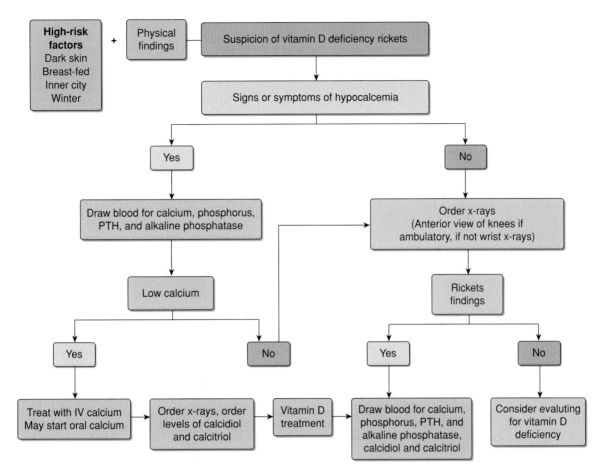

Figure 79–2. Algorithm for diagnosis of vitamin D-deficient rickets.

repetitive firing of individual motor units. These symptoms may include paresthesias, muscle cramping, carpopedal spasm, and laryngospasm, with resultant stridor and apnea. Hypocalcemia, particularly in infants, may present with symptoms of an upper airway obstruction.[22-24] With the many common causative factors for stridor and apnea in infants, hypocalcemic tetany may not be initially considered. Subclinical tetany may be induced by Chvostek's or Trousseau's signs. Cardiac contractility may be reduced, with prolongation of electrical systole as measured by the QT interval. Neurologic findings include seizures, irritability, memory loss, and affective disorders. There are several reports of congenital rickets presenting with hypocalcemic seizures. In these cases, the mother was found to have Vitamin D deficiency.[25,26]

Systemic findings observed in children with rickets may include hypotonia, muscular weakness, delay in walking, anorexia, and increased susceptibility to infection, especially pneumonia.[27] A state of deficiency occurs months before rickets is obvious on physical examination. Some site-specific findings of rickets are shown in Table 79–4.

LABORATORY EVALUATION

In vitamin D-deficient rickets, calcium is low in the early and late stages, but it can be normal. The phosphorus level is low in the vast majority of cases. Alkaline phosphatase levels are

▶ **TABLE 79–4. SITE SPECIFIC FINDINGS OF RICKETS**

Head
  Craniotabes (posterior flattening of the skull)
  Frontal bossing and square forehead (caput quadratum)
  Widened cranial sutures
Teeth
  Delayed dental eruption
  Enamel hypoplasia
Thorax
  Rachitic rosary—bulging of costochondral junction
  Prominent sternum
  Harrison groove—indentation of the lower anterior
    thoracic wall
Arms
  Bowing of the long bones
  Thickening of the wrist at the level of the epiphysis
Legs
  Bowing of the long bones
  Genu varum, because of weight bearing
    Anterior bowing of the tibia (saber shin deformity)
    Knock-knees (genu valgum)
    Thickening at the level of the ankle

▶ TABLE 79–5. **RICKETS BECAUSE OF VITAMIN D DEFICIENCY OR ABNORMAL METABOLISM OF VITAMIN D**

Laboratory Evaluation	Calcium	Phosphorus	Calcidiol	Calcitriol	PTH	Alkaline Phosphatase
Vitamin D deficiency	↓	↓	↓	N or ↓	↑	↑
Liver disease	↓	↓	↓	↓	↑	↑
Renal disease	↓	↑	N	↓	↑	↑
Vitamin D-dependent rickets (1α- hydroxylase deficiency)	↓	↓	N	↓	↑	↑
Vitamin D-resistant rickets (abnormal or absent vitamin D receptor)	↓	↓	N	↑	↑	↑

almost always elevated. Calcidiol levels are low and PTH levels are elevated. Calcitriol levels are normal or high because of PTH activity. Calcidiol, calcitriol, and PTH levels may take days to be reported and will not be available during emergency department evaluation. Table 79–5 summarizes the laboratory evaluation of the suspected rickets patient.

IMAGING

The most rapidly growing bones show the most striking abnormalities. The best radiograph for infants and children younger than 3 years is an anterior view of the knee showing the metaphyseal ends and epiphyses of the femurs and tibiae. Radiologic findings in rickets may include osteopenia with visible coarsening of trabeculae (Fig. 79–3) and cortical thinning. The metaphyses may show fraying, widening and cupping because of their exaggerated normal concavity and irregular calcification (Figs. 79–3 and 79–4).

When healing occurs, the metaphysis may have a brush border appearance (Fig. 79–4). Along the shaft, the uncalcified osteoid may cause the periosteum to appear separated from the diaphysis.[27]

▶ TREATMENT

Vitamin D is well stored in the body and released gradually over many weeks. Treatment of vitamin D deficiency may be administered gradually, over a extended period of time, or in a single day. Single-day dosing has the advantage of avoiding compliance issues. Vitamin D can be given as a single oral dose of 300 000 to 600 000 IU of vitamin D[28,29] or a single intramuscular injection at a dose of 600 000 IU.[20]

If a more gradual method is chosen, vitamin D can be given as a monthly intramuscular injection of 10 000 to 50 000 IU of vitamin D for 3 to 6 months[5,10]; oral vitamin D at a dose of 50 000 IU once a week for 8 weeks, followed by 50 000 IU

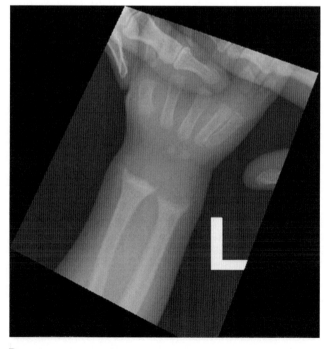

A   B

Figure 79–3. Frontal views (A and B) of the wrists show metaphyseal widening, cupping, and fraying consistent with rickets.

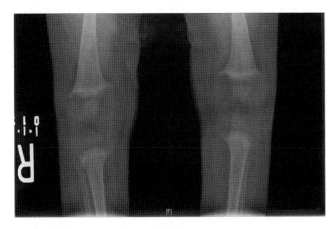

Figure 79–4. AP view of the knees show widening of the metaphysis. Brush border appearance of the metaphysis is consistent with healing rickets. There are unsharp, smudged-appearing trabecular markings consistent with osteomalacia.

every 2 to 4 weeks; or oral vitamin D at a dose of 1000 to 2000 IU/d for several weeks.[8,20] Some sources recommend up to 4000 IU daily in older children[8] Some authors also recommend 400 IU of vitamin D daily for 6 to 12 months after treatment for rickets.[29]

Calcium must be given along with vitamin D to avoid hypocalcemia because of "hungry bone" syndrome.[30] Calcium is given at a daily dose of 40 mg/kg of elemental calcium.[20] For symptomatic hypocalcemia, intravenous calcium may be administered cautiously. Calcium gluconate 10% (50–100 mg/kg/dose) or calcium chloride 10% (10–20 mg/kg/dose) is infused slowly over at least 12 to 15 minutes.

Orthopedic referral may be needed if severe deformities are present.

MONITORING

Serial measurements of alkaline phosphatase and appropriate x-rays are recommended to evaluate healing and resolution of the rachitic lesions.[20] Treatment is continued until healing is well established and the alkaline phosphatase concentration approaches the normal range. Serial levels of calcium, phosphorus, PTH, 25-hydroxyvitamin D, and urine calcium are not always recommended, but may be useful in specific cases.

▶ PREVENTION

Adequate sunlight exposure in infants and children is difficult to determine and new guidelines advocate for decreased sunlight exposure to decrease the risk of photoaging and skin cancer. To prevent vitamin D deficiency and rickets in healthy infants and children, the National Academy of Sciences recommends a supplement of 200 IU of vitamin D per day for the following:

- Breast-fed infants unless they are weaned to at least 500 mL/d of vitamin D-fortified formula or milk, beginning during the first 2 months of life.

- All non-breast-fed infants who are ingesting less than 500 mL/d of vitamin D-fortified formula or milk, beginning during the first 2 months of life.
- Children and adolescents who do not get regular sunlight exposure, do not ingest at least 500 mL/d of vitamin D-fortified milk, or do not take a daily multivitamin supplement containing at least 200 IU of vitamin D.

These guidelines are based on data mostly from the United States, Norway, and China, which show that an intake of at least 200 IU/d of vitamin D will prevent physical signs of vitamin D deficiency and maintain serum 25-hydroxy-vitamin D at or above 11 ng/mL.[15] Other sources recommend 400 IU, 1000 IU, or 2000 IU of vitamin D daily as a preventive dose for infants through 18 years of age.[6,11,19,20,31]

REFERENCES

1. Klein GL. Nutritional rickets and osteomalacia. In: Favus MJ, ed. *Primer on the Metabolic Bone Diseases and Disorders of Mineral Metabolism.* 4th ed. Philadelphia, PA: Lippincott Williams & Wilkins; 1999:315–319.
2. Thatcher T, Fischer P, Strand M, et al. Nutritional rickets around the world: causes and future directions. *Ann Trop Paediatr.* 2006;26:1–16.
3. Wharton B, Bishop N. Rickets. *Lancet.* 2003;362:1389–1400.
4. Welch TR, Bergstrom WH, Tsang RC. Vitamin D-deficient rickets: the re-emergence of a once-conquered disease. *J Pediatr.* 2000;137:143.
5. Rajakumar K. Vitamin D, cod-liver oil, sunlight, and rickets: a historical perspective. *Pediatrics.* 2003;112:e132–e135.
6. Holick MR. Resurrection of vitamin D deficiency and rickets. *J Clin Invest.* 2006;116:2062–2072.
7. Weisberg P, Scanlon K, Li R, et al. Nutritional rickets among children in the United States: review of cases reported between 1986 and 2003. *Am J Clin Nutr.* 2004;80(suppl):1697S–1705S.
8. Huh SY, Gordon CM. Vitamin D deficiency in children and adolescents: epidemiology, impact and treatment. *Rev Endocr Metab Disord.* 2008;9(2):161–170.
9. Dawson HB, Heeney RP, Holick MF, et al. Estimates of optimal vitamin D status. *Osteoporos Int.* 2005;16:713–716.
10. Vieth R, Bischoff-Ferrari H, Boucher BJ, et al. The urgent need to recommend an intake of vitamin D that is effective. *Am J Clin Nutr.* 2007;85:649–650.
11. Holick MF. Vitamin D deficiency. *NEJM.* 2007;357:266–281.
12. Bodnar LM, Simhan HN, Powers PW, et al. High prevalence of vitamin D insufficiency in Black and White pregnant women residing in the Northern United States and their neonates. *J Nutr.* 2007;137:447–452.
13. Dawodu A, Wagner CL. Mother-child vitamin D deficiency: an international perspective. *Arch Dis Child.* 2007;92:737–740.
14. Holick MF, MacLaughlin JA, Clark MB, et al. Photosynthesis of vitamin D3 in human skin and its physiologic consequences. *Science.* 1980;210:203–205.
15. Gartner LM, Greer FR. Prevention of rickets and vitamin D deficiency: new guidelines for vitamin D intake. *Pediatrics.* 2003;111:908–910.
16. Loomis WF. Skin-pigment regulation of vitamin-D biosynthesis in man. *Science.* 1967;157:501.
17. Hollis BW, Wagner CL. Assessment of dietary vitamin D requirements during pregnancy and lactation. *Am J Clin Nutr.* 2004;79:717–726.
18. Rigo J, Pieltain C, Salle B, et al. Enteral calcium, phosphate and vitamin D requirements and bone mineralization in preterm infants. *Acta Paediatr.* 2007;96:969–974.

19. Calvo MS, Whiting SJ, Barton CN. Vitamin D fortification in the United States and Canada: current status and data needs. *Am J Clin Nutr.* 2004;80:1710S–1716S.

20. Root AW, Diamond FB. Disorders of calcium metabolism in the child and adolescent. In: Sperling MA, ed. *Pediatric Endocrinology.* Philadelphia, PA: Saunders; 2002:645–652.

21. De Cristofaro JD. Tsang RC. Calcium. *Emerg Med Clin North Am.* 1986;4:207–221.

22. Sharief N, Matthew DJ, Dillon MJ. Hypocalcemic stridor in children: how often is it missed? *Clin Pediatr (Phila).* 1991;30:51–52.

23. Frankel A, Gruber B, Schey WL. Rickets presenting as stridor and apnea. *Ann Otol Rhinol Laryngol.* 1994;103:905–907.

24. Buchanan N, Pettifor JM, Cane RD, Bill PL. Infantile apnea due to profound hypocalcemia associated with vitamin D deficiency. A case report. *S Afr Med J.* 1978;53:766–767.

25. Orbak Z, Karacan M, Doneray H, et al. Congenital rickets presenting with hypocalcaemic seizures. *West Indian Med J.* 2007;56(4):364–367.

26. Erdeve O, Atasay B, Arsan S, Siklar Z, Ocal G, Berberoglu M. Hypocalcemic seizure due to congenital rickets in the first day of life. *Turk J Pediatr.* 2007;49(3):301–303.

27. Joiner TA, Foster C, Shope T. The many faces of vitamin D deficiency rickets. *Pediatr Rev.* 2000;21:296–302.

28. Cesur Y, Caksen H, Gundem A, et al. Comparison of low and high dose of vitamin D treatment in nutritional vitamin D deficiency rickets. *J Pediatr Endocrinol Metab.* 2003;16:1105–1109.

29. Shah BR, Finberg L. Single-day therapy for nutritional vitamin D-deficiency rickets: a preferred method. *J Pediatr.* 1994;125:487–490.

30. Key LL Jr. Nutritional rickets trends. *Endocrinol Metab.* 1991; 2:81.

31. Greer FR. Issues in establishing vitamin D recommendations for infants and children. *Am J Clin Nutr.* 2004;80:1759S–1762S.

CHAPTER 80

Fluid and Electrolyte Disorders

Susan A. Kecskes

▶ HIGH-YIELD FACTS

- Fluid therapy is guided by knowledge of the composition, distribution, and movement of body water.
- Fluid requirements are divided into three parts:
  - maintenance fluids
  - deficit replacement
  - replacement of ongoing losses
- Correction of circulatory failure with isotonic crystalloid or appropriate colloid is the first step in fluid management.
- Hypernatremia should generally be corrected gradually to avoid the complication of cerebral edema.
- Aggressive treatment of hyponatremia may lead to the osmotic demyelination syndrome.
- Therapy for hyperkalemia is aimed at halting intake, stabilizing cellular membranes, intracellular translocation, and enhancing elimination.
- Hypokalemia should be corrected orally, if possible. Extreme caution should be exercised during intravenous replacement to avoid hyperkalemia.

The initial approach to acutely ill children includes an assessment of their fluid and electrolyte status. The ability to maintain homeostasis and correct disturbances requires knowledge of the composition of the fluid spaces of the body and their changes with age and disease. This chapter discusses the physiologic basis of fluid management, some of the common disturbances, and an approach to management.

▶ FLUIDS

FLUID COMPARTMENTS

Total body water (TBW) is divided into the intracellular and extracellular compartments, with the extracellular compartment subdivided into intravascular and extravascular compartments. The relative size of these compartments varies with age (Fig. 80–1).[1] TBW is approximately 79% of body weight at birth, decreasing to the adult proportion of 55% to 60% over the first year of life. This primarily relates to a drop in extracellular fluid (ECF). Postnatal diuresis, as well as growth in cellular tissue, is responsible for the majority of the change. Additionally, blood volume decreases from 80 mL/kg at birth toward the adult value of 60 mL/kg. By the time the child is 1 year of age, TBW comprises approximately 60% of body weight and is approaching the adult distribution of one-third in the extracellular compartments and two-thirds in the intracellular compartments. Body water exists as a complex solution of salts, organic acids, and proteins. The exact composition varies with body compartment (Fig. 80–2).[2]

MOVEMENT OF FLUID

Cellular membranes form the barrier between the extracellular and intracellular spaces (Fig. 80–3). They are freely permeable to water, but impermeable to electrolytes and proteins, except by active transport. Although the specific osmoles differ in the two compartments, the osmolality is equal. Water distributes across this barrier by osmotic pressure. A rise in extracellular osmolality, as occurs with a sodium load, results in movement of water from the intracellular space to the extracellular space. Conversely, water intoxication leads to the movement of water from the extracellular space to the intracellular space.

The vascular endothelium forms the barrier between the intravascular and interstitial spaces. It is permeable to water and electrolytes, but not to protein. Two forces regulate fluid movement. Hydrostatic pressure, created by the propulsion of blood through vessels, favors movement of fluid from the intravascular space to the interstitial space. This pressure falls as blood travels from the arterioles through the capillary bed to the lower pressure veins. Oncotic pressure, exerted primarily by albumin found in the vascular space, favors water movement from the interstitium into the vascular space. Under normal conditions, there is a balance in the movement of water and electrolytes from the vascular space to the endothelium at the arteriolar side and in the reverse direction at the venous side.

These factors guide the selection of fluid to be administered to a patient. Free water added to the vascular space will distribute proportionally to all three compartments. Isotonic crystalloid distributes throughout the extracellular space. Isoncotic fluid will remain in the vascular space, with the exception of a small distribution to the interstitial space because of the increase in hydrostatic pressure.

FLUID REQUIREMENTS

Fluid requirements can be divided into three categories:

- Maintenance fluids, which replace routine daily fluid losses.
- Replacement of a fluid deficit, if needed.
- Ongoing excessive losses.

Maintenance fluids include insensible losses and routine outputs of urine and stool. These are proportional to the body

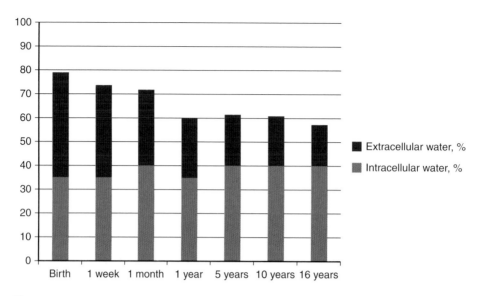

Figure 80–1. Distribution of total body water based on body weight at various ages. Both total body water and extracelluar water decline significantly over the first year of life.

surface area. Since infants and children have a higher body surface area per kilogram, they also have proportionally higher fluid requirements.[3] There are four common methods to calculate maintenance fluids (Table 80–1). Patients in renal failure should have maintenance fluids calculated as insensible loss plus urine replacement.

Common maintenance fluids are D_5 0.2% NaCl with 20 mEq/L of KCl in infants and young children and D_5 0.45% NaCl with 20 mEq/L of KCl in older children and adults. There is, however, increasing evidence that hospitalized patients receiving parenteral fluids are vulnerable to the development of hyponatremia.[4] This is likely related to antidiuretic hormone (ADH) excess that may be seen in many conditions seen in

the ER including hypovolemia, pneumonia, asthma, congestive heart failure (CHF), meningitis, and head injury. There have also been numerous reports of significant morbidity and mortality related to iatrogenic hyponatremia following surgery. For this reason, a number of experts are advocating the use of isotonic solutions (with or without dextrose, tailored to individual patient needs) as maintenance parenteral fluid outside the neonatal period. This remains an area of controversy.[4,5]

Many patients have fluid deficits that require replacement. In pediatrics, the most common cause is gastrointestinal disease associated with vomiting and diarrhea. The first priority in patients with fluid deficits is to restore circulation. To begin, the adequacy of the patient's perfusion is determined (Table 80–2). Mental status, urine output, skin character, capillary refill, and vital signs are assessed. Serum electrolytes, blood urea

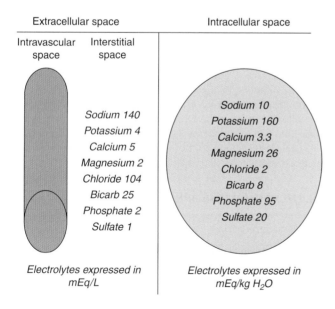

Figure 80–2. Electrolyte composition of intracellular space vs. extracellular space.

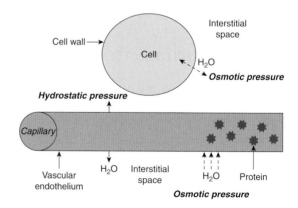

Figure 80–3. Osmotic pressure controls the movement of water across cell walls. Oncotic pressure promotes water retention in the vascular space. Hydrostatic pressure promotes water movement from the vascular space to the interstitial space.

▶ **TABLE 80-1. FOUR METHODS FOR MAINTENANCE FLUID CALCULATIONS**

Body Surface Area Method
    1500 mL/BSA (m^2)/d

100/50/20 Method

Weight (kg)	Fluid
0–10	100 mL/kg/day
11–20	100 mL + 50 mL/kg/day for every kg > 10 kg
>20	1500 mL + 20 mL/kg/day for every kg > 20 kg

4/2/1 Method

Weight (kg)	Fluid
0–10	4 mL/kg/h
11–20	40 mL + 2 mL/kg/h for every kg > 10 kg
>20	60 mL + 1 mL/kg/h for every kg > 20 kg

Insensible + Measured Losses Method
    400–600 mL/BSA (m^2)/d + urine output (mL/mL) + L other measured losses (mL/mL)

nitrogen, creatinine, acid–base status, urinalysis, and urine sodium concentration may be useful. If the patient's perfusion is inadequate, fluid resuscitation should be initiated. An initial bolus of 20 mL/kg of isotonic crystalloid (0.9% NaCl or lactated Ringer's [LR] solution) is given intravenously for more than 20 minutes. The patient is reassessed and further boluses are given until perfusion is adequate. Pediatric patients commonly require >60 mL/kg of resuscitation fluid to restore perfusion. If required, blood products may be substituted for some of the bolus fluid. Additional therapy, such as inotropes or pressors, may be added if the circulatory failure is not solely related to fluid deficit.

Once circulation has been stabilized, the remaining deficit needs to be replaced. The magnitude of dehydration is divided into mild (water loss < 5% TBW), moderate (water loss 5%–10% TBW), and severe (water loss > 10% TBW). Fluid deficit can also be estimated from changes in body weight (assuming all loss is due to fluid loss):

[premorbid body weight (kg) – morbid body weight (kg)] × 1000 = fluid loss (mL)

Resuscitation fluids may be subtracted from the calculated deficit and the remainder replaced over 24 hours if the patient is in a normal osmotic state. Typically, the remaining deficit would be replaced with a hypotonic fluid, such as D_5 0.45% NaCl with 20 mEq/L of KCl or an oral rehydration solution.

Replacement solutions should be adjusted to the electrolyte status of the individual patient.

Some patients may require replacement of ongoing fluid losses not included in normal maintenance requirements (Table 80–3). Continuing emesis and diarrheal losses require replacement along with losses through external drains. Fever increases the water requirement by 10% for each degree elevation over 37.8°C. Ongoing third space loss should be estimated and replaced. The type of fluid should be tailored to the content of the fluid lost. A standard solution with a composition close to the fluid being replaced is usually adequate to maintain homeostasis in patients with intact renal function. If more precision is required, the electrolyte content of the fluid being lost may be measured and replaced.

▶ SODIUM

The concentration of sodium reflects the total body store of sodium and its relation to total body water. In both hyponatremia and hypernatremia, the total body store of sodium may be high, low, or normal. It is the amount of TBW relative to total body sodium that determines sodium concentration. Sodium is found in highest concentration in the extracellular compartment and is normally maintained between 135 and 145 mEq/L.

▶ **TABLE 80-2. SIGNS AND SYMPTOMS OF DEHYDRATION**

	Mild (5% Total Body Weight)	Moderate (10% Total Body Weight)	Severe (15% Total Body Weight)
Mental status	Alert	Irritable; drowsy	Lethargic
Skin turgor	Brisk retraction	Mild delay	Prolonged retraction
Anterior fontanel	Normal	Minimally sunken	Sunken
Eyes	Moist; + tears	Dry; – tears	Sunken; – tears
Mucous membranes	Moist	Dry	Very dry
Pulses	Normal	Rapid; weak peripherally	Rapid; weak centrally
Capillary refill	< 2 s	2–5 s	> 5 s
Respiration	Normal	Rapid	Deep and rapid
Urine output	>1 mL/kg/h	< 1 mL/kg/h	Minimal or absent
Blood pressure	Normal	Low normal	Hypotension

▶ TABLE 80–3. **ADJUSTMENTS TO MAINTENANCE FLUIDS**

Fever	Increase maintenance fluids by 10% for each degree > 37.8°C.
Tachypnea *(nonhumidified environment)*	Increase maintenance fluids by 5%–10%.
Vomiting and gastric loss	Replace with 0.45% NaCl with 10 mEq/L KCl.
Stool loss	Replace with LR with 15 mEq/L KCl or 0.45% NaCl with 20 mEq/L KCl and 20 mEq/L NaHCO₃.
Cerebrospinal fluid	Replace with LR or 0.9% NaCl.
Pleural fluid, peritoneal fluid, wound drainage (serous)	Replace with LR or 0.9% NaCl; may need to replace albumin periodically—base replacement on measured serum albumin levels.
Blood	≤25% blood volume: replace with LR or 0.9% NaCl; assess hematocrit and physiologic status for administration of blood.
	> 25% blood volume: replace one-half to two-thirds of loss as whole blood and reassess. Alternatively, use "3-for-1" and replace 3 × the blood loss with LR or 0.9% NaCl.
Third-space losses	Estimate based on patient's physiologic status. Replace with LR or 0.9% NaCl.

One of the primary regulatory mechanisms is ADH. ADH is secreted by the posterior pituitary gland in response to stimulation of osmoreceptors residing in the anterior hypothalamus, baroreceptors in the great vessels, and volume receptors in the left atrium. The release of ADH results in increased water absorption by the renal tubule. Osmoreceptors detect increasing osmolarity, with sodium being the primary ion responsible for extracellular osmolarity. Baroreceptors and volume receptors regulate the intravascular volume. In cases of decreasing intravascular volume and diminishing osmolarity (due to body water in excess of body sodium), the volume receptors will override the osmoreceptors, resulting in ADH secretion and water retention, despite decreasing concentrations of sodium.[6]

HYPERNATREMIA

Hypernatremia is defined as serum sodium > 150 mEq/L. It may result from intake of sodium in excess of water or, more commonly, from loss of water in excess of sodium (Table 80–4). Primary sodium excess is usually associated with iatrogenic causes, such as inadequately diluted infant formula, excessive sodium bicarbonate administration, or intravenous hypertonic saline administration. More frequently encountered is hypovolemic hypernatremia, in which water loss exceeds sodium loss. The most common cause in pediatrics is gastroenteritis with diarrhea and vomiting. Other causes include increased insensible water loss (i.e., fever, use of radiant warming devices, burns), diabetes mellitus (solute diuresis), or inadequate access to free water.

Diabetes insipidus (DI) is a less common cause of hypovolemic hypernatremia. The essential feature is a functional lack of ADH, resulting in urinary water loss despite increasing osmolarity and hypovolemia. It may be caused by insufficient production and release of ADH (central DI) or end-organ unresponsiveness to ADH (nephrogenic DI). Disruption of the hypothalamic-pituitary axis by tumors, head trauma, hypoxic–ischemic brain injury, or neurosurgical procedures results in

central DI. It is frequently seen in children near brain death. Nephrogenic DI is a congenital (X-linked recessive) disorder in which the ADH receptors in the renal tubules are defective and unable to respond to ADH. It is present at birth and can be life-threatening if unrecognized. Very dilute urine (osmolarity < 150 mOsm/L or specific gravity < 1.005), serum hyperosmolarity (osmolarity > 295 mOsm/L), and hypernatremia characterize both central and nephrogenic DI. In acute situations, they may be differentiated by their responsiveness (central DI) or lack thereof (nephrogenic DI) to vasopressin.

As the serum sodium rises, ECF becomes relatively hyperosmolal compared to intracellular fluid (ICF). Water moves from the intracellular space to the extracellular space to equilibrate the osmolality. The assessment of decreased intravascular volume status is associated with a greater TBW deficit in

▶ TABLE 80–4. **TABLE 80–4. CAUSES OF HYPERNATREMIA**

Sodium Excess
   Inadequately diluted infant formula
   Excessive administration of sodium bicarbonate
   Excessive administration of hypertonic saline

Water Deficit
   Vomiting and diarrhea
   Increased insensible water loss
   Inadequate access to water
   Diabetes mellitus (osmotic diuresis)
   Diabetes insipidus

Central
   –Brain tumors (i.e., craniopharyngioma)
   –Head trauma
   –Hypoxic–ischemic brain injury

Nephrogenic
   –Congenital (X-linked recessive)
   –Renal disease (renal dysplasia, reflux, polycystic disease)

hypernatremia than in isotonic or hypotonic states. The brain attempts to conserve water by an increase in glucose, electrolytes, and idiogenic osmoles.[7] This process occurs over approximately 48 hours. Thus, although the intracellular space is relatively volume depleted in hypernatremia, the brain preserves its volume status.

Clinical manifestations of hypernatremia depend on the volume status of the patient. In primary sodium excess, the skin is often described as "doughy." In hypovolemic hypernatremia, the signs and symptoms of dehydration are manifested. In both, the central nervous system is adversely affected. Irritability and lethargy can progress to coma and seizures. Hyperreflexia and spasticity may also occur. Concomitant laboratory findings may include hyperglycemia and hypocalcemia.

Initial therapy of hypovolemic hypernatremia is focused on correction of circulatory failure, if present (Fig. 80–4). Subsequent restoration of TBW should be gradual, for ≥48 hours. Fatal cases of cerebral edema have occurred with correction over 24 hours, as fluid enters the already volume-repleted brain.[8] A gradual correction allows the brain to reduce the idiogenic osmoles and equilibrate with the ECF. The goal is to reduce the serum sodium at a rate of 0.5 to 1 mEq/L/h.[9] The higher the serum sodium and the longer the time of accumulation, the slower the rate of correction should be. Typically, the correction is started with isotonic crystalloid for stabilization of the circulatory system and completed with hypotonic crystalloid, such as D_5 0.45% NaCl. Maintenance fluids and replacement of ongoing losses must be provided in addition to the

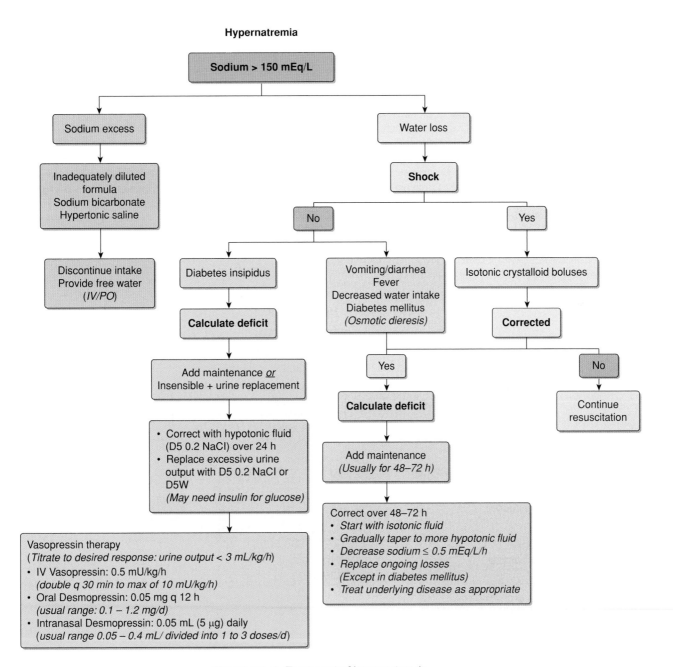

Figure 80–4. Treatment of hypernatremia.

deficit correction. Plasma electrolytes and osmolality should be monitored frequently.

In patients in whom DI is suspected, a trial of vasopressin should be attempted. The drug of choice is aqueous pitressin by continuous infusion beginning at 0.5 mU/kg/h and titrated every 30 minutes (maximum dose 10 mU/kg/h) to produce urine osmolality greater than serum osmolality. Alternatively, desmopressin (DDAVP) may be given via intermittent dosing. For oral administration, the initial dose is 0.05 mg po twice per day (titrate up to a maximum of 0.4 mg/dose, up to three times per day). The initial intranasal dose is 0.05 mL (5 μg), once per day (titrate up to a maximum of 0.4 mL/d over 1–3 doses).[10] Primary sodium excess is treated by removal of excess sodium. At first, the sodium intake is curtailed. In patients with intact renal function, provision of free water via the gastrointestinal tract or hypotonic fluids parenterally will aid correction. Patients with renal failure require dialysis.

HYPONATREMIA

Hyponatremia is defined as a serum sodium concentration < 130 mEq/L and reflects excess body water relative to body sodium. Depending on etiology, total body sodium may be decreased, increased, or normal (Fig. 80–5). Hyponatremia with decreased total body sodium occurs when sodium loss exceeds water loss. These losses may be extrarenal or renal. The most common extrarenal losses in children are vomiting and diarrhea. Other causes include burns, peritonitis, and pancreatitis. Extrarenal etiologies are associated with renal sodium conservation (urine sodium < 20 mEq/L).

Renal losses include diuretic use, osmotic diuresis, and salt-losing renal disease. Thiazide diuretics are more common culprits in hyponatremia than loop diuretics. Osmotic diuresis

may be produced iatrogenically with mannitol or glucose administration. It is also associated with glucosuria in diabetes mellitus. Hyperglycemia and mannitol induce urinary sodium and water loss along with osmotic water movement from ICF to ECF, further lowering serum sodium. Salt-wasting renal diseases include nephritis, obstructive uropathy, renal tubular acidosis, and adrenal insufficiency (congenital adrenal hyperplasia, Addison's disease). Renal causes of hyponatremia with decreased total body sodium are associated with ongoing urinary sodium loss (urine sodium > 20 mEq/L).

Hyponatremia with increased total body sodium occurs when the increase in TBW exceeds sodium retention. Common etiologies include CHF and renal failure. In CHF, decreased cardiac output leads to decreased GFR. The kidney then conserves water and sodium in an attempt to increase intravascular volume and improve renal perfusion. Water is conserved in excess of sodium. In renal failure, decreased urine output is unable to maintain sodium balance in the face of excess water intake.

Hyponatremia with normal total body sodium is commonly associated with two etiologies in children. First, the syndrome of inappropriate antidiuretic hormone (SIADH) leads to a dilutional hyponatremia. ADH is excreted in the absence of a physiologic stimulus for its secretion, leading the kidney to retain water. This syndrome is associated with diverse causes including central nervous system disorders, pulmonary disease, postoperative states, malignancies, glucocorticoid deficiency, and hypothyroidism. The most frequent etiology in the pediatric emergency room is meningitis. Urinary osmolarity (>200 mOsm/L) and sodium concentration (>20 mEq/L) are inappropriately elevated for the hypotonicity and sodium concentration of the serum. The second common etiology of hyponatremia with normal total body sodium is water intoxication. With isotonic crystalloid syndrome occurs when small infants are fed with overly dilute formula or excess

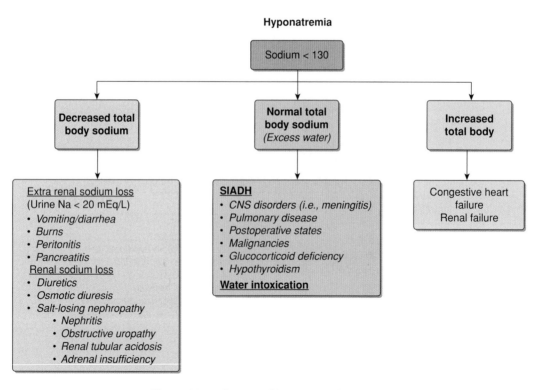

Figure 80–5. Causes of hyponatremia.

water.[11] Inappropriately hypotonic replacement of fluid losses is an iatrogenic cause of water intoxication. In both, the intake of free water exceeds the ability of the body to eliminate it.

The clinical manifestations of hyponatremia depend on the volume status of the patient, the rapidity of development, and degree of hypoosmolality. In hypovolemic hyponatremia, the symptoms of dehydration and acute circulatory failure prevail. Hyponatremia produces a decrease in the osmolarity of the ECF. Water flows into the ICF to maintain homeostasis. Rapid changes result in brain edema and CNS pathology. Symptoms range from lethargy to coma. Brain herniation may occur in the most severe cases. Hyponatremia is a common cause of afebrile seizures in children younger than 6 months.[12] More gradual onset of hyponatremia allows the brain to extrude electrolytes and other osmoles to prevent brain swelling and diminish the CNS pathology.

Treatment of hyponatremia begins with an assessment of the patient's volume status and correction of hypovolemic shock, if present (Fig. 80–6). Correction of the hyponatremia requires a loss of water in excess of sodium. This must be undertaken with care, as aggressive correction may lead to the osmotic demyelination syndrome.[13] Just as the brain can generate idiogenic osmoles to maintain cellular volume in hyperosmolal states, it can rid itself of osmoles in hypoosmolal states to prevent brain edema. Once rid of these osmoles, too rapid a correction of sodium can result in cell desiccation and myelinolysis.[14] Gradual correction allows the brain time to equilibrate with a reduction in neurologic sequelae. In hyponatremia of acute onset (<48 hours), it appears safe to correct the sodium over 24 hours. In hyponatremia of more gradual onset, sodium correction should not exceed a rate of 0.5 mEq/L/h. Therapy can be initiated with isotonic crystalloid at rates determined by the volume status of the patient. In euvolemic or hypervolemic patients, this may be at maintenance or fluid-restricted rates. Fluid restriction to two-thirds maintenance, or even insensible fluid loss, is the mainstay of therapy for SIADH. In hypovolemic patients, the deficit needs to be assessed and the correction timed to the desired rise in sodium concentration (approximately 10 mEq/L/24 h). Although most patients will correct gradually with isotonic crystalloid, more aggressive partial correction may be desired in patients with severe neurologic symptoms, such as seizures. A rise in serum sodium of 5 mEq/L can be produced by intravenous infusion of 6 mL/kg of 3% sodium chloride over 1 to 2 hours. A single bolus is usually sufficient to reduce acute symptoms and the remainder of the correction should be undertaken more gradually. Loop diuretics, such as furosemide, have been used as an adjunct to therapy to increase free water clearance. In all types of hyponatremia, the underlying pathology should be identified and appropriate treatment initiated.

▶ POTASSIUM

While only 2% of total body potassium is in the ECF, potassium is the main cation in ICF. Normal potassium concentration in the ECF is 3.5 to 5.5 mEq/L, compared to approximately 160 mEq/L in the ICF. The sodium–potassium ATPase pump in the cell membrane maintains this large concentration gradient.

Potassium homeostasis is managed through the use of both translocation and excretion. The majority of potassium excretion occurs in the kidney. The kidney can adjust urinary potassium excretion from <5 to >1000 mEq/24 h. Approximately 10% of daily potassium intake is lost through the gastrointestinal tract in stool.

As only 50% of a potassium load is excreted in the first 4 to 6 hours, translocation allows the body to maintain stable ECF potassium. In the first hours after ingestion, potassium is translocated into cells, primarily in the liver and muscle. Potassium uptake is regulated by insulin, epinephrine, aldosterone, and acid–base balance.[15] Insulin stimulates the sodium–potassium ATPase pump to promote potassium uptake in the liver and muscle. Catecholamines cause an initial rise in serum potassium as it is released from the liver. Subsequently, serum potassium falls as catecholamines promote movement to ICF. Aldosterone acts through both renal and extrarenal mechanisms to reduce serum potassium. Acid–base changes may result in potassium shifts. Acidemia promotes movement of potassium to the ICF, whereas alkalosis favors movement of potassium to the ECF.

HYPERKALEMIA

Hyperkalemia is defined as serum potassium >5.5 mEq/L and can result from increased potassium intake, decreased potassium loss, or from redistribution from the ICF. Increased potassium intake rarely results in an elevation of serum potassium unless iatrogenic or simultaneously associated with decreased excretion. Iatrogenic causes include excessive intravenous administration of potassium, administration of large quantities of cold stored blood, large doses of the potassium salts of penicillin, or oral intake of potassium-containing salt substitutes. Acute renal failure is the primary cause of decreased excretion. Less commonly, adrenal insufficiency may result in hyperkalemia due to decreased mineralocorticoid activity. Use of potassium-sparing diuretics is also associated with decreased potassium excretion.

Redistribution of potassium from the ICF to the ECF may occur via cell destruction or translocation from intact cells. In patients with trauma, burns, rhabdomyolysis, massive intravascular coagulopathy, or tumor necrosis, injured cells release stores of intracellular potassium into the circulation. Hematomas in the newborn and gastrointestinal bleeding may result in large volumes of hemolyzing cells and elevated potassium levels. Potassium can be quickly shifted from the ICF to the ECF in response to metabolic acidosis. The ICF is a major part of the body's buffering system, with extracellular hydrogen ions being exchanged for intracellular potassium ions.

Pseudohyperkalemia is a common occurrence and must be considered in the differential diagnosis of hyperkalemia. It is associated with hemolysis from the blood draw. Causes include prolonged tourniquet use, heel squeezing, or use of small-gauge needles. When pseudohyperkalemia is suspected, specimens should be repeated with attention to avoiding such mechanical factors.

Most patients with hyperkalemia are relatively asymptomatic. Neuromuscular symptoms begin with paresthesias and progress to muscle weakness and, ultimately, flaccid paralysis. Cardiac abnormalities are much more likely to produce life-threatening situations. Characteristic changes in the electrocardiogram (ECG) include peaked T waves, prolongation of the PR interval, and progressive widening of the QRS complex.

Treatment of Hyponatremia

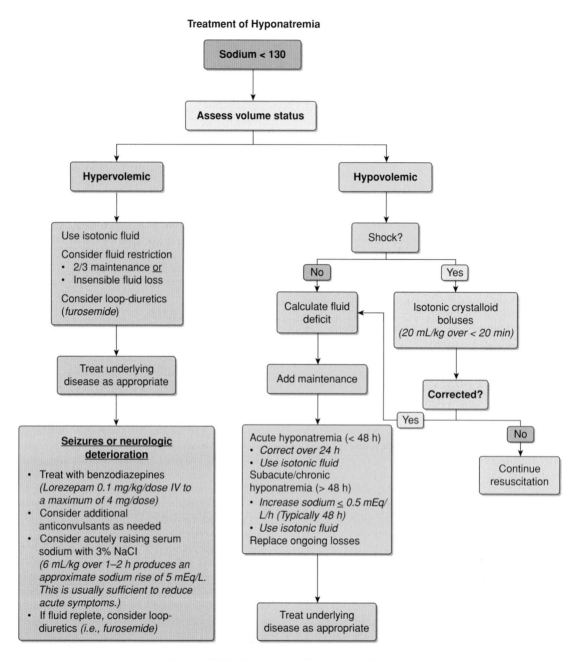

Figure 80–6. Treatment of hyponatremia.

As potassium continues to rise (typically, >8 mEq/L), the classic "sine wave" of hyperkalemia appears (Fig. 80–7). This may rapidly degenerate to asystole or ventricular fibrillation.

An ECG should always be obtained when hyperkalemia is suspected, to confirm the clinical severity. Serum electrolytes, renal indices (BUN, creatinine, and urinalysis), a complete blood count (CBC), and acid–base status should be measured. Urinary potassium levels may help evaluate the cause of the hyperkalemia. All patients with serum potassium levels >6.5 mEq/L should have continuous ECG monitoring and frequent laboratory follow-up.

Treatment of hyperkalemia depends on the level of serum potassium, along with the clinical symptoms and renal status of the patient. In all cases, intake of potassium and potassium-

sparing medication should be halted. In asymptomatic patients with intact renal function and modest (<7 mEq/L) levels of serum potassium, halting intake and follow-up of serum potassium levels may be all that is required (Fig. 80–8). For patients with renal dysfunction, the addition of the potassium-binding agent, sodium polystyrene sulfonate (Kayexalate, 1–2 g/kg po, ng, or pr), or dialysis should be considered to enhance elimination.

Those patients with serum potassium levels >7 mEq/L or who are symptomatic require aggressive intervention to stabilize the cellular membrane, shift potassium intracellularly, and increase potassium elimination. Membrane stabilization is effected by intravenous administration of calcium. Calcium gluconate, 10%, in a dose of 50 to 100 mg/kg, or calcium chloride,

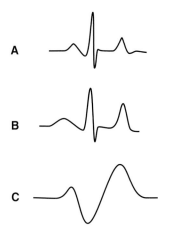

Figure 80–7. ECG changes in hyperkalemia. (A) Normal ECG. (B) ECG with peaked T waves, prolonged PR interval, and widened QRS, seen in moderate hyperkalemia (potassium >7.0 mEq/L). (C) "Sine wave" ECG seen at potassium levels >8 mEq/L.

10%, in a dose of 10 to 25 mg/kg, may be administered over 2 to 5 minutes with continuous ECG monitoring. Onset of action is immediate and the stabilizing effects last 30 to 60 minutes. Potassium may be shifted intracellularly to temporarily reduce serum potassium levels. Administration of sodium bicarbonate (1–2 mEq/kg intravenously over 5–10 minutes) has an onset of action of 5 to 10 minutes and duration of 1 to 2 hours. The dose may be repeated if necessary. Insulin administered in conjunction with glucose effectively shifts potassium to the ICF as well. Dextrose (1 g/kg) may be combined with insulin (0.25 U/kg) and infused over 2 hours. Inhalation of β_2-agonists is an attractive alternative for patients with delayed intravenous access.[16] Nebulized albuterol, in a dose of 2.5 mg for patients <25 kg and 5 mg for patients of 25 kg, has been reported to reduce potassium in adult patients with chronic renal failure and is likely to have a similar effect in pediatric patients. It should not be a substitute for appropriate intravenous therapy, but may be used while access is obtained. None of these methods alter total body potassium, so the time they buy should be utilized to enhance elimination of potassium from the body. In the absence of renal failure, loop diuretics and/or thiazides will enhance renal elimination of potassium. Sodium polystyrene sulfonate is a resin that exchanges sodium for potassium at a 1:1 ratio. It is administered through the gastrointestinal tract and may be used in patients with and without renal failure. In patients with renal failure or severely symptomatic cases, dialysis is the definitive therapy. Although hemodialysis is more effective than peritoneal dialysis, the peritoneal route is more readily available and may be instituted more quickly in many locations.

HYPOKALEMIA

Hypokalemia is defined by a serum potassium level <3.5 mEq/L and can result from decreased intake, increased renal excretion, increased extrarenal losses, or a shift of potassium from the ECF to the ICF. A low-potassium diet, eating

disorders such as anorexia nervosa, and prolonged administration of intravenous fluids without potassium may all lead to hypokalemia. Increased renal excretion may result from the use of diuretics, osmotic diuresis, hyperaldosteronism, Bartter syndrome, magnesium deficiency, and renal tubular acidosis. Extrarenal losses occur primarily through the gastrointestinal system.[15] Vomiting and nasogastric losses may lead to hypokalemia, both from the direct loss of potassium and from secondary hyperaldosteronism associated with hypovolemia. Diarrhea is associated with large potassium losses. Movement of potassium into the cells from the ECF can occur with correction of acidosis, alkalosis, administration of insulin, administration of β_2-agonists, or familial hypokalemic periodic paralysis.

Clinical manifestations of hypokalemia are related to its rapidity of onset and degree of severity. Muscle contraction is dependent on membrane polarization and requires a rapid influx of sodium into cells and a comparable efflux of potassium. Hypokalemia impairs this process. The result is alteration of nerve conduction and muscle contraction. Clinical symptoms include muscle weakness, ileus, areflexia, and autonomic instability, often manifested as orthostatic hypotension. Respiratory arrest and rhabdomyolysis can also occur. The ECG can show flattening of the T wave, ST segment depression, U waves, premature atrial and ventricular contractions, and dysrhythmias, especially in patients who are on digitalis. The kidney has a reduced ability to concentrate urine in hypokalemia, resulting in polyuria. Laboratory data should include serum electrolytes, including magnesium, serum pH, and urine potassium. Urine potassium concentration of <15 mEq/L indicates renal conservation and suggests extrarenal loss. An ECG should be done looking for the alterations just noted.

Since serum potassium levels only measure extracellular potassium concentration, total body concentration may be decreased or normal. Also, potassium must cross the smaller extracellular space to the larger ICF, where the majority of potassium is stored. Both of these factors lead to concern of "overshoot hyperkalemia" during correction. In the patient without life-threatening complications, hypokalemia should be corrected gradually with oral supplementation or, in those patients with a contraindication to oral intake, an increase in the maintenance potassium concentration in the intravenous fluids. Underlying conditions that accompany the hypokalemia, such as alkalosis or hypomagnesemia, should be corrected. Sources of ongoing potassium loss are identified. The loss is then measured and replaced. An effort should be made to determine the cause of the loss and, if possible, treat it. If hypokalemia is associated with digoxin use or life-threatening complications, such as cardiac dysrythmias, rhabdomyolysis, extreme muscle weakness, or respiratory arrest, intravenous therapy is required. Extreme care should be exercised in the ordering, preparation, and administration of intravenous potassium. Recommendations for dosage of potassium chloride in pediatric patients range from 0.5 to 1 mEq/kg/dose (maximum dose: 40 mEq) to infuse at 0.3 to 0.5 mEq/kg/h (maximum rate: 1 mEq/kg/h).[10] Potassium must be diluted prior to intravenous administration. In peripheral lines, the maximum concentration is 80 mEq/L. The maximum recommended central line concentration is 200 mEq/L (usually reserved for severely fluid restricted patients). Continuous ECG monitoring, along with frequent assessment of serum potassium levels, is essential during intravenous correction of hypokalemia.

Treatment of Hyperkalemia

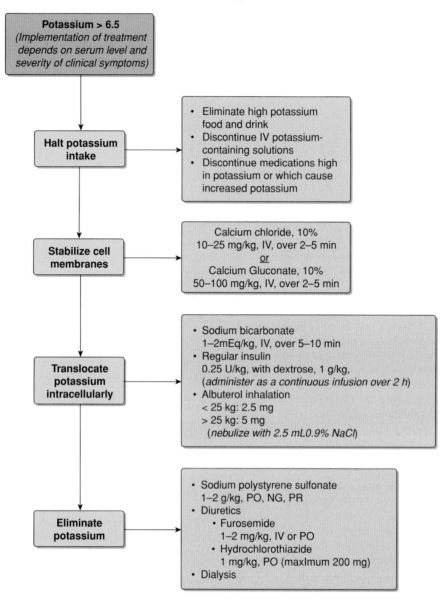

Figure 80–8. Treatment of Hyperkalemia.

► CALCIUM

Calcium is one of the most abundant and important minerals in the body, with 99% of body calcium stored in bone. Of the 1% present in the circulation, 40% is bound to proteins such as albumin, 15% is complexed with anions such as phosphate and citrate, and 45% is physiologically free and ionized.[17] Parathyroid hormone, vitamin D, and calcitonin interact to regulate calcium in a narrow range by controlling intestinal absorption, renal excretion, and skeletal distribution. Calcium is responsible for cellular depolarization, muscle excitation/contraction, neurotransmitter release, hormonal secretion, and the function of both leukocytes and platelets.

A serum calcium level measures both ionized and protein-bound calcium. Since approximately half of serum calcium is bound to albumin, the serum calcium level may need to be adjusted for alterations in the albumin level. For every 1 g/dL decrease in serum albumin, true serum calcium may be estimated by adding 0.8 mg/dL. Alternatively, ionized calcium levels are widely available.

HYPERCALCEMIA

Hypercalcemia is defined as a serum calcium level >10.5 mg/dL. Although often asymptomatic, complaints may include constipation, anorexia, vomiting, abdominal pain, or pancreatitis. Rarely, lethargy, depression, psychosis, or coma may occur. ECG changes may include QT segment shortening, bradycardia, heart block, and sinus arrest. Nephrolithiasis can be an important consequence of hypercalcemia.

The conditions in adults that are commonly associated with hypercalcemia (hyperparathyroidism and malignancies of the breast, lung, kidney, and head and neck) are rare in children. In children, hypercalcemia with malignancy is associated with bone metastasis or tumor lysis syndrome. Other causes in children include primary or tertiary hyperparathyroidism, hyperthyroidism, vitamin D intoxication, immobilization, thiazide diuretics, milk-alkali syndrome, and sarcoidosis.

Laboratory investigation should include total and/or ionized serum calcium, serum albumin and total protein, electrolytes (including magnesium and phosphorus), BUN, creatinine, CBC, ECG, and urinalysis. Hyperchloremic metabolic acidosis suggests primary hyperparathyroidism.

In symptomatic patients or those with levels >14 mg/dL, therapy is aimed at expansion of ECF, calcium excretion, increased bone storage, and definitive treatment of the underlying cause. Volume expansion begins with normal saline and is followed by diuresis with furosemide to promote calcium excretion. Hemodialysis may be required in the setting of renal insufficiency or life-threatening dysrythmias. Calcitonin, glucocorticoids, mithramycin, and indomethacin have all been used to suppress bone resorption, although the onset of action is > 24 hours.

HYPOCALCEMIA

Hypocalcemia is defined as serum calcium <9 mg/dL. Major etiologies are hypoparathyroidism and vitamin D deficiency. Hyperphosphatemia and magnesium deficiency may be associated with hypocalcemia. Additional etiologies are massive transfusion of citrated blood, phosphate enema toxicity, pancreatitis, and sepsis.

Nonspecific symptoms, including nausea, weakness, paresthesias, and irritability, are typical. Classic physical findings of neuromuscular irritability are Chvostek's and Trousseau's signs. In more severe cases, tetany, seizures, laryngospasm, and psychiatric manifestations may be seen.

The ECG may show prolongation of the QT interval, bradycardia, and dysrythmias. Laboratory tests include ionized and total calcium, magnesium, phosphorus, albumin and total protein, BUN, creatinine, and alkaline phosphatase. Vitamin D and parathyroid hormone levels may help elucidate the etiology, as may urine calcium and phosphorus levels.

For significant or symptomatic hypocalcemia, intravenous calcium may be administered cautiously with continuous ECG monitoring. Calcium gluconate, 10% (50–100 mg/kg/dose), or calcium chloride, 10% (10–25 mg/kg/dose), may be administered over 2 to 5 minutes.[10] Intravenous calcium is very irritating to tissues and veins. It should be diluted prior to administration. The maximum concentration of calcium gluconate should be 50 mg/mL and of calcium chloride be 20 mg/mL. It is preferably given through a central line or very secure peripheral venous access. It should never be given intramuscularly, subcutaneously, or via an endotracheal route, as tissue necrosis and sloughing will occur. Intravenous calcium predisposes to digitalis toxicity and precipitates when mixed with bicarbonate. Hyperphosphatemic patients are at risk of metastatic calcium deposition with calcium administration and require treatment aimed at lowering phosphorus levels. When hypomagnesemia is present, oral or intravenous correction should be undertaken. Magnesium sulfate may be administered intravenously at a dose of 25 to 50 mg/kg, diluted to a maximum concentration of 200 mg/mL, over 2 to 4 hours.[10]

REFERENCES

1. Friis-Hansen BJ. Body water compartments in children. *Pediatrics.* 1961;28:171.
2. Hill LL. Body composition and normal electrolyte concentrations. *Pediatr Clin North Am.* 1990;37:244.
3. Holliday MA, Segar WE. The maintenance need for water in parenteral fluid therapy. *Pediatrics.* 1957;19:823.
4. Moritz ML, Ayus JC. Prevention of hospital-acquired hyponatremia: a case for using isotonic crystalloid. *Pediatrics.* 2003;111:227.
5. Holliday MA, Ray PE, Friedman AL. Fluid therapy for children: facts, fashions and questions. *Arch Dis Child.* 2007;92:546.
6. Zerbe RL, Robertson GL. Osmotic and nonosmotic regulation of thirst and vasopressin secretion. In: Maxwell MH, Kleeman CR, Narins RG, eds. *Clinical Disorders of Fluid and Electrolyte Metabolism.* 4th ed. New York, NY: McGraw-Hill; 1987:68.
7. Lee JH, Arcinue E, Ross BD. Brief report: organic osmolytes in the brain of an infant with hypernatremia. *N Engl J Med.* 1994;331:439.
8. Finberg L. Hypernatemia (hypertonic) dehydration in infants. *N Engl J Med.* 1973;289:196.
9. Androgue HJ, Madias NE. Hypernatremia. *N Engl J Med.* 2000;342:1493.
10. Taketomo CK, Hodding JH, Kraus DM. *Pediatric Dosage Handbook.* 14th ed. Hudson, OH: Lexi-Comp; 2007.
11. Keating JP, Schears GH, Dodge PR. Oral water intoxication in infants: an American epidemic. *Am J Dis Child.* 1991;145:985.
12. Farrar HC, Chande VT, Fitzpatrick DF, et al. Hyponatremia as the cause of seizures in infants: a retrospective analysis of incidence, severity and clinical predictors. *Ann Emerg Med.* 1995;26:42.
13. Sterns RH, Riggs JE, Schochet SS Jr. Osmotic demyelination syndrome following correction of hyponatremia. *N Engl J Med.* 1986;314:1535.
14. Adrogue HJ, Madias NE. Hyponatremia. *N Engl J Med.* 2000;342:1581.
15. Gennari FJ. Current concepts: hypokalemia. *N Engl J Med.* 1998;339:451.
16. Allon M, Dunlay R, Copkney C. Nebulized albuterol for acute hyperkalemia in patients on hemodialysis. *Ann Intern Med.* 1989;110:426.
17. Lynch RE. Ionized calcium: Pediatric perspective. *Pediatr Clin North Am.* 1990;37:373.

CHAPTER 81

Inborn Errors of Metabolism

George E. Hoganson

▶ HIGH-YIELD FACTS

- Inborn errors of metabolism (IEM) that are more likely to present in the emergency department (ED) can be classified into a number of categories:
  ○ select amino acid disorders
  ○ urea cycle defects
  ○ disorder of carbohydrate metabolism
  ○ organic acid disorders
  ○ fatty acid oxidation defects
- Age of presentation is often related to the specific IEM and can vary from the newborn period to later in life, even into adulthood.
- With expanded newborn screening for IEM, more patients with one of these disorders will present to the ED with a known diagnosis. In these cases, information on associated clinical metabolic problems, indicated laboratory testing, and treatment for the condition is available.
- Patients with IEM can present with no prior history of medical problems. Precipitating events include febrile illness, gastroenteritis, poor oral intake, dietary change (EG, increased protein intake, or addition of fructose to the diet), or exercise.
- Clinical symptoms of IEM include vomiting, altered mental status/lethargy, seizures, hypotonia, and tachypnea.
- Hypoglycemia, anion gap acidosis, hyperammonemia, and ketosis are some of the metabolic consequences of IEM. Presence of these problems should lead to the inclusion of IEM in the patient's differential diagnosis.
- Initial medical management of patients with IEM in the ED requires suspicion that an IEM may be present, diagnosis of the possible metabolic problems, such as hypoglycemia or acidosis, and treatment of the problems found.
- Special biochemical genetics diagnostic testing is usually required to confirm the diagnosis.
- General laboratory testing to consider in a patient with a suspected IEM includes glucose, ammonia, liver function, creatine kinase, electrolytes, blood gas, uric acid, urinalysis, and urine-reducing substance.

Inborn errors of metabolism (IEM) or biochemical genetic disorders represent a diverse group of genetically determined diseases.[1] The majority of these conditions are inherited in an autosomal recessive pattern. A subset of these disorders has an X-linked recessive mode of inheritance. A family history of siblings with similar problems may suggest the presence of one of these disorders. In the case of an X-linked recessive disorder, there may be a history of affected males related through the maternal family. An example of this situation would occur in a family with ornithine transcarbamylase deficiency resulting in affected male infants with hyperammonemia.[2] A history of unexplained neonatal deaths in male infants would support this diagnosis. In the majority of suspected IEM cases, the family history is negative depending on an autosomal recessive inheritance pattern with a 25% risk for affected siblings. A history of recurrent illnesses or developmental delays may indicate an IEM. Table 81–1 lists categories and examples of some IEM that may present in the ED.

▶ PRESENTATION

The ED presentation of patients with IEM will be related to the underlying metabolic defect as well as the patient's age, health, and nutritional status. Neonatal presentation typically occurs when a severe metabolic defect is present.[3,4] Infants may present during the first weeks of life after an uneventful neonatal hospital course. A number of organic acidemias, urea cycle defects, and maple syrup urine disease (MSUD) can present in this manner. When severe neonatal forms of these disorders are present, symptoms related to the disorder are expected to develop within hours or days after birth. While neonatal problems can occur in most of the IEM, the absence of problems does not exclude the diagnosis.

In the majority of patients with an IEM, there is a relationship between onset of symptoms and a patient's health and nutritional status. The presence of an acute illness, typically viral, is often associated with the development of metabolic problems related to the IEM. An infant with glycogen storage disease will present with hypoglycemia when the feeding interval increases. Catabolism, depletion of glycogen stores, and increased production of toxic metabolites are some of the pathophysiologic mechanisms that can explain this association.[1]

A change in diet can precipitate biochemical change. For example, symptoms can develop in a patient with impaired protein metabolism who has been transitioned to cow's milk at the age of 1 year due to the higher protein content of milk, or after introduction of fructose/sucrose to the diet in a patient with hereditary fructose intolerance.

Intermittent forms of some disorders occur, where a patient may experience repeated episodes with vomiting and dehydration. Patients respond to treatment and return to their baseline state of health only to have the pattern repeat with the next illness. In some cases, the child is healthy during the first years of life and the initial presentation occurs much later in life. Given the diverse nature of IEM with the varied symptoms, clinical history, course, and laboratory findings, it is important

▶ TABLE 81-1. EXAMPLES OF INBORN ERRORS OF METABOLISM

Amino Acid Disorders	Organic Acidemias	Fatty Acid Oxidation Defects (FAOD)	Disorders of Carbohydrate Metabolism	Mitochondrial Disorders
Maple syrup urine disease (MSUD)	Isovaleric acidemia	Medium chain acyl-CoA dehydrogenase deficiency (MCAD)	Glycogen storage disease Ia, Ib, III (GSD)	Disorders of pyruvate metabolism
Tyrosinemia type I	Methylmalonic acidemia	Very long chain acyl-CoA dehydrogenase deficiency (VCLAD)	Hereditary fructose intolerance	Mitochondrial myopathies
Phenylketonuria does not cause acute metabolic problems	Propionic acidemia	Long chain hydroxyl acyl-CoA dehydrogenase deficiency (LCLAD)	Galactosemia	Electron transport chain defects
Urea cycle defects Ornithine transcarbamylase deficiency Citrullinemia Argininosuccinic acidemia Carbamyl phosphate synthetase deficiency	Glutaric acidemia Type I	Carnitine palmitoyl transferase I, II deficiency (CPT I, CPT II)		
		Carnitine deficiency		

that biochemical genetic disorders be considered in the differential diagnosis of ED patients with findings consistent with an IEM.[1-5]

Patients with an IEM may present with common symptoms including vomiting, diarrhea, and febrile illness. In these situations, the severity and presence of other symptoms or laboratory abnormalities may suggest the presence of an IEM. Examples of findings that are suggestive of IEM include unusual odors (present in an organic acidemia or MSUD) and more severe acidosis or ketosis than would be predicted based on the history or hypoglycemia. Table 81-2 lists symptoms associated with IEM. In other cases, patients may present to the ED with severe life-threatening problems including coma, severe acidosis, seizures, cardiomyopathy, or hypoglycemia. The first step in the evaluation for IEM begins in the ED with the physician considering the possibility that one of these conditions is present and is responsible for the symptoms and problems.

▶ DIAGNOSTIC TESTING

The second step in the evaluation is to identify which general laboratory testing to perform. This step is critical not only

▶ TABLE 81-2. PRESENTING SYMPTOMS OF IEM AND ASSOCIATED IEM

	Organic Acidemia	FAOD	MSUD	GSD	Urea Cycle Defect	Amino Acidopathy	Tyrosinemia	Fructose Intolerance	Homocysteinuria/ Cobalamin Defect
Hypoglycemia	×	×		×					
Anion gap acidosis	×		×						
Ketosis	×		×						
Vomiting	×		×		×				
Seizures	×		×	×	×				
Altered mental status/coma	×	×		×	×	×			
Hypotonia		×		×					
Hepatomegaly	×	×		×					
Hepatic failure		×					×	×	
Cardiomyopathy		×		×					
Thrombocytopenia	×								
Thrombotic events								×	×

FAOD, fatty acid oxidation deficiency; MSUD, maple syrup urine disease; GSD, glycogen storage disease.

▶ **TABLE 81-3. GENERAL LABORATORY TESTING TO CONSIDER IN CASE OF SUSPECTED IEM**

Glucose: hypoglycemia
Blood gas: acid/base states
Comprehensive metabolic panel: renal/liver/electrolyte
Lactate: lactic acidosis
Uric acid: elevated in organic acidemia/MSUD
Ammonia: hyperammonemia in urea cycle defect, FAOD, organic acidemia
Creatine kinase: increased with rhabodomyolysis
Urinanalysis: ketones, blood/myoglobin
Urine reducing substances: simple sugars, fructose, galactose
Complete blood count: neutropenia, thrombocytopenia

to obtain laboratory data to assist in the diagnosis but also, and potentially of greater immediate importance, to identify special areas requiring treatment. For example, in urea cycle defects, organic acid disorders, and fatty acid oxidation defects, it is important to obtain the blood ammonia level to diagnose hyperammonia. Definitive diagnosis of one of these disorders typically requires special biochemical diagnostic testing, which is not performed in many hospital laboratories. However, initiating this testing following an ED visit or subsequent hospitalization can greatly facilitate the diagnosis of one of these conditions and assist in the patient's medical management.

General laboratory testing can assist in determining if an IEM is present. Table 81-3 lists some of the general laboratory testing performed in this clinical setting. Testing performed in most situations would include glucose levels, evaluation of acid/base status, urinanalysis including urine ketones, complete blood count, and evaluation of renal and liver function. Additional testing may be indicated. For example, lactate level to assess for lactic acidosis and ammonia level for hyperammonemia is indicated in cases of acidosis or altered mental status, respectively. If evidence of myopathy, muscle weakness, or myalgia is present in an older patient, especially with an elevation in AST/ALT, a creatine kinase level is indicated to evaluate for a myopathic process and rhabdomyolysis as is present in some fatty acid oxidation deficiencies (FAOD).[1,6] The presence of blood on urinanalysis with normal urine RBC count in this setting may be indicative of myoglobinuria.

Initial laboratory testing is usually guided by the problem present at the time of presentation to the ED. In some situations, the order of testing may be influenced by both the clinical state of the patient and results of initial testing. Figure 81–1 outlines a possible approach for evaluation of hypoglycemia in a case of a suspected IEM. Hypoglycemia with negative ketone levels may indicate the presence of a FAOD; while the presence of acidosis, hypoglycemia, and ketosis is more suggestive of an organic acid disorder.

It is important to recognize that complicating factors present at the time of the patient's initial presentation may impact test results and their interpretation. A severely dehydrated child with poor perfusion may also have a secondary lactic acidosis. The patient's clinical course including laboratory results and response to treatment usually allows for a

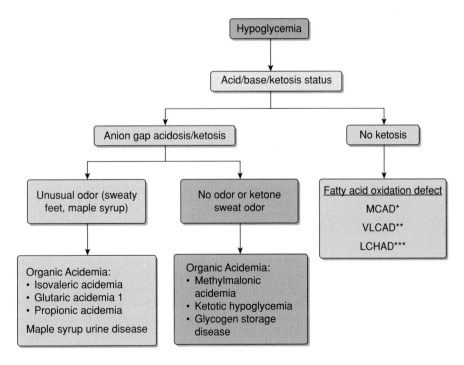

*MCAD: medium chain acyl-CoA dehydrogenase deficiency

**VLCAD: very long chain acyl-CoA dehydrogenase deficiency

***LCHAD: long chain hydroxyl acyl-CoA dehydrogenase deficiency

Figure 81–1. Possible IEM explanations for hypoglycemia.

▶ **TABLE 81–4. BIOCHEMICAL GENETIC TESTING UTILIZED IN THE DIAGNOSIS AND MANAGEMENT OF IEM**

Analyte determination
   Plasma amino acids
   Urine organic acids
   Blood carnitine level
   Blood acylcarnitine profile
Enzyme determination
Molecular diagnostics
   Common mutation detection
   Gene sequencing

determination as to whether the abnormalities are secondary or the consequence of an IEM. Initial treatment of identified laboratory findings usually follows general recommendations.

Table 81–4 lists some of the specialized biochemical genetic testing considered in the evaluation of IEM. Specific testing to be performed is often determined in consultation with the biochemical/clinical geneticist or other metabolic specialist. In many situations, biochemical genetic testing performed at the time of an acute illness can evaluate for specific abnormalities helpful in the IEM diagnostic evaluation. In some situations, diagnostic test results may only be detectable during an acute illness.

▶ NEWBORN SCREENING

With the implementation of tandem mass spectrometry in the diagnosis of IEM through neonatal screening, many of the conditions referred to thus far can be diagnosed in the newborn period. This allows for presymptomatic detection and the institution of a corresponding treatment regimen. Three groups of biochemical genetic disorders are screened for using this technology: amino acid disorders, organic acidemias, and fatty acid oxidation defects. Galactosemia testing is also included on most newborn screening panels. It is important to note that some disorders cannot be detected with this screening, because either biochemical markers of the disorder are not present or newborn screening does not detect the disorder in all cases. Under optimal conditions, it is expected that newborn screen testing will be completed and reported to the birth hospital and primary MD within 7 days of birth. While guidelines recommend which disorders should be included on newborn screening disease panels, not all state programs test for all disorders.[7,8] Therefore, it is important for physicians caring for newborns and pediatric patients to know which disorders are included in the newborn screen testing panel for their state and how to obtain the test results for an infant.[8] This information is usually not available at night or on weekends, but some data may be obtained from the birth hospital or primary physician. Newborn screen ACT sheets are available from the American College of Medical Genetics; these sheets summarize information on newborn screening diseases and medical response to a report of a positive result.[9] A newborn screen

result can provide important information to assist in the evaluation and treatment of a young infant, but a normal newborn screen result does not exclude the diagnosis of an IEM.

The early diagnosis of some IEM through newborn screening has resulted in another category of ER visits for patients with IEM. This group of diagnosed IEM patients is instructed by their treating physicians to take proactive and preventative steps at times of illness, or if there is a change in the child's condition. These instructions as well as testing recommendations and treatments are often summarized in an "emergency protocol." The emergency protocol typically provides the diagnosis, acute medical problems associated with the disorder, and treatment recommendations. The treating ED physician in this setting evaluates the child for problems and initiates the recommended evaluations and indicated treatments. In some situations, hospitalization is required to continue the appropriate supportive treatment and to prevent worsening of the patient's metabolic disorder. For many disorders, intravenous caloric support with dextrose can prevent or treat metabolic problems, such as ketosis in organic acid disorders and hypoglycemia in fatty acid oxidation disorders. In general, patients with these disorders cannot be discharged from the ED unless metabolic problems have been resolved and the patient can maintain an adequate oral caloric intake. For some disorders, patients must also be able to take prescribed medications. Arginine and ammonia-conjugating medication (Buphenyl) are needed to control blood ammonia levels in urea cycle defects.[2] In cases where metabolic problems are present, consultation with the treating metabolic specialist is required to determine the most appropriate course of treatment.

▶ TREATMENT

Initial treatment is determined by the patient's presentation. If the diagnosis of IEM is known, targeted evaluation can be initiated to determine the presence of specific problems associated with the specific IEM. Clinical and laboratory evaluation will identify areas requiring treatment. Additional general laboratory testing should be performed (Table 81–3) to evaluate the patient for associated medical problems. This approach will also increase the likelihood that medical problems such as hyperammonemia or rhabdomyolysis, which require further evaluation and specialized treatment, will be detected. In general, the initial treatment of medical problems in patients with IEM follows recommendations outlined in the respective chapters. In some clinical situations, it is necessary to address multiple problems simultaneously. For example, treatment of dehydration and hypoglycemia in a patient with an FAOD requires administration of fluids with high dextrose content. Consultation with a metabolic specialist, such as a biochemical/clinical geneticist, may be indicated for determining the most appropriate course of treatment and diagnostic evaluation.

When serious medical problems or complications are present, hospitalization, potentially in a PICU, is indicated. Hospitalization is often required to address medical problems resulting from the acute illness and to prevent worsening of the patient's condition. Typically, ED patients with an IEM who have responded well to initial treatment and have remained stable during a period of observation are capable of resuming their normal routine of diet and medication at home. If there is clinical evidence to suggest that problems might recur, hospitalization is indicated.

REFERENCES

1. Scriver CR, Beadet AL, Sly WS, et al., eds. *The Metabolic and Molecular Bases of Inherited Disease.* 8th ed. New York, NY: Mcgraw-Hill; 2001.

2. Nassogne MC, Heron B, Touati G, Rabier D, Saudubray JM. Urea cycle defects: management and outcome. *J Inherit Metab Dis.* 2005;28(3):407–414.

3. Leonard JV, Morris AA. Diagnosis and early management of inborn errors of metabolism presenting around the time of birth. *Acta Paediatr.* 2006;95(1):6–14.

4. Burton BK. Inborn errors of metabolism in infancy: a guide to diagnosis. *Pediatrics.* 1998;102(6):E69.

5. Saudubray JM, Sedel F, Walter JH. Clinical approach to treatable inborn metabolic diseases: an introduction. *J Inherit Metab Dis.* 2006;29(2–3):261–274.

6. Vockley J, Singh RH, Whiteman DA. Diagnosis and management of defects mitochondrial beta-oxidation. *Curr Opin Clin Nutr Metab Care.* 2002;5(6):601–609.

7. Watson MS et al. Newborn screening: toward a uniform screening panel and system—executive summary. *Pediatrics.* 2006;117(5):S296–S307.

8. National Newborn Screening Status report. National Newborn Screening and Genetics Resource Center(NNSGRC). http://genes-r-us.uthscsa.edu/nbsdisorders.pdf.

9. American College of medical genetics Website, Newborn Screening ACT Sheets and Confirmatory Algorithms. http://www.acmg.net/resources/policies/ACT/condition-analyte-links.htm.

SECTION XII

GENITOURINARY EMERGENCIES

CHAPTER 82

Male Genitourinary Problems

John W. Williams and Marianne Gausche-Hill

► HIGH-YIELD FACTS

- Acute scrotal pain is usually caused by testicular torsion, epididymitis, or torsion of the appendix testis.
- Testicular torsion is the most serious common cause of acute scrotal pain in children. Pain is abrupt and severe. Prompt urologic consultation must be obtained in each case.
- Torsion of an appendix is usually less severe and localized.
- Epididymitis is caused by urinary tract infections in young children and by sexually transmitted disease in older children and adolescents. Antibiotic treatment is based on age and presentation.
- Color Doppler ultrasound is the diagnostic test of choice for evaluation of the acute scrotum.
- A genitourinary examination should be performed on all children with abdominal or genitourinary complaints, as signs and symptoms may be nonspecific and abdominal pain may be caused by testicular torsion, inguinal hernia, epididymitis, and, rarely, testicular tumor.
- The emergency department can reduce up to 95% of inguinal hernias.
- Varicoceles are generally benign and most are left sided; however, persistent scrotal swelling and a "bag of worms" appearance indicates possible obstruction from tumor.
- With normal growth and stretching of the prepuce, it will become retractable in 90% of children by the age of 6 years.
- The evaluation of children with paraphimosis must begin by establishing that the children have not been circumcised and by eliminating the possibility of hair tourniquet syndrome. Treatment is manual reduction of the prepuce over the glans penis.
- Priapism can be divided into two mechanisms: low flow or ischemic as in sickle cell vasoocclusion and high flow or engorgement.

► TESTICULAR PAIN/SCROTAL MASSES

Acute scrotal pain and swelling in children has many causes; in most cases the emergency physician (EP) can determine the etiology by the history and physical examination and by considering the age of the patient. Scrotal swelling may be painful or painless (Table 82–1). The most common diagnoses for an acute scrotum are testicular torsion, torsion of the appendix testis or epididymis, and epididymitis. In all cases, the possibility of a surgical emergency must be considered and the

► TABLE 82-1. CAUSES OF SCROTAL SWELLING IN CHILDREN

Painful	Painless
Testicular torsion	Testicular tumor, leukemia
Torsion of the appendix testis or epididymus testis	Hydrocele
Epididymitis	Varicocele
Incarcerated hernia	Inguinal hernia
Idiopathic scrotal edema (dermatitis, angioedema, insect bite)	Idiopathic scrotal edema
Trauma (testicular rupture)	Henoch–Schonlein purpura
Scrotal cellulitis or abscess	Anasarca
Orchitis	
Renal colic	

evaluation and management must proceed accordingly. Color Doppler ultrasound is the examination of choice for imaging scrotal pathology.

TESTICULAR TORSION

Testicular torsion can occur anytime from infancy to adulthood. Its incidence is bimodal, first in the neonatal period and with peak incidence in adolescence.[1,2] Torsion of the testes is a urologic emergency and results in a significant amount of legal action against EPs for missed diagnosis. The EP must suspect this diagnosis in any child with complaint of scrotal pain or signs of scrotal swelling on physical examination.

Pathophysiology

The classic description of the anatomic abnormality associated with torsion is the "bell-clapper" deformity that is often bilateral and causes the testes to have a horizontal lie within the scrotal sac (Fig. 82–1). The testicular attachments to the intrascrotal subcutaneous tissue of the tunica vaginalis are abnormal, allowing the testis to twist within the scrotal sac along with the spermatic cord and associated testicular artery. If the torsion is complete, vascular compromise ensues and eventually the testis will necrose and atrophy. Intermittent torsion may spare the testes for a longer time interval, thus the actual duration of symptoms may not necessarily predict the viability of the testis. After 4 hours of pain, the salvage rate is 96%, but drops to 20% after 12 hours of pain, and below 10% at 24 hours. Patients with symptoms for more than 24 hours are unlikely to have a viable testis; beyond 48 hours, testicular salvage is poor.[1]

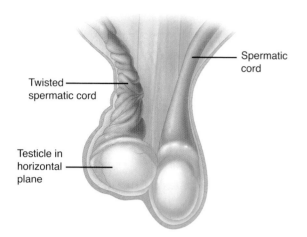

Figure 82–1. Bell-clapper deformity in testicular torsion results from the twisting of the spermatic cord and causes the testis to be elevated, with a horizontal lie. The lack of fixation of the tunica vaginalis to the posterior scrotum predisposes the freely movable testis to rotation and subsequent torsion. An elevated testis with a horizontal lie may be seen in asymptomatic patients at risk for torsion.

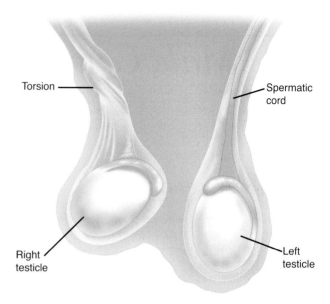

Figure 82–2. Torsion of the right testicle. The testicle lies horizontally and in a higher position than the normal testicle.

Signs and Symptoms

Patients usually present with sudden onset of unilateral scrotal or testicular pain, followed by vomiting. Pain may also be intermittent, which may represent recurring torsion with interval resolution. The history may include blunt scrotal trauma or a recent diagnosis of epididymitis. Associated symptoms of abdominal or flank pain are common. Patients may also relate a history of previous symptoms on the other side, and the EP should be alerted to the possibility of bilateral testicular torsion. Unilateral lower abdominal pain may indicate an undescended testis that has torsed, and indeed, undescended testes are more likely to torse than fully descended ones.

Physical examination often reveals a swollen, erythematous, and exquisitely tender hemiscrotum (Fig. 82–2). The testicle may be high riding when compared to the contralateral side and lying horizontally within the scrotum, a classic presentation that should prompt immediate urologic consultation.[1] With delay, the examination may become more difficult as edema, erythema, and a reactive hydrocele may develop.[1] Tenderness of the affected testis is diffuse, and the cremasteric reflex may be absent.[3] Elevating the testis will cause further pain (Prehn's sign) instead of the relief that can be seen in epididymitis; however, this cannot reliably include or exclude torsion. A focal area of tenderness over the superior testis or the epididymis may suggest epididymitis.[4]

Diagnostic Evaluation

Some studies may aid in the diagnosis of testicular torsion; however, prompt urologic consultation should not be delayed to obtain tests. Urinalysis that shows pyuria or bacteruria suggests UTI, epididymitis, or orchitis but does not rule out torsion. Other laboratory studies such as complete blood count and chemistries may be requested preoperatively but rarely help diagnosis, and should not delay definitive management.

High-resolution ultrasound with color-flow Doppler is rapid and readily available, and provides information about testicular blood flow. Sensitivity is 90% and specificity above 98% in experienced hands, with a false-positive rate of less than 1%.[4] Moreover, anatomic structure and relationships are displayed with ultrasound. Radionuclide imaging of the scrotum was the traditional test of choice but can take precious time, is not always available, requires IV access, and exposes the patient to ionizing radiation. Its has been reported to have an accuracy of 90%.[2] Further diagnostic evaluation is reserved for those patients in which the diagnosis of torsion is in question, and in which any delay in obtaining studies will not result in increased morbidity.

Management

Rapid urologic consultation should be obtained early on all patients with suspected torsion. Manual detorsion of the torsed testes may be attempted by the EP to reduce the ischemic time while awaiting the arrival of the urologist. Patients are sedated, and the testicle is detorsed by turning the testicle outward toward the thigh, like "opening a book" (Fig. 82–3). This should provide sudden relief, and the testicle may drop lower in the scrotum.[4] In some cases this may not help, and detorsion in the opposite direction may be attempted. Prompt surgical exploration is indicated, and bilateral orchiopexy is necessary to avoid recurrence. In all cases of torsion, the affected testicle is untwisted and the contralateral testis is also fixed. Orchidectomy of the affected testicle is often recommended.

TORSION OF THE APPENDIX TESTIS

Testicular appendices are common and may occur on the testicle, the spermatic cord, or the epididymis. The hydatid of Morgagni or appendix testis is the most common of the

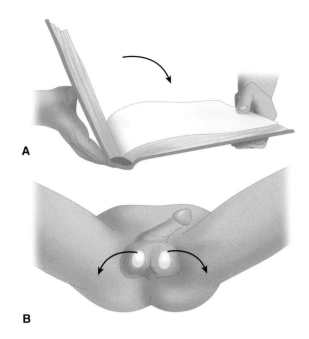

Figure 82-3. Testicular detorsion. This procedure is best done standing at the foot of or on the right side of the patient's bed. (A). The torsed testis is detorsed in a fashion similar to opening a book. (B). The patient's right testis is rotated counterclockwise, and the left testis is rotated clockwise.

vestiges to torse. Torsion of the appendix testis is often diffi-cult to distinguish from torsion of the spermatic cord. While it can occur in adolescents, it is more common in prepubertal boys.[4,5]

Signs and Symptoms

Signs and symptoms of torsion of the appendix testis are usu-ally less severe but may be indistinguishable than those of testicular torsion. Systemic symptoms such as nausea and vom-iting are uncommon, and the physical examination may reveal diffuse testicular enlargement and pain or only a focal ten-derness in the upper pole of the testis. A "blue-dot" sign is occasionally noted in children when the necrotic appendage casts a blue hue under the scrotal skin (Fig. 82–4).

Diagnostic Evaluation

Laboratory evaluation is not helpful, and the urinalysis is nor-mal. Color Doppler ultrasonography (US) is normal or reveals increased flow to the testicle, and only occasionally is diagnos-tic and shows a discrete appendage.[4]

Management

Once the diagnosis of torsion of the appendix testis is made, bed rest, urologic follow-up, and analgesia are recommended. Surgical intervention is sometimes indicated in cases in which the diagnosis of testicular torsion cannot be reliably excluded. The condition is self-limited, most patients improve with anal-gesics and bed rest within a few days; complications are rare.

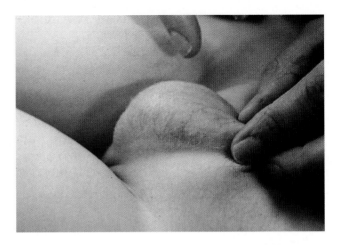

Figure 82-4. Blue-dot sign is caused by torsion of the testicular appendix. It is best seen with the skin held taut over the testicular appendix.

EPIDIDYMITIS

Epididymitis is more common in adolescents and adults than young children; however, it is the most common misdiagnosis for testicular torsion. It occurs in approximately one-third of children who present to the ED with acute scrotal pain. Epi-didymitis is rare in infants.[6]

Pathophysiology

Epididymitis is often caused by spread of infection from the urethra or bladder. In children younger than 6 years, urinary tract anomalies may be present and predispose to infection. Pathogens causing UTIs such as *Escherichia coli* can lead to local inflammation and swelling of the epididymis. In the ado-lescent it is unusual to find anatomic abnormalities, and epi-didymitis is often caused by sexually transmitted diseases such as *Neisseria gonorrhoeae* and *Chlamydia trachomatis*. Epi-didymitis may also be viral and occur after other infections such as upper respiratory infections, or possibly as a chemical inflammation caused by reflux of sterile urine into the ejacula-tory ducts.[6]

Signs and Symptoms

A careful history must be elicited, in particular, the time course of the symptoms; any history of trauma; recent sexual activity; and urinary symptoms such as dysuria, frequency, urgency, nocturia, incontinence, or hematuria. A history of vomiting, fever, and previous scrotal pain is also obtained.

The primary symptom is increasing dull unilateral scro-tal pain.[6] Symptoms in young children may be vague and nonspecific. In infants, caregivers may notice scrotal swelling. Fever and vomiting may preceed swelling of the hemiscro-tum. The onset may be gradual, with scrotal pain and swelling worsening over several days.[4] In the older child, the onset of pain is often insidious and isolated to the hemiscrotum; it later becomes diffuse, perhaps radiating into the lower abdomen. Fever and urinary symptoms from a preceding urethritis may also be present.

▶ **TABLE 82–2.** ANTIBIOTIC THERAPY FOR EPIDIDYMITIS IN CHILDREN

Antibiotic	Dose	Route
Outpatient management		
Nonsexually active		
Trimethoprim-sulfamethoxazole, or	8–10 mg/kg per 24 h	PO bid for 10–14 d
Cephalexin	25–50 mg/kg per 24 h	PO qid for 10 d
Sexually active		
Ceftriaxone, plus (if >8 y)	250 mg	IM
Doxycycline, or	100 mg	PO bid for 10 d
Erythromycin	50 mg/kg per 24 h	PO qid for 10 d
Inpatient management		
Ampicillin	100 mg/kg per 24 h	IV q 6 h
Plus gentamicin, or	7.5 mg/kg per 24 h	IV q 8 h
Cefotaxime, or	50–150 mg/kg per 24 h	IV q 6 h
Ceftriaxone	50–100 mg/kg per 24 h	IV q 12–24 h

PO, orally; bid, twice daily; qid, 4 times daily; IM, intramuscularly.
Note: ceftriaxone IV is incompatible and possibly lethal with calcium-containing parenteral solutions, and its use is being reconsidered for in-patient pediatrics; do not use it in hyperbilirubinemic neonates.

Physical examination reveals an erythematous, warm, swollen epididymis, testicle, and scrotum. A careful examination might reveal tenderness at the superior aspect of the testicle. The testicle itself is nontender and should have a normal lie. Prehn's sign—relief upon elevation of the scrotum—may be present but is not reliable in distinguishing epididymitis from testicular torsion. Likewise, patients usually have a normal cremasteric reflex.

Diagnostic Evaluation

In prepubescent children, epididymitis is difficult to distinguish clinically from testicular torsion. A urinalysis may show signs of urinary tract infection with increased white blood cells and bacteria, but pyuria is present in less than half the cases of epididymitis. A complete blood cell count may reveal an elevated white blood cell count with left shift; however, it is often normal in epididymitis. Because the consequences of a missed testicular torsion are dire, the EP should obtain prompt urologic consultation when the cause of the scrotal pain is unclear. Color Doppler US should be performed, and will reveal normal or increased flow to the affected testis if the patient has epididymitis. There may be a higher rate of indeterminate studies in infants and young children.

Once the diagnosis of epididymitis is confirmed, the evaluation for young children or adolescents in whom a concomitant UTI is suspected includes a urine culture. In sexually active adolescents, a urethral swab for *N. gonorrhoeae* and *Chlamydia* cultures and a VDRL or RPR are indicated. Bacterial epididymitis may be associated with a positive urine or STD culture. Viral infections are common and diagnosed presumptively.[4] After the infection is treated, appropriate imaging may include an US of the bladder and kidneys or a voiding cystourethrogram.[4] A noncontrast computed tomography (CT) of the abdomen may show urinary tract anomalies or renal stones causing obstruction.

Management

Management is dependent upon the age and clinical condition of the patient. Children younger than 1 month with associated UTI should be admitted to the hospital and receive IV antibiotics. This approach should be considered for infants 3 months of age or younger as well. Older infants and children younger than 2 years may also require admission depending on associated signs and symptoms. Older children and adolescents can usually be treated as outpatients with antibiotics and analgesics, bed rest, and scrotal elevation/support.

Inpatient antibiotic therapy for infants and children with a suspected urinary source should include ampicillin and an aminoglycoside or cefotaxime (Table 82–2). For the nonsexually active child, trimethoprim-sulfamethoxazole (TMP-SMX) orally for 10 to 14 days is the drug of choice, although drug resistance is on the rise. Cephalexin may also be used in this age group. For the sexually active adolescent, especially if there is urethral discharge, antibiotic treatment should include ceftriaxone, 250 mg intramuscularly, followed by doxycycline, 100 mg orally twice a day for 10 days. Patients < 9 years of age should be treated with erythromycin, 50 mg/kg/d divided four times a day. Prompt urologic consultation and subsequent follow-up is recommended for all of these patients.

SCROTAL AND TESTICULAR TRAUMA

Trauma to the scrotum can occur by many mechanisms, including child abuse. Most often, the mechanism is blunt trauma as a result of play in which the patient sustained a direct blow or a straddle injury, or a motor vehicle crash. The resulting injury is a scrotal hematoma and, rarely, testicular rupture.

Testicular rupture occurs when the testis is crushed against the bony pelvis. Rupture into a testicular tumor must be considered in patients with a scrotal hematoma after minor trauma. Bleeding into the scrotum occurs, and the scrotum may be ecchymotic or tense with blood. The testis may be difficult to palpate and may have an irregular border or be ill-defined. If testicular rupture is suspected, prompt evaluation of the integrity of the testis by US is essential. Ultrasonography can also locate a dislocated testicle secondary to major trauma. Urologic consultation sought immediately once the diagnosis of testicular rupture is made.

Scrotal hematomas and testicular contusions are treated with bed rest, scrotal support, ice packs, and analgesics. Testicular rupture is treated by surgical exploration and repair, although testicular salvage rates are poor.

TESTICULAR TUMORS

Testicular tumors are rare in childhood. They are more common in whites and less common in African Americans. Types of testicular tumors include teratomas, embryonal carcinomas, yolk sac, choriocarcinomas, Leydig cell, and Sertoli cell. Lymphoma and leukemia can metastasize to the testis and present as a testicular mass. An undescended testis is up to a 50 times more likely than a descended testes to contain a tumor, especially if it is located intra-abdominally.

Signs and Symptoms

Most often children and young adults have a feeling of fullness, tugging, or increased weight to the scrotum. Patients or their caregivers may feel a mass. On physical examination, the mass is firm, smooth, or nodular, and does not transilluminate. Tumors are generally painless, but bleeding into the tumor can cause sudden testicular pain or referred pain to the abdomen or flank. A thorough physical examination should be performed including evaluation for lymphadenopathy, an abdominal mass, hepatosplenomegaly, a petechial rash, and gynecomastia.

Diagnostic Evaluation

A urinalysis should be performed, as well as a complete blood cell count and test for α-fetoprotein levels. A rapid urine pregnancy test may be positive for human chorionic gonadotropin, since this hormone is often produced by germ cell tumors. Ultrasonography may confirm the presence and location of a mass, and differentiate between benign and malignant tumors.[1]

Management

Urologic consultation and prompt biopsy or removal of the mass is necessary to establish tumor type and subsequent treatment options for patients.

INGUINAL HERNIA

Pathophysiology

Indirect inguinal hernia repair is the most common pediatric surgery. Approximately 2% of children have an inguinal hernia (range 0.8%–4.4%) and the incidence increases with prematurity.[2,8,9] It occurs when peritoneal or pelvic contents herniate through a patent processus vaginalis into the scrotal sac.[10] Indirect hernias are usually right-sided. Males are up to 10 times more likely than females to have an inguinal hernia.[2,8]

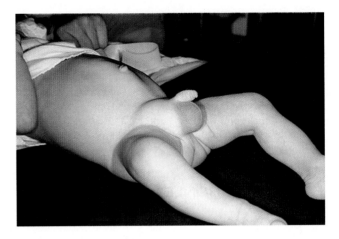

Figure 82–5. This infant presented with inconsolable crying and vomiting. Inguinal hernia may be either unilateral or bilateral. This patient's hernia could not be reduced into the abdominal cavity and the patient required surgical repair.

Signs and Symptoms

Inguinal hernias most often present in the first year of life when parents note an intermittent bulge into the scrotal sac when the infant cries or coughs. Most inguinal hernias are asymptomatic, but some parents report that the infant is fussy. Children may note a pulling feeling or heaviness in the groin and also note a bulge, which increases with intra-abdominal pressure. Systemic signs of fever, abdominal pain, poor feeding, or nausea and vomiting should alert the clinician to the possibility of incarceration of the hernia. Other signs of incarceration include a firm, painful, tender, and nonreducible mass in the inguinal area and scrotum. Incarcerated hernias can rapidly progress to strangulation, with ensuing vomiting, abdominal distention, peritonitis, and shock.[10] Approximately 10% of inguinal hernias incarcerate. Most incarcerations occur in children younger than 1 year,[8] particularly within the first 2 months.[10]

Diagnostic Evaluation

Inguinal hernias can usually be diagnosed from history and physical examination (Fig. 82–5). Transillumination of the scrotum should distinguish a hydrocele from an incarcerated inguinal hernia and from solid masses such as a swollen lymph node or a tumor. Undescended or retracted testes may mimic inguinal hernias. Both testicles should be palpated during the assessment of a possible inguinal hernia.[8] If the diagnosis is in question, an ultrasound may be helpful, particularly in differentiating among other causes of inguinal masses; accuracy approaches 98%.[9,10] It is the modality of choice in distinguishing a hernia from other inguinal masses such as an abscess, tumor, or hydrocele.[10] Abdominal radiographs are usually not helpful, except to establish the presence of an intestinal obstruction.

Management

Incarcerated hernias can be reduced up to 95% of the time with firm finger pressure on the internal inguinal ring, analgesics or sedation, ice pack to the area, and placement of patients in the

Trendelenburg position. If the hernia is reduced easily, then patients can be discharged to home with close follow-up with a surgeon for definitive repair. Patients with hernias that do not reduce easily, but still can be reduced, should be admitted for observation and delayed surgical repair. Patients with hernias that remain incarcerated or patients that demonstrate signs of peritonitis or bowel perforation must be taken immediately to the operating room. In these cases, stabilization of patients with fluid resuscitation and antibiotics should be initiated in the ED.

HENOCH–SCHÖNLEIN PURPURA

Henoch–Schönlein purpura (HSP) is a systemic vasculitis that often results in abdominal pain, gastrointestinal bleeding, purpuric rash, nephritis, arthritis, and hematuria. It is more common in children younger than 7 years. One-third of patients may have scrotal pain, swelling, or erythema,[4] and a purpuric rash on the scrotum may be seen. In some cases, it is impossible to clinically distinguish HSP from testicular torsion. The EP must then assume that the patient has testicular torsion, consult a urologist, and obtain color Doppler US. If the diagnostic evaluation is negative and the patient has other features of HSP, surgical exploration may not be necessary.

HYDROCELE

A hydrocele is formed from a patent processus vaginalis that normally regresses to form the tunica vaginalis. The hydrocele may communicate with the peritoneal cavity and can be associated with an indirect inguinal hernia. Fluid is noted adjacent to the testis and may result in a swollen and bluish-appearing scrotum. Transillumination of the swelling reveals that the mass is fluid filled, but it may be difficult to distinguish hydrocele from indirect inguinal hernia. If the hydrocele presents as a painful swelling, then the physician must consider intraperitoneal pathology, such as a ruptured appendix, or testicular torsion, otherwise a nonpainful hydrocele may be observed for 6 months to 1 year of age for spontaneous resolution. If the hydrocele persists past the first year of life, a patent processus vaginalis is surgically repaired.

VARICOCELE

Varicoceles usually present in the adolescent male as painless scrotal swelling. Incompetent valves in the testicular veins and the pampiniform plexus of the spermatic cord result in venous dilatation and a scrotum that looks and feels like a "bag of worms." Varicoceles occur in approximately 15% of the population and 85% are left-sided.[2] They are usually benign in nature, but could represent obstruction at the level of the renal vein from a tumor. Right-sided varicoceles may indicate obstruction by tumor at the level of the inferior vena cava (IVC). Patients should be examined in the standing position, which often exaggerates the findings of scrotal enlargement and "bag of worms" appearance, as well as in the supine position in which these findings are minimal or absent. Patients in whom the scrotal swelling persists in the supine position

should be evaluated for obstruction at the level of the renal vein on the left or the IVC on the right by renal ultrasound, IVP, or angiography. Surgical repair may be necessary for cases of testicular atrophy, lesions causing proximal obstruction, or patients with significant pain. Although there is an association between adolescent varicoceles and adult infertility, there is insufficient evidence that surgical repair is effective in most patients.[11,12]

OTHER CAUSES OF SCROTAL PAIN OR SWELLING

Other causes of scrotal swelling with and without pain include scrotal cellulitis, idiopathic scrotal edema, and lymphadenitis. Idiopathic scrotal edema is more common in prepubertal boys and characterized by thickening and erythema of the scrotum not involving the testes. It is not always painful and may be pruritic. Minor trauma, inlcuding insect bites, localized irritation, or contact dermatitis results in idiopathic scrotal edema. Treatment usually consists of antihistamines or topical steroids, and antibiotics if cellulitis is a concern.[4] Orchitis is an uncommon cause of scrotal pain and swelling; it is often viral mediated and is associated with mumps.

Fournier's Gangrene

There have been cases of Fournier's gangrene in children reported. It is infectious in origin and results in necrotizing fasciitis. Fournier's gangrene may initially present as cellulitis, balanitis, balanoposthitis, or scrotal pain and swelling. Patients may appear relatively nontoxic even when obvious gangrene appears in the perineum. Although staphylococcal and streptococcal organisms are the most common organisms to be cultured, management includes broad-spectrum antibiotic therapy to cover anaerobic and aerobic, gram-positive and -negative organisms. Prompt surgical consultation and operative incision and drainage of infected tissue with excision of necrotic tissue are paramount. Generally, the prognosis in children is better than it is in adults, and more conservative surgical debridement is recommended.

▶ PENILE EMERGENCIES

The differential diagnosis for males who present to the ED with a swollen, erythematous penis includes phimosis, paraphimosis, balanitis, posthitis, hair tourniquet syndrome, and insect bite.[1]

PHIMOSIS

Pathophysiology

Phimosis occurs when the distal prepuce is unable to be retracted over the glans penis. Normally, the prepuce cannot be retracted over the glans in infants and it should not be forced. With normal growth and stretching of the prepuce, it will become retractable in 90% of children by the age of 6 years. Local irritation or infection (balanoposthitis) can cause an abnormal constriction of the prepuce, preventing its ability to retract normally.

Signs and Symptoms

Phimosis may be noted on routine physical examination or may be reported by parents. Pain and swelling can occur with associated infections of the glans. Urinary stream in some cases may be diverted to one side or children may have hematuria.

Physical examination generally establishes the diagnosis. The EP will find a constricted distal prepuce that is unable to be retracted over the glans penis. Patients will sometimes have concomitant balanitis or balanoposthitis.

Diagnostic Evaluation

The diagnosis is established clinically; however, examination of the urine for UTI may be warranted in selected cases. If patients demonstrate signs of urinary tract obstruction, such as inability to urinate, abdominal fullness, or urinary frequency, then renal function studies should be obtained. Renal US may define the degree of obstruction.

Management

As most cases are not a result of a pathologic condition but a result of normal growth and development, reassurance and an explanation of the natural course of this condition to parents is often all that is needed. Betamethasone valerate, 0.6% cream applied twice daily for 2 weeks, has been used to treat phimosis and may be prescribed in cases in which the phimosis is not anatomic but pathologic. Patients with recurrent balanitis, balanoposthitis, UTI, or obstruction should be referred to a urologist for circumcision.

PARAPHIMOSIS

Pathophysiology

Paraphimosis is a condition in which the foreskin or prepuce of the uncircumcised male is retracted over the glans and becomes trapped and unable to move back into its normal position (Fig. 82–6). Once the prepuce is retracted, its constriction proximal to the coronal sulcus causes venous congestion of the glans that further prevents reduction. Ischemic injury to the glans may ensue.

Signs and Symptoms

Patients have pain and edema of the distal penis and prepuce. If the child has not been circumcised, then a thorough examination to look for possible hair tourniquets and penile foreign bodies must follow.

Management

The management of this condition focuses on retracting the prepuce over the head of the glans. Without anesthesia, most children poorly tolerate ice packs to the groin. The physician may place a penile block by injecting lidocaine 1% without

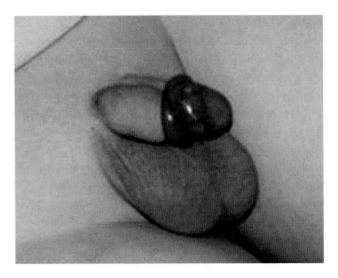

Figure 82–6. Paraphimosis: moderate edema of retracted foreskin, which is entrapped behind the coronal sulcus.

epinephrine around the base of the penis. This will effectively reduce the pain. Ice packs can then be placed for 10 minutes after which manual reduction should be attempted (Fig. 82–7). The physician's index fingers are placed on the leading edge of the edematous foreskin, and the thumbs are placed on the glans. Thumb pressure is directed inward toward the body as the prepuce is pushed back over the glans. Successful reduction following compression of the glans and distal penis by wrapping with a small ace bandage starting distally and working toward the base of the penis has also been described.[13] The Perth-Dundee method uses a 26-G needle to make multiple (up to 20) holes in the edematous foreskin, which is then manually compressed to express fluid, permitting reduction. As a last resort, it may be necessary to incise the constricting ring of tissue. General anesthesia may be required in young children. In most cases, subsequent circumcision is not necessary.[13]

Once reduction is complete, the prepuce should lie over the end of the glans and the urethral opening should not be visible. If retraction of the prepuce is successful and the child is able to urinate spontaneously, then the child can be discharged with urologic follow-up. If the prepuce cannot be retracted, then emergent urologic consultation is needed for surgical division of the phimotic ring, and eventually, circumcision.

BALANITIS AND BALANOPOSTHITIS

Balanitis (infection of the glans) and balanoposthitis (infection of the glans and foreskin) are more common in the uncircumcised male (approximately 6%) but may also be found in circumcised children (Fig. 82–8). It frequently presents during the preschool-age years and rarely prior to toilet training.

Pathophysiology

Balanitis may be caused by entrapment of organisms under a poorly retractable foreskin. The etiology is often related to inadequate hygiene or chemical irritation from soaps or bubble baths, or persistent manual manipulation.[1] Gram-negative

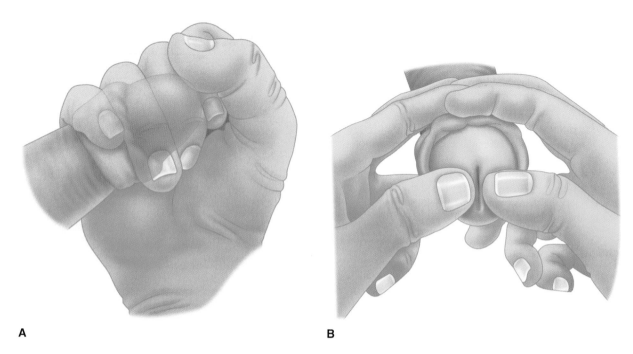

A   **B**

Figure 82–7. Reduction of paraphimosis. (A) Manual compression of the glans and foreskin to reduce the edema of the foreskin. (B) Manual reduction of a paraphimosis. The thumbs push the glans proximally while the fingers provide countertraction to slip the phimotic ring over the glans.

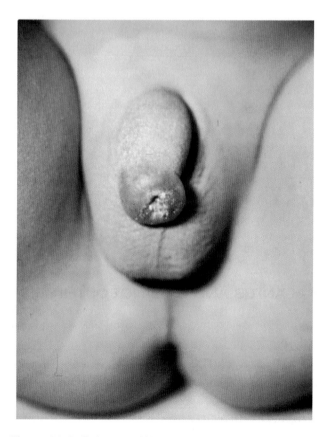

Figure 82–8. Balanoposthitis: note the erythema, localized edema, and significantly constricted preputial orifice of the distal penis.

or -positive bacterial organisms may be causative, and Group A β-hemolytic streptococcus has been implicated. Candidal infections are also associated with balanoposthitis in infants. In adolescents, sexually transmitted diseases must be considered as a cause. Chronic balanitis or phimosis may result in balanitis xerotica obliterans, a sclerotic disease of the prepuce noted histologically.

Signs and Symptoms

Signs and symptoms include swelling, erythema, penile discharge, dysuria, bleeding, and, rarely, ulceration of the glans. Phimosis can occur but is uncommon. A careful examination of the base of the penis should be performed to look for a strand of hair that may cause strangulation and edema.

Diagnostic Evaluation

Balanitis is diagnosed clinically. In selected cases, the clinician may wish to obtain a urinalysis and send cultures of the penile discharge.

Management

Local care with soaks (Sitz baths), gentle cleaning of the foreskin sulcus, and topical antibiotic ointment are recommended. Application of 0.5% hydrocortisone cream may be helpful.[1] The addition of oral antibiotics, such as cephalexin, for 5 to 7 days, may be reserved for the more severe cases. The presence of a purulent discharge, fiery-red erythema, and moist exudate might suggest a streptococcal etiology.[1] Urethral discharge should prompt STD cultures. Patients should be followed within 2 days to assure that symptoms have resolved. Children with repeated episodes may be referred to a urologist for elective circumcision.

PRIAPISM

Priapism is a prolonged (over 4 hours), painful erection unrelated to sexual stimulation. It is relatively uncommon in childhood except in patients with sickle cell disease. In this group, priapism occurs in up to 10% of patients. Priapism is rare in the neonatal period where polycythemia and trauma are presumed etiologies.

Pathophysiology

Pathophysiology of priapism can be divided into two mechanisms:

1. Low-flow or ischemic mechanism: there is little or no cavernous blood flow, and the penis is painful and tender to palpation; it is a urologic emergency seen in sickle cell disease and polycythemia
2. High-flow or engorgement mechanism: not ischemic, the penis is typically not fully rigid or painful; preceeding trauma is the most common etiology.[14,15]

Either mechanism results in engorgement of the corpora cavernosum with a flaccid corpora spongiosum and glans. This engorgement leads to inflammation, increased stasis of cavernous blood, deoxygenation, acidosis, further sludging, thrombosis, fibrosis, and impotence if unrelieved. Drugs of abuse such as alcohol, marijuana, cocaine, and amphetamines have also been implicated. Fortunately, most cases of priapism can be treated medically and do not result in impotence.

Factors that may precipitate priapism in patients with sickle cell anemia are infection, trauma, acidosis, hypoxia, sexual intercourse, and masturbation. Other etiologies of priapism include trauma (genital, pelvic, or perineal, such as a straddle injury), drugs (antihypertensives and vasoactive agents, anticoagulants, antidepressants or psychoactives, and alprostadil), leukemia, Kawasaki's disease, and polycythemia. When used as directed, phosphodiesterase-5 inhibitors commonly used for erectile dysfunction (such as sildenafil and tadalafil) have rarely been associated with priapism.[14]

Signs and Symptoms

Patients often have delayed presentation, possibly a result of embarrassment. Patients are noted on physical examination to have an erect penis, which is firm on the dorsal surface (corpora cavernosum) and soft on the ventral surface (corpora spongiosum) and glans. Patients should be asked about previous history of priapism and its treatment, duration and degree of pain, and placement of urethral and penile foreign bodies. The bladder should be palpated for signs of urinary retention, which can be easily relieved by placement of a urinary catheter.

Diagnostic Evaluation

Priapism is a clinical diagnosis based on physical examination. However, the physician may wish to order a complete blood count, looking for evidence of leukemia or anemia, and a sickle cell preparation and hemoglobin electrophoresis. Renal function studies are indicated if there has been significant urinary retention. If patients have suffered perineal trauma, a retrograde cystourethrogram may be indicated. Color Doppler US may be used to determine if the priapism is secondary to a low-flow or a high-flow state.

Management

Treatment is based on the presumed etiology. Providing oxygen, hydration, and analgesics to patients with sickle cell disease may alleviate the priapism. If not, an exchange transfusion in consultation with a hematologist is considered. Patients with leukemia may receive hydration and analgesics and appropriate treatment for their cancer. A urinary catheter should be inserted to relieve bladder distension. Once medical management is initiated, patients should be admitted for observation.

Urologic consultation is recommended in all cases. The timing of surgical management of priapism is controversial. Although some clinicians prefer to attempt medical management initially, the American Urological Association recommends that surgical treatment be initiated concurrent with systemic treatment for ischemic priapism.[14] Initial intervention uses therapeutic aspiration with or without irrigation, followed by intracavernous injection of a sympathomimetic vasoconstrictor such as phenylephrine. If unsuccessful, surgical shunting of blood from the cavernosum to the spongiosum or the glans may be performed.[14] Intravenous ketamine hydrochloride has been used to treat priapism in the newborn. Parenteral vasodilators, including hydralazine or terbutaline (0.25 to 0.5 mg IV every 4 hours), have been used to treat priapism with varying success. Aspiration and sympathomimetic agents are not used for nonischemic priapism emergently.[14]

REFERENCES

1. Leslie JA, Cain MP. Pediatric urologic emergencies and urgencies. *Pediatr Clin North Am.* 2006;53:513–527.
2. Haynes JH. Inguinal and scrotal disorders. *Surg Clin North Am.* 2006;86:371–381.
3. Gatti JM, Murphy JP. Current management of the acute scrotum. *Semin Pediatr Surg.* 2007;16:58–63.
4. Munden MM, Trautwein, LM. Scrotal pathology in pediatrics with sonographis imaging. *Curr Probl Diagn Radiol.* 2000;29:183–205.
5. Marcozzi D, Suner S. The nontraumatic acute scrotum. *Emerg Med Clin North Am.* 2001;19:547–567.
6. Brenner JS, Ojo A. Causes of scrotal pain in children and adolescents. www.uptodate.com 2008
7. D'Agostino JD. Common abdominal emergencies in children. *Emerg Med Clin North Am.* 2002;20(1):139–153.
8. Graf JL, Caty MG, Martin DJ, Glick PL. Pediatric hernis. *Semin Ultrasound CT MR.* 2002;23:197–200.

9. Louie JP. Essential diagnosis of abdominal emergencies in the first year of life. *Emerg Med Clin North Am.* 2007;15:1009–1040.

10. Bong GW, Koo HP. The adolescent varicocele: to treat or not to treat. *Urol Clin North Am.* 2004;31(3) 509–515.

11. Cayan S, Woodhouse CRJ. The treatment of adolescents presenting with a varicocele. *BJU Int.* 2007;100:744–747.

12. Little B, White M. Treatment options for paraphimosis. *Int J Clin Pract.* 2005;59(5):591–593.

13. Montague DK, Jarow J, et al. Guideline on the management of priapism (expert panel recommendations and practice guidelines). *Am Urol Assoc.* 2003.

14. Kadish H, Bolte R. A retrospective review of pediatric patients with epididymitis, testicular torsion, and torsion of testicular appendages. *Pediatrics.* 1998;102:73–76.

15. Mulhall JP, Honig SC. Priapism: etiology and management. *Acad Emerg Med.* 1996;3:810–816.

CHAPTER 83

Urinary Tract Diseases

John W. Williams and Marianne Gausche-Hill

▶ HIGH-YIELD FACTS

- Signs and symptoms of urinary tract infection (UTI) may be nonspecific in young infants, and even older children may not complain of dysuria.
- In the evaluation of infants and children with fever without a source, up to 7% of patients will be found to have a UTI.
- Urinary catheterization is the method of choice for obtaining the urine specimen in febrile infants and young children.
- Bacteria on a Gram stain and leukocyte esterase on urine dipstick are highly indicative of a UTI, but urine culture is the gold standard for diagnosis.
- Seventy-five percent of infants < 3 months of age with fever and a UTI are bacteremic. This number drops to 5% in older infants and children.
- Antibiotic choice for UTI must be guided by local resistance patterns and effectiveness against *Escherichia Coli*.
- Approximately 90% of renal stones are radiopaque.
- Computed tomography (CT) scan of the abdomen without contrast is the test of choice for the evaluation of children with renal stones.

▶ URINARY TRACT INFECTION

Urinary tract infection (UTI) is a frequent cause of fever in infants and young children and one of the most common bacterial infections.[1,2] It is important to identify and treat UTIs because of the morbidity associated with progression to pyelonephritis or sepsis, and chronic conditions such as hypertension. Fever may be the sole manifestation of a UTI. Febrile children younger than 24 months with no other identifiable source for fever on examination were found to have a 7% probability of UTI (range <1%–16%), which is higher than the likelihood of occult bacteremia (<1%) among fully immunized children.[3,4] The prevalence of UTI varies with age and gender, with some studies showing a higher risk of UTI in male neonates than age-matched females, particularly in the first 3 months of life[3,5]; uncircumcised boys have up to a 10-fold greater risk of UTI than circumcised.[6] Before the end of the first year and thereafter, females are diagnosed approximately 10 times more often than males.

According to various studies, UTIs are found in 5% to 13.6% of febrile infants and children.[6] In a febrile neonate younger than 2 months, the likelihood of a UTI is 4.6% in general, but is less in patients in whom a definite source of fever is present and higher if no source of fever is identified.[5,7] The prevalence of UTI in children older than 2 months but younger than 2 years is approximately 5%, even without a fever or other localizing signs.[8] The prevalence of UTI in older children with symptoms of a UTI is approximately 9%.[4] Thus the risk of a UTI in a febrile child is significant, especially if there is no source or only a presumptive source of fever. Another risk factor is fever higher than 39°C.[9]

PATHOPHYSIOLOGY

Escherichia coli causes 85% of UTIs in children; other gram-negative organisms include *Klebsiella* spp., *Proteus* spp., *Enterobacter, and Pseudomonas.* Some gram-positive pathogens include group B streptococci, *Enterococcus* spp., and *Staphylococcus aureus.*[4,10] Viruses may cause lower UTIs, and fungal UTIs occur in immunocompromised patients or those on long-term antibiotic therapy. Bacteria enter the urinary tract by the fecal-perineal-urethral route, with retrograde ascent into the bladder. In infants, UTIs can result from bacteremia. In fact, half of infants younger than 3 months with a UTI are bacteremic. After 3 months, the risk of sepsis drops to less than 5%.

The main defense mechanism against UTI is constant anterograde flow of urine from the kidneys with intermittent complete emptying of the bladder which washes out pathogens. In addition, the urine and the mucosal wall of the collecting system have antimicrobial qualities.[11] Bacteria that cause UTIs, such as *E. coli* species, often exhibit distinctive virulence factors that overcome the normal defenses. Dysfunctional elimination is another important and often overlooked factor associated with UTIs.

SIGNS AND SYMPTOMS

UTIs are divided into two overlapping categories. Cystitis and urethritis characterize uncomplicated lower UTIs, while ureteritis, pyelitis, and pyelonephritis are upper tract infections.[5] Signs and symptoms vary with the age of the patient. Neonates and infants younger than 3 months may have nonspecific symptoms with or without fever, including vomiting, diarrhea, lethargy or irritability, oliguria, poor feeding, or failure to thrive. Newborns may exhibit asymptomatic jaundice. Children younger than 2 years may exhibit fever, vomiting, or anorexia. Patients between 2 and 5 years of age may complain of fever and abdominal pain. In the older child, symptoms may become more specific, including dysuria, frequency, urgency, suprapubic discomfort, hematuria, and flank or back pain.[11] Up to 75% of children younger than 5 years with a UTI and fever have pyelonephritis documented on a renal cortical scan.

A thorough history in the patient suspected of having a UTI may uncover dysfunctional voiding. Symptoms include infrequent or incomplete bladder emptying, withholding maneuvers, daytime urgency-frequency syndrome, and enuresis or incontinence. In some children, constipation represents an equivalent to dysuria.[5] Abnormal elimination of bladder and bowel is an often overlooked factor in the pathophysiology of UTI, particularly in school-age children. Dysfunctional elimination is also a risk factor for vesicoureteral reflux (VUR) and renal scarring. Up to 40% of toilet-trained children with their first UTI and 80% of patients with recurrent UTIs have abnormal elimination.[4] Females have a trimodal-age distribution for UTI: highest in the first year, at the time of toilet training, and when sexual activity begins.

Patients with abdominal or flank pain, high fever, vomiting, or other systemic signs must be evaluated for pyelonephritis. Fever may be the predominant symptom, often without dysuria, even in older children.[5] Moreover, a UTI should be considered in all patients with serious illness even if there is evidence of other infection. All children should have a genital examination, looking for vaginal or penile discharge or foreign bodies, epididymitis or orchitis, or anatomic abnormalities.

DIAGNOSTIC EVALUATION

Urine culture from an adequate urine sample is the most important diagnostic test to establish the diagnosis of UTI. Results of a urinalysis are helpful but can be misleading. Although more than 50% of patients with UTI have pyuria, many other entities can cause pyuria including vaginitis, masturbation, appendicitis, gastroenteritis, acute glomerulonephritis, and bubble bath soap.

While urine culture is the gold standard for diagnosing a UTI, a urinalysis revealing more than 5 WBCs per HPF on microscopic examination of spun urine and/or Gram stain positive for bacteria are the most accurate rapid laboratory tests available, with sensitivity and specificity up to 95%.[6,10] The presence of bacteria on Gram stain is perhaps the single best indication of infection. WBC casts are pathognomonic of pyelonephritis.[6] Urine dipstick testing revealing the presence of either leukocyte esterase or nitrites also has good overall accuracy, but urine culture should be sent to detect the approximately 12% of UTIs that will be missed by this test.[10,12]

Methods of obtaining a urine sample include "bagging" the perineum, a "clean catch" of mid-stream urine, urinary tract catheterization, and suprapubic aspiration. Although bagging the perineum is easy and noninvasive, it is the least reliable method, with false-positive rates up to 85%. Screening for UTI with bagged urine is only useful as a screening test if it is negative. Circumcised boys older than 1 year are unlikely to have a UTI and very unlikely to have reflux. Therefore, the American Academy of Pediatrics (AAP) recommends that a bagged specimen is adequate to screen urine in this age group. If the urinalysis reveals signs of infection, urine obtained by catheterization or suprapubic aspiration should be sent for culture.

In all infants younger than 1 year, and in uncircumcised boys and in girls younger than 2 years, a urinary specimen should be obtained by catheterization. If bagged urine is sent and is consistent with a UTI, the AAP recommends that a follow-up urine obtained by catheterization or suprapubic as-

piration be obtained for culture. Catheterization is usually more acceptable to parents than suprapubic aspiration; it is also more likely to be successful but is more time-consuming.[13] Confirmation of sufficient bladder volume with bedside ultrasound improves the success rate in catheterization[14] as well as suprapubic aspiration. Complications of suprapubic aspiration are uncommon, but include hematuria, bowel perforation, cystitis, and abdominal wall hematoma or infection.[15] Older children are usually able to provide an adequate "clean catch" specimen.

Electrolytes and renal function tests should be obtained on all patients with signs of dehydration or toxicity as well as all infants, all males, and patients with signs of upper tract infection. Consideration may be given to obtaining a procalcitonin (PCT) plasma level, as correlations between pyelonephritis and increased plasma concentrations of PCT have been well demonstrated; higher levels reflect an increased likelihood of renal parenchymal infection and scarring.[6]

MANAGEMENT AND RADIOLOGIC EVALUATION OF THE URINARY TRACT

The management and radiologic evaluation of suspected UTI is dependent upon several factors (see algorithm in Fig. 83–1). Empiric antibiotic therapy for UTI is directed at the presumed infecting organism until results of the urine culture are obtained (Table 83–1). The choice should be guided by local resistance patterns and include coverage of *E. coli*. There is widespread resistance to ampicillin and amoxicillin, and resistance to trimethoprim-sulfamethoxazole (TMP-SMX) and to first-generation cephalosporins is growing. Appropriate first-line agents include second- and third-generation cephalosporins and aminoglycosides.[16] Children older than 6 years may benefit from the addition of phenazopyridine (Pyridium) for pain control. Pyridium can be given 10 mg/kg/d in three divided doses for 2 to 3 days or until patients are less symptomatic.

All neonates or infants younger than 2 months, infants with pyelonephritis, immunocompromised patients, and those with known urinary tract obstruction should be admitted for intravenous antibiotics. Criteria for admission are listed in Table 83–2. Intravenous antibiotic therapy that includes an aminoglycoside, such as gentamicin, continues until the sensitivity of the organism is known and the patient's clinical status is improved. Stable patients may be discharged on the appropriate oral antibiotic. Patients who are unable to tolerate oral medications and fluids should be considered for admission for IV antibiotics. Patients at risk for inadequate follow-up or with unreliable caretakers should also be considered for admission.

Complicated UTIs are usually treated for 10 to 14 days. This includes males, children younger than 2 years, patients with recurrent UTI, and all admitted patients. Some physicians recommend prophylactic antibiotics until imaging tests are completed. Older children with uncomplicated cystitis are usually treated for 5 to 7 days.[16]

Children with UTIs should be evaluated for urinary tract abnormalities that predispose to infection. Up to 57% of these patients will show anatomic anomalies that may benefit from some form of intervention. Neonates, females with recurrent UTI or with pyelonephritis, and males of any age should undergo radiologic evaluation for urinary tract abnormalities.

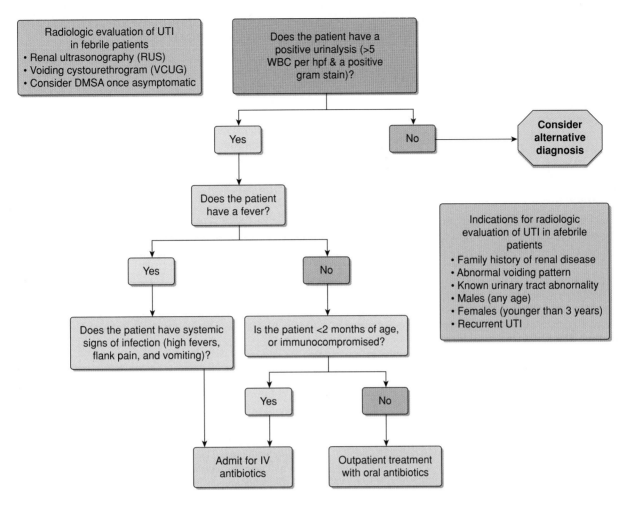

Figure 83–1. Algorithm showing evaluation and management of suspected urinary tract infection (UTI). WBC, white blood cells; hpf, high power field.

Table 83–3 summarizes the types of diagnostic tests, their indications, and limitations.

Renal ultrasonography (RUS) can identify hydronephrosis, anatomic abnormalities, and nephrolithiasis, but is not reliable to detect reflux and renal scarring or inflammation. Since it is noninvasive and involves no radiation, it is still favored in children.

The most common anatomic abnormality of the urinary tract is VUR. It is usually diagnosed in the first decade of life and resolves spontaneously in most cases. Voiding cystourethrogram (VCUG) has been the diagnostic test of choice for boys and girls with suspected urethral pathology. However, VUR,

especially when mild or moderate, is not associated with an increased incidence of UTI or morbidity in most cases, and the studies to identify reflux are now being questioned. Isotope cystography (IC) also assesses VUR, bladder anatomy, and the posterior urethra in boys with greater specificity and sensitivity and with far less radiation than VCUG. It is often used to evaluate children with UTI at low risk of complicating factors.

Radionuclide scanning (or renal cortical scintigraphy) using technetium-99m dimercaptosuccinic acid (DMSA) is the test of choice for diagnosis of upper tract infections. DMSA is injected intravenously and uptake by the kidneys is measured several hours later; areas of decreased uptake represent

▶ **TABLE 83–1. ANTIBIOTIC THERAPY FOR TREATMENT OF URINARY TRACT INFECTIONS IN CHILDREN**

Outpatient Management		Inpatient Management	
Cotrimoxazole (trimethoprim-sulfamethoxazole)	10 mg/kg per 24 h (based on TMP component) divided bid	Ampicillin *plus*	100 mg/kg per 24 h divided qid
Cefixime	8 mg/kg per 24 h divided bid	Cefotaxime	150 mg/kg per 24 h divided tid
Cephalexin	50 to 100 mg/kg per 24 h divided qid	Ceftriaxone*	75 mg/kg per 24 h
		Ceftazidime	150 mg/kg per 24 h divided qid
		Gentamicin	5–7.5 mg/kg per 24 h divided tid

Bid, twice daily; qid, 4 times daily; tid, 3 times daily.
*Ceftriaxone should be used with caution in neonates and infants; read latest CDC guidelines.

▶ **TABLE 83-2. ADMISSION CRITERIA FOR CHILDREN WITH URINARY TRACT INFECTION**

Neonate
Pyelonephritis (infants)
Known urinary tract abnormality
Urinary tract obstruction (stone)
Ureteral stents or other urinary tract foreign bodies
Immunocompromised state
Intractable vomiting and dehydration
Renal insufficiency
Toxic-appearing infant or child

pyelonephritis or scarring. DMSA has multiple advantages over intravenous urography, which is no longer routinely used in children. A negative DMSA scan, performed during the acute infection or months later, suggests that scarring in the future is unlikely.[6,17,18]

Current recommendations are to obtain a RUS and VCUG for any child with a febrile UTI (some recommend only <5 years), girls younger than 2 to 3 years, and boys of any age with a first UTI. Children with recurrent UTI or a first UTI associated with known urinary tract abnormalities, voiding dysfunction, hypertension, poor growth, or family history of renal disease are also candidates for a RUS and VCUG.[6,16] Some recommend that children who do not respond promptly to therapy have a RUS to determine the presence of a renal abscess or obstruction.[6]

▶ UROLITHIASIS

Urolithiasis refers to stone formation in the bladder, ureter, or kidney. It is less common in children than it is in adults, but nevertheless occurs in approximately 1 case per 7500 pediatric hospital admissions. The incidence of stones is highest in the southeastern and western United States. Most urinary calculi are calcium oxalate or calcium phosphate (58%). Urolithiasis

▶ **TABLE 83-4. CAUSES OF UROLITHIASIS IN NORTH AMERICAN CHILDREN**

Cause	Number (%)
Metabolic	162 (32.9)
Idiopathic hypercalciuria	
Cystinuria	
Myeloproliferative disorders	
Hyperoxaluria	
Renal tubular acidosis	
Primary hyperparathyroidism	
Hypercortisolism	
Other	
Endemic (urate)	10 (2.2)
Developmental anomalies of the genitourinary tract	160 (32.5)
Infection	21 (4.3)
Idiopathic	139 (28.3)

is less common in blacks but equally as common in girls as in boys, with a mean age of 9 years at presentation.

PATHOPHYSIOLOGY

Urinary stasis from anomalies of the urinary tract, concentrations of calcium, oxalate, uric acid, cystine in the urine, presence of urinary infection, and concentrated urine promote stone formation. There are many causes of urolithiasis in children. The most common causes are metabolic disorders and developmental anomalies of the urinary tract (Table 83–4).

SIGNS AND SYMPTOMS

Forty-four percent of patients with urolithiasis present with abdominal or flank pain, 38% with hematuria, 15% with fever, and

▶ **TABLE 83-3. DIAGNOSTIC IMAGING FOR URINARY TRACT INFECTIONS**

Study	Indication	Comments
Renal ultrasonography (RUS)	Hydronephrosis, nephrolithiasis	Shows general kidney anatomy No radiation Not invasive
Renal scintigraphy using DMSA (cortical scan)	Febrile UTI, pyelonephritis	Shows renal scarring and pyelonephritis Okay in neonates and adolescents Okay in renal insufficiency Little radiation
Voiding cystourethrogram (VCUG)	Initial UTI evaluation to rule out VUR Bladder and lower tract	Allows grading of reflux + Radiation + Catheterization
Isotope cystography (IC)	Initial UTI evaluation to rule out VUR Bladder and lower tract	Decreased radiation Increased sensitivity and specificity over VCUG Good screening examination
Computed tomography (CT)	Nephrolithiasis	+ Radiation
Intravenous pyelogram (IVP)	Renal or ureteral trauma	RUS preferred for routine GU evaluation

Table of diagnostic imaging tests for urinary tract infections, their indications, and limitations.

18% with other complaints related to the urinary tract. Flank pain is not as common in children as in adults, especially in patients less than 5 years of age. The emergency physician should solicit a history of recurrent UTIs, frequent bouts of abdominal pain, a family history of stones, a history of microscopic or gross hematuria, and passage of stones or gravel in the urine. Patients are questioned about their diet, including intake of vitamins C and D. A physical examination should be performed including evaluation of the blood pressure and growth parameters.

DIAGNOSTIC EVALUATION

Urinalysis, urine culture, and renal function studies should be obtained on all children with possible urinary tract stones. Urinalysis may reveal hematuria or be entirely normal. A complete blood cell count, renal function tests, electrolytes, uric acid, total protein, and albumin may also be obtained. Once the diagnosis is suspected from history, physical examination findings, and laboratory analysis, a CT scan of the abdomen without contrast should be performed. Since as many as 90% of renal stones in children are radiopaque, they should be visible on plain radiographs; however, computed tomography delineates underlying congenital abnormalities and degree of obstruction. Renal ultrasound may be useful in those patients who are pregnant, have renal insufficiency, or are allergic to contrast media. Ultrasound cannot distinguish obstructive from nonobstructive causes of hydronephrosis.

MANAGEMENT

In the emergency department, patients are evaluated for signs of infection and given adequate hydration. Morphine sulfate or other narcotic agents may be necessary to control pain. A nonsteroidal anti-inflammatory agent may be given to older children. Further diagnostic studies will need to be initiated but are not emergent and should be done in consultation with a pediatric urologist.

Patients with complete urinary obstruction, intractable pain, dehydration, a solitary kidney, renal insufficiency, or inability to tolerate oral fluids should be admitted. In the past, most children with urinary tract stones required surgical removal. Today, with extracorporeal shock wave lithotripsy,

medical management for urolithiasis may predominate. Sixteen percent of pediatric patients with urinary stones will have a recurrence, so close follow-up and outpatient dietary management are critical.

REFERENCES

1. Wald E. Urinary tract infections in infants and children: a comprehensive overview. *Curr Opin Pediatr.* 2004;16:85–88.
2. Mak RH, Huo HJ. Pathogenesis of urinary tract infection: an update. *Curr Opin Pediatr.* 2006;18:148–152.
3. Shaikh N, Morone NE, Lopez J, et al. Does this child have a urinary tract infection? *JAMA.* 2007;298:2895–2904.
4. Shaikh N, Hoberman A. Epidemiology and risk factors for urinary tract infections in children. 2007, www.uptodate.com.
5. Santen SA, Altieri MF. Pediatric urinary tract infection. *Emerg Med Clin North Am.* 2001;19:675–690.
6. Bauer R, Kogan BA. New developments in the diagnosis and management of pediatric UTIs. *Urol Clin North Am.* 2008;35:47–58.
7. Hoberman A, Chao HP, Keller DM, et al. Prevalence of urinary tract infection in febrile infants. *J Pediatr.* 1993;123:17–23.
8. Shaw KN, Gorelick MH. Urinary tract infection in the pediatric patient. *Pediatr Clin North Am.* 1999;46:1111–1124.
9. Hellerstein S. Acute urinary tract infection, evaluation and treatment. *Curr Opin Pediatr.* 2006;18:134–138.
10. Zorc JJ, Kiddoo DA, Shaw KN. Diagnosis and management of pediatric urinary tract infections. *Clin Micro Rev.* 2005;18:417–422.
11. Chang SL, Shortliffe LD. Pediatric urinary tract infections. *Pediatr Clin North Am.* 2006;53:379–400.
12. Shaikh N, Hoberman A. Clinical features and diagnosis of urinary tract infections in children. www.uptodate.com, 2007.
13. Bajaj L, Bothner J. Urine collection techniques in children. 2007, www.uptodate.com.
14. Baumann BM, McCans K, Stahmer SA, et al. Volumetric bladder ultrasound performed by trained nurses increases catheterization success in pediatric patients. *Am J Emerg Med.* 2008;26:18–23.
15. Buys H, Pead L, Hallett R, et al. Suprapubic aspiration under ultrasound guidance in children with fever of undiagnosed cause. *BMJ.* 1994;308:690.
16. Shaikh N, Hoberman A. Acute management, imaging, and prognosis of urinary tract infections in children. www.uptodate.com, 2007.
17. Biassoni L, Chippington S. Imaging in urinary tract infections: current strategies and trends. *Semin Nucl Med.* 2007;38:56–66.
18. Keren R. Imaging and treatment strategies for children after first urinary tract infection. *Curr Opin Pediatr.* 2007;19:705–710.

CHAPTER 84

Specific Renal Syndromes

Roger M. Barkin

▶ HIGH-YIELD FACTS

- Edema, hematuria, and oliguria suggest acute glomerulonephritis.
- Children with nephrotic syndrome are usually immunocompromised and at risk for life-threatening infection.
- Patients with hemolytic uremic syndrome are at risk for hypertension and seizures.
- Hemodialysis may be needed for fluid overload in patients with acute renal failure who are refractory to medical management.

▶ ACUTE GLOMERULONEPHRITIS

Glomerulonephritis is a histopathologic diagnosis acutely associated with clinical findings of hematuria, edema, and hypertension. It commonly follows a pharyngitis caused by group A β-hemolytic *Streptococcus* in children between 3 and 7 years of age. Patients < 2 years are rarely affected. Timely treatment of pharyngitis does not clearly decrease the incidence of acute glomerulonephritis.

Glomerulonephritis probably results from the deposition of circulating immune complexes in the kidney. These immune complexes are deposited on the basement membrane, reducing glomerular filtration.[1]

DIAGNOSTIC FINDINGS

There is usually a preceding streptococcal infection or exposure 1 to 2 weeks before the onset of glomerulonephritis. An interval of less than 4 days may imply that the illness is an exacerbation of preexisting disease rather than an initial attack. Fever, malaise, abdominal pain, and decreased urine output are often noted.

The physical findings reflect the duration of illness. Initial findings may be mild facial or extremity edema only, with a minimal rise in blood pressure. Patients uniformly develop fluid retention and edema and commonly have hematuria (90%), hypertension (60%–70%), and oliguria (80%). Fever, malaise, and abdominal pain are frequently reported. Anuria and renal failure occur in 2% of children. Circulatory congestion, as well as hypertensive encephalopathy, may be noted.

ANCILLARY DATA

Urinalysis reveals microscopic or gross hematuria. Erythrocyte casts are present in 60% to 85% of hospitalized children. Proteinuria is generally less than 2 g/m² per 24 hours. Hematuria (Fig. 84–1) and proteinuria (Fig. 84–2) may present independently and require a specific evaluation.[2] Leukocyturia and hyaline and granular casts are common.

The fractional excretion of sodium as a reflection of renal function may be reduced (Table 84–1). The blood urea nitrogen (BUN) level is elevated disproportionately to the creatinine level.

Total serum complement and specifically C_3 is reduced in 90% to 100% of children during the first 2 weeks of illness, returning to normal within 3 to 4 weeks. Ongoing low levels suggest the presence of chronic renal disease. The antistreptolysin (ASO) level is elevated, consistent with a previous streptococcal infection. Anemia, hyponatremia, and hyperkalemia may be present.

MANAGEMENT

Fluid and salt restriction is essential to normalize intravascular volume. Diuretics are often required. Elevated blood pressure may require specific pharmacologic management. Specific complications, such as congestive heart failure, renal failure, and hyperkalemia, must be anticipated and treated.[3]

Recovery is usually complete. More than 80% of patients recover without residual renal damage. Children without evidence of hypertension, congestive heart failure, or azotemia may be followed closely at home. A nephrologist is usually consulted.

▶ NEPHROTIC SYNDROME

Historically known as lipoid nephrosis, childhood nephrosis, foot process disease, nil disease, minimal change nephrotic syndrome, and idiopathic nephrotic syndrome, nephrotic syndrome is associated with increased glomerular permeability, which produces massive proteinuria. Hypoalbuminemia results, producing a decrease in the plasma osmotic pressure. The shift of fluids from the vascular to interstitial spaces shrinks the plasma volume, thereby activating the renin-angiotensin system and enhancing sodium reabsorption. Edema develops.

The etiology is generally idiopathic, but has been associated with glomerular lesions. Intoxications, allergic reactions,

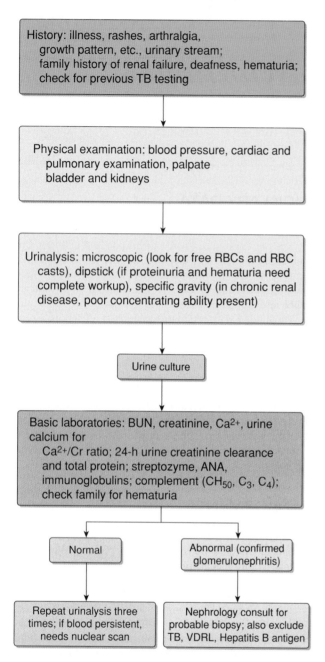

Figure 84–1. Evaluation for hematuria. TB, tuberculosis; RBC, red blood cell; BUN, blood urea nitrogen; Ca, calcium; Cr, creatinine; ANA, antinuclear antibody. (With permission from Barkin RM, Rosen P, eds. *Emergency Pediatrics: A Guide to Ambulatory Care.* 6th ed. St. Louis, MO: Mosby; 2003:269.)

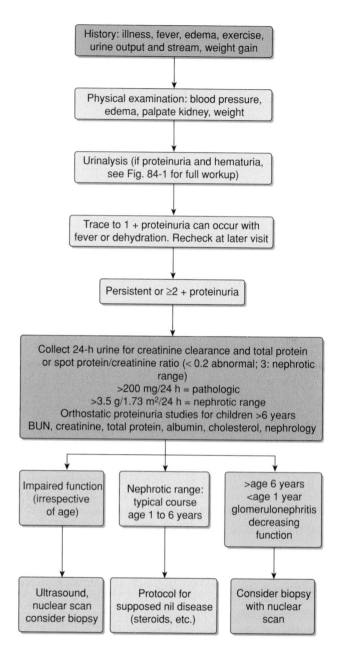

Figure 84–2. Evaluation for proteinuria. BUN, blood urea nitrogen. (With permission from Barkin RM, Rosen P, eds. *Emergency Pediatrics: A Guide to Ambulatory Care.* 6th ed. St. Louis, MO: Mosby; 2003:269.)

infection, and other entities have also been associated with the syndrome (Table 84–2). It may be a primary pathologic process or associated with a systemic disease.

Males are affected more frequently, but this equalizes in adulthood. Primary nephrotic syndrome occurs more commonly in children younger than 5 years while secondary nephrotic syndrome is more common in older children.

The renin-angiotensin-aldosterone system produces increased reabsorption of sodium chloride and worsens the edema state. Serum cholesterol levels rise and remain high even after resolution of urinary protein loss.[4]

DIAGNOSTIC FINDINGS

Patients frequently have edema, often with a history of a preceding flu-like syndrome. Edema initially is present periorbitally and may become generalized, associated with weight gain. Ascites may be caused by edema of the intestinal wall, often associated with abdominal pain, nausea, and vomiting. Pleural effusion or pulmonary edema may occur. Malnutrition may be noted secondary to protein loss.

▶ TABLE 84–1. EVALUATION OF RENAL FAILURE

Prerenal	Intrarenal	Postrenal
Ultrasound: normal	Ultrasound: can have increased renal density or slight swelling	Ultrasound: dilated bladder or kidney
Serum BUN:creatinine ratio >15:1		History and examination may be diagnostic
Urine Na$^+$ <15 mEq/L	Urine Na$^+$ > 20 mEq/L	Indexes not helpful
Urine osmolality >500 mOsm/kg H$_2$O	Urine osmolality <350 mOsm/kg H$_2$O	
Urine: plasma creatinine ratio > 40:1	Urine: plasma creatinine ratio < 20:1 (often <5:1)	
Fractional excretion of Na$^+$ < 1 (<2.5 in neonates)	Fractional excretion of Na$^+$ > 2 (>2.5 in neonates)	

$$\text{Fractional excretion of Na}^+ = \frac{\text{Urine Na}^+ \text{(mEq/L)}}{\text{Plasma Na}^+ \text{(mEq/L)}} \times \frac{\text{Plasma creatinine (mg/dL)}}{\text{Urine creatinine (mg/dL)}}$$

With permission from Barkin RM, Rosen P, eds. *Emergency Pediatrics: A Guide to Ambulatory Care.* 6th ed. St. Louis, MO: Mosby–YearBook; 2003:830.

Blood pressure may be decreased if the intravascular volume is depleted or increased in the presence of significant renal disease. Blood pressure is elevated in approximately 5% to 10% of these patients. Renal failure may develop.

Infection is probably the most common complication, related to the increased risk of peritonitis and concomitant immunosuppression due to the steroid therapy. Immune protein levels, including IgG, are low due to urinary losses. Children's blood is hypercoagulable, leading to an increased risk of thromboembolism. Renal vein thrombosis is probably underrecognized but should be suspected if hematuria, flank pain, and decreased renal function occur.

Hypoalbuminemia is common, as well as proteinuria and hyperlipidemia. A 24-hour urine collection reveals a protein excretion of >3.5 g /1.73 m^2 per 24 hours. A spot protein:creatinine ratio of >3.0 is noted, and BUN and creatinine levels are elevated in 25% of children. Serum complement is decreased. Plasma cholesterol carriers (low-density lipoprotein and very-low-density lipoprotein) are increased. Elevated lipids result from increased synthesis, as well as catabolism of phospholipid. Imaging studies, especially ultrasound, should document normal renal structure.

A renal biopsy should be considered if the following poor prognostic signs are present:

- Age more than 10 years
- Azotemia
- Decreased complement
- Hematuria
- Persistent hypertension
- No response to steroids

DIFFERENTIAL DIAGNOSIS

Other causes of edema should be excluded, including congestive heart failure, vasculitis, hypothyroidism, starvation, cystic fibrosis, protein-losing enteropathy, and drug ingestions (such as steroids or diuretics).

MANAGEMENT

The majority of patients should be hospitalized initially, usually in consultation with a nephrologist. Treat hypovolemia with albumin and fluids. Monitor closely and treat hypertension if it occurs.

After diagnosis and stabilization, patients without complications (<10 years, normal complement, no gross hematuria, no large protein loss) are started on prednisone at a dose of

▶ TABLE 84–2. NEPHROTIC SYNDROME: ETIOLOGY

Primary renal disorders	Nil or minimal change disease
	Focal segmental glomerulosclerosis
	Membranoproliferative glomerulonephritis
	Membranous glomerulonephritis
Intoxication	Heroin
	Mercury
	Probenecid
	Silver
Allergic reaction	Poison ivy or oak, pollens
	Bee sting
	Snake venom
Infection	Bacterial
	Viral: Hepatitis B, cytomegalovirus, Epstein–Barr virus
	Protozoa: Malaria, toxoplasmosis
Neoplasm	Hodgkin's disease, Wilms' tumor, etc.
Autoimmune disorder	Systemic lupus erythematosus
Metabolic disorder	Diabetes mellitus
Cardiac disorders	Congenital heart disease
	Congestive heart failure
	Pericarditis
Vasculitis	Henoch–Schönlein purpura
	Wegener's granulomatosis

2 mg/kg per 24 hours up to 80 mg per 24 hours and tapered once a response is noted. Nearly 75% of patients will respond within 14 days. Limited response to initial steroid therapy is generally predictive of a poor outcome. Treatment continues for approximately 2 months but is reinstituted if relapse is noted. Specific protocols exist for multiple relapses or resistance to steroid management. Other pharmacologic agents may ultimately be needed. Salt and water restriction should be initiated.

Diuretics may be needed if there is pulmonary edema or respiratory distress. However, they must be used judiciously to avoid vascular volume depletion and electrolyte abnormality. Loop diuretics such as furosemide, 1 to 2 mg/kg/d, may be helpful to decrease edema in cases of mild hypertension. Severe fluid overload requires specific management.

Watch for signs of infection since these patients are considered immunocompromised. Avoid deep vein punctures if possible to avoid triggering a deep vein thrombosis.

▶ HEMOLYTIC UREMIC SYNDROME

Nephropathy, microangiopathic hemolytic anemia, and thrombocytopenia are found in patients with hemolytic uremic syndrome (HUS). This syndrome commonly occurs in children younger than 5 years following an episode of gastroenteritis or respiratory infection. Siblings may also develop the disease due to a familial genetic component. The illness has an acute onset with rapid progression to renal failure and thrombocytopenia.

Hemolytic uremic syndrome results from endothelial damage of the renal microvasculature. A microangiopathic hemolytic anemia develops as a result of mechanical damage and sequestration of red blood cells. Platelet aggregation may produce microthrombi and hypoxia in the kidney. Decreased C_3 may result from deposition of complement in the lumina of the glomeruli.

ETIOLOGY

Associated infections can be found. *Escherichia coli* serotype 0157:H7 is the most commonly found organism, producing a cytotoxin that inhibits protein synthesis leading to cell death in gastrointestinal organs.[5]

Shigella, *Salmonella*, and group A *Streptococcus* may be associated with HUS, as well as coxsackievirus, influenza, and respiratory syncytial virus (RSV).

DIAGNOSTIC FINDINGS

Patients usually have a history of gastroenteritis with vomiting, bloody diarrhea, and crampy abdominal pain within 2 weeks of the onset of HUS. Children who develop HUS without a prodrome of gastroenteritis have a poor prognosis. Low-grade fever, pallor, hematuria, oliguria, and gastrointestinal bleeding occur. Central nervous system deterioration can occur with a spectrum from irritability to seizures or coma.

There is a tremendous spectrum of severity of clinical disease ranging from mild elevation of BUN with anemia to to-

tal anuria due to acute nephropathy with severe anemia and thrombocytopenia.

Ultimately, patients may develop hypertension; anemia with pallor, petechiae, and easy bruising; hepatosplenomegaly; and edema. Hypertension occurs in up to 50% of patients. Irritability or lethargy may develop. Seizures occur in 40% of the cases. Hyponatremia and hypocalcemia are common. Acute abdominal conditions including intussusception, bowel perforation, and toxic megacolon can occur. Hepatic and pancreatic injury can occur in HUS. There may be cardiac involvement with cardiomyopathy, myocarditis, or high-output failure. Recurrences may occur, often without a prodrome, and may be associated with a high mortality rate.

Laboratory evaluation should include assessment of renal function including electrolyte, BUN, and creatinine levels and urinalysis. Hematologic studies reveal low hemoglobin with a microangiopathic, hemolytic anemia. Burr cells are common. Platelets are usually decreased below 50 000/mm³. C-reactive protein is commonly elevated. Coagulation studies are usually normal.

MANAGEMENT

Initial stabilization is followed by admission to an appropriate medical center. Volume overload may occur secondary to anemia. Hypertension may occur and appears to be caused by increased renin levels. Treatment is recommended if the diastolic pressure is above 120 mm Hg. A variety of agents may be used, including nifedipine, labetolol, captopril, and hydralazine. Renal failure requires meticulous balancing of intake and output with specific treatment of hyperkalemia, acidosis, hypocalcemia, hyperphosphatemia, and other metabolic abnormalities. Peritoneal dialysis may be required, especially when the BUN is more than 100 or when congestive heart failure, encephalopathy, or hyperkalemia are present. Peritoneal dialysis is also indicated when anuria has been present for 24 hours.[6–8]

A serum hemoglobin < 5 g/dL or hematocrit < 15% generally requires treatment with packed red blood cells, infused slowly. Platelet survival is shortened and platelet infusions may be required in children with active bleeding. Seizures require specific management and are usually caused by hypertension or uremia. Acute treatment includes stabilization and anticonvulsants, as well as a consideration of emergency dialysis. Heparin and streptokinase have been tried without significant success.

▶ ACUTE RENAL FAILURE

Impairment of the kidney's ability to regulate urine volume and composition produces problems with hemostasis. This is usually associated with a decreased glomerular filtration rate (GFR).

The etiology of acute renal failure may be categorized on the basis of the type of renal injury. It may be prerenal (decreased perfusion of the kidney), intrarenal (damage to the actual nephron), or postrenal (downstream obstruction of the urinary tract; Table 84–1).

Prerenal patients have decreased perfusion of the kidney. Dehydration is usually the cause and may be secondary to vomiting, diarrhea, diabetic ketoacidosis, or decreased intravascular volumes associated with nephrotic syndrome, burns, or shock.

Intrarenal failure results from direct, intrinsic damage to the nephrons caused by glomerulonephritis (hematuria, proteinuria, edema, and hypertension), HUS, nephrotoxic exposures, crush injuries, sepsis, or disseminated intravascular coagulation.

Obstruction leads to postrenal failure and may be accompanied by symptoms, although blockage may be insidious and without symptoms. Causes of postrenal obstruction include posterior urethral valves, ureteropelvic junction abnormalities, renal stones, and trauma. Abdominal pain and an abdominal mass due to hydronephrosis may be noted.[9-10]

DIAGNOSTIC FINDINGS

The history may reflect the underlying disease and the category of renal failure. The physical examination will help determine the mechanism. It is essential to evaluate for hypovolemia, volume overload, hypertension, or obstruction.

Patients may have oliguria with urine output less than 1 mL/kg/h or be nonoliguric with an output excessive for the volume status. Azotemia may be noted.

Laboratory evaluation should include electrolytes, studies of renal function, and a search for the underlying pathology. The creatinine clearance is a good measure of GFR and is useful in initial assessment and ongoing monitoring. A 24-hour urine is normally needed.

$$\text{Creatinine clearance (mL/min/1.73 m}^2) = \frac{UV}{P} \times \frac{1.73}{SA}$$

Where U = urinary concentration of creatinine (mg/dL);

V = volume of urine divided by the number of minutes in collection period (24 hours = 1440 min) (mL/min);

P = plasma concentration of creatinine (mg/dL);

SA = surface area (m²)

A rapid approximation can be made using the formula:

$$\text{Creatinine clearance (mL/min/1.73 m}^2) - \frac{0.55 \times ht \text{ (cm)}}{P}$$

Normal values are the following:

- Newborn and premature: 40 to 65 mL/min/1.73 m²

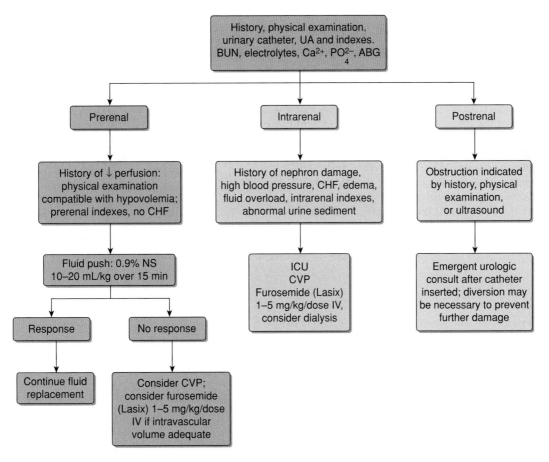

Figure 84–3. Acute renal failure: initial assessment and treatment. UA, urine analysis; BUN, blood urea nitrogen; Ca, calcium; po, orally; ABG, arterial blood gas; CHF, congestive heart failure; NS, normal saline; ICU, intensive care unit; CVP, central venous pressure; IV, intravenous. (With permission from Barkin RM, Rosen P, eds. *Emergency Pediatrics: A Guide to Ambulatory Care.* 6th ed. St. Louis, MO: Mosby; 2003:826.)

- Normal child: female, 109 mL/min/1.73 m^2 or male, 124 mL/min/1.73 m^2
- Adult: female, 95 mL/min/1.73 m^2 or male, 105 mL/min/1.73 m^2

A single-voided urine in adults has been of some use in assessing renal function. In patients with stable renal function, a spot protein:creatinine ratio of >3.0 represents nephrotic range proteinuria (a ratio of <0.2 is normal). Ultrasonography is also important in the evaluation of these patients. Combining data from serum, urine, and ultrasonography helps differentiate among prerenal, intrarenal, and postrenal failure (Table 84–1).

MANAGEMENT

Initial management must focus on stabilization with correction of fluid imbalance (Fig. 84–3). If the intravascular volume is adequate or overloaded, urine output may be enhanced with furosemide, usually in an initial dose of 1 mg/kg increased up to 6 mg/kg/dose. Mannitol may be administered if there is no response to furosemide. The dose is 0.5 to 0.75 mg/kg/dose IV. Do not use these agents if obstruction is present.

In oliguric or anuric patients with decreased intravascular volume, fluid may be administered slowly, often in conjunction with monitoring of the central venous pressure. Low-dose dopamine occasionally may be used to increase renal blood flow and GFR. Those with high urine output must receive a significant amount of fluid to avoid hypovolemia.

Hypertension may be caused by fluid overload or high renin secretion. Children having acute hypertension with a diastolic pressure more than 100 mm Hg should be treated parenterally because of the risk of seizures, encephalopathy, and other sequelae. Only a mild reduction is needed, usually to the diastolic range of approximately 100 mm Hg. Nitroprusside and nifedipine are useful for reduction of pressure.

Hyperkalemia causes membrane excitability with possible cardiac dysrhythmias. A potassium level >6.5 mEq/L can cause elevation of the T wave. Specific and immediate treatment for a potassium level >7.0 mEq/L is required. Treatment may include calcium chloride, 20 to 30 mg/kg slowly; sodium bicarbonate, 1 to 2 mEq/kg/dose; or glucose and insulin infusion of 1 mL/kg of D$_{50}$W followed by 1 mL/kg of D$_{25}$W and 0.5 U/kg of regular insulin per hour to keep serum glucose between 120 to 300 mg/dL. Kayexalate at 1 g/kg/dose every 4 to 6 hours mixed with 70% sorbitol, orally or rectally, may be useful after initial stabilization. Other abnormalities that may need specific treatment include anemia, metabolic acidosis, hyponatremia, and hyperphosphatemia.

Dialysis may be required for unresponsive fluid overload, severe hyperkalemia, severe hyponatremia or hypernatremia, unresponsive metabolic acidosis, BUN > 100 mg/dL, or altered level of consciousness secondary to uremia. Such patients obviously require hospitalization.

REFERENCES

1. Simckes AM, Spitzer A. Poststreptococcal acute glomerulonephritis. *Pediatr Rev.* 1995;16:278.
2. Wingo CS, Clapp WL. Proteinuria: potential causes and approach to evaluation. *Am J Med Sci.* 2000;320:188–194.
3. Roy S, Stapleton FB. Changing perspective in children hospitalized with post streptococcal acute glomerulonephritis. *Pediatr Nephrol.* 1990;4:585.
4. Warshaw BL. Nephrotic syndrome in children. *Pediatr Ann.* 1994;23:495.
5. Brandt JR, Fouser LS, Watkins SL, et al. *E. coli* 0157: H7–associated hemolytic-uremic syndrome after ingestion of contaminated hamburgers. *J Pediatr.* 1994;125:519.
6. Garg AX, et al. Long term renal prognosis of diarrhea associated hemolytic-uremic syndrome. *JAMA.* 2003;290:1360.
7. Kelles A, Van Dyck M, Proeshan W. Childhood haemolytic uraemic syndrome: long-term outcome and prognostic features. *Eur J Pediatr.* 1994;153:38.
8. Siegler RC, Milligan MK, Burningham TH, et al. Long-term outcome and prognostic indicators in the hemolytic uremic syndrome. *J Pediatr.* 1991;118:195.
9. Sehic A, Chesney RW. Acute renal failure: diagnosis, therapy. *Pediatr Rev.* 1995;16:101, 137.
10. Thadhani R, Pascual M, Bonventre JV. Acute renal flow. *N Engl J Med.* 1996;334:1448.

SECTION XIII

DERMATOLOGIC EMERGENCIES

CHAPTER 85

Petechiae and Purpura

Malee V. Shah and Robert A. Wiebe

▶ HIGH-YIELD FACTS

- Although purpura itself is not dangerous, it may be a sign of an underlying life-threatening illness that requires immediate attention.
- Petechiae above the nipple line with a history of cough or vomiting may be benign and caused by increased venous pressure.
- Purpura is present in almost all patients with Henoch–Schonlein purpura (HSP), but it may not always be the presenting sign. This can cause a delay in the diagnosis.
- Think of idiopathic thrombocytopenic purpura (ITP) in a non-toxic-appearing child with absence of splenomegaly and a normal hemoglobin and white blood cell count
- Child abuse should be suspected if bruising occurs to non-bony prominences or in areas not normally subjected to injury, or if the history is not consistent with the physical findings.

Purpura results from the extravasation of blood from vasculature into the skin or mucous membranes. A careful evaluation of a patient with a purpuric rash will help differentiate a benign illness from a life-threatening disorder (Fig. 85–1). Laboratory tests are helpful, but a thorough history and physical examination can offer the most information to identify the cause. This section gives an overview of the main causes of petechiae and purpura in children.

▶ PETECHIAE CAUSED BY SEPSIS

ETIOLOGY

Purpura fulminans secondary to sepsis is a life-threatening condition characterized by hemorrhagic infarction of the skin and multiorgan dysfunction. It may be caused by acute severe gram-negative bacterial or other infections. The organism most commonly implicated in pediatric patients is *Neisseria meningitidis* (>90%), followed by *Streptococcus pneumoniae* and group A and B streptococci.[1,2] Most cases of *Staphylococcus aureus* sepsis are reported as toxic shock syndrome. Outbreaks occur in semiclosed communities, such as child care centers, college dormitories, and military bases. Transmission occurs by direct contact with secretions or fomites carrying the offending organism.

PATHOPHYSIOLOGY

The septic lesions are thought to be initiated by local intradermal release of endotoxin leading to an inflammatory reaction and increased vascular permeability. The same endotoxin, 12 to 24 hours later, causes widespread microvascular thrombosis, hemorrhagic infarction of the skin, and necrotizing vasculitis. It does so by causing a disturbance in the anticoagulant and procoagulant pathways leading to disseminated intravascular coagulation (DIC).[1]

RECOGNITION

The sepsis-induced cutaneous lesions are similar regardless of the causative organism. The clinical course of skin necrosis begins with a region of dermal discomfort that quickly progresses to petechiae within minutes to hours. The petechiae, which can be found anywhere on the body, will usually distribute acrally over the hands and feet. They then coalesce to form purpura (Fig. 85–2). Hemorrhagic infarction and subsequent skin necrosis can occur at this point without initiation of aggressive therapy. Frank skin necrosis and gangrene are associated with more than 50% morbidity and mortality.[1] Even though the purpuric rash is the principle feature of purpura fulminans, it is a late sign of the disease. Instead, children may initially portray other signs and symptoms such as fever, malaise, vomiting, poor perfusion, altered mental status, and even hypotension. Most, but not all, patients will be ill-appearing.

It is important to keep in mind that in a patient who presents with petechiae just over the face, neck, and upper trunk above the nipple line, the history of violent coughing or vomiting may likely be owing to increased venous pressure rather than an infectious cause.

MANAGEMENT

The majority of affected patients develop septic shock and DIC.[1] Early recognition of the disease state and timely treatment is crucial and will decrease mortality. Aggressive systemic organ support is paramount for survival of these patients. Supplemental oxygen and mechanical ventilation help reduce metabolic demands by taking away the work of breathing. Aggressive fluid resuscitation is required to restore intravascular volume. Crystalloid solutions are the first-line choice

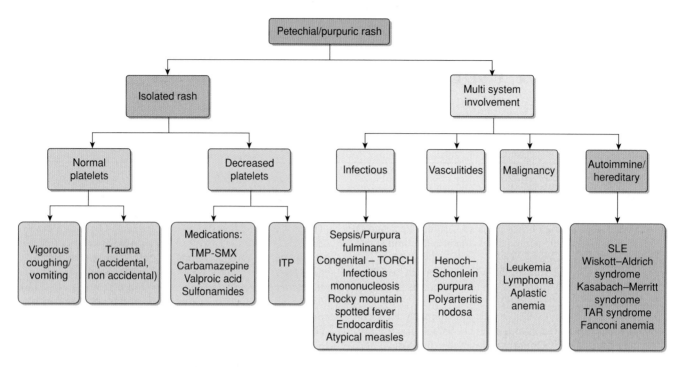

Figure 85–1. Differential diagnosis of petechiae and purpura.

in fluid repletion. Hypotension may arise despite aggressive fluid resuscitation, and ionotropic support may be necessary. Administration of antibiotics should also be initiated soon after diagnosis. Empiric coverage should include a third-generation cephalosporin, since it provides good coverage against *N. meningitidis* and streptococcus. Vancomycin should be added if methicillin-resistant *Staphylococcus aureus* is suspected. Once a causative organism is identified with antibiotic sensitivities, the coverage can be narrowed. Purpura fulminans almost always leads to full-thickness skin loss; thus, the treatment is similar to that of a burn patient.[1] The complications are

also the same, including secondary infection and compartment syndrome. Debridement of the necrotic tissue and eventually grafting may be required. When the tissue necrosis is extensive, limb amputation may be necessary (see Chapter 25 for a detailed discussion of the management of shock).

ANCILLARY STUDIES

A blood culture is valuable regardless of whether antibiotics have been given prior to obtaining it. Other cultures that should be obtained once the patient is stabilized are cerebrospinal fluid and urine cultures. Laboratory studies that may be useful are blood gas, DIC panel, lactate, and complete blood count. It is crucial to remember that getting the supplementary studies are not the priority. Highly sensitive rapid polymerase chain reaction (PCR) tests are available for detection of the most common serotypes of *N. meningitidis,* which can be performed on blood, urine, and cerebrospinal fluid.[3]

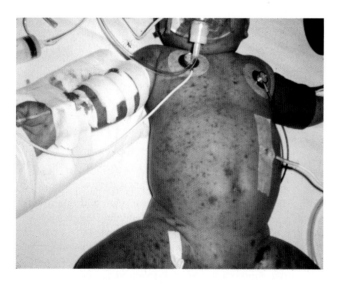

Figure 85–2. Patient with petechiae and purpura from gram-negative sepsis.

► HENOCH–SCHONLEIN PURPURA

ETIOLOGY

The triggers of the immune complex cascade causing HSP are mostly infectious. Mild viral respiratory infections (i.e., parvovirus), bacterial pharyngitis caused by group A β-hemolytic streptococcus, and certain vaccines have been implicated as possible offenders. Upper respiratory tract infections precede HSP in 30% to 50% of the cases.[4,5] Positive strep cultures have been reported in 10% to 30% of cases, antistreptolysin O titers are raised in 20% to 50%.[6]

EPIDEMIOLOGY

The incidence of HSP in children is approximately 10 to 20 cases per 100 000 children per year, and the median age is 4 to 6 years.[5,7] Boys are affected more often than girls.[6] The severity of symptoms tends to be milder in patients younger than 2 years, and becomes more severe in older patients.

PATHOPHYSIOLOGY

HSP is an IgA-mediated systemic small-vessel vasculitis of childhood. It is characterized by immune system activation, which includes the development of autoantibodies against endothelial cells and increased cytokines. These immune complexes deposit in the small blood vessels causing a nonthrombocytopenic purpura. The vasculitis can affect the vessels of the skin, joints, kidneys, gastrointestinal tract, and brain. The immune complexes are theorized to produce the purpuric lesions through their interaction with the complement and clotting systems.[8]

RECOGNITION

A prodromal event can usually be identified a couple of weeks prior to the onset of symptoms. Cutaneous involvement includes 1 to 10 mm palpable purpuric lesions and pinpoint petechiae distributed symmetrically over the lower extremities (Fig. 85–3A) and buttock region (Fig. 85–3B). Though the purpura are usually concentrated over the lower half of the body, they are not restricted to those areas. These purpuric lesions are unrelated to any underlying coagulopathy. Occasionally,

the systemic symptoms occur before the lesions appear which can cause a delay in diagnosis. Almost, if not all, patients with HSP will develop purpura during the course of the disease.[5–7]

Joint manifestations are the second most common feature of HSP and can be seen in up to 80% of patients.[6,8] The vasculitis typically causes arthralgia and arthritis of the knees and ankles. The involvement can be so severe that it may restrict walking. Interestingly, arthritis may precede the onset of purpura by a week in 15% to 25% of patients.[6]

Renal involvement is common and can be seen in up to 70% of children with HSP.[8] It can manifest within a few days to 4 weeks after the onset of other symptoms. Although most patients have asymptomatic microscopic hematuria, some may present with an acute nephritic/nephritic syndrome. Of the patients who develop HSP nephritis, 1% to 7% will likely advance to end-stage renal disease.[7] The risk factors for developing HSP nephritis are children older than 4 years, those with gastrointestinal bleeding, factor XIII activity less than 80% of normal, and/or those treated with factor XIII concentrate.[5]

The long-term morbidity of HSP is largely attributed to renal involvement. Another genitourinary complication that should be considered is orchitis, as 10% to 20% of males with HSP may have testicular pain.[6] Testicular torsion, though unlikely, should still be considered.

Abdominal pain is the most common gastrointestinal symptom; however, patients may also complain of vomiting, hematemesis, and bloody stools. The abdominal pain can be very severe, but usually does not last more than 24 hours. The stool can have either occult or gross blood. Gastrointestinal manifestations may precede purpura by up to 2 weeks.[6] Because of this, a workup for appendicitis may be initiated. Intussusception has been reported in 1% to 5% of patients.[6] Rarely, there can be cerebral involvement causing seizures, paresis, or coma.

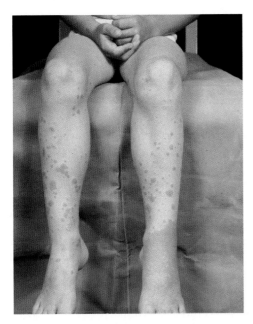

A

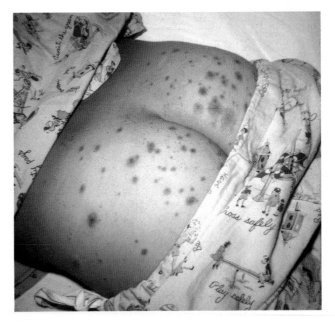

B

Figure 85–3. (A) Henoch–Schoenlein purpura on lower extremities. (B) Henoch–Schoenlein purpura on buttocks.

MANAGEMENT

HSP is usually a self-limited condition. Supportive care, such as analgesia, is required for patients with skin involvement only. Treatment and follow-up can be done on an outpatient basis.

When there is internal organ involvement, inpatient therapy may be necessary. Pulse therapy with intravenous corticosteroids may be beneficial for children with joint pain to the point of being unable to walk or with considerable abdominal pain.[6] Patients may also require intravenous fluids and nutrition if unable to eat. Rarely blood transfusions may be needed in those patients with severe blood loss through the GI tract. The efficacy of corticosteroids is unknown for the long-term prognosis of renal disease.[4] The use of plasmapheresis, immunosuppressive agents (cyclophosphamide, azathioprine), and intravenous immunoglobulin therapy may be of benefit when used in conjunction with corticosteroids for the more severe forms of nephritis.[4,8]

ANCILLARY STUDIES

There are no specific diagnostic tests for HSP; however, certain laboratory findings will help the clinician with the diagnosis as well as the identification of specific organ system involvement. A complete blood count will reveal whether or not the cutaneous lesions are secondary to thrombocytopenia. In HSP, platelet counts are normal. Serum IgA concentrations may be elevated. A urine analysis with microscopy will show the extent of renal involvement. Serum C3 and C4 concentrations are low in a few patients. Stool guaiac will help to identify presence of gastrointestinal bleeding. Other laboratory and radiographic studies are useful to exclude other conditions that may mimic HSP before the purpuric lesions appear (i.e., septic joint, appendicitis, testicular torsion).

▶ IDIOPATHIC THROMBOCYTOPENIC PURPURA

ETIOLOGY

Numerous viral infections including Epstein–Barr virus and cytomegalovirus have been implicated in causing ITP.[9]

EPIDEMIOLOGY

The incidence of ITP is approximately 3 to 8 per 100 000 children per year, making it one of the most common acquired bleeding disorders in pediatrics.[9] It affects males and females equally.

PATHOPHYSIOLOGY

ITP occurs secondary to an immune response to a viral infection. Antiplatelet antibodies are formed and cross-react with platelet antigens. These IgG antibodies bind to normal circulating platelets. The spleen subsequently destroys the antibody-covered platelets. The isolated thrombocytopenia that develops is the only cell line that is depressed and there is absence of other diseases causing thrombocytopenia. Because the bone marrow is functioning appropriately, it compensates by increasing platelet turnover and releasing younger, larger platelets into the bloodstream.

RECOGNITION

Patients that present with ITP are typically healthy and only complain of easy bruising and spontaneous bleeding. About one-third of patients will have nosebleeds and gingival bleeding as part of their initial complaint.[9] Other organ system involvement includes the gastrointestinal tract and urinary tract. Another possible, but rare, presentation is intracranial hemorrhage. This is seen when the platelet counts are extremely low ($<10\,000/mm^3$).[9] The mortality rate for intracranial hemorrhage is approximately 1% in children. Besides petechiae and bleeding of mucous membranes, the physical examination should be normal including the absence of hepatosplenomegaly and lymphadenopathy. ITP is classified as acute and chronic where the latter persists for more than 6 months. Patients with chronic ITP may have underlying autoimmune disorders and usually are in the adolescent age group. Acute ITP is more commonly seen in children younger than 10 years.

MANAGEMENT

Approximately 80% to 90% of cases are self-limited and will demonstrate recovery within 6 months without treatment.[9] Patients who have platelet counts less than 20 000/mm^3 and/or have significant mucous membrane bleeding should have consultation and follow-up with a hematologist. Therapeutic options are controversial and include intravenous gamma globulin and/or corticosteroids. Although both have advantages and disadvantages, they may improve total platelet counts within 24 to 72 hours. A second-line option is anti-Rh(D). It is only useful in patients who are Rh-positive. Splenectomy should be considered in those patients with chronic ITP refractory to pharmacologic measures. Long-term remission is only guaranteed in 60% to 90% of patients that undergo a splenectomy.[9]

ANCILLARY STUDIES

Although, bone marrow aspiration is the gold standard for diagnosing ITP, clinical examination and other less invasive tests usually suffice. Bone marrow examination is only needed when the diagnosis is uncertain and there are other systemic findings that are not typical of ITP. Laboratory findings on a complete blood count should be an isolated thrombocytopenia ($<150\,000\ mm^3$). When other cell lines are decreased, other diseases, specifically leukemia should be considered. Because there is normal bone marrow function, microscopic examination of a peripheral blood smear may demonstrate large young platelets and occasional megakaryocytes in response to the rapid platelet destruction. Coagulation studies are usually not needed when the diagnosis of ITP is evident as they are likely to be normal. If a bleeding time is performed, it will be prolonged.

► CHILD ABUSE

ETIOLOGY

Bruising caused by maltreatment is a consequence of blunt trauma inflicted on the patient. This can occur when caretakers attempt to discipline the child or when their anger is displaced on the child as bodily harm. Children that are abused are usually too young to protect themselves or fight back.

EPIDEMIOLOGY

It is estimated that each year more than 3 million children are victims of abuse, and as a result, an estimated 2000 children die.[10] Multiple factors contribute to the risk of child abuse. Children who are younger than 4 years or those who have comorbid conditions such as learning disabilities, chronic illnesses, conduct disorder, and mental retardation are at highest risk. Prematurity is another important risk factor. Caretakers who are likely to abuse are those who were abused themselves as children, and young, single, nonbiological parents.

RECOGNITION

Appropriate diagnosis of child abuse is achieved by a thorough history and physical as well as laboratory studies and imaging modalities. It is beneficial to interview caretakers individually because different stories may be given for the same injury. It is also important to be familiar with medical conditions and cultural practices (coining, cupping) that mimic child abuse (Fig. 85–4). The pattern of distribution and location of the traumatic lesions will help differentiate nonintentional from intentional trauma. Bruising over bony prominences often signify noninflicted trauma of a mobile child; however, bruising over the back, earlobes, buttocks, or other protected areas may suggest abuse. Bruising in the shape of teeth marks, belt marks, or hands should also increase your suspicion of maltreatment as should burns. Human bites, compared to animal bites, are more often crush injuries. Animal bites usually produce a puncture wound or cause tearing of the skin. Siblings may be used as scapegoats for a bite mark, but a bite width of more than 4 cm is indicative of an adult bite.[11] Another key piece to evaluation is noting the various stages of bruising. Fresh bruises implicate that abuse is ongoing. Aging bruises using standardized aging charts is no longer used. Any unexplained bruising in infants younger than 6 to 12 months should raise suspicion of abuse (see Chapter 145 for a detailed discussion of child abuse).

MANAGEMENT

In all states, physicians and other professionals (health care providers, teachers, and law enforcement personnel) are mandated by law to report suspected child abuse to the child protective services or law enforcement.[10] Consultation with other health professionals and Child Protective Services may be needed in cases where the physician is uncertain about the likelihood of abuse. The main goal is to safeguard the child from further harm. If the patient cannot be immediately placed in another home, admission is warranted until disposition to a foster family is completed. Other children in the offender's home may require removal as well. Medical clearance is needed prior to placement.

ANCILLARY STUDIES

It is important to consider any noninjury related causes of bruising. A complete blood count will help delineate a platelet abnormality. Coagulation studies may aid in ruling out a bleeding disorder. A skeletal survey helps identify subtle fractures that may need to be addressed. When a patient presents with decreased level of consciousness, a computed tomography of the head may reveal an intracranial bleed.

REFERENCES

1. Betrosian AP, Berlet T, Agarwal B. Purpura fulminans in sepsis. *Am J Med Sci.* 2006;332(6):339–345.
2. Hazelzet JA. Diagnosis meningococcemia as a cause of sepsis. *Pediatr Crit Care Med.* 2005;6(3):S50-S54.
3. Aber CA, Connelly EA, Schachner LA. Fever and rash in a child: when to worry? *Pediatr Ann.* 2007;36(1):30–38.
4. Gonzalez MA, Garcia C, Pujol RM. Clinical approach to cutaneous vasculitis. *Curr Opin Rheumatol.* 2005;17(1):56–61.
5. Ting TV, Hashkes PJ. Update on childhood vasculitides. *Curr Opin Rheumatol.* 2004;16(5):560–565.
6. Saulsbury FT. Clinical update: Henoch-Schonlein purpura. *Lancet.* 2007;369:976–978.
7. Chang W, Yang Y, Wang L, et al. Renal manifestations in Henoch-Schonlein purpura: a 10-year clinical study. *Pediatr Nephrol.* 2005;20:1269–1272.
8. Wetson WL, Lane AT, Morelli JG. *Color Textbook of Pediatric Dermatology.* 3rd ed. St. Louis, MO: Mosby-Year Book; 2002.
9. Chu Y, Korb J, Sakamoto KM. Idiopathic thrombocytopenic purpura. *Pediatr Rev.* 2000;21:95–104.
10. Swerdlin A, Berkowitz C, Craft N. Cutaneous signs of child abuse. *J Am Acad Dermatol.* 2007;57:371–392.
11. Cohen BA. *Pediatric Dermatology.* 2nd ed. St. Louis, MO: Mosby-Year Book; 1999.

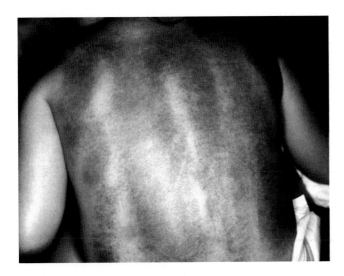

Figure 85–4. Purpura from "coining," a cultural practice for fever management.

CHAPTER 86

Pruritic Rashes

Malee V. Shah and Robert A. Wiebe

▶ HIGH-YIELD FACTS

- In infant atopy, cheeks and extensor surfaces of the legs are most commonly affected. Later in childhood, the antecubital and popliteal fossae are effected.
- Sudden onset of severe itching with similar complaints from other family members should raise your suspicion of scabies even if burrows are not visible.
- Urticaria tend to disappear and reappear over different areas of the body; whereas, erythema multiforme are fixed lesions. Subcutaneous epinephrine clears urticaria; however, it does not affect erythema multiforme.
- Stevens–Johnson syndrome and toxic epidermal necrolysis differ from erythema multiforme in that there is mucosal involvement and systemic symptoms are present. All three entities can be caused by a variety of drugs and infections.

▶ ATOPIC DERMATITIS

ETIOLOGY

Atopic dermatitis affects approximately 15% of children in the United States and accounts for up to 4% of all emergency department visits.[1] The causal basis of atopic dermatitis is uncertain. It is evident however, that patients with a personal history and/or a family history of asthma and other allergies are more prone to atopic dermatitis.[2] Patients with a genetic predisposition have a 90% chance of developing atopic dermatitis by the age of 5 years and a 95% chance by the age of 15 years.[3]

PATHOPHYSIOLOGY

Atopic dermatitis, also known as eczema, is thought to result from chronic inflammation of the skin. The exact mechanism is unknown; however, it is known that the skin barrier (stratum corneum) functions are defective. One hypothesis that exists is that there are genetic, environmental, pharmacologic, and immunologic triggers that induce hypersensitivity of the skin.[1,3] It generally presents in infancy. The course of the disease is unpredictable, but the symptoms in most children will resolve before adulthood.

RECOGNITION

Diagnosis can be made by the presence of pruritis, typical morphology and distribution of the rash, and a strong fam-

ily history of atopy. The rash usually presents after 4 to 6 weeks of life, where it characteristically involves the cheeks, trunk, and extensor surfaces (Fig. 86–1). Infants usually present with exudative lesions. In children, the distribution is over the flexor surfaces, including the antecubital and popliteal fossae. They present with areas of hypopigmentation and diffuse scaly patches. By adolescence, the involvement is the same with the addition of the face, neck, hands, and feet. Lichenification and hyperpigmentation are findings characteristic of chronicity. The clinical course of atopic dermatitis is characterized by relapsing episodes of symptom flares.

MANAGEMENT

Since there is no definitive treatment, education, reduction of symptoms, and prevention are the key. Avoidance of non-specific skin irritants such as synthetic fabrics, wool, and nonessential, highly fragranced toiletries is the first step. Keeping the skin moisturized as much as possible helps reduce inflammation and flare-ups. This can be achieved by limiting the time of bathing, using a mild moisturizing cleanser, and applying emollients frequently.[3]

Low- and medium-potency topical corticosteroids are the mainstay of therapy.[3,4] They should be used to control mild-to-moderate exacerbations; whereas, severe flare-ups may occasionally require a short course of systemic steroids.[1] Topical tacrolimus and pimecrolimus are nonsteroidal topical immunosuppresants that have proven to be safe and effective for moderate-to-severe flare-ups.[1,4] They should be used as second-line treatment. Several systemic immunomodulators such as cyclosporine and interferon-γ have shown efficacy, but their usefulness have been limited by side effects and the concerns about potential long-term adverse effects.[4] H1 antihistamines have not been shown to relieve pruritis from atopic dermatitis, but their sedative effects are useful for sleep disturbances secondary to scratching.[1] Although the skin of affected individuals is colonized with *Staphylococcus aureus* and *Streptococcus pyogenes*, oral and topical antibiotics are only indicated for active, secondary bacterial infection.[3]

ANCILLARY STUDIES

Although elevated serum IgE levels and eosinophilia are seen in 70% to 80% of patients, they are not specific to this disease process and need not be routinely used to diagnose atopic dermatitis.[1] Skin testing is also of little value and certain dietary restrictions are difficult in this age group. Diagnosis is by clinical observation and a good history.

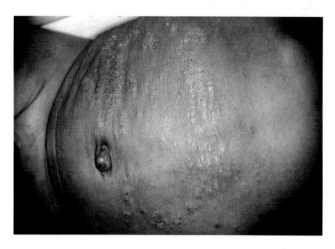

Figure 86–1. Atopic dermatitis seen over the trunk of an infant.

▶ CONTACT DERMATITIS

ETIOLOGY

Common allergens include nickel (jewelry, watches), chemicals in elastic, latex, tanning chemicals in leather, fabric dyes, and rhus (i.e., poison ivy, oak, and sumac). Contact dermatitis affects approximately 20% of all children at some time and occurs more in fair-skinned individuals.[5]

PATHOPHYSIOLOGY

Contact dermatitis is a type IV cell-mediated hypersensitivity reaction to an antigenic material that comes in direct contact with the skin. On initial contact with the irritant, the T lymphocytes go through an immunologic cascade and become sensitized. On subsequent exposures, the sensitized T lymphocytes combine with the antigen and cause the release of lymphokines. There is usually a 24-hour delay from the time of antigenic stimulation to onset of symptoms.

RECOGNITION

Contact dermatitis is characterized by the onset of an erythematous, papulovesicular eruption in the distribution of where skin contact with the irritant occurred. Bullae may also be present. With chronic exposure to the allergen, an individual will present with scaling, fissuring, and lichenification. Diagnosis is easily made when there is recognition of the pattern of dermatitis at the site of exposure to the offending agent (Table 86–1). An eczematous rash localized to the infraumbilical area may be suggestive of nickel dermatitis caused by the metal securing on pants. Elastic around the border of a diaper can cause diaper dermatitis. Shoe contact dermatitis may be caused by the dyes and tanning leather used for manufacturing them. When the reaction is to the Rhus group of plants, which include poison ivy, poison oak, and poison sumac, the rash may appear linear from contact with the edge of the leaf or the stem.

▶ TABLE 86–1. PATTERN OF DISTRIBUTION FOR CONTACT DERMATITIS

Distribution of Lesions	Contactant
Face, eyelids	Cosmetics
Ears	Earrings, eyeglasses
Neck	Necklaces, perfumes
Axillae	Deodorant
Wrists	Watch, bracelets
Extremities (linear patterns)	Rhus (i.e., leaf edge or stem)
Infraumbilical	Metal snap of pants, belt buckle
Feet	Leather and dyes from shoes

MANAGEMENT

Removal and avoidance of the causative material is the key management strategy. Mild, localized dermatitis responds well to cool compresses. For small areas of moderate contact dermatitis, potent topical steroids should be used twice daily for 2 to 3 weeks. The new topical immunomodulators such as tacrolimus and pimecrolimus are second-line therapies.[5] Antipruritic lotions, such as calamine, and oral antihistamines are also useful for pruritis and impaired sleep. For severe cases with more than 20% to 30% body involvement, a 5- to 7-day course of systemic corticosteroids is indicated.[1,6] The rash may last several weeks despite treatment.

ANCILLARY STUDIES

Patch testing may be done to elicit a reaction for confirmation of the diagnosis, but it should be avoided during an acute episode.[1,7] Biopsies are of little diagnostic help.

▶ PEDICULOSIS

ETIOLOGY

Pediculosis, or louse infestation, are generally site specific. *Pediculus humanus capitus* (head louse), *Pediculus humanus humanus* (body louse), and *Pthirus pubis* (crab louse) are the three types that infect humans. They are six-legged, wingless insects approximately 1 to 2 mm in length. Although it is not a reportable disease, an estimated 6 to 12 million people per year are affected in the United States.[8]

PATHOPHYSIOLOGY

The female louse attaches her eggs to the hair shaft. Nits remain on the hair after the eggs hatch. Lice feed on human blood by biting into the patient's skin. This action causes pruritis; however, some patients may remain asymptomatic allowing more time for transmission. Spread from person to person is achieved by close contact. Sharing of hats and combs facilitates the transmission.

RECOGNITION

Pruritis to the scalp, especially behind the ears and at the nape of the neck, is highly suggestive of head louse infestation. The presence of nits alone is not diagnostic of active infestation; however, direct visualization of the live louse confirms the diagnosis. Although nits are more easily found than lice, they may often be confused with dandruff.

MANAGEMENT

Curative treatment is achieved by 1% permethrin, 0.3% pyrethrin cream rinse, or 0.5% malathion to destroy the louse. A second treatment is recommended 7 to 10 days after the initial course to eliminate any recently hatched lice.[8] Viable eggs and nits may then be mechanically removed by combing through wet hair with a fine-toothed comb. Topical application of petroleum jelly or mayonnaise, both louse suffocants, may be considered.[7,8] A course of trimethoprim-sulfamethoxazole is also an effective second-line treatment for resistant disease.[7,8] Washing clothes and bedding are necessary to destroy nits that may be attached. All close contacts should be checked for lice and treated simultaneously.

▶ SCABIES

ETIOLOGY

Scabies is caused by the arachnid, *Sarcoptes scabiei*. These 8-legged mites may be up to 0.4 mm in length. Worldwide, the annual incidence of scabies is estimated to be around 300 million cases.[9]

PATHOPHYSIOLOGY

The female mite burrows into the skin and lays her eggs. Once infestation has occurred, it takes approximately 1 month for the classic skin manifestations to appear. This is the most contagious period since only casual contact is needed to spread the mite from person to person.

RECOGNITION

Sudden onset of severe itching is the hallmark of scabies. Involvement of other family members should be another clue to diagnosis. Patients may present with red, excoriated papular eruptions that are notably distributed in the folds of the body (beltline, gluteal folds, axillae), and the interdigital webs (Fig. 86–2). In contrast to older children and adults, infants may also develop eczematous papules over the head and face. The classic linear burrows may not commonly be present, but when they are, it is considered diagnostic.

MANAGEMENT

Treatment includes a head-to-toe application of permethrin 5% cream, which should be left on for 8 to 14 hours and

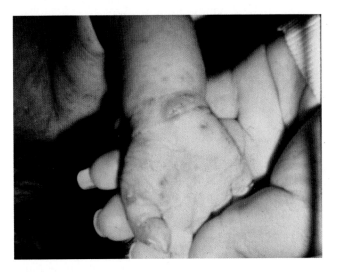

Figure 86–2. Excoriated, papular eruptions characteristic of scabies.

then washed off with soap and water.[2,7] In patients with extensive involvement, a repeat application may be needed a week after the initial treatment. Systemic therapy with oral ivermectin should be considered in widespread outbreaks in schools, nursing homes, or prisons for better disease control.[9] All caregivers and other close contacts of the household should be treated simultaneously. Bedding and clothing should be washed in hot water as heat eliminates scabies most effectively. Anticipatory guidance is important when treating patients and families for scabies because pruritis may persist for 1 to 2 weeks after treatment, even if the infection has resolved.

ANCILLARY STUDIES

Scabies is a clinical diagnosis, but confirmation of the diagnosis is possible by direct microscopic visualization of the mite, eggs, or feces of the mite. Samples should be obtained by scraping the linear burrows caused by the mites.

▶ PAPULAR URTICARIA

ETIOLOGY

Papular urticaria is a complication of insect bites often seen in preadolescent children. Dog and cat fleas are common offenders. Other less common sources include mosquitoes, grass mites, gnats, and bedbugs. The lesions tend to be more evident during the summer and spring months. It is predominantly seen in patients 18 months to 7 years of age.[2]

PATHOPHYSIOLOGY

The eruptions are caused by a type I delayed hypersensitivity reaction to a variety of biting and stinging arthropods. The bite releases the antigen into the bloodstream of patients who are susceptible to the disease, causing the rash. Immunoglobulin and complement then deposit on superficial dermal layers.

This is why the lesions can present anywhere throughout the body instead of just at the inoculation site.

RECOGNITION

These lesions are characterized by crops of symmetrically distributed pruritic erythematous papules surrounded by an urticarial wheal. They are frequently arranged in clusters over the shoulders, upper arms, and other exposed areas. Crops last 2 to 10 days, but recurrence is common and the eruptions may persist for 3 to 9 months.[2] Scratching may produce erosions and ulcerations, causing secondary impetigo or pyoderma.

MANAGEMENT

The management of papular urticaria is mostly conservative. Dogs and cats should be treated for fleas. When going outdoors, patients should be reminded to wear long sleeve shirts as well as other protective clothing. DEET-containing insect repellents are also useful. Carpets and furniture may require a thorough cleaning with the use of commercialized insecticides. When symptoms are severe, relief is achieved with topical medium-potency glucocorticosteroid creams applied three times daily.[2] An antihistamine may be helpful to control the itching.

► URTICARIA

ETIOLOGY

There are a variety of causes for urticaria, including foods (i.e., berries, nuts, shellfish), drugs (i.e., penicillins, cephalosporins), bites and stings, infections (i.e., viral, streptococcal), and certain systemic diseases. In most cases, no causative agent is identified. Approximately 2% to 3% of the pediatric population will develop urticaria at some point in their life.[2]

PATHOPHYSIOLOGY

IgE, after antigenic stimulation, causes degranulation of mast cells, releasing numerous vasoactive mediators (including histamine, cytokines, and prostaglandins) into the bloodstream These chemical mediators cause vasodilation of the small blood vessels and increased leakage of fluid into the dermis.

RECOGNITION

These lesions are commonly referred to as "hives" and appear suddenly as erythematous, raised, pruritic wheals with a pale center and serpiginous borders. They can involve any part of the body. They tend to disappear and reappear on different parts of the body (not fixed), and generally do not last more than 24 hours. These features help differentiate an urticarial lesion from erythema multiforme. Urticaria is considered chronic when it persists longer than 6 weeks. A major difference between chronic and acute urticaria is that there are no con-

cerns for airway compromise or hemodynamic instability in chronic urticaria. Acute urticaria is a reactive phenomenon, while chronic urticaria is an autoimmune process.[10]

MANAGEMENT

Treatment is dictated by the severity of the condition and presence or absence of airway involvement. Mild cases without airway involvement can be resolved with oral antihistamines, specifically diphenhydramine, an H1 blocker. For severe cases with airway involvement, establishing a patent airway is the first priority. This can be achieved with intramuscular epinephrine (1:1000) 0.01 mL/kg. Repeat doses may be required every 5 to 15 minutes. Adjunctive therapies include nebulized β-agonists, H1 and H2 antihistamines, as well as corticosteroids once the patient is stabilized. It is also important to identify and avoid any precipitating agents in the future.

For chronic urticaria, initial treatment consists of non- or low-sedating antihistamines. Patients should be advised that stress and fatigue may exacerbate recurrent symptoms. Most patients maintain control of symptoms with antihistamines alone but, often, minor flares may require a short course of oral corticosteroids. For uncontrollable disease, immunomodulators such as cyclosporine, methotrexate, tacrolimus, or intravenous immunoglobulins may be an option. Plasmapheresis can be considered in the most severe cases.[10]

► ERYTHEMA MULTIFORME

ETIOLOGY

Erythema multiforme (EM) has been linked to a variety of drugs and infections. Herpes simplex virus and *Mycoplasma pneumoniae* infections are the most common precipitants. The offending drugs causing EM include sulfonamides, penicillins, anticonvulsants, and nonsteroidal anti-inflammatory agents. More than 50% of cases will not have a causal agent that can be identified.[11]

PATHOPHYSIOLOGY

EM is an acute, T-cell mediated hypersensitivity reaction triggered by bacterial, viral, or chemical antigens. The immune response eventually may cause cutaneous and mucosal necrosis. Stevens–Johnson syndrome was once considered to be an extreme variant of EM, but recent evidence suggests that they have different etiologies and require different treatments. Stevens–Johnson syndrome and toxic epidermal necrolysis are now considered to be severity variants of a single entity.[12] The latter two mucocutaneous disorders encompass a clinical continuum of the same disease process of epithelial necrosis and subsequent denudation.

RECOGNITION

The distinctive lesions are characterized as round, fixed, and erythematous, appearing symmetrically on the skin. They are

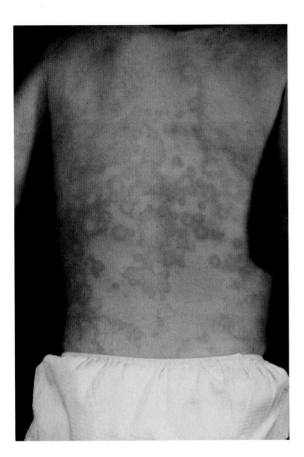

Figure 86–3. The classic target-like appearance of erythema multiforme with red borders and a central clearing.

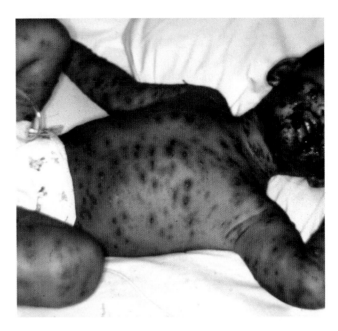

Figure 86–4. Stevens–Johnson syndrome seen with ocular and oral mucosal involvement.

often described as "target" lesions because of their central dusky area (Fig. 86–3). The lesions are distributed acrally but are often found on the trunk. They remain for a minimum of 1 week and can persist up to 2 to 3 weeks. Although uncommon, EM can have mucosal involvement, and when present, it usually involves the oral mucosa only.

In Stevens–Johnson syndrome, unlike EM, the systemic symptoms are severe, including fever, malaise, headache, vomiting, and diarrhea. The areas of epithelial and mucosal necrosis are more extensive, involving at least two mucosal surfaces (eyes, nose, mouth, upper airway, gastrointestinal, and genitourinary tracts) (Fig. 86–4). Stomatitis and conjunctivits are the most common mucosal concerns.[11] The initial lesions progress rapidly from central blistering and erosions to severe epidermal necrosis to sloughing and denuded skin. The cutaneous findings may extend beyond the extremities to the trunk and face. The area of involvement is usually less than 10% of the body surface. The course of symptoms ranges from 2 to 6 weeks. Patients with Stevens–Johnson syndrome may progress to toxic epidermal necrolysis.[12]

Toxic epidermal necrolysis is characterized by a morbilliform rash and multiple large blisters that coalesce to form bullae. They are predominantly found on the face and trunk, and involve more than 30% total body surface area. This is followed by epidermal detachment of the skin and mucosa. Similar to Stevens–Johnson syndrome, constitutional symptoms and mucosal involvement often precede the cutaneous lesions by 24 hours. Ocular scarring can be severe and extensive.[12]

MANAGEMENT

EM is usually a self-limited process and treatment usually is unnecessary. Supportive care with cool compresses and antihistamines suffices. For painful oral lesions, patients may benefit from soothing mouthwash. Acyclovir is not generally indicated but should be considered in patients who have recurrent EM secondary to HSV.[11] There is no evidence to support the use of corticosteroids. Discontinuing any recent medications or any possible causative agent is of utmost importance.

For patients with Stevens–Johnson syndrome and toxic epidermal necrolysis, treatment is similar to that of burn patients. They require either admission to a burn or intensive care unit. It is important to closely monitor their electrolyte and fluid status, prevent any secondary bacterial infection, and provide parenteral nutrition if needed.[12] Systemic corticosteroid use is controversial because of increased susceptibility to infection, but the use of intravenous immunoglobulin may help shorten the disease process.[11] An ophthalmologic consultation should be obtained when there is eye involvement. Precipitating medications should also be discontinued.

ANCILLARY STUDIES

A skin biopsy or frozen section of the lesions will reveal epidermal damage with perivascular lymphatic infiltration and edema. This may help distinguish toxic epidermal necrolysis from other disease processes, such as staphylococcal scalded skin syndrome.

REFERENCES

1. Ong PY, Boguniewicz M. Atopic dermatitis and contact dermatitis in the emergency department. *Clin Pediatr Emerg Med.* 2007;8:81–88.

2. Wetson WL, Lane AT, Morelli JG. *Color Textbook of Pediatric Dermatology*. 3rd ed. St. Louis, MO: Mosby-Year Book; 2002.

3. Eichenfield LF, Hanifin JM, Luger TA, et al. Consensus conference on pediatric atopic dermatitis. *J Am Acad Dermatol*. 2003;49:1088–1095.

4. Hanifin JM, Cooper KD, Ho VC, et al. Guidelines of care for atopic dermatitis. *J Am Acad Dermatol*. 2004;50:391–404.

5. Wetson WL, Bruckner AL. Allergic contact dermatitis. *Pediatr Clin North Am*. 2000;47:897–907.

6. Bruckner AL, Wetson WL. Allergic contact dermatitis in children: a practical approach to management. *Skin Therapy Lett*. 2002;7:3–5.

7. Fleisher GR, Ludwig S, Henretig FM. *Textbook of Pediatric Emergency Medicine*. 5th ed. Philadelphia, PA: Lippincott Williams & Wilkins; 2006.

8. Ko CJ, Elston DM. Pediculosis. *J Am Acad Dermatol*. 2004;50:1–12.

9. Hengge UR, Currie BJ, Jager G, et al. Scabies: a ubiquitous neglected skin disease. *Lancet Infect Dis*. 2006;6:769–779.

10. Altman LC. Autoimmune urticaria. *Pediatr Asthma, Allergy Immunol*. 2007;20(3):196–200.

11. Aber CA, Connelly EA, Schachner LA. Fever and rash in a child: when to worry? *Pediatr Ann*. 2007;36(1):30–38.

12. Williams PM, Conklin RJ. Erythema multiforme: a review and contrast from Stevens–Johnson syndrome/toxic epidermal necrolysis. *Dent Clin North Am*. 2005;49(1):67–76.

CHAPTER 87

Superficial Skin Infections

Malee V. Shah and Robert A. Wiebe

▶ HIGH-YIELD FACTS

- Poststreptococcal glomerulonephritis is caused by nephritogenic strains of streptococci which can cause skin infections and pharyngitis. It presents a couple of weeks after the primary infection.
- Staphylococcal scalded skin syndrome (SSSS) is characterized by an erythematous rash followed by diffuse epidermal exfoliation. Patients are managed similarly to a burn patient. The mortality rate is low unless associated with sepsis.
- Methicillin-resistant *Staphylococcus aureus* (MRSA) is responsible for many serious skin and soft tissue infections as well as bacterial pneumonia.
- Tinea corporis can be treated effectively with topical antifungals, but tinea capitis requires systemic antifungal therapy.

▶ IMPETIGO

ETIOLOGY

Staphylococcus aureus and group A β-hemolytic *Streptococcus* are the organisms that are most commonly isolated from skin infections. MRSA can be isolated from 70% to 80% of impetigo in certain areas of the United States.[1]

PATHOPHYSIOLOGY

Pathogens colonize the skin surface and occasionally invade the damaged epidermal layer and replicate within the skin. Breaks in the skin can be caused by trauma and from scratching atopic skin. Transmission occurs through direct contact; therefore, new lesions may be seen on the patient with no apparent break in the skin. The depth of invasion provides a clinical continuum for impetigo and ecthyma.

RECOGNITION

Impetigo refers to a superficial bacterial infection of the epithelium. It usually occurs in younger children who may be exposed to poor skin hygiene. They initially present as small vesicles and pustules that eventually rupture. The lesions become eroded and progress to areas of honey-crusted lesions. Exposed areas such as the face and extremities are more commonly affected (Fig. 87–1A).

Ecthyma describes the bacterial infections that affect the deeper layers of the epidermis. They are characterized by firm, dark crust that usually contains purulent exudate. The surrounding area is erythematous and indurated (Fig. 87–1B). Neonatal pyoderma is usually a result of a superficial staphylococcal infection and is manifested by variable-sized pustules and bullae (Fig. 87–1C).

MANAGEMENT

Topical mupirocin ointment can be used for uncomplicated, localized lesions. Areas with larger involvement require oral antibiotics. When systemic antibiotics are needed, the choice of antibiotics should be determined by local resistance patterns. A 10-day course of penicillin or cephalosporins may be sufficient coverage for gram-positive organisms in some areas.[1] Erythromycin is used for penicillin- or cephalosporin-allergic patients, but has little coverage for MRSA. Clindamycin has maintained its sensitivity for MRSA in some areas, and therefore, is a good choice when resistance is recognized. Good hand washing and other simple measures of personal hygiene may reduce the likelihood of spread.

ANCILLARY STUDIES

In recurrent or persistent infections, lesions should be cultured to determine if an antibiotic-resistant organism is present. Gram stain of the fluid will reveal many polymorphonuclear white blood cells and gram-positive cocci but is of little use for planning antibiotic choices.

▶ STAPHYLOCOCCAL SCALDED SKIN SYNDROME

ETIOLOGY

SSSS is caused by an exfoliative exotoxin-producing strain of *S. aureus*. This is not a skin infection, but rather a complication from toxin producing bacteria that may be present in the nasopharynx. It most commonly presents in infants and children younger than 5 years.[2]

PATHOPHYSIOLOGY

The exotoxin is carried through the circulation to the skin, where it targets the epidermal granular cells and activates a specific protein. Keratinocyte damage results in epidermal separation.

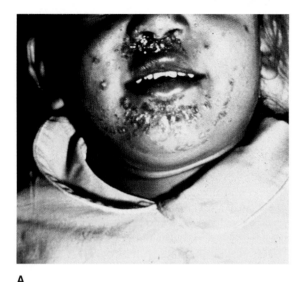

A

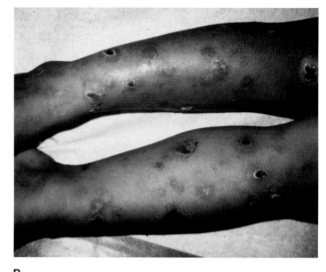

B

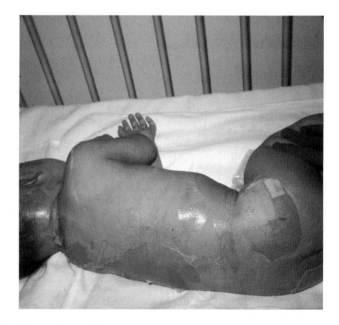

C

Figure 87-1. (A) Classic "honey-crusted" lesions of impetigo. (B) Chronic impetigo. (C) Neonatal pyoderma.

RECOGNITION

SSSS usually starts with prodromal symptoms including pharyngitis and conjunctivitis and is soon followed by fever, malaise, and a blistering skin eruption. The area rapidly enlarges and coalesces appearing similar to a sunburn which usually starts over the face, neck, axillae, and groin. Large, superficial bullae then form over the erythematous areas and rupture. The skin is exquisitely tender and fragile. Gentle rubbing of the skin results in desquamation of the epidermis, exposing a moist red base with the characteristic scalded appearance (Fig. 87–2). In infants and preschool children, the lesions are limited to the upper body, but in newborns, the entire cutaneous surface is involved (Ritter's disease).

MANAGEMENT

Patients with severe SSSS are managed similar to burn patients because of the increased risk of fluid and electrolyte losses through the exposed skin and secondary infection. The mainstay of treatment for SSSS is the rapid initiation of antibiotics.

Figure 87-2. Diffuse erythema and desquamation are the typical features of SSSS.

Intravenous nafcillin is the drug of choice since it adequately treats infections caused by penicillinase-producing staphylococci. Other options for antibiotic therapy include cephazolin and clindamycin. Skin tenderness can be relieved by analgesia, minimal handling, pressure-relieving mattresses, and emollient lubrication. Corticosteroids are contraindicated.[3] SSSS carries an 11% mortality rate in children with severe extensive skin involvement; however, the majority of the cases occur without sequelae or scarring.[2]

ANCILLARY STUDIES

Blood cultures as well as cultures from the nose, nasopharynx, conjunctivae, and external ear canal help isolate the offending pathogen.

▶ FUNGAL INFECTIONS

ETIOLOGY

Microsporum canis and *Trichophyton* species are the most common dermatophytes associated with the tinea infections of the skin and scalp.

PATHOPHYSIOLOGY

These dermatophytes invade and multiply within keratinized tissues such as skin, nails, and hair causing infection.

RECOGNITION

Tinea capitis infection can present with as little as dry, scaly patches resembling seborrheic or atopic dermatitis to irregular areas of scaling alopecia with broken-off hairs, giving the appearance of "black dots". They can progress to folliculitis suppuration or kerion formation, which are erythematous, boggy masses with overlying hair loss. A Wood's lamp may help differentiate tinea from other scaly lesions because it exudes a blue-green fluorescence. It is important to remember that not all dermatophyte lesions illuminate under a Wood's lamp.[4]

Tinea corporis can be found anywhere on the body. The lesions are characterized as sharply circumscribed scaly patches with central clearing and an elevated border (Fig. 87–3).

MANAGEMENT

Tinea capitis must be treated with systemic therapy. Griseofulvin (microcrystalline) for 6 to 8 weeks is first-line therapy. The concomitant use of topical agents such as 2.5% selenium sulfide shampoo may facilitate the response to therapy.[5]

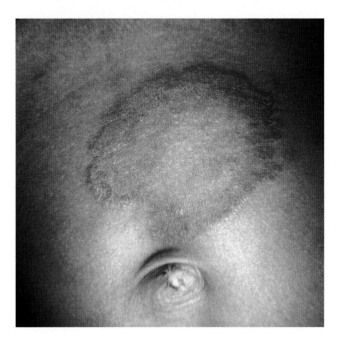

Figure 87–3. Tinea corporis seen with an elevated, sharply demarcated border and a scaly center.

Second-line oral therapy includes itraconazole, terbinafine, and fluconazole.[4]

Tinea corporis may be treated with topical antifungal agents, such as clotrimazole, miconazole, econazole, terbenafine, and butenafine. Improvement will be seen in about a week, but therapy should be continued for two weeks. If the treatment is ineffective, systemic griseofulvin should be added.[5]

ANCILLARY STUDIES

Although usually a clinical diagnosis, tinea infections can be evaluated by scraping the lesion and examining it under direct microscopy with potassium hydroxide (KOH) preparation. A culture to identify the exact causative agent may help in deciding treatment options when resistance occurs.[4]

REFERENCES

1. Wetson WL, Lane AT, Morelli JG. *Color Textbook of Pediatric Dermatology.* 3rd ed. St. Louis, MO: Mosby-Year Book; 2002.
2. Blyth M, Estela C, Young AE. Severe staphylococcal scalded skin syndrome in children. *Burns.* 2008;34:98–103.
3. Aber CA, Connelly EA, Schachner LA. Fever and rash in a child: when to worry? *Pediatr Ann.* 2007;36(1):30–38.
4. Gupta AK, Tu LQ. Dermatophytes: diagnosis and treatment. *J Am Acad Dermatol.* 2006;54:1050–1055.
5. Fleisher GR, Ludwig S, Henretig FM. *Textbook of Pediatric Emergency Medicine.* 5th ed. Philadelphia, PA: Lippincott Williams & Wilkins; 2006.

CHAPTER 88

Exanthems

Robert A. Wiebe and Malee V. Shah

► HIGH-YIELD FACTS

- Most childhood exanthemas are benign, self-limited, and require no treatment, but hidden in this presentation is an occasional myocarditis, encephalitis, or pneumonia.
- Worldwide, rubeola is still a major cause of morbidity and mortality. Early recognition can control spread.
- Roseola infantum is a common cause of febrile seizures in infants. A full fontanelle may be present in up to 25%.
- Children with varicella that may benefit from antiviral agents include patients on corticosteroids or chronic salicylates, immunocompromised patients, and those older than 12 years.
- Neonatal herpes has three presentations in the first 6 weeks of life: encephalitis with seizures, disseminated with a "neonatal sepsis" appearance, and those localized to the skin, eye, and mouth. Early treatment with acyclovir will prevent progression.

► INTRODUCTION

The vast majority of childhood exanthems are a result of nonspecific viral illnesses. Most are benign and self-limited and resolve without any therapeutic measures. The enterovirus group including echovirus and coxsackievirus consist of nearly 80 human host infections that may cause childhood exanthemas.[1] Although they rarely cause serious or life-threatening disease, some enterovirus infections can result in serious sequelae such as encephalitis and myocarditis. The clinician should always be vigilant to recognize associated symptoms that suggest life-threatening complications when examining children with exanthemas. Medication misadventures, bacterial and rickettsial disease can also cause recognizable clinical patterns. This chapter will describe recognizable childhood exanthemas, discuss risks of exposure, and provide an understanding of complications to expect and serious sequelae to consider.

► RUBEOLA (MEASLES)

Measles still remains a leading cause of preventable childhood morbidity and mortality worldwide. Although most cases today are limited to immunocompromised patients and in developing countries where poverty and malnutrition is a factor, outbreaks still occur in developed nations.

EPIDEMIOLOGY/PATHOPHYSIOLOGY

Measles is one of the most contagious diseases known to man with a 90% transmission rate to the unimmunized household contact. It remains a significant cause of morbidity and mortality in developing countries. In 2006, it resulted in 242 000 deaths worldwide. More than 95% of deaths occur in developing countries. Widespread use of live virus vaccine for immunization during the past 40 years has dramatically reduced the incidence of the disease in developed countries.[2] Infants are usually immunized between 12 and 15 months of age. Maternally acquired antibodies usually are sufficient to protect against clinical exposure in infants younger than 1 year of age.

Transmission of the virus is by aerosol exposure or contact with respiratory fluids. It enters the body through the respiratory tract. The incubation period ranges from 7 to 18 days after exposure, and patients are contagious for approximately 5 days starting with onset of symptoms.

CLINICAL FINDINGS

The characteristic rash associated with measles is preceded by 3 days of fever to 40°C and the characteristic "three Cs," cough, coryza, and conjunctivitis. Intense mucoid nasal drainage, hacking cough, and marked scleral and paplebral nonpurulent conjunctivitis are always present prior to the onset of rash. Koplik spots (Fig. 88–1A) are usually present during the early febrile period, but may be absent by the time the rash appears. This characteristic enanthema is typically present 24 hours before onset of the rash, and are blue-white discreet papules on the lateral buccal mucosa. By the time rash appears, Koplik spots may have coalesced into a white granular appearance or may be completely absent.

The rash of measles is a maculopapular erythematous rash that first appears on the face and spreads cephalocaudal to involve the trunk and extremities. At onset, it is discreet and maculopapular, but by the third day, begins to coalesce and becomes confluent as it turns from red to a yellow-brown color (Fig. 88–1B). The fever will resolve within 3 days of onset of rash, and in uncomplicated cases, all symptoms will resolve within 7 to 8 days.

ANCILLARY TESTS

When rubeola is suspected, confirmatory diagnostic testing is necessary and can be done through contact with state public health laboratories, or the Centers for Disease Control and

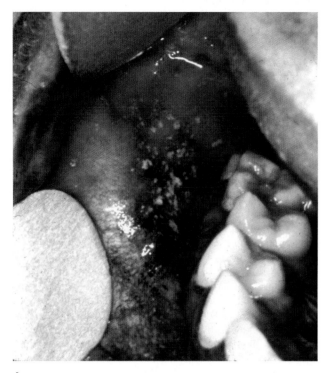

A

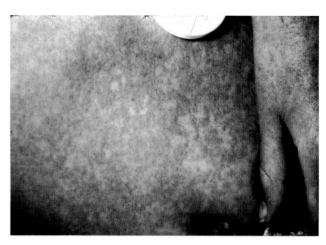

B

Figure 88–1. **(A)** Koplik spots present 24 hours before and remain 24 hours after onset of rash. **(B)** Rubeola exanthema at 3 days with coalescence.

Prevention (CDC). Measles IgM is usually present within 72 hours of the onset of rash and persists for at least 1 month.[3] Examination of the saliva for measles-specific IgA and serum testing for a rise in IgG antibodies can also be used for diagnosis. Measles virus can be isolated from respiratory secretions during the febrile period.

COMPLICATIONS

The most common complication is otitis media, occurring in up to 25% of children. Encephalitis will occur in approximately 1:1000 cases with outbreaks in developed countries. Serious complications such as pneumonia, diarrhea with dehydration, and blindness can be as high as 10% in poorly nourished children and 30% in the immunocompromised. Subacute sclerosing panencephalitis (SSPE) is a rare central nervous system degenerative disease that has virtually disappeared from the United States since widespread vaccination programs have been introduced.

MANAGEMENT

Management is nonspecific supportive care for the uncomplicated patient. There are no antiviral agents proven to modify the course of measles. Vitamin A supplementation may be helpful in preventing corneal ulcerations and blindness in malnourished children. When given within 72 hours of exposure, live virus vaccine may be beneficial in modifying the disease course. Susceptible children exposed to measles should receive intravenous immunoglobulin 0.25 mL/kg within 6 days of exposure. For children with history of immunodeficiency syndromes and HIV, 0.5 mL/kg is recommended.[3]

▶ RUBELLA (GERMAN MEASLES)

According to the Communicable Disease Center, rubella has not been seen in the United States since 2004. Outbreaks still occur in developing countries and with international travel; therefore, the clinician should be aware of the presentation and potential complications. Postnatally acquired rubella is generally mild and self-limited. The effects of virus exposure on the fetus in the first 20 weeks of gestation (congenital rubella syndrome) have made it an important cause of congenitally acquired fetal morbidity and mortality.

EPIDEMIOLOGY

Postnatal rubella is transmitted by airborne droplets from the upper respiratory tract. The virus can be isolated from respiratory secretions, urine, feces, and skin. A single infection will induce lifetime immunity. Man is the only known host for transmission of the virus. The virus has been shown to replicate in the nasopharynx and lymph nodes. Transmission of disease can occur for approximately 1 week before the onset of rash until up to 14 days after symptoms appear. Widespread use of live attenuated virus vaccine has proven to be highly successful in reducing the morbidity associated with rubella.

Congenital rubella syndrome is acquired by transplacental transfer of virus to the developing fetus during the first 20 weeks of gestation. The risk associated with serious morbidity

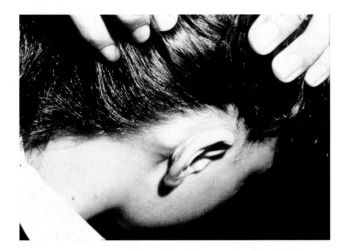

Figure 88-2. Post-auricular adenopathy of rubella infection.

and mortality is only from exposure of pregnant females in the first 20 weeks of gestation. Young mothers born outside the United States should be screened to assess immunity to rubella.

CLINICAL FINDINGS

The symptoms associated with postnatal rubella are usually mild and may be asymptomatic. The typical presentation is with mild cough, coryza, conjunctivitis, and a maculopapular erythematous rash that starts on the face and progresses cephalocaudal. Low-grade fever to 39°C is often present. The symptom complex can be differentiated from rubeola by the presence of a rash appearing at or near the onset of fever and the mild nature of symptoms. Headache and transient polyarthralgias and polyarthritis are common in older children and adults. Symptoms usually resolve in 3 to 4 days. Pea-sized postauricular lymphadenopathy is usually seen by the time the rash appears (Fig. 88-2).

Congenital rubella syndrome is recognized by the presence of hepatosplenomegaly, a "blueberry muffin rash," microcephaly, and low birth weight. Cardiac anomalies, especially patent ductus arteriosus, are common. Cataracts, glaucoma, and retinopathy may be seen on eye examination. Hearing loss, mental retardation, growth delays, and learning disabilities may present later.

ANCILLARY TESTS

Rubella-specific IgM antibody titers are the most commonly used tests to detect recent infection. False-negatives and false-positives do occur. Congenital rubella can be confirmed by persistent rubella-specific IgG antibody. IgG antibody titers can also be used to screen females of childbearing age. Assays for detecting rubella immunity include enzyme immunoassay tests, immunofluorescent assay, and latex agglutination tests.[3]

COMPLICATIONS

Complications from postnatal acquired rubella are rare. Thrombocytopenia occurs in approximately 1:3000 cases. Encephali-

tis occurs in 1:5000 cases with headache, vomiting, stiff neck, and lethargy. These symptoms are usually self-limited and not serious. Transplacentally acquired infections can result in fetal death or congenital rubella syndrome.

MANAGEMENT

Symptomatic treatment is all that is necessary for postnatal rubella. Isolation from child care or school should be recommended for 7 days after onset of rash. Intramuscular immunoglobulin (0.55 mL/kg) may reduce viral load and be beneficial for treating susceptible pregnant females who choose not to terminate pregnancy.[3]

▶ ROSEOLA (EXANTHEM SUBITUM)

EPIDEMIOLOGY/PATHOPHYSIOLOGY

Human herpesvirus 6 and 7 (HHV-6, HHV-7) have been found to cause the symptoms of roseola. The virus is transmitted through respiratory secretions from asymptomatic individuals and during the febrile viremic phase of the illness. Maternally transferred antibodies provide protection for the first 3 to 6 months of life. By the age of 4 years, virtually all children have serologic evidence of prior infection from HHV-6. The incubation period is approximately 9 to 10 days.

CLINICAL FINDINGS

Sudden onset of high fever to 40°C with fever spikes persisting for 72 hours followed by a transient erythematous maculopapular truncal rash in an infant from 6 months to 2 years of age is the classic presentation. The rash may occur up to 24 hours before or after the fever resolves. It presents on the trunk, but often progresses to involve the extremities. Skin manifestations of roseola may be so transient that they escape detection, but the rash usually lasts approximately 24 hours. Infants with fever are rarely ill-appearing and look remarkably well for the high fever. Large postoccipital lymph nodes are characteristic and their presence in an infant with high fever can predict roseola as the cause of fever. A bulging fontanelle has been found in up to 25% of infants infected with HHV-6. If the infant is alert, playful, and when bounced on the caretakers lap, does not cry or arch their back, meningitis is very unlikely.

COMPLICATIONS

Febrile convulsions have been seen in up to 20% to 30% of infants with roseola due to the sudden rise in body temperature.[4] Fatigue, irritability, and anorexia are reported occasionally. Pneumonia, encephalitis, hepatitis, and hemophagocytic syndrome have been rarely reported in immunocompromised individuals.

MANAGEMENT

Management is supportive and fever may be treated for comfort.

► FIFTH DISEASE (ERYTHEMA INFECTIOSUM)

EPIDEMIOLOGY

Erythema infectiosum is caused by the human parvovirus B19. Humans are the only known host for carrying and transmitting the disease. Infection can occur at any age, but is most common in mid-to-late childhood. The virus is mainly transmitted through contact with respiratory secretions, but can be carried through blood products and from maternal–fetal transmission.

PATHOPHYSIOLOGY

Replication of virus in red cell precursors causes a transient reduction in red blood cell formation during the viremic phase. This is unimportant in an otherwise healthy child with a normal red cell survival of 120 days, but can cause serious symptoms when the normal red cell lifespan is short as occurs in the child with hemolytic anemia, or in early fetal development.

Viremia occurs approximately 1 to 2 weeks after exposure and lasts 3 to 5 days. By the time the rash appears, the patient is no longer contagious. This is important because patients with hemolytic disease when presenting with an aplastic crises are shedding virus and can transmit disease to others. They are not, however, at risk for getting the virus from patients who exhibit the characteristic rash.

CLINICAL FINDINGS

The characteristic rash consists of bright erythema of the cheeks giving a "slapped cheek" appearance, and a fine, lacy reticular rash on the extremities and trunk. The rash may resolve in a few days, only to reappear with exposure to sun or warm baths, and may recur for several weeks. Low-grade fever, arthralgia, headache, and myalgia may be seen in some children as a prodrome before the rash appears. Arthritis is rare in children but common in adults.

Other presentations of infection with parvovirus B19 include the papulopurpuric glove-and-sock syndrome. This consists of pruritic or painful petechiae and purpura limited to the hands and feet. Some investigators have isolated parvovirus B19 from occasional patients with Henoch-Schoenlein Purpura.

ANCILLARY TESTS

The diagnosis is usually made by clinical observation, but antibody testing by radioimmunoassay or enzyme-linked immunosorbent assay may be used to identify presence of IgM during the acute phase of the illness or IgG antibody titer rise 2 to 3 weeks after the symptoms resolve. In the immunocompromised host, demonstration of the virus by polymerase chain reaction (PCR) assay is preferred.

COMPLICATIONS

In a healthy host, complications are rare and limited to transient arthritis or arthralgias. Children with hemolytic disease and short red cell survival are at risk for aplastic crises with often critical drops in hemoglobin with no compensatory rise in reticulocyte counts during the viremic phase. Pregnant women, especially during the first trimester are at risk for hydrops fetalis with spontaneous abortion.

MANAGEMENT

Supportive care is all that is necessary in healthy children. Patients with hemolytic anemia and aplastic crisis may require blood transfusions.

► VARICELLA (CHICKEN POX)

Widespread childhood immunization programs since 1995 have dramatically reduced the prevalence of varicella infection in children in the United States. Varicella-zoster virus is the cause of both chicken pox and shingles. Varicella-zoster virus or human herpes virus 3 (HHV-3) is a member of the herpesvirus family.

EPIDEMIOLOGY

Man is the only known reservoir for this highly contagious virus. It enters through the respiratory tract or conjunctivae, and is transferred from person-to-person by air or contact with fluid from vesicles. The incubation period is 10 to 21 days, and infected patients are most likely to be infectious to others from 2 days before the onset of rash until the lesions are crusted and dry.

CLINICAL FINDINGS

A prodrome of nonspecific symptoms precedes the rash by 1 to 2 days. These can include nasal congestion, conjunctival injection, headache, malaise, anorexia, cough, and low-grade fever. The rash begins as erythematous macules that rapidly progress to papules and eventually form the characteristic vesicles on an erythematous base (dew drops on a rose petal). Within 6 to 24 hours the vesicles become pustules that break and dry into crusts. New crops of lesions develop with all stages of lesions present on the skin at the same time. In a normal host the lesions resolve in 5 to 7 days. The rash is often pruritic and is found mainly on the head, trunk, and to a lesser extent, the extremities (Fig. 88–3).

ANCILLARY TESTS

When confirmatory testing is necessary, PCR or direct fluorescent antibody of vesicles is preferred.

COMPLICATIONS

The most common minor complication is secondary bacterial infection of the skin lesions. Serious complications include varicella pneumonia, encephalitis, secondary bacterial

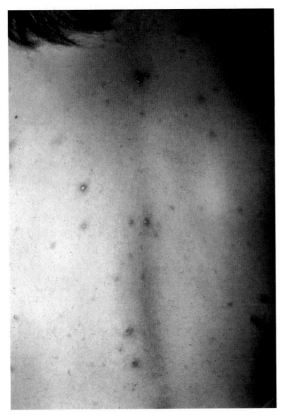

A

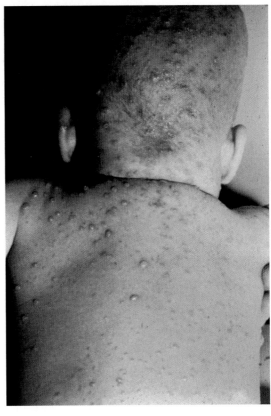

B

Figure 88–3. **(A)** Characteristic varicella rash with papules, vesicles, pustules, and crusting. **(B)** Varicella in an infant.

pneumonia, cellulites, necrotizing fasciitis, and sepsis. The disease is more severe in adolescents and adults. Immunocompromised children and those on chronic corticosteroids are also at greater risk. Congenital varicella syndrome with brain and eye anomalies, limb hypoplasia, and intrauterine growth retardation can occur in 0.4% to 2% of susceptible pregnant women who are infected during the first 20 weeks of gestation.[5]

MANAGEMENT

Uncomplicated varicella in the normal host requires only symptomatic treatment to control itching. In healthy children, virus replication ends within 72 hours of onset of the rash, making late treatment with antiviral agents of no value. Early use of acyclovir may be used in low-risk children in order to modify the disease course. For children who are at high risk of complications, specifically those on chronic corticosteroids and immunosuppressives, intravenous antiviral therapy should be started early. Intravenous immunoglobulin, or preferably, varicella-zoster immunoglobulin may modify the disease if given early after exposure.[3] Oral acyclovir is indicated in moderate-risk children with chronic cutaneous or pulmonary disease, those on long-term salicylate therapy, children on short, intermittent oral or aerosol corticosteroids, and children older than the age of 12 years. Table 88–1 provides

treatment doses and antiviral agent options. Varicella vaccine, when administered within 36 hours of exposure, can be useful in preventing disease and providing postexposure prophylaxis.[6]

▶ HERPES ZOSTER (SHINGLES)

Herpes zoster should be considered a common complication resulting from a prior varicella-zoster virus exposure. As the primary varicella infection resolves, virus remains latent in spinal sensory nerve root ganglia. Zoster is rare in children, but incidence increases with age and may have a lifetime incidence of 10% to 50%.

CLINICAL FINDINGS

A prodrome of tingling pain may precede the onset of rash. Crops of vesicles occur, usually limited to a specific dermatome nerve distribution. Eruptions can occur anywhere, but are most commonly in a unilateral distribution over the thoracic or lumbosacral regions. The lesions start as crops of vesicles, but may burst and leave shallow ulcers that crust over with time (Fig. 88–4). In adolescents and adults, shingles can be extremely painful, but in children, pruritis rather than pain is often the chief complaint.

▶ **TABLE 88-1. ANTIVIRAL AGENTS FOR THE TREATMENT OF VARICELLA-ZOSTER AND HERPES SIMPLEX**

Host Condition	Age	Age	Drug Route	Dose
Varicella, immunocompetent with "at-risk" conditions	>2 y	Acyclovir	po	80 mg/kg/d in 3 divided doses for 5 d (max 3200 mg/d)
Varicella, immunocompromised host	All ages	Acyclovir	IV	30 mg/kg/d in 3 divided doses for 7–10 d
Zoster, immunocompromised host	<12 y	Acyclovir	IV	60 mg/kg/d in 3 divided doses for 7–10 d
	>12 y		IV	30 mg/kg/d in 3 divided doses for 7 d
Neonatal herpes simplex	Birth–3 mo	Acyclovir	IV	60 mg/kg/d in 3 divided doses for 14–21 d
Herpes encephalitis	3 mo–12 y	Acyclovir	IV	60 mg/kg/d in 3 divided doses for 14–21 d
	>12 y			30 mg/kg/d in 3 divided doses for 14–21 d
HSV, immunocompromised host	<12 y	Acyclovir	IV	30 mg/kg/d in 3 divided doses for 7–14 d
	>12 y			15 mg/kg/d in 3 divided doses for 7–14 d
HSV prophylaxis in immunocompromised host	>2 y	Acyclovir	po	600–1000 mg/kg/d in 3–5 divided doses for risk period
Genital HSV, primary infection	>12 y	Acyclovir or	po	400 mg 3 times daily for 7–10 d
				1 g twice daily for 7–10 d
		Valacyclovir or	po	250 mg 3 times daily for 7–10 d
		Famcyclovir	po	
Genital HSV, recurrent (episodic treatment)	>12 y	Acyclovir or	po	400 mg 3 times daily for 5–10 d
				1 g once daily for 5 d (1 g twice daily for 5–10 d for immunocompromised)
		Valacyclovir or	po	
		Famcyclovir	po	125 mg twice daily for 5 d (500 mg twice daily for 5–10 d for immunocompromised)

Adapted from: American Academy of Pediatrics. Herpes Simplex. In: Pickering LK, Baker CJ, Long SS, McMillan JA, eds. *Red Book: 2006 Report of the Committee on Infectious Diseased.* 27th ed. Elk Grove Village, IL. American Academy of Pediatrics; 2006:361–371, and Fatahzadeh M, Schwartz RA. Human herpes simplex virus infections: epidemiology, pathogenesis, symptomatology, diagnosis and management. *J Am Acad Dermatol.* 2007:57(5):737–763.

COMPLICATIONS

Cranial nerves are rarely involved, but when present, corneal ulceration can be serious. Pain can persist for weeks to months, and may continue to recur without the presence of rash. Serious complications can occur in immunosuppressed patients and patients on chronic corticosteroids. Treatment guidelines for management of shingles are the same as for chicken pox. Famciclovir or valacyclovir are preferred for treatment of adults. Table 88–1 provides treatment options.

▶ HERPES SIMPLEX

Herpes simplex virus (HSV) has affected up to 95% of the population. Clinical manifestations are highly variable and include primary and secondary presentations. The virus can result in encephalitis and serious systemic symptoms, self-limited simple mucocutaneous signs, or asymptomatic infection.

EPIDEMIOLOGY/PATHOPHYSIOLOGY

Clinical disease in humans is caused by two members of the Herpesviridae family, HSV1 and HSV2. There is an overlap in clinical expression of the viruses, and both can remain latent in cells after primary infection. Herpes virus enters the host through epithelial cells and may undergo replication at the site of invasion. After the primary infection has occurred, HSV travels through the periaxonal sheath of sensory nerves to ganglia of the host nervous system. The cervical and lumbosacral sensory ganglia are particularly vulnerable. The virus replicates in ganglia and may persist for life. Periods of virus latency may be interrupted by reactivation. An asymptomatic person can shed virus, but during primary infection and reactivation, virus shedding is increased. Reactivation of virus can occur as a result of a variety of external and internal triggers including fever, immunosuppression, local trauma, menstruation, stress, fatigue, temperature changes, and exposure to sunlight.[7]

CLINICAL FINDINGS

HSV1 is mainly associated with infections involving the mouth, pharynx, and eyes, while HSV2 primarily shows genital mucosal symptoms, but there is overlap and both viruses can enter the central nervous system and cause encephalitis and systemic disease. Figure 88–5 shows herpes progenitalis in an infant.

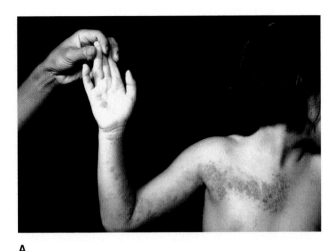

A

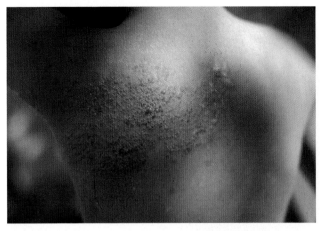

B

Figure 88–4. (A and B) Two examples of herpes zoster with characteristic dermatome distribution.

The most common manifestation of HSV1 is primary herpetic gingivostomatitis. This is seen in young children older than 6 months of age and may be subclinical. A prodrome of fever, irritability, malaise, and loss of appetite lasting 1 to 2 days is followed by vesicles on the oral mucosa and tongue that rapidly rupture and become superficial and painful ulcers. Perioral extension of the ulcers is common. An intense gingivitis is almost always present and helps to distinguish HSV from coxsakievirus enanthems. Tender submandibular adenopathy is usually present. Symptoms may last up to 2 weeks (see Chapter 97 for the review of genital herpes simplex).

Neonatal herpes occurs in 1:3000 to 1:20 000 births.[3] Most infections arise from intrapartum transfer of virus, but can be contracted postnatally from oral, genital, or hand contact from a caregiver or from contaminated fomites. Three distinct clinical entities can result. Disseminated herpes presents in the first 1 to 4 weeks of life with a clinical presentation similar to bacterial sepsis and a mortality rate of 25% with antiviral treatment. Herpes encephalitis may present with seizures in the neonatal period and, if untreated, will progress to systemic disease. Neonatal herpes with involvement limited to the skin, eye, and mouth can result in minimal morbidity if treated early with antiviral agents. Symptoms may occur as late as 6 weeks of life.

Congenital HSV infection is rare, but presents as a small for gestational age infant, usually premature, and with microcephaly, retinitis, and vesicular rash.

Eczema herpeticum (Kaposi's varicelliform eruption) is an uncommon but serious primary manifestation of HSV in children with atopic dermatitis and breaks in skin integrity. The virus is usually transmitted from a labial lesion on the caregiver to the eczematous eruption (Fig. 88–6).

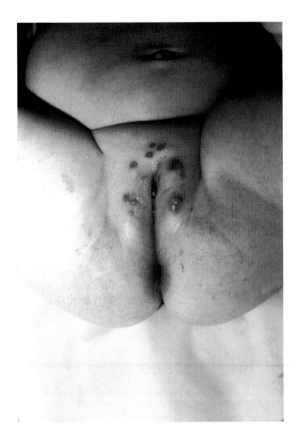

Figure 88–5. Herpes progenitalis in an infant.

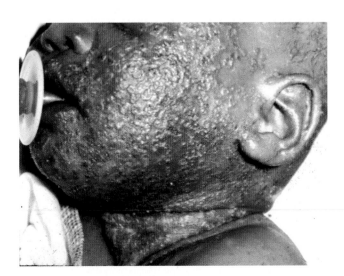

Figure 88–6. Eczema herpeticum.

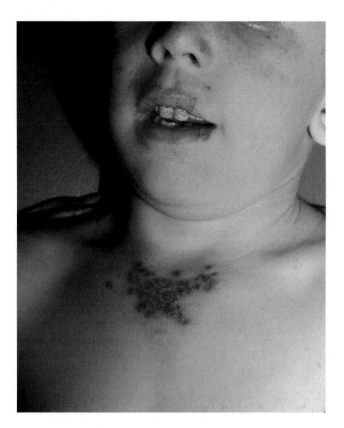

Figure 88-7. Cutaneous herpes simplex.

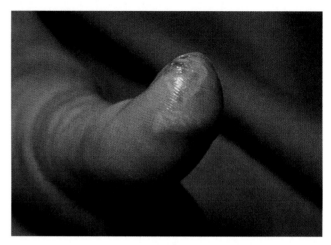

Figure 88-8. Herpetic whitlow.

There are a number of distinct secondary manifestations of herpes simplex. Patches of cutaneous herpes simplex occur commonly from contact of abraded skin with active oral or other herpes lesions actively shedding virus (Fig. 88–7). Outbreaks among athletes have been termed "herpes gladiatorum." Herpetic whitlow is caused by secondary inoculation of virus from mouth to fingers. This is common in children with primary herpetic gingivostomatitis who suck their thumbs or fingers (Fig. 88–8). To the untrained eye, a whitlow can be confused with paronychia, and attempts at drainage can cause bad cosmetic results. This is a self-limited problem with complete resolution in 2 to 3 weeks. Other manifestations include ocular herpes or herpes keratoconjunctivitis, a major cause of blindness worldwide. Conjunctivitis can be unilateral or bilateral and result in corneal ulcerations. Herpes meningoencephalitis may occur at any age and have no skin manifestions at presentation.

The most common presentation of HSV is recurrent orofacial herpes, commonly referred to as "fever blisters." This secondary phenomenon occurs in 15% to 40% of patients who have had symptomatic or asymptomatic primary herpetic oral infections. Reactivation of virus decreases with age. There may be a prodrome of pain or pruritis before emergence of the labial ulcer. Less frequently, intraoral vesicles may recur.

Erythema multiforme (EM) has been associated with HSV reactivation and possibly with primary infections. In some series, presence of HSV with EM has been as high as 75%.[8] Recurrent EM with recrudescence of HSV can occur repeatedly with attacks lasting up to 2 weeks. The characteristic acral EM rash (erythematous and of multiform) occurs within 10 days of reactivation and may last 2 weeks (see Chapter 86).

ANCILLARY TESTS

Uncomplicated HSV infection can be diagnosed clinically. When necessary, DFA of skin lesions provides quick and reliable results. PCR of the cerebrospinal fluid is particularly useful in diagnosing neonatal HSV and herpes encephalitis. Use of the Tzanck smear for diagnosis should be discouraged. There is a high incidence of false-negatives, and the Tzanck test cannot distinguish HSV from varicella-zoster virus. Culture from lesions or body fluids will grow in vitro in 1 to 15 days.

COMPLICATIONS

Serious complications are mainly limited to the immunocompromised host, the neonate, and those with involvement of the eye or central nervous system. Scarring is uncommon, but can occur, especially with eczema herpeticum or children with chronic cutaneous conditions.

MANAGEMENT

Antiviral agents can suppress virus replication and modify the clinical course but cannot irradicate the virus. Topical antiviral agents such as docosanol 10%, penciclovir 1%, and acyclovir 5% creams have been shown to reduce the symptoms of recurrent labial herpes when started early during the prodrome. Acyclovir is the mainstay for systemic disease in neonates, infants, and young children. Its poor bioavailability and short plasma half-life make newer but more expensive options attractive for treatment of adolescents and immunosuppressed hosts. These include drugs with greater bioavailability such as valacyclovir and famciclovir (see Table 88–1 for therapeutic options).

► ENTEROVIRUSES

Although most enteroviral infections have nonspecific clinical presentations, a few are associated with clinically distinguishable exanthemas and/or enanthems.

CLINICAL FINDINGS

Hand-foot-mouth syndrome is associated with infection from coxsackievirue A16 and enterovirus 71. There is a prodrome of low fever, malaise, and abdominal pain that may precede the skin and mucosal manifestations. Small vesicles appear on the palms and soles and frequently rupture leaving fine erythematous macules. The skin lesions occasionally may be found on the buttocks and trunk. Vesicles appear on the tongue, palate, and buccal mucosa. The symptoms resolve in less than a week in a normal host. The clinical picture can be distinguished from herpetic gingivostomatitis by a lack of intense gingivitis. Complications are rare, but myocarditis, pneumonia, and meningoencephalitis have been reported.

Herpangina is caused by coxsackievirus A1 to A8 and A12. Examination of the oropharynx reveals small erythematous vesicles localized to the soft palate and anterior tonsillar fossae. This is mainly a disease of infants and toddlers with refusal to eat, low-grade fever, and irritability as the presenting symptoms. Diagnosis is made by clinical examination and needs no further testing.

► SCARLET FEVER

PATHOPHYSIOLOGY

Scarlet fever is a childhood exanthema caused by specific erythrogenic toxin producing types of streptococcus pyogenes. The source of infection is usually from pharyngitis with group A β-hemolytic *Streptococcus* (GABHS), but rarely skin, soft tissue, and surgical wound infections can be a source for toxin production. The peak incidence is at 4 to 8 years of age, and it is rarely seen before 2 years of age or in adolescents. Less than 10% of the clinical cases of streptococcal pharyngitis will manifest the exanthema.

CLINICAL FINDINGS

Fever to 40°C, fatigue, sore throat, abdominal pain, vomiting, and headache will precede the rash by 12 to 48 hours. The exanthema is a fine, erythematous, rough ("sandpaper") rash that blanches on pressure (Fig. 88–9). It is generalized with increased intensity in the skin folds (Pastia's lines) with circumoral pallor and facial flushing. The enanthem may include red macules on the hard and soft palate (Forchheimer spots) and a "strawberry" tongue. The rash fades over 3 to 4 days with desquamation that may continue for 1 to 6 weeks. Early treatment with antibacterial agents may reduce the desquamation process.

ANCILLARY TESTS

Culture of the pharynx or source of infection is recommended and can give results in 24 hours. Several rapid screening tests are commonly used as a surrogate to culture, but false-negatives do occur. Specificity of rapid tests is high and if positive, does not require confirmation with culture.

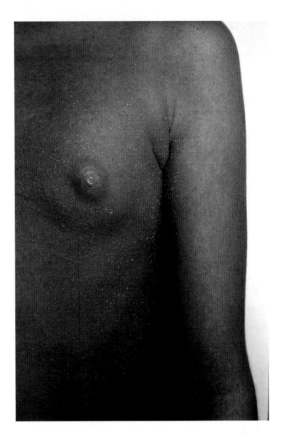

Figure 88–9. Scarlet fever.

COMPLICATIONS

The risk of post-streptococcal sequelae, acute rheumatic fever, and acute glomerulonephtitis is the same for scarlet fever as for simple GABHS pharyngitis. Sepsis, meningitis, pneumonia, and toxic shock are rare complications but have been reported.

MANAGEMENT

Penicillin V is the oral treatment of choice for both scarlet fever and GABHS pharyngitis. Oral therapy may be given 250 mg three times daily for children less than 27 kg, and 500 mg three times daily for children more than 27 kg.[3] Intramuscular penicillin G at 25 000 U/kg to a maximum adult dose of 1.2 million units is an acceptable alternative. In the penicillin allergic patient, clindamycin or erythromycin may be used. Isolation from school or day care for 24 hours after starting treatment will prevent spread.

► PITYRIASIS ROSEA

Pityriasis rosea is a benign, self-limited exanthema that does appear in clusters, but there is no evidence of person-to-person spread and the cause is unknown. It occurs most commonly in adolescents and young adults. Clinical presentation starts with the "herald patch," an oval, scaly, 2 -to 5-cm lesion that is often confused with a fungal dermatitis, and occurs 1 to 20 days before onset of a generalized rash. This is followed by multiple rose-pink ovoid macules that have a "Christmas tree" distribution over the back and may involve the trunk and extremities to a lesser degree. The face is usually spared. The rash lasts 2 to 6 weeks and may be associated with no symptoms or low-grade fever, headache, malaise, nausea, and pruritis. Treatment is supportive to control itching, if present. Limiting sun exposure may reduce symptoms. The rash resolves untreated without sequelae.

REFERENCES

1. Mancini AJ. Childhood exanthemas: a primer for the dermatologist. *Adv Dermatol.* 2000;16:3–37.

2. World Health Organization. http://www.who.int/mediacenter/factsheets/fs286/en/. Accessed October 1, 2008.

3. American Academy of Pediatrics. Herpes Simplex. In: Pickering LK, Baker CJ, Long SS, McMillin JA, eds. *Red Book: 2006 Report of the Committee on Infectious Diseases.* 27th ed. Elk Grove Village, IL. American Academy of Pediatrics; 2006: 361–371.

4. Hall CB, Long CE, Schnabel KC, et al. Human herpesvirus-6 infection in young children. *N Engl J Med.* 1994;331:432–438.

5. Andrews JI. Diagnosis of fetal infections. *Curr Opin Obstet Gynecol.* 2004;16(2):163–166.

6. Watson B, Seward J, Yang A, et al. Post exposure effectiveness of varicella vaccine. *Pediatrics.* 2000;105:84–88.

7. Fatahzadeh M, Schwartz RA. Human herpes simplex virus infections: epidemiology, pathogenesis, symptomatology, diagnosis, and management. *J Am Acad Dermatol.* 2007;57(5):737–763.

8. Weston WL. Herpes-associated erythema multiforme. *J Invest Dermatol.* 2005;124:200, xv–xvi.

CHAPTER 89

Infant Rashes

Robert A. Wiebe and Malee V. Shah

▶ HIGH-YIELD FACTS

- Seborrheic dermatitis can be recognized clinically by the presence of greasy scales and erythematous plaques.
- Diaper dermatitis is usually caused by irritation of the skin from prolonged contact with feces and urine. Sparing of the skin folds is diagnostic.
- Multiple café au lait spots of neurofibromatosis increase the risk for auditory and CNS tumors.
- Vascular malformations in a "beard distribution" on the face are associated with airway hemangiomas.

▶ BENIGN INFANT RASHES

When the newly born infant leaves the protection of the intrauterine fluid environment, the skin and its complex organs must adapt quickly to the continually changing environment of the *real world*. As sebaceous and sweat glands in the skin adapt to the changes, transient and benign rashes commonly appear.[1] Although clinically insignificant, these rashes cause high anxiety in young, new parents.

Milia are small, discreet white papules usually limited to the face and scalp. They are small inclusion cysts that arise from sebaceous glands at the base of hair follicles. Milia consist of keratinized debris. No treatment is necessary, and the lesions resolve spontaneously in weeks to months.

Miliaria are lesions caused by obstruction of eccrine sweat glands. These are particularly common in warm climates. Very superficial sweat gland obstruction results in *miliaria crystallina* which results from sweat being trapped in the intracorneal layer of the skin producing tiny clear vesicles. *Miliaria rubra* or *heat rash* is common in febrile or overheated infants.

These are erythematous small papules that are most commonly found on the upper trunk and head.

Erythema toxicum is present in up to 50% of newborn infants. They usually appear shortly after discharge from the hospital at 24 to 48 hours and last approximately 1 week. These are pinpoint, papulopustular lesions on an erythematous base that appear on the face, trunk, and extremities. The lesions are at the opening of sebaceous ducts. A scraping performed with Wright stain will reveal sheets of eosinophils.

Pustular melanosis is found almost exclusively in African American infants, and the lesions are usually present at birth. These are very superficial pustules that become scaly brown macules as they resolve. A Wright stain of the contents will show a predominance of neutrophils. If necessary, they can be differentiated from neonatal pyoderma by the absence of bacteria on Gram stain. As they resolve, the subcorneal pustules may persist as hyperpigmented small brown macules for months. There are a variety of vesiculopustular lesions that can be confused with pustular melanosis that may have serious complications (Table 89–1).[2]

Seborrheic dermatitis in infants usually has its onset within the first 4 weeks of life. The scalp is the first to show signs with the appearance of greasy yellow scales, occasionally with loss of hair (Fig. 89–1). Erythematous plaques develop and skin creases are often involved. The retroauricular area may have weeping or scaly denuded areas of involvement. It is not uncommon for candida to complicate the rash. Overproduction of sebum causes the accumulation of greasy scales, but the cause is still unclear. Treatment consists of low-potency topical corticosteroids to treat inflammation. Mild tar shampoo and oatmeal baths will help resolution. When severe, consider the possibility of histiocytosis (Letterer–Siwe disease) or Leiner's disease with generalized erythroderma and failure to thrive. Seborrhea can occasionally be confused with atopic dermatitis,

▶ TABLE 89–1. VESICULOPUSTULAR AND BULLOUS LESIONS WITH SYSTEMIC COMPLICATIONS[2]

Condition	Cause	Diagnosis	Complications
Bacterial infections	*Staphylococcus, Streptococcus*	Gram stain of lesions	Sepsis; see Chapter 85
Neonatal herpes	Herpes Simplex, 1 or 2	DFA, PCR	See Chapter 86
Fetal, neonatal varicella	Varicella–Zoster virus	DFA, PCR	See Chapter 86
Incontinentia pigmenti	X-linked inherited	Skin biopsy	Neurologic sequelae, seizures
Mastocytosis	Unknown	Clinical, biopsy	Histamine release
Acrodermatitis enteropathica	Defect in zinc uptake from GI tract	Serum zinc level	Diarrhea, Irritability, FTT
Methylmalonic academia	Defect in valine, isoleucine metabolism	Plasma amino acids	Lethargy, FTT, hypotonia
Epidermolysis bullosum	Autosomal recessive and dominant forms	Skin biopsy	Multiple comorbidities

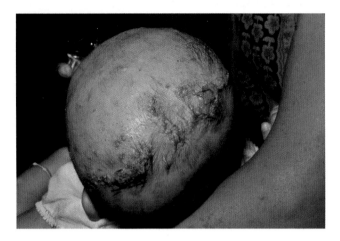

Figure 89-1. Seborrheic dermatitis in infant.

but with atopic dermatitis, the diaper area is spared and intense pruritis is always present (see Chapter 86).

Diaper dermatitis encompasses all causes of skin irritation localized to the diaper area. Irritant dermatitis is the most common cause and may be related to prolonged skin contact with urine and feces or from soaps and chemicals present in the diaper. Absorbable disposable diapers have decreased to incidence of this problem. Irritant dermatitis can usually be recognized by erythema and scaling of the skin with sparing of the skin folds. Secondary infection with Candida can confuse the appearance with involvement of the skin folds and presence of satellite lesions extending beyond the area of erythema (Fig. 89–2). Candida skin infections may be secondary to excessive use of oral antibiotics. Diffuse erythema involving the perineal area with scaling and satellite lesions is the characteristic presentation. Treatment includes topical antifungal agents such as nystatin, ketoconazole, or clotrimazole.

► DISORDERS OF PIGMENTATION

Dermal melanosis or Mongolian spots are diffuse blue–grey patches of melanocytes located in the dermis. They are most commonly found on the buttocks and sacral region of the lower back and slowly resolve over a few years. When they are present on the extremities, shoulders, and face they may persist. Mongolian spots should not be confused with bruising.

Neurofibromatosis is a group of inherited neurocutaneous disorders manifested by multiple café au lait spots. Presence of six or more lesions measuring >5 mm in an infant or the presence of axillary "freckling" (Fig. 89–3) is diagnostic. These disorders are associated with a high incidence of optic gliomas, acoustic neuromas, and a variety of other CNS tumors.[3] The patient with neurofibromatosis who presents with headache or focal neurologic signs must be evaluated for an intracranial mass lesion. Other causes of café au lait spots include *McCune–Albright syndrome,* which is characterized by polyostotic fibrous dysplasia and multiple endocrine abnormalities.

Urticaria pigmentosa can present in the first few months of life as red-brown macules. *Type 1,* a solitary mastocytoma is of no consequence. *Type 2,* can present with multiple pigmented macules or papules that when scraped with a blunt object will produce a wheal and flare termed *Darier's sign.* (Fig. 89–4) This condition is caused by populations of mast cells in the cutaneous tissue. When irritated by scratching, they release histamine, thereby, producing the characteristic wheals and occasionally blisters. With temperature changes, metabolic insults, such as fever or viral illnesses, large numbers of the degranulating lesions can produce flushing and systemic symptoms from histamine release.

Incontinentia pigmenti is an X-linked disorder occurring in females and is usually present at birth (Fig. 89–5). It is a neurocutaneous syndrome with four overlapping stages of skin presentation. The first stage is manifested by linear blisters surrounded by erythema. The second stage presents usually before 6 months of age as the blisters evolve into warty plaques. As the plaques disappear, they become whorles of hyperpigmentation during stage three. The final stage occurs later in adulthood with hypopigmentation and loss of hair and sweat

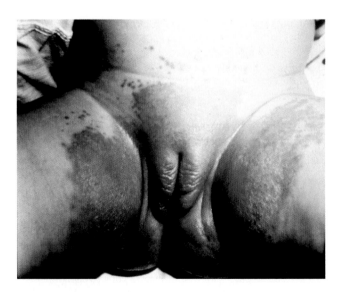

Figure 89-2. Irritant dermatitis with Candida overgrowth.

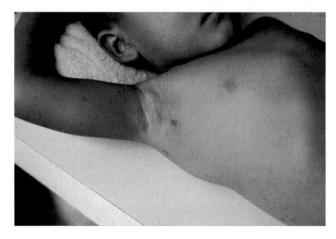

Figure 89-3. Neurofibromatosis with axillary freckling. (Crowe sign).

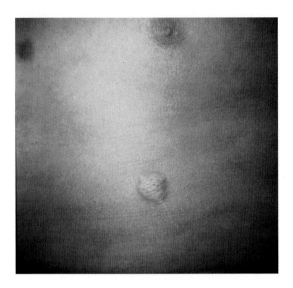

Figure 89-4. Darier's sign for urticaria pigmentosa.

glands. Approximately 20% of patients will have seizures, various neurologic deficits, and mental retardation.

► VASCULAR LESIONS OF INFANCY

Cutis marmorata is a vascular instability caused by cold ambient temperature and may be present in an unclothed infant

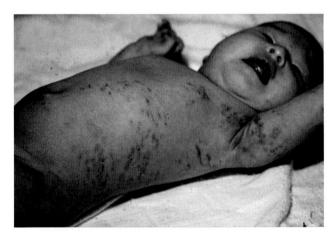

Figure 89-5. Incontinentia pigmenti.

for the first few months of life. A reticulated, blanching rash is characteristic, and this may be confused with mottling. Acrocyanosis, cyanosis of the hands and feet, may also be present. Keeping the infant warm and in a neutral thermal environment will resolve the color changes in minutes.

Vascular malformations are common skin presentations at birth or in the first few months of life. They can be secondary to abnormalities of the capillary, venous, arterial, or lymphatic systems. Most are benign and self-limited, but a few may herald serious systemic consequences.[4] The *salmon patch* is a common capillary malformation usually located on the forehead and upper eyelids and is present at birth. These usually resolve within 1 to 2 years, but if present on the back of the neck, may persist for life. *Nevus flammus, or Port wine stains,* are generally benign capillary malformations, but may persist for life. When present in the area innervated by the ophthalmic branch of the facial nerve (includes the upper eyelid and forehead), it is associated with *Sturge–Webber syndrome,* a neurocutaneous disorder with vascular malformations of the brain and intractable seizures.

Simple capillary hemangiomas are the most common vascular tumors in infancy. They may be unrecognized at birth, but appear early in the neonatal period as a small, red telangiectasia that rapidly grows to become the characteristic strawberry hemangioma over the first 6 months to 1 year, then slowly regress and disappear over the first decade. Multiple capillary hemangiomas may be associated with deep tissue and parenchymal involvement. Vascular malformations of the skin over the "beard distribution" of the face in an infant presenting with stridor or upper airway involvement suggests airway hemangiomas.

There are a number of hereditary conditions with vascular, hyper- and hypopigmented lesions that are beyond the scope of this text.

REFERENCES

1. Eichenfeld LF, Frieden IJ, Esterly NB. *Textbook of Neonatal Dermatology.* Philadelphia, PA: WB Saunders Company; 2001.
2. Van Praag MG, Van Rooij RG, Folkers E, et al. Diagnosis and treatment of pustular disorders in the neonate. *Pediatr Dermatol.* 1997;14:131–143.
3. Yohay K. Neurofibromatosis types 1 and 2. *Neurologist.* 2006;12(2):86–93.
4. Blei F. Basic science and clinical aspects of vascular anomalies. *Curr Opin Pediatr.* 2005;17(4):501–509.

SECTION XIV

OTOLARYNGOLOGIC EMERGENCIES

CHAPTER 90

Ear and Nose Emergencies

Raemma Paredes Luck and Evan J. Weiner

▶ HIGH-YIELD FACTS

- *Pseudomonas aeruginosa* is the cause of almost all cases of malignant otitis externa.
- The diagnosis of otitis media is based on the rapid onset of signs and symptoms of middle ear inflammation in the presence of middle ear effusion.
- Pneumatic otoscopy is an essential component of the ear examination.
- *Streptococcus pneumoniae* is the most common cause of bullous myringitis.
- Worsening otitis media, while on antibiotics, may be a sign of a suppurative complication.
- Sinusitis should be considered in patients with severe rhinitis and in patients with persistent or worsening URI symptoms after 10 days.
- Hospitalization for intravenous antibiotics, sinus imaging, and subspecialty consultation are indicated in patients with sinusitis with orbital or intracranial extension.

▶ ACUTE OTITIS EXTERNA

Otalgia is a frequent presenting complaint in the emergency department. An algorithm on the conditions that can cause otalgia is presented in Figure 90–1. A large subset of these patients will have inflammatory conditions of the external ear. Most external ear infections are easy to recognize and to treat. However, it is important to differentiate a simple otitis externa from other conditions.

PATHOPHYSIOLOGY

The external ear, consisting of the pinna and the external auditory meatus, ends as a blind sac at the tympanic membrane. The medial two-thirds, or the osseous portion, lacks subcutaneous tissue and has a thin skin that tightly covers the bone. The cartilaginous portion or lateral third contains hair follicles, subcutaneous tissue, and ceruminous glands overlying the perichondrium and cartilage.

The fragile skin of the external auditory canal is easily infected when it is disrupted by any trauma or inflammation. Aggressive removal of the protective cerumen barrier can allow the normal ear flora (*Staphylococcus* spp., *Streptococcus* spp., diptheroids, and *Pseudomonas aeruginosa*) to invade the tissue. In addition, heat, humidity, and moisture promote the

development of infection (thus the term "swimmer's ear"). Such an infection manifests as a diffuse cellulitis affecting the skin of the external auditory canal and pinna, underlying tissue, and regional lymph nodes[1] (Fig. 90–2).

DIAGNOSIS

In acute uncomplicated cases of acute otitis externa, the diagnosis is a clinical one. A history of local trauma, swimming, and travel to a warm climate may or may not be present. Depending on the severity of the infection, most patients will present with localized ear pain and itching. The pinna should be normal in appearance; however, manipulation of the pinna or tragus or movement of the jaw usually elicits pain. Redness and edema of the ear canal can be seen along with an exudate. If the infection is due to a fungus (predominantly *Aspergillus* spp.), white or gray masses composed of hyphae may be noted in the canal. Local lymphadenopathy may also be present.

Special mention should be made of malignant or necrotizing otitis externa. This condition, most commonly caused by *P. aeruginosa*, is characterized by a severe cellulitis of the external canal with osteomyelitis of the underlying bone. Inpatient hospitalization for intravenous antipseudomonal antibiotics and otolaryngology consultation are indicated. Imaging with a CT scan or MRI is often necessary to define the extent of any bony and soft tissue involvement.[2] Necrotizing otitis externa and otomycosis are two conditions predominantly seen among patients who are immunocompromised or have diabetes.[1]

DIFFERENTIAL DIAGNOSIS

Other conditions can mimic acute otitis externa. A furuncle (abscess) may develop at a hair follicle in the lateral canal. Depending on the degree of fluctuance, a combination of antistaphylococcal topical or oral antibiotics and incision and drainage should be employed. Retained ear foreign bodies may also be mistaken for an external ear infection. Conditions affecting the skin of the ear, such as atopic dermatitis, seborrheic dermatitis, and contact dermatitis, may also lead to itching and inflammation of the external canal. Ramsay Hunt syndrome (herpes zoster) may present with vesicles at the external ear canal and pinna.[3] Because of the large amount of debris and exudate, an acute otitis media with perforation may be indistinguishable from acute otitis externa.

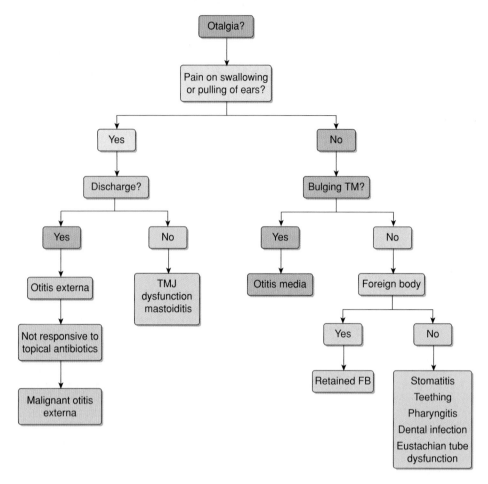

Figure 90-1. Algorithm for otalgia.

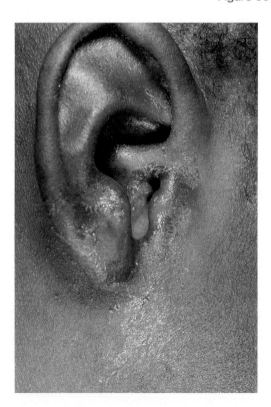

Figure 90-2. Picture showing otitis externa.

MANAGEMENT

Treatment of uncomplicated acute otitis externa consists of a combination of topical antimicrobial preparations and external ear cleaning. Antibiotic drops that target *P. aeruginosa* are the drugs of choice. Options include acetic acid, a combination of polymyxin B and neomycin, quinolones, and aminoglycosides. Many current preparations also include a topical steroid. Recent studies indicate that the antibiotic-steroid preparations may lead to faster and better cure rates.[4,5] Often the amount of ear canal debris and edema limits the ability to instill the eardrops. Cleaning of the ear canal with suctioning, irrigation, and dry swabbing may be necessary. If significant edema exists, application of an ear wick can help deliver the topical medications to the infection. The wick should be removed within 2 days. If one suspects a perforated eardrum, then prescribe a topical antimicrobial suspension as the solution may damage the middle ear.

▶ ACUTE OTITIS MEDIA AND MASTOIDITIS

Middle ear infections are an extremely common entity in childhood. Most are easily treated and have good outcomes.

However, it is important to recognize the changing treatment approaches to this disorder as well as possible suppurative complications.

PATHOPHYSIOLOGY

The middle ear is the space located behind the tympanic membrane that facilitates sound transfer to the inner ear structure. It is part of a continuous space that extends from the eustachian tube to the mastoid air cells. Normally, the eustachian tube functions to equilibrate middle ear pressure, clear the middle ear of secretions (via the action of ciliated epithelium), and protect the middle ear from the nasopharynx. Any alteration of these eustachian tube functions due to obstruction, inflammation, or excessive compliance can lead to effusion and subsequent infection in the middle ear. In addition, the eustachian tubes of children are much more horizontal in orientation than those of adults, possibly impeding drainage.[5] Common conditions predisposing to otitis media include upper respiratory infections, allergic rhinitis, supine bottle-feeding, and exposure to tobacco smoke.[6] Breast-feeding has been shown to decrease the occurrence of otitis media.[7] Young age (less than 2 years) exposure to tobacco smoke and attendance at day care also increases the risk of middle ear infections. Otitis media with effusion refers to a collection of serous fluid in the middle ear, which may commonly occur in a viral upper respiratory infection. However, acute otitis media indicates superinfection with bacteria from the nasopharynx. *Streptococcus pneumoniae* (25%–50%), *Haemophilus influenzae* (15%–30%), and *Moraxella catarrhalis* (3%–20%) represent the major bacterial pathogens. The routine use of the heptavalent pneumococcal vaccine in infants is changing the epidemiology of otitis media.[6] A large number of *H. influenzae* and *M. catarrhalis* isolates produce β-lactamases, which affect therapeutic options. *S. pneumoniae* resistance is increasingly common, particularly penicillin resistance, because of altered penicillin-binding proteins.

DIAGNOSIS

The diagnosis of acute otitis media is a clinical one and is based on the rapid onset of signs and symptoms of middle ear inflammation in the presence of middle ear effusion.[6] Patients often present with ear symptoms such as pain or fullness. Otorrhea may be present if the tympanic membrane has perforated. Other symptoms may include fever, rhinorrhea, nasal congestion, and fussiness. Middle ear effusion is highly suggested by a bulging tympanic membrane with decreased mobility and should be confirmed by pneumatic otoscopy (Fig. 90–3). Redness and dullness of the eardrum can indicate infection but are less predictive.[6] A crying or febrile child can cause erythema of the tympanic membranes but should have normal mobility on pneumatic otoscopy. Routine tympanocentesis or cultures are not necessary in the diagnosis of uncomplicated otitis media.

DIFFERENTIAL DIAGNOSIS

Otitis media with effusion should be differentiated from acute otitis media, since the former indicates middle ear fluid with-

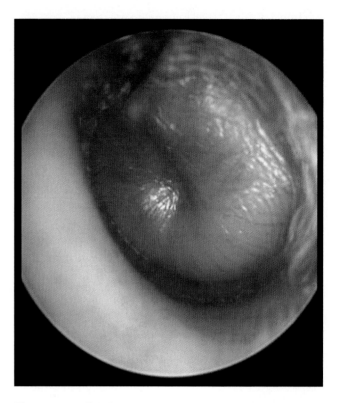

Figure 90–3. Bulging tympanic membrane in otitis media. (Courtesy of Glenn Issacson, MD.)

out infection. Bullous myringitis is an infection of the tympanic membrane that occurs alone or in combination with a middle ear infection. It characteristically presents with bullae on the tympanic membrane. Traditionally, the condition has been associated with *Mycoplasma pneumoniae.* However, a recent study showed that the pathogens causing these infections are similar to the pathogens causing otitis media, particularly *S. pneumoniae.*[8] Acute otitis externa may be difficult to differentiate from acute otitis media with perforation, unless the membrane can be well visualized after suctioning. Differentiating erythematous tympanic membranes due to fever or crying from true acute otitis media is a challenge. The instillation of anesthetic eardrops may help distinguish crying due to otalgia from other more serious conditions like meningitis.

COMPLICATIONS

Suppurative complications from otitis media, although decreasing in incidence, still occur. An important complication to recognize is acute mastoiditis, an infection of the mastoid bone. The patient usually presents with postauricular erythema, tenderness, and lateral displacement of the pinna. Computerized tomography of the temporal bones is crucial to determine the extent of infection and to detect sinus thrombosis or brain abscess[9] (Fig. 90–4). Other complications of acute otitis media include tympanic perforation, cholesteatoma, facial paralysis, and labyrinthitis. Intracranial suppurative complications such as meningitis, brain abscess, encephalitis, and lateral sinus thrombosis, although rare, should be suspected in patients

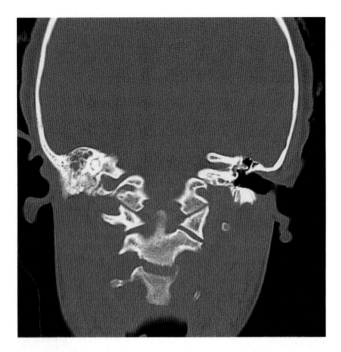

Figure 90–4. CT scan showing mastoiditis and cholesteatoma.

with worsening ear pain while taking antibiotics, persistent headache, intractable emesis, or behavior change.

MANAGEMENT

Treatment approaches for acute otitis media have changed in recent years. As expected, antibiotics play no role in the treatment of otitis media with effusion. However, the role of antibiotics in the treatment of acute bacterial otitis media is evolving. There is evidence that most cases of acute otitis media resolve on their own without antibiotics.[6,10] There is also concern that the overuse of antibiotics contributes to increasing bacterial resistance. One new approach advocated by the American Academy of Pediatrics is a period of observation for 48 to 72 hours without antibiotics in select patients with uncomplicated otitis media. Candidates for this option include patients older than 6 months with an *uncertain* diagnosis of otitis media and without severe symptoms; and those older than 2 years with otitis media but without severe symptoms (fever less than 39°C and mild otalgia).[6]

In cases where antibiotics are indicated, high-dose amoxicillin (80–90 mg/kg/d) remains the initial first-line medication.[6] For patients with non-type-1 penicillin allergy, cefdinir (14 mg/kg/d in one or two divided doses), cefuroxime (30 mg/kg/d in two divided doses), or cefpodoxime (10 mg/kg/d) may be used. For patients with type 1 allergic reaction to penicillin (urticaria or anaphylaxis), azithromycin (10 mg/kg on day 1 then 5 mg/kg on days 2 to 5 days as a single dose), or clarithromycin (15 mg/kg in two divided doses) may be used. For treatment failure after 48 to 72 hours of amoxicillin or for severe otitis media as initial treatment, high-dose amoxicillin-clavulanate (90 mg/kg/d in two divided doses) or a second- or third-generation cephalosporin as outlined above is appro-

priate. There is also evidence that a single dose of ceftriaxone (50 mg/kg) is equal in efficacy to 10 days of oral amoxicillin.[11] Alternatively, patients who fail to improve after 48 to 72 hours can also receive a series of three daily intramuscular doses of ceftriaxone. Patients with persistent treatment failures as well as those with recurrent middle ear infections should consult with an otolaryngologist due to the potential chronic effects on hearing and development.

Mastoiditis is a serious complication of otitis media and should be treated aggressively. The most common causative agent is *S. pneumoniae* with an increasing proportion of isolates showing resistance to penicillin.[12] Management strategies consist of intravenous antibiotics, with or without myringotomy and, in select cases, mastoidectomy to remove necrotic bone.[13]

► FOREIGN BODY OF THE NOSE AND EAR

Foreign bodies lodged in the ear and noses are common presenting complaints in the emergency department. Although a wide variety of foreign bodies have been described in the literature, hair beads, toy parts, eraser tips, food, and insects are commonly encountered. Most of these objects are self-inserted either in play or as a response to an itch or irritation. While children may report insertion of a foreign body, many foreign bodies are accidentally discovered by parents and occasionally by physicians during routine examination.

DIAGNOSTIC FINDINGS

Foreign bodies are usually apparent on direct visualization. In the absence of a clear history, helpful clues include epistaxis, pain, discharge, and alteration of sense of smell or hearing. Bleeding and purulent discharge can impede the physical examination. Foreign bodies can masquerade as chronic infections, tumors, recurrent epistaxis, and generalized body odor (bromidrosis).

COMPLICATIONS

Complications can occur as a result of the foreign body itself or during removal. Blockage of the external auditory canal or nares can interfere with normal function. Aural foreign bodies can predispose to otitis externa, cellulitis, tympanic membrane perforation, or vertigo. Undiscovered nasal foreign bodies may present with recurrent epistaxis, a unilateral foul-smelling discharge, sinusitis, or periorbital cellulitis. During removal, these foreign bodies may be lodged further where it is harder to retrieve and may cause bleeding, laceration, perforation, or aspiration. Button batteries, in particular, can cause tissue necrosis, ossicular disruption, perforation, and facial nerve paralysis.[14]

MANAGEMENT

Depending on the material, length of time lodged, and location, the removal of nasal and aural foreign bodies can be difficult. Refer the patient to an otolaryngologist if there is a low

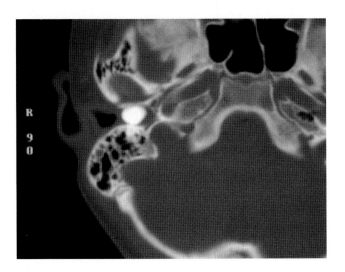

Figure 90–5. CT scan showing a retained rock in the ear canal necessitating removal in the operating room. (Courtesy of Glenn Issacson, MD.)

probability of successful removal in the emergency department (Fig. 90–5). Explain to the parents the procedure, the need for immobilization with or without sedation, possible complications, as well as other options. To ensure success in the first attempt, appropriate equipment, supplies, and lighting must be present and the child adequately immobilized. See Table 90–1 for the equipment necessary to have in the removal of aural or nasal foreign bodies. Multiple attempts may cause bleeding, mucosal edema, and movement of the object to a less accessible area. Application of a topical vasoconstrictor on the nasal mucosa may reduce intranasal tissue edema and aid foreign body removal.

Foreign body shape, location, and composition as well as physician preference influence the removal technique and instrument employed. Forceps removal, irrigation, and suctioning are the three most common techniques used. It is generally recommended that insects be killed with mineral oil, antipyrine/benzocaine drops, or alcohol before removal is attempted. Wood and other vegetable matter tend to swell when wet and are best removed before irrigating the ear canal. When possible, forceps are used to grasp the foreign body. Round, fragile objects may be more successfully removed by placing a wire loop curette or a right-angle hook behind the foreign body or by using super-glue-type adhe-

▶ TABLE 90–1. EQUIPMENT FOR EXAMINATION
   AND REMOVAL OF A NASAL OR AURAL
   FOREIGN BODY

Immobilization device (sheet or papoose board)
Otoscope for instrumentation under direct visualization
Nasal speculum
Headlight (optional)
Topical vasoconstrictor (phenylephrine 0.125%–0.5%,
   cocaine 4%, or epinephrine 1:1000)
Alligator or Hartman forceps
Wire loop or right angle curette
Suction apparatus, including catheters of various sizes

sive on a cotton-tipped applicator.[15] If the canal is traumatized, prophylactic topical antibiotics for acute otitis externa should be considered.

Small aural foreign bodies close to the tympanic membrane may be removed with body temperature tap water or saline irrigation using a large 60-mL syringe attached to a plastic infusion catheter. A foreign body that completely occludes the nares can be removed by using positive pressure ventilation through a bag valve mask applied to the mouth while occluding the noninvolved nare.[16] Alternatively, the caregiver may apply mouth-to-mouth pressure as well. Since children may pack a nose or ear with several objects at once, a thorough check for other objects is advisable after a foreign body is removed.

▶ EPISTAXIS

Although nosebleeds are a common occurrence in the pediatric age group, they are alarming to both parent and child. Most of these nosebleeds are mild and stop spontaneously on their own without medical attention. Unlike in adults where posterior nasal bleeds are more common, majority of nosebleeds in children and adolescents are anterior in location.[17] These occur at the nasal vestibule or the plexus of vessels on the anteroinferior portion of the nasal septum (Little's area, Kiesselbach's plexus).

ETIOLOGY

The etiology of epistaxis can be divided into local or systemic causes. In children, epistaxis digitorum, or "nose picking," is the most frequent cause followed by mucosal irritation due to decreased humidity, especially during the winter months.[17] Recurrent upper respiratory infections and allergic rhinitis increase the vascularity of the nasal mucosa and coupled with frequent nose blowing predispose to nosebleeds. Nasal foreign bodies, chronic inhaled steroid use, cocaine or heroin sniffing, and nasal fractures are some of the traumatic causes of epistaxis. Tumors such as angiofibromas, hemangioma, or pyogenic granuloma are rare causes of epistaxis. Bleeding disorders from acquired or congenital coagulopathy and platelet or blood vessel abnormalities should be suspected in patients who have prolonged nosebleeds with minor trauma, spontaneous and frequent nosebleeds, or have a positive family history of bleeding disorders. The most common bleeding disorder associated with recurrent epistaxis is von Willebrand disease.[18]

DIAGNOSTIC FINDINGS

If the patient is stable and the nosebleed is minimal or has stopped, the etiology of the bleeding is usually apparent in the history and physical examination. Determine the severity of the epistaxis by asking about its frequency, duration, estimated amount, and whether the bleeding involves one or both nares. Obtain any history of recent trauma to the face, upper respiratory illness, or exposure to dry air. Ascertain use of any medication such as aspirin, nonsteroidal anti-inflammatory agents, nasal steroids, recreational drugs, or use of complementary therapies. A foul-smelling odor emanating from the patient's face may suggest a retained foreign body in the nose. Allergic shiners, allergic salute, and a cobblestoned pharynx suggest allergic rhinitis as the cause of recurrent epistaxis. Pallor, weakness, resting tachycardia, or orthostatic dizziness is indicative of significant blood loss.

MANAGEMENT

It is important that the patient be rapidly assessed for any respiratory compromise, hemodynamic instability, or change in mental status that require airway intervention or fluid resuscitation.[17,19] If the patient is stable, identifying the source of the nosebleed and initiating measures to stop it should be done at the same time. Equipment and supplies, including a suction apparatus and suction tips, gauzes, and topical medications, should be ready before attempting evaluation or immobilization of the child (Table 90–1). Positioning small children in their parent's lap with manual restraint is often helpful. Optimal examination is facilitated by the use of a headlamp and a nasal speculum. Removal of blood with a Fraser suction tip can aid in localizing the bleeding point.

No treatment is required for patients whose bleeding resolved spontaneously or with direct pressure.[17,19] However, the emergency physician should allay the anxiety of both patient and parent by identifying the cause and providing advice to prevent recurrences. Measures that help in keeping the nasal mucosa moist include running a cool mist humidifier at night and application of saline drops, petroleum jelly, or antibiotic cream into the nasal septum and orifice.[19] Fingernails should be cut short.

For active anterior nosebleeds, continuous firm compression of the nasal alae for 5 to 10 minutes will usually stop the bleeding. Intermittent compression will not allow sufficient blood clot to form on the Kiesselbach's plexus. The child should be sitting up, breathing through his mouth, and leaning forward with his face down to prevent blood from dripping into the hypopharynx or oral cavity. Application of a topical nasal decongestant such as oxymetazoline or phenylephrine prior to compression causes local vasoconstriction and helps stop the bleeding.[17,20]

If compression does not control the bleeding, chemical cautery with silver nitrate sticks may be attempted, especially in the cooperative patient. A cotton pledget soaked in phenylephrine (0.125%–0.5%), 1% lidocaine, or cocaine (4%) can be applied to the bleeding area prior to the application of silver nitrate. The tip of the stick should be in contact with the site for a few seconds and repeated as necessary until a grayish-white coloration is noted. Continued bleeding may necessitate the use of an electrocautery device after local anesthesia. Care should be applied to the use of cautery devices as these can cause mucosal injury and, in rare cases, nasal ulceration or perforation.[17,20]

Recently, the use of topical thrombin, fibrin, or hemostatic sealants was reported to be more effective in controlling bleeding, easier to use and better tolerated by patients with anterior epistaxis compared to cautery or packing.[21,22]

If the techniques above are not sufficient to control the bleeding, anterior nasal packing in consultation with an otolaryngologist is the next step. However, this technique is poorly tolerated by children in the emergency department. Packing materials currently in use include nonresorbable (Vaseline™ or Xeroform™) gauge, Merocel™ sponge) and resorbable (Gelfoam®, Surgicel) agents. Packing should be removed within 1 to 2 days. A course of antibiotics effective against staphylococcus and streptococcus is usually prescribed.[17,20] Other techniques such as posterior nasal packing, balloon catheter insertion, arterial ligation, pterygopalatine fossa block, and embolization are rarely needed in a child. Refractory bleeding necessitates reevaluation of the etiology, otolaryngology consultation, and hospital admission for further workup and management.

▶ SINUSITIS

Sinusitis is inflammation of the paranasal sinuses. Viral infection of the nasal passages and sinuses (viral rhinosinusitis) and allergic rhinitis are the two most common predisposing factors for sinusitis.[23] With children averaging 6 to 8 upper respiratory infections per year, it is estimated that 6% to 13% of these infections are complicated by bacterial sinusitis.[24] Acute bacterial sinusitis is defined as bacterial infection of the sinuses with resolution of symptoms in less than 30 days.[29] Subacute bacterial sinusitis is present when symptoms last more than 30 days but less than 90 days. Chronic sinusitis is defined by the persistence of symptoms for more than 90 days. Recurrent sinusitis is present when the patient has had 3 episodes of acute sinusitis in 6 months or 4 episodes in a year.[23,25]

ANATOMY AND PATHOPHYSIOLOGY

While the maxillary and ethmoid sinuses are present at birth, the sphenoid sinuses do not become pneumatized until after 5 years of age. The frontal sinuses appear by 6 to 8 years but do not reach complete development until adolescence.[23] The sphenoidal and posterior ethmoidals drain into the ostium of the superior meatus on the lateral wall while the maxillary, frontal, and anterior ethmoidals drain into the middle meatus. Normal function of the paranasal sinuses depends on patency of the sinus ostia, function of the ciliary apparatus, and the nature of sinus secretions. Abnormality of any of these will predispose to bacterial infection.

ETIOLOGY

Aside from viral rhinosinusitis and allergic rhinitis, other predisposing factors for sinusitis include mucosal irritants such as tobacco smoke, dry air, foreign bodies, craniofacial abnormalities, septal deviation, adenoidal hypertrophy, and polyps secondary to allergies or cystic fibrosis (Fig. 90–6). Conditions that cause ciliary dysfunction and changes in atmospheric pressure can also cause sinusitis. Day care attendance increases the risk for sinusitis.[26]

DIAGNOSTIC FINDINGS

Symptoms of viral rhinosinusitis such as nasal congestion, rhinorhea, and cough can last about a week but should be

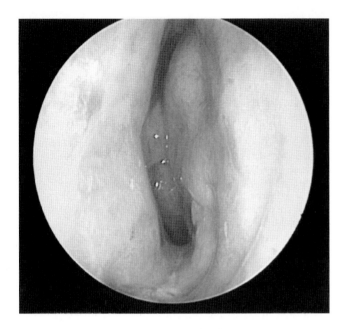

Figure 90–6. Nasal polyp.

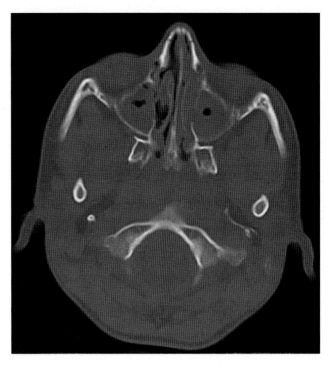

Figure 90–7. CT scan showing pansinusitis.

resolving by 10 days. Fever usually occurs in the first 24 to 48 hours of the illness. A more severe clinical picture in the first week, or persistence or worsening of symptoms beyond the first week, signals the development of bacterial sinusitis. The nasal discharge can be clear or purulent and the cough is frequently worse at night. Presence of headache, facial pain, and halitosis is variable and less common in children.[25] Fatigue, malaise, and decreased appetite are sometimes noted.

On physical examination, there is anterior or postnasal drainage and swelling of the nasal mucosa. Signs of allergic rhinitis such as allergic shiners, allergic salute, and cobblestoning of the posterior pharynx may be present. Periorbital swelling suggests ethmoidal sinusitis. Transillumination is of limited value in children.

RADIOLOGIC EVALUATION

Radiologic evaluation of the sinuses by either plain films or computed tomography has variable reliability, especially in the younger age group. Normal studies are helpful in ruling out sinusitis. Radiographic findings are frequently found even in patients with rhinosinusitis alone.[27] Hence, abnormal studies need to be correlated to the patient's clinical course and presentation. Findings in plain films or computed tomography consistent with sinusitis include complete opacification of the sinus, mucoperiosteal thickening of more than 4 mm, and presence of air-fluid levels[28] (Fig. 90–7).

According to the American Academy of Pediatrics, the diagnosis of acute uncomplicated bacterial sinusitis in children younger than 6 years can be made on clinical grounds alone.[23] Although controversial, plain radiographs of the sinuses (anteroposterior, lateral, and occipitomental views) may be obtained in children older than 6 years to confirm the diagnosis before treatment or in those who do not improve after a course of antibiotics. A patient suspected to have orbital or intracranial complications should undergo contrast enhanced computed tomography of the sinuses and of the orbits or brain.[25]

DIFFERENTIAL CONSIDERATIONS

Other conditions with similar symptoms to sinusitis include recurrent rhinitis, enlarged adenoids, and allergic rhinitis. Foreign body, neoplasm, or polyp commonly causes unilateral drainage and obstruction and predispose to the development of sinusitis. Other causes of persistent cough such as pertussis or reactive airway disease should be considered.

COMPLICATIONS

Sinusitis can seed the systemic circulation resulting in bacteremia or septicemia. Local extension can result in facial cellulitis, facial abscess, periorbital and orbital cellulitis, osteomyelitis of the skull (Pott's puffy tumor), cavernous sinus thrombosis, epidural abscess, subdural empyema, meningitis, and brain abscess.[25]

MANAGEMENT

The pathogenesis and microbiology of acute bacterial sinusitis are similar to acute otitis media. *S. pneumoniae*, nontypeable *H. influenzae*, and *M. catarrhalis* are the most common causes. Although some children with sinusitis will improve gradually, antibiotic therapy is indicated to hasten resolution of symptoms and to prevent complications. Amoxicillin (45–90 mg/kg/d divided twice a day) remains the drug of choice because of its effectiveness, safety, and tolerability. However, patients should be assessed for risk factors for bacterial resistance to amoxicillin such as (1) age younger than 2 years (2) day care attendance, and (3) antibiotic use within the past 90 days. In the presence of these risk factors or more severe symptoms, amoxicillin with clavulanate (80–90 mg/kg/d in two divided doses), cefdinir (14 mg/kg/d in one or two doses), cefuroxime (30 mg/kg/d), or cefpodoxime (10 mg/kg/d) can be used. For patients with non-type-1 hypersensitivity reactions to penicillin, cefdinir, cefuroxime, and cefpodoxime can be used. Those with type-1 hypersensitivity reaction to penicillin can be prescribed clarithromycin (15 mg/kg/d in two divided doses), azithromycin (10 mg/kg on day 1 and 5 mg/kg per dose once a day on days 2–5), or clindamycin (30–40 mg/kg/d in three divided doses).[23,25] For patients who are vomiting, a single dose of ceftriaxone (50 mg/kg/d intramuscularly or intravenously) can be used with initiation of oral antibiotics 24 hours later once vomiting has subsided. Oral antibiotics can be given for a minimum of 10 days and extended depending on the clinical response. Most patients will have improvement in their symptoms within 48 to 72 hours.

Patients who have severe symptoms, clinical deterioration while on oral antibiotics, orbital or intracranial involvement, or immunodeficiency should be hospitalized for intravenous antibiotics and sinus imaging studies. CT scan of the sinuses with contrast is the modality of choice in the emergency department. Consultation with an otolaryngologist should be initiated. Parenteral antibiotic regimen that provides coverage against resistant pneumococci, *H. influenzae*, and *M. catarrhalis* includes cefotaxime (100–200 mg/kg/d divided every 6 hours) or ceftriaxone (100 mg/kg/d divided every 12 hours).[23,25]

Other adjunctive therapies such as antihistamines, decongestants, and nasal steroids have limited efficacy and are not recommended.[25] Saline nose drops, however, may be useful in liquefying nasal secretions.

REFERENCES

1. Hirsch BE. Diseases of the external ear. In: Bluestone CD, Stool SE, Kenna MA, eds. *Pediatric Otolaryngology*. Philadelphia, PA: W. B. Saunders; 1996:378–382.
2. Handzel O, Halperin D. Necrotizing (malignant) otitis externa. *Am Fam Physician*. 2003;68:309–312.
3. Aizawa H, Ohtani F, Furuta Y, Sawa H, Fukuda S. Variable patterns of varicella-zoster virus reactivation in Ramsay Hunt Syndrome. *J Med Virol*. 2004;74:355–360.
4. Van Balen HAM, Smit WM, Zuithoff NPA, Verheij TJM. Clinical efficacy of three common treatments in acute otitis externa in primary care: randomized control trial. *BMJ*. 2003;327:1201–1205.
5. Pistorius B, Westberry K, Drehobl M. Prospective, randomized, comparative trial of ciprofloxacin otic drops, with or without hydrocortisone, vs. polymyxinB-neomycin-hydrocortisone otic suspension in the treatment of acute diffuse otitis externa. *Infect Dis Clin Pract*. 1999l;8:387–395.
6. Subcommittee on Management of Acute Otitis Media. Diagnosis and management of acute otitis media. *Pediatrics*. 2004;113:1451–1465.
7. Paradise JL, Rockette HE, Colborn DK, et al. Otitis media in 2253 Pittsburgh-area infants: prevalence and risk factors during the first two years of life. *Pediatrics*. 1997;99:318–333.
8. Palmu AAI, Kotikoski MJ, Kaijalainen TH, Puhakka HJ. Bacterial etiology of acute myringitis in children less than two years of age. *Pediatr Infect Dis J*. 2001;20:607–611.
9. Smith JA, Danner CJ. Complications of chronic otitis media and cholesteatoma. *Otolaryngol Clin North Am*. 2006;39:1237–1255.
10. Del Mar C, Glasziou P, Hayem M. Are antibiotics indicated as initial treatment for children with acute otitis media? A meta-analysis. *BMJ*. 1997;314:1526–1529.
11. Green SM, Rothrock SG. Single-dose intramuscular ceftriaxone for acute otitis media in children. *Pediatrics*. 1993;91:23–30.
12. Kaplan S, Mason E, Wald ER, et al. Pneumococcal Mastoiditis in children. *Pediatrics*. 2000;106:695–699.
13. Talor MF, Berkowitz RG. Indications for mastoidectomy in acute mastoiditis in children. *Ann Otol Rhinol Laryngol*. 2004;113:69–72.
14. Kavanagh KT, Litovitz T. Miniature foreign bodies in auditory and nasal cavities. *JAMA*. 1986;255:1470–1472.
15. Hanson RM, Stephens M. Cyanoacrylate-assisted foreign body removal from the ear and nose in children. *J Paediatr Child Health*. 1994;30:77.
16. Finkelstein JA. Oral ambu-bag insufflation to remove unilateral nasal foreign bodies. *Am J Emerg Med*. 1996;14:57–58.
17. Massick D, Tobin E. Epistaxis. In: Flint P, Haughey B, Robbins KT, Thomas JR, eds. *Cummings Otolaryngology: Head and Neck Surgery*. Philadelphia, PA: Mosby Elsevier; 2005.
18. Sandoval C, Dong S Visintainer P, et al. Clinical and laboratory features of 178 children with recurrent epistaxis. *J Pediatr Hematol Oncol*. 2002;24:47–49.
19. Up to Date: Management of epistaxis in children. Messner, Anna. http://www.utdol.com/utd/content/topic. Accessed January 18, 2008.
20. Bernius M, Perlin D. Pediatric ear, nose and throat emergencies. *Pediatr Clin North Am*. 2006;53:195–214.
21. Vaiman M, Segal M, Eviatar E. Fibrin glue treatment for epistaxis. *Rhinology*. 2002;40:88–91.
22. Mathiasen R, Cruz R, Cruz R. Prospective randomized clinical trial of a novel hemostatic sealant in patients with acute anterior epistaxis. *Laryngoscope*. 2005;115:899–902.
23. Clinical Practice Guideline. Management of Sinusitis. *Pediatrics*. 2001;108:798–808.
24. Wald ER, Guerra N, Byers C. Upper respiratory tract infections in young children:duration of and frequency of complications. *Pediatrics*. 1991;87:129–133.
25. Up to date: Clinical features, evaluation, and diagnosis of acute bacterial sinusitis in children. http://www.utdol.com/utd/content/topic. Accessed February 28, 2008.
26. Wald ER, Dashefsky B, Byers C, et al. Frequency and severity of infections in daycare. *J Pediatr*. 1988;112:540–546.
27. Glasier CM, Mallory GB, Steele RW. Significance of opacification of the maxillary and ethmoid sinuses in infants. *J Pediatr*. 1989;114:45–50.
28. Diament MJ. The diagnosis of sinusitis in infants and children: x-ray, computed tomography, and magnetic resonance imaging. Diagnostic imaging of pediatric sinusitis. *J Allergy Clin Immunol*. 1992;90:442–444.
29. Up to date: Microbiology and Treatment of acute bacterial sinusitis in children. http://www.utdol.com/utd/content/topic. Accessed February 28, 2008.

CHAPTER 91

Emergencies of the Oral Cavity and Neck

Daryl Williams and Gregory Garra

▶ HIGH-YIELD FACTS

- Avulsed primary teeth should not be replaced. Avulsed permanent teeth should be reimplanted as soon as possible.
- Always consider aspiration when a tooth/tooth fragment cannot be located.
- Fractures of primary teeth may be a sign of child abuse. The presence of *Neisseria gonorrhoeae* pharyngitis in a child suggests sexual abuse.
- Physicians should maintain a high index of suspicion for carotid injury in a patient with trauma to the oropharynx.
- Uncomplicated dental infections are treated on an outpatient basis. Deep fascial space infections often require hospitalization, IV antibiotics, and surgical drainage.
- Suppurative complications of pharyngitis include peritonsillar abscess, Lemierre's postanginal sepsis, and Ludwig's angina.
- Needle aspiration may be employed diagnostically to differentiate between peritonsillar cellulitis and peritonsillar abscess. Definitive treatment may be achieved via aspiration, incision and drainage, or tonsillectomy in selected cases.
- Airway assessment is important in suspected cases of peritonsillar abscess, retropharyngeal abscess (RPA), and Ludwig's angina. Definitive management of unstable airways is best achieved in the operating room with the assistance of an anesthesiologist or an ENT specialist. Emergency airway equipment should be available at the bedside.

Emergencies pertaining to the oral cavity and neck can be broadly divided into four categories: dental trauma, oropharyngeal trauma, dentoalveolar infections, and soft tissue infections. Facial and neck trauma are covered in Chapters 34 and 19, respectively.

▶ ORAL AND DENTAL ANATOMY

Tooth development begins in utero, with completion of mineralization of all primary (deciduous) teeth prior to birth. Eruption of the primary teeth begins with the lower central incisors between 6 and 10 months of age. The primary dentition consists of 20 teeth with eruption usually completed by 33 months. Eruption of the secondary (permanent) teeth begins with the lower central incisors at approximately 6 years of age. Full secondary teeth eruption is usually completed by 21 years of age and consists of 32 permanent teeth.

A tooth is composed of a neurovascular center, or pulp, which is surrounded by dentin (Fig. 91–1). The exterior surface of the tooth, or crown, is covered by enamel. The root of the tooth is protected by cementum and is attached to alveolar bone by the periodontal ligament (PDL).

The oral cavity is lined by mucosa composed of stratified squamous epithelium. The superior portion is formed by the hard and soft palates, while the inferior portion is formed by the tongue and its supportive structures. The oral cavity is bordered laterally by the cheeks which are supported by buccinator muscles. The vestibule is the space between the cheeks/lips and teeth. Gingiva covers the alveolar surfaces of the maxilla and mandible.[1]

▶ DENTOALVEOLAR TRAUMA

Approximately 30% of preschool-aged children suffer injuries of the primary dentition, equally distributed between males and females.[2] Among school-aged children, trauma to permanent incisors occurs in approximately 23% of boys and 13% of girls.[3] Falls are the most common cause of injury in the preschool and school-aged group. Among older children and teenagers, males are twice as likely to suffer dental trauma and commonly results from motor vehicle collisions, sports-related injuries, and altercations.[4] The maxillary central incisor is the most commonly injured dental structure.[3] Dental trauma may be a marker for child abuse.[5,6]

DIAGNOSTIC FINDINGS

Trauma to the tooth can result in loosening, avulsion, or fracture. Luxations are injuries which result from damage to the supporting structures of the teeth (PDL and alveolar bone). Luxations are defined in terms of the lie of the tooth. The distinct types of luxation injuries are described in Table 91–1.

Dental fractures may involve the tooth and/or supporting structures. The Ellis classification system has been widely used in emergency medicine texts to characterize these fractures; however, this system is not recognized by the dental community. The more uniform and widely recognized classification of dental fractures, adopted from the World Health Organization's

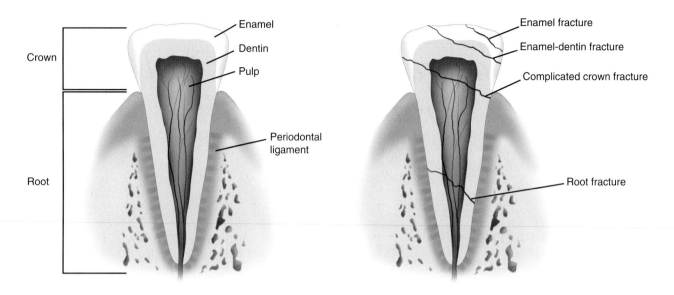

Figure 91–1. Dental anatomy.

Application of the International Classification of Diseases to Dentistry and Stomatology, are listed in Table 91–2.[7]

COMPLICATIONS

While dental trauma is rarely life-threatening, associated maxillofacial injuries and complications thereof may result in airway compromise, injury to surrounding nerves and blood vessels, penetration of anatomic planes of the neck with subsequent subcutaneous emphysema, pneumomediastinum, or mediastinitis.

Trauma to the primary teeth may result in a number of complications including: infection of the tooth, pulp necrosis with subsequent discoloration, displacement, premature loss, or problems with root resorption. Intrusion injuries to primary teeth are particularly concerning because of the anatomic proximity to secondary teeth. The frequency of anomalous permanent tooth development resulting from primary tooth injury ranges from 16% to 60%.[8]

Injuries to permanent teeth, including avulsion, can also result in pulp necrosis with subsequent color change, as well as abscess formation. The prognosis for avulsed permanent teeth is inversely proportional to the extraoral dry time. If the extraoral dry time is more than 60 minutes, the prognosis for saving the tooth is poor because of necrosis of the PDL.

MANAGEMENT

Emergency physicians generally do not have the equipment available for dental radiography (panoramic, periapical, and bitewing radiographs). Therefore, all but the most minor cases should be referred to a dentist for evaluation and radiographic documentation. Definitive treatment is largely dependent upon the type of tooth involved, primary versus secondary.

Analgesia is indicated for all dentoalveolar injuries. NSAIDs have been shown to be as effective as narcotics for the treatment of dental pain.[9]

▶ **TABLE 91–1. LUXATION INJURIES**

Category	Description
Concussion	Tender but immobile and no displacement is present
Subluxation	Abnormally loose but not displaced
Lateral luxation	Displacement of the tooth in a nonaxial direction
Extrusive luxation	Partial avulsion or dislodgement of a tooth from the alveolar bone
Intrusive luxation	Compression of the tooth into its socket
Avulsion	Complete displacement of the tooth from its socket

▶ **TABLE 91–2. DENTAL FRACTURE TERMINOLOGY**

Category	Description
Dental Infraction	An incomplete fracture (crack) of the enamel without loss of tooth substance
Enamel fracture	A fracture with loss of tooth substance that is confined to the enamel
Enamel–dentin fracture	A fracture with loss of tooth substance confined to enamel and dentin, but not involving the pulp
Complicated crown fracture	A fracture involving enamel and dentin, and exposing the pulp
Uncomplicated crown-root fracture	A fracture involving enamel, dentin, and cementum, but not exposing the pulp
Complicated crown-root fracture	A fracture involving enamel, dentin, and cementum, and exposing the pulp

Primary teeth: Enamel and enamel–dentin fractures are treated with smoothing of sharp edges and dental referral. Complicated crown fractures require capping with calcium hydroxide, pain management, and dental referral. Treatment of root, crown-root, and alveolar fractures are individualized. Therefore, prompt dental referral is indicated. Luxation injuries generally heal without any treatment. Removal of severely loosened teeth is indicated if there is a high risk of aspiration. Reimplantation of an avulsed primary tooth is not recommended.

Permanent teeth: Uncomplicated crown fracture should be covered with glass ionomer. Reattachment of the tooth fragment can be performed on an outpatient basis. Complicated crown fractures require prompt capping with calcium hydroxide if available, analgesia, and prompt dental referral. Maintaining the integrity of the PDL is the primary goal in the treatment of luxation injuries. Concussion injuries require no treatment. All other luxation injuries should be repositioned, splinted, and referred to dental services for definitive care. Avulsion injuries of the permanent teeth require immediate reimplantation or placement in a nutritive storage media (milk, saliva, or Hanks balanced salt solution). Figure 91–2 describes the procedure for reimplantation of an avulsed tooth. Gingival lacerations should be sutured as needed. Antibiotic prophylaxis with penicillin is appropriate for contaminated avulsions. Tetanus status should be assessed and updated when indicated. Prompt dental referral is indicated.

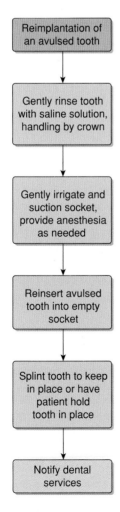

Figure 91–2. Procedure for tooth reimplantation.

▶ OROPHARYNGEAL TRAUMA

Soft palate or lateral pharyngeal wall trauma may present as avulsions, lacerations, and impalement. The major concern with oropharyngeal trauma is injury to the carotid artery resulting in thrombosis and neurologic sequelae. Based on case series, less than 1% of children with oropharyngeal trauma develop this serious complication.[10] While the incidence of neurologic complications is exceedingly low, the sequelae can be devastating, mandating a thorough assessment and high index of suspicion on the part of the clinician caring for these patients.

DIAGNOSIS

Injuries to the oropharyngeal soft tissues may present with bleeding, erythema, swelling, visible breaches in mucosal integrity, or presence of foreign bodies. Much of the data on the diagnostic evaluation of oropharyngeal injury are derived from small case series. There is no definitive diagnostic protocol. Carotid angiography is considered the gold standard for diagnosis of carotid injury but is invasive. Carotid ultrasound, CT scan, and MRA are other imaging modalities that can be considered. The utility of these studies in detecting thrombosis in the asymptomatic patient has not been demonstrated.[11]

COMPLICATIONS

Most soft tissue oropharyngeal injuries heal without complications. However, severe complications of seemingly innocuous injuries have been reported. Carotid artery injury, presumably arising from compression of the vessel, may result in an intimal tear with subsequent carotid and cerebrovascular thrombosis. The appearance of neurologic signs can be delayed for up to 60 hours. The size of the lesion does not seem to correlate with vascular injury, and there are no reliable clinical factors which help identify patients at increased risk for neurologic sequelae.[11–13]

MANAGEMENT

There is no clear consensus on the management of oropharyngeal injuries. The treatment of diagnosed carotid injuries is variable, thus necessitating the expertise of neurosurgery and/or vascular surgery.[14] A systematic approach to management of palatal injuries is provided in Figure 91–3.

▶ DENTOALVEOLAR INFECTIONS

Dentoalveolar infections include infections of the teeth and/or supporting structures (periodontium, bone). These infections

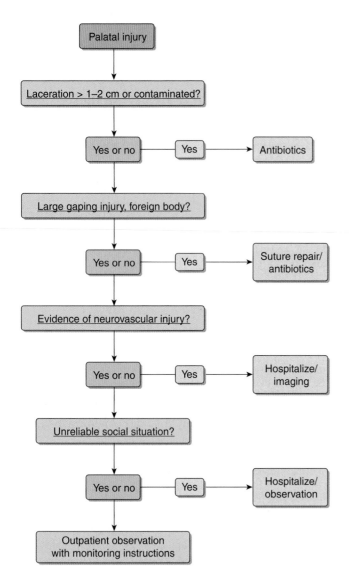

Figure 91–3. Algorithm for management of palatal injury. (With permission from Randall DA, Kang DR. Current management of penetrating injuries of the soft palate. *Otolaryngol Head Neck Surg.* 2006;135(3):356–360.)

include dentoalveolar abscesses and periodontal infections (gingivitis, periodontitis, pericoronitis).

Dental abscesses may be classified as endodontic or periodontic. Endodontic (periapical) abscesses are located at the apex of the tooth and typically originate from dental caries which results in acute inflammation (pulpitis) followed by necrosis of the pulp. Untreated necrosis may lead to cellulitis and/or bacterial invasion of surrounding bone. Endodontic abscesses are the most common type of dental abscess in children.

Periodontal abscesses are those that involve supportive tooth structures (PDL or alveolar bone) and form following infection of the periodontal tissues. This infection may occur from many proposed etiologies which include trauma, foreign body such as food debris, and surrounding gingival disease. These abscesses are more common in adults.

Pericoronitis is an acute, localized infection of the opercula of partially erupted or impacted teeth. Typically, the third

molars (wisdom teeth) are involved, but the condition may affect any tooth.

ETIOLOGY

Dentoalveolar infections are characteristically polymicrobial in nature, typically involving three or four species which are usually endogenous to the oral cavity. Commonly isolated organisms include *Prevotella, Porphyromonas, Fusobacterium* spp., and anaerobic streptococci.[15] Infections less than 3 days duration tend to be caused by penicillin-sensitive aerobic streptococci. Infections present for longer than 3 days tend to involve anaerobes. Infections involving fascial planes reportedly involve an average of two to six organisms.[16]

DIAGNOSIS

The clinical presentation of dentoalveolar infections depend on the virulence of the causative organism, location of infection and surrounding anatomical structures, host defense mechanisms, degree and nature of spread to adjacent structures, and underlying host factors such as diabetes, corticosteroid use, malignancy, and neutropenia. Reversible pulpitis presents as transient pain in response to thermal stimulation. Irreversible pulpitis manifests as persistent, throbbing pain exacerbated by heat and relieved by cold. Extension of the infection beyond the tooth to the periapical tissues is suggested by exquisite pain on chewing, touch or percussion of the teeth, and usually requires pain medication in addition to local therapy. Fever, lymphadenopathy, tooth mobility, or edema of the soft tissues suggests the presence of a periapical abscess. An erythematous, fluctuant mass (parulis) extending toward the buccal side of the gum overlying the affected tooth may be seen.

Local extension and deep space involvement is common in patients with delayed presentations of odontogenic pain. Swelling of deep spaces may represent simple cellulitis or abscess. Figure 91–4 illustrates the different deep spaces associated with space infection.

Periapical, bitewing, or panoramic radiography may demonstrate radiolucencies where abscesses are located. In patients with signs and symptoms of local extension, a CT scan with IV contrast may be necessary to differentiate deep space cellulitis from abscess.

COMPLICATIONS

Most complications of dentoalveolar infections result from direct spread of infection to deep spaces. In addition to the aforementioned abscesses, sequelae such as maxillary sinusitis and orbital cellulitis are reported. Spread to osseous structures, most commonly the mandible, may result in osteitis or osteomyelitis.

Ludwig's angina is an extensive, life-threatening cellulitis of the submandibular, sublingual, and submental spaces. Patients present with erythema and a characteristic brawny, boardlike swelling of the anterior neck. There is usually associated pain, edema, and elevation of the tongue as well. These

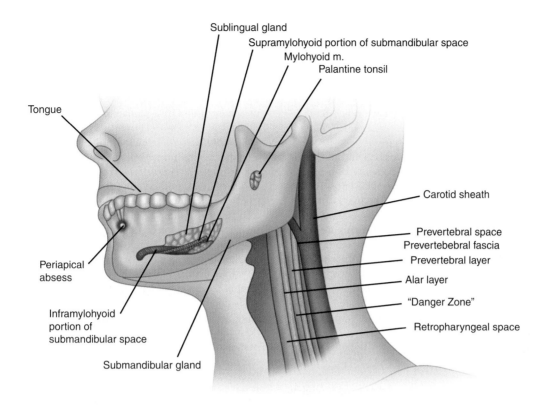

Figure 91–4. Deep spaces of the face and neck.

patients often appear toxic and dehydrated because of inability to swallow.

Indirect spread via lymphatic or hematogenous routes may also occur and may result in regional lymph node involvement producing painful regional lymphadenopathy. Deep fascial spread may also result in cavernous sinus thrombosis.

MANAGEMENT

Treatment for the majority of these disorders is generally rendered on an outpatient basis except in cases of life-threatening infections of the deep fascial planes. Analgesic therapy is a mainstay of treatment. NSAIDs are as effective as narcotics for treating dental pain.[9]

Simple, uncomplicated dental caries require analgesia and dental referral. Pulpitis and irreversible pulpitis are treated by removal of infected pulpal tissue (root canal or dental extraction when irreversible). Periapical and periodontal abscesses are treated by drainage; achieved by I&D, root canal therapy, or tooth extraction.

Antibiotics are indicated in cases where local or systemic spread of infection is suspected. Penicillin or amoxicillin are effective against the majority of endodontic infections. Infections present for more than 3 days have a higher incidence of anaerobic agents. Therefore, clindamycin or penicillin plus metronidazole are appropriate regimens.

Pericoronitis and periodontitis are treated with irrigation, debridement of the opercula, and removal of retained debris.

Localized cases that do not respond to mechanical therapy, and more severe cases where cellulitis is present may be managed with antibiotics and pain management. Prompt dental referral should be advised.

Systemically ill patients with infections of deep fascial planes require close attention. Admission to the hospital for airway monitoring, intravenous antibiotics, and surgical drainage is indicated. Involvement of anesthesia and otolaryngologic specialists is advised in patients with spread to the floor of the mouth.

▶ INFECTIONS OF THE ORAL SOFT TISSUE

Infections and ulcerative lesions of the oral mucosa are common. Recurrent aphthous stomatitis (RAS) is the most common mucosal disease in North America.[17] Importantly, oral mucosal infections may be a sign of systemic disease and thus should be carefully evaluated. Oral candidiasis and angular cheilitis are the most common oral manifestations of children with HIV infection.

ETIOLOGY

Primary herpetic gingivostomatitis is caused by herpes simplex virus type 1, with 30% to 40% of infected patients developing recurrent symptoms.[17] The etiology of RAS is unknown but may be precipitated by trauma, stress, menstruation, nutritional deficiencies, food allergies, and endocrinopathies.

DIAGNOSTIC FINDINGS

Infants and toddlers with pharyngitis may have nonspecific irritability, poor feeding, anorexia, and drooling. Older children who can verbalize may localize pain.

Herpangina causes small vesicular lesions and punched-out ulcers in the posterior pharynx. The presence of posterior pharyngeal ulcers is likely to represent Coxsackie virus. Buccal and lingual vesicles and maculovesicles on the hands and feet (hand-foot-mouth disease) are also caused by enteroviruses (Coxsackie A5, 10, and 16). Primary herpes simplex infection usually manifests with high fever and swollen, red, friable gums with diffuse oropharyngeal mucosal lesions that may become confluent. The stomatitis of candida produces curdy or velvety white plaques on the tongue and/or oral mucosa.

Laboratory evaluation is generally not indicated in most oral soft tissue infections unless systemic illness is suspected.

MANAGEMENT

Treatment of soft tissue infections of the oral mucosa is largely symptomatic. Children with stomatitis, ulcers, or severe sore throat may benefit from gargling or careful oral administration of a combination of Kaopectate or Maalox, diphenhydramine, and viscous lidocaine. One must use appropriate caution when prescribing viscous lidocaine as overtreatment can result in toxicity. Candida infection usually responds to oral nystatin. Acyclovir is recommended for herpes simplex virus infections in immunocompromised hosts at a dose of 15 to 30 mg/kg/d in three divided doses for 7 to 14 days. Limited data suggest that acyclovir may also be useful in preventing future recurrences in immunocompetent individuals.[18]

▶ PHARYNGITIS

Pharyngitis is defined as inflammation of the mucous membranes and underlying structures of the throat. It is one of the most common illnesses for which children visit primary care physicians. The peak incidence of viral and bacterial pharyngitis occurs in children aged from 4 to 7 years, and approximately 10% of children seek medical care for pharyngitis annually. Most cases occur during colder months of the year when viruses are prevalent, and spread among family members in the home is a prominent feature.[19]

ETIOLOGY

Viruses, bacteria, spirochetes, *Chlamydia, Mycoplasma,* mycobacteria, fungi, and parasites can all cause pharyngitis. Forty to sixty percent of cases are viral in origin. Commonly involved viruses include adenovirus, parainfluenza virus, rhinovirus, herpes simplex, respiratory syncytial virus, Epstein–Barr virus, influenza virus, Coxsackie virus, echo virus, coronavirus, and cytomegalovirus.

Group A β-hemolytic *Streptococcus* (*S. pyogenes,* GAS) is the most common bacterial cause of pharyngitis in children, responsible for 15% to 30% of cases.[19] Other, less common bacterial causes to consider include groups C and G streptococci, *Mycoplasma pneumoniae,* and *Corynebacterium diphtheriae. Corynebacterium hemolyticum* causes pharyngitis accompanied by a scarlatiniform rash similar to GAS. Pneumococcus, *Staphylococcus aureus, Neisseria meningitides,* and *Haemophilus influenzae* are thought to cause pharyngitis, usually after a viral upper respiratory infection. In sexually active adolescents, *Neisseria gonorrhoeae, Chlamydia trachomatis,* and syphilis should be considered.

Noninfectious causes of pharyngitis include postnasal drip, sinusitis, and respiratory irritants such as tobacco smoke or caustic ingestions. Agranulocytosis, lymphoma, and lymphocytic leukemia, though rare, can present with pharyngeal inflammation and symptoms.

Uvular inflammation may result from bacterial infection, trauma (usually medical instrumentation), and allergy. Uvulitis is most worrisome when associated with epiglottitis or angioneurotic edema, both potentially life-threatening conditions. Bacterial pathogens than can cause uvulitis are group A hemolytic streptococcus, *H. influenzae* type B, and *Streptococcus pneumoniae.*

DIAGNOSTIC FINDINGS

Acute GAS pharyngitis commonly presents as sore throat, fever, and odynophagia. Examination typically reveals tonsillopharyngeal erythema with or without exudate. Headache, vomiting, abdominal pain, and scarlatiniform rash (fine, erythematous sandpaperlike) commonly accompany streptococcal pharyngitis. Respiratory symptoms such as clear rhinorrhea, cough, hoarseness, or mucosal ulcers, suggest a viral etiology. Epstein–Barr virus and cytomegalovirus infection often have associated pharyngeal inflammation, diffuse lymphadenopathy, and hepatosplenomegaly. Low-grade fever, follicular conjunctivitis, sore throat, and cervical lymphadenopathy characterize pharyngoconjunctival fever.

Pharyngitis accompanied by rash, joint pain, and urethral or vaginal discharge may indicate gonorrhea. Syphilis in the primary stage may present with diffuse pharyngeal erythema and a chancre. Secondary syphilis may manifest with gray oropharyngeal patches and a rash. Diphtheria presents as an adherent, grayish pharyngeal membrane with bull neck and toxic appearance. History of exposure to the tissue or secretions of infected small animals may suggest tularemia.

Rapid *Streptococcus* detection by latex agglutination or enzyme immunoassay is useful when positive. False-positives with latex agglutination are uncommon (specificity approximately 95%), but false-negatives occur more frequently (sensitivity 80%–90%).[19] Current recommendations suggest culture confirmation of negative rapid strep tests. Swabbing of tonsillar tissue yields the most success in detection of streptococci.

CBC, EBV titers (Monospot), syphilis screening tests, and/or cultures for *N. gonorrhoeae* are indicated for unusual presentations or recurrent disease. The presence of positive gonococcal culture in a young child is a marker for sexual abuse and must be reported to the appropriate authorities.

► TABLE 91–3. **JONES CRITERIA**

Major manifestations	Carditis
	Chorea
	Erythema marginatum
	Polyarthritis
	Subcutaneous nodules
Minor manifestations	Clinical
	Arthralgia
	Fever
	Laboratory
	Elevated acute-phase reactants (ESR, leukocyte count)
	ECG
	Prolonged PR interval
Evidence of antecedent GAS infection	Elevated or rising streptococcal antibody titers
	Positive throat culture or rapid antigen test
	Recent scarlet fever

COMPLICATIONS

Suppuration can spread to contiguous tissues causing peritonsillar abscess, life-threatening Lemiere's postanginal sepsis (aerobic or anaerobic bacteremia from septic thrombophlebitis of the tonsillar vein), and Ludwig's angina. Hematologic spread may result in mesenteric adenitis, meningitis, brain abscess, cavernous sinus thrombosis, suppurative arthritis, endocarditis, osteomyelitis, sepsis, and septic embolization to the lung.

Nonsuppurative complications of GAS include scarlet fever, acute rheumatic fever (ARF), and glomerulonephritis (PSGN). ARF typically begins 1 to 5 weeks after GAS infection and is suggested by the presence of clinical features outlined in the Jones criteria (Table 91–3). Management of ARF involves confirmation of the diagnosis and limiting the sequelae of chronic valvular pathology. Treating acute GAS pharyngitis within 10 days of the illness can prevent ARF. Once diagnosed, patients with ARF should be managed by pediatric cardiology and infectious disease to prevent recurrent ARF and further damage to the heart valves. PSGN tends to occur in outbreaks associated with virulent strains of GAS. Symptoms typically appear 1 to 3 weeks after pharyngitis, and 3 to 6 weeks after scarlet fever or impetigo. The most common presentation is dark urine and edema. Hypertension is seen in 60% to 70% of cases. C3 levels are almost always diminished secondary to activation of the complement system. The clinical course is usually benign; management of edema and hypertension with fluid restriction and furosemide is recommended. There is no evidence that treatment of GAS pharyngitis prevents PSGN.

MANAGEMENT

Current recommendations for GAS pharyngitis support treatment of cases where clinical suspicion is high or diagnosis is confirmed by rapid-antigen testing or culture. Penicillin (oral or IM) is the first-line agent in most cases. Advanced macrolide antibiotics such as azithromycin may be used in penicillin-

allergic patients. Cephalosporins have also been advocated for the management of GAS pharyngitis, but there is insufficient evidence to support their use as first-line agents at this time.[19]

Other bacterial causes require specific and supportive management. If diphtheria is suspected, diphtheria antitoxin is given along with penicillin or erythromycin to eradicate the organism.

► PERITONSILLAR ABSCESS

Peritonsillar abscess (PTA) is the most common deep infection of the head and neck, typically seen in children older than 12 years.[20] It is usually a complication of bacterial tonsillitis. PTA usually begins as an episode of acute tonsillitis. Occlusion of tonsillar crypts and bacterial invasion of the peritonsillar area results in peritonsillar cellulitis. Pus collection in the supratonsillar fossa results in PTA.

ETIOLOGY

Most peritonsillar abscesses are polymicrobial infections. Group A streptococci are predominate; *Peptostreptococcus, Fusobacterium,* and other normal mouth flora, including anaerobes, may also be detected.[21] Uncommonly, *H. influenzae, S. pneumoniae,* and *S. aureus* are cultured.

DIAGNOSIS

Patients with PTA usually present with fever, gradually increasing pharyngeal discomfort, ipsilateral otalgia, trismus, and dysarthria. Drooling is not unusual. The voice has a muffled "hot potato" quality, and patients often appear toxic.

Examination of the oropharynx may sufficiently distinguish peritonsillar cellulitis from an abscess. Cellulitis is commonly associated with diffuse swelling and edema in the peritonsillar region. An abscess causes varying degrees of trismus because of mass effect and involvement of the internal pterygoid muscle. Inferomedial displacement of the tonsil, contralateral shifting of the uvula, and ipsilateral cervical adenopathy are typically identified in patients with PTA.

The white blood cell count may be elevated. The throat culture will often document a streptococcal infection. Needle aspiration of purulent material is the diagnostic gold standard and useful for directing antibiotic therapy. CT scan of the neck with contrast can be used to differentiate PTA from peritonsillar cellulitis and delineate extension of the disease to adjacent structures. The reported sensitivity and specificity of CT scan for PTA are 100% and 75%, respectively.[22] Intraoral ultrasound has also been used but has demonstrated a lower sensitivity than CT scan.[22]

COMPLICATIONS

Most complications of PTA result from direct spread and invasion of adjacent tissue. Septicemia, parapharyngeal abscess, glottic edema, and airway obstruction are reported. The lateral pharyngeal recess provides a natural communication to the anterior chest which could result in mediastinitis, lung abscess, thrombophlebitis, or necrotizing fasciitis.

MANAGEMENT

There is no consensus on the management of PTA and several treatment options exist. All patients with PTA should receive IV hydration and parenteral antibiotics. Penicillin is the drug of choice. Clindamycin or a second- or third-generation cephalosporin are recommended in cases involving β-lactamase organisms. Similar cure rates have been documented in patients managed by I&D or 3-point permucosal needle aspiration. Needle aspiration and antibiotic therapy is effective in 85% to 90% of cases. Needle aspiration has several advantages. It can be performed safely in cooperative patients by emergency personnel, provides immediate relief of symptoms, and confirms diagnosis with minimal trauma. I&D has been documented to be more effective in rapidly relieving symptoms and may prevent recurrence of the disease.

▶ RETROPHARYNGEAL ABSCESS

RPA is a local infection with accumulation of pus in the prevertebral soft tissue of the neck; commonly seen in children aging between 2 and 6 years.[23] RPA frequently originates from infection of the nose, paranasal sinuses, or nasopharynx with subsequent spread to retropharyngeal lymph nodes. RPA can also result from direct inoculation of the space from penetrating oropharyngeal trauma or spread from contiguous spaces (parapharyngeal and submandibular).

ANATOMY AND PHYSIOLOGY

The retropharyngeal space is a pocket of connective tissue that extends from the base of the skull to the tracheal carina. It lies posterior to the pharynx and is bordered anteriorly by the buccopharyngeal fascia, posteriorly by the prevertebral fascia, and laterally by the carotid sheaths. It harbors two paramedian chains of lymphoid tissue that drain the nasopharynx, adenoids, and posterior paranasal sinuses. The lymphatic chains begin to atrophy around the third or fourth year of life. Fifty percent of cases of RPA occur between 6 and 12 months of age, and 96% occur in children younger than 6 years.[23,24] Bacterial infections of the areas drained by the retropharyngeal nodes may result in suppuration of the nodes and abscess formation.

ETIOLOGY

S. Aureus and group A hemolytic streptococci are the most common pathogens. *H. influenzae* and anaerobes (*Bacteroides, Peptostreptococcus,* and *Fusobacterium* spp.) are also pathogenic. The incidence of β-lactamase production is high, with one study reporting up to 22%.[25]

DIAGNOSTIC FINDINGS

There is usually a prodrome of nasopharyngitis progressing to the abrupt onset of high fever, dysphagia, refusal of feeding, severe throat pain, and neck pain or torticollis. Irritability, fever, and decreased appetite are described in infants and toddlers. Respirations may be labored; drooling and stridor may be present. Stiff neck with sore throat, dysphagia, stridor, and "hot potato" voice suggests retropharyngeal space infection. Meningismus may result from irritation of the paravertebral ligaments. Airway obstruction by RPA may mimic epiglottitis or croup, peritonsillar abscess, and infectious mononucleosis.

An elevated white cell count, with a left shift is noted, but is usually not needed for a therapeutic decision. Soft tissue lateral neck radiography will usually demonstrate retropharyngeal mass in stable patients. In children younger than 15 years, the prevertebral space is normally <7 mm anterior to C2 and <14 mm anterior to C6 or <40% of the anteroposterior diameter of the C3 or C4 vertebral bodies. Neck flexion during plain radiography can cause false-positive results.

IV contrast-enhanced CT scan of the neck is very sensitive at demonstrating RPAs and will provide further information on local structures.[25] Cultures and Gram's stain of purulent material obtained from incision and drainage is essential.

COMPLICATIONS

The most serious acute complications are airway obstruction and aspiration. The abscess may rupture into the esophagus, mediastinum, or lungs resulting in pneumonia, empyema, and mediastinitis. Blood vessels may be eroded resulting in severe hemorrhage. Spread of infection to adjacent spaces and structures may also occur resulting in mediastinitis, osteomyelitis, and jugular vein thrombosis. Inadequate drainage can allow reformation of the abscess.

MANAGEMENT

A standard approach to airway maintenance is vital since airway obstruction and aspiration can occur at any time. Patients require hospitalization for hydration, intravenous antibiotics, analgesia, and surgical drainage. The optimal antibiotic regimen has not been established. Most resources recommend use of a penicillinase-resistant penicillin with addition of clindamycin, metronidazole, and/or a third-generation cephalosporin for additional gram-negative coverage. One regimen includes intravenous penicillin G or nafcillin. A third-generation cephalosporin such as ceftriaxone or cefotaxime may also be added. Duration of treatment remains controversial. Emergent surgical intervention and drainage may be necessary with particular attention to the airway and ventilation.

▶ ORAL PIERCINGS

Piercing of the tongue, lips, and cheeks has become an increasingly popular form of body art among adolescents, particularly in the last 10 years. Because of the largely unregulated nature of the piercing profession, these piercings are often performed by unlicensed personnel with little knowledge of oral anatomy or the potentially serious medical conditions, which may result from the piercing. The tongue is the most frequently pierced oral structure. The type of piercing generally utilized consists of a stud with two balls screwed at each end.

Complications from oral piercing are reported in 17% to 70% of subjects and may be either acute (early) or chronic (late).[26] Acute complications usually arise within 24 hours and include severe bleeding, infection, pain, and swelling of the tongue, changes in speech, galvanic current generation between the jewelry and resident metallic fillings, and allergy to metal. Chronic complications include traumatic injury to the teeth such as chipping, fractures, and pulpal damage, localized tissue overgrowth, various mucogingival defects, and aspiration of the jewelry fragments. Life-threatening complications such as Ludwig's angina have been described. Transmission of hepatitis B and HIV has also been reported.[27]

Tongue inflammation should be treated with removal of the piercing, local debridement, antibiotic therapy, and chlorhexidine mouthwashes. Dental injuries and infections of the fascial planes and spaces of the oral cavity and neck (e.g., Ludwig's angina) should be treated as previously described.

REFERENCES

1. Martini FH, Timmons MJ, McKinley MP. The digestive system. In: Corey PF, ed. *Human Anatomy.* 3rd ed. New Jersey: Prentice Hall; 2000:656.

2. Andreasen JO, Ravn JJ. Epidemiology of traumatic dental injuries to primary and permanent teeth in a Danish population sample. *Int J Oral Surg.* 1972;1(5):235–239.

3. Kaste L, Gift H, Bhat M, et al. Prevalence of incisor trauma in persons 6 to 50 years of age: United States, 1988–1991. *J Dent Res.* 1996;75 Spec No:696–705.

4. Forsberg CM, Tedestam G. Etiological and predisposing factors related to traumatic injuries to permanent teeth. *Swed Dent J.* 1993;17(5):183–190.

5. Becker DB, Needleman HL, Kotelchuck M. Child abuse and dentistry: orofacial trauma and its recognition by dentists. *J Am Dent Assoc.* 1978;97(1):24–28.

6. da Fonseca MA, Feigal RJ, ten Bensel RW. Dental aspects of 1248 cases of child maltreatment on file at a major county hospital. *Pediatr Dent.* 1992;14(3):152–157.

7. Vinson DR. The Ellis fracture: an anachronistic eponym in dentistry. *Ann Emerg Med.* 1999;33(5):599–600.

8. Sennhenn-Kirchner S, Jacobs HG. Traumatic injuries to the primary dentition and effects on the permanent successors— a clinical follow-up study. *Dent Traumatol.* 2006;22(5): 237–241.

9. Cooper SA, Engel J, Ladov M. Analgesic efficacy of an ibuprofen-codeine combination. *Pharmacotherapy.* 1982;2(3): 162–167.

10. Hellmann JR, Shott SR, Gootee MJ. Impalement injuries of the palate in children: review of 131 cases. *Int J Pediatr Otorhinolaryngol.* 1993;26(2):157–163.

11. Randall DA, Kang DR. Current management of penetrating injuries of the soft palate. *Otolaryngol Head Neck Surg.* 2006;135(3):356–360.

12. Soose RJ, Simons JP, Mandell DL. Evaluation and management of pediatric oropharyngeal trauma. *Arch Otolaryngol Head Neck Surg.* 2006;132(4):446–451.

13. Suskind DL, Tavill MA, Keller JL, et al. Management of the carotid artery following penetrating injuries of the soft palate. *Int J Pediatr Otorhinolaryngol.* 1997;14;39(1):41–49.

14. Altieri M, Brasch L, Getson P. Antibiotic prophylaxis in intraoral wounds. *Am J Emerg Med.* 1998;4(6):507–510.

15. Kuriyama T, Karasawa T, Nakagawa K, et al. Bacteriologic features and antimicrobial susceptibility in isolates from orofacial odontogenic infections. *Oral Surg Oral Med Oral Pathol Oral Radiol Endod.* 2000;90(5):600–608.

16. Stefanopoulos PK, Kolokotronis AE. The clinical significance of anaerobic bacteria in acute orofacial odontogenic infections. *Oral Surg Oral Med Oral Pathol Oral Radiol Endod.* 2004;98(4):398–408.

17. Oh TJ, Eber R, Wang HL. Periodontal diseases in the child and adolescent. *J Clin Periodontol.* 2002;29(5):400–410.

18. Amir J, Harel L, Smetana Z, et al. Treatment of herpes simplex gingivostomatitis with aciclovir in children: a randomised double blind placebo controlled study. *BMJ.* 1997;314(7097):1800–1803.

19. Gerber MA. Diagnosis and treatment of pharyngitis in children. *Pediatr Clin North Am.* 2005;52(3):729–747.

20. Schraff S, McGinn JD, Derkay CS. Peritonsillar abscess in children: a 10-year review of diagnosis and management. *Int J Pediatr Otorhinolaryngol.* 2001;57(3):213–218.

21. Brook I. Microbiology and management of peritonsillar, retropharyngeal, and parapharyngeal abscesses. *J Oral Maxillofac Surg.* 2004;62(12):1545–1550.

22. Scott PM, Loftus WK, Kew J, et al. Diagnosis of peritonsillar infections: a prospective study of ultrasound, computerized tomography and clinical diagnosis. *J Laryngol Otol.* 1999;113(3):229–232.

23. Tannebaum RD. Adult retropharyngeal abscess: a case report and review of the literature. *J Emerg Med.* 1996;14(2):147–158.

24. Coulthard M, Isaacs D. Retropharyngeal abscess. *Arch Dis Child.* 1991;66(10):1227–1230.

25. Ungkanont K, Yellon RF, Weissman JL, et al. Head and neck space infections in infants and children. *Otolaryngol Head Neck Surg.* 1995;112(3):375–382.

26. Levin L, Zadik Y, Becker T. Oral and dental complications of intra-oral piercing. *Dent Traumatol.* 2005;21(6):341–343.

27. De Moor RJ, De Witte AM, Delmé KI, et al. Dental and oral complications of lip and tongue piercings. *Br Dent J.* 2005; 199(8):506–509.

SECTION XV

OPHTHALMOLOGIC EMERGENCIES

CHAPTER 92

Eye Trauma

Jeremiah J. Johnson and Stephen A. Colucciello

▶ HIGH-YIELD FACTS

- A history of exposure to power tools or metal striking metal should raise the suspicion of an intraocular foreign body.
- Children with sickle cell disease or coagulopathy are more likely to suffer complications associated with a hyphema.
- Visual acuity is the vital sign of the eye and should be documented in every child with an ocular injury or visual complaint.
- Be concerned about the appearance of a corneal abrasion in the absence of known trauma as this may represent herpetic dendrites rather than corneal abrasions.
- Obtain an ophthalmology consultation in the emergency department on all patients with hyphemas, suspected globe rupture, or significant visual impairment.
- A caustic injury to the eye (acid or alkali) is one of the few situations in which treatment must occur prior to examination and visual acuity testing. Copious irrigation with normal saline takes precedence over all but lifesaving interventions and should begin at the time and site of exposure.

Ocular trauma is the leading cause of noncongenital blindness in individuals younger than 20 years. Every year in the United States approximately 840 000 children injure an eye with an estimated cost of more than $88 million. Motor vehicle crashes account for the majority of hospitalized eye injuries. Recreational and sports injuries are more prevalent in the pediatric population than they are in adults. In addition, ocular trauma may occur as a consequence of child abuse. In preschool children, most injuries are due to falls, motor vehicle collisions, and accidental blows to the eye. In adolescents and teenagers, ocular trauma occurs twice as often in male patients.[1] This is also the age group in which sports-related injuries become an important factor, especially baseball, ice hockey, racquet sports, soccer, archery, and fishing injuries.[2] Fireworks and gun-related eye injuries have decreased in incidence in the last 10 years but remain significant causes of pediatric eye injury.[3,4]

▶ HISTORY

Obtain a full history and note any preexisting eye abnormality and whether or not the child normally wears glasses or contacts. A history of exposure to power tools or metal striking metal should raise the suspicion of an intraocular foreign body. Inquire as to whether the child is having double vision. If so, determine whether the diplopia is monocular or binocular. Monocular double vision implies a problem with the lens

or retina, whereas double vision that occurs only with both eyes open is associated with periorbital fractures, extraocular muscle injury, or palsy.

Past medical history is also important. Children with sickle cell disease or coagulopathy are more likely to suffer complications associated with a hyphema. Children with osteogenisis imperfecta have fragile sclera and are more prone to open globe injuries from trauma.[5]

▶ PHYSICAL EXAMINATION

The physical examination of the eye should be performed early in the emergency department (ED) course, after any life-threatening injuries have been excluded or addressed. Progressive lid edema can prevent an adequate examination of the eye.

VISUAL ACUITY

Visual acuity is the vital sign of the eye and should be documented in every verbal and conscious child with an ocular injury or visual complaint. In trauma, the best predictor of ultimate visual outcome is initial visual acuity. Assessment should be done *before* intervention, except in the case of major trauma or caustic exposure. Topical anesthetic given before testing visual acuity decreases pain and blepharospasm and assists in diagnosis (Fig. 92–1).

If the child wears glasses, measure acuity with the glasses on. If the glasses have been lost or damaged, correct refractive error by having the child look through a pinhole in a piece of paper. Lack of correction with pinhole testing suggests significant pathology.

Evaluate preliterate children with an Allen or "E" chart and move a toy or a light to test the young child's ability to track with each eye. If the child is unable to read an eye chart, ask him or her to finger count at 6 ft; if that fails, due to visual loss, assess for light perception.

Test visual fields in older children in the usual fashion. Younger children will glance toward a toy brought into the field of view. Assess for symmetrical ocular motion and symptoms of diplopia.

ADNEXAE

To avoid missing subtle signs of trauma, begin the examination with the lids and periorbital structures and work centrally

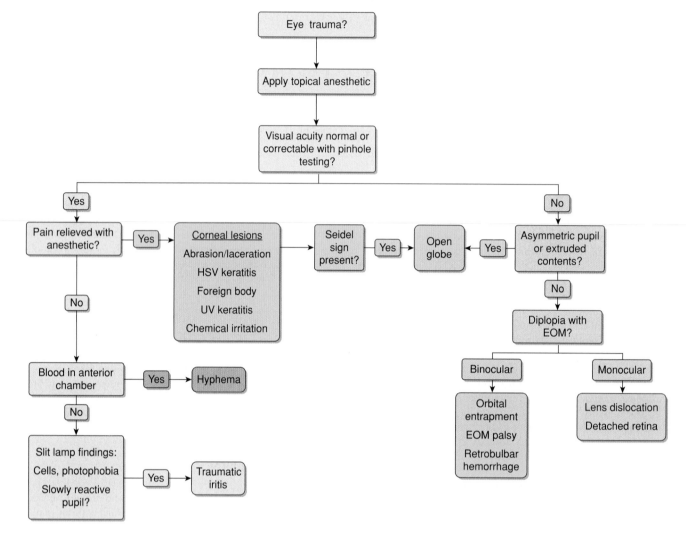

Figure 92–1. Diagnostic algorithm for ocular trama.

in a focused fashion. Examine the lids for swelling or pene-trating injury and inspect for ecchymosis. Retract swollen lids with a finger, being careful not to put pressure on the affected eye. Lid retractors or bent paper clips can be used in the case of massive lid edema. Periorbital soft tissue air indicates fracture into a sinus or nasal antrum and is most commonly seen with a blowout fracture. Examine the eye for normal lacrimal drainage. Lid lacerations involving the medial third of the eyelid often involve the cannilicular system and injured ducts may require stenting by an ophthalmologist. *Epiphora*, tears spilling over the lid margins, may be secondary to injury of the canalicular system.

CONJUNCTIVA AND SCLERA

Examine the conjunctiva for injection and presence of ciliary flush around the iris (perilimbal injection), which may indicate iritis. Check for chemosis (edema of the conjunctiva), which can be seen in globe rupture. Look at the sclera carefully for any disruption or penetration. The location of any subconjunctival hemorrhage should be documented.

PUPILS, IRIS, LENS, AND ANTERIOR CHAMBER

Evaluate the pupils for any asymmetry or irregularity. A pointing pupil indicates iris detachment and possible extrusion (Fig. 92–2). Congenital anisocoria may be detected by obtaining history from the parents or by checking a photograph of the child to see if the asymmetry was preexisting. Pupillary dilatation may occur with direct blows to the eye (posttraumatic mydriasis), with anticholinergic medication, or with a third nerve palsy. A dilated pupil in a conscious patient is not due to a herniation syndrome. Pilocarpine drops will constrict a pupil that is dilated secondary to a third nerve lesion but will have no effect on pharmacologic mydriasis. The emergency physician should also never overlook the possibility of a glass eye.

The lens should be transparent and the margins should not be visible. Examine the anterior chamber for abnormal shallowness or depth. To specifically assess optic nerve function, perform the swinging flashlight test. Swing the flashlight from eye to eye. A pupil that initially dilates when illuminated by light (even if it later constricts) has a sensory (afferent) defect (Marcus Gunn pupil).

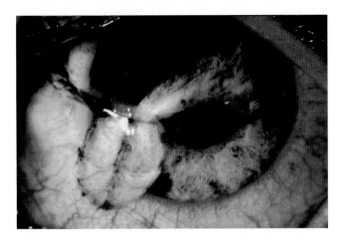

Figure 92-2. Ruptured globe with extravasation of ocular contents. (With permission from Khaw PT, Shah P, Elkington AR. Injury to the eye. *BMJ*. 2004;328:36–38.)

FUNDOSCOPIC EXAMINATION AND INTRAOCULAR PRESSURE

The vitreous should be clear, allowing visualization of the retina. However, visualization of the retina does not completely exclude retinal detachment, as many cases are anterior and thus undetectable with a direct ophthalmoscope. Do not measure intraocular pressure if globe rupture or penetrating injury is apparent, as this may herniate ocular contents. Normal intraocular pressure is between 15 and 20 mm Hg.

▶ EQUIPMENT

The basic equipment for a standard pediatric eye examination includes the following:

- Visual acuity charts (Snellen and Allen "E" chart)
- Pen light
- Ophthalmoscope
- Wood's lamp
- Slit lamp
- Ocular spud
- Fluorescein strips
- Shiotz tonometer or Tono-Pen
- Morgan lens
- Metal eye shields

▶ MEDICATIONS

Topical anesthetics, such as 0.5% tetracaine or proparacaine, have an onset of action within 1 minute and typically last for 15 to 20 minutes. Topical anesthetics should never be prescribed for home use, as prolonged lack of sensation and loss of normal protective reflexes may lead to corneal damage. Cycloplegics such as homatropine (2%–5%) and cyclopentolate hydrochloride (1%–2%) dilate the eye and decrease pain by overcoming ciliary spasm. Always document the use of such medications to avoid later confusion regarding the etiology of

an unreactive pupil. Avoid atropine due to its extremely long duration of action.

Steroids are useful in some inflammatory conditions but may lead to glaucoma, cataract formation, and acceleration of fungal and herpetic infections, resulting in visual loss. Never use ocular steroids without first consulting an ophthalmologist. Evaluate the need for tetanus prophylaxis in all patients with ocular injuries. To administer medications to young or uncooperative children, lay them down in a dark room, secure the head, and place the drop in the medial canthus. The child will open the eyes and the medication will reach the conjunctiva.

▶ SPECIFIC INJURIES

LID LACERATIONS

Minor lacerations, superficial to the tarsal plate, that do not involve the lid margins and with no suggestion of injury to deeper structures may be repaired by the emergency physician. Other lacerations require specialty repair.

Consider the possibility of globe penetration or injury to deeper structures whenever an eyelid is lacerated. Because eyelids have no subcutaneous fat, the appearance of fat in a wound suggests underlying globe injury. Significant lacerations involving the medial third of the upper or lower lids may involve the lacrimal system and should be referred to an ophthalmologist for repair. One way to detect injury of the lacrimal system is to instill fluorescein in the eye and then use a Wood's lamp to check the wound for fluorescence.

Injuries to the lid margins are also problematic as they may result in deformity of the lids and abnormal lid movement if repair is not precise. If the levator palpebrae muscle is injured and not repaired, posttraumatic ptosis will result. Trauma involving the tarsal plate (which only exists in the upper lid as a dense band of fibrous tissue) indicates a complex laceration. Plastic surgery or ophthalmologic consultation should be obtained for repair of any of these lacerations described above. For isolated eyelid lacerations, delayed surgical repair of 12 to 36 hours will not affect the outcome of closure and may allow a better repair due to decreased swelling.[6]

SUBCONJUNCTIVAL HEMORRHAGE

The most important aspect of the evaluation of subconjunctival hemorrhage is to rule out other, more serious injury. With significant blunt trauma, a subconjunctival hemorrhage may hide a scleral rupture or provide evidence of periorbital fracture. Clues to severe globe injury include decreased visual acuity, severe pain, photophobia, and extension of hemorrhage beyond the limbus. Evaluate for the presence of Seidel's sign indicating open globe injury with fluorescein (see later). Consider the possibility of a periorbital fracture in patients with traumatic subconjunctival hemorrhage. Lateral hemorrhages in particular are frequently associated with zygomatic fractures (tripod fractures).

In the more common instances when the etiology involves minor trauma with no evidence of severe globe injury, coughing or sneezing spells, or spontaneous subconjunctival hemorrhage, parents should be reassured, told that spontaneous resolution will occur over 2 weeks, and informed of the dramatic color changes that may occur.

CORNEAL ABRASION

Children with corneal abrasions complain of a foreign body sensation, pain, and photophobia and present with marked blepharospasm and a red eye. Infants may present with only crying. Use tetracaine or proparacaine prior to examination to decrease blepharospasm and pain.

A few drops of fluorescein placed in the conjunctival sac followed by examination under a Wood's lamp or the cobalt blue light of a slit lamp will result in marked fluorescence of corneal abrasions. Make sure that no foreign body is present and that there is no evidence of penetration of the sclera. Multiple vertical striations (ice-rink sign) usually indicate a retained foreign body under the upper lid. Careful examination with lid eversion should reveal the offending agent.

Be concerned about the appearance of a corneal abrasion in the absence of known trauma. This may represent herpetic dendrites rather than corneal abrasions. If this finding is present, test to see whether the corneal reflex is equally brisk in each eye by gently touching the cornea with a wisp of cotton (either before topical anesthesia or after the anesthesia has worn off). Herpetic lesions may decrease the corneal reflex in the involved eye. Patients may have concurrent oral or genital herpes. In the case of herpes keratitis, ophthalmologic consultation is required.

Treat corneal abrasions with ophthalmic antibiotics to prevent secondary infection. The multiple layers of the cornea normally provide a barrier against infection from common organisms such as *Pseudomonas* sp. and *Staphylococcus aureus*, and injury to this barrier may lead to secondary infection. One drop of antibiotic solution applied every 4 to 6 hours for 4 days is sufficient. Ointment in young children and infants can be given at the same frequency by applying a 1-cm length inside the lower eyelid. Several drops of a mydriatic agent such as cyclopentolate 1% or homatropine 5% applied two to three times a day for 1 to 2 days will decrease ciliary spasm and provide comfort.

Eye patching is not recommended for mild to moderate corneal abrasions. It has not been shown to speed healing or decrease pain, and it may increase infection risk if prophylactic antibiotics are not given due to the patch.[7,8] Corneal abrasions associated with Bell's palsy or other causes of incomplete lid closure should be patched to protect the eye from further injury. Any patch should be rechecked and removed in 24 hours. Some centers suggest that all abrasions should be rechecked in 24 to 48 hours to assess healing. Others tell patients to return if they are still symptomatic after 48 hours. Symptoms and redness should gradually decrease each day. If not, secondary infection, retained foreign body, or corneal erosion should be suspected.

TRAUMATIC IRITIS

Patients with posttraumatic iritis usually present 1 to 2 days after blunt trauma to the eye, complaining of photophobia, pain, and tearing. They often have marked blepharospasm and perilimbal injection (ciliary flush). Test for pain on accommodation by having the patient first look across the room at a distant object and then quickly focus on the examiner's finger held several inches away. If near gaze causes pain, there is a high probability of iritis. The pupil may be large or small. Posttraumatic miosis develops secondary to spasm of the pupillary sphincter muscle, whereas posttraumatic mydriasis results when sphincter fibers are ruptured. Slit lamp examination will usually reveal cells in the anterior chamber, the hallmark of iritis.

Treat with a long-acting topical cycloplegic, such as 5% homatropine, four times a day for 1 week, oral anti-inflammatory medication, and dark sunglasses to decrease pain. Symptoms may persist for up to 1 week. Although ocular steroids decrease inflammation, prescribe them only after consultation with the ophthalmologist who will see the patient in follow-up.

HYPHEMA

A hyphema is defined by blood in the anterior chamber (see Fig. 92–3). Hyphemas are almost always secondary to blunt trauma. The blood may layer out or may present initially as a diffuse red haze that takes hours to settle. Hyphemas are described by the percentage of the anterior chamber that is filled with blood. A 100% hyphema, known as an "eight ball," may cause complete loss of light perception. Hyphemas are easily overlooked in cases of massive lid edema, and for this reason, early lid retraction is necessary for the diagnosis. Older children with hyphemas usually complain of pain, whereas young children may present with somnolence. However, decreased mental status should not be attributed to the hyphema until intracranial injury has been ruled out. Other injuries associated with hyphema include lens dislocation, vitreous hemorrhage, and retinal damage. A large untreated hyphema may result in permanent corneal staining with subsequent loss of visual acuity and deprivational amblyopia. Often it is not the initial hyphema that causes serious morbidity but the rebleed that can occur in several days as the clot breaks down. Rebleeding occurs

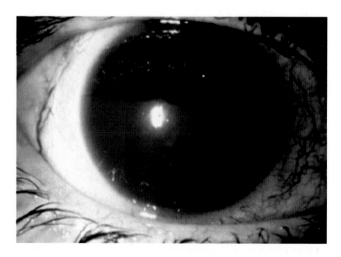

Figure 92–3. Hyphema. (With permission from Khaw PT, Shah P, Elkington AR. Injury to the eye. *BMJ*. 2004;328: 36–38.)

in up to 16% to 25% of patients and may obstruct the aqueous outflow system, causing increased intraocular pressure. Patients with rebleeding have a significantly worse prognosis. Because hemoglobinopathies, particularly sickle cell disease, sickle cell trait, and sickle thalassemia, predispose to rebleeding and other complications, it is critical to determine whether any of these conditions exist in the child with hyphema.

Initial treatment involves bed rest with the head elevated at 30 degrees. Shield the involved eye, taking care not to touch or apply pressure to the eye. Obtain an ophthalmology consultation in the ED on all patients with hyphemas.

The subsequent treatment of hyphemas is controversial. Traditionally, all patients have been admitted and placed on strict bed rest. However, older children and reliable adults are now being treated with bed rest at home if they have only a microhyphema (circulation of red blood cells only, with no layering) and if daily reexamination for 5 days is possible. Some specialists utilize antifibrinolytics such as aminocaproic acid to reduce rebleeding.[9] The decision as to use of mydriatics, ocular steroids, osmotic agents, or acetazolamide should be left to the ophthalmologist. Acetazolamide or osmotic agents are contraindicated in patients with sickle cell disease due to increased risk of bleeding. Patients should avoid aspirin or other platelet-active medications, as these increase the risk of rebleeding.

LENS INJURY

Blunt ocular trauma may result in lens subluxation or dislocation. Subluxation may cause monocular diplopia, whereas dislocation results in profoundly blurred vision. The lens may sublux either posteriorly or anteriorly, resulting in a deep or shallow anterior chamber and a visible lens margin. *Iridodonesis* is a shimmering or shaking of the iris provoked by rapidly changing gaze and is associated with posterior dislocation.

Acute blunt trauma to the eye can cause a cataract if the capsule of the lens is disrupted. The lens subsequently absorbs fluid, taking on a cloudy appearance. Lens injuries should be referred to an ophthalmologist.

RETINAL INJURY

Retinal trauma often occurs in conjunction with other eye injuries. Older children with retinal injury complain of light flashes or a "curtain" over the visual field. Central vision will be spared if the macula remains unaffected.

Fundoscopy may reveal a variety of hemorrhage patterns or may be normal with direct fundoscopy. Preretinal hemorrhages are boat shaped, with a horizontal "deck," whereas superficial hemorrhages are flame shaped. Deep hemorrhages are round, with a purple-gray color. The shaken baby syndrome causes linear retinal hemorrhages and associated exudates. Any suspicion of retinal detachment or injury requires ophthalmology consultation.

RETROBULBAR HEMORRHAGE

Bleeding behind the globe may result in deficits in extraocular motion and lead to proptosis or bulging of the eye. Subsequent compromise of the optic nerve produces an afferent pupillary defect (Marcus Gunn pupil). In cases of severe proptosis, progressively worsening vision, and potential optic nerve injury surgical decompression may be necessary. In rare instances, a lid release procedure (lateral canthotomy) may be required in the ED.

CONJUNCTIVAL AND SCLERAL LACERATIONS

Perform a slit lamp examination on all children with conjunctival lacerations to assess for deeper scleral violation. Scleral rupture from blunt trauma often occurs at the insertions of the intraocular muscles or at the limbus. Clues to the presence of scleral disruption include decreased visual acuity, an abnormal anterior chamber, low intraocular pressure (<6), and a positive Seidel's test. To perform the Seidel's test for scleral laceration, place fluorescein on the cornea and observe the suspicious area under the cobalt blue light of the slit lamp. A swirling dilution of fluorescein secondary to leaking aqueous denotes scleral disruption.[10] If a scleral laceration is seen, tonometry is contraindicated. The additional pressure against the eye from the tonometer can extrude the iris.

Treat small conjunctival lacerations with topical antibiotic drops alone. Sutures are not usually necessary. If the patient has deeper injury (i.e., scleral laceration), place an eye shield on the child, administer intravenous antibiotics, provide adequate sedation, and obtain an ophthalmology consultation.

CORNEAL AND SCLERAL FOREIGN BODIES

Patients with a superficial foreign body are in pain. Their eye is usually red and tearing, and verbal children will complain of "something in my eye." Corneal abrasions, however, will present in a similar mode.

Perform a thorough examination in all patients by doubly everting the lids after anesthetizing the cornea. This may be done with a cotton swab placed on the middle of the upper lid and folding the lid upward over the swab. Look carefully for a foreign body on the inner surface of the lids. Attempt removal with a cotton applicator soaked in topical anesthetic. In older cooperative children, remove more tenacious foreign bodies under slit lamp guidance using an eye spud or 25-gauge needle on a tuberculin syringe. A foreign body sensation may persist even after removal due to an underlying corneal abrasion. Iron-containing foreign bodies may leave rust rings that may result in photophobia and decreased visual acuity. Some emergency physicians refer these to a specialist, whereas others use an ophthalmic burr to remove superficial rings.

After removing a foreign body, check for additional foreign bodies and abrasions. Instill both a mydriatic agent and a topical antibiotic and recheck the child in 24 hours. Prescribe appropriate analgesia including narcotic agents if appropriate. If a foreign body penetrates the corneal stroma or the sclera (Fig. 92–4), consult an ophthalmologist for evaluation in the ED.

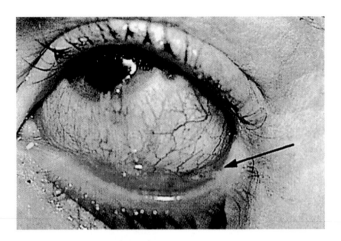

Figure 92–4. Intraocular foreign body. Note foreign body at arrow. Also note perforation of globe with asymmetric pupil and leaking vitreous. (With permission from Khaw PT, Shah P, Elkington AR. Injury to the eye. *BMJ.* 2004;328: 36–38.)

INTRAOCULAR FOREIGN BODY

Intraocular foreign bodies are vision-threatening injuries that may be easily overlooked. The key to identification of an intraocular foreign body is to consider it. Ask specific questions about risk factors. Exposure to power tools and metal striking metal, such as a hammer on a nail, predisposes to occult intraocular foreign body.

Certain foreign bodies place the patient at greater risk than others. Iron (siderosis) and copper (chalcosis) are particularly toxic to the eye, whereas glass and plastic are less inflammatory. Organic foreign bodies pose a high risk for intraocular infection.

Children with intraocular foreign bodies may have decreased visual acuity, pupillary distortion, and relatively little pain. A foreign body penetration through the cornea may damage the iris, causing a teardrop-shaped pupil that will "point" to the perforation site.

A number of imaging modalities can detect intraocular foreign bodies. Although larger metallic objects may be seen by routine radiography, a computed tomography scan of the orbit provides greater resolution if the foreign body is small. Ocular ultrasound is highly sensitive for both metallic and nonmetallic penetrations. Magnetic resonance imaging (MRI) accurately detects organic, plastic, and glass particles but may cause further injury if mistakenly used in the case of metal objects. In such cases, the MRI magnet may move the foreign body, causing greater damage.

Cover the involved eye with a metal eye shield and keep the child at rest. Administer broad-spectrum intravenous antibiotics, such as vancomycin and ceftazidime.[11]

Topical antibiotics are not indicated with penetrating globe injuries and, in particular, antibiotic ointments should be avoided as they can produce intraocular granulomas and obscure examination.

Should a child with penetrating globe injury require emergency intubation, some authorities suggest a nondepolarizing blocker, such as rocuronium, in place of succinylcholine. Succinylcholine and ketamine may increase intraocular pressure and could theoretically extrude intraocular contents. However, if a difficult airway is anticipated, then succinylcholine may be the agent of choice.[6]

FOREIGN BODIES IN SITU

Foreign bodies that protrude from the eye, such as a nail or wire, must be left in place and removed in the operating room. Cover the affected eye with a cup to prevent further manipulation of the eye and patch the unaffected eye closed to prevent extraocular movement.

CHEMICAL INJURIES TO THE EYE

A caustic injury to the eye (acid or alkali) is one of the few situations in which treatment must occur prior to examination and visual acuity testing. Copious irrigation with normal saline takes precedence over all but lifesaving interventions and should begin at the time and site of exposure. Extent of caustic injury is dependent on the quantity, the pH, and the duration of the exposure (i.e., time to irrigation). Alkali injuries result in the most serious damage to the eye by causing liquefaction necrosis with saponification of ocular tissues and deep penetration. Acids produce a coagulation necrosis resulting in a protein barrier that blocks further penetration. Complications of caustic injuries include blindness, perforation, corneal neovascularization, secondary glaucoma, cataract formation, and retinal damage.

Begin irrigation in the prehospital setting immediately after injury. Upon arrival at the ED, the child may require sedation with a rapidly acting intramuscular or intravenous agent to allow irrigation of the eye, but topical anesthesia alone may be adequate. If particulate matter remains in the eye, pour liter bottles of irrigant into the eye while retracting the lids to wash the particles out. Perform double lid eversion to expose the fornices and irrigate or swab out any caustic particulate matter. When irrigating the eyes, a Morgan lens (a contact lens connected to intravenous tubing) is useful. An alternative to the Morgan lens is a nasal oxygen cannula placed on the bridge of the nose, which can be connected to intravenous bags of normal saline. This allows bilateral irrigation of the eyes through the nasal prongs.

Never attempt to neutralize acids with alkalis, or vice versa, because the resultant heat release will further damage the eye. Lavage the eyes for at least 20 minutes, ideally with 2 L of normal saline. Irrigation may be beneficial for up to 24 hours after alkali exposure. In cases of serious alkali exposure, continuously irrigate the eyes until stopped by the ophthalmologist. Use litmus paper to check the pH in the conjunctival sac after 20 minutes of irrigation, and continue irrigation until the pH is between 7.4 and 7.6. If irrigation is stopped, recheck the pH after 10 minutes to ensure a stable level.

Hydrofluoric acid exposure is a unique situation and may require irrigation with a magnesium oxide solution. Consult a poison center for the latest recommendations.

ULTRAVIOLET KERATITIS

Ultraviolet keratitis occurs when children are exposed to prolonged glare from snow, water, or white sand or when they stare at an eclipse. Unprotected vision of an eclipse can also cause severe retinal damage and blindness. Older children who watch a welder's torch or use tanning booths without special glasses may also suffer this injury. Photophobia and eye pain usually occur 8 to 12 hours after exposure and, for this reason, patients with ultraviolet keratitis generally present at night. They exhibit both scleral and perilimbal injection accompanied by tearing and blepharospasm. Slit lamp examination using fluorescein shows thousands of punctate, shallow lesions on the cornea (keratitis), which looks as if it had been sandblasted. Treat with cycloplegia and oral analgesia. Ultraviolet keratitis is usually bilateral and generally heals in 24 to 48 hours.

THERMAL BURNS

Because of reflex blinking, lids are more often damaged from thermal injury than is the globe. Eyelashes and eyebrows are often burned. Evaluate for corneal injury with the slit lamp in the usual fashion with and without fluorescein staining, and apply topical antibiotics to burned lids. Third-degree burns to the eye and periorbital tissues require admission.

▶ CONCLUSIONS

The emergency physician is often the first and only physician to evaluate ocular trauma. Proper identification depends primarily on the consideration of the potential for injury, and on the performance of a thorough, systematic examination. Unfortunate sequelae can often be avoided through timely identification and appropriate specialty consultation. Any eye injury regardless of acuity should be considered an opportunity for physicians to inform parents and patients about protective eyewear and risk reduction behavior.

REFERENCES

1. Brophy M, Sinclair S, Hosteler SG, Xiang H. Pediatric eye injury-related hospitalizations in the United States. *Pediatrics.* 2006;117:e1263–e1271.
2. McGwin G Jr, Owsley C. Incidence of emergency department-treated eye injury in the Unitied States. *Arch Ophthalmol.* 2005;123:662–666.
3. McGwin G Jr, Xie A, Owsley C. Gun related eye injury in the United States, 1993–2002. *Ophthalmic Epidemiol.* 2006;13:15–21.
4. Witsaman RJ, Comstock RD, Smith GA. Pediatric fireworks related injuries in the United States: 1990–2003. *Pediatrics.* 2006;118:293–303.
5. Pirouzian A, O'Halloran H, Scher C, et al. Traumatic and spontaneous scleral rupture and uveal prolapse in osteogenisis imperfecta. *J Pediatr Ophthalmol Strabismus.* 2007;44:315–317.
6. Salvin J. Systematic approach to pediatric ocular trauma. *Curr Opin Ophthal.* 2007;18:366–372.
7. Burnette DD. Opthalmology. In: Marx JA, ed. *Rosen's Emergency Medicine: Concepts and Clinical Practice.* Philadelphia,PA: CV Mosby; 2006:70.
8. Turner AR. Patching for corneal abrasion. *Cochrane Database Syst Rev.* 2006;(2):CD004764.
9. Rocha KM, Martins EN, Melo LA Jr, et al. Outpatient management of traumatic hyphema in children: prospective evaluation. *J AAPOS.* 2004;8:357–361.
10. Pokhrel PK, Loftus SA. Ocular emergencies. *Am Fam Physician.* 2007;76:829–836.
11. Waheed NK, Young LH. Intraocular foreign body related endophthalmitis. *Int Opthalmol Clin.* 47:165–171.

CHAPTER 93

Eye Emergencies in Childhood

Lauren P. Ortega, Katherine M. Konzen, and Ghazala Q. Sharieff

▶ HIGH-YIELD FACTS

- Normal visual acuity is 20/40 in a 3-year-old, 20/30 in a 4-year-old, and 20/20 in a 5- to 6-year-old child.
- Steroids should not be used for patients with iritis or keratitis until herpes simplex is excluded.
- Glaucoma should be suspected in patients who have eye pain and nausea and vomiting. Bilateral eye pressures should be checked immediately.
- Neonates with suspected gonococcal conjunctivitis should undergo a complete sepsis work-up, including a lumbar puncture. These patients should be admitted for intravenous antibiotics.
- Physical examination of patients with iritis reveals a miotic pupil, perilimbal injection, and an aqueous flare and cells on slit lamp examination.
- Chemical alkali burns to the eye can result in liquefactive necrosis and should be irrigated until the eye pH is between 6 and 8.

Children with eye disorders often come to the emergency department (ED). It is imperative that the emergency physician performs a complete eye examination in order to avoid overlooking potentially debilitating ophthalmologic injuries. The physician must remember certain important guidelines when facing patients with ocular disease.

- The cardinal rules of resuscitation are *A*irway, *B*reathing, and *C*irculation. In patients with multiple trauma or severe systemic disease, the life-threatening conditions must be evaluated and managed first. The eye must be protected from further damage. In patients with blunt head trauma, the mechanism of injury must be considered and treated appropriately. Problems should be anticipated ahead of time.
- A thorough and complete history must be taken. Have there been previous eye problems or surgeries? Are there underlying health problems? Does the patient wear glasses or contact lenses? If a traumatic injury has occurred, when and where did it occur? Who saw it? What type of instrument was involved? Who else was involved? What was done for the patient prior to arrival in the ED? In the absence of trauma, is eye pain present? Has there been eye discharge or exposure to others with similar conditions? Has there been use of systemic or topical medications?
- The visual acuity in both eyes must always be checked. Information about the unaffected eye can help guide one in the assessment of the affected eye.

- A general physical examination should be performed and rapport should be built with the child. Physicians should look for other underlying injuries or signs of systemic illness. The eye examination should be performed in a logical, methodical manner. Patients should be observed for any facial asymmetry. Toys or other objects that hold the interest of the child and allow proper evaluation of the visual fields should be used. The eye should be touched and dilated only after a thorough systemic examination, and only if indicated.
- If the possibility of a globe perforation exists, manipulation of the eye should not be performed. A metal shield should be used to protect the eye; a pressure patch is contraindicated. If there is concomitant head trauma, pupils should not be dilated.
- Physicians must know when to stop and when to consult an ophthalmologist.

▶ PHYSICAL EXAMINATION OF THE EYE AND DIFFERENTIAL CONSIDERATIONS

A thorough and systematic eye examination is divided into six major categories: vision, lids and orbit, anterior segment, pupils and extraocular movements, posterior segment, and intraocular pressure.

VISION

Some method of testing visual acuity must be available for both preverbal and verbal children. For very young children, the ability to focus on an object such as a toy may give a rough assessment of visual acuity. A newborn can fixate on a close object and a 1-month-old infant should be able to follow a moving object. For older children, Snellen letters or Allen figures are useful to check visual acuity in both eyes. Normal visual acuity is 20/40 in a 3-year-old, 20/30 in a 4-year-old, and 20/20 in a 5- to 6-year-old child. Vision can be impaired from any obstruction of the visual pathway.

LIDS AND ORBIT

The lids must be examined by testing the ability to raise and lower the eyes and noting any erythema, edema, lacerations, or ecchymosis. Children with periorbital cellulitis will often have significant edema and erythema of both the upper and lower eyelids. The upper lid must be everted to rule out the presence of a foreign body by firmly grasping the lashes at the lid margin and everting the lid against countertraction at the superior tarsal margin using a cotton-tip applicator. Lacerations involving the medial canthus may result in a lacrimal duct injury and should be repaired by an ophthalmologist.

Examination of the orbit includes palpation for defects in the orbital bony structure or for subcutaneous emphysema. Orbital fractures are often accompanied by ecchymosis, lid swelling, proptosis, and limitation in extraocular movements. Herniation and entrapment of the inferior rectus muscle within the orbital floor fracture results in paralysis of upward gaze. Sinus fractures may be associated with subcutaneous emphysema. Physicians should note the presence of exophthalmos or enophthalmos.

ANTERIOR SEGMENT

Inspect the sclera and conjunctiva for swelling, erythema, foreign bodies, hemorrhage, or discharge. Diseases of the cornea and conjunctiva are divided into two main categories of infection or trauma. The history should lead one to the most likely problem. Infections are of bacterial, viral, or fungal etiologies. Conjunctival infections often begin unilaterally but may spread to the other eye within a few days. Crusting and exudate are usually present. In North America, the most common corneal infection causing permanent visual impairment is herpes simplex. Throughout the rest of the world, the most common agent is trachoma. Traumatic injuries to the cornea should be considered in even the youngest of children and can be the cause of a crying infant. Fluorescein examination for a corneal abrasion may be appropriate during the initial examination. Evaluate the corneal light reflex for both briskness and adequacy of response. Self-inflicted thermal wounds from curling irons, microwave popcorn bags, or other mechanism should be thoroughly evaluated.

The anterior chamber comprises the aqueous humor, iris, and lens. Acute iritis (anterior uveitis) is rare in children and may be associated with juvenile rheumatoid arthritis or sarcoidosis. One should consider the possibility of iritis in children who have unilateral, sudden onset of pain, photophobia, and redness. Physical examination reveals a miotic pupil and perilimbal injection. Aqueous flare and cells are seen on slit lamp examination. Treatment includes early ophthalmologic consultation, cycloplegics, and steroid drops if recommended by the specialist. Infections of the uvea can be caused by bacteria, fungi, viruses, or helminths. Measles, mumps, and pertussis may be associated with a uveitis; however, this is not due to direct invasion.

Trauma can cause damage to the anterior chamber. A hyphema occurs when there is hemorrhage in the anterior chamber. Complications of hyphemas include rebleeding, increased intraocular pressure, glaucoma, and corneal bloodstaining. Optic nerve atrophy can occur in patients with sickle cell disease. Since these complications may result in permanent loss of vision, an ophthalmologist should be consulted. The iris should be evaluated for shape and contour. Under penlight or direct ophthalmoscopic examination, the lens should be clear. If opacification is present, cataracts should be considered. Depending on the type of trauma, cataract formation can occur

within days or years of an injury. For further discussion of eye trauma, see Chapter 92.

Aniridia presents as an apparent absence of the iris but has many variations. The pupil appears as large as the cornea while the iris remains as a small residual structure. The visual acuity for patients with aniridia is extremely poor due to macular hypoplasia; nystagmus and photophobia are often present. Two-thirds of patients have a hereditary autosomal dominant condition, while one-third are sporadic cases. Approximately 20% of infants with sporadic aniridia develop a Wilms' tumor, other genitourinary defects, or mental retardation. Other ocular defects associated with aniridia include a displaced lens, cataracts, corneal epithelial dystrophy, and glaucoma.

PUPILS AND EXTRAOCULAR MOVEMENTS

Pupils should be black, round, symmetric, and equally reactive to light. Changes in the anterior chamber, lens, or vitreous may result in a pupil that is not black. A ruptured globe or intracranial process can lead to pupillary asymmetry. Assess extraocular movements in all visual fields and clearly document all deficits (Fig. 93–1). Pupillary assessment includes evaluation for an afferent pupillary defect known as a Marcus Gunn pupil in which pupillary constriction is delayed and diminished in both eyes when light is shone in the affected eye as compared to the normal eye. A Marcus Gunn pupil is the evidence of injury to the anterior visual system and is a poor prognostic sign.

A white spot on the pupil, leukocoria, can be due to congenital cataract, coloboma, retinopathy of prematurity, retinal dysplasia, congenital toxoplasmosis, old vitreous hemorrhage, retinoblastoma, or retinal detachment, in addition to a wide variety of other hereditary, developmental, inflammatory, and miscellaneous conditions. It is essential for patients with leukocoria to have a thorough fundoscopic examination by an ophthalmologist.

POSTERIOR SEGMENT

The posterior segment comprises the vitreous, retina, and optic nerve. Direct ophthalmoscope can be used to examine for

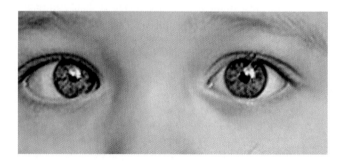

Figure 93–1. This patient has a left cranial nerve 6 (abducens nerve) palsy. CN 6 innervates the lateral rectus muscle that is responsible for eye abduction. (Photo courtesy of Dr. Shira Robbins, University of California, San Diego.)

papilledema, hemorrhages, retinal detachment, and intraocular foreign bodies. Chronic conditions including uveitis can cause deposits in the vitreous. Endophthalmitis (infections inside the eye) may result from penetrating injury, worsening superficial infection, or surgery. Children will have unilateral severe pain in or around the eye and compromised vision. Purulent exudate in the vitreous will show up as a greenish color on the ophthalmoscopic examination. Often a hypopyon (pus in the anterior chamber) is seen.

Blunt or penetrating trauma to the eye can lead to a vitreous hemorrhage. Other causes of hemorrhage include diabetes mellitus, hypertension, sickle cell disease, leukemia, retinal tears, central retinal vein occlusion, and tumor. These patients typically present with sudden loss of vision.

Retinal artery and retinal vein obstruction are relatively uncommon in the pediatric population and etiologies include trauma and other systemic entities. Retinal artery occlusion is a true ocular emergency and can be due to emboli in patients with endocarditis and systemic lupus erythematosus or result from hypercoagulability in patients with sickle cell disease. When central retinal artery occlusion occurs, there is sudden, painless loss of vision in one eye. Ophthalmoscopic examination reveals the cherry-red spot of the fovea, a pale optic nerve, and markedly narrowed arteries. A Marcus Gunn pupil may be present. Ophthalmology consultation should be immediately obtained for possible paracentesis of the anterior chamber to decompress the globe. Temporizing measures include ocular digital massage, topical beta-blocker (Timoptic 0.5%), Diamox, and CO_2 rebreathing by having patients blow into a paper bag for 5 to 10 minutes.

Retinal vein obstruction also leads to sudden painless loss of vision that varies depending on the extent of the obstruction. Retinal hemorrhages and a blurred, reddened optic disk may be seen. These findings are often described as a "blood and thunder" fundus. Arteries are often narrowed, veins are distended, and there may be white exudates. Retinal vein obstruction can occur in trauma as well as leukemia, cystic fibrosis, and retinal phlebitis. An ophthalmologist should be consulted. Aspirin therapy may be initiated to inhibit further thrombosis.

Retinal tears can lead to vitreous hemorrhage causing diminished vision in the affected eye. Retinal detachment may take years to develop after a tear. As the detachment progresses, patients may have a visual field deficit or may complain of flashing lights or a "curtain" draping over the affected eye. Ophthalmoscopic examination will reveal a light-appearing retina in the area of detachment.

The optic nerve is responsible for the transmission of visual information to the cortex. Disruptions in this transmission can lead to visual loss. Optic neuritis is usually due to inflammation or demyelination. It is characterized by an abrupt, rapid, unilateral loss of vision while pain is variable. Rarely does optic neuritis present as a separate entity in children. Most often it is caused by meningitis, viral infections, encephalomyelitis, and demyelinating diseases. Lead poisoning and long-term chloramphenicol therapy are other known culprits.

Various toxins have been associated with impaired vision. Most act on the ganglion cells of the retina or optic nerve causing visual defects. Methyl alcohol can cause sudden, permanent blindness. Other recognized toxins include sulfanilamide, quinine, quinidine, and halogenated hydrocarbons.

Finally, one must consider that visual loss can result from impedance within the visual cortex of the brain. Head trauma, hypoglycemia, leukemia, cerebrovascular accidents, and anesthetic accidents can all be associated with cortical blindness.

INTRAOCULAR PRESSURE

Either infection or injury to the anterior chamber can lead to increased intraocular pressure. Glaucoma can manifest any time after an insult to the eye. Pain and blurred vision should alert one to the possibility of glaucoma. The pupil is nonreactive and dilated, and patients may complain of seeing halos around objects. Accurate measurement is accomplished by slit lamp tonometry or with a handheld tonometer. This should not be undertaken, however, if the possibility of a ruptured globe exists. In patients with acute glaucoma, rough tactile measurement of intraocular pressure can be made by gentle palpation of the globes with the fingers through the eyelids. An extremely firm eye can easily be detected. Normal eye pressure in children ranges from 10 to 22 mm Hg. An ophthalmologist must be immediately involved in the care and treatment of children with suspected glaucoma. Immediate medical management includes a combination of topical pilocarpine 1% to 2% once the intraocular pressure is below 40 mm Hg, adrenergic agents, mannitol 1 to 2 g/kg IV, and carbonic anhydrase agents. Diamox is most often used at an oral dose of 15 mg/kg/d.

► ERRORS TO AVOID

In managing eye emergencies, physicians should avoid some common mistakes:

- Forgetting to examine the unaffected eye
- Not thoroughly examining the injured eye
- Failing to consider and recognize globe perforation
- Prescribing topical anesthetics and steroids
- Using eye drops or ointment when a perforation exists
- Failure to ensure proper follow-up for patients

► COMMON EYE COMPLAINTS

THE RED EYE

History is extremely important in differentiating the etiology of the red eye. Although conjunctivitis is common in childhood, other etiologies must be thoroughly considered prior to arriving at the diagnosis. Time of onset, exposure to chemicals or noxious stimuli, exposure to other children with similar problems, presence of systemic illness, history of trauma, photophobia, and excessive tearing are all important in the consideration of the differential diagnosis. The differential diagnosis for the red eye is listed in Table 93–1.

EYE PAIN

Two fiber systems are involved in the transmission of eye pain. Myelinated fibers transmit the sharp transient pain while unmyelinated fibers transmit the dull aching sensations. Pain

▶ **TABLE 93–1. DIFFERENTIAL DIAGNOSIS OF THE RED EYE**

Conjunctivitis
  Bacterial
  Viral herpes simplex
  Other viral etiology
  Chemical
  Allergic (including vernal)
  Neonatal ophthalmia
Corneal abrasion and corneal ulcer
Foreign bodies
Glaucoma
Hordeolum or chalazion
Iritis
Keratitis, episcleritis, scleritis
Periorbital or orbital cellulitis
Systemic disorders
  Ataxia-telangiectasia
  Collagen vascular disease
  Infectious disease—mumps, measles, rubella, otitis media,
    influenza, EBV, CMV, coxsackie, Perinaud oculoglandular
    syndrome
  Inflammatory bowel disease
  Juvenile rheumatoid arthritis
  Kawasaki disease
  Lyme disease
  Leukemia
  Stevens–Johnson syndrome
Trauma
  Chemical burns and thermal burns
  Ruptured globe
  Subconjunctival hemorrhage
  Hyphema

fibers innervating the eye and periorbital structures arise from the trigeminal or fifth cranial nerve. The first (ophthalmic) division is the most important one responsible for eye pain. It innervates the globe, forehead, lacrimal gland, canaliculi, and the lacrimal sac, as well as the frontal sinus, upper lid, and side of the nose. The second major branch (maxillary nerve) supplies the cheek, lower eyelid, and a small lower segment of the cornea, upper lip, side of the nose, maxillary sinus, roof of the mouth, and temporal region. The third division of the trigeminal nerve (mandibular) supplies sensation to other areas of the cheek in addition to the preauricular region. Referred pain can occur if the sensory pathway is stimulated in other regions. Interestingly, the cornea represents one of the areas of greatest density of pain nerve endings in the body.

Eye pain often can be difficult to characterize in young children. Superficial eye pain is frequently associated with such epithelial abnormalities as a corneal abrasion, whereas deep eye pain is more often associated with increased intraocular pressure or uveitis. Eye pain associated with burning makes one consider dry eyes, allergies, or irritation secondary to chemicals or noxious stimuli. Pain caused by bright light is associated with iritis, uveitis, and glaucoma.

Eye pain in children results from a variety of causes including foreign bodies, corneal abrasions, conjunctivitis, epis-

cleritis, acute dacryocystitis, congenital glaucoma, uveitis, optic neuritis, hordeolum, herpes zoster, and a wide array of trauma. Physicians should attempt to characterize the pain and then thoroughly search for the underlying etiology. Eye pain secondary to chemical alkali burns (lye or ammonia) result in a liquefactive necrosis that can cause permanent damage to the iris and lens. Acid burns result in a coagulative necrosis, and, therefore, the depth of the burn is self-limiting. Immediate treatment for both types of injuries includes irrigation with a minimum of 1 to 2 L of normal saline. The irrigation should be continued until the eye pH, measured by litmus paper, is between 6 and 8. Fluorescein examination should then be performed. If there is no epithelial deficit, erythromycin ointment or drops can be initiated four times a day with ophthalmologic consultation within 48 hours. If there is a corneal epithelial deficit, ophthalmology consultation and referral within 24 hours is warranted. These patients benefit from a cycloplegic agent, erythromycin ointment, and possibly eye patching for comfort.

EXCESSIVE TEARING

Usually noted in infants, excessive tearing can be due to nasolacrimal obstruction (dacryostenosis) or may be secondary to bacterial, viral, or allergic conjunctivitis. Sometimes infants with a corneal abrasion or glaucoma will have tearing.

EYE DISCHARGE

Purulent eye discharge is most often associated with bacterial conjunctivitis. Viral and allergic conjunctivitis are more often associated with mucoid discharge. Patients with blepharitis have crusting in addition to the discharge.

▶ NONTRAUMATIC EYE DISORDERS

EYELID INFECTIONS

Eyelid infections are frequent throughout childhood. The glands of Zeis are sebaceous glands attached directly to the hair follicles; the Meibomian glands are sebaceous glands that extend through the tarsal plate. Eyelid infections (blepharitis) often involve one of these glands. The most common infections of the eyelid include chalazion, hordeolum, impetigo contagiosa, and herpes simplex.

Clinical Findings

An external hordeolum or stye is a suppurative infection of the glands of Zeis, whereas an internal hordeolum or chalazion is an acute infection of a Meibomian gland. A chalazion presents as a painless, hard nodule and is often located in the midportion of the tarsus, away from the lid border caused from obstruction of the gland duct. Chalazions are uncommon during infancy but frequently occur during childhood. Initially, the swelling may be diffuse but usually becomes localized to the lid margin. Impetigo contagiosa is a pyoderma usually presenting with vesicles; it then develops a yellowish crust, which occurs due to local invasion by staphylococci or streptococci. In patients with impetigo, there can often be an underlying seborrheic dermatitis. Herpes simplex can present on the eyelids of children and can lead to latent infection, which may persist throughout life and be reactivated. Recurrent infection often involves the cornea. Herpetic blepharitis is characterized by the formation of vesicles, which break down and form a yellowish-crusted surface.

Differential Diagnosis

The differential diagnosis of an external hordeolum includes contact dermatitis and allergic conjunctivitis. Itching is a more prominent feature in the latter two entities and is not usually associated with a hordeolum. The differential diagnosis of a chalazion includes rhabdomyosarcoma, capillary hemangiomas, dermoids, orbital cysts, molluscum contagiosum, sarcoidosis, fungal infections, foreign bodies, and juvenile xanthogranuloma. Differentiation is made by lack of response to local therapy and/or biopsy. Impetigo contagiosa and herpes simplex can be easily confused. Cultures should be obtained to ascertain etiology.

Management

The management of hordeolum includes warm compresses and eyelid hygiene using baby shampoo on a washcloth. Twice-daily application of an antistaphylococcal antibiotic ointment (erythromycin ophthalmic ointment or polymyixin B sulfate) or ophthalmic drops should also be initiated. A chalazion is initially managed in the same manner, and antibiotic treatment should be continued for several days after rupture of the chalazion to prevent recurrence. If there is a lack of response to medical treatment, surgical incision and drainage under general anesthesia is recommended for young children. Recurrence commonly results from autoinoculation and inattention to good hygienic care.

Impetigo contagiosa should be treated by removing crusts and with topical antistaphylococcal and streptococcal antibiotics. A cotton-tip applicator soaked in baby shampoo can be used to clean the lid margins. Bacitracin ophthalmic ointment is often effective; however, topical erythromycin and gentamicin can be used. If systemic impetigo is present, oral antibiotics should be initiated.

Herpes simplex blepharitis should be treated with trifluorothymidine topical drops. Oral acyclovir should be considered but may be of limited value. Treatment of herpes simplex will be discussed in further detail in the following sections.

CELLULITIS OF THE PERIORBITAL AND ORBITAL REGION

Periorbital infections are common in childhood and usually resolve with appropriate therapy and without sequelae. A review of the sinuses and classification of this infection is helpful in considering the correct diagnosis. The anatomic development of the sinuses in children is thought to play a major role in the development of orbital and periorbital infections.

Periorbital infections, particularly sinusitis, may cause infection or severe inflammation in the orbital tissues thus leading to a preseptal or orbital cellulitis. The proximity of the paranasal sinuses to the orbital walls and the interconnection between the venous system of the orbit and the face allow infection to spread from the sinuses to the orbit either directly or via the bloodstream. The orbital venous system is devoid of valves so that two-way communication is allowed with the venous system of the nose, face, and pterygoid fossa. The superior and inferior ophthalmic veins drain directly from the orbit and empty into the cavernous sinus. Orbital and facial infections can lead to cavernous venous thrombosis.

The orbital periosteum and septum are important anatomic structures, which help to limit direct spread of infection. The orbital periosteum acts as a barrier to the spread of infection from the sinuses; however, it may become eroded if a periorbital abscess develops. The orbital septum may also limit the spread of infection from the preseptal space to the orbit. The following classification has been described for orbital infections

- *Class I:* Periorbital or preseptal cellulitis (Fig. 93–2)—Cellulitis is confined to the anterior lamella tissue because of a lack of flow through the drainage ethmoid vessels. Lid edema and erythema may be mild or severe. The globe ordinarily is not involved and so vision and function remain normal.
- *Class II:* Orbital cellulitis—Orbital tissue is infiltrated with bacteria and cells, which extend through the

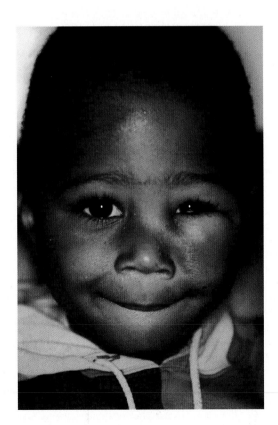

Figure 93–2. A patient with an insect bite and associated preseptal cellulitis. (Photo courtesy of Dr. Katherine Konzen, Rady Children's Hospital, San Diego.)

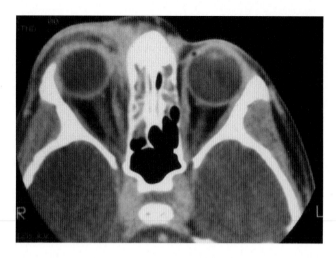

Figure 93-3. CT scan demonstrating sinus disease with inflammation of preseptal (lid) structures as well as purulent material in the periosteal space, causing lateral displacement of the globe. (Image Courtesy of Dr. Melvin Senac, Rady Children's Hospital, San Diego.)

septum into the orbital fat and other tissues. Manifestations usually include proptosis, impaired or painful movement, and periocular pain. Visual acuity may be impaired and septicemia may be present.

- *Class III:* Subperiosteal abscess (Fig. 93–3)—Purulent material collects between the periosteum and the orbital wall. Medial wall involvement causes the globe to be displaced inferiorly or laterally. Symptoms include edema, chemosis, and tenderness with ocular movement, while vision loss and proptosis vary in severity.
- *Class IV:* Orbital abscess—When pus accumulates within the orbital fat inside or outside the muscle cone, an orbital abscess has developed. The infectious process becomes localized and encapsulated, unlike orbital cellulitis, which tends to be more diffuse. Exophthalmos, chemosis, ophthalmoplegia, and visual impairment are generally severe; systemic toxicity may be impressive.
- *Class V:* Cavernous sinus thrombosis—Thrombosis results from extension of an orbital infection into the cavernous sinus. Nausea, vomiting, headache, fever, pupillary dilation, and other systemic signs may be present. There is marked lid edema and early onset of third, fourth, and sixth cranial nerve palsies.

The bacteriology involved in orbital infections depends on the age of the patient and the underlying problem. In newborn infants and in those up to the age of 5 years, *Haemophilus influenzae, Streptococcus pneumoniae,* and *Moraxella catarrhalis* are predominant, particularly in children with upper respiratory tract infections, conjunctivitis, sinusitis, or otitis media. The incidence of infections due to *H. influenzae* type B has dropped since the advent of routine vaccination against this pathogen.[1] In patients with a history of skin infections or trauma, *Staphylococcus aureus* and streptococcal species are the main offending agents. The incidence of infections with community-acquired Methicillin-resistant *S. aureus* continues to increase.[2] Polymicrobial and anaerobic infections are more common in older children. Children with cystic fibrosis are susceptible to infections with *Pseudomonas aeruginosa.*

Fungal orbital cellulitis is uncommon in children. A slowly progressive course of orbital swelling in children with vomiting or dehydration may indicate an underlying fungal infection; immunocompromised and diabetic children may be at greatest risk. *Rhizopus* and *Mucor* are the most common fungi causing infections.

Clinical Findings

Most of the clinical findings are described with each class of infection. Preseptal or periorbital cellulitis is marked by periorbital edema, erythema, and tenderness but is not accompanied by proptosis, ophthalmoplegia, or loss of visual acuity. Chemosis and conjunctivitis may be present, as well as fever and leukocytosis. In young children who have fever and other systemic signs, a lumbar puncture and intravenous antibiotics should be considered because of the possibility of underlying meningitis. In young children, *H. influenzae* type B can produce a distinctive type of bluish–purple hue to the eyelid. It is often accompanied by fever, irritability, otitis media, and bacteremia.

Patients with orbital cellulitis present similarly but have further development of ophthalmoplegia, proptosis, pain on eye movement, worsening chemosis, and changes in vision. Fever and leukocytosis are often seen. Blood cultures are positive in up to 25% of patients. If the orbital cellulitis is secondary to sinusitis, headache, rhinorrhea, and swelling of the nasal mucosa may also be present. At times, swelling of the eyelid may be so severe that further evaluation is necessary. Computed tomography (CT) has been useful in the delineation of periorbital cellulitis from orbital cellulitis. It, however, has its limitations in making a definitive diagnosis of a subperiosteal abscess from reactive subperiosteal edema.

Management

In patients with mild periorbital cellulitis and no history of fever or other systemic illness, a thorough physical examination is recommended but laboratory investigation may be unnecessary. Mild cases of preseptal cellulitis due to local trauma or conjunctivitis can be treated with oral antibiotics such as amoxicillin-clavulanate (20–40 mg/kg/d) to cover against *S. aureus.* Cellulitis associated with an upper respiratory infection may also be treated with amoxicillin-clavulanate or with cefuroxime. For cellulitis secondary to bug bites, oral antihistamines and warm compresses may also be helpful. Close follow-up is mandatory.

For patients requiring hospitalization, a complete blood cell count, lumbar puncture, cultures of the blood, nasal mucosa, throat and conjunctiva, and CT of the head may be warranted. A lumbar puncture should be considered to rule out meningitis if patients appear toxic and are younger than 2 years or if infection with *H. influenzae* is suspected. The following management scheme has been recommended by several authors:

- All patients hospitalized for orbital inflammation should receive ophthalmologic and otolaryngology consultation.
- Broad-spectrum antimicrobial therapy should be instituted at once while awaiting blood or intraoperative culture results. Children younger than 5 years of age,

without a history of trauma, should be placed on appropriate coverage against *H. influenzae* type B, *S. pneumoniae*, and group A streptococcus. A suggested initial regimen consists of ceftriaxone, 100 mg/kg/d, with the addition of vancomycin, 40 mg/kg/d in severe cases. Children older than 5 years, or those fully immunized with the Haemophilus vaccine, do not generally require coverage for Haemophilus; appropriate antimicrobials are similar to those used for treatment of severe sinusitis.

- Attempts must be made to delineate if the cellulitis is of preseptal or postseptal origin. CT of the head is a helpful diagnostic aid but may not differentiate between subperiosteal abscess and reactive periosteal edema.
- Surgical indications include diminishing visual acuity, lack of improvement despite adequate antibiotics, or spiking fevers suggesting possible development of orbital abscess or cavernous venous thrombosis.

Posttraumatic suppurative cellulitis is treated by early incision and drainage of the infected space, coupled with parenteral antibiotics. Tetanus prophylaxis should be considered. Sufficient coverage for *S. aureus* and *Streptococcus pyogenes* is necessary. Anaerobic coverage should be instituted following animal and human bites. Intravenous antibiotics are recommended for a minimum of 48 to 72 hours, and then consideration of oral therapy may be appropriate.

Orbital cellulitis secondary to sinusitis should be managed with the consultation of ophthalmology and otolaryngology. Intravenous antibiotics should consist of a third-generation cephalosporin and a penicillinase-resistant penicillin. If the potential for an anaerobic infection exists, clindamycin may be substituted for the penicillinase-resistant penicillin. Frequent ophthalmologic examination with thorough clinical reassessment is warranted to determine response to treatment and need for surgical intervention (Fig. 93–4).

Complications

In addition to the previously mentioned complications of cavernous venous thrombosis and meningitis, blindness has been associated with postseptal cellulitis. In the pre-antibiotic era, up to 20% of patients with postseptal inflammation developed blindness. Alarmingly, recent studies report a 10% incidence of blindness resulting from orbital complications of sinusitis. Clearly, broad-spectrum antibiotics and modern surgical techniques have not totally alleviated this devastating complication. In fact, negative or equivocal CT findings often contributed to an inappropriate delay in surgical intervention. CT of the head cannot solely determine patient management; clinical judgment must prevail.

SCLERITIS AND EPISCLERITIS

The sclera, made up mainly of collagen and connective tissue, is the thick vascular covering of the eye. Scleritis is uncommon but can be associated with juvenile rheumatoid arthritis or various infectious processes including herpes simplex, varicella zoster, mumps, syphilis, and tuberculosis.

The thin vascular membrane between the sclera and conjunctiva is called the episclera. Inflammation of this area produces some irritation but not the severe pain associated with scleritis. Episcleritis is also associated with a variety of diseases including varicella zoster, syphilis, Henoch–Schonlein purpura, erythema multiforme, and penicillin sensitivity. Episcleritis often presents as a distinct area of injected conjunctiva with dilated vessels in the involved layer of tissue. Differentiation may be helpful with the administration of topical phenylephrine, which constricts vessels dilated by conjunctivitis but not those vessels involved in scleritis or episcleritis. Management consists of treating the underlying disease and some combination of oral nonsteroidal anti-inflammatory agents, topical corticosteroids, and cycloplegics.

CONJUNCTIVITIS

Diagnostic Terms

A review of certain diagnostic terms is cardinal to this discussion. *Hyperemia* is due to an increase in the number, caliber, and the tortuosity of vessels in the conjunctiva resulting in a reddish appearance to the conjunctiva occurring in both acute and chronic conjunctival processes. Edema often accompanies hyperemia. *Congestion* is caused by diminished conjunctival drainage, producing a dusky red discoloration secondary to prolonged circulation time within the conjunctival vessels. Congestion is most often seen in allergic conjunctivitis where the conjunctiva takes on a jelly-like appearance. *Exudates* are the by-products produced from conjunctival inflammation and may be purulent, watery, catarrhal, ropy, mucoid, or bloody. They collect in the lid margin and corners of the eyes and are viewed best when the lids are pulled away from the eye. *Follicles* are collections of lymphocytes within the conjunctiva and are often associated with allergy, viral conjunctivitis, and toxicity to topical medications. Vessels are usually located on the outside of each follicle. *Papillae* are elevations of the conjunctiva that have a central vascular core; around the core is a clear area of conjunctival swelling. Small ones produce a velvety appearance on the surface of the conjunctiva. Large papillae are easily seen without magnification and are associated with contact lens wear, irritation from surgical sutures, and vernal conjunctivitis. *Membranes and pseudomembranes* are coagulum formed by inflammatory reaction to an infection. Pseudomembranes are very fine coagula covering the conjunctival surface and, when removed, do not damage the underlying conjunctiva and hence do not cause bleeding. Membranes differ in that they are coagula firmly attached to the underlying conjunctiva and, when removed, cause bleeding. Pseudomembranes are seen in epidemic keratoconjunctivitis, primary herpes simplex conjunctivitis, streptococcal conjunctivitis, alkaline burns, and erythema multiforme. Membranes are associated with diphtheria and less frequently with streptococcal conjunctivitis, adenovirus types 8 and 19, alkali burns, and erythema multiforme.

OPHTHALMIA NEONATORUM

Conjunctivitis in newborn infants (first 28 days of life) is not uncommon (Table 93–2). Because of the potential complications from ocular infections in infancy, neonates with symptoms mandate a thorough evaluation. Important guidelines for evaluation include the following:

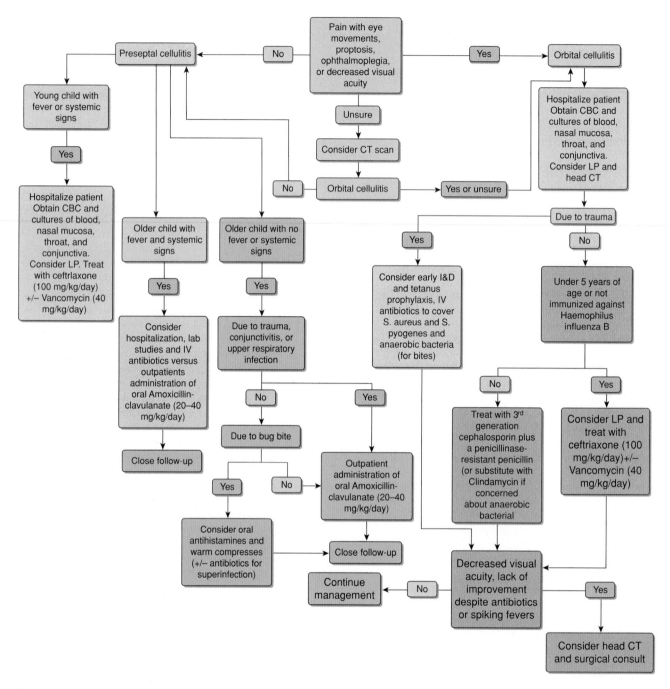

Figure 93–4. Algorithm delineating the inpatient and outpatient diagnosis and management of preseptal and orbital cellulitis. (Algorithm courtesy of Dr. Lauren P. Ortega, Medical City Hospital, Dallas, TX.)

- Obtaining a detailed maternal history including prenatal care, history of or exposure to venereal disease, duration of rupture of membranes, type of delivery, agent used for ocular prophylaxis at birth, recent exposure to conjunctivitis, and timing of onset of symptoms. History should also include a description of excessive tearing, type and amount of exudate, and elucidation of systemic signs of illness in the baby, such as fever, vomiting, irritability, or lethargy.
- Physical examination must be thorough, including a comprehensive eye examination searching for evidence of eyelid erythema, edema, discharge, corneal ulcera-

tion, globe perforation, or foreign body. In addition, general physical examination must be complete; special attention must focus on the skin, respiratory, and genitourinary system for evidence of concomitant systemic involvement.
- Conjunctival scrapings should be obtained for Gram's stain, Giemsa's stain, and viral and bacterial cultures including *Neisseria*. A rapid antigen test is sensitive and specific for *Chlamydia* and can be obtained easily from the conjunctiva. Culture is usually not necessary. Multiplex PCR is now available at many centers to test for viruses such as HSV 1 and 2, HHV-6, CMV, EBV, and

▶ TABLE 93–2. OPHTHALMIA NEONATORUM

	Chemical Conjunctivitis	*Chlamydia*	Bacterial	*Neisseria*	Herpes Simplex	Viral
Onset	0–2 days	1–2 weeks	1–4 weeks	0–30 days	2–14 days	0–30 days
Discharge	−	+	+	+++	+	+
Unilateral/bilateral hyperemia	B	U	U/B	B	U/B	U/B
Fever	−	±	−	±	±	−
Diagnosis	Negative Gram's stain, few WBCs	Rapid antigen, Giemsa's stain, or culture	Gram's stain culture	Gram's stain culture	Fluorescein staining, multinucleated giant cells, intranuclear inclusion cells, fluorescent antigen tests	History of contact exposure, negative Gram's stain, and viral culture
Treatment	None	Systemic oral erythromycin, 2–3 weeks	Topical antimicrobial	Intravenous third-generation cephalosporin	Intravenous acyclovir, topical trifluorothymidine	Topical antimicrobial
Associated findings	None	Pneumonia, otitis media	None	Rhinitis, anorectal infection, arthritis, meningitis	Skin lesions, septicemia	Upper respiratory tract infection
Long-term complications	None	Conjunctival scarring, micropannus formation	None	Blindness	Keratitis, cataracts, chorioretinitis, optic neuritis, others	None

− = absent; ± = may or may not be present; + = mild; ++ = moderate; +++ = severe; WBC, white blood cells.

VZV, all of which can cause a conjunctivitis. Studies have shown that use of fluorescein and topical anesthetics may reduce the accuracy of PCR tests. The eye should be rinsed with saline after the use of these agents and before PCR samples are obtained.[3]

Differential Diagnosis
Chemical Conjunctivitis
Chemical conjunctivitis caused by silver nitrate drops in the immediate newborn period occurs in almost 10% of newborns. Signs of this type of conjunctivitis include bilateral conjunctival hyperemia and mild discharge that begin in the first 24 hours of life and usually subside within 48 hours. Gram's stain reveals no organisms and only a few white blood cells. The inflammation is typically quite mild and does not require intervention.

Chlamydia Trachomatis
Chlamydia infections have a typical incubation period of 1 to 2 weeks, but can occur earlier if there was premature rupture of membranes. Onset of symptoms may be delayed in babies who received prophylaxis at birth. The overall incidence of chlamydial ophthalmia is approximately 20 to 40 cases per 1000 births annually. The prevalence of chlamydial infections in pregnant women ranges from 2% to 23%; transmission rates from infected mothers range from 23% to 70%. Typically, the conjunctiva becomes hyperemic and edematous with the palpebral conjunctiva more involved than is the bulbar conjunctiva. Unilateral, purulent involvement is characteristic. Neonates may

also have evidence of a concomitant otitis media or afebrile pneumonia. Samples are obtained by scraping the palpebral conjunctiva of the lower lid. The diagnosis is confirmed by identification of chlamydial antigen, detection of intracellular inclusions from Giemsa's stain, or isolation of the organism. Antigen detection tests are rapid, sensitive, and specific and are the most efficient means of confirming the diagnosis. Gram's stain is not helpful in confirming the diagnosis.

Management
Systemic therapy is absolutely essential in the treatment of this condition. The treatment of choice is oral erythromycin (40–50 mg/kg/d) for a 2- to 3-week course to eliminate both conjunctival and nasopharyngeal colonization. Administration of a topical agent is unnecessary. Since chlamydia is the most frequent sexually transmitted disease, prevention by detection of infection in the mother prior to delivery is essential. Treatment of the affected infant's mother and her partner(s) is also recommended. Early studies suggested that the administration of erythromycin ointment prophylaxis in newborns was effective in preventing chlamydia conjunctivitis but not in altering the rate of development of pneumonia or nasopharyngeal infection. Subsequent studies have revealed that neonatal ocular prophylaxis with erythromycin does not reduce the incidence of chlamydial conjunctivitis. Chlamydial conjunctivitis can lead to chronic changes such as conjunctival scarring and micropannus formation. Fortunately, these long-term ocular sequelae are quite rare. In some cases, chlamydial conjunctivitis may resolve spontaneously without treatment; however, these

infants are at risk for reoccurrence of infection involving not only the eyes, but the pharynx, rectum, and lungs as well.

Bacterial Conjunctivitis

The role of other bacteria in the newborn period is not quite as clear and can be caused by *S. aureus, Haemophilus* spp., *S. pneumoniae,* and *Enterococci.* Many studies have also shown that these bacteria, in addition to *Corynebacterium, Propionibacterium, Lactobacillus,* and *Bacteroides* can be normal flora. Typically, the conjunctiva is red and edematous with some amount of exudate. Diagnosis is made by Gram's stain and culture. Broad-spectrum topical antimicrobial therapy is initiated, although there are no good studies in this population to document the necessity or efficacy of topical therapy. If cultures have been obtained, antimicrobial therapy can be tailored to treat the offending organism. Untreated cases of bacterial conjunctivitis could potentially progress to corneal ulceration, perforation, endophthalmitis, and septicemia.

Neisseria gonorrhoeae

Historically, gonococcal ophthalmia neonatorum has been of greatest concern because of its serious complications. In the early 1900s, approximately 25% of children admitted to American schools for the blind acquired their disability from *N. gonorrhoeae.* By the late 1950s, 0.5% were blind as a result of *Neisseria.* With the onset of antibiotics and postnatal prophylaxis, the current incidence in the United States is thought to be 2 to 3 cases per 10 000 live births. The mean incubation period is 6.5 days with a range of 1 to 31 days. Gonococcal ophthalmia neonatorum classically presents as a purulent, bilateral conjunctivitis. Conjunctival hyperemia, chemosis, eyelid edema, and erythema may also be seen. This entity is diagnosed by Gram's stain, revealing gram-negative intracellular diplococci. Cultures should be sent immediately on blood and chocolate agar, because the organisms die rapidly at room temperature. Cultural growth usually occurs within 2 days. Infants with conjunctivitis may have other manifestations of localized disease including rhinitis, anorectal infection, arthritis, and meningitis. Neonates with suspected gonococcal conjunctivitis or any neonate with fever and conjunctivitis should have a sepsis evaluation, including a lumbar puncture. Gonococcal conjunctivitis is considered an ophthalmologic emergency.

Management

Treatment must be systemic; there is no role for oral or topical antibiotics. Neonates without meningitis should be treated for 7 days with either ceftriaxone or cefotaxime. If meningitis is present, treatment continues for 10 to 14 days. If the organism is sensitive to penicillin, penicillin G can be substituted. Treatment must also include frequent saline irrigation of the eyes. Parents should be screened for gonococcal disease. An infant born to a mother with known active gonococcal infection should receive one dose of ceftriaxone immediately after delivery.

Herpes Simplex

Most neonates with herpes simplex become colonized during the birth process. Neonatal herpes simplex may occasionally present first as conjunctivitis. The onset is generally 2 to 14 days after birth. Characteristics are not clinically distinctive;

however, unilateral or bilateral epithelial dendrites are virtually diagnostic. Fluorescein staining reveals these defects. Parental history of herpes is important to obtain. Often conjunctivitis leads to further disseminated infections that carry a high morbidity and mortality rate. The conjunctivitis can be diagnosed with conjunctival scrapings looking for multinucleated giant cells and intranuclear inclusions. A fluorescent antibody test should be obtained followed by a viral culture.

Management

Treatment should consist of intravenous acyclovir for 10 days and topical trifluorothymidine. Parents must be aware of the high risk of recurrence of keratitis later in life; an ophthalmologist should follow these children closely. Recurrences are treated with topical therapy alone. Neonatal herpes simplex can lead to the development of keratitis, cataracts, chorioretinitis, and optic neuritis in addition to numerous other ocular problems. Long-term follow-up studies have shown that more than 90% of neonates with neurologic sequelae from herpes simplex infection also have some type of ocular abnormality.

Viral Etiologies (Nonherpetic)

Other viral causes of conjunctivitis in neonates are infrequent. Conjunctivitis in a sibling or parent is the most likely source of infection. Hands or fomites are the modes of transmission. Diagnosis is made by history of recent exposure and clinical findings. Usually infections are self-limited; often topical antimicrobials are prescribed to avoid secondary infection but are probably of limited value. Education regarding hand-washing and not sharing of washcloths and towels is necessary.

Obstructed Nasolacrimal Duct

Congenital nasolacrimal duct obstruction, or dacryostenosis, is often only recognized when infants have a history of recurrent ocular infections. The blockage is frequently caused by failure to canalize a membrane called the *valve of Hasner,* which is located at the lower end of the nasolacrimal duct. Affected infants often have pooling of tears onto the lower lid and cheeks and maceration of the eyelids. Upon crying, tears fail to arrive at the external nares. It is important to differentiate nasolacrimal duct obstruction from congenital glaucoma. Congenital glaucoma presents with tearing, photophobia, and a cloudy, enlarged cornea. Redness is not a major feature of nasolacrimal duct obstruction. Conservative treatment consists of massaging the lacrimal sac, suppressive topical antimicrobials, and warm compresses. Probing of the nasolacrimal system is not recommended until after 1 year of age because 95% of children younger than 13 months will experience spontaneous opening of the lacrimal duct (Fig. 93–5).

Noninfectious Etiologies

The differential diagnosis of the red eye in neonates should also include noninfectious etiologies. Corneal abrasions can be detected in infants and may often be secondary to a scratch from their fingernail. Conjunctival hyperemia may be present; fluorescein staining is diagnostic. Linear abrasions on the superior aspect of the cornea should alert the physician to an upper eyelid foreign body. Trauma to the eye during delivery can also cause a corneal abrasion or laceration. Foreign bodies

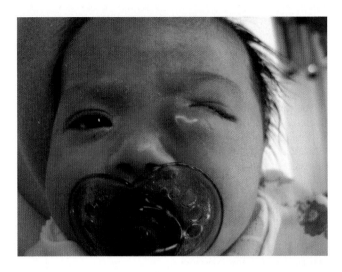

Figure 93–5. A newborn infant with congenital lacrimal duct stenosis causing dacryocystitis. (Photo courtesy of Dr. Shira Robbins, University of California, San Diego.)

in the neonatal period are rare but should be considered in the evaluation.

CONJUNCTIVITIS BEYOND THE NEONATAL PERIOD

Conjunctivitis is a frequently encountered entity in children (Table 93–3). Considerations in management include the following:

- Age
- Onset of conjunctivitis (acute being <2 weeks, chronic lasting >2 weeks)
- Previous history of conjunctivitis
- Trauma
- Type of eye discharge
- Unilateral versus bilateral symptoms
- Photophobia
- Lacrimation
- Pain
- Change in visual acuity
- History of herpes simplex
- Exposure to conjunctivitis
- Associated systemic symptoms of fever, sore throat, or rash

▶ **TABLE 93–3. CONJUNCTIVITIS IN CHILDHOOD**

	Bacterial	Pharyngo-conjunctival	Acute Hemorrhagic	Herpes Simplex	Gonococcal	Allergic
Organism	See text	Adenovirus	Enterovirus 70, coxsackie A24	Herpes simplex	*Neisseria gonorrhoeae*	None
Discharge	++	+	+++	±	+++	−
Unilateral/bilateral hyperemia	U/B	U/B	B	U	U/B	B
Fever	−	+	+	++	±	−
Diagnosis	History and Gram's stain, culture if necessary	History and associated symptoms, rapid antigen and viral culture if necessary	Subconjunctival hemorrhages and viral culture	Antifluorescent test Gram's stain, culture	Gram's stain, culture	History, physical examination
Treatment	Topical antimicrobial Oral antibiotic for conjunctivitis-otitis syndrome	Topical antimicrobial to prevent secondary infection	Topical antimicrobial to prevent secondary infection	Topical trifluorothymidine	Intramuscular ceftriaxone	Topical antihistamine, vasoconstrictors, and/or glucocorticoids
Associated findings	Otitis media with *Haemophilus*	Upper respiratory infection, regional adenopathy	Malaise, myalgias, upper respiratory infection	Eyelid vesicles, preauricular adenopathy	Periorbital inflammation	Atopy
Long-term complications	None	None	None	Corneal ulcerations, cataracts	Blindness, septicemia	None

−, absent; ±, may or may not be present; +, mild; ++, moderate; +++, severe.

It is crucial to identify conjunctivitis from more serious conditions. Conjunctivitis in older children is characterized by normal vision, a gritty sensation in the eye, diffuse injection, and exudate. Photophobia and lacrimation are not usually associated with conjunctivitis. Keratitis and iritis typically are associated with impaired vision, true pain, photophobia, and lacrimation.

Clinically, viral conjunctivitis is difficult to distinguish from bacterial conjunctivitis. Marked exudate, severe injection, and lid matting is more typical of bacterial or chlamydial infections. Preauricular adenopathy is often associated with viral infections. Follicles on the palpebral conjunctivae are more indicative of viral or chlamydial infections.

Bacterial Conjunctivitis

The bacteriology of conjunctivitis in children is expansive and includes *H. aegyptius, S. pneumoniae, S. aureus, N. gonorrhoeae* and *meningitides, Escherichia coli, P. aeruginosa, Proteus* spp., *viridans streptococci, S. pyogenes, Corynebacterium diphtheria, Chlamydia trachomatis,* and *M. catarrhalis.* Outbreaks of acute catarrhal conjunctivitis, also known as "pink eye," may occur in day care or among school-aged children. The offending organisms are most frequently *S. pneumoniae* or *H. aegyptius.* Outbreaks are more often seen in the winter months. Results from prospective studies indicate that the organisms most significantly associated with conjunctivitis in childhood are *H. influenzae, S. pneumoniae,* and adenoviruses. The role of *S. aureus* in nontraumatic conjunctivitis is difficult to determine because it occurs frequently in asymptomatic patients. In addition, *Haemophilus* has been associated with concomitant otitis media, and subsequent studies have coined the term *conjunctivitis-otitis syndrome* when the two occur together. The otitis associated with this syndrome may be asymptomatic, but when detected should be treated with oral antibiotics. The addition of topical antibiotics may not increase efficacy of treatment.

Pseudomonas is an infrequent pathogen that can cause an acutely advancing necrotizing picture, so it must be recognized and treated aggressively. Children with cystic fibrosis and those who wear contact lenses are at highest risk for infection with *Pseudomonas.* These patients should be evaluated by an ophthalmologist to assess for the presence of corneal ulceration. *Phlyctenular* conjunctivitis is a rare manifestation of active primary infection with *Mycoplasma tuberculosis* associated with a high degree of hypersensitivity. Notably small grayish nodules are present on the bulbar conjunctiva accompanied by intense pain and photophobia. Skin testing is recommended and culture for other bacteria is important because of the high incidence of secondary bacterial infections.

Although most types of acute bacterial conjunctivitis are self-limited, the use of topical antibiotic therapy is thought to shorten the clinical course and more quickly eradicate the organism, thereby decreasing the amount of time patients are contagious. Routine Gram's stain and culture usually is unnecessary unless there is a history of copious mucopurulent exudate (*Neisseria*) or a chronic history of conjunctivitis.[4]

Treatment is empiric with topical antimicrobial ointments or ophthalmic drops. Specific drugs include tobramycin drops, ciprofloxacin drops or ointment, ofloxacin drops, polymyxin B sulfate drops, erythromycin ointment, trimethoprim-polymyxin drops, or gentamicin drops.

Contact lenses can cause conjunctivitis and corneal abrasions. Lens wear should be discontinued; storage and cleaning solutions must be replaced to prevent further contamination. Although patching is no longer recommended in these patients, topical antibiotics to avoid *Pseudomonas* or secondary bacterial infection may be initiated. An aminoglycoside such as tobramycin (Tobrex) drops or a fluoroquinolone such as ciprofloxacin (Ciloxan) or ofloxacin (Ocuflox) should be administered four times a day for 5 to 7 days. Corneal ulcers should always be considered in patients who wear contact lenses and have a red eye. These patients should be referred to an ophthalmologist.

Viral Conjunctivitis

Adenoviruses are the most common cause of viral conjunctivitis in children. There are a few clinical syndromes associated with this group of viruses including pharyngoconjunctival fever, epidemic keratoconjunctivitis, and nonspecific follicular conjunctivitis. Pharyngoconjunctival fever is most common in children and is associated with an upper respiratory tract infection, regional lymphadenopathy, and fever. The illness is usually self-limited, lasting 1 to 2 weeks, and is due to serotypes 3, 4, and 7. It can spread by droplet transmission although numerous epidemics have been linked to swimming pools. Epidemic keratoconjunctivitis is more common in the second to fourth decades of life and causes preauricular lymphadenopathy with diffuse superficial keratitis. Serotypes 3, 8, and 19 are associated. Instruments in eye clinics have been linked to its transmission.

Enteroviral infections from particular coxsackie viruses and echoviruses may cause conjunctivitis but are often associated with other clinical signs including rash or aseptic meningitis. Acute hemorrhagic conjunctivitis is caused by enterovirus 70 or coxsackie A24 and also occurs in epidemics. Transmission is by direct contact with an incubation of <2 days. Clinically, patients present with sudden onset of unilateral ocular redness, excessive tearing (epiphora), photophobia, pain, purulent discharge, and eyelid swelling, which develop in a span of 6 to 12 hours. Patients may complain of a burning pain often described as a foreign body sensation that is thought to be due to discrete patches of epithelial keratitis (diagnosed with fluorescein staining). In 80% of the cases, the other eye becomes involved within 24 hours. Some patients develop subconjunctival hemorrhages, which are usually located beneath the superior bulbar conjunctiva. Malaise, myalgias, fever, headache, and upper respiratory tract symptoms may also accompany conjunctivitis. Conjunctival scrapings for a viral culture yield identification of the virus. Ophthalmologic sequelae are rare: <5% of cases develop a secondary bacterial conjunctivitis.

Management

Treatment is symptomatic with cool compresses. Many physicians prescribe a topical antimicrobial to prevent secondary bacterial infection, but this practice has not been proven to be effective. Patients with epidemic keratoconjunctivitis should be kept out of school for 2 weeks to prevent an outbreak.

Herpes Simplex and Varicella-Zoster

Vesicular lesions on the eyelid can be due to herpes simplex, varicella-zoster, impetigo, or contact dermatitis. History and a general physical examination should aid in the diagnosis. Of all herpes simplex infections, 1% involve the eye. Infections are characterized by unilateral, follicular conjunctivitis with vesicles localized to the eyelids. Preauricular lymphadenopathy is commonly present. Fifty percent of the patients develop keratitis within 2 weeks. The virus remains latent in the sensory ganglion and lacrimal glands. Approximately 25% of all children will have recurrences; these usually begin with corneal involvement. Long-term complications include necrotizing stromal disease, diffuse retinitis, and scarring. Herpes simplex is the most common cause of severe corneal ulceration in children and is second only to trauma as a cause of corneal blindness in children.

Ocular involvement with varicella is relatively uncommon, occurring in <5% of cases. In chicken-pox, the conjunctiva can become involved through two mechanisms: eyelid vesicles can slough virus into the conjunctival cul-de-sac or vesicle formation can take place on the conjunctival surface. Occasionally, the cornea is involved. Fluorescein staining of the cornea and conjunctiva is necessary.

Zoster is uncommon in children, with only 5% of all cases occurring in children younger than 5 years of age. Zoster infections of the eye notably follow the distribution of the first division of the trigeminal nerve. Lesions are usually located on the forehead and upper eyelid and can be located on the tip of the nose.

Trifluorothymidine is the preferred agent for the treatment of herpes simplex because of its increased solubility, diminished toxicity, and lack of viral resistance.[5] Approximately 95% of the corneal ulcers treated with it are cured within 2 weeks; however, treatment should be extended for 1 additional week after resolution of the lesions. Rarely corneal debridement is required. For herpetic eye lesions, systemic acyclovir is not recommended because the drug does not penetrate the avascular cornea (Figs. 93–6 and 93–7).[6]

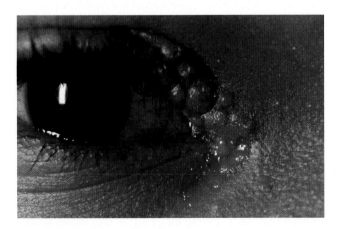

Figure 93–6. Ocular Herpes Simplex. This 10-year-old has had recurrent ocular herpes simplex since age 6 years. Vesicles should not be mistaken for hordeola. Reproduced with permission from Knoop et al. *Atlas of Emergency Medicine.* 3rd ed. New York: McGraw-Hill; 2010. (Photo contributed by Lawrence B. Stack, MD.)

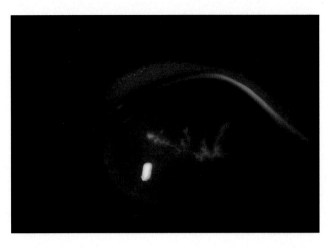

Figure 93–7. This microscopic view of a patient with herpes keratits demonstrates the stereotypical conjunctival dendrite (branching ulceration) seen with this infection. (Photo courtesy of Dr. Shira Robbins, University of California, San Diego.)

Neisseria gonorrhoeae

Gonococcal eye infections can occur in prepubertal children. A nonvenereal mode of transmission has been suggested. Certain patients have a negative history and physical examination suggestive of abuse. Some of these patients have occasionally shared a bed with a parent. Interestingly, isolates collected from selected patients have identical sensitivities to that obtained from a parent. Intravenous antibiotics are still recommended for this age group.

Gonococcal conjunctivitis can occur in sexually active children and adolescents; the mode of transmission is similar to that of adults. Treatment may consist of ceftriaxone, 1 g IM plus saline irrigation. Alternatively, ceftriaxone 1 g IM or IV may be administered for 5 days along with saline irrigation.

Occasionally a *Neisseria* conjunctivitis is attributable to *Neisseria meningitides*. The eye may act as a portal and patients may develop meningococcemia and/or meningitis. These patients should be treated with ceftriaxone and their contacts given prophylaxis with Rifampin.

Chlamydia trachomatis

Chlamydial eye infections can occur outside of the newborn period. Infection of children and adolescents may warrant an investigation for child sexual abuse and/ or other concomitant sexually transmitted infections. Treatment consists of systemic oral erythromycin for 2 to 3 weeks. Children aged 1 and older may be treated with a single oral dose of azithromycin (20 mg/kg with a maximum dose of 1 g).[7]

Allergic Conjunctivitis

Seasonal and Perennial Allergic Conjunctivitis

Itching is frequently the hallmark of allergic conjunctivitis. Seasonal allergic conjunctivitis has its onset of symptoms in either the fall or spring. Patients with sensitivity to grass have more symptoms in the spring, while individuals sensitive to ragweed

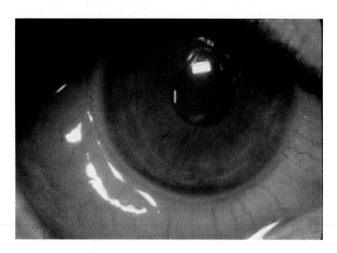

Figure 93–8. This patient is suffering from chemosis associated with allergic conjunctivitis. (Photo courtesy of Dr. Eli O. Meltzer, Allergy and Asthma Medical Group and Research Center, San Diego, California.)

have more symptoms in the fall. Patients often complain of bilateral itchy, watery eyes with a burning sensation. The conjunctiva is mildly inflamed with varying degrees of edema. Perennial allergic conjunctivitis is a variant with symptoms on a year-round basis and often allergens such as dust, mites, animal dander, and feathers are responsible for it. This conjunctivitis represents a type I hypersensitivity reaction.

Management

Treatment consists of a combination of topical vasoconstrictors (naphazoline-antazoline and naphazolinepheniramine), antihistamines (levocabastine 0.05%, emedastine difumarate 0.05%, azelastine hydrochloride 0.05%, ketotifen fumarate 0.025%, and olopatadine 0.1%), topical steroids (rimexolone 1% or loteprednol etabonate 0.2%), and anti-inflammatory agents (ketorolac 0.5% or diclofenac 0.1%). Systemic antihistamines such as loratidine may be of some benefit. Mast cell stabilizers (Cromolyn sodium 4%, nedocromil 2%, pemirolast potassium 0.1%, and lodoxamide tromethamine 0.1%) eye drops have also been shown to be effective when used as a prophylactic agent (Fig. 93–8).

Vernal Conjunctivitis

Vernal keratoconjunctivitis is a rare condition mainly affecting children under the age of 10. It is common in warm, dry climates, and occurs most commonly in males (male-to-female ratio of 2:1). Often there is a significant history of atopy. Peak incidence is between April and August. Patients usually have a history of bilateral itching, foreign-body sensation, clear mucoid discharge, photophobia, and injection. The giant papillae involve the upper tarsal conjunctiva and consist of large "cobblestone" papillae. The pathophysiology is not entirely clear; IgE and IgG are thought to play a role. The mainstay of treatment consists of mast cell stabilizers and topical antihistamines. Systemic antihistamines, anti-inflammatory drops, and steroid drops may also

be added. Cyclosporine drops are reserved for steroid-resistant disease.[8]

Special Forms of Conjunctivitis

Patients with Stevens–Johnson syndrome may have severe conjunctival involvement. In the acute phase of the disease, the palpebral and ocular conjunctiva can scar together. Often goblet cells are lost in the conjunctival epithelium and the mucous layer of tear film is lost. Since mucus allows tear film to stick to the surface of the eye, the dry-eye state of Stevens–Johnson syndrome is characterized by abundant tears that do not cover the surface of the eye because they are unable to adhere to it. Treatment consists of a combination of topical lubricants and antibiotics.

Kawasaki disease is associated with a bilateral bulbar, nonexudative conjunctivitis. This diagnosis should be suspected in patients who have fever for >5 days and have conjunctivitis, strawberry tongue, cervical adenopathy, fissuring of the lips, diffuse oral injection, erythema and induration of the hands and feet, rash, and desquamation of the fingers and toes. Not all symptoms are required to make the diagnosis.

A chronic blepharoconjunctivitis can be caused by *Pthirus pubis* when the eyelashes are infected by nits or by the bug itself. The only recognized lice to infect the eyelashes are pubic lice. Family members should be screened. The type of conjunctivitis seen with lice results from a hypersensitivity reaction. Systemic treatment of the organism is necessary for successful eradication. Eye ointments have been used for treatment because they are thought to paralyze and smother the lice. A cotton-tip applicator should be used for debridement prior to the placement of the ointment.

Molluscum contagiosum can cause conjunctivitis when the virus is shed into the eye. Typically, it causes a chronic conjunctivitis that does not respond to topical antimicrobials. The problem results from the virus protein, which is toxic to the eye. One may see lesions on the eyelids that are often buried between the eyelashes. Eradication of the virus requires that the lesions be opened with a needle and the central core of the umbilicated region be removed. Bleeding into the core is considered definitive treatment.

Other viral syndromes can be associated with nonspecific conjunctivitis. These include rubella, influenza, mumps, measles, infectious mononucleosis, and cytomegalovirus. Papillomavirus can cause eyelid warts, which shed on the conjunctiva, causing a type of conjunctivitis similar to that described for molluscum contagiosum.

Perinaud oculoglandular syndrome is a rare manifestation of cat scratch disease that occurs when the conjunctiva is directly inoculated with *Bartonella henselae* or *Afipia felis*. The condition manifests as a unilateral granulomatous or follicular conjunctivitis. Lymphadenopathy in the preauricular, cervical, and/or submandibular regions is common. Treatment consists of oral doxycycline, erythromycin, or ciprofloxacin. A similar syndrome can be caused by infections with *Francisella tularensis, Sporothrix schenckii, Mycobacterium tuberculosis,* or *Treponema pallidum.*

Other systemic diseases presenting with eye findings mimicking conjunctivitis include ataxia-telangiectasia, where large tortuous vessels are noted on the bulbar conjunctiva. Patients with Lyme disease may develop nonspecific conjunctivitis with or without eye pain.

▶ CONCLUSION

Patients with a red eye should have a thorough history and physical examination. Appropriate testing should include fluorescein staining and culture swabs for leukocytes and organisms depending on the circumstance. Patients with conjunctivitis should be instructed concerning good hygiene, and the physician should adhere to good hand-washing techniques as well as thoroughly cleaning instruments between patients.

REFERENCES

1. Ambati B, Ambati J, Azar N, et al. Periorbital and orbital cellulitis before and after the advent of *Haemophilus influenzae* type B vaccination. *Ophthalmology.* 2000;107:1450–1453.
2. Blomquist PH. Methicillin-resistant *Staphylococcus aureus* infections of the eye and orbit. *Trans Am Ophthalmol Soc.* 2006;104:322–345.
3. Goldschmilt P, Rostane H, Saint-Jean C. Effects of topical anaesthetics and fluorescein on the real-time PCR used for the diagnosis of herpesviruses and acanthamoeba keratitis. *British J Ophthalmol.* 2006;90:1354–1356.
4. Everitt HA, Little PS, Smith PWF. A randomised controlled trial of management strategies for acute infective conjunctivitis in general pediatrics. *BMJ.* 2006;333:321.
5. Kaufman H, Varnell E, Thompson H. Trifluridine, cidofovir, and penciclovir in the treatment of experimental herpetic keratitis. *Arch Ophthalmol.* 1998;116:777–780.
6. Herpetic Eye Disease Study Group: Oral acyclovir for herpes simplex virus eye disease. *Arch Ophthalmol.* 2000;118:1030–1036.
7. Soloman A, Holland M, Alexander N. Mass treatment with a single dose of azithromycin for trachoma. *N Engl J Med.* 2004;351:1962–1971.
8. Kilic A, Gurler B. Topical 2% cyclosporin A in preservative-free artificial tears for the treatment of vernal keratoconjunctivitis. *Can J Ophthalmol.* 2006;41:693–698.

SECTION XVI

GYNECOLOGIC EMERGENCIES

CHAPTER 94

The Adolescent Pregnant Patient

Adriana M. Rodriguez, Pamela J. Okada, and Jeanne S. Sheffield

▶ HIGH-YIELD FACTS

- Since preeclampsia is present in up to 7% of pregnancies, always check the blood pressure and screen for proteinuria.
- HELLP syndrome includes hemolysis, elevated liver enzymes, and low platelet counts; the lower the platelet count, the higher the mortality.
- Bleeding in the first trimester should alert the physician to ectopic pregnancy or threatened/spontaneous abortion. In later trimesters, consider placenta previa and abruption.
- With placenta previa, examination of the cervix can exacerbate hemorrhage.
- Placental abruption classically presents with vaginal bleeding, abdominal pain, uterine tenderness, and contractions. Bleeding may be concealed and does not correlate with severity of abruption.
- Ultrasonography is insensitive and unreliable for diagnosis of placental abruption.
- Ectopic pregnancy is the leading cause of maternal mortality during the first half of pregnancy in the United States, and should be suspected in any patient with abdominal pain and vaginal bleeding.
- Symptomatic deep vein thrombosis may be difficult to diagnose clinically because the pregnant patient often has leg swelling and discomfort during normal pregnancy.
- In the pregnant trauma patient, shock may be difficult to diagnose because during pregnancy, blood volume is increased, as is respiratory rate and heart rate.

Teenage pregnancies and children born to adolescents have a great impact on society. Pregnant teens are less likely to receive prenatal care and are more likely to partake in high-risk behaviors such as smoking and consumption of alcohol during pregnancy. Teen mothers are at risk of not completing their education and living in poverty as compared to their peers.

Although the overall rate of teenage pregnancy has declined over the past decade, there are still more than 850 000 teen pregnancies a year.[1] From 1990 to 2002, the teen pregnancy rate decreased from 38.6 to 21.4 per 1000 pregnancies. Although this is a significant improvement, certain ethnic groups continue to have a disproportionately high incidence of pregnancy in teens, from ages 15 to 17 years. The non-Hispanic black and Hispanic teenagers continue to have greater than 85 per 1000 pregnancies in this age group, as compared to non-Hispanic white teens who average 25 per 1000.[2] The decline in teen pregnancy is due to an increase in the use of contraception, a decrease in sexual activity, and effective pregnancy prevention programs.[3]

Emergency medicine physicians who routinely care for adolescents must therefore have the basic knowledge and skills to care for the adolescent pregnant patient, as well as resources to ensure appropriate treatment and follow-up. It is important that the emergency physician be able to recognize, stabilize, and treat complications of pregnancy, to recognize signs and symptoms that require immediate obstetrical referral, and to access appropriate and timely medical follow-up and resources unique to the needs of the adolescent patient.

▶ PREECLAMPSIA

Preeclampsia, or toxemia of pregnancy, complicates 2% to 7% of all pregnancies.[4] Preeclampsia is defined as hypertension with a blood pressure of 140/90 mm Hg or greater associated with proteinuria, and/or edema during pregnancy greater than 20 weeks gestation. Preeclampsia is further divided into mild and severe presentations. In mild preeclampsia, the patient is asymptomatic with blood pressure less than 160/110 mm Hg. Mental status, reflexes, abdominal examination, liver function, and coagulation studies are normal. In severe preeclampsia, diastolic blood pressures may exceed 110 mm Hg and may be associated with visual blurring, headache, abdominal pain, coagulaopathy, hyperreflexia, disseminated intravascular coagulation, or vaginal bleeding (Table 94–1). The exact etiology is not known.

Ultimately, the most effective therapy is delivery of the infant. The treatment goal is to prevent seizures and permanent maternal end organ damage as well as to protect the health of the infant. Therapy includes controlling seizures with magnesium sulfate, lowering blood pressure with hydralazine or labetolol, and affecting delivery of the fetus (Table 94–2).

Laboratory studies such as a CBC, platelet count, liver function transaminases, and creatinine level should be obtained to assess maternal organ injury. Monitor urine output closely. A cranial head computed tomography (CT) or MRI should be considered if there is a change in mental status, presence of seizures, or if lateralizing neurologic signs are evident.

▶ ECLAMPSIA

Eclampsia is the occurrence of seizures that cannot be attributed to other causes in a pregnant woman with preeclampsia. Complications associated with eclampsia include abruption placentae, disseminated intravascular coagulaopathy, pulmonary edema, acute renal failure, aspiration pneumonia, and

► **TABLE 94–1. MILD AND SEVERE PREECLAMPSIA DIAGNOSTIC CRITERIA[5]**

Mild preeclampsia
  Systolic blood pressure ≥140 mm Hg or diastolic blood
    pressure ≥90 mm Hg (in women with previously normal
    blood pressure)
  Proteinuria: ≥300 mg/L in 24 h or ≥1+ urine dipstick

Severe preeclampsia
  Systolic blood pressure ≥160 mm Hg or diastolic blood
    pressure ≥110 mm Hg
  Proteinuria: urinary excretion of 2 g or more on 24-h urine
    collection or 3+ protein on urine dipstick on two random
    urine samples 4 h apart
  Serum Cr ≥1.2 mg/dL (in patients with otherwise normal
    renal function)
  Oliguria <500 cc of urine in 24 h
  Cerebral/visual disturbance
  Pulmonary edema
  Hemolysis
  Epigastric or RUQ pain
  Elevation of liver transaminases
  Thrombocytopenia (platelets <100 000)
  Fetal growth restriction
  Headache

cardiopulmonary arrest. Perinatal death rate ranges from 5.6% to 11.8%. The treatment is the same as listed for preeclampsia. While ensuring prevention of maternal injury and supporting respiratory and cardiovascular functions, immediate obstetrical support should be called for.[6]

► HELLP SYNDROME

HELLP syndrome is defined as hemolysis (microangiopathic hemolytic anemia), elevated liver enzymes, and low platelets (<100 000/mm³). HELLP syndrome is a part of the spectrum of preeclampsia; however, hypertension can be absent in 10% to 15% of cases. Of note, the lower the platelets, the higher the

► **TABLE 94–2. TREATMENT FOR SEVERE PREECLAMPSIA[5]**

Systolic BP ≥160 mm Hg or diastolic BP ≥110 mm Hg:
  Hydralazine 5–10 mg doses at 15–20 min intervals OR
  Labetolol 10 mg and reevaluate in 10 min, increase to
    20 mg in 10 min, then 40 mg, followed by another 40 mg,
    then another 80 mg, if not effective. Total dosage not to
    exceed 220 mg
Seizure prophylaxis: Magnesium sulfate IV load with 4–6 g over
  15–20 min, then 2 g/h for desired levels of serum Mg of
  4.8–8.4 mg/dL
Fluid resuscitation for oliguria (urine output <30 cc/h)
  500 cc of crystalloid IV bolus
  Provide maximum of 3× 500 cc crystalloid IV boluses and
    MIVF rate of 100–125 cc/h
Delivery of infant

maternal and fetal morbidity and mortality.[7] Mortality resulting from the HELLP syndrome ranges from 2% to 24% of cases. The treatment is the same as preeclampsia and requires immediate obstetrical support.

► VAGINAL BLEEDING IN PREGNANCY

Pregnant adolescents who present with vaginal bleeding represent a high-risk population. Bleeding in the first trimester occurs in 20% to 25% of patients. Common etiologies include ectopic pregnancy, threatened abortion, spontaneous abortion, sexually transmitted infection, and trauma. Other causes of vaginal bleeding more common in the later trimesters include placenta previa and placental abruption.

PLACENTA PREVIA

Placenta previa is defined according to the proximity of the implantation of the placenta to the cervical os (Table 94–3). Placenta previa is seen in approximately 0.5% of births in the United States.[8] It is the primary cause of painless third trimester bleeding. Risk factors include maternal age more than 35 years, smoking, minority race, multiparity, cocaine use, prior placenta previa, and prior cesarean section. Damage to the endometrium is thought to be the cause of placenta previa. Each pregnancy damages the endometrium at the implantation site, making multiparity a risk factor for placenta previa.

The classic presentation of placenta previa is painless, bright red bleeding from the vagina. The uterus usually remains soft; however, contractions may occur in up to 20% of patients. Diagnosis of placenta previa requires extreme care, since examination of the cervix may exacerbate hemorrhaging by further tearing of the placenta. Digital examination is contraindicated, and thus the use of ultrasonography is necessary to make the diagnosis. Transvaginal ultrasonography is controversial because of the risk of further tearing the placenta, but if carefully performed, is more sensitive than transabdominal ultrasonography. Occasionally, an MRI is necessary to determine invasion into the myometrium (placenta accreta).

Management of known placenta previa that is not bleeding in the emergency department is typically expectant and includes pelvic rest, limiting long-distance travel, and maintaining a safe hemoglobin level. Patients with hemorrhage should be stabilized with insertion of two large-bore IV catheters and given crystalloid fluids and blood transfusions, if needed. Cesarean delivery is required in cases of placenta previa because

► **TABLE 94–3. CLASSIFICATION OF PLACENTA PREVIA[9]**

Complete: placenta completely covers internal cervical os
Incomplete: inferior edge of placenta partially covers or
  encroaches upon internal os
Marginal: edge of placenta just reaches the internal os, but does
  not cover it
Low lying placenta: extends into the lower uterine segment but
  does not reach the internal os

of increased risk for hemorrhage from the implantation site. Delivery may ultimately lead to a hysterectomy.[8,9] Placenta previa will triple the rate of neonatal mortality secondary to an increase in preterm delivery. Thus, obstetric consultation and transfer to a facility capable of managing the mother and newly born should be initiated early.

PLACENTAL ABRUPTION

Placental abruption is the premature separation of a normally implanted placenta. The separation can be total or partial. The hemorrhage may be concealed or present as vaginal bleeding. Placental abruption accounts for 30% of bleeding during the latter half of pregnancy, is seen in 1% of all pregnancies, and accounts for more than 20% of perinatal mortality.[9,10] Maternal risk factors include advanced maternal age, hypertension, advanced parity, tobacco use, poor nutrition, cocaine use, premature rupture of membranes (PROM), diabetes, preeclampsia, trauma, polyhydramnios, and chorioamnionitis.[11]

The classic presentation of placental abruption typically includes vaginal bleeding, abdominal pain, uterine tenderness, and contractions. Bleeding is dark in color and the amount of bleeding does not correlate with the severity of abruption. The degree of separation can be minimal to severe. In more severe cases of placental abruption, severe hemorrhage, uterine tetany and tenderness, maternal hypotension, coagulopathy, and fetal distress can be seen. Unlike placenta previa, ultrasonography is insensitive and unreliable in the diagnosis of placental abruption. In most mild cases, the diagnosis is made postpartum on inspection of the placenta.

The management of a patient with suspected placenta abruption includes stabilizing the airway, 100% oxygen, two large-bore IV catheters, fluid resuscitation, and careful monitoring of the mother and fetus. Laboratory evaluation includes a CBC, platelet count, coagulation studies, fibrinogen, fibrin degradation products, prothrombin and partial thromboplastin time and type and cross for matched blood. Complications of placental abruption include preterm delivery, low birth weight, intrauterine growth restriction, stillbirth, and perinatal death. Again, early obstetric consultation and transfer to facility capable of caring for the mother and newly born must be initiated early.[9–11]

▶ ECTOPIC PREGNANCY/ THREATENED ABORTION

Ectopic pregnancy is the leading cause of maternal mortality during the first half of pregnancy in the United States, and should be suspected in any patient with vaginal bleeding or abdominal pain. An ectopic pregnancy is defined as the implantation of the blastocyst outside the endometrial lining of the uterine cavity. The incidence of ectopic pregnancies is 2 in 100 pregnancies.[12] The mortality rate for African American and other minority women remains more than twice that for white women, and the highest mortality rate occurs in the 15- to 19-year-old age group.[13] The higher mortality rate in adolescents is largely due to delays in seeking medical care. Greater than 95% of ectopic pregnancies are in the fallopian tube.[14] Risk factors include prior ectopic pregnancy, previous salpingitis (history

▶ **TABLE 94–4. DIAGNOSIS OF ECTOPIC PREGNANCY[15]**

Serum beta-HCG: positive
Transvaginal ultrasound showing an empty uterus ± adnexal mass
Serum progesterone: >25 ng/mL → not likely ectopic < 5 ng/mL → nonviable fetus (ectopic vs. dead fetus)
CBC for hemoglobin and leukocytosis

of trauma or inflammation to the fallopian tube), pelvic inflammatory disease (PID), and intrauterine device. Since many of these risk factors increase with sexual maturity, adolescents are at lower risk.[12]

Clinical presentation of ectopic pregnancies varies, but most cases present within the first 8 weeks of gestation with abdominal pain or abnormal vaginal bleeding. Most commonly, the patient complains of pelvic or abdominal pain and exquisite tenderness. Others present with amenorrhea and vaginal bleeding, which is often confused with menses. The vaginal bleeding is usually scant and dark in color. In the case of intra-abdominal hemorrhage and hypovolemia, the clinical presentation may include dizziness and/or presyncope.[15]

The classic physical examination of a patient with an ectopic pregnancy includes tenderness on abdominal examination, shock, and an adnexal mass; however, this presentation is rare. More commonly, the abdominal examination may be unremarkable or there may be adnexal and/or cervical motion tenderness. Unfortunately, the history and physical examination are insufficient to detect an unruptured ectopic pregnancy, and the emergency medicine physician must rely on other modalities to aid in the diagnosis (Table 94–4).

Emergency management of the patient with an ectopic pregnancy begins with stabilization. Provide attention to airway, breathing and circulation, placement of two large-bore IV catheters, fluid resuscitation with crystalloid and packed red blood cell transfusions, and early obstetric consultation for surgical management and transfer of care. Additionally, the Rh negative patient requires Rh immunoprophylaxis with 50 μg anti-D immune globulin intramuscularly.

In the hemodynamically stable patient, methotrexate, a folic acid antagonist, can be used for the medical management of an early ectopic pregnancy. Methotrexate when compared to laparoscopy showed no difference in tubal preservation of patency, but reduced hospitalization and overall costs. Factors that favor improved success with methotrexate are outlined in Table 94–5. Contraindications to medical management include unstable vital signs, active bleeding, tubal rupture, or contraindications to methotrexate. If medical management

▶ **TABLE 94–5. FACTORS ASSOCIATED WITH IMPROVED SUCCESS RATE OF METHOTREXATE FOR ECTOPIC PREGNANCIES[16]**

No maternal hemorrhage
Beta-HCG <15 000 mIU/mL
Less than 4 cm product of pregnancy
Less than 6 wk' gestation

► **TABLE 94–6. RISK FACTORS FOR THROMBOTIC EVENTS IN PREGNANCY[17]**

Cesarean section delivery
Operative vaginal delivery
Maternal age (advancing age yields increasing risk)
Thrombophilias
Antiphospholipid antibodies
Obesity
Trauma
Infection
Prolonged bed rest

► **TABLE 94–7. RISK FACTORS FOR PULMONARY EMBOLISM[20]**

Prior DVT
Anti-phospholipid antibody
Hereditary thrombophilias
Familial hypercoaguability state
Trauma/prolonged hospitalization
Mechanical heart valve
Atrial fibrillation

is contraindicated or not desired, surgical management is appropriate.[16]

► DEEP VEIN THROMBOSIS AND PULMONARY EMBOLISM IN PREGNANCY AND POSTPARTUM

Deep vein thrombosis (DVT) and pulmonary embolism (PE) are significant causes of morbidity and mortality during pregnancy and the puerperium. The risk for developing a DVT and/or subsequent PE is five times greater during this period. Thrombotic events are seen as often as 1 in 1000 pregnancies.[17] Of these thrombotic events, up to 15% will result in PE. PE causes up to 15% of maternal death during pregnancy or puerperium and is the primary cause of direct maternal death.[18,19]

Factors that contribute to the increase incidence of thrombotic events during pregnancy and the puerperium include venous stasis, blood vessel trauma, and hypercoaguability (Table 94–6). Venous stasis is compounded by compression of the inferior vena cava and pelvic veins by a gravid uterus.[17] Hypercoaguability is due to physiologic changes during pregnancy, which include increase in circulating clotting factors and decreasing amounts of protein S.

The left lower extremity is the most common site for a DVT; however, the pelvic veins are the most common source for PE.[18,20] PE is preceded by symptomatic DVT in less than half of the cases.[17] DVT is more common in the antenatal period, whereas PE is more common in the postpartum period. The clinical presentation of DVT include leg pain or discomfort especially on the left, swelling, tenderness, increased temperature and edema, and/or lower abdominal pain. Many DVTs can be asymptomatic. Symptomatic DVTs present similarly in pregnant or postpartum women as they do in nonpreg-

nant women and are particularly difficult to diagnose clinically since leg swelling and discomfort are common features of normal pregnancy. Compression ultrasonography with or without color Doppler is used for the diagnosis of DVT. Magnetic resonance venography or venography can also be performed if compression ultrasonography does not provide a definite diagnosis.

PE arises from DVT, but many DVTs are not recognized prior to the occurrence of a PE. Recognizing the risk factors for venous thromboembolism, timely diagnosis, and appropriate treatment are important to the emergency medicine physician caring for the pregnant patient (Table 94–7). The diagnosis of PE requires a high index of suspicion. Signs and symptoms may vary and can be difficult to diagnose. Most common symptoms are dyspnea and tachypnea, seen in up to 90% of cases (Table 94–8). Hemoptysis is seen in less than 10% of the cases.

The diagnosis of PE can be difficult and a high index of suspicion is necessary. Arterial blood gas, chest radiograph, and ECG changes will be seen only variably. Ventilation/perfusion (V/Q) lung scan is safe throughout pregnancy; however, it has low specificity. The current first line diagnostic test is a spiral chest CT. The use of serum D-dimer for the diagnosis of DVT or PE is not presently recommended because of decreased sensitivity in pregnancy. In pregnancy, D-dimer can be increased secondarily to the physiologic changes in the coagulation system, especially if there is preeclampsia. MRI has no significant advantage over the spiral CT.

When a DVT or PE is suspected clinically, treatment with unfractionated heparin or low-molecular-weight heparin should be started until the diagnosis is excluded, unless anticoagulation is contraindicated (Table 94–9). In patients with DVT, elevate the leg and apply thromboembolic deterrent stockings. In patients with PE, analgesia for pleuritic pain and oxygen are beneficial. Early obstetric consultation and transfer is recommended.

► **TABLE 94–8. CLINICAL PRESENTATION OF PULMONARY EMBOLISM[21]**

Dyspnea
Chest pain
Cough
Tachypnea
Tachycardia
Hemoptysis

► **TABLE 94–9. TREATMENT OF ACUTE PE[22]**

Intravenous heparin bolus 5000 units
Continuous infusion of 30 000 or more units of heparin over 24 h to prolong the PTT to 1.5–2.5 times control
Continue anticoagulation for 5–7 d
Therapeutic heparinization with subcutaneous dosing for ≥3 mo
May use low molecular weight heparin or Coumadin (if postpartum) after initial intravenous dosing

▶ TABLE 94-10. CLASSIFICATION OF HYDATIDIFORM MOLES[23]

Complete Hydatidiform Mole	Partial Hydatidiform Mole
No embryo–fetus	Often present embryo-fetus
Diffuse villous edema	Amnion/fetal red blood cells present
Slight to severe trophoblasts	Karyotype 69, XXX or 69 XXY
Karyotype 46, XX or 46, XY	
Clinical presentation	*Clinical presentation*
Molar gestation	Missed abortion
50% large for dates	Small for dates
Frequent medical complications	Rare medical complications
18%–28% chance of gestational trophoblastic neoplasia	<5% chance of gestational trophoblastic neoplasia

▶ HYDATIDIFORM MOLE

Hydatidiform mole is a proliferative abnormality of trophoblastic tissue or abnormality of chorionic villi that consist of trophoblastic proliferation and edema of villous stroma. The incidence of hydatidiform moles is 1 in 1500 pregnancies.[23] Hydatidiform moles are classified as complete or partial molar pregnancies (Table 94–10). Risk factors for hydatidiform mole are maternal age younger than 15 years or older than 45 years and previous molar pregnancies. The signs and symptoms of a hydatidiform mole include abnormal uterine bleeding, large uterine size, no fetal activity, gestational hypertension or preeclampsia prior to 24 weeks gestation, hyperemesis, thyrotoxicosis, and embolization.

The diagnosis of hydatidiform mole is made with a serum beta-HCG level that is higher than expected for estimated gestation and evidence of a molar pregnancy on ultrasonography. Treatment includes immediate evacuation of mole with uterine dilation and curettage. Subsequent evaluation for persistent trophoblastic proliferation or malignant change is also necessary.

▶ EMERGENCY CONTRACEPTION

Approximately 3 million of the 6 million pregnancies in the United States are unintended. Emergency contraception (EC) is defined as a drug or device used to prevent pregnancy after sexual intercourse or after recognition of contraception failure.[24] In the United States, the two most common and available methods include Levonogestrel 1.5 mg (Plan B®) and copper IUD containing 380 mm of copper (Paragaurd®). Plan B became available without need of prescription in August 2006. There is currently no data available to determine the impact on unplanned pregnancies since this EC was made available.

EC is intended as a back-up method of contraception and should be used only occasionally. Both of these methods can be used up to 5 days after sexual intercourse. Levonogestrel is

noted to have improved effectiveness if used within the first 48 hours. The directions for Plan B are to take 0.75 mg tablet of Levonogestrel every 12 hours for a total of two doses. Studies have also shown that taking one dose totaling 1.5 mg of Levonogestrel is equally as effective as splitting the dose as described above. Because nausea and vomiting can be significant side effects, if vomiting is experienced within 1 to 2 hours after taking Plan B, the dose(s) should be repeated. Side effects include nausea, vomiting, irregular bleeding, dizziness, fatigue, breast tenderness, headache, and abdominal pain. The copper IUD does not have reduced effectiveness between 48 and 120 hours after sexual intercourse. Placement of an IUD as an EC has the same risk factors as in a person using it for conventional contraception.

▶ TRAUMA IN PREGNANCY

Trauma in pregnancy complicates up to 1 in 12 pregnancies and is the most common cause of nonobstetrical morbidity and mortality.[25] Motor vehicle crashes are the number one cause followed by assaults, falls, and intimate partner violence (IPV). A much smaller number of cases are from homicide, burns, and electrical injury. As the uterus and fetal size increases with gestational age, the risk of injury increases from 10% to 15% in the first trimester to 50% to 54% during the third trimester. Pregnant adolescents are at the highest risk of IPV and are at an increased risk of vaginal bleeding, poor weight gain, alcohol or drug abuse, and death.[26]

The approach to the traumatized pregnant patient requires an understanding of anatomic and physiologic changes in pregnancy. Such changes include an increased respiratory rate, heart rate and cardiac output, a relative hypotension, an increased blood volume by 50%, and a relative decrease in hematocrit. These physiologic changes make the diagnosis of shock difficult.

The general management and assessment of a pregnant patient is similar to that of all trauma patients. The priorities of resuscitation follow ATLS guidelines. Special precautions are important to remember. As compared to the nonobstetric patient, pregnant women are at higher risk for aspiration from delayed gastric emptying. There should be no hesitation in protecting the airway. Oxygen saturation should always be optimized. Placement of a chest tube thoracostomy needs to be 1 to 2 intercostal spaces higher than usual. Hemodynamic instability can be difficult to diagnose because in pregnancy maternal blood volume is increased. As in all trauma cases, two large-bore IV catheters are necessary. Deflection of the uterus to the left side, once the airway is secured, is important to limit aortocaval compression and to improve venous return. In addition to the mother's vital signs, fetal heart tones should be monitored. Shock may occur with minimal change in pulse or blood pressure, and fetal distress may be the first sign of maternal hemodynamic instability. If vasopressor support is indicated, ephedrine and mephentermine are preferred. Early obstetric and surgical consultation is essential in maximizing outcome.

Laboratory tests may include a CBC, type and cross matching, urinalysis, serum bicarbonate level or blood gas analysis, and fibrinogen levels. Radiographs should not be withheld because of concerns of radiation exposure to the fetus. Plain radiographs of the cervical spine, chest, and pelvic can be obtained while shielding the uterus. CT of the head and chest are generally safe. As a general rule, avoid abdominal CTs in early pregnancy and consider other diagnostic modalities such as ultrasound or diagnostic peritoneal lavage (DPL). Ultrasonography can be used to locate free intraperitoneal fluid, guide for DPL, establish gestational age, placental localization, aid in diagnosis of placental abruption, and estimate amniotic fluid volume.

Disposition after trauma in pregnancy varies with severity of injury and gestational age. Generally, patients that are greater than 20 weeks with blunt abdominal trauma should be monitored for at least 4 to 6 hours. Evidence of fetal distress requires urgent obstetric assistance and may require emergency cesarean section.[27] In cases of maternal cardiopulmonary arrest or death, emergent cesarean section within the first 4 minutes is recommended for potential fetal survival. Indicators of poor prognosis include vaginal bleeding, abdominal tenderness, postural hypotension, fetal heart abnormalities, and frequent uterine contractions.[28]

▶ Rh SENSITIZATION

Rh sensitization occurs when an Rh negative mother is exposed to Rh positive fetal blood. It can occur after trauma, spontaneous or therapeutic abortions, or ectopic pregnancy. Anytime there is mixing of maternal and fetal blood, anti-D immune globulin (RhoGAM) is indicated and can be given at a dose of 50 μg intramuscularly (IM) prior to 12 weeks gestational age or 300 μg IM after 12 weeks gestational age.[29]

REFERENCES

1. Trends from 1976–2003 in pregnancy, birth and abortion rates in teens 15–17 years. *MMWR Morb Mortal Wkly Rep.* 2005;54 (04):100.
2. Ventura SJ, Abma JC, Mosther WD, et al. *Recent Trends in Teenage Pregnancy in the United States, 1990–2002.* National Center for Health Statistics; 2006. http://www.cdc.gov/nchs/products/pubs/pubd/hestats/teenpreg1990–2002/teenpreg1990–2002.htm.
3. Santelli JS, Lindberg LD, Finer LB, et al. Explaining recent declines in adolescent pregnancy in the United States: the contributions of abstinence and improved contraceptive use. *Am J Pub Health.* 2007;97(1):150–156.
4. Sibai BM. Diagnosis and management of gestational hypertension and preeclampsia. *Obstet Gynecol.* 2003;102(1):181–192.
5. Cunningham FG, Leveno KJ, Bloom SL, et al. Hypertensive disorders in pregnancy. In: Rouse D, Rainey B, Spong C, Wendel GD. *Williams Obstetrics.* New York, NY: McGraw-Hill; 2005: 761–808.
6. Sibai BM. Diagnosis, prevention, and management of eclampsia. *Obstet Gynecol.* 2005;105(2):402–410.
7. Leduc L, Wheeler JM, Kirshon B, et al. Coagulation profile in severe preeclampsia. *Obstet Gynecol.* 1992;79(1):14–18.
8. Cunningham FG, Leveno KJ, Bloom SL, et al. Obstetrical hemorrhage. In Rouse D, Rainey B, Spong C, Wendel GD, eds. *Williams Obstetrics.* New York, NY: McGraw-Hill; 2005:809–854.
9. Baron F, Hill WC. Placenta previa, placenta abruptio. *Clin Obstet Gynecol.* 1998;41(3):527–532.
10. Hladky K, Yankowitz J, Hansen WF. Placental abruption. *Obstet Gynecol Surv.* 2002;57(5):299–305.
11. Saftlas AF, Olson DR, Atrash HK, et al. National trends in the incidence of abruptio placentae, 1979–1987. *Obstet Gynecol.* 1991;78:1081–1086.
12. Ectopic pregnancy—United States, 1990–1992. *MMWR Morb Mortal Wkly Rep.* 1995;44(3):46–48.
13. Lawson HW, Atrash HK, Saftlas AF, et al. Ectopic pregnancy in the United States, 1970–1986. *MMWR CDC Surveill Summ.* 1989;38(2):1–10.
14. Bouyer J, Coste J, Fernandez H, et al. Sites of ectopic pregnancy: a 10 year population-based study of 1800 cases. *Hum Reprod.* 2002;17(12):3224–3230.
15. Mukul LV, Teal SB. Current management of ectopic pregnancy. *Obstet Gynecol Clin N Am.* 2007;34(3):403–419.
16. Ory SJ; American College of Obstetricians and Gynecologists (ACOG). Medical management of tubal pregnancy. Washington (DC): American College of Obstetricians and Gynecologists. *ACOG Practice Bulletin.* 1998;(3):7.
17. Lindqvist P, Dahlbäck B, Marś ál. Thrombotic risk during pregnancy: a population study. *Obstet Gynecol.* 1999;94(4):595–599.
18. Gherman RB, Goodwin TM, Leung B, et al. Incidence, clinical characteristics, and timing of objectively diagnosed venous thromboembolism during pregnancy. *Obstet Gynecol.* 1999;94:730–734.
19. Rutherford SE, Phelan JP. Deep venous thrombosis and pulmonary embolism in pregnancy. *Obstet Gynecol Clin N Am.* 1991;18:345–369.
20. Greer IA. Prevention and management of venous thromboembolism in pregnancy. *Clin Chest Med.* 2003;24(1):123–137.
21. Greer IA, Thomson AJ. Management of venous thromboembolism in pregnancy. *Best Pract Res Clin Obstet Gynaecol.* 2001;15(4):583–603.
22. Lowe GDO. Treatment of venous thrombotic embolism. *Baill Clin Obstet and Gynaecol.* 1997;11:511–521.
23. Garner EI, Goldstein DP, Feltmate CM, et al. Gestational trophoblastic disease. *Clin Obstet Gynecol.* 2007;50(1):112–122.
24. Allen RH. Goldberg AB. Emergency contraception: a clinical review. *Clin Obstet Gynecol.* 2004;50(4):927–936.
25. Shah AJ, Kilcline BA. Trauma in pregnancy. *Emerg Med Clin N Am.* 2003;21:615–629.
26. Gunter J. Intimate partner violence. *Obstet Gynecol Clin N Am.* 2007;34:367–388.
27. Pearlman MD, Tintinalli JE, Lorenz RP. A prospective controlled study of outcome after trauma during pregnancy. *Am J Obstet Gynecol.* 1990;162:1502–1510.
28. Atta E, Gardner M. Cardiopulmonary resuscitation in pregnancy. *Obstet Gynecol Clin N Am.* 2007;34:585–597.
29. Bowman J. Thirty-five years of Rh prophylaxis. *Transfusion.* 2003;43:1661–1666.

CHAPTER 95

Gynecologic Disorders of Infancy, Childhood, and Adolescence

Geetha M. Devdas and Maria Stephan

▶ HIGH-YIELD FACTS

- An understanding of the anatomic and physiologic variations among various age groups is essential to managing childhood gynecological disorders. It is important to take a detailed history and remain compassionate toward the young female prior to and during the physical examination.
- An external examination of the genitalia and specimen collection, if indicated, is often all that is needed for prepubescent patients. A standard speculum examination is indicated in those patients who are sexually active, those who have bleeding from trauma or a suspected foreign body.
- Congenital vaginal obstruction may present as an abdominal mass or bulging mass at the introitus. In severe cases, urinary tract infection, obstructive uropathy, and/or septicemia may result from secondary infection of a vaginal obstruction.
- Treatment of labial adhesions is usually not indicated if the patient is asymptomatic. If treatment is indicated for symptomatic relief of local inflammation and irritation, estrogen cream is the first line of therapy. Surgery is rarely indicated, but necessary if symptoms persist and become severe despite medical treatment.
- Urethral prolapse occurs most commonly in prepubertal African American female patients. Therapy with estrogen cream has been reported to be successful to reduce swelling of urethral tissue. If symptoms persist despite medical management, surgery to excise the redundant tissue may be indicated.

The emergency physician will have encounters with infants, prepubescent children, and adolescents who present with gynecological disorders. The pathologic processes in infants and young children differ significantly from that of the adolescent female patients. It is important to have knowledge of basic anatomic and physiologic variations among various age groups, as well as be able to provide compassionate and quality care to young female patients. Additionally, it is very important to take a thorough history, including any irritants or medications a child may be using, as well as a careful review of the social setting in which the child inhabits.

▶ EVALUATION OF PREMENARCHEAL PATIENTS

INFANT AND TODDLER

The female infant is under the influence of maternal estrogens for the first 8 weeks of life. As a result, the labia majora appears full and there is thickening and enlargement of the labia minora.[1] Hymenal tissue stays thick, redundant, and elastic throughout infancy. The hymen tends to surround the vaginal orifice and appears circumferential[2] (Fig. 95–1 illustrates the genital morphology). Estrogen levels continue to fall until about 1.5 to 2 years of age.[1]

YOUNGER SCHOOL-AGE CHILDREN (AGES 3–6)

As the estrogen levels reach their lowest levels between 3 and 9 years of age, the appearance of the female genitalia changes.[2] The clitoris is less prominent and the labia become flatter.[1] The hymen generally becomes thinner and may appear translucent, while also leaving a "crescentic" appearance as the hymen tissue recedes from the anterior vaginal orifice. There is a high degree of variability, with some of these changes occurring earlier in some children and later in others. The vaginal pH during this time is alkaline.[2]

OLDER SCHOOL-AGE CHILDREN (AGES 7–12)

The labia continue to develop and the hymen thickens, while the vagina elongates to about 8 cm. The vaginal mucosa thickens and the vaginal pH becomes acidic. A thin white vaginal discharge, also known as physiologic leukorrhea, may be noted.[1,2]

APPROACH TO THE PHYSICAL EXAMINATION

A successful examination requires adequate lighting and an environment in which the child feels extremely relaxed and

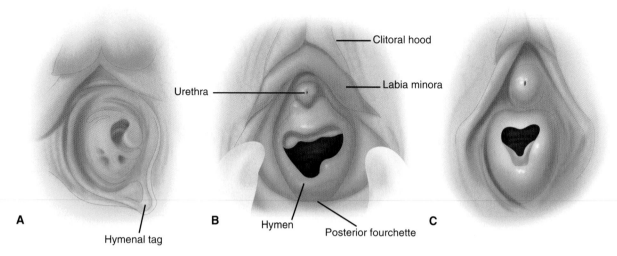

Figure 95–1. Developmental changes in gential morphology. (A) Infant: hymen circumferential and redundant. (B) Preschool through school age: rudimentary labia minora, thinner hymen. (C) Early puberty: labia minora develop and hymen thickens.

as comfortable as possible. During the examination, it is very important to address any concerns or fears the child may have, especially in cases of sexual assault. When beginning the evaluation of the child, it is important to assess the stage of sexual development by examining the breasts and looking for any indication of puberty[3] (Table 95–1). A standard speculum examination is used in patients who are sexually active or if there is bleeding from trauma. In prepubertal girls, external visualization is often all that is needed to make the diagnosis. This should be performed in a methodical manner with careful notations of abnormalities or variations. The frog-leg position is commonly used and allows easy visualization of the genitalia. This is sometimes performed with the child in the mother's lap. Another useful position for examination is the knee-chest position in which the child lies with her knees pulled to her chest on the examination table, supporting her weight on her knees, with her buttock elevated.[2] A good view of the vaginal introitus can be accomplished using labial traction, which consists of grasping the labia with the thumb and forefinger and gently pulling the labia toward the examiner.[2]

(Figs. 95–2 and 95–3 show examination techniques.) If there is a suspected abdominal mass, a rectal examination may be useful.

An internal examination may be indicated if there is a suspected foreign body, vaginal bleeding or discharge, or suspected tumor. In prepubertal girls, it is sometimes necessary to perform an internal examination under general anesthesia using various instruments such as a vaginoscope, cystoscope, hysteroscope, or endoscope with irrigating properties.[1]

Specimen collection is indicated if there is any vaginal discharge. The specimen should be sent for Gram stain, culture, and wet mount preparation. A sample can be collected from the vaginal introitus with a swab that has been moistened with normal saline. In a very young or uncooperative child, a large bore intravenous catheter can be used to flush 1 to 2 mL of saline that can then be sent for further studies.[4] After initial fluid collection, irrigating the vagina with larger amounts of saline is sometimes useful for washing out small foreign bodies.[1] In cases of suspected sexual abuse, specific specimens should be collected. For example, specimens should be

▶ TABLE 95–1. **STAGES OF SEXUAL DEVELOPMENT**

Sexual Maturity Rating (SMR)	Breast Development	Pubic Hair Development
1	Elevation of papilla	No pubic hair
2	Breast buds appear, areola appears as small mound	Straight hair extends along labia
3	Breast enlargement with protrusion of papilla or nipple	Darker and increased in quantity on pubis and remains in triangle
4	Breast enlargement with projection of areola and nipple as secondary mound	Darker, more coarse and curly, adult distribution but not as abundant
5	Adult configuration with no projection of areola as secondary mound	Adult pattern with extension of hair into medial aspect of thigh

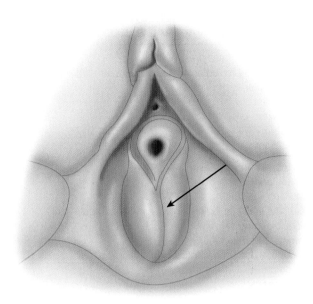

Figure 95–2. External hymenal ridge (arrow) and sleeve-like hymen—a normal variant.

sent for cultures of *Neisseria gonorrhoeae* and *Chlamydia trachomatis*, as well as slide preparations for *Trichomonas*. (See Chapter 144 for more detail on sexual abuse examination and testing.)

▶ GYNECOLOGIC DISORDERS OF INFANCY AND CHILDHOOD

NEONATAL PHYSIOLOGIC VARIANTS

In infancy, the newborn girl is affected by circulating maternal estrogens. As a result of these estrogens, it is not uncommon to see breast buds, sometimes with a milky discharge from the nipple. Additionally, neonates may also experience transient vaginal secretions that result from exposure to maternal estrogens. The maternal estrogens stimulate mucoid secretions in the neonate and these secretions may appear as a whitish or clear mucous discharge, and occasionally as a bloody discharge. This transient discharge should subside after about 2 weeks as maternal estrogen levels in the neonate decline, so only reassurance is required as the condition is self-limited. If the vaginal discharge or bleeding persists beyond 2 weeks, further evaluation should be initiated.[1]

CONGENITAL VAGINAL OBSTRUCTION

Etiology

Congenital vaginal obstruction can present at variable times during infancy and childhood. The two most common types of obstruction are due to an imperforate hymen or a transverse vaginal septum, also known as vaginal atresia. A transverse

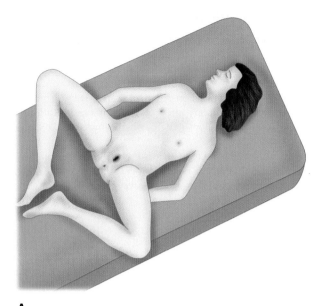

A

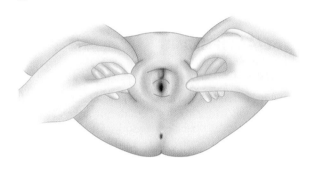

B

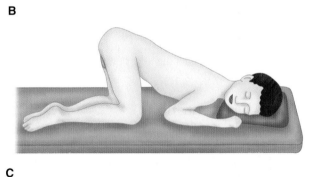

C

Figure 95–3. Physical examination positions.

vaginal septum is thought to result from failure in canalization of the vaginal plate at various levels. An imperforate hymen is a remnant of the urogenital membrane. Other lesions, such as cloacal malformation and common urogenital sinus, result from an interruption of the normal differentiation of the hindgut. The vaginal plate and sinovaginal bulbs subsequently do not develop and the upper vagina and rectum enter the urogenital sinus.[5,6] These lesions can lead to obstruction of normal mucoid secretions and cause hydrocolpos, which is distension of the vagina (colpos), or hydrometrocolpos, which is distension of the uterus (metro) and vagina.

Clinical Presentation

Hydrocolpos in the newborn period may present as an abdominal mass or a bulging mass at the introitus.[2,7] On rare occasions, vaginal obstruction can lead to recurrent urinary tract infections, obstructive uropathy, and renal failure secondary to compression by the mass on other structures. There have also been reports of secondary infection and septicemia leading to accumulation of purulent material in the mass that requires emergent drainage.[8,9]

An imperforate hymen that is not diagnosed in infancy may present at puberty as primary amenorrhea and intermittent lower abdominal pain that worsens every month. On physical examination, a bluish bulge, also known as hematocolpos, may be seen at the introitus.

Management

Treatment of vaginal atresia and imperforate hymen is surgical correction of the anomaly. In cases of hydrocolpos or hydrometrocolpos, surgical drainage is necessary to relieve the obstruction.[1]

LABIAL ADHESIONS

Etiology

Labial adhesions, also known as labial agglutination, usually begin posteriorly and extend superiorly toward the clitoris, often leaving a small opening anteriorly. There is usually a thin line or demarcation that represents the fused portion.[1] It is reported to have a prevalence of 1.8% to 3.3% with a peak incidence in the 13- to 23-month age group,[10] but commonly occurring in ages from 1 to 6 years. The etiology is unknown, but some theories suggest that the adhesions are due to an estrogen deficiency in the prepubertal period and inflammation that results in thinning of the superficial mucosal layers.[1]

Clinical Presentation

A parent may bring a child in after noticing that the vaginal area appears to be "closing." A physician may also notice labial adhesions during routine physical examination of a child. Occasionally, the adhesions may be mistaken for congenital absence of the vagina or imperforate hymen. The two can be distinguished by the raphe or vertical line connecting the adhesions.

Management

Most cases of labial adhesions resolve on their own and only reassurance is required, especially in asymptomatic cases. If the child has symptoms such as pain, inflammation, or urinary tract infections, first-line therapy is estrogen cream applied to the fine thin raphe twice a day for 2 weeks followed by once daily application for 2 weeks. This may be repeated in 6-month to 1-year intervals if there is recurrence.[1] If the adhesions and symptoms persist, surgical separation may be indicated.[11,12] Manual separation is not recommended because of the physical and emotional trauma to the child.

▶ **TABLE 95–2. DIFFERENTIAL DIAGNOSIS OF PREPUBERTAL VAGINAL BLEEDING**

Visible lesion or mass present
Traumatic injury including sexual assault, straddle injury
Urethral prolapse
Lichen sclerosis
Genital warts or ulcers
Neoplasm
Hemangioma

No visible lesion or mass
Vaginal foreign body
Infectious vaginitis
Traumatic injury including sexual assault, straddle injury
Rectal bleeding
Premature menarche
Exogenous hormone withdrawal
Hematuria
Coagulopathy
Neoplasm

▶ PUBERTAL VAGINAL BLEEDING

VAGINAL FOREIGN BODY

Etiology

There are a variety of causes for prepubertal vaginal bleeding (Table 95–2). One of the most common causes of bleeding is a vaginal foreign body. Often the foreign body is a small toy or more commonly small pieces of toilet paper. It is important to take a detailed history and evaluate for sexual abuse if there is any suspicion for sexual misconduct.[2]

Clinical Presentation

A child may present with persistent, foul-smelling, brown or bloody discharge. There may be complaints of dysuria and pelvic or abdominal pain. The child may also have some vulvar or vaginal irritation.[12]

Management

The treatment for a retained vaginal foreign body is removal of the foreign body. If the foreign body is small and visible, a warm saline irrigation may be used to wash it out. This is especially useful for small pieces of toilet paper. In some cases, a plain radiograph may be used to distinguish whether or not the foreign body is too large to be manually removed. If the foreign body is too large, not visible, or too deeply implanted, it may be necessary to remove it while the child is under general anesthesia.[12]

URETHRAL PROLAPSE

Etiology

Urethral prolapse is protrusion of urethral mucosa through the urethral meatus. The etiology is unclear, but is thought to occur

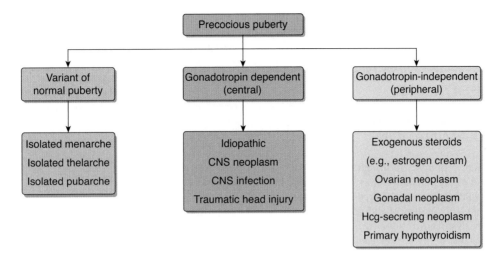

Figure 95–4. Algorithm of precocious puberty.

secondary to increased intra-abdominal pressure in association with poor attachments between smooth muscle layers of the urethra. It is an uncommon problem, but tends to occur more often in prepubescent African Americans girls.[13]

Clinical Presentation

On physical examination, the vaginal orifice may be obscured and a ring of congested and edematous tissue may be seen at the introitus. The mucosa appears red or purple and some areas may even appear black and necrotic. A child may present with painless bleeding.[2,13]

Management

Clinicians have reported good response with topical estrogen cream. Cream is applied to the area once daily for 1 week and then every other day for another 1 week. In addition, a sitz bath may also be helpful. If the child is constipated, stool softeners can be prescribed to prevent straining with defecation, which may make the prolapse worse. Other published reports of treatments include topical steroid or antibiotic cream. If conservative medical treatment fails, patients can be treated surgically by excising redundant tissue.

PRECOCIOUS PUBERTY

Etiology

Precocious puberty is defined as the onset of secondary sexual characteristics at an age that is greater than 2.5 standard deviations below the mean age of pubertal onset for the population. In the past decade, there has been much controversy regarding the normal age for the onset of puberty in young girls. In the United States, the estimated incidence of precocious puberty is 0.01% to 0.05% per year. It is more common in African American girls than Caucasian girls.[14] Traditionally, physicians have been using the age of 8 years as the normal year for onset of puberty and have been doing full evaluations on girls below this age. More recent data based on a study of more than

17 000 girls aged 3 to 12 years by the Pediatric Researchers in Office Setting (PROS) investigators shows that this age cutoff is younger and varies with regard to race. For example, the data from the study shows that African American girls can have an onset of puberty as early as 6 years and in Caucasian girls at the age of 7.[15] Most physicians, however, still use the 8-year age range as the cut-off pending the development of other prospective studies.[16]

Clinical Presentation

There are various causes of precocious puberty and it is often described as either gonadotropin-dependent precocious puberty (GDPP) or gonadotropin-independent precocious puberty (GIPP) (Fig. 95–4). GDPP occurs secondary to activation of the hypothalamic–pituitary–gonadal axis and GIPP occurs secondary to steroid production, regardless of gonadotropin secretion. Some young girls may present with isolated menarche, thelarche, or pubarche that may be a variant of normal puberty.

Specific clinical symptoms will relate to the particular disease process. For example, girls with GDPP, also known as central precocious puberty, may present with pubertal changes such as vaginal bleeding, breast and pubic hair growth, acne as well as neurologic abnormalities such as headaches, seizures, focal deficits, polyuria, polydipsia, vision changes, or galactorrhea.

Girls with GIPP, or peripheral precocious puberty, may present with thyroid and abdominal or uterine masses. There may be a history of estrogen cream use. Clinicians should also pay attention to skin findings such as acne, or café au lait spots that could be consistent with McCune–Albright syndrome.[14,16]

Management

It is important for the emergency physician to determine whether there is a disease process that needs immediate attention versus a disorder that can be referred from the emergency department (ED) to a pediatrician or a pediatric endocrinologist. If there is any suspicion for trauma, a malignant neoplasm, or CNS abnormality, an evaluation should be initiated in the ED.

▶ GYNECOLOGIC DISORDERS OF ADOLESCENCE

ADOLESCENT HISTORY AND PHYSICAL EXAMINATION

The adolescent patient requires a thorough sexual and menstrual history because it is important to screen for the possibility of pregnancy or sexually transmitted infections. It is also important to note if there is any history of abdominal pain, vaginal discharge, pruritis, or dysuria. Any adolescent with these complaints and a positive history for sexual activity should always receive a pregnancy test. If there is a suspicion of a sexually transmitted infection, a standard speculum and bimanual examination may be necessary. It is sometimes difficult for a patient to discuss sexual history in front of a parent, so it is recommended that history be obtained without the parent present and to maintain confidentiality. Additionally, it is also important to reduce anxiety prior to the examination by explaining the procedure and providing reassurance as it is sometimes a very difficult and uncomfortable examination for the adolescent female patients.

OVARIAN TORSION

Etiology

It has been reported that about 15% of ovarian torsion occurs during childhood. It can occur in the prepubertal girls, but occurs more frequently in the adolescent female patients.[17] The ovary twists on its pedicle, which is made up of lymphatic and vascular structures that form an axis between the abdominal wall and uterus. Infarction of the ovary ensues when the arterial supply is compromised.[18]

Clinical Manifestations

Patients may present with abdominal pain, nausea, vomiting, and fever. They may have symptoms that are similar to other pelvic and abdominal disease processes such as pelvic inflammatory disease, ruptured ovarian cyst, ectopic pregnancy, appendicitis, and gastroenteritis. Some studies have shown that torsion occurs more commonly on the right than the left. It is hypothesized that this may be due to the protective effect that the sigmoid colon has on the left side.[17]

Management

Several studies have shown that the diagnosis of ovarian torsion can be made by evidence of an abnormal ovary on ultrasound. This may be done with or without Doppler flow studies. Normal blood flow through an ovary does not exclude the diagnosis. If diagnosis is not made by ultrasound, laparoscopy or laparotomy should be done.[17] Early diagnosis is very important because salvage of the ovary depends on the duration of symptoms. Although data on pediatric ovarian

torsion is limited, one study from 2001 reports that an ovary can be salvaged if surgery is done within 8 hours of onset of symptoms; however, all patients in this study underwent bilateral salpingo-oophorectomy.[19] A more recent pediatric study in 2005 reports the salvage rate within 8 hours of symptoms to be 40% and within 24 hours of symptoms to be 33%. Those operated beyond 24 hours had no salvageable ovaries.[18] Thus, the timing of diagnosis and operative management is critical for salvaging ovaries.

BARTHOLIN ABCESS

Etiology

Bartholin glands are located on the labia minora at the 4-o'clock and 8-o'clock position on the vestibule. These glands drain into a duct that is about 2.5 cm long. Bartholin gland cysts are usually asymptomatic, but occasionally may become enlarged or infected if the duct that it is draining into becomes obstructed.[20]

Clinical Manifestation

Patients may complain of pain when walking or sitting, dyspareunia, or vulvar pain. Normally the gland cannot be palpated, but if it is enlarged, the patient may notice a new bulge or it may be discovered during the gynecologic examination (Fig. 95–5).

Management

Incision and drainage of the abscess often results in recurrence. Definitive treatment involves treatment with a Word catheter or marsupialization. A Word catheter is a catheter with a rubber tip that can be inserted into the incision and inflated with water or jelly. The loose end of the catheter can be inserted into the vagina. The catheter is then left in the drained cyst for about 4 weeks to promote complete epithelialization. Marsupialization involves incision and removal of a portion of the cyst and a part of the vestibular wall with approximation of the remaining

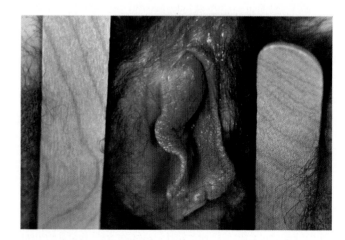

Figure 95–5. Inflammation of Bartholin's gland. (*Credit to CDC/Susan Lindsley.*)

▶ **TABLE 95-3. DIFFERENTIAL DIAGNOSIS OF PELVIC PAIN IN THE ADOLESCENT FEMALE PATIENT**

Ectopic pregnancy
Ovarian torsion
Mittelschmerz
Imperforate hymen
Endometriosis
Pelvic inflammatory disease, tubo-ovarian abcess
Urinary tract infection, urolithiasis
Dysmenorrhea
Appendicitis

vestibular skin with the adjacent cyst wall with sutures, making a new tract that will epithelialize and form a new duct orifice.[20]

ACUTE PELVIC PAIN

Etiology

Adolescent females often present with complaints of acute lower abdominal or pelvic pain. There are a variety of causes that include gastrointestinal, urological, and gynecological reasons for pelvic pain (Table 95–3). Mittelschmerz is thought to occur during mid-menstrual cycle when a follicle ruptures during ovulation. Minor bleeding from the follicle into the abdominal cavity may lead to irritation of the peritoneum and subsequently cause lower abdominal pain. This pain should usually last a few hours or less.[21,22]

Although ovarian cysts are usually benign and painless, a ruptured ovarian cyst may cause lower abdominal pain secondary to hemoperitoneum. This can sometimes be severe and confused with appendicitis. Other causes including expansion of a cyst, hemorrhagic corpus luteum cyst can also cause peritoneal irritation secondary to blood or tissue contact.[21,22]

Management

The evaluation of pelvic pain in the adolescent patient should always begin with a pregnancy test. Other diagnostic tools may be obtained including a urinalysis to identify urinary tract infection or urolithiasis. A CBC may be useful to look for evidence of anemia or bleeding, a basic metabolic profile to assess renal function, and abdominal labs including tests for hepatitis and pancreatitis. If there is a history of fever, sexual activity, or vaginal discharge, a pelvic examination to identify STDs and pelvic inflammatory disease (PID) should be considered. Imaging studies such as pelvic or transvaginal ultrasound and CT scan of the abdomen and pelvis are also useful to look for etiologies such as appendicitis, ovarian torsion, tubo-ovarian abscess, or urolithiasis[21] (Fig. 95–6).

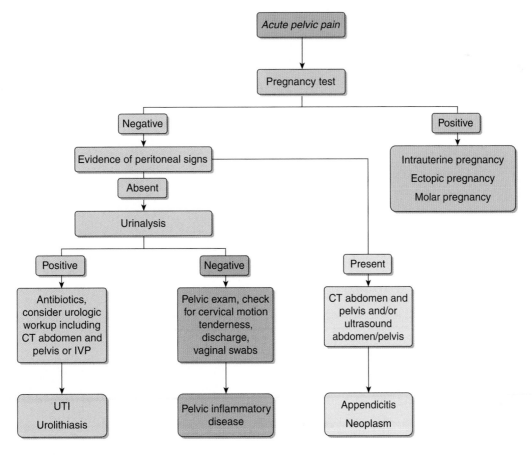

Figure 95-6. Algorithm of acute pelvic pain.

REFERENCES

1. Kass-Wolff JH, Wilson EE. Pediatric gynecology: assessment strategies and common problems. *Semin Reprod Med.* 2003;21: 329–338.

2. Sugar MF, Graham EA. Common gynecologic problems in prepubertal girls. *Pediatr Rev.* 2006;27:213–222.

3. Carswell JL, Stafford DE. Normal physical growth and development. In: Neinstein NS, Gordon CM, Katzman DK, Rosen DS, Woods ER, eds. *Adolescent Healthcare: A Practical Guide.* Lippincott Williams & Wilkins; 2007.

4. Farrington, PF. Pediatric vulvo-vaginitis. *Clin Obstet.* 1997;40: 135–140.

5. Laufer MR, Goldstein DP, Hendren WH. Structural anomalies of the female reproductive tract. In: Emans SJH, Laufer MR, Goldstein DP, eds. *Pediatric and Adolescent Gynecology.* Philadelphia, PA: Lippincott; 2005:334–416.

6. Edmonds DK. Congenital malformations of the genital tract. *Obstet Gynecol Clin North Am.* 2000;27:49–62.

7. Zafar N, Raheela RM, Rahat N, Qureshi RN, Zarrish SK, Zarak K. Congenital vaginal obstructions: varied presentation and outcome. *Pediatr Surg Int.* 2006;22:749–753.

8. Imamoglu M, Cay A, Sarihan H, Kosucu P, Ozdemir O. Two cases of pyometrocolpos due to distal vaginal atresia. *Pediatr Surg Int.* 2004;21:217–219.

9. Dursun I, Gunduz Z, Kucukaydin M, Yildirim A, Yilmaz A, Poyrazoglu H. Distal vaginal atresia resulting in obstructive uropathy accompanied by acute renal failure. *Clin Exp Nephrol.* 2007;11:244–246.

10. Leung AK, Robson WL, Tay-Uyboco J. The incidence of labial fusion in children. *J Paediatr Child Health.* 1993;29:235–236.

11. Kumetz LM, Quint EH, Fisseha S, Smith YR. Estrogen treatment success in recurrent and persistent labial agglutination. *J Pediatr Adolesc Gynecol.* 2006;19:381–384.

12. Someshwar J, Lutfi R, Nield LS. The missing "Bratz" doll: a case of vaginal foreign body. *Pediatr Emerg Care.* 2007;23:897–898.

13. Valerie E, Gilchrist BF, Frischer J, Scriben R, Klotz H, Ramenofsky ML. Diagnosis and treatment of urethral prolapse in children. *Urology.* 1999;54:1082–1084.

14. Muir A. Precocious puberty. *Pediatr Rev.* 2006;27:373–381.

15. Herman-Giddens ME, Slora EJ, Wasserman RC, Bourdony CJ, Bhapkar MV, Koch GG. Secondary sexual characteristics and menses in young girls seen in office practice: a study from the pediatric research in office setting network. *Pediatrics.* 1997; 99:505–512.

16. Nield Linda S, Cakan N, Kamat D. A practical approach to precocious puberty. *Clin Pediatr.* 2007;46:299–306.

17. Servaes S, Zurakowski D, Laufer MR, Feins N, Chow JS. Sonographic findings of ovarian torsion in children. *Pediatr Radiol.* 2007;37:446–451.

18. Anders JF, Powell EC. Urgency of evaluation and outcome of acute ovarian torsion in pediatric patients. *Arch Pediatr Adolesc Med.* 2005;159:532–535.

19. Kokoska ER, Keller MS, Weber TR. Acute ovarian torsion in children. *Am J Surg.* 2002;183:95–96.

20. Hill DA, Lense JJ. Office management of Bartholic gland cysts and abcesses. *Am Fam Physician.* 1998;57:1611–1620.

21. Ganong WF. Physiology of reproduction. In: Pernoll ML, ed. *Current Obstetric and Gynecologic Diagnosis and Treatment.* Norwalk, CT: Appleton & Lange; 1991:125.

22. Samraj GP, Curry WR. Acute pelvic pain: evaluation and management. *Compr Ther.* 2004;30:173–184.

CHAPTER 96

Vaginitis

Geetha M. Devdas and Maria Stephan

▶ HIGH-YIELD FACTS

- Vulvovaginitis is the most common gynecological disorder in childhood; its causes include physical and chemical irritants and a variety of infectious agents.
- Group A β-hemolytic *Streptococcus* and *Hemophilus influenza* can be self-inoculated from nose and mouth to the vulvar region.
- Candidal vaginitis is rare in prepubertal children and should raise suspicion of diabetes mellitus or depressed immune function.
- Enterobius vermicularis (pinworms) can be a source of irritant vaginitis.
- A prepubertal child with Gardnerella vaginitis should be evaluated for potential sexual abuse.

▶ VULVOVAGINITIS

Vulvovaginitis, or inflammation of the vulvar and vaginal tissues, is the most common gynecological disorder of children.[1] This inflammation may be caused by physical, chemical, or infectious irritants.[2] In recent studies, only one-third of girls who presented with vulvovaginitis were found to have bacterial causes.[2] The majority of cases were found to be due to nonspecific or irritant vulvitis (Table 96–1). The differential diagnosis of childhood vaginitis varies with age and the symptoms may include vaginal discharge with or without vaginal bleeding, itching, or dysuria.[3]

Historical considerations include an overview of nutritional and hygienic practices such as the use of irritating soaps or constrictive clothing, underlying medical disorders (immunocompromised state), and the potential for sexual abuse. (A comprehensive discussion on sexually transmitted infections is covered in Chapter 97.) History should include an assessment for the presence of pruritis and odor, the character and amount of discharge, and the patient's menstrual and sexual history.

▶ NONSPECIFIC VULVOVAGINITIS

ETIOLOGY

The pathogenesis of vulvovaginitis may be associated with an alteration of the vaginal flora with an overgrowth of fecal aerobic bacteria or an overabundance of anaerobic bacteria found in the vaginal flora. Vaginal cultures may reveal organisms con-

sidered to be normal vaginal flora such as diptheroids, enterococci, and lactobacillus. The presence of *Escherichia coli* is often found on vaginal culture, which suggests contamination with bowel flora.[3]

MANAGEMENT

Treatment recommendation includes proper hygiene measures (Table 96–2). Sometimes, a child may become part of a "scratch and itch" cycle where discharge and inflammation has led to pruritis with subsequent scratching that leads to bacterial superinfection. In these cases, antibiotics such as amoxicillin, amoxicillin/clavulinic acid, or cephalosporin for 7 to 10 days may be helpful.[3]

▶ VAGINITIS DUE TO UPPER RESPIRATORY INFECTIONS

ETIOLOGY

Vaginitis may be caused by bacterial pathogens. The most common bacteria isolated are respiratory pathogens, with group A β-hemolytic *Streptococcus* (GAS) being the most commonly identified.[2] Another common pathogen is *Haemophilus influenzae*. The mode of transmission is likely to be caused by self-inoculation by hand from the nose and mouth to the vulvar region.[2] There have been rare case reports of recurrent vulvovaginitis with GAS and the proposed mechanism is thought to be secondary to continued asymptomatic, bacterial carriage of the bacteria in the nasopharynx.[4]

CLINICAL PRESENTATION

In addition to vaginal discharge, a dramatic erythematous dermatitis is often seen involving the vulva and perianal tissues.[2,5]

MANAGEMENT

Treatment is antibiotic therapy directed toward the specific bacteria. Empiric therapy with penicillin for 10 days may be started if symptoms and discharge are profuse once cultures are taken.[5] Treatment with penicillin should be adequate for treatment of GAS vulvovaginitis, but for recurrent cases clindamycin or penicillin with rifampin may be considered for a 10-day course.

▶ **TABLE 96–1. CAUSES OF NONSPECIFIC VULVOVAGINITIS IN CHILDREN**

Poor hygiene, including inadequate front-to-back wiping
Small labia minora, with a short distance from anus to vagina
Vulvovaginal epithelium that is thin and not well estrogenized, making the area more prone to irritation
Foreign body including toilet paper, small toys, pieces of cloth
Chemical irritants including soap, shampoo, bath oils, deodorant soaps, bubble baths
Eczema and seborrhea
Chronic disease or immunodeficiency
Sexual abuse

▶ CANDIDAL VAGINITIS

ETIOLOGY

Candidal vaginitis occurs more frequently in adolescents than younger girls because *Candida albicans* colonizes the vagina after the onset of puberty, when estrogen is present to promote fungal growth. Candidal infections are therefore uncommon in the prepubertal girl, except in the presence of diabetes mellitus, immunodeficiency, or antibiotic use.[6] Diabetes mellitus and depressed immune function should be considered in the prepubertal girl with frequent infections with candida.

CLINICAL PRESENTATION

The symptoms of candidal vaginitis include inflammation of the vulva and perianal region, and a thick, whitish discharge. Satellite lesions and white plaques may sometimes be identified. A wet mount with a potassium hydroxide preparation is used to make the diagnosis. If the diagnosis is still in question, specific cultures for yeast may be sent.[7]

MANAGEMENT

Treatment includes topical antifungals including imidazoles. Many of these medicines come with intravaginal applicators, but for premenarchal children applying the cream to the vulva

▶ **TABLE 96–2. TREATMENT OF NONSPECIFIC VULVOVAGINITIS**

Improve local hygiene, including using front-to-back wiping after a bowel movement, and keeping the vulvar area clean and dry
Sitz bath (lukewarm bathwater with 2 tbsp baking soda)
Discontinue bubble baths, deodorant soaps, lotions and use mild bath soap instead
Use unscented toilet paper
Wash hands before and after using toilet
Remove wet bathing suit soon after leaving a swimming area

alone is adequate.[6] If the child has a reaction to the topical application or is immunosuppressed, treatment with oral fluconazole may be considered.[7]

▶ SHIGELLA VAGINITIS

CLINICAL PRESENTATION

Enteric pathogens including enterococci, escherichia, and shigella may be a cause of vaginitis in the prepubertal child. *Shigella flexneri* can cause a mucopurulent, bloody discharge sometimes seen after an episode of diarrhea.[3]

MANAGEMENT

Diagnosis is made by culture of the vaginal discharge. Rectal cultures are sometimes positive.[6] Treatment should be directed toward antibiotic sensitivities. Empiric treatment is trimethoprim-sulfamethoxazole for 10 to 14 days.

▶ PARISITIC VULVOVAGINITIS

CLINICAL PRESENTATION

Pinworms, or *Enterobius vermicularis*, can cause another type of irritant vulvitis. These 1-cm long, thin white worms can crawl from the anus to the vulvar introitus and cause severe pruritis.

MANAGEMENT

Diagnosis is made by either anal pinworm preparation or an application of transparent adhesive tape to the anal region in the morning to identify eggs.[2] Treatment is mebendazole 100 mg orally once and repeated in 1 week.[3]

▶ GARDNERELLA VAGINITIS

ETIOLOGY

Gardnerella vaginitis, also known as bacterial vaginosis, is a result of an overgrowth of mixed flora and occurs when the vaginal pH is above 4.5. It tends to occur more frequently in sexually active women and is relatively uncommon in the prepubertal girl.[6] Thus, a prepubertal child with a suspected diagnosis of gardnerella vaginitis should be evaluated for potential sexual abuse.

CLINICAL PRESENTATION

Bacterial vaginosis is characterized by a grayish-white malodorous vaginal discharge and a fishy, amine-like odor released when 10% potassium hydroxide solution is added to the sample of discharge. Additionally, "clue" cells, which are vaginal epithelial cells with adherent coccobacilli, are characteristically seen on a wet mount preparation. In prepubertal children, however, there is physiologic absence of lactobacilli, which makes diagnosis more challenging.[8]

TREATMENT

Treatment is with oral metronidazole for 7 to 10 days.

REFERENCES

1. Mroueh J, Muram D. Common problems in pediatric gynecology: new developments. *Curr Opin Obstet Gynecol.* 1999;11:463–466.
2. Sugar MF, Graham EA. Common gynecologic problems in prepubertal girls. *Pediatr Rev.* 2006;27:213–222.
3. Kass-Wolff JH, Wilson EE. Pediatric gynecology: assessment strategies and common problems. *Semin Reprod Med.* 2003;21:329–338.
4. Hansen MT, Sanchez VT, Eyster K, Hansen KA. *Streptococcus pyogenes* pharyngeal colonization resulting in recurrent, prepubertal vulvovaginitis. *J Pediatr Adolesc Gynecol.* 2007;20:315–317.
5. Mogielnicki NP, Schwartzman JD, Elliot JA. Perineal group A streptococcal disease in a pediatric practice. *Pediatrics.* 2000;106:276–281.
6. Hettler J, Paradise J. Pediatric and adolescent gynecology. In: Fleisher GR, Ludwig S, Henretig FM, eds. *Textbook of Pediatric Emergency Medicine.* Philadelphia, PA: Lippincott Williams & Wilkins; 2006:1126–1127.
7. Farrington PF. Pediatric vulvo-vaginitis. *Clin Obstet.* 1997;40:135–140.
8. Kohlberger P, Bancher-Todesca D. Bacterial colonization in suspected sexually abused children. *J Pediatr Adolesc Gynecol.* 2007;20:289–292.

CHAPTER 97

Sexually Transmitted Diseases

Geetha M. Devdas and Maria Stephan

► HIGH-YIELD FACTS

- Chlamydia and gonorrhea are most common among 15- to 19-year-old women.
- Throughout the United States, medical care for STDs can be provided to all adolescents without parental consent or knowledge.
- Adolescent HIV testing and counseling can be performed without parental consent in the majority of U.S. states.
- STDs in children may require official investigation for potential sexual abuse, if acquired after the neonatal period.
- The presence of genital ulcers has been associated with an increased risk for HIV infection.
- Many STDs occur concurrently. Therefore, evaluate and treat the patient appropriately at the initial examination.
- Symptomatic trichomoniasis occurs primarily in women, but men may be silent carriers.
- Treat sexual contacts of patients with primary, secondary, or early latent syphilis without waiting for clinical symptoms or a positive serologic test.
- Diagnosis of genital herpes should not be based on clinical examination alone as other genital ulcerative lesions may have a similar appearance.
- HIV screening is recommended for patients seeking STD treatment in all health care settings. The patient should be notified that testing will be performed unless the patient declines (opt-out screening).
- Separate written consent for HIV testing should not be required. General consent for medical care should be considered sufficient consent for HIV testing.
- If the cause of urethritis is unknown, treat with ceftriaxone 250 mg IM plus 10-day course of doxycycline.
- Prepubertal boys presenting with epididymitis should be referred for investigation of congenital abnormalities of the urinary tract (i.e., vesicoureteral reflux).
- Treatment of PID must include effective treatment of sex partners; HIV infection may be as high as 20%.

► CHLAMYDIA

ETIOLOGY

Chlamydia is the most common sexually transmitted disease (STD) after human papillomavirus (HPV). It is the most common treatable STD in the United States, occurring in 10% or more of sexually active adolescent female patients attending STD clinics,[1,2] with higher prevalence in patients living in inner cities or with lower socioeconomic status. Approximately 33% to 45% of patients with gonorrhea are co-infected with *Chlamydia trachomatis*. Patients with chlamydial infections are at increased risk of acquiring HIV infection.[1]

CLINICAL MANIFESTATIONS

Presentation of symptoms is variable, but most women and many men are asymptomatic. Vaginal discharge, mild abdominal pain, dysuria, urinary frequency, or postcoital/intermenstrual bleeding is observed in women. Physical examination reveals pyuria without bacteriuria, cervical edema, erythema, easily induced cervical bleeding, and mucopurulent discharge. In men, symptoms include dysuria, urethral itching, or clear to whitish urethral discharge. Often the discharge may be slight and noted as stained underwear in the morning resulting from minimal overnight discharge. Physical examination in men demonstrates meatal edema, erythema, and a whitish/clear discharge. Pyuria is common.[3]

DIAGNOSIS

Culture of cervical swabs from women and urethral swabs in men for *C. trachomatis* remain the standard for diagnosis, but are labor-intensive and have variable sensitivity. It is still required for cases with medicolegal implications (i.e., sexual assault). When obtaining specimens, do not use swabs with a wooden shaft as wood may contain substances toxic to Chlamydia. For prepubertal female patients, vaginal rather than cervical specimens should be taken. Specificity for this test is virtually 100%.

DNA probes for detection of *C. trachomatis* from collected swabs of cervical or male urethral sites are also available. In this test, the DNA probe hybridizes to chlamydial rRNA from a cervical or urethral swab specimen and detects *C. trachomatis* by chemiluminescence. It is also highly specific and the specimen can also be used for testing gonorrhea. Direct fluorescent antibody testing is highly specific. Material from the swab is stained with fluorescent monoclonal antibody that binds to chlamydial elementary bodies, which are identified by fluorescence microscopy. Results can be obtained in 30 minutes. Nucleic acid amplification tests—polymerase chain reaction (PCR), ligase chain reaction (LCR), and transcription-mediated amplification (TMA)—may all be performed on urine specimens. They are more sensitive than culture for *C. trachomatis*.[1]

TREATMENT

Treatment in adolescents and adults is a single oral dose of azithromycin or a 7-day course of oral doxycycline. Other options include a 7-day course of erythromycin, ofloxacin, or levofloxin. For preadolescent children, treatment includes oral erythromycin for 14 days in children weighing less than 45 kg, a single dose of azithromycin in children weighing at least 45 kg but younger than 8 years, and a single oral dose of azithromycin or a 7-day course of oral doxycycline in children 8 years or older (Table 97–1).

▶ GENITAL WARTS

ETIOLOGY

External genital warts are caused by an infection of HPV. This is a DNA-containing virus, which is spread by skin-to-skin contact, causing external growths in the perigenital and perianal areas.[2] The incubation period is 1 to 6 months. Treatment may not eradicate the HPV infection and recurrences are common. Other common names for genital warts are condyloma acuminata, anogenital wart, verruca acuminata, and venereal

▶ **TABLE 97–1. SUMMARY TABLE OF SEXUALLY TRANSMITTED DISEASES**

Disease	Etiology	Clinical Manifestations	Diagnosis	Therapy	Treatment Administration
Chlamydia	*Chlaymidia trachomatis*	Vaginal discharge, dysuria, abdominal or testicular pain, or asymptomatic	NAAT, culture	po	Azithromycin 1 g **or**
				po	Doxycycline 100 mg bid × 7 d **or**
				po	EES base 500 mg qid × 7 d **or**
				po	EES ethylsuccinate 800 mg qid × 7 d **or**
				po	Ofloxacin 300 mg bid × 7 d **or**
				po	Levofloxacin 500 mg qid × 7 d **Children** <**45 kg**: EES (base or ethylsuccinate) 50/kg/dose × 14 d
				po	**Children** >**45 kg** + <**8 y:** Azithromycin 1 g × 1 **Children** >**45 kg** + >**8 y:** Adult dosing
Gonorrhea	*Neisseria gonorrhoeae*	Asymptomatic, dysuria, penile or vaginal discharge, abdominal pain, rash	NAAT, culture, DNA probe	IM	Ceftriaxone 125 mg × 1 **or**
				po	Cefixime 400 mg × 1 **or**
				po	Ciprofloxacin 500 mg × 1 **or**
				po	Ofloxacin 400 mg × 1 **or**
				po	Levofloxacin 250 mg × 1
				IM	**Children** >**45 kg**: adult dosing used on above medications **Children** <**45 kg**: Ceftriaxone 125 mg × 1 **Add treatment for chlamydia if not ruled out**
Trichomoniasis	*Trichomonas vaginalis* (protozoan)	Asymptomatic (men & women) or frothy, odorous vaginal discharge, dyspaurenia, urgency	Saline wet prep, culture, rapid antigen testing	po	Metronidazole 2 g × 1 **or**
				po	Tinidazole 2 g × 1

(continued)

▶ TABLE 97–1. (CONTINUED) SUMMARY TABLE OF SEXUALLY TRANSMITTED DISEASES

Disease	Etiology	Clinical Manifestations	Diagnosis	Therapy	Treatment Administration
Genital warts	Human papilloma virus (HPV), types 6,11, 16,18	Asymptomatic or pain, itching, bleeding, or obstructive effects from wart size	Visual exam, biopsy,	Topical	Podofilox 0.5% gel/solution bid × 3 d **or** Imiquimod 5% cream qhs 3 times/wk × 16 wk
				Specialist administered	Cryotherapy, intralesional interferon, podophyllin, laser & surgical removal
Genital Ulcers Syphilis	*Treponema pallidum*	Chancre, genital ulceration Secondary: lymphadenopathy rash, condyloma lata Latent Syphilis: no evidence of disease Teriary: neuropathy, dementia, tabes dorsalis, aoritis, gumma of skin	Dark-field DAT, serologic testing (treponemal & nontreponemal)	IM IM po po IM IM	Benzathine penicillin G 2.4 million units × 1 **Children:** Benzathine penicillin G 50,000 U/kg up to adult dose × 1 Alternatives: doxycycline 100 mg bid × 14 d Tetracycline 500 mg qid × 14 d. Not recommended for children <8 y. Ceftriaxone 1 g qid × 8–10 d Secondary syphilis treatment: same as primary **Late Latent disease:** Benzathine penicillin G 2.4 million units q wk × 3 wk **Children:** Benzathine penicillin G 50,000 U/kg up to adult dose q wk × 3 wk
Herpes Simplex	Herpes simplex virus type 2	Painful genital ulcers, dysuria, dyspaurenia	Viral culture-specific antibody assays	po po po po po po po po po po	*First clinical episode* Acyclovir 400 mg tid 7–10 d **or** Acyclovir 200 mg 5 × d × 7–10 d **or** Famciclovir 250 mg tid × 7–10 d **or** Valacyclovir 1 g bid × 7–10 d **Episodic treatment for recurrent infections** Acyclovir 400 mg tid × 5 d **or** Acyclovir 800 mg bid × 5 d **or** Acyclovir 800 mg tid × 2 d **or** Famciclovir 125 mg bid × 5 d **or** Famciclovir 1000 mg bid × 1 d **or** Valacyclovir 500 mg tid × 3 d **or** Valacyclovir 1 g qid × 5 d

Adapted from CDC guidelines, *MMWR Recomm Rep.* 2006;55(RR-11):1–95.

warts. HPV serotypes 6 and 11 commonly cause external genital warts. Types 16 and 18 cause endocervical wart infections and may predispose to cervical cancer.[1]

The prevalence of HPV is approximately 1% of the entire adult population.[4] Ten to twenty percent of sexually active women are infected annually. It is three times more common than genital herpes. Its occurrence is most common in 15 to 30-year-olds and equally common in men and women. Perinatal transmission of HPV also occurs.[1,4]

CLINICAL MANIFESTATIONS

HPV is usually asymptomatic. Pain, itching, irritation, and bleeding may occur depending on the size and location of the warts. Difficulties in urination and defecation have been reported secondary to their local obstructive effects. In female patients, physical examination may reveal lesions on the external genitalia, cervix, vaginal wall, urethra, or perianal region (Figs. 97–1 and 97–2). In male patients, lesions are noted in the subpreputial area, on the coronal sulcus or penile shaft, and in the urethra. The conjunctiva, nose, mouth, and larynx may also be affected.[4] Intra-anal warts may be seen in male and female patients who have had receptive anal sex. The appearance of external genital warts is variable. They may be soft, pink or gray, occurring in clusters; cauliflower-shaped, domed-shaped or flat. Keratotic papules are genital warts that have a thick horny layer and may resemble common warts or seborrheic keratosis.[4]

Other conditions that may be confused with genital warts include pearly penile papules, molluscum contagiosum, Bowenoid papules, and condyloma lata. Bowenoid papules are usually flat-topped papules and associated with HPV type 16, which predisposes to genital neoplasia. Condyloma lata are flat warty lesions secondary to syphilis. Often they are adjacent to the previous chancre site. An aspirate of this lesion will show spirochetes on dark-field microscopy. Serologic tests for syphilis will be positive.[4]

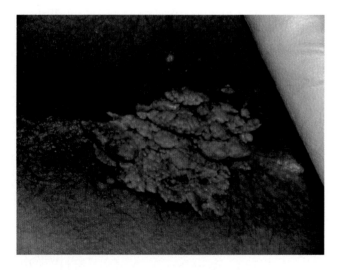

Figure 97–1. Perianal human papillomavirus. (Photo courtesy of Matthew Cox, MD.)

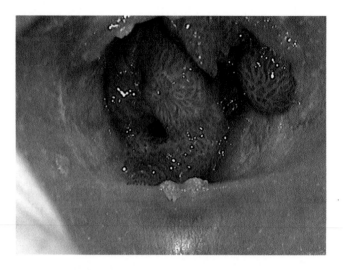

Figure 97–2. Prepubertal human papillomavirus. (Photo courtesy of Matthew Cox, MD.)

DIAGNOSIS

Diagnosis is visual examination. Biopsy can be used to confirm the diagnosis. There are no commercially available serologic tests and the organism cannot be grown in culture. However, diagnostic testing should include evaluation for other STDs, including serologic testing for syphilis (VDRL & RPR).[1,4]

TREATMENT

The patient should be referred to a specialist who can provide definitive care. Several options are available. Podofilox, a keratolytic, and antimitotic is applied to external genital warts. It is not indicated for treatment of mucous membrane warts. Imiquimod is an immunomodulator that enhances the immune response to viral infections and tumors by inducing immune system cells, cytokine, and interferon. This also is indicated for the treatment of external genital warts in patients 12 years of age or older. Other treatment options requiring professional administration include cryotherapy, podophyllin, intralesional interferon alfa-2b, surgical removal, and laser therapy.

Genital warts in children should prompt investigation to exclude sexual abuse. Genital warts in adolescents should prompt questioning as to whether sexual contact was forced. Genital warts during pregnancy may increase in size and are always referred to obstetrics/gynecology for treatment.

▶ GONORRHEA

ETIOLOGY

Gonorrhea is an infection in the epithelium of the urethra, cervix, rectum, pharynx, or eyes by *Neisseria gonorrhoeae*, a gram-negative, kidney-shaped diplococci. It is second only to chlamydia in the number of STD cases reported to the CDC.[1] The incidence is highest in urban areas in persons younger than 24 years of age with multiple sex partners. Nontreatment

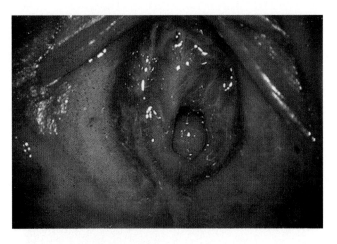

Figure 97–3. Prepubertal gonorrhea. (Photo courtesy of Matthew Cox, MD.)

may lead to bacteremia and septic complications. Disseminated gonococcal bacteremia can manifest as pustular lesions on the hands and feet, tenosynovitis and polyarthritis. It can also cause septic arthritis and endocarditis. In male patients, orchitis and epididymitis are seen.[5] Resistance to *N. gonorrhoeae* has continued to increase in the United States. Quinolone resistance has increased to 6.7% in 2006.[6]

CLINICAL MANIFESTATIONS

In female patients, symptoms begin 7 to 21 days postexposure. Eighty percent of women are asymptomatic. Symptoms described include vaginal discharge, dysuria, urinary frequency, and abdominal/pelvic pain. Gonococcal pharyngitis is usually asymptomatic in both sexes. Gonococcal proctitis, however, may be very painful with purulent rectal discharge, pain, itching, and rectal spasm. Skin lesions and arthritis may occur in disseminated gonococcal infection, occurring in both male and female patients. On examination, the cervix may be red and friable with a mucopurulent discharge. A purulent discharge may be seen from the urethra, Skene's ducts, or Bartholin's glands. Salpingitis is a common complication[1,5] (Fig. 97–3).

In male patients, symptoms occur 2 to 14 days post exposure. Symptoms described include dysuria, urethral discharge, urinary frequency, and urgency as the disease spreads to the posterior urethra. Although symptoms usually present earlier in men, the asymptomatic period may last up to 45 days. On examination, a purulent yellow-green urethral discharge is noted. The meatus may appear red and swollen.[2]

Rectal gonorrhea in both sexes may be asymptomatic, or appear with pain, painful defecation, and rectal discharge. Gonococcal pharyngitis from orogential contact may be asymptomatic or painful. The oropharyngeal area may be reddened and purulent.[5]

In preadolescent children, vaginitis is the most common manifestation of infection. Sexual abuse is the most common cause. Parents may give a history of dysuria or staining on underpants. On examination, irritation, erythema of the vulva, or purulent vaginal discharge may be noted.[1]

DIAGNOSIS

Diagnosis is made by culture of the urethra (men) or endocervix (women), rectum, and pharynx for *N. gonorrhoeae*. This requires special media for culture. This is the only method to test antibiotic sensitivity. In children, culture is the standard for diagnosis, as usually legal implications are present. Other tests available include nucleic acid hybridization, ligase chain reaction, DNA probe, and microscopic examination of Gram-stained specimen from the urethra or endocervix. Ligase chain reaction, a DNA amplification method, has not been studied for use in rectal or pharyngeal infection. It is also recommended to perform syphilis and HIV testing at the same time.[1]

TREATMENT

Management of uncomplicated gonococcal infections of the cervix, urethra, and rectum is a single dose of a cephalosporin (e.g., ceftriaxone, 125 mg IM or cefixime 400 mg po). The dose for children weighing less than 45 kg is ceftriaxone 125 mg IM or cefixime 8 mg/kg (maximum 400 mg) as a single dose. Children weighing 45 kg or more should be treated with the adult regimen. For disseminated gonococcal infection, the adult dosing regimen is ceftriaxone 1 g intravenous or intramuscular every 24 hours, continue until improvement is seen, and then switch to oral therapy with cefixime 400 mg every 12 hours for 7 days. For disseminated gonococcal infections in children, treatment is ceftriaxone 25 to 50 mg/kg/dose intravenous every 12 hours for 7 days. Treat for 14 days for meningitis. For ophthalmia neonatorum, treatment is ceftriaxone 25 to 50 mg/kg/day as a single dose.[1] Flouroquinolones have not been recommended for patients less than 18 years of age.[1]

▶ TRICHOMONIASIS

ETIOLOGY

Trichomoniasis is caused by the flagellated protozoan, *Trichomonas vaginalis*. The incubation period is 3 to 28 days. Eight million new cases are reported annually in North America.[2] It is the most common nonviral STD in the world.[7]

CLINICAL MANIFESTATION

Fifty percent of women are symptomatic. The classic presentation in women is frothy white or green foul-smelling vaginal discharge, puritus, and erythema. Abdominal pain, dyspaurenia, and urinary urgency may also occur. On examination, the classic "strawberry cervix" and vulva are noted in 1% to 2%,[7] in addition to a malodorous discharge. In male patients, the infection is often asymptomatic, but can produce urethritis.[7]

DIAGNOSIS

Diagnosis is made by viewing the flagellated organism on microscopy of saline preparations (wet prep) of vaginal discharge or urine. This has a sensitivity of 70%.[1] Additionally, the pH of the vaginal discharge is elevated. Other available diagnostic tests include culture, nucleic acid amplification and probe test, enzyme immunoassay, immunofluorescence, and immunochromatographic capillary flow dipstick techniques.[1]

TREATMENT

Metronidazole, 2 g orally as a single dose, is the standard of treatment. It is curative in 95% of the cases.[1] It is safe in the second trimester of pregnancy. Treatment of the partner is necessary to prevent recurrence.

▶ SYPHILIS

ETIOLOGY

Syphilis is caused by the spirochete *Treponema pallidum*. It is solely a human pathogen. Transmission occurs via penetration through mucous membranes and abrasions on epithelial surfaces. It can also be acquired via placental transmission and blood transfusions.[8] The incubation time is about 3 weeks but ranges from 10 to 90 days.[2] It is more common in men. Incidence is 0.32/100 000.[8] Tertiary syphilis develops in 8% to 40% of untreated patients over several decades following primary infection.[1]

CLINICAL MANIFESTATIONS

The primary lesion of syphilis is the chancre developing within 3 weeks after contact. During this stage, spirochetes can be isolated from the surface of the ulcer. Whether treated or not, healing occurs in 3 to 12 weeks. The manifestations of secondary syphilis are variable. It is located on the glans, corona, or perianal area in men and the labial or anal area in women. Commonly nontender bilateral inguinal/regional lymphadenopathy may be present.[8] Figure 97–4 demonstrates a primary syphilitic

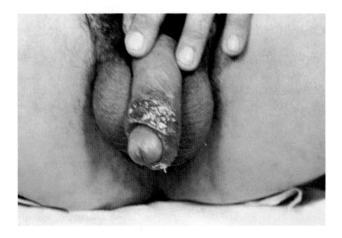

Figure 97–4. Primary syphilitic penile chancre. (From the CDC, Public Health Image Library.)

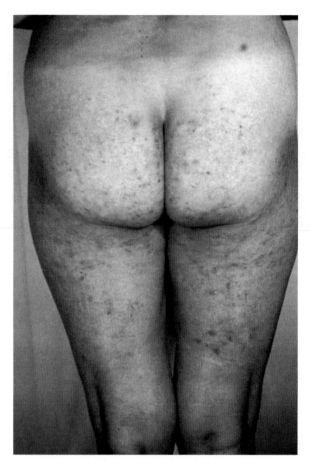

Figure 97–5. Exanthem of secondary syphilis. (From the CDC, Public Health Image Library.)

penile chancre. Latent syphilis, defined as those patients without clinical manifestations, is detected by serological testing.[1]

Secondary syphilis occurs weeks to months after resolution of the primary lesion. It is characterized by the development of a rash and lymphadenopathy (Fig. 97–5).

The rash is usually generalized, nonpuritic, maculopapular beginning on the trunk/arms and spreading to the palms and soles.[8] Mucous membrane involvement includes oral lesions and condyloma lata (cauliflower-like growths that are infectious) usually occurring in the anogenital region (Fig. 97–6). Patchy alopecia may develop. Systemic systems of fever, malaise, anorexia, arthralgias, hepatitis, and generalized lymphadenopathy are described.[8]

DIAGNOSIS

Diagnosis in the first or second stage is by dark-field and direct fluorescent antibody (DAT) of the treponemes from the chancre of condyloma lata or oral lesions. Serologic tests include nontreponemal VDRL or RPR and treponemal FTA-ABS. Sensitivity is 78% for RPR and 86% for VDRL in primary syphilis and 100% in secondary syphilis.[2] These tests become negative 1 year after treatment. The treponemal tests stay positive for life and do not correlate with disease activity.[2]

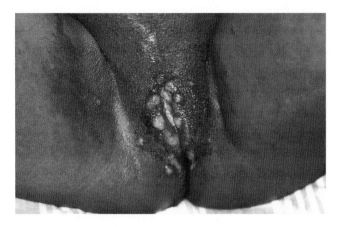

Figure 97–6. Vaginal ulcer from secondary syphilis. (From the CDC, Public Health Image Library.)

TREATMENT

Penicillin G, administered parenterally, is the preferred drug for treatment of all stages of syphilis.[1] Benzathine penicillin G 2.4 million units IM as a single dose remains the treatment of choice for the primary and secondary uncomplicated infections. Doxycycline, tetracycline, and ceftriaxone remain alternatives[1] (Table 97–1).

   Children with syphilis should have CSF examination to detect asymptomatic neurosyphilis. Treatment for children is benzathine penicillin G 50 000 units/kg intramuscularly up to the adult dose as a single injection[1] (Table 97–1).

▶ HERPES SIMPLEX INFECTION

ETIOLOGY

Genital herpes is most commonly caused by herpes simplex virus (HSV) type 2 in 90% of cases, with the remaining 10% caused by HSV type 1 and is the most common cause of genital ulcer infections in the industrialized world. Up to 75% of infections are asymptomatic and thus the virus may easily be spread to partners.[9] Nongenital infections of HSV-1 during childhood may be protective to some extent against subsequent genital HSV-2 infections in adults.[2]

CLINICAL MANIFESTATIONS

The incubation period is about 1 week. At that time, painful ulcers or vesicles develop on the genitalia and anus. Tender inguinal lymphadenopathy and constitutional systemic symptoms of fever and myalgias may also develop. Dysuria, dyspaurenia, and urinary retention may occur. Aseptic meningitis occurs in 30% of patients. Resolution occurs within 3 weeks with crusting of the ulcers. With recurrent infections, symptoms are milder[2,10] (Figs. 97–7 and 97–8).

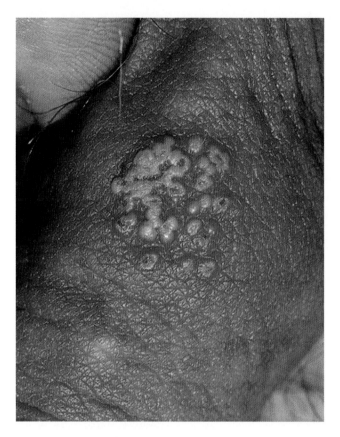

Figure 97–7. Herpes simplex penile lesion in adult. (Photo courtesy of Matthew COX, MD.)

DIAGNOSIS

The diagnosis should be confirmed by viral culture. Glycoprotein specific antibody assays that identify antibodies to HSV glycoprotein G-1 and G-2, which evoke a type-specific antibody response, have been FDSA approved.[11] Point of care testing can provide results for HSV-2 antibodies from capillary blood or serum during a health care visit.[1]

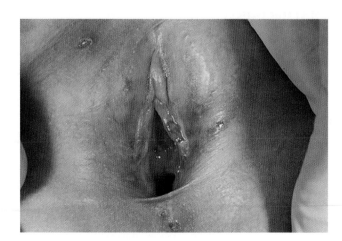

Figure 97–8. Prepubertal herpes simplex. (Photo courtesy of Matthew COX, MD.)

TREATMENT

Acyclovir, valacyclovir, and famciclovir are the antivirals recommended for treatment. Recurrence can be treated with episodic or suppressive approaches. Daily suppressive therapy has been shown to prevent 80% of recurrences[1,2] (Table 97–1).

► HUMAN IMMUNODEFICIENCY VIRUS AND ACQUIRED IMMUNODEFICIENCY DISEASE SYNDROME

ETIOLOGY

Acquired immunodeficiency disease syndrome (AIDS) is caused by the human immunodeficiency virus (HIV). Modes of transmission include homosexuality, heterosexuality, bisexuality, intravenous drug use, needle sticks, blood transfusion before 1985, and maternal–neonatal transmission. The majority of adolescents and adults infected remain asymptomatic for a median time period of 10 years.[1] Viral replication continues during all stages of infection. Prompt diagnosis will allow early treatment and hopefully prevent further spread.

Most HIV infections in the United States are HIV-1. HIV-2 infections are endemic in West Africa. Therefore, risk factors of receiving blood transfusions, unsterile needle sticks, or sex partners from West Africa may alert the physician to perform appropriate testing.[1]

CLINICAL MANIFESTATIONS

The disease spectrum is variable from primary infection, asymptomatic carrier, to AIDS with life-threatening complications. Fever, malaise, lymphadenopathy, and skin rash occur with several weeks of infection.[1] Other manifestations include adenopathy, failure to thrive or weight loss, hepatosplenomegaly, opportunistic infections, and malignancies.

DIAGNOSIS

The diagnosis is made with testing for antibodies against HIV-1 using enzyme immunoassay (EIA) or rapid test, usually within one hour. If positive, confirmatory testing with either Western blot or immunoflourescence assay (IFA) is performed. Referral to a health care provider knowledgeable in HIV management is recommended. Combination testing for HIV-2 is also available.[1] Make sure to complete a thorough investigation for the etiology of fever, if it is a presenting symptom. It is recommended to perform testing for other STDs at this time as they can occur concomitantly.

TREATMENT

Available retroviral medications include zidovudine, didanosine, zallcitabine, stravudine, inidinaavir, and ritonavir. How-

ever, newly diagnosed patients need to be referred to specialist at this time for appropriate counseling, treatment strategy, and psychosocial evaluation.[1]

► CLINICAL PRESENTATIONS OF STD

GENITAL ULCERS

Both primary syphilis and herpes simplex will present with genital ulcers.

URETHRITIS, EPIDIDYMITIS, AND CERVICITIS

Urethritis is the inflammation of the urethra, most commonly caused by *N. gonorrhoeae* and *C. trachomatis*. Other causes include *Ureaplasma urealyticum* and *Mycoplasma genitalium*, Trichomonas, herpes, and papillomavirus. Noninfectious causes may be symptoms of systemic diseases, topically applied agents, foods, and others that cause irritation.[12]

In men, dysuria, mucopurulent, or purulent penile discharge may be seen. Hematuria is uncommon. Women often are symptomatic, but dysuria, urinary frequency, and vaginal discharge or cervicitis may exist.[12] In men, the diagnosis of gonoccoal urethritis is made by finding gram-negative diplococci on Gram stain. Also consider use of nucleic acid amplification methods. Treatment should be per recommendations of STD guidelines outlined in Table 97–1.

Epididymitis is inflammation of the epididymis. Causative agents vary with patient age. The most common infectious etiologies in perpubertal boys are due to *Escherichia coli* or *Hemophilus influenzae* and in men younger than 35 years due to STDs (*N. gonorrhoeae* and *C. trachomatis*).[13] Noninfectious causes include trauma, vigorous physical activity leading to an inflammatory response to sterile urine refluxing through the ejaculatory ducts and vas deferens into the epididymus.[14] Scrotal pain may be dull or sharp. Swelling, edema, reactive hydrocoele, a palpable abnormality or systemic signs of fever, and tachycardia may be identified.[2,14] Testicular torsion must be first ruled out by Doppler ultrasound if indicated.

Laboratory diagnosis includes the presence of pyuria, bacteriuria, positive urine culture, and leukocytosis. The CDC recommends that evaluation of epididymitis in men is similar to the evaluation of urethritis including Gram stain of urethral secretions with >5 WBC/oil immersion field or positive leukoesterase on first-void specimen or first-void urine with >10 WBC/oil immersion field.[1,2] Gonoccoal infection is confirmed by finding gram-negative diplococci on the smear. Also consider use of nucleic acid amplification methods. Treatment should be as per recommendations of STD guidelines. Additionally, analgesia, rest, scrotal elevation, and warm tub baths to ease pain are recommended (Table 97–1).

Cervicitis, defined as inflammation of the cervix with a mucopurulent endocervical discharge, is most commonly caused by STD. On speculum examination, a friable bleeding cervix, mucopurulent or purulent endocervical discharge is seen. Evaluate for STDs using culture or nucleic acid amplification testing.[1,12] Treatment should be as per recommendations of STD guidelines (Table 97–1).

▶ PELVIC INFLAMMATORY DISEASE

Pelvic inflammatory disease (PID) is a disease of sexually active women. Infection is usually due to *C. trachomatis* and *N. gonorrhoeae*. The infection ascends the female genital tract to involve the uterus, fallopian tubes, ovaries, and pelvic peritoneum leading to pelvic abscesses.[15] The vaginal flora becomes infected with facultative organisms such as *E. coli*, *Bacteroides* spp, anaerobic cocci, *H. influenzae*, group A strep, *Mycoplasma hominis*, and *Ureaplasma urealyticum*. Therefore, treatment must be with broad spectrum antibiotic coverage. Twenty to thirty percent of cases are in sexually active adolescents with the peak incidence in 15 to 24 year olds.[15]

The clinical presentation is with pelvic pain, vaginal discharge, abnormal uterine bleeding, dysuria, and dyspaurenia. Some women are asymptomatic. Fever, mucopurulent endocervical discharge, adnexal and cervical motion tenderness on palpation are considered the "classic" examination findings.[15,16]

Diagnosis is difficult as the presentation is variable. Diagnostic criteria include fever >38.3°C (101°F), abnormal cervical or vaginal discharge, elevated ESR and C-reactive protein, confirmed gonococcal or chlamydial infection of the cervix, saline microscopy of vaginal fluid with increased WBCs. Definitive criteria for diagnosis include ultrasound showing tubo-ovarian abscess, laparoscopic abnormalities consistent with PID, or endometrial biopsy.[1,15] Ectopic pregnancy must always be excluded.

Oral antibiotics are recommended for mild to moderately severe acute PID. Patients usually respond within 72 hours. Outpatient oral treatment recommended by the CDC is a single dose of a third-generation cephalosporin (ceftriaxone or cefoxitin) plus oral doxycycline plus oral metronidazole to complete a 14-day course.[1]

Inpatient treatment is reserved for patient presenting with high fever, ill appearing, patients with uncertain diagnosis (i.e., appendicitis), those who cannot tolerate or comply with oral medication, failed outpatient management, and pregnancy or tubo-ovarian abscesses. Parenteral management includes cefotetan or cefoxitin plus oral or intravenous doxycycline. An alternative treatment option is clindamycin plus gentamicin. Intravenous treatment is continued until there is clinical improvement for 24 hours, then switch to an oral outpatient regimen.[1,15,16]

REFERENCES

1. Workowski K, Berman S. Sexually transmitted diseases treatment guidelines 2006. *MMWR Recomm Rep.* 2006;55(RR-11): 1–95.
2. Frenkl T, Potts. Sexually transmitted infection. *Urol Clin North Am.* 2008;35:33–46.
3. Miller JE. Diagnosis and treatment of *Chlamydia trachomatis* infection. *Am Fam Physician.* 2006;73:1411–1416.
4. Wiley D, Douglas J, Buener K, et al. External genital warts: diagnosis, treatment, and prevention. *Clin Infect Dis.* 2002; 35(suppl 2):S210–S224.
5. Miller KE. Diagnosis and treatment of *Neissera gonorrhoeae* infections. *Am Fam Physician.* 2006;73(10):1779–1784.
6. Van Vranken M. Prevention and treatment of sexually transmitted diseases: an update. *Am Fam Physician.* 2007;76(12):1827–1832.
7. Wendel K, Workowski K. Trichomoniasis: challenges to appropriate management. *Clin Infect Dis.* 2007;44(suppl 3):S123–S129.
8. French P. Syphilis. *BMJ.* 2007;34:143–147.
9. Langenberg A, Corey L, Ashley R, et al. A prospective study of new infections with herpes simplex virus type 1 and type 2. Chiron HSV vaccine study group. *N Eng J Med.* 1999;341:1432–1438.
10. Sen P, Barton S. Genital herpes and its management. *BMJ.* 2007;334:1048–1052.
11. Wald A, Ashley-Morrow R. Serological testing for herpes simplex virus (HSV)-1 and HSV-2. *Clin Infect Dis.* 2002;35(suppl 2):S173–S182.
12. Simpson Y, Oh M. Urethritis and cervicitis in adolescents. *Adol Med Clin.* 2004;15(2):253–271.
13. Berger R, Alexander G, Harnisch J, et al. Etiology, manifestations and therapy of acute epididymitis: prospective study of 50 cases. *J Urol.* 1979;121:750–754.
14. Galejs LE, Kass E, Diagnosis and treatment of the acute scrotum. *Am Fam Phy.* 1999;59:817.
15. Crossman S. The challenge of pelvic inflammatory disease. *Am Fam Phy.* 2006;73:859–864.
16. Banikarim C, Chacko M. Pelvic inflammatory disease in adolescents. *Adol Med Clin.* 2004;15(2):273–285.

CHAPTER 98

Dysmenorrhea and Dysfunctional Uterine Bleeding

Mercedes Uribe and Pamela J. Okada

▶ HIGH-YIELD FACTS

- Dysmenorrhea is the most common cause of school/work absenteeism.
- The pain of dysmenorrhea may be experienced in the pelvis, lower back, or anterior thighs.
- Nonsteroidal anti-inflammatory drugs are the *first-line* treatment for dysmenorrhea.
- In a normal menstrual cycle there is an average of 35 to 80 mL of blood loss.
- Dysfunctional uterine bleeding is a diagnosis of exclusion and involves any disturbance in regularity, frequency, duration, or volume of menstrual flow.
- Up to 20% of adolescents with dysfunctional uterine bleeding will have a coagulopathy.
- The hallmark of dysfunctional uterine bleeding is a negative pelvic examination.

▶ DYSMENORRHEA

DEFINITION

Dysmenorrhea is defined as cyclic menstrual cramps and pain associated with menstruation. Dysmenorrhea may be classified by pathophysiology (primary or secondary) or by intensity (mild, moderate, or severe)[1] (Table 98–1). The term primary dysmenorrhea refers to pain with menses in the absence of pelvic pathology, and usually begins early in adolescence once the regular ovulatory cycle has been established. Secondary dysmenorrhea is usually associated with underlying pelvic pathology, occurs at any time after menarche, and is most often seen in older women.[2,3]

INCIDENCE

A systematic review of the literature from 1996 to 2001 estimates the prevalence of primary dysmenorrhea to be 43% to 93%; the lowest prevalence is among the younger adolescents and the greatest severity in the older adolescent girls.[4–6] According to one study, only 14% of US adolescents aged 12 to 17 years with dysmenorrhea sought help from a physician and 30% to 60% of girls report at least occasionally self-medicating with over-the-counter preparations.[7]

The societal impact of dysmenorrhea is great. Dysmenorrhea is the most common cause of school and work absenteeism and results in limitations on social, academic, and sporting activities. As per data from various studies, 38% of adolescent girls miss school, 51% of women with primary dysmenorrhea limit their activities, and 17% miss work because of secondary dysmenorrhea.[4–8]

PATHOPHYSIOLOGY

The cause of primary dysmenorrhea is unclear but is associated with prostaglandin F2 release in the endometrium during menstruation. Sloughing endometrial cells release prostaglandins, causing myometrial contraction and vasoconstriction and resulting in pain and cramping. The involvement of vasopressin is still controversial but is postulated to be increased in menstrual fluids and having a similar role as prostaglandins. Hormones, cervical morphology, nerves, and psychologic factors may also play role, but they, too, act through prostaglandins.[9] In secondary dysmenorrhea, prostaglandins also play a role, but by definition concomitant pelvic pathology must also be present.

ETIOLOGY/RISK FACTORS

Primary dysmenorrhea affects women of all races. Women at increased risk are those with a history of smoking or exposure to environmental smoke, early menarche before age 11 years, nulliparity or women with a previous abortions, nonoral contraceptive use, poor mental health, severe distress, single, younger age of marriage, sexual violence, alcohol use, anxiety, depression, infertility, obesity, longer menstrual cycles, or heavy menstruation flow[5,6,8,10–13] (Table 98–2). Risk of secondary dysmenorrhea is increased if there is a history of sterilization, sexual assault, intrauterine device, or presence of pelvic pathology as described previously (Table 98–1). Decreased risk of dysmenorrhea is found in women with oral contraceptive use, increased fish intake, higher physical activity, higher parity, and those married or in a stable relationship.[10,14]

▶ **TABLE 98-1. CLASSIFICATION OF DYSMENORRHEA**

Pathophysiology	Severity
Primary	**Mild**
No pelvic pathology	No systemic symptoms
Secondary	Medication rarely required
Endometriosis	Work rarely affected
Uterine fibroids and	
adenomyosis	**Moderate**
Ovarian cyst or tumors	Few systemic symptoms
Pelvic inflammatory disease	Medication required
Abnormal pregnancy	Work moderately affected
Intrauterine device use	
Gastrointestinal disorders:	**Severe**
irritable bowel disease,	Multiple symptoms
celiac disease	Poor medication response
Malformation of the Mullerian	Work inhibited
ducts	
Obstruction of menstrual flow:	
bicornuate or septate	
uterus, vaginal septum,	
imperforate hymen	

CLINICAL PRESENTATION

The pain of dysmenorrhea may be experienced in the pelvis, lower back, or anterior upper legs. In primary dysmenorrhea, pain usually begins within the first 6 months after menarche and once ovulatory cycles are established and occurs at the onset of menses lasting 8 to 72 hours (median duration of 2 days).[5,14] Other associated symptoms include headache, diarrhea, nausea, fatigue, dizziness, and vomiting.[4] In secondary dysmenorrhea, pain usually occurs in the older population after painless menstrual cycles have been established. In addition, some women experience infertility, dyspareunia, itch-

▶ **TABLE 98-2. RISK FACTORS FOR DYSMENORRHEA**

Smoking or passive smoking
Early menarche, age <11 y
Nulliparity
Prior abortions
Nonoral-contraceptive use
Poor mental health
Severe distress
Single or younger age of marriage
Sexual violence
Alcohol use
Anxiety
Depression
Obesity
Infertility
Heavy menstrual flow
History of sterilization
Intrauterine device

▶ **TABLE 98-3. DIAGNOSTIC MODALITIES FOR SECONDARY DYSMENORRHEA**

Laparoscopy: Endometriosis, pelvic adhesion, pelvic inflammatory disease
Hysteroscopy and saline sonohysterography: Endometrial polyps and submucosal leiomyomas, obstructing mullerian malformation
Sonography: Pelvic mass, ovarian cyst
MRI: Adenomyosis

iness, vaginal discharge, irregular bleeding, heavy bleeding, and dysuria during times other than menses.

DIAGNOSTIC EVALUATION

Primary dysmenorrhea is usually benign in nature and requires little diagnostic evaluation other than a careful history.[2–15] Secondary dysmenorrhea requires a more detailed assessment to determine the underlying pathology and may include a complete blood count (CBC), urinalysis, pregnancy test, gonococcal and chlamydial cervical cultures, and an erythrocyte sedimentation rate (ESR).

Imaging studies are not helpful in the evaluation of primary dysmenorrhea. For secondary dysmenorrhea, abdominal and transvaginal ultrasonography is recommended to identify anatomic abnormalities. Other modalities such as laparoscopy, hysteroscopy, and saline sonohysterography may be indicated depending on the suspected underlying pathology (Table 98–3).

MANAGEMENT

Pharmacologic Treatment

Nonsteroidal anti-inflammatory drugs (NSAIDs) are the first line of treatment for dysmenorrhea. NSAIDs reduce prostaglandin production via cyclooxygenase inhibition and this in turn also decreases menstrual flow. Adverse side effects include gastrointestinal disturbance such as gastritis, indigestion, and drowsiness.[2,15]

A newer class of NSAIDs, the cyclooxygenase-2 (COX-2) inhibitors, inhibits the cyclooxygenase-2 enzyme, which aids in the metabolism of arachidonic acid to prostaglandin. Its efficacy was confirmed by Sahin et al. demonstrating significant decrease in pain of primary and secondary dysmenorrhea but concerns of the gastrointestinal and cardiovascular side effects of these agents were raised[2,3,16,17] (Table 98–4).

Oral contraceptive pills (OCPs) are an off-label method of treatment for dysmenorrhea. OCPs work by inhibiting ovulation and reducing the endometrial lining of the uterus. Menstrual fluid volume and prostaglandin production are both decreased. Hendryx et al. reported greater reduction of cramping with the use of low-dose desogestrel versus placebo.[18,19] Treatment to suppress the menstrual cycle with Danazol (an androgen) and Leuprolide acetate (a gonadotropin releasing hormone) may be considered in refractory cases. And finally,

▶ **TABLE 98-4. PHARMACOLOGY MEDICATIONS FOR DYSMENORRHEA**

Nonsteroidal anti-inflammatory drugs
Ibuprofen 400–600 mg bid–qid
Naproxen 250–500 mg bid
Mefenamic acid 250 mg daily or qid
Ketoprofen 25–75 mg qid
Diclofenac 25–75 mg tid
Etodolac 200 mg bid
Indomethacin 25 mg tid
Fenoprofen 200 mg bid
Nimesulide 100–200 mg daily
Flufenamic acid 200 mg bid
Piroxicam 20–40 mg daily

COX-2 Inhibitors
Celecoxib 200 mg bid

bid, (twice per day); qid, (4 times per day); tid, (3 times a day).

preliminary data evaluating oral nifedipine and intravenous terbutaline have shown promise in reducing myometrial contractions; however, prospective clinical trials still need to be done.

Nonpharmacologic Treatment

The efficacy of conventional treatment using NSAIDs is considerable; however, the failure rate is still 20% to 25%. Consumers are now seeking alternatives to conventional medicine. Herbal and dietary therapies such magnesium, vitamin B6, vitamin B1, omega-3 fatty acids, fish oil, and Japanese herbals have been shown to reduce pain during menses. Vitamin E did not show any effect.[3,20] Behavioral interventions such as pain management training, relaxation, imagery, and biofeedback may improve symptoms. Studies suggest that this results in less time absent from school and work.[3,21] Finally interventions such as chiropractic-spinal manipulative therapy and acupuncture have been used anecdotally, but little research has been published to establish efficacy.

Treatment of secondary dysmenorrhea depends upon an accurate diagnosis of the cause of pain. In the absence of a clear diagnosis, nonacute pain can be managed empirically for a short period of time using the interventions previously mentioned. Surgical intervention with referral to a gynecologist for laparoscopy, presacral neurectomy, laparoscopic uterosacral nerve ablation, or hysterectomy may be considered in refractory cases.[3]

▶ DYSFUNCTIONAL UTERINE BLEEDING

DEFINITIONS

The normal menstrual cycle consists of the follicular (or proliferative) phase, the ovulation phase, and the luteal (or se-

cretory) phase. During the first 5 days of the follicular phase menstruation occurs secondary to the disintegration and sloughing of the functionalis layer of the endometrium. From the fifth to fourteenth day, this phase is characterized by endometrial proliferation caused by estrogen produced by the ovarian follicle under the influence of follicle stimulating hormone (FSH). This period ends as estrogen production peaks. This triggers the FSH and luteinizing hormone (LH) surge. After 24 to 36 hours of the LH surge, the ovarian follicle ruptures releasing the ovum. This process is known as the ovulation phase. From day 15 to 28, the luteal phase occurs, which is characterized by the proliferation of progesterone and estrogen by the corpus luteum (formed by luteinization of the follicular cells). Here the endometrium increases in thickness and the stroma becomes edematous. If pregnancy does not occur, the corpus luteum will regress and estrogen and progesterone levels will decrease. This feedback will cause an increase in FSH and LH, initiating the next cycle[22,23,24] (Fig. 98–1).

In a normal menstrual cycle, menstruation occurs every 21 to 35 days, lasts from 2 to 7 days, and produces an average of 35 to 80 mL of blood loss. Dysfunctional uterine bleeding (DUB) is a diagnosis of exclusion and involves any disturbance in regularity, frequency, duration, or volume of menstrual flow that occurs only when organic and structural causes for abnormal vaginal bleeding have been ruled out[25,26] (Table 98–5).

INCIDENCE

Women with DUB account for 20% of all gynecologic visits. Of these, 20% are adolescents and 50% are women aged 40 to 50 years.[26,27]

PATHOPHYSIOLOGY

Anovulatory Cycle

Approximately 90% of DUB results from anovulation, with adolescent and perimenopausal women being the most affected. In adolescents, specifically during the first 2 years post menarche, anovulatory estrogen breakthrough bleeding is common secondary to immaturity of the hypothalamic–ovarian axis. The LH surge is unable to respond to rising estradiol levels causing failure to induce ovulation. As a result, the corpus luteum is not formed and the progesterone level remains low or absent, allowing the endometrium to proliferate under the influence of unopposed estrogen. Ultimately, the endometrium outgrows the blood supply and architectural support, resulting in menometrorrhagia.[23,25,26]

In perimenopausal women, anovulatory estrogen withdrawal bleeding occurs secondary to a shortened follicular phase. The ovarian follicles secrete less estradiol leading to insufficient endometrial proliferation with irregular and light menstrual bleeding. This also occurs in prepubertal girls.[23,26]

Ovulatory Cycle

Approximately 10% of DUB occurs in women of reproductive age (15–35 years) who have normal ovulatory cycles. This

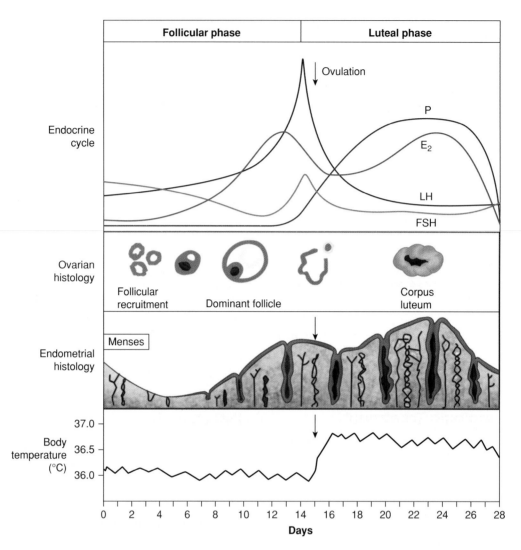

Figure 98–1. Normal menstrual cycle.

is characterized by regular menses but heavy menstrual loss. There is no disturbance of pituitary–ovarian axis and the hormonal profile is normal.

ETIOLOGY/RISK FACTORS

The cause of abnormal vaginal bleeding is extensive. As previously mentioned, the most common cause is anovulatory bleeding. It may be associated with sports, stress, eating disorders, and endocrinopathies such as hypothyroidism, hyperthyroidism, and diabetes mellitus. Patients with polycystic ovary syndrome (PCOS) may experience heavy bleeding with very long or short cycles. PCOS is often associated with type 2 diabetes, overweight, insulin resistance, hirsutism, acanthosis nigricans, and a family history of PCOS.[28] Other pathologic causes of DUB are described in Table 98–6.

In up to 20% of adolescents with DUB, there is an associated underlying systemic disease; 50% of these will have a coagulopathy such as thrombocytopenia, von Willebrand disease

▶ **TABLE 98–5. PATTERNS OF MENSTRUAL BLEEDING**

Menorrhagia	Excessive bleeding (>80 mL) at regular intervals
Metrorrhagia	Prolonged bleeding (>7 d) and irregular intervals
Menometrorrhagia	Excessive, prolonged, and irregular bleeding (>80 mL for >7 d)
Oligomenorrhagia	Interval of 35 d to months
Polymenorrhea	Interval less than 21 d
Hypermenorrhea	Regular menses for more than 7 d duration
Amenorrhea	No uterine bleeding for 6 mo or longer
Intermenstrual bleeding	Spotting, variable amounts between regular menstrual periods

▶ TABLE 98–6. PATHOLOGIC CAUSES OF DYSFUNCTIONAL UTERINE BLEEDING

Systemic
- Coagulopathies:
  Thrombocytopenia, von Willebrand disease, leukemia
- Liver disease
- Sepsis
- Endocrinopathies:
  Diabetes mellitus, polycystic ovarian syndrome, Addison's disease, hypothyroidism, congenital adrenal hyperplasia, Cushing's disease, Turner's syndrome, hyperprolactinemia
- Others:
  Hypertension, cystic fibrosis, inflammatory bowel disease

Miscellaneous
- Stress
- Excessive exercise
- Excessive weight gain
- Poor nutritional status

Iatrogenic
- Intrauterine contraceptive device (IUCD)
  Medications: Oral contraceptive, steroids, tamoxifen anticoagulants, antihistamines, metoclopramide, methyldopa, and phenothiazine
- Trauma to cervix, vulva, or vagina
- Foreign body
- Sexual abuse

Reproductive Tract
- Myomas:
  Adenomyosis, endometriosis, polyps, fibroids, ovarian cyst
- Carcinoma of the vagina, cervix, uterus, and ovaries
- Condyloma, cervicitis, vaginitis, endometritis, oophoritis
- Pregnancy related: Threatened, incomplete, missed abortion, molar or ectopic pregnancy, placenta previa, and abruption

(vWD), or leukemia. A retrospective study of 10- to 19-year-old adolescents with DUB found that 13% had thrombocytopenia, 11% had an inherited blood disorder (such as vWD or a platelet function defect), and 35% were anemic.[29] Another review of the literature found the prevalence of vWD in women with DUB to be 5% to 20%. Of women with vWD, 60% to 95% reported DUB.[30]

CLINICAL PRESENTATION

History

A detailed and complete menstrual history is critical and should include age of menarche, frequency, amount, and duration of menses, pain with menses, impact on life, and last menstrual period. Sexual history including number of partners and history of sexually transmitted diseases, medications use, reproductive history, and family history should also be included.

During the review of signs and symptoms, pay particular attention to signs of hypovolemia including hypotension, tachycardia, diaphoresis, or pallor. Look for symptoms of bleeding such as epistaxis, easy bruising, or a history of excessive bleeding with surgical interventions or dental procedures. Look for signs of PCOS, such as acne, hirsutism, acanthosis nigricans, and ask about symptoms often seen in thyroid disorders, such as weight gain, cold or heat intolerance, or hair loss.[26,31,32]

Physical Examination

A complete physical examination should begin with vital signs and ABCs to assess for hemodynamic stability. In the stable patient, assess for evidence of pathological causes of DUB. A pelvic examination must be performed to exclude sexually transmitted infection; if the adolescent is not sexually active, the pelvic examination may be deferred. The hallmark of DUB is a negative pelvic examination.[26,31,32]

DIAGNOSTIC EVALUATION

Laboratory Studies

In the patient with unstable vital signs, perform a CBC with platelets, prothrombin time (PT), activated thromboplastin time (aPTT), type and cross-match, and pregnancy test. In stable patients, a pregnancy test and CBC should be considered. The hemoglobin and hematocrit are helpful in estimating blood loss and severity of bleeding. A platelet count helps rule out thrombocytopenia.[33]

Pregnancy, including ectopic pregnancy, threatened or spontaneous abortion, and complications of a recent induced abortion can present with vaginal bleeding. It is important to rule out pregnancy in all adolescents who present with unexplained heavy bleeding, especially in those with previously regular cycles.[34] Sexually transmitted diseases such as *Chlamydia trachomatis* and *Neisseria gonorrhoeae* are also associated with cervicitis and endometrial intermenstrual bleeding. Screen for gonorrhea and chlamydia infections by urine nucleic acid amplification tests (NAATs) or cervical cultures.

To test platelet function, the platelet function analysis (PFA) is the study of choice. Historically, bleeding times were obtained, but were found to be nonspecific. The platelet function analysis-100 (PFA-100) was found to be superior, showing 96% sensitivity and 98% specificity for measuring platelet function.[35] Evaluation of vWD includes obtaining a ristocetin cofactor assay of von Willebrand's factor (vWF), vW antigen, and a factor 8 (FVIII) level.[30] Finally, consider thyroid function tests to rule out thyroid disease and FSH, LH, testosterone, and DHEAS levels to rule out PCOS. A detailed work up for DUB is beyond the scope of the ED but the history and physical examination can be used to guide the choice of additional laboratory tests.

Imaging Studies

Generally, patients with DUB can be managed appropriately without the use of expensive imaging studies. Pelvic

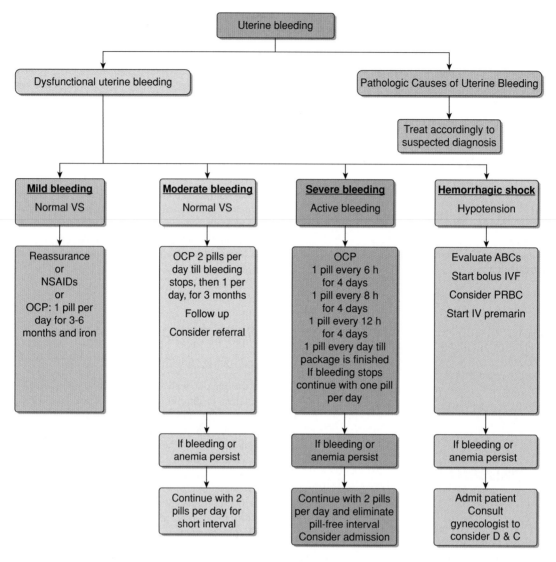

Figure 98–2. Treatment of dysfunctional bleeding. VS (vital signs), NSAIDs (nonsteroidal anti-inflammatory drugs), Hgb (hemoglobin), ABCs (airway, breathing, circulation), PRBC (packed red blood cells), OCP (oral contraceptive), IVF (intravenous fluids), D&C (dilation and curettage).

sonography is often performed to rule out anatomical or structural pathology of the reproductive tract such as benign or malignant tumors or PCOS.

MANAGEMENT OF DYSFUNCTIONAL UTERINE BLEEDING

The first step in the management of any patient with bleeding is the assurance of hemodynamic instability.[36] Patients in hemorrhagic shock, with severe anemia (hemoglobin <7 g/dL) or with heavy bleeding are hemodynamically unstable. Evaluate the airway, breathing, circulation, and address priorities of resuscitation according to the established Pediatric Advanced Life Support (PALS) guidelines. Obtain vascular access and begin rapid infusion of isotonic crystalloid. After 2 or 3 boluses, consider a packed red blood cell transfusion (PRBC) and administer intravenous estrogen (Premarin) in a dose of 25 mg every 4 to 6 hours until bleeding stops for 24 hours. Once bleeding

is controlled, start the patient on an OCP with a strong progestin. If bleeding is not controlled, consider admission and consult a gynecologist for further treatment such as dilatation and curettage.[32,36]

Patients who are hemodynamically stable can be managed with OCPs, NSAIDs, and referred to the gynecologist for outpatient management (Fig. 98–2 and Table 98–7).

In summary, to manage patients with mild bleeding, provide reassurance and offer NSAIDs, a monophasic OCP, and iron. For patients with moderate bleeding, consider starting OCPs at a higher dose (2 pills per day) until the bleeding stops and then 1 pill per day for 3 to 6 months. Patients with heavy bleeding will benefit from starting 1 pill every 6 hours for 4 days, followed by 1 pill every 8 hours for 4 days, and a tapering schedule for the rest of the month. Once bleeding is controlled, the patient should take 1 pill per day for 3 to 6 months.

OCPs are useful for cycle regulation, contraception, and prevention of associated prolonged unopposed estrogen stimulation of the endometrium. OCPs are contraindicated in

▶ **TABLE 98-7. TREATMENT OF DYSFUNCTIONAL UTERINE BLEEDING**

Oral contraceptive pills (OCPs)

Mild bleeding
- 30 μg ethinyl estradiol plus 0.3 mg norgestrel one pill per day
- 30 μg ethinyl estradiol plus 0.15 mg levonorgestrel one pill per day
- 20–35 μg ethinyl estradiol plus a progestin one pill daily

Moderate bleeding
- 35 μg ethinyl estradiol plus progestin twice to every 6 h for 5–7 d followed by one pill to completion of 28 d pack; then one pack per month for 3–6 mo.

Severe bleeding
- 35 μg ethinyl estradiol plus progestin one pill every 6 h for 4 d, one pill every 8 h for 4 d, one pill every 12 h for 4 d, one pill to completion of 28 d-pack; then one pack per month for 3–6 mo

Intravenous conjugated estrogens

Hemorrhagic shock (Premarin): 25 mg IV every 4–6 h for 24 h

Progestins
- Medroxyprogesterone acetate 10 mg per day for 12–14 d per month
- Norethindrone acetate 5 mg per day for 12–14 d per month
- Micronized progesterone 200 mg per day for 12 d per month

Elemental iron 60 mg three times per day for 8 wk

Nonsteroidal anti-inflammatory drugs
- Ibuprofen 400–600 mg bid–qid
- Mefenamic acid 250 mg qd–qid
- Naproxen 250–500 mg bid

smokers, women older than 35 years, and those with high risk of thromboembolism. In these women, progestins are recommended.[37,39]

Treatment of stable patients with ovulatory DUB includes NSAIDs, levonorgestrel-releasing intrauterine systems (LNG IUS), OCPs, androgens, antifibrinolytics, desmopressin, and surgery. A detailed explanation of these therapies is outside the scope of this book, but there are many excellent reviews available to the reader.[38–42]

REFERENCES

1. Durain D. Primary dysmenorrhea: assessment and management update. *J Midwifery Women's Health.* 2004;49:520–528.
2. Proctor M, Farquhar C. Diagnosis and management of dysmenorrhoea. *BMJ.* 2006;332:1134–1138.
3. Guylaine L, Odette P. Primary dysmenorrhea consensus guidelines. *J Obstet Gynaecol. Can.* 2005;27:1117–1130.
4. Tomislav S, Bukovic D, Pavelic, et al. Anthropological and clinical characteristics in adolescent women with dysmenorrhea. *Coll Antropol.* 2003;27:707–711.
5. Siobán H, Meekyong P. A longitudinal study of risk factors for the occurrence, duration and severity of menstrual cramps in a cohort of college women. *BJOG.* 2006;103(11):1134–1142.
6. Patel V, Tank Sale V, Sahasrabhojanee M. The burden and determinants of dysmenorrhoea: a population-based survey of 2262 women in Goa, India. *BJOG.* 2006;113:453–463.
7. Chantay B, Chacko M, Kelder S. Prevalence and impact of dysmenorrhea on Hispanic female adolescents. *Arch Pediatr Adoles. Med.* 2000;154:1226–1229.
8. Burnett MA, Antao V, Black. A prevalence of primary dysmenorrhea in Canada. *J Obstet Gynaecol Can.* 2005;27:765–770.
9. Dawood Y. Primary dysmenorrhea advances in pathogenesis and management. *Obstet Gynecol.* 2006;108:428–441.
10. Changzhong C, Sung C, Andrew D, et al. Prospective study of exposure to environmental tobacco smoke and dysmenorrhea. *Environ Health Perspect.* 2000;108:1019–1022.
11. Harlow SD, Campbell OM. Epidemiology of menstrual disorders in developing countries: a systematic review. *BJOG.* 2004; 111:6–16.
12. Wang L, Wang X, Wang W, et al. Stress and dysmenorrhoea: a population based prospective study. *Environ Med.* 2004;61: 1021–1026.
13. Latthe P, Mignini L, Gray R, et al. Factors predisposing women to chronic pelvic pain: systematic review. *BMJ.* 2006;332:749–755.
14. Davis R, Carolyn L. Primary dysmenorrhea in adolescent girls and treatment with oral contraceptives. *J Pediatr Adolesc Gynecol.* 2001;14:3–8.
15. Majoribanks J, Proctor ML, Farquhar C. Non steroidal anti-inflammatory drugs for primary dysmenorrheal. *Cochrane Database Syst Rev.* 2003;4:CD001751.
16. Sahin I, Saracoglu F, Kurban Y. Dysmenorrhea treatment with a single dose of rofecoxib. *Int J Gynecol Obstetrics.* 2003;83:285–291.
17. U.S. The Food and Drug Administration center for drug evaluation and research. *COX-2 Selective and Non-Selective Non-Steroidal Anti-Inflammatory Drugs.* Created April 7, 2005, updated July 18, 2005. http://www.fda.gov/cder/drug/infopage/COX2/default.htm.
18. Proctor ML, Roberts H, Farquhar CM. Combined oral contraceptive pill (OCP) as treatment for primary dysmenorrhoea. *Cochrane Database Syst Rev.* 2001, Issue 2. Art. No: CD002120. DOI:10.1002/14651858.CD002120.
19. Hendrixa S, Alexander N. Primary dysmenorrhea treatment with a desogestrel-containing low-dose oral contraceptive. *Contraception.* 2002;66:393–399.
20. Proctor ML, Murphy PA. Herbal and dietary therapies for primary and secondary dysmenorrhoea. *Cochrane Database Syst Rev.* 2001, Issue 2. Art. No: CD002124. DOI:10.1002/14651858.CD002124.
21. Proctor ML, Murphy PA, Pattison HM, et al. Behavioral interventions for primary and secondary dysmenorrhoea. *Cochrane Database Syst Rev.* 2007, Issue 3. Art. No: CD002248. DOI:10.1002/14651858.CD002248.pub3.
22. Albers J, Hull S, Wesley R. Abnormal uterine bleeding. *Am Fam Physician.* 2004;69:1931–1932.
23. Scott S. Abnormal bleeding in the pediatric patient. *Postgrad Obstet Gynecol.* 2006;26:1–6.
24. Disorders of the ovary and female reproductive tract. In: *Harrison's Principles of Internal Medicine*, 16th ed. Details 2005: chap 326.
25. Livingstone M, Fraser I. Mechanism of abnormal uterine bleeding. *Hum Reprod. Update.* 2002;8:60–67.
26. Shwayder J. Pathophysiology of abnormal uterine bleeding. *Obstet Gynecol Clin North Am.* 2000;27:219–234.
27. Nicholson W, Ellison S, Grason, H, et al. Patterns of ambulatory care use for gynecologic conditions: a national study. *Am J Obstet Gynecol.* 2001;184:523–530.
28. Ehrmann D. Polycystic ovary syndrome. *N Engl J Med.* 2005; 352:1223–1236.
29. Bevan J, Kelly Maloney, Hillery, C, et al. Bleeding disorders: a common cause of menorrhagia in adolescent. *J Pediatr.* 2001;138:856–861.
30. Kujovich J. Von Willebrand's disease and menorrhagia: prevalence, diagnosis, and management. *Am, Hematol.* 2005;79:220–228.

31. Hayden S, Emans J. Abnormal vaginal bleeding in adolescents. *Pediatr Rev.* 2007;28:175–182.

32. Slap G. Menstrual disorders in adolescent. *Best Pract Res Clin Obstet Gynecol.* 2003;17:75–92.

33. Dilley A, Drews C, Lally C, et al. A survey of gynecologist concerning menorrhagia: perceptions of bleeding disorders as possible cause. *J Womens Health Gend Based Med.* 2002;11:39–44.

34. Guttmacher Institute. *U.S. Teenage Pregnancy Statistics National and State Trends and Trends by Race and Ethnicity.* New York, NY: Guttmacher Institute; 2006:1–3.

35. Kouides P. Menorrhagia from a haematologist's point of view. Part I: initial evaluation. *Haemophilia.* 2002;8:330–338.

36. PALS subcommittee. *Shock. Pediatric Advanced Life Support.* Provider manual: chapter 5, 2006.

37. Hickey M, Balen A. Menstrual disorders in adolescent: investigation and management. Hum. *Reprod Update.* 2003;9:493–504.

38. Lethaby AE, Cooke I, Rees M. Progesterone or progestogen-releasing intrauterine systems for heavy menstrual bleeding. *Cochrane Database Syst Rev.* 2005, Issue 4. Art. No: CD002126. DOI:10.1002/14651858.CD002126.pub2.

39. Munro M, Mainor N, Basu R. Oral medroxyprogesterone acetate and combination oral contraceptives for acute uterine bleeding. *Obstet Gynecol.* 2006;108:924–929.

40. Grimes DA, Hubacher D, Lopez LM, et al. Non-steroidal anti-inflammatory drugs for heavy bleeding or pain associated with intrauterine-device use. *Cochrane Database Syst Rev.* 2006, Issue 4. Art. No: CD006034. DOI:10.1002/14651858.CD006034.pub2.

41. Beaumont H, Augood C, Duckitt K, et al. Danazol for heavy menstrual bleeding. *Cochrane Database Syst Rev.* 2007, Issue 3. Art. No: CD001017. DOI:10.1002/14651858.CD001017.pub2.

42. Lethaby A, Farquhar C, Cooke I. Antifibrinolytics for heavy menstrual bleeding. *Cochrane Database Syst Rev.* 2000, Issue 4. Art. No: CD00249. DOI:10.1002/14651858.CD000249.

SECTION XVII

HEMATOLOGIC AND ONCOLOGIC EMERGENCIES

CHAPTER 99

Anemia

Audra L. McCreight and Jonathan E. Wickiser

▶ HIGH-YIELD FACTS

- The mean hemoglobin concentration for normal newborns is 18 g/dL, after which it falls to a nadir of 11.5 g/dL (mean concentration) at 2 to 3 months of life. Although mean hemoglobin concentrations in children continue to vary somewhat by age, 11 g/dL defines the lower limits of normal for the prepubertal patient population.
- Anemias are most easily classified based on red blood cell (RBC) size and degree of bone marrow activity. The size of RBCs is measured as mean corpuscular volume (MCV), with the lower limit of normal for the MCV equaling 70 plus the age in years; bone marrow activity is reflected by the reticulocyte count.
- The most common cause of microcytic anemia in childhood is iron deficiency, usually due to excess intake of whole cow's milk.
- Thalassemias are inherited defects resulting in the inability to synthesize sufficient quantities of various globin chains of the hemoglobin molecule. Thalassemia trait produces marked microcytosis out of proportion to the degree of anemia.
- If the reticulocyte count is high in the presence of a normocytic anemia, blood loss or a hemolytic process must be considered.
- A low reticulocyte count in the face of significant anemia indicates bone marrow underproduction. If the abnormality is isolated to the RBC line, the primary considerations are transient erythroblastopenia of childhood (TEC) or an aplastic crisis complicating an underlying hemolytic anemia.
- Thrombocytopenia or white blood cell (WBC) abnormalities associated with normocytic anemia and poor reticulocyte response suggests a marrow infiltrative process such as leukemia or acquired aplastic anemia.
- Macrocytic anemia is uncommon in pediatric patients. Folate and vitamin B_{12} deficiencies are rare in otherwise healthy children.

Physiologically, anemia occurs when the hemoglobin level is too low to meet cellular oxygen demands. Practically, anemia is defined as a hemoglobin concentration more than 2 standard deviations below the mean for a comparable population. The normal hemoglobin concentration varies by age and, in the postpubertal population, by sex. Hemoglobin values are high at birth and slowly fall to a nadir at 2 to 3 months of age. This nadir is deeper and occurs at a younger age in premature infants. Although mean hemoglobin concentrations in children continue to vary somewhat by age, 11 g/dL plus 0.1 times the age in years defines the lower limits of normal for the prepubertal patient population. After puberty, normative data for adult populations apply and gender differences become apparent.

Patients with mild anemia are usually asymptomatic, and the anemia is most commonly discovered on a routine complete blood count (CBC). Even children with moderate to severe anemia may be asymptomatic if the problem develops slowly, compensating well for even severely low hemoglobin levels. When the hemoglobin becomes low enough to produce symptoms, patients may present with fatigue, irritability, or shortness of breath on exertion. Physical examination may reveal pallor, tachycardia, jaundice, and systolic ejection murmur owing to an increased cardiac output. With a rapid drop in hemoglobin, the child may develop dizziness, orthostatic hypotension, or high-output cardiac failure.

Important history to obtain when evaluating anemia includes the patient's diet, prior blood counts, and prior episodes of jaundice. A family history of anemia, splenectomy, jaundice, or gallstones might suggest a hemoglobinopathy or a hereditary membrane disorder. Knowledge of any chronic disorders such as kidney disease, cardiovascular disease, or underlying inflammatory processes is necessary. Physical examination should assess for signs of jaundice, lymphadenopathy, splenomegaly, or skeletal anomalies.

Laboratory evaluation of anemia should begin with a CBC, reticulocyte count, and review of the peripheral blood smear. Further diagnostic evaluation, if needed, is determined by the results of these tests. Causes of anemia are most easily classified based on red blood cell (RBC) size (microcytic, normocytic, or macrocytic) and degree of bone marrow activity. The size of RBCs is measured as the mean corpuscular volume (MCV), the normal values of which vary with age. The lower limit of normal for the MCV equals 70 plus the age in years up to the normal adult low of 80. Bone marrow activity is reflected by the reticulocyte count. Table 99–1 summarizes the basic interpretation of a screening CBC for the cause for anemia. Table 99–2 reviews the interpretation of the peripheral smear examination of RBC morphology to help determine the cause of anemia.

▶ MICROCYTIC ANEMIA

The most common cause of microcytic anemia in children is iron deficiency. Thalassemia, anemia of inflammation, hemoglobin C disease, hemoglobin E disease, and sideroblastic anemia may also lead to microcytic anemia. Table 99–3 reviews a method for sorting out the common causes of microcytic anemia.

▶ TABLE 99–1. **ANEMIA SCREENING TESTS FOR CAUSE**

Mean corpuscular volume (MCV)
- Microcytic?
- Normocytic?
- Macrocytic?

Reticulocyte count
- Low—Decreased production
- High—Increased destruction or blood loss

Red cell distribution width (RDW)—iron deficiency (high) vs. thalassemia (low)

Peripheral smear examination (see Table 99–2)

▶ TABLE 99–2. **PERIPHERAL SMEAR INTERPRETATION**

Fragmented RBCs, shistocytes, burr cells
- Hemolytic uremic syndrome
- Thrombotic thrombocytopenic purpura
- Disseminated intravascular coagulopathy

Spherocytes
- Hereditary spherocytosis
- ABO incompatibility

Eliptocytes: Hereditary eliptocytosis
Target cells
- Thalassemia
- Hemoglobinopathies

Sickle cells: Sickle hemoglobinopathies
Basophilic stippling: Lead poisoning
Variation in size and shape: See interpretation of MVC and RDW

IRON DEFICIENCY

Risk factors for iron deficiency anemia include age between 6 months and 2 years, decreased prevalence or duration of breast-feeding, lack of use of iron-fortified formulas, early introduction of whole cow's milk into the diet, and low socioeconomic status. Whole cow's milk is deficient in bioavailable iron but rich in calories. Excess intake produces iron deficiency by its inherent lack of iron, by reducing appetite and intake of iron-rich foods, and leading to occult gastrointestinal bleeding from the effect of unmodified cow's milk proteins on gastrointestinal mucosa.[1] During fetal life, most of the total body iron is absorbed during the last trimester, so premature infants are at greater risk for iron-deficiency anemia. They deplete their reduced iron stores early and have an even greater need than full-term infants for iron supplementation.

Iron deficiency anemia develops slowly and patients rarely present with acute symptoms. Even with drastically reduced hemoglobin levels, patients are usually well compensated and hemodynamically stable. The diagnosis is usually made on the basis of the history, with CBC results showing anemia and significant microcytosis. The reticulocyte count is low or normal, when it should be elevated in response to the level of anemia. Thrombocytosis is common in iron deficiency anemia, but thrombocytopenia may also be seen. If necessary, further diagnostic testing will reveal a reduced serum iron, an elevated total iron binding capacity (TIBC), and a reduced ferritin level. Ferritin, however, is an acute-phase reactant and in the face of infection or inflammation may be elevated despite the presence of iron deficiency anemia. A trial of iron therapy is both diagnostic and therapeutic. Ferrous sulfate is administered in an amount sufficient to provide 4 to 6 mg/kg of elemental iron per day in two divided doses for 3 to 4 months. Multivitamins with iron, such as poly-vi-sol with iron, do not provide adequate amounts of iron to correct iron deficiency. An increase in the reticulocyte count is typically seen in a matter of days, and the hemoglobin level increases in 1 to 2 weeks. Identification and elimination of the cause of the iron deficiency is also necessary and is usually accomplished with appropriate dietary counseling.

THALASSEMIA

Thalassemias are inherited defects resulting in the absence or decreased production of normal hemoglobin, leading to a microcytic anemia. The condition is most common in people of Mediterranean, Southeast Asian, and African ancestry and is the most common single gene disease worldwide.[2] In general, the disease is classified by the number of abnormal globin genes. The heterozygous form of thalassemia is often referred to as thalassemia trait. Thalassemia trait produces marked microcytosis out of proportion to the degree of anemia. There is typically a high total RBC count and narrow RDW, which helps differentiate thalassemia trait from iron deficiency anemia. Unlike

▶ TABLE 99–3. **DIFFERENTIATING MICROCYTIC ANEMIA**

Parameter	Iron Deficiency	Thalassemia	Anemia of Chronic Disease
History	Prematurity or high milk intake	None or family history	Chronic inflammation or disease
Reticulocyte count	Low	Normal	Low
MCV	Low	Very low	Normal to low
RDW	High	Low	Normal to high
Serum ferritin	Low	Normal	High
Serum iron	Low	Normal or elevated	Low
TIBC	High	Normal	Low

MCV, mean corpuscular volume; RDW, red cell distribution width; TIBC, total iron binding capacity.

iron deficiency, the reticulocyte count in thalassemia should be normal or slightly elevated.

α-Thalassemia results from a decreased production of α-globin because of a deletion or mutation in one or more of the four α-globin genes. Patients will have a normal hemoglobin electrophoresis outside of the newborn period. The silent carrier state results from a defect in a single gene and patients have no anemia and normal-appearing red cells. α-thalassemia trait refers to a defect in two genes, resulting in mild microcytic anemia. Hemoglobin H disease occurs when there is only one normal α-globin gene. These patients have moderate anemia in the 8 to 10 g/dL range, but may have increased hemolysis with stress or infection. A defect in all four α-globin genes results in α-thalassemia major, a condition leading to severe fetal complications.

β-Thalassemia results from a decreased production of β-globin because of a mutation or deletion in one or more of the two β-globin genes. In β-thalassemia trait, the hemoglobin concentration is often 2 to 3 g/dL below normal values. A hemoglobin electrophoresis will demonstrate an elevated A_2 component and in some cases an elevated level of fetal hemoglobin (Hgb F). In β-thalassemia intermedia, patients maintain a hemoglobin of 6 to 8 g/dL and do not require chronic transfusion. β-thalassemia major produces severe hemolytic anemia with marked microcytosis and reticulocytosis. It usually presents within the first year of life. Pallor, jaundice, and hepatosplenomegaly are often present. Because patients require lifelong transfusion therapy, the use of uncrossmatched blood is avoided, except in the most dire circumstances. The major side effect of long-term transfusion therapy is iron overload, which adversely affects multiple organs, especially the pancreas, liver, and heart.

LEAD POISONING

While microcytic anemia may be seen in children with lead poisoning, the anemia is actually owing to iron deficiency. Lead poisoning must be considered in the child with microcytic anemia. Iron deficiency leads to pica and the ingestion of lead. Iron deficiency also increases absorption of lead from the gastrointestinal tract.

▶ NORMOCYTIC ANEMIA

Although normocytic anemia is less common than microcytic anemia, the differential diagnosis in childhood is extensive (Table 99–4). The primary determinant in establishing a differential is whether the anemia is owing to decreased production, increased destruction, or blood loss. Most diagnosis may be made based on history, reticulocyte count, and review of RBC morphology.[3]

NORMOCYTIC ANEMIA WITH HIGH RETICULOCYTE COUNT

If the reticulocyte count is high in the presence of a normocytic anemia, blood loss must be considered. If there is no evidence

▶ **TABLE 99–4. DIFFERENTIAL DIAGNOSIS FOR NORMOCYTIC ANEMIA**

Blood loss (high reticulocyte count)

Hemolytic anemia (high reticulocyte count)
Immune
  Autoimmune hemolytic anemia
  Neonatal–maternal blood group incompatibility
Nonimmune
  Microangiopathic
    Disseminated intravascular coagulation (DIC)
    Hemolytic uremic syndrome (HUS)
  Macroangiopathic
    Artificial cardiac valve
    Membrane abnormalities
    Spherocytosis
    Elliptocytosis
  Metabolic abnormalities
    G6PD deficiency
    Pyruvate kinase deficiency
  Hemoglobinopathies

Nonhemolytic anemia (low or normal reticulocyte count)
Abnormality isolated to red cell line
  Chronic hemolytic anemia with concurrent aplastic crisis
    Transient erythroblastopenia of childhood (TEC)
  Chronic disease
    Renal insufficiency
    Diamond–Blackfan anemia
Abnormality affecting other cell lines
  Bone marrow infiltration
    Leukemia
    Lymphoma
    Tumor metastasis
  Acquired aplastic anemia

of blood loss, a hemolytic anemia is likely. The workup for a patient with hemolytic anemia includes a Coombs or Direct Anti-globulin Test (DAT) to determine whether the hemolytic anemia is immunologic in nature. Immune hemolytic anemia may be the result of a drug reaction, infection, collagen vascular disorder, or malignancy, but commonly no etiology is determined.

Patients often present acutely with severe anemia, pallor, jaundice, and hemoglobinuria. Transfusions may be necessary with severe symptomatic anemia, but may be difficult owing to the circulating antibody causing "incompatibility" in vitro and rapid destruction of transfused RBCs in vivo. Immunosuppression with corticosteroid is frequently adequate to diminish RBC destruction so that the patient's brisk reticulocytosis can repair the anemia. In severe or refractory cases, plasmapheresis or IVIG may be necessary.

The differential diagnosis for nonimmune hemolytic anemia includes micro and macroangiopathic destruction, membrane disorders, metabolic abnormalities, and hemoglobinopathies. Sickle cell anemia is discussed in detail in Chapter 100.

Microangiopathic RBC destruction can occur with disseminated intravascular coagulation (DIC), thrombotic thrombocytopenic purpura (TTP), and hemolytic uremic syndrome. The peripheral smear will demonstrate schistocytes, burr cells, and other RBC fragments.

Hereditary spherocytosis (HS) and elliptocytosis (HE) result from inherited mutations in a variety of proteins making up the red cell membrane. The incidence of HS is estimated at 1 in 5000 in the United States. Most cases are inherited in an autosomal dominant pattern, making family history important in the diagnosis. However, up to 25% of cases may arise in patients with no family history.[4] Hemolytic anemia occurs due to splenic destruction of abnormally shaped RBCs. The disease often presents as jaundice and anemia in infancy. The degree of anemia varies widely, but is often consistent within affected family members. Laboratory studies reveal anemia, reticulocytosis, and hyperbilirubinemia. The diagnosis is made by reviewing the peripheral smear and possibly family history; osmotic fragility studies are confirmatory. The major hematologic crisis is aplastic anemia, which is usually secondary to a parvovirus infection. Patients may also have an increased rate of hemolysis with stress or infection. Splenectomy is curative and is considered in patients with severe hemolysis leading to frequent transfusion or hospitalization. Spherocytes may be seen in the peripheral smear of conditions other than HS, including neonates with ABO incompatibility, patients with clostridial sepsis, severe burns, and spider, bee, or snake bites.

Inherited metabolic disorders, such as pyruvate kinase and glucose-6-phosphate dehydrogenase (G6PD) deficiencies, also cause chronic hemolysis. There are multiple variants of G6PD deficiency, with varying degrees of severity. The A-variant is seen in approximately 10% of African American males and becomes symptomatic only after a significant challenge from a drug or infection. Enzyme levels are higher in young cells, so normal levels of G6PD may be obtained when assayed from G6PD-deficient patients during periods of brisk reticulocytosis. The assay may have to be repeated when the acute hemolysis has passed. Treatment involves blood transfusion with severe anemia and counseling regarding avoidance of oxidant stressors.

NORMOCYTIC ANEMIA WITH LOW RETICULOCYTE COUNTS

A low reticulocyte count in the face of significant anemia indicates bone marrow underproduction. If the abnormality is isolated to the RBC line, the primary considerations are transient erythroblastopenia of childhood (TEC) and an aplastic crisis complicating an underlying hemolytic anemia.

TEC is an acquired pure RBC aplasia; WBC and platelet counts are normal. It typically affects children between 1 and 4 years of age. There is seasonal clustering and an associated history of preceding viral illness, but no causative viral agent has been identified. Supportive therapy is usually sufficient as patients are typically hemodynamically stable and recover spontaneously over several weeks. Transfusion may be necessary in symptomatic patients. Steroids have not been shown to speed recovery.

Other entities in the differential of normocytic anemia with low to normal reticulocyte counts and no abnormalities of other cell lines include anemia of chronic disease, inflammatory processes, and decreased erythropoietin from renal insufficiency. Anemia of chronic disease (ACOD) occurs in patients with acute or chronic immune activation, resulting in disorder iron hemostasis and blunted erythropoietin response.[5] ACOD is usually a mild normocytic, normochromic anemia; but may be microcytic in long-standing cases, making it difficult to differentiate from iron deficiency (see Table 99–1). Diamond–Blackfan anemia is a congenital RBC aplasia that usually presents in the first year of life with severe anemia. The age of onset of anemia may help to differentiate Diamond–Blackfan from TEC. Occasionally, other congenital abnormalities are associated, such as cleft palate, skeletal anomalies, and congenital heart disease.

Thrombocytopenia or WBC abnormalities associated with normocytic anemia and poor reticulocyte response suggests marrow infiltration or acquired aplastic anemia. Marrow infiltration is most commonly due to leukemia. Leukemic blasts may be apparent in the peripheral blood. Atypical lymphocytes from Epstein–Barr virus or other viral infections can appear similar to lymphoblasts. Lymphoma and other tumors with potential to metastasize to the bone marrow may also cause failure of production, with resultant decreases in multiple cell lines.

Acquired aplastic anemia in the absence of an underlying hemolytic anemia has been associated with drugs and infections. Often no etiology is determined. The prognosis is quite poor and bone marrow transplantation is often required. Blood transfusion is performed judiciously for patients who are candidates for bone marrow transplantation because of the risk of sensitization.

► MACROCYTIC ANEMIA

Macrocytic anemia is relatively uncommon in pediatric patients. Aplastic anemia or leukemia, although usually causing normocytic anemia, can result in macrocytosis. Because of the large size of reticulocytes, marked reticulocytosis can lead to a high MCV, although mature RBCs may be of a normal size. Folate and vitamin B_{12} deficiencies can result in megaloblastic anemia. These are rare in otherwise healthy children, but should be considered in children with underlying gastrointestinal pathology. Goat's milk contains little folate, and infants maintained on this alone may develop microcytic anemia. Some drugs, notably AZT, can cause macrocytosis.

REFERENCES

1. Booth IW, Aukett MA. Iron deficiency anaemia in infancy and early childhood. *Arch Dis Child.* 1997;76:549–554.
2. Lo L, Singer ST. Thalassemia: current approach to an old disease. *Pediatr Clin North Am.* 2002;49(6):1165–1169.
3. Segel GB, Hirsh MG, Feig SA. Managing anemia in pediatric office practice: part 1. *Pediatr Review.* 2002;23(3):75–84.
4. Shah S, Vega R. Hereditary spherocytosis. *Pediatr Review.* 2004;25(5):168–172.
5. Weiss G, Goodnough LT. Anemia of chronic disease. *NEJM.* 2005;352(10):1011–1023.

CHAPTER 100

Sickle Cell Disease

Audra L. McCreight and Jonathan E. Wickiser

► HIGH-YIELD FACTS

- Sickle cell disease (SCD) is a chronic hemolytic anemia that is most common among African Americans, of whom approximately 1 in 600 are affected with homozygous hemoglobin SS, the most severe of the sickle syndromes. Patients with a single abnormal gene for HbS have sickle cell trait and remain essentially asymptomatic.
- Acute vasoocclusive events, or painful "crisis," are the most common complication of SCD and are the most frequent cause of emergency department visits.
- A complete blood count and reticulocyte count should be obtained every time a patient with SCD presents to the emergency department.
- Patients with SCD presenting with a new infiltrate on chest radiograph and chest pain, fever, and/or respiratory symptoms have acute chest syndrome (ACS). Therapy for ACS consists of antibiotics, pain control, respiratory support, and possibly transfusion. All children with ACS should be admitted to the hospital.
- A blood culture should be obtained and parenteral antibiotic given to every patient with SCD and fever due to the risk of sepsis from encapsulated bacteria, especially *Streptococcus pneumoniae*.
- Splenic sequestration crisis occurs when RBCs become entrapped in the spleen, resulting in a rapidly enlarging spleen and a sudden drop in Hgb. The mainstay of therapy is blood transfusion.
- Stroke occurs in 10% of patients with sickle cell anemia under 18 years of age. Patients with signs and symptoms concerning for stroke should have neuroimaging performed (preferably MRI and MRA) and consultation with a hematologist as soon as possible.

Hemoglobin S (Hgb S) is a variant resulting from a single nucleotide mutation in the sixth codon of the β-globin gene leading to the substitution of hydrophobic valine for the normal hydrophilic glutamic acid. Sickle cell disease (SCD) occurs when an individual is homozygous for Hgb S or is a compound heterozygote for Hgb S and another interacting β-globin variant. The most common combination of hemoglobins leading to SCD are Hgb SS (sickle cell anemia), Hgb SC (hemoglobin SC disease), and Hgb S-β thalassemia (either β^0 or β^+). Although there is wide variability in individual severity of illness, patients with double heterozygous states such as Hgb SC, Hgb Sβ^+ thalassemia, and Hgb SD are typically less seriously affected than those with Hgb SS or Hgb Sβ^0 (no hemoglobin A production). Approximately 8% of the African American population are sickle trait carriers, with 1 in 600 having sickle cell anemia.[1] However, Hgb S also occurs in people of Mediterranean, Indian, Central and South American, and Middle Eastern descent.

Patients with a single abnormal gene for HbS have sickle cell trait. The concentration of HbS is typically 40%, and the large percentage of normal hemoglobin allows the patients to remain asymptomatic except under the most severe hypoxic stress. Sickle trait should be considered a benign condition. Patients with SCD experience a number of complications that are likely to bring them to the emergency department (ED).

► VASOOCCLUSIVE CRISIS

Acute vasoocclusive events, or painful "crisis," are the most common complication of SCD and are the most frequent cause of ED visits.[2] Pain episodes result from the obstruction of blood flow in the microcirculation leading to tissue ischemia and microinfarction. Vasoocclusion occurs via a combination of sickle cell interactions with endothelial cells and obstruction from nondeformable sickled cells.

Dactylitis, or hand–foot syndrome, is vasoocclusion in marrow of the metacarpal or metatarsal bones (Fig. 100–1). This is often the earliest presentation of SCD, usually occurring between 6 and 18 months of life. Infants present with hand and foot swelling and tenderness, which may lead to refusal to walk and irritability. Dactylitis declines with age as hematopoiesis shifts to the long bones.

Older patients typically experience vasoocclusive events in the long bones, back, joints, and abdomen. Pain events may be precipitated by dehydration, hypoxia, cold exposure, or infection. However, often no instigating factor is identified. There is a great deal of individual variation in number and severity of painful crises. On average, patients with SCD experience 0.8 hospitalizations per patient-year, but 5% of patients have frequent pain crises and account for approximately one-third of all medical contacts for painful crisis.[2] Figure 100–2 outlines the management of severe acute pain in the ED.

As there is no diagnostic test or clinical finding that will identify patients in vasoocclusive crisis, the diagnosis is made on the basis of history alone. Patients with SCD and pain should be evaluated for other disease processes such as traumatic injuries, osteomyelitis, septic arthritis, and surgical abdominal problems. The formation of gallstones due to chronic hemolysis may lead to cholecystitis or pancreatitis and abdominal pain. A complete blood count (CBC) and reticulocyte count is indicated in every encounter with SCD patients. Typically, patients

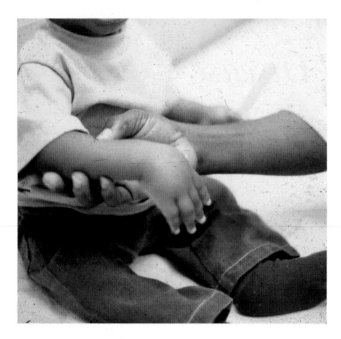

Figure 100–1. Child with sickle cell anemia and dactylitis.

remain at baseline levels of Hgb during a painful event. Hydration at maintenance should be initiated to correct and prevent dehydration. Overhydration may lead to acute chest syndrome (ACS) and should be avoided. Oxygen has not been shown to be beneficial in the management of pain crises unless hypoxemia is present.

Pain should be assessed at least every 30 minutes using standardized pain scales. Pain relief is achieved with a variety of analgesics, depending on the severity of the crisis and what the patient has required in past crisis. Oral agents such as acetaminophen, nonsteroidal anti-inflammatory drugs (NSAIDs), and codeine used separately or in combination are the mainstays of treatment for mild to moderate pain. Usually, patients have unsuccessfully tried these therapies on a scheduled basis at home prior to presenting to the ED. For patients who have not attempted oral therapy at home, this should be initiated first. Parenteral opioids, preferably morphine or hydromorphone, are often necessary for severe pain. Anxiety about giving children narcotics leads to undertreatment of pain, which should be avoided. Although meperidine has commonly been used in the past, the availability of other potent analgesics has made it a poor choice for SCD pain. Extended use of meperidine will result in the buildup of normeperidine, a toxic metabolite with poor analgesic effect. Normeperidine can cause dysphoria and increases the risk of seizures.

Typically, patients in the ED receive scheduled oral opioid and NSAID and parenteral opioid analgesics and are observed for 3 or 4 hours. Patients will often require further doses of parenteral opioid. If the patient remains comfortable without further need for parenteral opioid, he or she may be discharged with continued scheduled oral opioid and NSAID at home. If adequate pain relief is not achieved, the patient is admitted for further parenteral analgesia. Analgesia should be provided at frequent regular time intervals to avoid breakthrough pain. PRN pain medications should be avoided in a crisis. When pain recurs between doses, the recurring pain is more difficult to control. Patient-controlled analgesia (PCA) with a morphine drip allows baseline levels of pain relief, and the patient may titrate pain relief as needed for activity or other painful times. Hypoventilation as a result of opiate use may increase the risk of developing ACS. Incentive spirometry should be encouraged in order to decrease this risk.

► ACUTE CHEST SYNDROME

Acute chest syndrome (ACS) is the presence of a new lobar or segmental pulmonary infiltrate in the presence of fever, respiratory symptoms, and/or chest pain (Fig. 100–3). Various causes may contribute to ACS including infection, pulmonary infarction due to vasoocclusion, and fat emboli from marrow infarction.[3] Chest pain from vasoocclusion may cause splinting and hypoventilation, leading to the development of ACS in a patient who initially presents with a painful episode. It is difficult to differentiate vasoocclusion from pneumonia in patients with ACS, since both etiologies cause similar manifestations. Infectious organisms associated with ACS include *S. pneumoniae* in younger children and *Mycoplasma* or *Chlamydia* in adolescents. ACS may present with or rapidly progress to respiratory failure requiring mechanical ventilation.

All patients with ACS should be admitted to the hospital. Laboratory evaluation should include a CBC, reticulocyte count, and blood culture. Antibiotic therapy directed at *S. pneumoniae* and atypical organisms such as a third-generation cephalosporin and a macrolide should be initiated. A type and crossmatch should be considered as red cell transfusion may be necessary. A chest radiograph is adequate; lung scans are not useful in establishing a diagnosis. Room air oxygen saturation should be checked and supplemental oxygen initiated via face mask or nasal cannula in hypoxemic patients. Analgesia for chest pain should be provided, but managed carefully to prevent hypoventilation. Hydration should be limited to 1 to 1.25 times maintenance po + IV in order to avoid fluid overload. Patients with hemoglobin >2 g below baseline, hypoxia, or a rapidly progressing process will require blood transfusion. Transfusion may be either simple or by exchange depending on the severity of symptoms and level of anemia compared to the patient's baseline hemoglobin. Transfusion will decrease the percentage of Hgb S and increase the blood's oxygen-carrying capacity. Bronchodilators may be beneficial in patients with a history of reactive airway disease.

► INFECTION

Patients with SCD are at high risk for infection primarily due primarily to functional asplenia. The major risk comes from encapsulated bacteria, especially *S. pneumoniae*. Although prophylactic penicillin and vaccines for pneumococci and *Haemophilus influenzae* type B have reduced the incidence of sepsis in this vulnerable population, overwhelming pneumococcal sepsis remains a significant cause of death in children with SCD. Children younger than 3 years are particularly susceptible to bacteremia, which can occur as commonly as nine bacteremic events per 100 patient-years.[4] The fatality rate

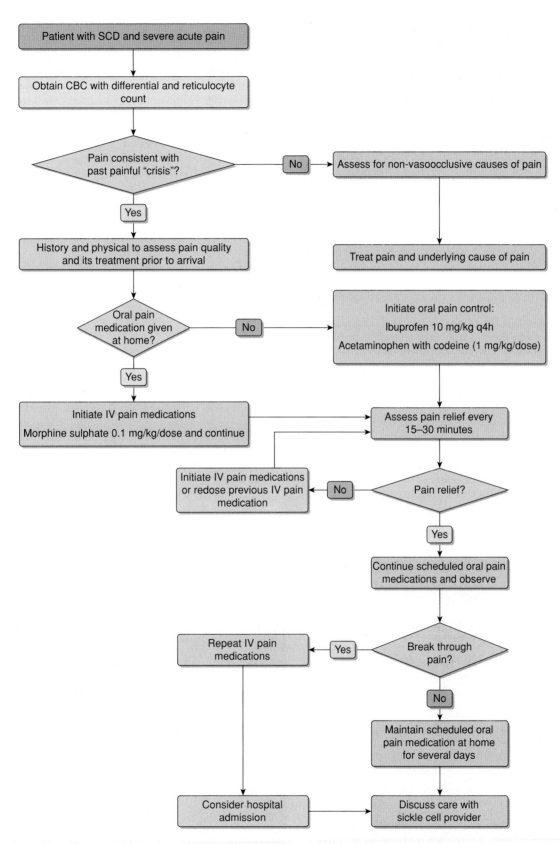

Figure 100–2. Algorithm for the management of sickle cell disease.

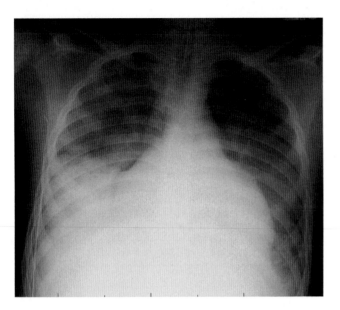

Figure 100–3. Chest film of a 14-year-old boy with sickle cell anemia who presented to the ED with chest pain and fever. X-ray shows presence of new right lower lobe infiltrate.

is high, even though many of these children appear well at initial presentation.

Children with SCD who present to the ED with fever (>38.5°C) are at highest risk for bacteremia. After obtaining a CBC and blood culture, all persons with SCD should be promptly treated with parenteral antibiotics effective against *S. pneumoniae* and, if unimmunized, *H. influenzae* B. Meningitis does occur in children with SCD, but lumbar puncture in the absence of meningeal signs is not warranted. Hospital admission is necessary for any toxic-appearing child. Hospitalization should be considered in patients presenting with a temperature >40°C, a WBC count >30 000 per mm³, thrombocytopenia, hemoglobin significantly below baseline value, or in a situation where follow-up is uncertain or unlikely. Some institutions use a long-acting cephalosporin, such as ceftriaxone, along with close outpatient follow-up in nonseptic-appearing children. The risk for infection in SCD persists into adulthood; all patients should be evaluated as above regardless of age.

In addition to overwhelming sepsis, children with SCD are susceptible to other infections such as pneumonia, meningitis, and osteomyelitis. The etiology is most frequently encapsulated organisms. Unlike the general population, the most common organism identified as the cause of osteomyelitis in patients with SCD is *Salmonella*.

▶ STROKE (CEREBROVASCULAR ACCIDENTS)

Stroke occurs in approximately 10% of children with sickle cell anemia before 18 years of age, but is rare in children with Hgb SC and Hgb Sβ⁺. Most strokes in children are ischemic events, involving large arteries. Hemorrhagic events are more common in adults, but may be seen in adolescents. Common presenting signs and symptoms of infarctive stroke include hemiparesis, refusal to use an arm or leg, aphasia, dysphasia, seizures, cranial nerve palsy, or coma. Initial management should include a careful history, focusing on any previous neurologic events and results of previous neuroimaging. A CBC, reticulocyte count, and type and crossmatch should be drawn. An MRI and MRA (Fig. 100–4) with diffusion-weighted imaging should be obtained as soon as possible, a noncontrast enhanced CT is only necessary if there will be a delay in obtaining MRI.

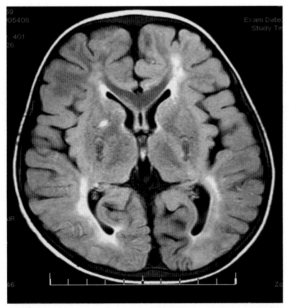

A

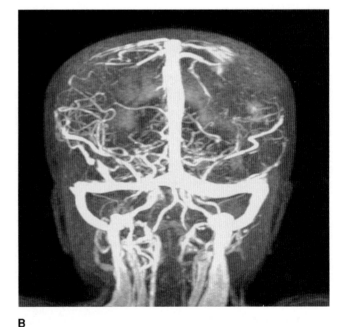

B

Figure 100–4. (A) MRI and (B) MRA of a 3-year-old with sickle cell anemia, who presented to the ED with aphasia and multiple motor defects. Imaging revealed acute ischemic stroke and evidence of previous subacute stroke.

Results of neuroimaging may be normal early in the event and the diagnosis of stroke may be made clinically. While there is no treatment proven to change the acute outcome, exchange or simple transfusion to reduce Hgb S to less than 30% is the management of choice. Care must be taken to maintain the patient's hemoglobin below 11 g/dL until Hgb S is known to be below 30%. Chronic transfusion to maintain Hgb S below 30% has been shown to reduce recurrent stroke events.

▶ SPLENIC SEQUESTRATION

Acute splenic sequestration crisis (ASSC) occurs when red cells become trapped in the spleen, resulting in a rapidly enlarging spleen, a sudden drop in Hgb, and the potential for shock. ASSC occurs most often in patients with Hgb SS between 3 months and 5 years of age. Repeated infarctions of the spleen in patients with Hgb SS lead to autosplenectomy by 3 to 5 years of age, decreasing the risk of ASSC. In patients with Hgb SC and Hgb Sβ+, ASSC is less common, but persistent splenomegaly may occur in adolescence or adulthood. ASSC may present with the sudden onset of weakness, pallor, tachycardia, tachypnea, or abdominal fullness. Parents of children with SCD are taught to palpate the spleen regularly at home and present to the ED for a newly palpable spleen or enlargement of a chronically enlarged spleen. Laboratory studies demonstrate marked anemia, an elevated reticulocyte count, and often thrombocytopenia.

The mainstay of therapy is simple blood transfusion. If the patient is unstable, fluid expansion may be used in the initial stages of resuscitation while waiting for blood to be available, but it must be used carefully as volume overload and congestive heart failure can result. Blood transfusion should be considered with a decline in hemoglobin of 2 g or more below baseline, hemoglobin below 5 g/dL, or in any patient with signs of cardiovascular compromise. Transfusion will support oxygen-carrying capacity, decrease the percent of Hgb S, and result in sequestered red cells being released from the spleen. Thus the goal of transfusion is hemoglobin of 9 g/dL. Sequestration frequently recurs, with up to 50% of children having a second ASSC.[5] Splenectomy may be necessary in children with recurrent ASSC.

▶ APLASTIC CRISIS

Infections with Parvovirus B19 may cause transient red cell aplasia. In normal children whose RBC lifespan is 120 days, brief marrow suppression will not lead to a significant drop in Hgb. However, the shortened lifespan of the RBC in sickle cell anemia (10–25 days) may lead to a significant drop in hemoglobin with even a short period of red cell aplasia. With Parvovirus, reticulocytopenia begins 5 days post exposure and continues for 7 to 10 days. Patients may have fever, upper respiratory symptoms, nausea and vomiting, arthralgias, or myalgias, but may also have minimal symptoms. Fatigue, pallor, tachycardia, and tachypnea may be present with severe anemia. A CBC will reveal a drop in the hemoglobin from baseline and a decreased reticulocyte count (usually <1%). Patients presenting in the recovery phase may have a high reticulocyte count and numerous nucleated RBCs noted on the blood smear. Mildly anemic and asymptomatic children can be managed with supportive care and close outpatient observation pending marrow recovery. Simple transfusion of RBCs is necessary in patients with hemoglobin below 5 g/dL or with cardiovascular compromise. Children with Hgb SC or Sβ+ rarely require transfusion with aplastic crisis because of the higher baseline hemoglobin and longer lifespan of the RBCs in these conditions. It is important to remember the patient is infectious and proper isolation procedures must be followed. Parents should be made aware of the risk to siblings or other family members with SCD.

▶ PRIAPISM

Priapism, a prolonged painful erection of the penis, may occur in up to 50% of boys with SCD before 21 years of age.[6] Priapism may occur in stuttering episodes that last less than 2 hours but with frequent recurrence, or may occur as a sudden event lasting for hours. If episodes are prolonged, priapism may lead to impotence. No specific therapy is necessary for a single episode of stuttering priapism. Maneuvers such as hydration, warm showers or baths, opioid pain medication, or frequent urination may end an episode. Oral adrenergic agents such as pseudoephedrine may treat brief episodes, and are often used prophylactically in patients with frequent events. Events lasting longer than 2 hours require immediate medical management and evaluation by an experienced urologist.

REFERENCES

1. Steinberg MH. Drug therapy: management of sickle cell disease. *N Engl J Med.* 1999;340:1021–1030.
2. Platt OS, Thorington BD, Brambilla DJ, et al. Pain in sickle-cell disease. Rates and risk factors. *N Engl J Med.* 1991;325:11–16.
3. Vichinsky EP, Neumayr LD, Earles AN, et al. Causes and outcomes in acute chest syndrome in sickle cell disease. *N Engl J Med.* 2000;342:1855–1865.
4. Gill FM, Sleeper LA, Weiner SJ, et al. Clinical events in the first decade in a cohort of infants with sickle cell disease. Cooperative study of sickle cell disease. *Blood.* 1995;86:776–783.
5. Topley JM, Rogers DW, Stevens MCG, et al. Acute splenic sequestration and hypersplenism in the first five years in homozygous sickle cell disease. *Arch Dis Child.* 1981;56:765–769.
6. Rogers ZM. Priapism in sickle cell disease. *Hematol/Oncol Clin North Am.* 2005;19:917–928.

CHAPTER 101

Bleeding Disorders

Audra L. McCreight and Jonathan E. Wickiser

▶ HIGH-YIELD FACTS

- Aggressive treatment of hemophilia patients with head trauma is imperative as signs and symptoms of intracranial bleeding may be delayed. Even though initial imaging studies may be normal, factor replacement is indicated and careful monitoring of the patient is crucial to detect subtle changes in mental status.
- Patients with hemophilia and inhibitors remain challenging management cases and are best cared for in conjunction with a hematologist.
- Treatment of bleeding episodes in von Willebrand patients may include DDAVP, cryoprecitate, or factor VIII concentrates rich in vWf.
- Young children with idiopathic thrombocytopenic purpura and a platelet count <20 000 are at risk for bleeding complications such as intracranial hemorrhage.
- Treatment options for ITP are based on the clinical severity of bleeding, Consultation with a hematologist is indicated for patients with bleeding complications or platelet counts <20 000.

▶ HEMOPHILIA

Hemophilia is an X-linked recessive disorder of coagulation caused by deficiency of factor VIII (hemophilia A) or factor IX (hemophilia B). The incidence of hemophilia A is 10 to 20 cases per 100 000 births. The percentage of factor present determines the severity of disease. Five to twenty-five percent denotes mild disease with no tendency for spontaneous hemorrhage and bleeding occurring usually only with surgery or severe trauma. Two to five percent implies moderate disease with bleeding following mild trauma. Less than 1% is severe disease with proclivity to spontaneous hemorrhage. Two-thirds of male patients with hemophilia have severe disease. In both hemophilia A and B, the prothrombin time (PT) is normal and partial thromboplastin time (PTT) is prolonged. The same types of bleeding occur in both factor VIII and factor IX deficiency. Bruising, hemarthroses, and intramuscular hematomas predominate. Intracranial hemorrhage is less common but can be devastating. It is important to listen to the patient and their parents as the initial presentation of bleeding may not be dramatic.

ACUTE HEMARTHROSIS

Knees, elbows, ankles, hips, and shoulders are the most commonly affected joints (Fig. 101–1). Older patients may be aware of a bleed prior to the onset of pain and swelling, whereas younger patients may present with new onset limp or limited range of motion. It is generally agreed that even if joint bleeding cannot be confirmed, treatment is indicated. This philosophy is based on the potentially crippling sequelae of hemarthrosis. Intraarticular bleeding provokes a strong synovial inflammatory reaction causing erosion of the cartilage, synovial hypertrophy, and friability. Muscle atrophy around the joint leads to instability, which increases the likelihood of more frequent hemarthroses. Unless treated early and adequately, repeated bleeding into a "target joint" can lead to complete cartilaginous destruction causing secondary osteoarthritis. Joint swelling that is persistent and associated with fever may indicate a septic joint. Aspiration preceded by appropriate factor replacement may be necessary, but should only occur after discussion with the child's hematologist. Joint aspiration is not recommended for most cases of bleeding.

Symptomatic treatment of hemarthroses consists of splinting, ice, immobilization, elastic bandages, and analgesia with acetaminophen with or without codeine. A single factor infusion to raise levels to 30% to 50% is usually sufficient to terminate bleeding. A joint that has bled repeatedly may require several doses of factor. Range of motion and physical therapy are instituted as soon as possible. Bleeding into the hip is especially worrisome because pressure within the joint can lead to aseptic necrosis of the femoral head. Factor replacement to 80% to 100% levels with subsequent daily replacement to 50% may be necessary.

INTRAMUSCULAR BLEEDING

Such hemorrhage usually affects the large weight-bearing muscles such as the iliopsoas, calf, gluteal, and forearm muscles, but can affect any muscle of the body (Fig. 101–2). Bleeding is often slow, occurring over extended periods of time before symptoms of pain, tenderness, and swelling appear. Therefore, such hemorrhages often present as a large hematoma. Treatment consists of factor replacement to a level of 30% to 50%. Forearm, calf, and hand bleeding can result in a compartment syndrome. Vascular compromise or nerve paralysis may occur if not treated promptly. Iliopsoas hemorrhage, which can be massive, presents with flexion of the thigh, groin, or iliac fossa pain, and paresthesias along the anterior thigh from femoral nerve compression. This characteristic triad of symptoms is secondary to femoral nerve compression by the swollen iliopsoas muscle as it passes under the anterior ligament. Ultrasound or computed tomography (CT) can confirm the diagnosis. Compartment syndromes and psoas hemorrhages are treated with

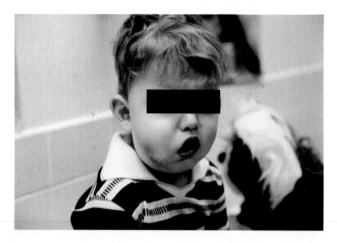

Figure 101–1. A child with severe factor VIII deficiency and buccal hematoma.

correction to achieve factor levels of 80% to 100% and require admission for observation and continued factor replacement.

INTRACRANIAL HEMORRHAGE

Intracranial bleeding may be traumatic or spontaneous. Minor trauma may present with neurologic changes days after the event. Symptoms include headache, lethargy, loss of consciousness, vomiting, and seizures. Forceful blows to the head, regardless of symptoms, are empirically treated with factor replacement. If intracranial hemorrhage is suspected, immediate factor replacement to a 100% level is necessary. Factor infusion should not be delayed for imaging studies.

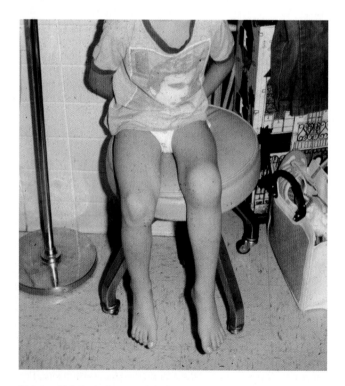

Figure 101–2. A 5-year-old with severe factor VIII deficiency and acute left knee hemarthrosis.

OTHER BLEEDING MANIFESTATIONS

Subcutaneous hemorrhage, abrasions, and lacerations that do not require sutures do not require factor replacement. However, factor replacement is necessary prior to laceration repair, lumbar puncture, surgery, and dental extractions. Men with hemophilia can also present with painless, gross hematuria. An anatomic source of the bleeding is often not found and treatment with factor may or may not be necessary. Prednisone is advocated by some to decrease the duration and degree of hematuria. In cases such as this, close consultation with the child's hematologist is invaluable. Intramuscular injections, aspirin, and jugular and femoral venipuncture are to be avoided in this patient population. Simple peripheral venipuncture is followed by at least 5 minutes of pressure to the site.[1]

MANAGEMENT ISSUES

Factor replacement for hemophilia A or B is accomplished by transfusion with a variety of factor VIII or IX concentrates, respectively. These products are made from either pooled donor plasma-derived or recombinant proteins. The purest of the plasma-derived products are monoclonal antibody purified. Recombinant products may contain human albumin and are not necessarily superior. The amount of factor to be delivered will be dependent on the nature and severity of the bleeding episode. For minor bleeding, target factor level is 30% to 40%. For major bleeding or prior to surgery a minimum of 50% factor level is required. For life- or limb-threatening bleeds, 80% to 100% factor level is needed, and treatment with factor replacement is required every 12 hours or by continuous infusion until healing occurs.

The following formulas may be used to calculate factor replacement:

- Factor VIII (units) = weight (kg) × 0.5 × desired increment (percent) of factor VIII level (i.e., 1 U/kg of factor VIII raises the level by 2%).
  - Example: To achieve 50% factor VIII level in an 80-kg patient

    80 × 0.5 × 50 = 2000 units of factor VIII given as a bolus

- Factor IX (units) = weight (kg) × 1.0 × desired increment (percent) of factor IX level (i.e., 1 U/kg of factor IX raises the level by 1%–1.5%).
  - Example: To achieve a 50% factor IX level in an 80-kg patient

    80 × 1.0 × 50 = 4000 units of factor IX given as bolus

Patients and parents often present with their home supply of factor and this may be utilized. Always give an entire vial of factor even if it results in a higher than calculated dose per weight, as any leftover factor must be wasted.

Approximately 20% of patients with severe factor VIII deficiency develop an inhibitory IgG antibody against factor VIII. Treatment of patients with inhibitors can be problematic, as the infused factor VIII is immediately neutralized by the circulating antibody. Treatment of bleeding episodes in these children depends on inhibitor titer and the severity of the bleeding. Children with low titers and serious hemorrhage may respond to large doses (up to 100–200 U/kg) of factor VIII. Some children with inhibitors demonstrate an anamnestic response (high responders) with high titers of antibody appearing rapidly after factor VIII administration. Alternatives for treating patients with high titers of inhibitor include prothrombin complexes (which bypass the need for factor VIII through the presence of factors II, VII, and X), and recombinant factor VIIa. rFVIIa has a very short half-life and must be given every 2 hours. The response to these therapies is judged by the patient's clinical response.

Purified factor VIII concentrate prepared from pooled plasma donations transmitted hepatitis virus and human immunodeficiency virus (HIV) to 95% of hemophilia patients in the United States in the 1970s and early 1980s. Current concentrates, through a combination of mandatory donor screening and viral attenuation techniques, have greatly reduced, but not completely eliminated, viral transmission. No cases of HIV-1 transmission from clotting factor concentrates have been documented since 1986.

Adjuncts to therapy in hemophilia are available in certain situations. Some centers use corticosteroids for the management of hematuria or recurrent joint bleeds. Epsilon aminocaproic acid (Amicar) and tranexamic acid (Cyklokapron) are clot stabilizers used for the prevention or treatment of oral hemorrhage. Both can be administered orally or intravenously. Desmopressin (DDAVP) increases factor VIII levels in patients with mild hemophilia and may be useful for minor bleeds in patients who have shown prior adequate response to this therapy. DDAVP is administered intravenously over 30 minutes (0.3 μg/kg) or intranasally (150 μg or one metered dose for children <50 kg and 300 μg or two metered dose sprays for children >50 kg).

▶ VON WILLEBRAND DISEASE

Von Willebrand factor (vWf) is the carrier protein in plasma for factor VIII and it also acts as a bridge between platelets and subendothelial collagen fibers. Von Willebrand disease exists when there are decreased levels of or defective vWf proteins. The condition is heterogeneous with respect to its genetic, molecular biology, clinical manifestations, and laboratory values. Unlike the sex-linked hemophilias, von Willebrand disease is typically transmitted as an autosomal dominant trait showing variable expression and penetrance. Classification systems separate quantitative deficiencies of vWf (type 1, classic) from qualitative abnormalities (types 2A and 2B) and type 3 in which plasma vWf and factor VIII levels are not measurable or are <5 U/dL.

Most patients present as young adults with clinical manifestations including epistaxis, easy bruising, menorrhagia, prolonged oozing from superficial cuts, and bleeding after dental extraction. Posttraumatic and postsurgical hemorrhage can occur, but hemarthroses are uncommon. Many people exhibit no clinical problems with bleeding in spite of biochemical abnormalities. Typical laboratory findings include a normal PT and platelet count, with a prolonged bleeding time and a PTT that may be normal or prolonged. Measurement of antigenic vWf (vWf:Ag) and ristocetin cofactor (vWf R:Co) activity can usually confirm the diagnosis. Both are decreased in most von Willebrand patients.

Of the subtypes, approximately 80% of patients have Type I von Willebrand disease, which is often amenable to DDAVP

therapy. DDAVP stimulates the endogenous release of vWf. The dose is 0.3 μg/kg intravenously infused over 20 to 30 minutes. This can be repeated every 4 to 6 hours for continued bleeding. Stimate (1.5 mg/mL) is a concentrated intranasal preparation of desmopressin that has demonstrated effectiveness. In teens and adults, the dose is 150 μg/nostril, with a total dose of 300 μg. For children <50 kg, the total dose is 150 μg.

Treatment with a factor VIII concentrate rich in vWf is sometimes necessary for patients who do not respond to desmopressin or in whom its use in contraindicated. Loading dose of concentrate is 40 to 60 IU vWf/kg with follow-up doses administered every 12 to 24 hours to maintain vWf ristocetin cofactor activity >0.5 IU/mL. All currently available concentrates are plasma derived and undergo a viral inactivation step making it unlikely to transmit viruses such as hepatitis and HIV.[3]

▶ ACQUIRED COAGULOPATHIES

Acquired abnormalities of coagulation include vitamin K deficiency, liver disease, disseminated intravascular coagulation (DIC), thrombocytopenia, and platelet dysfunctions. Vitamin K deficiency leads to decreases in the vitamin K-dependent factors (II, VII, IX, and X) and prolongation of the PT. It can be seen in malabsorption syndromes, such as cystic fibrosis and celiac disease, biliary obstruction, and prolonged diarrhea. Children with poor nutrition who receive broad-spectrum antibiotics are also at risk. Drugs, such as diphenylhydantoin, phenobarbital, isoniazid, and coumadin may cause vitamin K deficiency as a side effect. Vitamin K deficiency can lead to hemorrhagic disease of the newborn unless supplementation is provided routinely at delivery. Administration of vitamin K is safest by the subcutaneous route. A dose of 10 mg of vitamin K given subcutaneously will correct the PT within 24 hours. Rare but severe anaphylactoid reactions are described with intravenous infusion. The liver is the primary site of production of clotting factors, and severe liver disease may lead to coagulation defects that can mimic DIC.[2]

DISSEMINATED INTRAVASCULAR COAGULATION

Disseminated intravascular coagulation (DIC) is an acquired syndrome characterized by simultaneous activation of coagulation and fibrinolysis within the microvasculature. Microthrombi form in small blood vessels, leading to vessel occlusion, tissue ischemia, and end organ damage. Excessive bleeding occurs due to thrombocytopenia, consumption of clotting factors, and fibrinolysis. In pediatric patients, the leading cause of DIC is overwhelming infection. However, conditions that can precipitate DIC are numerous and include tissue injuries, such as burns, multiple trauma, and crush injuries, severe head trauma, abruption placenta and eclampsia, tumors, hemolytic transfusion reactions, myocardial infarctions, giant hemangiomas, respiratory distress syndrome, snake bites, and heat stroke or hypothermia. Although bleeding is the predominant symptom, thrombotic damage can occur in most organ systems. Common ischemic complications include hemorrhagic necrosis of the skin, renal failure, seizures, coma, hypoxemia, and pulmonary infarcts. Laboratory findings in DIC are variable but usually include hemolytic anemia with schistocytes, thrombocytopenia, prolonged PT and PTT, and decreased levels of factor V, factor VIII, and fibrinogen with increased fibrin split products. There is also usually a marked decrease in protein C, protein S, and antithrombin III.

Management consists of treating the underlying disorder; antibiotics for sepsis, volume expanders for shock, and oxygen for hypoxemia. In addition, therapy is also directed to control the abnormalities of hemostasis. Therapeutic options include factor replacement, anticoagulants, and antifibrinolytics. Factor replacement may be accomplished with fresh frozen plasma (10–20 mL/kg) to keep the PT in the normal range. Cryoprecipitate provides increased concentration of fibrinogen, factor VIII, and vWf. Persistent oozing may be due to severe thrombocytopenia. Platelet transfusion may be considered to keep platelet counts >50 000.

PLATELET DISORDERS

Normally functioning platelets are a necessary component of the clotting process. Platelet activation, adherence, recruitment, and aggregation and binding of fibrinogen result in the cellular clot that is responsible for primary hemostasis following a disruption of a vessel wall. A deficit in platelet number or function can lead to excessive bleeding following injury. Congenital platelet dysfunction can affect a variety of platelet functions, such as receptor defects, platelet–vessel wall adhesion, platelet–platelet interactions to name just a few. Acquired platelet dysfunction is caused most commonly by aspirin, which inhibits production of thromboxane A_2 and causes decreased platelet aggregation and vessel constriction. Patients with congenital platelet dysfunction typically present with severe bleeding diatheses early in life. Even minor platelet dysfunction can result in easy bruisability and significant bleeding from mucosal membranes.

Deficits in platelet number are much more common in pediatric patients. Thrombocytopenia is defined as a platelet count less than 150 000/μL, although it is rare to develop any abnormal bleeding with counts greater than 50 000/μL. Platelet counts below 20 000/μL indicate severe thrombocytopenia; in that range there is increased risk for life-threatening hemorrhage and intracranial bleeding.

In the emergency department, thrombocytopenia is often an unexpected finding on a complete blood count obtained for unrelated reasons. Symptomatic patients may present as well-appearing children with a petechial or purpuric rash. At times the extensive ecchymoses in the absence of a history of significant trauma can wrongly suggest child abuse. With lower counts, patients may develop significant bleeding and bruising from minor trauma, mucosal bleeding, hematuria, or hematochezia. In addition to the skin findings, the physical examination should focus on evidence of systemic disorders such as recent weight loss, hypothyroidism, lymphadenopathy, and hepatosplenomegaly as these findings help establish the differential diagnosis. Involvement of other bone marrow elements also help guide the workup.

The differential diagnosis of thrombocytopenia is extensive, but the single most common cause in the well-appearing child is immune thrombocytopenic purpura (ITP). Other causes include autoimmune diseases such as systemic

lupus erythematosus, in which anemia and lymphopenia are usually seen, and secondary immune destruction of platelets from infectious agents such as hepatitis B and Epstein–Barr viruses. Sepsis can cause destruction of platelets with or without the presence of DIC.

Bone marrow infiltration from leukemia, lymphoma, and other malignancies may initially present with thrombocytopenia but will often have associated hepatosplenomegaly, anemia, and abnormalities of the white blood cells. Cancer chemotherapy agents also cause suppression of all cell lines, including platelets. Thrombocytopenia may be the initial presentation of aplastic anemia. Idiosyncratic immune reactions leading to thrombocytopenia may be seen following administration of various agents, most commonly valproic acid, phenytoin, and trimethoprim/sulfamethoxazole.[3]

HEMOLYTIC UREMIC SYNDROME

Hemolytic uremic syndrome presents with a triad of acute renal failure, microangiopathic hemolytic anemia, and thrombocytopenia; it is discussed in more detail in Chapter 84. The thrombocytopenia is usually mild to moderate. The typical presentation is that of a pale, somewhat lethargic young child with a prodromal history of a gastrointestinal infection. Abdominal pain, vomiting, and bloody diarrhea are common, as are acute renal failure and neurologic manifestations. Laboratory examination typically reveals anemia with schistocytes, thrombocytopenia, electrolyte and acid–base disturbances, and elevated serum creatinine. Management consists of early dialysis to treat the effects of renal failure and reduce the fluid overload and hyperkalemia associated with the frequent blood transfusions that are necessary.

IMMUNE THROMBOCYTOPENIC PURPURA

Immune thrombocytopenic purpura (ITP) is the most common cause of thrombocytopenia in a well-appearing young child. The peak age of diagnosis is 2 to 4 years, occurring equally in

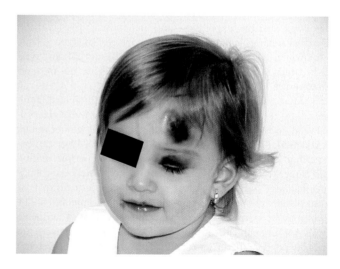

Figure 101–3. A child with ecchymosis associated with immune-mediated thrombocytopenia.

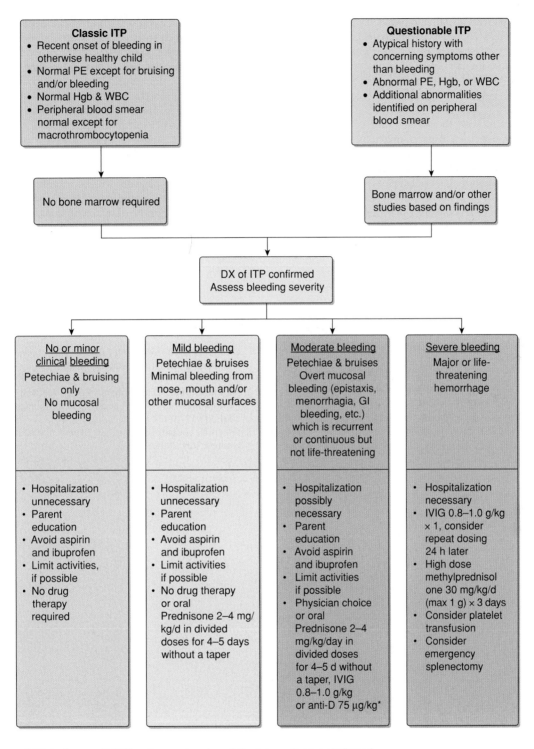

* IVIG 1 g/kg or anti-D 75 µg/kg may be given if Prednisone is contraindicated or according to physician discretion. Repeat CBC is recommended at 72 hours to document response. Anti-D can be given only when Hgb is within normal limits and patient is Rh+.

Figure 101–4. Algorithm for the diagnosis and treatment of ITP during childhood.

female and male patients. Children typically have a history of a preceding viral illness, although the link to the development of antiplatelet antibodies is not clear. The platelet surface is covered with increased amounts of IgG and the spleen removes the affected platelets from the circulation. Platelet production is increased in the bone marrow, but not enough to offset the rapid destruction.

Patients present with the acute onset of bruising, petechiae, and purpura; they have normal physical examinations other than for skin findings (Fig. 101–3). Mucosal or gastrointestinal bleeding can occur. The most serious complication intracranial hemorrhage occurs in less than 0.1% to 0.5% of patients.

The diagnosis of ITP is likely when the complete blood count reveals thrombocytopenia in association with normal red and white blood cell numbers and morphology. Definitive diagnosis by bone marrow aspirate is not necessary in cases with thrombocytopenia and absence of signs, symptoms, or blood count results suggesting another diagnosis. Such children usually do not require hospitalization and can be followed as outpatients. The natural history of the condition is that 85% of children make a full recovery within 6 months. Of the 15% with persistently low platelets, bleeding symptoms are rare and splenectomy is rarely needed. Treatment of patients with ITP is controversial, consultation with a pediatric hematologist is recommended. An algorithm for the suggested management of ITP is provided in Figure 101–4. Therapeutic options include corticosteroids, intravenous immune globulin (IVIG), and anti-Rh(D) immunoglobulin (WinRho-SD). Corticosteroids or IVIG may promptly increase the platelet count in patients with profound thrombocytopenia. Both modalities are presumed to block reticuloendothelial destruction of platelets. However, there is currently no evidence that treatment diminishes the risk of major bleeding and, therefore, it is uncertain if the benefits of treatment outweigh its risks. Infusion of anti-Rh(D) immunoglobulin in Rh-positive individuals results in immune clearance of the antibody-coated red cells and coincident prolonged survival of autoantibody-coated platelets. Anti-D appears to be as safe and effective as IVIG in Rh-positive patients.[3] Anti-D may only be administered in Rh-positive patients who have a normal hemoglobin level. Transfused platelets will be rapidly destroyed due to the immune response and have no role in the management of patients except in life-threatening hemorrhage. In that circumstance, platelet transfusion along with intravenous gamma globulin and high-dose intravenous steroids are administered. Emergency splenectomy may be required with life-threatening bleeding.

REFERENCES

1. Gionia KP et al. *Congenital Bleeding Disorders: Principles and Practices.* Hemophilia Nursing Alliance. King of Prussia, PA. 2000.
2. Mannucci PM, Tuddenham EGD. Medical progress: the hemophilias—from royal genes to gene therapy. *N Engl J Med.* 2001;344:1773–1779.
3. Green D, Ludlam CA. *Bleeding Disorders.* Oxford: Health Press Limited; July 2004.

CHAPTER 102

Blood Component Therapy

Audra L. McCreight and Jonathan E. Wickiser

▶ HIGH-YIELD FACTS

- It is common to underestimate quantitative blood loss in the setting of trauma. Careful and frequent monitoring of vital signs and hematocrit is critical in the detection of severe hemorrhage.
- Massive transfusion protocols exist to supply O-negative blood and other essential blood products for the resuscitation of the hemodynamically unstable trauma patient.
- Mild to severe reactions can occur during the transfusion process including fever, chills, nausea, hypotension, or shock. Whether this is caused by blood type incompatibility, antibodies to donor cells, or blood product contamination, the transfusion must be stopped immediately and the symptoms of the reaction treated aggressively.

Transfusion of blood and blood components is often necessary in the emergency department (ED). Whole blood, packed red blood cells (PRBCs), platelets, granulocytes, fresh frozen plasma, cryoprecipitate, specific clotting factors, albumin, and immunoglobulins each have specific indications and risks associated with their use. As blood for transfusion is a scarce commodity, the component that will specifically address the patient's need is generally transfused.

▶ WHOLE BLOOD

Transfusion of whole blood is rarely performed but may be indicated for prompt restoration of red cells and volume after trauma or surgery. After 24 hours of storage, platelets and granulocytes contained within whole blood have lost function. Activity of labile clotting factors V and VIII is also diminished greatly within 3 to 5 days. The risk of transfusion reactions with whole blood is doubled owing to the volume of foreign proteins and antibodies that it contains.[1]

▶ PACKED RED BLOOD CELLS

PRBC units contain approximately 30 to 50 mL of plasma and have a hematocrit ranging from 55% to 80%, depending on the preservative used for storage. Units are stored in solution with anticoagulant and preservative for up to 42 days. There are no functional platelets or granulocytes in this preparation. For patients with a previous history of febrile reactions to transfusions or if the risk of cytomegalovirus (CMV) transmission is to be particularly avoided, filtered, leukocyte-poor red cells are

recommended. Leukocyte depleted preparations contain $<10^7$ leukocytes per unit. In many institutions all PRBC units are routinely leukocyte depleted.[2]

▶ PLATELET CONCENTRATE

Platelet concentrates are obtained by either pooling multiple individual platelet concentrates from approximately four to eight individual whole blood donors (commonly known as a "6-pack") or from plateletpheresis of a single donor. There may be advantages to the reduced donor exposure of single donor product; however, platelet product choice varies by institution and availability. Both preparations contain approximately 5.5×10^{10} platelets in approximately 50 mL of plasma. They should be ABO and Rh compatible, but crossmatching is not necessary. In children, the dose is estimated at 0.1 to 0.2 U/kg of random donor platelets required to raise the platelet count by 50 000 to 100 000/μL. Platelet transfusions are indicated for patients with thrombocytopenia or platelet dysfunction who are actively bleeding. Counts above 20 000/μL rarely result in spontaneous bleeding, but at counts below 10 000/μL, the risk is severe. Patients with immune thrombocytopenia or thrombotic thrombocytopenic purpura do not benefit from platelet transfusions except in cases of life-threatening hemorrhage, since the ongoing antibody mediated disease process destroys the transfused platelets rapidly.[2]

▶ GRANULOCYTE CONCENTRATES

Transfusion of white cells is indicated only in a severe, prolonged neutropenic patient with documented or strongly suspected antibiotic resistant sepsis. The use of granulocyte infusions is controversial and should only be done under the advisement and supervision of a pediatric hematologist.

▶ FRESH FROZEN PLASMA

Fresh frozen plasma (FFP) is produced by freezing plasma within 8 hours of collection. It consists of the noncellular components of blood including procoagulant clotting factors such as factors V and VIII, the anticoagulants protein S, protein C, and antithrombin III. ABO compatibility is important, but crossmatching is not necessary. The most common indications for using FFP include situations where multiple factor deficiencies are present simultaneously. Table 102–1 reviews the indications for use of FFP. It is used at a dose of 10 to

- Disseminated intravascular coagulopathies
- Acute blood loss (trauma)
- Unknown factor deficiencies
- Chronic liver disease
- Vitamin K deficiency
- Treatment of excessive warfarin of dicumarol therapy

20 mL/kg infused to gravity. The risk of disease transmission is similar to that of whole blood transfusion and allergic reactions are possible. FFP is not indicated for acute volume expansion.[2]

▶ CRYOPRECIPITATE

Cryoprecipitate is prepared by slow thawing of FFP at 4°C and subsequent refreezing for storage of the protein precipitate, which is rich in fibrinogen, factor VIII:vWf, and factor XIII. This is a purely procoagulant preparation as compared to FFP, which also contains physiologic anticoagulants protein C and protein S. Cryoprecipitate does not require crossmatching. It is indicated for treatment of hypo- or a-fibrinogenemia. It has also been used as a treatment for von Willebrand disease, though other therapies are now considered preferable. In pediatrics, one unit of cryoprecipitate is given per 5 kg of body weight.[2]

▶ FACTORS VIII AND IX

Highly purified concentrates of factors VIII and IX are now produced by monoclonal antibody techniques and by recombinant DNA technology. A number of such products are available and have replaced single donor products such as FFP in the treatment of hemophilia because they avoid or greatly diminish the risk of infectious disease transmission.

▶ ALBUMIN

Available in both 5% and 25% solutions, albumin is most frequently used for blood volume expansion in shock, trauma, burns, and surgery. Heat and chemical treatment eliminates the infectious transmission risk and it contains no blood group antibodies. Only the 5% solution is isosmotic with plasma, and the 25% solution is never used to treat shock without other fluids.

▶ IMMUNE GLOBULINS

These antibody-rich preparations are occasionally used in the ED to treat conditions such as rabies and tetanus, as postexposure disease prophylaxis. It is also a mainstay of therapy in other immune mediated diseases such as Kawasaki's disease.[2]

▶ INDICATIONS FOR TRANSFUSION

The most common scenario in the ED requiring blood transfusion is the hemodynamically unstable trauma patient. Most other anemic patients are hemodynamically compensated, and transfusion can be carried out after admission. The rapidly exsanguinating trauma patient has both quantitative and qualitative transfusion requirements. Recently, several institutions have developed massive transfusion protocols to address these needs. Massive transfusion generally refers to the replacement of a patient's total blood volume in less than 24 hours, or as the acute replacement of more than half the patient's estimated blood volume in any 4-hour period. These protocols were designed to support rapid transfusion in the ED with O-negative blood (universal donor) and blood products such as platelets and FFP that are released from the blood bank automatically upon provider request. The risks of minor blood group incompatibility causing hemolysis or recipient sensitization to red blood cell antigens are overshadowed in this situation. Failure to provide sufficient volume and coagulation support increases the risk of mortality in the trauma patient.[3]

Conversely, patient-specific blood typing should be done in the hemodynamically stable patient. Blood typing (for ABO and Rh) is a rapid screening process for antibodies and crossmatching, finding donor blood that the patient's body will accept. This process usually takes 60 minutes or more.

In general,

- if Hgb >10 g/dL, transfusion is rarely indicated
- if Hgb <5 g/dL, transfusion is usually necessary
- if Hgb is between 5 and 10 g/dL, clinical status is helpful in determining transfusion requirements

The decision to transfuse is ultimately determined by clinical status. In general, the history of blood loss in a given patient is often inaccurate and the initial hemoglobin may not reflect losses, so it is crucial to monitor heart rate and blood pressure for changes of early shock.[4]

▶ COMPLICATIONS

There are several types of transfusion reactions, which range from mild to life threatening. In the event of a reaction, the transfusion is stopped and the blood bank is notified. Care in collecting and labeling specimens for the blood bank is crucial.

ACUTE HEMOLYTIC TRANSFUSION REACTIONS

Acute hemolytic transfusion reactions (AHTR) occur when a patient's anti-A or anti-B antibodies bind to incompatible transfused red cells. These reactions are seen immediately and are almost always the result of errors in labeling of specimens. The transfused cells are lysed, releasing inflammatory mediators.

Symptoms usually begin with an increase in body temperature and pulse rate. Other symptoms may include chills, back or flank pain, nausea and vomiting, dyspnea, flushing, abnormal bleeding, and hypotension. Disseminated intravascular coagulation, shock, renal failure, and death may ensue.

Laboratory finding can include hemoglobinemia, and/or hemoglobinuria, an increased serum bilirubin, and a positive direct antibody test. Aggressive fluid resuscitation with normal saline to maintain blood pressure and urine output should be initiated, as well as specific therapies to correct any associated coagulopathy.[2]

DELAYED HEMOLYTIC TRANSFUSION REACTIONS

Delayed hemolytic transfusion reactions (DHTR) are caused by sensitization to non-ABO antigens from a previous transfusion. The most prominent signs and symptoms are unexplained anemia, jaundice, fever, back pain, and rarely, hemoglobinemia and/or hemoglobinuria. DHTR are detected 3 to 14 days after transfusion, the previously transfused patient's hemoglobin is below expected values with a history of fever and jaundice. No treatment is usually required.[2]

FEBRILE NONHEMOLYTIC TRANSFUSION REACTIONS

Febrile or nonhemolytic transfusion reactions (FNHTR) are benign and self-limiting; they account for the great majority of transfusion reactions and occur most commonly in the multiply transfused patient. Symptoms include fever and chills that may be difficult to distinguish from AHTR; therefore, if the patient is very uncomfortable, the transfusion should be stopped. Antipyretics may be given. FNHTR are caused by recipient antibodies to antigens on donor leukocytes and platelets. There are no laboratory tests available to predict or prevent these reactions; however, the parent or the patient can often give a history of previous FNHTRs, allowing intervention with antipyretics if prior reactions were severe or frequent.[2]

ALLERGIC TRANSFUSION REACTION

Allergic transfusion reactions are of three types, each with different etiologies:

- Urticarial reactions may involve allergens, cytokines, or histamine in stored blood products. The transfusion must be interruped and the patient watched closely for signs and symptoms of anaphylaxis. An antihistamine such as diphenhydramine (1 mg/kg) should be administered. When the urticaria fades, transfusion can be resumed.
- Anaphylactic reactions are severe urticarial reactions that commonly occur in patients with congenital IgA deficiency who have high-titer IgG anti-IgA antibodies. Activation of a complement and chemical mediator cascade precipitates increased vascular permeability, resulting in angioedema, respiratory distress, urticaria, and shock. The transfusion is stopped, epinephrine is administered (0.01 mg/kg 1:1000 subcutaneously), and blood pressure is stabilized with crystalloid and vasopressive agents if necessary.

- Transfusion-related acute lung injury (TRALI) occurs when the permeability of the pulmonary microvasculature is acutely increased, which leads to massive pulmonary edema, usually within 6 hours of transfusion. It is thought to be related to the presence of granulocyte antibodies in either the donor product or the recipient, although the specific mechanism is still unknown. Therapy consists of rapid and aggressive pulmonary support.[4]

COMPLICATIONS OF MASSIVE TRANSFUSIONS

Disturbances in coagulation can occur with massive transfusion therapy. Table 102–2 summarizes complications that may occur when large amounts of whole blood or PRBCs are given rapidly. Dilutional thrombocytopenia can be seen when 1.5 times the blood volume must be replaced or when there is preexisting thrombocytopenia or disseminated intravascular coagulation (DIC). Each unit of packed red blood cells contains approximately 3 g of citrate, which will bind ionized calcium. In a healthy patient, the liver will metabolize 3 g of citrate every 5 minutes. At transfusion rates greater than one unit per 5 minutes or with impaired liver function, citrate toxicity occurs leading to hypocalcemia causing tetany or hypotension. Hyperkalemia can occur with rapid transfusion of PRBCs because the concentration of potassium in stored blood increases with storage. Hypokalemia is also common as transfused red blood cells begin active metabolism and intracellular reuptake of potassium. Other complications that can occur include hypothermia if a blood warmer is not used, disturbances in acid/base status, and acute respiratory distress syndrome (ARDS).[2]

INFECTIOUS COMPLICATIONS

Donated blood is routinely screened for HIV-1 and -2, HTLV, hepatitis B surface antigen, hepatitis B core antibody (a surrogate marker for non-A, non-B hepatitis), hepatitis C virus, and syphilis. The current estimated risk of transmitting HIV through a blood transfusion is 1 in 2 135 000 units transfused; hepatitis B, 1 in 205 000 units transfused; and hepatitis C, 1 in 1 935 000 units transfused.[5]

Bacterial contamination of blood products can occur and accounts for other transfusion reactions and fatalities. Fever, chills, rigor, vomiting, and hypotension present soon after the transfusion is begun. Blood cultures should be sent from the patient and from the blood product. AHTR is in the differential if the patient is receiving red blood cells, and samples (blood

▶ **TABLE 102–2. COMPLICATIONS OF MASSIVE TRANSFUSION THERAPY**

- Dilutional thrombocytopenia
- Citrate-induced hypocalcemia
- Hyperkalemia
- Hypokalemia
- Acid/base disturbances
- Acute respiratory distress syndrome

and first voided urine) should be sent to the blood bank to check for hemolysis.[1]

REFERENCES

1. Dodd RY, Notari EP, Strainer SL. Current prevalence and incidence of infectious disease markers and estimated window period risk in the American Red Cross Blood Donor Population. *Transfusion.* 2003;42:975–979.

2. Miller Y, Bachowski G, Benjamin R, et al. *Practice Guidelines for Blood Transfusion: A Compilation from Recent Peer-Reviewed Literature.* 2nd ed. Washington, DC: American Red Cross; April 2007.

3. Trauma.org. *Transfusion for Massive Blood Loss.* http://www.traum.org/archive/resus/massive.html. Accessed July 2008.

4. American Association of Blood Banks. *Technical Manual.* 15th ed. Bethesda, MD: AABB Press 2005. http://www.aabb.org. Accessed July 2008.

5. *Transfusion Transmitted Diseases.* http://www.bloodbook.com/trans-tran.html. Accessed July 2008.

CHAPTER 103

Oncologic Emergencies

Audra L. McCreight and Jonathan E. Wickiser

▶ HIGH-YIELD FACTS

- Acute leukemia is the most common malignancy in childhood and may present with a variety of symptoms including fever, fatigue, bleeding, adenopathy, or bone pain.
- Complications of childhood cancer result from the disease itself or from the therapy aimed at treating the cancer. Most oncologic emergencies arise from metabolic, hematologic, structural, or toxic chemotherapy effects.
- Infection is one of the most common complications of the treatment of children with cancer, and is a significant cause of morbidity and mortality. Findings associated with inflammation may be absent in the neutropenic patient, with fever the only sign of serious infection.
- Infection may progress rapidly in the neutropenic host; evaluation and initiation of antibiotic therapy must be done urgently.
- Initial antibiotic coverage usually includes an aminoglycoside and a beta-lactam penicillin or cephalosporin, but must be tailored to local bacterial sensitivities.
- Tumor lysis syndrome results from the death of tumor cells and release of their intracellular contents leading to hyperuricemia, hyperphosphatemia, and hyperkalemia.
- Mediastinal compression from the tumors may result in superior vena cava syndrome or superior mediastinal syndrome. Management of these patients may be difficult as airway collapse from tumor compression may occur.

Approximately 10% of childhood deaths are related to cancer.[1] The leukemias, central nervous system (CNS) tumors, and lymphomas account for more than one-half of all childhood malignancies (Table 103–1). Advances in cancer treatment have led to improvements in survival. However, much of this progress has come with increased intensity of treatment regimens. It is important for the emergency physician to be aware of the common malignancies that occur in children and to be ready to treat the complications of cancer at presentation and during treatment.

▶ COMMON PEDIATRIC MALIGNANCIES

ACUTE LEUKEMIAS

Leukemia is a condition in which there is uncontrolled, clonal proliferation of an immature white blood cell within the bone marrow, with subsequent suppression of normal hematopoiesis. Acute leukemia is the most common childhood malignancy, representing approximately 30% of newly diagnosed cancers.[2] Acute lymphoblastic leukemia (ALL) accounts for approximately 75% of pediatric leukemia, with acute myelogenous leukemia (AML) accounting for the other 25%. Chronic leukemia is rare in pediatrics, with chronic myelogenous leukemia (CML) accounting for less than 1% of all childhood cancers.

The peak incidence of ALL in children occurs between the ages of 3 and 5 years. Overall, 75% to 80% of patients survive more than 5 years beyond diagnosis, with many patients considered cured of disease. Unlike ALL, the incidence of AML is relatively constant throughout childhood and has a much poorer prognosis with approximately 50% of patients surviving at 5 years from diagnosis.

The signs and symptoms of acute leukemia reflect replacement of bone marrow or extramedullary collections of leukemic blasts. Common presentations include pallor, fatigue, petechiae, purpura, and infection as a result of defective hematopoiesis from marrow replacement. Lymphadenopathy, hepatomegaly, splenomegaly, and mediastinal or testicular masses may represent extramedullary involvement. Bone pain results from leukemic involvement of the periosteum and bone, causing patients to limp or even refuse to walk. Leukemia may be present in the CNS, leading to cranial nerve deficits, headache, or changes in vision. Other nonspecific symptoms such as anorexia, fever, and irritability may also be present in a variety of nonmalignant conditions, making the diagnosis of leukemia dependent on a high level of suspicion.

The leukocyte count at diagnosis varies greatly, and may be high or low. Even in the absence of neutropenia at diagnosis, patients should be considered immunocompromised as the white blood cells produced may not be functional. Most patients will be anemic and/or thrombocytopenic.

Despite hematologic abnormalities in the peripheral blood, the diagnosis of leukemia must be confirmed by evaluation of the bone marrow. Further morphologic and cytogenetic characterization of the leukemic blasts determines the particular treatment regimen. Treatment consists of multiagent systemic chemotherapy with CNS preventive therapy. Length and intensity of therapy varies by type of leukemia.

HODGKIN DISEASE

Hodgkin disease is a malignancy of the lymph nodes. The Reed–Sternberg cell is considered to be the malignant cell. The normal counterpart to the Reed–Sternberg cell has not been identified, but current theories propose a B lymphocyte

▶ **TABLE 103–1. CANCER INCIDENCE RATES IN CHILDREN AGED 0 TO 14 YEARS: SEER 2000–2004**

Cancer	Rate*
Leukemia	4.9
Acute lymphocytic	3.8
Brain and other nervous system tumors	3.2
Lymphoma	1.4
Soft tissue	1.0
Kidney	0.8
Bone and Joint	0.7

*Annual incidence rates per 100 000 children aged 0 to 14 years. Data from Ries LAG, Melbert D, Krapcho M, et al, eds. *SEER Cancer Statistics Review, 1975–2005.* Bethesda, MD: National Cancer Institute; http://seer.cancer.gov/csr/1975_2005.

lineage. Approximately 5% of pediatric malignancies are Hodgkin disease, with a peak incidence in adolescents and young adults.[1]

The majority of pediatric patients have painless supraclavicular or cervical lymphadenopathy. Nodes are rubbery, matted, and, unlike reactive nodes, do not decrease in size. A lymph node is considered enlarged if it is >10 mm at its greatest diameter, with the exception of an epitrochlear node, which is considered enlarged at 5 mm, and an inguinal node, at 15 mm. The abdominal examination may reveal hepatomegaly or splenomegaly. Mediastinal involvement is common and a chest radiograph should be obtained on any patient suspected of having Hodgkin disease. Systemic or "B" symptoms may occur in one-third of the patients and include unexplained fever, weight loss, and night sweats.

The differential diagnosis of Hodgkin disease includes other causes of lymphadenopathy, such as infectious mononucleosis, mycobacterial infections, or other metastatic malignancies. Abnormalities may be seen on CBC secondary to metastatic disease in the bone marrow. Biopsy of an effected lymph node is required for diagnosis.

Once the diagnosis of Hodgkin disease is confirmed and histologically classified, patients undergo further workup for staging. Exploratory laparotomy and splenectomy are no longer performed in the routine staging or treatment of Hodgkin disease. Treatment regimens include multidrug chemotherapy and/or radiation, with 5-year survival rates of >90%.

NON-HODGKIN LYMPHOMAS

Non-Hodgkin lymphomas (NHL) are a heterogeneous group of malignancies of lymphatic tissue. Unlike Hodgkin lymphoma there is no peak age incidence, but cases increase steadily with age. Compared to the indolent nature of many adult lymphomas, childhood NHLs are rapidly proliferating and are often disseminated in extranodal tissues at the time of presentation. The most common types of NHL seen in children are Burkitt's, Burkitt's-like, and large B cell lymphoma (all of mature B cell

origin), lymphoblastic lymphoma (predominately of precursor T cell origin), and anaplastic large cell lymphoma (ALCL).

Clinically, children with NHL present with clinical symptoms that correlate with the histologic subtype. Lymphoblastic lymphomas often present with a mediastinal mass or supraclavicular adenopathy leading to cough, wheeze, chest pain, airway obstruction, or signs and symptoms of superior vera cava obstruction. Burkitt's lymphomas most often present with abdominal involvement causing pain, nausea, vomiting, distension, ascites, or bowel obstruction. Right lower quadrant pain reflects distal ileal, appendiceal, or cecal involvement and may mimic appendicitis. Abdominal lymphoma may be a lead point for an intussusception. Bone, bone marrow, and the CNS are common sites of metastasis. ALCL have a broad spectrum of clinical presentations including lymphadenopathy, skin, and bone involvement. Patients presenting with NHL often require emergency management owing to the rapid doubling time and growth rate of the tumor (Burkitt's lymphoma) or owing to tumor mass encroachment on vital structures (lymphoblastic lymphoma).

Initial laboratory studies include a CBC to assess for marrow involvement as well as electrolytes, creatinine, calcium, phosphorous, and uric acid to evaluate for tumor lysis syndrome (discussed later). Chest radiograph may reveal a mediastinal mass (Fig. 103–1). Table 103–2 lists the most common malignant mediastinal tumors by location. Patients with isolated nodal enlargement suspicious of lymphoma are referred to an appropriate facility for biopsy. Patients with an abdominal mass are evaluated with abdominal ultrasound or

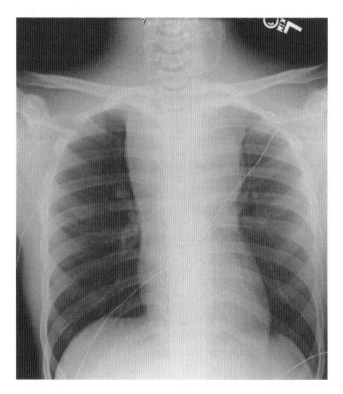

Figure 103–1. Large mediastinal mass in an 11-year-old boy. Lymphoblasts were seen in the peripheral blood, confirming the diagnosis of T-cell lymphoblastic lymphoma.

▶ **TABLE 103–2. MALIGNANT MEDIASTINAL TUMORS IN CHILDREN**

Anterior Mediastinum	Middle Mediastinum	Posterior Mediastinum
Non-Hodgkin lymphoma	Non-Hodgkin lymphoma	Neuroblastoma
Hodgkin disease	Hodgkin disease	Ganglioneuroblastoma
Germ cell tumor	Rhabdomyosarcoma	Ewing's sarcoma
Thymoma	Germ cell tumor	Pheochromocytoma
Sarcoma		Non-Hodgkin lymphoma

computed tomography (CT) scan. Multiagent chemotherapy with/without radiation is the mainstay of treatment, with up to 80% or higher long-term, disease-free survival depending on histologic type.

CENTRAL NERVOUS SYSTEM TUMORS

Tumors of the CNS represent the second most common pediatric cancer diagnosis.[3] Factors increasing the risk of developing a CNS malignancy include various genetic disorders, such as neurofibromatosis or tuberous sclerosis, and exposure to ionizing radiation.

Classification of CNS tumors is generally based on histologic type. Tumors arising in the supratentorial region include cerebral astrocytoma, optic glioma, and craniopharyngioma. These more commonly occur in neonates and infants. Infratentorial tumors such as cerebellar astrocytoma, medulloblastoma, ependymoma, and brain stem glioma are more commonly seen after 2 years of age.

The clinical presentation depends on the site and extent of involvement of the tumor. Supratentorial tumors may cause headache, seizures, or visual impairment. However, compared to adults, seizure is rarely the initial presenting sign of a CNS tumor. Truncal ataxia or incoordination is typical of infratentorial tumors. Impingement of the brain stem may lead to cranial nerve palsies or Horner's syndrome. Raised intracranial pressure (ICP) in infants and toddlers may manifest as vomiting, anorexia, irritability, developmental regression, or impaired upward gaze ("sunsetting" sign). There may be excessive enlargement of the head circumference and persistently palpable cranial sutures. Parents may note a change in behavior or personality in their child. Older children may complain of headache, fatigue, or vomiting. Headaches are rarely due to a CNS malignancy. Headaches that are recurrent, intense, associated with vomiting, or that awaken patients from sleep should raise the suspicion of a malignancy. In addition, patients may have back pain, bladder, or bowel dysfunction, or focal neurologic deficits that suggest spinal cord or cauda equina involvement.

Other conditions that may present with raised ICP or neurologic deficits include brain abscess, chronic subdural hematoma, and vascular malformations. Tumors of the CNS may be diagnosed by CT; however, magnetic resonance imaging (MRI) is more sensitive. Specific tissue diagnosis is achieved through biopsy. Treatment is multimodal, utilizing surgical resection, chemotherapy, and radiation therapy.

WILMS' TUMOR

Wilms' tumor (nephroblastoma) arises from embryonal renal cells. The peak age of diagnosis is 2 to 3 years with most cases diagnosed before 5 years of age. Most children appear well at diagnosis with a nontender abdominal mass. Systemic symptoms are rare. Hematuria is uncommon with Wilms' tumor, and if present is usually microscopic. Other uncommon features at diagnosis include pain, hypertension, polycythemia, or an acquired von Willebrand disease. Rarely, cases are associated with an underlying genetic predisposition syndrome such as Beckwith–Wiedemann, Denys–Drash, or Wilms' tumor, aniridia, genitourinary anomalies, mental retardation (WAGR).[4] Tumor may be present in both kidneys at diagnosis in 5% to 10% of cases.

The differential diagnosis includes other conditions that present with abdominal or pelvic mass. Initial workup includes a CBC, urinalysis, and imaging of the chest and abdomen. Ultrasound or CT will often reveal a large, encapsulated mass arising from the kidney (Fig. 103–2). Patients suspected of having

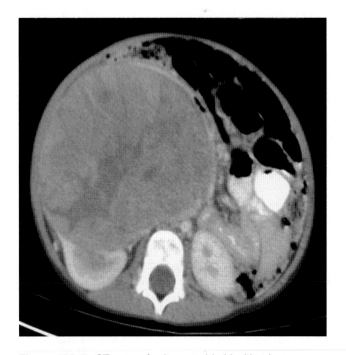

Figure 103–2. CT scan of a 3-year-old girl with a large encapsulated mass arising from the right kidney. The patient underwent a right nephrectomy and pathology confirmed the diagnosis of Wilms' tumor.

a Wilms' tumor are referred for further evaluation and management, which includes surgical resection and chemotherapy or radiation. Nephrectomy or biopsy should only be performed by a surgeon experienced with Wilms' tumor in order to avoid rupture and subsequent upstaging of the tumor.

NEUROBLASTOMA

Neuroblastoma is a malignant tumor arising from neural crest cells, originating anywhere along the sympathetic chain or the adrenal medulla It is the most common extracranial solid tumor in childhood, with almost all cases diagnosed before 5 years of age.[4] Presenting signs and symptoms are most often related to the local effects of the primary or metastatic tumor. Two-thirds of neuroblastomas arise in the abdomen and pelvis and may present as an abdominal mass. Impingement of renal vasculature may lead to renin-mediated hypertension. Cervical or thoracic primary tumors are more often seen in infants. Horner's syndrome, with unilateral ptosis, miosis, and anhidrosis, may occur with cervical or high thoracic involvement. Tumors of the paraspinal ganglia may grow around and through the intervertebral foramina, causing spinal cord or nerve root compression. Metastatic disease may be present at diagnosis in up to half of cases, most often in bone, bone marrow, liver, or skin. Lung or brain involvement is rare and usually represents end-stage or relapsing disease. Retrobulbar involvement can cause proptosis or periorbital ecchymosis. Bone pain and limping may be related to bone and bone marrow disease. Massive hepatomegaly due to liver involvement, more common in infants, can cause respiratory compromise or liver failure. Skin manifestations appear as bluish, nontender subcutaneous nodules. Opsoclonus-myoclonus is a paraneoplastic syndrome characterized by myoclonic jerking and random eye movements seen in a small percentage of neuroblastoma patients at diagnosis.

A CBC may reveal cytopenias due to marrow involvement. Abdominal ultrasound or CT scan may reveal a suprarenal mass, often with calcifications (Fig. 103–3). Lytic lesions and periosteal reaction may be seen on radiographs of painful areas of bone. The catecholamine metabolites homovanillic acid and vanillylmandelic acid are elevated and detectable in the urine in greater than 90% of patients. Tissue from either a primary or metastatic site is necessary for diagnosis. Therapy is stage dependent, with low-stage tumors curable with surgical resection and multimodal therapy with a combination of surgery, chemotherapy, and radiation for higher stage tumors.

MUSCULOSKELETAL TUMORS

Common musculoskeletal tumors in children include osteosarcoma, Ewing's sarcoma, and rhabdomyosarcoma.[5] Rhabdomyosarcoma is a malignant solid tumor from mesenchymal tissue that normally forms striated muscle, and may arise anywhere. Osteosarcoma is the most common malignancy of bone, with a predilection for the metaphysis of long bones, particularly the distal femur and proximal tibia. Ewing's sarcoma occurs equally between long bones and flat bones; it may also present as a soft tissue mass without bone involvement.

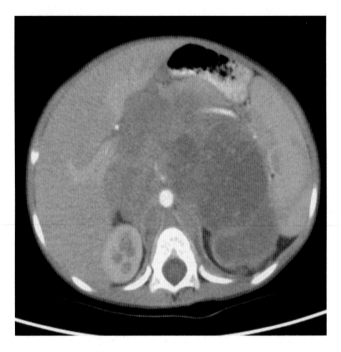

Figure 103–3. CT scan of a 2-year-old boy who presented with 2 weeks of bruising, pallor, and abdominal distension. Compared to the Wilms' tumor shown in Fig. 103–2, this mass is not encapsulated and displaces normal structures (note the position of the abdominal aorta). Biopsy confirmed the diagnosis of neuroblastoma.

Rhabdomyosarcoma most often presents as a painless mass, and signs and symptoms are location dependent. Genitourinary tract involvement may manifest with hematuria or urinary obstruction. Vaginal tumors may present with hemorrhagic discharge and may mimic a foreign body. The most common presenting symptom of osteosarcoma and Ewing's sarcoma is pain in a bone or joint, often after an injury. Other presentations include a palpable mass or pathologic fracture.

Initial imaging of a soft tissue mass suspected to be rhabdomyosarcoma is dependent on location. Plain radiographs should be the first step in the initial evaluation of a suspected bone tumor. In osteosarcoma, the tumor may extend through the periosteum, causing new malignant bone deposition resulting in the characteristic radiographic "sunburst" pattern (Fig. 103–4). Ewing's sarcoma may cause a multilaminar periosteal reaction resulting in an "onionskin" appearance on plain film (Fig. 103–5). Each of these tumors may metastasize to the lung. Rhabdomyosarcoma and Ewing's sarcoma may metastasize to the bone marrow.

Patients with radiographic changes suggestive of a musculoskeletal tumor are referred to a pediatric cancer center for biopsy and further management. Treatment is multimodal, utilizing chemotherapy and surgery or radiation depending on tumor type and location.

RETINOBLASTOMA

Retinoblastoma is the most common intraocular tumor of childhood. It is strongly linked to deletions of the RB1 gene on

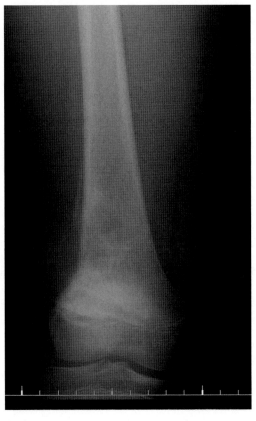

A

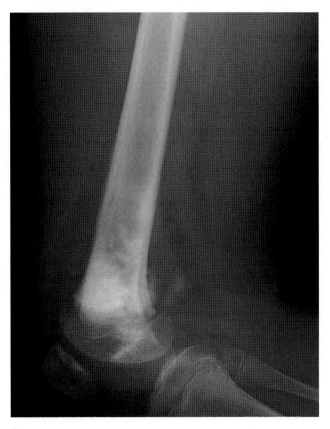

B

Figure 103–4. Radiographs of the distal femur of a 13-year-old girl with osteosarcoma. There is a poorly marginated diffuse bony lesion present in the femoral metaphysis extending to the growth plate. Note the aggressive periosteal reaction with a Codman's triangle along the lateral aspect of the distal femur. There is tumoral bone formation posteriorly.

chromosome 13, with 40% of cases associated with a germ line mutation in RB1.[6] Disease may be bilateral in 30% of cases. Most cases are diagnosed before 4 years of age. Retinoblastoma most commonly presents with leukocoria or strabismus. The disease may be localized to the orbit, or it may metastasize to the brain, liver, kidneys, and adrenals. A CT or MRI is needed to determine the presence of choroidal or optic nerve spread and orbital, subarachnoid, or intracranial involvement. Unilateral disease is treated with enucleation. Depending on the extent of disease, other therapy beyond surgery, including radiation, chemotherapy, thermotherapy, and cryotherapy, may be necessary.

▶ COMMON COMPLICATIONS OF CHILDHOOD CANCER

The emergencies encountered in children with cancer may arise at any time in the course of care, from the initial diagnosis through treatment to the time of tumor recurrence. Complications may result from the tumor itself or treatment directed at the malignancy.

METABOLIC EMERGENCIES

Tumor Lysis Syndrome

Tumor lysis syndrome (TLS) results from the death of tumor cells and the subsequent release of intracellular contents into circulation. The result is hyperuricemia, hyperphosphatemia, and hyperkalemia. TLS occurs most often with hematologic malignancies, particularly Burkitt's lymphoma and T-cell lymphoma or leukemia. TLS is rare with nonlymphomatous solid tumors. TLS may occur prior to initiation of therapy, but usually begins within the first few days of treatment. TLS may be precipitated by the administration of corticosteroids to a patient not initially thought to have a malignancy.

The breakdown of released nucleic acids from tumor cells leads to hyperuricemia. With hyperuricemia, uric acid may crystalize within the renal tubules leading to obstruction, oliguria, and renal failure. The release of intracellular potassium leads to hyperkalemia, which may be exacerbated by declining renal function. Hyperkalemia may lead to life-threatening arrhythmias. Hyperphosphatemia will lead to secondary hypocalcemia. Severe hypocalcemia may cause tetany, seizures, and arrhythmias. Precipitation of calcium phophate crystals in the renal tubules leads to renal failure.

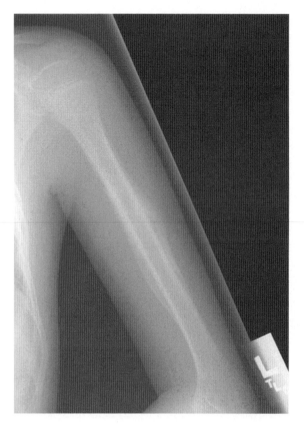

Figure 103–5. Radiographic appearance of a Ewing's sarcoma of the humerus with periosteal elevation and "onionskin" appearance. Ewing's sarcoma of the long bones is more often located in the diaphyses, whereas osteosarcoma most often involves the metaphyses.

Signs and symptoms of TLS are nonspecific and are related to declining renal function and electrolyte abnormalities. All patients with possible TLS require the following studies: CBC, creatinine, electrolytes, glucose, calcium, phosphate, and uric acid. An electrocardiogram should be obtained if hyperkalemia is found.

Early recognition or anticipation of TLS is important. Hydration is the most important initial intervention, facilitating uric acid and phosphate excretion. Intravenous fluid is administered at a minimum of twice the patient's maintenance rate with 5% dextrose in ¼ normal saline with 40 mEq of sodium bicarbonate per liter, aiming to produce a urine pH of 7.0 to

7.5. Alkalinization of the urine increases uric acid solubility and excretion. Over alkalinization may lead to crystallization of calcium phosphate in the kidneys. Fluids should not contain potassium unless symptomatic hypokalemia exists. Allopurinol inhibits xanthine oxidase, the enzyme that promotes the degradation of purine to uric acid, and may be used to prevent hyperuricemia. Recombinant urate oxidase (0.2 mg/kg) given intravenously will convert uric acid to allantoin, and may be indicated in the place of allopurinol in patients with an elevated uric acid, tumors of a high proliferative rate such as Burkitt's lymphoma, or with a large tumor burden. Calcium supplementation for hypocalcemia is indicated only in patients who are severely symptomatic with a normal serum phosphate. Giving calcium in the face of hyperphosphatemia may increase the precipitation of calcium phosphate. Hyperkalemia may be reduced by calcium gluconate, sodium bicarbonate, and insulin along with dextrose (Table 103–3). Sodium polystyrene sulfonate (Kayexalate) should not be an initial choice for hyperkalemia due to its slow onset of action and desire to avoid per rectum route of administration in neutropenic patients. Dialysis is indicated with persistent oliguria or electrolyte abnormalities that do not correct with medical management.

Hypercalcemia

Although hypercalcemia is more commonly associated with adult malignancies, it may occur with ALL, NHL, neuroblastoma, and Ewing's sarcoma. Disruptions in calcium homeostasis or excessive bone resorption by parathyroid hormone secreting tumors are the usual causes. Clinically, patients may experience constipation, weakness, polyuria, and drowsiness. Treatment begins with intravenous hydration with normal saline, followed by furosemide to promote calcium excretion.

HEMATOLOGIC COMPLICATIONS

Hematologic complications include anemia, hemorrhage, and hyperleukocytosis. Management of anemia includes transfusion therapy with packed red blood cells (PRBC). Patients who are symptomatic will often have a hemoglobin of <6 to 8 g/dL and experience malaise, decreased activity, headache, or irritability due to reduced oxygen-carrying capacity. They warrant transfusion with 10 to 12 mL/kg PRBC given over 3 to 4 hours. Those with a hemoglobin <5 g/dL that has developed gradually may require transfusion with multiple smaller aliquots

▶ TABLE 103–3. **MANAGEMENT OF HYPERKALEMIA**

Purpose	Agent	Dose	Rate of Administration
Improve membrane stability	Calcium gluconate	1 mL/kg of 10% solution	Intravenous over 10–15 min
Shift potassium into cells	β-agonist	5–20 mg	Nebulized with 5 L oxygen
	Sodium bicarbonate	0.5 mg/kg per dose	Intravenous over 10–15 min
	Glucose	0.5 g/kg	Intravenous over 30 min
	Insulin	0.1 U/kg	
Enhanced elimination	Kayexalate	1–2 g/kg	Per rectum may be contraindicated in immunocompromised patients
	Dialysis		Done in coordination with nephrology

(3–5 mL/kg) to avoid congestive heart failure. Patients with signs of fluid overload may be given furosemide. Blood products given to chemotherapy or stem cell transplant patients should be irradiated and leukoreduced. Blood-product irradiation helps minimize the occurrence of posttransfusion graft-versus-host disease by inhibiting the mitotic activity of lymphocytes in donor blood products. Leukoreduction decreases the occurrence of transfusion reactions as well as the transmission of CMV.

Hemorrhage may occur due to thrombocytopenia secondary to leukemia, chemotherapy, or DIC. Petechiae, bruising, and mucosal bleeding may be seen with platelet counts <20 000/mm^3, but significant spontaneous hemorrhage is more likely with platelet counts <10 000/mm^3. Platelet transfusions are warranted for patients who have significant bleeding, such as epistaxis, gingival bleeding, or gross gastrointestinal hemorrhage. Prophylactic use of platelet transfusions for nonbleeding patients with a platelet count <20 000/mm^3 is controversial but may be justified in the presence of infection or prior to an invasive procedure.

Hemorrhage can also be secondary to disseminated intravascular coagulation, which causes a prolongation of the prothrombin time and partial thromboplastin time, reduced fibrinogen level, thrombocytopenia, and elevated fibrin degradation products. Disseminated intravascular coagulation may occur in the setting of sepsis, newly diagnosed or relapsing acute myelogenous leukemia, and hyperleukocytosis. Initial management includes treatment of the underlying condition and replacement of coagulation factors with fresh frozen plasma (10 mL/kg). Platelet and PRBC transfusions may be necessary.

Hyperleukocytosis may be seen with acute leukemia. Unlike RBCs and platelets, WBCs are larger and not easily deformed, contributing significantly to blood viscosity. Leukemia cells tend to aggregate and impair tissue perfusion. Patients may be dyspneic, confused, agitated, or experience blurred vision. The level of leukocytosis leading to symptoms is variable and depends on the type of leukemia. Patients with AML may be symptomatic at a lower WBC than those with ALL; symptomatic hyperleukocytosis is rarely seen in CML despite very high WBC counts. Physical examination may reveal plethora, cyanosis, papilledema, retinal hemorrhage, ataxia, priapism, or focal findings on neurologic examination. The CBC will confirm an elevated peripheral WBC count. The chest radiograph may show a diffuse interstitial infiltrate. Patients with hyperleukocytosis are at risk for TLS. Thrombocytopenia is corrected to a platelet count of at least 20 000/mm^3, as there is a significant risk of intracranial hemorrhage with hyperleukocytosis. Leukopheresis prior to initiation of chemotherapy will decrease viscosity and help correct electrolyte abnormalities, and may be indicated in patients with symptomatic hyperleukocytosis.

INFECTIOUS COMPLICATIONS

Infection is one of the most common complications in the treatment of children with cancer and is a significant cause of morbidity and mortality. The single most important factor is the development of neutropenia due to replacement of healthy bone marrow by malignant cells or from myelosuppressive chemotherapy, which often produces granulocytopenia 8 to 16 days posttherapy. The best estimate of production of neutrophils is the absolute neutrophil count (ANC), calculated as the total WBC count multiplied by the sum of the percentages of band cells plus polymorphonuclear neutrophils:

$$\text{ANC} = \text{total WBC} \times (\% \text{ Bands} + \% \text{ PMNs})$$

Patients are defined as being neutropenic if their ANC is <500/mm^3 or if it is <1000/mm^3 with predicted decline to <500/mm^3. Fever is defined as a single oral temperature of ≥38.3°C (101°F) or a temperature of ≥38.0°C (100.4°F) for ≥1hour.[7] These patients are at significant risk of bacteremia or fungemia. There are also qualitative abnormalities of granulocyte function that result from chemotherapy or radiation therapy. Impaired cell–mediated immunity results in a greater risk for fungal, mycobacterial, and viral infections. In addition, mechanical barriers such as the skin and mucous membranes may be broken down by infection, chemotherapy, or long-term indwelling venous access devices (IVAD). Patients are at risk of infection from their own endogenous flora, as well as nosocomial pathogens from recent hospitalizations. It is important to promptly evaluate and treat immunocompromised patients with fever, since their infections can be life threatening. The common pathogens are listed in Table 103–4.

Evaluation of children with cancer and fever includes a careful history and physical examination. Particular attention is paid to occult sites of potential infection, such as the oropharynx, axillae, groin, perineum, and sites of previous procedures, as well as along the tract of any IVAD. It is important to note that fever may be the only positive sign. Because of a decreased number of neutrophils, the inflammatory response is blunted; hence, other findings, such as exudates, adenopathy, fluctuance, warmth, and swelling, may be absent. Children with early pneumonia may not have cough or sputum production.

Initial investigations include a creatinine, CBC, and blood cultures sent for bacterial and fungal culture. A chest

TABLE 103–4. COMMON PATHOGENS IN CHILDREN WITH CANCER

Bacteria			
Gram-positive	**Gram-negative**	**Fungi**	**Viruses**
• *Staphylococcus aureus* • Coagulase-negative staphylococci • Alpha-hemolytic streptococci • *Enterococcus faecalis*	• *Escherichia coli* • *Klebsiella* species • *Pseudomonas aeruginosa*	• *Candida* species • *Aspergillus* species	• HSV • Varicella • CMV • EBV • RSV • Influenza

▶ **TABLE 103–5. EMPIRIC ANTIBIOTIC THERAPY FOR FEBRILE NEUTROPENIC PATIENTS**

Monotherapy	Combination Therapy		
• Cefepime	Aminoglycoside		
• Ceftazadime	• Amikacin		
• Imipenem	• Tobramycin		
• Meropenem	• Gentamicin		
	PLUS		
	Extended spectrum cephalosporin	Anti-pseudomonal penicillin	Carbapenem
	• Cefepime	• Piperacillin-tazobactam	• Imipenem
	• Ceftazadime	• Ticarcillin-clavulanate	• Meropenem

radiograph is required if respiratory symptoms are present. If an IVAD is present, a blood culture should be obtained from the line. Debate exists as to whether a culture from a peripheral vein as well as from the IVAD is necessary. Institutional standards should be followed. An aspirate for Gram stain and culture is sent from any other areas suggestive of focal infection.

Prompt initiation of empiric antibiotic therapy in febrile neutropenic children is critical as infection may progress rapidly. All febrile neutropenic patients are admitted to the hospital for continuation of intravenous antibiotics. The outpatient management of the febrile neutropenic child is not well established, and should only be done in coordination with a pediatric oncologist and in the context of a clinical trial. The choice of antibiotic regimen must consider the microbial sensitivity patterns in the institution. Combination therapy has been the usual approach to provide broad-spectrum antibiotic coverage (Table 103–5), which includes an aminoglycoside and an antipseudomonal beta lactam. The development of broad-spectrum antibiotics has made monotherapy an option in some institutions. Ceftazidime, imipenem, cefepime, and meropenem have good activity against *Pseudomonas aeruginosa*, and may be as efficacious as the standard combination therapy. The routine use of vancomycin in the initial empiric regimen has not shown to be of added benefit. However, vancomycin is warranted if there is evidence of intravenous catheter-related infection, methicillin-resistant *Staphylococcus aureus* colonization, severe chemotherapy-induced mucosal damage, fluoroquinolone prophylaxis, recent administration of high dose cytarabine, or septic shock.

Modifications to Therapy

Patients with a focus of infection may require modifications in therapy. Signs or symptoms suggestive of an infection along the gastrointestinal tract warrant extended anaerobic coverage with either metronidazole or clindamycin. The presence of a pulmonary infiltrate may represent a bacterial, viral, fungal, or parasitic infection.

Fungal Infections

Cancer patients who are febrile and neutropenic are at risk for fungal infections, particularly *Candida* and *Aspergillus* species. In pediatric patients, the oral cavity is the most common site for fungal infection. It may present asymptomatically as punc-

tate foci or diffuse erythematous mucosal plaques and ulcerations. Any patient with difficulty breathing, hoarseness, or stridor should be considered to have epiglottic or laryngeal candidiasis. A scraping from the base of a lesion is sent for fungal and viral culture. Neutropenic patients who are afebrile and able to tolerate oral medication may be treated with topical antifungal agents such as clotrimazole. Empiric intravenous antifungal therapy is not initially indicated for febrile patients, but may be added after several days of fever in a persistently neutropenic patient.

Viral Infections

Herpes simplex virus (HSV) infections tend to be localized, even in the immunocompromised patient, and commonly involve the mouth, nares, esophagus, genitals, and perianal region. Pain is the predominant presenting symptom. Disruption of the mucosa may promote secondary bacterial infection. Immunocompromised patients with mild mucocutaneous disease may be started on oral acyclovir. Patients with moderate or severe HSV infection should be admitted for intravenous acyclovir therapy.

Varicella zoster virus (VZV) infections in immunocompromised patients are associated with significant morbidity and mortality, including potential dissemination. Diagnosis of VZV infection is usually based on the characteristic vesicular lesions and history of recent exposure. Laboratory confirmation is by positive culture of the virus from scraping of the base of the lesions. A chest radiograph is obtained to assess for pneumonia. Immunocompromised patients with VZV infection are admitted for intravenous acyclovir.

Parasitic Infections

Pneumocystis carinii is the infectious organism that causes pneumocystis carinii pneu-monia—the most common parasitic infection in immunocompromised patients. Children with hematologic malignancies are at the highest risk. Typically, patients will have fever, dry cough, tachypnea, and intercostal retractions without detectable rales. Hypoxia may be present and out of proportion to the degree of tachypnea. The chest radiograph may be normal in early disease, but later progresses to bilateral alveolar infiltrates. Diagnosis is confirmed by bronchoalveolar lavage or open lung biopsy. Immunocompromised patients should be started on empiric therapy with TMP-SMX pending definitive diagnosis. The incidence of infections caused by *P. carinii* has been greatly reduced with the routine use of prophylaxis with TMP-SMX, pentamidine, or dapsone in immunocompromised patients.

Fever in the Nonneutropenic Oncology Patient

The evaluation of the nonneutropenic oncology patient should be the same as that for the neutropenic patient. Nonneutropenic patients remain at risk for infection from an IVAD and therapy related immune dysfunction outside of neutropenia. If the nonneutropenic febrile patient has an IVAD, antibiotic therapy with a third-generation cephalosporin such as ceftriaxone (75 mg/kg q24h) should be given. The patient should be observed for some time after receiving antibiotics, and if stable, outpatient management may be arranged with the child's oncologist. Hospitalization may be warranted in children whose ANC is expected to decline below 500 in the next few days or in the septic appearing patient. In the absence of an IVAD or focus of infection, the febrile nonneutropenic patient may be observed after obtaining a blood culture without the initiation of an antibiotic.

SUPERIOR VENA CAVA SYNDROME AND SUPERIOR MEDIASTINAL SYNDROME

Several pediatric malignancies, including non-Hodgkin lymphoma, Hodgkin lymphoma, neuroblastoma, germ cell tumors, and acute lymphoblastic lymphoma may present with a mediastinal mass. Mediastinal compression from the tumors may result in Superior Vena Cava Syndrome (SVCS) or Superior Mediastinal Syndrome (SMS). SVCS refers to the signs and symptoms resulting from obstruction, compression, or thrombosis of the SVC. SMS occurs with compression of the narrow, more compliant trachea in children. SMS and SVCS usually occur together in pediatrics. Patients may present with edema and plethora of the face, conjunctivae, neck, and upper torso. Tortuous collateral veins can appear on the chest and upper abdomen. Headache, papilledema, seizures, coma, cerebral hemorrhage, and engorgement of retinal veins may result from cerebral venous hypertension. Compression of the tracheobronchial tree may cause tachypnea, wheezing, stridor, orthopnea, or cyanosis. Death may occur as a result of airway obstruction, cerebral edema, or cardiac compromise.

Chest radiography reveals superior mediastinal widening and occasionally a pleural or pericardial effusion (Fig. 103–6). The trachea may appear deviated or narrowed. A CBC with differential may show evidence of leukemia or lymphoma. Electrolytes may show evidence of tumor lysis.

Management of these patients is challenging as complete obstruction of the airway may be precipitated. Securing the airway may be difficult, particularly if the obstruction is at or below the distal trachea. Attempts at intubation (either tracheal or selective bronchial intubation) or emergent tracheostomy after airway collapse may not be possible. Even if intubation is achieved, collapse of the airway below the level of the endotracheal tube may lead to inadequate ventilation and

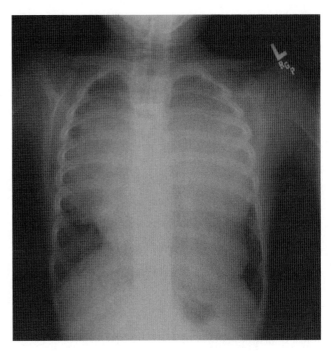

Figure 103–6. Chest radiograph of a 6-year-old boy who presented with wheezing and tachypnea. The large mediastinal mass is causing deviation of the trachea and compression of the lower airway. The child became hypoxic in the supine position. Chemotherapy was begun emergently. Biopsy of the mass several days later confirmed the diagnosis of T-cell lymphoblastic lymphoma.

life-threatening ventilation perfusion mismatch. Several cases of death due to airway collapse at induction of anesthesia have been reported. Peak expiratory flow rates and CT determined tracheal cross sectional area have been suggested as means to judge anesthetic risk. However, patients with a critical mass may not tolerate the supine positioning needed for the CT scan or cooperate with obtaining flow rates. If intubation is required, it is recommended that the patient should be awake with spontaneous respiration. The use of extracorporeal membranous oxygenation has been reported in patients at high risk of lower airway collapse.[8] Patients with significant respiratory compromise may require the initiation of therapy with either radiation or chemotherapy prior to definitive tissue diagnosis.

Supportive therapy includes minimizing cerebral hypertension by elevation of the head of the bed. Intravenous hydration may be more efficient through a low-pressure lower extremity vein. Upper extremity phlebotomy should be avoided as these veins are under high pressure and may bleed excessively. Correction of electrolyte abnormalities and treatment of hyperuricemia should be initiated.

SPINAL CORD COMPRESSION

Spinal cord compression may occur with extradural metastatic tumors such as soft tissue sarcomas, neuroblastoma, germ cell tumors, and Hodgkin disease, or rarely with an intradural cord tumor. Pain is the most common initial presenting symptom. The pain is usually worse when supine; there may be tenderness with palpation. Muscle weakness, which is usually symmetric, is a later finding. Most patients with weakness will already have extradural spinal cord compression at the time of diagnosis. Sensory deficits are less common than weakness and present with ascending numbness and paraesthesias. Changes in bladder or bowel function may also occur. Hydrocephalus may result from physical obstruction of cerebrospinal fluid flow. Most patients will usually have objective neurologic deficits at the time of presentation.[9]

Plain spine radiographs will show an abnormality in some patients with spinal cord compression; however, an MRI provides a more definitive study.

Spinal cord compression is a true neurologic emergency. Consultation with an oncologist and neurosurgeon should be obtained immediately. Treatment begins with dexamethasone to reduce tumor-related edema. MRI should be done immediately in those patients with progressive neurologic deficit. Patients should be promptly referred for possible surgery or radiation therapy. Chemotherapy is an option for chemotherapy-sensitive diseases such as Hodgkin disease, NHL, neuroblastoma, or germ cell tumors.

CENTRAL NERVOUS SYSTEM EMERGENCIES

Children with cancer may have CNS complications, such as altered mental status, intracranial hemorrhage, and seizures. Electrolyte abnormalities, hypoxia, renal or hepatic failure, disseminated intravascular coagulation, hyperleukocytosis, and sepsis may lead to altered level of consciousness. Primary CNS tumors and metastatic lesions may present with acute mental status changes. Cerebrovascular accidents may complicate acute leukemia as a result of thrombosis or hemorrhage. Occasionally, hemorrhage can occur at the site of intracerebral metastases. Subdural and subarachnoid hemorrhage may occur due to thrombocytopenia or coagulopathy. Thrombosis may occur after CNS irradiation or chemotherapy. Seizures may arise from electrolyte abnormalities, infection, metastatic disease, or as a complication of CNS therapy.

The initial evaluation of a child with a neurologic emergency should include a detailed history and neurologic examination. Recent administration of chemotherapeutic agents, either intravenous or intrathecal, such as methotrexate, cytarabine, corticosteroids, and ifosfamide may cause neurologic toxicity. Laboratory evaluation includes a CBC, electrolytes, glucose, creatinine, phosphate, calcium, uric acid, magnesium, blood culture, and coagulation studies. A CT scan of the head without contrast should be done to quickly assess for tumor or intracranial bleeding. MRI may be performed when the child is stable.

Treatment for patients with altered mental status begins with support and protection of the airway and breathing. If necessary, endotrachial intubation is performed utilizing medications that do not increase intracranial pressure in conjunction with lidocaine. If raised ICP is suspected, controlled ventilation to a Pco_2 of 30 to 35 mm Hg will cause cerebral vasoconstriction and thereby help reduce cerebral blood flow. Corticosteroid is given to patients with an intracranial tumor in order to

decrease cerebral edema. Hyperosmolar agents, such as mannitol and 3% saline, may help to reduce cerebral edema by creating an osmotic gradient between the blood and the brain with an intact blood–brain barrier. Use of a diuretic (furosemide) in conjunction with mannitol may enhance the reduction in ICP. Prompt neurosurgical consultation is recommended. If meningitis is suspected, lumbar puncture is deferred but antibiotics are initiated prior to the CT scan. Thrombocytopenia and coagulopathy are corrected, especially in the presence of an intracranial hemorrhage.

GASTROINTESTINAL EMERGENCIES

Pediatric cancer patients are at risk for a number of unique conditions leading to acute abdominal pain as a result of immunosuppresion, cancer therapy, tumor invasion or compression. Esophagitis, typhlitis, enterocolitis, and perirectal abscess may occur as a result of immunosuppresion and infection. Typhlitis is a severe necrotizing colitis of the cecum in neutropenic patients; it may mimic signs and symptoms of acute appendicitis. Gastrointestinal hemorrhage can result from thrombocytopenia, coagulopathy, mucosal ulceration, or abnormal tumor vessels. The use of high-dose corticosteroids in the treatment of leukemia and lymphoma places patients at high risk of upper GI bleeding. Obstruction may be caused by tumor mass at presentation, adhesions from previous resection of an abdominal tumor, or paralytic ileus from medications such as vincristine. The use of asparaginase in the treatment of leukemia may cause pancreatitis. Venoocclusive disease presents with tender hepatomegaly, ascites, weight gain, and hyperbilirubinemia. It most often occurs during stem cell transplant, but may be a complication of some chemotherapy regimens. Common causes of an acute abdomen, such as appendicitis, must also be considered.

Determining the etiology of the abdominal pain may be difficult in neutropenic or immunosuppressed patients. The inflammatory response may be reduced due to leukopenia and normally localized processes may be generalized. The abdominal examination begins with careful observation, gentle palpation, auscultation, and serial reexamination. Examination of the perineum and rectum is important in detecting pelvic and perirectal disease, neutropenia is not necessarily a contraindication to this maneuver.

Laboratory workup includes a CBC, blood and urine cultures, urinalysis, electrolytes, glucose, amylase, and lipase. A chest radiograph is done to assess for pneumonia, while abdominal films may reveal bowel obstruction, perforation, or pneumatosis intestinalis. An abdominal CT may be helpful if plain films are nondiagnostic.

Patients with an acute abdomen should be admitted and started on intravenous hydration. Nonneutropenic patients with esophagitis and presumptive gastric stress ulcers may benefit from H_2 antagonists. Thrombocytopenia and coagulopathies are corrected in the presence of hemorrhage. Patients with typhlitis must be started on broad-spectrum antibiotics to cover both gram-negative pathogens as well as gastrointestinal anaerobes. Early surgical consultation is recommended. Indications for laparotomy with typhlitis include evidence of perforation, persistent gastrointestinal hemorrhage despite correction of existing coagulopathies, and clinical deterioration.

REFERENCES

1. Smith MA, Gloeckler Ries LA. Childhood cancer: incidence, survival, and mortality. In: Pizzo PA, Poplack DG, eds. *Principles and Practice of Pediatric Oncology.* 4th ed. Philadelphia, PA: Lippincott Williams & Wilkins; 2002.
2. Pearce JM, Sills RH. Childhood leukemia. *Pediatr Rev.* 2005; 26(3):96–104.
3. Strother DR, Pollack IF, Fisher PG, et al. Tumors of the central nervous system. In: Pizzo PA, Poplack DG, eds. *Principles and Practice of Pediatric Oncology.* 4th ed. Philadelphia, PA: Lippincott Williams & Wilkins; 2002.
4. Golden CB, Feusner JH. Malignant abdominal masses in children: quick guide to evaluation and diagnosis. *Pediatr Clin N Am.* 2002;49(6):1369–1392.
5. Arndt CAS, Crist WM. Common musculoskeletal tumors of childhood and adolescence. *N Engl J Med.* 1999;341 (5):342–352.
6. Melamud A, Rakhee P, Singh A. Retinoblastoma. *Am Fam Physician.* 2006;73(6):1039–1044.
7. Hughes WT, Armstrong D, Bodey GP, et al. 2002 guidelines for the use of antimicrobial agents in neutropenic patients with cancer. *Clin Infect Dis.* 2002;34:730–751.
8. Wickiser JE, Thompson M, Leavey PJ, et al. Extracorporeal membrane oxygenation (ECMO) initiation without intubation in two children with mediastinal malignancy. *Pediatr Blood Cancer.* 2007;49(5):751–754.
9. Prasad D, Schiff D. Malignant spinal-cord compression. *Lancet Oncol.* 2005;6(1):15–24.

SECTION XVIII

NON-TRAUMATIC BONE AND JOINT DISORDERS

CHAPTER 104

Infectious Musculoskeletal Disorders

Kemedy K. McQuillen

▶ HIGH-YIELD FACTS

- *Staphylococcus aureus* predominates as the cause of septic arthritis and osteomyelitis. Other bacteria commonly implicated, especially in younger patients, include *Kingella kingae*, pneumococcus, and group A *Streptococcus*.
- Neonates and young infants are particularly vulnerable to infection of the hip. In older infants and children, the knee is more commonly affected.
- No single test or finding is sufficient to predict the presence of a septic joint but a history of fever, the inability to bear weight, elevated erythrocyte sedimentation rate or C-reactive protein, and an elevated white blood cell count are suggestive of the diagnosis.
- The mainstay in the diagnosis of septic arthritis is analysis of joint fluid. Fluid is usually obtained by percutaneous aspiration. In the hip, aspiration is facilitated by sonographic guidance.
- Treatment of septic arthritis consists of antibiotic therapy and drainage of the involved joint. Drainage may be by aspiration or surgical intervention.
- Ultrasound is able to detect subperiosteal abscesses early in osteomyelitis and may be the only imaging test required in uncomplicated cases. Magnetic resonance imaging has the highest sensitivity and specificity for detecting osteomyelitis.
- Intervertebral diskitis is an acute infection of the vertebral disk usually seen in children younger than 5 years. The lumbar area is most commonly involved.

Musculoskeletal diseases are frequently encountered in pediatric patients. They vary in significance from minor, self-limited illnesses to serious systemic diseases. Limb-threatening complications can occur. In the case of infants and young children, the evaluation of musculoskeletal complaints is complicated by the patient's inability to articulate the problem and the inherent difficulty of performing a sufficient physical examination in an uncooperative patient.

▶ SEPTIC ARTHRITIS

Septic arthritis is an infection within a joint space. Bacterial pathogens are common in patients with acute septic arthritis, whereas fungal and mycobacterial pathogens tend to be associated with chronic septic arthritis. Acute septic arthritis occurs in all age groups but is more common in children; 75% of cases occur in children younger than 5 years, with the peak incidence being between 6 and 24 months of age. Boys are affected twice as frequently as girls.[1] The infection involves a joint of the lower extremity in 75% of cases, with the knee and hip being most commonly involved. Other affected joints, in order of involvement, include the ankle, elbow, shoulder, and wrist. More than 90% of cases are monoarticular.

ETIOLOGY

Seeding of the joint with bacteria occurs either by hematogenous spread, direct inoculation of infected material into the joint capsule, or from an adjacent site of infection. In children, it most commonly results from hematogenous spread as bacteria pass into the synovial space through the highly vascular synovial membrane. Infection secondary to trauma most commonly affects the knee. Contiguous spread of infection from osteomyelitis to the joint space occurs in approximately 10% of cases and is more common in newborns and young infants. In these children, blood vessels cross the physis and thereby connect the metaphysis and epiphysis and allow bacteria direct access into the joint space. Additionally, the joint capsules of the hip and shoulder overlie the bony metaphyses of the femur and humerus, facilitating direct extension of osteomyelitis into these joint spaces.

The most common bacterial causes of septic arthritis are listed in Table 104–1. In all age groups, *S. aureus* is the most common cause of septic arthritis and infection with community-acquired methicillin-resistant *S. aureus* (CA-MRSA) is becoming more common.[2,3] In addition to the organisms listed in Table 104–1, additional causative organisms include *Neisseria gonorrhoeae* in neonates and sexually active adolescents, *Pseudomonas aeruginosa* and *Candida* species in intravenous drug abusers, *Salmonella* species in children with sickle cell disease, and gram-negative bacteria in immunosuppressed children. *Kingella kingae*, a fastidious gram-negative coccobacillus that colonizes the respirtory and oropharyngeal tract in children, has also been implicated as a common cause of osteoarticular infections in young children.[4,5] In one study 40% to 50% of culture-negative septic arthritis cases in children younger than 2 years were attributable to *K. kingae*.[4] Fortunately, *K. kingae* is susceptible to a wide array of antibiotics that are usually given empirically to young children for septic arthritis.

CLINICAL PRESENTATION

The clinical picture of septic arthritis varies with age. Clinically, infants tend to have fever, failure to feed, lethargy, pseudoparalysis of the extremity, and pain with diaper changes.

▶ **TABLE 104–1. PATHOGENS AND TREATMENT OF SEPTIC ARTHRITIS AND OSTEOMYELITIS***

Age or Comorbidity	Organisms	Initial Antibiotics
0 mo to 2 mo	Group B *Streptococcus* *S. aureus* Gram-negative rods *Candida*† *N. gonorrhoeae*	Nafcillin 50 mg/kg and Cefotaxime 50 mg/kg
2 mo to 5 y	*S. aureus* Group A *Streptococcus* *S. pneumoniae* *K. kingae* *Haemophilus influenzae* type b‡	Nafcillin 50 mg/kg and Cefotaxime 50 mg/kg or Ceftriaxone 50 mg/kg or Cefuroxime 50 mg/kg
5 y to 12 y	*S. aureus* *S. pyogenes* *Haemophilus influenzae* type b‡	Nafcillin 50 mg/kg or Cefazolin 25 mg/kg
>12 y	*N. gonorrhoeae* *S. aureus*	Ceftriaxone 50 mg/kg
Immunocompromised	Gram-negative enteric bacilli *S. aureus* *P. aeruginosa*	Ceftazidime 50 mg/kg and Vancomycin 10 mg/kg
Sickle cell disease	*Salmonella* spp. Gram-negative enteric bacilli *S. aureus*	Ceftriaxone 50 mg/kg and Nafcillin 50 mg/kg
Puncture wounds of the foot	*P. aeruginosa* *S. aureus*	Ceftazidime 50 mg/kg and Nafcillin 50 mg/kg

*If MRSA is a concern or local rates are >5% to10%, use intravenous vancomycin; consider supplementing with gentamicin +/− rifampin for synergy if ICU admission.
†Neonates with indwelling catheters.
‡If unimmunized.

Neonates (younger than 1 month), however, can have less fever and fewer systemic signs of illness than older infants, thus making the diagnosis even more difficult.[6] In older infants and children, the knee is more commonly affected. Older infants and children have systemic symptoms of fever, malaise, poor appetite and irritability, as well as localized symptoms of pain and limp or refusal to walk. With septic arthritis, the onset of symptoms is more acute than with osteomyelitis. Physical examination of joints, other than the hip, reveals local erythema, warmth, and swelling. If the hip is affected, it is often held in flexion, abduction and external rotation that allows for maximum opening of the joint capsule and helps relieve pressure. Range of motion is decreased because of pain and muscle spasm and passive joint movement is painful. In infants, joint dislocation may be observed.

Gonococcal arthritis presents in postpubertal patients with joint pain and fever. It usually accompanies asymptomatic disease of the genitourinary tract. In the early stages, patients may complain of fever, chills, and polyarthralgia that subsequently progresses to monoarticular or polyarticular arthritis. The knees, ankles, wrists, hands, and fingers are affected. Some patients develop tenosynovitis. A rash may develop that can consist of petechiae, papules, and pustular lesions with erythematous halos.

DIAGNOSTIC EVALUATION

The laboratory evaluation of suspected septic arthritis includes a complete blood count, erythrocyte sedimentation rate (ESR), C-reactive protein (CRP), blood culture, and joint fluid analysis. In most patients, the white blood count, ESR and CRP will be elevated although the CRP can be normal, especially with *K. kingae* infection.[2] Blood cultures are positive in 20% to 50% of cases. Neonates and young infants are more likely to have positive blood cultures.

It should be noted that the ESR rises 24 hours or more after the onset of signs and symptoms of infection, so it may not be helpful during the first day of illness. CRP may be a better monitor of septic arthritis than the ESR. It is a simpler test that requires only a finger stick sample of blood; it rises more quickly than the ESR does, is typically elevated at initial evaluation and, with appropriate therapy, will normalize within a week. In contrast, the ESR will not normalize for more than a month.[8]

If *N. gonorrhoeae* is suspected, special media is required for cultures of joint fluid, blood, pharynx, skin lesions, cervix, urethra, vagina, and rectum. Urine, urethral, cervical, and vaginal specimens can also be obtained for nucleic amplification testing. If the patient has signs or symptoms of pharyngitis, a

▶ TABLE 104–2. **ANALYSIS OF JOINT FLUID**

	Character	WBC Count (/μL)	PMNs (%)	Glucose (Synovial/Blood)	Other
Normal	Clear; yellow	<200	<10	>50	Good mucin clot
JRA	Turbid	250–50 000	50–70	>50	Fair to poor mucin clot 50% with low complement
Reactive arthritis	Clear or turbid	1000–150 000	50–70	>50	Fair to poor mucin clot Elevated complement
Lyme arthritis	Turbid	500–100 000	>50	>50	Poor mucin clot
Septic arthritis	Turbid; white-gray	10–250 000	>75	<50	Poor mucin clot High lactate

JRA, juvenile rheumatoid arthritis; PMN, polymorphonuclear leukocytes; WBC, white blood cell count.

throat culture for *Streptococcus pyogenes* should be sent. Antibody titers to antistreptolysin O and anti-DNAase B may also be helpful in establishing a causative organism.

Evaluation of synovial fluid is the mainstay for diagnosing septic arthritis. Fluid is usually obtained by percutaneous aspiration into a heparinized syringe. With a septic hip joint, aspiration is facilitated by sonographic guidance. Joint fluid should be sent for Gram stain, aerobic and anaerobic cultures, cell count with differential, glucose determination, and a mucin clot test. The synovial fluid in patients with septic arthritis tends to be turbid or grossly purulent. Although there is considerable overlap in the cell count between bacterially mediated arthritis and other causes of joint inflammation, the white blood cell count in a septic joint is generally >50 000 cells/mm³ and has a predominance of polymorphonuclear cells. Synovial glucose may be low (synovial fluid/blood glucose less than 0.5) and protein and lactate elevated (Table 104–2). Joint fluid should be inoculated directly into blood culture bottles to enhance identification of fastidious organisms such as *K. kingae*. Cultures may need to be incubated for a week or more. Culture of the joint fluid is positive in approximately 60% of patients[8] except in the case of gonococcal arthritis, in which the culture is usually negative. Up to 50% of patients have a positive Gram stain.

Multiple studies have attempted to define criteria to help differentiate septic arthritis from transient synovitis. Clinical decision rules have included the presence or absence of fever, the ability to bear weight, white blood cell (WBC) counts, inflammatory markers (ESR and CRP), side-to-side differences in the width of the joint space on radiographs and prior visits to a health care provider. Kocher and colleagues found four independent multivariant predictors of septic arthritis: fever, inability to bear weight, ESR greater than or equal to 40 mm/h and a serum WBC greater than 12 000 cells/mm³. Patients with three of the four predictors had a 93% chance of having septic arthritis and those who had all four, had a 99% likelihood of pyarthrosis.[9] A subsequent study to validate their findings showed that patients with zero of the predictors had a 2% probability of septic arthritis, those with one of four criteria had a 9.5% probability, those with two of four had a 35% probability, those with three of four had a 73% probability and patients who had all four predictors had a 93% probability of septic arthritis.[10] However, when this algorithm was tested at another institution the presence of all four Kocher criteria predicted septic arthritis only 59% of the time.[11] In general, in children with septic arthritis and transient synovitis, the overlap of laboratory values and historical features is too great to provide a foolproof diagnostic algorithm.[12]

In patients with septic arthritis, plain films may demonstrate a widened joint space but plain films are most useful in ruling out other conditions such as fractures, Legg–Calve–Perthes disease, and slipped capital femoral epiphysis. Normal plain films do not rule out a septic joint. Ultrasonography is much more sensitive than plain radiography in detecting hip effusion and provides direct visualization of the fluid (Fig. 104–1A and B) and needle during joint aspiration. Radionuclide scanning can be helpful in difficult cases. It is diagnostic of

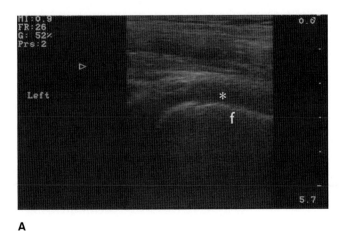

A

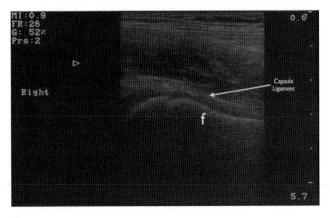

B

Figure 104–1. (A) Ultrasound image showing hip effusion. (B) Ultrasound image of a normal hip for comparison.

septic arthritis earlier than other imaging techniques and is a useful adjunct in identifying associated osteomyelitis or avascular necrosis of the femoral head. Magnetic resonance imaging (MRI) can be helpful in differentiating septic arthritis from transient synovitis.[13]

DIFFERENTIAL DIAGNOSIS

The differential diagnosis of septic arthritis includes transient synovitis, cellulitis, traumatic hemarthrosis, osteomyelitis, and a multitude of processes that can cause sterile joint inflammation, such as collagen vascular diseases and Henoch–Schönlein purpura. It is also common for children with acute leukemia to have bone or joint pain. In the hip, a number of problems specific to that joint must be considered. These include Legg–Calvé–Perthes disease, slipped capital femoral epiphysis, psoas abscess, obturator internus abscess and diskitis. In the knee, the possibility of referred pain from the hip must be considered. Nonbacterial causes of infectious arthritis include viral, mycoplasmal, mycobacterial, and fungal etiologies. Fungal etiology is a greater consideration for premature infants and for those with central venous catheters. Reactive arthritides following streptococcal infections, gastrointestinal problems, and viral hepatitis may be especially difficult to diagnose since the interval between the inciting illness and the reactive arthritis may be 2 weeks or more.

TREATMENT

Septic arthritis requires immediate admission, antibiotics, and drainage of the involved joint. Drainage options range from needle aspiration to open surgical drainage, but no randomized controlled trials have compared these two treatment approaches. Emergent surgical drainage is recommended for septic arthritis of the hip. Infants with septic arthritis of the shoulder are also treated with emergent surgical drainage. When other joints are affected, daily aspiration may be sufficient. If there is a large amount of pus or debris in the joint, loculated fluid, recurrence of joint fluid after four or five aspirations or lack of clinical improvement within 3 days, surgical drainage is recommended.

Empiric antibiotic therapy for septic arthritis is directed against the most likely organisms based on patient age and comorbid conditions (Table 104–1). Treatment may then be changed after culture and sensitivity results are known. To maximize culture results, antibiotics should not be given until a specimen of joint fluid is obtained. Initial treatment is parenteral to ensure adequate serum antibiotic concentrations. After the patient's clinical condition is stabilized, oral antibiotic therapy can be instituted. In general, doses two to three times those used for mild infections are sufficient. Response to therapy is measured by clinical improvement and acute phase reactants, such as ESR and CRP.

With drainage and appropriate antibiotic therapy, improvement should be rapid. Shorter courses of antibiotic therapy are now used for these infections, but a minimum of 21 days of therapy is recommended for *S. aureus* and gram-negative infections; 14 days for group A *Streptococcus*, pneu-

mococcus, and *H. influenzae* type B; and 7 days for *N. gonorrhoeae*.

The mortality rate associated with septic arthritis has fallen to less than 1%, but the morbidity remains significant. Sequelae include leg length discrepancy, persistent pain, limited range of motion, and ischemic necrosis of the femoral head.

► OSTEOMYELITIS

Osteomyelitis is an infection of the bone. In the pediatric age group, it is most common between the ages of 3 and 12 years with 50% of cases occurring in the first 5 years of life.[2] Boys are more commonly affected than are girls. Although any bone may be affected, the long bones of the lower extremity are most commonly involved. A history of preceding trauma is elicited in 30% of cases.[2]

PATHOPHYSIOLOGY

In children, osteomyelitis is most commonly caused by acute hematogenous spread after an episode of asymptomatic bacteremia. It can also result from direct inoculation after trauma, puncture wounds, surgery, or from local invasion from a contiguous focus of infection, such as an infected sinus, mastoid bone, adjacent joint, or dental abscess. Neonates subjected to invasive procedures in the setting of the intensive care unit are especially prone to develop osteomyelitis.

Osteomyelitis most commonly begins in the metaphysis of long bones. The metaphysis possesses a rich capillary network with loops that have few anastomotic connections. This may result in sluggish circulation that can promote seeding with bacteria. In addition, fenestrations present in metaphyseal cortical bone are potential sites for seeding by bacteria. Infection usually develops in the metaphysis and may spread along the bone. In children younger than 18 months, the metaphyses are vascularized by transphyseal vessels.[2] These vessels enter the epiphysis and ultimately the joint space making younger children more likely to develop septic arthritis as a complication of osteomyelitis; up to one-third of patients will have septic joint involvement.

ETIOLOGY

S. aureus is the most common etiology of osteomyelitis and accounts for 70%–90% of infections: MRSA is becoming an increasingly common pathogen. Table 104–2 lists the most common pathogens associated with acute osteomyelitis. As in septic arthritis, *K. kingae* is being implicated in osteomyelitis more frequently. It is part of normal respiratory flora and is often found as the cause of osteomyelitis following an upper respiratory tract infection or stomatitis. *S. pyogenes* causes up to 10% of cases of acute hematogenous osteomyelitis with a peak incidence in preschool and early school-age children. Children with *S. pyogenes* infection often have a recent history of varicella infection and present with more pronounced fevers and higher WBC counts than do those with *S. aureus*.[2] Children with *S. pneumoniae* osteomyelitis tend to be younger than those with osteomyelitis due to *S. aureus* and *S. pyogenes* and they are more likely to have joint involvement. Because of the small proportion of bone infections caused by *S. pneumoniae* (1%–4%), the impact of the heptavalent pneumococcal vaccination is limited. Additionally, *H. influenzae* should be considered in infants and toddlers if they have not been adequately immunized. Puncture wounds of the foot can be complicated by osteomyelitis due to *Pseudomonas*, *S. aureus*, enteric gram-negative bacteria, anaerobes, skin flora, and, when the puncture is due to a used toothpick, oral flora. *Salmonella* is a consideration in patients with sickle cell anemia. *S. aureus*, *E. coli*, Hib, *Shigella*, and *S. pneumoniae* have also been implicated. Anaerobic osteomyelitis is uncommon but can occur as a result of a bite, chronic sinusitis, mastoiditis, or dental infection. Polymicrobial infection is rare and occurs most commonly with puncture wounds or other trauma.[8]

CLINICAL MANIFESTATIONS

The presentation of osteomyelitis varies according to age. Neonates may demonstrate few clinical findings other than irritability, fever and resistance to movement, with or without redness and swelling over the affected area. In neonates, disseminated infection involving multiple bones and contiguous joints and soft tissue is common.

Older infants and children tend to have focal infection and they are more able to localize discomfort over the affected site. Their pain is acute, persistent, and progressive. Limp is a common finding in ambulatory patients. In some cases, the physical examination reveals erythema, warmth, and swelling over the area of bone involvement, but more subtle presentations are common. Fever and bacteremia are more common in children than in adults.

Pelvic osteomyelitis, which accounts for up to 11% of cases of acute hematogenous osteomyelitis, typically affects older children. Symptoms, including hip, buttock, low back, and abdominal pain, are often nonspecific and poorly localized. Physical examination may elicit tenderness of the pelvic bones, pain with movement of the hip, decreased range of motion of the hip, and refusal/inability to bear weight. Fever may be absent. The ilium tends to be most commonly affected but any pelvic bone may be involved.

Chronic recurrent multifocal osteomyelitis is characterized by recurrent bone pain and fever. Girls are more commonly affected and associated findings include psoriasis and palmoplantar pustulosis. Radiographs show multiple, often symmetric bone lesions, with the long bones and clavicles being most frequently involved.

DIAGNOSTIC TESTING

Blood tests are often supportive but not diagnostic for osteomyelitis. Laboratory assessment includes a complete blood count, ESR, CRP, blood cultures, and radiographs of the affected area. The white blood cell count may be normal or elevated. The ESR is increased in 80% to 90% of cases and the CRP is elevated in 98% of cases.[2] Blood cultures are positive approximately 50% to 60% of the time.[14] Needle aspiration yields an organism in approximately two-thirds of cases.[8] There is enhanced isolation of *K. kingae* by polymerase chain reaction

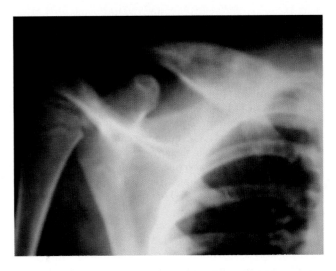

Figure 104–2. Osteomyelitis of the clavicle.

(PCR) or by culture if bone aspirates are inoculated into blood culture bottles.

Although plain radiographs may show only soft tissue swelling or obscuration of tissue planes during the first week to 10 days of the illness, they are helpful in eliminating fracture or malignancy as the cause of the patient's pain. Mottling and demineralization of the bone are usually observed a week after the initial symptoms. Periosteal and lytic changes are not usually seen for 10 to 21 days after the onset of symptoms (Fig. 104–2).

Nuclear scintigraphy with technetium-99m is often utilized because it is more sensitive than plain radiography early in the course of disease. Increased uptake is usually observed within 1 to 2 days after the onset of infection. False-negative studies do occur, however, in up to 25% of patients, particularly in infants and young children. Other processes, such as cellulitis, trauma, and tumors, may also result in increased uptake, simulating osteomyelitis. Gallium-67 or indium-111 bone scan may be useful when technetium-99m scans are inconclusive. Ultrasound is able to detect subperiosteal abscesses accurately and simply early in the course of the disease and may be the only imaging test required in uncomplicated cases. Currently, MRI is the most sensitive modality for detecting bony changes consistent with acute osteomyelitis. It is also helpful in detecting contiguous myositis or pyomyositis. MRI is the imaging study of choice if pelvic or vertebral osteomyelitis is suspected.[2] CT is also useful and can be considered when MRI is unavailable or impractical.

The diagnosis is confirmed by needle aspiration of infected material. A steel needle is needed to penetrate the cortex. Aspiration of subperiosteal or metaphyseal pus confirms the diagnosis and provides an excellent specimen for culture.

TREATMENT

Children with osteomyelitis should be admitted and, after samples are taken for culture, treated with antibiotics. Antibiotic coverage for *S. aureus* is always indicated. Other antibiotic coverage depends on the age of the patient and the clinical situation. Table 104–2 lists antibiotic coverage for osteomyelitis under various circumstances. Sequential intravenous to oral therapy is effective and safe with the duration of each therapy dependant upon the extent of the infection, clinical response, and underlying risk factors. In general, 3 to 6 weeks of antibiotics are required.

In infants and children who receive appropriate therapy, there are few long-term sequelae. Recurrence occurs in 5% of cases with risk factors for recurrence including delayed diagnosis, abbreviated antibiotic therapy, and young age. Neonates, however, have a higher complication rate with sequelae occurring in 6% to 50% of patients.[2] Sequelae include disturbances in bone growth, limb-length discrepancies, arthritis, abnormal gait, and pathologic fractures.

Chronic osteomyelitis occurs in <5% of children after an episode of acute osteomyelitis. It is more frequent if osteomyelitis is from contiguous spread. *S. aureus* and gram-negative enterics are the most common pathogens. Patients may present with chronic symptoms of swelling, pain, and intermittent drainage with acute exacerbations of fever, swelling, and redness over the bone. Bone necrosis and fibrosis ultimately develop. With chronic osteomyelitis, surgery may be required to evacuate pus or to excise necrotic tissue. Surgical management is augmented by a prolonged course of antibiotics.

A Brodie abscess is a subacute form of osteomyelitis that results in a collection of necrotic bone and pus in a fibrous capsule. It tends to occur in the long bones of adolescents. It can be seen on plain films and MRI. Laboratory evaluation reveals a normal or elevated ESR. Treatment includes surgical drainage and antibiotics.

▶ INTERVERTEBRAL DISKITIS

Intervertebral diskitis is an acute infection of the vertebral disk occasionally seen in children. Affected patients are usually younger than 5 years and the lumbar area is most commonly involved. The most common pathogen is *S. aureus* although, less commonly, pneumococcus and gram-negative organisms are involved. Rarely, the infection results from tuberculosis. Diagnosis is often delayed with one study finding a mean duration of symptoms of 33 days (range: 5 days to 3 months).[15]

Most cases of intervertebral diskitis are preceded by an upper respiratory infection. Symptoms include irritability and refusal to sit or walk in infants and toddlers, respectively. Older children may complain of back or leg pain or may limp. If the lesion occurs at the lower thoracic or upper lumbar area, the child may have gastrointestinal symptoms.

Physical examination may show a loss of lordosis. If the cervical vertebrae are involved, torticollis can occur. Tenderness along the vertebrae, mild fullness of the paraspinal muscles secondary to irritation, and occasionally hip pain and stiffness can occur. Fever may be present.

Laboratory abnormalities include an elevated ESR. In approximately 40% of cases, blood cultures are positive. Radiographs of the involved area may demonstrate a narrowing of the disk space and, eventually, erosion of the vertebral end plates (Fig. 104–3). Technetium-99m bone and MRI scans are also diagnostic and more sensitive early in the course of the disease.

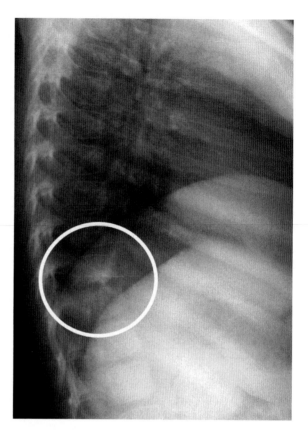

Figure 104–3. Diskitis between T10 and T11 in a 3-year-old child.

Affected children can usually be managed as outpatients, with antibiotic therapy directed against *S. aureus*. Despite treatment, older children commonly develop spontaneous spinal fusion.

▶ LYME DISEASE

Lyme disease is the most common tick-born illness in North America and Europe. In the United States, Lyme disease is caused by the spirochete *Borrelia burgdorferi* and is most often acquired from the bite of the *Ixodes scapularis* tick, commonly known as the deer tick. The initial presentation is with a skin lesion known as erythema migrans. If not treated, 60% will go on to develop monoarticular or oligoarticular arthritis. For further discussion of Lyme disease, (see Chapter 65).

▶ ACUTE SUPPURATIVE TENOSYNOVITIS

Acute suppurative tenosynovitis usually begins as a localized infection that then extends to involve the synovial sheath surrounding the flexor tendon of the finger. If infection penetrates beyond the synovial sheath, it can spread to the deep spaces of the palm. When infection is limited to the tendon sheath, physical examination of the hand reveals erythema and tenderness along the course of the sheath. Patients hold the affected finger in a flexed position and active or passive extension provokes intense pain. The affected finger is diffusely swollen.

The most common bacterial etiologies are *S. aureus* and group A *Streptococcus*. In adolescents and sexually abused children, *N. gonorrhoeae* is also a possibility. Management consists of antibiotics and surgical drainage.

REFERENCES

1. Lampe RM. Osteomyelitis and suppurative arthritis. In: Behrman RE, Kliegman RM, Jenson HB, eds. *Nelson Textbook of Pediatrics*. 17th ed. Philadelphia, PA: WB Saunders, 2004.

2. Gutierrez K. Bone and joint infections in children. *Pediatr Clin North Am*. 2005;52:779.

3. Arnold SR, Elias D, Buckingham SC, et al. Changing patterns of acute hematogenous osteomyelitis and septic arthritis. *J Pediatr Orthop*. 2006;26:703.

4. Osteomyelitis/septic arthritis caused by *Kingella kingae* among day care attendees-Minnesota, 2003. *MMWR Morb Mortal Wkly Rep*. 2004;53:244.

5. Chometon S, Benito Y, Chaker M, et al. Specific real-time polymerase chain reaction places *Kingella kingae* as the most common cause of osteoarticular infections in young children. *Pediatr Infect Dis J*. 2007;25:377.

6. Klein DM, et al. Sensitivity of objective parameters in the diagnosis of pediatric septic hips. *Clin Orthop*. 1997;338:153.

7. Kallio MJT, et al. Serum C-reactive protein, erythrocyte sedimentation rate and white blood cell count in septic arthritis of children. *Pediatr Infect Dis J*. 1997;16:411.

8. Frank G, Mahoney HM, Eppes SC. Musculoskeletal infections in children. *Pediatr Clin North Am*. 2005;52:1083–1106.

9. Kocher M, Zurakowski D, Kasser J. Differentiating between septic arthritis and transient synovitis of the hip in children. An evidence-based clinical prediction algorithm. *J Bone Joint Surg Am*. 1999;81:1662.

10. Kocher M, Mandiga R, Zurakowski D, et al. Validation of a clinical prediction rule for differentiation between septic arthritis and transient synovitis of the hip in children. *J Bone Joint Surg Am*. 2004;86:1629.

11. Luhmann S, Jones A, Schootman M, et al. Differentiation between septic arthritis and transient synovitis of the hip in children with clinical prediction algorithms. *J Bone Joint Surg Am*. 2004;86:956.

12. Frick SL. Evaluation of the child who has hip pain. *Orthop Clin North Am*. 2006;37:133.

13. Yang WJ, Im SA, Lim GY, et al. MR imaging of transient synovitis: differentiation from septic arthritis. *Pediatr Radiol*. 2006;36:1154.

14. Kaplan SL. Osteomyelitis in children. *Infect Dis Clin North Am*. 2005;19:787–797.

15. Fernandez M, Carrol CL, Baker CJ. Discitis and vertebral osteomyelitis in children: an 18-year review. *Pediatrics*. 2000;105:1299–1304.

CHAPTER 105

Inflammatory Musculoskeletal Disorders

Kemedy K. McQuillen

► HIGH-YIELD FACTS

- Toxic synovitis of the hip is an inflammatory process that often follows an upper respiratory infection. The disorder is usually seen in children between the ages of 3 and 6 years of age. The most common complaint is a refusal to walk.
- In the absence of fever, an elevated white blood cell count, or elevated erythrocyte sedimentation rate, septic joint is unlikely and the diagnosis of transient synovitis can be made without obtaining joint fluid.
- Systemic lupus erythematosus (SLE) is an autoimmune inflammatory disease that affects multiple organ systems. Fifteen to twenty percent of cases of SLE begin in childhood or adolescence.
- Therapy for SLE is directed primarily at ameliorating the underlying inflammatory process. NSAIDs, glucocorticoids, immunosuppressants, and biologic agents are treatment options.
- The diagnosis of acute rheumatic fever (ARF) is made by utilizing a combination of clinical and laboratory findings summarized in the revised Jones criteria.
- Patients with suspected ARF are admitted to the hospital. Penicillin is indicated to eradicate any residual carriage of group A β-hemolytic *Streptococcus*.
- Spondyloarthropathies include enthesitis-related arthritis (formerly known as juvenile ankylosing spondylitis), psoriatic arthritis, inflammatory bowel disease–related arthropathies, and reactive arthritis.
- Enthesitis-related arthritis is a rheumatic disorder that can present in later childhood or adolescence. The disorder is predominantly characterized by involvement of the sacroiliac joints and lumbar spine, but patients may also have peripheral arthritis.
- The treatment of reactive arthritis is with anti-inflammatory agents: the role of antibiotic treatment is unclear; however, it may be helpful if *Chlamydia trachomatis* is the inciting infection.
- In juvenile idiopathic arthritis (JIA), polyarticular disease involves more than four joints and rheumatoid factor may be present or absent.
- Pauciarticular JIA involves four or fewer joints. Leg joints are most commonly affected, but hip involvement is unusual.
- Systemic onset JIA occurs throughout childhood. Intermittent spiking fever may be the initial manifestation of disease.
- The treatment of JIA consists of aggressive therapy with NSAIDs. For pauciarticular disease, intra-articular steroids may be used. Systemic steroids, cytotoxic drugs, and biological medications may also be effective.

► TRANSIENT SYNOVITIS

Transient synovitis, also known as toxic synovitis, is the most common cause of hip pain in childhood.[1] It is a self-limited inflammatory condition caused by a nonpyogenic inflammatory response of the synovium. Its peak incidence is between 3 and 6 years of age. Transient synovitis of the hip affects boys more commonly than girls and has a slight predilection for the right side. Less than 5% of cases are bilateral. Though most commonly affecting the hip, transient synovitis can also affect the knee. The etiology of transient synovitis is unknown. Current theories imply an association with active or recent infection, trauma, or allergic hypersensitivity. At least half the children with transient synovitis have or recently have had an upper respiratory illness.[2]

In transient synovitis, hip or groin pain is the most common initial symptom, but referred pain to the medial aspect of the thigh or knee is found in 10% to 30% of patients. Affected patients either walk with a limp or, with severe pain, refuse to walk at all. The leg is held in flexion with slight abduction and external rotation. On examination, passive movement is usually pain-free; however, there may be pain and a slightly decreased range of motion with extreme internal rotation or abduction. Although most children with transient synovitis tend to otherwise be well, some will have a low-grade fever and malaise.

The diagnosis of transient synovitis is one of exclusion and relies on the history and physical examination in combination with limited laboratory testing and radiographs (AP and "frog-leg" lateral views of the pelvis). Laboratory tests are used to help differentiate children with transient synovitis from those with septic arthritis. In transient synovitis, laboratory values may be normal or may reveal mild elevations in the white blood cell count and erythrocyte sedimentation rate (ESR). Clinical decision rules have been developed to help differentiate transient synovitis from septic arthritis. These rules are based on the presence or absence of fever, the ability to bear weight, white blood cell (WBC) counts, inflammatory markers (ESR and CRP), side-to-side differences in the width of the joint space on radiographs, and prior visits to a health care provider.[3,4] Although the overlap of laboratory values is too great to provide a foolproof diagnostic algorithm to differentiate transient synovitis from septic arthritis, patients with septic arthritis tends to be more febrile and have significantly elevated WBC and ESR. In the absence of fever and without elevated WBC and ESR, septic joint is unlikely and the diagnosis of transient synovitis can be made without obtaining joint fluid. If there is any doubt about the diagnosis, immediate orthopedic consultation is necessary.

Although radiographs of the hip and pelvis tend to be normal in transient synovitis, they are helpful in excluding other diseases. Radiographic findings consistent with transient synovitis include medial joint space widening, an accentuated pericapsular shadow, and Waldenström's sign, which is lateral displacement of the femoral epiphysis with surface flattening secondary to effusion. However, these findings are also apparent in Legg–Calvé–Perthes (LCP) disease and, if present, mandate close follow-up or further investigation with MRI. If joint aspiration is necessary to clarify the diagnosis, ultrasonography can be used to guide hip joint aspiration. Effusions are present in 60% to 70% of cases of transient synovitis; however, they are also present in septic arthritis, osteomyelitis, acute slipped capital femoral epiphysis (SCFE), LCP disease, rheumatoid and infectious arthritis, malignancy, and osteoid osteoma. Therefore, the presence of an effusion on ultrasonography cannot be used to distinguish transient synovitis from other causes of hip pain.[5]

Treatment of transient synovitis is twofold: (1) rest via non–weight bearing or, in cases of extreme pain, bed rest and (2) reduction of synovitis with anti-inflammatory medications. Temperatures should be monitored closely and any fever should be reported to the physician. Children are allowed a gradual return to activity as the pain subsides and full, unrestricted activity is permitted when the hip is completely pain free with no evidence of a limp. Repeat examination is recommended for all children within 12 to 24 hours and then again after 10 to 14 days if the symptoms have not resolved.

The prognosis for children with transient synovitis is excellent. Up to 75% of patients have complete resolution of pain within 2 weeks and 88% within 4 weeks. The remainder may have less intense, but persistent pain for up to 8 weeks. Relapse is possible, though infrequent, and usually occurs within 6 months.

▶ SYSTEMIC LUPUS ERYTHEMATOSUS

Systemic lupus erythematosus (SLE) is a chronic but often episodic multisystem autoimmune disease with protean manifestations. Fifteen to twenty percent of cases of SLE are diagnosed in childhood with a median age of 12.2 years.[6] SLE is rare in those younger than 5 years.[7] The time from symptom onset to diagnosis ranges from 1 month to 3.3 years with a median of 4 months.[6] Female patients are preferentially affected with a female:male ration of 3:1 prepuberty and 9:1 after puberty. Native Americans, Hispanics, Chinese, and Filipinos are more susceptible to developing SLE and greater disease severity in seen in African Americans and Hispanics. SLE is a multigenic disease. Patients with lupus are more likely to have a relative with either lupus or another autoimmune disease such as thyroiditis or insulin-dependent diabetes.

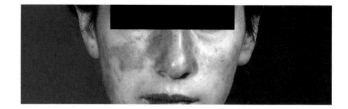

Figure 105–1. The characteristic malar rash of systemic lupus erythematosus. Note the extension across the cheeks and the nasal bridge with sparing of the nasolabial folds.

The most common presenting signs of pediatric SLE (pSLE) are rash, mucositis, and arthritis. Common constitutional symptoms include fever, fatigue/malaise, and weight loss. Skin, musculoskeletal and renal systems are the most common organ systems involved in pSLE. Skin manifestations have been reported in 50% to 80% of patients at the time of diagnosis and occur in approximately 85% of patients during the course of the disease. Mucocutaneous findings include malar rash (Fig. 105–1), photosensitivity, vasculitic lesions with nodules or ulcerations, palmar and plantar erythema, alopecia, and, less commonly, discoid lupus or lupus profundus. The appearance of a malar rash often heralds a disease flare. Oral and nasal mucosa may manifest hyperemia, petechial rashes on the hard palate or painless ulcerations. Sun exposure can exacerbate the skin disease of lupus and can also cause a systemic flare. Avoidance of sunbathing and the use of protective clothing and sunscreen are recommended.

Most patients with pSLE will have musculoskeletal involvement such as arthritis, arthralgia, myalgia, diffuse muscle weakness, tenosynovitis, periostitis, and, less commonly, myositis. The arthritis of pSLE tends to be nonerosive and nondeforming. It is painful, symmetric, and polyarticular and can affect small or large joints. Clinically, the patient's pain and tenderness may be disproportionately greater than the degree of swelling would suggest. This is in contrast to most patients with JIA, who often have markedly swollen joints but complain of only mild discomfort. With joint involvement, prolonged morning stiffness is also common.

Approximately 10% of patients with pSLE also develop avascular necrosis due to the illness itself or as a consequence of steroid therapy. Hips and knees are most commonly affected. Lupus and steroid therapy may also cause osteoporosis and vertebral fractures.

Approximately 75% of children with pSLE will have renal involvement, usually within 2 years of disease onset. Renal disease is the leading cause of serious morbidity and mortality in SLE. Early findings include microscopic hematuria and proteinuria; however, hypertension, decreased glomerular filtration rate, azotemia, and renal failure may develop. Lupus nephritis classification is based on histopathology and can range from normal by light microscopy (class I) to advanced sclerotic nephritis (class VI). It is difficult to predict the histologic lesion based on clinical and laboratory findings. Since treatment differs for differing forms of SLE nephritis, renal biopsy is warranted. Most patients with lupus nephritis have constitutional symptoms that may include fever, malaise, anorexia, and weight loss. Renal flares are common and can frequently be detected by increasing proteinuria before constitutional symptoms develop.

Central nervous system (CNS) disease is the second leading cause of serous morbidity and mortality in SLE and is difficult to diagnose because of vague and varied complaints. Headache is the most common neuropsychiatric manifestation. Severe unremitting headache may reflect vasculitis, cerebral vein thrombosis (CVT), CNS infection, pseudotumor cerebri or organic brain syndrome. CVT may present without other CNS manifestations and is almost always associated with the presence of lupus anticoagulant. Other neuropsychiatric manifestations of pSLE include psychosis, altered mental status, cognitive dysfunction, cerebrovascular disease, seizures, movement disorders, neuropathy, and transverse myelitis.

Hematologic abnormalities include anemia, which may be from hemolysis, but most commonly reflects the presence of chronic disease. Thrombocytopenia can occur, as can leukopenia. Involvement of serosal membranes, including the pleura, peritoneum, and pericardium, is a prominent aspect of SLE and leads to complications that include pleuritis with or without pleural effusion, peritonitis, and pericarditis. Pericarditis can occasionally result in a clinically significant pericardial effusion. Cardiac complications include myocarditis, endocarditis, and premature atherosclerosis causing coronary artery disease. Pulmonary disease includes pneumonitis and, infrequently, pulmonary hemorrhage or pulmonary hypertension. Shrinking lung syndrome may also occur and results from diaphragmatic dysfunction that elevates the lung, resulting in decreased lung volume. Gastrointestinal disease is uncommon in pSLE but may include pancreatitis, mesenteric vasculitis, and hepatitis.

The differential diagnosis of SLE is vast, and it is unlikely that the initial diagnosis will be made in the emergency department. To confirm SLE, it is necessary to integrate data from the history, physical, and laboratory results. Important disorders to exclude in the emergency department are malignancies, especially leukemia, acute rheumatic fever, JIA, and infectious processes. Drug-induced lupus is seen in children as well as adults. The medications most commonly implicated are anticonvulsants (phenytoin and carbamazepine), isoniazid, and minocycline.[8] If a patient with SLE symptoms is taking these medications, they should be stopped immediately.

In all patients with suspected SLE, a complete blood count, prothrombin time (PT), international normalized ratio (INR), partial thromboplastin time (PTT), serum electrolytes, blood urea nitrogen, creatinine, erythrocyte sedimentation rate (ESR), and C-reactive protein (CRP) are indicated. Urinalysis will often reveal microscopic hematuria and proteinuria. If there is evidence of coagulopathy, lupus anticoagulant and antiphospholipid antibody tests are indicated. Antinuclear antibody (ANA), other autoantibodies, rheumatoid factor, complement studies, and quantitative immunoglobulins are indicated, but the results will not be available in the emergency department. ANA is a good screening test for SLE because it is positive in almost all patients who have active disease. Unfortunately, it is not specific and may be positive in up to 33% of healthy patients. Antibodies to double-stranded DNA (anti-ds DNA) are more specific to SLE and are found in 60% to 70% of patients with SLE.[6]

Over the course of the illness, children with SLE develop malar rash, neurologic features (headache, chorea, seizures), and renal disease more frequently than do adults. Hematologic and renal involvement tends to be worse in pediatric SLE than in adult SLE. Over the past several years, the overall prognosis of patients with pSLE has improved due to earlier diagnosis and improved treatments.[9] Pediatric SLE now has a 92% 5-year survival rate and an 85% 10-year survival rate.[7] The primary causes of death are renal disease, infection, and CNS disease.

Treatment of SLE includes NSAIDs, steroids, immunosuppressants, and biologic agents; the choice of medication depends on the extent of organ system involvement. Mild skin and joint manifestations may be controlled with NSAIDs and hydroxychloroquine.[9] Hydroxychloroquine can also be used to reduce fatigue, mucocutaneous symptoms, and alopecia. Methotrexate can be used for more extensive arthritis. Internal organ system disease, especially CNS, renal, and hematologic disease, requires the use of glucocorticoids, often in high doses. Patients with acute, severe symptoms may require high-dose pulse therapy with intravenous glucocorticoids. Intravenous immunoglobulin may be helpful for chorea and thrombocytopenia. In extremely severe cases, such as rapidly progressive renal disease, immunosuppressive agents, such as cyclophosphamide or azathioprine, are added to glucocorticoid therapy. Mycophenolate mofetil (MMF), an immunosuppressant that inhibits B and T lymphocyte proliferation, is also beneficial. Many biologic agents are being tested for the treatment of SLE. These medications target specific cytokines and costimulatory molecules or attempt to enhance B-cell tolerance. Autologous stem cell transplant has also been used successfully in adults with severe, refractory SLE.

▶ RHEUMATIC FEVER

Acute rheumatic fever (ARF) is an autoimmune systemic inflammatory response to infection with group A β-hemolytic *Streptococcus* (GAβHS). ARF occurs after GAβHS pharyngitis but is not associated with streptoccocal infections of the skin. In developing areas of the world, the incidence of ARF exceeds 50 per 100 000 children with rates as high as 350 per 100 000 children in aboriginal children of northern Australia.[10] Worldwide, rheumatic heart disease (RHD), a complication of ARF, is the most common form of acquired heart disease in all age groups and accounts for up to 50% of all cases of cardiovascular disease in many developing countries.[11] In the United States, the rate of ARF are less than 10 per 100 000 children. By the early 1980s, some areas of the United States had an annual incidence as low as 0.5/100 000 children. Beginning in the mid-1980s, however, there have been outbreaks of ARF in Salt Lake City, Ohio, western Pennsylvania, Tennessee, New York City, Missouri, and Texas, as well among military recruits in San Diego and at the Fort Leonard Wood Training base in Missouri.[11]

The incidence of ARF peaks between 5 and 15 years of age.[11] Only 5% of episodes arise in children younger than 5 years and the disease is almost unheard of in children younger than 2 years.[10] It is most common during the winter and spring. Although ARF generally develops 2 to 4 weeks following the inciting infection, it may present weeks to months later. One-third of children do not recall an antecedent sore throat. ARF is more common in girls.

The main clinical features of ARF are outlined in the modified Jones Criteria (Table 105–1).[12] The World Health Organization (WHO) has also developed criteria to aid in diagnosing

▶ **TABLE 105–1. DIAGNOSIS OF RHEUMATIC FEVER (REVISED JONES CRITERIA)**[*†]

Evidence of Antecedent GAβHS Infection
Positive throat culture or rapid antigen test for GAβHS
Raised or rising streptococcal antibody titer (antistreptolysin O, anti-DNase B or antihyaluronidase)

Major Manifestation: J♥NES
J: Joints (Polyarthritis)
♥: Carditis
N: Nodules (subcutaneous nodules)
E: Erythema marginatum
S: Sydenham chorea

Minor Manifestation
Arthralgia
Fever
Elevated ESR or CRP concentrations
Prolonged PR interval on electrocardiogram

Recurrent Acute Rheumatic Fever
One major or several minor manifestations *plus*
evidence of antecedent GAβHS infection

---

[*]Diagnosis requires two major *or* one major and two minor manifestations *plus* evidence of antecedent GAβHS infection.
[†]Chorea and indolent carditis do not require evidence of antecedent GAβHS infection.

ARF (Table 105–2). The WHO criteria are less stringent than the revised Jones criteria to reflect the increased incidence of ARF in developing countries. The Jones and the WHO criteria are only diagnostic guidelines and can be adapted. This is especially important in populations at high risk for ARF so that there is greater sensitivity for disease detection. There are five major and four minor Jones manifestations as well as an absolute requirement for evidence of a recent GAβHS infection. The diagnosis of ARF can be established by the Jones criteria with two major manifestations or one major and two minor manifestations PLUS, in both instances, evidence of recent GAβHS infection. In two instances, ARF can be diagnosed

▶ **TABLE 105–2. DIAGNOSIS OF RHEUMATIC FEVER (WHO CRITERIA)**[*]

First episode
As per Jones criteria

Recurrent episode
Patients without established rheumatic heart disease:
  As per first episode
Patients with established rheumatic heart disease:
  2 minor manifestations

plus
  Evidence of antecedent GAβHS infection
    Positive throat culure or rapid antigen test for GAβHS
    Raised or rising streptococcal antibody titer
    (antistreptolysin O, anti-DNase B or antihyaluronidase)
    Recent scarlet fever

---

[*]Chorea and indolent carditis do not require evidence of antecedent GAβHS infection.

without strict adherence to the Jones criteria: chorea and indolent carditis that is diagnosed months after the onset of ARF.

Joint complaints are common in ARF and range from arthralgias to frank arthritis. Arthralgia is a minor manifestation of ARF in the absence of arthritis as a major criterion. The arthralgias are especially intense at night and can wake children from sleep. Pain is out of proportion to the clinical findings. Arthritis is a major manifestation of ARF and occurs in approximately 75% of cases. Classically, it involves larger joints, especially the knees, ankles, wrists, and elbows and is migratory (moves from joint to joint). Monoarticular arthritis is less common but may occur, especially with early use of anti-inflammatory medications. Synovial fluid in ARF usually has 10 000 to 100 000 white blood cells/mm^3 with a predominance of neutrophils, protein of ≥ 4g/dL, normal glucose, and the ability to form a good mucin clot.[11] ARF arthritis responds dramatically to salicylates. There tends to be an inverse relationship between the severity of the arthritis and the severity of carditis. Joint symptoms of ARF tend to resolve within a month and leave no permanent damage.

Patients with arthritis that is not typical of ARF but who have recently had a streptococcal infection may have post-streptococcal reactive arthritis (PSRA). PSRA typically develops 3 to 14 days after streptococcal pharyngitis. It is nonmigratory and can affect small and large joints as well as the axial skeleton. It responds poorly to anti-inflammatory treatment and is unaffected by antimicrobial therapy. PSRA may last from 1 week to 8 months with a mean duration of 2 months.[13] Laboratory evaluation of patients with PSRA shows a normal WBC count with an elevated ESR. Throat culture or rapid antigen test for GAβHS may be positive. Antibodies suggestive of a recent streptococcal infection may or may not be present at presentation but should manifest 3 to 4 weeks after initial evaluation. Approximately 5% of patients with PSRA develop carditis and some authors suggest echocardiography at presentation and one year later. Because of the risk of carditis, patients with PSRA should receive antimicrobial prophylaxis with penicillin or erythromycin, to prevent recurrent streptococcal infection, for one year if carditis is not detected and for a minimum of 5 years if carditis develops.[13]

Carditis occurs in 50% to 60% of cases of ARF. Rheumatic carditis is characterized by pancarditis, with inflammation of the peri-, myo- and endocardium. Endocarditis (valvulitis) is universal while the presence of myocarditis and pericarditis is variable. Carditis and the resultant rheumatic heart disease (RHD) account for most of the morbidity and mortality associated with ARF. The carditis can be clinically silent or severe enough to result in congestive heart failure. Acute rheumatic carditis usually presents with tachycardia and a cardiac murmur related to valvulitis. The mitral valve is most commonly involved, with or without involvement of the aortic valve. Valvular insufficiency is characteristic of acute and convalescent stages of ARF with valvular stenosis appearing years to decades after the acute illness. Echocardiographic findings in acute ARF may include pericardial effusion, decreased ventricular contractility, or mitral and/or aortic regurgitation. Echocardiographic demonstration of valvular insufficiency without auscultatory corroboration does not satisfy the Jones criteria for carditis. Patients with valvulitis are at risk for developing infective endocarditis.

Sydenham chorea, which is due to an autoimmune insult to the basal ganglia,[14] occurs in 10% to 15% of patients and may be the only manifestation of ARF. Chorea usually presents as involuntary choreiform movements and facial grimacing that are exacerbated by stress and disappear with sleep. Mild cases may present with restlessness and clumsiness. The motor movements may be unilateral. Symptoms are often preceded by behavioral disturbances including emotional lability, personality changes, anxiety, and poor school performance. Some patients may have "Sydenham speech" that is characterized by bursts of dysarthric speech. The time to development of chorea (1–6 months) is longer than for arthritis or carditis, and because of the insidious onset of symptoms and delays in diagnosis, streptococcal antibodies may be decreasing or undetectable when the patient presents. Physical findings of chorea include irregular contractions of the hands when squeezing the examiner's finger (milkmaid's grip), spooning and pronation of the hands when the arms are extended and wormian movements of the tongue upon protrusion. The patient and family may also notice alterations in handwriting. The duration of chorea varies, but it is a self-limited process. Recurrence has been reported in 20% to 60% of patients and usually occurs within 2 years of initial presentation.[14] Sixty-three to ninety-four percent of patients with Sydenham chorea will also have cardiac involvement.[14]

The dermatologic manifestations of ARF are infrequent and include erythema marginatum and subcutaneous nodules. Erythema marginatum is a nonpruritic, erythematous, serpiginous macule with a pale center. It occurs on the trunk and extremities and tends to spare the face. It is accentuated by warming the skin.[11] Subcutaneous nodules are firm, painless nodules along the extensor surface of the tendons near bony prominences. They are approximately 1 cm in diameter.

The differential diagnosis of ARF is extensive and variable based on the findings at the time of presentation. ARF arthritis may mimic findings associated with septic arthritis, juvenile idiopathic arthritis, reactive arthritis, serum sickness, malignancies, systemic lupus erythematosus, Lyme disease, idiopathic juvenile arthritis, and sickle cell disease.

Diagnostic evaluation for ARF includes throat culture and rapid antigen testing for GAβHS, titers for antistreptolysin O, anti-DNase B, antihyaluronidase, ESR, and CRP. An electrocardiogram is indicated as is an echocardiogram to assess heart size as well as the structural and functional integrity of the valves. A chest radiograph can exclude congestive heart failure.

Patients with suspected ARF are admitted to the hospital. Ten days of orally administered penicillin or erythromycin or a single intramuscular injection of benzathine penicillin is indicated to eradicate GAβHS infection. Patients with arthritis but without carditis are managed with high-dose aspirin (100 mg/kg/d in four divided doses). Consideration should be given to withholding anti-inflammatories if arthralgia or atypical arthritis is the only manifestation of presumed ARF. Acetaminophen or another pain medication can be used while the patient is observed for more definitive signs of ARF. Patients with carditis and cardiomegaly or congestive heart failure are treated with prednisone (2 mg/kg/d in four divided doses). Digoxin, fluid and salt restriction, diuretics, and oxygen may also be beneficial. Chorea may respond to haloperidol, thorazine, valproic acid, or carbamazepine.

Patients with ARF are vulnerable to recurrent attacks that may cause or exacerbate valvular damage. Recurrent attacks can be prevented by prophylactic administration of antibiotics, most commonly by injections of benzathine penicillin administered every 3 to 4 weeks. Alternatively, oral penicillin may be used if careful compliance can be ensured. First attacks can be prevented by prompt treatment of streptococcal pharyngitis, but care should be given to avoid inappropriate overtreatment of non-streptococcal infections with antibiotics.

► SPONDYLOARTHROPATHIES

Spondyloarthropathies include enthesitis-related arthritis (formerly known as juvenile ankylosing spondylitis), psoriatic arthritis, inflammatory bowel disease–related arthritis, and reactive arthritis. The typical characteristics of each entity are outlined in Table 105–3. The spondyloarthropathies are characterized by inflammation of joints of the axial skeleton and limbs, the presence of enthesitis, and by the absence of rheumatoid factor. Tenosynovitis and periostitis may also occur. Enthesitis is characterized by chronic inflammation at the sites of tendon, ligament, fascia, and capsule attachment to bone. Tenderness from enthesitis may be noted in the chest wall, iliac crest, ischial tuberosity, posterior or plantar surface of the heel, metatarsophalangeal area, and anterior tibial tuberosity. The

► TABLE 105–3. CHARACTERISTICS OF SPONDYLOARTHROPATHIES

Type	Gender	Age	Type of Inflammation	Joints	Other
Enthesitis-related arthritis (juvenile ankylosing spondylitis)	M >> F	Adolescence, adulthood	Oligoarthritis Enthesitis	Axial skeleton SI joints Legs > arms	HLA-B27(+) > 90%
Psoriatic arthritis	F >> M	Childhood	Oligoarthritis	Extremities	HLA-B27(−)
Inflammatory bowel disease arthropathies	M > F	Any age	Polyarthritis	Extremities	Reflects activity of GI inflammation HLA-B27(−)
Inflammatory bowel disease arthropathies	M > F	Any age	Oligoarthritis	SI joints Extremities	Independent of GI inflammation HLA-B27(+)
Reactive arthritis	M > F	Any age	Oligoarthritis	Legs > arms	HLA-B27 (+) ~30%–50% (16)

inflammatory changes result in calcification of ligaments and fusion of joints in adulthood.

ENTHESITIS-RELATED ARTHRITIS (JUVENILE ANKYLOSING SPONDYLITIS)

Although enthesitis-related arthritis in children tends to have a greater frequency of extra-axial symptoms than in adults, it is still considered to belong to the group of spondyloarthropathies. Involved joints may include the spine (see Fig. 105–3), sacroiliac joints, and lower extremities, including the hips. During the first 6 months of disease, hip joint arthritis may be the only finding. Patients often complain of hip, back, and thigh pain that is worse at night and improves with movement. Upper extremity involvement is uncommon and more suggestive of another type of juvenile idiopathic arthritis. Systemic symptoms include fatigue and low-grade fever. Enthesitis at characteristic locations around the foot and knee is common and is part of seronegative enthesitis and arthritis (SEA) syndrome with seronegativity referring to the absence of rheumatoid factor. SEA is probably the most common initial presentation of enthesitis-related arthritis.[15] Physical examination of patients with enthesitis-related arthritis may reveal tenderness over the sacroiliac joints and loss of range of motion of the lumbar spine. Radiographic evidence of sacroiliitis is absent until late in the disease. MRI is able to identify sacroiliitis much earlier. Acute, painful iridocyclitis occurs in up to 25% of patients with enthesitis-related arthritis. Less commonly, patients may have low-grade fever, aortic valve insufficiency, aortitis, muscle weakness, or atlantoaxial subluxation. The course of the disease is characterized by long periods of active disease interspersed with long periods of remission. Over the long term, the enthesitis-related arthritis may cause fusion of the spine and SI joints with significant disability.

PSORIATIC ARTHRITIS

Although psoriatic arthritis is most commonly an asymmetric oligoarthritis that affects the knees, ankles, and small joints of the hands and feet, it may present with symmetric distal interphalangeal joint disease or HLA-B27-associated sacroiliitis. The presence of a psoriatic rash, nail pitting, dactylitis, oncholysis, or a family history of psoriasis supports the diagnosis. Chronic iridocyclitis occurs in approximately 15% of children with psoriatic arthritis. Antinuclear antibodies may be present in up to 50% of affected patients. Psoriatic arthritis tends to be a chronic unremitting disease.

INFLAMMATORY BOWEL DISEASE–RELATED ARTHROPATHIES

Ulcerative colitis and Crohn disease may be complicated by two types of arthritis: a peripheral polyarthritis that is not a true spondyloarthropathy and is reflective of GI inflammation or, less commonly, an HLA-B27-associated spondyloarthropathy of the sacroiliac and peripheral joints that is independent of GI inflammation. Associated findings may include ery-

▶ **TABLE 105–4. FINDINGS ASSOCIATED WITH REACTIVE ARTHRITIS[16],[17]**

Constitutional Symptoms	Musculoskeletal
Fever	Arthritis
Malaise	Tenosynovitis
Weight loss	Periostitis
	Enthesitis
Skin	Sacroiliitis
Keratoderma blennorrhagica	Dactylitis
Balanitis circinata	
Oral ulcers	*Genitourinary*
Hyperkeratosis	Urethritis
Subungual keratosis	Cervicitis
Nail pits	Cystitis
Onycholysis	Hematuria
Cardiac	*Ocular*
Aortitis	Conjunctivitis
Aortic insufficiency	Acute anterior uveitis
Heart block	
Pericarditis	

thema nodosum, pyoderma gangrenosum, fever, weight loss, and anorexia. Although the peripheral arthritis of inflammatory bowel disease is usually controlled when the GI symptoms are controlled, the HLA-B27-associated arthritis tends to be more chronic.

REACTIVE ARTHRITIS

Reactive arthritis is usually preceded by a gastrointestinal infection with *Salmonella, Yersinia, Campylobacter,* or *Shigella,* or a GU infection with *Chlamydia trachomatis.* Although it is considered a sterile synovitis, bacterial degradation products and even bacterial DNA have been isolated in affected joints. Reactive arthritis is usually oligoarticular and may be associated with considerable pain, swelling, and erythema with symptoms starting 1 to 4 weeks after the inciting infection.[16] Associated findings are listed in Table 105–4. Approximately half of affected patients have resolution of symptoms within 6 months while the rest develop a chronic reactive arthritis that may exhibit a relapsing course.[16] Enthesitis may be prominent. HLA-B27 positive patients may develop sacroiliitis. Patients with post enteric reactive arthritis may develop mild chronic diarrhea.[16]

The diagnosis of spondyloarthropathy is based on historical and clinical features; laboratory evaluations are helpful in excluding other etiologies. Laboratory findings may include elevated markers of inflammation (ESR and CRP) as well as mildly elevated WBC and platelet counts. Rheumatoid factor is negative and antinuclear antibodies are absent except in psoriatic arthritis. HLA-B27 is very common in enthesitis-related arthritis (>90% of patients) and may also be found in the other spondyloarthropathies, especially if sacroiliitis or anterior uveitis is present. Radiographic changes may include periarticular osteoporosis, changes associated with enthesitis (loss of sharp cortical margins, erosions, bony spurs), indistinct margins and erosions of the SI joints, sclerosis on the iliac side of

Figure 105–2. Erythema marginatum: one of the major manifestations of acute rheumatic fever.

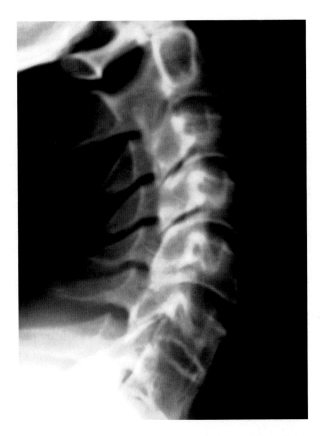

Figure 105–3. Radiograph of patient with enthesitis-related arthritis. Note the narrowed joint spaces between C6/C7 and C7/T1 with ankylosing of C6 to T1 vertebral bodies.

the joint, and squaring of the corners of the vertebral bodies (Fig. 105–2).

The primary treatment goals of the spondyloarthropathies are to control inflammation, minimize pain, and preserve function. NSAIDs, such as naproxen, may be sufficient. Sulfasalazine and intra-articular steroid injections may also be helpful. Although etanercept is approved for JIA as well as ankylosing spondylitis and psoriatic arthritis in adults, it is not yet approved for use in the pediatric spondyloarthropathies. The role of antibiotic treatment for reactive arthritis is unclear but may be beneficial when *Chlamydia trachomatis* is the inciting cause.[16,17] Physical therapy, along with education and exercise, plays an important role in maintaining function and flexibility. Patients with foot and ankle enthesitis may also benefit from custom fitted insoles.

▶ JUVENILE IDIOPATHIC ARTHRITIS

Juvenile idiopathic arthritis is a term that encompasses all forms of arthritis that begin before the age of 16 years, persist for more than 6 weeks, and have no identifiable cause. It is a diagnosis of exclusion.[18] The term juvenile idiopathic arthritis (JIA) has been adopted to replace juvenile rheumatoid arthritis in North America and juvenile chronic arthritis in Europe. The American College of Rheumatology (ACR), European League Against Rheumatism (EULAR), and International League of Associations for Rheumatology (ILAR) use three separate systems to classify patients. Developed in 1997, the ILAR classification system is the most recent and includes seven disease categories based on the features present in the first 6 months of illness (Table 105–5). JIA is the most common chronic rheumatic disease in childhood. Although its cause is unclear, it appears to be a complex genetic illness that involves multiple genes related to immunity and inflammation.

Polyarticular disease involves five or more joints during the first 6 months of disease. It is further categorized as rheumatoid factor-positive (RF[+]) or rheumatoid factor-negative (RF[–]) with RF[–] polyarthritis having at least three distinct subsets. RF[+] polyarthritis includes the presence of IgM rheumatoid factor on at least two occasions, at least 3 months apart. RF[+] polyarthritis is the same as adult RF[+] polyarthritis and is mainly seen in adolescent female patients. At presentation, small joints of the hands and feet tend to be affected; if large joints are affected, it is usually in association with small joint disease. Many patients have involvement of the axial skeleton including the cervical spine; severe cases can result in atlantoaxial instability. Some patients have involvement the cricoarytenoid joint, where it can result in hoarseness of the voice. The temporomandibular joint may also be affected. Boutonniere deformities (proximal interphalangeal joint flexion and distal interphalangeal joint hyperextension) and swan-neck deformities (proximal interphalangeal joint hyperextension and distal interphalangeal joint flexion) are common. Extra-articular manifestations include rheumatoid nodules in approximately 30% of patients and, much less frequently, aortic regurgitation.

RF[–] polyarthritis has a biphasic age of onset with an early peak between 2 and 4 years and a late peak between 6 and 12 years. Subsets include an early onset asymmetric arthritis that is associated with positive anti-nuclear antibodies (ANA), an

▶ **TABLE 105-5. JUVENILE IDIOPATHIC ARTHRITIS (JIA): THE ILAR CLASSIFICATION SYSTEM**[19,20]

Type	Frequency	Age at Onset	Gender	Arthritis	Joints
Systemic arthritis	10%–20%	Childhood	F = M	Symmetrical Polyarticular	Large and small
Oligoarthritis	50%–60%	Early childhood (<6 y)	F >>> M	Asymmetric	Lower extremities
RF [+] polyarthritis	5%–10%	Late childhood/ adolescence	F >> M	Symmetric	Small joints (+/– large joints)
RF [–] polyarthritis	20%–30%	Childhood	F >> M	Asymmetric or symmetric	Large and small
Enthesitis-related arthritis	1%–7%	Late childhood/ adolescence	M >> F	Oligoarticular	Lower extremities Axial skeleton SI joints
Psoriatic arthritis	2%–15%	Childhood		Asymmetrical	Small and large
Undifferentiated arthritis	11%–21%			Oligoarticular	

ILAR, International League of Associations for Rheumatology; RF, rheumatoid factor.

increased risk of iridocyclitis, and a strong HLA association; a polyarthritis that presents in school-aged children with symmetric large and small joint disease, an increased ESR, and a negative ANA; and a "dry synovitis" that is characterized by negligible joint swelling with significant joint stiffness, flexion contractures, and a normal or minimally elevated ESR.[18]

In RF[+] and RF[–] polyarthritis, affected joints are swollen and warm, with minimal or no erythema. Although there is discomfort on range of motion, joint pain is generally not severe. Systemic involvement in polyarticular disease includes fever, irritability, and occasional hepatomegaly. In severe cases, significant growth disturbances can occur. RF[+] polyarticular disease is characterized by progressive, diffuse joint involvement with early radiographic changes, especially in the hands and feet. RF[–] polyarticular disease has a variable outcome depending on its subtype.

Oligoarticular arthritis involves four or fewer joints during the first 6 months of disease. In the ILAR criteria, patients are excluded from this category if they have psoriasis, a family history of psoriasis and HLA B27-associated illness in a first degree relative, a positive RF test or if the disease occurs in a male patient older than 6 years. Knees are most commonly affected followed by the ankles. Fifty percent of patients will present with monoarticular disease affecting only the knee.[19] Acute phase reactants may be normal or moderately increased; infrequently ESR is very high. Patients with oligoarticular arthritis are frequently ANA positive (70%–80%), may develop an asymptomatic iridocyclitis (30%), and have a strong association with some HLA alleles.[18] Systemic manifestations of disease are generally mild. Patients may have persistent oligoarthritis, in which the disease remains confined to four or fewer joints, or they may develop an extended oligoarthritis, in which more than four joints become involved after the first 6 months. Risk factors for the development of extended oligoarthritis include ankle, wrist, or hand involvement, symmetric arthritis, arthritis of two to four joints and an elevated ANA titer and ESR.[18,19] The overall remission rate for oligoarthritis is 12% in patients with extended disease and 75% in patients with persistent disease.[19]

Systemic onset disease occurs throughout childhood. Diagnosis of systemic arthritis requires the presence of arthritis accompanied or preceded by at least 2 weeks of quotid-

ian fever plus typical evanescent rash (discrete, circumcised, salmon-colored, 2- to 10-mm macules on the trunk and proximal extremities that typically coincide with fever), hepatomegaly, splenomegaly, generalized lymphadenopathy, or serositis. The onset of joint disease may be significantly delayed, which can obscure the diagnosis of JIA. Patients may be ill-appearing and have myalgias and abdominal pain during episodes of fever. Laboratory findings include leukocytosis with a preponderance of neutrophils, elevated liver enzymes, microcytic anemia, thrombocytosis, and very high ESR and CRP concentrations. The ANA titer is rarely positive.[19] In approximately 50% of cases, systemic-onset JIA is associated with a relapsing-remitting course in which arthritis accompanies episodes of fever and remits when systemic features are controlled. In the other 50% of patients, it is associated with an unremitting, debilitating arthritis with few systemic symptoms. Other complications include the development of pericarditis, which in some cases can result in a clinically significant pericardial effusion, myocarditis, or pleuritis. Very infrequently, patients develop amyloidosis.

A rare but life-threatening complication of systemic JIA is macrophage activation syndrome. This syndrome is characterized by the sudden onset of sustained fever, pancytopenia, hepatosplenomegaly, liver insufficiency, coagulopathy, and neurologic symptoms. Laboratory findings include pancytopenia, prolonged prothrombin and partial thromboplastin times, elevated fibrin split products, hypertriglyceridemia, hyponatremia, and increased ferritin concentrations. The ESR is often low.

The differential diagnosis of JIA includes ARF, SLE, bacterial arthritis, reactive arthritis, and neoplastic diseases, especially leukemia. In the emergency department, the workup of suspected JIA includes a complete blood count, renal function studies, and a rapid streptococcal screen. Tests for antinuclear antibodies and rheumatoid factors are indicated even though results are not immediately available. If a pyogenic arthritis is suspected, analysis of joint fluid is indicated. Patients with systemic-onset disease with evidence of myocarditis or pericarditis require an electrocardiogram and echocardiogram. It is difficult to make the diagnosis of JIA in the emergency department; consultation with a pediatric rheumatologist may be necessary. Especially in the case of systemic onset disease, hospitalization may be necessary.

Although JIA tends to be a chronic illness, there has been great improvement in functional outcome over the past decade. Indicators of poor outcome include greater severity or extension of arthritis at onset, symmetrical disease, early wrist or hip involvement, presence of RF, persistent active disease, and early radiographic changes.[20]

The treatment of JIA consists of physical and occupational therapy to maintain and improve range of motion, muscle strength, and skills for daily activities. Splints may be used to prevent contractures. Aggressive treatment with NSAIDs is the initial treatment for most patients with JIA. For pauciarticular disease, intraarticular steroids may be used. For cases that do not respond to NSAIDs, glucocorticoids, cytotoxic drugs such as methotrexate or biological medications such as etanercept and infliximab may be effective.[21,22] Sulfasalazine is effective in patients with extended oligoarticular JIA[21,22] and juvenile spondyloarthropathies. Patients with severe pericarditis or myocarditis, which can occur in systemic onset disease, may respond to therapy with prednisone. Macrophage activation syndrome is treated with high-dose steroids and cyclosporin.

REFERENCES

1. Mac Ewen GD, Dehse R. The limping child. *Pediatr Rev.* 1991;12:268.
2. Koop S, Quanbeck D. Three common causes of childhood hip pain. *Pediatr Clin North Am.* 1996;43:1053.
3. Kocher M, Zurakowski D, Kasser J. Differentiating between septic arthritis and transient synovitis of the hip in children. An evidence-based clinical prediction algorithm. *J Bone Joint Surg Am.* 1999;81:1662.
4. Luhmann S, Jones A, Schootman M, et al. Differentiation between septic arthritis and transient synovitis of the hip in children with clinical prediction algorithms. *J Bone Joint Surg Am.* 2004;86:956.
5. Zamzam MM. The role of ultrasound in differentiating septic arthritis from transient synovitis of the hip in children. *J Pediatr Orthop B.* 2006;15:418.
6. Benseler SM, Silverman ED. Systemic lupus erythematosus. *Pediatr Clin North Am.* 2005;52:443.
7. Gottlieb BS, Ilowite NT. Systemic lupus erythematosus in children and adolescents. *Pediatr Rev.* 2006;27:323.
8. Tucker LB. Making the diagnosis of systemic lupus erythematosus in children and adolescents. *Lupus.* 2007;16:546.
9. Kone-Paut I, Piram M, Guillaume S, et al. Lupus in adolescence. *Lupus.* 2007;16:606.
10. Carapetis JR, McDonald M, Wilson NJ. Acute rheumatic fever. *Lancet.* 2005;366:155.
11. Gerber MA. Group A Streptococcus. In Behrman RE, Kliegman RM, Jenson HB, eds. *Nelson Textbook of Pediatrics.* 17th ed. Philadelphia, PA: WB Saunders; 2004.
12. Special writing group of the committee on rheumatic fever. Guidelines for the diagnosis of acute rheumatic fever: Jones criteria, 1992 update. *JAMA.* 1992;268:2069.
13. Ahmed S, Ayoub EM. Poststreptococcal reactive arthritis. *Pediatr Infec Dis J.* 2001;20:1081.
14. Weiner SG, Normandin PA. Sydenham chorea: a case report and review of the literature. *Pediatr Emerg Care.* 2007; 23:20.
15. Miller ML, Petty RE. Ankylosing spondylitis and other spondyloarthropathies. In Behrman RE, Kliegman RM, Jenson HB, eds. *Nelson Textbook of Pediatrics.* 17th ed. Philadelphia, PA: WB Saunders; 2004.
16. Carter JD. Reactive arthritis: defined etiologies, emerging pathophysiology, and unresolved treatment. *Infect Dis Clin North Am.* 2006;20:827.
17. Flores D, Marquez J, Garza M, et al. Reactive arthritis: newer developments. *Rheum Dis Clin North Am.* 2003;29:37.
18. Hannu t, Inman R, Granfors K, et al. Reactive arthritis or postinfectious arthritis? *Best Prac Res Clin Rheum.* 2006;20:419.
19. Ravelli A, Martini A. Juvenile idiopathic arthritis. *Lancet.* 2007;369:767.
20. Weiss JE, Ilowite NT. Juvenile idiopathic arthritis. *Pediatr Clin North Am.* 2005;52:413.
21. Ravelli A, Martini A. Early predictors of outcome in juvenile idiopathic arthritis. *Clin Exp Rheumatol.* 2003;21:S89.
22. Hashkes PJ, Laxer RM. Medical treatment of juvenile idiopathic arthritis. *JAMA.* 2005;294:1671.
23. Guthrie B, Rouster-Stevens KA, Reynolds SL. Review of medications used in juvenile rheumatoid arthritis. *Pediatric Emerg Care.* 2007;23:38.

CHAPTER 106

Nonmalignant Tumors of Bone

Kemedy K. McQuillen

▶ HIGH-YIELD FACTS

- Many benign bone tumors are painless and are incidental findings on radiographs. They may also present with pain from the tumor or from a pathologic fracture.
- Osteoid osteoma is a relatively common benign tumor. It frequently causes pain that is worse at night and is exquisitely responsive to NSAIDs.
- Nonossifying fibromas are common fibrous lesions. They are often incidental findings but can also cause chronic pain.
- Osteochondromas tend to present as a bony, nonpainful mass. Radiographically they appear as sessile or pedunculated lesions of the long bones.
- Patients with enchondromas may present with a mass or pathologic fracture, but most are asymptomatic. The hands are most commonly involved.
- Solitary bone cysts in the lower extremity are prone to fracture and require excision.
- Aneurysmal bone cysts commonly involve the long bones. They are associated with rapidly progressive pain and swelling and can cause significant morbidity.

A number of histologically benign tumors of bone present in childhood. Many of these tumors are painless and are found incidentally on routine radiographs. Alternatively, they may present with pain from either the tumor itself or from a pathologic fracture.

▶ OSTEOID OSTEOMAS

Osteoid osteoma is a very common benign tumor of bone and accounts for 2% to 3% of all bone tumors and 10% to 20% of benign bone tumors.[1] It is two to three times more frequent in men and is most common between 5 and 20 years of age. Osteoid osteoma most commonly involves the long bones of the lower extremities but may occur in any bone including the spine and the short bones of the hands.

Pain is the most common presentation of osteoid osteoma and point tenderness at the site is usual. Patients initially have mild intermittent bone pain that becomes continuous and severe. The pain tends to be worse at night. The pain of osteoid osteoma is mediated by the proliferation of nerve endings in the tumor and a high level of prostaglandins in the nidus. This accounts for the exquisite responsiveness of the pain to nonsteroidal anti-inflammatory drugs (NSAIDs).[2] Patients may have point tenderness, a swollen limb, and/or a tender palpable mass. Alternatively, patients may present with a painless limp.

Osteoid osteomas in the joints may mimic arthropathy while those in the spine may present with stiff scoliosis, torticollis, hyperlordosis, or kyphoscoliosis. Osteoid osteomas that are close to the growth plates may lead to growth disturbance and limb length discrepancies or angular deviations. If the diagnosis of osteoid osteoma is delayed, patients may present with chronic pain or limping as well as atrophy of the affected limb.

Clinical history and standard radiographs are usually sufficient to diagnose osteoid osteoma. The typical radiographic appearance of a cortical osteoid osteoma is of a small (<1 cm) radiolucent round or oval area of osteolysis (nidus), surrounded by a regular ring of bony sclerosis (Fig. 106–1). The entire entity rarely exceeds 1.5 cm. In some cases, the center of the nidus may have an irregular nucleus of bone density giving a cockade appearance. The bone circumference may be increased. Cortical diaphyseal lesions may produce an oblong thickening to one side of the shaft. In these lesions, the nidus lies at the center of the thickening and may be contained within the primary cortex or oriented toward the endosteal or periosteal side of the bone. The surrounding reactive bone may be sufficiently dense as to obscure the nidus. With a medullary osteoid osteoma, osteosclerosis may be minimal or absent because of the lack of adjacent periosteum as the absence of periosteum limits the bone's ability to mount a proliferative response. If osteosclerosis is present with a medullary osteoid osteoma, it may be located away from the lesion. Joint space widening may occur in the presence of synovitis. Osteoid osteomas of the spine typically involve the posterior elements and may be difficult to visualize on plain radiographs; films may be normal or demonstrate only osteosclerosis.[2]

If conventional radiography is insufficient, computed tomography (CT) and isotope bone scans may aid in the diagnosis of osteoid osteoma. CT using bone windows will show the nidus of the osteoid osteoma as a well-defined, rounded area of decreased attenuation with a smooth periphery. This is surrounded by a variable amount of reactive sclerosis. The hypervascular nidus of an osteoid osteoma may also be demonstrated on a contrast-enhanced CT scan. Because of the small size of the tumor, however, the CT scan should be performed in thin sections (1–2 mm). On bone scans, osteoid osteomas exhibit a small, rounded area of intense uptake (the nidus) centered in a less intensely positive and more diffuse halo (peripheral hypervascularization and sclerosis). This is called the double density sign and is best visualized using a pinhole magnification at the site of increased uptake. Magnetic resonance imaging (MRI) is inferior to CT in diagnosing osteoid osteomas and is rarely necessary.[3,4]

When clinical and radiographic data are typical of an osteoid osteoma there is no need for histologic confirmation.

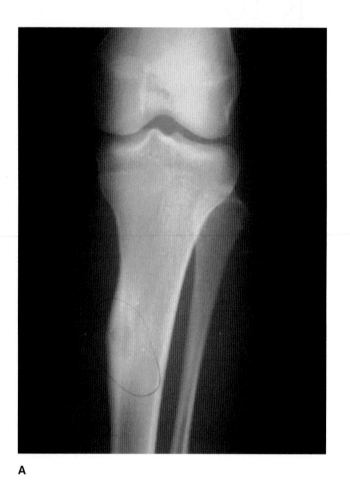

A

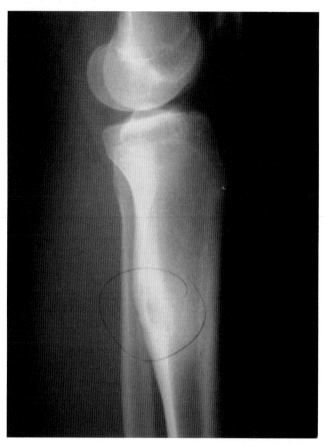

B

Figure 106–1. Osteoid osteoma of the proximal tibia.

Osteoid osteomas tend to be nonprogressive and may resolve over the course of several years. Medical management with prolonged use of NSAIDs is an option but, in many cases, severe pain, intolerance of NSAIDs, and disuse muscle atrophy mandates removal of the nidus. Surgical removal of the lesion is curative. Techniques include wide surgical excision, intralesional excision with minimal bone removal, arthroscopic, CT and MRI-guided core drill excision, injection of ethanol, interstitial laser photocoagulation, radiofrequency ablation, and a variety of minimally invasive surgeries. If the nidus is not removed completely, the patient may have persistent pain.

▶ NONOSSIFYING FIBROMAS

Nonossifying fibromas (NOF), also known as fibrous cortical defects, metaphyseal fibrous defects, and cortical desmoids, are extremely common fibrous lesions seen in up to 40% of preadolescents and adolescents.[5] They are rarely found in adults and, when followed radiographically over time, usually fill in with normal bone during adolescence.[6] They tend to be asymptomatic and are usually discovered incidentally but occasionally present with pain from a pathologic fracture. Infrequently, the fibroma may cause chronic pain. NOFs may occur in multiple bones.

Radiographs reveal an eccentric lucency in the metaphyseal cortex that has sharp margins and surrounding sclerosis. Lesions may be multilocular and expansile with extension into the medullary bone.[5] The long axis of the fibroma parallels the long axis of the bone. With an overlying stress fracture and associated periosteal reaction, NOFs may be mistaken for osteogenic sarcomas. NOFs may also have an atypical appearance if they are discovered as they are filling in with normal bone. CT scanning may be helpful if plain radiographs are not diagnostic. NOFs with a characteristic radiographic appearance do not require biopsy.[5]

Routine follow-up for asymptomatic NOFs is controversial. Fibromas found in young children may increase in size relative to the growth of the adjacent bone and place the bone at risk for fracture. For this reason, yearly or semi-annual radiographs may be considered in younger patients until the lesion is stable in size relative to the involved bone. NOFs discovered in adolescence do not require follow-up.

The majority of NOFs do not require treatment. Because of the risk of associated pathologic fracture, some authors advocate that lesions >50% the width of the bone or smaller lesions in areas of high stress be considered for curettage and bone grafting.[6] Injection, extensive burring, chemical, thermal or other adjuvants are not required. Recurrence is rare.

► OSTEOCHONDROMAS

Osteochondromas, also called cartilaginous exostoses, are the most common benign bone tumor in children and adolescents.[5] Most osteochondromas occur in the metaphysis of long bones, particularly the proximal tibia, proximal humerus, and distal femur. They are cartilaginous in growing children, enlarge during skeletal growth, and ossify at skeletal maturity. Osteochondromas are usually discovered between 5 and 15 years of age and present as a bony, nonpainful mass.[5] If pain is present, it is usually owing to friction or pressure on the adjacent structures. Occasionally, exostoses have been associated with pseudoaneurysms, vascular obstruction, and nerve damage.

Although most exostoses occur singly, some patients have multiple hereditary exostoses (MHE)—a rare disorder with autosomal dominant transmission—resulting in multiple osteochondromas.[6] Although the degree of involvement tends to run in families, phenotypic expression is variable. Severely affected individuals may have short stature, limb length discrepancies, premature partial physeal arrests, extremity deformities, and deterioration of the hip joint.

Radiographs demonstrate sessile or pedunculated projections arising from the surface of the bone usually directed away from the joint (Fig. 106–2). The lesion's cartilage cap, which can be more than 2-cm thick in childhood, is not seen on x-ray,

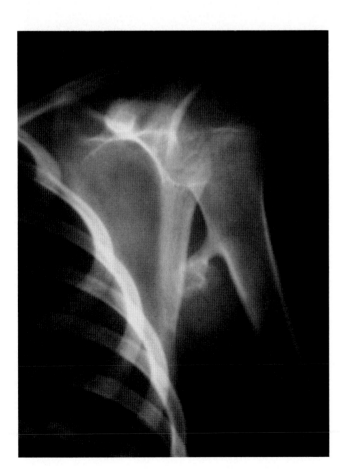

Figure 106–2. Osteochondroma of the proximal humerus.

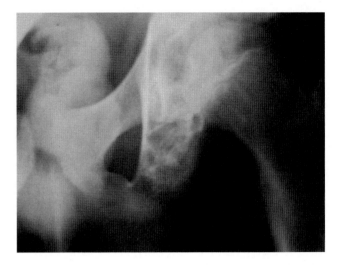

Figure 106–3. Enchondroma of the pelvis.

making the osteochondroma appear smaller on radiographs than it is on physical examination. The cortex and marrow space of the involved bone are continuous with the lesion. CT or MRI may be needed to demonstrate it clearly. The radiographic appearance is usually pathognomonic and biopsy is rarely needed to establish the diagnosis.[6]

Resection of osteochondromas may be considered for cosmetic reasons or for pain relief. Osteochondromas are also removed if they cause growth retardation, vascular obstruction, or pseudoaneurysms.

Malignant transformation of a single lesion is exceptionally rare. In families with MHE, however, there is a 1% to 8% lifetime risk of developing chondrosarcomas in the exostoses. Malignant transformation occurs in adulthood.[7]

► ENCHONDROMAS

Enchondroma is a benign lesion of hyaline cartilage that occurs centrally in the bone and most commonly affects the hands.[5] The majority of lesions are asymptomatic but some patients may present with a mass or pathologic fracture. Radiographs show a radiolucent, sharply marginated lesion in the medullary canal with associated thinning of bone and cortical bulging (Fig. 106–3). Punctate or stippled calcification may be seen; however, this finding is more common in adults.

Most enchondromas are solitary with a low risk for malignant transformation. The risk of malignant transformation is much greater in the multifocal enchondromas of Ollier disease (enchondromas, bony dysplasia, short stature, limb length abnormalities, and joint deformity) (Fig. 106–4) and Maffucci syndrome (enchondromas and soft tissue angiomas). Orthopedic consultation is indicated since curettage and bone grafting may be considered for large or symptomatic lesions.

► UNICAMERAL BONE CYSTS

Unicameral bone cysts, also known as simple or multiloculated bone cysts, are expansile, usually serous fluid-containing

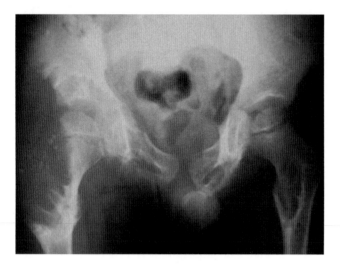

Figure 106–4. Pelvis radiograph in a patient with Ollier's disease. Note the stippled calcification.

defects of tubular and flat bones. Ninety-four percent of unicameral bone cysts occur in the proximal humerus and proximal femur with the humerus being affected two to three times more frequently than the femur.[8] They can occur at any age but tend to be discovered in children between 3 and 14 years of age with an average age of 9. Men are affected twice as frequently as women. In most patients, only one bone is affected. Because their location and lack of symptoms, cysts that occur in the flat bones tend to be found later in life (between 12 and 72 years of age) with an average patient age at discovery of 32.[8]

Unicameral bone cysts start near the epiphyseal plate and extend toward the diaphysis during growth. They tend to be active in children younger than 10 years and inactive in children beyond 10 years of age. Active cysts have a higher recurrence rate than do inactive cysts.

Unicameral bone cysts can be asymptomatic and found incidentally or may be discovered as a result of a pathologic fracture from a minor trauma. Patients may also present with pain, limp, or failure to use the extremity normally.

Radiographically, long bone unicameral cysts are seen as concentrically located lytic lesions in the medullary cavity of the metaphysis with expansion in all directions (Fig. 106–5). This creates an expanded, thinned but unpenetrated cortex. Cysts in the flat bones are centered between the inner and outer tables of the ilium and midportion of the superior pubic ramus. The long axis of the lesion tends to exceed its width. Unicameral bone cysts do not induce a periosteal reaction and, if one is seen, it suggests an associated fracture. The "fallen leaf" sign is pathognomonic of a multiloculated bone cyst and represents a broken piece of cortex that has fallen into the fluid-containing cavity of the cyst. If the radiographic diagnosis is in question, CT scanning can be helpful. Houndsfield units can differentiate fluid within the cystic defect (2–18 U) from a lipoma (0 to –200 U).

These lesions are prone to fracture and require excision, especially in the lower extremity. Orthopedic consultation is indicated. Injection of steroid into the lesion is also therapeutic

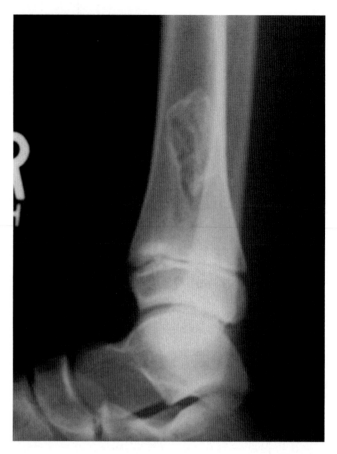

Figure 106–5. Unicameral bone cyst of the distal tibia.

but two to three injections may be required for complete healing. More recently, a single percutaneous injection of demineralized bone matrix has been found to result in cyst resolution in 80% to 90% of patients.[6] Regardless of treatment regimen, children older than 10 years heal at a higher rate (90%) than those younger than 10 years (60%).[8] Radiographs may never normalize and the goal of treatment is a functionally stable bone, not a normal-appearing x-ray.

▶ ANEURYSMAL BONE CYSTS

Aneurysmal bone cyst (ABC) is a rare, rapidly growing, destructive bone tumor that most commonly involves the humerus, femur, tibia, fibula, pelvis, or spine. Although they are benign, ABCs have the potential to cause significant morbidity. Most ABCs present in the first two decades of life and are slightly more common in female patients.[9] Most patients present with pain or a mass. Less frequently, they are discovered after a child sustains a pathologic fracture. Patients with an ABC arising in the spine may present with neurologic deficits. Less than 10% of patients will have involvement of multiple bones. Up to 30% of ABCs may arise with a coexisting bone lesion; the most common underlying lesions include fibrous dysplasia, chondroblastoma, giant cell tumor, and osteosarcoma.[10]

On plain radiographs, ABCs demonstrate an eccentric, fusiform, aneurysmal dilation of the bone with a thin rim of

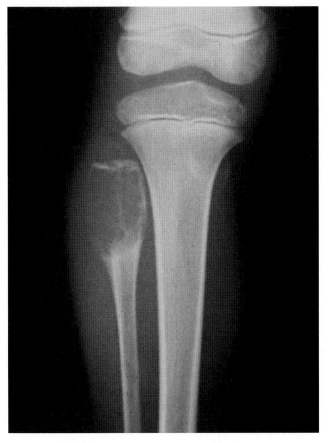
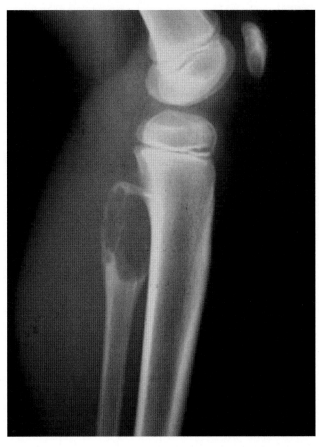

A **B**

Figure 106–6. Aneurysmal bone cyst of the proximal fibula. Note the faint trabeculations that give it a "soap bubble" appearance.

cortical bone seen peripherally (Fig. 106–6). They are often located near the end of the metaphysis and may penetrate into the epiphysis through the growth cartilage. In most instances, there is aggressive lytic bony destruction and, in the long bones, laminated periosteal reaction is common. Faint trabeculations are usually present giving the tumor a "soap bubble" appearance. ABCs may also demonstrate a soft tissue mass extending out of the bone into the soft tissues.

ABCs are filled with blood and, on cross-sectional imaging, fluid–fluid levels may be seen as red cells and serous components separate when the patient lies still for the examination. Fluid–fluid levels may also be seen in telangiectatic osteosarcoma, giant cell tumor, and simple cyst with fracture so, although they are highly suggestive of ABCs, they are not pathognomonic.

The pathologic diagnosis is based on a biopsy done at the time of definitive surgery.[11] The mainstay of treatment is curettage and bone grafting and/or cementation.[10] A high-speed burr may be used intraoperatively to remove microscopic disease. The use of adjuvants, such as phenol and liquid nitrogen, is not routine although they may be considered for recurrent lesions. Surgical treatment of ABCs may be complicated by copious bleeding. In patients with lesions that are central or difficult to access, preoperative embolization should be considered.[6]

Low-dose radiation therapy is used for incompletely resectable, aggressive, or recurrent ABCs with local control in 90% of cases.[10]

Ten to fifty percent of ABCs will recur,[6] with recurrence being more common in younger patients. Most recurrences are seen within 2 years of treatment. Recurrent lesions are treated with surgery or radiation.

REFERENCES

1. Ghanem I. The management of osteoid osteoma: updates and controversies. *Curr Opin Pediatr.* 2006;18:36–41.
2. Chan K, Myers S, Monu JUV. Osteoid osteoma:diagnosis and management. *Contemp Diag Radiol.* 2006;29(25):1–5.
3. Hosalkar HS, Garg S, Moroz B, et al. The diagnostic accuracy of MRI versus CT imaging for osteoid osteoma in children. *Clin Orthop Related Research.* 2005;433:171–177.
4. Lefton DR, Torrisi JM, Haller JO. Vertebral osteoid osteoma masquerading as a malignant bone or soft-tissue tumor on MRI. *Pediatr Radiol.* 2001;31(2):72–75.
5. Arndt CAS. Benign tumors and tumor-like processes of bone. In: Behrman RE, Kliegman, RM, Jenson HB, eds. *Nelson Textbook of Pediatrics.* 17th ed. Philadelphia, PA: Saunders, 2004.

6. Biermann JS. Common benign lesions of bone in children and adolescents. *J Pediatr Orthop*. 2002;22(2):268–273.

7. Kivioja A, Ervasti H, Kinnunen J, et al. Chondrosarcoma in a family with multiple hereditary exostoses. *J Bone Joint Surg [Br]*. 2000;82:261–266.

8. Baig R, Eady J. Unicameral (simple) bone cysts. *Southern Med J*. 2006;99(9):966–976.

9. Leithner A, Windhager R, Lang S, et al. Aneurysmal bone cyst. *Clin Orthop Related Research*. 1999;363:176–179.

10. Mendenhall WM, Zlotecki RA, Gibbs CP, et al. Aneurysmal bone cyst. *Am J Clin Oncol* 2006;29:311–315.

11. Cottalorda J, Bourelle S. Modern concepts of primary aneurysmal bone cyst. *Arch Orthop Trauma Surg*. 2007;127:105–114.

SECTION XIX

TOXICOLOGIC EMERGENCIES

CHAPTER 107

General Approach to the Poisoned Pediatric Patient

Timothy B. Erickson

► HIGH-YIELD FACTS

- Many pediatric patients with ingestions present with common toxic syndromes or "toxidromes."
- In asymptomatic children presenting with nontoxic ingestions, observation alone is adequate.
- Ipecac is no longer considered useful in pediatric ingestions in either the home or the emergency setting.
- Activated charcoal is the safest mode of gastrointestinal decontamination method and has the fewest side effects.
- Cathartic agents are not necessary in the pediatric patient; multiple doses can result in significant dehydration and electrolyte disturbances.
- Whole bowel irrigation with an osmotically neutral and electrolyte safe polyethyleneglycol solution may be indicated with certain pediatric toxic ingestions.
- There are specific antidotes available for a limited number of pediatric toxic exposures.

► EPIDEMIOLOGY

There has been a 94% decline in the number of pediatric poisoning deaths in the United Sates in children <6 years of age over the past four decades, with 450 reported deaths in 1960 and 29 in 2006. During this latest year, pediatric fatalities accounted for 2.4% of all poisoning deaths.[1] Child-resistant product packaging, heightened parental awareness of potential household toxins, and more sophisticated medical intervention at the poison control and emergency and intensive care levels have all contributed to reduce morbidity and mortality. Nonetheless, poisoning continues to be a preventable cause of pathology in children and adolescents. It is imperative that the pediatric emergency physician be familiar with the general approach to poisoned children, as well as the latest treatment modalities available.

Two-thirds of poisonings reported to the American Association of Poison Control Centers (AAPCC) occur in individuals younger than 20 years. Specifically, children younger than 3 years were involved in 38% of exposures and 51% occurred in children younger than 6 years in 2006.[1] Most exposures in this age group are accidental and result in minimal toxicity. The majority of these poisonings result from ingestions. They may also result from inhalation, intravenous, dermal, ocular, and environmental exposure. Nonaccidental causes of drug toxicity include recreational drug abuse, suicide attempts, and Munchausenby-proxy.[2]

► HISTORY

Although it may be difficult to obtain an accurate and complete history regarding a recent ingestion, this is an essential part of the proper evaluation of poisoned pediatric patients. All sources of information are explored in children who are comatose or too young to provide details. The history includes the toxin or medication to which the children were exposed, the time of the exposure or ingestion, what other medications were available to the children, and how much was taken. It is prudent to assume the worst-case scenario.[2–4]

► PHYSICAL EXAMINATION

A comprehensive physical examination may provide valuable clues regarding the ingestion or exposure. Since many drugs and toxic agents have specific effects on the heart rate, temperature, blood pressure, and respiratory rate, monitoring the vital signs may direct the clinician toward the proper diagnosis (Table 107–1). Additionally, the level of consciousness, pupillary size, and potential for coma or seizures may be directly affected by the poison in a dose-dependent fashion (Tables 107–2 and 107–3). Other diagnostic clues are obtained in the skin examination and breath odor (Tables 107–4 and 107–5). Several groups of toxins consistently present with recognizable patterns or signs. Recognizing these toxic syndromes or toxidromes may expedite not only the diagnosis of the toxic agent but also its management (Table 107–6).[5]

► DIAGNOSTIC AIDS AND LABORATORY STUDIES

In children with a significant or unknown ingestion, baseline laboratory studies include a complete blood cell count, BUN and creatinine, serum electrolytes, glucose, and a venous or arterial blood gas. In patients with a known ingestion who have no overt signs of toxicity, a more selective approach to diagnostic studies is acceptable. If a venous or arterial blood gas value reveals a metabolic acidosis, calculating the anion gap can assist in formulating a differential diagnosis. A metabolic acidosis with an increased anion gap results from the presence

▶ **TABLE 107–1. DIAGNOSING TOXICITY FROM VITAL SIGNS**

Bradycardia (PACED)

Propranolol (β-blockers), poppies (opiates), propoxyphene, physostigmine

Anticholinesterase drugs, antiarrhythmics

Clonidine, calcium channel blockers

Ethanol or other alcohols

Digoxin, digitalis

Tachycardia (FAST)

Free base or other forms of cocaine, Freon

Anticholinergics, antihistamines, antipsychotics amphetamines, alcohol withdrawal

Sympathomimetics (cocaine, caffeine, amphetamines, PCP), solvent abuse, strychnine

Theophylline, TCAs, thyroid hormones

Hypothermia (COOLS)

Carbon monoxide

Opioids

Oral hypoglycemics, insulin

Liquor (alcohols)

Sedative-hypnotics

Hyperthermia (NASA)

Neuroleptic malignant syndrome, Nicotine

Antihistamines, alcohol withdrawal

Salicylates, sympathomimetics, serotonin syndrome

Anticholinergics, antidepressants, antipsychotics

Hypotension (CRASH)

Clonidine, calcium channel blockers

Rodenticides (containing arsenic, cyanide)

Antidepressants, aminophylline, antihypertensives

Sedative-hypnotics

Heroin or other opiates

Hypertension (CT SCAN)

Cocaine

Thyroid supplements

Sympathomimetics

Caffeine

Anticholinergics, amphetamines

Nicotine

Rapid respiration (PANT)

PCP, paraquat, pneumonitis (chemical), phosgene

ASA and other salicylates

Noncardiogenic pulmonary edema, nerve agents

Toxin-induced metabolic acidosis

Slow respiration (SLOW)

Sedative-hypnotics (barbiturates, benzos)

Liquor (alcohols)

Opioids

Weed (marijuana)

of organically active acids and is characteristic of several toxins and various other disease states (Table 107–7). Normal anion gap acidosis results from loss of bicarbonate (diarrhea and renal tubular acidosis) or from addition of chloride-containing compounds (NH_4Cl and $CaCl_2$). The anion gap can be calculated from serum electrolytes as follows: Anion gap calculation $= Na - (Cl + HCO_3)$. The normal anion gap ranges from 8 to 12 mEq/L.

If ingestion of a toxic alcohol, such as methanol or ethylene glycol, is suspected, calculation of the osmolal gap is recommended. The osmolal gap is the difference between the actual osmolality, best measured by freezing-point depression, and that calculated from major osmotically active molecules in the serum (sodium, glucose, and blood urea nitrogen).

$$\text{Calculated osmolality} = 2(Na) + \text{glucose}/$$
$$18 + BUN/2.8\ ETOH/4.6$$

$$\text{Osmolal gap} = \text{measured osmol} - \text{calculated}$$
$$\text{osmol (normal} <10)$$

When a particular drug or toxin is known or highly suspected, blood or serum can be tested for specific drug levels.

▶ **TABLE 107-2. AGENTS THAT AFFECT PUPIL SIZE**

Miosis (**COPS**)	Mydriasis (**SAW**)
Cholinergics, clonidine, carbamates	**S**ympathomimetics
Opiates, organophosphates,	**A**nticholinergics
Phenothiazines (antipsychotics), pilocarpine, pontine hemorrhage	**W**ithdrawal
Sedative-hypnotics	

These levels confirm the ingestion and often guide medical management. Commonly available tests are listed in Table 107–8.

Toxicology screening can be helpful in the diagnosis of the unknown ingestion if the clinician is aware of its limitations. Even when a drug has been ingested, blood toxicology

▶ **TABLE 107–3. AGENTS THAT CAUSE COMA OR SEIZURES**

COMA (LETHARGIC)	SEIZURES (OTIS CAMPBELL*)
L-Lead, lithium	**O**rganophosphates, oral hypoglycemics
E-Ethanol, ethylene glycol, ethchlorvynol	**T**ricyclic antidepressants
T-Tricyclic antidepressants, thallium, toluene	**I**soniazid, insulin
H-Heroin, hemlock, hepatic encephalopathy, heavy metals, hydrogen sulfide, hypoglycemics	**S**ympathomimetics, strychnine, salicylates
A-Arsenic, antidepressants, anticonvulsants, antipyschotics, antihistamines	**C**amphor, cocaine, carbon monoxide, cyanide, chlorinated hydrocarbons
R-Rohypnol (sedative hypnotics), risperidone	**A**mphetamines, anticholinergics
G-GHB	**M**ethylxanthines (theophylline, caffeine), methanol
I-Isoniazid, insulin	**P**hencyclidine (PCP), propranolol
C-Carbon monoxide, cyanide, clonidine	**B**enzodiazepine withdrawal, botanicals (water hemlock, nicotine), bupropion, GHB
	Ethanol withdrawal, ethylene glycol
	Lithium, lidocaine
	Lead, lindane

*Famous T. V. "town drunk" on the Andy Griffith Show.

▶ TABLE 107-4. **AGENTS THAT CAUSE SKIN SIGNS**

Diaphoretic skin (SOAP)	**Flushed or red appearance**
Sympathomimetics	Anticholinergics, niacin
Organophosphates	Boric acid
Acetylsalicylic acid or other salicylates	Carbon monoxide (rare)
Phencyclidine	Cyanide (rare)
Dry Skin	**Cyanosis**
Antihistamines, anticholinergics	Ergotamine
	Nitrates
	Nitrites
	Aniline dyes
	Phenazopyridine
	Dapsone
	Any agent causing hypoxemia, hypotension, or methemoglobinemia.
Bullae	**Acneiform rash**
Barbiturates and other sedative-hypnotics, **B**ites: **S**nakes and spiders	**B**romides **C**hlorinated aromatic hydrocarbons

screens may be negative if the drug has a short half-life and the specimen is not obtained immediately after the exposure. The urine toxicology screen may be of greater value, since the drug's metabolites continue to be excreted in the urine for 48 to 72 hours following the ingestion. Toxicology panels typically screen for drugs of abuse such as narcotics, amphetamines, cannabinoids, phencyclidine (PCP), and cocaine. However, since most of these screens are qualitative, the mere detection of a drug does not necessarily entail toxicity. A grave error can also occur if the physician assumes the child ingested nothing simply because the toxicology screen is reported as negative and the actual drug ingested has not been included in the screen.

Radiological testing can prove valuable with certain ingestions, particularly those that are radiopaque on abdominal studies or those that may induce a noncardiogenic pulmonary edema or chemical pneumonitis (Table 107–9).[6]

▶ TABLE 107-5. **ODORS THAT SUGGEST THE DIAGNOSIS**

Odor	Possible Source
Bitter almonds	Cyanide
Carrots	Cicutoxin (water hemlock)
Fruity	Diabetic ketoacidosis, isopropanol
Garlic	Organophosphates, arsenic, dimethyl sulfoxide (DMSO), selenium
Gasoline	Petroleum distillates
Mothballs	Naphthalene, camphor
Pears	Chloral hydrate
Pungent aromatic	Ethchlorvynol
Oil of wintergreen	Methylsalicylate
Rotten eggs	Sulfur dioxide, hydrogen sulfide
Freshly mowed hay	Phosgene

▶ TABLE 107-6. **COMMON TOXIDROMES**

Cholinergic	**Opioid**
Examples: organophosphates, carbamates, pilocarpine)	Examples: heroin, morphine, codeine, methadone, fentanyl, oxycodone, hydrocodone
(DUMBELLS)	
Diarrhea, diaphoresis	Miosis
Urination	Bradycardia
Miosis	Hypotension
Bradycardia, bronchosecretions	Hypoventilation
Emesis	Coma
Lacrimation	
Lethargic	
Salivation	
Nicotinic	
M-Mydriasis	
T-Tachycardia	
W-Weakness	
T-Tremors	
F-Fasciculations	
S-Seizures	
S-Somnulent	
Anticholinergic	**Withdrawal**
Examples: antihistamines, cyclic antidepressants, atropine, benztropine, phenothiazines, scopolamine	Diarrhea
	Mydriasis
	Goose flesh
	Tachycardia
	Lacrimation
Hyperthermia (HOT as a hare)	Hypertension
Flushed (RED as a beet)	Yawning
Dry skin (DRY as a bone)	Cramps
Dilated pupils (BLIND as a bat)	Hallucinations
Delirium, hallucinations (MAD as a hatter)	Seizures (with ETOH and benzodiazepine withdrawal)
Tachycardia	
Urinary urgency and retention	
Sympathomimetic	
Examples: cocaine, amphetamines, ephedrine, phencyclidine, pseudoepedrine	
Mydriasis	
Tachycardia	
Hypertension	
Hyperthermia	
Seizures	

▶ MANAGEMENT

STABILIZATION

The cornerstone of management of patients with a suspected overdose is supportive care, with particular attention to the airway, breathing, and circulation. Resuscitative measures are instituted prior to antidotal therapy or gastric decontamination (Fig. 107–1).

In children with an altered level of consciousness or in whom a bedside glucose oxidase test documents hypoglycemia, the physician should administer intravenous

▶ **TABLE 107-7. AGENTS CAUSING METABOLIC ACIDOSIS/ELEVATED ANION GAP**

METAL
Methanol, metformin, massive overdoses
Ethylene glycol
Toluene
Alcoholic ketoacidosis,
Lactic acidosis

ACID
Acetaminophen (large ingestions)
Cyanide, carbon monoxide, colchicine
Isoniazid, iron, ibuprofen (large ingestions)
Diabetic ketoacidosis

GAP
Generalized seizure-producing toxins
Acetylsalicyclic acid or other salicylates
Paraldehyde, phenformin

dextrose at 0.5 to 1.0 g/kg, given as 2 to 4 mL/kg of D_{25} W in children or 50 mL (1 ampul) of D_{50} W in the adolescent. If intravenous access is difficult or unobtainable, glucagon, 1 mg, is administered intramuscularly.

In addition to dextrose, naloxone is given to children or adolescents with lethargy or coma. Naloxone is a specific opiate antagonist with minimal side effects. Agitation and signs of withdrawal may develop in opiate-dependent adolescents or in neonates whose mothers are narcotic addicts or on methadone during pregnancy. The initial dose is 0.1 mg/kg intravenously or 2 mg for children weighing >20 kg. Often, additional doses of naloxone are required for certain opiates, such as fentanyl, codeine, methadone, and propoxyphene, which have high potency and a prolonged half-life.[7] If an intravenous line cannot be established, naloxone may be administered via the endotracheal tube, intramuscularly, intralingually, or subcutaneously.[8]

GASTRIC DECONTAMINATION

Gastrointestinal decontamination is one of the more controversial topics in toxicology. Whether patients are managed with gastric lavage, whole bowel irrigation, or activated charcoal alone depends on the toxicity of the particular drug, the quantity and time of ingestion, and patient's condition. If children ingest a nontoxic agent or a very small amount of a poison unlikely to cause toxicity, no gastric decontamination measures are necessary. However, if the ingestion is recent and the child

▶ **TABLE 107-8. AGENTS INCREASING THE OSMOLAR GAP**

ME DIE
Methanol
Ethylene glycol
Diuretics (mannitol), diabetic ketoacidosis (acetone)
Isopropyl alcohol
Ethanol

▶ **TABLE 107-9. AGENTS VISIBLE ON ABDOMINAL RADIOGRAPHS**

COINS
Chloral hydrate, cocaine packets, calcium
Opium packets
Iron, other heavy metals such as lead, arsenic, mercury
Neuroleptic agents
Sustained-released or enteric coated agents

DRUGS CAUSING ACUTE LUNG INJURY OR PULMONARY EDEMA
MOPS
Meprobamate, methadone
Opioids
Phenobarbital, propoxyphene, paraquat, phosgene
Salicylates

is symptomatic, or the ingested toxin may cause delayed toxicity, gastric decontamination is generally recommended. Several clinical trials have been conducted to determine which of the gastric decontamination modalities are most efficacious. However, the investigations either involve adult volunteers, who ingested subtoxic amounts of an agent and received decontamination at a set postingestion time, or involve mild-to-moderately poisoned patients, and exclude patients with significant overdoses. Few children have been included in these trials. Therefore, these studies must be critically interpreted prior to their definitive application in the clinical setting, especially in the pediatric patient. Most treatment modalities have focused on stomach evacuation, while the ultimate goal should be to decontaminate the entire gastrointestinal tract.[9,10]

INDUCTION OF EMESIS

Historically, syrup of ipecac was the most commonly used gastric decontamination agent (Fig. 107-2). It is a mixture of alkaloids consisting of emetine and cephaeline, which are strong emetic agents that stimulate the gastric mucosa as well as the brain's chemoreceptor trigger zone. Ipecac gained popularity for home use in pediatric poisonings in the 1960s.[11,12]

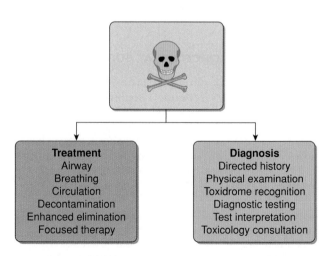

Treatment	Diagnosis
Airway	Directed history
Breathing	Physical examination
Circulation	Toxidrome recognition
Decontamination	Diagnostic testing
Enhanced elimination	Test interpretation
Focused therapy	Toxicology consultation

Figure 107-1. General approach to the poisoned patient.

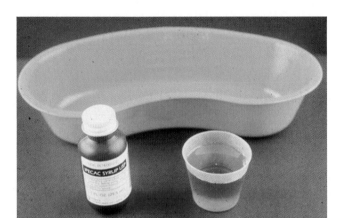

Figure 107–2. Routine induction of emesis with syrup of ipecac is no longer recommended.

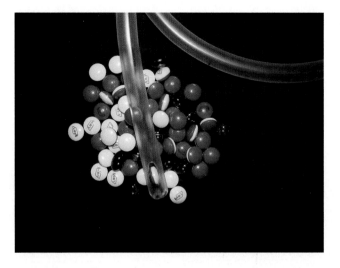

Figure 107–3. Even large-bore gastric lavage tubes may not have sufficient size to aspirate pills and medication fragments.

However, its use has fallen out of favor in the emergency department and prehospital settings and is no longer advocated in the heath care setting for treatment of the acutely poisoned patient. In 1985, it was given in 15% of all oral exposures reported to poison control centers. In 2006, it was administered in only 0.1% of the cases.[1]

Ipecac can be expected to induce vomiting within 20 to 60 minutes. The recovery of ingested material in the vomitus is approximately 30% if ipecac is administered within 5 minutes of ingestion, and far less if delayed beyond 1 hour. Most children will experience up to three episodes of vomiting, which often delays the administration of activated charcoal. In human volunteer studies, ipecac was not able to significantly decrease absorption of drugs after 30 to 60 minutes and was inferior when compared to activated charcoal alone.

Ipecac is contraindicated in children younger than 6 months, in patients with evidence of a diminished gag reflex and potential for coma or seizures, and in the ingestion of most hydrocarbons, acids, alkalis, and sharp objects. Complications following ipecac use that have been reported in the literature include aspiration pneumonia, dehydration due to protracted vomiting, diaphragmatic rupture and death, Mallory-Weiss tears of the esophagus, and gastric rupture.[13-15]

The use of ipecac is no longer recommended by the American Academy of Pediatrics or the American Association of Poison Centers for use in the emergency setting. Research has demonstrated no improvement in clinical outcome with its use.[15] There is also no accepted role for syrup of ipecac in the prehospital management of poisonings. The American Academy of Pediatrics issued a statement that ipecac should no longer be used routinely as a home treatment strategy, that existing ipecac in the home should be disposed of safely.[16] There has been no reduction in resource usage or improvement in patient outcome from the use of syrup of ipecac at home.[13]

GASTRIC LAVAGE

Ideally, gastric lavage mechanically removes toxins from the stomach through a large-bore orogastric tube. In pediatric patients, the size of the lavage tube ranges from 16 to 32 Fr, depending on the age of the patient. In fact, gastric lavage re-

moves, at best, up to 40% of the ingested toxin. In some cases, the holes at the end of the evacuation tube are too small to allow pill fragments to be suctioned into the lavage tube lumen (Fig. 107–3). It is important to note that gastric lavage does not remove toxic agents from the intestinal tract, where the majority of drug absorption occurs. It is also important to realize that there have been no clinical trials evaluating the efficacy of gastric lavage in small children.[10]

Gastric lavage should not be routinely performed in overdosed pediatric patients.[17] Gastric lavage may be considered if a patient has ingested a potentially life-threatening amount of a toxin and presents within 1 hour of ingestion.[17-21] However, even in this scenario, there is no clear evidence that its use improves clinical outcome. Airway protection by endotracheal intubation prior to the lavage is indicated in children with a depressed level of consciousness to order to avoid aspiration pneumonitis. In these cases, the risk of intubation must be weighed against the potential benefits of gastric lavage. Gastric lavage should never be used as a punitive measure in cases of nontoxic overdoses or forced on pediatric patients who are combative or otherwise uncooperative. Additionally, endotracheal intubation solely to perform gastric lavage is discouraged; the decision to intubate should be independently of the decision to perform gastric lavage.

With gastric lavage, after verifying proper orogastric tube placement, the stomach contents are aspirated, then irrigated with 50 to 100 mL aliquots of normal saline until the returned lavage fluid is clear; in adolescents, 250 mL aliquots are recommended. In patients in whom lavage may be indicated, it is theoretically attractive to give charcoal down the tube immediately upon insertion, followed by lavage, followed by charcoal. This obviously would not apply to drugs not bound to charcoal, but it does address the concern that process of lavage moves drugs from the stomach into the small intestine, thereby enhancing absorption. Theoretically, the charcoal administered prior to lavage binds to drug that would be forced through the pylorus by the lavage fluid, limiting the drug's absorption.

If the child has recently ingested an elixir or liquid, a simple nasogastric tube is adequate in order to avoid orogastric injury from traumatic insertion of a large-bore tube. Although controversial, there may be some efficacy for lavage beyond 1 hour when the agent ingested slows gut motility, such as with anticholinergics or opioids, or when the toxin forms concretions, such as with iron and salicylates. However, this has never been substantiated in the toxicology literature.[10]

Gastric lavage is contraindicated in ingestions of most hydrocarbons, acids, alkalis, and sharp objects. Although relatively safe when performed properly, it is not a benign procedure and complications including aspiration, esophageal perforation, bleeding, electrolyte imbalance, and hypothermia have been described. Therefore, the clinician must have adequate rationale to perform this gastric decontamination procedure.

ACTIVATED CHARCOAL

The majority of poisoned children who are not critically ill can be managed safely and effectively in the emergency department setting with charcoal alone. Activated charcoal is an odorless, tasteless, fine black powder that is effective in adsorbing many toxins.[22] Recent charcoal products have been "superactivated" resulting in large surface areas of up to 3000 m^2/g, allowing for maximum absorptive power.

Activated charcoal is the most frequently used and most effective gastrointestinal decontamination agent. Evidence suggests that activated charcoal is more effective than induced emesis or gastric lavage for gastric decontamination.[23] Activated charcoal can be administered rapidly and is most beneficial when administered within 1 hour after the ingestion. The absorptive properties of activated charcoal are effective beyond the gastric mucosa; absorbing drugs throughout the small intestine. While studies have demonstrated reduced drug absorption with activated charcoal use, it is important to note that there is no evidence that administration of activated charcoal ultimately improves patient outcome.[23,24] Its routine administration in nontoxic ingestions is not indicated.

Most young children will refuse to drink charcoal due to its gritty texture and threatening appearance (Fig. 107–4). Children can be distracted by administrating the charcoal in an opaque styrofoam cup with a lid and straw, or by adding favoring to enhance its palatability. Additionally, medical personnel may allow reliable parents to administer the charcoal to the child. Occasionally, a patient may be unable to or may refuse to drink charcoal. In these scenarios, when charcoal is clearly indicated, a small nasogastric tube may need to be inserted in order to facilitate its administration.

Although most sources recommend an activated charcoal dose of 1 mg/kg, if the amount of drug ingested is known, a more accurate dose of activated charcoal can be calculated using a 10:1 ratio of charcoal to the ingested toxin. However, even this 10:1 ratio, although adequate in most scenarios, has never been shown to be as efficacious or superior to larger ratios. Practically speaking, most pediatric patients will not tolerate larger doses of activated charcoal.

For some drugs, such as theophylline, phenobarbital, and carbamazepine, multiple dosing of activated charcoal may enhance elimination due primarily to enteroenteric circulation of

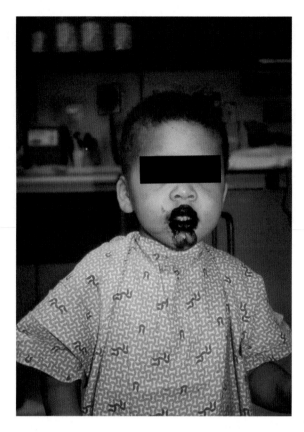

Figure 107–4. Although safe and effective, activated charcoal administration may be a challenge in younger pediatric patients.

the drug (Table 107–10).[25] Repeated use of charcoal preparations premixed with cathartics such as sorbitol is to be avoided, since dehydration and electrolyte imbalance may result.

Activated charcoal is the preferred mode of gastrointestinal decontamination when the history of the overdose or time of ingestion is unclear, since delayed administration may be beneficial, with minimal adverse side effects. Rare cases of vomiting, constipation, obstruction, and aspiration have been reported, but the incidence, particularly in pediatric cases, is

▶ **TABLE 107–10. AGENTS RESPONSIVE TO MULTIPLE DOSES OF ACTIVATED CHARCOAL**

Substances adsorbable by activated charcoal (ABCD)
Antimalarials (quinine), **A**minophylline (theophylline)
Barbiturates (phenobarbital)
Carbamazepine
Dapsone

Substances not adsorbable by activated charcoal (PHAILS)
Pesticides, potassium
Hydrocarbons
Acids, alkali, alcohols
Iron, insecticides
Lithium
Solvents

extremely low.[24,26,27] The administration of activated charcoal in the home or prehospital setting is gaining popularity as a superior substitute for syrup of ipecac.[2,28] Activated charcoal is neither effective nor indicated in heavy metal poisonings, such as with iron, lithium, or borates; ingestions of ethanol containing products; or following ingestion of acids or alkalis where gastric visualization or endoscopy may be required (Table 107–10).

CATHARTICS

Cathartics are osmotically active agents that eliminate toxins from the gastrointestinal tract by inducing diarrhea. The most common agents are sorbitol, magnesium citrate, and magnesium sulfate (Fig. 107–5). Historically, it was recommended that one dose of a cathartic be administered with the first dose of charcoal in order to reduce the gastrointestinal transit time of the toxin–charcoal mixture. However, the efficacy of cathartic use in reducing the absorption or increasing the elimination of toxins has not been established.[29] There is no published data demonstrating an improved outcome with cathartic use alone or combined with activated charcoal.[29] Studies investigating the use of sorbitol in combination with activated charcoal have found that it enhances charcoal's palatability. As a result, younger children are more accepting of its oral administration. In the pediatric population, cathartic agents have been reported to result in hypermagnesemia, severe dehydration, and electrolyte imbalances if used excessively or in repetitive

doses.[30] In young children, it is recommended that activated charcoal be administered with water only, without any cathartic agent.

WHOLE BOWEL IRRIGATION

Originally used as a preoperative bowel preparation, whole bowel irrigation (WBI) is now used in the overdose setting to "flush" the toxin through the gastrointestinal tract and prevent further absorption. In theory, it may also produce a concentration gradient that allows previously absorbed toxins to diffuse back into the gastrointestinal tract.[31] The solution used is nonabsorbable, isotonic polyethylene glycol electrolyte (PEG) solution that, unlike cathartic agents, does not appear to create fluid or electrolyte disturbances (Fig. 107–6). The dose is 100 to 200 mL/h for small children and 1 to 2 L/h for adolescents. The irrigation process is continued until the rectal effluent is clear, usually within 4 to 6 hours.

While volunteer studies have demonstrated decreased bioavailability of certain drugs using WBI, there is currently no conclusive evidence that WBI improves clinical outcome of poisoned patients.[32] Although much of the evidence for WBI is anectdotal, this modality has been used in the pediatric population with minimal to no side effects. In patients who are hemodynamically stable and have normal bowel function and anatomy, it is reasonable to consider using WBI with specific ingestions. In case reports, it has been effective in ingestions not well absorbed by activated charcoal such as iron tablets,[33–35] lead paint chips,[36] lithium,[37] and sustained released calcium channel blockers.[38] With these cases, an abdominal radiograph demonstrating radioopacities can be followed in a serial manner to document the effectiveness of WBI. In addition, its use has been documented following cocaine and opiate packet ingestions. In agents well absorbed by charcoal, WBI is discouraged as it may actually decrease the efficacy of activated charcoal.[39]

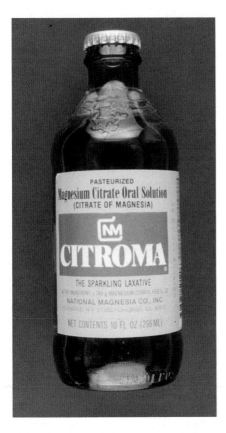

Figure 107–5. Cathartic agents can cause severe electrolyte and fluid disturbances and are not recommended in children.

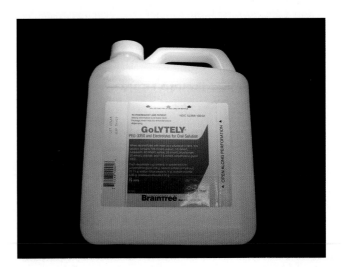

Figure 107–6. Polyethylene glycol solution is an osmotically neutral and electrolyte safe solution used for whole bowel irrigation with selected poisons.

▶ **TABLE 107–11. ANTIDOTES AND THEIR INDICATIONS**

Antidote	Indication (agent)
N-acetylcysteine	Acetaminophen
Ethanol/fomepizole (4-MP)	Methanol/ethylene glycol
Oxygen/hyperbarics	Carbon monoxide
Naloxone/Nalmefene	Opioids
Physostigmine	Anticholinergics
Atropine/pralidoxime (2-PAM)	Organophosphates
Methylene blue	Methemoglobinemia
Nitrites/Hydroxycobalamine	Cyanide
Deferoxamine	Iron
Dimercaprol (BAL)	Arsenic, lead
Succimer (DMSA)	Lead, mercury
CaEDTA	Lead
Fab fragments	Digoxin, Crotalids, Colchicine,
Glucagon	β-Blockers, Calcium channel blockers
Sodium bicarbonate	Tricyclic antidepressants
Calcium/insulin/dextrose	Calcium channel antagonists
Dextrose, glucagons, octreotide	Oral hypoglycemics

4-MP, 4-methylpyrazone; EDTA, calcium ethylenediamine tetraacetate; BAL, British antilewisite; DMSA, dimercaptosuccinic acid; 2-PAM, 2-pralidoxime.

ANTIDOTES

Although the majority of poisonings in the pediatric population respond to supportive care and gastric decontamination alone, there are a few toxins that require antidotes.[40] The purpose of antidotal therapy is to reduce the agent's toxicity by inhibiting the toxin at the effector site or target organ, to reduce the toxin's concentration, or to enhance its excretion. The number of effective antidotes is limited (Table 107–11) and is not for indiscriminate use. Antidotal therapy should be used carefully and in clinical circumstances when specifically indicated. Newly approved antidotes include fomepizole for toxic alcohols,[41,42] CroFab for pit viper envenomations,[43,44] dextrose–insulin therapy for calcium channel blockers,[45,46] and hydroxycobalamin administration for cyanide poisoning.[47,48]

ENHANCED ELIMINATION

Enhancing elimination is the process of removing a toxin from the body once absorption has already occurred. Methods of enhanced elimination include multiple-dose-activated charcoal, urinary alkalinization, and extracorporeal elimination. The role of multiple-dose-activated charcoal was discussed previously. Urinary alkalinization involves the use of an intravenous sodium bicarbonate infusion and promotes urinary elimination of substances that are weak acids. It is important to maintain a normal potassium level when performing alkalinization, since appropriate alkalinization cannot be achieved when hypokalemia is present. A common use of urinary alkalinization is in the salicylate-poisoned patient. Another use may be in patients who overdose on phenobarbital. As an aside, urinary acidification has been recommended in the past as a method of

▶ **TABLE 107–12. TOXINS ACCESSIBLE TO HEMODIALYSIS**

UNSTABLE
Uremia
No response to conventional therapy
Salicylates
Theophylline
Alcohols (isopropanol, methanol)
Boric acid, barbiturates (phenobarbital)
Lithium
Ethylene glycol

Enhanced elimination by charcoal hemoperfusion
Theophylline
Barbiturates
Carbamazepine
Paraquat
Glutethamide

enhanced elimination with poisoning by weak bases, such as phencyclidine and amphetamine. This procedure is no longer recommended because of the high risk of myoglobinuria and rhabdomyolysis.[3]

HEMODIALYSIS AND HEMOPERFUSION

Although hemodialysis is recommended for a wide variety of toxins, it is necessary in only a few severely poisoned patients.[49] Drugs that may be adequately dialyzed include those with a low molecular weight, low volume of distribution, low protein binding, and high water solubility. Examples include isopropanol, salicylates, theophylline, uremia-causing agents, methanol, barbiturates, lithium, and ethylene glycol (Table 107–12). Theophylline is also responsive to charcoal hemoperfusion. If children have a severe overdose that may require dialysis, early consultation with a nephrologist is critical.

▶ DISPOSITION

Disposition of poisoned pediatric patients is not always straightforward and depends on the clinical condition of the children, as well as the potential toxicity of the agent. Clearly, all children demonstrating clinical instability are best monitored in an intensive care setting. Emergency department observation for 6 to 8 hours is adequate if patients demonstrate no overt signs of toxicity and the ingestion does not involve agents with known delayed or prolonged onset of action. Such agents include sustained release products, calcium channel antagonists, theophylline, lithium, methadone, Lomotil, monoamine oxidase inhibitors, and oral hypoglycemic agents. Overdose with these substances may require up to 24 hours of continuous observation.[50] If children have ingested a potentially dangerous toxin,[51,52] are manifesting mild-to-moderate toxicity, require antidotal therapy, or their home environment is not considered safe, a general pediatric admission is indicated. In the setting of any accidental overdose, the parents are counseled and educated regarding proper poison prevention in the home. In the case of adolescents with recreational drug abuse, drug rehabilitation programs are encouraged. If the adolescents are suicidal, psychiatric consultation is obtained once they are stabilized medically.

REFERENCES

1. Bronstein A, Spyker D, Cantilena L, et al. 2006 Annual Report of the American Association of Poison Control Centers' National Poison Data System (NPDS)'. *Clin Toxicol.* 2007;45(8):815–917.
2. Eldridge DL, Van Eyk J, Kornegay C. Pediatric toxicology. *Emerg Med Clin North Am.* 2007;25(2):283–308.
3. Erickson T. Toxicology: ingestions and smoke inhalation. In: Gausche-Hill M, Fuchs S, Yamamoto L, eds. *APLS: The Pediatric Emergency Medicine Resource. AAP and ACEP.* 4th ed. Boston, MA: Jones and Bartlett; 2004:234–267.
4. Henretig FM. Special considerations in the poisoned pediatric patient. *Emerg Clin North Am.* 1994;12:549–567.
5. Erickson T, Thompson T, Lu J. The approach to the patient with an unknown overdose. *Emerg Med Clin North Am.* 2007;25:249–281.
6. Sporer KA, Dorn E. Heroin-related noncardiogenic pulmonary edema: a case series. *Chest.* 2001;120(5):1528–1530.
7. Schumann H, Erickson T, Thompson T, Zautcke J. Deadly Fentanyl Epidemic in Chicago and surrounding Cook County, Illinois. *Clin Toxicol.* 2008, in press.
8. Wanger K, Brough L, Macmillan I, Goulding J, MacPhail I, Christenson JM. Intravenous vs subcutaneous naloxone for out-of-hospital management of presumed opioid overdose. *Acad Emerg Med.* 1998;5:293–299.
9. Kulig K. Initial management of toxic substances. *N Engl J Med.* 1992;326:1677–1681.
10. Erickson T, Kulig K. Gastric Decontamination. In: *Pediatric Toxicology: Diagnosis and Management of the Poisoned Child.* New York, NY: McGraw-Hill; 2005.
11. Arnold FJ, Hodges JB, Barta PA, et al. Evacuation of the efficacy of lavage and emesis in the treatment of salicylate poisoning. *Pediatrics.* 1959;23:286.
12. Corby DC, Decker W. Clinical comparison of pharmacologic emetics in children. *Pediatrics.* 1968;42:361.
13. Bond GR. Home syrup of ipecac use does not reduce emergency department use or improve outcome. *Pediatrics.* 2003;112(5):1061–1064.
14. Shannon M. The demise of ipecac? *Pediatrics.* 2003;112(5) 1180–1181.
15. American Academy of Clinical Toxicology. Position paper: Ipecac syrup. *J Toxicol Clin Toxicol.* 2004;42:133–143.
16. American Academy of Pediatrics. Committee on Injury, Violence, and Poison Prevention: poison treatment in the home. *Pediatrics.* 2003;112(5):1182–1185.
17. American Academy of Clinical Toxicology. Position paper: gastric lavage. *J Toxicol Clin Toxicol.* 2004;42:933–943.
18. Bosse GM, Barefoot JA, Pfeifer MP, Rodgers GC. Comparison of three methods of gut decontamination in tricyclic antidepressant overdose. *J Emerg Med.* 1995;13:203–209.
19. Merigian KS, Woodard M, Hedges JR, Roberts JR, Stuebing R, Rashkin MC. Prospective evaluation of gastric emptying in the self-poisoned patient. *Am J Emerg Med.* 1990;8(6):479–483.
20. Pond SM, Lewis-Driver DJ, Williams GM, Green AC, Stevenson NW. Gastric emptying in acute overdose: a prospective randomised controlled trial. *Med J Aust.* 1995;163:345–349.
21. Kulig K, Bar-Or D, Cantrill SV, Rosen P, Rumack BH. Management of acutely poisoned patients without gastric emptying. *Ann Emerg Med.* 1985;14:562–567.
22. Holt LE, Holz PH. The black bottle. *Pediatrics.* 1963l;63:306.
23. Chyka PA, Seger D, Krenzelok EP, Vale JA. Position paper: single-dose activated charcoal. *Clin Toxicol (Phila).* 2005;43: 61–87.
24. Seger D. Single-dose activated charcoal-backup and reassess. *J Toxicol Clin Toxicol.* 2004;42:101–110.
25. American Academy of Clinical Toxicology. Position statement and practice guidelines on the use of multidose activated charcoal in the treatment of acute poisoning. *Clin Toxicol.* 1999;37(6):731–751.
26. Moll J, Kerns Wn, Tomaszewski C, Rose R. Incidence of aspiration pneumonia in intubated patients receiving activated charcoal. *J Emerg Med.* 1999;17:279–283.
27. Gomez HF, Brent JA, Munoz DC IV, et al. Charcoal stercolith with intestinal perforation in a patient treated for amitriptyline ingestion. *J Emerg Med.* 1994;12:57–60.
28. Greene SL, Kerins M, O'Connor N. Prehospital activated charcoal: the way forward. *Emerg Med J.* 2005;22:734–737.
29. American Academy of Clinical Toxicology. Position paper: cathartics. *J Toxicol Clin Toxicol.* 2004;42:243–253.
30. Nejman G, Hoekstra J, Kelley M. Journal club: gastric emptying in the poisoned patient. *Am J Emerg Med.* 1990;8:265–269.
31. Tenenbein M. Whole bowel irrigation for toxic ingestions. *Clin Toxicol.* 1985;23:177.
32. American Academy of Clincial toxicology. Position paper: whole bowel irrigation. *J Toxicol Clin Toxicol.* 2004;42:843–854.
33. Tenenbein M. Whole bowel irrigation in iron poisoning. *Pediatrics.* 1987;111:142.
34. Everson GW, Bertaccini EJ, O'Leary J. Use of whole bowel irrigation in an infant following iron overdose. *Am J Emerg Med.* 1991;9:366.
35. Kaczorowski JM, Wax PM. Five days of whole bowel irrigation in a case of pediatric iron ingestion. *Ann Emerg Med.* 1996;27:258.
36. Roberge RJ, Martin TG. Whole bowel irrigation in acute oral lead intoxication. *Ann Emerg Med.* 1992;10:577.
37. Smith SW, Ling LJ, Halstenson CE. Whole-bowel irrigation as a treatment for acute lithium overdose. *Ann Emerg Med.* 1991;20:536.
38. Buckley N, Dawson AH, Howarth D, et al. Slow-release verapamil poisoning: Use of polyethylene glycol whole bowel irrigation lavage and high dose calcium. *Med Aust.* 1993;158:202.
39. Rosenberg PJ, Livingstone DJ, McLellan BA. Effect of whole-bowel irrigation on the antidotal efficacy of oral activate charcoal. *Ann Emerg Med.* 1988;17:681.
40. Calello DP, Osterhoudt KC, Henretig FM. New and novel antidotes in pediatrics. *Pediatr Emerg Care.* 2006;22:523–530.
41. Brent J, McMartin K, Phillips S, et al. Fomepizole for the treatment of ethylene glycol poisoning. *N Engl J Med.* 1999;340:832–838.
42. Megarbane B, Borron SW, Baud FJ. Current recommendations for treatment of severe toxic alcohol poisonings. *Intensive Care Med.* 2005;31:189–195.
43. Dart RC, McNally J. Efficacy, safety, and use of snake antivenoms in the United States. *Ann Emerg Med.* 2001;37:181–188.
44. Offerman SR, Bush SP, Moynihan JA, Clark RF. Crotaline Fab antivenom for the treatment of children with rattlesnake envenomation. *Pediatrics.* 2002;110:968–971.
45. Lheureux PE, Zahir S, Gris M, Derrey AS, Penaloza A. Bench-to-bedside review: hyperinsulinaemia/euglycaemia therapy in the management of overdose of calcium-channel blockers. *Crit Care.* 2006;10:212.
46. Yuan TH, Kerns WP, Tomaszewski CA, et al. Insulin-glucose as adjunctive therapy for severe calcium channel antagonist poisoning. *J Toxicol Clin Toxicol.* 1999;37:463–474.
47. Borron SW, Baud FJ, Barriot P, et al. Prospective study of

hydroxocobalamin for acute cyanide poisoning in smoke inhalation. *Ann Emerg Med.* 2007;49(6):794–801.

48. Kerns W, Beuhler M, Tomaszewski C. Hydorxocobalamin versus thiosulfate for acute cyanide poisoning. *Ann Emerg Med.* 2008;51(3):338–339.

49. Pond SM. Extracorporeal techniques in the treatment of poisoned patients. *Med J Aust.* 1991;154:617–622.

50. Bosse GM, Matyunas NJ. Delayed toxidromes. *J Emerg Med.* 1999;17:679–690.

51. Liebelt EL, Shannon MW. Small doses, big problems: a selected review of highly toxic common medications. *Pediatr Emerg Care.* 1993;9:292–297.

52. Koren G. Medications which can kill a toddler with one tablet or teaspoonful. *Clin Toxicol.* 1993;31:407–414.

PART 1
ANTIPYRETIC ANALGESICS

CHAPTER 108

Acetaminophen

Leon Gussow

▶ HIGH-YIELD FACTS

- Widely available in both prescription and OTC products, acetaminophen is a leading cause of pediatric poisoning.
- Acetaminophen toxicity is a potentially preventable cause of hepatic failure.
- *N*-acetylcysteine (NAC) is the antidote for acetaminophen overdose.
- NAC should be utilized in any case of acetaminophen-induced hepatotoxicity, regardless of the time elapsed since ingestion.

Death caused solely by acetaminophen ingestion is rare in the pediatric population. In 2006, only seven deaths associated with acetaminophen in patients younger than 19 years were reported to poison control centers in the United States.[1] All of these cases involved teenagers, the majority of whom had also ingested other drugs. The small number of fatalities in this population can be explained by the availability of a very effective antidote, NAC, as well as the fact that young children are relatively resistant to acetaminophen-induced hepatotoxicity.

Young children are more likely to be administered liquid acetaminophen preparations, which are absorbed more rapidly than pills, or rectal suppositories, which have prolonged and unpredictable absorption. Adolescents often are not aware that acetaminophen ingestion can be lethal, and may unknowingly take a life-threatening amount as a suicidal gesture.[2]

▶ PATHOPHYSIOLOGY

Acetaminophen (also called APAP or paracetamol) is a synthetic analgesic and antipyretic that lacks the anti-inflammatory effects found in salicylates and nonsteroidal agents. The ther-

apeutic dose of APAP in children is 15 mg/kg given every 4 to 6 hours, with a maximum recommended total daily dose of 75 mg/kg (or five doses). Therapeutic serum levels are 10 to 20 μg/mL.[3] Acetaminophen is well absorbed after an oral therapeutic dose, with peak levels generally occurring at 30 to 60 minutes. However, after overdose, the peak level may be delayed for up to 4 hours. Absorption of liquid elixir is more rapid than that of tablets or caplets. Following gastrointestinal absorption, APAP is taken up by the liver, where tissue concentrations are high. Normal serum half-life is 1 to 3 hours after a therapeutic dose, but may be prolonged significantly following toxic ingestion.

Acetaminophen is eliminated primarily by hepatic pathways. After a therapeutic dose, 90% of the drug is metabolized to inactive sulfate and glucuronide conjugates. In young children, unlike in adults and adolescents, the sulfate conjugate predominates. Less than 5% is excreted unchanged in the urine. The remaining 2% to 4% is metabolized by the cytochrome P450 mixed-function oxidase (MFO) system to the toxic intermediate NAPQI. In the presence of adequate hepatic stores of glutathione, NAPQI is rapidly converted to nontoxic conjugates. In overdose, the sulfate and glucuronide pathways become saturated, and increased amounts of acetaminophen are shunted through the MFO system. Glutathione becomes depleted and free NAPQI attacks hepatocytes, causing acute liver failure. Drugs that induce activity of the MFO system (for example, isoniazid) may increase the risk of toxicity after acetaminophen overdose.[4]

Acute ingestion of more than 140 mg/kg of acetaminophen is potentially toxic and requires emergent evaluation. It is important to remember that acetaminophen is found in many combination products. For example, if a patient presents to the emergency departmant comatose after taking an oxycodone-acetaminophen preparation, the clinician should not neglect to measure an acetaminophen level, and begin treatment if indicated. It is essential not to overlook this aspect of the case while dealing with the more evident and dramatic opioid effects.

▶ CLINICAL PRESENTATION: THE FOUR STAGES OF ACETAMINOPHEN TOXICITY

STAGE I (0–24 HOURS AFTER INGESTION): GASTROINTESTINAL IRRITATION

Although patients in this initial stage may be asymptomatic, young children frequently vomit after acetaminophen overdose. Hepatic enzymes are in the normal ranges. Atypical findings such as lethargy, coma, or acidosis should prompt consideration of possible coingestants.

STAGE II (24–48 HOURS AFTER INGESTION): LATENT PERIOD

As nausea and vomiting resolve, patients appear to improve, but rising transaminase levels reveal evidence of hepatic necrosis. On physical examination, hepatic tenderness and enlargement may be apparent. Increased aspartate aminotransferase (AST) is the most sensitive indicator of liver toxicity.[3]

STAGE III (72–96 HOURS AFTER INGESTION): HEPATIC FAILURE

Severe hepatotoxicity presents with jaundice, hypoglycemia, renewed nausea and vomiting, right upper quadrant pain, coagulopathy, encephalopathy, hyperbilirubinemia, and markedly elevated transaminase levels. In this stage, acetaminophen-induced hepatotoxicity is usually accompanied by an AST >1000 IU/L. In fulminant hepatic failure, AST can rise to levels of 20 000 or 30 000 IU/L. It is very unusual, but not unprecedented, for children younger than 6 years to develop fulminant effects from acute APAP ingestion.

STAGE IV (4–14 DAYS AFTER INGESTION): RECOVERY OR DEATH

Patients who ultimately recover show improvement in laboratory parameters of hepatic function starting on about day 5, and eventually recover completely. Follow-up histology is normal. Less fortunate patients develop progressive encephalopathy, renal failure, coagulopathy, and hyperammonemia. The prognosis is poor for patients with these findings unless liver transplantation is performed.

▶ LABORATORY STUDIES

The Rumack-Matthew nomogram (Fig. 108–1) allows the clinician to predict the probability that hepatic toxicity will occur after single acute acetaminophen ingestion. A blood acetaminophen level is drawn 4 hours after the acute ingestion, or immediately if more than 4 hours have elapsed since the time of ingestion. Levels drawn earlier than 4 hours may not represent the peak serum concentration and thus may be mislead-

ingly low. This level is plotted on the nomogram against hours postingestion. If the point falls above the potential toxicity line, treatment with the antidote NAC is indicated. It is important to realize that this nomogram cannot be used in cases of chronic toxicity or when the time of ingestion is not well established. If treatment with NAC is indicated, additional laboratory values that may influence management include liver enzymes, bilirubin, electrolytes, creatinine, and coagulation profile.

▶ MANAGEMENT

GASTROINTESTINAL DECONTAMINATION

Induction of emesis with syrup of ipecac is contraindicated. Gastric lavage is generally not indicated but can be considered if the patient presents within 1 hour of ingestion and has taken a life-threatening overdose of another drug in addition to acetaminophen. Standard doses of activated charcoal can be given if the patient arrives within 1 hour of ingesting APAP alone, or if other toxic substances are also involved.

ANTIDOTE

NAC helps restore the liver's ability to detoxify NAPQI and can prevent hepatonecrosis. It is most effective if started within 8 hours after an acute overdose.[5] However, there is now good evidence that NAC has some benefit even if started very late, possibly even up to days after ingestion when hepatic failure is evident.[6] NAC should not be withheld on the basis of an arbitrary time limit.

The Rumack-Matthew nomogram indicates which patients require treatment following a single, acute APAP ingestion occurring at a known time (Fig. 108–1). It was devised using data from a relatively small number of adult patients, but is also applied to children. The original studies indicated that 60% of patients whose levels are above the probable toxicity line after a single acute APAP overdose would go on to develop severe hepatotoxicity (serum AST >1000 IU/L). The lower "possible toxicity" line was added to give a margin of safety. It is current practice to treat any patient who has an APAP level that falls in the range of possible or probable hepatotoxicity. In cases where the patient has not taken a single acute overdose, but rather has taken multiple doses or overdoses of APAP, or has ingested APAP chronically, the nomogram cannot be used to predict hepatotoxicity or need for treatment with NAC.

The oral NAC protocol long used in the United States for treating APAP toxicity consists of a loading dose of 140 mg/kg followed by 17 additional doses of 70 mg/kg given at 4-hour intervals. The commercial 20% solution (Mucomyst, Mead Johnson & Company) is unpalatable and should be diluted with three parts fruit juice or soda. If vomiting occurs within 1 hour of treatment, the dose is repeated. Persistent vomiting that interferes with therapy can be suppressed with metoclopromide (0.25 mg/kg IV over 5 minutes) or ondansetron (0.15 mg/kg over 5 minutes). If necessary, NAC can be infused slowly through a nasogastric tube. If activated charcoal has been administered, the usual dose of NAC does not need to

Acetaminophen nomogram

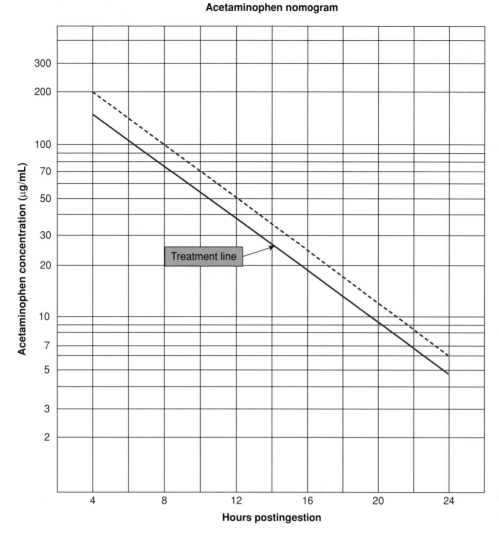

Figure 108–1. The Rumack-Matthew nomogram predicts the probability that hepatic toxicity will occur after a single acute acetaminophen ingestion.

be increased, but is best given at least 30 to 60 minutes after the charcoal.

In a review of APAP toxicity over the first 35 years of the drug's use, Rumack describes how the NAC treatment regimen was originally derived from theoretical calculations, with individual doses and length of treatment tripled to provide a margin of safety.[7] Rumack states "The 72-hour oral NAC protocol is probably unnecessary in many cases where the drug has a shorter half-life [than 4 hours] and disappears before the full dosage is completed." Based on a retrospective chart review of 75 mostly adult patients, Woo and coworkers suggested that, because evidence of APAP-induced hepatotoxicity is apparent within 36 hours of acute ingestion, treatment could be stopped at that time if liver enzymes were normal and APAP levels undetectable.[8] Some poison centers have been using this guideline for years.

Expanding on this idea of abbreviated therapy, Dart and Rumack recently proposed the concept of "Patient-Tailored Acetylcysteine Administration."[9] They suggested that treatment with NAC should be continued, not for an arbitrary period of time or number of doses, but until a specific clinical endpoint is reached. They reported that their practice at the Rocky Mountain Poison Center was to start treatment with the loading dose of NAC, and then continue maintenance doses until three criteria were met: (1) acetaminophen level was zero or near zero (usually this means <10 μg/mL), (2) alanine aminotransferase (ALT) level was normal or clearly improving, and (3) the patient was clinically well. They point out that an advantage of this goal-oriented therapy is that it can be used in all situations: acute overdose, repeated (chronic) supratherapeutic ingestion, unknown time of ingestion, and cases where the pattern of ingestion is not known. Although this protocol has not been tested in a large prospective controlled study, there is no reason to think it would not be safe and effective, and every reason to believe it would drastically simplify the approach to these cases. Recently, Betten et al. reported good outcomes in a series of more than 200 patients with potentially toxic acute APAP ingestions treated with oral NAC for at least 20 hours.[10] After this time, treatment was stopped if serum APAP was less than 10 μg/mL and liver enzymes and coagulation studies were

► TABLE 108–1. **ACETYLCYSTEINE DOSAGE GUIDELINES PEDIATRIC (WEIGHT <40 kg)**

| Body Weight | | Loading Dose | | Second Dose | | Third Dose | |
kg	lb	Acetadote (mL)	D5W (mL)	Acetadote (mL)	D5W (mL)	Acetadote (mL)	D5W (mL)
30	66	22.5	100	7.5	250	15	500
25	55	18.75	100	6.25	250	12.5	500
20	44	15	60	5	140	10	280
15	33	11.25	45	3.75	105	7.5	210
10	22	7.5	30	2.5	70	5	140

Loading dose: 150 mg/kg over 60 min; second dose: 50 mg/kg over 4 h; third dose: 100 mg/kg over 16 h.
Source: Package insert, Acetadote, Cumberland Pharmaceuticals.

normal. However, only five of these patients were ≤5 years of age.

Intravenous NAC had been used for decades in Europe and Canada to treat APAP toxicity. Finally, in 2004, the Food and Drug Administration approved IV NAC for use in the United States. (Acetadote, Cumberland Pharmaceuticals). After Acetadote was marketed in the United States, it became apparent that the recommended procedure for administering the product had two problems. First, the suggested interval for infusing the loading dose (15 minutes) caused an increased risk for anaphylactoid reactions. Second, the suggested method for diluting the supplied 20% NAC resulted in small children receiving excessive free water, risking hyponatremia and seizures. In February 2006, the package insert was revised to minimize these risks (Table 108–1).

Indications for the use of IV NAC include inability to tolerate oral NAC, intractable vomiting that does not respond to antiemetics, intestinal pathology (such as bowel obstruction or GI bleeding), encephalopathy, and neonatal acetaminophen toxicity secondary to maternal overdose. Some physicians prefer the IV preparation in almost all circumstances. With the 21-hour IV protocol, abbreviated treatment options are not necessary. However, in some cases treatment with NAC may have to be extended beyond 21 hours. White and Liebelt proposed a reasonable protocol for treating acute APAP overdose with IV NAC:

1. Draw acetaminophen level and plot on Rumack-Matthew nomogram.
2. If APAP level falls above the "possible toxicity" line, begin therapy with NAC.
3. Draw AST/ALT, PT/INR, electrolytes, BUN, creatinine, and CBC.
4. At the end of the infusion, draw PT/INR, AST/ALT, BUN/creatinine. If any of laboratory results are abnormal, infusion should be continued at a rate of 6.3 mg/kg/h until liver function improves (Note: this is equivalent to 100 mg/kg over 16 hours).
5. Consult with medical toxicologist regarding duration of therapy.
6. If the patient develops hepatic injury/failure secondary to acetaminophen, NAC therapy should be continued until liver function and/or clinical status improves.[11]

Adverse reactions to IV NAC—which usually occur during administration of the loading dose—are generally anaphylac-

toid and include rash, itching, and wheezing. These will often resolve if the infusion is temporarily suspended and the patient treated with an antihistamine. Very rarely life-threatening reactions have been reported in children with preexisting asthma. When considering the use of IV NAC, it is good practice to seek toxicology consultation through the local poison center.

► DISPOSITION

An asymptomatic patient whose APAP level falls below the "possible toxicity" line on the Rumack-Matthew nomogram can be medically cleared, but should not be discharged home until appropriate interventions have been accomplished. These may include psychiatric assessment in the case of suicidal gesture or attempt, social service consultation for suspected abuse, or counseling of parents or caregivers about the principles of poison prevention. If the APAP level is above the "possible toxicity" line, the patient should be admitted for treatment with NAC.

Asymptomatic patients with suspected chronic APAP overdose can be medically cleared if their liver enzymes are normal and APAP levels essentially undetectable. Any patient with evidence of fulminant hepatic failure (encephalopathy, hypoglycemia, coagulopathy, or acidosis) is admitted to intensive care. All patients whose exposure results from an attempt at self-harm need psychiatric evaluation and adequate suicide precautions.

REFERENCES

1. Bronstein AC, Spyker DA, Cantilena LR, et al. 2006 Annual Report of the American Association of Poison Control Centers' National Poison Data System. *Clin Toxicol.* 2007;45:815.
2. Huott MA, Storrow AB. A survey of adolescents' knowledge regarding toxicity of over-the-counter medications. *Acad Emerg Med.* 1997;4:214.
3. Marzullo L. An update of *N*-acetylcysteine treatment for acute acetaminophen toxicity in children. *Curr Opin Pediatr.* 2005;17:239.
4. Kozer E, Koren G. Management of paracetamol overdose: current controversies. *Drug Safety.* 2001;24:503.
5. Prescott L. Oral or intravenous *N*-acetylcysteine for acetaminophen poisoning? *Ann Emerg Med.* 2005;45:409.

6. Tucker JR. Late-presenting acute acetaminophen toxicity and the role of *N*-acetylcysteine. *Pediatr Emerg Care.* 1998;14:424.

7. Rumack BH. Acetaminophen hepatotoxicity: the first 35 years. *Clin Toxicol.* 2002;40:3.

8. Woo OF, Mueller PD, Olson KR, et al. Shorter duration of oral *N*-acetylcysteine therapy for acute acetaminophen overdose. *Ann Emerg Med.* 2000;35:363.

9. Dart RC, Rumack BH. Patient-tailored acetylcysteine administration. *Ann Emerg Med.* 2007;50:280.

10. Betten DP, Cantrell FL, Thomas SC, et al. A prospective evaluation of shortened course oral *N*-acetylcysteine for the treatment of acute acetaminophen poisoning. *Ann Emerg Med.* 2007;50:272.

11. White ML, Liebelt EL. Update on antidotes for pediatric poisoning. *Pediatr Emerg Care.* 2006;22:740.

CHAPTER 109

Aspirin

Michele Zell-Kanter

▶ HIGH-YIELD FACTS

- Despite improvements in packaging, toxic ingestions of aspirin continue to occur.
- Children with aspirin toxicity can rapidly develop metabolic acidosis without a respiratory alkalosis.
- Treatment of mild-to-moderate aspirin overdose consists primarily of supportive management and alkalinization of the urine.
- The decision to treat is predicated on the patient's symptoms.

Acetylsalicylic acid (aspirin, ASA) is easily accessible and is commonly used in suicide attempts. Accidental overdoses continue to occur despite improved packaging. Patients who are acutely poisoned with aspirin generally exhibit less toxicity than patients who receive aspirin chronically, such as individuals taking high doses of aspirin for chronic inflammatory conditions.[1] Individuals poisoned from chronic aspirin administration may present with signs consistent with sepsis and/or dementia. Annual data from the 2006 American Association of Poison Control Centers reported more than 17 000 exposures to aspirin alone, with 3600 of these occurring in children younger than 6 years.[2]

▶ PHARMACOKINETICS

Aspirin is rapidly absorbed from the stomach and small intestine. If taken in large amounts, absorption can be delayed by the formation of concretions. Enteric coated preparations will also have delayed absorption.[3]

In therapeutic doses, aspirin's metabolism is first-order, but in the overdose setting pharmacokinetics change to zero-order enzyme saturable, in which a small increase in dose will result in a large increase in plasma salicylate level. Thus, there is a very narrow therapeutic range for aspirin when it is used in higher doses.

Ingestions of <150 mg/kg are generally nontoxic.[4] With ingestions of 150 to 300 mg/kg mild-to-moderate toxicity occurs, and overdoses of >300 mg/kg can be lethal. It is crucial to know the concentration of the preparation ingested in order to estimate the potential for toxicity. Infant aspirin bottles are limited to 36 tablets of 81 mg each. Oil of wintergreen, on the other hand, contains 100% methyl salicylate and can be lethal in extremely small amounts.

▶ PATHOPHYSIOLOGY AND CLINICAL PRESENTATION

Children have a quicker onset of toxicity from salicylate poisoning and exhibit more severe signs than adults. This can occur in part because salicylate is distributed more rapidly into organs such as the brain, kidney, and lungs. Patients may complain of tinnitus and impaired hearing. Direct stimulation of respiratory centers causes tachypnea, which in turn results in an early respiratory alkalosis. Uncoupling of the Krebs cycle results in anaerobic metabolism and ketonemia causing the characteristic anion gap metabolic acidosis. The acidosis can be exacerbated by hypovolemia as a result of vomiting, increased insensible losses from tachypnea and perspiration, and an osmotic diuresis. Fluid losses are especially severe in young children. In pediatric patients, the onset of metabolic acidosis tends to occur more rapidly than in adults, and a respiratory alkalosis may not occur.

An acidotic environment facilitates salicylate distribution into the brain, where it can cause agitation, delirium, seizures, and coma. Rhabdomyolysis can occur and can cause acute renal failure.

Patients can develop noncardiogenic pulmonary edema, most likely because of a toxic effect of salicylates on pulmonary endothelium. Risk factors for this include CNS toxicity, metabolic acidosis, and chronic salicylate ingestion. Uncoupling of oxidative phosphorylation can result in hyperthermia, which generally indicates significant toxicity.

Commonly observed electrolyte abnormalities include hypo- or hypernatremia, hypokalemia, and hypocalcemia. In children, hypoglycemia is more common than hyperglycemia. Salicylate-induced ventricular dysrhythmias are infrequent and indicative of a poor prognosis.[5] Dysrhythmias may result from acid–base and/or electrolyte abnormalities, or a direct effect on the myocardium (Table 109–1).

▶ LABORATORY STUDIES

Required initial laboratory studies include a complete blood count, serum electrolytes, creatinine, glucose, and arterial or venous blood gases.

Plasma salicylate levels are easily obtainable and are best drawn 6 hours postingestion, when they reflect peak concentration. However, since the history of ingestion is often inaccurate, a plasma salicylate level should be drawn upon presentation, and repeated every 2 hours to ensure that the level is decreasing. Plasma levels following ingestion of enteric

Acetylsalicylic acid (aspirin, ASA)
Bismuth subsalicylate
Choline salicylate
Magnesium choline salicylate (Trilisate)
Magnesium salicylate
Methyl salicylate
Salsalate (Disalcid)
Sodium salicylate

coated or extended release preparations will reflect delayed absorption.[3] When a concretion is present, levels can continue to increase after they have appeared to level off, or have slightly decreased. Patients with toxicity from chronic ingestion generally have a worse prognosis and clinical findings are more predictive of toxicity than the plasma level.

▶ MANAGEMENT

Goals in the management of the salicylate-intoxicated patient are

- fluid replacement
- correction of metabolic disturbances
- prevention of further absorption of the toxin
- enhancement of elimination

Intravascular volume is restored by boluses of crystalloid at doses of 10 to 20 mL/kg until adequate perfusion is assured. After urine output is established, potassium is added to the intravenous fluid for patients who are hypokalemic.

Large amounts of aspirin have a tendency to form concretions in the stomach. Whole bowel irrigation is of theoretical benefit. It can be considered for stable patients in whom a concretion is observed on radiograph, or for patients who have ingested sustained-release preparations.

Activated charcoal is effective in adsorbing ingested aspirin. Studies evaluating multiple doses of activated charcoal (MDAC) are inconclusive, and MDAC use is not recommended by the American Academy of Clinical Toxicology.[6] The efficacy of whole bowel irrigation with activated charcoal is unknown.[7]

Salicylate elimination is enhanced by systemic alkalinization. Alkalemia increases the ionized fraction of salicylate and decreases its entry into the brain and other tissues. The goal of alkalinization is to increase the urine pH to 7.5 to 8. This is accomplished by administering sodium bicarbonate in an initial bolus of 1 to 2 mEq/kg, followed by a bicarbonate drip titrated to the urine pH. Serial arterial blood gases are obtained to assure that the patient is not overalkalinized.

Hypokalemia is common in salicylism. This can impair attempts to alkalinize the urine since potassium is exchanged for hydrogen in the tubular fluid when serum potassium is low. In hypokalemic patients, potassium is added to the intravenous solution once urine output is adequate. Complications of alkalinization include congestive heart failure secondary to volume load, excessive alkalemia, and hypernatremia.

For patients with extreme toxicity, hemodialysis should be considered. Hemodialysis removes salicylate three to five times faster than systemic alkalinization. Indications for its use include congestive heart failure, noncardiogenic pulmonary edema, CNS depression, seizure, metabolic acidosis refractory to alkalinization, hepatic failure, or coagulopathy. The salicylate level is not useful as a sole criterion for dialysis unless it is >80 mg/dL in an acute ingestion. The threshold for dialysis is lower for patients chronically on salicylates since these patients exhibit more severe toxicity.

REFERENCES

1. Gaudreault P, Temple AR, Lovejoy FH. The relative severity of acute versus chronic salicylate poisoning in children: a clinical comparison. *Pediatrics*. 1982;70:566–569.
2. Bronstein AC, Spyker DA, Cantilena LR, et al. 2006 Annual report of the American Association of Poison Control Centers' National Poison Data System (NPDS). *Clin Toxicol*. 2007;45:815–917.
3. Rivera W, Kleinschmidt KC, Velez LI, et al. Delayed salicylate toxicity at 35 hours without early manifestations following a single salicylate ingestion. *Ann Pharmacother*. 2004;38:1186–1188.
4. Notarianni L. A reassessment of the treatment of salicylate poisoning. *Drug Saf*. 1992;7:292–303.
5. Kent K, Ganetsky M, Cohen J, et al. Non-fatal ventricular dysrhythmias associated with severe salicylate toxicity. *Clin Toxicol (Phila)*. 2008;46:297–299.
6. American Academy of Clinical Toxicology and European Association of Poisons Centres and Clinical Toxicologists. Poison statement and practice guidelines on the use of multi-dose activated charcoal in the treatment of acute poisoning. *J Toxicol Clin Toxicol*. 1999;37:731–751.
7. Mayer AL, Sitar DS, Tenenbein M. Multiple-dose charcoal and whole bowel irrigation do not increase clearance of absorbed salicylate. *Arch Intern Med*. 1992;152:393–396.

CHAPTER 110

Nonsteroidal Anti-inflammatory Drugs

Michele Zell-Kanter

▶ HIGH-YIELD FACTS

- Nonsteroidal anti-inflammatory agents (NSAIDs) are relatively devoid of toxicity in the overdose setting.
- Typically, patients who ingest NSAIDs exhibit only central nervous system (CNS) and/or gastrointestinal (GI) toxicity.
- Long-term use of NSAIDs is associated with nephrotoxicity, including acute tubular necrosis, acute interstitial nephritis, and acute renal failure. Renal toxicity is not associated with acute overdose.
- Infrequently, overdose of NSAIDs has been associated with an anion-gap acidosis. For patients with severe clinical symptoms, an arterial blood gas is indicated.
- After the patient is stabilized, activated charcoal is administered

There are many drugs in use today that are categorized as NSAIDs (Table 110–1). These drugs function largely by inhibiting cyclooxygenase,[1] the enzyme needed to convert arachidonic acid to prostaglandin. NSAIDs are typically non-toxic in the overdose setting. The 2006 Annual Report of the American Association of Poison Control Centers listed one death secondary to ibuprofen, although there were more than 71 000 ingestions, of which more than 39 000 occurred in children younger than 6 years. There were 13 000 ingestions of other NSAIDs, resulting in one death.[2]

▶ CLINICAL PRESENTATION

Typically, patients who ingest NSAIDs exhibit only CNS and/or GI toxicity. Symptoms are generally seen within 4 to 6 hours of ingestion.

Common symptoms of CNS toxicity can include drowsiness, dizziness, and lethargy.[3] The mefenamic acid compound, Ponstel, has a propensity to cause seizures.[4] Other NSAIDs associated with seizures include piroxicam, naproxen, and ketoprofen. Headache is more likely to occur after ingestion of indomethacin than other NSAIDs. Aseptic meningitis has been reported with NSAIDs, most typically with ibuprofen.[5,6]

Symptoms of GI toxicity include nausea, vomiting, and epigastric pain, all of which can occur at therapeutic doses.[3] The gastritis associated with NSAIDs probably occurs secondary to inhibition of prostaglandin synthesis.

Cardiovascular complications of NSAID overdose are generally limited to tachycardia and hypotension, usually secondary to volume depletion.[7] Respiratory complications include hyperventilation and apnea, which are rare.

Long-term use of NSAIDs is associated with nephrotoxicity, including acute tubular necrosis, acute interstitial nephritis, and acute renal failure. Renal papillary necrosis has been reported in children being treated with NSAIDs for juvenile rheumatoid arthritis. Renal toxicity is not associated with acute overdose.

Other long-term complications of NSAID use include hepatocellular injury and cholestatic jaundice.

▶ LABORATORY STUDIES

Assay procedures for measuring plasma ibuprofen levels are available. There is a poor correlation between the absolute level and toxicity. Therefore, there is negligible clinical utility in obtaining an ibuprofen level.[8]

Laboratory tests include a complete blood count, electrolytes, glucose, creatinine, and coagulation profile.

▶ TABLE 110–1. CURRENTLY AVAILABLE NSAIDS

Cox-1 Inhibitors
Acetic Acids Derivatives
   Diclofenac (Voltaren)
   Etodolac (Lodine)
   Indomethacin (Indocin)
   Ketorolac (Toradol)
   Nabumetone (Relafen)
   Sulindac (Clinoril)
   Tolmetin (Tolectin)
Fenamic Acid Derivatives
   Meclofenamate (Meclomen)
   Mefenamic acid (Ponstel)
Oxicams
   Piroxicam (Feldene)
Propionic Acid Derivatives
   Fenoprofen (Nalfon)
   Flurbiprofen (Ansaid)
   Ibuprofen (Advil, Motrin, and others)
   Ketoprofen (Orudis)
   Naproxen (Anaprox, Naprosyn, and others)
   Oxaprozin (Daypro)

Cox-2 Inhibitors
Celecoxib (Celebrex)
Meloxicam (Mobic)

Infrequently, overdose of NSAIDs has been associated with an anion-gap acidosis. For patients with severe clinical symptoms, an arterial blood gas is indicated.

► MANAGEMENT

Gastric decontamination with activated charcoal is indicated after the patient is stabilized. At the present time, there are no data to support multiple doses of activated charcoal.

The high protein binding of NSAIDs renders extracorporeal methods of elimination ineffective.

REFERENCES

1. Vane JR, Botting RM. Anti-inflammatory drugs and their mechanism of action. *Inflamm Res*. 1998;47(suppl 2):S78–S87.

2. Bronstein AC, Spyker DA, Cantilena LR Jr, et al. 2006 Annual Report of the American Association of Poison Control Centers' National Poison Data System (NPDS). *Clin Toxicol*. 2007;45:815–917.

3. Skeith KJ, Wright M, Davis P. Differences in NSAID tolerability profiles: fact or fiction? *Drug Saf*. 1994;10:183–195.

4. Smolinske SC, Hall AH, Vandenburg SA, et al. Toxic effects of nonsteroidal antiinflammatory drugs in overdose. *Drug Saf*. 1990;5:252–274.

5. Nguyen HTV, Juurlink DN. Recurrent ibuprofen-induced aseptic meningitis. *Ann Pharmacother*. 2004;38:408–410.

6. Martinez R, Smith DW, Frankel LR. Severe metabolic acidosis after acute naproxen sodium ingestion. *Ann Emerg Med*. 1989;18:1102–1104.

7. Wood DM, Monaghan J, Streete P, et al. Fatality after deliberate ingestion of sustained-release ibuprofen: a case report. *Crit Care*. 2006;10;R44–R49.

8. McElwee NE, Veltri JC, Bradford DC, et al. A prospective, population-based study of acute ibuprofen overdose: complications are rare and routine serum levels are not warranted. *Ann Emerg Med*. 1990;19:657–662.

PART 2
HOUSEHOLD CHEMICALS

CHAPTER 111

Toxic Alcohols

Timothy B. Erickson

▶ HIGH-YIELD FACTS

- Ethanol overdose in children may result in hypoglycemia.
- Methanol ingestion is associated with visual disturbance, metabolic acidosis, and possibly multiorgan system failure.
- Ethylene glycol poisoning is associated with metabolic acidosis, renal failure, and possibly death.
- Isopropanol may cause CNS depression but does not usually cause metabolic acidosis.
- All of the toxic alcohols can produce an osmolal gap.
- Fomepizole is the only FDA approved antidote for ethylene glycol and methanol toxicity.
- Hemodialysis is indicated in severe toxic alcohol ingestions not responsive to conventional medical therapy, or with evidence of end-organ damage or severe acidosis.

▶ ETHANOL

According to a recent 2-year prospective study in Norway, of those pediatric poisonings reported in children aging from 8 to 15 years, 46% involved ethanol.[1] In addition to alcohol-containing beverages such as beer, wine, and hard liquors, children have access to more than 700 ethanol containing medicinal preparations, colognes and perfumes, as well as mouthwashes that can contain up to 75% ethanol. There has been increasing legislation in the United States regulating child-resistant packaging and product-warning labels on mouthwash products containing ethanol. Since these interventions were instituted in 1995, improved outcomes have been documented in regards to these ingestions in children.[2,3]

PHARMACOKINETICS AND PATHOPHYSIOLOGY

Ethanol undergoes hepatic metabolism via two metabolic pathways: alcohol dehydrogenase and the microsomal ethanol-oxidizing system (MEOS). Alcohol dehydrogenase pathway is the major metabolic pathway and the rate-limiting step in con-
verting ethanol to acetaldehyde. In general, nontolerant individuals metabolize ethanol at 10 to 25 mg/dL/h and alcohol tolerant metabolize up to 30 mg/dL/h. Children may ingest large amounts of ethanol in relation to their body weight, resulting in rapid development of high blood alcohol concentrations. In children younger than 5 years, the ability to metabolize ethanol is diminished because of immature hepatic dehydrogenase activity.

CLINICAL PRESENTATION

Ethanol is a selective CNS depressant at low concentrations, and a generalized depressant at high concentrations. Initially, ethanol produces exhilaration and loss of inhibition, which progresses to lack of coordination, ataxia, slurred speech, gait disturbances, drowsiness, and, ultimately, stupor, and coma. The intoxicated child may demonstrate a flushed face, dilated pupils, excessive sweating, gastrointestinal distress, hypoventilation, hypothermia, and hypotension. Death from respiratory depression may occur at serum ethanol concentrations >500 mg/dL. Convulsions and death have been reported in children with acute ethanol intoxication owing to alcohol-induced hypoglycemia. Hypoglycemia results from inhibition of hepatic gluconeogenesis and is most common in children younger than 5 years. It does not appear to be directly related to the quantity of alcohol ingested.[4]

LABORATORY STUDIES

In symptomatic, pediatric patients who have suspected ethanol intoxication, the most critical laboratory tests are the serum ethanol and glucose concentrations.[5] Although blood ethanol concentrations roughly correlate with clinical signs, the physician must treat patients based on their clinical status, not the absolute level. If the ethanol level does not correlate with the clinical picture, coingestants or other causes of altered mental status should be considered. If children have experienced fluid losses, serum electrolytes are monitored.

MANAGEMENT

The majority of children with accidental acute ingestions of ethanol respond to supportive care. Attention is directed toward management of the patient's airway, circulation, and glucose status. A bedside glucose is obtained; younger hypoglycemic patients should receive 2 to 4 mL/kg of D25 W; older children and adolescents receive 1 amp of D50 W. Serial glucose levels are followed to detect recurrent hypoglycemia. In obtunded patients, naloxone 2 mg IV push is indicated to rule out opiate toxicity.

In ethanol ingestions, gastric decontamination is unnecessary. Activated charcoal is probably not efficacious in isolated ethanol ingestions. Since hemodialysis increases ethanol clearance by three to four times, it may be considered in massive ethanol ingestions in patients do no respond to conventional therapy.[4]

DISPOSITION

Any infant with significantly altered mental status following acute ethanol ingestion is admitted for observation of respiratory status, fluid resuscitation, and glucose monitoring. Asymptomatic patients may be discharged home with reliable caretakers. Adolescent patients should be referred for counseling in an alcohol addiction program if a recurrent pattern of ethanol abuse is suspected.

▶ METHANOL

Methanol is present in a variety of substances found around the home and workplace, including paint solvents, gasohol, gasoline additives, canned heat products, windshield washer fluid, and duplicating chemicals.

PHARMACOKINETICS AND PATHOPHYSIOLOGY

Methanol is rapidly absorbed following ingestion. Peak serum levels can be reached as early as 30 to 90 minutes postingestion. As with ethanol, methanol is primarily metabolized by hepatic alcohol dehydrogenase. The half-life of methanol may be as long as 24 hours, but in the presence of ethanol or fomepizole, it is longer. In one report of methanol poisoning in an infant, methanol metabolism demonstrated first order elimination kinetics.[6] Methanol itself is harmless; however, its main metabolite, formic acid, is extremely toxic. Fatalities have been reported after ingestion of as little as 15 mL of a 40% methanol solution, although 30 mL is generally considered a minimal lethal dose. Ingestion of only 10 mL can lead to blindness. Adults have survived ingestions of 500 mL.

CLINICAL PRESENTATION

The onset of symptoms following methanol ingestion varies from 1 to 72 hours. Patients may have the classic triad consisting of visual complaints, abdominal pain, and metabolic acidosis. Eye signs and symptoms are generally delayed and include blurring of vision, photophobia, constricted visual fields, snowfield vision, and hyperemia of the optic disk. Although the blindness is usually permanent, recovery has been reported.[7]

Patients also typically complain of nausea and vomiting and can experience gastrointestinal bleeding and acute pancreatitis. Unlike with the other alcohols, these patients often lack the odor of ethanol on their breath, and typically have a clear sensorium. Methanol toxicity should be suspected in patients with altered mental status and metabolic acidosis of unclear etiology, especially if they have complaints involving their vision.[8]

LABORATORY STUDIES

Baseline laboratory data include a complete blood cell count, serum electrolytes and blood glucose, amylase, blood urea nitrogen (BUN) and serum creatinine, a urinalysis, and an arterial blood gas. Classically, methanol-intoxicated patients develop an elevated anion gap metabolic acidosis, although this may not be present if the patient presents before a significant quantity of formic acid has been generated.[9] The anion gap should be calculated using the equation:

$$(Na) - (Cl + HCO_3).$$ The normal anion gap is 8 to 12 mEq/L.

Another valuable clue in establishing the diagnosis is the presence of an elevated osmolal gap, which is the difference between measured and calculated serum osmolarity. An elevated osmolal gap indicates that a highly osmotic compound not normally found in the serum is present in a significant quantity. The most accurate determination of the measured osmolality is made using a freezing point depression method, since the standard vapor pressure analysis volatizes alcohols and can produce erroneous results.

The formula for calculating serum osmolality is:
$$2(NA) + glucose/18 + BUN/2.8 + ETOH/2.4.$$

Normally, the difference between the measure serum osmolality and the calculate serum osmolality is less than 10 mOsm. Other toxicologic causes of elevated osmolal gaps include ethylene glycol, ethanol, and isopropanol poisoning, all of which are highly osmotically active compounds. Although the osmolal gap is a useful clue, cases of significant methanol and ethylene glycol overdoses have been reported with normal osmolal gaps.

Measurement of methanol and ethanol levels is critical in diagnosing these poisonings. Generally, levels <20 mg/dL result in no effects. It is generally stated, but undocumented, that CNS effects appear with levels >20 mg/dL and peak levels >50 mg/dL indicate serious toxicity. Ocular effects occur at levels >100 mg/dL, and fatalities have been reported in untreated victims with levels >150 mg/dL.[10] One problem in interpreting levels is the time of ingestion versus the time of patient presentation and serum level assessment. Patients with low serum methanol concentrations may still be significantly poisoned and acidotic if they present late in their clinical course.

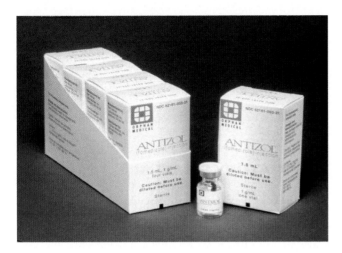

Figure 111–1. Antizole (4-MP).

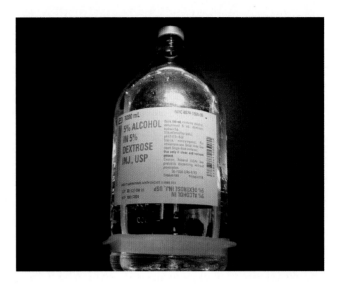

Figure 111–2. A 5% intravenous alcohol solution.

MANAGEMENT

Gastrointestinal decontamination may be efficacious for patients presenting within 1 hour of ingestion, although this is unlikely, particularly with a rapidly absorbed agent such as methanol. Although the utility of activated charcoal and cathartics in preventing absorption of the toxic alcohols has not been well established, 1 g/kg can be administered, particularly if a coingestion is suspected.

If a significant ingestion of methanol is likely, empiric treatment with the intravenous alcohol dehydrogenase inhibitor fomepizole is recommended,[11,12] even if laboratory tests are unavailable. Fomepizole (Fig. 111–1) competitively binds hepatic alcohol dehydrogenase 500 to 1000 times more avidly than methanol, and prevents the formation of the toxic metabolite formic acid. Other indications for fomepizole therapy include serum methanol levels >20 mg/dL or acidemia (pH < 7.20). A fomepizole loading dose of 15 mg/kg should be administered, followed by doses 10 mg/kg every 12 hours for four doses, until methanol levels are 20 mg/dL. Fomepizole is the only FDA approved antidote for methanol poisoning.[13] A recent investigation demonstrated that oral administration of fomepizole produced similar blood levels as an identical intravenous dose.[14]

If fomepizole is unavailable, ethanol may be administered in an attempt to block alcohol dehydrogenase[15] (Fig. 111–2). To inhibit toxic metabolite formation, ethanol levels are maintained between 100 and 150 mg/dL. An intravenous solution of 10% ethanol in D5 W is optimal, with a loading dose of 0.6 g/kg. A simplified approximation of the loading dose is 1 mL/kg of 10% diluted absolute ethanol. Close monitoring of the ethanol level every 1 to 2 hours is necessary in order to adjust the maintenance infusion rate for each individual patient. If IV ethanol preparations are unavailable, oral ethanol therapy can be instituted. Since hypoglycemia is a complication of toxic ethanol levels in young children, serum glucose levels are closely monitored.

Continued therapy with fomepizole or ethanol is recommended until methanol level falls below 20 mg/dL. Although there is no clinical outcome data confirming the superiority of either of these antidotes, there are significant disadvantages

with ethanol therapy. These include difficulty in maintaining therapeutic concentrations, induced hypoglycemia, and CNS depression that may require endotracheal intubation, particularly in children. Unlike ethanol, fomepizole does not cause CNS depression and hypoglycemia. In pediatric cases, minimal side effects make fomepizole the antidote of choice.

Additional therapies for methanol poisonings may include bicarbonate if the serum pH falls below 7.20. Folate, the active form of folic acid, is a coenzyme in the metabolic step converting the toxic metabolite formate to CO_2 and H_2O, and is indicated in the methanol-poisoned patient. Up to 50 mg of folate can be given intravenously every 4 hours, until the acidosis is corrected and methanol levels fall below 20 mg/dL.

Hemodialysis effectively removes methanol and formic acid. Indications for dialysis include visual impairment, metabolic acidosis not corrected with bicarbonate administration, renal failure, and methanol levels >50 mg/dL (with or without clinical signs or symptoms). It is important to note that ethanol and fomepizole are readily dialyzed, so the rate of IV administration may have to be increased during dialysis. For fomepizole, the recommendation is increasing the frequency of dosing to every 4 hours during hemodialysis.[16]

DISPOSITION

Any patients who are comatose and have abnormal vital signs, visual complaints, metabolic acidosis, or high methanol levels need admission to a pediatric intensive care unit. Asymptomatic patients without an evidence of acidosis and with a methanol level <20 mg/dL may be discharged from after observation in the emergency department.[4]

► ETHYLENE GLYCOL

Ethylene glycol is an odorless, sweet-tasting compound that is found in antifreeze products, coolants, preservatives, and glycerin substitutes.

PHARMACOKINETICS AND PATHOPHYSIOLOGY

Ethylene glycol undergoes rapid absorption from the gastrointestinal tract, and initial signs of intoxication may occur as early as 30 minutes postingestion. It undergoes hepatic metabolism via alcohol dehydrogenase to form the toxic metabolites glycolaldehyde, glycolic acid, and ultimately oxalate, which is excreted through the kidney. The hallmarks of ethylene glycol toxicity are a severe anion gap metabolic acidosis because of accumulation of glycolic acid, hypocalcemia, and renal failure, which results from the precipitation of calcium oxalate crystals in the kidney.[17]

CLINICAL PRESENTATION

The clinical effects of ethylene glycol toxicity can be divided into three stages:

- Stage I occurs within the first 12 hours of ingestion, with CNS symptoms similar to that experienced with ethanol. This stage is characterized by slurred speech, nystagmus, ataxia, vomiting, lethargy, and coma. Patients may suffer convulsions, myoclonic jerks, and tetanic contractions because of hypocalcemia. As with methanol toxicity, patients can demonstrate an anion gap acidosis with an elevated osmol gap. In approximately one-third of cases, calcium oxalate crystals will be discovered in the urine, a finding considered strongly suggestive of ethylene glycol poisoning (Fig. 111–3). These types of crystals are also found in the urine of patients ingesting certain vegetable diets.
- Stage II occurs within 12 to 36 hours after ingestion, and is characterized by rapidly progressive tachypnea, cyanosis, pulmonary edema, adult respiratory distress syndrome, and cardiomegaly.
- Death is most common during this stage.

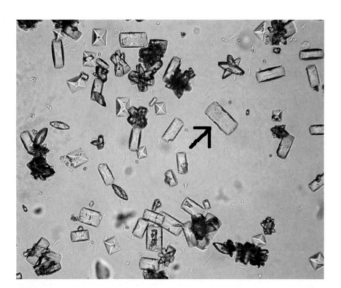

Figure 111–3. Calcium oxalate crystals found with ethylene glycol poisoning.

- Stage III occurs 2 to 3 days postingestion and is heralded by flank pain, oliguria, proteinuria, anuria, and renal failure.

Ethylene glycol poisoning is possible in any inebriated patient lacking an odor of ethanol who has severe acidosis, oxalate crystalluria, hematuria, or renal failure. In a child with a metabolic acidosis of an unclear etiology, this diagnosis should be considered.[18]

LABORATORY STUDIES

Indicated laboratory studies include complete blood cell count, serum electrolytes, blood glucose, calcium, creatine kinase, serum ethanol and ethylene glycol, an arterial blood gas, BUN and serum creatinine, serum osmolarity, and urine for crystals, protein, and blood. Both anion and osmolal gaps are calculated. Because of the potential for severe cardiopulmonary toxicity, a chest radiograph and an electrocardiogram are recommended. Since fluorescein is present in many antifreeze products, fluorescence of the patient's urine, gastric aspirate, or perioral area when exposed to light from a Wood's lamp can be a valuable diagnostic clue, although the clinical efficacy and practicality of this test has been challenged in the recent literature.

MANAGEMENT

Gastric lavage may be useful in patients presenting within 1 hour of ingestion. Syrup of ipecac is contraindicated. Activated charcoal can be administered, although there are no studies documenting its effectiveness in ethylene glycol toxicity. Patients who develop seizures are treated with standard doses of benzodiazepines and phenobarbital.

The alcohol dehydrogenase inhibitor fomepizole has been FDA approved for treatment of ethylene glycol poisoning.[13,19] Indications include a metabolic acidosis (pH less than 7.20 of unknown cause) or an ethylene glycol level >20 mg/dL. In cases where a significant ingestion is suspected, therapy should not be delayed pending an ethylene glycol level.

Ethanol competitively binds alcohol dehydrogenase with an affinity 100 times greater than ethylene glycol and slows the accumulation of toxic metabolites; it is an alternative to therapy with fomepizole.[15] If an intravenous preparation of ethanol is unavailable, patients can be loaded orally to achieve an ethanol level of 100 to 150 mg/dL. Since toxic ethanol levels result in profound hypoglycemia in small children, serial glucose measurements are monitored.

Bicarbonate administration is recommended for patients with pH >7.20. Serum calcium levels are monitored and hypocalcemia is treated with 10% calcium gluconate if the patient has clinical signs of hypocalcemia. Calcium replacement is not indicated for hypocalcemia alone, since this will encourage the formation of calcium oxalate crystals. Additionally, thiamine and pyridoxine (vitamin B$_6$) are recommended in ethylene glycol poisonings in order to shunt or reroute the metabolism of ethylene glycol toward less toxic metabolites (Table 111–1).

Hemodialysis effectively removes ethylene glycol, as well as its major circulating toxic metabolite, glycolic acid. It is

▶ TABLE 111–1. **TOXIC ALCOHOL ANTIDOTES**

Methanol	Ethylene Glycol
Fomepizole	Fomepizole
Folate	Thiamine
	Pyridoxine
Ethanol	Ethanol

▶ TABLE 111–2. **COMPARISONS OF TOXIC ALCOHOLS**

Parameter	Methanol	Ethylene Glycol	Isopropanol
Anion gap Acidosis	+	+	−
Osmolal gap	+	+	+
CNS depression	+	+	+
Eye findings	+	−	−
Renal failure	−	+	−
Ketones	−	−	+
Oxalate crystals	−	+	−

indicated in the setting of metabolic acidosis not responsive to bicarbonate administration, pulmonary edema, renal failure. Serum ethylene glycol levels >50 mg/dL, regardless of clinical signs, is an indication for hemodialysis in patients who are being treated with ethanol.[20] Recent data have suggested that hemodialysis may not be necessary for cases of ethylene glycol poisoning that can be treated with fomepizole as blocking therapy before acidosis or renal dysfunction develops.[21]

▶ ISOPROPANOL

Isopropanol is a common solvent and disinfectant with CNS-depressant properties similar to ethanol. The majority of pediatric exposures (up to 90%) occur in children younger than 6 years. Exposure from isopropyl alcohol occurs more frequently in these children than ethanol, methanol, or ethylene glycol ingestions. Toxicity results from both accidental and intentional ingestions, as well as inhalation and dermal exposures in young children given "rubbing alcohol" sponge baths for fever.

PHARMACOKINETICS AND PATHOPHYSIOLOGY

Isopropanol is rapidly absorbed across the gastric mucosa, with acute intoxication occurring within 30 minutes of ingestion. It is metabolized by alcohol dehydrogenase, but, unlike the other alcohols, is not metabolized to an acidic end product. Rather, isopropanol is converted to the CNS depressant acetone. Respiratory elimination of the acetone causes a fruity-acetone odor on the patient's breath similar to diabetic ketoacidosis. Since 70% isopropanol is a potent inebriant that is about twice as intoxicating as ethanol, a level of 50 mg/dL is comparable to an ethanol level of 100 mg/dL.

CLINICAL PRESENTATION

Isopropanol-intoxicated patients are classically lethargic or comatose, hypotensive, and tachycardiac, with the characteristic breath odor of rubbing alcohol or acetone. Coma develops at levels >100 mg/dL. Hypotension results from peripheral vasodilation and cardiac depression. Gastrointestinal irritation with acute abdominal pain and hematemesis can also occur. With isopropanol, unlike the other toxic alcohols, acidosis, ophthalmologic changes, and renal failure are absent. However, like ethanol, methanol, and ethylene glycol, isopropanol can produce a significant osmolal gap[9] (Table 111–2).

LABORATORY STUDIES

Patients are tested for the presence of acetonemia and acetonuria. Unlike diabetic ketoacidosis, the acetone is typically found in the absence of glucosuria, hyperglycemia, or acidemia. Indicated laboratory studies include a complete blood cell count, serum electrolytes, an arterial blood gas, blood glucose, serum ethanol and isopropanol levels, serum osmolarity, and BUN and creatinine. Isopropanol levels >400 mg/dL correspond to severe, life-threatening toxicity.

MANAGEMENT

Patients are managed with particular attention paid to the integrity of the airway. Hypotension is treated with intravenous crystalloid. Since isopropanol is so rapidly absorbed from the gastrointestinal tract, gastric decontamination with a nasogastric tube is unlikely to be of any benefit. Activated charcoal may be administered if there is a coingestion. The efficacy of activated charcoal for isopropanol poisoning alone is questionable. No alcohol dehydrogenase inhibition is indicated since the metabolite acetone is relatively nontoxic and excreted through the lungs. Hemodialysis is effective in removing isopropanol, but is reserved for prolonged coma, hypotension, and isopropanol levels >400 to 500 mg/dL. Typically, patients progress well with supportive care alone.[22]

DISPOSITION

Isopropanol-intoxicated patients who are lethargic should be admitted, while asymptomatic children may be observed in the emergency department. Ingestion of more than three swallows (15 mL) of 70% isopropanol by a 10-kg child (1.5 mL/kg) is an indication for several hours of observation.[4]

REFERENCES

1. Rajka T, Heyerdahl F, Hovda K, et al. Acute child poisonings in Oslo: a 2 year prospective study. *Acta Pediatr.* 2007;96(9): 1355–1359.
2. Mrvos R, Krenzelok EP. Child-resistant closures for mouthwash: do they make a difference? *J Emerg Med.* 2007;23(10): 713–715.

3. Massey C, Shulman J. Acute ethanol toxicity from ingesting mouthwash in children younger than age 6, 1989–2003. *J Pediatr Dent.* 2006;28(5):405–409.
4. Haymond MW. Hypoglycemia in infants and children. *Endocrinol Metab Clin North Am.* 1989;18:211–252.
5. Erickson T, Brent J. Toxic Alcohols. In: Erickson T, Ahren W, Aks S, et al., eds. *Pediatric Toxicology Diagnosis and Management of the Poisoned Child.* 1st ed. New York, NY: McGraw-Hill; 2005:326–332.
6. Wu AB, Kelly T, McKay C, et al. Definitive identification of an exceptionally high methanol concentration in an intoxication of a surviving infant: methanol metabolism by first order elimination kinetics. *J Forensic Sci.* 1995;40:315–320.
7. Erickson T. Toxic alcohol poisoning: when to suspect and keys to diagnosis. *Consultant.* 2000;40:1845–1856.
8. Brent J, Lucas M, Kulig, Rumack BH. Methanol poisoning in a 6 week old infant. *J Pediatr.* 1991;118:644–646.
9. Kraut J, Kraut I. Toxic alcohol ingestions: clinical features, diagnosis and management. *Clin J Am Soc Nephrol.* 2008;3(1):208–225.
10. Liu JJ, Daya MR, Carrasquill O, et al. Prognostic factors in patients with methanol poisoning. *J Toxicol Clin Toxicol.* 1998;36:175.
11. Brent J, McMartin K, Phillips S, et al. Fomepizole for the treatment of methanol poisoning. *N Engl J Med.* 2001;344:424–429.
12. Brown MJ, Shannon MW, Woolf A, et al. Childhood methanol ingestion treated with 4-MP and hemodialysis. *Pediatrics.* 2001;108:77–79.
13. White ML, Liebelt EL. Update on antidotes for pediatric poisoning. *Pediatr Emerg Care.* 2006;22(11):740–746.
14. Marraffa J, Forrest A, Grant W, et al. Oral administration of fomepizole produces similar blood levels as identical intravenous doses. *Clin Toxicol.* 2008;46(3):11–16.
15. Jacobsen D, McMartin KE. Antidotes for methanol and ethylene glycol poisoning. *J Toxicol Clin Toxicol.* 1997;35:127.
16. Barceloux DG, Bond RG, Krenzelok EP, et al. American Academy of Clinical Toxicology Ad Hoc Committee: AACT practice guidelines on the treatment of methanol poisoning. *J Toxicol Clin Toxicol.* 2002;40(4):415–446.
17. Saladino R, Shannon M. Accidental and intentional poisoning with ethylene glycol in infancy: diagnostic clues and management. *Pediatr Emerg Care.* 1991;7:93–96.
18. Woolf AD, Wynshaw-Boris A, Rinaldo P, et al. Intentional infantile ethylene glycol poisoning presenting as an inherited metabolic disorder. *J Pediatr.* 1992;120:421–424.
19. Brent J, McMartin K, Phillips S, et al. Fomepizole for the treatment of ethylene glycol poisoning. *N Engl J Med.* 1999;340:832–838.
20. Barceloux DG, Krenzelor E, Olson K, et al. American Academy of Clinical Toxicology Ad Hoc Committee: guidelines on the treatment of ethylene glycol poisoning. *J Toxicol Clin Toxicol.* 1999;37:537–560.
21. Velez L, Sheperd G, Lee Y, et al. Ethylene glycl ingestion treated with only fomepizol. *J Med Toxicol.* 2007;3(3):125–128.
22. Burkhart KK, Kulig KW. The other alcohols: methanol, ethylene glycol and isopropanol. *Emerg Clin North Am.* 1990;8:913–928.

CHAPTER 112

Organophosphates and Carbamates

Leon Gussow

- Organophosphates inactivate the enzyme acetylcholinesterase, causing increased levels of acetylcholine at cholinergic receptor sites in muscles, glands, and neural ganglia.
- The early muscarinic manifestations of organophosphate toxicity include salivation, lacrimation, diarrhea, vomiting, and miosis.
- Although organophosphate exposure can often present with seemingly nonspecific respiratory, gastrointestinal, or neurologic manifestations, the combination of miosis and increased salivation should prompt serious consideration of the diagnosis.
- The antidotes atropine and pralidoxime are used to treat organophosphate exposure, while atropine alone is used for carbamate toxicity.
- Nicotinic manifestations are common in organophosphate exposure, but uncommon in carbamate toxicity.

More than 50% of exposures to organophosphate and carbamate pesticides involve children younger than 6 years. Several factors make these pediatric cases difficult to diagnose. Often the child is too young to give a history, and the parents might not suspect that oral or topical pesticide exposure has occurred. In addition, the typical respiratory and gastrointestinal symptoms of the cholinergic syndrome may be mistaken for those of common childhood illnesses: bronchitis, pneumonia, upper respiratory infection, or gastroenteritis. Finally, some studies have indicated that well-recognized manifestations of cholinergic toxicity in adults—for example, bradycardia and muscle fasciculations—occur in only a minority of pediatric cases, whereas tonic-clonic seizures occur more frequently in children.[1] A high index of suspicion allows early diagnosis, which will not only facilitate optimal treatment for the individual patient but may also provide early warning of contamination in the child's home or environment.[2,3]

▶ **PATHOPHYSIOLOGY**

Acetylcholine is the chemical messenger at junctions where nerves connect to skeletal and smooth muscle, and to secretory glands. Organophosphates poison acetylcholinesterase; the enzyme breaks down and inactivates acetylcholine. This causes a buildup of acetylcholine and hyperstimulation of areas of the nervous system that contain cholinergic receptors.[3] There are two major classifications of cholinergic receptors: (1) muscarinic receptors, found on glands and involuntary smooth muscle, and (2) nicotinic receptors, found on voluntary skeletal muscle and some autonomic ganglia. There are also central cholinergic receptors found within the brain. When thinking of the clinical presentation of organophosphate toxicity, it is helpful to break down the signs and symptoms according to the three different types of receptors: muscarinic, nicotinic, and central.

▶ **CLINICAL PRESENTATION**

The initial signs and symptoms of cholinergic toxicity are often muscarinic. A helpful mnemonic to remember these muscarinic manifestations is DUMBELS:

- *D*iarrhea, *D*iaphoresis
- *U*rination
- *M*iosis
- *B*ronchorrhea, *B*ronchospasm
- *E*mesis
- *L*acrimation
- *S*alivation

Although miosis and the overall increase in secretions—saliva, sweat, and tears—can help suggest the diagnosis, the life-threatening effects are really bronchospasm and bronchorrea—the so-called "killer Bs." As the airway fills with secretory fluid and constricts, oxygenation and ventilation may be difficult or impossible unless adequate antidote is administered.

Nicotinic effects of excess acetylcholine at the neuromuscular junction include muscle spasm and fasciculations, followed by weakness or paralysis as the muscle fatigues. Bronchorrhea, bronchospasm, and respiratory muscle weakness can combine to cause respiratory failure requiring intubation and assisted ventilation.

Central nervous system effects of organophosphate exposure range from agitation and delirium to seizure activity and coma. Because of the different types of cholinergic receptors, vital signs at presentation can vary. The patient may be bradycardic because of a parasympathetic cardiac effect, or tachycardic because of hypoxia or nicotinic action on sympathetic ganglia.[4] Likewise, the patient may be hypotensive or hypertensive. In addition, presenting symptoms may be affected by the route of exposure. External dermal exposure can initially cause localized sweating and fasciculations. Inhalation can present with predominant respiratory manifestations—the killer Bs. Ingestion can cause early vomiting, diarrhea, and abdominal distress. A review of 37 cases of children diagnosed with organophosphate or carbamate toxicity found that the following signs and symptoms occurred most frequently:

- Miosis (73%)
- Excessive salivation (70%)
- Muscle weakness (68%)
- Lethargy (54%)
- Tachycardia (49%).

Only 8 of the 37 (22%) children had fasciculations, and only 7 (19%) had bradycardia.[1] In addition to acute effects, several delayed neurologic syndromes follow apparent recovery from acute organophosphate exposure. *Organophosphate-induced delayed neuropathy* has been described with an onset 1 to 3 weeks after the acute phase. This often starts with leg cramping, followed by weakness and diminished deep tendon reflexes in the lower extremities; this is predominantly a distal motor polyneuropathy. Cranial nerves and the muscles of respiration are usually spared.[5] An "intermediate syndrome" has also been reported, starting 1 to 3 days after acute toxicity, with weakness of neck flexors, proximal limb and respiratory muscles, and muscles innervated by cranial nerves. Respiratory failure can occur. This syndrome has not been well described in children.

▶ LABORATORY STUDIES

History, suggestive clinical signs and symptoms, and a high index of suspicion are the keys to making the diagnosis of organophosphate toxicity. The combination of miosis and increased salivation is relatively specific for exposure to a cholinergic agent such as organophosphate. There is no readily available laboratory test that can indicate the diagnosis during initial management.

That being said, certain tests can confirm the diagnosis in retrospect. Decreased levels of plasma (serum) cholinesterase and red blood cell cholinesterase are consistent with organophosphate exposure. Many hospital laboratories do not perform these tests and must send them to an outside facility. Although a decreased level of plasma cholinesterase supports the diagnosis, the level itself does not seem to have prognostic significance.[6] Red blood cell cholinesterase—although more difficult to measure—more closely reflects levels of enzyme activity in the central and peripheral nervous systems, and more accurately tracks clinical severity.

Other laboratory tests can be obtained if clinically indicated. Pulse oximetry can help evaluate oxygenation status. The cardiac monitor can detect tachycardia or bradycardia, either of which can be seen following organophosphate exposure. A chest radiograph may show aspiration pneumonitis, which is especially likely if the organophosphate preparation included a hydrocarbon vehicle. Noncardiogenic pulmonary edema may also be seen.

▶ TREATMENT

Adequate external decontamination of a patient with organophosphate toxicity is critical to prevent continued exposure. All clothing and jewelry should be removed and placed in well-sealed plastic bags. Contaminated skin should be irrigated with copious amounts of water, or *gently* washed with soap and water. Vigorous scrubbing should be avoided, since it might actually increase systemic uptake of the toxin.

To prevent secondary contamination, all members of the medical team who are directly treating or decontaminating the patient should wear adequate protective gear. Simple surgical masks and gowns do *not* provide sufficient protection. Butyl rubber gloves and aprons are more effective options. If the patient is vomiting, gastric contents may contain the organophosphate agent and be a source of secondary contamination.

Neither gastric lavage nor activated charcoal has any demonstrated benefit in the setting of organophosphate ingestion. Either intervention would be expected to increase the risk of pulmonary aspiration. The clinician is probably better off devoting his or her full attention to basic support of airway, breathing, and circulation, and to administration of sufficient antidote.

The immediate life-threat in severe organophosphate poisoning is respiratory failure from the combined muscarinic effects of bronchospasm and bronchorrhea. Both of these can be alleviated by the antimuscarinic antidote atropine sulfate. The initial dose of atropine is 0.02 mg/kg intravenously (IV). In severe cases, this dose should be doubled every 5 minutes until pulmonary secretions dry up, bronchospasm resolves, and the child can be oxygenated and ventilated. It is important to realize that tachycardia is *not* a contraindication to the administration of atropine. In resuscitation algorithms, airway and breathing take precedence over circulation. Often a rapid heart rate will actually decrease after atropine is given as the respiratory status improves. It is also important to note that there is no maximum dose of atropine. Frequently, in these cases, surprisingly large doses are required.

The antidote pralidoxime chloride should be given to treat moderate-to-severe cholinergic toxicity from organophosphates or an unknown agent. The dose is 25 to 50 mg/kg IV over 30 minutes. Pralidoxime regenerates acetylcholinesterase by removing organophosphate from the enzyme's active site. The dose can be repeated at 6 hours intervals, or a continuous infusion of 10 mg/kg/h can be started after the initial load. Pralidoxime is not indicated in known carbamate exposure, but should be administered in cases of significant cholinergic toxicity where the exact agent is not known.

Diazepam is the treatment of choice for organophosphate-induced seizures. Studies indicate that it may also be beneficial in any patient with evidence of severe central cholinergic toxicity, such as those who are comatose or minimally responsive. If a patient needs to be paralyzed to facilitate endotracheal intubation, the clinician should bear in mind that the rapidly acting depolarizing agent succinylcholine is normally metabolized by plasma cholinesterase. Since this enzyme is inactivated by organophosphates, administration of succinylcholine may result in markedly prolonged paralysis and is best avoided.[7,8]

▶ CARBAMATES

Carbamate insecticides such as Aldicarb and Carbaryl (Sevin) also inactivate cetylcholinesterase. Unlike organophosphates, however, this inactivation is not permanent. Functional enzyme activity is often largely restored within 8 hours, with red blood cell cholinesterase completely restored within 48 hours.

Carbamate toxicity is primarily restricted to muscarinic effects. Carbamates are much less likely than organophosphates to cause CNS effects, since they do not penetrate the blood–brain barrier well. Nicotinic manifestations are also uncommon. However, children with severe carbamate poisoning can develop mental status depression and occasionally seizures.

The initial management of the muscarinic effects of carbamate toxicity is similar to that for organophosphates, with stabilization of the airway and breathing, and adequate decontamination of the patient. Atropine is administered as indicated for muscarinic manifestations. Because carbamates have a relatively short duration of action, pralidoxime is unlikely to be of benefit.

REFERENCES

1. Zweiner RJ, Ginsburg CM. Organophosphate and carbamate poisoning in infants and children. *Pediatrics*. 1988;81:121.

2. Karr CJ, Solomon GM, Brock-Utne AC. Health effects of common home, lawn, and garden pesticides. *Pediatr Clin North Am*. 2007;54:63.

3. O'Malley M. Clinical evaluation of pesticide exposure and poisoning. *Lancet*. 1997;349:1161.

4. Nel L, Hatherill M, Davies J, et al. Organophosphate poisoning complicated by a tachyarrhythmia and acute respiratory distress syndrome in a child. *J Paediatr Child Health*. 2002;38:530.

5. Aiuto LA, Pavlakis SG, Boxer RA. Life-threatening organophosphate-induced delayed polyneuropathy in a child after accidental chlorpyrifos ingestion. *J Pediatr*. 1993;122:658.

6. Aygun D, Doganay Z, Altintop L, et al. Serum acetylcholinesterase and prognosis of acute organophosphate poisoning. *J Toxicol Clin Toxicol*. 2002;40:903.

7. Selden BS, Curry SC. Prolonged succinylcholine-induced paralysis in organophosphate insecticide poisoning. *Ann Emerg Med*. 1987;16:215.

8. Sener EB, Ustun E, Kocamanoglu S, et al. Prolonged apnea following succinylcholine administration in undiagnosed acute organophosphate poisoning. *Acta Anaesthesiol Scand*. 2002;46:1046.

CHAPTER 113

Caustics

Jenny J. Lu and Trevonne M. Thompson

▶ HIGH-YIELD FACTS

- Alkali burns cause *liquefaction necrosis*, a deep penetration injury associated with a pronounced exothermic reaction.
- Acid burns cause *coagulation necrosis* with severe injury to superficial tissues; penetration to deeper tissues is limited by the formation of an eschar.
- Induction of emesis in caustic ingestions is contraindicated.
- Ophthalmic exposures require urgent and copious irrigation with tap water if necessary; a delay of a few minutes can dramatically alter outcome.
- Endoscopy helps to define the severity of the injury and aids in determining prognosis.
- A battery lodged in the esophagus requires urgent removal.
- In a significant number of caustic exposures, the product is not in the original or appropriate container.

On direct contact with tissues, caustics cause immediate functional and histologic injury. Acids, alkalis, and antiseptics such as iodine, concentrated hydrogen peroxide, phenol, and formaldehyde are all capable of causing injury. Other common exposures include drain cleaners, household ammonia, automatic dishwasher detergents, and hair relaxer products. Although improvements in safety packaging, child-resistant caps, and federal regulations lowering the maximum concentration for many household caustics have decreased the overall incidence of unintentional pediatric caustic exposures, thousands of accidental exposures occur annually.[1] Acids are frequently reported, but the severe pain caused on initial contact usually limits the amount swallowed by small children. In contrast, intentional caustic ingestions by adolescents and adults may involve significantly larger quantities, which generally have a worse outcome. Long-term survivors of moderate and severe esophageal caustic injuries have a 1000-fold risk of esophageal carcinoma.[2]

▶ PATHOPHYSIOLOGY

Regardless of whether the caustic is an acid or an alkali, the severity of injury depends on:

- the type, concentration, volume, pH, and titratable acid (or alkaline) reserve of the agent
- duration of contact with tissues
- presence or absence of contents in the stomach
- tonicity of the pyloric sphincter
- esophageal reflux after the ingestion

Solids and liquids have different effects on the nature of the injury. Solids tend to produce intense localized oral pharyngeal or upper esophageal injury, while liquids, especially strong bases, tend to produce circumferential lesions in the distal esophagus. Areas of anatomic narrowing may be subject to longer contact time and suffer greater injury. Theoretically, the presence of stomach contents can decrease tissue injury by exerting a buffering effect. Pylorospasm prevents gastric emptying which increases contact time of the corrosive with the stomach and results in more severe gastric injury. Any reflux of ingested material back into the esophagus reexposes the tissues to further caustic damage. The titratable acid or alkaline reserve (TAR) is the amount of a xenobiotic required to neutralize or raise the pH of a caustic to that of physiologic tissues. This neutralization results in an exothermic reaction, which can produce or worsen injury.[2,3] There are three major pathophysiologic phases of both acid and alkali injuries[3]:

- Phase 1 is an acute inflammatory stage in which vascular thrombosis occurs. Cellular necrosis peaks on days 1 to 2. Sloughing of the necrotic mucosa on approximately days 3 to 4 results in ulceration.
- Phase 2 is the latent granulation phase, in which fibroplasia and granulation tissues develop in the ulcer during the middle of the first week. By the end of the first week, collagen starts to replace the granulation tissue. Perforation is most likely during this phase when the gastrointestinal wall is the weakest. This phase may continue for 2 weeks.
- Phase 3 is the chronic cicatrization phase. It begins during weeks 2 to 4, producing variable degrees of scar formation and contractures.

ALKALI BURNS

Alkali burns cause *liquefaction necrosis*, fat saponification, and protein disruption, which result in a deep penetration injury associated with a pronounced exothermic reaction. Tissue destruction continues until the compound is sufficiently neutralized by the tissue or until the concentration of the compound is greatly decreased.

In one 10-year retrospective analysis of childhood exposures, the most common caustic ingestion was found to be household bleach, 11% of which resulted in burns.[3] Grade II and III injuries tend to occur in patients with large ingestions of concentrated products. Most accidental ingestions of household grade bleach appear to do well with supportive care.[2,3]

Lye refers to a specific alkali, commonly sodium hydroxide or potassium hydroxide. Liquid lye can cause severe esophageal injuries with minimal associated oropharyngeal findings. Injuries following liquid lye ingestion tend to be more severe than those from solid lye because they are circumferential and can lead to stricture formation.

Small quantities of an ingested base can cause severe damage without ever reaching the stomach, which is involved only approximately 20% of the time. The gastric acid in the stomach does not neutralize a strong base.

ACID BURNS

Acid burns cause *coagulation necrosis* with severe injury to superficial tissues. Penetration to deeper tissues is limited by the formation of an eschar. Unlike liquid alkali, which tends to produce injury very rapidly, acid injury may continue for up to 90 minutes after the ingestion. In most cases of acid ingestion, both the esophageal and gastric mucosa are affected. On occasion, due to rapid esophageal transit time, an acid can reach the stomach without being significantly buffered in the esophagus and can cause severe gastric injury, including perforation.[2] Injury to the small bowel can also occur, especially if the pyloric sphincter is relaxed at the time of ingestion.

▶ PRESENTATION AND DIAGNOSIS

An accurate history is important if a patient is suspected of having ingested a caustic. Caretakers should be asked to bring the container, including labels, of the ingested agent, as substances are often placed in beverage or other containers and the contents may be different from what is listed on the package label. Manufacturers can sometimes be contacted to identify ingredients. Material safety data sheets (MSDS) can often be found on the internet for various compounds. The poison control center can assist with identifying the ingredients of a brand name product or chemical compound. Many other resources are also available (Table 113–1).

The child with a caustic ingestion may be completely asymptomatic in fulminant respiratory distress or shock. The gastrointestinal tract, respiratory tract, eyes, and skin are potential sites for harm. Dysphagia, drooling, vomiting, hematemesis, chest and abdominal pain, and melena are indicative of severe injury. Many caustics, including highly alkaline laundry detergents, can cause life-threatening airway edema. Stridor, dyspnea, and dysphonia, all indicate upper airway compromise. Patients with upper airway obstruction should be intubated under direct visualization; severe edema precluding oral intubation may require a surgical airway. Blind nasotracheal intubation is contraindicated.

Patients without immediate airway issues should be observed for excessive crying, drooling, or refusal to eat or drink, all of which may indicate a significant injury. The oral cavity should be evaluated for signs of intraoral burns. The chest should be visualized for retractions and auscultated for wheezes or rhonchi indicating aspiration. The abdomen should be examined for distention, tenderness, or rigidity, which suggest the possibility of gastrointestinal tract perforation.

▶ MANAGEMENT

Airway management and recognition of esophageal or gastric perforation are the highest priorities. Fluid resuscitation and supportive care are critical to the treatment of the patient with a caustic exposure. Patient should not be fed until it is deemed safe to do so.

LABORATORY AND RADIOLOGY STUDIES

In patients with signs of respiratory distress, oxygen saturation or arterial blood gases along with a chest radiograph should be obtained, since many caustics are powerful emetics and, if aspirated, can cause severe pneumonitis or noncardiogenic pulmonary edema.

Laboratory studies should include blood pH, complete blood count, electrolytes, renal function, coagulation profile, and serum lactate. Patients with abdominal pain or tenderness also require radiologic evaluation to exclude the presence of free air. The initial evaluation immediately following a caustic ingestion is esophagoscopy; a contrast esophogram may be useful to identify strictures at a later point.[2]

DILUENTS AND BUFFERS

Some medical sources and product labels may still advocate neutralization of caustics with acidic substances such as lemon juice or vinegar after an alkali ingestion, or sodium bicarbonate following an acid ingestion. Most authors, however, now advise against neutralization of a caustic due to the concern that attempting to buffer a strong acid or alkali may lead to an exothermic reaction and worsen tissue destruction. There may be a role for diluents, however, in the ingestion of a weak acid since such injuries are usually purely caustic and there is no risk of thermal injury. Studies demonstrate limited effects of diluents and extrapolation of these studies suggests that dilutional therapy is probably most beneficial in the first seconds or minutes after ingestion.[2,3] Milk or water dilution may be indicated in an attempt to move particulate material out of the oropharynx and esophagus. The amount given should be easily tolerated by the child; gastric distention from too much

▶ TABLE 113–1. **INTERNET RESOURCES**

Household Products Database (National Institutes of Health)	http://householdproducts.nlm.nih.gov/index.htm
OSHA/EPA Occupational Chemical Database	http://www.osha.gov/web/dep/chemicaldata/
Agency for Toxic Substances and Disease Registry	http://www.atsdr.cdc.gov/toxfaq.html
THOMSON POISONDEX® System	http://www.micromedex.com/products/poisindex/

fluid can precipitate emesis. Dilutional therapy should be limited only to those patients with no airway compromise, no drooling or vomiting, and no chest or abdominal pain. There is probably no value in administering diluents in liquid alkali ingestions because the injury is likely to be complete in a very short time.[3]

GASTRIC DECONTAMINATION

Induction of emesis in caustic ingestions is absolutely contraindicated, since increased tissue damage can occur as the esophagus is reexposed to the offending agent. Violent episodes of emesis can increase risk of both pulmonary aspiration and esophageal perforation.

In general, there is no role for gastric emptying in accidental caustic ingestions. Risks include induction of emesis, aspiration, or perforation. Cautious placement of a small bore nasogastric tube in a massive intentional ingestion of a potentially lethal acid could potentially be considered if the benefits are judged to greatly outweigh the risks. However, these situations are very rare and should be seriously considered only in massive ingestions where the patient presents within minutes to the hospital.[2] The administration of charcoal is not recommended because caustics are poorly adsorbed by charcoal, and charcoal creates a problem with visualization for the endoscopist.

ENDOSCOPY

The challenge in managing the child with a caustic ingestion is in identifying the patient who is at risk for a serious injury. Several studies indicate that the clinical manifestations of caustic ingestion injuries are poor predictors of the severity of injuries. There is no correlation between the presence or absence of oral burns and the presence of esophageal or gastric injuries. Crain et al. found that 33% of patients with evidence of oral cavity burns had esophageal burns.[4] Dogan et al. found that 61% of 389 patients with no oral burns had esophageal lesions.[5] Wijburg et al. found esophageal lesions in 39% of children who were suspected of having ingested a caustic agent.[5] In Gandreault's study of 378 children with caustic ingestions, 10 of 80 children who were asymptomatic had grade II lesions on endoscopy. If two of the three symptoms of vomiting, drooling, or stridor are present, the likelihood of gastrointestinal burns is high. Of the three, vomiting is the most powerful predictor of severe esophageal injury.[6]

Endoscopy should ideally be performed within 12 hours and no later than 24 hours after the ingestion, because the risk of perforation begins a few days and continues for 2 to 3 weeks after the exposure.[2] Early endoscopy helps to define the extent of the injury and to establish a prognosis.[7] Caustic injury is categorized as first, second, and third degree, based on appearance at endoscopy. Any child with a history of a potentially significant ingestion, with oral lesions, or who is otherwise symptomatic, warrants endoscopy. Most intentional ingestions warrant endoscopy. For asymptomatic patients with accidental ingestions of household bleach, ammonia, or nonphosphate detergents, observation may be acceptable. Evidence of perforation or shock is a clear contraindication to endoscopy.

SURGICAL INTERVENTION

Immediate surgical involvement is advised if endoscopy demonstrates evidence of perforation. Other signs in which surgical consultation is warranted include severe abdominal tenderness or rigidity, hematemesis or melena, worsening acidemia, hypotension, or shock.

STEROIDS

Steroids remain a controversial aspect of management of caustic ingestions. Theoretically, steroids decrease the incidence of esophageal strictures in patients with severe burns; they have been shown to decrease the incidence of strictures in animal models.[3] In humans, studies show conflicting results.[8] Steroids are not indicated for first-degree burns, because they do not form strictures. Third-degree burns invariably develop strictures, and since steroids may significantly increase complications, they are not recommended. Steroids may be of benefit in second-degree burns. Potential adverse effects of steroids include risk of infection and perforation. The potential benefit of steroids in this setting must be weighed against the risks.

ANTIBIOTICS

Antibiotics should be reserved for suspected or documented infections. If systemic steroids are administered, prophylatic antibiotics are often given concurrently.[3]

WOUND CARE

Dermatologic burns are treated with debridement, topical antibiotic ointments, and sterile nonadherent dressings. Silver sulfadiazine can be used for second-degree burns. Deep second- or third-degree burns, especially to the face or hands, should be evaluated by a burn specialist.

SPECIAL CONCERNS

Caustic Eye Injuries

Caustic eye injuries can have devastating consequences, including blindness. The alkaline by-products of sodium azide released in automobile air bags can cause ophthalmic injury. The cornerstone of management of ophthalmologic exposure is immediate irrigation of the eye for a minimum of 15 to 20 minutes with 0.9% saline, lactated Ringer's solution, or tap water. Irrigation is intended to dilute the offending xenobiotic, remove the xenobiotics, remove any foreign bodies, and normalize the pH. Delays of just a few minutes can affect outcome dramatically. After exposure to acids or alkalis, normalization of the conjunctival pH is often suggested as a useful end point. Full extent of injury may not be evident for 48 to 72 hours. Ophthalmologist evaluation is recommended for all ophthalmic caustic injuries.

▶ **TABLE 113–2. REPLACEMENT THERAPY FOR HYPOCALCEMIA***

Dose	Calcium chloride (Repeat q 10 min as needed; follow QTc, labs, and clinical condition)	Calcium gluconate (Repeat q 10 min as needed; follow QTc, labs, and clinical condition)
Adult	1 amp (10 mL of 10%) over 5 min	10–30 mL of 10% IV over 5 min
Pediatric	10–25 mg/kg up to 1 amp per dose	30–75 mg/kg over 5 min, up to 1 g/dose

*Caravati EM. In: Dart RC, ed. *Medical Toxicology*. 3rd ed. Philadelphia, PA: Lippincott Williams & Wilkins; 2004:167–168.

Button Batteries

Button batteries are frequently swallowed by children. The batteries contain a metallic salt in a concentrated alkaline medium. Although the vast majority of patients do well, this ingestion poses a unique injury, and rare deaths have occurred. In Litovitz's study of 2382 cases of battery ingestion, 2 patients had life-threatening symptoms; both had batteries lodged in the esophagus. The study also showed that 61% of the batteries passed spontaneously within 48 hours and 86% within 96 hours.[9] Historically, leakage of battery contents was a legitimate concern; new production techniques are much more effective at preventing leakage of battery contents.

Pressure necrosis at the site where the battery becomes lodged can occur. Lodging is most likely to occur at regions of anatomic narrowing, such as the cricopharyngeus, where the aorta or carina cross the esophagus, or in gut malformations such as Meckel's diverticulum. Rarely, if the battery does break open, the caustic contents may cause ulceration, perforation, or rarely fistula formation. Heavy metal absorption may occur, although clinical toxicity from battery ingestion has not been reported. Finally, injury from electrical current can also occur.

A battery lodged in the esophagus or airway requires urgent removal. Burns have been reported as early as 4 hours after ingestion, and perforation in as early as 6 hours.[9] The preferred method of extraction is endoscopy, which allows direct visualization of any esophageal injury. Buttons lodged in nasal passages should also be removed immediately.

If a swallowed battery has passed through the esophagus, as apparent from radiographs, watchful waiting is acceptable, unless there are signs and symptoms of intra-abdominal injury. A large battery ingested by a small child may also require removal. If a battery greater than 15 mm in diameter ingested by a child younger than 6 years of age has not passed the pylorus within 48 hours, it is unlikely to do so.

An asymptomatic patient with a battery that has passed the esophagus can be discharged and followed as an outpatient with serial radiographs to document passage of the battery. Daily radiographs are also recommended. Passage of the battery can be followed by straining the stool. Whole bowel irrigation is an option.

Hydrofluoric Acid

Hydrofluoric acid (HF) is a weak acid found in some cleaning and rust-removing products. External contact can result in severe dermal or ocular injury. Death has been reported with exposures affecting as little as 2.5% of the body surface area. Severe pain and deep penetration despite minimal skin findings is the hallmark of a hydrofluoric acid burn. The mechanism of injury involves liquefaction necrosis and the formation of insoluble calcium and magnesium salts. Oral ingestions are frequently fatal. In cases of significant burns, systemic acidosis, hypocalcemia, hypomagnesemia, and hyperkalemia are common. Renal failure and hemolysis have also been reported to occur.[10]

En route to the emergency department, decontamination of all burned areas with copious irrigation is indicated. Calcium gluconate gel (2.5%) can be applied topically to HF burns. If unavailable, it can be prepared using 3.5 g of calcium gluconate powder and 150 mL of a sterile water-soluble lubricant (K-Y Jelly), or 25 mL of 10% calcium gluconate in 75 mL of sterile water lubricant. Persistent pain may be alleviated by intradermal injection of calcium gluconate. Calcium chloride or calcium carbonate can be substituted for calcium gluconate. Intra-arterial infusion of calcium gluconate can be considered for refractory cases or cases involving HF burns to arms or legs. Hypocalcemia from ingestions of HF are often refractory to treatment and may require large amounts of calcium (Table 113–2). Ocular HF exposures require immediate copious irrigation with 0.9% normal saline or tap water, if available. One percent calcium gluconate ophthalmic drops have been suggested, although calcium salts may be very irritating to the eye.

REFERENCES

1. Lai MW, Klein-Schwartz W, Rodgers GC, et al. 2005 Annual Report of the American Association of Poison Control Centers' National Poisoning and Exposure Database. *Clin Toxicol (Phila)*. 2006;44(6–7):803–932.
2. Fulton JA, Rao RB. Caustics. In: Flomenbaum NE, Goldfrank LR, Hoffman RS, Howland MA, Lewin NA, Nelson LS, eds. *Goldfranks' Toxicologic Emergencies*. 8th ed. New York, NY: McGraw Hill; 2006:1405–1416.
3. Caravati EM. Caustics. In: Dart RC, ed. *Medical Toxicology*. 3rd ed. Philadelphia, PA: Lippincott Williams & Wilkins; 2004:1294–1303, 1304–1309.
4. Crain EF, Gershel JC, Mezey AP. Caustic ingestions: symptoms as predictors of esophageal injury. *Am J Dis Child*. 1984;138:863–865.
5. Dogan Y, Erkan T, Cokugras FC. Caustic gastroesophageal lesions in childhood: an analysis of 473 cases. *Clin Pediatr (Phila)*. 2006;45(5):435–438.
6. Gaudreault P, Parent M. Predictability of esophageal injury from signs and symptoms: a study of caustic ingestions in 378 children. *Pediatrics*. 1983;71:767–770.
7. Poley J-W, Steyerberg EW, Kuipers EJ, et al. Ingestion of acid and alkaline agents: outcome and prognostic value of early upper endoscopy. *Gastrointest Endosc*. 2004;60(3):372–377.
8. Anderson KD, Rouse TM, Randolph JG. A controlled trial of corticosteroids in children with corrosive injury of the esophagus. *N Engl J Med*. 1990;323:637–640.

9. Litovitz T, Schmitz BF. Ingestion of cylindrical and button batteries: an analysis of 2382 cases. *Pediatrics*. 1992;89:747–757.

10. Caravati EM. Acute hydrofluoric acid exposure. *Am J Emerg Med*. 1988;6:143–150.

SUGGESTED READING

Ford M, Delaney KA, Ling LJ, Erickson T, eds. *Clinical Toxicology*. Philadelphia, PA: Saunders; 2001:1002–1038.

Homan CS, Singer A, Henry MC, et al. Thermal effects of neutralization and water dilution for acute alkali exposures in canines. *Acad Emerg Med*. 1997;4:27.

Howell JM. Alkaline ingestions. *Ann Emerg Med*. 1986;15:820–825.

Penner GE. Acid ingestion: toxicology and treatment. *Ann Emerg Med*. 1980;9:374–379.

Previtera C, Giuisti F, Guglielmi M. Predictive value of visible lesions (cheeks, lips, oropharynx) in suspected caustic ingestion: may endoscopy reasonably be omitted in completely negative pediatric patients? *Pediatr Emerg Care*. 1990;6:176–178.

CHAPTER 114

Hydrocarbons

Trevonne M. Thompson

▶ HIGH-YIELD FACTS

- Hydrocarbon-containing products are ubiquitous in daily life.
- Viscosity, surface tension, and volatility are three important properties to assess the toxicity of liquid hydrocarbons.
- The primary concern after hydrocarbon ingestion is pulmonary toxicity.
- Clinical manifestations of hydrocarbon ingestion depend on the amount and route of exposure.
- Coughing, gagging, chocking, and vomiting after hydrocarbon ingestion is presumptive of aspiration.
- The mainstay of treatment for hydrocarbon exposure is supportive care.

The term hydrocarbon is used to describe a large number of organic molecules that contain mostly hydrogen and carbon atoms. Hydrocarbons are primarily derived from petroleum distillates but may also be derived from other sources such as plants, animal fats, and natural gas. Hydrocarbon-containing products are pervasive in daily life (Table 114–1).

In 2006, the National Poison Data System reported nearly 50 000 pediatric hydrocarbon exposures in the United States.[1] Eighty-seven percent of those exposures were unintentional. The most common exposures reported were gasoline, fluorochlorocarbons/propellant, lubricating/motor oil, lighter fluid, lamp oil, diesel fuel, and kerosene. Young children tend to have accidental exposures; adolescent exposures tend to represent the abuse of volatile hydrocarbons or suicidal attempts/gestures. Fortunately, deaths from hydrocarbon exposures are rare.

▶ CLASSIFICATION AND PROPERTIES

There are two basic types of hydrocarbon molecules. The aliphatic compounds consist of a branched or straight chain structure; the cyclic hydrocarbons consist of a closed ring. Each of these basic types have many subtypes, all with varying characteristics such as hydrogen or carbon substitutions, the presence of one or more double covalent bond, multiring structures, etc.

The length of the hydrocarbon chain affects the chemical properties of the molecule. Short-chain molecules, such as butane, are gases at room temperature. Intermediate length chains, which encompass the majority of chemical exposures,

are liquids at room temperature. The long-chain hydrocarbons, such as paraffin and tar, are solids at room temperatures.

Viscosity, surface tension, and volatility are three important physical properties used to assess the toxicity of liquid hydrocarbons. Viscosity is the measurement of a liquid's resistance to flow. Volatility describes the tendency of a liquid to become a gas. Surface tension describes the property of adherence of a liquid compound along a surface. These three properties are used to assess the risk of pulmonary toxicity from hydrocarbon ingestion.

▶ PATHOPHYSIOLOGY

Pulmonary toxicity is the primary concern after hydrocarbon ingestions. The exact pathogenesis of hydrocarbon-induced pulmonary toxicity is debated in the literature; however, aspiration of hydrocarbons can lead to direct injury of lung tissue.[2] The viscosity, surface tension, and volatility of hydrocarbons determine the risk of aspiration during ingestion. Compounds with low viscosity, low surface tension, and high volatility have a higher risk of aspiration and subsequent pulmonary toxicity.

Inhalation of hydrocarbon vapor can lead to CNS depression. This effect may be desirable in drug abusers and lead to behaviors such as sniffing, huffing, and bagging. Sniffing is the direct inhalation of a hydrocarbon vapor. Huffing is the practice of saturating a cloth with a liquid hydrocarbon and inhaling the vapors from the cloth. Bagging is placing a hydrocarbon source inside a plastic bag and placing the open end of the bag at the mouth and/or nose while inhaling. The exact mechanism of CNS depression from hydrocarbons is unclear. In cases of hydrocarbon-induced pulmonary toxicity, hypoxia may contribute to the CNS effects.

Hydrocarbon exposure via any route may induce cardiac toxicity manifested by ventricular dysrhythmias. Although halogenated hydrocarbons are most often implicated in cardiac toxicity, other hydrocarbons have also been reported to cause similar effects.[3] Sudden sniffing death syndrome is a sudden cardiac death associated with volatile hydrocarbon abuse.[4,5] Such deaths tend to occur when physical exertion or excitation occur immediately after inhaling hydrocarbon vapors.

▶ CLINICAL PRESENTATION

The clinical manifestations of hydrocarbon poisoning depend on the route and amount of the exposure. Patients may present asymptomatically or in fulminate respiratory distress. Many fall on a continuum between the two.

► **TABLE 114–1. COMMON HYDROCARBON PRODUCTS**

Lighter fluid
Gasoline
Paint thinner
Pine oil
Mineral oil
Aerosol propellants
Kerosine
Lamp oil
Camphor
Turpentine
Correction fluid
Paraffin
Solvents

Coughing, gagging, choking, and vomiting after an ingestion of a hydrocarbon is presumptive of aspiration. Signs of pulmonary toxicity may include tachypnea, crackles, bronchospasm, hemoptysis, hypoxia, acute lung injury, or respiratory failure. The respiratory signs typically progress over one to several days and then resolve. Fortunately, death is rare.

The radiographic findings of pulmonary toxicity are protean. They range from increased bronchovascular markings to definite consolidations. There may be involvement of one lung lobe or segment or multilobular findings. The cardiac findings range from mild tachycardia to ventricular tachydysrhythmias. Victims of sudden sniffing death syndrome may present in full cardiac arrest. Myocardial depression may also occur. The typical CNS finding is mental status depression, although this may be preceded by a brief period of CNS excitation. The CNS depression may be profound. Seizures have also been reported. Chronic volatile hydrocarbon abuse has been associated with a leukoencephalopathic syndrome that can include neurobehavioral abnormalities such as ataxia and dementia.[6].

► MANAGEMENT

The mainstay of treatment for a hydrocarbon exposure is supportive care. Special attention should be given to maintaining a patent airway, providing adequate ventilation, and addressing tachydysrhythmias. All patients who ingested a hydrocarbon and have a history of choking, coughing, gagging, vomiting, or any respiratory signs or symptoms should have chest radiography performed. Asymptomatic patients do not need early radiography. Supplemental oxygen and bronchodilating agents may provide some relief in symptomatic patients.

Gastric decontamination is controversial in hydrocarbon ingestions. In the majority of pediatric exposures, gastric decontamination will not be necessary. In the case of a large volume, highly toxic hydrocarbon ingestion, the decision to attempt decontamination with lavage should be made in conjunction with a medical toxicologist. The use of activated charcoal is typically unnecessary as hydrocarbons adsorb poorly to it.

The use of antibiotics and corticosteroids are also controversial in patients with pulmonary toxicity from hydrocarbons. If bacterial superinfection is suspected, appropriate antibiotics may be indicated. Based on the currently available evidence, the use of corticosteroids is generally not recommended.[7]

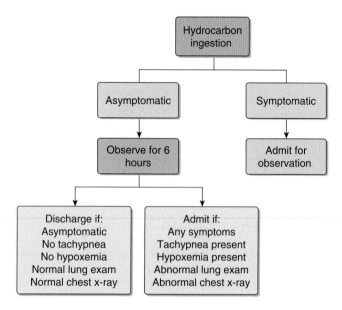

Figure 114–1. Disposition algorithm.

► DISPOSITION (Figure 114–1)

An asymptomatic patient should be observed for 6 hours after the ingestion. If there is no tachypnea, no hypoxia, no abnormal pulmonary findings, and a normal chest radiograph after this 6-hour period, the patient may be safely discharged.[8] Any symptomatic patient should be admitted and observed until symptom resolution. Patients with significant signs of pulmonary toxicity should be considered for an intensive care admission. Figure 114–1 illustrates the disposition algorithm for patients who have ingested a hydrocarbon. A psychiatric evaluation may be indicated in adolescents who ingest a hydrocarbon as a suicide attempt or gesture.

REFERENCES

1. Bronstein AC, Spyker DA, Cantilena LR, et al. 2006 Annual report of the American Association of Poison Control Centers' National Poison Data System (NPDS). *Clin Toxicol.* 2007;45:815–917.
2. Dice WH, Ward G, Kelley J, et al. Pulmonary toxicity following gastrointestinal ingestion of kerosene. *Ann Emerg Med.* 1982;11:138–142.
3. Bass M. Death from sniffing gasoline. *N Engl J Med.* 1978;299:203.
4. Bass M. Sudden sniffing death. *N Engl J Med.* 1970;212:2075–2079.
5. Kulig K, Rumack B. Hydrocarbon ingestion. *Curr Top Emerg Med.* 1981;3:1–5.
6. Filley CM, Franklin GM, Heaton RK, et al. White matter dementia: clinical disorders and implications. *Neuropsychiatry Neuropsychol Behav Neurol.* 1988;1:239–245.
7. Marks MI, Chicoine L, Legere G, et al. Adrenocorticosteroid treatment of hydrocarbon pneumonia in children—a cooperative study. *J Pediatr.* 1972;81:366–369.
8. Anas N, Namasonthi V, Ginsburg CM. Criteria for hospitalizing children who have ingested products containing hydrocarbons. *JAMA.* 1981;246:840–843.

CHAPTER 115

Rodenticides

Michael S. Wahl and Anthony Burda

► HIGH-YIELD FACTS

- The labels of all currently US Environmental Protection Agency (EPA) approved indoor rodenticides contain a registration number, active ingredients, concentration, instructions for use, warnings, and first-aid information.
- An accidental ingestion or "taste" by pediatric patients of currently marketed indoor rodenticides, such as the long-acting anticoagulants, bromethalin, cholecalciferol, or zinc phosphide, are not likely to result in serious toxicity.
- Measures such as GI decontamination, prophylaxis with vitamin K_1, or laboratory monitoring are unwarranted following accidental tastes of long-acting coagulant rodenticides.
- A single large ingestion or repeated small ingestions of long-acting anticoagulant ("superwarfarin") compounds may cause serious bleeding. Phytonadione (vitamin K_1) is the specific antidote. Active bleeding may require treatment with fresh frozen plasma (FFP).
- Very large ingestions of bromethalin may cause neurologic toxicity attributed to increased intracranial pressure. Cholecalciferol (vitamin D_3) may cause hypercalcemia. Zinc phosphide is converted to phosphine gas in the GI tract, and may result in pulmonary edema and multiorgan injury.
- Ingestions of any amount of very old, illegal, or unapproved products for indoor use should be considered extremely serious as these products may contain arsenic, cyanide, strychnine, sodium mono-fluoroacetate, thallium, white phosphorus, aldicarb, or other highly toxic chemicals.

Ingestion of rodenticides by children account for a significant number of exposures reported to poison centers around the country. These exposures are compiled in the National Poison Data System (NPDS) by the American Association of Poison Control Centers (AAPCC). For the 8-year period, 2000 to 2007, NPDS reported a total of 124 127 rodenticide exposures in patients younger than 6 years of age. Trivial, unintentional pediatric ingestions resulted in no clinical effects in the overwhelming majority of cases.

The risk of toxicity following unintentional ingestion of a "taste" or small amount of a rodenticide is determined by its composition and concentration of active ingredients. The EPA currently approves four rodenticides for indoor use: anticoagulants, cholecalciferol, bromethalin, and zinc phosphide. An ingestion of a few granules of these chemicals by a small child is unlikely to cause toxicity (Table 115–1). However, ingestion of even a small quantity of outdated, illegal, or unapproved products designed for indoor use can pose a significant danger to children and pets. Examples of these highly toxic products include strychnine, arsenic, white phosphorus, and sodium mono-fluoroacetate (Table 115–2).

This chapter will primarily focus on the anticoagulant products, as these are the most common rodenticides encountered by children. Clinicians should not assume however, that all exposures will involve these products. The Federal Insecticide Fungicide and Rodenticide Act (FIFRA) requires all pesticide labels to contain the following information: an EPA registration number, active ingredients and concentration, first-aid statement, restrictions on usage, environmental hazards, physical and chemical hazards, directions for use, net contents, and name and address of registrant. An improperly packaged and labeled poison or products obtained by other than legitimate means should raise suspicion for a potentially highly toxic chemical.

► DEVELOPMENTAL CONSIDERATIONS

The NPDS data shows that children younger than 6 years comprise the largest population at risk of rodenticide poisoning. Toddlers are attracted to the colorful appearance (usually green) of the pellets or cakes. Bait stations or trays are generally not child resistant, and these products are often transferred from their original container to food bowls or dishes placed in reachable areas. Children with developmental delay or those with a history of pica are at greater risk of a large scale or chronic ingestion.

Adolescents and young adults may consume rodenticides intentionally in a suicide attempt. Mentally ill patients have been known to chronically eat these products as well. As a result, these two groups of patients are more prone to serious toxicity from a rodenticide exposure (Fig. 115–1).

► PATHOPHYSIOLOGY

Prior to 1980, most anticoagulant rodenticide exposures involved a warfarin-containing product. Two problems arose with warfarin use as a pesticide, which made it progressively less effective: (1) Several feedings of bait over a number of days by the target animal were required to reach a lethal dose; and (2) a genetic selection process led to the emergence of warfarin-resistant rats. These problems were overcome by the development and introduction of the superwarfarin, or long-acting anticoagulant products that are approximately 100 times more potent than warfarin, and could kill the target animal with

▶ **TABLE 115–1. OTHER NON-ANTICOAGULANT INDOOR RODENTICIDES**

Rodenticide	Toxicology/Clinical Findings	Management/Antidotes

Bromethalin
Bait 0.01%
Assault®, Clout All
  Weather Bait®,
  Fastrac®, Real Kill Rat
  and Mouse Killer®, Top
  Gun®, Vengeance®
	Uncouples oxidative phosphorylation resulting in decreased ATP production and increased fluid accumulation which interrupts nerve impulse conduction with resultant increased pressure on nerve axons; there is no established human lethal dose. SX: large ingestions may cause headaches, confusion, tremors, myoclonic jerking, seizure, cerebral edema, or coma. Toxicity may be delayed 8–12 h or longer due to conversion to a more active metabolite	Activated charcoal following ingestion of a large amount; no specific antidote; supportive care including measures to correct cerebral edema, i.e., hyperventilation, mannitol or furosemide, dexamethasone; benzodiazepines/ phenobarbital for seizures; monitor cerebral spinal fluid pressure

Cholecalciferol Bait 0.075% Quintox®, Rampage®	Mobilizes calcium from bones producing hypercalcemia, osteomalacia, and metastatic calcification of the cardiovascular system, kidneys, stomach, and lungs; toxicity may occur from a single large ingestion or chronic consumption; death occurs in animals in 2–5 d; however, serious human poisonings or fatalities from these rodent baits have yet to be reported. SX: anorexia, nausea, vomiting, diarrhea or constipation, headache, fatigue, weakness, hypercalcemia, hyperphosphatemia, cardiac dysrhythmias, myocardial infarction, renal tubular injury	Treat for hypercalcemia as clinically indicated

Zinc phosphide
Granules 2%
Eraze®, Mole Nots®, and
  Mr. Rat Guard®
Note: aluminum
  phosphide is a
  fumigant not sold for
  household use
	Converted to phosphine gas when in contact with acid or moisture; direct cellular toxin causing multiorgan injury by inhibiting cytochrome C oxidase, thus blocking the electron transport chain. In one case series of 21 patients, those ingesting under 1 g had a favorable outcome; lethal dose: 4 g in an adult; SX: nausea, profuse vomiting and diarrhea which may be bloody, a decaying fish odor may be noted, headache, cough, tachypnea, dyspnea, dizziness, tremulousness, hypotension, shock, hypocalcemia, tetany, pulmonary edema, convulsions, cardiac dysrhythmias, renal damage, hepatotoxicity, acute pancreatitis, coma; death may occur in 12–24 h	GI decontamination is controversial; lavage may release phosphine gas; activated charcoal may be given but is of questionable value; antacids, H2 blockers, and proton pump inhibitors may be considered; ED staff should work in a well-ventilated area; no specific antidote; provide intensive supportive care including intubation at earliest sign of pulmonary edema, which may be delayed 24–72 h; give benzodiazepines/phenobarbital for seizures; monitor electrolytes, glucose, calcium, renal and hepatic function tests, magnesium, ABGS or pulse oximetry, chest x-rays

a single feeding. These superwarfarins are also much more potent in humans. The long-acting anticoagulants are classified in two groups: the 4-hydroxy coumarins and the indandiones (Table 115–3).

Both short-acting and long-acting anticoagulants inhibit the activity of vitamin K_{2-3} epoxide reductase, an enzyme involved in the synthesis of the active form of vitamin K. This leads to reduction of vitamin K-dependent blood clotting factors II, VII, IX, and X. The onset of coagulopathy is delayed until existing stores of active vitamin K are depleted and circulating factors are reduced. Factor VII has the shortest half-life, which is approximately 5 hours. The anticoagulant effects will become evident after three to four factor VII half-lives (15–20 hours) after ingestion.

Anticoagulants also damage capillaries and increase their permeability, thereby increasing the risk of hemorrhage. Indandione derivatives have caused cardiopulmonary and neurologic toxicity in animals. In rats, the minimal amount of brodifacoum to depress PT activity is 0.1 mg/kg. Extrapolating to humans, the minimum toxic amount would be approximately 1.5 mg for a 10-kg child or 20 to 30 g of a 0.005% bait (Fig. 115–2).

▶ PHARMACOLOGY/ TOXICOKINETICS

These agents are well absorbed orally. Toxicity following dermal exposure to low-concentration solid baits is unlikely; however, percutaneous absorption of concentrated industrial-strength products can result in toxicity. Warfarin undergoes extensive hepatic metabolism and has a therapeutic half-life of 35 hours. High lipid solubility and high concentrations in the liver account for the prolonged duration of action of the superwarfarins. The half-life of brodifacoum is approximately 124 days in dogs and 6.5 days in rats. In one adult patient, the terminal half-life was 56 days. The half-life of chlorophacinone in four adult poisonings ranged from 6 to 11 days. Because of

▶ TABLE 115-2. OUTDATED, ILLEGAL, AND UNAPPROVED RODENTICIDES FOR INDOOR USE

Rodenticide*	Toxicology/Clinical Findings	Management/Antidotes
α-naphthylthiourea (2) ANTU Bait 1%–3% Bontu®	Damages pulmonary epithelium causing pulmonary edema; human lethal dose is estimated to be more than 4 g/kg with no known reported human fatalities; SX: dyspnea, cyanosis, noncardiogenic pulmonary edema and effusions, hypothermia; pulmonary edema may be delayed by 24–72 h	Activated charcoal; no known antidote; symptomatic care with oxygen and ventilatory support; monitor ABGs
Arsenic (1) Arsenic trioxide	Combines with sulfhydryl (-SH) groups in many essential cellular proteins and enzymes; estimated fatal dose 1–4 mg/kg; SX: garlic like breath odor, profuse vomiting and diarrhea, hypotension and shock, cardiac dysrhythmias, renal tubular damage, pulmonary edema, delirium, seizures, coma; delayed SX: peripheral neuropathy, alopecia, Mees lines, blood dyscrasias	Consider orogastric lavage as indicated, activated charcoal; whole bowel irrigation if abdominal radiograph is positive; obtain blood, spot urine, and 24 h urine for arsenic; monitor electrolytes, EKG, renal function tests, CBC; antidotes: IM dimercaprol or po succimer; supportive care with IV fluids, pressors, antidysrhythmics, hemodialysis
Barium carbonate (1)	Soluble barium salts lower serum potassium and raise intracellular potassium; estimated lethal dose 20–30 mg/kg; barium sulfate is nontoxic; SX: nausea, vomiting, diarrhea, paresthesias, weakness, paralysis, hypoglycemia, rhabdomyolysis, dysrhythmias, cardiac/respiratory failure	Consider orogastric lavage as indicated; frequent serum potassium levels with IV potassium replacement as necessary; supportive care with antidysrhythmics; no specific antidote; barium level may confirm diagnosis
Chloralose (2) (α-chloralose)	Has sedative effects similar to chloral hydrate and stimulant effect similar to strychnine; human toxic dose: 1–4 g, infants: 20 mg/kg; SX: increased salivation, sedation, coma, respiratory depression, myoclonis, seizures, hypotension, hypo- or hyperthermia, acidosis	Activated charcoal; no specific antidote; supportive care for respiratory failure, hypotension, rhabdomyolysis; benzodiazepines/phenobarbital for seizures
Calcium cyanide	This solid fumigant rodenticide reacts with moisture in the air to form highly toxic HCN gas. CN inhibits cytochrome oxidase enzymes halting aerobic cellular respiration. Estimated lethal dose of HCN: 50–100 mg. SX: skin flushing, anxiety, tachypnea, tachycardia, headache, progressing to bradycardia, hypotension, agitation, stupor, coma, seizures, and lactic acidosis	Administer 100% oxygen and provide ventilatory support. Consider activated charcoal following ingestion of CN salts. Antidotes to consider include the CN Antidote Kit or the Cyanokit.
Phosphorus (1) White or Yellow Stearns Chemical Paste® 2.5%	Protoplasmic poison causing direct cell injury leading to multiorgan failure; lethal dose: 1 mg/kg; mixed with peanut butter as bait; (note: red phosphorous found in matches is nontoxic) SX: bloody emesis, burns to GI tract, vomitus and stools may appear "smoking" or luminescent and have a garlic like odor, delirium, coma, shock, hypocalcemia, hypoglycemia, pulmonary edema, hemorrhage, cardiovascular collapse; delayed SX: myocardial, hepatic, and renal damage; dermally may cause partial and full thickness burns	Lavage and activated charcoal are usually not performed as phosphorous is corrosive; no specific antidote; supportive care with IV fluids and blood products; standard burn care; administer narcotics (e.g., morphine) for pain control; N-acetylcysteine may be hepatoprotective; ED staff must wear personal protective equipment to avoid contact with phosphorous
PNU (1) N-3-pyridylmethyl-N'-p-nitro-phenyl urea, Vacor® Bait 0.5%, 2%	Destroys pancreatic β cells via interference with niacinamide (nicotinamide) metabolism; lethal dose: 5 mg/kg; product introduced in 1975 and withdrawn in 1979; SX: nausea, vomiting (peanut odor), hyperglycemia, diabetic ketoacidosis, sensory motor and autonomic neuropathies, GI perforation, cardiac dysrhythmias; permanent SX: insulin-dependent diabetes mellitus and postural hypotension	Orogastric lavage and activated charcoal; antidote: early IM or IV niacinamide (nicotinamide) may prevent toxicity, however, parenteral products are not available in the United States; niacin (nicotinic acid) may not be effective; treat hyperglycemic ketoacidosis with insulin; monitor for GI perforation; mineralocorticoids (e.g., fludrocortisone) for persistent postural hypotension

(continued)

▶ TABLE 115–2. (CONTINUED) OUTDATED, ILLEGAL, AND UNAPPROVED RODENTICIDES FOR INDOOR USE

Rodenticide*	Toxicology/Clinical Findings	Management/Antidotes
Red Squill (3) Urginea maritima Bait 100%, or as 4.5% extract in bait	Contains scillaren A and B, which are cardiac glycosides; two bulbs have been fatal to an adult; intensely nauseating causing rapid vomiting which limits toxicity; SX: large amounts may cause nausea, vomiting, hyperkalemia, A-V block dysrhythmias, however, cardiac toxicity is rare	Activated charcoal following large ingestions; monitor vital signs, serum potassium, and EKG; antidotes: atropine and digoxin immune Fab
Sodium mono-fluoroacetate (1) Compound 1080® and Sodium fluoro-acetamide Compound 1081®	SMFA is converted to fluorocitric acid which blocks the tricarboxylic cycle of the Krebs cycle; estimated lethal dose 2–10 mg/kg, however, 1 mg may cause serious toxicity; SMFA is a white crystalline powder combined with nigrosin black dye as a colorant; SX: nausea, vomiting, diarrhea, seizures, acidosis, cardiac dysrhythmias, hypotension, hypocalcemia, hypokalemia, respiratory depression, coma	Orogastric lavage and activated charcoal; supportive care for hypotension, acidosis, dysrhythmias, and seizures; IV calcium gluconate for hypocalcemia; no known effective antidote.
Strychnine (1) Bait 0.3%–0.5%	Acts by antagonizing glycine, an inhibitory neurotransmitter in the postsynaptic motor neurons of the spinal cord; lethal dose 1–2 mg/kg, but may be as low as 5–10 mg in a child; SX: rapid onset of nausea, vomiting, apprehension, painful tonic-tetanic spasms, trismus, opisthotonos, "risus sardonicus" (facial grimacing), seizures, respiratory paralysis, lactic acidosis, rhabdomyolysis, hyperthermia, cardiac arrest; patient is conscious with normal mentation until hypoxia or acidosis leads to CNS depression	Activated charcoal; avoid any stimulus that may trigger seizures; treat seizures with benzodiazepines, phenobarbital; severe cases may need paralyzing agents with ventilator support; supportive care for acidosis, respiratory failure, rhabdomyolysis, and renal failure; no specific antidote, multiple dose activated charcoal possibly beneficial
Rodenticide: TETS (3) Tetramine (tetramethylenedisulfote-tramine) Dushuqiang	TETS binds noncompetitively and irreversibly to GABA receptors on neuronal cell membranes and blocks chloride channels. Illegally imported from China. Two samples were analyzed to have 6.4% and 13.8%, respectively. LD50 in mammals: 0.10–0.3 mg/kg; 7–10 mg is lethal in humans. SX: Refractory seizures, coma, and possible ischemic changes on EKG	Information is limited. No specific antidote is available. Supportive care. Seizures were refractory to benzodiazepines and phenobarbital in one pediatric case. Animal studies in China suggest benefit from IV pyridoxine and DMSA. Patients in China have been treated with charcoal hemoperfusion and hemodialysis
Thallium sulfate (1)	Interferes with oxidative phosphorylation by binding with mitochondria sulfhydryl groups; banned in 1965; lethal dose 1 g; SX: nausea, bloody vomiting, and diarrhea followed by ileus, painful sensory neuropathy, respiratory failure, delirium, seizures, renal failure, optic neuritis, muscle weakness, lethargy, coma; delayed SX: alopecia, Mees lines, neuropathies	Orogastric lavage and activated charcoal as clinically indicated; thallium may appear radio-opaque on an abdominal radiograph, obtain blood and 24 h urine collection for thallium; Prussian blue (Radiogardase®) interrupts enterohepatic and enteroenteric circulation and enhances fecal elimination; multiple dose charcoal may also enhance elimination; supportive care including IV fluids, blood products, hemodialysis
Tres Pasitos (1) Aldicarb	Acts as a reversible inhibitor of cholinesterase enzymes; product is an approved carbamate insecticide sold illegally as a rodenticide; smuggled into the United States from the Dominican Republic; LD_{50} in rats: 1 mg/kg; Muscarinic SX: "SLUDGEBAM;" Nicotinic SX: tachycardia, mydriasis, weakness, fasciculations, respiratory failure; CNS SX: coma, seizures	Activated charcoal; antidotes: IV atropine sulfate to reverse muscarinic symptoms, benzodiazepines for seizures.

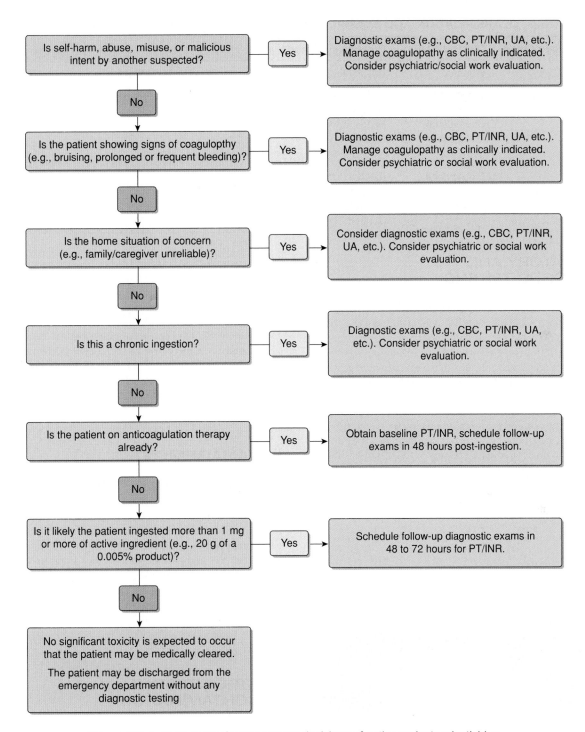

Figure 115–1. Flow chart of management decisions of anticoagulant rodenticides.

these extremely long half-lives, large, symptomatic ingestions require weeks to months of medical care.

▶ CLINICAL FINDINGS

Bleeding diathesis following unintentional ingestion of anticoagulant rodenticides by pediatric patients is unlikely, although mild PT prolongation has been noted. Clinical evidence of bleeding may occur, however, following acute intentional ingestions of large amounts or repeated, chronic ingestions as in the case of pica, child abuse, or Munchausen syndrome, by proxy.

Signs and symptoms may range from minor to life-threatening bleeding. These include epistaxis, easy bruising, gingival bleeding, petechiae, hematuria, hematemesis, melena, hemoptysis, extremity pain associated with compartment syndrome, vaginal bleeding, and intracerebral hemorrhage.

▶ **TABLE 115–3. CLASSIFICATION AND EXAMPLES OF ANTICOAGULANT RODENTICIDES**

Anticoagulant Class	Generic Name	Proprietary Brand
Coumarin	Warfarin	D-Con Mouse Prufe, Fumarin, Hot Shot Rat and Mouse Killer, Kypfarin, Warfarin Plus
4-Hydroxycoumarin	Brodifacoum Bromodiolone Coumatetralyl Difenacoum	D-Con Mouse Prufe II, Enforcer Rat Kill II, Final, Havoc, Talon-G Bromone, Contrac, Maki, Ratimus, Super-Caid, Endox, Endrocid, Endrocide, Racumin Ratack
Indandiones	Chlorophacinone Diphacinone Pindone	Caid, Drat, Enforcer Rat Bait V, Liphadione, Microzul, Ramucide, Ratomet, Raviac, Rozol Contrax-D, Diaphacin, Ditrac, Liqua-Tox, Promar, Ramik, Tomcat Contract-P, Pival, Pivacin, Pivalyn, Tri-Ban

LABORATORY AND DIAGNOSTIC TESTING

No coagulation studies or other laboratory testing is necessary in the asymptomatic pediatric patient following a single unintentional ingestion of a small amount of an anticoagulant rodenticide. In the asymptomatic patient presenting soon after a single large intentional ingestion of an anticoagulant product, obtain a baseline prothrombin time (PT) and international normalized ratio (INR) and then reevaluate the patient at 24 and 48 hours. If an abnormal PT/PTT or INR is obtained from a clinically asymptomatic child, consider repeating the test to rule out a falsely elevated value from incomplete filling of the citrated blue-top tube. In symptomatic patients or those demonstrating abnormal coagulation profiles, consider obtaining the following:

- PT/PTT or INR every 6 to 12 hours until the patient is stabilized.
- Serial hemoglobins and hematocrits.
- Urinalysis to assess for hematuria.
- Stool hemoccult test.
  Type and screen; order type and cross if significant bleeding is present.

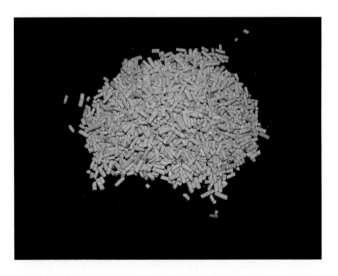

Figure 115–2. This green-colored, brodifacoum-containing rodenticide is commonly found in the home.

- Liver function tests to rule out hepatotoxicity as a cause of coagulopathy.
- Assays for long-lasting anticoagulants may be performed by some reference laboratories. They may aid in confirmation of the diagnosis, but they are not routinely followed or used to guide therapy. Consider factor analysis if the cause of the coagulopathy is unknown; anticoagulants depress factors II, VII, IX, and X.
- Head CT, if mental status changes are present.
- Endoscopy may be considered for the assessment of significant GI bleeding.

▶ MANAGEMENT

IDENTIFICATION OF PRODUCT

It is imperative that every effort be made to identify the product involved in a rodenticide poisoning, including brand name, active ingredients, and concentration. Patients who ingest any amount of the highly toxic rodenticides listed in Table 115–2 must be immediately evaluated and treated as clinically appropriate. A child presenting soon after a rodenticide exposure who has a rapid onset of gastrointestinal, neurologic, or cardiovascular symptoms should raise the suspicion of a very old, illicit, or highly toxic pesticide.

GASTROINTESTINAL DECONTAMINATION

Generally, no GI decontamination procedures are necessary following accidental trivial ingestions of these products. For patients presenting soon after intentional ingestions of large amounts, give one dose of activated charcoal without a cathartic. Do not perform gastric lavage or induce vomiting in any patient actively bleeding or demonstrating an elevated PT or INR.

ENHANCED ELIMINATION

No definitive, clinically proven method of enhanced elimination exists for these agents.

ANTIDOTAL THERAPY: VITAMIN K₁

Vitamin K_1 is a specific antidote for warfarin toxicity. It is a necessary cofactor that competes with warfarin and the long-acting anticoagulants to initiate formation of depleted clotting factors II, VII, IX, and X. Vitamin K_1 therapy is indicated for any patient experiencing active bleeding or with a significantly elevated PT or INR.

Prophylactic therapy is not indicated in asymptomatic patients with normal coagulation studies. Vitamin K_1 administration would merely provide a false sense of security for the prescribing physician, and only serve to delay the onset of anticoagulant effect of the rodenticide due to its much longer duration of action. It is crucial to note that the only effective form of vitamin K is K_1 phytonadione (AquaMEPHYTON®, Mephyton®), which is the active form of the vitamin. Other forms of vitamin K, including vitamin K_3 menadione (Synkayvite®), are ineffective and should not be used.

Oral vitamin K_1 is the safest method of administration and has an onset of effect ranging from 6 to 12 hours. Vitamin K_1 is usually administered three to four times daily, since it has a short therapeutic half-life. Following any adjustment in dose, the patients PT or INR should be checked.

Phytonadione may also be given parenterally, intramuscularly (IM), subcutaneously (SC), or intravenously (IV). IM administration poses the risk of hematoma; therefore, the SC route may be a safer alternative. IV phytonadione offers the fastest onset of action (as little as 1–2 hours). However, due to the potential to cause anaphylactoid reactions, IV administration is rarely used except for the most severe cases; in these situations, FFP will generally have a faster effect in correcting the coagulopathy, with potentially fewer adverse reactions. Untoward reactions, which may occur even at correct dosages and rates, include flushing, hypotension, cyanosis, dizziness, diaphoresis, dyspnea, cardiac and/or respiratory arrest. If vitamin K_1 is given by the IV route, be prepared to resuscitate with epinephrine, antihistamines, and corticosteroid should the patient have a serious adverse effect. Caution is advised in neonates since high doses of phytonadione (10–20 mg) may cause hyperbilirubinemia and severe hemolytic anemia. Following large ingestions of superwarfarin products, antidotal therapy with large doses of vitamin K_1 (phytonadione), i.e., 50 to 100 mg/d, may be required for weeks to months.

FFP AND BLOOD PRODUCTS

For clinically significant active bleeding, FFP is essential to replenish all clotting factors except platelets. The pediatric FFP dose is 10 to 25 mL/kg. The adult FFP dose is 2 to 4 U. This dose may be repeated as needed. Packed red cells, which do not supply clotting factors, may be given to correct severe anemia secondary to hemorrhage.

▶ DISPOSITION

The asymptomatic pediatric patient with a reliable history of a "taste" amount of anticoagulant may be discharged with instructions provided to caregivers to observe for signs of bleeding or easy bruising for next few days.

In the case of the pediatric patient suspected of ingesting large amounts of anticoagulant bait, consider GI decontamination with charcoal followed by a 48-hour outpatient evaluation of coagulation status. The adolescent patient who presents soon after the intentional ingestion of a large amount of anticoagulant bait is a candidate for activated charcoal, admission to a noncritical or psychiatric care unit, and monitoring of coagulation profile for 24 to 48 hours.

For the asymptomatic patient presenting several days after a large acute ingestion, or in a patient with a history of chronic consumption with an abnormal coagulation profile, admission to a noncritical care unit with frequent coagulation studies is reasonable. Initiate vitamin K_1 therapy as indicated. For any symptomatic patient who is actively bleeding, admit to a critical care unit for definitive care with FFP and vitamin K_1.

Upon discharge from the hospital, severly poisoned patients and their family members must be educated about the importance of full compliance with outpatient oral vitamin K_1 regimens and outpatient coagulation monitoring, since the half-life of the long-acting rodenticides far exceeds that of vitamin K. A social services investigation should be pursued following any suspicion of child neglect, abuse, or Munchausen syndrome, by proxy.

Product identification and clinical management recommendations are available through the regional poison control center at 1–800–222–1222, 24 hours a day. Another valuable resource is the National Pesticide Information Center (NPIC) at 1–800–858–7378 (http://npic.orst.edu/). The NPIC is operated by Oregon State University and the EPA from 6:30 AM to 4:30 PM Pacific time, 7 days a week, excluding holidays. This service provides information including pesticide products, recognition and management of pesticide poisoning, toxicology, and environmental chemistry.

REFERENCES

1. Amr MM, Abbas EZ, El-Samra GM, et al. Neuropsychiatric syndromes and occupational exposure to zinc phosphide in Egypt. *Environ Res.* 1997;73:200–206.
2. Babcock J, Hartman K, Pedersen A, et al. Rodenticide induced coagulopthy in a young child: a case of Munchausen syndrome by proxy. *Am J Pediatr Hematol Oncol.* 1993;15(1):126–130.
3. Barrueto F, Nelson LS, Hoffman RS, et al. Poisoning by an illegally imported Chinese rodenticide containing tetramethylenedisulfotetramine—New York City. *MMWR Morb Mortal Wkly Rep.* 2003;52(10):199–201.
4. Binks S, Davies P. Oh Drat!—a case of transcutaneous superwarfarin poisoning and its recurrent presentation. *Emerg Med J.* 2007;24(4):307–308.
5. Blondell J. Epidemiology of pesticide poisonings in the United States with special reference to occupational cases. *Occ Med.* 1997;12(2):209–220.
6. Blondell J. Decline in pesticide poisonings in the United States from 1995 to 2004. *Clin Toxicol.* 2007;45(5):589–592.
7. Caravati EM, Erdman AR, Scharman EJ, et al. Long-acting anticoagulant rodenticide poisoning: an evidence-based consensus guideline for out-of-hospital management. *Clin Toxicol.* 2007;45(1):1–22.
8. Chau CM, Leung AK, Tan IK. Tetramine poisoning. *Hong Kong Med J.* 2005;11(6):511–514.

9. Chugh SN, Aggarwal HK, Mahajan SK. Zinc phosphide intoxication symptoms: analysis of 20 cases. *Int J Clin Pharmacol Ther.* 1998;36(7):406–407.

10. Favus MJ. Treatment of vitamin D intoxication. *NEJM.* 1970; 283(26):1468–1469.

11. Ingels M, Lai C, Manning BH, et al. A prospective study of acute, unintentional pediatric superwarfarin ingestions managed without decontamination. *Ann Emerg Med.* 2002;40(1): 73–78.

12. Jibani M, Hodges NH. Prolonged hypercalcaemia after industial exposure to vitamine D₃. *BMJ.* 1985;290:748–749.

13. Johnson D, Kubic P, Levitt C. Accidental ingestion of Vacor rodenticide. *Am J Dis Child.* 134:161–164, 180.

14. Kanabar D, Volans G. Accidental superwarfarin poisoning in children—less is better. *Lancet.* 2002;360:963.

15. Mullins ME, Brands BL, Daya MR. Unintentional pediatric superwarfarin exposures: do we really need a prothrombin time? *Pediatrics.* 2000;105(2):402–404.

16. National Poison Data System: https://www.npds.us/

17. Nelson LS, Perrone J, DeRoos F, et al. Aldicarb poisoning by an illicit rodenticide imported into the United States: Tres Pasitos. *J Toxicol Clin Toxicol.* 2001;39(5):447–452.

18. Ramon A, Dong P, Perrone J, et al. Poisonings associated with illegal use of aldicarb as a rodenticide—New York City, 1994–1997. *MMWR Morb Mortal Wkly Rep.* 1997;46(41):961–964.

19. Robinson RF, Griffith JR, Wolowich WR, et al. Intoxication with sodium monofluoroacetate (compound 1080). *Vet Hum Toxicol.* 2002;44(2):93–95.

20. Rodengerg HD, Chang CC, Watson WA. Zinc phosphide ingestion: a case report and review. *Vet Hum Toxicol.* 1989;31(6): 559–562.

21. Sheperd G, Klein-Schwartz W, Anderson B. Acute, unintentional pediatric brodifacoum ingestions. *Pediatr Emerg Care.* 2002;18(3):174–178.

22. Talcott PA, Mather GG, Kowitz EH. Accidental ingestion of a cholecalciferol-containing rodent bait in a dog. *Vet Hum Toxicol.* 1991;33(3):252–255.

23. Travis SF, Warfield W, Greenbaum BH, et al. Clinical and laboratory observations: spontaneous hemorrhage associated with accidental brodifacoum poisoning in a child. *J Pediatr.* 1993;122(6):982–984.

24. Valentina O, Lopez C. Brodifacoum Poisoning with Toxicokinetic Data. *Clin Toxicol.* 2007;45(5):487–489.

25. Van Lier RB, Cherry LD. The toxicity and mechanism of action of bromethalin: a new single-feeding rodenticide. *Fundam Appl Toxicol.* 1988;11:664–672.

26. Watts RG, Castleberry RP, Sadowski JA. Accidental Poisoning with a superwarfarin compound (brodifacoum) in a child. *Pediatrics.* 1990;86(6):883–887.

PART 3
PRESCRIPTION DRUGS

CHAPTER 116

Cardiotoxins

Allan R. Mottram and Jerrold B. Leikin

► β-ADRENERGIC BLOCKING AGENTS

► HIGH-YIELD FACTS

- β-Blockers are rapidly absorbed with the onset of symptoms as soon as 30 minutes after ingestion. Cardiovascular manifestations include hypotension, bradycardia, heart block, and heart failure.
- Absorption of β-blockers can be decreased by the administration of activated charcoal.
- Glucagon may reverse the toxic effects of β-blockers.
- Patients who do not respond to glucagon are treated with aggressive fluid resuscitation, vasopressors, and atropine. Refractory cases may require invasive supportive measures.
- A patient who ingested a non–sustained-release β-blocker can be discharged home after 8 hours of observation if they have a normal exam, mental status, vital signs, and EKG.
- A history of sustained-release β-blocker preparation ingestion requires admission to a monitored setting for 24 hours.

The mortality rate following β-blocker overdose is much than that for calcium channel blockers or digoxin, but in terms of absolute numbers they are the second leading cause of death from cardiovascular medications.[1] American Association of Poison Control Centers data from 2006 indicates 18 853 β-blocker exposures. Two thousand eight hundred and twelve of these involved children younger than 6 years and 712 involved 6- to 19-year-olds. β_1- and β_2-receptor antagonism, intrinsic sympathomimetic activity, and membrane-stabilizing activity are responsible for the clinical effects of these drugs. α-antagonist activity is seen with labetalol and carvedilol.[2]

PHARMACOLOGY

The pharmacologic effects of β-blocking drugs are mediated through modulation of intercellular signals and calcium secondary to inhibited adrenergic activation.[3] β_1-Antagonism causes decreased cardiac contractility and conduction. β_2-

Antagonism causes increased smooth muscle tone which may manifest as bronchospasm, increased peripheral vascular tone, and increased gut motility. Although many β-blockers are β_1-selective at therapeutic doses, these drugs have both β_1- and β_2-effects in overdose.

Intrinsic sympathomimetic properties of some β-blockers causes agonist–antagonist activity, which may blunt the bradycardic response in some patients.[2,4] Drugs with intrinsic sympathomimetic activity include acebutolol, carteolol, oxprenolol, penbutolol, and pindolol. The membrane-stabilizing activity characteristic of some β-blockers is a quinidine-like effect, resulting in inhibition of fast sodium channels, decreased contractility, and ventricular arryhythmias.[5] This effect is additive to the β_1-toxic effects.

β-Blockers with increased intrinsic sympathomimetic activity and decreased membrane-stabilizing properties demonstrate less toxicity than those with increased membrane-stabilizing properties.[5–8] Drugs with significant membrane-stabilizing properties include propranolol, acebutolol, betaxolol, and oxprenolol.[9]

Sotalol is a β-blocker which has class III antiarrhythmic properties.[10] In overdose, it may prolong the QT interval, resulting in ventricular arrhythmias, including torsades de pointes. Each different β-blocker may have only some of the described activities, and the clinical manifestations may vary.

PHARMACOKINETICS

The absorption, distribution, and elimination of β-blockers vary with the preparation. Extended-release formulations of β-blockers can have a marked delay in the onset of toxic effects. Conversely, standard release β-blockers are rapidly absorbed, with 30% to 90% bioavailability. The elimination half-life varies from 2 to 24 hours, but can be significantly increased in overdose.

PATHOPHYSIOLOGY

Toxicity from acute β-blocker overdose largely results from suppression of the cardiovascular system. Negative inotropic and chronotropic effects result in bradycardia and hypotension. Respiratory compromise in β-blocker overdose can result from cardiogenic shock, decreased respiratory drive, or β$_2$-antagonist effects. β$_2$-Blockade causes bronchospasm, and usually affects patients with previously diagnosed asthma. Hypoglycemia can occur secondary to β$_2$-mediated decrease in glycogenolysis and gluconeogenesis; however, it is not common unless there are associated comorbidities or coingestants.[11] CNS depression can be caused by direct toxicity, hypoxia, hypoglycemia, or shock.

CLINICAL PRESENTATION

The onset of symptoms can be as rapid as 30 minutes after ingestion, but most commonly occurs within 1 to 2 hours. Cardiovascular manifestations include hypotension, bradycardia, heart block, and congestive heart failure. Electrocardiographic manifestations of toxicity include sinus bradycardia, prolongation of the PR interval, second- and third-degree AV blockade, and interventricular conduction delays.[6,12] The QRS may be prolonged with ingestions of β-blockers with membrane-stabilizing effects. Propranolol and sotalol have been associated with ventricular arrhythmias.[12] Deaths from β-blockers toxicity are associated with bradydysrhythmias and asystole; ventricular arrhythmias are less common. Respiratory toxicity includes noncardiogenic pulmonary edema, pulmonary edema, exacerbation of asthma, and decreased respiratory drive. Patients may also present with CNS depression or seizures.

LABORATORY EVALUATION

All patients with a history of β-blocker ingestion are placed on a cardiac monitor and receive an electrocardiogram (ECG). Laboratory tests for blood levels of β-blockers are available from reference laboratories but are not helpful in the acute setting. Serum electrolytes are obtained. Serum glucose is assessed. Arterial blood gas and chest radiograph may be useful in the patient with respiratory signs or symptoms.

MANAGEMENT

The effects of β-blocker ingestion range from negligible to catastrophic. A well-looking patient should not be reassuring, since they can decompensate quickly. Patients with normal mental status should be decontaminated with activated charcoal. Gastric lavage has limited utility, and should only be used in patients with potentially life threatening ingestions who present within 1 hour of ingestion. In the event of significant toxicity, standard PALS resuscitation techniques including advanced airway management should be utilized, followed by focused therapies for β-blocker toxicity.

Glucagon is the agent of choice in β-blocker ingestions resulting in hypotension and/or bradycardia.[13,14] Glucagon binds to its own receptor site, triggering cAMP signaling pathways, bypassing the cellular lesion at the β-receptor.[15] An initial bolus of glucagon is administered intravenously at a dose of 0.05 to 0.15 mg/kg IV over 1 minute. If symptoms recur, a repeat

bolus is given. An infusion can be started following the bolus dose, with the effective bolus dose infused per hour. The initial effect is seen within several minutes, and should persist for 10 to 15 minutes. Nausea and vomiting are common side effects of glucagon, which can complicate the management of a patient who may subsequently require intubation.

Adrenergic agents are often effective in increasing heart rate, contractility, and peripheral vascular resistance. In cases of severe cardiovascular drug toxicity, large doses may be required.[16] If the response to glucagon is inadequate, epinephrine and dopamine may improve both heart rate and blood pressure.[8] Norepinephrine is effective in situations with low systemic vascular resistance, however with the myocardial depression seen with severe β-blockade, alternative agents may be more efficacious.[16] Atropine, 0.02 mg/kg IV (minimum single dose 0.1 mg; maximum cumulative dose 1 mg) may be useful for bradycardia.

Bradycardia and hypotension refractory to pharmacologic intervention may benefit from temporary pacing, although this will not reverse the myocardial depression in severe overdose.[17,18] Interventions such as intra-aortic balloon pump, extracorporeal membrane oxygenation (ECMO) or cardiac bypass are considerations for patients with toxicity refractory to all other therapy.[18,19] Hemodialysis, hemofiltration, and hemoperfusion are rarely useful in the setting of β-blocker overdose. Most of the β-blockers have a large volume of distribution and are highly protein bound, making drug removal by hemodialysis impractical. A few drugs, such as nadolol, sotalol, atenolol, and acebutolol, can be dialyzed, but experience is limited to case reports.[19–21] Hemodialysis can be considered in the setting of renal failure and hemodynamic instability in a drug with low volume of distribution and low protein binding.

DISPOSITION

A patient with a history of immediate-release β-blocker ingestion is observed on a cardiac monitor for 8 hours after ingestion.[22,23] Patients who have signs of cardiovascular, respiratory, or CNS toxicity are admitted to an intensive care setting. Patients with a history of ingestion of extended-release preparations or sotalol are admitted and monitored for 24 hours. A patient who ingested an immediate release β-blocker can be medically cleared after the 8 hour observation period if there are no signs of toxicity found by clinical examination, ECG, or cardiac monitoring.

► CALCIUM CHANNEL BLOCKERS

► HIGH-YIELD FACTS

- Onset of symptoms in calcium channel blocker overdose can be as soon as 30 minutes after ingestion. Time to onset can be greatly increased with sustained-release preparations.
- Absorption of calcium channel blockers can be decreased by the administration of activated charcoal.
- In all cases of calcium channel blocker overdose, cardiovascular effects predominate.

- For calcium channel blocker overdose with hypotension that persists despite the administration of fluids, calcium salts and glucagon, therapy with vasopressors is indicated.
- High-dose insulin therapy is effective in the management of refractory calcium channel blocker overdose.
- An asymptomatic patient who ingested a non–sustained-release calcium channel blocker can be medically cleared after an 8-hour observation period.
- Ingestion of a sustained-release calcium channel blocker preparation requires admission and monitoring for at least 24 hours.

The American Association of Poison Control Centers annual report indicated 10 031 calcium channel blocker exposures in 2006. 1363 exposures occurred in children younger than 6 years and 234 occurred in those aging between 6 and 19 years. Because of recognition of this poisoning in conjunction with intensive management, deaths due to calcium channel blocker overdose have been declining in recent years and rarely occur in the pediatric setting.

PHARMACOLOGY

Calcium channel blockers are classified as dihydropyridines, phenylalkylamines, or benzothiazepines. Dihydropyridines include nifedipine, isradipine, amlodipine, felodipine, nimodipine, nisoldipine, and nicardipine. Verapamil is a phenylalkylamine, and diltiazem is a benzothiazepine. Calcium channel blockers work at the L-type calcium channel, effecting automaticity at the sinoatrial node, conduction through the atrioventricular node, excitation–contraction coupling in cardiac and smooth muscle, as well as pancreatic insulin secretion.[3,24]

The clinical effects of the three classes of calcium channel blockers differ for several reasons. They bind at different locations on calcium channel receptor subunits, have preference for different resting cell membrane potentials, and bind as a function of channel state.[25–27] Receptor selectivity translates into the dihydropyridines primarily resulting in vasodilation; the nondihydropyridines have more pronounced effects on cardiac conduction. Verapamil affects myocardial contractility, AV node conduction, peripheral vascular resistance, and is one of the more toxic calcium channel blockers in overdose. Diltiazem slows AV node conduction and causes coronary artery dilatation; it has less effect on peripheral vasculature and myocardial contractility. Nifedipine, a dihydropyridine, has the greatest effect on peripheral vascular resistance. It also decreases cardiac contractility, but has minimal effect on AV node conduction. In overdose all classes of calcium channel blockers can cause significant peripheral vasodilatation, decreased AV conduction, and decreased myocardial contractility.

PHARMACOKINETICS

Most calcium channel blockers undergo hepatic metabolism with extensive first pass effect, have a large volume of distribution, and are highly protein bound.[24,28] The onset of action for immediate release preparations is 30 minutes, with a half-life from 3 to 7 hours; this can be greatly increased in the setting of overdose and with sustained-release preparations. It is important to be aware that the onset of life-threatening effects from sustained-release preparations may also be delayed because of their prolonged absorption time.

PATHOPHYSIOLOGY

The clinical effects of calcium channel blocker overdose can be life threatening. Slowing of the sinus node causes bradycardia. Slowing of conduction can cause heart blocks or asystole. Decreased contractility can cause heart failure and shock. Lowered peripheral vascular resistance leads to hypotension, which may exacerbate the hypotension associated with bradycardia, bradyarrhythmias, and heart failure. Hyperglycemia occurs frequently with significant overdoses, and may correlate with the severity of poisoning.[29] Patients with cardiac disease and those on other medications that suppress heart rate and contractility may develop severe toxic effects after mild overdose, or even at therapeutic doses.

CLINICAL EFFECTS

The different pharmacologic profile of calcium channel blockers will cause variation in toxic effects, but in all cases cardiovascular effects predominate. Verapamil and diltiazem typically cause bradycardia and hypotension. Hypotension may be caused by sinoatrial node depression, atrioventricular node depression leading to AV blocks, or decreased peripheral vascular resistance. Nifedipine primarily affects the arterioles, causing decreased peripheral vascular resistance, which leads to hypotension and reflex tachycardia.

Neurologic and respiratory findings are usually secondary to cardiovascular toxicity and shock. Respiratory effects include decreased respiratory drive, pulmonary edema, and ARDS. Neurologic sequelae include depressed sensorium, cerebral infarction, and seizures. Nausea, vomiting, and constipation can occur.

LABORATORY EVALUATION

Drug levels for calcium channel blockers are available by reference laboratories but are not helpful in an acute overdose. An ECG is obtained. Electrolytes are evaluated, specifically Na^+, Ca^{2+}, Mg^{2+}, and K^+. Glucose is evaluated since decreased insulin release can lead to hyperglycemia. Chest radiographs are obtained for patients with respiratory signs or symptoms. An abdominal radiograph may be useful in patients with a history of ingesting sustained-release tablets, since some calcium channel blockers are radiopaque, and concretions can occur.

MANAGEMENT

The effects of calcium channel blocker ingestion range from negligible to catastrophic. A well-looking patient should not be reassuring, since they can decompensate quickly. Patients with normal mental status should be decontaminated with activated charcoal. Gastric lavage has limited utility, and should only be used in patients with potentially life threatening ingestions who present within 1 hour of ingestion. Whole bowel irrigation can be considered for asymptomatic patients who present early after overdosing on a sustained-release formulation, but it should be used with great caution as there is no evidence of improved outcomes with whole bowel irrigation, and it may complicate the management of patients who subsequently become hypotensive. In the event of significant toxicity, standard PALS resuscitation techniques, including advanced airway management, apply, followed by focused therapies for calcium channel blocker toxicity.

Following initial resuscitation, therapy focuses on enhancing calcium channel function. However, treatment may have little effect when the calcium channel is severely poisoned.[30–33] Calcium salts increase extracellular calcium concentration, and may reverse hypotension because of vasodilation, especially in less severe overdoses. However, improvement is usually transient in the serious overdose setting, and there is little or no effect on heart rate or conduction. Atropine may be helpful for patients with symptomatic bradycardia or heart block. Isoproterenol or pacemaker devices may be useful. A trial of glucagon is reasonable when coingestion with a β-blocker is suspected. It is not as effective for calcium channel blocker poisoning as it is for β-blocker poisoning. Nausea and vomiting are frequent side effects of glucagon. This becomes relevant in the patient who may subsequently require intubation.

Vasopressors should be utilized early for patients who do not respond to intravenous fluid, calcium, and atropine. An agent with combined α- and β-effects, such as high-dose dopamine or norepinephrine, is appropriate. Phenylephrine and dobutamine may also be effective. More than one agent may be required.

Hyperinsulinemia–euglycemia therapy (HIE) should be considered early in the critically ill patient. Efficacy of HIE is likely attributable to the metabolic effects of insulin which result in improvement in blood pressure, systolic and diastolic myocardial performance, and survival time.[34] The evidence in support of HIE is limited to animal studies, adult case reports and case series.[9,35–39] Despite this limitation, given the lack of alternative therapies, HIE should be utilized early for severe calcium channel blocker overdose.[16,36,41]

The protocol for HIE is 1 unit/kg regular insulin intravenous bolus followed by 0.5 units/kg/hr intravenous infusion.[41] An intravenous dextrose bolus of 0.25 gm/kg, followed by an infusion of 0.5 g/kg/h may be initiated, however patients with significant poisoning are not expected to develop hypoglycemia. Serial blood sugar determinations are followed, and the dextrose infusion adjusted accordingly. Potassium is monitored and replaced to maintain serum potassium levels at 2.8 to 3.2 mEq/L.

Interventions such as intra-aortic balloon pump, extracorporeal membrane oxygenation (ECMO) or cardiac bypass are considerations for patients with toxicity refractory to all other therapy.[42–44] Hemodialysis, hemofiltration, and hemoperfusion are unlikely to be effective for calcium channel blocker overdose. Most calcium channel antagonists have a large volume of distribution, are highly protein bound, and subject to hepatic metabolism making them poor candidates for extracorporeal removal.

Patients who have signs of cardiovascular, respiratory, or CNS compromise are admitted to an intensive care unit. Patients with a history of sustained-release ingestion are observed for at least 24 hours. Those patients with no signs of toxicity, no history of sustained-release ingestion, and no ECG abnormalities can be observed for 8 hours after the time of ingestion. If they do not develop any signs of toxicity or ECG abnormalities during this period, they may be medically cleared.

▶ DIGOXIN

▶ HIGH-YIELD FACTS

- Plants that contain cardiac glycosides include foxglove, oleander, lily of the valley, and red squill.
- Digoxin acts by poisoning the Na^+-K^+ ATPase pump in the heart. High serum potassium may be seen after acute overdose.
- A toxic dose of greater than 0.1 mg/kg may be an indication for antidotal therapy.
- Both hyperkalemia and hypokalemia can predispose to digoxin-induced cardiac dysrhythmias.
- Almost any cardiac dysrhythmia may be seen with digoxin toxicity. Accelerated junctional rhythms, premature ventricular contractions (PVCs), paroxysmal atrial tachycardia, and atrioventricular blocks are more commonly seen rhythms in this setting.
- Atropine is effective for digoxin-induced bradycardia.
- Calcium chloride, potassium, and bretylium should be avoided in treating digoxin toxicity.
- Digoxin immune Fab fragments are indicated in any patient exhibiting a life-threatening dysrhythmia, regardless of the digoxin level.

Digoxin is used today for the treatment of congestive heart failure and supraventricular dysrhythmias. In addition, there are several plants that contain cardiac glycosides (digoxinlike substances), including foxglove, oleander, lily of the valley, and red squill.

Historically, mortality because of digoxin overdose has been related to the type of cardiac arrhythmia induced by toxicity and the degree of associated hyperkalemia. Mortality rates of 68% for patients exhibiting digoxin-induced sustained ventricular tachycardia and 100% for ventricular fibrillation were noted prior to the development of digoxin immune Fab fragments. According to the American Association of Poison Control Centers, in 2007 there were a total of 2610 cardiac glycoside ingestions. Of these 293 were in children aging 6 years, 52 were in children between the ages of 6 and 19 years, and there were a total of 22 deaths in all age groups (accounting for almost half of all deaths because of cardiovascular drug ingestions)[1]

PHARMACOLOGY/ PATHOPHYSIOLOGY

Digoxin is a positive inotrope that increases the force and velocity of myocardial contractions. In the failing heart, it can increase the cardiac output and decrease elevated end-diastolic pressures.

On the cellular level, digoxin presumably functions by binding to and inactivating the Na^+-K^+ ATPase pump in the heart. This results in increased intracellular sodium concentration. In addition, enhanced contractility depends on intracellular ionized calcium concentrations during systole. At toxic concentrations, it is felt that intracellular calcium concentrations are markedly increased, and that the membrane potential is unstable, which leads to dysrhythmias.

There are numerous factors that predispose the patient to digoxin toxicity, the most common of which is electrolyte imbalance.[45] Both hypokalemia and hyperkalemia can increase the possibility of developing digoxin toxicity. Hyperkalemia in particular can result in significant conduction delays. Hypokalemia is common in patients on diuretic therapy and can predispose patients to the effects of chronic digoxin toxicity. Hypomagnesemia, hypercalcemia, renal insufficiency, and underlying heart disease all predispose to digoxin toxicity.[46]

CLINICAL PRESENTATION

The presentation of digoxin toxicity is highly varied, and depends largely on whether it results from an acute overdose or is a manifestation of chronic toxicity.[46]

In the acute setting, patients tend to have more dramatic, clinical, and laboratory parameters than in chronic toxicity. Symptoms can be abrupt, with severe nausea, vomiting, and diarrhea. Associated complaints include weakness, headache, paresthesias, and altered color perception. Cardiovascular symptoms include palpitations and dizziness that may be secondary to hypotension. Movement disorders may also be present.[47]

Patients with chronic toxicity tend to have more vague complaints, although many of the symptoms of acute overdose also occur. Malaise, anorexia, and low-grade nausea and vomiting are common. Patients with chronic toxicity tend to be more symptomatic at lower levels than those with acute overdoses.

Cardiovascular toxicity is the most important factor in determining morbidity and mortality. There are multiple dysrhythmias associated with digoxin toxicity, the most common being frequent premature ventricular beats. Other dysrhythmias can be supraventricular, nodal, or ventricular. Common disturbances are junctional escape beats and accelerated junctional rhythm, paroxysmal atrial tachycardia with AV block, and AV block of varying degrees. There is no single pathognomonic rhythm. Lethal cardiac disturbances rarely occur in children with normal hearts, but serious AV conduction disturbances can occur.[48]

DIAGNOSIS

A history of the exact amount of digoxin ingested is extremely helpful. A dose greater than 0.1 mg/kg is an indication that serious consequences can occur.

A serum digoxin level is indicated whenever there is clinical suspicion of toxicity.[46,49] In an overdose situation, the level is most accurate if obtained ≥6 hours after the ingestion. The therapeutic digoxin range is between 0.8 and 1.8 ng/mL. Unfortunately, there is poor correlation between the digoxin level and clinical manifestations. In an acute overdose, a level as high as 2.6 ng/mL does not correlate well with toxicity. In a chronic overdose, toxicity can occur at lower levels. The fatality rate approaches 50% when the serum digoxin level exceeds 6 ng/mL.

Other necessary laboratory studies include a complete blood count, serum electrolytes, calcium, magnesium, blood urea nitrogen, and creatinine. Cardiac monitoring is essential, as is a 12-lead electrocardiogram.

MANAGEMENT

Digoxin-intoxicated patients can be highly unstable. All patients require a secure airway, intravenous access, and cardiac monitoring. (See Fig. 116–1 for initial evaluation and treatment of digoxin toxicity.)

Gastric Decontamination

Syrup of ipecac is contraindicated and should not be used because of the potential for sudden hemodynamic instability, deterioration of consciousness, and the subsequent potential for vomiting and aspiration. Gastric lavage has limited utility, and should only be used in patients with potentially life-threatening ingestions who present within 1 hour of ingestion. Activated charcoal is indicated as a single dose. Multiple doses of charcoal have been reported to be of value for digitoxin preparations in which there is avid enterohepatic circulation, and may be of value for digoxin. However, the advent of Digibind has supplanted consideration for enhanced elimination with MDAC. Whole-bowel irrigation should be avoided in patients with potential for hemodynamic instability.

Antidotal Therapy

Digoxin immune Fab fragments are specific antidigoxin antibodies derived from sheep. In order to decrease the risk of immunogenicity, only the Fab fragment is used.[50] Specific indications include an ingestion of greater than 0.1 mg/kg, a digoxin level of greater than 10.0 ng/mL, potassium greater than 5 mEq/L, or the presence of a life-threatening dysrhythmia. In chronic digoxin poisoning significant toxicity may occur at much lower serum levels. Standard modalities to treat hyperkalemia may also be used, with the exception of calcium salts. In the face of digoxin toxicity the administration of calcium may exacerbate the development of dysrhythmias.

The dose of Fab fragments is based either on the amount ingested or on the serum level. Each vial of Fab fragments contains 38 mg of protein that will bind 0.6 mg of digoxin. Specific guidelines for dosing Fab fragments are available on the package insert.

Allergic reactions to Fab fragments are rare.[50] Skin testing can be performed, but is usually not necessary. In cases where Fab fragments have been effective, results have been achieved 30 minutes to 4 hours after administration. After administration of Fab fragments, subsequent digoxin levels will be falsely elevated for several days, because the bound digoxin is measured along with the free drug.[51] Certain laboratories can assay free digoxin levels which avoids this problem.

In addition to the administration of Fab fragments, standard treatment of dysrhythmias or AV blocks is indicated.

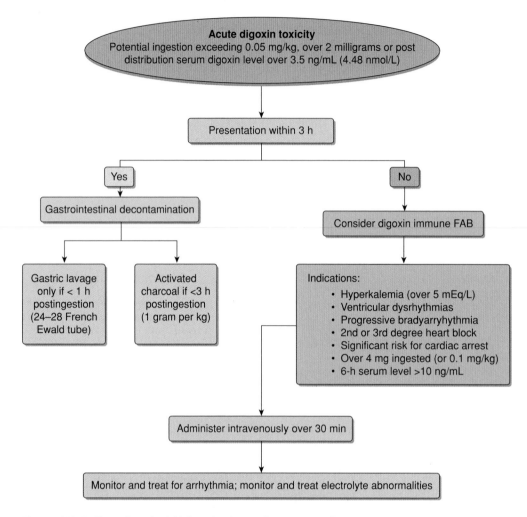

Figure 116–1. Flow chart for initial evaluation and treatment of acute digoxin toxicity.

Atropine or temporary pacing may be necessary to temporize while Fab fragments are taking effect. Cardioversion and lidocaine are appropriate in the event of ventricular tachycardia or fibrillation. Treatment with intravenous phenytoin or magnesium sulfate has been shown to be useful in digoxin-induced tachydysrhythmias. Drugs to avoid in the treatment of digoxin-induced cardiac toxicity include calcium, bretylium tosylate, sotalol, isoproterenol, and quinidine. Direct-current cardioversion should only be used as a last resort for unstable, life-threatening arrhythmias. If utilized, it should be dosed at the lowest energy possible.

Diuresis, hemodialysis, and hemoperfusion do not aid in the removal of digoxin or digitoxin. Plasma exchange is also not expected to be useful.

DISPOSITION

Children with trivial ingestions (less than 0.05 mg/kg) who are asymptomatic and have no detectable levels of digoxin 4 hours after the ingestion can be discharged from the emergency department after 6 hours of observation. Any child with signs or symptoms of toxicity is admitted to a pediatric intensive care unit.

REFERENCES

1. Bronstein AC, Spyker DA, Cantilera LR Jr, et al. 2006 Annual Report of the American Association of Poison Control Centers' National Poisoning and Data System (NPDS). *Clin Toxicol (Phila)*. 2007;45:815–917.
2. Frishman WH. Clinical differences between beta-adrenergic blocking agents: implications for therapeutic substitution. *Am Heart J.* 1987;113(5):1190–1198.
3. Katz AM. Selectivity and toxicity of antiarrhythmic drugs: molecular interactions with ion channels. *Am J Med.* 1998;104 (2):179–195.
4. Frishman WH. Clinical significance of beta 1-selectivity and intrinsic sympathomimetic activity in a beta-adrenergic blocking drug. *Am J Cardiol.* 1987;59(13):33F–37F.
5. Henry JA, Cassidy SL. Membrane stabilising activity: a major cause of fatal poisoning. *Lancet.* 1986;1(8495):1414–1417.
6. Love JN et al. Electrocardiographic changes associated with beta-blocker toxicity. *Ann Emerg Med.* 2002;40(6):603–610.
7. Frishman W et al. Clinical pharmacology of the new beta-adrenergic blocking drugs. Part 8. Self-poisoning with beta-adrenoceptor blocking agents: recognition and management. *Am Heart J.* 1979;98(6):798–811.
8. Weinstein RS. Recognition and management of poisoning with beta-adrenergic blocking agents. *Ann Emerg Med.* 1984;13(12):1123–1131.

9. Brubacher J. β-Adrenergic agonists. In: Hoffman RS, Nelson LS, Howland M, et al., eds. *Goldfrank's Toxicologic Emergencies.* 8th ed. McGraw-Hill; 2007: chap 59.

10. Hohnloser SH, Woosley RL. Sotalol. *N Engl J Med.* 1994;331(1): 31–38.

11. Reith DM et al. Relative toxicity of beta blockers in overdose. *J Toxicol Clin Toxicol.* 1996;34(3):273–278.

12. Delk C, Holstege CP, Brady WJ. Electrocardiographic abnormalities associated with poisoning. *Am J Emerg Med.* 2007;25 (6):672–687.

13. Pollack CV Jr. Utility of glucagon in the emergency department. *J Emerg Med.* 1993;11(2):195–205.

14. Taboulet P et al. Pathophysiology and management of self-poisoning with beta-blockers. *J Toxicol Clin Toxicol.* 1993;31 (4):531–551.

15. Yagami T. Differential coupling of glucagon and beta-adrenergic receptors with the small and large forms of the stimulatory G protein. *Mol Pharmacol.* 1995;48(5):849–854.

16. Kerns W II. Management of beta-adrenergic blocker and calcium channel antagonist toxicity. *Emerg Med Clin North Am.* 2007;25(2):309–331; abstract viii.

17. Kenyon CJ et al. Successful resuscitation using external cardiac pacing in beta adrenergic antagonist-induced bradyasystolic arrest. *Ann Emerg Med.* 1988;17(7):711–713.

18. Lane AS, Woodward AC, Goldman MR. Massive propranolol overdose poorly responsive to pharmacologic therapy: use of the intra-aortic balloon pump. *Ann Emerg Med.* 1987;16(12): 1381–1383.

19. Rooney M et al. Acebutolol overdose treated with hemodialysis and extracorporeal membrane oxygenation. *J Clin Pharmacol.* 1996;36(8):760–763.

20. Saitz R, Williams BW, Farber HW. Atenolol-induced cardiovascular collapse treated with hemodialysis. *Crit Care Med.* 1991;19(1):116–118.

21. Salhanick SD, Wax PM. Treatment of atenolol overdose in a patient with renal failure using serial hemodialysis and hemoperfusion and associated echocardiographic findings. *Vet Hum Toxicol.* 2000;42(4):224–225.

22. Love JN. Beta blocker toxicity after overdose: when do symptoms develop in adults? *J Emerg Med.* 1994;12(6):799–802.

23. Love JN et al. Acute beta blocker overdose: factors associated with the development of cardiovascular morbidity. *J Toxicol Clin Toxicol.* 2000;38(3):275–281.

24. Pitt B. Diversity of calcium antagonists. *Clin Ther.* 1997;19 (suppl A):3–17.

25. Taira N. Differences in cardiovascular profile among calcium antagonists. *Am J Cardiol.* 1987;59(3):24B–29B.

26. Barrett TD et al. Mechanism of tissue-selective drug action in the cardiovascular system. *Mol Interv.* 2005;5(2):84–93.

27. Hondeghem LM, Katzung BG. Antiarrhythmic agents: the modulated receptor mechanism of action of sodium and calcium channel-blocking drugs. *Annu Rev Pharmacol Toxicol.* 1984;24:387–423.

28. Leikin JB, Palouchek FP, eds. *Poisoning and Toxicology Handbook.* 3rd ed. Lexi-Comp, Inc; 2002.

29. Levine M et al. Assessment of hyperglycemia after calcium channel blocker overdoses involving diltiazem or verapamil. *Crit Care Med.* 2007;35(9):2071–2075.

30. Yuan TH et al. Insulin-glucose as adjunctive therapy for severe calcium channel antagonist poisoning. *J Toxicol Clin Toxicol.* 1999;37(4):463–474.

31. Caulfield MP, Birdsall NJ. International Union of Pharmacology. XVII. Classification of muscarinic acetylcholine receptors. *Pharmacol Rev.* 1998;50(2):279–290.

32. Wolf LR, Spadafora MP, Otten EJ. Use of amrinone and glucagon in a case of calcium channel blocker overdose. *Ann Emerg Med.* 1993;22(7):1225–1228.

33. Haddad LM. Resuscitation after nifedipine overdose exclusively with intravenous calcium chloride. *Am J Emerg Med.* 1996;14(6):602–603.

34. Kline JA et al. Insulin improves heart function and metabolism during non-ischemic cardiogenic shock in awake canines. *Cardiovasc Res.* 1997;34(2):289–298.

35. Boyer EW, Shannon M. Treatment of calcium-channel-blocker intoxication with insulin infusion. *N Engl J Med.* 2001;344(22): 1721–1722.

36. Boyer EW, Duic PA, Evans A. Hyperinsulinemia/euglycemia therapy for calcium channel blocker poisoning. *Pediatr Emerg Care.* 2002;18(1):36–37.

37. Rasmussen L, Husted SE, Johnsen SP. Severe intoxication after an intentional overdose of amlodipine. *Acta Anaesthesiol Scand.* 2003;47(8):1038–1040.

38. Marques M, Gomes E, de Oliveira J. Treatment of calcium channel blocker intoxication with insulin infusion: case report and literature review. *Resuscitation.* 2003;57(2):211–213.

39. Harris NS. Case records of the Massachusetts General Hospital. Case 24–2006. A 40-year-old woman with hypotension after an overdose of amlodipine. *N Engl J Med.* 2006;355(6):602–611.

40. Ortiz-Munoz L, Rodriguez-Ospina LF, Figueroa-Gonzalez M. Hyperinsulinemic-euglycemic therapy for intoxication with calcium channel blockers. *Bol Asoc Med P R.* 2005;97(3)(Pt 2): 182–189.

41. Lheureux PE et al. Bench-to-bedside review: hyperinsulinaemia/euglycaemia therapy in the management of overdose of calcium-channel blockers. *Crit Care.* 2006;10(3):212.

42. Holzer M et al. Successful resuscitation of a verapamil-intoxicated patient with percutaneous cardiopulmonary bypass. *Crit Care Med.* 1999;27(12):2818–2823.

43. Frierson J et al. Refractory cardiogenic shock and complete heart block after unsuspected verapamil-SR and atenolol overdose. *Clin Cardiol.* 1991;14(11):933–935.

44. Hendren WG, Schieber RS, Garrettson LK. Extracorporeal bypass for the treatment of verapamil poisoning. *Ann Emerg Med.* 1989;18(9):984–987.

45. Williamson KM, Thrasher KA, Fulton KB, et al. Digoxin toxicity: an evaluation in current clinical practice. *Arch Intern Med.* 1998;158:2444–2449.

46. Kelly RA, Smith TW. Recognition and management of digitalis toxicity. *J Am Coll Cardiol.* 1991;17:590.

47. Sekkul EA, Kaminer S, Sethi KD. Digoxin-induced chorea in a child. *Mov Disord.* 1999;14(5):877–879.

48. Wells TG, Young RA, Kearns GL. Age-related differences in digoxin toxicity and its treatment. *Drug Saf.* 1992;7:135–151.

49. Lewis RP. Clinical use of serum digoxin concentrations. *Am J Cardiol.* 1992;69:97G–107G.

50. Woolf AD, Wenger TL, Smith TW, et al. Results of multicenter studies of digoxin-specific antibody fragments in managing digitalis intoxication in the pediatric population. *Am J Emerg Med.* 1991;9(2)(suppl 1):16–20.

51. Valdes R Jr, Jortani SA. Monitoring of unbound digoxin in patients treated with anti-digoxin antigen-binding fragments: a model for the future? *Clin Chem.* 1998;44:183–185.

CHAPTER 117

Antidepressants

Timothy Meehan and Steven E. Aks

▶ HIGH-YIELD FACTS

- The quinidinelike effect of the tricyclic antidepressants (TCAs) produces QRS and QT abnormalities.
- A clinical hallmark of tricyclic antidepressant overdoses is that patients may appear to be clinically well, then suddenly deteriorate in the first 2 hours after presentation.
- Clinical signs and symptoms are the best way to diagnose tricyclic antidepressant toxicity. Blood levels are generally not helpful.
- The serotonin syndrome is manifested by mental status changes, rigidity, hyperthermia, hyperreflexia, and tremor.
- Unlike the selective serotonin reuptake inhibitors (SSRIs), the atypical antidepressants may cause adverse cardiac and hemodynamic effects in overdose.

Antidepressants are powerful modulators of the monoamine pathways of the CNS and are found in many households. According to CDC data, in 2005 approximately 20% of all prescriptions were for antidepressants.[1] The wide availability of this class of pharmaceuticals underscores the risk of either intentional or unintentional pediatric ingestions.

According to the 2005 report of the American Association of Poison Control Centers (AAPCC), there were 13 804 ingestions in patients younger than 6 years and 18 703 in patients between 6 and 19 years of age. The vast majority of these ingestions were because of SSRIs (18 940), with 2590 because of cyclic antidepressants. However, the cyclic antidepressants resulted in more hospitalizations and serious outcomes.[2] This is likely because of the narrow therapeutic index with TCAs in children compared to the SSRIs. Dosing as low as 10 to 20 mg/kg of a TCA can result in serious toxicity, whereas most adults can tolerate up to 1000 mg before encountering life-threatening consequences. Therefore, it is worthwhile to discuss both TCAs and SSRIs, as well as the newer atypical antidepressants (Table 117–1).

▶ TRICYCLIC ANTIDEPRESSANTS

The TCAs, exert their therapeutic effects primarily through presynaptic reuptake inhibition of norepinephrine and serotonin. TCAs are primarily used in the pediatric population for behavior-related problems such as enuresis or obsessive compulsive disorder that are refractory to the SSRIs.

The TCAs can have a direct or indirect effect on a myriad of physiologic systems. Cardiac effects are directly mediated by quinidinelike effects that slow phase 0 of depolarization and clinically manifest as widened QRS and QTc intervals. However, the most commonly encountered EKG abnormality is sinus tachycardia. Norepinephrine reuptake inhibition leads to tachycardia and can cause hypertension. However, upon depletion of norepinephrine stores hypotension can occur. α blockade can also cause hypotension by decreasing peripheral vasomotor tone. Finally, antimuscarinic effects can cause an anticholinergic syndrome. This leads to decreased GI motility and may contribute to toxicity by prolonging absorption because of an increase in contact time with the intestinal mucosa.[3] Seizures are often short-lived and often self-limited, but treatment with benzodiazepines may be necessary.

A key point to be emphasized is that patients who have overdosed on TCAs may present to the ED appearing clinically stable and may then suddenly deteriorate. The majority of patients who develop life-threatening problems do so within 2 hours of arrival in the ED. Qualitative drug screens may establish a diagnosis, but quantitative levels are of little help unless they are very high. Attending to the clinical signs and symptoms is the best way to make the diagnosis. If a possible TCA overdose is in the differential, then continuous cardiac monitoring and obtaining an EKG are essential first steps in the assessment. Sinus tachycardia may herald later clinical deterioration.

Several electrocardiographic parameters have been identified as markers of significant TCA toxicity. The QRS duration has received much attention as a marker for overdose. While not fully studied in the pediatric population, adult EKG analysis has revealed that a QRS duration between 100 and 160 ms is associated with seizures and dysrhythmias, and a QRS greater than 160 ms with a high risk of seizures and dysrhythmias.[4] When confronted with a QRS of >120 msec, 1 to 2 mEq/Kg boluses of sodium bicarbonate should be administered. If the patient is intubated, relative hyperventilation should be done to achieve a target pH of 7.5. If additional episodes of QRS widening occur, more bicarbonate boluses can be given. If the cardiac rhythm devolves into ventricular tachycardia despite aggressive treatment with bicarbonate lidocaine can be given.

▶ SELECTIVE SEROTONIN REUPTAKE INHIBITORS

SSRIs were developed in response to toxicity of the TCAs.[5] They act primarily on serotonin reuptake, and thereby interact with norepinephrine and dopamine metabolism. However, the mechanism by which they alleviate symptoms of depression is unclear. Unlike TCAs, they have minimal interaction on the cholinergic/adrenergic systems, GABA systems, and sodium

▶ **TABLE 117–1. ANTIDEPRESSANT CLASS**

TCA
Amitriptyline
Imipramine
Nortriptyline

SSRI
Citalopram
Escitalopram
Fluoxetine
Fluvoxamine
Paroxetine
Sertraline

Atypicals

SNRI (Serotonin Norepinephrine Reuptake Inhibitor)
Duloxetine
Venlafaxine

NDRI (Norepinephrine Dopamine Reuptake Inhibitor)
Bupropion

Miscellaneous
Trazodone (serotonin agonist, α-antagonist)
Mirtazepine (SSRI and α_2-blocker)

channels. They are considered first-line treatment for depression and many behavioral disorders. However, concern exists about the increase in suicidal ideation in the adolescent population taking SSRIs. This effect is thought to be because of the activating properties of SSRIs, which manifest before antidepressant effects are seen. Recent studies have suggested, however, that actual suicide completion rates are lowered by SSRI treatment, which leaves this controversy still unanswered.[6]

In overdose, SSRIs can present with a nebulous constellation of symptoms which are because of serotonergic excess.[7] These symptoms involve the GI (nausea/vomiting), cardiovascular (sinus tachycardia), and CNS (dizziness, blurry vision, MS changes) systems. Treatment is largely supportive. An EKG should be obtained to screen for coingestants such as TCAs, but also because citalopram and escitalopram have been associated with QRS and QTc changes. The mechanism is similar to TCAs and atypical antipsychotics, respectively.[8] They should be managed in the same way as those agents.

The most severe consequence of SSRI overdose is a state of extreme serotonin excess which as been termed the serotonin syndrome. This syndrome is manifested by hyperactivity of multiple physiologic systems, and includes mental status changes, hyperreflexia, tremor, rigidity, and hyperthermia. In combination, these clinical problems can lead to profound multiorgan failure. This includes rhabdomyolysis, renal hepatic failure, and possibly hyperthermia-induced cellular dysfunction.[9]

Treatment of serotonin syndrome involves reducing the tremors and hyperthermia through the use of benzodiazepines and aggressive external cooling. There are data that suggests a role for cyproheptadine, a serotonin antagonist, in the setting of serotonin syndrome in adults. However, its benefit beyond supportive care is unproven. The adult dose is 4 to 8 mg orally.

▶ **ATYPICAL ANTIDEPRESSANTS**

The atypical antidepressants are derived from SSRIs. Consequently, they all act on serotonin receptors as well as other CNS receptors.

Venlafaxine and duloxetine are classified as serotonin-norepinephrine reuptake inhibitors (SNRIs), and can present with nonspecific symptoms including tachycardia, vomiting, dizziness, stupor, or seizures. Rarely, a quinidinelike effect can occur similar to that caused by TCAs; it is treated with sodium bicarbonate.

Buproprion, a norepinephrine-dopamine reuptake inhibitor (NDRI), is a unicyclic compound. In overdose symptoms include tachycardia, hypertension, vomiting/diarrhea, agitation, and CNS depression. It can lower the seizure threshold, and seizures should be treated initially with benzodiazepines. In addition, widened-QRS tachycardia can occur, and should be treated with sodium bicarbonate. In one case series involving children, most buproprion overdoses were noted to be accidental.[10] Children should be observed for 24 hours for the development of seizures or other signs of toxicity, particularly after the ingestion of sustained-release preparations.

Trazodone is a serotonin agonist as well as an α-antagonist. Overdoses tend to result in CNS depression (serotonin) and orthostatic hypotension (α-antagonism). Priapism has been reported rarely as a side effect.

Mirtazapine acts as an SSRI as well as an α_2-blocker which increases norepinephrine and serotonin levels in the synaptic cleft. It interferes with negative feedback on presynaptic dopaminergic and adrenergic neurons, and overdoses manifest with tachycardia and mental status changes.

REFERENCES

1. Cherry DK, et al. National Ambulatory Medical Care Survey: 2005 Summary. US Dept. of Health and Human Services, National Center for Health Statistics. http://www.cdc.gov/nchs/data/ad/ad387.pdf. Accessed May 10, 2008.
2. Lai MW, et al. 2005 Annual Report of the American Association of Poison Control Centers' National Poisoning and Exposure Database. *Clin Toxicol (Phila)*. 2006;44(6–7):803–932.
3. Adams BK, et al. Prolonged gastric emptying half-time and gastric hypomotility after drug overdose. *Am J Emerg Med*. 2004;22(7):548–554.
4. Boehnert MT, Lovejoy FH. Value of QRS duration versus the serum drug level in predicting seizures and ventricular arrhythmias after an acute overdose of tricyclic antidepressants. *N Engl J Med*. 1985;313(8):474–479.
5. Finley PR. Selective serotonin reuptake inhibitors: pharmacologic profiles and potential therapeutic distinctions. *Ann Pharmacother*. 1994;28:1359–1369.
6. Gibbons RD, et al. The relationship between antidepressant prescription rates and rate of early adolescent suicide. *Am J Psychiatry*. 2006;163:1898–1904.
7. Borys DJ, et al. Acute fluoxetine overdose: report of 234 cases. *Am J Emerg Med*. 1992;10:115–120.
8. Catalano G, et al. QTc interval prolongation associated with citalopram overdose: a case report and literature review. *Clin Neuropharmacol*. 2001;24(3):158–162.
9. Sternbach H. The serotonin syndrome. *Am J Psychiatry*. 1991; 148:705–713.
10. Balit CR, et al. Bupropion poisoning: a case series. *Med J Aust*. 2003;178(2):61–63.

CHAPTER 118

Neuroleptics

Timothy B. Erickson

▶ HIGH-YIELD FACTS

- Depending on chemical class, neuroleptics cause varying degrees of CNS depression, anticholinergic symptoms, cardiac toxicity, and movement abnormalities.
- Movement disturbances, known as extrapyramidal symptoms (EPS), include acute dystonic reactions, Parkinson dyskinesias, akathisia, and tardive dyskinesia. Many EPS reactions respond to administration of an anticholinergic agent such as diphenhydramine or benztropine mesylate.
- Cardiac conduction disturbances, most notably a prolonged QT interval, are significant complications associated with thioridazine and haloperidol.
- Neuroleptic malignant syndrome (NMS) is a life-threatening condition associated with chronic medication therapy and acute drug overdose characterized by hyperthermia, skeletal muscle rigidity, and altered mental status.
- Newer "atypical neuroleptics" offer therapeutic advantages of lowered incidences of EPS and NMS. Toxicity from these agents may include blood dyscrasias, CNS and respiratory depression, hypotension, and reflex tachycardia.

Neuroleptics or phenothiazines are a group of major tranquilizers or antipsychotic drugs that are designed to treat schizophrenia and other psychiatric disorders.

▶ PHARMACOLOGY

There are several classes of typical neuroleptics (Table 118–1),[1] all of which have the same basic three-ringed structure. Although all classes exhibit similar therapeutic and adverse effects, modification of the basic structure results in variable degrees of toxicity.[2] Neuroleptics include broadly diverse chemical classes. These entities differ in the degree to which they cause anticholinergic, cardiovascular, or EPS reactions.

▶ PATHOPHYSIOLOGY

Neuroleptics act by blocking dopaminergic, α-adrenergic, muscarinic, histaminic, and serotonergic neuroreceptors. Blockade of the dopamine receptors results in the desired behavior modification, but also produces extrapyramidal side effects, such as dystonic reactions. α-adrenergic blockade produces peripheral vasodilation and orthostatic hypotension. Muscarinic blockade results in anticholinergic properties such as sedation, tachycardia, flushed or dry skin, urinary retention, and delayed GI

motility. Neuroleptics also cause a membrane-depressant action or quinidinelike effect that alters myocardial contractility, and can result in conduction defects. Although the mechanism of toxicity in neuroleptics resembles that of tricyclic antidepressants, serious cardiac dysrhythmias, refractory hypotension, respiratory depression, and seizures are uncommon.[3]

▶ DYSTONIC REACTIONS

CLINICAL PRESENTATION

Acute dystonia is an unpredictable side effect of neuroleptics that occurs in approximately 10% of overdoses. It can also occur as an idiosyncratic reaction following a single therapeutic dose of a neuroleptic. Dystonic reactions are characterized by slurred speech, dysarthria, confusion, dysphagia, hypertonicity, tremors, and muscle restlessness. Other reactions or dyskinesias include oculogyric crisis (upward gaze), torticollis (neck twisting), facial grimacing, opisthotonos, and tortipelvic gait disturbances. Symptoms usually begin within the first 5 to 30 hours after ingestion. Dystonic reactions are relatively common in infants and adolescents.

Of the neuroleptics, prochlorperazine most often causes acute dystonia. In recent years, several new neuroleptic agents have become very popular, including clozapine, olanzapine, risperidone, quetiapine, ziprasidone, aripiprazole, and paliperidone (Table 118–2). This group of agents produces a lower incidence of extrapyramidal side effects than previous agents.

MANAGEMENT

If a child exhibits signs of acute muscular dystonia, intravenous or intramuscular diphenhydramine is rapidly administered. Alternatively, the patient can be given benztropine intramuscularly. Improvement usually occurs within 15 minutes.[4,5] Doses exceeding 8 mg over a 24-hour period can result in severe anticholinergic symptoms.

▶ ACUTE OVERDOSE

CLINICAL PRESENTATION

Following an acute overdose of neuroleptics, mild CNS depression is common, usually occurring within 1 to 2 hours of the ingestion. Children are more susceptible to sedative effects

▶ **TABLE 118–1. COMMON TYPICAL NEUROLEPTICS**

Chemical Class	Generic Name	Proprietary Name
Phenothiazines		
Aliphatics	Chlorpromazine	Thorazine
	Promethazine	Phenergan
	Acepromazine (veterinary)	Aceprotabs
Piperazines	Prochlorperazine	Compazine
	Trifluoperazine	Stelazine
	Fluphenazine	Prolixin
	Perphenazine	Trilafon
Piperidines	Mesoridazine	Serentil
	Thioridazine	Mellaril
Butyrophenones	Droperidol	Inapsine
	Haloperidol	Haldol
Thioxanthenes	Thiothixene	Navane
Indoles	Molindone	Mobane
Dibenzoxazepines	Loxapine	Loxitane
Diphenylbutylpiperidines	Pimozide	Orap

than adults. In the overdose setting, respiratory depression can occur, but rarely requires aggressive airway management. Phenothiazines tend to lower a patient's seizure threshold, although the actual incidence of seizures in acute overdose is low.

Like the tricyclic antidepressants, poisoning from neuroleptics can result in orthostatic hypotension and cardiac dysrhythmias, particularly with the piperidine and aliphatic phenothiazines. Sinus tachycardia is the most common dys-

rhythmia, but QT interval prolongation can sometimes be noted on electrocardiogram. Other clinical effects in the acute overdose setting include pupillary miosis, which in one study was observed in 72% of children with high-grade coma following ingestion of a phenothiazine. Because of the anticholinergic properties of the neuroleptics, the patient may also exhibit decreased GI motility, urinary retention, hyperthermia, and dry or flushed skin. Mydriasis may occur; however, miosis is common because of α-adrenergic blockade.

Hypothermia can be noted but is rarely clinically significant. Therapeutic phenothiazine use has been associated with sleep apnea and sudden death in infants.

LABORATORY TESTS

Although serum phenothiazine levels can be obtained to confirm ingestion, levels correlate poorly with clinical effects, making their utility negligible. Baseline laboratory tests include complete blood count, electrolytes, renal function, and glucose. Urine should be collected for myoglobin, particularly if the patient is hyperthermic.

The urine can be qualitatively tested with a 10% ferric chloride solution. Ten to fifteen drops of ferric chloride will change the urine to a deep burgundy color if phenothiazines are present. Because of potential neuroleptic-induced cardiotoxicity, an electrocardiogram is indicated.[6,7]

MANAGEMENT

Initial management of an acute neuroleptic overdose includes stabilizing the airway and circulation. If the patient remains

▶ **TABLE 118–2. ATYPICAL NEUROLEPTIC AGENTS**

Chemical Class	Generic Name	Proprietary Name
Unclassified	Aripiprazole	Abilify
Dibenzodiazepines	Clozapine	Clozaril
	Olanzapine	Zyprexa
Dibenzothiazepines	Quetiapine	Seroquel
Benzisoxazoles	Risperidone	Risperdal
Benzisothiazoyl	Ziprasidone	Geodone
Unclassified	Paliperidone	Invega

Atypical Neuroleptics	
Aripiprazole	During clinical trials, one case of an 18-mo-old child ingesting 15 mg of aripiprazole and 2 mg of Ativan was reported to be "uneventful."
Clozapine	Case reports of as little as 50 mg in children, ranging in age from 21 mo to 4 y, have resulted in CNS depression, ataxia, and tachycardia. Death was reported in a 15-y-old following an intentional overdose of an unknown amount of clozapine.
Olanzapine	Case reports of 10–100 mg ingestions in children have resulted in agitation, CNS depression, EPS, and hypersalivation. A 15-y-old required intubation following ingestion of 115 mg of olanzapine along with carbamazepine. In one report, onset of symptoms did not occur until 10 h postingestion.
Quetiapine	A single case report of a 1300 mg ingestion in an 11-y-old resulted only in mental status changes.
Risperidone	Several published series and case reports of pediatric risperidone ingestions, in doses ranging from 1 to 110 mg, revealed somnolence, agitation, hypotension, tachycardia, and EPS to be the most common symptoms of overdose.
Ziprasidone	During premarketing trials, there were 10 accidental or intentional poisonings, with the highest dose reported as 3240 mg. That patient only experienced mild sedation, slurred speech, and transient hypertension.

hypotensive despite adequate amounts of IV fluid, a vaso-pressor with α-agonist activity, such as norepinephrine, may be considered. Vasopressors with both α- and β-agonist activity, such as dopamine, may actually exacerbate hypotension because of unopposed β-adrenergic stimulation, during which α-receptors are being blocked by the neuroleptic. Because of the potential cardiotoxicity of phenothiazines, patients require close monitoring. α_1-Receptor blockade, along with direct myocardial depression, may cause significant hypotension following overdose. Patients may also have orthostatic hypotension because of α-receptor antagonism while receiving therapy at standard doses. Sinus tachycardia is the most common dysrhythmia associated with neuroleptic toxicity, however, supraventricular and ventricular tachydysrhythmias can occur. Many agents, most notably the piperidine phenothiazines and the butyrophenones, have quinidinelike effects on the myocardium.[1,6,7]

Since phenathiazine toxicity classically demonstrates CNS depression and pupillary miosis, naloxone can be administered to treat potential coexistent opioid toxicity. Activated charcoal may be administered following a recent ingestion. No specific antidote exists for acute neuroleptic poisoning, and hemodialysis is not efficacious. Most children presenting after acute neuroleptic toxicity do well with supportive care alone.

▶ NEUROLEPTIC MALIGNANT SYNDROME

CLINICAL PRESENTATION

Less than 1% of patients exhibit the life-threatening extrapyramidal dysfunction known as the NMS, characterized by skeletal muscle rigidity, coma, and severe hyperthermia following the use of phenothiazines or haloperidol. This syndrome can occur following acute overdose, during chronic therapy, or idiosyncratically following a single dose of a neuroleptic. Patients with NMS will present with a constellation of clinical manifestations, including features from each of the following symptom groups[8]:

- Temperature dysregulation: fever, which may be life-threatening.
- Altered mental status: agitation, confusion, and delirium, which may be insidious in onset, and ultimately leading to lethargy, obtundation, and coma.
- Autonomic instability: fluctuating vital signs, including tachycardia and hypotension or hypertension.
- Musculoskeletal: generalized "lead pipe" rigidity, myoclonus, and tremors.
- Others: diaphoresis, dehydration, tachypnea, respiratory failure, rhabdomyolysis, and renal failure.

MANAGEMENT

The neuroleptic syndrome has a high mortality rate and is treated aggressively with rapid cooling and administration of dantrolene, at 0.8 to 3.0 mg/kg intravenously every 6 hours, up to 10 mg/kg/d. Dantrolene acts peripherally by treating skeletal muscle rigidity.

Oral bromocriptine, a direct-dopamine agonist, has been successfully used alone and in conjunction with dantrolene to successfully treat adult patients with NMS.[9,10]

DISPOSITION

Any symptomatic child presenting with acute neuroleptic poisoning is admitted and observed for CNS and respiratory depression, as well as for cardiotoxicity or thermoregulatory problems. Patients with minor, asymptomatic ingestions can be observed for up to 6 hours. If the patient is discharged, care takers are advised to watch for signs of delayed dystonic reactions. If the child has been treated successfully for acute dystonia with either diphenhydramine or benztropine, a 2- to 3-day course of oral diphenhydramine is indicated, since many of the neuroleptics have a long duration of action.

▶ ATYPICAL ANTIPSYCHOTICS

The existing pharmacovigilance data reports indicate these medications are relatively safe when taken in overdose, particularly when coingestants are not involved.[11] They generally have a safer therapeutic and overdose profile than first-generation antipsychotic medications, but many adverse and toxic effects still need to be considered in therapeutic monitoring and overdose management[1,12] (Table 118–2). Toxicologic exposures and fatalities associated with atypical antipsychotics continue to increase in the United Sates and the toxicologic potential of these agents in children may be underestimated.[13]

CLOZAPINE

Clozapine can cause salivation, CNS depression, agitation, seizures, and rarely cardiac disturbances. It is known for its potential to precipitate clinically significant agranulocytosis during chronic therapy and following acute overdose.[11,14]

OLANZAPINE

In an overdose setting, olanzapine can cause CNS depression, which may be prolonged, miosis, QT interval prolongation, and ketosis.[15]

QUETIAPINE

Quetiapine toxicity results in agitation, combativeness, depressed sensorium, hypotension, and tachycardia. QT interval prolongation has been reported in large overdoses.[16,17]

RESPERIDONE

Transient lethargy, hypotension, and tachycardia have been reported in adolescents in the setting of overdose.[18]

ZIPRASIDONE

Overdose of ziprasidone may cause sedation and QT interval prolongation. Serious neurologic or cardiovascular complications are uncommon, but morbidity and mortality has been reported with mixed ingestions.[19]

ARIPIPRAZOLE

Overdose in children may cause several hours of sedation in children, drooling, flaccid facial muscles, mild hypotension, ataxia, tremor, and vomiting. Toxicity is generally not associated with QT interval prolongation, dysrhythmias, or seizures.[20]

PALIPERIDONE

This new atypical antipsychotic was FDA approved in 2007. It increases prolactin levels and is available in extended-release forms. Side effects include restlessness, movement disorders, tachycardia, and insomnia.[12]

REFERENCES

1. Burda A, Lipscomb J. Neuroleptics. In: Erickson T, Ahrens W, Aks S, et al., eds. *Pediatric Toxicology: the Diagnosis and Management of the Poisoned Child.* 1st ed. New York, NY: McGraw Hill; 2005.
2. Deroos FJ. Neuroleptics. In: Ford M, Delaney K, Ling L, Erickson T. eds. *Clinical Toxicology.* Philadelphia, PA: Saunders; 2001:539–545.
3. Raggi MA. Atypical antipsychotics: pharmacokinetics, therapeutic drug monitoring pharmacological interactions. *Curr Med Chem.* 2004;11(3):279–296.
4. Raja M. Managing antipsychotic induced acute and tardive dystonia. *Drug Saf.* 1998;19:57–72.
5. Van Harten PN, Hoek H, Kahn RS. Acute dystonia induced by drug treatment. *BMJ.* 1999;319:623–626.
6. Kao LW. Drug-induced QT prolongation. *Med Clin North Am.* 2005;89(6):1125.
7. Buckley NA. Cardiovascular effects of antipsychotics used in bipolar illness. *J Clin Psychiatry.* 2002;63(4):20–23.
8. Rusyniak DE. Toxin-induced hyperthermic syndrome. *Med Clin North Am.* 2005;89(6):1277–1296.
9. Buckley P, Hutchinson M. Neuroleptic malignant syndrome. *J Neurol Neurosurg Psychiatry.* 1995;58:271–273.
10. Kwol JS, Chan TK. Recurrent heat-related illnesses during antipsychotic treatment. *Ann Pharmacother.* 2005;39(11):1940–1942.
11. Antia S, Sholevar E, Baron D. Overdoses and ingestions of second generation antipsychotics in children and adolescents. *J Child Adolesc Psychopharmacol.* 2005;15(6):970–985.
12. Reilly T, Kirk M. Atypical antipsychotics and newer antidepressants. *Emerg Clin North Am.* 2007;25:477–497.
13. Dubois D. Toxicology and overdose of atypical antipsychotic medications in children: does newer necessarily mean safer? *Curr Opin Pediatr.* 2005;17(2):227–233.
14. Borzutzky A, Avello E, Rumie H, et al. Accidental clozapine intoxication in a ten year old child. *Vet Hum Toxicol.* 2003;45(6):309–310.
15. Torry EF, Swalwell CI. Fatal olazepine–induced ketoacidosis. *Am J Psychiarty.* 2003;160(12):224.
16. Juhl G, Benitez J, McFarland S. Acute quetiapine overdose in an eleven year old girl. *Vet Hum Toxicol.* 2002;44(3):163–164.
17. Catalano G, Catalano M, Nunez C, et al. Atypical antipsychotic overdose in the pediatric population. *J Child Adolesc Psychopharmacol.* 2001;11(4):425–434.
18. Catalano G, Catalano M, Augstines R, et al. Pediatric quetiapine overdose: a case report and literature review. *J Child Adolesc Psychopharmacol.* 2002;12(4):355–361.
19. Burton S. Ziprasidone overdose. *Am J Psychiatry.* 2000;157:835.
20. Lofton A, Klein-Schwartz W. Atypical experience: a case series of pediatric aripiprazole exposures. *Clin Toxicol (Phila).* 2005;43(3):151–153.

CHAPTER 119

Isoniazid Toxicity

Jenny J. Lu and Theodore Toerne

▶ HIGH-YIELD FACTS

- Isoniazid toxicity (INH) should be considered in any patient with metabolic acidosis and seizures refractory to conventional therapy.
- Altered sensorium, slurred speech, ataxia, coma, and seizures can occur rapidly after ingestion of INH ingestion.
- INH has a half-life of approximately 180 minutes in slow acetylators and 70 minutes in fast acetylators.
- INH toxicity is associated with a profound metabolic acidosis and increased lactate levels.
- The antidote for INH overdose is pyridoxine (B_6), given in a gram-for-gram dose to the amount of INH ingested. With ingestions involving unknown quantities, 70 mg/kg (up to a total of 5 gram) of pyridoxine should be given IV and repeated if seizures continue.

For the last several decades, INH has been used as a first-line treatment against active tuberculosis (TB) and as prophylactic therapy for positive tuberculin skin test reactions. Globally, the burden of TB continues to be enormous. The World Health Organization reported an estimated 9.2 million new cases of TB in 2006, an increase from 9.1 million cases in 2005.[1] Within the United States, the 2005 Annual Report of the Poison Control Centers Toxic Exposure Surveillance System reported 354 INH exposures, of which 76 were in children younger than 6 years, and 127 cases in children between the ages of 6 and 19 years.[2] A high index of suspicion of INH toxicity by the health care provider, coupled with prompt, aggressive treatment, is needed to prevent morbidity and mortality in the overdose scenario.

▶ PHARMACOLOGY

Isoniazid, or isonicotinic acid hydrazide, is an antimycobacterial agent whose mechanism of action is thought to be the disruption of mycolic acid synthesis, which is essential to the mycobacterial cell wall. The pyridine ring is a critical component of its antituberculous activity. Structurally, INH is similar to the metabolic cofactors nicotinic acid (niacin), nicotinamide-adenosine dinucleotide (NAD), and pyridoxine (vitamin B6). Ninety percent of ingested INH is readily absorbed from the gastrointestinal tract, with serum concentrations usually peaking within 2 hours. Peak cerebrospinal fluid levels reach approximately 10% of serum levels. INH is highly water-soluble, with an apparent volume of distribution of 0.6 L/kg. It exhibits less than 10% protein binding.[3]

Metabolic degradation of INH is complex and occurs primarily by hepatic acetylation. The ability to inactivate INH by acetylation via the enzyme N-acetyltransferase is genetically determined in an autosomal dominant fashion. Slow acetylators are autosomal recessive for the acetylation gene. Fifty to sixty percent of Caucasians and blacks are slow acetylators, while up to 90% of Asians and Inuits are rapid inactivators.[3,4] The effectiveness of the drug is not significantly affected by the rate of acetylation, although slow acetylation can lead to higher peak plasma concentrations, potentially increasing the risk for toxic side effects. The elimination half-life in fast acetylators is approximately 70 minutes, compared to 180 minutes in slow acetylators.[3,4] Following acetylation, the INH metabolites are excreted into the urine, with 50% to 95% of a single dose eliminated within 24 hours.[3,4]

INH can inhibit several cytochrome P450-mediated functions, such as demethylation, oxidation, and hydroxylation. INH has been associated with interactions with several drugs, including theophylline, phenytoin, warfarin, valproate, and carbamazepine.[3,5] For example, phenytoin intoxication can occur because of INH inhibition of phenytoin metabolism.[6] It is also believed that INH use may potentially increase risk of acetaminophen-induced hepatotoxicity.[3]

▶ PATHOPHYSIOLOGY

The process by which INH toxicity occurs is complex but includes two main mechanisms which have the overall effect of depleting gamma-aminobutyric acid (GABA), the primary inhibitory neurotransmitter in the CNS. First, INH creates a functional deficiency of pyridoxine by inhibiting pyridoxine phosphokinase, which converts pyridoxine to its active form, pyridoxal-5′-phosphate. Pyridoxal-5′-phosphate is a necessary cofactor in the conversion of glutamic acid to GABA. INH itself also combines with pyridoxine-5′-phosphate, forming inactive INH pyridoxal hydrazones, which are renally excreted.[3,4,6]

Second, INH inhibits the enzyme glutamic acid decarboxylase which, along with pyridoxine-5′-phosphate, is also required for the synthesis of GABA. Depletion of GABA leading to increased CNS excitability is believed to be the etiology of INH-induced seizures (Fig. 119–1).[3,4,6]

The metabolic acidosis associated with INH toxicity appears to be caused by increased serum lactate levels, secondary to intense seizure-induced muscle activity. Clearance of lactate may be slower than in non-INH-induced seizures, as a result of a blockade in the conversion of lactate to pyruvate. Other theories for the INH-associated lactic acidosis include generation

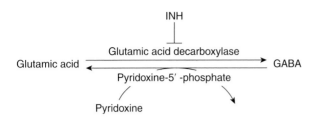

Figure 119–1. Mechanisms of INH toxicity.

of acidic INH metabolites and increased serum ketoacids from increased fatty acid oxidation.[3]

The toxic dose of INH is highly variable. The normal pediatric therapeutic dose is 10 to 20 mg/kg/d, up to 300 mg/d. Acute ingestion of as little as 1.5 gram of INH can lead to neurotoxicity, 6 to 10 gram may be fatal, and more than 10 grams is usually fatal without medical intervention.[4] Doses larger than 30 mg/kg often produce seizures. Ingestion of more than 80 to 150 mg/kg can lead rapidly to death.[7] Patients with underlying seizure disorders may develop seizures with ingestions of lower doses.

► DIAGNOSIS

CLINICAL PRESENTATION OF ACUTE TOXICITY

Because of rapid gastrointestinal absorption, symptoms of INH toxicity typically occur within 30 minutes to 1 hour postingestion. Initial symptoms and signs include nausea, vomiting, fever, dizziness, ataxia, altered sensorium, and slurred speech. Toxicity can quickly progress to the triad of refractory seizures, metabolic acidosis, and coma. Seizures are often the presenting sign and can persist until GABA stores are replenished. Hyperthermia, hypotension, hyperglycemia, ketonemia, and ketonuria have also been observed in overdose. INH toxicity may initially be confused with diabetic ketoacidosis.[4] The duration of coma can be protracted, lasting as long as 24 to 36 hours after the termination of seizures and resolution of acidemia. The diagnosis of a toxic INH ingestion in the convulsing pediatric patient is frequently missed and the antidotal treatment delayed. A high index of suspicion for INH toxicity is necessary in the evaluation of any child or adolescent who presents with acute-onset seizures, especially when the seizures are refractory to conventional therapy.

In the acute ingestion, quantitative INH levels are typically unavailable. Levels may be helpful in confirming the diagnosis, but treatment of toxicity should never be withheld while awaiting results. A serum level of 10 mg/ml, a level greater than 3.2 mg/ml 2 hours after ingestion, or a level greater than 0.2 mg/ml after 6 hours are considered toxic.[4,6] Other causes of altered mental status, seizures, or anion gap acidosis should be considered as part of the patient's complete evaluation.

► TREATMENT

STABILIZATION

Airway control, stabilization of breathing and circulation, and seizure management in an environment of attentive supportive care are the priorities in caring for the symptomatic patient with INH toxicity.

DECONTAMINATION

Even in patients who appear to be asymptomatic initially, orogastric lavage is contraindicated because of the potential risk for seizures and consequent complications in an unprotected airway. Activated charcoal could be considered if the patient presents *within minutes* after an ingestion, although the risk of seizures and aspiration exists. Endotracheal intubation should never be performed for the sole purpose of administering activated charcoal. There is no role for whole bowel irrigation.

ANTIDOTAL THERAPY

Correction of GABA deficiency through the administration of Pyridoxine (B_6) is the cornerstone of treatment in INH toxicity. Commercially available in 1 g/10 mL vials, pyridoxine is mixed in a 5% or 10% solution with D_5 W. If the INH dose is known, the amount of pyridoxine administered should equal the amount of INH ingested on a gram-for-gram basis, administered over 5 to 10 minutes. If the dose of INH ingested is unknown, pyridoxine is given initially at 70 mg/kg up to a total of 5 gram, and repeated at 5 to 10 minute intervals until the seizures are controlled. If the parenteral form of pyridoxine is unavailable or in inadequate supply, similar doses of crushed pyridoxine tablets may be given orally or as a slurry through a nasogastric tube.[6] A minimum of 10 gram of pyridoxine, the upper limit necessary to treat an ingestion of a therapeutic 1-month supply of INH, should be stocked and readily available. The severe acidosis seen in INH overdose may require sodium bicarbonate administration, but in most cases control of seizures with pyridoxine, benzodiazepines, and adequate fluid resuscitation will improve acidemia. Bicarbonate therapy is reserved for severe, persistent acidosis (pH < 7.1). Electrolytes, specifically sodium, should be carefully followed in the pediatric patient if bicarbonate therapy is administered.

In general, for toxicant-induced seizures, benzodiazepines such as diazepam and lorazepam are the first line of treatment. Phenytoin is not recommended as a first line anticonvulsant for toxicant-induced seizures, since it appears to be more effective in seizures with an anatomic focus; toxicant-induced seizures are generally global in nature. In INH-induced seizures, because of depletion of GABA, pyridoxine may be the only effective therapy. Short-acting barbiturates or inhaled anesthetics (in consultation with an anesthesiologist) could be considered if the seizures are unresponsive to benzodiazepines or pyridoxine. It should be noted that paralytic agents control only the muscular activity seen with convulsive seizures and that the electrical hyperactivity in the brain may continue despite muscular paralysis. EEG monitoring should be in place if use of paralytics is required.

ENHANCED ELIMINATION

INH is dialyzable, but hemodialysis is usually unnecessary if adequate doses of pyridoxine and benzodiazepines have been given. Hemodialysis, hemoperfusion, and exchange transfusion have all been described in case reports as useful, but are reserved for the most severe, refractory cases, or for patients with renal failure.[8]

DISPOSITION

All patients suspected of ingesting INH require close observation in a setting with capabilities for rapid airway and seizure management. Asymptomatic patients who remain completely symptom-free after 8 hours following an alleged isolated ingestion with INH may be medically cleared in the ED. Symptomatic patients require admission to an intensive care unit. Psychiatric evaluation should be obtained for all intentional ingestions.

▶ CHRONIC TOXICITY

Chronic INH toxicity is uncommon in the normal pediatric population and is usually restricted to children receiving active or prophylactic treatment. The appearance of nausea, vomiting, fever, abdominal pain, or pruritus may herald hepatic insult that, if not treated, can progress to fulminant hepatic failure. Chronic INH use has also been associated with optic neuritis, hepatitis, peripheral neuropathy, a pellagralike syndrome of dermatitis, diarrhea, dementia, and a variety of psychological reactions. During treatment or prophylaxis of TB with INH, serum transaminase levels should be evaluated periodically to screen for early signs of hepatotoxicity.

REFERENCES

1. Global Tuberculosis Control: surveillance, planning, financing: WHO report 2008, c. World Health Organization. Geneva, Switzerland: WHO press; 2008. http://www.who.int/tb/publications/global_report/2008/pdf/fullreport.pdf. Accessed May 15, 2008.
2. Lai, MW, Klein-Schwartz W, Rodgers GC, et al. 2005 Annual Report of the American Association of Poison Control Centers' National Poisoning and Exposure Database. *Clin Toxicol (Phila)*. 2006;44(6–7).
3. Boyer EW. Antituberculous agents. In: Goldfrank LR, Flomenbaum NE, Lewin NA, et al., eds. *Goldfrank's Toxicologic Emergencies*. 8th ed. Stamford, CT: Appleton & Lange; 2006:1308–1324.
4. Maw G, Aitken P. Isoniazid overdose: a case series, literature review and survey of antidote availability. *Clin Drug Investig*. 2003;23(7):479–485.
5. Preziosi P. Isoniazid: metabolic aspects and toxicological correlates. *Curr Drug Metab*. 2007;8(8):839–851.
6. Shah BR, Santucci K, Sinert R, et al. Acute isoniazid neurotoxicity in an urban hospital. *Pediatrics*. 1995;95:700–704.
7. Romero JA, Kuczler FJ. Isoniazid overdose. Recognition and management. *Am Fam Physician*. 1998;57:749–752.
8. Cash JM, Zawada ET Jr. Isoniazid overdose—successful treatment with pyridoxine and hemodialysis. *West J Med*. 1991;155:644–646.
9. Parish RA, Brownstein D. Emergency department management of children with acute isoniazid poisoning. *Pediatr Emerg Care*. 1986;2:88–90.
10. Caksen, H, Odabas D, Mehmet E, et al. Do not overlook acute isoniazid poisoning in children with status epilepticus. *J Child Neurol*. 2003;18;142.

SUGGESTED READING

Orlowski JP, Paganini EP, Pippenger CE. Treatment of a potentially lethal dose isonizid ingestion. *Ann Emerg Med*. 1988;17:73–76.

Sullivan EA, Geoffrey P, Weisman R, et al. Isoniazid poisonings in New York City. *J Emerg Med*. 1998;16:57–59.

CHAPTER 120

Carbon Monoxide Poisoning

Sean M. Bryant

▶ HIGH-YIELD FACTS

- Carbon monoxide (CO) poisoning is commonly due to smoke inhalation, but also results from exposure to malfunctioning of or improperly vented heating and cooking appliances, automobile exhaust fumes, and methylene chloride, a component of paint strippers.
- The toxic effects of CO poisoning result from tissue hypoxia and reperfusion injury in the brain.
- Clinical signs and symptoms of CO poisoning are notoriously nonspecific and correlate only roughly with the COHb concentration.
- Any illness affecting more than one member of a family or group from a common environment requires that CO poisoning be ruled out.
- The half-life of COHb is decreased to 90 minutes with an F_{IO_2} of 100%, and 23 minutes with hyperbaric oxygen (HBO) therapy.

Carbon monoxide (CO) has historically been the most common etiology of poison-related deaths. Three thousand to four thousand cases of CO-related deaths occur yearly in the United States. According to poison center data, in 2006 there were roughly 16 000 reported cases of CO toxicity, with approximately 25% attributed to victims younger than 19 years; there were 1829 cases in children younger than 6 years.[1] Overall, CO was responsible for 46 deaths.[1] While mortality secondary to CO is significant, morbidity from delayed cognitive sequelae is a significant problem, especially in the unintentionally poisoned patient.

▶ PATHOPHYSIOLOGY

Carbon monoxide is an insidious poison because it is colorless, odorless, tasteless, and nonirritating. CO is formed as a byproduct of the incomplete combustion of fossil fuels or materials such as wood or charcoal. Children and family members are commonly exposed to CO from malfunctioning furnaces, generators, or charcoal grills. Motor exhaust from automobiles and houseboats are also sources of significant exposure. Methylene chloride, a hydrocarbon commonly found in paint stripping chemicals, is metabolized to CO by the liver, and can result in delayed CO poisoning after respiratory, dermal, or gastrointestinal exposure.[2]

One effect of CO poisoning is the production of a functional anemia. CO binds to hemoglobin with 240 times the affinity of oxygen, displacing oxygen from its normal binding site. In doing so, the hemoglobin molecule is altered, resulting in increased affinity for any oxygen already bound. The oxyhemoglobin dissociation curve is therefore shifted to the left, resulting in tissue hypoxia.

Carbon monoxide also binds to metalloproteins such as myoglobin and cytochromes C oxidase, and P-450 oxidase. Cytochrome inhibition results in disruption of electron transport and interference with cellular respiration. Myocardial myoglobin can be affected, resulting in reduction of contractility and cardiac output, further reducing tissue oxygen delivery.

Ischemic–reperfusion injury to the brain after CO poisoning is an area of great interest and ongoing research. Interaction with the free radical nitric oxide results in a cascade of events including endothelial injury and leukocyte adherence. Activated lymphocytes may cause the conversion of xanthine dehydrogenase to xanthine oxidase, which promotes the formation of oxygen free radicals. The final common pathway is the development of delayed lipid peroxidation and apoptosis in the brain.[3]

Tissues of the body most sensitive to oxygen deprivation, especially the central nervous system and cardiovascular system, are notoriously susceptible to CO exposure. Because of their increased metabolic rate, children may be more sensitive than adults to the effects of CO. Symptomatology can result in children at lower concentrations of CO than in adults. The developing fetus is particularly vulnerable to CO toxicity, especially while undergoing organogenesis. The fetal oxyhemoglobin dissociation curve lies further to the left than that of the adult, the normal oxygen content of fetal blood is quite low, and the half-life of carboxyhemoglobin (COHb) is prolonged in the fetus. These factors result in an exaggerated hypoxic effect in the fetus exposed to CO.

▶ CLINICAL PRESENTATION

Clinical signs and symptoms of CO poisoning are notoriously nonspecific, and correlate only roughly with the COHb level at the scene of exposure (Table 120–1). It cannot be overemphasized that there is a great degree of overlap between COHb levels and corresponding symptoms noted in the table. For example, a child may be in comatose state or die with an unexpectedly low COHb level simply because of the delay in presentation from time of exposure.

While many poisons cause a characteristic signs and symptoms that are easily detected, CO toxicity is an infamously problematic diagnosis to make. Having a high index of suspicion is of supreme importance. Multiple patients presenting

► TABLE 120–1. CLINICAL MANIFESTATIONS OF CARBON MONOXIDE TOXICITY

COHb Level (%)	Signs and Symptoms
5	None
10	Slight headache or dyspnea with extreme exertion
20	Headache, dyspnea with exertion
30	Severe headache, dizziness, nausea, vomiting, fatigue, irritability
40–50	Confusion, tachypnea, tachycardia, lethargy
50–60	Syncope, seizures, coma
60–70	Coma, hypotension, respiratory failure, death
>70	Rapidly fatal

simultaneously to the emergency department (ED) with vague complaints such as headache, dizziness, and nausea, should arouse the suspicion of CO poisoning. Viral syndrome or influenza are the most common misdiagnoses when CO toxicity is missed.[4] Although CO poisoning is more common during the winter months, it can occur any time of the year. In infants, the only suggestion of toxicity may be irritability or difficulty feeding. Other situations in which CO poisoning should be considered include unexplained alteration of mental status, nonspecific neurologic abnormalities, and metabolic acidosis. Children, by and large, have symptoms similar to those of adult patients. However, because of higher minute ventilation, they can become symptomatic sooner. Acute gastroenteritis is a common misdiagnosis in children with CO toxicity. Delayed neurologic sequelae and hydrocephalus have been noted in children poisoned by CO.[5,6]

The physical examination is often unrevealing, and vital sign abnormalities are nonspecific. An abnormal mental status or comatose state signifies significant exposure. The cherry red skin regularly associated with CO poisoning is usually only appreciated in the morgue, and bullous lesions have been rarely noted. Retinal hemorrhages are suggestive of CO poisoning but are infrequently present. Cardiac toxicity most commonly manifests as tachydysrhythmias, but in older patients CO may precipitate angina or an acute myocardial infarction. Pulmonary edema, rhabdomyolysis, and renal failure occur rarely.

► LABORATORY STUDIES

Either arterial or venous measurement of COHb via co-oximetry helps confirm exposure to CO. This laboratory value quantifies the percentage of CO bound to hemoglobin. While providing an excellent marker of exposure, it must be interpreted with great caution, as it may not correlate with degree of clinical toxicity. The severity of poisoning is better related to factors such as concentrations of CO at the scene of exposure, the duration of exposure, and the activity level of the patient when exposed. Some patients can be quite ill despite low COHb levels simply because there is delay in obtaining a COHb after exposure. Normal levels generally are less than

5%, resulting from the endogenous production of CO that occurs during heme metabolism. Heavy smokers may have levels up to 10%.

Other diagnostic tests may be indicated. Arterial or venous blood gas analysis provides information concerning acid–base status. Since CO does not affect the P_{O_2}, it will be normal, but measured oxygen saturation will be decreased. Oxygen saturation via a pulse oximeter is problematic as it records falsely normal values in CO poisoning. In severe cases of CO poisoning, the electrolytes can reveal an anion gap metabolic acidosis. In victims of structural fires, elevated serum lactate indicates serious CO poisoning or concomitant cyanide toxicity. Hemoglobin values may be useful to assess premorbid oxygen-carrying capacity. Urinary myoglobin and creatinine phosphokinase values are indicated for patients with prolonged unconsciousness, or those who are otherwise at risk for rhabdomyolysis.

An electrocardiogram and cardiac enzymes are useful to detect ischemia in adults, but their value in children is unknown. No specific changes are noted on chest radiographs in CO poisoning. Computed tomography and/or magnetic resonance imaging of the brain can reveal characteristic low-density changes in the globus pallidus and subcortical white matter in cases of CO poisoning.

► TREATMENT

Just as with any poisoned patient, general treatment always begins with aggressive supportive care. Addressing concomitant injuries or illnesses such as burns, smoke inhalation, seizures, or trauma is important. Airway management and intubation follow standard indications.

High-flow supplemental oxygen is the cornerstone of treatment in the CO-poisoned patient (Fig. 120–1). Since short-term administration of high concentrations of oxygen is nearly risk-free, it is indicated as soon as the diagnosis of CO poisoning is entertained. While the half-life of COHb ranges from 4 to 6 hours while breathing room air, it is decreased to 90 minutes with the administration of 100% oxygen via a tight fitting, non-rebreather face mask or via a ventilator in intubated patients. Normobaric supplemental oxygen is sufficient in the majority of cases. The endpoint of this focused therapy is when the COHb level falls below 5%, and there are no clinical manifestations of toxicity. Therapy for pregnant women treated with normobaric oxygen should be five times longer than usual because of the more avid binding and prolonged elimination of CO by fetal hemoglobin.

In more significantly poisoned patients or those at high risk for central nervous system toxicity, hyperbaric oxygen (HBO) therapy may be indicated. HBO reduces the half-life of COHb to an average of 23 minutes, and increases the amount of oxygen dissolved in the plasma by 2 vol% for every atmosphere. HBO at 3 atm increases the concentration of dissolved oxygen to 6 to 7 vol%, an amount sufficient to support the oxygen demands of the body until the oxygen-carrying capacity of hemoglobin is restored. In patients with central nervous system toxicity and cerebral edema, HBO may also lower intracranial pressure. Advocates of HBO for the treatment of CO poisoning cite a reduction in neuronal disruption and apoptosis

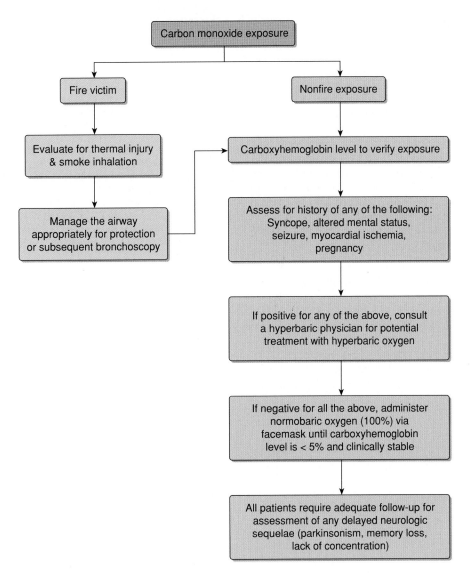

Figure 120–1. Diagnostic and treatment algorithm.

from reperfusion injury.[7,8] Two randomized double-blinded clinical trials report conflicting data pertaining to the ability of HBO to prevent cognitive and delayed neurologic sequelae.[9,10] These studies differed greatly in their methods and, therefore, are impossible to compare with other clinical trials via a meta-analysis. While one study concluded that HBO is not beneficial and should not be utilized, the other study revealed a reduction in the incidence of delayed neurologic complications in patients treated with HBO when compared to those treated with normobaric oxygen.[9,10] Thus, controversy continues to exist among clinicians concerning the use of HBO for CO-poisoned patients. Further research is needed to define which patient population might benefit the most from HBO.

Specific indications for HBO vary among centers with hyperbaric chambers. While the COHb is not a great indicator as to the severity of poisoning, levels greater than 25% often meet a hyperbaric center's indication for treatment. Generally accepted clinical indications include coma or other signs

of neurologic impairment, any period of unconsciousness including syncope, and evidence of myocardial ischemia. HBO therapy is also a consideration for the pregnant patient with any evidence of significant exposure, especially when there is evidence of fetal distress. Aggressive use of HBO should also be considered in neonates and infants, given their greater vulnerability to the effects of CO poisoning and the difficulty in assessing the degree of toxicity. A useful strategy may be to treat young children based on the symptoms of older victims of the same exposure. The risks of HBO are minimal. They include increased pressure in the sinuses and middle ear, and rarely pneumothorax and seizures.

The closest HBO center can be located by contacting the regional poison center (1–800–222–1222). When in doubt as to whether a patient is in need of HBO, it is best to consult with a hyperbaricist to discuss the situation. The risks of transferring an ill patient must be weighed against the potential benefits of HBO.

▶ DISPOSITION

Children who are asymptomatic can be discharged after oxygen therapy has decreased COHb levels to <5%. Effort should be made to locate and eliminate the source of CO. Parents and/or caretakers should be advised of the potential for delayed neuropsychiatric sequelae, including persistent headaches, memory lapses, irritability, and personality changes. Occasionally, gait disturbances or incontinence can occur. Since it is difficult to predict which children will develop sequelae, it may be useful to recommend psychometric testing in any patient with a history of significant toxicity 3 to 4 weeks after exposure. Follow-up for all patients discharged for neurologic reassessment is important.

Patients who require admission to the hospital include children with the following:

- An unsafe environment at home.
- Any history of syncope or abnormal neurologic examination.
- Acidosis or end-organ injury.
- COHb levels greater than 25% (relative indication for admission).
- Requirement for HBO and still symptomatic.
- Pregnant females who were symptomatic after CO exposure, have levels greater than 15%, and require fetal monitoring.

REFERENCES

1. Bronstein AC, Spyker DA, Cantilena LR, et al. 2006 Annual Report of the American Association of Poison Control Centers' National Poison Data System (NPDS). *Clin Toxicol.* 2007;45: 815–917.
2. Rioux JP, Myers RA. Methylene chloride poisoning: a paradigmatic review. *J Emerg Med.* 1988;6:227–238.
3. Thom SR. Carbon monoxide-mediated brain lipid peroxidation in the rat. *J Appl Physiol.* 1990;68:997–1003.
4. Dolan MC, Haltom TL, Barrows GH, et al. Carboxyhemoglobin levels in patients with flu-like symptoms. *Ann Emerg Med.* 1987;16:782–786.
5. Lacey DJ. Neurologic sequelae of acute carbon monoxide intoxication. *Am J Dis Child.* 1981;135:145–147.
6. So GM, Kosofsky BE, Souther JF. Acute hydrocephalus following carbon monoxide poisoning. *Pediatr Neurol.* 1997;17:270–273.
7. Thom SR. Antagonism of CO-mediated brain lipid peroxidation by hyperbaric oxygen. *Toxicol Appl Pharmacol.* 1990;105:340–344.
8. Thom SR. Functional inhibition of leukocyte beta2 integrins by hyperbaric oxygen in carbon monoxide-mediated brain injury in rats. *Toxicol Appl Pharmacol.* 1993;123:248–256.
9. Scheinkestel CD, Bailey M, Myles PS, et al. Hyperbaric or normobaric oxygen for acute carbon monoxide: a randomized controlled clinical trial. *Med J Aust.* 1999;170:203–210.
10. Weaver LK, Hopkins RO, Chan KJ, et al. Hyperbaric oxygen for acute carbon monoxide poisoning. *N Engl J Med.* 2002;347: 1057–1067.

PART 4
DRUGS OF ABUSE

CHAPTER 121

Opioids

Timothy B. Erickson

▶ HIGH-YIELD FACTS

- The classical triad of central nervous system depression, respiratory depression, and pinpoint pupils characterizes opioid toxicity.
- Some opioids, such as methadone and diphenoxylate-atropine (Lomotil), can have delayed or prolonged effects.
- Certain opioids can cause acute lung injury or noncardiogenic pulmonary edema in severe overdoses.
- Toxicity from proxyphene, meperidine, and tramadol, as well as neonatal opioid withdrawal, can result in seizure activity.
- Airway management and the use of the pure opioid antagonist naloxone are the mainstays of opioid toxicity treatment.
- Longer-acting opioid antagonists, such as nalmefene, may be effective in nonopioid-dependent children.

▶ INTRODUCTION

Opioids are naturally occurring or synthetic drugs that have activity similar to that of opium or morphine. The term opiate refers only to those drugs derived from natural opium, which includes morphine, codeine, and thebaine. The term narcotic is derived from the Greek word for stupor, and was originally used to describe any drug that could induce sleep, but became erroneously associated with opioids alone. Some have defined narcotics as those substances that bind opiate receptors, while others refer to any illicit substances as narcotics. The poppy plant *Papaver* somniferum is the source of all opium alkaloids.[1]

Opioids are used clinically for analgesia, anesthesia, as cough suppressants, and to alleviate diarrhea. These drugs are widely available for medical and illicit use in oral, inhalational, parenteral, transdermal, and suppository forms.

▶ AGE AND DEVELOPMENTAL CONSIDERATIONS

Neonates can experience lethargy at birth if there was recent maternal opioid use, or if large doses of an opioid agent were iatrogenically administered to the mother during labor. Additionally, the neonate is prone withdrawal symptoms during the newborn period if the mother exhibited chronic dependency during her later prenatal stages. Toddlers are prone to opioid poisoning if their environment permits exposure, most often from unintentional ingestions. For example, powdered heroin, methadone[2] and codeine tablets, long-acting morphine derivatives, and fentanyl patches[3] may be readily available to the younger child. Methadone is one of the more potentially toxic opioids to toddlers; the incidence of accidental ingestion is on the rise, resulting in serious poisonings with small doses.[4,5] Chronically exposed newborn, withdrawal symptoms are rarely encountered in younger children unless the child is using opioids for chronic pain management.

A survey by the National Institute on Drug Abuse (NIDA) documented an 80% increase in opioid use among high school students over the past decade, heralding a resurgent heroin epidemic in the adolescent population.[6] Adolescents tend to experiment with different routes of exposure, such as inhalational (smoking),[7] intranasal (snorting), ingestion, or intravenous administration.[8] In a suicide attempt, they are potentially exposed to life-threatening doses. In addition, opioids may have synergistic effects with other drug combinations such as ethanol, benzodiazepines, and GHB (γ-hydroxybutyrate), or opposing effects when mixed with sympathomimetic agents like cocaine and amphetamines. Chronically addicted teenagers are also prone to acute withdrawal states, particularly when treated with naloxone.[1]

▶ PHARMACOLOGY/ TOXICOKINETICS

Opium is broken down into alkaloid constituents. These alkaloids are divided into two distinct chemical classes, phenanthrenes and isoquinalines. The principle phenanthrenes are morphine, codeine, and thebaine. The isoquinolines have no significant central nervous system effects and are not federally regulated. Opioids produce clinical effects by interacting with specific receptors located throughout the central and peripheral nervous system and the gastrointestinal tract. Opioid activity resembles the body's three endogenous opioid peptides: enkephalins, endophins, and dynophins. The three main receptors are mu (m), kappa (k), and delta (d).[9] Most analgesia results from supraspinal m_1 receptors. It is the only opioid receptor in the brain and is primarily responsible for the opioid-induced euphoria and sedation. M_2 is responsible for spinal analgesia, respiratory depression, miosis, physical dependence, and decreased gut motility. Kappa$_1$ produces spinal analgesia and miosis (although less pronounced than m_2). Kappa$_2$ results in dysphoria and disorientation. The delta receptor produces spinal analgesia and is the least defined of the three receptors.[10]

The pharmakokinetics for morphine and morphine derivatives in children aged 1 to 15 years are comparable to adults.[11] Most opioids are completely absorbed from the gastrointestinal tract and peak within 60 to 90 minutes, with a duration of effect lasting 3 to 6 hours. Exceptions range from fentanyl, with a duration of effect approximating 1 hour, to methadone, which lasts up to 24 to 48 hours. Many of the other oral agents, such as codeine, sustained release morphine, (e.g., MS-Cotin, Oxycontin), oxycodone,[12] and Lomotil (an antidiarrheal agent containing diphenoxylate and atropine)[13,14] will also demonstrate a delayed effect of up to 4 to 12 hours. Pharmacokinetics are also dependent of the route of exposure. For example, intravenous users experience a peak effect within 1 to 5 minutes, but have a duration of effect of approximately 30 minutes. Fentanyl, a synthetic opioid approximately 80 times more potent than morphine, causes toxicity with extremely small doses.[15] Fentanyl is available in intravenous form, as a transdermal patch, and as fentanyl citrate on a "popsicle" stick. See Table 121–1 for commonly prescribed opioid compounds listed with their generic and trade names.[6]

The development of tolerance is characterized by a shortened duration and a decreased intensity of analgesia, euphoria, and sedation, which creates the need to consume progressively larger doses to attain the desired effect. Tolerance does not develop uniformly for all actions of these drugs, giving rise to a number of toxic effects. Physical dependence refers to physiologic and psychological changes, which necessitate the continued presence of a drug in order to prevent a withdrawal syndrome. The intensity and character of the physical symptoms experienced during withdrawal are directly related to the particular drug of abuse, the total daily dose, the interval between doses, the duration of use, and the underlying health of the user. In general, shorter-acting narcotics tend to produce shorter, more intense withdrawal symptoms, while longer-acting narcotics produce a withdrawal syndrome that is protracted but tends to be less severe. Although unpleasant, withdrawal form narcotics is rarely life-threatening.[1]

▶ PATHOPHYSIOLOGY

Opioid-induced respiratory depression is primarily mediated through the m_2 receptors. When opioid agonists bind to these receptors, the ventilatory drive is reduced by diminishing the sensitivity of the medullary chemoreceptors to hypercapnia. Acute lung injury, classically described with severe opioid

▶ **TABLE 121–1. COMMON OPIOIDS WITH GENERIC AND TRADE NAMES**

Generic	Trade Names
Morphine	MS-Contin, Oramorph SR, MSIR, Roxanol, Kadian, RMS
Hydromorphine	Dilaudid
Codeine	Tylenol #3, #4, Tylenol with codeine
Oxycodone	OxyContin, Oxyl, Percodan (ASA) Percocet (APAP)
Hydrocodone	Anexsia, Hycodan, Hycomine, Lorcet, Lortab, Tussinex, Tylox, Vicodin, Vicoprofen
Meperidine	Demeral, Mepergan, MPPP, MPTP
Methadone	Dolophinel, ORLMM
Buprenophine	Buprenex
Propoxyphene	Darvon
Pentazocine	Talwin, Talwin Nx (with naloxone)
Butorphanol	Stadol, Torbugesic, Torbutol
Fentanyl	Sublimaze (80× more potent than morphine)
Fentanyl patch	Durgesic patch
Fentanyl citrate	Actiq (solid on a stick for oral use)
Sufentanil	Sufenta (1000× more potent than morphine)
Carfentanil	Wildnil (10 000× more potent than MS)

overdose, results from hypoxia secondary to ventilatory compromise, which causes precapillary pulmonary hypertension. This results in increased pulmonary capillary permeability, which causes an extensive fluid leak. This variation of acute lung injury (described in other sources as "noncardiogenic pulmonary edema") may also be due to direct hypersensitivity or alveolar membrane toxicity.[10]

The mechanism by which opioids induce miosis is controversial. Morphine specifically causes stimulation of parasympathetic pupilloconstrictor neurons in the oculomotor nerve. Other opioids mediate inhibitory neurotransmission, causing hyperpolarization of inhibitory neurons to the parasympathetic neurons, causing the classic "pinpoint pupil" associated with opioid use. Constipation is a common side effect of both therapeutic and recreational opioid use. This is mediated by the m_2 receptors within the smooth muscle of the intestinal wall.

Opioid-induced seizure activity[16] is most often secondary to profound hypoxia. However, a proconvulsant effect has also been demonstrated in animal models treated with morphine, which is not inhibited by naloxone, suggesting that the mechanism may be unrelated to opioid receptor binding. Morphin-induced seizures in neonates may also be related to incomplete formation of the newborn blood–brain barrier, resulting in greater central nervous system toxicity. Certain opioids cause cardiotoxicity via conduction system dysfunction. Propoxyphene blocks myocardial sodium channels, with a quinidine-like effect similar to cyclic antidepressants. As a result, propoxyphene is consistently listed among the leading causes of drug overdose-related fatalities by forensic medical examiners.

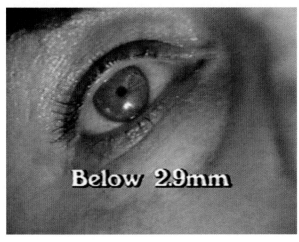

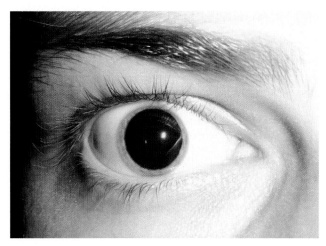

A

B

Figure 121–1. Miotic (pinpoint pupils) (A) versus mydriatic (dilated) pupils (B). (www.drugabuserecognition.com/sitebuilder/imag. www.drugabuserecognition.com/about_us.html.)

▶ CLINICAL PRESENTATION

Opioid poisoning classically presents with an altered level of consciousness. The triad of acute toxicity consists of CNS depression, respiratory depression, and pupillary constriction or "pinpoint pupils" (Fig. 121–1A). CNS depression ranges from mild sedation to stupor and coma. Patients are typically hypotensive, hypothermic, bradycardic, and hyporeflexic. Many patients experience central-mediated vomiting. This, coupled with respiratory depression and a diminished gag reflex, places the patient at risk for aspiration pneumonitis. Other respiratory effects may also include brochospasm from histamine release induced by insufflating or inhaling fumes of opioid compounds cut with impurities or adulterants. In massive overdoses, the respiratory toxicity can also cause severe hypoxia, hypercarbia, and acute lung injury.

While miotic or "pinpoint" pupils are a classic opioid-induced clinical finding, mydriasis or pupillary dilation (Fig. 121–1B) has been described with meperidine, propoxyphene and diphenoxylsate-atropine (Lomotil) overdoses. With Lomotil overdose, a two-phase toxicity has been described. Phase I manifests with anticholinergic symptoms such as dry mouth, flushing, and mydriasis, while phase II consists of opioid effects causing respiratory and central nervous system depression, with associated miosis.

Less common effects of opioid toxicity include generalized seizure activity following overdose of propoxyphene, meperidine, tramadol,[17] fentanyl, or pentazocine. Neonates receiving continuous intravenous morphine can also suffer seizures from toxicity or during acute opioid withdrawal.[16]

Dermatologic effects include flushing and pruritus secondary to histamine release. Gastrointestinal effects include decreased gut motility and constipation. Finally, medical complications common among chronic users arise from adulterants found in street drugs and the nonsterile practices of injecting drugs. Patients who chronically use opioids intravenously or by "skin popping" can contract bacterial endocartitits, septic pulmonary emboli, skin infections, tetanus, wound botulism, hepatitis, and human immunodeficiency virus infection.

LABORATORY AND DIAGNOSTIC TESTING

Patients presenting with suspected opioid toxicity should have their oxygenation status continually monitored. If severe respiratory compromise and hypoxia continue despite antidote therapy and oxygen administration, an arterial blood gas analysis is obtained to rule out hypercarbia and acidosis. If a child presents with a depressed level of consciousness, a rapid bedside serum glucose is measured to rule out hypoglycemia. If head trauma is suspected, a CAT scan of the brain is indicated. With severe respiratory distress, acute lung injury or aspiration pneumonitis should be suspected, and confirmed with a chest radiograph. With a propoxyphene overdose, an electrocardiogram and QRS complex is assessed.

Toxicology screens are not helpful in the initial management of the opioid overdosed child. Serum assays may only detect opioid compounds for up to 6 hours. Urinary qualitative screens may be useful in ruling out an opioid exposure in a child presenting with altered mental status. These are typically positive for up to 48 to 72 hours postingestion. Most urinary screens lack sensitivity and may not detect many of the synthetic opioids including methadone, hydrocodone, and propoxyphene. In addition, routine screens may not detect potent opioids such as fentanyl, since standard detection or "cutoff" limits are usually set at around 2000 ng/mL. Toxicology screens may also result in "false-positive" screens following dietary ingestion of poppy seeds. Along with other routine baseline laboratory tests, serum acetaminophen and salicylate levels should be measured, since many opioid compounds like hydrocodone and codeine also contain these common analgesics.[10]

► MANAGEMENT

The primary management of opioid poisoning includes stabilization of the airway and administration of the pure opioid antagonist naloxone[18–20] (Fig. 121–2). If adequate doses of this antidote are given in a timely fashion, intubation can be avoided, since the onset of action for naloxone is usually within 1 minute of administration. However, if there is no response to naloxone, and oxygenation cannot be maintained with bag-valve-mask ventilations, the patient's airway is secured by endotracheal intubation.[1,10]

According to the most recent American Association of Poison Control Centers (AAPCC) database, naloxone was the third most commonly administered antidote. Naloxone is derived from thebaine, a minor constituent of opium. In addition to intravenous administration, naloxone can be given via the endotracheal tube, subcutaneously, intramuscularly, intranasally,[21] or by nebulizer, with a comparably rapid onset of action. Clinical trials have demonstrated that slower absorption via the subcutaneous route was offset by the delay in establishing intravenous access, particularly in young children.[22] Intramuscular administration has also been demonstrated to be safe and efficacious in an urban prehospital adult patient population. In the overdose setting, the dose of naloxone is 0.1 mg/kg in children from birth to 5 years of age or in children weighing less than 20 kg. In older children, or in the setting of life-threatening toxicity, a rapid 2-mg dose is recommended.[23] Naloxone can be administered in any intravenous fluid in varying concentrations. If there is no response, repeat doses of 2 mg every 2 to 3 minutes can be given to older children and adolescents, up to a maximum of 10 mg. If no response occurs, other causes for CNS and respiratory depression should be considered. Naloxone doses up to 4 mg/kg have been given to human adult volunteers with minimal to no adverse side effects.[24] An exception to this rule is in the chronic opioid abusing adolescent, in whom an acute withdrawal syndrome can be precipitated. In this setting, doses of 0.1 to 0.4 mg can be given to relieve the respiratory depression without precipitating florid withdrawal symptoms. If the patient experiences acute withdrawal symptoms, general supportive care measures are indicated, since opioid withdrawal is not a life-threatening situation. In the newborn setting, however, withdrawal seizures have been well documented in neonates born to opioid-dependent mothers.

Naloxone's duration of action is 20 to 30 minutes, which is shorter than most opioid agents, except fentanyl. Thus, repeated doses may be indicated, particularly when dealing with opioids with longer duration of action,[25] such as oxycodone,[26,27] methadone, and Lomotil (diphenoxylate).[28,29] Titrated doses administered every 3 to 5 minutes may be initially required. If repeat doses of naloxone are necessary, a continuous intravenous infusion of naloxone can be instituted.[30] The drip rate can be calculated by using two-thirds of the initial dose required to reverse the patient's respiratory depression and administering this amount hourly.[31] The infusion rate may vary depending on the specific opioid and the patient's level of physical dependence.

The new longer-acting antagonist nalmefene may be useful in younger, non–opioid-dependent children who are exposed to longer-acting agents. Although studies of this agent in the pediatric population are limited, it has been safely administered in the clinical setting by reversing iatrogenically induced opioid sedation in children, with no reported adverse side effects.[32,33] Doses of 0.5 to 2.0 mg have been reported to be safe and effective, with a duration of effect up to 8 hours.[34] Nalmefene would be most clinically efficacious in younger children not experiencing withdrawal symptoms. In the setting of chronically addicted adolescents, a shorter-acting antagonist like naloxone would be a more humane approach, since withdrawal symptoms would be shorter in duration.

An initial dose of activated charcoal is advised following any oral ingestion, particularly in opioids that have delayed absorption, such as diphenoxylate-atropine (Lomotil) and sustained-relaease morphine products.

As with cyclic antidepressant overdose, cardiotoxicity from propoxyphene[35] demonstrating a widened QRS complex may be responsive in intravenous administration of sodium bicarbonate.

Children who present as body packers[36] or stuffers of heroin or opioid-containing drugs may require gastrointestinal decontamination with whole-bowel irrigation using PEG (polyethylene glycol) solution to enhance elimination of drug packets. The PEG dose is 25/mL/kg/h, which often requires orogastric tube insertion. Contraindications to whole-bowel irrigation include unstable vital signs, respiratory compromise, and lack of bowel sounds or gut motility. Activated charcoal should be given prior to whole bowel irrigation to adsorb any leaking drug from the packets. Charcoal in the rectal effluent indicates successful whole-bowel irrigation.

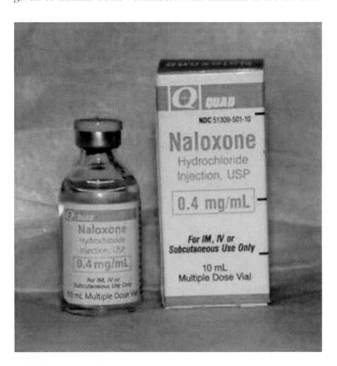

Figure 121–2. Naloxone is the most commonly administered opioid antagonist.

► DISPOSITION

Any young pediatric patient presenting with CNS and respiratory depression from opioid poisoning that is responsive to naloxone should be admitted for observation, since most of the opioids demonstrate longer duration of action than naloxone, and repetitive dosing or continuous naloxone infusion may be required. Long-acting agents such as methadone and the antidiarrheal agent Lomotil are much more likely to demonstrate recurrence of central nervous system and respiratory depression.[4] Because of the potential delays in toxicity, young children should be observed in a monitored setting for at least 24 hours. However, most recurrences will be evident within 2 hours of presentation. Adolescent patients presenting with CNS depression from heroin overdose who quickly respond to naloxone administration can be discharged home with reliable caretakers after 4 to 6 hours of observation. It would be prudent to observe patients who continue to demonstrate respiratory compromise or who require repeated doses of naloxone for a longer period of time. In patients demonstrating chronic addiction patterns, detoxification programs and appropriate counseling referrals should be arranged.[1]

REFERENCES

1. Erickson T. Opioids. In: Erickson T, Ahrens W, Aks S, et al., eds. *Pediatric Toxicology: Diagnosis and Management of the Poisoned Child.* 1st ed. New York, NY: McGraw-Hill; 2005.
2. Binchy JM, Molyneux EM, Manning J. Accidental ingestion of methadone by children in Merseyside. *Br Med J.* 1994;308:1335.
3. Behrman A, Goertemoieller S. A sticky situation: toxicity of clonidine and fentanyl transdermal patches in pediatrics. *J Emerg Nurs.* 2007;33(3):290–293.
4. Sachdeva D, Standnyk J. Are on or two dangerous? Oral exposure I toddlers. *J Emerg Med.* 2005;29(1):77–84.
5. Michael J, Sztajnkrycer M. Deadly pediatric poisons: nine common agents that kill at low doses. *Emerg Med Clin North Am.* 2004;22(4):1019–1050.
6. U.S. Drug Enforcement Administration (DEA) web site: http://www.dea.gov/pubs/abuse/index.html. Section on Narcotics: 2007. Accessed July 1, 2007.
7. De la Fuente L, Barrio G, Royuela L. Heroin smoking by "chasing the dragon": its evolution in Spain. *Addiction.* 1998;93:444–446.
8. Sporer KA. Acute heroin overdose. *Ann Intern Med.* 1999;130:584–590.
9. Minami M, Satoh M. Molecular biology of the opioid receptors: structures, functions and distributions. *Neurosci Res.* 1995;23:121–145.
10. Nelson L. Opioids. In: Goldfrank LR, Flomenbaum NE, Lewin NA, et al., eds. *Goldfrank's Toxicologic Emergencies.* 7th ed. Philadelphia, PA: McGraw-Hill; 2002:901–923.
11. Glare PA, Walsh TD. Clinical pharmakokinetics of morphine. *Ther Drug Monit.* 1991;13:1–23.
12. Cone EJ, Fant RV, Rohay JM, et al. Oxycodone involvement in drug deaths: a DAWN-based classification scheme applied to an oxycodone postmortem database containing over 1000 cases. *J Anal Toxicol.* 2003;27(2):57–67.
13. Cutler EA, Barrett GA, Craven PW, et al. Delayed cardiopulmonary arrest after Lomotil ingestion. *Pediatrics.* 1980;65:157–158.
14. Rumack BH, Temple AR. Lomotil poisoning. *Pediatrics.* 1974;53:495–500.
15. Glick C, Evans OB, Parks BR. Muscle rigidity due to fentanyl infusion in the pediatric patient. *South Med J.* 1996;889:1119–1120.
16. Koren G, Butt W, Pape K, et al. Morphine-induced seizures in newborn infants. *Vet Hum Toxicol.* 1985;27:519.
17. Meyer FP, Rimasch H, Glaha B, et al. Tramadol withdrawal in a neonate. *Eur J Clin Pharmacol.* 1997;53:159–160.
18. Chamberlain JM, Klein BL. A comprehensive review of naloxone for the emergency physician. *Am J Emerg Med.* 1994;12:650–660.
19. Moore RA, Rumack BH, Conner CS, et al. Naloxone. *Am J Dis Child.* 1980;134:156–158.
20. Sporer KA, Kral AH. Prescription naloxone: a novel approach to heroin overdose prevention. *Ann Emerg Med.* 2007;49(2):172–177.
21. Kerr D, Dietze P, Kelly AM. Intranasal naloxone for the treatment of suspected heroin overdose. *Addicition.* 2008;102(3):379–386.
22. Wagner K, Brough L, MacMillan I, et al. Intravenous vs subcutaneous naloxone for out-of-hospital management of presumed opioid overdose. *Acad Emerg Med.* 1998;5:293–299.
23. Kauffman RE, Banner W, Blumer JL, et al. Naoloxone dosage and route of administration for infants and children. *Pediatrics.* 1990;86:484.
24. Cohen MR, Cohen RM, Pickar D, et al. Behavioral effects after high-dose naloxone administration to normal volunteers. *Lancet.* 1981;2:1110.
25. Watson WA, Steele MT, Muelleman RL, et al. Opioid recurrence after an initial response to naloxone. *Clin Toxciol.* 1998;36:11–17.
26. Medical Letter. Oxycodone and oxycontin. *Med Lett Drugs Ther.* 2001;43(1113):80–81.
27. Schneir AB, Vadeboncoeur TF, Offerman SR, et al. Massive oxycontin ingestion refractory to naloxone therapy. *Ann Emerg Med.* 2002;40(4):425–428.
28. Ginsburg CM. Lomotil (diphenoxylate and atropine) intoxication. *Am J Dis Child.* 1973;125:241–242.
29. McCarron MM, Challoner RR, Thompson GA. Diphenoxylateatropine (Lomotil) overdose in children; an update. *Pediatrics.* 1991;87:694–700.
30. Lewis JM, Klein-Shwartz W, Benson BE, et al. Continuous naloxone infusion in pediatric narcotic overdose. *Am J Dis Child.* 1984;138:944–946.
31. Goldfrank L, Weisman RS, Errick JK, et al. A dosing nomogram for continuous infusion intravenous naloxone. *Ann Emerg Med.* 1986;15:566–570.
32. Chumpa A. Nalmefene hydrochloride. *Pediatr Emerg Care.* 1999;15:141–143.
33. Chumpa A, Kaplan RL, Burns MM, Shannon MW. Nalmefene for elective reversal of procedural sedation in children. *Am J Emerg Med.* 2001;19(7):545–548.
34. Kaplan JL, Mark JA, Calabro JJ, et al. Double-blind, randomized study of nalmefene and naloxone in emergency department suspected narcotic overdose. *Ann Emerg Med.* 1999;34:42–50.
35. Stork CM, Redd JT, Fine K, Hoffman RS. Proxyphene-induced wide QRS complex dysrhythmia responsive to sodium bicarbonate: a case report. *Clin Toxicol.* 1995;33:179–183.
36. Utecht MJ, Stone AF, McCarron MM. Herion body packers. *J Emerg Med.* 1993;159:750–754.

CHAPTER 122

Cocaine Toxicity

Steven E. Aks

▶ HIGH-YIELD FACTS

- Myocardial ischemia has been reported in patients with normal coronary arteries as young as 17 years old after the use of cocaine.
- Other causes of chest pain after cocaine use must be differentiated. Consider asthma, pulmonary infarction, pneumomediastinum, aortic dissection, and pneumothorax.
- Benzodiazepines are the first-line agents for agitation, tremulousness, mild hypertension, and tachycardia from cocaine use.
- Activated charcoal and possibly whole bowel irrigation are indicated for orally ingested cocaine, as in the case of body stuffers.

Cocaine abuse and toxicity continue to be pervasive problems (Fig. 122–1).[1] Adolescents and adults predominantly use cocaine as a recreational drug. Children usually suffer toxicity when exposed to cocaine being used by others.[2] Seizures have been reported in children who accidentally ingest cocaine, and toxicity has occurred in toddlers who inhale cocaine being "freebased" by nearby adults.[3] Convulsions have been reported in a breast-fed infant whose mother abused cocaine. Cocaine, multiple-drug ingestions, and tricyclic antidepressants are among the most prominent causes of cardiac arrest for patients younger than 40 years.[4]

According to data obtained by the Drug Abuse Warning Network (DAWN) in 2005, there were a total of 1.4 million emergency department (ED) visits related to drug abuse or misuse. There were 448 481 involving cocaine. In children aged 0 to 5 years, there were 212 ED visits, and this increased to 992 ED visits in the 12 to 17-year age range.[1] In one study, 2.4% of children in a group of inner city preschoolers tested positive for the cocaine metabolite benzoylecgonine in their urine.[3]

▶ PHARMACOLOGY AND PATHOPHYSIOLOGY

Chemically, cocaine is benzoylmethylecgonine, a naturally occurring local anesthetic. It is derived from the plant *Erythroxylum coca* and is rapidly absorbed from mucous membranes, lung tissue, and the gastrointestinal tract.

Pharmacologically, cocaine is a sympathomimetic that blocks fast sodium channels. The primary target organs are the central nervous system (CNS), cardiovascular system, lungs, gastrointestinal tract, skin, and thermoregulatory center.

Clinically, cocaine causes CNS stimulation that can result in agitation, hallucinations, abnormal movements, and convulsions. Paradoxically, children may present with lethargy. Both ischemic and hemorrhagic strokes have been reported.[5]

Cardiovascular manifestations of cocaine toxicity include sinus tachycardia and both supraventricular and ventricular dysrhythmias. Elevation in blood pressure can range from mild to fulminant hypertension associated with strokes. Myocardial ischemia, including myocardial infarction, has been described in otherwise healthy individuals as young as 17 years old with normal coronary arteries.[6]

Multiple pulmonary effects from inhalation of cocaine have been described, including exacerbation of asthma, pulmonary infarction, pneumomediastinum, pneumothorax, and respiratory failure.

Orally ingested cocaine can cause ischemic complications in the gastrointestinal tract that include acute abdominal pain, hemorrhagic diarrhea, and shock.

In association with agitation and hypertension, cocaine-induced hyperthermia can occur. A potential complication of hyperthermia is acute rhabdomyolysis.[7] Cocaine-induced rhabdomyolysis can also occur in the absence of hyperthermia.

The dermatologic manifestations of cocaine abuse are primarily related to intravenous injection and "skin popping." These include localized areas of necrosis or infection.

▶ DIAGNOSIS

Cocaine toxicity is likely in a patient who exhibits signs and symptoms consistent with sympathomimetic stimulation. Occasionally, the sympathomimetic toxidrome is difficult to distinguish from that caused by anticholinergic toxicity. Both toxidromes are associated with CNS excitation, mydriasis, tachycardia, hypertension, and hyperthermia. Unlike sympathomimetic toxicity, however, anticholinergics will cause urinary retention and decreased bowel sounds. Also, sympathomimetic toxicity is often associated with diaphoresis, while anticholinergic overdose is associated with dry skin.

Orally ingested cocaine by body stuffers or body packers may be difficult to diagnose without a direct history. Body stuffers ingest poorly wrapped packets hurriedly in order to avoid arrest.[8] Body packers by contrast ingest well-wrapped packets with much higher content of drug in order to smuggle.

▶ LABORATORY STUDIES

For patients in whom cocaine toxicity is suspected, a urine toxicology screen can confirm the ingestion. Benzoylecgonine, a cocaine metabolite, can be detected in the urine for up to 72 hours after ingestion. Blood levels of cocaine and cocaine

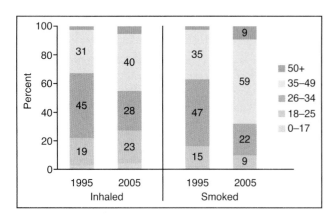

Figure 122–1. Primary cocaine admissions, by age at admission and route of administration: 1995 and 2005.

metabolites correlate poorly with signs and symptoms. Cardiac monitoring is essential to evaluate the patient for dysrhythmias. Patients who complain of chest pain require a 12-lead electrocardiogram, and possibly cardiac enzymes. For patients with chest pain, a radiograph is also useful to exclude pneumothorax, pneumomediastinum, or infiltrate.

Laboratory studies help establish a baseline and are useful for patients with significant toxicity. They include a complete blood count, serum electrolytes, glucose, blood urea nitrogen, and creatinine. If a urine dipstick is positive for blood but microscopy is negative for red blood cells, the patient is evaluated for rhabdomyolysis with a serum creatine kinase and urine myoglobin.

For patients with severe headache or neurological deficit, a computed tomographic (CT) scan of the brain is indicated to rule out the possibility of a cocaine-induced cerebrovascular accident.

Plain radiographs are helpful in body packers, but are not useful for body stuffers. A CT scan with and without contrast may visualize packets in body stuffers if confirmation of the diagnosis is necessary.

▶ MANAGEMENT

Mildly toxic patients generally require no specific therapy. Moderate-to-severe agitation responds to benzodiazepines, which are also the drugs of choice for seizures. Persistent seizure activity may require treatment with high-dose benzodiazepines or phenobarbital. Rarely, status epilepticus requires paralysis. Patients with persistent seizures may suffer from a structural CNS lesion or toxicity from a coingestant. Benzo-diazepines are also effective treatment for most patients with mild-to-moderate hypertension. In more severe cases, agents including sodium nitroprusside or phentolamine may be used. In general β-blockers are contraindicated in the presence of cocaine-induced sympathetic overdrive, since unopposed α-stimulation can exacerbate hypertension.

Patients with severe hyperthermia are treated with aggressive cooling, and the urine may be alkalinized in patients with rhabdomyolysis.

Activated charcoal adsorbs unpackaged orally ingested cocaine and is useful for the treatment of gastric contamination in body stuffers and body packers.[9] Whole bowel irrigation has been used for body stuffers and packers, but its usefulness and necessity is unproven.[10]

▶ DISPOSITION

In asymptomatic or mild cases of cocaine toxicity, 4 to 6 hours of observation in the ED is adequate. Patients with moderate-to-severe symptoms are admitted to a monitored bed.

REFERENCES

1. *Drug Abuse Warning Network, 2005: National Estimates of Drug-related Emergency Deparment Visits.* DAWN Series D-29, DHHS Publication No. (SMA) 07-4256, Rockville, MD; 2007.
2. Lustbader AS, Mayes LC, McGee BA, et al. Incidence of passive exposure to crack/cocaine and clinical findings in infants seen in an outpatient service. *Pediatrics.* 1998;102(1):e5.
3. Kharasch SJ, Glotzer D, Vinci R, et al. Unsuspected cocaine exposure in young children. *Am J Dis Child.* 1991;145:204–206.
4. Richman PB, Nashed AH. The etiology of cardiac arrest in children and young adults: special considerations for ED management. *Am J Emerg Med.* 1999;17:264–270.
5. Seaman ME. Acute cocaine abuse associated with cerebral infarction. *Ann Emerg Med.* 1990;19:34–37.
6. Minor RL, Scott BD, Brown DD, et al. Cocaine-induced myocardial infarction in patients with normal coronary arteries. *Ann Intern Med.* 1991;115:797–806.
7. Roth D, Alarcon FJ, Fernandez JA, et al. Acute rhabdomyolysis associated with cocaine intoxication. *N Engl J Med.* 1988;319:673–677.
8. Aks SE, Vanden Hoek TL, Hryhorczuk DO, et al. Cocaine liberation from body packets in an in vitro model. *Ann Emerg Med.* 1992;21:1321–1325.
9. Tomaszewski C, Vorhees S, Wathen J, et al. Cocaine adsorption to activated charcoal in vitro. *J Emerg Med.* 1992;10:59–62.
10. June R, Aks SE, Keys N, et al. Medical outcome of cocaine bodystuffers. *J Emerg Med.* 2000;18:221–224.

CHAPTER 123

Phencyclidine and Ketamine Toxicity

Christopher Hoyte and Steven E. Aks

▶ HIGH-YIELD FACTS

- Phencyclidine (PCP) is a dissociative anesthetic structurally similar to ketamine.
- Street names of PCP include angel dust, peace pill, wickey weed, wacky weed, illy, Sherman, monkey tranquilizer, and embalming fluid.
- Bidirectional nystagmus is a classic finding of PCP or ketamine intoxication
- A urine dipstick positive for blood but negative for RBCs should prompt the diagnosis of rhabdomyolysis in PCP intoxicated patients.
- Urinary acidification is contraindicated in PCP intoxication because it can cause precipitation of myoglobin in the tubules.

Phencyclidine (PCP) first came to the market as a surgical anesthetic and sedative in the 1950s. It was introduced as *Sernyl* by Parke Davis Pharmaceutical Company; however, the drug was removed from the market due to adverse side effects such as hallucinations. In the late 1960s, however, PCP made its return to commercial use as a veterinary tranquilizer. In the same year, PCP was first reported as an illicit drug used for recreational purposes in San Francisco, where it was called the "Peace Pill." The Controlled Substance Analogue Enforcement Act of 1986 made PCP and its derivatives illegal. Its precursor, piperidine, requires mandatory reporting. According to data collected by the Drug Abuse Warning Network in 2005, there were 7535 emergency department (ED) visits for PCP.[1] This places it below cocaine and heroin in frequency of use. The drug carries various street names such as "angel dust," "hog," "horse tranquilizer," "crystal joint," and "illy."[2]

Ketamine is a legal analogue of PCP used in humans for sedation and anesthesia. Ketamine is also a drug of abuse; it is used regularly at raves and nightclubs by adolescents and young adults for its hallucinatory, out of body experiences. In this arena, the drug carries street names such as "Special K," "K," "KitKat," and "Vitamin K." It has a relatively short duration of action (15–45 minutes) and has only one-tenth the potent toxic effect of PCP. Because of its abuse potential, ketamine is in the Controlled Substance Act of 1999.[3]

▶ PATHOPHYSIOLOGY

PCP is classically categorized as a dissociative anesthetic because when anesthetized, the patient is conscious, yet experiences a feeling of dissociation from themselves—the "out of body" experience.

After ingestion, absorption occurs in the upper intestine. The drug has an enterogastric circulation such that PCP is secreted by the stomach and then absorbed in the small intestine. Because the drug recirculates in this way, it typically produces a cyclical symptomatology.[4]

The drug interacts at many receptor sites, including N-methyl-D-aspartic acid type glutamate receptors, the neuronal dopamine/norepinephrine/serotonin (DA/NE/5HT) reuptake complex site, and the sigma opiate receptor complex.[5]

As mentioned above, ketamine is an anesthetic agent that is commonly used for sedation prior to painful procedures. Because it is a bronchodilator, it is also often used as an induction in the patient with status asthmaticus or COPD exacerbation who requires intubation. The induction dose is 1 to 4.5 mg/kg IV over 1 minute. In the setting of conscious sedation, the dose is 1 mg/kg IV. The onset of action is rapid; the dissociative state is achieved within seconds. While laryngeal reflexes usually remain intact, depression of the cough reflex is not uncommon. This, coupled with ketamine's potential to increase salivary secretions, has been reported to obstruct the airway. Administration of anticholinergic agents minimizes the increase in salivation.

▶ CLINICAL FINDINGS

The clinical presentation in the ED after PCP use depends on the dose, route of administration, concomitant drug use, and the patient's susceptibility to the drug. Typically, abnormal vital signs and psychomotor abnormalities are present. Mild elevations in blood pressure, tachycardia, and hyperthermia can all be present. Respiratory drive is not compromised and hypoventilation is rare unless extremely high doses are used. The risk of laryngeal and pharyngeal reflex hyperactivity in the pediatric population has been documented.[6] Horizontal, vertical, and rotary nystagmus can be present with PCP toxicity. Pupils may be miotic or mydriatic, but react to light. A fluctuating level of consciousness is typical of PCP intoxication. In addition, the patient may exhibit remarkable strength, and completely disregard lacerations, fractures, or other traumatic injuries.[4]

Ketamine causes a similar clinical presentation to PCP. Respiratory drive remains intact and hypoventilation is uncommon.[3] The rare cases of respiratory depression and apnea reported have been associated with rapid infusion. Infusing ketamine over 1 to 2 minutes decreases this risk.

▶ LABORATORY

PCP exposures are most often diagnosed clinically. Diagnostic testing is required only in cases where child abuse or foul play is suspected. Qualitative tests are available as a part of the urine toxicology screen. In an acute PCP exposure, urinary metabolites are present for 7 days; in cases of chronic exposure metabolites can be present for up to 4 weeks. There is also a serum test for quantitative testing. The latter is not routinely used, because serum concentrations do not correlate with toxicity. Useful laboratory studies include blood urea nitrogen and creatinine to assess renal function and creatine phosphokinase and myoglobin to screen for rhabdomyolysis. The white blood cell count is frequently be elevated. A blood glucose should be obtained to exclude hypoglycemia.[4]

Ketamine may cross-react with PCP on urine immunoassay.[7] Other drugs that can cause a false-positive result are dextromethorphan, diphenhydramine, ibuprofen, imipramine, meperidine, mesoridazine, metamizol, methyphenidate, thioridazine, and venlafaxine.[7,8]

▶ MANAGEMENT

The acute care of the patient's airway, circulation, and thermoregulation are of utmost importance. Potential airway threats caused by PCP or ketamine toxicity include increased salivation, increased tracheobronchal tree secretions, and laryngospasm. These may require intubation. Emergence reactions and agitation have been reported and can be treated with benzodiazepines. Emergence reactions are more frequent in older patients.

Patients arriving in the ED soon after the ingestion of PCP or ketamine may benefit from activated charcoal. In an agitated or somnolent patient charcoal administration can increase the risk of aspiration.

Urinary acidification to enhance renal elimination is not recommended. The benefit of the minor increase in renal clearance of PCP from ion trapping of the weak base is far outweighed by the potential harm created by systemic academia. With acidification of urine myoglobin excretion is decreased, which may cause acute tubular necrosis. Adequate hydration, supportive care, and symptomatic treatment are the mainstays of therapy.[9]

▶ DISPOSITION

Monitoring in the ED or the ICU is appropriate for the patient experiencing adverse reactions to PCP or ketamine until the signs and symptoms resolve. Supportive care is the recommended therapy. Patients with recreational exposures should be discharged with follow-up that includes referral for drug counseling.

REFERENCES

1. Drug Abuse Warning Network, 2005: *National Estimates of Drug-related Emergency Department Visits.* DAWN Series D-29, DHHS Pub. No. (SMA) 07–4256, Rockville, MD; 2007.
2. McCarron MM, Schulze BW, Thompson GA, et al. Acute phencyclidine intoxication: incidence of clinical findings in 1000 cases. *Ann Emerg Med.* 1981;10:237–242.
3. Moriarty AL. What's "new" in street drugs: "Illy." *J Pediatr Health Care.* 1996;10:41–42.
4. Weiner AL, Vieira L, McKay CA. Ketamine abusers presenting to the emergency department: a case series. *J Emerg Med.* 2000;18:447–451.
5. Hahn I-H. Phencycline and Ketamine. In: Erickson TB, Ahrens WR, Aks SE, et al., eds. *Pediatric Toxicology: Diagnosis and Management of the Poisoned Child.* New York, NY: McGraw-Hill; 2005:423–428.
6. Schwartz RH, Einhorn A. PCP intoxication in seven young children. *Pediatr Emerg Care.* 1986;2:238–241.
7. Shannon M. Recent ketamine administration can produce a urine toxic screen which is falsely positive for phencyclidine. *Pediatr Emerg Care.* 1998;14:180.
8. Marchei E, Pellegrini M, Pichini S, et al. Are false-positive phencyclidine immunoassay instant-view multi-test results caused by overdose concentrations of ibuprofen, metamizol, and dextromethorphan? *Ther Drug Monit.* 2007;5:671–673.
9. Patel R, Connor G. A review of thirty cases of rhabdomyolysis-associated acute renal failure among phencyclidine users. *Clin Toxicol.* 1985;23:547–556.

CHAPTER 124

Amphetamines

James W. Rhee

▶ HIGH-YIELD FACTS

- Amphetamine toxicity results from generalized sympathetic stimulation
- Manifestations of toxicity include tachycardia, diaphoresis, hypertension, tachypnea, tremor, and possibly seizures
- Seratonin syndrome and hyponatremia are associated with MDMA use
- Moderate amphetamine toxicity is treated with benzodiazepines
- Benzodiazepines are the first line treatment for amphetamine associated seratonin syndrome and seizures.

▶ BACKGROUND

Amphetamines have been used for medicinal and recreational purposes over the past century. Initially developed as a treatment for respiratory conditions, they were also noted to have stimulant properties. These stimulant properties were exploited to enhance alertness and decrease sleepiness in soldiers during World War II. The "high" that is often experienced with amphetamines made these drugs popular for recreational use. Modifications to amphetamines have led to the development of compounds with hallucinogenic effects enhancing their appeal to the recreational users.

Strictly, the term "amphetamine" is an acronym used to describe the phenylethylamine stimulant **a**lpha-**m**ethyl**ph**enyl-**et**hyl**amine**. Over time, a number of different modifications to the phenylethylamine molecule have spawned many other amphetamine-related compounds with a variety of stimulant and hallucinogenic effects, including methamphetamine and 3,4-methylenedioxymethamphetamine (MDMA). Collectively, these compounds are often referred to as "amphetamines" as well (Fig. 124–1).

Over the past 30 years, amphetamines have been gaining increasing popularity. Methamphetamine has taken over as the leading drug of abuse in the western United States,[1] and MDMA has become a leading drug of abuse among adolescents and young adults. MDMA is especially popular at dance parties (e.g., "raves") and other social gatherings.[2] This increased popularity of amphetamines in illicit drug activities has led to the creation of laws that limit access to some over-the-counter decongestants. These medications are structurally related to the amphetamine compounds and were used as part of the production of certain amphetamines—particularly methamphetamine.

In 2006, there were 12 021 amphetamine, 1932 hallucinogenic amphetamine, and 1186 methamphetamine exposures reported to the American Association of Poison Control Centers National Poison Database System (NPDS)—over half of these exposures occurred in patients younger than 19 years.[3] Despite the reported numbers to the NPDS, the true prevalence of amphetamine toxicity is likely much higher.

▶ PHARMACOLOGY

In general, amphetamines are relatively lipophilic and cross the blood–brain barrier readily. The serum half-life of amphetamine varies from 8 to 30 hours, that of methamphetamine from 12 to 34 hours, and that of MDMA from 5 to 10 hours. Frequent use may lead to an accumulation of drug in the body prolonging the half-life and duration of effect.

Amphetamines act to increase the amount of monoamines released for neurosynaptic transmission leading to the indirect general activation of monoamine receptors—notably adrenergic and dopaminergic receptors. The mechanisms by which these amphetamines elicit this response are very complex and are not completely elucidated.[4] Some of the clearer mechanisms include amphetamine-induced exchange diffusion, reverse transport, and channel-like transport phenomena. The weak base properties of amphetamine may also contribute to increased monoamine availability. In addition, amphetamines may affect monoamine transporters through phosphorylation, transporter trafficking, and the production of reactive oxygen and nitrogen species.[5]

Generalized monoamine release results in increased activation of monoamine receptors—notably, dopamine and adrenergic receptors. This occurs in both the central nervous system and the peripheral nervous system. MDMA can lead to significant activation of serotonin receptors as well.

▶ CLINICAL MANIFESTATIONS

The clinical manifestations of amphetamine toxicity are generally derived from their indirect activation of monoamine receptors. Activating peripheral adrenergic receptors leads to a generalized sympathetic stimulation resulting in a constellation of symptoms similar to other sympathomimetic agents. These symptoms include tachycardia, diaphoresis, hypertension, tremor, tachypnea, and mydriasis. Central monoamine receptor activity can cause agitation, hallucinations, euphoria, and paranoia.

Extraneous motor activity is sometimes noted with amphetamine exposures. Classically, MDMA can induce bruxism—grinding of the teeth. Some users address this effect by chewing on objects such as pacifiers. These extraneous motor

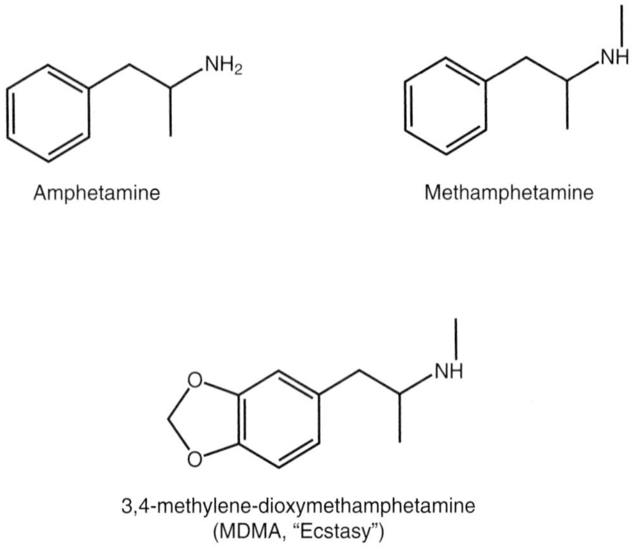

Amphetamine

Methamphetamine

3,4-methylene-dioxymethamphetamine
(MDMA, "Ecstasy")

Figure 124–1. Chemical structures of common amphetamines.

findings are likely a result of increased dopamine receptor activity.

Serotonin syndrome has been described with MDMA use. This syndrome of neuromuscular excitability with associated autonomic instability, altered mental status, and hyperthermia is due to an excess of serotonergic activity. A patient presenting with evidence of clonus or hyperreflexia in the setting of MDMA use should alert the clinician to the possibility of serotonin syndrome.[6]

Hyponatremia is a recognized complication of MDMA use. MDMA can elicit the increased release of vasopressin that results in the increased retention of free water by the body. This effect is compounded by the behavior of drinking an excessive amount of water while at a "rave" party. These factors lead to a fast decline in serum sodium concentrations. When extreme, the ensuing hyponatremia can cause cerebral edema, seizures, and death.

Protracted and extreme toxicity can cause many other severe complications including rhabdomyolysis, hyperthermia, seizures, stroke, intracerebral hemorrhage, acute coronary syndrome, and malignant cardiac dysrhythmias.

▶ DIAGNOSTIC TESTING

Routine laboratory and other diagnostic studies are generally not helpful in diagnosing amphetamine toxicity. The clinical examination has much more utility in this regard. However, diagnostic studies may be useful to identify complications from amphetamine toxicity.

When amphetamine exposure results in clinically significant symptoms, the patient should be placed on a cardiac monitor. Diagnostic studies including electrolytes, glucose, blood urea nitrogen, creatnine, complete blood count, creatine phosphokinase, and an electrocardiogram may be performed to assess for complications of amphetamine toxicity.

In the setting of altered mental status, a computed tomography of the head and follow-up lumbar puncture with cerebrospinal fluid analysis should be performed to evaluate for intracerebral hemorrhage and to exclude other etiologies of the patient's condition.

A urine drug screen may help confirm amphetamine exposure, but care should be taken to interpret the results carefully. A number of agents can cause a positive amphetamine screen including pseudoephedrine, phenylpropanolamine, selegiline, and ephedra. Additionally, some of the modified amphetamines may not cross-react reliably with the immunoassay used in the urine drug screen, thus causing a negative result. It is best to consult with the drug screen manufacturer to understand the limitations of the specific amphetamine immunoassay used at a particular institution.

▶ MANAGEMENT

As with all poisoned children, initial management should focus on measures to support airway patency, adequate respirations, and effective circulation. These measures should take priority over any other intervention and by themselves are the most critical in the care of the child exhibiting amphetamine toxicity.

The administration of activated charcoal (1 gm/kg) should be considered in children who present within an hour of an oral exposure to amphetamines. This may help decrease the amount of amphetamine available of absorption. Activated charcoal is best administered to an awake, alert, and cooperative patient to minimize the risk of aspiration. If these conditions are not met, the administration of activated charcoal should be held unless adequate protection of the patient's airway is otherwise ensured.

Moderate toxicity manifesting with symptoms including tachycardia, hypertension, and agitation can be managed with benzodiazepines (e.g., diazepam 0.2–0.5 mg/kg intravenously, lorazepam 0.05–0.1 mg/kg intravenously). The administration of these benzodiazepines should be repeated every five minutes as needed for effect. Significant toxicity manifesting as severe hypertension, tachycardia, and agitation may warrant a large amount of benzodiazepines. β-adrenergic receptor antagonists are generally avoided in the setting of amphetamine toxicity as it is in cocaine toxicity.

Benzodiazepines are also the first-line agent for serotonin syndrome and amphetamine-induced seizures. For protracted seizure activity, another sedative-hypnotic agent such as phenobarbital or propofol may be needed. Endotracheal intubation may be needed in this setting. Phenytoin, while it is often considered a second-line agent for the treatment of status epilepticus, is generally not effective for toxin-induced seizures.[7]

Evaluation for hyponatremia is warranted in seizing patients with a history of MDMA exposure, as seizures may be the only outward sign of this complication. The treatment in this setting, after controlling seizure activity, is the correction of the underlying hyponatremia.

Hyperthermia in the setting of amphetamine toxicity is a very poor prognostic sign and should be attended to immediately. Aggressive active cooling measures should be instituted to bring the core temperature to a normal range. These measures may include the use of evaporative cooling with fans and mist or cool water immersion.[8] Sedation with benzodiazepines or other sedative-hypnotic agent is necessary to limit the body's heat production. In extreme conditions, neuromuscular blockade with a nondepolorizing paralytic agent may be necessary to decrease motor hyperactivity. The airway must be definitively secured beforehand. Continuous bedside electroencephalography should be performed whenever neuromuscular blockade is administered in this setting to monitor for seizure activity.

Rhabdomyolysis, stroke, intracerebral hemorrhage, acute coronary syndrome, and malignant cardiac dysrhythmias are all other complications that may occur with amphetamine toxicity and other than the general avoidance of β-blockers, there is little deviation from the standard management of these conditions.

▶ DISPOSITION

Children who are asymptomatic or with mild toxicity should be observed in a controlled medical setting for 4 to 6 hours. Circumstances surrounding the exposure of these patients should be considered when planning the subsequent disposition of these children. Patients with moderate-to-severe symptoms and those exhibiting complications from toxicity warrant admission for further observation and management.

REFERENCES

1. Maxwell JC, Rutkowski BA. The prevalence of methamphetamine and amphetamine abuse in North America: a review of the indicators, 1992–2007. *Drug Alcohol Rev.* 2008;27:229–235.
2. Green AR et al. The pharmacology and clinical pharmacology of 3,4-methylenedioxymethamphetamine (MDMA, "ecstasy"). *Pharmacol Rev.* 2003;55:463–508.
3. Bronstein AC et al. 2006 Annual Report of the American Association of Poison Control Centers' National Poison Data System (NPDS). *Clin Toxicol (Phila).* 2007;45:815–917.
4. Sulzer D et al. Mechanisms of neurotransmitter release by amphetamines: a review. *ProgNeurobiol.* 2005;75:406–433.
5. Fleckenstein AE et al. New insights into the mechanism of action of amphetamines. *Ann Rev Pharmacol Toxicol.* 2007;47:681–698.
6. Boyer EW, Shannon M. The serotonin syndrome. *N Engl J Med.* 2005;352:1112–1120.
7. Wills B, Erickson T. Drug- and toxin-associated seizures. *Med Clin North Am.* 2005;89:1297–1321.
8. Rusyniak DE, Sprague JE. Toxin-induced hyperthermic syndromes. *Med Clin North Am.* 2005;89:1277–1296.

CHAPTER 125

Gamma-Hydroxybutyrate

Jenny J. Lu and Timothy B. Erickson

► HIGH-YIELD FACTS

- The clinical picture of an abrupt onset of coma followed by rapid recovery within a few hours should arouse suspicion for GHB intoxication.
- GHB levels are rarely available in a timely fashion.
- Coingestions with alcohol and ecstasy are commonly associated with the recreational use of GHB.
- Exposures to solvents or other products containing GHB precursors may lead to delayed GHB intoxication.
- From a legal perspective, GHB levels are problematic

Gamma-hydroxybutyrate (GHB) was originally investigated in the 1960s as a general anesthetic. Adverse effects such as seizure-like activity and an unpredictable duration of anesthesia precluded its widespread acceptance in the United States. During the 1980s, GHB became popular with bodybuilders as a purported anabolic steroid alternative, and was available in gymnasiums and health food stores. After several reports of GHB toxicity were released, nonprescription sales of GHB in nutritional supplements were banned by the FDA. Despite this ban, however, in the 1990s, recreational use of GHB by adolescents and young adults at rave parties became an increasingly common problem, particularly in Europe. GHB gained notoriety in recent years as a drug used to facilitate sexual assault, because of its ability to cause rapid intoxication and amnesia. In addition, it is nearly colorless and odorless. In 2002, GHB was approved for the treatment of cataplexy in patients with narcolepsy, which remains its main clinical use today. It has dual status as a Schedule I and Schedule III drug of the Controlled Substances Act. Recently, some toys were found to have a coating containing 1,4-butanediol (1–4 BD), a GHB precursor which, after conversion to GHB, accidental intoxication in some children.[1]

GHB is sold illicitly under various street names (Table 125–1). Intentionally obscure synonyms for the chemical names of GHB and its precursors help to conceal the identity of illicit GHB products. Two common precursors of GHB include gamma-butyrolactone (GBL) and 1–4 BD, which can be found in industrial solvents such as paint thinners, floor strippers, and consumer nail care products. Sales of "chemistry kits" containing GHB precursors were an attempt to circumvent the GHB restriction. Currently, both GBL and 1–4 BD are listed as controlled substance analogues.

► PHARMACOLOGY

GHB is available as a clear liquid, white powder, tablet, or capsule. Oral ingestion is the route most commonly used. For oral ingestions, peak concentrations occur within 25 to 45 minutes. The presence of gastric contents may decrease bioavailability. Duration of effect is approximately 1 to 2.5 hours after anesthetic doses of 50 to 60 mg/kg and 2.5 hours after accidental overdoses. Plasma levels are usually undetectable within 4 to 6 hours after therapeutic doses. Volume of distribution is variable owing to saturable absorption and elimination. GHB is not protein bound.[2]

► PATHOPHYSIOLOGY

GHB is a naturally occurring neuromodulator with a number of effects, including the inhibition of dopamine release and an increase in endogenous opioids throughout the brain. Structurally, it is an analog of the inhibitory neurotransmitter gamma-aminobutyric acid (GABA) with the ability to traverse the blood–brain barrier and cause agonist activity at the GHB and GABA (B) receptors.[3] Endogenous and exogenously administered GHB demonstrate distinct pharmacologic profiles, because of the specific receptors on which they exert their action; exogenous GHB is mediated more by the GABA (B) receptor. Abrupt loss of consciousness and apnea caused by exogenous GHB, and subsequent complications including aspiration and pulmonary edema, can potentially lead to serious morbidity or death. Several GHB analogues and precursors exist, but common precursors include gamma-butyrolactone and 1,4-butanediol, both of which can be metabolized to GHB and cause similar, but delayed, clinical effects. Synthetic precursors include gamma-valerolactone and tetrahydrofuran.

► DIAGNOSIS

CLINICAL PRESENTATION OF ACUTE TOXICITY

GHB rapidly crosses the blood–brain barrier and enters the central nervous system. It has a steep dose–response curve, and overdose resulting in coma can easily occur with illicit use. Other signs and symptoms of GHB overdose include vomiting,

► **TABLE 125–1. "STREET" AND CHEMICAL NAMES FOR GAMMA-HYDROXYBUTYRATE**

Common Street Names	Common Chemical Names
Liquid X	4-hydroxy butyrate
Grievous Bodily Harm	Gamma hydrate
Cherry Meth	Gamma-hydroxybutyrate
Organic Quaalude	sodium
Easy Lay	Gamma-hydroxybutyric acid
Georgia Home Boy	Gamma-OH
Insom-X	Sodium oxybate
Liquid E	Sodium oxybutyrate
Gamma G	

sedation, and respiratory depression, which may be associated with loss of the gag reflex. Depression of mental status and respiratory drive may be severe enough to warrant endotrachial intubation. However, unpredictable spontaneous sudden wakening just prior to insertion of an endotracheal tube in patients who have overdosed on GHB has been anecdotally described. Although GHB is classically considered to be a CNS depressant, agitation, excitement, and combativeness have been reported following its use. In some cases, periods of agitation alternating with somnolence have been described. Patients who have overdosed on GHB may present to the emergency department with a history of recreational drug use, an accidental exposure to a GHB precursor-containing product, or as the victim of an alleged poisoning for the purposes of sexual assault. A high index of suspicion regarding the possibility of GHB intoxication is required to make the diagnosis. As with all toxic exposures, other causes of altered mental status and coma should be considered.

Coingestions with intentional exposures to GHB are frequently reported. Ecstasy and ethanol are common coingestants.[4] Ethanol, fasting, and other depressants may enhance GHB's effects. Urine toxicology screens may be helpful in identifying coingestants if the clinical picture is not entirely clear.

Laboratory studies employing gas chromatography/mass spectrometry to measure blood and urine concentrations of GHB are not routinely available, thus most routine hospital toxicology screens do not test for GHB or its precursors. Blood and urine specimens must be sent to one of a few national reference laboratories, although results are unlikely to return in a timely enough fashion to be clinically useful.[5] In addition, interpreting results can be challenging. Appropriate cutoff levels must be selected and careful interpretation of results is required in order to distinguish between endogenous and exogenous GHB concentrations.[6] Because of its rapid metabolism and elimination, the window for detection of GHB is very narrow and GHB concentrations may have returned to endogenous levels by the time a specimen is obtained. This brief window of detection can make proof of GHB poisoning problematic in cases of alleged sexual assault. A "normal" or "negative" GHB test could potentially be detrimental to an alleged victim's case by misleading a jury into believing that there was no evidence of GHB poisoning.

Serum and urine GHB levels may be normal or undetectable by 8 and 12 hours, respectively, following an ingestion.[7] Depending on when a patient presents to the emergency department, determining levels may not be useful. In one case of alleged sexual assault, hair testing demonstrating GHB exposure was documented 1 month after the exposure.[8] Ideally, hair testing should complement serum and urine testing, rather than substitute for one or the other.

► **TREATMENT**

STABILIZATION

Attentive supportive care, airway control, and stabilization of breathing and circulation should be the priorities in caring for the symptomatic patient with GHB intoxication.

DECONTAMINATION

There is essentially no role for gastric lavage or activated charcoal administration for isolated ingestions of GHB, since significant amounts of the drug are unlikely to be present in the stomach by the time of presentation. Additionally, there is a risk of pulmonary aspiration from the abrupt loss of consciousness observed with GHB intoxication. Activated charcoal for other coingestions can be considered if the patient's airway is protected and the patient is not combative. Endotracheal intubation solely for the purpose of decontamination is not recommended.

ANTIDOTAL THERAPY

No specific antidote is available for GHB poisoning. Treatment is centered around supportive care.

Reversal agents such as naloxone, flumazenil, and physostigmine have not been conclusively demonstrated to be effective in reversing GHB-induced coma. The use of physostigmine has been associated with adverse cardiovascular effects.[9,10] Dextrose and thiamine should be given as clinically indicated.

ENHANCED ELIMINATION

There is no role for hemodialysis or hemoperfusion for the isolated overdose with GHB. Cases involving coingestants must be evaluated on an individual basis.

DISPOSITION

Patients who require ventilatory support or other significant interventions should be admitted for further observation and management. Patients whose symptoms have completely resolved and who are accompanied by reliable family members can potentially be considered for discharge after a period of observation. Patients with coingestants may require further observation and management. Arrangements should be made for appropriate counseling for substance use/abuse, psychiatric issues, and follow-up. Consultation with a poison center is prudent for management and disposition issues.

REFERENCES

1. "Toys linked to 'Date Rape' Drug Pulled," CBS News, Nov 8, 2007, http://www.cbsnews.com/stories/2007/11/07/health/main3469765.shtml. Accessed June 5, 2008.
2. Dyer JE. Gamma-hydroxybutyrate (GHB). In: Olsen KR, ed. *Poisoning & Drug Overdose*. 5th ed. New York, NY: McGraw-Hill; 2007:209–212.
3. Tunnicliff G. Sites of action of gamma-hydroxybutyrate (GHB)—a neuroactive drug with abuse potential. *J Txicol Clin Toxicol*. 1997;35(6):581–590.
4. Couper FJ, Thatcher JE, Logan BK. Suspected GHB overdoses in the emergency department. *J Anal Toxicol*. 2004;28(6)481–484.
5. Drasbek KR, Christensen J, Jensen K. Gamma-hydroxybutyrate—a drug of abuse. *Acta Neurol Scand*. 2006;114(3):145–156.
6. Crookes CE, Faulds MC, Forrest AR, et al. A reference range for endogenous gamma-hydroxybutyrate in urine by gas chromatography-mass spectrometry. *J Anal Toxicol*. 2004;28(8):644–649.
7. Sporer KA, Chin RL, Dyer JE, et al. γ-Hydroxybutyrate serum levels and clinical syndrome after severe overdose. *Ann Emerg Med*. 2003;42(1):3–8.
8. Kintz P, Cirimele V, Jamey C, et al. Testing for GHB in hair by GC/MS/MS after a single exposure. Application to document sexual assault. *J Forensic Sci*. 2003;48(1):195–200.
9. Li J, Stokes SA, Woeckener A. A tale of novel intoxication: a review of the effects of gamma-hydroxybutyric acid with recommendations for management. *Ann Emerg Med*. 1998;31(6):729–736.
10. Zvosec DL, Smith SW, Litonjua R, et al. Physostigmine for gamma-hydroxybutyrate coma: inefficacy, adverse events, and review. *Clin Toxicol*. 2007;45(3):261–265.

SUGGESTED READING

Cumpston K, Aks S. Drug-facilitated sexual assault. In: Erickson T, Ahrens W, Aks S, et al., eds. *Pediatric Toxicology: Diagnosis and Management of the Poisoned Child*. 1st ed. New York, NY: McGraw-Hill; 2005:416–422.

Li J, Stokes SA, Woeckener A. A tale of novel intoxication: seven cases of γ-hydroxybutyric acid overdose. *Ann Emerg Med*. 1988;31(6):723–728.

Nicholson KL, Balster RL. GHB: a new and novel drug of abuse. *Drug Alcohol Depend*. 2001;63(1):1–22.

O'Connell T, Kaye L, Plosay JJ III. Gamma-hydroxybutyrate (GHB): a newer drug of abuse. *Am Fam Physician*. 2000;62(11):2478–2483.

CHAPTER 126

Lead Poisoning

Mark B. Mycyk

► HIGH-YIELD FACTS

- Lead poisoning causes multisystem clinical effects: headache, abdominal pain, constipation, vomiting, clumsiness, irritability, and drowsiness.
- Laboratory evaluation may demonstrate anemia, basophilic stippling, elevated erythrocyte protoporphyrins (EP), zinc protoporphyrins (ZPP), and elevated blood lead level (BLL).
- Management requires identification and removal of the source of exposure.
- Chelation with $CaNa_2EDTA$, BAL, or succimer is dictated by BLL and severity of symptoms.

The average blood lead level of American children has decreased by more than 80% since the 1970s because of early screening initiatives and environmental hazard reduction.[1,2] In spite of this progress, it is estimated that almost 1 million children still have some degree of lead poisoning.[3] Several long-term studies have shown an association of lead levels previously thought to be nontoxic with impaired growth and behavioral and neurocognitive development.[4] Before 1970, the lead intervention level was 60 μg/dL, but the Centers for Disease Control and Prevention revised the action downward several times to its current level of 10 μg/dL in 1991.[1] Lead poisoning affects people of all ages and classes, but the prevalence of lead poisoning remains highest in inner-city underprivileged children.[5,6]

► SOURCES

Despite frequent media reports of lead discovered in children's toys (mostly imported from overseas), ingestion of leaded household paint is the most common and clinically relevant source of lead poisoning in children.[6,7] Most homes built before 1978 were painted with lead-based paint.[8] A small paint chip containing 50% lead can produce acute lead poisoning in a toddler. Renovation of old buildings and poorly controlled lead abatement pose a risk for lead poisoning through inhalation and ingestion of contaminated dust and soil.[9] Lead exposure can also occur through drinking water contaminated by lead in plumbing, from living in close proximity to stationary air pollution sources such as lead smelters, from lead brought home from a parent's workplace, drinking from improperly fired lead-glazed pottery, some folk remedies, bullets lodged in joint spaces, and other unusual sources. The phaseout of leaded gasoline has had a major impact in reducing exposure to lead.[8]

► PHARMACOKINETICS/ PATHOPHYSIOLOGY

Up to 50% of lead ingested can be absorbed by the gastrointestinal tract in infants and children.[6] Iron deficiency and dietary calcium deficiency increase the absorption of lead in the gut. Up to 30% of lead dust and fumes can be absorbed through the respiratory tract, while percutaneous absorption of lead is less than 0.1% of the applied quantity. Lead readily crosses the placental barrier, and fetal exposure is cumulative until birth.[10] Although distribution of absorbed lead in the body is complex, the emergency physician should think of lead using a three-compartment model: blood, soft tissue, and bone. Acutely 99% of the lead in blood is attached to red blood cells. Under chronic exposure conditions, the bone serves as a storage organ for 70% of the pediatric lead burden and can release lead back into the blood and soft tissues. Absorbed lead is eliminated primarily in the urine and bile. In adults, the elimination of lead is first-order and triphasic with elimination half-lives of 1 week, 1 month, and 10 to 20 years. Pediatric data are sparse, but some reports indicate that the biologic half-life of blood lead in 2-year-old children is approximately 10 months.[11]

Lead toxicity results from interaction of lead with sulfydryl and other ligands on enzymes and other macromolecules.[2] The major target organs of lead are the bone marrow, central nervous system, peripheral nervous system, and kidneys. Lead inhibits heme synthesis through inhibition of ALA-dehydratase, coproporphyrin utilization, and ferrochelatase, resulting in the buildup of aminolevulinic acid, coproporphyrins, and free erythrocyte protoporphyrin. Lead also inhibits the enzyme pyrimidine-5-nucleotidase. Clinically, inhibition of heme synthesis is manifested as anemia. Lead encephalopathy occurs from demyelinization and precipitation of ribonucleoprotein with resulting cell death, tissue necrosis, vascular damage, and cerebral edema. Peripheral neuropathy results from demyelinization of peripheral nerves. Renal insufficiency results from disturbed mitochondrial respiration and phosphorylation.

► CLINICAL MANIFESTATIONS

Symptoms and signs of lead toxicity are often subtle, non-specific, and sometimes not noticeable.[2,6] With improvements in preventing childhood lead poisoning in the United States, the most likely cause for ED referral is a high blood lead level (BLL) found during a screening program in asymptomatic children. Symptomatic lead poisoning, on the other hand, is characterized by one or more of the following: decrease in

▶ **TABLE 126–1. CLASS OF CHILD, TOXIC EFFECT, AND RECOMMENDED ACTION ACCORDING TO BLOOD LEAD MEASUREMENT**

Class	Blood Lead Level (μg/dL)*	Toxic Effect	Recommended Action
I	0–5	No noticeable effect	
	5–9	Inhibition of ALAD	
IIA	10–14		Rescreen every 3 mo; educate parents
IIB	15–19	Inhibition of ferrochelatase	Retest in 3 mo, nutritional and educational intervention, environmental investigation
III	20–44	Reduced growth, hearing, nerve conduction, neuropsychological deficits, reduced heme synthetase, increased EP, urine d-ALA	All of the above plus retest 1 wk–1 mo
IV	45–69	Anemia, abdominal colic, reduced IQ, lead lines in x-ray	All of the above plus chelation: oral DMSA or IV CaNa$_2$EDTA
V	>70	Encephalopathy risk, nephropathy (>100 μ/dL)	Medical emergency: chelate with BAL plus EDTA, increased ICP precautions

*Conversion factor: 1.0 μg/dL = 0.04826 mmol/L.
ALAD, aminolevulinic acid dehydratase; EP, erythrocyte protoporphyrin; ALA, aminolevulinic acid.
With permission from Centers for Disease Control and Prevention. Screening young children for lead poisoning: Guidance for state and local public health officials. US Dept. of Health and Human Services, Public Health Service, *Federal Register*, February 21, 1997.

play activity, irritability, drowsiness, anorexia, sporadic vomiting, intermittent abdominal pain, constipation, regression of newly acquired skills (particularly speech), sensorineural hearing loss, clumsiness, and slight attenuation of growth. It is not uncommon for some children to be seen by a health practitioner several times with these nonspecific symptoms before lead poisoning is even considered. Lead toxicity is grossly correlated with BLL (Table 126–1), but is more pronounced in young children and in those with prolonged exposure to lead.

Overt lead encephalopathy may ensue after days or weeks of symptoms and present with ataxia, forceful vomiting, lethargy, or stupor, and can progress to coma and seizures. Although seen less commonly than in the past, lead encephalopathy is a medical emergency. It may occur with a BLL >70 μg/dL, but is generally associated with BLLs in excess of 100 μg/dL. Permanent brain damage may result in 70% to 80% of children with lead encephalopathy, even with adequate treatment (Fig. 126–1). Peripheral neuropathy is rare under the age of 5, and consists mainly of motor weakness in lower limbs or upper limbs (e.g., wrist drop).

Microcytic anemia frequently coexists with lead poisoning. Lead nephropathy can result in a Fanconi-like syndrome and acute tubular necrosis, but is rare in children.

Since lead poisoning is so frequent and may present with a variety of signs and symptoms, a high index of suspicion is required to make the diagnosis. This is particularly true among populations at risk, such as children with pica, inner city dwellers, nonwhites, children of families with limited economic means, recent immigrants or adoptees from overseas, and those who live in old houses that have been recently renovated.[6,9]

The definitive diagnosis of lead poisoning and assessment of its severity and chronicity depends on laboratory evaluation of a whole BLL (Table 126–1). Periodic screening is important in all children aged 6 months to 2 years who live in houses built before 1970s, who live near active lead smelters or other lead-related industries, in those who have siblings with lead

poisoning, or with parents who have lead-related occupations or hobbies.[2,6]

If screening done on capillary blood indicates a high BLL, a confirmatory venous BLL is obtained because of potential

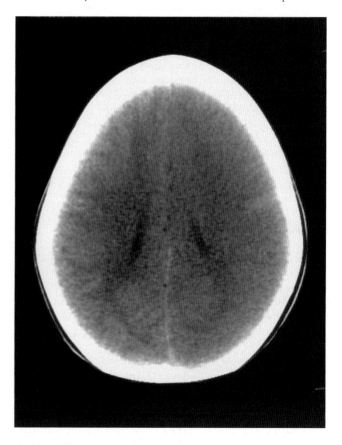

Figure 126–1. Computerized tomography scan of the brain reveals diffuse cerebral edema and loss of gray-white matter differentiation. (Courtesy of Department of Radiology, St. Christopher's Hospital for Children, Philadelphia, PA.)

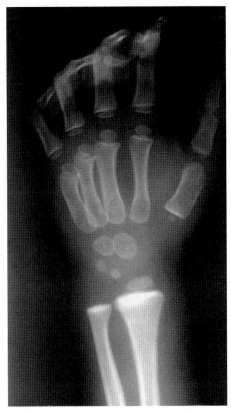 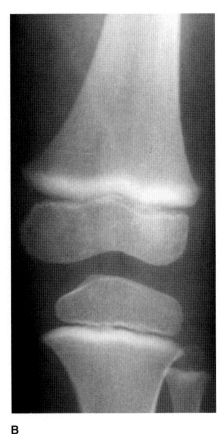

A   B

Figure 126–2. (A) Radiograph of the wrist reveals increased bands of calcification: "lead lines." (Courtesy of Department of Radiology, St. Christopher's hospital for children, Philadelphia, PA.) (B) Similar radiographic findings in another patient at the knee. (Courtesy of Richard Markowitz, MD, Department of Radiology, Children's hospital of Philadelphia, Philadelphia, PA.)

lead dust skin contamination in capillary samples. Definition of lead poisoning classes, the toxic effects of lead at various levels, and the recommended actions are outlined in Table 126–1. Elevation in BLL is followed by a rise in the free erythrocyte protoporphyrin (EP) or zinc protoporphyrin (ZPP). Since an elevated EP or ZPP reflects inhibited heme synthesis and affects only newly formed RBCs, this effect occurs at BLL >25 μg/dL and lags behind the initial rise in BLL by 2 to 3 weeks. Thus, low EP or ZPP and high BLL suggest recent acute exposure, whereas elevated EP or ZPP with high BLL suggests chronic exposure.

Radiographic evidence of lead poisoning consists of bands of increased density at the metaphyses of long bones that are best seen in radiographs of the distal femur and proximal tibia and fibula (Fig. 126–2). The popular term "lead lines" is a misnomer, since the increased radiopacity is caused by abnormal calcification from the disrupted metabolism of bone matrix rather than actual deposition of lead in the metaphysis. The formation of lead lines requires a few months of BLLs >45 μg/dL, and their width grossly correlates with the duration of lead poisoning. Radiopaque foreign material seen in the intestine by a flat abdominal film suggests a recent (<48 hours previously) ingestion of lead-containing paint chips, but ingestion of lead-laden dust in old homes where renovation has been done may not be visible on x-ray studies (Fig. 126–3).

Other essential tests include measurement of hemoglobin and hematocrit, evaluation of the patient's iron status, and a urinalysis to exclude glycosuria or proteinuria.[12]

Basophilic stippling may be seen on peripheral smear but is not diagnostic for plumbism. A spinal tap should be avoided in children with presumed lead encephalopathy due to the concern for herniation.

A new method for evaluating the total body lead burden by x-ray fluorometry (XRF) of bone lead has been introduced in adults and is being studied in children. This technique may eventually supersede blood lead screening in populations with low blood levels.

▶ MANAGEMENT

The principles of management in lead poisoning include environmental identification of the lead source, removing the patient from the source, correction of nutritional deficiencies that enhance lead absorption, and pharmacologic chelation.[12–14]

For patients with lead levels between 10 and 20 μg/dL, treatment consists of environmental management, nutritional evaluation, and follow-up BLL testing within 3 months. Removal of lead-based paint from the home should be done by professional deleaders. Nutritional intervention consists of a

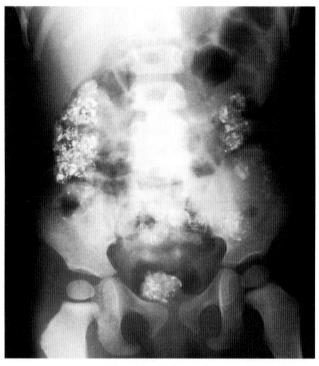

A

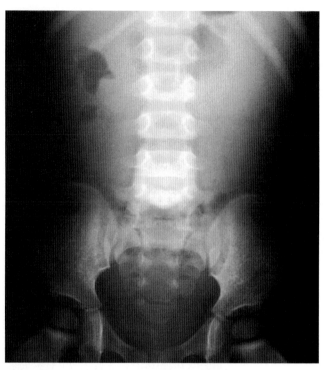

B

Figure 126–3. (A) Abdominal radiograph of a child who had massive paint chip ingestion. (B) Follow-up radiograph after whole-bowel irrigation. (Courtesy of Department of Radiology, St. Christopher's Hospital for Children, Philadelphia, PA.)

review of the child's diet and correction of deficiencies of iron, calcium, and zinc.

For patients with BLLs between 20 and 44 μg/dL, environmental and nutritional evaluation are required and repeat BLL testing within the month. Pharmacologic chelation is no longer routinely recommended at these levels because long-term clinical benefits have not been confirmed in recently published studies, but chelation at these levels does reduce body lead burden.[5,12,15]

Children with *asymptomatic* lead poisoning and BLLs 45 to 69 μg/dL may be treated as an outpatient with oral dimercaptosuccinic acid (DMSA) or admitted to the hospital for chelation therapy with either IV CaNa$_2$EDTA or DMSA.[13]

Oral DMSA is currently the only treatment approved for oral chelation of childhood lead poisoning.[16] DMSA is chemically similar to British antilewisite (BAL) and produces a lead diuresis comparable to that produced by CaNa$_2$EDTA without depletion of other metals. It is given 30 mg/kg/d in three divided doses for the first 5 days, then 20 mg/kg/d in two divided doses for 14 more days. It has a bad odor and may cause nausea and vomiting, rashes, and transient elevation of liver enzymes. For patients who do not tolerate DMSA, oral d-penicillamine has been shown to be an effective alternative even though not currently approved by the FDA for this indication.[17] Side effects include leukopenia, thrombocytopenia, transient elevation of liver enzymes, vomiting, and, rarely, nephrotoxicity. It must not be given to patients allergic to penicillin. Iron supplements are avoided in patients treated with d-penicillamine, since they can block its absorption.

Patients with BLLs >70 μg/dL or *symptomatic* lead poisoning require hospitalization and treatment with BAL at a dose of 25 mg/kg/d in six divided doses each day given by deep intramuscular injection. Once the first dose is given and adequate urine flow is established, CaNa$_2$EDTA is added as a continuous intravenous infusion at 50 mg/kg/d in dextrose or saline. When treating a child with encephalopathy, the intramuscular route for CaNa$_2$EDTA with procaine 0.5% is preferred to reduce the amount of fluid administered. This combined treatment is given for 5 days, with daily monitoring of blood urea nitrogen (BUN), creatinine, liver enzymes, and electrolytes. Side effects of CaNa$_2$EDTA include fever and transient renal dysfunction reflected in a rise in BUN, proteinuria, and hematuria. BAL may cause nausea and vomiting, transient hypertension, fever, transient elevation in liver enzymes, and hemolysis in G6PD-deficient patients. BAL is prepared in peanut oil and caution is warranted in those with a peanut allergy. Iron can form a toxic complex with BAL and is not administered simultaneously.

Lead encephalopathy should always be considered in young children with mental status changes and no other clinical evidence of infection. In addition to pharmacologic chelation, lead encephalopathy is treated with fluid restriction, mechanical hyperventilation, and diuretics. Dexamethasone may have a salutary effect in improving vascular integrity. Seizures are controlled with diazepam. Patients with lead encephalopathy are best managed in an intensive care unit.

Lead poisoning is most commonly a consequence of chronic exposure, and a rebound elevation of BLL is expected after each course of chelation therapy as lead is mobilized from body stores.[12] Repeat BLLs 2 weeks after the completion of chelation gives a reasonable peak rebound level. Since successful management of lead poisoning demands environmental, nutritional, and pharmacological intervention over a prolonged time course, these children should be followed by clinicians who are familiar with the multiple aspects of this disease and can provide a multidisciplinary team approach. The importance of removing the child from the source of lead exposure cannot be overemphasized.

REFERENCES

1. Lanphear BP, Hornung R, Khoury J, et al. Low-level environmental lead exposure and children's intellectual function: an international pooled analysis. *Environ Health Perspect.* 2005;113(7):894.
2. Needleman H. Lead poisoning. *Annu Rev Med.* 2004;55:209.
3. Pirkle JL, Kaufmann RB, Brody DJ, et al. Exposure of the U. S. population to lead, 1991–1994. *Environ Health Perspect.* 1998;106(11):745.
4. Canfield RL, Henderson CR Jr, Cory-Slechta DA, et al. Intellectual impairment in children with blood lead concentrations below 10 microg per deciliter. *N Engl J Med.* 2003;348(16):1517.
5. Rogan J, Dietrich KN, Ware JH, et al. The effect of chelation therapy with succimer on neuropsychological development in children exposed to lead. *N Engl J Med.* 2001;344:1421–1426.
6. Bellinger DC. Lead. *Pediatrics.* 2004;113(4 suppl):1016.
7. VanArsdale JL, Leiker RD, Kohn M, et al. Lead poisoning from a toy necklace. *Pediatrics.* 2004;114(4):1096.
8. Pirkel JL, Brody DJ, Gunter EW, et al. The decline in blood lead levels in the United States—The National Health and Nutrition Examination Surveys (NHANES). *JAMA.* 1994;272:284–291.
9. Amitai Y, Graef JW, Brown MJ, et al. Hazards of "deleading" homes of children with lead poisoning. *Am J Dis Child.* 1987;141(7):758.
10. Shannon M, Graef JW. Lead intoxication in infancy. *Pediatrics.* 1992;89:87–90.
11. Manton WI, Angle CR, Stanek SL, et al. Acquisition and retention of lead by young children. *Environ Res.* 2000;82:60–80.
12. Woolf AD, Goldman R, Bellinger DC. Update on the clinical management of childhood lead poisoning. *Pediatr Clin North Am.* 2007;54(2):271.
13. American Academy of Pediatrics Committee on Environmental Health. Lead exposure in children: prevention, detection, and management. *Pediatrics.* 2005;16(4):1036.
14. Angle CR. Childhood lead poisoning and its treatment. *Ann Rev Pharmacol Toxicol.* 1993;33:409–434.
15. Gracia RC, Snodgrass WR. Lead toxicity and chelation therapy. *Am J Health Syst Pharm.* 2007;64(1):45.
16. Liebelt EL, Shannon MW. Oral chelators for childhood poisoning. *Pediatr Ann.* 1994;23:616–626.
17. Shannon M, Grace A, Graef JW. Use of penicillamine in children with small lead burdens. *N Engl J Med.* 1989;321(14):979.

CHAPTER 127

Iron Poisoning

Steven E. Aks

▶ HIGH-YIELD FACTS

- When calculating the amount of iron ingested, one must convert to elemental content. More than 40 mg/kg is associated with significant toxicity and more than 60 mg/kg with death.
- Phase II of iron toxicity is the quiescent or danger phase of the overdose. The patient will appear to be better clinically, which may falsely reassure the clinician.
- Serum iron concentrations should be obtained between 2 and 6 hours after ingestion.
- The "vin rose" urine occurs after deferoxamine treatment. It represents the ferrioxamine complex being excreted in the urine.
- Whole bowel irrigation should be considered if multiple radiopaque iron tablets are seen on abdominal radiography.
- The preferred route of deferoxamine administration is intravenously at a rate of 15 mg/kg/h.

Iron is one of the most important pediatric toxins. It is an extremely common cause of poisoning and has a high potential for morbidity and mortality. According to data from the American Association of Poison Control Centers (AAPCC), from 1983 through 1990 iron was the most common cause of pediatric unintentional ingestion death, accounting for 30.2% of reported cases.[1] From 1985 through 1989, there were more than 11 000 reported exposures to iron in children.

The FDA has required unit dose packaging (blister-packs) for most products containing more than 30 mg elemental iron per tablet. Since this change in packaging the rate of serious iron ingestions reported has plummeted. In 2006, only 3953 iron ingestions were reported to the AAPCC. There were no fatalities.[2] This change in packaging has had a tremendous effect in saving lives.

▶ PATHOPHYSIOLOGY

Iron is absorbed through the gastrointestinal mucosa in the ferrous (Fe^{2+}) state. It is oxidized to the ferric (Fe^{3+}) state and is bound to transferrin. Toxicity occurs when the transferrin-binding capacity is exceeded. Iron is a potent catalyst of free radical generation, which is the chief mechanism of iron toxicity. Circulating free iron can damage blood vessels and can cause transudation of fluids from the intravascular space, resulting in hypotension. Hypotension is potentiated by the release of ferritin, a potent vasodilator. Other target organs include the gastrointestinal tract, heart, and lungs. Autopsy findings include cloudy swelling, fatty degeneration, and necrosis of hepatocytes. Iron deposits can be found in hepatocytes and the reticuloendothelial cells of the liver and spleen. Fatty degeneration occurs in the heart and renal tubules. The lungs may reveal congestive changes.

▶ TOXICITY AND ESTIMATING RISK

It is important to identify the specific preparation because the content of elemental iron varies (Table 127–1). If the preparation and the number of tablets are known, the total dose of elemental iron can be calculated. A dose exceeding 60 mg of elemental iron per kilogram of body weight is associated with life-threatening toxicity. Table 127–2 reflects poison center-based triage guidelines.

▶ CLINICAL PRESENTATION

Patients commonly present to the emergency department with a history of having ingested iron tablets, liquids, or vitamins containing iron.[3] If the amount of elemental iron ingested cannot be closely approximated, a worst-case scenario is assumed. It is useful to describe iron overdose in terms of the known stages of toxicity. The stages are generally sequential, although there can be overlap.

STAGE 1

This stage begins at the time of ingestion and lasts for about 6 hours. Mild cases demonstrate nausea and vomiting. More severe ingestions suffer vomiting, diarrhea, hematemesis, altered mental status, and possibly hypotension.

STAGE 2

Stage 2 occurs from about 6 to 12 hours postingestion, and is referred to as the quiescent or "danger" phase because the patient can appear to be improving, or may even be asymptomatic. A meticulous history is vital to diagnosing a patient in this stage, with emphasis on stage 1 symptoms, especially vomiting and diarrhea. A blood gas at this time may reveal a mild metabolic acidosis.

► **TABLE 127–1. IRON PREPARATIONS**

Iron Preparation	Elemental Iron (%)
Ferrous sulfate	20
Ferrous fumarate	33
Ferrous gluconate	12

STAGE 3

The period, from about 12 to 24 hours postingestion, marks stage 3, in which the patient can exhibit major signs of toxicity. Gastrointestinal hemorrhage and cardiovascular collapse can occur. Patients may develop altered mental status ranging from lethargy to coma. Both renal and hepatic failure can occur, and patients can develop a severe metabolic acidosis. Although hypoperfusion is a contributor, it is mostly because of the hydration of non–transferrin-bound iron by the reaction $Fe^{3+} + 3H_2O \rightarrow FeOH^3 + 3H^+$. Thus, one ferric ion generates three protons.

STAGE 4

This is the hepatotoxic phase. It usually occurs in the first 48 hours of a severe overdose. Transaminases greater than 2000 to 4000 are an ominous sign. Shock and followed by hepatic failure are the most common causes of death from iron poisoning.[4,5]

STAGE 5

At 4 to 6 weeks after the ingestion, the patient may develop symptoms of an obstruction. This is due to strictures that develop typically at the level of the pylorus.

► DIAGNOSIS

The most important laboratory tests to obtain include a basic metabolic profile, measurement of acid–base status, a serum iron concentration, and an abdominal radiograph. A basic metabolic profile demonstrating an anion gap is extremely important. An elevated anion gap along with a metabolic acidosis is suggestive of mitochondrial dysfunction due to iron toxicity.

► **TABLE 127–2. POISON CENTER-BASED TRIAGE GUIDELINES**

Ingested Dose (mg/kg)	Treatment Recommendation
<30	Observe at home
>30–40	If symptomatic, refer to a health care facility
>40 mg/kg	Refer to health care facility

With permission from Klein-Schwartz W, Oderga GM, Gorman RL, et al. Assessment of management guidelines in acute iron ingestion. *Clin Pediatr.* 1990;29:316–321.

Historically, a white blood cell count (WBC) greater than 15 000 mm^3 and a serum glucose greater than 150 mg/dL have been correlated with serum iron levels greater than 300 µg/dL. More recent studies have cast doubt on the predictive value of these markers. Normal WBC and serum glucose do not rule out iron toxicity.

Iron levels should be obtained between 2 and 6 hours after ingestion, but are optimally drawn at 4 hours postingestion. Levels greater than 500 µg/dL are typically associated with toxicity and levels greater than 1000 µg/dL are potentially fatal.

Measurement of the total iron-binding capacity (TIBC) has been used historically to determine the presence of a toxic ingestion, based on the assumption that toxicity occurs when serum iron exceeds the TIBC. However, it is not a reliable indicator, since ingesting iron will raise the measured TIBC level when it is done by standard colorimetric methods.[6] The TIBC is not useful in the acute management of iron ingestion and should not be used.

Abdominal radiographs can locate iron-containing tablets in the gut, and may reveal the presence of concretions. If pills are identified, the patient is at risk for delayed absorption of iron. Obtaining serial levels every 2 to 4 hours until the iron level peaks is appropriate. A positive radiograph after gastric lavage has recently been suggested as an indication for whole bowel irrigation.[7]

► TREATMENT

The preferred method of GI decontamination is whole bowel irrigation (WBI). Activated charcoal does not adsorb iron. Neither syrup of ipecac nor gastric lavage have been shown to be effective.

Whole bowel irrigation with polyethylene glycol electrolyte lavage solution (PEG-ELS) should be initiated if pills are seen on abdominal radiographs. PEG-ELS is given by nasogastric tube at a rate of 25 mL/kg/h in small children and 1 to 2 L/h in adolescents and adults. The end point of therapy is a clear rectal effluent. It is also useful to obtain a postirrigation abdominal x-ray to confirm the absence of pills. Active gastrointestinal bleeding, ileus, and bowel obstruction are contraindications to whole bowel irrigation.[7] Whole bowel irrigation has been given safely in the pregnant iron poisoned patient.[8]

Previous recommendations suggested complexation of iron in the stomach with bicarbonate, phosphate, or deferoxamine. All these methods should not be attempted as they are either ineffective or dangerous.

Even moderately poisoned children require meticulous supportive care to ensure a positive outcome. For patients in shock, large volumes of IV fluids and sodium bicarbonate are required to maintain fluid, electrolyte, and acid–base parameters.

Chelation with deferoxamine is used for significant iron ingestions. Indications are the presence of significant symptoms or signs of iron poisoning, a serum iron concentration greater than 500 µg/dL, and metabolic acidosis. Historically, deferoxamine was given as an intramuscular challenge test; however, this test has not been validated. Significant poisoning should be treated with intravenous deferoxamine.

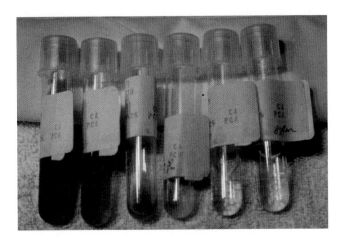

Figure 127–1. A rare example of the progression of coloration of vin rose urine (from the excreted ferrioxamine complex) over 15 hours of chelation with deferoxamine.

Intravenous deferoxamine should be administered at a rate of 15 mg/kg/h. The duration of chelation therapy is variable; there are no reliable end points (Fig. 127–1).[9] Serum iron determinations during the course of iron poisoning do not reflect clinical toxicity, and they are often unreliable during deferoxamine therapy.

Using a return of urine color to normal is not recommended as an end point for chelation therapy. It has never been validated and pigmentation of urine (vin rose urine) is concentration and pH dependent. The most useful criterion for continued chelation is the presence of a metabolic acidosis despite satisfactory perfusion. This indicates the presence of non–transferrin-bound iron in the plasma. Deferoxamine is rarely required beyond the first 24 hours after iron ingestion.

Hypotension is the most common side effect of intravenous therapy. In a dog model, hypotension has been observed at infusion rates of 100 mg/kg/h. It is not reported at the usually recommended rate in humans, 15 mg/kg/h. Hypotension can be treated by slowing down the drip or making the solution more dilute. Delayed pulmonary toxicity with symptoms resembling those of acute respiratory distress syndrome has been reported in patients who received prolonged chelation (>24 hours).[10]

Allergic reactions are rare. Renal failure can be seen in ill-hypovolemic patients. For patients undergoing chronic therapy, visual and hearing deficits and *Yersinia* infections have been reported.

▶ DISPOSITION

Children with peak serum iron levels less than 500 μg/dL approximately 4 hours postingestion and without symptoms of toxicity may be discharged in the care of reliable caretakers. Children requiring intravenous chelation with deferoxamine will need to be in an intensive care unit. Associated metabolic acidosis, hypotension, or shock will also require meticulous intensive care. All patients attempting suicide will need to be evaluated by a psychiatrist. Upon complete resolution of the metabolic consequences of iron toxicity, the patient can be discharged. However, follow-up should be assured to recognize any delayed scarring that may occur in phase V, stricture formation.

REFERENCES

1. Litovitz TL, Manoguerra A. Comparison of pediatric poisoning hazards: an analysis of 3.8 million exposure incidents: a report from the American Association of Poison Control Centers. *Pediatrics.* 1992;89:999–1006.
2. Bronstein AC, Spyker DA, Cantilena LR, et al. 2006 Annual Report of the American Association of Poison Control Centers' National Poison Data System (NPDS). *Clin Toxicol.* 2007;45:815–917.
3. Finkelstein Y, Wahl MS, Bentur Y, et al. Universal versus selective iron supplementation for infants and the risk of unintentional poisoning in young children: a comparative study of two populations. *Pharmacother.* 2007;41:414–419.
4. Tenebein M, Kopelow ML, DeSai DJ. Myocardial failure secondary to acute iron poisoning. *Vet Hum Toxicol.* 1986;28:491.
5. Tenenbein M. Hepatotoxicity in acute iron poisoning. *J Toxicol Clin Toxicol.* 2001;39:721–726.
6. Burkhart KK, Kulig KW, Hammond KB, et al. The rise in total iron-binding capacity after iron overdose. *Ann Emerg Med.* 1991;20:532–535.
7. Position paper: whole bowel irrigation. *J Toxicol Clin Toxicol.* 2004;42:843–854.
8. Turk J, Aks S, Ampuero F, Hryhorczuk DO. Successful therapy of iron intoxication in pregnancy with intravenous deferoxamine and whole bowel irrigation. *Vet Hum Toxicol.* 1993;35:441–444.
9. Tenenbein M. Benefits of parenteral deferoxamine for acute iron poisoning. *J Toxicol Clin Toxicol.* 1996;34:485–489.
10. Tenenbein M, Kowalski S, Sienko A, et al. Pulmonary toxic effects of continuous desferioxamine administration in acute iron poisoning. *Lancet.* 1992;339:699–701.
11. Klein-Schwartz W, Oderga GM, Gorman RL, et al. Assessment of management guidelines in acute iron ingestion. *Clin Pediatr.* 1990;29:316–321.

PART 5
ENVIRONMENTAL POISONS

CHAPTER 128

Cyanide Poisoning

Mark B. Mycyk

► HIGH-YIELD FACTS

- Cyanide poisoning causes profound tissue hypoxia.
- Poisoning causes rapid onset of central nervous system and cardiovascular toxicity.
- Helpful laboratory clues include lactic acidosis and a diminished arterial–venous O_2 difference.
- Antidotal therapy with nitrites and sodium thiosulfate or with hydroxocobalamin needs to be considered early.

Cyanide poisoning is unusual in the United States and very rare among children, although its contribution to toxicity and death may be underestimated in victims of smoke inhalation from building fires.[1] Hydrogen cyanide gas is formed as a combustion product of wool, silk, synthetic fabrics, and building materials in fires and is now recognized as a major cause of toxicity among fire victims previously thought to be poisoned by carbon monoxide.[2,3] Acetonitrile, or methyl cyanide, is found in agents used to remove sculpted nails and has caused cyanide poisoning in children.[4] Pediatric cyanide poisoning has also occurred from ingestion of cyanide-containing metal cleaning solutions imported from Asia and cyanogenic glycosides, like amygdalin, found in the seeds and pits of certain plants such as apples, apricots, and peaches.[5]

► TOXICOKINETICS

Hydrogen cyanide gas is rapidly absorbed in the lungs and may cause profound toxicity within seconds. Ingested cyanide salts, such as sodium cyanide and potassium cyanide, are also rapidly absorbed across the gastric mucosa and may result in toxicity within minutes. Acetonitrile appears to release cyanide through oxidative metabolism by the hepatic cytochrome P450 system, thus delaying clinical manifestations of toxicity for 2 to 6 hours from the time of ingestion. Ingestion of amygdalin and other cyanogenic glycosides requires hydrolysis to release cyanide, so toxicity may also be delayed up to several hours after ingestion.

The endogenous enzyme rhodanase (sulfurtransferase) converts cyanide to nontoxic thiocyanate: this mechanism is augmented in the presence of thiosulfate. In the presence of hydroxocobalamin (vitamin B_{12a}), cyanide is converted to cyanocobalamin (vitamin B_{12}), which is also nontoxic.

► PATHOPHYSIOLOGY

Cyanide primarily causes tissue hypoxia by binding with ferric iron (Fe^{3+}) in cytochrome a-a₃ of the mitochondrial cytochrome oxidase. Inhibition of cytochrome oxidase prevents efficient cellular oxygen use and disrupts ATP production, which results in anaerobic metabolism and severe lactic acidosis (Fig. 128–1). Cyanide also shifts the oxygen-hemoglobin dissociation curve to the left, further impairing oxygen delivery to the tissues. Cyanide inhibits a wide variety of other iron- and copper-containing enzymes, although their contribution to clinical toxicity is uncertain. The critical targets of cyanide are those organs most dependent on oxidative phosphorylation, namely, the brain and the heart.[6]

► CLINICAL PRESENTATION

The clinical presentation depends on the route and dose of exposure. Inhalation of cyanide gas causes loss of consciousness within seconds, whereas symptoms from an oral exposure develop anywhere from 30 minutes to several hours. Initial symptoms in victims not experiencing rapid loss of consciousness include headache, anxiety, confusion, blurred vision, palpitations, nausea, and vomiting. With progression of toxicity, patients may experience a feeling of neck constriction, suffocation, and unsteadiness. Early clinical signs of cyanide poisoning are CNS stimulation or depression, tachycardia or bradycardia, hypertension, dilated pupils, bright red retinal veins on funduscopy, and declining mental status. Late signs of poisoning are seizures, coma, apnea, cardiac arrhythmias, and complete cardiovascular collapse. The characteristic smell of bitter almonds may be detected in some cases, but the ability to detect this is a genetically determined trait not possessed by every examiner.

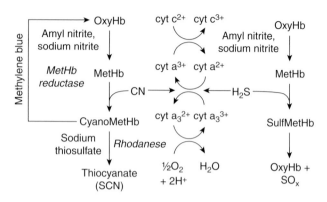

Figure 128–1. Pathway of cyanide and hydrogen sulfide toxicity and detoxification.

Although cyanide poisoning causes tissue hypoxia, the presence of cyanosis is a relatively late finding.[6] Since cyanide poisoning typically causes a leftward shift of the oxygen dissociation curve, the absence of cyanosis in a patient with clinical evidence of severe hypoxia should prompt the examiner to consider the diagnosis of cyanide poisoning.

▶ LABORATORY EVALUATION

Whole blood cyanide levels may be ordered from the ED, but these results are not available emergently and will therefore be of little value in guiding therapy. However, blood gas analysis and serum chemistries may be helpful in the acute setting. Arterial blood gases will typically show a marked metabolic acidosis. Obtaining a simultaneous venous blood gas analysis for comparison may demonstrate a diminished arterial–venous O_2 difference ($AO_2 - VO_2$ approaching zero) since the tissues' ability to extract oxygen from the blood is severely impaired.[7] Serum chemistries may demonstrate an elevated anion gap due to the presence of a lactic acidosis from anaerobic metabolism.[5]

Numerous electrocardiographic changes may occur in cyanide toxicity. Sinus bradycardia may be noted early, and later sinus tachycardia may be seen, as well as atrial fibrillation, atrioventricular block, ventricular ectopy, and ventricular dysrhythmias. A shortened QT segment or T waves originating high on the R wave may be seen.

▶ TREATMENT

The management of cyanide poisoning requires immediate supportive care as well as specific antidotal therapy. Airway management with 100% oxygen should be initiated and an intravenous line established in all patients. Fluid resuscitation should be administered to patients with hypotension, and sodium bicarbonate should be considered in profound acidosis. Mouth-to-mouth resuscitation by primary rescuers should be avoided because of the theoretical risk of secondary cyanide exposure.

CYANIDE ANTIDOTES

Although some victims of cyanide poisoning have survived with supportive care alone, early antidotal therapy clearly im-

proves survival and shortens the recovery period.[8] Two options now exist in the United States for cyanide treatment: the Taylor Antidote Kit, which contains amyl nitrite perles, sodium nitrite solution, and sodium thiosulfate, or intravenous hydroxocobalamin.

Taylor Kit

Methemoglobin produced by the nitrite components of the Taylor Kit binds cyanide to form the relatively nontoxic cyanomethemoglobin. Several experimental and clinical findings suggest that methemoglobin formation is not the sole mechanism of benefit from nitrites, especially since clinical benefit is often seen before peak methemoglobin levels. Some authors suggest that the vasodilatory effect of nitrites allows for greater endothelial enzymatic degradation of cyanide.[9]

Amyl nitrite perles held near the nose are used first while establishing an intravenous line and preparing the sodium nitrite solution. After an IV is established, sodium nitrite (9 mg/kg, or 0.3 mL/kg of a 3% solution, not to exceed 10 mL) is administered at a rate of 2.5 mL/min. In an unstable or hypotensive patient, or when there is concomitant CO poisoning, the dose may be given more slowly. Methemoglobin levels should be monitored periodically after the infusion and should not exceed 12% to 15%.[9] Side effects of nitrite administration include headache, blurred vision, nausea, vomiting, and hypotension.

Sodium thiosulfate provides a sulfur donor for the rhodanase-mediated conversion of cyanomethemoglobin to methemoglobin and thiocyanate. Thiocyanate is minimally toxic and is excreted by the kidneys.

Sodium thiosulfate may be administered following nitrite therapy or concurrently at a separate site. The pediatric dose is 1.65 mL/kg of a 25% solution up to 50 mL (12.5 g). Thiosulfate itself is relatively safe, but accumulation of thiocyanate, especially in patients with impaired renal excretion, may be associated with nausea, vomiting, arthralgias, and psychosis.

Hydroxocobalamin

Hydroxocobalamin, a precursor to vitamin B_{12}, detoxifies cyanide by binding it to form cyanocobalamin, a nontoxic compound excreted in the urine. Hydroxocobalamin was first approved for use in France in 1996 and approved in the United States in 2007.[10] Although it has been studied primarily in adults, a case series of pediatric patients with smoke inhalation in France demonstrated a significant reduction in mortality when hydroxocobalamin was used at a dose of 70 mg/kg.[11] Hydroxocobalamin is not associated with the complications of hypotension or excessive methemoglobinemia as has been seen with nitrite therapy.[10] Red discoloration of the skin seems to be the primary adverse effect. Future studies may show a benefit to combining hydroxocobalamin with sodium thiosulfate.[12,13]

▶ SMOKE INHALATION

Several studies suggest a correlation between elevated carboxyhemoglobin levels and cyanide levels in smoke inhalation victims.[1] Thus, when an elevated carboxyhemoglobin level is found in a severely ill fire victim, cyanide poisoning is possible, needs to be considered early, and treated appropriately. This is particularly true in a fire victim who requires intubation or has a persistent metabolic acidosis, abnormal mental status, or cardiovascular instability not resolving with conventional high-dose oxygen therapy for carbon monoxide poisoning.

▶ DISPOSITION

Patients who are asymptomatic and whose exposure has apparently been minimal are observed for 4 to 6 hours. Those who have ingested cyanogenic glycosides are observed for at least 6 hours for evidence of the onset of toxicity. Those ingesting acetonitrile-containing compounds are observed for 12 to 24 hours. Patients requiring antidotal treatment are cared for in an intensive care unit where vital signs, mental status, arterial blood gases, methemoglobin, and carboxyhemoglobin levels can be checked frequently. Following recovery, patients are observed for 24 to 48 hours. Rarely, late neurologic syndromes have been reported following cyanide toxicity, and periodic outpatient follow-up is advised.

REFERENCES

1. Baud FJ, Barriot P, Toffis V, et al. Elevated blood cyanide concentrations in victims of smoke inhalation. *N Engl J Med*. 1991; 325:1761.

2. American Academy of Pediatrics. Committee on Injury and Poison Prevention: reducing the number of deaths and injuries from residential fires. *Pediatrics*. 2000;105:1355.

3. Clark CJ, Campbell D, Reid WH. Blood carboxyhemoglobin and cyanide levels in fire survivors. *Lancet*. 1981;1:1332.

4. Caravati EM, Litovitz TL. Pediatric cyanide intoxication and death from an acetonitrile-containing cosmetic. *JAMA*. 1988; 260:3470.

5. Geller RJ, Barthold C, Saiers JA, Hall AH. Pediatric cyanide poisoning: causes, manifestations, management, and unmet needs. *Pediatrics*. 2006;118(5):2146.

6. Hall AH, Rumack BH. Clinical toxicology of cyanide. *Ann Emerg Med*. 1986;15:1067.

7. Johnson RP, Mellors JW. Arteriolization of venous blood gases: a clue to the diagnosis of cyanide poisoning. *J Emerg Med*. 1988;6:401.

8. Berlin CM. The treatment of cyanide poisoning in children. *Pediatrics*. 1970;46:793.

9. Kirk MA, Gerace R, Kulig KW. Cyanide and methemoglobin kinetics in smoke inhalation victims treated with the cyanide antidote kit. *Ann Emerg Med*. 1993;22:1413.

10. Borron SW, Baud FJ, Barriot P, et al. Prospective study of hydroxocobalamin for acute cyanide poisoning in smoke inhalation. *Ann Emerg Med*. 2007;49(6):794.

11. Haouach H, Fortin JL, LaPostolle F. Prehospital use of hydroxocobalamin in children exposed to fire smoke [abstract]. *Ann Emerg Med*. 2005;46:S30.

12. Shepherd G, Velez LI. Role of hydroxocobalamin in acute cyanide poisoning. *Ann Pharmacother*. 2008;42(5):661.

13. Hall AH, Dart R, Bogdan G. Sodium thiosulfate or hydroxocobalamin for the empiric treatment of cyanide poisoning? *Ann Emerg Med*. 2007;49(6):806.

CHAPTER 129

Mushroom Poisoning

Steven E. Aks

▶ HIGH-YIELD FACTS

- Most potentially life-threatening mushrooms will cause symptoms more than 6 to 8 hours, or even longer, after ingestion.
- Cyclopeptide (*Amanita phalloides*), Monomethylhydrazine (*Gyromitra spp.*) mushrooms can cause life-threatening hepatotoxicity.
- The majority of toxic mushrooms taken belong to the gastrointestinal irritant group.
- *A. muscaria* mushrooms do not cause significant muscarinic symptoms. They belong to the Ibotenic acid/muscimol group, and the name is a misnomer.

▶ INTRODUCTION/EPIDEMIOLOGY

Most toxic mushroom species fall into one of nine distinct classifications or groups. These groups contain specific chemical toxins that give rise to distinct clinical syndromes that are characterized by the time to onset after ingestion, and the nature of the symptoms.

The more severely toxic and potentially life-threatening species generally have a delayed onset of symptoms. For Groups I and II, symptoms usually begin 6 to 24 hours after ingestion; Group VIII can cause symptoms 24 hours to 2 weeks after ingestion. Less toxic species, comprising Groups III to VII, usually cause symptoms within 30 minutes to 3 hours after ingestion (Fig. 129–1). When identification of a particular mushroom is necessary, an expert mycologist can be located by contacting a regional poison center.[1]

GROUP I: CYCLOPEPTIDE-CONTAINING MUSHROOMS

This is one of the major groups of mushrooms that can lead to life-threatening toxicity. Some examples of mushrooms in this group include *A. phalloides* (Fig. 129–2), *A. verna, A. virosa*, and certain species of *Galerina* and *Lepiota*. These mushrooms contain amatoxins, phallatoxins, and virotoxins. Only the amatoxins are considered significant in human poisoning. Amatoxins are felt to cause toxicity by interfering with RNA polymerase reactions.

Initial toxic effects primarily include nausea, vomiting, and abdominal pain; they are characteristically delayed 6 to 24 hours postingestion. This is an important clinical distinction from the very large group of GI irritants (Group VII). Other clinical effects include fluid and electrolyte derangement, hypotension, CNS depression, seizures (rare), fulminant hepatic failure, and coagulopathy. After the period of initial GI distress, the patient may seem to improve clinically while having a subclinical deterioration in hepatic status. Fulminant hepatic failure is the most important consequence of cyclopeptide toxicity, and is seen approximately 3 days postingestion.[2]

Treatment generally centers on supportive care and replacement of fluid and electrolytes. Activated charcoal is generally recommended. There are a number of interventions that have been attempted for cyclopeptide poisoning, including hemoperfusion, high-dose penicillin, high-dose cimetidine, *N*-acetylcysteine, silibinin, and thioctic acid. None of these therapies have been subjected to controlled studies in humans, and the data regarding their clinical efficacy is conflicting and controversial.[2] Liver transplantation has been used successfully in cases of cyclopeptide-induced fulminant hepatic failure.[3]

GROUP II: MONOMETHYLHYDRAZINE-CONTAINING MUSHROOMS

The monomethylhydrazine-containing group is clinically important because ingestion can lead to life-threatening hepatotoxicity. This group contains the "false morels." The true morel or *Morchella* species is a choice edible mushroom found throughout North America. The *Gyromitra* species of mushrooms can be confused with this delicacy, hence the term "false morel." These mushrooms contain the toxin gyromitrin, which is converted to monomethylhydrazine (MMH) and *N*-methyl-*N*-formylhydrazine (MFH).

As in the Group I mushrooms, the onset of gastrointestinal symptoms may be delayed for 6 to 12 hours. Nausea, vomiting, diarrhea, and abdominal cramps are common. Hepatic failure can occur.[4] Important hematologic effects include hemolysis and methemoglobin production. The mechanism of toxicity of the hydrazine-containing mushrooms is similar to that of isoniazid, which is well known to cause seizures in overdose.

Treatment is primarily focused on supportive care. Seizures can be managed with vitamin B_6 (pyridoxine). An infusion of 1 g can be initiated in children. In older teenagers and adults, a dose of 5 g can be administered. Benzodiazepines can be used synergistically with vitamin B_6 for seizures. For symptomatic methemoglobinemia, methylene blue can be utilized.

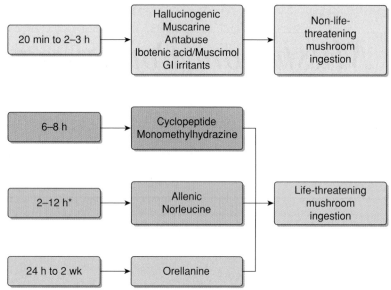

Time of onset to symptoms, mushroom group and risk of life-threat
*Allenic norleucine violates the rule that life-threatening mushrooms must have a delay in
symptom onset

Figure 129–1. Timeline algorithm after ingestion.

GROUP III: MUSCARINE-CONTAINING MUSHROOMS

The muscarine-containing mushrooms cause a cholinergic tox-idrome. The onset of symptoms is early, usually between 30 minutes to 2 hours. A useful mnemonic to recall the clinical effect of muscarinic poisoning is SLUGBAM:

Salivation

Lacrimation

Urination

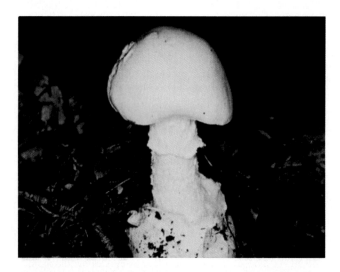

Figure 129–2. *Amanita phalloides,* the "death cap" produces amatoxins and accounts for most of the fatalities due to mushroom ingestion. (With permission from Knoop et al. *Atlas of Emergency Medicine*, 2nd ed. McGraw-Hill; 2002.)

Gastrointestinal distress

Bronchorrhea, bradycardia, bronchospasm

Abdominal cramping

Miosis

Some muscarine-containing species include *Clitocybe dealbata,* certain other species of *Clitocybe,* and numerous species of *Inocybe.* Treatment is generally supportive and usually no specific antidotes need to be administered. Rarely, atropine may be administered for excessive muscarinic effects.

GROUP IV: *COPRINUS* SPECIES (ANTABUSE)

Several species of *Coprinus* contain the toxins coprine and 1-aminocyclopropanol. The representative mushroom,*Coprinus atramentarius,* is also known as the "alcohol inky cap" because it turns into a puddle of inky-like liquid as it decomposes. The toxin acts as an inhibitor of aldehyde dehydrogenase and can therefore lead to an antabuse reaction when consumed with alcohol.[5] Treatment of toxicity is supportive.

GROUP V: IBOTENIC ACID/MUSCIMOL

This category of mushrooms has previously been felt to cause anticholinergic effects; however, more recent information shows that toxicity is caused by GABA and glutamate effects. Some representative species of this group include *A. muscarina* and *A. pantherina.* Effects of glutamate agonism include central nervous system (CNS) excitation, while GABA agonist effects include CNS depression. Symptoms of overdose begin as early as 30 minutes and up to 3 hours after ingestion.

The patient may exhibit ataxia, hallucinations, hysteria or hyperkinetic behavior, CNS depression, myoclonic jerking, and seizures. Vomiting is rare. Treatment of this mushroom group is focused on supportive care.[6]

GROUP VI: HALLUCINOGENIC MUSHROOMS

Clinicians may encounter this group of mushrooms due to recreational use by adolescents or young adults at rock concerts or other venues. Some representative examples of these mushrooms include certain species of *Conocybe, Gymnopilus, Panaeolus, and Psilocybe.* The toxins are indole alkaloids, such as psilocybin and psilocin.

Clinically, patients will present with delirium, visual hallucinations, psychosis, and erratic behavior. On physical examination, the patient may have mydriasis, tachycardia, flushing, vomiting, tremors and, rarely, seizures. Treatment is supportive. Patients can be placed in a quiet darkened room to decrease stimulation; adjunctive treatment benzodiazepines may be helpful.[7]

GROUP VII: GASTROINTESTINAL IRRITANTS

This group comprises the largest group of toxic mushrooms. Most of these cause symptoms within 3 hours of ingestion in contrast to mushrooms in groups I, II, and VIII. Examples of GI irritants include *Chlorophyllum molybdites, Omphalotus olearius,* certain species of Agaricus, Boletus, Gomphus, Hebeloma, Lactarius, Lepiota, Tricholoma, etc., and a few species of Amanita (Fig. 129–3).

The cornerstone of management is properly identifying and distinguishing this classification of mushrooms from those that can result in serious toxicity. Patients usually suffer from vomiting and diarrhea. Maintaining adequate hydration and fluid and electrolyte balance is essential.[8]

GROUPS VIII & IX: RENAL TOXINS

There are two groups of mushrooms that are potentially renal toxic. They are the *Cortinarius orellanus* group and the recently described *A. smithiana.* The *Cortinarius* species contain the toxins orellanine and orelline, which cause renal toxicity. Like the Group I and II mushrooms, Group VIII species cause delayed symptoms, which can occur 24 hours to 2 weeks after ingestion. Renal failure is estimated to occur in 30% to 45% of ingestions. While some of these species are found in the United States, reported cases of poisoning have occurred in Europe, and no deaths due to ingestion of mushrooms in this group have been reported in North America.

A newly appreciated nephrotoxic mushroom is *A. smithiana.* This mushroom is found in the Pacific Northwest of the United States. The toxins in this mushroom include allenic norleucine and chlorocrotylglycine. These toxins specifically lead

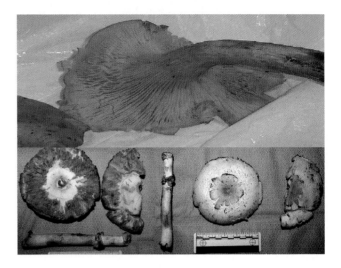

Figure 129–3. Gastrointestinal irritant mushrooms: Jack O'Lantern (Omphalotusolearius) and Chlorophyllum sp. (With permission from Erickson et al. *Pediatric Toxicology.* McGraw-Hill; 2005.)

to renal toxicity. In one series, the time to onset of symptoms ranged from 20 minutes to 12 hours.[9] Therefore, this species is an exception to the general rule of mushroom poisoning, because serious manifestations of toxicity occur soon after ingestion. The treatment for both of these mushroom groups is supportive. Hemodialysis should be instituted for patients developing worsened renal failure.

REFERENCES

1. Fischbein C, Mueller G, Leacock P, Wahl M, Aks S. Digital imaging: a promising tool for mushroom identification. *Acad Emerg Med.* 2003;10(7):808–811.
2. Enjalbert F, Rapior S, Nouguier-Soule J, et al. Treatment of Amatoxin poisoning: 20-year retrospective analysis. *J Toxicol Clin Toxicol.* 2002;40:715–757.
3. Klein AS, Hart J, Brems JJ, et al. Amanita poisoning: treatment and the role of liver transplantation. *Am J Med.* 1989;86:187–193.
4. Stolpe HJ, Hentschel H, Hein C, et al. Hepatic Injury after ingestion of *Gyromitra esculenta* in children. *J Toxicol Clin Toxicol.* 2000;38:260.
5. Michelot D. Poisoning by *Coprinus atramentarius. Nat Toxins.* 1992;2:73–80.
6. Benjamin DR. Mushroom poisoning in infants and children: the *Amanita pantherina/muscaria* group. *J Toxicol Clin Toxicol.* 1992;30:13–22.
7. Miller PL, Gay GR, Ferris KC, et al. Treatment of acute, adverse psychedelic reactions: "I've tripped and I can't get down." *J Psychoactive Drugs.* 1992;24:277–279.
8. Stenklyft PH, Augenstein WL. *Chlorophyllum molybdites*—sever mushroom poisoning in a child. *Clin Toxicol.* 1990;28:159–168.
9. Warden CR, Benjamin DR. Acute renal failure associated with suspected *Amanita smithiana* mushroom ingestions: a case series. *Acad Emerg Med.* 1998;8:808–812.

CHAPTER 130

Poisonous Plants

Ejaaz A. Kalimullah and Andrea G. Carlson

▶ HIGH-YIELD FACTS

- Since the vast majority of plant exposures are unintentional and involve small quantities, most patients do not develop any symptoms.
- Gastrointestinal upset is the most common manifestation of symptomatic exposure.
- *Dieffenbachia* and *Philodendron* are houseplants and are common causes of symptomatic plant ingestions. They can cause oral and pharyngeal pain from injection of insoluble calcium oxalate crystals.
- During the Christmas holidays, children are often exposed to poinsettia, mistletoe, and holly.
- Foxglove, oleander, and lily of the valley are among several species of plants that contain cardiac glycosides and may cause toxicity similar to digoxin intoxication.
- Water hemlock is easily confused with the wild carrot. The potential for serious toxicity is significant and patients may progress to status epilepticus, rhabdomyolysis, respiratory distress, and death.

Evaluation of a patient with a plant exposure presents several challenges to the health care provider. Significant geographical variation in plant species exists. Historical information regarding the species of plant as well as the amount ingested is often lacking. The degree of toxicity expected may depend on the particular part of the plant structure ingested such as seeds, fruit, stem, or root. Plants vary in toxicity during different stages of their growth cycle. Mechanical preparation of the plant material may also affect the overall toxicity. Furthermore, there is considerable overlap in the clinical manifestations of toxicity of many plants. Although the majority of plants do not cause clinical toxicity, a small number are mildly toxic and a few are harmful with even a small exposure.

▶ EPIDEMIOLOGY

According to American Association of Poison Control Center (AAPCC) data, 64 236 human exposures to plants were reported in 2006, accounting for 2.7% of the catalogued human exposures. The clear majority of these exposures occurred in pediatric patients, with 44 710 plant exposures reported in children ≤5 years of age.[1] The majority of plant ingestions are fairly benign events, with only a single fatality attributed to a plant or herbal/botanical product in the 2006 AAPCC National Poison Data System (NPDS) annual report.[1] With regard to pediatric cases, two common scenarios exist. Nearly 70% of plant in-

gestions are by children younger than 6 years.[1] Toddlers and other young children may ingest plant material while exploring their environment. Many of these ingestions involve small or insignificant amounts. In the second common scenario, older children and adolescents may intentionally consume specific plant species for their purported psychoactive effects. Despite the fact that the latter group of ingestions may carry a higher risk of morbidity, significant toxicity is relatively rare.

▶ IDENTIFICATION OF PLANTS

Plant name and/or accurate species information may not always be readily available to the clinician. Historical information to be elicited includes whether the plant is an indoor or outdoor variety and a description of the plant's flower, stem, leaves, height, and location. Consultation with a botanist, medical toxicologist, or poison control center is highly recommended whenever assistance is needed in identifying an unknown plant. Transmission of digital color or facsimile images can be used to assist consultants.[2] When expert consultation is unavailable, rough recognition of taxonomic families of poisonous plants and/or comparison of the species in question with pictures from a field guide may help exclude potentially life-threatening plant exposures. In general, it is useful to consider clinically relevant plants according to the predominant and most serious manifestations of toxicity.

▶ SPECIFIC TOXIC PLANTS

MUCOSAL IRRITANTS

When ingested, a wide variety of plant species causes mucous membrane irritation due to microscopic needle-shaped bundles of calcium oxalate (raphides) present throughout the plant structures. When masticated, the rhaphides release the calcium oxalate crystals, which damage mucous membranes and, in conjunction with unclarified additional mediators, cause immediate burning and inflammation. Commonly encountered plants containing calcium oxalate include philodendron (*Philodendron* sp.), dumb cane (*Dieffenbachia*) (Fig. 130–1), peace lily (*Spathiphyllum* sp.), pothos (*Epipremnum aureum*), caladium (*Caladium bicolor*), calla lily (*Zantedeschia aethiopica*), Jack-in-the-pulpit (*Arisaema triphyllum*), elephant's ear (*Colocasia esculenta*), and skunk cabbage (*Symplocarpus foetidus*).[3] Of the species listed above, *Philodendron* and *Dieffenbachia* have historically accounted for the highest percentage of exposures.[4] While oropharyngeal irritation and

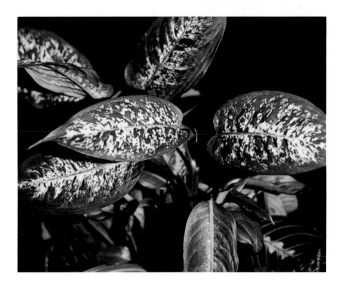

Figure 130–1. Leaves of *Dieffenbachia* plant.

localized swelling can last for several days following oral exposure, one retrospective case review reported only 4/188 (2.1%) symptomatic cases, with only minor oral symptoms developing within 5 minutes of exposure.[5] Although case reports exist of severe airway edema requiring tracheostomy in an adult,[6] esophageal injury complicated by delayed death in a pediatric patient,[7] and even aortoesophageal fistula,[8] such events are exceedingly rare. A recent review of the thousands of *Dieffenbachia* exposures reported to poison control centers revealed that only about a third of patients developed documented symptoms, of which oral irritation was most common (18.2%). There were no reports of respiratory obstruction or death.[9] For such plants, treatment is symptomatic with demulcents such as milk, popsicles, and cool drinks. Analgesics may be required and associated pruritis or dermal irritation may respond to antihistamines.

Exposures to various *Capsicum* species such as the chili pepper (*Capsicum annuum*) continue to constitute an important source of plant exposures. In addition, the 2006 AAPCC NPDS annual report listed "pepper mace" as one of the 25 most frequent plant exposures.[1] Both the *Capsicum* plants and "pepper spray" or "pepper mace" contain capsaicin, which is the toxin responsible for causing symptoms. Symptomatic exposures often occur after handling or ingesting the fruits or seeds of the *Capsicum* plants. Capsaicin causes release of substance P from nociceptive type C nerve fibers.[10] Clinical effects consist of intense burning pain, hyperalgesia, irritation, and erythema. Profuse lacrimation and conjunctival inflammation may occur with ocular exposure. Capsaicin does not cause chemical burns and vesication is not seen.[3,10] In some cases, contact dermatitis can develop and symptoms can persist for hours to days depending on the duration of exposure. Treatment is focused on decontamination and pain control, and exposure does not result in long-term injury. Although cold-water irrigation can provide relief, capsaicin is poorly soluble.[10] A number of remedies have been suggested in the medical literature, including vinegar, topical antacids, vegetable oil, and 2% lidocaine gel.[11–14]

GASTROINTESTINAL IRRITANTS

American Mistletoe (*Phoradendron serotinum, Phoradendron leucarpum*)

Although often thought of as highly toxic by laypersons, reports of significant toxicity from mistletoe involve *Viscum album* (European mistletoe), which contains cardiovascular toxins (viscotoxins) and a toxalbumin (viscumin).[3,15] Based on reviews of poison center data, it seems that pediatric accidental ingestions of American mistletoe are largely asymptomatic, with essentially no major morbidity.[16] Reported symptoms are mostly gastrointestinal upset, with symptoms developing within 6 hours of exposure.[15] Treatment is supportive, and decontamination for small ingestions is unnecessary. In the absence of significant GI symptoms, most cases can be managed at home. Intentional or large ingestions of >20 berries or >5 leaves should be referred to the ED.[16]

Poinsettia (*Euphorbia pulcherrima*)

The 2006 AAPCC NPDS annual report listed the poinsettia as the second most common plant exposure.[1] Similar to American mistletoe, the poinsettia is erroneously thought of as a highly toxic plant by laypersons, possibly because of an apocryphal report of a pediatric fatality dating from the early 20th century.[17] A review of 22 793 poison center cases confirmed the relatively benign nature of poinsettia exposures. Most were accidental pediatric exposures; 96.1% were managed without ED referral and most (92.4%) remained asymptomatic. No fatalities were reported.[17] Management of these exposures requires no more than supportive care and GI decontamination has not been shown to be of benefit.

Holly (*Ilex* sp.)

Ilex species accounted for the third largest group of plant exposures in the 2006 AAPCC NPDS annual report. *Ilex opaca* (American holly) and *Ilex aquifolium* (English holly) are most frequently encountered due to their use as Christmas decorations. The plants produce green berries, which mature into red berries that highlight the foliage and are attractive to small children. It is thought that the berries are responsible for toxicity and large ingestions can cause nausea, vomiting, abdominal cramping, and diarrhea.[3] Cases involving small (≤2 berries) accidental ingestions are expected to produce minimal if any symptoms. Basic supportive care with attention to hydration status is sufficient.

Pokeweed (*Phytolacca americana*)

Pokeweed exposures have been fairly commonly reported to the AAPCC; the most recent annual report lists pokeweed as one of the top 25 plant exposures.[1] Pokeweed contains toxic saponins (phytolaccatoxin, phytolaccagenin), as well as a lymphotropic mitogen.[18] All parts of the plant, particularly the root, are toxic. Most human exposures result from consumption of leaves ("poke salad"), or from mistaking the roots for horseradish or parsnips.[3] Although parboiling is traditionally used to lower the toxin content when preparing "poke salad," cases of symptomatic poisoning have nonetheless occurred.[19] Pokeweed poisoning primarily causes nausea, vomiting, abdominal cramps, and diarrhea. Symptoms generally begin within 2 to 4 hours after ingestion and usually resolve within 24 to 48 hours. Severe cases with heme positive stools, tachycardia, and hypotension have also been reported.[19] Rare cases with electrocardiographic (EKG) changes have been reported in adults with significant GI symptoms, although the mechanism for the EKG findings may not be related to pokeweed itself.[19,20] Contemporary medical literature includes a single case of fatal ventricular fibrillation in an 18-year-old male following the ingestion of a 4 to 5 in piece of pokeweed root.[21] Supportive care is the mainstay of treatment. Decontamination with activated charcoal may be considered in nonvomiting patients who present after potentially significant ingestions. Antiemetics and intravenous fluid therapy may be necessary. Admission may be required for observation and continued care in the setting of large or markedly symptomatic ingestions.

SYSTEMIC TOXINS

Plants Containing Anticholinergic Substances

Jimsonweed (*Datura stramonium*) (Fig. 130–2), deadly nightshade (*Atropa belladonna*), and black henbane (*Hyoscyamus niger*) are some of the plants that contain muscarinic antagonist alkaloids such as atropine, hyoscyamine, and scopolamine. Jimsonweed, also called locoweed and devil's trumpet, is a tall plant with a musty odor and spiny seedpods. The plant grows wild throughout the United States, and its seeds have been abused by adolescents and teenagers due to its psychotropic effects.[22,23] Patients with significant ingestion will manifest an anticholinergic toxidrome: tachycardia, mydriasis, dry skin and mucous membranes, hypoactive bowel sounds, urinary retention, and hyperthermia. Central anticholinergic effects result in altered mental status, ranging from somnolence to severe agitation and delirium with hallucinations.[23] Symptoms usually

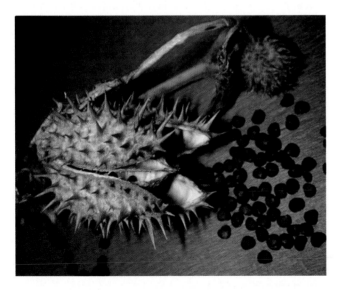

Figure 130–2. Seedpod and seeds from jimsonweed (*Datura stramonium*).

arise within 30 to 60 minutes of ingestion and can last for 24 to 48 hours.[18] Decontamination with activated charcoal may be considered in cooperative individuals. Agitation should be initially treated with benzodiazepines. Hyperthermia should be treated supportively with cooling measures. Physostigmine has been safely and effectively used as an antidote in cases of anticholinergic plant poisoning.[24–26] Physostigmine is generally reserved for patients with refractory delirium, hyperthermia, seizures, or significant arrhythmias; there is ongoing controversy regarding its effect on clinical course and outcome.[27,28] Physostigmine can be given in pediatric doses of 0.02 mg/kg IV over the course of several minutes with concurrent cardiac and blood pressure monitoring. If there is no improvement, readministration after 5 to 10 minutes may be attempted, to a total of 2 mg. The dose for adolescents and adults is 1 to 2 mg IV administered slowly over 4 minutes ($\leq$0.5 mg/min). Physostigmine's effects typically last 30 to 60 minutes and repeat dosing may be required. Patients with marked delirium, seizures, cardiopulmonary instability, or those treated with physostigmine should be admitted to an intensive care unit.

Plants Containing Solanine

Plants containing solanaceous alkaloids grow throughout the United States, and include the black nightshade (*Solanum nigrum*), Jerusalem cherry (*Solanum pseudocapsicum*), bittersweet (*Solanum dulcamara*), and potato (*Solanum tuberosum*). While all parts of the black nightshade and bittersweet plants are poisonous, it is the unripe berries that are the most toxic. Ingestion of sun-greened potatoes or uncooked potato sprouts may also cause illness as they contain α-solanine and the related glycoalkaloid, α-chaconine. The mechanism of solanine toxicity remains unclear. Small ingestions of these plants generally result in no more than self-limited gastrointestinal effects. Severe intoxications can manifest with CNS and respiratory depression, hyperthermia, bradycardia, hypotension, and tachycardia. The clinical picture may be clouded by the concurrent presence of anticholinergic agents in some of these plants, which may dominate the initial presentation.[29,30]

Plants Containing Cardiac Glycosides

Foxglove (*Digitalis purpurea*) (Fig. 130–3), lily-of-the-valley (*Convallaria majalis*), common oleander (*Nerium oleander*), and yellow oleander (*Thevetia peruviana*) all contain digitalis-like glycosides.[3] Ingestion of yellow oleander results in the most significant degree of toxicity and, of plants containing digitalis-like glycosides, is responsible for the greatest number of fatalities worldwide. All parts of these plants, particularly the seeds in the case of yellow oleander, are potentially toxic. While children with small exploratory ingestions of whole plant material from lily-of-the-valley or common oleander are unlikely to develop toxicity, ingestion of only a few yellow oleander seeds can produce life-threatening poisoning. Patients may present with nausea, vomiting, dizziness, diarrhea, and abdominal pain.[18] EKG findings following yellow oleander poisoning have been found to primarily consist of sinus bradycardia and conduction defects affecting the sinus or AV node.[31] Hyperkalemia may also be noted, as well as a detectable serum digoxin level. While the serum digoxin level can help prove exposure, the absolute level cannot be

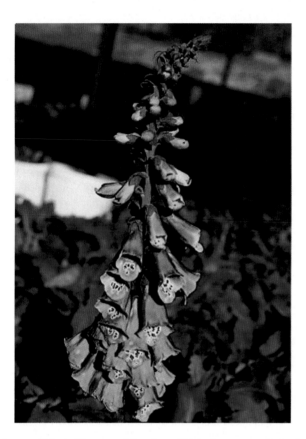

Figure 130–3. Flowers of foxglove (*Digitalis purpurea*) plant.

used to guide antidotal therapy. Treatment with antidigoxin Fab fragments is safe and effective for patients with significant cardiac arrhythmias.[32] It has been shown to restore sinus rhythm, correct bradycardia, and ameliorate hyperkalemia. The exact dose required is unknown and is likely much higher than those used to treat digoxin overdose.[32] Decontamination with a single dose of activated charcoal is reasonable in patients not at risk for aspiration. However, the therapeutic value of multidose-activated charcoal in yellow oleander ingestion remains unclear.[33,34] Patients who are asymptomatic following nontrivial ingestions should have serial EKGs, repeat electrolyte determinations, and be observed for 12 hours.

Plants Containing Sodium Channel Activators

Monkshood (*Aconitum* sp.), false hellebore (*Veratrum* sp.), azalea (*Rhododendron* sp.), rhododendron (*Rhododendron* sp.), and mountain laurel (*Kalmia latifolia*) all contain various toxins capable of stabilizing the open form of voltage-dependent sodium channels within the excitable membranes of neuronal and cardiac tissues.[3] Aconitine is the toxic alkaloid found in *Aconitum* sp., while the steroidal veratrum alkaloids are contained in *Veratrum* sp. Exposure to grayanotoxins, found in the *Rhododendron* and *Kalmia* sp., can occur after ingestion of the leaves or via honey made from flower nectar. The resulting clinical syndromes are fairly similar, with vomiting, paresthesias, muscle weakness, hypotension, and, rarely, seizures. Bradydysrhythmias, conduction blocks, and

tachydysrhythmias have been described.[18] Symptom onset is generally rapid in patients with significant ingestions and often resolves within 24 to 48 hours. No antidote exists and therapy is supportive. Decontamination with activated charcoal should be initiated provided that it can be safely performed. Intubation and circulatory support with fluids and vasopressors may be needed. Aconitine has been associated with various ventricular dysrhythmias, including bidirectional ventricular tachycardia. Both lidocaine and electrical cardioversion performed poorly in published case series; amiodarone or flecainide may be reasonable alternatives.[35] Bradycardia or AV block may respond to atropine, although temporary pacing has been required.[18] While death is rare even in adults, and large ingestions are less likely in children, pediatric cases with significant toxicity have been reported.[36]

Yew (*Taxus* sp.)

Yew plants are short evergreen shrubs commonly used in landscaping designs. The seeds and leaves of the plant, but not the fleshy red aril, contain the cardiotoxic alkaloids taxine A and B. Yew exposures in children likely result from the attractive appearance of the red aril surrounding the seed. While deaths have been reported in the medical literature, they are typically in the setting of suicidal ingestions.[37] A poison center review of >11 000, largely pediatric, yew exposures revealed that the majority of cases (92.5%) were asymptomatic and no deaths were reported.[38] The most frequently encountered symptoms were GI upset (65.5%), dermal irritation (8.3%), hypotension or arrhythmias (6%), and seizures (6%). There is no antidote and treatment is supportive care–driven.

Tobacco (*Nicotiana* sp.)

Cases of significant morbidity from tobacco exposure reported in the literature resulted from exposure to green tobacco leaves or highly concentrated nicotine preparations. Most pediatric exposures involve the exploratory ingestion of cigarettes, cigarette butts, or nicotine gum.[39] Symptoms usually develop within 30 to 90 minutes in children who ingest tobacco products. Patients who ingest ≥2 whole cigarettes or ≥6 cigarette butts are more likely to develop symptoms.[40] Vomiting is commonly seen and patients without spontaneous vomiting in the first hour are unlikely to have ingested a toxic amount. Clinical response to nicotine intoxication may follow a biphasic course. Tachycardia, mydriasis, hypertension, tremor, and seizures may be seen. The stimulatory phase is then followed by autonomic and neuromuscular blockade from persistent stimulation, resulting in fasciculations and skeletal muscle paralysis. Death is usually because of respiratory arrest or cardiovascular collapse. Treatment is supportive, and most patients may be safely discharged after brief observation.

Poison Hemlock (*Conium maculatum*)

Poison hemlock can be found throughout the United States. The plant can be identified by the "mousy" odor it emits. The plant contains coniine as well as other nicotinic alkaloids, which are found particularly in the roots and seeds. Most human ingestions result from misidentification, because of its similarity to wild carrot (*Daucus carota*). Manifestations of toxicity

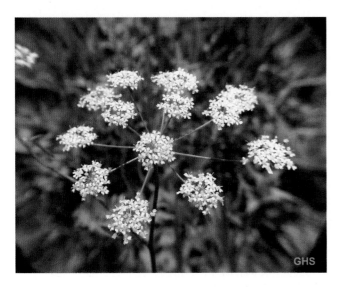

Figure 130–4. Flowering top of water hemlock (*Cicuta maculata*) plant.

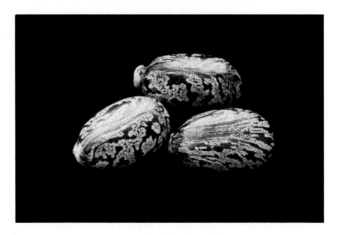

Figure 130–5. Castor beans from *Ricinus communis* plant.

are similar to those seen with nicotine, with an initial stimulatory phase that may include tachycardia, diaphoresis, tremor, and seizures. The subsequent depressant phase may involve bradycardia, hypotension, muscular paralysis, and coma. Initial gastrointestinal symptoms are often prominent. Meticulous supportive care is the mainstay of therapy. While death occurs rarely, it usually results from respiratory compromise.[41] Asymptomatic patients who present with a possible ingestion should be observed for 4 to 6 hours.

Water Hemlock (*Cicuta* sp.)

Water hemlock is easily confused with the wild carrot (*D. carota*) or water parsnip (*Pastinaca sativa*), and may be mistaken for an edible tuber. The plant is often found growing along the borders of freshwater lakes and streams (Fig. 130–4). The plant contains cicutoxin and other toxic C_{17}-polyacetylenes throughout, with the highest concentrations in the root. Cicutoxin is a highly potent convulsant due to its antagonism of $GABA_A$ (gamma-aminobutyric acid (subtype A)) receptors. Water hemlock is thought to be the most toxic plant in North America. Patients may suffer gastrointestinal symptoms and then rapidly develop seizures, respiratory distress, and rhabdomyolysis. Death may result from cardiopulmonary arrest complicating status epilepticus. Treatment consists of aggressive supportive care with early attention to definitive airway management and rapid escalation of anticonvulsant therapy. Benzodiazepines and phenobarbital should be used; phenytoin is unlikely to be beneficial.[42] Early decontamination should be performed whenever it can be safely accomplished. Symptomatic patients should be admitted to an intensive care unit; at least 4 to 6 hours of observation is indicated for all patients with suspected ingestions.

Plants Containing Toxalbumins

The castor bean (*Ricinus communis*) (Fig. 130–5) and rosary pea or jequirty bean (*Abrus precatorius*) contain the toxalbumins ricin and abrin, respectively. Less potent toxalbumins are also found in the physic nut (*Jatropha curcas*), black locust tree (*Robinia pseudoacacia*), and European mistletoe (*Viscum album*).[3] Castor beans are used in the production of castor oil, and are cultivated commercially and as garden ornamentals throughout the United States.[3] The bright scarlet and black seed of the rosary pea is very appealing to children, and is used for jewelry and in the making of maracas in the tropics. Because of reported fatalities after the ingestion of small numbers (range ~2–20) of castor beans, ricin is regarded as highly toxic.[43] However, the seeds of both plants have a thick waxy shell and must be chewed to liberate the toxin. Seeds swallowed whole are unlikely to produce toxicity. Ricin and abrin both inhibit ribosomal protein synthesis and exert pronounced effects on the GI tract. After oral exposure, vomiting and diarrhea leading to dehydration and delayed shock may occur. Castor bean ingestion has also been associated with GI bleeding and hemolysis. Onset of symptoms after ingestion is usually within 4 to 6 hours, but may take up to 10 hours.[44] There is no antidote available, but oral castor or jequirty bean ingestions are rarely fatal in the presence of appropriate supportive care. Decontamination should be attempted in patients who are not at risk for aspiration. Symptomatic patients will require aggressive fluid resuscitation and may need vasopressor support.

Plants Containing Colchicine

Both the autumn crocus (*Colchicum autumnale*) and the glory lily (*Gloriosa superba*) are members of the Lily family, which contain the antimitotic agent, colchicine.[3] All parts of these plants contain colchicine. Poisoning, although rare, is serious and potentially fatal. Acutely, nausea, vomiting, abdominal pain, and diarrhea may result. In more severe intoxications, delayed effects may be seen, including GI hemorrhage, bone marrow suppression, multiorgan failure, and cardiovascular collapse. Fatalities have been reported in modern medical literature after the mistaken ingestion of colchicine-containing plants.[45] There is no commercially available antidote, and prolonged supportive care may be required in severely poisoned patients. ED care entails circulatory support and early decontamination whenever possible, given the potential for significant morbidity and lack of an available antidote. Given the variable onset of symptoms (2–12 hours), even asymptomatic patients merit observation for an extended period.

Ackee (*Blighia sapida*)

Ackee fruit is a staple of the Jamaican diet and is grown in the West Indies, Florida, and Hawaii. The unripe fruit and seeds contain the toxins, hypoglycin A, and B, which inhibit metabolic pathways and can cause profound hypoglycemia.[3] Toxicity, which also manifests severe gastrointestinal distress and CNS derangements, is known as Jamaican vomiting sickness. Lethargy, metabolic acidosis without ketonemia, seizures, and coma may occur.[46] Patients can develop hepatic steatosis similar to that of Reye's syndrome. Fatalities are more common in children, possibly because of lower liver glycogen stores and a greater tendency to hypoglycemia. Treatment requires hospital admission, careful attention to blood glucose levels, antiemetics, hydration, and symptom-driven supportive care.

PSYCHOACTIVE PLANTS

A variety of plants and plant products have been abused by adolescents and teenagers for their hallucinogenic effects. The seeds of morning glory (*Ipomea violacea*), Hawaiian baby woodrose (*Argyreia nervosa*), and Hawaiian woodrose (*Merremia tuberosa*) contain lysergic acid amides and can cause effects similar to lysergic acid diethylamide. Approximately 250 morning glory seeds must be chewed in order to achieve a psychedelic effect.[47] Peyote (*Lopophora williamsii*) is a small, spineless cactus found in the southwestern United States and northern Mexico. The tops of the cactus are sliced off and dried, forming brown "buttons" that have a high content of mescaline. *Salvia divinorum* is a herb native to southern Mexico, which contains the potent hallucinogen salvinorin A. Most cases of hallucinogen intoxication are self-limited and symptoms generally subside in 4 to 6 hours.[47] Intoxication may cause agitation and anxiety, requiring sedation with benzodiazepines. Patients should receive supportive treatment in a quiet, nonthreatening environment.

REFERENCES

1. Bronstein AC, Spyker DA, Cantilena LR Jr, Green J, Rumack BH, Heard SE. 2006 Annual Report of the American Association of Poison Control Centers' National Poison Data System (NPDS). *Clin Toxicol (Phila)*. 2007;45(8):815–917.
2. McKinney PE, Gomez HF, Phillips S, Brent J. The fax machine: a new method of plant identification. *J Toxicol Clin Toxicol*. 1993;31(4):663–665.
3. Nelson LS, Shih RD, Balick MJ. *Handbook of Poisonous and Injurious Plants*. 2nd ed. New York, NY: Springer; 2007.
4. Krenzelok EP, Jacobsen TD. Plant exposures...a national profile of the most common plant genera. *Vet Hum Toxicol*. 1997;39(4):248–249.
5. Mrvos R, Dean BS, Krenzelok EP. Philodendron/dieffenbachia ingestions: are they a problem? *J Toxicol Clin Toxicol*. 1991;29(4):485–491.
6. Cumpston KL, Vogel SN, Leikin JB, Erickson TB. Acute airway compromise after brief exposure to a Dieffenbachia plant. *J Emerg Med*. 2003;25(4):391–397.
7. McIntire MS, Guest JR, Porterfield JF. Philodendron—an infant death. *J Toxicol Clin Toxicol*. 1990;28(2):177–183.
8. Snajdauf J, Mixa V, Rygl M, Vyhnánek M, Morávek J, Kabelka Z. Aortoesophageal fistula—an unusual complication of esophagitis caused by Dieffenbachia ingestion. *J Pediatr Surg*. 2005;40(6):e29-e31.
9. Pedaci L, Krenzelok EP, Jacobsen TD, Aronis J. Dieffenbachia species exposures: an evidence-based assessment of symptom presentation. *Vet Hum Toxicol*. 1999;41(5):335–338.
10. Williams SR, Clark RF, Dunford JV. Contact dermatitis associated with capsaicin: hunan hand syndrome. *Ann Emerg Med*. 1995;25(5):713–715.
11. Weinberg RB. Hunan hand. *N Engl J Med*. 1981;305(17):1020.
12. Vogl TP. Treatment of Hunan hand. *N Engl J Med*. 1982;306(3):178.
13. Jones LA, Tandberg D, Troutman WG. Household treatment for "chile burns" of the hands. *J Toxicol Clin Toxicol*. 1987;25(6):483–491.
14. Herman LM, Kindschu MW, Shallash AJ. Treatment of mace dermatitis with topical antacid suspension. *Am J Emerg Med*. 1998;16(6):613–614.
15. Krenzelok EP, Jacobsen TD, Aronis J. American mistletoe exposures. *Am J Emerg Med*. 1997;15(5):516–520.
16. Spiller HA, Willias DB, Gorman SE, Sanftleban J. Retrospective study of mistletoe ingestion. *J Toxicol Clin Toxicol*. 1996;34(4):405–408.
17. Krenzelok EP, Jacobsen TD, Aronis JM. Poinsettia exposures have good outcomes... just as we thought. *Am J Emerg Med*. 1996;14(7):671–674.
18. Froberg B, Ibrahim D, Furbee RB. Plant poisoning. *Emerg Med Clin North Am*. 2007;25(2):375–433.
19. Roberge R, Brader E, Martin ML, Jehle D, et al. The root of evil–pokeweed intoxication. *Ann Emerg Med*. 1986;15(4):470–473.
20. Hamilton RJ, Shih RD, Hoffman RS. Mobitz type I heart block after pokeweed ingestion. *Vet Hum Toxicol*. 1995;37(1):66–67.
21. Brooker J, Obar C, Courtemanche L. A fatality from Phytolacca Americana (pokeweed) root ingestion. *J Toxicol Clin Toxicol*. 2001;39(5):549–550.
22. Tiongson J, Salen P. Mass ingestion of Jimson Weed by eleven teenagers. *Del Med J*. 1998;70(11):471–476.
23. Spina SP, Taddei A. Teenagers with Jimson weed (Datura stramonium) poisoning. *CJEM*. 2007;9(6):467–468.
24. Orr R. Reversal of Datura stramonium delirium with physostigmine: report of three cases. *Anesth Analg*. 1975;54(1):158.
25. Sopchak CA, Stork CM, Cantor RM, Ohara PE. Central anticholinergic syndrome due to Jimson weed physostigmine: therapy revisited? *J Toxicol Clin Toxicol*. 1998;36(1–2):43–45.
26. Donovan JW. Anticholinergic plants. In: Brent J, Wallace KL, Burkhart KK, et al., eds. *Critical Care Toxicology*. Philadelphia, PA: Elsevier Mosby; 2005:1335–1343.
27. Rodgers GC Jr, Von Kanel RL. Conservative treatment of jimsonweed ingestion. *Vet Hum Toxicol*. 1993;35(1):32–33.
28. Salen P, Shih R, Sierzenski P, Reed J. Effect of physostigmine and gastric lavage in a Datura stramonium-induced anticholinergic poisoning epidemic. *Am J Emerg Med*. 2003;21(4):316–317.
29. Ceha LJ, Presperin C, Young E, Allswede M, Erickson T. Anticholinergic toxicity from nightshade berry poisoning responsive to physostigmine. *J Emerg Med*. 1997;15(1):65–69.
30. Parisi P, Francia A. A female with central anticholinergic syndrome responsive to neostigmine. *Pediatr Neurol*. 2000;23(2):185–187.
31. Eddleston M, Ariaratnam CA, Sjöström L, Jayalath S, et al. Acute yellow oleander (Thevetia peruviana) poisoning: cardiac arrhythmias, electrolyte disturbances, and serum cardiac

glycoside concentrations on presentation to hospital. *Heart*. 2000;83(3):301–306.

32. Eddleston M, Rajapakse S, Rajakanthan, Jayalath S, et al. Anti-digoxin Fab fragments in cardiotoxicity induced by ingestion of yellow oleander: a randomised controlled trial. *Lancet*. 2000;355(9208):967–972.

33. de Silva HA, Fonseka MM, Pathmeswaran A, Alahakone DG, et al. Multiple-dose activated charcoal for treatment of yellow oleander poisoning: a single-blind, randomised, placebo-controlled trial. *Lancet*. 2003;361(9373):1935–1938.

34. Eddleston M, Juszczak E, Buckley NA, Senarathna L, et al. Multiple-dose activated charcoal in acute self-poisoning: a randomised controlled trial. *Lancet*. 2008;371(9612):579–587.

35. Lin CC, Chan TY, Deng JF. Clinical features and management of herb-induced aconitine poisoning. *Ann Emerg Med*. 2004;43(5):574–579.

36. Dunnigan D, Adelman RD, Beyda DH. A young child with altered mental status. *Clin Pediatr (Phila)*. 2002;41(1): 43–45.

37. Van Ingen G, Visser R, Peltenburg H, Van Der Ark AM, et al. Sudden unexpected death due to Taxus poisoning. A report of five cases, with review of the literature. *Forensic Sci Int*. 1992;56(1):81–87.

38. Krenzelok EP, Jacobsen TD, Aronis J. Is the yew really poisonous to you? *J Toxicol Clin Toxicol*. 1998;36(3):219–223.

39. Johnson DW, Wilkins V. Ingestion of tobacco products by children: a prospective study. *J Toxicol Clin Toxicol*. 1996;34(5): 600.

40. McGee D, Brabson T, McCarthy J, Picciotti M. Four-year review of cigarette ingestions in children. *Pediatr Emerg Care*. 1995;11(1):13–16.

41. Fiesseler FW, Shih RD. Poison hemlock. In: Brent J, Wallace KL, Burkhart KK, et al., eds. *Critical Care Toxicology*. Philadelphia, PA: Elsevier Mosby; 2005:1319–1323.

42. Cetaruk EW. Water hemlock. In: Brent J, Wallace KL, Burkhart KK, et al., eds. *Critical Care Toxicology*. Philadelphia, PA: Elsevier Mosby; 2005:1311–1317.

43. Challoner KR, McCarron MM. Castor bean intoxication. *Ann Emerg Med*. 1990;19(10):1177–1183.

44. Audi J, Belson M, Patel M, Schier J, Osterloh J. Ricin poisoning: a comprehensive review. *JAMA*. 2005;294(18):2342–2351.

45. Brvar M, Ploj T, Kozelj G, Mozina M, Noc M, Bunc M. Case report: fatal poisoning with Colchicum autumnale. *Crit Care*. 2004;8(1):R56–R59.

46. Joskow R, Belson M, Vesper H, Backer L, Rubin C. Ackee fruit poisoning: an outbreak investigation in Haiti 2000–2001, and review of the literature. *Clin Toxicol (Phila)*. 2006;44(3):267–273.

47. Traub SJ. Hallucinogens. In: Shannon MW, Borron SW, Burns MJ, eds. *Haddad and Winchester's Clinical Management of Poisoning and Drug Overdose*. 4th ed. Philadelphia, PA: Saunders Elsevier; 2007:793–802.

CHAPTER 131

Lethal Toxins in Small Doses

Leon Gussow

▶ HIGH-YIELD FACTS

- Camphor is present in many over-the-counter liniments and cold preparations. As little as 1 g has been reported to cause death in an 18-month-old child. Clinical camphor toxicity occurs rapidly, with onset 5 to 120 minutes after ingestion. Muscle twitching and fasciculation may herald the onset of seizures. Management of camphor ingestion is generally supportive, emphasizing airway protection and seizure control.
- Benzocaine, present in many local anesthetics, can cause methemoglobinemia, especially in infants younger than 4 months. Clinical signs and symptoms of benzocaine toxicity, which begin as early as 30 to 60 minutes after ingestion, include a characteristic cyanosis that does not respond to oxygen. Treatment of benzocaine-induced methemoglobinemia consists of general support and, in selected cases, administration of the antidote methylene blue.
- Lomotil is an antidiarrheal preparation that combines an opiate (diphenoxylate) with an anticholinergic (atropine). After ingestion, respiratory depression can recur as late as 24 hours and there appears to be no correlation between dose ingested and severity of symptoms. Therefore, any child with known or suspected ingestion of any amount of Lomotil is admitted and monitored for at least 24 hours, no matter what the initial clinical condition.
- Chloroquine, an antimalarial agent, is a powerful, rapidly acting cardiotoxin capable of causing sudden cardiorespiratory collapse. The interval between ingestion and cardiac arrest is often less than 2 hours.
- Methyl salicylate is a concentrated liquid that is absorbed quickly and can produce early-onset severe salicylate toxicity. Ingestion of less thanone teaspoon has been fatal in a child.

Fortunately, the overwhelming majority of toxic exposures in young children are not life-threatening. For example, using data from 2006, the National Poison Data System of the American Association of Poison Control Centers reported over a half a million exposures in children younger than 2 years of age, but only 16 fatalities.[1] In addition, most medications that cause serious consequences in toddlers do so only after ingestion of clearly excessive amounts. Because so many pediatric toxic exposures turn out to be innocuous, it is easy for the clinician to become complacent about these cases, especially if by history the child ingested at most 1U dose of a medication. However, there are a number of prescriptions and over-the-counter preparations that can cause extreme toxicity, even fatality, in

a toddler after ingestion of a single dose.[2,3] The emergency physician must be familiar with these highly toxic agents.

This chapter will not discuss certain nonmedicinal agents such as hydrocarbons, acetonitrile, caustics, methanol, selenious acid, or environmental toxins that can also be extremely toxic in small amounts. Additionally, it will not be an exhaustive discussion of all possible relevant pharmaceuticals. For example, some highly toxic drugs, such as β-blockers and calcium channel blockers are not discussed here, but are covered in separate chapters of this text.[4,5]

▶ CAMPHOR

Camphor is present in many over-the-counter liniments and cold preparations, such as Campho-Phenique, Ben-Gay, Vicks Vaporub, Absorbine, and Tiger Balm.[3,6,7] Camphor has long been used as an antipruritic, rubefacient, and antiseptic. A common source of serious toxicity in the past has been camphorated oil, which was sometimes mistaken for castor oil and administered to children in high doses. Fortunately, this product is no longer available.

Camphor has a strong, unmistakable odor and a pungent taste that some children find appealing. It is a rapidly acting neurotoxin, producing both CNS excitation and depression. As little as 1 g has been reported to cause death in a 19-month-old child. Major toxicity has not been reported for ingestions <30 mg/kg and is rare in ingestions <50 mg/kg. Ingestions of less than one teaspoon of topical liniments or cold preparations should not cause toxicity.[6]

Clinical symptoms begin rapidly with onset of symptoms 5 to 120 minutes after ingestion. Initially, a feeling of generalized warmth progresses to pharyngeal and epigastric burning. Mental status changes can follow: confusion, restlessness, delirium, and hallucinations. CNS depression with coma and hypoventilation can occur. Muscle twitching and fasciculations may herald the onset of seizures, which have also been reported to occur suddenly, without preceding symptoms. The epileptogenic potential of camphor was demonstrated in 1919 when a child care facility inadvertently administered camphorated oil to 20 children between 1 and 4 years of age. All the children developed symptoms and most developed seizures.

Management of ingestion of camphor consists of supportive care with an emphasis on airway protection and seizure control. The role of gastric aspiration with a nasogastric tube in this setting has not been studied, but because camphor is so rapidly absorbed it is not likely to be beneficial in most cases. For the same reason, activated charcoal is unlikely to improve clinical outcome. The use of ipecac is contraindicated.

Seizures not responsive to benzodiazepines can be treated with phenobarbital.[3] Asymptomatic patients should be observed for 6 hours after ingestion prior to discharge from the emergency department.[7]

► BENZOCAINE

Benzocaine is present in many local anesthetics, including first aid ointments and infant teething formulas. Baby Orajel contains 7.5% benzocaine, Baby Orajel Nighttime Formula 10%, and Americaine Topical Anesthetic First Aid Ointment 20%.[6] Exposure can be from oral ingestion or dermal absorption. Benzocaine is metabolized to aniline and nitrosobenzene, both of which can cause methemoglobinemia, especially in infants younger than 4 months, who are deficient in methemoglobin reductase. Methemoglobinemia has occurred in an infant after an ingestion of 100 mg of benzocaine, the amount in one-quarter teaspoon of Baby Orajel. Recently, reports have appeared in the medical literature of male infants developing methemoglobinemia from EMLA cream (lidocaine/prilocaine) utilized for analgesia during circumcision.[8]

Clinical signs and symptoms typically begin within 30 minutes to 6 hours after ingestion, with tachycardia, tachypnea, and a characteristic cyanosis that does not respond to oxygen. In more severe exposures, agitation, hypoxia, metabolic acidosis, lethargy, stupor, and coma may supervene. Seizures can also occur.[6]

Treatment of benzocaine exposure consists principally of general support, and, in selected cases, the administration of antidote. Neither gastric lavage nor administration of activated charcoal is mandatory in this setting, since they have not been demonstrated to improve clinical outcome.

The antidote for patients with methemoglobinemia is methylene blue. Indications for use include methemoglobin levels >30% or signs of respiratory distress or altered mental status. The dose—1 to 2 mg/kg IV over 5 minutes—is repeated in 1 to 2 hours if symptoms persist.[6] Isolated cyanosis is not an indication for methylene blue, because it often occurs at low methemoglobin levels, is usually well tolerated, and resolves spontaneously. There is a further discussion of the use of methylene blue in Chapter 98.

► LOMOTIL

Lomotil is an antidiarrheal preparation that combines an opiate (diphenoxylate) with an anticholinergic (atropine). Several unique properties make Lomotil poisoning potentially dangerous in the pediatric population. Respiratory depression can recur as late as 24 hours after ingestion, and there appears to be no correlation between the dose ingested and the severity of symptoms.[3] Therefore, any child with known or suspected ingestion of any amount of Lomotil is admitted and monitored for at least 24 hours, no matter what the initial clinical condition.[3,6]

Each tablet or 5 mL of liquid Lomotil contains 2.5 mg diphenoxylate hydrochloride and 0.025 mg atropine sulfate. Difenoxin is the major metabolite of diphenoxylate and is both more active and longer-acting than its parent drug.[9] This metabolite is probably responsible for the recurrent respiratory depression often seen in these overdoses.[6]

Ingestion of one-half to two tablets has been reported to cause toxic signs and symptoms. The lowest reported fatal dose is 1.2 mg/kg (diphenoxylate).[6] Both atropine and diphenoxylate are rapidly absorbed from the gastrointestinal tract, but since the anticholinergic effect from atropine can delay gastric emptying, intact tablets have been recovered as long as 27 hours after ingestion.

Although patients often present with a confusing mix of opioid and anticholinergic signs and symptoms, opioid effects are always seen in overdose and often predominate. Atropine-induced anticholinergic symptoms can occur before, during, or after opioid effects, or may not occur at all. Initial manifestations of Lomotil overdose in children include drowsiness, lethargy or excitement, dyspnea, irritability, miosis, hypotonia or rigidity, and urinary retention. In severe cases the patient may present with coma, respiratory depression, hypoxia, and seizures. Symptoms may not be related to the dose ingested, and can recur as late as 24 hours after ingestion. Death is often accompanied by cerebral edema.

Management of Lomotil poisoning includes admission of all patients and careful observation for 24 hours.[3] Syrup of ipecac is contraindicated since CNS depression may supervene and induced emesis will delay the administration of activated charcoal. The role of gastric lavage has not been studied in this setting, and there is no evidence suggesting it would be beneficial. Difenoxin undergoes enterohepatic circulation; if there are active bowel sounds, multiple-dose activated charcoal (1 g/kg every 4 hours) can be considered.[6] A Foley catheter may be needed to relieve urinary retention. Excessive hydration should be avoided to minimize the risk of cerebral edema. Respiratory depression and coma are treated with intravenous naloxone (0.1 mg/kg), which may have to be repeated frequently. A maintenance dose of naloxone can be given, starting with two-thirds of the bolus dose that initially produced the desired response administered each hour, titrated to clinical condition. When naloxone is given, anticholinergic symptoms may emerge.

► CHLOROQUINE AND HYDROXYCHLOROQUINE

Chloroquine has been used since the 1940s for the treatment and prevention of malaria. Additional uses currently include the treatment of extraintestinal amebiasis and some connective tissue diseases such as SLE and rheumatoid arthritis. Chloroquine is a powerful rapidly acting cardiotoxin capable of causing sudden cardiopulmonary collapse. The interval between ingestion and cardiac arrest is often less than 2 hours.[10] Even a small amount can be life-threatening in a toddler. Death has been reported after ingestion of as little as 300 mg.[10]

Chloroquine causes myocardial depression and vasodilation, producing sudden profound hypotension. Automaticity and conductivity of myocardium is also impaired, resulting in bradycardia and ventricular escape rhythms. The electrocardiogram can show sinus bradycardia, widened QRS, prolonged intraventricular conduction time, T-wave changes, ST depression, prolonged QT, complete heart block, ventricular tachycardia, or ventricular fibrillation. Neurotoxicity induced by chloroquine often presents as drowsiness and lethargy, followed by excitability. Seizures and coma can occur.

The physician treating chloroquine toxicity should be prepared to manage sudden cardiac or respiratory arrest. Intubation and supported ventilation may be required. Blood pressure is maintained with intravenous fluids and pressors. Class IA antiarrhythmics (quinidine, procainamide, disopyramide) are contraindicated. Because chloroquine is rapidly absorbed from the gastrointestinal tract, gastric lavage is unlikely to improve clinical outcome. Chloroquine is well absorbed by activated charcoal, which may be considered if it can be administered within 30 to 60 minutes of ingestion. As with theophylline toxicity, hypokalemia can occur because of ion transport into cells. Aggressive repletion of potassium in this setting has in some cases led to severe hyperkalemia. Recent evidence suggestions that early mechanical ventilation with administration of high-dose diazepam and epinephrine may be lifesaving in severe cases of chloroquine toxicity in adults. However, this therapy has not been well described in the pediatric population.[11]

Any child who has ingested chloroquine should be referred immediately to a medical facility for observation and cardiac monitoring. If no coingestants are involved, a patient who is asymptomatic for 6 hours can be safely discharged after consideration of the social situation and potential for repeat exposure. Any symptoms or EKG changes require admission. A poison control center should be consulted for all cases of chloroquine ingestion.

There is scant literature concerning hydroxychloroquine overdose in children. Although considered less toxic than chloroquine, hydroxychloroquine has similar cardiac and neurologic effects. The most prudent course would be to handle hydroxychloroquine ingestion with a similar approach to that outlined above for chloroquine.[10]

▶ METHYL SALICYLATE

Methyl salicylate is a concentrated liquid that is absorbed quickly and can produce early-onset severe salicylate toxicity. It is found in many topical liniments (Ben Gay, Icy Hot Balm) and in oil of wintergreen food flavoring. One teaspoon of oil of wintergreen contains 7 g of salicylate (equivalent to 21 aspirin tablets). Since ingestion of less than one teaspoon has killed a child, any ingestion of these preparations is potentially serious. Clinical presentation and treatment of this overdose is similar to that of other types of salicylate poisoning.[3,6]

▶ IMIDAZOLINE DECONGESTANTS

Imidazoline decongestants are found in a wide variety of over-the-counter nasal sprays and eye drops. Examples include tetrahydrozoline (Visine), naphazoline (Naphcon), and oxymetazoline (Afrin).[6] Significant toxicity with hypotension, lethargy, and respiratory depression requiring intubation has been reported in a toddler after ingestion of half a teaspoon of Visine eye drops.

Imidazolines are α_2 adrenergic agonists. When applied topically to the nasal mucosa or into the eye, their peripheral α-2 activity produces vasoconstriction. However, after ingestion, these lipophilic agents rapidly enter the CNS and reduce sympathetic outflow from the vasomotor center, causing hypotension, bradycardia miosis, CNS depression, and respiratory depression. These opioid-like effects are similar to those caused by the antihypertensive drug clonidine, also an α_2 agonist.[6] Because of the interplay between the central and peripheral actions of the imidazolines, overdose can present with a variable and changing clinical picture. Bradycardia can alternate with tachycardia, hypotension with hypertension, and lethargy with agitation. Hypoglycemia and hypothermia have both been reported.

Onset of symptoms is generally within 4 hours of ingestion, with resolution by 24 to 48 hours. Because these products are rapidly absorbed from the GI tract, it is unlikely that aspiration of stomach contents through a nasogastric tube or administration of activated charcoal would improve clinical outcome. As with clonidine toxicity, imidazoline-induced CNS depression may respond to naloxone. Clinically significant bradycardia can be treated with atropine. Asymptomatic children should be observed for 6 hours.[6]

REFERENCES

1. Bronstein AC, Spyker DA, Cantilena LR, et al. 2006 Annual Report of the American Association of Poison Control Centers' National Poison Data System. *Clin Toxicol.* 2007;45:815.
2. Bar-Oz B, Levichek Z, Koren G. Medications that can be fatal for a toddler with one tablet or teaspoonful: a 2004 update. *Pediatr Drugs.* 2004;6:123.
3. Michael JB, Sztajnkrycer MD. Deadly pediatric poisons: nine common agents that kill at low doses. *Emerg Med Clin North Am.* 2004;22:1019.
4. Love JN, Sikka N. Are 1–2 tablets dangerous? Beta-blocker exposure in toddlers. *J Emerg Med.* 2004;26:309.
5. Ranniger C, Roche C. Are one or two dangerous? Calcium channel blocker exposure in toddlers. *J Emerg Med.* 2007;33:145.
6. Liebelt EL, Shannon MW. Small doses, big problems: a selected review of highly toxic common medications. *Pediatr Emerg Care.* 1993;9:292.
7. Love JN, Sammon M, Smereck J. Are one or two dangerous? Camphor exposure in toddlers. *J Emerg Med.* 2004;27:49.
8. Couper RTL. Methaemoglobinaemia secondary to topical lignocaine/prilocaine in a circumcised neonate. *J Paediatr Child Health.* 2000;36:406.
9. McCarron MM, Challoner KR, Thompson GA. Diphenoxylate-Atropine (Lomotil) overdose in children: an update (report of eight cases and review of the literature). *Pediatrics.* 1991;87:694.
10. Smith ER, Klein-Schwartz W. Are 1–2 dangerous? Chloroquine and hydroxychloroquine exposure in toddlers. *J Emerg Med.* 2005;28:437.
11. Riou B, Barriot P, Rimailho A, et al. Treatment of severe chloroquine poisoning. *N Engl J Med.* 1988;318:1.

CHAPTER 132

Chemical Weapons: Nerve Agents and Vesicants

Leon Gussow

▶ HIGH-YIELD FACTS

- Nerve agents cause death by respiratory failure, primarily from the muscarinic effects of bronchorrhea and bronchospasm.
- The antidote atropine can counteract the muscarinic effects of nerve agents.
- Removing all clothing and jewelry will most likely constitute adequate decontamination of victims exposed to nerve agent vapor.

Planning for a medical response to terrorism has primarily focused around the needs of healthy military recruits or the population as a whole. There as been little discussion pertaining to vulnerable populations such as children. Unfortunately, entire communities are now at risk for terrorism. Children are even more susceptible than adults to the effects of chemical weapons, especially those that are inhaled or absorbed through the skin.[1] There are several reasons for this such as, a child's surface area relative to his or her body mass is greater than that of an adult, increasing effective dermal absorption of chemical agents, as well as the risk of fluid loss and hypothermia. The child's higher metabolic and respiratory rates would increase uptake of inhaled vapors. Metabolic pathways that detoxify or eliminate poisons may be underdeveloped. Many chemical agents, such as vesicants and the nerve agents, are heavier than air, producing increased concentrations closer to the ground. In addition, aspects of disaster planning and response such as mass decontamination of children and dosing of antidotes in the pediatric population would pose unique challenges.

▶ NERVE AGENTS

Nerve agents are highly toxic organophosphate compounds first developed in the years leading up World War II. They are, essentially, much more potent versions of the organophosphate insecticides. Although commonly called "nerve gases", these agents are actually liquids with variable volatility at room temperature. Nerve agents that have been manufactured and stockpiled in the past include tabun, sarin, and soman. VX is the most potent of these agents, with a potentially fatal liquid exposure involving as little as one drop applied to the skin of an adult; this lethal amount would be proportionally much less in children.

Nerve agents are powerful inhibitors of the enzyme acetylcholinesterase (AChE). This enzyme normally serves to modulate the actions of acetylcholine, a neurotransmitter that is found throughout the peripheral and central nervous systems. With the enzyme blocked, acetylcholine accumulates and the cholinergic receptors become overstimulated in an uncontrolled manner. There are three major classifications of cholinergic receptors and actions:

MUSCARINIC

These receptors are found at the neuromuscular junction of smooth (involuntary) muscles of the respiratory and gastrointestinal tracts, as well as in secretory glands. As acetylcholine builds up in these locations, smooth muscle contracts spasmodically and glands secrete uncontrollably. A convenient mnemonic to help remember the *muscarinic* actions of nerve agents is DUMBELS:

> *D*iaphoresis, *D*iarrhea
> *U*rination
> *M*iosis
> *B*ronchorrhea, *B*ronchospasm
> *E*mesis
> *L*acrimation
> *S*alivation, *S*weating

Victims of nerve gas exposure die from respiratory failure, primarily because of bronchorrhea and bronchospasm, the so-called "Killer Bs". These can make it difficult if not impossible to ventilate and oxygenate the victim unless antidote is first administered. Miosis and hypersalivation, although not life-threatening, can be important clues to the diagnosis of cholinergic syndrome.

NICOTINIC

Nicotinic receptors are found in skeletal (voluntary) muscle and in some ganglia. Manifestations of nicotinic stimulation include fasciculations, muscle weakness, and paralysis.

CENTRAL

Hyperstimulation of cholinergic receptors located in the brain causes seizures, coma, and central apnea. Note that bronchorrhea and bronchospasm, respiratory muscle weakness, and central apnea can combine to contribute to death from respiratory failure.

The major considerations in managing victims of nerve agent exposure include decontamination, supportive care, and treatment with appropriate antidotes. Although most emergency response plans call for victims to be decontaminated in the field, history teaches that in mass disasters the overwhelming majority of patients come to emergency departments on their own, not through the EMS system. It is extremely unlikely that patients who arrive walking and talking have significant liquid dermal exposure, or that they need "wet" decontamination with mass showers or copious water irrigation. However, the 1995 experience from the sarin release on the Tokyo subway system indicates that small amounts of vapor can be trapped in the clothing of people who were at the scene of an incident, and that in enclosed spaces this vapor can off gas and build up to levels sufficient to cause symptoms. This leads to two important points: (1) Not all patients who present to the hospital after a nerve agent mass contamination incident need be brought into the emergency department. Response plans should call for most of the "walking wounded" to be observed somewhere apart from the acute care area—preferably outdoors if weather permits. (2) In cases of pure vapor exposure, removing and bagging the patients' clothing before they are brought into an enclosed area will most likely accomplish adequate decontamination.

A discussion of the complexities of planning for and implementing "wet" decontamination is beyond the scope of this chapter.

There are three major antidotes for nerve agent exposure, which correspond to the three types of receptors and effects:

1 *Atropine* blocks the *muscarinic* effects of nerve agents, most importantly drying up respiratory secretions and relieving bronchospasm.[2] It does not affect the nicotinic manifestations. The initial dose is 0.05 to 0.10 mg/kg IV or IM (maximum 5 mg). This can be repeated every 5 minutes until ventilation and oxygenation are possible. The dose should not be titrated against heart rate or pupil size. Tachycardia is not a contraindication of use of atropine. Since there is evidence that administering IV atropine to a hypoxic nerve agent victim may induce ventricular fibrillation, initial doses in a seriously toxic patient should ideally be given IM using an autoinjector.[2] Pediatric atropine autoinjectors are now available with doses ranging from 0.25 to 2.0 mg (AtroPen, Meridian Medical Technologies). Some authors recommend that for children aging 1 year or older, the full-adult dose of atropine (2 mg) be administered by autoinjector, whereas for children younger than 1 year 0.5 mg be given if available.[1,3]

2 *Pralidoxime chloride (2-PAM)* removes nerve agent from the active site on acetylcholinesterase (AChE), reactivating the enzyme. This helps reverse the *nicotinic* effects of nerve agents such as muscle weakness.

The optimal dose in infants and children has not been determined, but 25 mg/kg (maximum 1 g) has been recommended.[2] This can be given IV or IM and repeated at 30 to 60 minutes. Pralidoxime is available in an autoinjector containing an adult dose (600 mg). There has been some concern about using this product on infants, especially since too-rapid administration of 2-PAM can cause significant hypertension. A recent review found few reports of adverse drug reactions to 2-PAM in the literature. The authors recommended that even children younger than 3 years could be treated with the adult autoinjector if that were the sole source of antidote.[4]

3 *Diazepam* is indicated not only to treat nerve agent-induced seizures, but also for any severe exposure with *central* manifestations. Animal data suggest that it may be neuroprotective in this setting. The dose is 0.1 to 0.3 mg/kg (maximum 5 mg).[2] If diazepam is not available, equivalent amounts of another benzodiazepine can be used.

▶ SULFUR MUSTARD

The blistering agent *sulfur mustard* is an oily liquid with an odor similar to that of garlic, horseradish, or mustard. Mustard quickly damages cellular components such as nucleic acids and proteins, causing cell death.[2] Rapidly dividing cells, such as the hematopoietic components of bone marrow and the linings of the gastrointestinal and respiratory tracts, are most sensitive to mustard's effects. The LD_{50} is approximately 1.5 teaspoons, which is enough to cause a 25% body surface area burn in adults.

Clinical effects are dose-dependent. At low doses, skin irritation and blistering occurs; at higher doses, systemic toxicity can also be seen. While tissue damage occurs within minutes of exposure, initial signs and symptoms are typically delayed for several hours. Skin findings include erythema that progresses to blister formation over 24 hours. Warm, moist areas such as the axillae and groin are particularly susceptible. Ocular manifestations are similarly delayed and include lid edema, conjunctival injections, and, with severe exposure, corneal ulceration. Respiratory involvement begins with sore throat, cough, and hoarseness, and can in rare instances of overwhelming exposure progress to pulmonary edema. Early tachypnea or dyspnea suggests a poor prognosis.

The diagnosis of vesicant toxicity is clinical. Treatment begins with immediate skin and eye decontamination. Although tissue damage occurs almost immediately upon contact with mustard liquid or vapor, late decontamination is still indicated to minimize systemic absorption and to prevent secondary contamination of rescue or medical personnel. Copious irrigation with water and a mild detergent constitutes appropriate dermal decontamination.

There are no specific antidotes for sulfur mustard exposure. As with thermal burns, aggressive airway, fluid, electrolyte, and pain management coupled with prevention of secondary infection with topical antibiotics and sterile dressing changes are the mainstays of therapy. In contrast to thermal burns, mustard injury does not generally cause massive fluid loss. Death most frequently occurs 5 to 10 days after exposure, usually from pulmonary insufficiency or infection.

REFERENCES

1. Foltin G, Tunik M, Curran J, et al. Pediatric nerve agent poisoning: medical and operational considerations for emergency medical services in a large American city. *Pediatr Emerg Care.* 2006;22:239.

2. Lynch EL, Thomas TL. Pediatric considerations in chemical exposures: are we prepared? *Pediatr Emerg Care.* 2004;20:198.

3. Baker MD. Antidotes for nerve agent poisoning: should we differentiate children from adults? *Curr Opin Pediatr.* 2007;19:211.

4. Quail MT, Shannon MW. Pralidoxime safety and toxicity in children. *Prehosp Emerg Care.* 2007;11:36.

SECTION XX

ENVIRONMENTAL EMERGENCIES

CHAPTER 133

Human and Animal Bites

David A. Townes

► HIGH-YIELD FACTS

- Bite wounds account for approximately 1% of emergency department (ED) visits each year in the United States.
- The majority of bite wounds occur in children.
- It is important to obtain a thorough history and perform a complete examination of bite injuries.
- Wound infection is the greatest potential complication of bite wounds.
- Thorough wound cleaning including adequate irrigation is the best method to prevent wound infection.
- Antibiotic treatment should be directed at the most likely infective agent.
- *Pasteurella* species are a common infective agent for both dog and cat bite wounds.
- *Eikenella corrodens* is a common infective agent in human bite wounds.
- Rabies and tetanus prophylaxis should be considered in animal bite injuries.
- Bite wounds treated on an outpatient basis should be reevaluated within 48 hours.

An estimated two million bite wounds are reported each year in the United States. The actual number is undoubtedly higher. Bite wounds account for approximately 1% of all ED visits and result in numerous hospitalizations. More than half of these injuries occur in children. Dog bites account for the majority, followed by cat bites, with the remainder divided among a variety of animal species (Fig. 133–1). Boys tend to be bitten more often than girls and bite injuries are clustered in the summer months. Because of the frequency of these injuries and the potential morbidity associated with them, it is important that the physician working in the ED be familiar with their management. The general approach to human and common animal bites is outlined in Figure 133–2.[1]

► HISTORY AND PHYSICAL EXAMINATION

Proper management of bite wounds begins with a thorough history and physical examination. It is important to obtain a complete history of the injury, including what type of animal caused the wound and the age of the wound. One must also elicit host factors that may affect wound healing. Especially important is a history of diabetes, peripheral vascular disease, chronic use of glucocorticoids, or other immunocompromised states.[2]

The physical examination should include a full examination and exploration of the wound. The type of wound (laceration, crush, or puncture) and the extent of involvement of deep structures must be determined. If the wound occurs over a joint, the joint should be examined through the full range of motion. When appropriate, radiographs should be obtained to look for fractures, foreign bodies, and air in the joint or soft tissues. One should keep in mind that the canine jaw can generate forces up to 450 pounds per square inch. In children, this force may be sufficient to penetrate the cranium. Computed tomography of the head should be considered in bite wounds to the scalp. Careful attention should be paid to signs of infection, including erythema, swelling, discharge, lymphadenopathy, or pain on passive range of motion.[2]

► WOUND CARE

The most common complication associated with bite wounds is wound infection. Numerous studies have been performed to determine the rate of infection of bite wounds. These have demonstrated infection rates as high as 30% for dog bites, 50% for cat bites, and 60% for human bites (Fig. 133–3). This is in comparison to an infection rate of approximately 15% for other wounds. It is therefore important to make every effort to minimize the risk of infection. One of the best methods of reducing the risk of infection is adequate irrigation of the wound. An acceptable method is to irrigate the wound with 1 to 2 L of normal saline through a 19- or 20-gauge vascular catheter. This will provide enough pressure to dislodge and wash away bacteria without inoculating organisms or further disrupting deeper tissues. The wound should be debrided as needed.[3]

The decision to close the wound depends on its age, type, and location. Under no circumstances should a wound that appears infected be closed. In most cases, bite wounds on the hand should be left open because of the high potential for morbidity if these wounds become infected. Dog bites may be safely closed if they are not located on the hands. Cat bites, which are usually puncture wounds, should not be closed because they cannot be adequately cleaned. The question of whether puncture wounds should be extended to better irrigate them remains controversial and should be decided on an individual basis. Cat bites that are lacerations rather than puncture wounds may be closed if they are not on the hands. In general, wounds that are more than 8- to 12-hours-old should be left open. Potentially disfiguring bite wounds on the face may be closed even when more than 12-hours-old (Fig. 133–4); however, these patients must be followed very carefully for

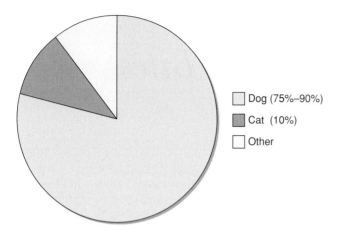

Figure 133–1. Distribution of bites by type of animal.

Dog (75%–90%)
Cat (10%)
Other

wounds treated on an outpatient basis should be reevaluated within 48 hours.[4]

▶ ANTIBIOTICS

Wounds that have evidence of infection should be treated with antibiotics. The use of antibiotics as prophylaxis remains controversial. The type of animal, location of the wound, and host factors must be considered. Wounds on the hands and feet should be treated with antibiotics, while those on the face and scalp are less likely to become infected and do not need prophylactic antibiotic coverage. In general, bite wounds caused by cats and humans should be treated prophylactically, while those caused by dogs and rodents may not need treatment with antibiotics. If the decision to treat with prophylactic antibiotics is made, the initial treatment should be for 3 days. If at the end of this time there is no evidence of infection, the wound is very unlikely to become infected and the antibiotics may be discontinued.[5]

In general, the organisms responsible for bite wound infections are from the animal's oral flora rather than the host's skin flora. More than 200 different organisms have been

evidence of infection. Surgical consultation should be obtained if there is a question concerning the management of these wounds.[4]

The decision to close any bite wound must be made after adequate exploration and cleaning of the wound. All bite

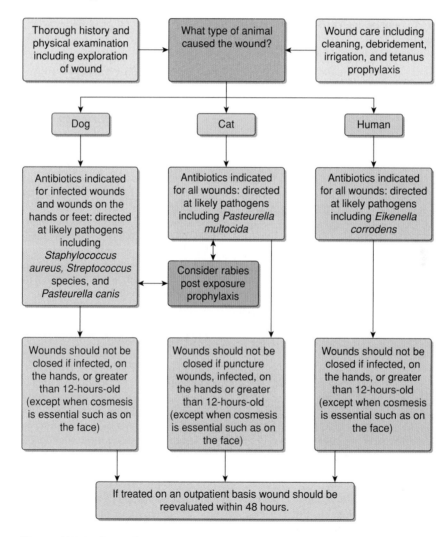

Figure 133–2. General approach to human and common animal bite wounds.

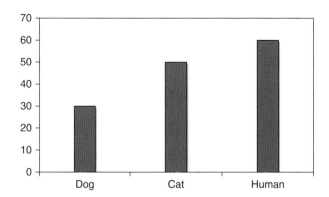

Figure 133–3. Rate (%) of bite wound infection by type of animal.

identified in bite wounds. Approximately one-third of wound infections demonstrate multiple organisms. One study of dog and cat bite wound infections demonstrated a median of five bacterial isolates per wound culture. The predominant organism in any bite wound will depend on the type of animal causing the wound.[5]

Dog bites tend to become infected with *Staphylococcus aureus, Streptococcus* species, and *Pasteurella canis,* but *Pseudomonas* species, *Enterobacter cloacae,* and many others have been identified. Cat bites are likely to become infected with *Pasteurella multocida.* In one study, *Pasteurella* species were the most common organisms isolated in both dog and cat bite wound infections (50% and 75%, respectively). These organisms cause a rapidly developing infection with signs and symptoms apparent in less than 24 hours. Delay in these findings for more than 24 hours should lead the physician to consider other etiologic agents such as *Staphylococcus* or *Streptococcus* species. Human saliva contains 10^8 bacteria per mL, with over 40 species represented. Human bite wounds tend to become infected with *S. aureus, Streptococcus* species, and *Eikenella corrodens. Pasteurella* species are unlikely infectious agents in human bite wounds.[6]

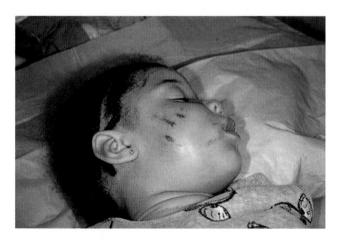

Figure 133–4. Cellulitis in a dog bite: Intense local tenderness, severe pain (greater than clinical signs indicated), and rapidly spreading erythema were seen in this febrile patient who came back to the ED 12 hours after being discharged from the ED following a bite by a German shepherd that was owned by the family.

Antibiotic coverage should be directed at the most likely infective organism. In the case of dog and cat bites *Staphylococcus* and *Streptococcus* species may be covered by dicloxacillin or a first-generation cephalosporin. With the increasing incidence of methicillin-resistant *Staphylococcus aureus* (MRSA), consideration may also be given to using trimethoprim–sulfamethoxazole or clindamycin. *Pasteurella* species are covered by penicillin, ampicillin, amoxicillin, amoxicillin/clavulanic acid, second- and third-generation cephalosporins, doxycycline, trimethoprim–sulfamethoxazole, clarithromycin, and azithromycin. In vitro, antistaphylococcal penicillins, first-generation cephalosporins, clindamycin, and erythromycin are less active against *Pasteurella* species. Empiric therapy for dog and cat bites should include a β-lactam antibiotic and a β-lactamase inhibitor, a second-generation cephalosporin with anaerobic activity, or a combination of penicillin and a first-generation cephalosporin. For human bite wounds, *Eikenella corrodens* is covered by penicillin or amoxicillin/clavulanic acid, and dicloxacillin can be used to cover *Staphylococcus* and *Streptococcus.* It may be necessary to use a two-antibiotic regimen for human bite wounds.[5,6]

▶ RABIES PROPHYLAXIS

Rabies infection should be considered in animal bite injuries. Rabies is a viral infection transmitted in the saliva of infected animals. It is caused by the rhabdovirus group and may lead to encephalomyelitis. The disease is almost universally fatal. Only 55 cases have been reported in the United States since 1960, but it continues to be a substantial problem in certain parts of the world. Rabies accounts for an estimated 30 000 deaths in Asia annually.[7,8]

In determining the need for rabies prophylaxis, the physician must consider the type of animal causing the injury and the prevalence of rabies in the region. If rabies is not suspected, no treatment is indicated. In the case of dogs, cats, and ferrets, the animal should be captured and quarantined for 10 days. If the animal remains healthy, no treatment is necessary. If the animal becomes ill or if rabies is suspected, the animal should be sacrificed and the brain examined for evidence of rabies. If the animal is infected, the child should be immediately vaccinated.[9]

Most other carnivores including skunks, raccoons, and foxes should be considered infected unless proven negative by laboratory testing. Livestock, large rodents, lagomorphs, and other mammals should be considered on an individual case basis. If the animal cannot be located, decisions regarding prophylaxis must be based on the prevalence of rabies in the area and the species of biting animal. Local animal control authorities may be helpful in obtaining this information. Postexposure prophylaxis is indicated for bite, scratch, or mucous membrane exposure to a bat if the animal cannot be collected and tested. Postexposure prophylaxis may be indicated in cases in which contact is likely to have occurred but is not documented. This includes a child sleeping in a room where a bat is found.[9]

Postexposure prophylaxis includes thorough cleaning of the wound, the administration of one of the available vaccines, and the administration of human rabies immune globulin (HRIG). The vaccine, such as human diploid cell vaccine (HDCV), is given in five 1-mL intramuscular injections on days

0, 3, 7, 14, and 28. It should be administered in the deltoid or anterolateral thigh. It should not be administered in the gluteal area. HRIG is dosed at 20 IU/kg. If feasible, the entire volume should be infiltrated into the wound and the surrounding area. Any remaining volume should be administered intramuscularly at a site remote from the vaccine administration. The same syringe should not be used to administer the vaccine and the HRIG.[9]

Preexposure prophylaxis is not indicated for children living in the United States. Typically, individuals receiving preexposure prophylaxis include veterinarians, laboratory workers, animal control officers/handlers, and spelunkers; however, the World Health Organization (WHO) has promoted the use of preexposure prophylaxis in toddlers and children living in highly endemic areas. Preexposure prophylaxis includes HDCV administered on days 0, 7, 21, or 28. Postexposure prophylaxis in these individuals includes HDCV administered on days 0 and 3. HRIG is not indicated in individuals who have been previously vaccinated.[9]

The recommended dosing and schedule for pre- and postexposure prophylaxis are shown in Table 133–1. A variety of alternative dosing and accelerated schedules are utilized.[9]

▶ TETANUS PROPHYLAXIS

Tetanus immunoprophylaxis should also be considered. Refer to Chapter 39 for guidelines.[4]

REFERENCES

1. Jackson SC. Mammalian bites. In: Surpure JS, ed. *Synopsis of Pediatric Emergency Care.* Boston, MA: Andover Medical; 1993:393–401.
2. Dire DJ. Emergency management of dog and cat wounds. *Emerg Med Clin North Am.* 1992;10:719.
3. Chen E, Hornig S, Shepherd SM, Hollander JE. Primary closure of mammalian bites. *Acad Emerg Med.* 2000;7:157–161.
4. Trott A. Bite wounds. In: Trott A, ed. *Wounds and Laceration: Emergency Care and Closure.* 3rd ed. St. Louis, MO: Mosby-Year Book; 2005:223–238.
5. Edwards MS: Infections due to human and animal bites. In: Geigin RD, Cherry JD, eds. *Textbook of Pediatric Infectious Diseases.* 5th ed. Philadelphia, PA: Saunders; 2003:3267–3274.
6. Talan DA, Citron DM, Abrahamian FM, et al. Bacteriologic analysis of infected dog and cat bites. *N Engl J Med.* 1999;340:85–92.
7. Wilkerson JA. Clinical updates in wilderness medicine—rabies update. *Wilderness Environ Med.* 2000;11:31–39.
8. Dodet B. An important date in rabies history. Meeting report of the Asian Rabies Expert Bureau (AREB). *Vaccine.* 2007;25:8647–8650.
9. Manning SE, Rupprecht VMD, Fishbein D, et al. Human Rabies Prevention—United States, 2008. Recommendations of the Advisory Committee on Immunization Practices (ACIP). *MMWR Recomm Rep.* 2008;57(RR03):1–26, 28.

▶ TABLE 133–1. RABIES PRE- AND POSTEXPOSURE PROPHYLAXIS

	HDCV (1.0 mL)	HRIG (20 IU/kg)
Preexposure prophylaxis	Day 0, 7, 21 or 28	None
Postexposure prophylaxis		
Not previously vaccinated	Day 0, 3, 7, 14, 28	Day 0
Previously vaccinated	Day 0, 3	None

CHAPTER 134

Snake Envenomations

Timothy B. Erickson and Andrew Zinkel

▶ HIGH-YIELD FACTS

- Pit vipers (crotalids) account for the majority of envenomations in pediatric patients. Because of their small body weight, young children are relatively more vulnerable to severe envenomation.
- Pit viper (Crotalidae) envenomations result in hematotoxicity while coral snakes (Eliapidae) cause neurotoxicity.
- Crotaline snakes are responsible for the vast majority of snake envenomations in the United States. Identification of exact species is not essential since treatment is the same for all indigenous American pit vipers.
- Prehospital management of snakebites includes immobilization of the bitten extremity, minimization of physical activity, fluid administration. No "first aid" technique has been demonstrated to improve outcome after envenomation. Rapid transport for administration of antivenom is the most important intervention in prehospital care.
- Antivenom, such as Crotaline Fab antivenom, consisting of highly purified papain-digested antibodies, is the current standard of care for treatment of crotaline snake envenomation.
- Antivenom dosing in pediatric patients is based on potential venom load, not kilogram size of the patient.

▶ EPIDEMIOLOGY

Worldwide, approximately 30 000 fatal snakebites are sustained each year.[1] Of the 120 snake species that are indigenous to the United States, approximately 20% are venomous (Table 134–1). Venomous snakes are classified into two families: Viperidae and Elapidae. Crotalinae is a subfamily of Viperidae better known as pit vipers due to the heat sensing organs on either side of the head. The Crotalinae subfamily includes three genera: *Crotalus* (rattlesnakes), *Agkistrodon* (copperheads and cottonmouths), and *Sistrurus* (massasauguas).[2] While copperhead (*Agkistrodon contortrix*) and cottonmouth (*Agkistrodon piscivoris*) snakes are primarily found in the southern and eastern United States,[3] several species of rattlesnake are found throughout the continental United States. Although snakebites are typically underreported, it is estimated that 8000 crotaline envenomations occur in the United States annually. Approximately 20% of these involve patients younger than 20 years with 5 to 6 annual fatalities.[1]

▶ PIT VIPERS

ANATOMY

A few anatomic characteristics differentiate venomous pit vipers from nonpoisonous snakes. Pit vipers possess a triangular or arrow-shaped head, whereas nonpoisonous North American snakes have a smooth, tapered body and narrow head. Crotalids have facial pits between the nostril and eye that serve as heat and vibration sensors, enabling the snake to locate prey (Fig. 134–1). While nonpoisonous snakes typically possess round pupils, pit vipers have vertical or elliptical pupils. Members of the genus *Crotalus* are further characterized by tail rattles and a single row of ventral anal scales.[4]

PATHOPHYSIOLOGY

Since snakes are defensive animals and rarely attack, they will remain immobile or even attempt to retreat if given the opportunity. Bites most commonly occur in small children who are paralyzed with fear or in individuals who handle and harass the snake. Because of their small body weight, infants and young children are relatively more vulnerable to severe envenomation. The severity of envenomation also depends on the location of the bite. Bites on the head, neck, or trunk are more severe than extremity bites.[5] Bites on the upper extremities are most common and potentially more dangerous than those on the lower extremities, whereas lower extremity bites may result in delayed clinical signs of toxicity. Male children are more likely than female children to suffer Crotaline snakebites that require antivenom therapy. Males are also more likely to be bitten in the upper extremities.[6] Direct envenomation into an artery or vein is associated with a much higher mortality rate.

It is important to remember that when envenomation occurs, the smaller pediatric patient is generally exposed to a larger milligram per kilogram venom load. Treating clinicians should anticipate a higher likelihood of systemic symptoms. As a result, the basic principles of treatment do not change depending on the child's age or developmental stage. Intravenous antivenom is always the first-line therapy and dosing should be targeted toward the potential venom load, as opposed to the patient's kilogram weight.[7]

The venom itself is a complex mixture of enzymes that primarily function to immobilize, kill, and digest the snake's prey. Proteolytic enzymes cause muscle and subcutaneous necrosis

▶ **TABLE 134–1. INDIGENOUS POISONOUS SNAKES OF THE UNITED STATES**

Southeast
  Eastern coral snake (*Micrurus fulvius fulvius*)
  Cottonmouths and copperheads (*Agkistrodon* spp.)
  Timber rattlesnake (*Crotalus horridus*)
  Eastern diamondback rattlesnake (*C. adamamteus*)
  Massasauga pygmy rattlesnake (*Sistrurus miliarius*)

East/Northeast
  Cottonmouths and copperheads (*Agkistrodon spp.*)
  Timber rattlesnake (*C. horridus*)
  Eastern massasauga (*S. catenatus*)

Mideast/Midwest/Central
  Cottonmouths and copperheads (*Agkistrodon* spp.)
  Timber rattlesnake (*C. horridus*)
  Western prairie rattlesnake (*C. viridus*)
  Eastern massasauga (*S. catenatus*)
  Massasauga pygmy rattlesnake (*S. miliarius*)

Southwest/West
  Cottonmouths and copperheads (*Agkistrodon* spp.)
  Western coral snake (*M. fulvius tenere*)
  Western diamondback rattlesnake (*C. atrox*)
  Western prairie rattlesnake (*C. viridus*)
  Great basin rattlesnake (*C. viridus lutosus*)
  Sidewinder rattlesnake (*C. cerastes*)
  Mojave rattlesnake (*C. scutulatus*)
  Timber rattlesnake (*C. horridus*)
  Rock rattlesnake (*C. lepidus*)
  Black-tailed rattlesnake (*S. molossus*)
  Twin-spotted rattlesnake (*C. pricet*)
  Red diamond rattlesnake (*C. ruber*)
  Speckled rattlesnake (*C. mitchelli*)
  Tiger rattlesnake (*C. tigris*)

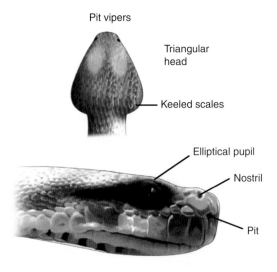

Pit vipers

Triangular head

Keeled scales

Elliptical pupil

Nostril

Pit

Figure 134–1. Pit vipers classically possess a triangular or arrow-shaped head and facial pits between the nostril and eye that serve as heat and vibration sensors, enabling the snake to locate prey. (From *Auebach PS. Wilderness Medicine.* 5th ed. Philadelphia: Mosby/Elsevier; 2007.)

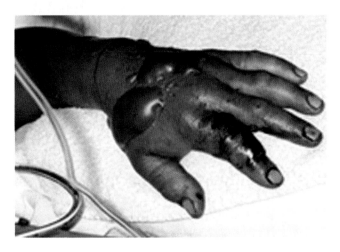

Figure 134–2. If the pit viper envenomation is severe, extremity swelling, edema, and hemorrhagic vesicles can appear within hours. ernursey.blogspot.com/ 2007archive.html.

as a result of a trypsinlike action. Hyaluronidase decreases the viscosity of connective tissue, phospholipase provokes histamine release from mast cells, and thrombinlike amino acid esterases act as defibrinating anticoagulants.[8] The major toxic effects occur within the surrounding tissue, blood vessels, and blood components.

CLINICAL PRESENTATION

Local cutaneous changes classically include one or two puncture marks with pain and swelling at the site, while nonvenomous snakes usually leave a horseshoe-shaped imprint of multiple teeth marks. Approximately 25% of all pit viper bites are considered "dry bites" resulting in no toxicity. If the envenomation is severe, swelling and edema may involve the entire extremity within 1 hour. Ecchymosis, hemorrhagic vesicles, and petechiae may appear within several hours (Fig. 134–2). Systemic signs and symptoms include paresthesias of the scalp, periorbital fasciculations, weakness, diaphoresis, nausea, dizziness, and a "minty" or metallic taste in the mouth. Severe bites can result in coagulopathies, thrombocytopenia, and disseminated intravascular coagulation (DIC).[9] Rapid hypotension and shock, with pulmonary edema and renal and cardiac dysfunction, can also result, particularly if the victim suffers a direct intravenous envenomation.

PREHOSPITAL MANAGEMENT

The victim's extremity should be immobilized and physical activity minimized. To maintain renal flow and intravascular volume, oral fluids are vigorously administered. Overaggressive first aid measures can be dangerous and may exacerbate limb morbidity. Incision and suction of the bite wound with the human mouth may result in tissue damage or infection. Mechanical suction devices exist and have been anecdotally reported to remove up to one-third of the venom if used immediately after envenomation, but no well-designed human clinical trials

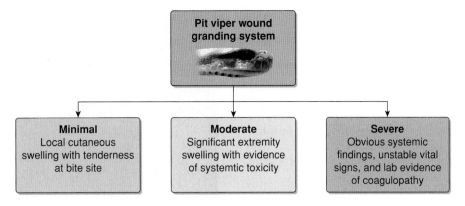

Figure 134–3. Pit viper wound grading system.

exist which support their use. A more recent study used a porcine model to examine the effects of the Sawyer extractor on local envenomation findings. These authors found no improvement in limb swelling when the extractor was used. In addition, 20% of the experimental animals developed localized skin necrosis at the extractor application site.[10] Cryotherapy can lead to further wound necrosis and is not currently recommended. Electric shock therapy was historically publicized as a first aid treatment of snakebites, but again case reports and animal studies have not documented any improvement with this prehospital technique.

Optimal therapy consists of placing the patient at rest with the affected extremity raised to the cardiac level. Emergency evacuation should be arranged as quickly as possible for transport to the closest facility with access to antivenom therapy. During transport, the wound site should be measured and leading edges marked, so that symptom progression can be judged upon hospital arrival. Intravenous access is obtained if possible and narcotic analgesics administered. The prehospital use of crotaline Fab antivenom may be available in the future. Currently, this intervention is unstudied, and cannot be recommended. Crotaline snakebite wounds are generally graded as minimal, moderate, and severe based on the degree of envenomation, which can ultimately guide therapy (Fig. 134–3).

DIAGNOSTIC STUDIES

Laboratory studies recommended in the assessment of rattlesnake bites include a complete blood count including platelets, prothrombin time or international normalized ratio (INR), partial thromboplastin time, fibrinogen level, and fibrin degradation products. Abnormal hematologic parameters are considered evidence of systemic toxicity and should be incorporated along with clinical examination into the decision to administer antivenom. If initial laboratory testing is normal and minor local tissue swelling and pain are present, it is acceptable to reevaluate these hematologic laboratory values in 2 to 6 hours. Other laboratory testing such as chemistry panels, creatinine phosphokinase (CPK), and urinalysis should be monitored if evidence of rhabdomyolysis, myoglobinuria, or renal insufficiency are present.

HOSPITAL MANAGEMENT

Patients presenting after rattlesnake envenomation should be given tetanus prophylaxis if indicated. Affected extremities should be elevated to the level of the heart and any previously placed constriction bands or wraps removed. Intravenous access in an unaffected extremity should be established for the delivery of antivenom as well as analgesic medications. The liberal use of narcotic agents is often necessary to control pain. Prophylactic antibiotics are generally not recommended since rattlesnake venom possesses its own bacteriostatic properties. However, evidence of infection or a history of human mouth suction to the wound may be indications for wound culture and initiation of a first-generation cephalosporin or amoxicillin-clavulanate.[11]

While prophylactic fasciotomy and digital dermatomy have been advocated as routine crotaline snakebite treatments in the past, these techniques are discouraged and rarely indicated. A true compartment syndrome is unlikely following rattlesnake envenomation.[1,12,13] Rattlesnake strikes generally place venom subcutaneously, not subfascially. The tense edema that is frequently apparent is usually a result of swelling and necrosis of the subcutaneous tissues. As a result, these bitten extremities should not be managed like other potential compartment syndromes. The preferred treatment for significant limb swelling is intravenous antivenom. Surgical therapy should only be considered in cases where elevated compartment pressures have been well documented despite aggressive intravenous antivenom therapy. Surgical debridement of devitalized tissues or amputation of necrotic digits may become necessary but should be delayed until complete wound stabilization.[14]

ANTIVENOM THERAPY

Crotalidae Polyvalent Antivenin (Wyeth-Ayerst, ACP). Equine-derived crotaline polyvalent antivenin is an older whole IgG preparation for the treatment of rattlesnake envenomation in North America and South America and is still available in many hospitals. The antivenin is a high-affinity antibody that binds to the venom proteins and enhances elimination. It is effective against envenomations from rattlesnakes, cottonmouths, copperheads, fer-de-lance, cantiles, and South American bushmasters. The amount of antivenin administered depends on the severity of the envenomation. Antivenin is packaged in vials containing 10 mL. In general, if the envenomation is rated as minimal, 5 vials are routinely administered; in moderate cases, 10 vials are used; and in severe cases, 15 to 20 vials are administered. The amount of antivenin administered can also vary depending on the species and geographic distribution of the snake. In comparison with adults, pediatric patients are given proportionately more antivenin, since children receive a greater amount of venom per kilogram of body weight.

Polyvalent antivenin is most efficacious if given within 4 to 6 hours of the bite. It is of less value if delayed for 8 hours, and is of questionable value after 24 hours. Prior to any antivenin administration, skin testing is done with dilute horse serum given subcutaneously (this is usually included in the antivenin kit). However, skin testing is often inconsistent and can produce false-negative and false-positive results. In the setting of a severe envenomation, patients with positive skin reactions can still receive the antivenin, although close monitoring for anaphylaxis and pretreatment with diphenhydramine and glucocorticoids is essential. Epinephrine should also be ready at the bedside.

Serum sickness, a flulike syndrome with fever, malaise, arthralgias, lymphadenopathy, rash, pruritus, and urticaria, usually develops 10 to 20 days after antivenin administration, with symptoms proportionate to the number of vials given. It is generally self-limited and effectively treated with antihistamines and a short course of methylprednisolone.

Crotaline Fab antivenom is an ovine (sheep serum) preparation that is highly purified and consists of only the smaller Fab antibody fragments. Crotaline Fab is equally effective and safer than the older polyvalent antivenin product resulting in a significant reduction in the rates of allergic reaction.[5,14–19] However, in the event that Fab antivenom is not available, therapy with the traditional equine formulation may still be instituted.

Crotaline Fab antivenom is administered intravenously. As with the older antivenin, it is important to remember that dosing is based on venom load as opposed to the kilogram weight of the patient. Patients with envenomation symptoms should initially receive four to six vials of Crotaline Fab regardless of the child's size. Antivenom doses are dissolved in 250 to 500 mL of normal saline and infused over 30 to 60 minutes. The vast majority of pediatric envenomations occur in children who are mobile and greater than 10 kg. As a result, Crotaline Fab doses placed into 250 mL of normal saline for infusion should not be problematic in these younger patients.[5,7] Symptoms should be reassessed hourly and antivenom redosed at two to four vials until symptoms have stabilized or improved.

While the severity of acute side effects associated with the new crotaline Fab antivenom appears to be much lower than that of equine-based antivenom, patients should still be observed closely for anaphylactoid reactions. Most of these reactions can be easily treated by slowing the infusion rate and administering intravenous diphenhydramine. The incidence of serum sickness is low when crotaline Fab is used regardless of the number of vials given in the course of treatment.[7]

When indicated, Fab antivenom should be administered first as a larger dose to gain initial control, and then as smaller maintenance doses to prevent local recurrence.[1] A phenom-

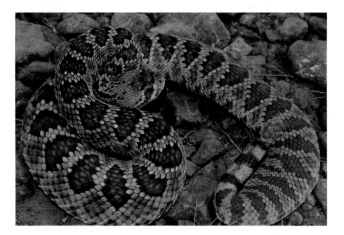

Figure 134–4. Mojave rattlesnake. www.elmerfudd.us/dp/pictures/animals.htm.

enon of recurrent venom effects has been observed following stabilization using crotaline Fab antivenom.[20] It is thought that this effect may be due to the rapid renal clearance of Fab antivenom in the face of depot venom at the wound site. Therefore, patients should be rechecked for recurrence of local and hematologic venom effects at 48 to 72 hours after stabilization. Recurrence is generally considered an indication for further antivenom dosing. Some clinicians and the product package insert recommend the administration of two additional vials of crotaline Fab every 6 hours for three doses to patients who develop laboratory evidence of coagulopathy or thrombocytopenia during the course of the envenomation. Persistent thrombocytopenia without clinical significance has been reported in one pediatric series.[16]

DISPOSITION

Asymptomatic patients presenting after a crotaline strike should be observed for a minimum of 8 hours following the injury. If no symptoms or signs of envenomation develop, the patient may be safely discharged with the diagnosis of a "dry" (nonenvenomated) bite. One exception to this rule would include patients with envenomation by a Mojave rattlesnake (*C. scutulatus scutulatus*) (Fig. 134–4). These snakes have been associated with delayed onset of significant neurotoxic symptoms.[21–23] Therefore, patients with presumed Mojave envenomation should be admitted and observed for a minimum of 24 hours.

All patients with symptoms of envenomation should be admitted for further antivenom therapy, wound care, and monitoring. These patients require admission to an intensive care setting that allows for frequent wound checks as well as frequent antivenom and analgesic dosing. Wound checks including extremity measurements should be performed hourly during the initial phase of treatment until symptoms have stabilized.

► CORAL SNAKES

Two members of the coral snake family (Elapidea) are indigenous to the United States. The western coral snake (*Micrurus euryxanthus*) found in Arizona and New Mexico and the more

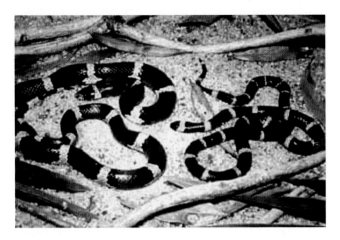

Figure 134–5. "Red on yellow, kill a fellow; red on black, venom lack" helps distinguish the venomous North American coral snake from the nonpoisonous scarlet king snake. http://www.tpwd.state.tx.us/learning/junior_naturalists/compare.phtml.

venomous eastern coral snake *(Micrurus fulvius fulvius)* found in the Carolinas and the Gulf states. Coral snakes account for only 1% to 2% of annual snakebites in the United States.

Coral snakes have rounded heads and circular pupils similar to many nonpoisonous species. The coral snake is often mistaken for certain varieties of the nonpoisonous king snake because both have red, yellow, and black rings. The old adage "red on yellow, kill a fellow; red on black, venom lack" helps distinguish the venomous coral snake from the nonpoisonous scarlet king snake (Fig. 134–5). Narrow yellow rings separate larger red and black bands on a coral snake while black rings are adjacent to red bands in the scarlet king snake. It is important to note that these distinguishing patterns are only accurate in North America. Highly venomous South American coral snakes and other snakes worldwide may have red and black adjacent bands. The much smaller fangs of a coral snake may leave little evidence of envenomation; therefore, any suspicion of an elapid bite warrants medical evaluation.

CLINICAL PRESENTATION

As with other Elapidae serpents, the venom of the coral snake is primarily neurotoxic. The bite site will initially exhibit local cutaneous edema, swelling, and tenderness. However, there have been reports of envenomation without evidence of actual tooth marks. Within several hours the patient may experience paresthesias, vomiting, weakness, diplopia, fasciculations, confusion, and occasionally respiratory depression. Convulsions have been observed in smaller children. The fatality rate from eastern coral snake bites is as high as 10%.[24]

MANAGEMENT

Coral snake bites are treated aggressively, since a significant bite can lead to neurologic and respiratory depression within 24 hours. Antivenin is administered early in the treatment course.[24] The coral snake antivenin is effective against bites

of the eastern coral snake, but not against western coral snake bites. Fortunately, the venom of the western coral snake is less toxic than that of its eastern counterpart. Three to five vials of the antivenin are generally recommended following skin testing. As with the *Crotalid* polyvalent antivenin, adverse side effects include anaphylaxis and serum sickness.

DISPOSITION

Any child who has sustained a documented bite from a coral snake is admitted to the intensive care unit for airway management and appropriate antivenin administration for a 24- to 48-hour period.

► EXOTIC SNAKES

Several bites occur each year from nonindigenous snakes.[25] Many of these snakes are illegally imported into the United States as exotic pets or purchased over the Internet from international distributors. Physicians encountering victims of exotic snake envenomation may receive assistance in treatment by calling the local zoo's herpetologist or regional poison control center. The general approach is local wound care, supportive treatment, and specific antivenin therapy, if available.

REFERENCES

1. Cox M, Reeves J, Smith K. Concepts in Crotalidae snake envenomation management. *Orthopedics.* 2006;29(12):1083–1087.
2. Sing KA, Erickson TB, Aks SE, et al. Eastern massassauga rattlesnake envenomations in an urban wilderness. *J Wild Med.* 1994;5:77.
3. Lawrence WT, Giannopoulos A, Hansen A. Pit viper bites: rational management in locales in which copperheads and cottonmouths predominate. *Ann Plastic Surg.* 1996;36:276–285.
4. Norris RL, Bush SP. North American venomous reptile bites. In: Auerbach PS, ed. *Wilderness Medicine.* 5th ed. St. Louis, MO: Mosby; 2007:1051–1085.
5. Richardson W, Barry J, Tri T, et al. Rattlesnake envenomation to the face of an infant. *Pediatr Emerg Care.* 2005;21(3):173–176.
6. Matteucci M, Hannum J, Riffenburgh R, Clark R. Pediatric sex group differences in location of snakebite injuries requiring antivenom therapy. *J Med Toxicol.* 2007;3(3):103–107.
7. Richardson W, Offerman S, Clark R. Snake envenomations. In: Ahrens T, Aks W, et al., eds. *Pediatric Toxicology Erickson.* 1st ed. New York, NY: McGraw-Hill; 2005:548–555.
8. Iyaniwura TT. Snake venom constituents: biochemistry and toxicology (part 1). *Vet Human Toxicol.* 1991;33:468–474.
9. Cruz NS, Albarez RG. Rattlesnake bite complications in children. *Pediatr Emerg Care.* 1994;10:30.
10. Bush SP, Hegewald KG, Green SM, Cardwell MD, Hayes WK. Effects of a negative pressure venom extraction device (extractor) on local tissue injury after artificial rattlesnake envenomation in a porcine model. *Wild Environ Med.* 2000;11:180–188.
11. Clark RF, Selden BS, Furbee B. The incidence of wound infection following crotalid envenomation. *J Emerg Med.* 1993;11:583–586.
12. Talen DA, Danish DC, Clark RF. Crotalidae polyvalent immune Fab antivenom limits the decrease in perfusion pressure of the anterior leg compartment in a porcine crotaline envenomation model. *Ann Emerg Med.* 2003;41:384–390.

13. Talen D, Danish D, Grice G, et al. Fasciotomy worsens the amount of myonecrosis in a porcine model of crotaline envenomation. *Ann Emerg Med.* 2004;44:99–104.

14. Corneille MG, Larson S, Stewet R, et al. A large single-center experience with treatment of patients with crotalid envenomations: outcomes with an evolution of antivenin therapy. *Am J Surg.* 2006;192:848–852.

15. Clark RF, Williams SR, Nordt SP, Boyer-Hassen LV. Successful treatment of crotalid-induced neurotoxicity with new polyvalent FAB antivenom. *Ann Emerg Med.* 1997;30:54–57.

16. Pizon A, Riley, B, LoVecchio, et al. Safety and efficacy of Crotalidae polyvalent immune Fab in pediatric crotaline envenomations. *Acad Emerg Med.* 2007;14:373–376.

17. Trinh H, Hack J. Use of Crofab antinvenin in the management of a very young pediatric copperhead envenomation. *J Emerg Med.* 2005;29(2):159–162.

18. Dart RC, McNally J. Efficacy, safety and use of snake antivenoms in the United States. *Ann Emerg Med.* 2001;37:181–188.

19. Offerman SR, Bush SP, Moynihan JA, Clark RF. Crotaline Fab antivenom for the treatment of children with rattlesnake envenomation. *Pediatrics.* 2002;110:968–971.

20. Seifert SA, Boyer LV. Recurrence phenomena after immunoglobulin therapy for snake envenomations: part I. Pharmacokinetics and pharmacodynamics of immunoglobulin antivenoms and related antibodies. *Ann Emerg Med.* 2001;37:189–195.

21. Farstad D, Thomas T, Chow T, Bush S, Stiegler P. Mojave rattlesnake envenomation in southern California: a review of suspected cases. *Wild Environ Med.* 1997;8:89–93.

22. Jansen PW, Perkin RM, Van Stralen D. Mojave rattlesnake envenomation: prolonged neurotoxicity and rhabdomyolysis. *Ann Emerg Med.* 1992;21:322–325.

23. Bush SP, Siedenburg E. Neurotoxicity associated with suspected Southern Pacific rattlesnake envenomation. *Wild Environ Med.* 1999;10:247–249.

24. Kitchens CS, Van Mierop LH. Envenomation by the eastern coral snake (*Micrurus fulvius fulvius*). A study of 39 victims. *JAMA.* 1987;258:1615–1618.

25. Chippaux JP. Snake bites: appraisal of the global situation. *Bull World Health Organ.* 1998;76:515–524.

CHAPTER 135

Spider and Arthropod Bites

Timothy B. Erickson and Renee King

► HIGH-YIELD FACTS

- Black widow spider bites result in painful muscle spasms, secondary to neurotoxicity, that are responsive to antivenin.
- Brown recluse spider bites result in hematotoxicity and manifest locally as skin necrosis.
- Scorpion stings cause severe localized pain with occasional systemic effects in children.
- Hymenoptera stings from bees and wasps can result in severe anaphylactic reactions and are responsible for more adverse outcomes and fatalities in children than any other arthropods.
- Fire ant stings can cause painful localized skin reactions.

In North America, bites and stings by arthropods occur frequently. Approximately 50 000 bites or stings by these species occur annually with about half of these specifically because of spiders. There are more than 30 000 species of spiders, most of which cannot inflict serious bites to humans because of their delicate mouthparts and impotent or prey-specific venoms.[1] Most exposures go unnoticed or do not need treatment. Spiders are not known to spread infectious diseases, but certain spiders are known to produce toxic venoms, which can lead to local diseases of the skin, systemic toxicities, or neurological sequelae.

► BLACK WIDOW SPIDERS

ANATOMY

The *Latrodoctus* genus is a common spider found in temperate and tropical areas of the world. The species most common in North America include *L. bishopi, L. geometricus, L. hesperus, L. variolus,* and *L. mactans.* Generally speaking, females are 20 times larger, darker in color, and more toxic than their male counterparts. Black widows are described as charcoal or black with eight eyes, eight legs, fangs, poison glands, and a characteristic red hourglass mark on the ventral aspect of the abdomen (Fig. 135–1). Black widows seem to be more prevalent during warmer periods of the year.

PATHOPHYSIOLOGY

The female black widow is generally considered poisonous to humans; whereas the males are not significantly poisonous due to their small jaws and a minimal number of poison glands.

Black widows spiders control the amount of venom they inject; an estimated 15% of bites to humans are nonenvenomating.[2] The venom's toxicity is due to the α-latrotoxin present in the spider's venom. This toxin facilitates exocytosis of synaptic vesicles and the release of the neurotransmitters norepinephrine, γ-aminobutyric acid, and acetylcholine.[3] The toxin also causes degeneration of motor end plates, resulting in denervation. The venom destabilizes nerve cell membranes by opening ion channels, causing a massive influx of calcium into the cell, which may lead to hypocalcemia.

CLINICAL PRESENTATION

Black widow bites usually produce a pinprick sensation but often they go unnoticed. Within the first two hours after the bite, the site may develop redness, cyanosis, urticaria, or a characteristic halo-shaped target lesion. These local symptoms may be followed by generalized symptoms of pain in regional lymph nodes, chest, abdomen, and lower back. Pain classically descends down the lower extremities with burning sensation on the soles of the feet. Abdominal rigidity and vomiting can be quite severe and may even be mistaken as a surgical emergency.[4] According to one study, signs and symptoms in infants were erythema on wound areas, irritability, constant crying, sialorrhea, agitation, and seizures. Elementary aged children and adolescents described pain on the wound site, abdominal and thoracic pain, muscle spasms, and fine tremors.[5]

Flexor spasm of the limbs can cause the patient to assume a fetal position while writhing in pain. Other severe symptoms include hypertension, sweating, salivation, dyspnea with increased broncho-secretions, and convulsions. If untreated, these symptoms may persist for up to several days, followed by muscle weakness and pain for several weeks. Less common effects include compartment syndrome of the upper extremity[6] and priapism.[7] Death is uncommon, although it may occur from respiratory or cardiac failure, with an overall mortality of <5%.[8]

MANAGEMENT

Local wound care is appropriate and pain at the bite site may be relieved with early application of ice. Tetanus prophylaxis should be updated, but antibiotics are unnecessary unless there is evidence of a wound infection. Oral analgesics may be of benefit and parenteral analgesics, such as morphine, may be used if the pain is severe. Muscle spasms may require oral or parenteral benzodiazepines.

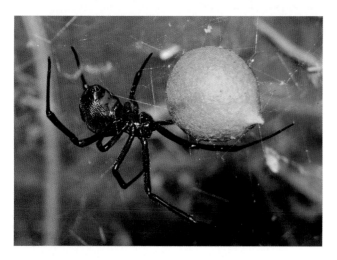

Figure 135–1. Female black widow spider with egg sac. www.prevailpest.com.

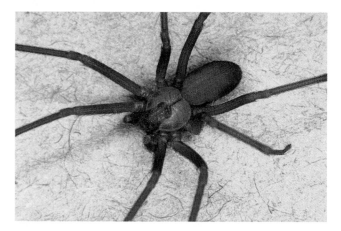

Figure 135–2. *Loxosceles reclusa*—also known as the Brown Recluse or "fiddle back" spider. www.deboradale. wordpress.com.

In the past, administration of calcium gluconate was considered because of concern for the development of hypocalcemia following black widow envenomation. This is currently not advocated as recent studies have proven no benefit to the administration of calcium.

In extreme cases with severe symptoms, latrodectus antivenin is recommended.[9] Antivenin is available in Australia and Arizona where envenomations occur most frequently. Since antivenin is derived from horse serum, the patient should be skin tested by injecting a 1:10 dilution subcutaneously to test for an anaphylactic reaction prior to administration of a full dose of the antivenin. Although this practice is recommended, the antivenin has been associated with a relatively low rate of allergic reactions.[10] The use of latrodectus-specific antivenin is restricted to patients with severe envenomation and no allergic contraindications and in whom opioids and benzodiazepines are ineffective. Young children[11] and elderly patients with severe toxicity should receive antivenin early in the clinical course, as well as patients with hypertensive and cardiac disease. Patients receiving antivenin may experience flu-like symptoms or serum sickness 1 to 3 weeks following treatment. This entity is generally self-limited and responsive to antihistamines and prednisolone.

DISPOSITION

Any symptomatic pediatric patient who has suffered a bite from a black widow spider is admitted for observation and pain control. If there is cardiopulmonary compromise or convulsions, the child is admitted to the intensive care unit for stabilization and antivenin administration.

► BROWN RECLUSE SPIDERS

The six species of recluse spiders in North America are *Loxosceles arizonica, L. deserta, L. devia, L. laeta, L. rufescens,* and *L. recluse. L. recluse* is the most common. The spiders are known to be reclusive nocturnal hunters and are more active from April to October. Their webs are scant and ill-

defined. Victims typically are bitten on the extremities while rummaging in confined spaces such as a closet or an attic, while putting on a shoe or using a blanket that a spider is trapped in.

ANATOMY

The brown recluse gets its name because of its brown or fawn colored body. It is approximately 1 to 5 cm in length, with a characteristic violin or fiddle-shaped marking on the dorsal cephalothorax (Fig. 135–2). They have long, slender legs and have six eyes rather than eight, which is the norm for spiders.[12]

PATHOPHYSIOLOGY

The venom of the recluse spider, per volume, is more potent than that of the rattlesnake and can cause extensive skin necrosis. The venom acts directly on the cell wall, causing immediate injury and cell death. It contains the calcium-dependent enzyme sphingomyelinase D which, along with C-reactive protein, has a direct lytic effect on red blood cells. Following cell wall damage, intravascular coagulation causes a cascade of clotting abnormalities and local polymorphonuclear leukocyte infiltration, culminating in a necrotic ulcer.

CLINICAL PRESENTATION

Most brown recluse bites occur in predawn hours and are often painless. The clinical response to loxoscelism ranges from cutaneous irritation (necrotic arachnidism) to a life-threatening systemic reaction. Most signs and symptoms of envenomation are localized to the bite area. The majority (90%) result in nothing more than a local reaction and resolve spontaneously.[13] Within a few hours, the patient experiences itching, swelling, erythema, and tenderness over the bite site. Classically, erythema surrounds a dull, blue-gray macule circumscribed by a ring or halo of pallor. The color difference is important in identifying necrotic arachnidism. Gradually, over 3 to 4 days, the wound forms a necrotic base with a central black eschar. In 7 to 14 days, the wound develops a full necrotic ulceration.[14] Some sources aver that the diagnosis of necrotic arachnidism secondary to brown recluse spiders is overreported in many case series due to inadequate documentation and call for stricter diagnostic criteria.[15–17]

The systemic reaction, which is much less common than the cutaneous reaction, is associated with a higher morbidity. The reaction rarely correlates with the severity of the cutaneous lesion. Within 24 to 72 hours following the envenomation, the patient experiences fever, chills, myalgias, and arthralgias. In severe systemic reactions, the patient may suffer coagulopathies, hypotension, jaundice, disseminated intravascular coagulation (DIC), convulsions, renal failure, and hemolytic anemia.[18,19] In rare cases, a patient may succumb to the systemic reaction.[13]

▶ HOBO SPIDER

The Hobo spider (*Tegenaria agrestis*), originally from Europe and central Asia, now resides in the Pacific Northwest region of the United States and Canada.[19] This spider should be included with *Loxosceles* species when discussing cases of necrotic arachnidism. Similar symptomatology leads many to incorrectly attribute hobo spider bites to that of the brown recluse, which is not indigenous to the northwest United States. This species exhibits an aggressive nature, biting with minor provocation.[20] Hobo spiders are brown with gray markings, have a 7- to 14-mm body length and 27- to 45-mm leg span (Fig. 135–3). They live in moist, dark environs such as woodpiles or basements.

MANAGEMENT

The proper management of envenomation by the brown recluse or hobo spider depends on whether the reaction is local or systemic. It is difficult to predict which type of wound

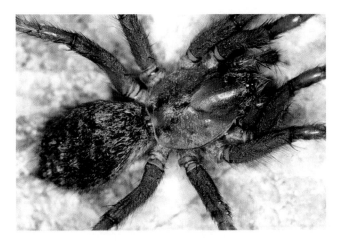

Figure 135–3. The Hobo spider (*Tegenaria agrestis*) can cause a necrotic skin lesion similar to a brown recluse spider. www.entomology.unl.edu.

will eventually progress to a disfiguring necrotic ulcer, so appropriate wound care should be done for all suspected brown recluse wounds. Proper care includes wound cleansing, immobilization, and elevation of the affected extremity to reduce pain and swelling. Early application of ice to the bite area will lessen the local wound reaction, whereas heat will exacerbate the symptoms. Tetanus immunization should be updated, but antibiotics are only indicated if there is a secondary wound infection. Antihistamines and analgesics prove to be beneficial, especially in children.

Early excision of ulcers and steroid injections are not recommended since studies have demonstrated that wound healing is slowed and scarring is more severe as a result those practices. Some complications of early surgical intervention include recurrent wound breakdown as well as long-term distal extremity dysfunction. Delayed excision of ulcers after the necrotic process has subsided (usually within 8 weeks), followed by secondary closure with skin grafting is the preferred way of dealing with necrotic ulcers due to brown recluse bites. With appropriate wound care, most bite wounds heal well with a 10% to 15% occurrence of major scarring.

Historically, the use of the polymorphonuclear leukocyte inhibitor, dapsone, was advocated to diminish scarring and subsequent surgical complications. Its use, however, has not proven effective in any large study with human or animal models.[21,22] Because of the potential for dapsone to induce methemoglobinemia and hemolytic anemia in children with G6PD deficiency, administration in pediatric patients is generally not advised. Another suggested method of treating expanding wound necrosis due to brown recluse spider bites is hyperbaric oxygen treatment. However, results with such treatment have been mixed and little evidence exists to support its use.[13,21]

Systemic effects of brown recluse spider bites are rare but can be life-threatening and should be treated aggressively. Although not proven in clinical trials, glucocorticoids may provide a protective effect on the RBC membrane, thus slowing hemolysis. The patient must be monitored closely for the development of DIC. Transfusion of RBCs and platelets may be necessary. Urine alkalinization with bicarbonate may lessen renal damage if the patient is experiencing acute hemolysis. Although it is not commercially available in the United States, there is ongoing research with brown recluse antivenom.[23] However, there is little evidence to support its efficacy, particularly against local effects.[10]

DISPOSITION

Patients with a rapidly expanding lesion or necrotic area with evidence of hemolysis are hospitalized. Patients who are asymptotic following a period of observation in the emergency department and have normal baseline laboratory values may be discharged home with close outpatient follow-up for wound care within 24 to 48 hours.

▶ TARANTULAS

Tarantulas are widely feared because they are the largest of all spiders (Fig. 135–4). Found predominantly in the deserts

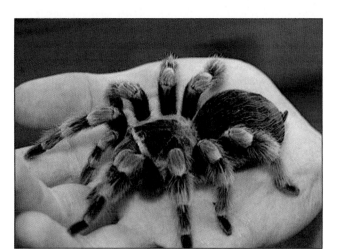

Figure 135–4. Common tarantulas are extremely shy and bite only when vigorously provoked or roughly handled. www.userbars.be.

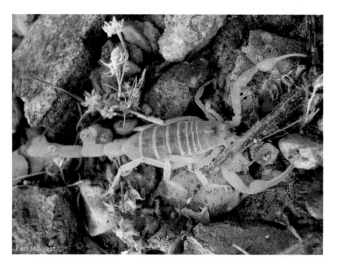

Figure 135–5. The bark scorpion or *Centruroides exilicauda* has a pair of anterior legs with pinchers, a segmented body, and a long, mobile tail equipped with a stinger. www.museum.utep.edu.

of the western United States, but spotted even as far east as the Mississippi River Valley, these large, hairy spiders are relatively harmless. They are extremely shy and bite only when vigorously provoked or roughly handled. Their bites usually cause minimal pain and surrounding edema with little or no necrosis and no serious systemic effects. While tarantula bites are usually of little consequence in humans, they can be more severe in household animals, especially canines. Treatment of bites consists of local wound care and tetanus prophylaxis. Involved limbs should be raised and immobilized and medication can be given to alleviate pain. If needed, the patient can be treated with antihistamines and topical glucocorticoids. The growing trade of these arachnids as exotic pets should prompt the clinician to inquire about this as a possible cause an unusual skin lesion.[24]

More concerning than tarantula bites is exposure to the hairs on their abdomen. These hairs can be flicked off in large numbers as a defense mechanism and are capable of producing urticaria and pruritis that may persist for several weeks. The hairs may also get into the eyes and cause keratoconjunctivitis or ophthalmia nodosa, a nodular, granulomatous lesion in the eye.[25] Patients with these complaints after exposure to a tarantula should be immediately referred to an ophthalmologist. Without appropriate care, these eye lesions may progress to keratitis, uveitis, retinitis, and even orbital cellulitis.

▶ SCORPIONS

Epidemiologically, scorpions are the most significant of all arachnid envenomations, potentially resulting in adult morbidity and pediatric mortality.[10] Worldwide, scorpions are responsible for thousands of deaths annually.[26,27] In the United States, there have been no reported deaths from scorpion stings in more than 25 years. Nevertheless, they remain a public health concern throughout the South and Southwest. Despite a steady decline in the number of deaths from scorpion stings over the past 20 years in Mexico, children younger than 5 years and the elderly remain the most vulnerable patient populations.[28]

ANATOMY

The scorpion has a pair of anterior legs with pinchers, a segmented body, and a long, mobile tail equipped with a stinger (Fig. 135–5). While members of the genera *Hadrurus*, *Vejovis*, and *Uroctonus* are capable of inflicting painful wounds, only the southwestern desert scorpion (*Centruroides exilicauda*, formerly *C. sculpturatus*) poses a serious health threat in the United States. Also called bark scorpions because they cling to the bottom of fallen brush and trees, they are brownish in color, vary in length from 1 to 6 cm, and are most active at night. The chitin shell of this scorpion will fluoresce under an ultraviolet or Wood's lamp, aiding in identification.

PATHOPHYSIOLOGY

Centruroides venoms cause spontaneous depolarization of nerves of both the sympathetic and parasympathetic nervous systems.

CLINICAL PRESENTATION

Unless the scorpion is identified, the diagnosis is based on clinical symptoms. Most victims will have only local pain, tenderness, and tingling; however, young children and those who suffer more serious envenomations may manifest the venom effects as overstimulation of the sympathetic, parasympathetic, and central nervous systems. Elevation of all the vital signs usually occurs within an hour of envenomation and tachydysrhythmias may develop during this time. Dysconjugate, "roving" eye movements are very common in children, along with other neurological findings including muscle fasciculations, weakness, agitation and opisthotonos. Less common findings are ataxia, respiratory distress, and seizures.

MANAGEMENT

The treatment of *Centruroides* envenomations is supportive. Cool compresses and analgesics are used for the local symptoms and pain. Wound care and tetanus prophylaxis are indicated. Tachydysrhythmias and hypertension may be treated with intravenous β-blockers, such as esmolol or labetalol. Benzodiazepines may be helpful for agitation and muscle spasms. Advanced life support and airway control are essential for more severe envenomations. Recently, a clinical score predicting the need for hospitalization in scorpion stings has been described.[29]

In the United States, a *Centruroides*-specific, goat-derived antivenom (Antivenom Production Laboratory, Arizona State University) has been available in very limited supply.[20,30] Scorpion antivenom directed against different species has been produced for research or clinical use in several other countries.[31] As with all animal-derived antivenoms, both immediate and delayed allergic reactions including serum sickness are possible.[32] For this reason, *Centruroides*-specific antivenom should be reserved for cases of severe systemic toxicity. Consultation with a toxicologist experienced in scorpion envenomation is recommended before using antivenom. Although investigations outside the United States have found no benefit in routine administration of antivenom for scorpion stings, one to two vials of antivenom, in cases of severe toxicity, can lead to rapid resolution of symptoms.[20]

▶ HYMENOPTERA

The order hymenoptera includes bees, vespids (hornets and wasps), and fire ants. These insects cause one-third of all reported envenomations in the United States and an estimated 50 to 150 annual deaths. While hymenoptera venoms possess intrinsic toxicity, it is their ability to sensitize the victim and cause subsequent anaphylactic reactions that makes them so lethal.

BEES AND VESPIDS

Honeybees (*Apis mellifera*) are fuzzy insects with alternating black and tan body stripes. Not intrinsically aggressive, they usually sting defensively when stepped on. Like that of other hymenoptera, the honeybee's stinger is a modified ovipositor (only females' sting) that is connected to a venom sac. Since honeybees lose their barbed stinger after stinging and die, they generally only sting in defense when provoked.

Africanized honeybees, or "killer bees," (*Apis mellifera scutellata*) (Fig. 135–6) are now found in Texas, Arizona, California, and most of the temperate southeastern and southwestern states.[33] In the 1950s, African bees were imported into Brazil for breeding experiments designed to improve honey production and disease resistance. Many escaped and subsequently mated with previously imported European honeybees.[34] These hybrids have since migrated northward along the coasts and temperate regions of the continent. Although the toxicity of their venom is equal to that of their native counterpart, they are far more aggressive. A hive can respond

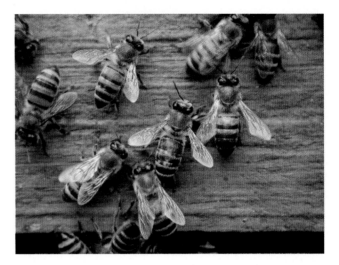

Figure 135–6. Africanized honeybees, or "killer bees" (*Apis mellifera scutellata*), are dangerous because they sting in large swarms. www.uni.uiuc.edu.

to a perceived threat with more than 10 times the number of bees than its typical native North American counterpart. Massive numbers of stings from an attack of Africanized bees can result in multisystem damage and death from severe venom toxicity. Most patients of massive envenomation suffer acute tubular necrosis or renal involvement with myoglobinuria.[35] In swarms, these bees can overwhelm and kill even healthy nonallergic victims.[36]

The most common hornets in the United States are the yellow jackets (*Vespa pennsylvanica*). They are usually seen around garbage cans, beverage containers, and various foods. They are extremely aggressive and sting with little provocation. Wasps (*Polistes annularis*, the paper wasp) have thin, smooth bodies and a formidable sting. They build their nests in the eaves of buildings. These vespids are carnivorous and able to use their smooth stingers multiple times, unlike honeybees, which lose their stingers after a single sting.[37,38]

Pathophysiology

Hymenoptera venoms contain enzymes that directly affect vascular tone and permeability. Although their enzymes are similar, there is little immunologic cross-reactivity between bee and vespid venoms. While a bee sting may not sensitize a person to yellow jacket venom, a yellow jacket sting would more likely sensitize one to wasp venom.[39] Four possible reactions are seen after hymenoptera stings: a local reaction, toxic reaction, systemic anaphylaxis, and a less common delayed-type hypersensitivity reaction.[20,40]

Local reactions are the most common reactions resulting from the vasoactive effects of the venom and are generally mild. The most common response includes pain, mild erythema, edema, and pruritus at the sting site. There are no systemic signs or symptoms, but a severe local reaction may involve one or more contiguous joints. Local reactions occurring in the mouth or throat can produce swelling that may lead to upper airway obstruction, especially in younger children.

Toxic reactions may occur when a patient suffers from multiple stings. Africanized bees are notorious for such attacks, but an aggressive native hive may elicit a similar response. The essential lethal dose is approximately 20 stings/kg in most mammals.[38] Symptoms of a toxic reaction may resemble anaphylaxis, but gastrointestinal manifestations (nausea, vomiting, and diarrhea) and sensations of light-headedness and syncope may also occur. Headache, fever, drowsiness, involuntary muscle spasms, edema without urticaria, and convulsions may ensue. Although urticaria and bronchospasm are not always present, severe envenomations may lead to respiratory insufficiency and arrest. Hepatic failure, rhabdomyolysis, and DIC have been reported in both adult and pediatric victims. Toxic reactions are believed to occur from a direct multisystem effect of the venom.

Anaphylactic reactions are aeneralized systemic allergic reactions that may occur after envenomation. Generalized systemic reactions to hymenoptera venom are thought to occur from an immunoglobulin E (IgE-) mediated mechanism, leading to the release of pharmacologically active mediators within mast cells and basophils. Symptoms are often mild, but severe reactions can lead to death within minutes. Unlike the toxic reaction, there is no correlation between systemic allergic reactions and the number of stings. The majority of allergic reactions occur within the first 10 to 15 minutes and nearly all occur within 6 hours. Fatalities that occur within the first hour of the sting usually result from airway obstruction or hypotension. Initial symptoms typically consist of ocular pruritus, facial flushing, and generalized urticaria. Symptoms may intensify rapidly with chest or throat constriction, wheezing, dyspnea, abdominal cramping, diarrhea, vomiting, vertigo, fever, laryngeal stridor, syncope, and shock.

Delayed reactions, appearing 1 to 2 weeks after a sting, consist of serum sickness-like signs and symptoms of fever, malaise, headache, urticaria, lymphadenopathy, and polyarthritis. This reaction is believed to be immune complex-mediated.[40]

Management

If present, the embedded stinger should be removed manually. Previous sources recommended cautiously scraping the stinger off with lateral pressure, rather than grasping it, in order to avoid compression of the venom sac resulting in further release of venom. However, recent studies have demonstrated that this is erroneous because the venom has likely been completely released within seconds of envenomation.[41] Treatment is symptomatic, with ice or cold compresses and an antihistamine. In more severe local reactions, there is a more sustained inflammatory response and the swelling may spread to the entire extremity and persist for several days. A short course of prednisone (1 mg/kg/d for 5 days) may decrease the duration of symptoms.

Toxic reactions reflect the effects of multiple stings (usually 25–50 stings or more). Gastrointestinal symptoms are the principal features; urticaria and bronchospasm are not usually present. Treatment is supportive. A novel Fab-based antivenom for the treatment of massive bee attacks is under investigation.[42]

Systemic reactions occur in approximately 1% of hymenoptera stings. They range from mild, non–life-threatening cutaneous reactions to classic anaphylactic shock. In all but the mildest of systemic reactions, the mainstay of treatment is

epinephrine. Epinephrine counteracts the bronchospastic and vasodilatory effects of histamine. Epinephrine can be given as a subcutaneous injection (0.01 mL/kg of 1:1000 solution; not to exceed 0.3 mL). In more severe reactions, the intravenous or endotracheal route is preferred (0.1 mL/kg of 1:10 000 solution). The dose may be repeated at 15-minute intervals as needed. Early intubation is indicated if there is evidence of severe laryngeal edema or stridor because airway obstruction is the leading cause of death in anaphylaxis. Antihistamines should be given early, but not as a substitute for epinephrine. An H_2-receptor blocker (e.g., cimetidine or ranitidine), in addition to an H_1-receptor blocker (diphenhydramine), may aid in inhibiting the vasodilatory effects of histamine. Adjunctive therapy for bronchospasm might include inhaled β_2-agonists (e.g., albuterol) and intravenous aminophylline. When hypotension is present, vigorous isotonic fluid resuscitation should be instituted. Glucocorticoids should be given for their anti-inflammatory effects as well as their effect in preventing the late-phase response.

A delayed serum sickness–like reaction may appear 10 to 14 days following the initial sting. This immune complex disorder may be treated with a short course of prednisone.

Venom immunotherapy desensitization is very effective in preventing further systemic reactions, with 95% to 100% protection after 3 months of treatment. Referral to an allergist is indicated for any child who has experienced life-threatening respiratory symptoms or hypotension. Children less than 16 years old who have only urticaria or angioedema do not require venom immunotherapy. Only 10% of these children will have systemic reactions with subsequent stings.[41]

Disposition

Essential to the treatment of any systemic reaction is the prevention of future reactions. Patients who have had a systemic reaction should be instructed to wear protective clothing and avoid hymenoptera-infested habitats. Portable epinephrine kits (Epi-Pen and Epi-Pen Jr) are available. They should be prescribed prior to the patient leaving the emergency department. The patient should be urged to carry the kit at all times and to use epinephrine for any systemic symptoms. Even if symptoms are mild, the patient should seek emergency care. The patient should also be instructed to wear a medical alert tag.

▶ IMPORTED FIRE ANTS

Five known species of fire ants belonging to the genus *Solenopsis* are found in the United States. Two of the species were imported into the United States, the red fire ant (*Solenopsis invicta*) and the black fire ant (*Solenopsis richteri*), of which *S. invicta* is the predominant species (Fig. 135–7). They were "imported" aboard ships from South America during World War II and subsequently spread throughout the Southeast. They are presently found in 13 southern states, from Florida to Texas; their geographic range apparently limited by soil, temperature, and moisture.[43]

S. invicta are 2 to 5 mm in size and red in color. They live in colonies and build large mounds up to 3 ft. in diameter, which are interconnected by underground tunnels up to 100-ft. long. These mounds are found most commonly in

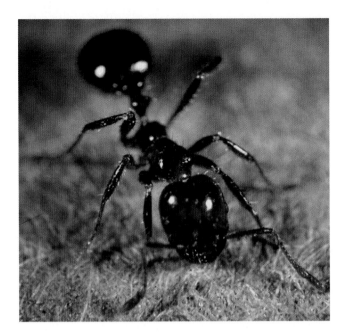

Figure 135–7. Fire ants (*Solenopsis*) are social insects that tend to attack in swarms, inflicting multiple stings. www.sbs.utexas.edu.

yards, playgrounds, and open fields.[44] Fire ants are aggressive insects with no natural enemies. They are social insects and tend to attack in swarms, with multiple stings the norm. In endemic areas, nearly 50% of the exposed population is stung each year. Stings are more common among children and occur most frequently on their ankles and feet during the summer months.

PATHOPHYSIOLOGY

Bee and wasp venoms are made of proteins. Conversely, fire ant venoms are 95% alkaloids.[38] Fire ants sting in a two-phase process. The ant first bites the victim with powerful mandibles, then, if undisturbed, will arch the body and swivel around the attached mandibles to sting the victim repeatedly with the stinger. This produces a characteristic circular pattern of papules/stings around two central punctures. Fierce fire ant attacks ensue in response to an alarming pheromone released by an individual or group of ants.

Fire ant venoms produce a sharp, burning sensation; hence the name. The venoms have cytotoxic, bactericidal, insecticidal, and hemolytic properties. They also activate the complement pathway and promote histamine release. Fire ant venoms are immunogenic and result in sensitization of the sting victim creating the risk of future anaphylaxis.

CLINICAL PRESENTATION

Clinical manifestations reflect the venom's effects and are predominantly local dermatologic reactions. The initial bites and stings cause burning pain associated with circular wheals or papules around the central hemorrhagic punctures. The wheal-and-flare reactions resolve within 1 hour, but then develop into sterile pustules within 24 hours. The pustules slough off over 48 to 72 hours, leaving shallow ulcerated lesions. The pustules are intensely pruritic and often become contaminated after the victim scratches the lesions. Secondary infections are usually minor but may cause considerable morbidity.

Between 15% and 50% of victims develop more severe local reactions, characterized by an exaggerated wheal-and-flare response, followed by the development of erythema, edema, and induration >5 cm in diameter. These lesions are intensely pruritic, may resemble cellulitis, and persist for 24 to 72 hours.[44]

MANAGEMENT

Topical glucocorticoid ointments, local anesthetic creams, and oral antihistamines may be useful for the itching associated with these reactions. No intervention has been shown to prevent or resolve the pustules. Treatment consists of local conservative measures including application of ice or cool compresses for symptomatic relief and gentle, frequent cleansing of the affected areas to prevent secondary infections.

Anaphylactic reactions have been estimated to occur after as many as 1% of fire ant stings. Anaphylaxis may occur several hours after a sting and is known to occur more frequently in children than in adults.

Immunotherapy may be appropriate for persons with severe hypersensitivity to fire ant venom or those who have had a previous anaphylactic reaction to a fire ant sting. The efficacy of immunotherapy has been variable, but it has been reported to provide as high as 98% protection.[43,45]

REFERENCES

1. Diaz J, Leblanc K. Common spider bites. *Am Fam Physician.* 2007;75(6):869–873.
2. Peterson ME. Black widow spider envenomation. *Clin Tech Small Anim Pract.* 2006;21(4):187–190.
3. Rash LD, Hodgson WC. Pharmacology and biochemistry of spider venoms. *Toxicon.* 2002;40:225–254.
4. Clark RF, Wethern-Kestner S, Vance MV, et al. Clinical presentation and treatment of black widow spider envenomation: a review of 163 cases. *Ann Emerg Med.* 1992;21:782–787.
5. Sotelo-Cruz N, Hurtado G, Gomez N. Poisoning caused by Latrodectus mactans (black widow) spider bite among children. clinical features and therapy. *Gac Med Mex.* 2006;142(2):103–108.
6. Cohen J, Bush S. Case report: compartment syndrome after a suspected black widow spider bite. *Ann Emerg Med.* 2005;45(4):414–416.
7. Hoover N, Fortenberry J. Use of antivenin to treat priapism after a black widow spider bite. *Pediatrics.* 2004;111(1):128–129.
8. Woestman R, Perkin R, Van Stralen D. The black widow: is she deadly to children? *Pediatr Emerg Care.* 1996;12(5):360–364.
9. Clark RF. The safety and efficacy of antivenin *Latrodectus mactans. Clin Toxicol.* 2001;39:125–127.
10. Isbister G, Graudins A, White J, et al. Antivenom treatment in archnidism. *J Toxciol Clin Toxicol.* 2003;41(3):291–300.
11. Reeves JA, Allison EJ, Goodman PE. Black widow spider bite in a child. *Am J Emerg Med.* 1996;14:469–471.
12. Erickson T, Hryhorczuk DO, Lipscomb J, et al. Brown recluse

spider bites in an urban wilderness. *J Wild Med.* 1990;1:258–264.

13. Tutrone W, Green K, Norris T, et al. Brown recluse spider envenomation: dermatologic application of hyperbaric therapy. *J Drugs Dermatol.* 2005;4(4):424–428.

14. Swanson D, Vetter R. Bites of brown recluse spiders and suspected necrotic arachnidism. *N Eng J Med.* 2005;352(7):700–707.

15. Vetter R, Swanson D. Of spiders and zeras: publications of inadequate documentation loxoscelism case reports. *J Am Acad Dermatol.* 2007;56(6):1063–1064.

16. Furbee R, Kao L, Ibrahim D. Brown recluse envenomation. *Clin Lab Med.* 2006;26(1):211–226.

17. Osterhoudt KC. Diagnosis of brown recluse spider bites in absence of spiders. *Clin Peadiatr.* 2003;42(6):406.

18. Elbahlawan L, Stidham G, Bugnitz M, et al. Severe systemic reaction to Loxosceles recluse spider bites in a pediatric population. *Pediatr Emerg Care.* 2005;21(3):177–180.

19. Anonymous (Center for Disease Control). Necrotic arachnidism—Pacific Northwest, 1988–1996. *MMWR Morb Mortal Wkly Rep.* 1996;45:433–436.

20. Tong T, Scheir A, Clark RF. Arthropod bites and stings. In: Erickson T, Ahrens W, Aks S, et al., eds. *Pediatric Toxicology: Diagnosis and Management of the Poisoned Child.* 1st ed. New York, NY: McGraw-Hill; 2005:556–566.

21. Philips S, Kohn M, Baker D, et al. Therapy of brown spider envenomation: a controlled trial of HBO, dapsone and cryoheptadine. *Ann Emerg Med.* 1995;25:363–368.

22. Vetter R, Bush S. Additional considerations in presumptive brown recluse spider bites and dapsone therapy. *Am J Emerg Med.* 2004;22(6):494–495.

23. deRoodt AR, Estevez-Ramirez J, Litwin S, et al. Toxicity from two North American loxosceles (brown recluse spiders) venoms and their neutralization by antivenoms. *Clin Toxicol.* 2007;45(6):678–687.

24. Saucier JR. Arachnid envenomation. *Emerg Clin North Am.* 2004;22(2):405–422.

25. Belyea DA, Tuman DC, Ward TP, Babonis TR. The red eye revisited: ophthalmia nodosa due to tarantula hairs. *South Med J.* 1998;91:565–567.

26. Bucaretchi F, Bacaracat EC, Nogueira RJ, et al. A comparative study of severe scorpion envenomation in children caused by Tityus bahiensis and Tityus serrulatus. *Rev Inst Med Trop Sao Paulo.* 1995;37:331–336.

27. Das S, Nalini P, Antakrishnan S, et al. Cardiac involvement and scorpion envenomation in children. *J Trop Pediatr.* 1995;41:338–340.

28. Celis A, Gaxiola RR, Sevilla GE, et al. Trends in mortality from scorpion stings in Mexico 1979–2003. *Rev Panam Salud Publica.* 2007;21(6):373–380.

29. Quan D, LoVecchio F. A clinical score predicting the need for hospitalization in scorpion envenomations. *Am J Emerg Med.* 2007;25(7):85–86.

30. Sofer S, Shahak E, Gieron M. Scorpion envenomation and antivenin therapy. *J Pediatr.* 1994;124:973–978.

31. Abroug F, ElAtrous S, Nouira S, et al. Serotherapy in scorpion envenomation: a randomized controlled trial. *Lancet.* 1999;354:906–909.

32. Lovecchio F, Welch S, Klemmens J, et al. Incidence of immediate and delayed hypersensitivity to centruroides antivenin. *Ann Emerg Med.* 1999;34:615–619.

33. Kim KT, Oguro J. Update on the status of Africanized honeybees in the western United States. *West J Med.* 1999;170:220–222.

34. Whitfield CW, Behura SK, Berlocher SH, et al. Thrice out of Africa: ancient and recent expansions of the honey bee, Apis mellifera. *Science.* 2006;314(5799):642–645.

35. Bourgain C, Pauti M, Fillastre J, et al. Massive poisoning by African bee stings. *Press Med.* 1998;27(22):1099–1101.

36. Bledsoe BE. Unwelcome visitors: is EMS ready for fire ants and killer bees. *Emerg Med Serv.* 2007;36(8):68–72.

37. Vetter RS, Visscher PK, Camizine S. Mass envenomation by honey bees and wasps. *West J Med.* 1999;170:223–227.

38. Fitzgerald KT, Flood AA. Hymeoptera stings. *Clin Tech Small Anim Pract.* 2006;21(4):194–204.

39. Hamilton RG. Diagnosis of hymenoptera venom sensitivity. *Curr Opin Allergy Clin Immunol.* 2002;2:347–351.

40. Lazoglu AH, Boglioli LR, Taff ML, et al. Serum sickness reaction following multiple insect stings. *Ann Allergy Asthma Immunol.* 1995;75:522–523.

41. Erickson T. North American arthropod envenomation and parasitism. In: Auerbach PS, ed. *Wilderness Medicine.* 5th ed. St. Louis, MO: Mosby; 2007:947–981.

42. Jones RGA, Corteling RL, To HP, et al. A novel Fab-based antivenom for the treatment of mass bee attacks. *Am J Trop Med Hyg.* 1999;61:361–366.

43. Rhoades R. Stinging ants. *Curr Opin Allergy Clin Immunol.* 2001;1:343–348.

44. Kemp SF, deShazo RD, Moffitt JE, et al. Expanding habitat of the imported fire ant (Solenopsis invicta): a public health concern. *J Allergy Clin Immunol.* 2000;105:683–691.

45. Cohen PR. Imported fire ant stings: clinical manifestations and treatment. *Pediatr Dermatol.* 1992;9:44.

CHAPTER 136

Marine Envenomations

Timothy B. Erickson and Armando Marquez

▶ HIGH-YIELD FACTS

- For most marine stings, local wound care, irrigation, tetanus immunization, wound exploration for foreign bodies, and selected antibiotic coverage are standard therapies.
- Hot water soaks are recommended for stingray, scorpion fish, echinoderm, and catfish stings.
- Dermatologic irrigation with vinegar, rubbing alcohol, household ammonia, baking soda, or papain will neutralize many coelenterate envenomations, including jellyfish.
- Antivenoms are available for stonefish, box jellyfish, and sea snake envenomations.

As more humans venture into aquatic environments for recreational activities, vacations, and an improved quality of life, the opportunity for children to encounter venomous marine life increases. Also, as more aquarists collect exotic marine life for display in the home, the incidence of bites and stings will rise regardless of the geographic locale.[1] Hazardous marine life can be classified into four major groups:

- Venomous bites and stings, such as those inflicted by scorpion fish and the Portuguese man-o'-war.
- Shock injuries, as from electric eels.
- Traumatogenic bites (such as from sharks and barracudas).
- Toxic ingestions or fish poisoning.[2]

This chapter will discuss venomous bites and stings.

Toddlers are most likely to be envenomed in shallow waters and are typically unable to give a detailed or reliable history. Young children may step on poisonous marine animals or handle them resulting in extremity stings. Adolescents are more adventurous and frequent deeper waters as surfers,[3] ocean swimmers, snorkelers, and scuba divers.[4] This age group is also more susceptible to intoxication with ethanol or recreational drugs.[1]

▶ COELENTERATES

Coelenterates (phylum Cnidaria) include jellyfish, sea anemones, and corals. Jellyfish stings are the most common marine envenomations, with an estimated 500 000 annual stings occurring in the Chesapeake Bay and 250 000 in Florida. A commonly encountered jellyfish is the sea nettle (*Chrysaora quinquecirrha*), which is widely distributed in temperate and tropical waters. One of the more feared jellyfishes is the Portuguese man-o'-war *(Physalia physalis).* This jellyfish is most commonly found in the Gulf of Mexico and off the Florida coasts between July and September. Its tentacles can reach up to 30 meters in length (Fig. 136–1). The deadliest and most venomous of coelenterates is the box jellyfish or sea wasp of Australia (Fig. 136–2).[5–7]

PATHOPHYSIOLOGY

Coelenterates envenomate with organelles called nematocysts, which contain venom-bearing threads that reside within specialized epithelial cells on the tentacles. Each nematocyst is a capsule with a folded eversible tubule, carrying a variety of toxins with neurologic, cytolytic, and enzymatic effects. Upon contact or when encountering a change in osmolality, these threads are everted from the nematocysts in order to be thrust into the prey (Fig. 136–3). When a human is stung, the penetration reaches into the innervated and vascular dermis. Both living and dead coelenterates can envenomate, as can fragmented tentacles and "unfired" nematocysts on the skin. Venoms vary, but generally contain histamine and kininlike factors capable of causing systemic as well as local tissue effects. The venom in nematocysts is potentially dermatonecrotic, myotoxic, cardiotoxic, neurotoxic, and hemolytic.

CLINICAL PRESENTATION

Mild coelenterate envenomation from true jellyfish or sea nettles generally causes local pruritus and characteristic linear, spiral, and painful urticarial lesions. The lesions often blister and there is localized surrounding edema. The pain and stinging sensation occurs instantly, peaks within 60 minutes, and may persist for hours. Systemic symptoms from Portuguese man-o'-war stings may include nausea, vomiting, dysphagia, muscle cramps, myalgias, arthralgias, diaphoresis, and weakness.[8] In addition, hemolysis and renal failure have been described following man-o'-war stings in pediatric patients.[9] Severe dyspnea and oral swelling as a result of a facial jellyfish envenomation in an adolescent patient has also been reported.[10] Other severe systemic symptoms include hemolysis, dysrhythmias, cardiovascular collapse, respiratory distress, paralysis, seizures, coma, and death.[11] The vast majority of *C. fleckeri* stings are not life-threatening with painful skin welts as the major finding. However, fatalities that do occur usually do so within 5 to 20 minutes of the envenomation.[12] Death in a child has been described in the literature following envenomation by the cuboid jellyfish *(Chiropsalmus quadrumanus)* which is found in the Atlantic and Indian Oceans.[13]

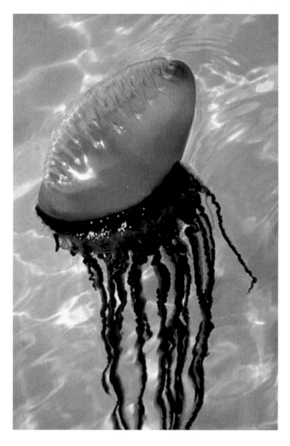

Figure 136–1. Portuguese man-o'-war. www.animals. nationalgeographic.com.

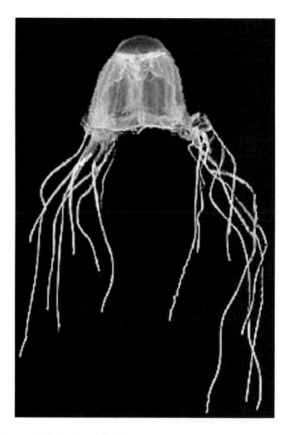

Figure 136–2. Box jellyfish or sea wasp. www.aimsgov.au.

MANAGEMENT

Treatment includes reassurance of the victim and immobilization of the injured part. Ice may provide some analgesia. The area is rinsed with sterile saline or seawater to maintain a condition isosmolar to seawater and to wash off unfired nematocysts. Fresh water is not recommended because it is hypoosmolar and often activates unfired nematocysts. As soon as possible apply a topical decontaminant. To inactivate nematocysts remaining on the skin, alter the pH by soaking the wounds with a weak acidlike household vinegar (5% acetic acid solution).[14] The inactivated nematocysts are then removed by gentle shaving or scraping. In the absence of a razor and shaving foam, one can also use the edge of a credit card or something like a popsicle stick or clamshell.[5]

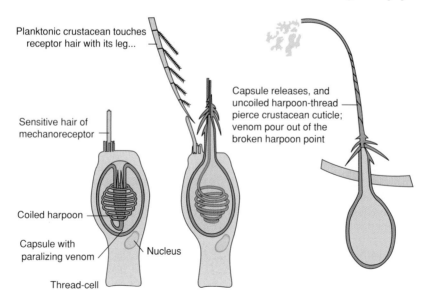

Planktonic crustacean touches receptor hair with its leg...

Sensitive hair of mechanoreceptor

Coiled harpoon

Capsule with paralizing venom

Nucleus

Thread-cell

Capsule releases, and uncoiled harpoon-thread pierce crustacean cuticle; venom pour out of the broken harpoon point

Figure 136–3. Coelenterate nematocysts.

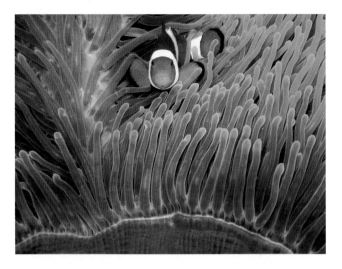

Figure 136–4. Sea anemone. www.tommyschultz.com.

If the victim shows signs and symptoms of anaphylaxis, treat appropriately. In most cases, analgesics and antihistamines are helpful. As a substitute for vinegar, one can apply household ammonia, rubbing alcohol, baking soda paste, or a slurry containing papain, which is commonly found in meat tenderizers.[10] Rubbing sand or pouring ethanol over the wounds has no proven efficacy. Human urine has actually been described as causing massive nematocyst discharge in *Chironex* tentacles and, contrary to popular belief, has little scientific basis for use.[15] Tetanus immunization is indicated, but prophylactic antibiotics are not.

Sea anemones (Fig. 136–4) and corals are sessile creatures that cause local urticarial reactions upon contact. Contact with hard (true) corals may cause lacerations that are treated with vigorous local wound care, topical antiseptics, and tetanus prophylaxis.

If a child is envenomated by an Australian box jellyfish, antivenom against Chironex is available in Australia and from major US city aquaria and certain theme parks, such as Sea World. The antivenom is ovine in derivation and has been administered safely in more than 75 episodes of envenomation. One ampule (20 000 units) can be administered IVPB, diluted in 1:5 ratio with crystalloid fluid, or it can be administered IM according to the manufacturer's instructions.[16] For the rapid onset of cardiotoxicity with severe envenomations, the antivenom should be given without delay and in proper doses to be life-saving.[12]

To prevent coelenterate stings, ocean bathers should wear proper skin protection, such as a neoprene "wet suit" or Lycra "dive skin." A commercially available jellyfish safe sun block is a topical sunscreen-jellyfish sting inhibitor combination that can be used to protect skin against stings and is recommended for anyone who will expose otherwise unprotected skin to jellyfish, fire corals, anemones, or other similar stinging creatures.[1,5]

DISPOSITION

Mild stings responsive to vinegar can be managed at home after a 3- to 4-hour observation. Children with systemic toxicity or inadequate pain control despite local wound treatment should be kept for observation. Any child envenomed by a box jellyfish should be kept for observation for 8 hours. Symptomatic patients may require antivenom.

▶ VENOMOUS FISH

There are more than 250 species of venomous fish, consisting mostly of shallow water reef or inshore fish. Stingrays are the most commonly encountered venomous fish, with more than 2000 stings reported annually. Eleven species of stingrays are found in US coastal waters.

On the West Coast, the round stingray (*Urolophus halleri*) is most commonly found; on the east coast and Caribbean, the southern stingray (*Dasyatis americana*) is most frequently encountered. They are flat, round-bodied fishes that burrow underneath the sand in shallow waters (Fig. 136–5). When startled or stepped on, the stingray thrusts its spiny tail upward and forward, driving its venom-laden stinging apparatus into the foot or lower extremity of the victim.

Varieties of scorpion fish include zebrafish and lionfish (*Pterois*), scorpion fish (*Scorpaena*), and stonefish (*Synanceja*), in increasing order of venom toxicity. Although more common in tropical waters of the Indo-Pacific, these fish are found in the shallow water reefs of the Florida Keys, Gulf of Mexico, southern California, and Hawaii. Lionfish are increasingly popular as aquarium pets (Fig. 136–6).[17,18]

Catfish are found in both fresh and salt water. Stings occur from spines contained within an integumentary sheath on their dorsal or pectoral fins. The hands and forearms of fishermen and seafood handlers are the most common sting sites.

PATHOPHYSIOLOGY

Stingrays have one to four venomous spines or barbs on the dorsum of a whiplike tail. The spines are retroserrated, so they anchor and may become difficult to remove (Fig. 136–7). As the sting is withdrawn, the sheath surrounding it ruptures and the venom is released. Parts of the sheath may be torn away and

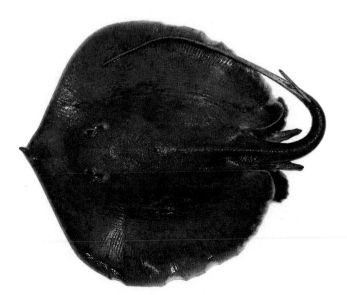

Figure 136–5. Sting ray.

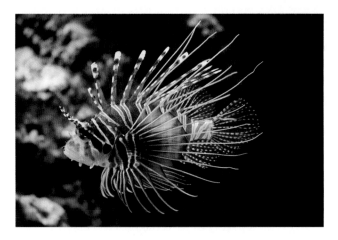

Figure 136–6. Lionfish.

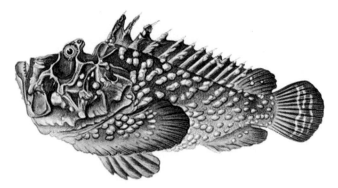

Figure 136–8. Stone fish.

remain in the wound. The venom is intensely active, partially heat-labile, and causes varying degrees of local tissue necrosis and cardiovascular disturbances. One death of a 12-year-old male is described in the literature from a stingray spine that directly penetrated the child's chest wall, heart and lung, resulting in myocardial necrosis and tamponade.[19]

Scorpionfish have venomous spines on the dorsal, anal, and pelvic fins. This venom is also partially heat-labile. Stonefish have 13 dorsal spines harboring one of the most toxic fish venoms (Fig. 136–8).[20] Analysis of stonefish venom re-

veals several toxic components including hyaluronidase, substances with hemolytic activity, and biogenic amines, such as norepinephrine. Cardiotoxicity is primarily from verrucotoxin, a negative chronotropic and ionotropic agent, that acts by inhibiting calcium channels.

For catfish spine stings, heat-labile venoms comprise dermatonecrotic, vasoconstrictive, and other bioactive agents produce symptoms similar to those of mild stingray envenomations. A unique parasitic catfish, the Amazonian Candiru (genus *Urinophilus*), may invade its victim by swimming "upstream" into the human urethra. Acute painful hemorrhage may result if forceful extraction of the catfish is attempted.[21]

CLINICAL PRESENTATION

With stingrays, intense pain out of proportion to the apparent injury is the initial finding, peaking within 1 hour and lasting up to 48 hours. Signs and symptoms are usually limited to the injured area, but weakness, nausea, anxiety, and syncope have been reported.

Envenomations from lionfish, scorpionfish, and stonefish cause immediate intense pain that peaks within 60 to 90 minutes and persists for up to 12 hours. Local erythema or blanching, edema, and paresthesias may persist for weeks. Systemic findings include nausea and vomiting, weakness, dizziness, and respiratory distress. Although similar to those of the other scorpion fish, stonefish stings are more severe. Stonefish venom, a potent neurotoxin, can cause dyspnea, hypotension, and cardiovascular collapse within 1 hour and death within 6 hours. Local necrosis and severe pain may persist for days.

With catfish stings, burning and throbbing sensation occurs immediately, but usually resolves within 60 to 90 minutes. The discomfort may last up to 48 hours. Systemic symptoms are rarely reported.

MANAGEMENT

Treatment of stingray wounds includes irrigation with sterile saline to dilute the venom and remove sheath fragments. The spine of the stingray including the venom gland is typically difficult to remove from the victim and radiographs may be necessary to locate the spine or retained fragments.[22] However, a recent large retrospective study of 119 sting ray injuries found

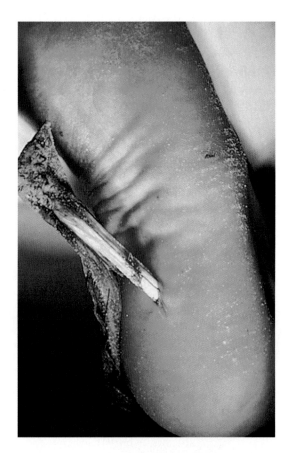

Figure 136–7. Embedded sting ray barb in foot. www.healthline.com.

no positive radiographic evidence of foreign bodies in any of their patients.[23]

The injured part should be immersed in hot water, no warmer than 113°F, for 30 to 90 minutes, to inactivate any heat-labile venom components.[15] Analgesics are usually required. Because of the penetrating nature of the envenomation, wounds are debrided and left open. Tetanus immunization is updated if needed. Treatment with a broad-spectrum prophylactic antibiotic such as trimethoprim–sulfamethoxazole (TMP–SMX), ciprofloxacin, or a third-generation cephalosporin is recommended because of concern for infection by *Vibrio* species, as well as *Staphylococcus* and *Streptococcus* spp.[3]

Treatment for scorpionfish and lionfish envenomation is immersion of the affected limb in hot water (113°F) for 30 to 90 minutes, or until pain is relieved. Some case reports have documented failure to respond to standard warm water immersion therapy at 45°C.[18] Wounds are irrigated with sterile saline, explored, and cleaned of debris. The wound is left open and treatment with prophylactic antibiotics is initiated.[24]

Local treatment for a stonefish sting is the same as that for envenomations by other scorpion fish, with special attention given to maintaining cardiovascular support.[4] There is a specific stonefish antivenom available in Australia.[25] The antivenom is an equine-derived product and carries the risk for inducing anaphylaxis. One 2 mL ampule of stonefish antivenom is diluted in 50 mL normal saline and given IVPB. A case series of eight patients suggests that the majority of stonefish envenomations do not result in significant morbidity or mortality and usually require only supportive management.[26] Another larger more recent series of 57 patients suffering stonefish envenomation noted severe pain in 95% of victims with half of the patients requiring hospital admission. All responded to analgesic medications and antibiotic coverage and there was no mention of antivenom administration.[27] It remains uncertain whether stonefish antivenom is efficacious in stings of other venomous fish.[12]

Catfish sting treatment is immediate immersion in hot water (no warmer than 113°F) for pain relief. Catfish spines may penetrate the skin and break off. Sometimes, the spines can be located by routine radiographs. Occasionally, MRI is necessary to locate a foreign body. The wound should be explored and debrided. Retained catfish spines should be removed by a qualified practitioner. The puncture wound is left open. Treatment with prophylactic, broad-spectrum antibiotics and tetanus prophylaxis are indicated.

DISPOSITION

Children with mild stings responsive to hot water soaks may be discharged after observation. Children not responsive to pain management may have a retained foreign body. Children envenomed by stonefish should be monitored in an intensive care setting. If it is available, antivenom administration is indicated in symptomatic patients.

► ECHINODERMS

Echinoderms are spiny invertebrates that include sea urchins, sea stars, starfish, sand dollars, and sea cucumbers. Of these,

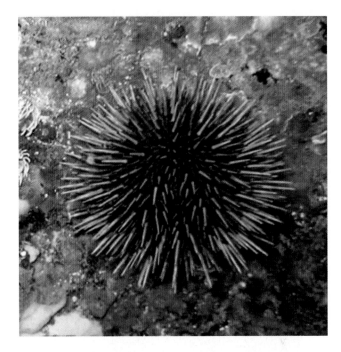

Figure 136–9. Sea urchin. www.withquiz.org.uk.

sea urchins most often cause medically significant envenomations. They are slow moving, colorful bottom dwellers found at various ocean depths (Fig. 136–9).

PATHOPHYSIOLOGY

The spines or pedicellariae of sea urchins produce painful puncture wounds, swelling, and localized erythema.

CLINICAL PRESENTATION

The spines can be up to 1 ft long in the needle-spined urchin (genus *Diadema*). They can easily puncture the skin, break off and be retained. Their venom can cause local pain that may persist for days.

MANAGEMENT

Treatment is immediate immersion in hot water (no warmer than 113°F), careful removal of pedicellariae and spines, and local wound care. Tetanus immunization and antibiotic prophylaxis are often indicated.[28,29]

DISPOSITION

Most sea urchin puncture victims can be discharged home with continued hot water soaks and antibiotic prophylaxis. If there is a retained foreign body, follow-up evaluation is prudent.

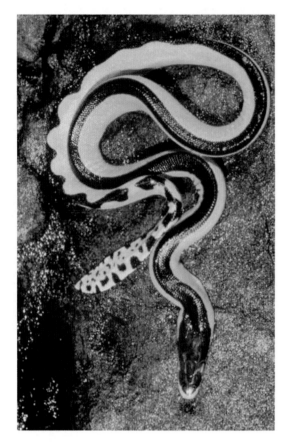

Figure 136–10. Venomous yellow-bellied sea snake.
www.susanscott.net.

► SEA SNAKES

Sea snakes of the family Hydrophiidae are encountered throughout the Indo-Pacific region. The yellow-bellied sea snake (*Pelamis platurus*) (Fig. 136–10) has the widest distribution ranging from the Indo-Pacific to Africa to Central America. Sea snakes are air-breathing reptiles with venomous anterior fangs. They are among the deadliest snakes in the world and may bite without provocation.[5,30] Most bites are associated with net fishing and inadvertent handling.

CLINICAL PRESENTATION

The venom of the sea snake has neurotoxic, myotoxic, and nephrotoxic effects. Most sea snake bites are dry bites with little venom injected. With true envenomations, symptoms usually manifest within 30 minutes to 3 hours. Initial symptoms may include muscle spasms and trismus. Severe envenomations may result in acute neurotoxicity with rapid muscular and respiratory paralysis.

MANAGEMENT

Apply pressure immobilization technique by wrapping the involved extremity with a compression bandage with immobilization until the victim is brought to definitive care. Respiratory support may be required. A polyvalent antivenom from Australia is commercially available.[12] Additionally, a monovalent antivenom designed for the Australian terrestrial tiger snake has been used successfully when the polyvalent sea snake antivenom is unavailable. If antivenom is administered, the patient should be closely monitored for signs of anaphylaxis and given appropriate doses of diphenhydramine, glucocorticoids, and epinephrine as needed.

DISPOSITION

All documented and suspected sea snake envenomation victims should be monitored in an intensive care setting for possible airway management and antivenom administration.

► SUMMARY

For an overview of management of marine envenomations, see Figure 136–11.

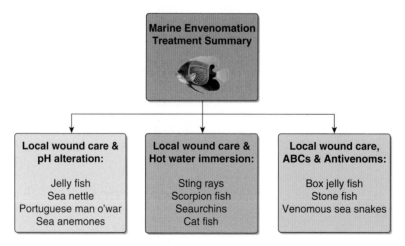

Figure 136–11. Marine envenomation treatment summary.

REFERENCES

1. Erickson T, Auerbach P. Marine envenomations and seafood poisoning. In: Erickson T, Ahrens W, Aks S, et al., eds. *Pediatric Toxicology: Diagnosis and Management of the Poisoned Child.* 1st ed. New York, NY: McGraw-Hill; 2005:524–532.

2. Brown CK, Shepherd SM. Marine trauma, envenomations and intoxications. *Emerg Med Clinic North Am.* 1992;10:385.

3. Taylor KS, Zoltan TB, Achar SA. Medical illnesses and injuries encountered during surfing. *Curr Sports Med Rep.* 2006;5(5): 262–267.

4. Lyon RM. Stonefish poisoning. *Wilderness Environ Med.* 2004; 15(4):284–288.

5. Auerbach P. Envenomation by aquatic animals. In: Auerbach PS, ed. *Wilderness Medicine.* 5th ed. St. Louis, MO: Mosby; 2007:1450–1487.

6. Auerbach PS. Marine envenomations. *N Engl J Med.* 1991;325: 486–493.

7. Hartwick R, Callanan V, Williamson J. Disarming the box jellyfish: nematocyst inhibition in Chironex fleckeri. *Med J Aust.* 1980;1:15.

8. Exton D, Moran PJ, Williamson J. Phylum echinodermata. In: Williamson JA, Fenner PJ, Burnett JW, et al., eds. *Venomous and Poisonous Marine Animals.* Sydney: University of South Wales; 1999:312–326.

9. Guess HA, Saviteer PL, Morris CR. Hemolysis and acute renal failure following a Potuguese man o' war sting. *Pediatrics.* 1983;70:979.

10. Armoni M, Ohali M, Hay E. Severe dyspnea due to jellyfish envenomation. *Pediatr Emerg Care.* 2003;19(2):84–86.

11. Fenner PJ, Williamson JA. Worldwide deaths and severe envenomation from jellyfish stings. *Med J Aust.* 1996;165:658.

12. Currie BJ. Marine antivenoms. *J Toxicol Clin Toxicol.* 2003;41 (3):301–308.

13. Bengston K, Nichols MM, Schnadig V, et al. Sudden death in a child following jellyfish envenomation (Chriopsalmus quadrumanus). Case Report and autopsy findings. *JAMA.* 1991; 266:1404.

14. Nimorakiotakis B, Winkel K. Marine envenomations Part 1-Jellyfish. *Aust Fam Physician.* 2003;32(12):969–974.

15. Atkinson PR, Boyle A, Hartlin D, et al. Is hot water an effective treatment for marine envenomation? *Emerg Med J.* 2006; 23(7):503–508.

16. Beadnell CE, Rider TA, Williamson JA, et al. Management of a major box jellyfish (Chironex fleckeri) sting. Lessons from the first minutes and hours. *Med J Aust.* 1992;156(9):655–658.

17. Aldred B, Erickson T, Lipscomb J, et al. Lionfish stings in an urban wilderness. *J Wilderness Environ Med.* 1994;4:291–296.

18. Vetrano SJ, Lebowitz JB, Marcus S. Lionfish envenomation. *J Emerg Med.* 2002;23(4):379–382.

19. Frenner PJ, Williamson JA, Skinner RA. Fatal and nonfatal stingray envenomation. *Med J Aust.* 1989;151:621.

20. Brenneke F, Hatz C. Stonefish envenomation-a lucky outcome. *Travel Med Infect Dis.* 2006;4(5):281–285.

21. Breault JL. Candiru: Amazonian parasitic catfish. *J Wilderness Med.* 1991;2:304.

22. Perkins RA, Morgan SS. Poisoning, envenomation and trauma from marine creatures. *Am Fam Physician.* 2004;69(4):885–890.

23. Clark RF, Girard RH, Roa D, et al. Stinray envenomation: a retrospective review of clinical presentation and treatment in 119 cases. *J Emerg Med.* 2007;33(1):33–37.

24. Auerbach PS, McKinney HE, Rees RS, et al. Analysis of vesicle fluid following the sting of a lionfish (Pterosis volitans). *Toxicon.* 1987;25:1350–1353.

25. Kreger AS. Detection of a cytolytic toxin in the venom of stonefish (Syanceia trachynis). *Toxicon.* 1991;29:733.

26. Lee JY, Teoh LC, Leo SP. Stonefish envenomations of the hand-a local marine hazard: a series of 8 cases and review of the literature. *Ann Acad Med Singapore.* 2004;33(4):515–520.

27. Grandcolas N, Galea J, Anada R, et al. Stonefish stings: difficult analgesia and notable risk of complications. *Presse Med.* 2008;3793:395–400.

28. Morocco A. Sea urchin envenomation. *Clin Toxicol.* 2005; 43(2):119–120.

29. Bedry R, de Haro L. Venomous and poisonous animals. V Envenomations by marine invertebrates. *Med Trop.* 2007; 67(3):223–231.

30. Bedry R, de Haro L. Venomous and poisonous animals. IV Envenomations by venomous aquatic vertebrates. *Med Trop.* 2007;67(2):111–116.

CHAPTER 137

Drowning

Julie Martino and Mark Mackey

► HIGH-YIELD FACTS

- Drowning is the second most common cause of nonintentional death in children and adolescents, with a bimodal distribution of peak incidence between the ages of 1 and 4 years and 11 and 14 years.
- While wet, dry, fresh water, and salt water drowning differ in pathophysiology, there is little difference in their clinical presentation and management.
- Early oxygenation and resuscitation, including establishment of an airway and provision of chest compressions, are the most important interventions in determining prognosis and survival.
- Poor prognostic indicators include prolonged submersion, asystole upon emergency department (ED) arrival, and delay in effective cardiopulmonary resuscitation.
- Hypothermia from immersion in extremely cold water may exert a protective effect, especially if the hypothermic event occurs before the immersion.
- Patients who have been asymptomatic and remain so, with a normal CXR and oxygenation, may be discharged after a 6-hour observation period.

In the past, there have been a number of terms associated with drowning that caused much confusion. Medical literature has used terms such as near-drowning (survival from a submersion event beyond 24 hours) and secondary drowning (drowning because of another abnormality that triggered the event).[1,2] In 2002, the World Congress on Drowning published the following consensus definition for drowning.

"Drowning is a process resulting from primary respiratory impairment from submersion/immersion in a liquid medium." Given this definition, duration of survival and initial cause of submersion are irrelevant. This chapter will use this definition for drowning and will identify mortality as "death from drowning."[3]

► EPIDEMIOLOGY

Drowning is the second leading cause of death from unintentional injuries in children aged from 1 to 14 years. It is the leading cause of death in children aged from 1 to 4 years. Males are more likely to drown than females in all age groups, with the highest rate in the 0 to 4 age group.[4]

► PATHOPHYSIOLOGY

Drowning occurs when airway submersion impairs respiration and causes hypoxia. The pathophysiology surrounding this event is complex and influenced by a number of factors (Table 137–1). Drowning medium, water temperature, associated trauma, and patient-specific factors are just a few of them. Despite the multitude of influencing variables, the primary insult is always hypoxia.

PULMONARY

After the patient is submerged, he or she aspirates a small amount of water causing reflex laryngospasm. Apnea leads to hypoxia and loss of consciousness. Once unconscious, most patients will aspirate a moderate amount of water. Approximately 10% of patients will maintain laryngospasm, causing what was previously described as "dry drowning."[5]

Aspirated fresh water and salt water cause different pathophysiologic effects on the pulmonary system but ultimately lead to the same result. Aspirated fresh water causes surfactant to washout, thus altering the surface tension properties of the alveolus. The alveoli collapse, preventing ventilation and causing an intrapulmonary shunt. Some of the fluid diffuses into the cell walls of the alveoli, leading to cell rupture and edema. Most water, however, is absorbed into the plasma volume. The ultimate effects of fresh water aspiration are ventilation–perfusion (V/Q) mismatch from alveolar collapse and shunt (Fig. 137–1).[5–9]

Salt water causes V/Q mismatch via a different mechanism. The aspirated hypertonic saltwater pulls fluid from the plasma into the alveolar spaces causing pulmonary edema. The fluid-filled alveoli thus are not ventilated, creating an intrapulmonary shunt (Fig. 137–1).[5–8,10]

NEUROLOGIC

Most neurologic sequelae are because of hypoxia and ischemia. Decreased ventilation causes hypoxemia. Cardiopulmonary arrest leads to decreased cerebral blood flow. The combination of hypoxemia and decreased cerebral perfusion rapidly leads to ischemia. The neuronal cell destruction that occurs with ischemia subsequently causes cerebral edema and increased intracranial pressure (ICP). Despite a number of trials in previous decades, monitoring of ICP following

▶ **TABLE 137-1. PATHOPHYSIOLOGY OF DROWNING**

System	Features
Pulmonary	Apnea Fresh water: surfactant washout and atelectasis Salt water: pulmonary edema V/Q mismatch and shunt
Neurologic	Cerebral ischemia caused by hypoxia Cerebral edema and increased ICP
Cardiovascular	Bradycardia Increased SVR Decreased cardiac output
Electrolytes	Metabolic acidosis Significant electrolyte changes are rare

drowning has not proven to influence management and thus is not recommended.[9,11,12] With cases of brain injury, tight glycemic control should be maintained.[6,11] Approximately 10% of drowning survivors will suffer severe neurologic sequelae.[5,6,7,9,11]

CARDIOVASCULAR

Cardiac arrhythmias normally occur as a consequence of hypoxia, acidosis, and hypothermia. Decreased oxygen tension sensed by the carotid bodies leads to activation of the autonomic nervous system and frequently results in bradycardia and peripheral vasoconstriction. Sinus bradycardia and atrial fibrillation are the most commonly observed rhythms.[2] Catecholamine release that accompanies the stress response also contributes to increased systemic vascular resistance.[2,9] The cardiovascular picture often resembles cardiogenic shock.[13] Decrease in cardiac output is usually related to the degree of hypoxemia and can be reversible with treatment of the underlying cause.[12,14]

ELECTROLYTES

Clinically, significant electrolyte derangements are uncommonly observed. Most patients who survive drowning aspirate less than 10 mL/kg water. Dog studies have shown that more than 11 mL/kg water need to be aspirated for fluid shifts and more than 22 mL/kg for significant electrolyte imbalances.[1,7] Acidosis that is commonly seen is initially because of apnea-related hypercarbia causing respiratory acidosis.

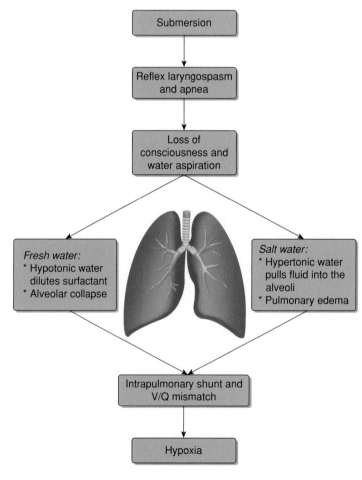

Figure 137-1. Pathophysiology of drowning.

Hypoxia-induced tissue ischemia can further contribute to acidosis, causing a mixed metabolic-respiratory acidosis.

RENAL

Renal failure can occur because of hypothermia and shock-induced acute tubular necrosis. Rhabdomyolysis can also occur, compounding the renal injury.[15]

HEMATOLOGIC

Disseminated intravascular coagulation (DIC) is uncommonly seen in the drowning victim and is a late finding when present.[2] Anemia can occasionally be seen in drowning victims. As the volume of aspirated water is rarely sufficient to cause hemodilution, any decrease in hemoglobin should be assumed to be because of blood loss.[1]

HYPOTHERMIA

Hypothermia (core body temperature <35°C) is often seen in drowning victims. It may contribute to bradycardia, ventricular fibrillation, acute respiratory distress syndrome (ARDS), and shock. Older literature has emphasized the importance of the "diving reflex." This occurs in mammals when the face contacts cold water. The body responds with breath holding, vasoconstriction, bradycardia, and decreased cardiac output. The outcome is increased blood flow to cardiac and cerebral tissues.

While there are a number of animals that exhibit this, it is not believed to play a significant role in humans.[9] There is recent data to suggest that induced hypothermia may exert neuroprotective properties on victims of cardiac arrest. While this is a promising avenue, further research needs to be performed in this area. Therapeutic hypothermia in the pediatric drowning victim cannot be universally recommended at this time.[16]

▶ MANAGEMENT

PREHOSPITAL

Since the outcome from drowning largely depends on the restoration of oxygenation and ventilation, rapid rescue and resuscitation is of prime consideration. Routine attempts at postural drainage or use of the Heimlich maneuver are not recommended. Suctioning is indicated in the event of vomiting which occurs in 66% of those receiving rescue breathing and 86% of those receiving chest compressions.[17] Coexistent cervical spine injury is rare in immersion injuries. Routine immobilization of the cervical spine is not recommended unless a potential high impact mechanism exists, such as diving into shallow water, boating accident, fall from a height, or the presence of alcohol.[18]

EMERGENCY DEPARTMENT

For those in cardiac arrest, reevaluation of the effectiveness of cardiopulmonary resuscitation (CPR) including intubation

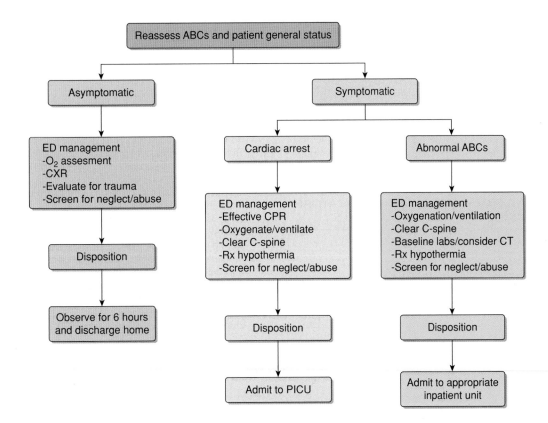

Figure 137–2. Management of pediatric drowning.

and ventilation and appropriate screening for cervical spine injuries are the management priorities. Early assessment for hypothermia should be performed with use of a low-reading rectal probe. The presence of severe hypothermia may dictate the duration of resuscitation and modify prognosis. Survival after prolonged submersion and cardiac arrest has been reported in cold water drowning.

Restoration of oxygenation in the victim who has a perfusing rhythm may require 100% oxygen and positive pressure treatment, such as continuous positive airway pressure (CPAP) or bilevel positive airway pressure (BiPAP). Intubation and ventilation with positive end-expiratory pressure (PEEP) are indicated for those with persistent hypoxia or ventilatory failure. Those with evidence of bronchospasm should be treated with β-agonists. Assessment of oxygenation and a baseline chest x-ray should be performed on all symptomatic patients. ARDS should be anticipated with significant fluid aspiration. There is no definitive evidence that empiric antibiotics or steroids have a positive affect on the incidence of ARDS or pneumonia.[7,9,10,19] Patients with altered mental status should be intubated for airway protection.

Obtain appropriate screening tests for alternate explanations of mental status changes including serum glucose, head CT scan, drug screening, and appropriate medication levels for patients with a history of seizures.[1] Serum electrolytes should be evaluated, but generally will not be affected without ingestion of a significant amount of water (>22 mL/kg).[7] Treatment of hypothermia is summarized in Chapter 125. Survival has been reported after prolonged cardiac arrest in hypothermic patients. Consider transferring the patient to a facility capable of cardiopulmonary bypass for victims who are severely hypothermic (<28°C).[20]

Please refer to Figure 137–2 for a summary of ED management of the drowning victim.

▶ PROGNOSIS

Most drowning victims either die or survive neurologically intact.[1] Of those patients who arrive to the ED awake and alert, survival approaches 100%. Good prognostic indicators include short submersion time and spontaneous pulse and respira-

tion. Approximately 10% of survivors have severe neurologic damage.[6,7,9,11] There are no signs or symptoms that can predict outcome with perfect accuracy. No one indicator should be used to decide upon treatment withdrawal.

Please refer to Table 137–2 for a list of poor prognostic indicators.

REFERENCES

1. Burford AE, Ryan LM, Stone BJ, et al. Drowning and near-drowning in children and adolescents. *Ped Emer Care.* 2005;21:610–616.
2. Hasibeder WR. Drowning. *Curr Opin Anaesthesiol.* 2003;16:139–146.
3. Idris AH, Berg RA, Bierens J, et al. Recommended guidelines for uniform reporting of data from drowning: the "Utstein style." *Circulation.* 2003;108:2565–2574.
4. Centers for Disease Control and Prevention. National Center for Injury Prevention and Control Web Based Injury Statistics Query and Reporting System. cdc.gov/ncipc/wisqars.
5. Quan L. Near-drowning. *Pediatr Rev.* 1999;20:255–260.
6. Moon RE, Long RJ. Drowning and near-drowning. *Emerg Med (Fremantle).* 2002;14:377–386.
7. Modell JH. Drowning. *NEJM.* 2003;328:253–256.
8. Giammona ST, Modell JH. Drowning by total immersion: effects on pulmonary surfactant of distilled water, isotonic saline, l and sea water. *Am J Dis Child.* 1967;114:612–616.
9. Ibsen LM, Koch T. Submersion and asphyxial injury. *Crit Care Med.* 2002;30:S402–S408.
10. van Berkel M, Bierens JJL, Lie RLK, et al. Pulmonary oedema, pneumonia, and mortality in submersion victims: a retrospective study in 125 patients. *Intensive Care Med.* 1996;22:101–107.
11. Bierens JJ, Knape JT, Gelissen HT. Drowning. *Curr Opin Crit Care.* 2002;8:578–586.
12. Orlowski JP, Szpilman D. Drowning: rescue, resuscitation and reanimation. *Pediatr Clin North Am.* 2001;48:627–646.
13. Hildebrand CA, Hartmann AG, Arcinue L, et al. Cardiac performance in pediatric near-drowning. *Crit Care Med.* 1988;16:331–335.
14. Orlowski JP, Abulleil MM, Phillips JM. The hemodynamic and cardiovascular effects of near-drowning in hypotonic, isotonic, or hypertonic solutions. *Ann Emerg Med.* 1989;18:1044–1049.
15. Bonnor R, Siddiqui M, Ahuja T. Rhabdomyolysis associated with near-drowning. *Am J Med Sci.* 1999;318:201.
16. American Heart Association. Part 10.3: Drowning. *Circulation.* 2005;112:IV-133-IV-135.
17. Manolios N, Mackie I. Drowning and near drowning on Australian beaches patrolled by life savers: a 10 year study, 1973–1983. *Med J Aust.* 1988;148:165–167, 170–171.
18. Watson RS, Cummings P, Quan L, et al. Cervical spine injuries among submersion victims. *J Trauma.* 2001;51:658–662.
19. Kennedy GA, Kanter RK, Weiner LB, et al. Can early bacterial complications of aspiration with respiratory failure be predicted? *Pediatr Emerg Care.* 1992;3:123–125.
20. Wollenek G, Honarwar N, Golej J. Cold water submersion and cardiac arrest in treatment of severe hypothermia with cardiopulmonary bypass. *Resuscitation.* 2002;52:255–263.

▶ **TABLE 137–2. POOR PROGNOSTIC INDICATORS IN DROWNING**

Prolonged submersion (>10 min)
Delay in effective CPR
Severe metabolic acidosis (pH <7.1)
Asystole on arrival in ED
GCS <5
Fixed, dilated pupils

CHAPTER 138

Pediatric Burns

Kavitha Reddy and Lisa Parke Maier

▶ HIGH-YIELD FACTS

- Burns are the fifth leading cause of unintentional injury-related death. Children younger than 4 years tend to have scalding-related injuries, whereas older children tend to suffer from exposure to flames.
- Most physicians use the classic Lund and Brower chart to estimate %BSA burned as it adjusts for the age of the patient. Because of the possibility for error in estimations, some physicians use the child's palm, considered approximately 1%, to measure the total %BSA burned.
- The primary survey should focus on the patency of the child's airway as well as the severity of the burn. Any carbonaceous sputum or singed nasal hairs should alert the physician to impending airway edema.
- Of particular importance are circumferential burns, which may cause both vascular and respiratory compromise. If vascular compromise is apparent, the patient should undergo an immediate escharotomy.
- The Parkland formula is widely used to estimate fluid requirements. This formula calls for an isotonic crystalloid solution (such as Lactated Ringers) to be given at 4 mL/kg/%BSA over a 24-hour period. Half of this fluid volume is given over the first 8 hours, and the second half is given over the next 16 hours.
- Pain management is an important consideration in burn management. Opioid analgesia is often required.
- Initial wound care in the emergency department should consist of covering the burns with a dry, sterile sheet. Antiseptic solutions such as povidone–iodine and topical antibiotics should be avoided in patients who are being transferred to a burn center until the primary service has had the opportunity to evaluate the wounds.
- Topical antibiotics are routine in outpatient burn care. One percent silver sulfadiazine is most commonly used.
- All burn patients should be reevaluated at 24 to 48 hours to ensure proper wound healing and to examine for signs of infection.

▶ EPIDEMIOLOGY

Burns account for the fifth leading cause of unintentional injury-related death. Between 1987 and 2000, the mortality rate for children younger than 14 years old has fallen by approximately 50%.[1] In 2002, there were about 90 000 visits to emergency departments related to pediatric burns.[2] Children younger than 4 years old tended to have scalding-related injuries, whereas older children tend to suffer from exposure to flames. In a recent study on mortality in pediatric burns, those with at least 60% total body surface area (TBSA) involved had a decrease in mortality rates from 33% to 14% over the last 20 years.[3] With earlier intervention, the morbidity and mortality related to thermal burns has decreased; however, there are still significant sequelae that increase with the amount of TBSA involved. The following chapter addresses common etiologies, clinical evaluation, management, and disposition of children who present to the emergency department with thermal injuries.

▶ ETIOLOGY

THERMAL

Many pediatric burns are unintentional and entirely preventable. Scald injuries are the most common cause of burns in children younger than 4 years old. These typically occur as a result of hot liquids that tip over or are accidentally spilled near a child. Children can sustain greater depth of injury to the skin with less contact time than adults. Prevention techniques such as keeping pot handles away from a child's reach or keeping bath water less than 120°F could greatly reduce unintentional burns.

FLASH

Accidental ignition of volatile substances, such as alcohol-based cleaners and liquids, can cause flash injuries to children. Because the time of exposure is so short, the result is usually a partial-thickness burn (Fig. 138–1).

FLAME

Flame injuries are the most common reason for burn-related injuries in older children. Young children can still sustain these types of burns, particularly with house fires, or even accidental ignition of clothing. In 2001, approximately 600 children died from unintentional fire-related incidents. Flames and burn injuries accounted for about a quarter of these deaths. These children can suffer from any type of burn ranging from partial-thickness to full-thickness burns. Complicating this process is the inhalation of toxic gases, including carbon monoxide and cyanide. Much has been done in the matter of fire prevention, including smoke-detector programs, as well as education in fire prevention and escape.

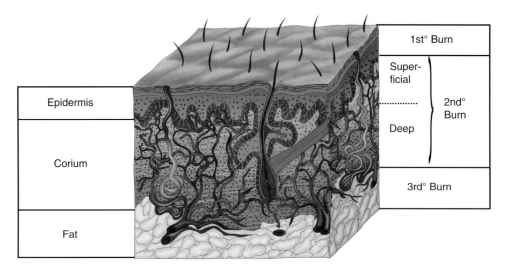

Figure 138–1. Depth of burn wounds.

CHILD ABUSE

Unfortunately, burn-related injuries are not only accidental. Any child with these injuries must be appropriately examined and family must be questioned to rule out potential abuse. The injury must match the mechanism described. For example, burns in a stocking distribution on the legs are highly suspicious for intentional scalding injuries in hot water. Appropriate authorities should be notified in these situations.

▶ PATHOPHYSIOLOGY

Burn injuries can range from simple first-degree burns to devastating fourth-degree burns. Tissues are destroyed by coagulation necrosis and the resulting inflammatory process. The injured cells begin to release vasoactive mediators that continue to cause injury even after the inciting agent is removed. Ischemia, necrosis, and thrombosis can occur. Later, the damaged capillaries become more permeable and leakage of protein and fluid into the interstitial space results in edema. Third-spacing of this fluid can result in profound intravascular hypovolemia and shock, especially in total-body burns. In addition to the potential for hemodynamic instability, injured tissue can serve as a nidus for bacterial infections. Given the potential for serious injury and complication, it is important to note the location, depth of injury, and percentage of body surface area involved. (Fig. 138–1)

FIRST DEGREE

First-degree burns involve the epidermis and sensation remains intact. There are no blisters. A good example is a sunburn. First-degree burns can easily be managed with pain medicine and usually heal in approximately 1 week (Fig. 138–2A).

SECOND DEGREE

Second-degree burns are also known as deep partial-thickness burns and involve the epidermis and part of the dermis. The skin will be edematous, often with blistering, weeping, and marked pain with palpation of the area (Fig. 138–2B). Scalding injuries are the most common etiologies. Healing time can be approximately 2 to 3 weeks.

THIRD DEGREE

Third-degree burns are also known as full-thickness burns. These injuries involve the entire extent of the epidermis and dermis. Nerve endings are damaged resulting in insensate skin, which can appear white, black, or dusky (Fig. 138–2C and 138–2D). There may be thin-walled blisters. The skin does not regenerate well and may require skin-grafting. Fluid losses can be severe with this type of injury.

FOURTH DEGREE

Fourth-degree burns are also full-thickness burns, but extend even further than the underlying dermis. The injury can involve muscles, tendons, and even bone, and obviously carries even more risk of fluid loss and infection compared with third-degree burns.

Burns can be classified by the above categories, or more commonly by either partial-thickness, deep-partial thickness, or full-thickness injury. It is important to note the type of burn involved, but even more important to note the location and percentage of body-surface area burned. This percentage becomes necessary to calculate fluid requirements, and the location of the burn will determine need for transfer to a burn center. This will be discussed further in the management section.

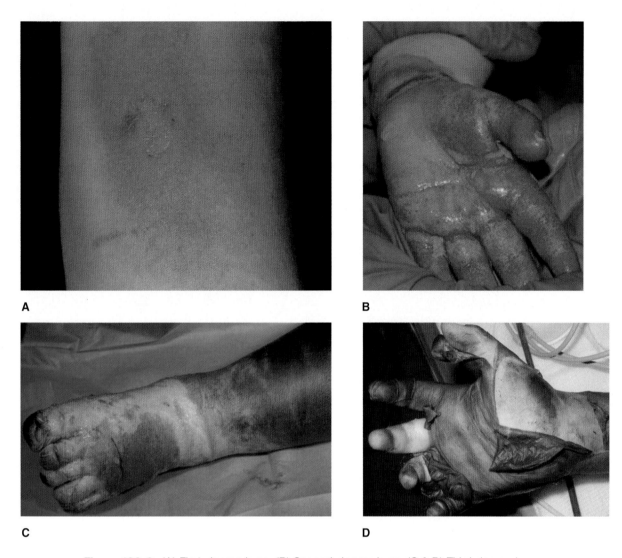

Figure 138–2. (A) First-degree burn. (B) Second-degree burn. (C & D) Third-degree burns.

The body surface area is generally calculated by using the "rule of nines." This is simply an estimate, generally more useful with adults. In this estimate, 9% surface area is given to the head and each upper extremity. Eighteen percent is given to the anterior chest and 18% is given to the posterior chest. Each lower extremity is worth 18% and finally, the perineal area and genitalia are 1%. Children have different proportions in their body parts, especially the head, and this can cause erroneous estimations. Most physicians use the classic Lund and Browder chart to estimate %BSA burned as it adjusts for the age of the patient (Fig. 138–3). Because of the possibility for error in estimations, some physicians use the child's palm, considered approximately 1%, to measure the total %BSA burned.

► CLINICAL EVALUATION

Of course, any evaluation begins with an initial history and physical examination. In the case of a severely burned child, time is of the essence. It is important to talk with the family, the child, and any witnesses to determine the cause of the burn and to rule out any possible physical abuse. If the patient was a victim of a fire, special considerations for potential carbon monoxide or cyanide toxicity, as well as smoke inhalation and hypoxia must be taken.

The primary survey should focus on the patency of the child's airway as well as the severity of the burn. Victims of fires are at increased risk for airway edema. Carefully examine the face including oral mucosa and nasal hairs. Any carbonaceous sputum or singed nasal hairs should alert the physician to impending airway edema. Because this process can occur quickly, early intubation is necessary.

If intubation is not deemed to be necessary, but the patient has some signs of bronchospasm or hypoxia, humidified oxygen can be supplied or PEEP/CPAP can be used. β-Adrenergic agonists, such as albuterol/levoalbuterol can improve bronchospasm. Monitor the patient with continuous cardiac monitoring and pulse oximetry.

A child with greater than 20%BSA burned will need further management with two large-bore intravenous lines. The amount of fluid needed will be discussed further in the management section. In addition to routine blood work the patient

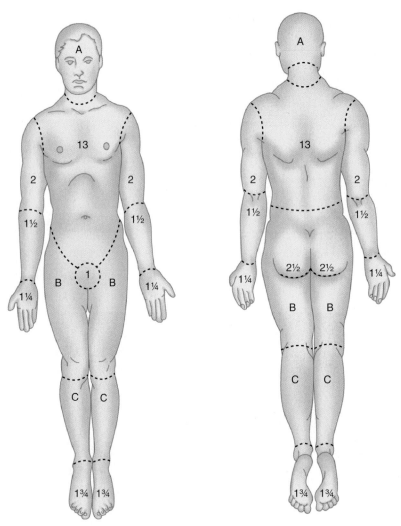

Relative percentages of areas affected by growth (age in years)

	0	1	5	10	15	Adult
A = half of head	9½	8½	6½	5½	4½	3½
B = half of one thigh	2¾	3¾	4	4¼	4½	4¼
C = half of one leg	2½	2½	2¾	3	3¼	3½

Second degree_____ and

Third degree_____ "

Total percent burned____

Figure 138–3. Classic Lund and Browder chart.

will need a chest x-ray, ABG to assess acid/base status, oxygenation, and carbon monoxide level, and type/cross-match if surgery or skin grafting will become necessary. A myoglobin level may be useful, as severely injured patients can have significant muscle injury and rhabdomyolysis.

The secondary survey should include a thorough physical examination. An examination of the eye using fluorescein stain should be considered to evaluate for corneal burns. The location and depth of burns should be recorded. Of particular im-

portance are circumferential burns, which may cause both vascular and respiratory compromise. Vascular perfusion should be carefully monitored using capillary refill and distal pulses, employing a Doppler evaluation if necessary. Signs of impending ischemia or compartment syndrome include pulselessness, paresthesias, and severe pain. If vascular compromise is apparent, the patient should undergo an immediate escharotomy, wherein a lateral incision is made through the depth of the eschar to relieve pressure. Escharotomy may also be indicated in circumferential burns of the thorax, which can mechanically impair chest wall expansion, leading to respiratory compromise.

▶ LABORATORY STUDIES

During the evaluation of a pediatric burn patient, it will be necessary to perform certain laboratory studies. The most important of these will include a complete blood count, basic metabolic panel, a myoglobin level, urinalysis, arterial blood gas, and coagulation studies along with a type and cross-match if surgical repair becomes necessary.

The white blood cell count in a burn victim will often be elevated initially because of acute demargination in response to injury, but it can become elevated because of infection and needs to be monitored closely. A patient can have a falsely elevated hemoglobin and hematocrit because of hemoconcentration from significant fluid loss, or can be low because of blood loss. It is important to assess the renal function in a burn patient in order to follow not only potential acidosis from volume loss, but also to see signs of acute tubular necrosis from myoglobinuria caused by muscle breakdown. The urine will show large blood without any evidence of red cells on microscopic analysis. Hyperkalemia can also develop from cell breakdown and a potential metabolic acidosis from hypovolemia and hypoperfusion can cause an extracellular shift of potassium. Continue aggressive hydration to avoid these potential complications.

Continual pulse oximetry monitoring, chest x-ray, and arterial blood gases with carbon monoxide levels can also help in assessing a patient's respiratory status, and are very necessary in patients with inhalation injuries, that is, fire victims.

▶ MANAGEMENT

After airway management has been addressed, the priority in burn patients is fluid resuscitation. Although there is controversy on the subject of resuscitation formulas, the Parkland formula is widely used. This formula calls for an isotonic crystalloid solution (such as Lactated Ringers) to be given at 4 mL/kg/%BSA over a 24-hour period. Half of this fluid volume is given over the first 8 hours, and the second half is given over the next 16 hours. BSA can be calculated using the Lund and Browder diagram (Fig. 138–3), with only second- and third-degree burns factoring into fluid resuscitation. Patients should be started on maintenance IV fluids as well, with adjustments to resuscitation made in order to maintain urine output of 1 mL/kg/h.[4,5]

Tetanus immunization should be administered to all patients without a complete immunizations series or who have not had a tetanus booster within 5 years.

Pain management is an important consideration in burn management. Burns, especially partial-thickness burns, can be extremely painful. Opioid analgesia is often required, preferably given intravenously because of fluid shifts and absorption irregularities from the oral and intramuscular routes. Morphine is the most commonly used analgesic, with a starting dose of 0.1 mg/kg IV.[6]

Initial wound care in the emergency department should consist of covering the burns with a dry, sterile sheet. The burn surface can be cleaned with a sterile saline solution, and debridement may be performed on devitalized tissue. Sterile saline-soaked dressings may be applied to small burns, but should be avoided in large burns because of the risk of developing hypothermia. Antiseptic solutions such as povidone–iodine and topical antibiotics should be avoided in patients who are being transferred to a burn center until the primary service has had the opportunity to evaluate the wounds.

Minor burns can be managed on an outpatient basis (Table 138–1). These burns should be cleaned with sterile saline solution. Ruptured blisters and devitalized tissue should be debrided. The management of intact blisters remains controversial; large or hemorrhagic blisters should be debrided but smaller blisters can be left intact.[7] Topical antibiotics are routine in outpatient burn care. One percent silver sulfadiazine is most commonly used, although it should be avoided in facial burns because of the risk of staining of the skin. Alternative agents include bacitracin or polymyxin B ointments, as well as commercially available dressings that contain silver.[8]

Sterile dressings should be applied. Conventional gauze dressings should be changed twice a day. Newer synthetic alternatives are available for smaller burns. Designed to act as a "second skin," these dressings do not require frequent changes and have been associated with improved patient compliance and outcomes.[9]

All burn patients should be reevaluated at 24 to 48 hours to ensure proper wound healing and to examine for signs of infection.

▶ TABLE 138–1. GUIDELINES FOR BURN TRIAGE AND DISPOSITION

Outpatient Management
  Partial-thickness burn—less than 10% body surface
  Full-thickness burn—less than 2% body surface

Inpatient Management
  Hospital (other than burn center)
    Partial-thickness burn—less than 25% body surface
    Full-thickness burn—less than 15% body surface
    Partial-thickness burn—face, hands, feet, perineum
    Questionable burn wound depth or extent
    Chemical burn, minor
    Significant coexisting illness or trauma
    Inadequate family support
    Suspected abuse
    Fire in an enclosed space
  Burn center
    Partial-thickness burn—more than 25% body surface
    Full-thickness burn—more than 15% body surface
    Full-thickness burn—face, hands, feet, perineum
    Respiratory tract injury
    Associated major trauma
    Major chemical and electrical burns

With permission from American Academy of Pediatrics; Dallas: American College of Emergency Physicians. Burns: thermal and electrical trauma. In Strange GR, ed. *APLS: The Pediatric Emergency Medicine Course.* Elk Grove Village, IL: American Academy of Pediatrics and Dallas: American College of Emergency Physicians; 1998:108.

▶ DISPOSITION

Indications for outpatient management, admission, and transfer to burn center are given in Table 138–1.

REFERENCES

1. National Center for Injury Prevention and Control; Centers for Disease Control and Prevention. Web-based injury Statistics Query and Reporting System (WISQARS) Fatal Injury Reports (Online). 2000 http://www.cdc.gov/ncipc/wisqars. Accessed February 29, 2008.
2. U S Consumer Product Safety Commission. Personal communiqué. Russ Regner. Bethesda, MD US CPSC, 2002 December.
3. Sheridan RL et al. Current expectations for survival in pediatric burns. *Arch Pediatr Adolesc Med.* 2000;154:245–249.
4. Barrow RE, Jeschke MG, Herndon DN. Early fluid resuscitation improves outcomes in severely burned children. *Resuscitation.* 2000;45:91.
5. Sheridan RL. Burns. *Crit Care Med.* 2002;30:S500.
6. Martin-Herz SP, Patterson DR, Honari S, et al. Pediatric pain control practices of North American burn centers. *J Burn Care Rehabil.* 2003;24:26.
7. Sargent RL. Management of blisters in the partial-thickness burn: an integrative research review. *J Burn Care Res.* 2006; 27:66.
8. Caruso DM, Foster KN, Blome-Eberwein SA, et al. Randomized clinical study of Hydrofiber dressing with silver or silver sulfadiazine in the management of partial-thickness burns. *J Burn Care Res.* 2006;27:298.
9. Whitaker IS, Worthington S, Jivan S, et al. The use of Biobrane by burn units in the United Kingdom: a national study. *Burns.* 2007;33(8):1015–1020. Epub 2007 Aug 30.
10. Gore DC et al. Assessment of adverse events in the demise of pediatric burn patients. *J Trauma.* 2007;63(4):814–818.

CHAPTER 139

Electrical and Lightning Injuries

Mary Ann Cooper

▶ HIGH-YIELD FACTS

- Even low-voltage electrical injuries can be fatal if the child's skin resistance is decreased by sweat or soapy bath water where the entire energy travels to vulnerable areas such as the heart. These often show no external or internal burns.
- Higher energy electrical injury can cause massive muscle damage and release of myoglobin. Without adequate early fluid resuscitation, myoglobinuric renal failure can occur.
- Standard burn formulas such as the Parkland formula cannot be used for electrical burn resuscitation, because the underlying deep tissue damage may have no relationship to overlying skin burns. Sufficient fluid should be administered to maintain a urine flow of 1 to 1.5 mL/kg/h.
- Very young children may suck on electrical cords, sustaining severe orofacial injuries that are often full-thickness, involving the lips and oral commissure. These burns are initially bloodless and nearly painless, but as the eschar separates in 1 to 2 weeks, severe bleeding can occur as the labial artery is uncovered.
- Both electrical and lightning injuries can result in postconcussion syndromes, which include GI symptoms and resistant headaches. Longer term sequelae include chronic pain syndromes, cognitive deficits, personality changes, sleep difficulties, and atypical seizures.
- No place outside is safe when thunderstorms are in the area. All camps and sports venues in lightning-prone areas should have lightning safety plans.
- Cardiac arrest at the time of the injury is the only cause of death. "Reverse triage" (resuscitation of the apparently dead) is the rule since victims who have a pulse and respirations will recover, even if they suffer permanent disabilities.
- Lightning injuries may occur indoors as children use hard-wired phones, game stations, and computers.
- Lightning causes neurologic and blunt musculoskeletal injury from secondary impact. Burns occur in less than one-third of the victims and are almost always quite superficial.

▶ ELECTRICAL INJURIES

Electrical injuries are not common but can be frightening, devastating, and life-changing. They may result in massive tissue destruction, changes in growth patterns, and neurologic injury, including chronic pain syndromes and permanent cognitive deficits, affecting the child's ability to learn and become a productive adult.

Children at most risk are exploring toddlers (12–30 months), who suck on extension cords or stick things into electrical outlets, and adventuresome adolescents. The majority of victims are male. Adolescents often use the outdoors fearlessly as a proving ground, incurring injuries from climbing utility poles and trees and trespassing into transformer substations, resulting in high-voltage injuries.[1]

ELECTROPHYSIOLOGY

The old teaching on electrical injuries involved consideration of voltage, amperage, tissue resistance, duration, current type, and pathway. Unfortunately, taken together, these factors are much too complex to be used in predicting the extent of an injury. When taken separately, they often give simplistic answers that are not borne out in the individual patient. However, these terms are still used in the literature and we will briefly consider them.

- *Voltage* is a measurement of the electrical "pressure" in a system. Injuries are divided into low (<1000 V) and high (>1000 V) voltage. High voltage tends to produce greater tissue destruction.
- *Amperage* is a measure of the rate of flow of electrons. There is a direct relationship between current and heat generated in the material through which current flows given a constant resistance.
- *Resistance* is a measure of the difficulty of electron flow through a given substance. Resistance is measured in ohms and is related to voltage and current by Ohm's law:

$$\text{current}\,(\text{amperes}) = \frac{\text{voltage}\,(\text{volts})}{\text{resistance}\,(\text{ohms})}$$

When electricity enters an extremity, it flows readily through all of the tissues, generating more heat in some and more coagulative damage and dessication in others. However, heat-generated tissue injury is roughly inversely proportional to the cross-sectional area of the conductor through which it passes. For a given energy, more severe injuries will occur in smaller cross-sectional areas than the same energy flowing through body parts with larger cross-sectional areas such as a thigh or the trunk. Damage to internal organs may be more diffuse and hard to appreciate initially because of the larger cross-sectional diameter of the torso.[2]

Regardless of overall tissue resistance differences, physical factors which affect skin resistance can be useful in explaining clinical or forensic findings in electrical injury. Skin is the primary resistor to electric current flowing into the body. Its resistance is affected by thickness, age, moisture, and cleanliness. In general, thickly calloused skin will have higher resistance and tends to sustain greater thermal damage at the site of contact but impedes the flow of energy internally. Skin that is wet with sweat or rainwater will have a tremendously lowered resistance. It may show no or little local thermal damage but allows the majority of the energy to flow internally to the heart or other vital structures. This explains why a "bath-tub" injury may show no external signs of injury while causing cardiac arrest.[2]

Increased *duration* tends to result in increased damage until such time as the tissue is coagulated, charred, or mummified.[2]

Current type may be either alternating or direct. Alternating current (AC) is much more dangerous than direct current (DC) at the same voltage. Household circuits in the United States (110/220 V) operate at 60 cycles per second (cps), a frequency at which neuromuscular function continues indefinitely, leading to tetany. Because the flexors of the hand are stronger than the extensors, the hand gripping an AC electrical source will tend to hold onto the source in a tetanic contraction. Flexion will tend to occur at the wrist, elbow, and shoulder, seeming to pull the victim into the energy source. Tetanic muscle contraction can "freeze" the victim to the current source, prolonging the duration of contact and amount of tissue destruction. The effect of tetanic contraction is also related to the amperage applied—the margin between the household amperage (0.001–0.01 A) that causes a buzz but usually little harm, and that capable of causing respiratory arrest (0.02–0.05 A) and ventricular fibrillation (0.05–0.10 A) is narrow.[2]

With AC injuries it makes little sense to speak of entry and exit burns. Source and ground are more appropriate terms. It is often impossible to determine where the *pathway* started from looking at the burn and neither classification matters, as the emergency physician and surgeon care for the outcome, not the mechanism.[2]

Electric field strength, not listed as one of the factors, is a more useful and accurate concept in explaining and predicting injuries from technical or man-made electricity than the classical Kouwenhoven factors that have traditionally been cited in the medical literature. When 20 kV is applied to a 6-ft man, causing current to ground, an internal electrical field strength of approximately 10 kV/m is generated. When a child chews on an electric cord and suffers a lip burn, the field strength is approximately the same: 110 volts applied to 1 cm of a child's lip generates a field strength of 11 kV/m. While no one would classify the child's injury as "high" voltage, it is a high electrical field strength and produces the same tissue destruction in a small localized area much as would a "high voltage" applied to a 6-ft man (Fig. 139–1).[2]

Not only can electricity cause heating, desiccation, coagulation, and immediate death of tissues due to its thermal effects, it can also cause cellular disruption without immediate death of the cell through the electrical field effect. When an electrical field is applied to a cell, the cell surface can become charged and the cell membrane can be disrupted as water molecules are forced into the bipolar lipid membrane (electroporation).[3,4]

The pores that are formed allow material and water to flow nearly unhindered across the cell membrane, threatening cellular integrity. As the cell struggles to maintain its intracellular milieu, it can expend tremendous energy and resources, swell, and eventually become exhausted and die over a more extended period of time.

MECHANISMS OF INJURY

There are several common mechanisms of injury (Table 139–1). Contact burns are probably the most common and result from direct contact with the electrical source or grounding points. Flash burns occur when the person is close to but not part of an electrical arc or explosion. They vary from very superficial injury with little underlying damage to extensive deep burns accompanied by blunt injury from the concussive force. Arc burns may occur when energy jumps from a source to a nearby person, making them part of the circuit. These injuries typically have deep and extensive tissue damage. Flame burns can occur if clothing or flammable chemicals in the area are secondarily ignited.

Concussive injury is not uncommon with electrical injuries, often due to explosion of electrical transformers and circuit boxes or from rapid heating of gases around the electrical source. Significant blunt injury may occur if a person is thrown or falls. Fractures or dislocations may occur from intense muscle contraction or from being thrown.

While electrical injuries are often classified under burns, higher energy injuries may more closely resemble crush injuries caused by muscle destruction, compartment syndromes, and myoglobin production. Some victims of electrical injury may have very little external damage while sustaining serious underlying tissue damage.

ANATOMIC SITES OF INJURY

Surface burns are found in many non-water-related electrical injuries. The most common areas of injury are the hand, skull, and foot. **Subcutaneous tissues, muscle, nerves, and blood vessels** also suffer thermal damage. **Skeletal muscle** damage is produced by heat or electrical breakdown of cell membranes. Tissue that initially appears viable may later die because of electroporation effects, as well as ischemia caused by vascular wall damage, edema, and thrombosis which may affect either inflow or outflow of blood to tissue.[5,6]

A common injury for very young children is incurred by sucking on the ends of extension cords resulting in severe **orofacial injuries**. Burns are often full thickness, involving the lips and oral commissure. These burns are initially bloodless and painless. As the eschar separates in 2 to 3 weeks, severe bleeding can occur from damage to the labial, facial, or even carotid arteries. There can be mandibular damage, growth retardation, devitalization of teeth, and microstomia from extensive scarring.[6]

Current passing directly through **the heart** can induce ventricular fibrillation. A wide variety of arrhythmias can occur, including supraventricular tachycardia, extrasystoles, right bundle branch block, and complete heart block. The most common electrocardiographic (ECG) abnormalities are sinus

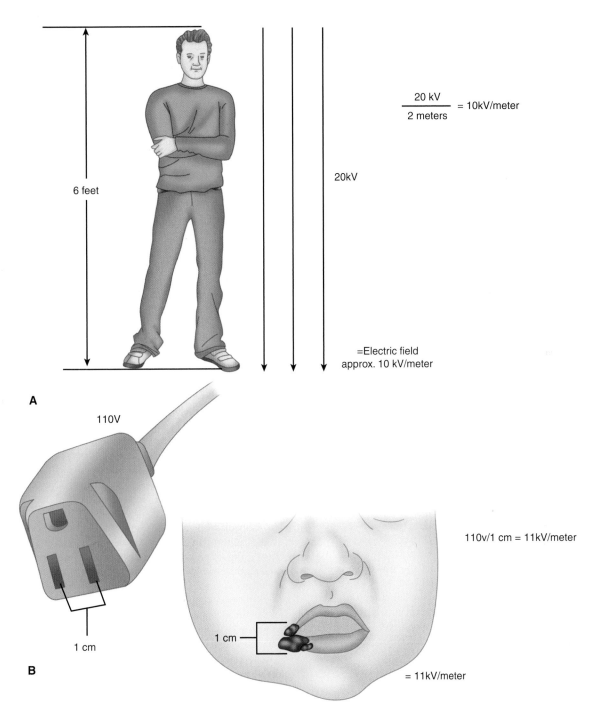

$$\frac{20\ kV}{2\ meters} = 10kV/meter$$

6 feet

20kV

=Electric field
approx. 10 kV/meter

A

110V

110v/1 cm = 11kV/meter

1 cm

1 cm

= 11kV/meter

B

Figure 139–1. Electrical field effect.

▶ **TABLE 139–1. MECHANISMS OF ELECTRICAL INJURY**

Contact injury
Flash burn
Arc burn
Secondary ignition
Concussive force
Blunt trauma

tachycardia and nonspecific ST-T wave changes. Most rhythm disturbances are temporary.[7] Myocardial infarction and ventricular perforation have been reported.

Vascular injuries include thrombosis, vasculitis with necrosis of large vessels, vasospasm, and late aneurysm formation. Maximal decrease in blood flow will occur in the first 36 hours. Strong peripheral pulses do not guarantee vascular integrity.

Acute renal failure may occur from myoglobin released by extensively damaged muscle or from hemoglobin resulting from hemolysis. Kidney damage may also occur from blunt trauma, hypotension, hypoxic ischemic injury, cardiac arrest, and hypovolemia. Oliguria, albuminuria, hemoglobinuria, and renal casts may be seen transiently.

Immediate **CNS** effects include loss of consciousness, agitation, amnesia, deafness, seizures, visual disturbance, and sensory complaints. Vascular and blunt injury damage may result in epidural, subdural, or intraventricular hemorrhage. Within several days, the syndrome of inappropriate antidiuretic hormone secretion (SIADH) may lead to cerebral edema and herniation. Peripheral nerve injury from vascular damage, thermal effect, or direct action of current may occur and be progressive. A variety of autonomic disturbances also occur. Late involvement of the spinal cord may produce ascending paralysis, amyotrophic lateral sclerosis, transverse myelitis, or incomplete cord transection. **Cataracts** can be seen in any electrical injury involving the head or neck.

Passage of current through the **abdominal** wall can cause Curling's ulcers in the stomach or duodenum. Other injuries described include evisceration, stomach or intestinal perforation, esophageal stricture, and electrocoagulation of the liver or pancreas.

Blunt trauma or tetanic muscle contractions can cause **fractures or dislocations**. Amputation of an extremity is necessary in 35% to 60% of survivors of high-energy injury caused by extensive underlying injuries. **Infections** frequently occur in gangrenous tissue. Prevalent organisms include *Staphylococcus, Pseudomonas,* and *Clostridium.*

Victims may suffer **depression, flashbacks, attention deficit disorder, sleep problems, and other cognitive difficulties** that can affect learning and school performance as well as social function within the family or school.

MANAGEMENT

Prehospital Care

Extrication is extremely dangerous until the power source is disconnected. Victims should be treated both as burn victims as well as blunt trauma patients, with special attention given to spinal immobilization. Aggressive fluid therapy is essential to sustain circulation and begin diluting myoglobin. Transport to a health care facility should not be delayed.[8,9]

Emergency Department Care

A victim of electrical injury should be approached in the same way as a victim of blunt trauma with a crush injury. The greatest threats to life include cardiac arrhythmias, renal failure from myoglobin and hemoglobin precipitants, and hyperkalemia from massive muscle breakdown. A thorough search for burns, other wounds, and hidden skeletal injuries is necessary.[8,9]

Lesser injuries and small burns can be treated conservatively with few or no laboratory tests or x-rays. Referral for appropriate follow-up may be all that is needed. Baseline ECG and cardiac monitoring is not indicated for children exposed to household current (120–240 V) unless there was loss of consciousness, tetany, wet skin, transthoracic current flow, or the event was unwitnessed.[8,9]

For more extensive injuries, laboratory tests may include arterial blood gases, complete blood count, serum electrolytes,

blood urea nitrogen, creatinine, glucose, blood type and crossmatch, and urinalysis for myoglobin. Creatine kinase (CK), although commonly drawn in these patients, is not predictive of the degree of injury. Although CK-MB (muscle brain) isoenzyme elevations can be seen, they may be from damaged skeletal muscle. Radiographs of the cervical spine, chest, and pelvis may be done. Other films may be obtained as dictated by physical examination. Electrocardiograms are routinely done in more serious injuries but may not be helpful. If the ECG is consistent with cardiac injury, further evaluation with echocardiography or nuclear scanning may be necessary.[8,9]

For the patient who requires fluid resuscitation and admission, the usual fluid replacement formulas utilized for burn patients often underestimate fluid requirements. Adequate fluids should be given to maintain a urine output of 1 to 2 mL/kg/h when pigmentation is present and less after it has cleared. Accurate measurement requires Foley catheter placement. Alkalinization of the urine with bicarbonate and administration of mannitol or furosemide may be needed to treat myoglobinuria. These therapies should be approached cautiously if coexisting head trauma is possible. Overzealous use of bicarbonate can result in metabolic alkalosis and hypernatremia. A decreasing level of consciousness, unexplained coma, lateralizing signs, or change in mental status necessitates cranial computed tomography (CT) scan to rule out intracranial damage.[8,9]

Extensive muscle damage may necessitate fasciotomy, particularly if the chest wall is involved. Compartment syndromes can occur if venous output is blocked by thrombosis and as tissue edema occurs. Debridement is best left to a burn surgeon and should be conservative for lip burns.[8,9]

Tetanus prophylaxis should be evaluated and given as needed in the emergency department. Nasogastric intubation may be required and antacids and cimetidine are administered.[8,9]

Consultations may be required, depending on the severity and type of injury. All children with oral injuries require plastic surgery and dental or orthodontic consults. Neurosurgical, ophthalmologic, and ear-nose-throat consults may also be necessary. Transfer to a burn center may be indicated.[8,9]

Infection remains the most common cause of death after electrical injury. Despite aggressive debridement and decompression, digit or limb loss may be unavoidable if tissue necrosis is extensive.[8,9]

Recommendations for admission are varied. It is generally agreed that admission is not required for nontransthoracic low-voltage injuries in the asymptomatic child without ECG abnormalities. All other patients require admission, close observation, and frequent neurovascular checks of the extremities to monitor for compartment syndromes. A multidisciplinary approach, including medical, psychiatric, and social services, is required.[8,9]

PREVENTION

Physicians can play an important role in prevention by educating patients and families. The following advice should be given:[10]

- Extension cords should be in good repair and not used to replace or avoid conduit wiring.

- Unused outlets should be covered with dummy plugs.
- Electrical appliances must be kept away from sinks and bathtubs.
- Electrically operated toys should be age-appropriate. Use of such toys should be supervised by adults.

Older children and adolescents can benefit from school safety programs that address the dangers of power lines and transformer substations.

▶ LIGHTNING INJURIES

Lightning kills more people annually in the United States than any other storm-related phenomenon except floods (Fig. 139–2).[11] Injuries are most common during high-thunderstorm months but not unheard of in the winter. More males are injured than females at nearly every age.[2,12,13] Deaths and injuries are underreported by as much as 30%.[2,14–16] Currently, there are less than 50 reported deaths per year and probably around 500 injuries per year. While 90% of those injured by lightning survive, a significant number may have disabilities from chronic pain or neurocognitive injury.

PHYSICS

Lightning is produced by the development of an electrical potential between a cumulonimbus cloud and the ground. Within a cloud, rising warm, humid air meets cooler air causing condensation. As ice crystals rise and fall within the cloud, charge separation occurs with primarily positive charges in the upper cloud layers and negative charges in the lower cloud layers.[2]

Around the area of the thundercloud, the negative charge in the bottom of the cloud induces the usually normally negatively charged earth to become positively charged. Eventually, static discharges occur between areas of charge separation in the cloud causing intracloud lightning, which makes up approximately 90% of lightning discharges. The remainder, cloud-to-ground lightning, is primarily responsible for personal injuries.

Opposite charges are also induced in structures on the ground, such as a tree, person, cow, or blade of grass. "Stream-

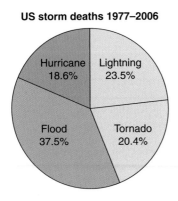

US storm deaths 1977–2006

Hurricane 18.6%
Lightning 23.5%
Flood 37.5%
Tornado 20.4%

Figure 139–2. Weather causes of U.S. storm deaths (1977–2006).

ers" or upward leaders of charge emanate from these structures toward the charged cloud that can be sufficient to injure even when a complete lightning channel is not formed.[17,18]

MECHANISMS OF INJURY

Lightning is dangerous for three reasons: electrical effects, heat production, and concussive force. In addition, lightning may injure indirectly via forest fires, house fires, explosions, or falling objects such as trees. Only direct injury by lightning will be discussed (Fig. 139–3). The distribution of injury by commonly accepted mechanisms is shown in Table 139–2.[19]

Direct strike occurs when a lightning discharge attaches directly to the victim. Despite media reports, which mention this as the mechanism, direct strike is actually one of the less common mechanisms. While it is intuitive that a direct strike might be the most likely to cause fatalities, this has not been shown in any studies.[19]

Contact potential occurs when a person is touching a fence, indoor plumbing, hard-wired telephone, game controller, or similar object attached to a conductor hit at a distance, which then transmits the lightning energy to the person.[19]

Side splash/flash occurs when a portion of the lightning energy separates from the primary conductor to injure a nearby person. Current divides itself between the two paths in inverse proportion to their resistances. Standing under or close to trees and other tall objects is a very common way in which people are splashed. Side flashes may also occur from person to person.[19]

Ground current injury occurs when lightning strikes the ground or an object near a victim and spreads out through the ground under the person. When the victim stands with feet apart, a potential difference between the feet allows current to flow through the body to the ground (stride potential or step current).[19]

Upward streamer/leader injury occurs when a streamer of charge induced by the thundercloud in a person is of sufficient magnitude to cause injury, even though a complete lightning channel is never formed.[19]

It is likely that a **combination** of these electrical mechanisms may occur, especially when multiple victims are involved.[20] **Blunt injury** may also occur with most of these mechanisms as the concussive wave of expanding air near the lightning strike impacts the individual or if the person is thrown by muscle contraction.[19]

TYPES OF INJURIES

Less than one-third of lightning survivors have any **external signs of burns**, probably due to the usually indirect mechanism of injury.[2] Skin damage is probably decreased by a combination of short duration of contact, lower skin resistance from rain or sweat and flashover, where the majority of the energy flows over the outside of the body rather than through it. **Deep muscle damage** is rare. Victims or observers may incorrectly interpret superficial external burns as "entry" or "exit" areas,

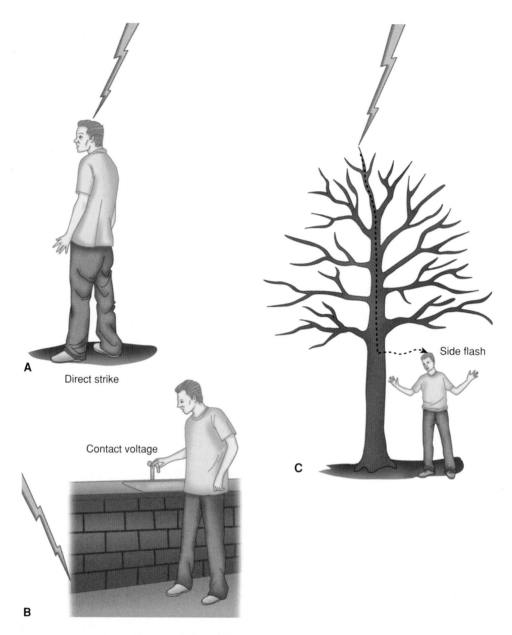

Figure 139–3. Mechanisms of lightning injury.

which rarely, if ever, occur with lightning. The most common types of skin injury are listed below:[2]

- Lichtenberg figures: These are arborescent, evanescent, spidery, erythematous streaks that are pathognomonic of lightning injury but unfortunately are rarely seen.

▶ **TABLE 139–2. ESTIMATED FREQUENCY OF MECHANISMS OF LIGHTNING INJURY**

Mechanism	Frequency (%)
Direct strike	3–5
Contact potential	15–25
Side splash/flash	20–30
Ground current	40–50
Upward streamer/leader	10–15

They most commonly disappear within hours of the injury.
- Linear burns: Linear burns are partial-thickness burns usually correlating to area of high sweat or water concentration on the body.
- Punctate burns: Cinderlike burns may occur singly or in linear or grouped patterns. They can be full- or partial-thickness burns.
- Thermal burns: Heating of metal objects or ignition of clothing can cause secondary thermal burns.

Cardiac arrest at the time of the injury is the only proximate cause of death from lightning, except in freak accidents such as someone falling from a cliff after being injured. It is unknown if the arrest is from CNS damage, autonomic nervous system injury, damage to conduction pathways or a combination of these, and other factors including the portion of the

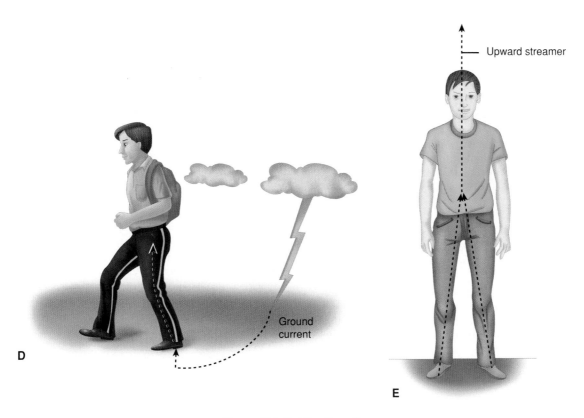

Figure 139–3. (*Continued*)

cardiac cycle in which the injury occurs. In some instances, **respiratory arrest** may be prolonged, again from unknown specific causes. Although the heart sometimes spontaneously resumes an organized rhythm, those with prolonged respiratory arrest have a poor prognosis with secondary hypoxia and ventricular fibrillation. **Congestive heart failure, cardiac contusions, and delayed rupture** have also been reported. ECG changes include nonspecific ST-T wave changes, T-wave changes, axis shift, QT prolongation, and ST-segment elevation. These usually resolve gradually. **Lung injuries** reported include pulmonary contusion, hemorrhage, pneumothorax, pulmonary edema, and aspiration secondary to altered mental status. **Arterial spasm and vasomotor instability** result in cool, mottled, pulseless extremities. This usually resolves in several hours.[2]

Transient loss of consciousness, retrograde amnesia, transient paralysis, and paresthesias are common. Keraunoparalysis (from the Greek keraunos, meaning lightning) is a flaccid paralysis accompanied by vasomotor changes, which may last several hours. **Other neurologic findings** may include seizures, skull fracture, intracerebral hemorrhages, elevated intracranial pressure, cerebellar ataxia, Horner's syndrome, SIADH, and peripheral nerve damage.[2]

Cognitive injury similar to other blunt head injury commonly occurs but may not be recognized acutely. Survivors of cardiac resuscitation may have typical **anoxic injury** as well. Direct or **blunt injury to the spinal cord** should always be ruled out, especially if symptoms do not resolve. **Postconcussive headaches** lasting weeks to months are common.[2]

Myoglobinuria is rare; however, hypotension from prolonged cardiac arrest can lead to **acute tubular necrosis**. The kidneys may rarely be damaged by **concussive force** or the person being thrown.[2]

Cataracts may occur, developing either immediately or over a prolonged recovery period. Some resolve spontaneously. **Fixed and dilated pupils** may be seen after lightning strike from other mechanisms including retinal or optic nerve damage. **Other eye injuries** reported include uveitis, hyphema, vitreous hemorrhage, macular holes, retinal detachment, and optic neuritis.[2]

Tympanic membrane rupture is common but is most often best treated nonsurgically. **Other aural complications** include burns to the ear, ossicular disruption, tinnitus, vertigo, and nystagmus.[2]

Gastric upset similar to postconcussive syndrome is not uncommon for weeks to months after the injury.[2]

Psychologic sequelae, including anxiety, sleep disturbances, nocturnal enuresis, depression, and cognitive disability, have all been reported.[2]

MANAGEMENT

Prehospital Care

Lightning injury victims should be approached as blunt multiple trauma patients with attention to advanced life-support protocols and cervical spine protection. Because of the unusual findings of transient, fixed, and dilated pupils, autonomic abnormalities, keraunoparalysis, and transient asystole with prolonged apnea, standard triage procedures should be ignored. Anyone who has not suffered a cardiac arrest is highly likely to survive, is unlikely to be unstable, and may be left for later care. Victims who appear to be dead should be treated aggressively. If the history of lightning strike is unclear, protocols for altered mental status should be followed, including administering glucose and naloxone. Bystanders may be helpful in providing history.[2]

It should be noted that, contrary to popular belief, lightning can strike twice in the same area. Emergency personnel can certainly be at risk when working with victims near active thunderstorms and should exhibit caution if the threat of lightning strike exists at the time of their arrival.[2]

Emergency Department Care

Treatment follows the same guidelines as for all severely injured patients. Amnesia suffered by the victim and lack of available bystanders may limit history taking. Clues that may lead to the diagnosis of lightning strike include recent thunderstorm, outdoor occurrence, clothing disintegration, typical arborescent burn pattern, tympanic membrane injury, and magnetization of metallic objects on the victim's body. A complete physical examination, after attention to the ABCs and cervical spine control, is indicated. A thorough search for blunt injuries is necessary. A baseline ECG is also required. Cardiac monitoring is only indicated if there was a cardiac arrest or abnormal initial ECG. Any arrhythmia should be treated by standard protocols. Fluid resuscitation must be approached cautiously; central-monitoring lines may be helpful.

Laboratory tests are likely to be completely normal except in the most severely injured and are probably not cost-effective. More severely injured patients who will be admitted may benefit from baseline tests including complete blood count, renal function tests, and urinalysis for myoglobin. Arterial blood gases, creatine kinase with isoenzymes, serum troponin, and serum chemistries may be indicated for more severe patients. In some cases, urine and blood should be sent for toxicology. Radiographs are done as indicated. Cranial CT scan is indicated for all unconscious patients.

Burns should be treated by protocol. Fasciotomy is rarely indicated, as the mottled, pulseless extremity associated with lightning injury often improves over several hours. Eye and ear examinations should not be overlooked. Tetanus prophylaxis may be indicated depending on the patient's immunization status.

DISPOSITION

The vast majority of lightning survivors can be discharged from the emergency department. Exceptions, of course, include postcardiac arrest, unstable or confused patients or those with inadequate home supervision, and close follow-up care. Appropriate consultation and documentation is necessary.

SEQUELAE

Long-term sequelae may include postconcussive syndrome, cognitive disability leading to school performance issues, chronic pain syndromes, delayed and often atypical seizures

▶ **TABLE 139–3. LIGHTNING INJURY PREVENTION GUIDELINES**

Know the weather forecast beforehand if outdoor activities are planned.

Change plans if thunderstorms or severe weather are in the forecast for the area and time of the activity.

If one must be outdoors, *have a safety plan* thought out that includes a safer place (substantial buildings or fully enclosed metal vehicles) for evacuation. Be sure there is time to reach it.

Have a "*weather eye*" to the sky to watch for threatening weather.

When Thunder Roars, Go Indoors!
(If thunder is heard, immediately seek a safer area.)

Do not resume outdoor activity until *thirty minutes after the last lightning* is seen or thunder heard.

When indoors, *do not touch conducting materials* such as hard-wired phones, game controllers, computers, and plumbing when thunderstorms are in the area.

Adults are always *responsible* for the safety of children in their care.

A wonderful teaching tool is the *Leon the Lightning Lion Safety Game*, written for preschoolers and nonreaders but also useful for older children and adults. This and other teaching materials, posters, public service announcements by prominent sports figures, and games are available at the *National Lightning Safety Week Web site.*

and disturbances in balance, coordination, mood, sleep, affect, and memory. Some of these may be especially difficult to appreciate in adolescents.

PREVENTION

No place outside is safe when thunderstorms are in the area. While no one can guard against the stray "bolt from the blue," the majority of lightning injuries are preventable if one knows and follows lightning injury prevention guidelines listed in Table 139–3.[21]

REFERENCES

1. Price TG, Cooper MA. Electrical and lightning injuries. In: Marx JA, Hockberger RS, Walls RM, eds. *Rosen's Emergency Medicine: Concepts and Clinical Practice.* 5th ed. Philadelphia, PA: Mosby-Elsevier; 2002:2267–2278.

2. Cooper MA, Andrews CJ, Holle RL. Lightning injuries. In: Auerbach PS, ed. *Wilderness Medicine.* 5th ed. St. Louis, MO: Mosby; 2007:67–108.

3. Lee RC, Gaylor DC, Prakah-Asante K, et al. Role of cell membrane rupture in the pathogenesis of electrical trauma. *J Surg Res.* 1988;44:709–719.

4. Lee RC. Cell injury by electric forces. *Ann NY Acad Sci.* 2005;1066:85–91.

5. Garcia CT, Smith GA, Cohen DM, et al. Electrical injuries in a pediatric emergency department. *Ann Emerg Med.* 1995;26:604–608.

6. Niazi ZV, Salzberg CA. Thermal, electrical and chemical injury to the face and neck in children. *Facial Plast Surg.* 1999;7:185–193.

7. Bailey B, Gaudreault P, Thivierge RL, et al. Cardiac monitoring of children with household electrical injuries. *Ann Emerg Med.* 1995;25:612–617.

8. Smith ML. Pediatric burns: management of thermal, electrical and chemical burns and burn-like dermatologic conditions. *Pediatr Ann.* 2000;29:367–378.

9. Zubair M, Besner GE. Pediatric electrical burns: management strategies. *Burns.* 1997;23:413–420.

10. Rabban JT, Blair JA, Rosen CL, et al. Mechanisms of pediatric electrical injury: new implications for product safety and injury prevention. *Arch Pediatr Adolesc Med.* 1997;151:696–700.

11. Roeder WP. Recent changes in lightning safety. Preprints, 3rd Conference. Meteor. Appl. Lightning Data, New Orleans, LA: *Amer Meteor Soc.* 2008:5.

12. Holle RL, López RE, Navarro BC. Deaths, injuries, and damages from lightning in the United States in the 1890s in comparison with the 1990s. *J App Meteorol.* 2005;44:1563–1573.

13. López RE, Holle RL. Fluctuations of lightning casualties in the United States: 1959–1990. *J Climate.* 1996;9:608–615.

14. Adekoya N, Nolte KB. Struck-by-lightning deaths in the United States. *J Environ Health.* 2005;67:45–50.

15. López RE, Holle RL, Heitkamp TA, et al. The underreporting of lightning injuries and deaths in Colorado. *Bull Am Meteorol Soc.* 1993;74:2171–2178.

16. Shearman KM, Ojala CF. Some causes for lightning data inaccuracies: the case of Michigan. *Bull Am Meteorol Soc.* 1999;80:1883–1891.

17. Anderson RB. Does a fifth mechanism exist to explain lightning injuries? *IEEE Eng Med Biol.* 2001:105–116.

18. Carte AE, Anderson RB, Cooper MA. A large group of children struck by lightning. *Ann Emerg Med.* 2002;39(6):665–670.

19. Cooper MA, Holle RL, Andrews CJ. Distribution of lightning injury mechanisms. In: Proceedings from International Lightning Detection *Conference*; 2008; Tucson, AZ.

20. Anderson RB, Jandrell IR, Nematswerami HE. The upward streamer mechanism versus step potentials as a cause of injuries from close lightning discharges. *Trans: The SA Inst Elec Eng.* 2002: 33–43.

21. National Lightning Awareness Week. http://www.lightningsafety.noaa.gov. 2008.

CHAPTER 140

Heat and Cold Illness

Heather M. Prendergast and Gary R. Strange

► HIGH-YIELD FACTS

- Children are more susceptible to extremes of temperature because of a greater area-to-body mass ratio, higher metabolic heat per mass unit, and a diminished ability to dissipate body heat by evaporation.
- Heat-related illnesses comprise a continuum of conditions ranging from minor entities such as heat cramps to more serious conditions including heat exhaustion and heatstroke. Heatstroke is the most severe form of heat illness, with reported mortality between 17% and 80%
- Heat exhaustion is a syndrome of dizziness, postural hypotension, nausea, vomiting, headache, weakness, and, occasionally, syncope, which may be associated with normal temperature or moderate temperature elevation (39°C–41.1°C). One hallmark is the absence of mental status changes.
- Heatstroke is a state of complete thermoregulatory failure and is an immediately life-threatening entity requiring aggressive management. Patients with heatstroke present with disorientation, seizures, or coma. After assessment and stabilization of the airway, breathing, and circulation, cooling should be instituted immediately, usually by spraying the skin with room-temperature water and directing an electric fan onto the patient's skin.
- The core temperature defines the presence and severity of hypothermia. Most thermometers for routine clinical use will record a temperature down to only 34.4°C. Special glass or electronic thermometers are required for accurate measurement of temperatures in hypothermic patients.
- Shivering will often be present in the older child or adolescent but ceases by the time the temperature reaches 31°C. The skin is typically cold, firm, pale, or mottled, and localized damage due to frostbite may be present.
- In moderate-to-severe cases of hypothermia, active rewarming is started as soon as possible. Heated, humidified oxygen and intravenous fluids heated to 40°C have been shown to be safe and efficacious and are used from the beginning.
- Extracorporeal rewarming is the most rapid method of rewarming and is indicated in hypothermic cardiac arrest and with patients who present with completely frozen extremities. Using this technique, young, otherwise healthy people have survived deep hypothermia with no or minimal cerebral impairment.

► HEAT ILLNESS

The spectrum of heat illness varies from mild, self-limited problems, such as heat cramps, to major, life-threatening problems, such as heatstroke. The annual average number of deaths from heat illness in the United States for 1999 through 2003 was 688, almost doubled from previous decades.[1] Infants are predisposed to the development of heat illness due to their poorly developed thermoregulatory systems.[2] Older children and adolescents are susceptible to heat illness when they exercise vigorously under hot, humid conditions.[3] Exercising children have a reduced ability to dissipate body heat because of a lesser sweating capacity.[3] Adolescent zeal for competitive athletics, coupled with an often-held belief among the young in their invulnerability, can lead to serious heat illness. A major contributing factor is acclimatization.[4] Acclimatization to a hot, humid environment allows the individual to perform harder and longer without developing heat illness.[4] The rate of acclimatization for pediatric patients is much slower than that of adults. Full acclimatization takes 3 to 4 weeks, during which the individual must limit exertion. The adjustment process involves alterations in sodium and water balance, which are mediated by aldosterone. When a person is acclimatized, increased aldosterone secretion leads to sodium retention and expansion of extracellular fluid volume.[5]

Heat illness is the second leading cause of death in athletes, after head and spinal injuries. Drug-related heat illness is also seen with increasing incidence in the adolescent population. Other factors associated with the development of heat illness in pediatric patients are dehydration, excessive clothing and bundling, infections, mental retardation, and obesity. An especially tragic situation, which is entirely preventable through parental education, is the development of heat illness in small children left in closed cars on hot days. Children with cystic fibrosis (see Chap. 45) are prone to develop a form of heat illness characterized by excessive electrolyte loss with sweating. Any patient who has had a previous episode of heatstroke is markedly predisposed to recurrence.[6]

PATHOPHYSIOLOGY

At rest, the body generates enough heat to raise the body temperature by approximately 1°C/h. Heavy exertion can increase heat production to 12 times this level. When the ambient temperature exceeds the body temperature, there is a net heat gain from the environment. The body can dissipate heat by radiation, conduction, convection, and evaporation[5] (Table 140–1).

TYPES OF HEAT ILLNESS

Heat-related illnesses comprise a continuum of conditions ranging from minor entities such as heat cramps to more

▶ **TABLE 140–1. PRIMARY MECHANISMS OF HEAT DISSIPATION RELATED TO HEAT ILLNESS**

Mechanism	Contribution to Heat Dissipation	Maximal Effectiveness	Conditions Rendering Less Effective
Radiation	Vasodilation can increase by a factor of 20	Ambient temperatures less than 20°C (68°F) Air temperature lower than body temperature	Environmental temperature exceeds 35°C (95°F)
Evaporation	Sweating accounts for greatest contribution; dependent upon physical conditioning	Ambient temperatures greater than 20°C (68°F) Dependent on humidity levels	Humidity levels >75%
Conduction	Immersion in cool water can increase by a factor of 32	Direct contact with cooler objects	Absence of wind Lack of movement Excessive subcutaneous fat Ambient temperature >35°C (95°F)
Convection	Wind currents and fanning can increase by a factor of 10	Rapid movement of air around the body	Ambient temperature >35°C (95°F)

serious conditions including heat exhaustion and heatstroke. Depending upon the condition, the management priorities are varied (Table 140–2).

Heat Cramps

With heavy exertion, the muscles that are working hardest may begin to go into spasm. Heat cramps are extremely painful and typically involve involuntary skeletal muscle spasms. This can occur regardless of whether exercise is performed in hot or cold weather. The underlying cause has long been described as dilutional hyponatremia, which usually occurs in conditioned athletes who replace fluid losses with water. However, there is no clear evidence that dilutional hyponatremia is the actual cause.[4] The most recent theory suggests that the underlying mechanism is due to alterations in the spinal neural reflex activity stimulated by fatigue in susceptible individuals.[5] The body temperature remains normal and there is associated sweating. There are no central nervous system signs. The pain associated with the muscle spasms can be resistant to narcotics in the absence of adequate fluid rehydration.[7]

Heat Exhaustion

Heat exhaustion is a syndrome of dizziness, postural hypotension, nausea, vomiting, headache, weakness, and, occasionally, syncope, which may be associated with normal temperature or moderate temperature elevation (39°C–41.1°C).[8] It tends to occur in unacclimatized individuals. The skin is usually wet from profuse sweating. The associated morbidity is low.[8]

The cause of heat exhaustion may be either salt or water depletion. Salt depletion occurs when fluid losses are replaced by water or other hypotonic solutions and hyponatremia results. Although severe hyponatremia can result in significant mental status changes and/or seizures, the mental status in heat exhaustion patients tends to be normal. Water depletion occurs when victims are unable to replace fluid losses, result-

ing in hypernatremic dehydration. This can occur in infants or mentally retarded children, who cannot communicate their thirst.[4,6,9]

HeatStroke

Heatstroke is the most severe form of heat illness and represents a state of complete thermoregulatory failure. The reported mortality for heatstroke ranges from 17% to 80%.[5–8] Patients with heatstroke present with disorientation, seizures, or coma. Classic heatstroke is typically seen at the extremes of age (infants and elderly) and develops over a period of days.[10] The skin is usually hot and dry. With exertional heatstroke, which is much more likely in the pediatric population, the skin may be dry or sweating may continue. The temperature ranges from 41.1°C to 42.2°C. There is no clear scientific evidence to indicate that heatstroke results from fluid and electrolyte abnormalities. In fact, the risk of developing exertional heatstroke appears greater in individuals performing high-intensity exercise for a relatively short time span.[5]

Predisposing conditions for classic heatstroke include dehydration, obesity, neurologic disorders, hyperthyroidism, extremes of age, alcohol consumption, sickle cell trait, and medications that interfere with heat dissipation (e.g., phenothiazines, anticholinergics, and diuretics).[6,7]

Complications are common, leading to the high mortality rate. These include neurologic dysfunction moderate-to-severe renal insufficiency secondary to acute tubular necrosis and low urine output, hepatic damage and disseminated intravascular coagulation, and adult respiratory distress syndrome. As heatstroke continues, signs consistent with multiorgan system dysfunction may develop.[5,8] These include encephalopathy, hemorrhagic complications, intestinal ischemia or infarction, rhabdomyolysis, and sepsis.[5,7] In-hospital mortality is reported at 21%, and 33% of patients have moderate-to-severe functional impairment at the time of hospital discharge. In follow-up, the functional impairment was found to persist at 1 year.[5,8] Whereas the outcome may be somewhat better for the young,

► TABLE 140-2. **SPECTRUM OF HEAT-RELATED ILLNESS**

Syndrome	At Risk Features/Groups	Pertinent Findings on History or Physical Examination	Management Priorities	Caveats
Heat cramps	Heavy exertion independent of ambient temperature	Normal body temperature Sweating present Absence of central nervous system signs	Rest in a cool environment Oral fluid replacement with isotonic solutions	Pain may be resistant to narcotics in the absence of adequate fluid rehydration
Heat exhaustion	Unacclimatized individuals Hyponatermic dehydration Salt or water depletion Hypernatremic dehydration More common in infants, mentally challenged	Dizziness Nausea Vomiting Headache Weakness Syncope Normal or slightly elevated body temperature Sweating present	Rest in a cool environment Rehydration with intravenous normal saline Rapid cooling measures not required	Patients should be observed for progression to heatstroke If symptoms have resolved during ED treatment and observation, discharge may be considered
Classic heatstroke	Elderly Infants Individuals with impaired mobility	Disorientation Seizures Coma Skin typically hot and dry Core body temperature >40°C (104°F) Shock Diarrhea	Airway, breathing, and circulation Rapid cooling 　Spray skin with room temperature water 　Ice packs to groin, axilla 　Directing electric fan onto patient Monitor core temperature closely Intravenous fluids at a rate of 20 mL/kg	Applying ice water to skin can cause vasoconstriction Antipyretics are ineffective Discontinue active cooling once core temperature reaches 39°C Tends to develop slowly over several days
Exertional heatstroke	Pediatric population Dehydration Unacclimatized individuals Risk appears greatest in individuals performing high intensity exercise for relatively short periods	Disorientation Seizures Coma Sweating present Core body temperature >40°C (104°F) Shock Diarrhea	Airway, breathing, and circulation Rapid cooling 　Spray skin with room temperature water 　Ice packs to groin, axilla 　Directing electric fan onto patient Monitor core temperature closely Intravenous fluids at a rate of 20 mL/kg	Applying ice water to skin can cause vasoconstriction Antipyretics are ineffective Discontinue active cooling once core temperature reaches 39°C Rapid onset with development in hours

otherwise healthy individual, mortality and morbidity are unquestionably significant.

MANAGEMENT

Prompt reversal of hyperthermia is the mainstay of heat-related illness treatment. Management is directed by proper identification of the suspected condition (Fig. 140–1 and Table 140–2).

Heat cramps are treated by removing the patient to a cool environment and providing rest and oral electrolyte solutions.

Salt tablets may cause gastrointestinal cramping and are not recommended. A solution of 1 tsp table salt in 500 mL water can be used if no prepared solutions are available. Avoid use of replacement fluids that contain caffeine or alcohol because of their diuretic effects.[5,7]

Heat exhaustion is also treated by removal to a cool environment and providing rest. Intravenous rehydration is recommended, starting with 20 mL/kg of normal saline over 30 minutes and continuing rehydration as outlined in Chapter 10. If hypernatremic dehydration is suspected on clinical or laboratory grounds, slower replacement is indicated.[6,9]

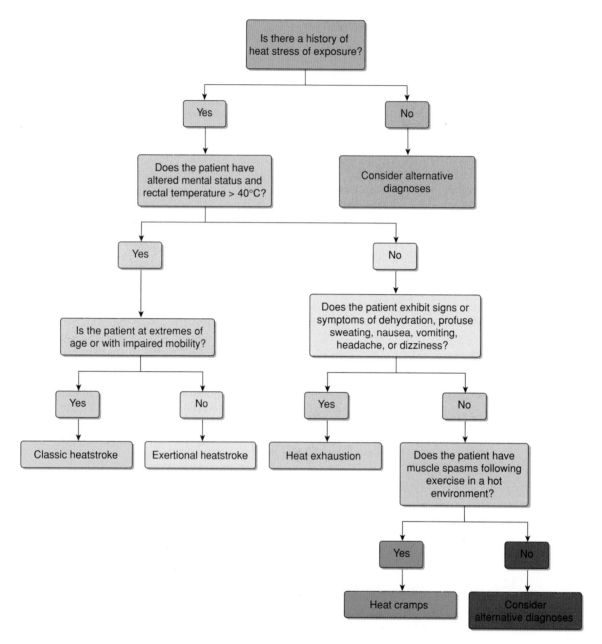

Figure 140–1. Approach to the patient with heat exposure.

Victims of heat exhaustion may require observation in the hospital. However, if all symptoms have resolved during emergency department treatment and observation, the patient may be released to continue rest and rehydration in a cool environment.

On the other hand, heatstroke is an immediately life-threatening entity and must be treated vigorously. After assessment and stabilization of the airway, breathing, and circulation, cooling should be instituted immediately.[11] Spraying the skin with room-temperature water and directing an electric fan onto the patient's skin will usually result in rapid reduction of the core temperature. Ice packs may be used in the groin and axilla, but ice water applied widely to the skin may cause vasoconstriction and impair the dissipation of heat. Submersion in cold water is very effective in lowering the temperature

but makes other resuscitative efforts practically impossible. Invasive lavage to lower the body temperature has not been adequately studied and is not currently recommended. Antipyretics are also ineffective.[3,7] Core temperature should be monitored continuously during treatment and active cooling should continue until the core temperature falls to 39°C.[5]

Diazepam, 0.2 to 0.3 mg/kg/dose IV, may be required to prevent shivering.

Intravenous fluids are required and should initially be given as isotonic crystalloid at a rate of 20 mL/kg over the first hour. Central venous or pulmonary artery catheters are frequently needed for adequate monitoring of fluid resuscitation.

Since the effects of heatstroke are widespread throughout essentially every system of the body and the differential diagnosis is broad (Fig. 140–1, Table 140–3), extensive diagnostic

▶ **TABLE 140–3. DIFFERENTIAL DIAGNOSIS OF HEATSTROKE: SYMPTOM COMPLEX—ALTERED MENTAL STATUS, HYPERTHERMIA**

Potential Diagnosis	Pertinent History	Pertinent Findings on Physical Examination	Pertinent Laboratory Data
Encephalitis and meningitis	Fever Prodromal illness Severe headache Chills	Temperature Neck stiffness Kernig and Brudzinski signs positive	Lumbar puncture: elevated WBCs, positive Gram's stain, cultures
Malaria	Exposure Travel history Previous history	Fever pattern Confusion	Peripheral blood smear
Typhoid fever, typhus	Exposure Travel history	Fever pattern	Titers: Well-Felix reaction, complement fixation
Sepsis	Fever Age extreme Immunocompromised	Fever Confusion Coma Focal infection	Chest x-ray WBC: elevated Cultures: blood, urine, spinal fluid
Hypothalamic hemorrhage	Hypertension Anticoagulant therapy	Coma Fever Focal neurologic findings	Brain CT: hemorrhage
Thyroid storm	Preexisting hyperthyroidism Risk factors Stress Surgery Trauma Infection Failure to take antithyroid medication	Goiter Tachycardia Seizures Hypotension	Thyroid function studies: T_3 and T_4
Malignant hyperthermia	Inhalation anesthetic Succinylcholine	Muscle fasciculation	Arterial blood gases: acidosis Electrolytes: hyperkalemia hypermagnesemia
Heatstroke	Risk factors Exposure to heat load Exercise	Hot, flushed skin Confusion Agitation Seizures Tachycardia Hypotension Vomiting Diarrhea Muscle tenderness	AST: elevated WBC: elevated Electrolytes: hyper- or hypokalemia, hyponatremia, hypocalcemia, hypophosphatemia Arterial blood gases: metabolic acidosis Urine: myoglobin Clotting factors: decreased Blood glucose: variable

With permission from Barreca RS. Heat illness. In: Hamilton GC, Sanders AB, Strange GR, Trott AT, eds. *Emergency Medicine: An Approach to Clinical Problem-Solving*. Philadelphia, PA: W. B. Saunders; 1991:402.

evaluation is indicated. Arterial blood gases are helpful in evaluating oxygenation, ventilation, and acid-base status. Changes in body temperature alter blood gas values, but whether corrections in the values are helpful before treatment decisions are made is controversial.[6,7]

The complete blood count will usually show an elevated white blood cell count. Counts $>20\,000/mm^3$ and elevated band counts are more consistent with an underlying infection and should prompt a complete septic workup. Hemoglobin and hematocrit values are usually elevated due to dehydration. Electrolyte studies may reveal abnormal sodium levels. Elevated potassium levels may indicate the development of rhabdomyolysis. Renal function tests may initially be elevated due to dehydration and may rise later, as renal failure develops. Urinalysis will often show a high specific gravity as a reflection of the hydration status. If the urine is positive for hemoglobin in the absence of red blood cells on the microscopic evaluation, rhabdomyolysis should be suspected. Liver enzymes may be elevated, since the liver is very sensitive to heat stress. Transaminase levels peak in 24 to 48 hours and correlate well with the severity of injury. Very high levels (aspartate transaminase >1000 IU) are predictive of severe illness and complications. Serum glucose levels are variable but should be monitored to assess the need for replacement or control. Coagulation studies are needed to detect the development of disseminated intravascular coagulation. Cultures are an integral part of the sepsis workup, which is essential to rule out an infectious etiology or concomitant infection.

Radiologic studies will usually include a chest radiograph as part of the sepsis workup. Computed tomographic scanning of the brain is indicated to rule out intracranial pathology, especially if the mental status does not promptly improve with lowering of the temperature.

An electrocardiogram is indicated to evaluate for myocardial ischemia, which can result from severe cardiovascular stress.

After evaluation and stabilization, patients with heatstroke are admitted to an intensive care setting for continued monitoring and aggressive treatment.

▶ COLD ILLNESS

On average, there are 700 deaths per year in the United States resulting from excessive environmental cold exposure.[12] Hypothermia is defined as an unintentional drop in core body temperature of <35°C. Hypothermia can be separated into three categories: mild (core body temperature 35°C–32°C), moderate (core body temperature 32°C–30°C), and severe (core body temperature less than 30°C).[13] A low body temperature may develop as a result of exposure to low ambient temperature or may be secondary to a disease process (Table 140–4).

Age is an important factor in determining the susceptibility to hypothermia and the morbidity and mortality associated with it. Neonates are at high risk for developing hypothermia due to their large surface area compared with body mass and the relative paucity of subcutaneous tissue.[14]

They have also been postulated to have poorly developed thermoregulatory systems. The evaporation of warm amniotic fluid from the skin of the newborn is a major source of heat loss that must be guarded against in all cases. Throughout in-

fancy and young childhood, children remain susceptible to hypothermia with exposure to cold, although less so with advancing age. Most cases of accidental hypothermia in older children and adolescents are associated with near drowning in cold water.[15] However, in recent years, there has been an increase in exposure-related hypothermia in older children and adolescents; this is believed to be associated with the increased popularity of winter sports.[15] The greater the environmental stress, the higher the potential for development of hypothermia.[13] Inexperience and lack of caution, which are common among adolescents, increase the likelihood of their becoming victims of hypothermia.

PATHOPHYSIOLOGY

Normal body temperature varies over a narrow 1°C range. The primary mechanisms of heat loss related to cold illness are outlined in Table 140–5. Exposure to cold stimulates skin receptors, resulting in peripheral vasoconstriction and conservation of heat. As the temperature of the blood declines, the preoptic anterior hypothalamus is stimulated. Heat production is then increased by shivering and by metabolic and endocrine means of thermogenesis, primarily mediated by thyroid and adrenal secretions (Fig. 140–2).[16]

The overall functioning of all organ systems are impaired by the cold (Fig. 140–3). The most prominent effects are seen in the cardiovascular, central nervous, respiratory, renal, and gastrointestinal systems.[13,17]

The effects of hypothermia on the cardiovascular system are often the most noticeable. After an initial tachycardia, the heart rate falls as temperature falls. Mean arterial pressure also falls progressively, along with cardiac output.[13,18,19] Atrial dysrhythmias commonly appear at temperatures

▶ **TABLE 140–4. CAUSES OF HYPOTHERMIA IN INFANTS AND CHILDREN**

Environmental factors	Cyclic antidepressants
Exposure	Narcotics
Near drowning	Phenothiazines
Infections	CNS disorders
Meningitis	Degenerative diseases
Encephalitis	Head trauma
Sepsis	Spinal cord trauma
Pneumonia	Subarachnoid hemorrhage
Metabolic and endocrine	Cerebrovascular accidents
factors	Intracranial neoplasm
Hypoglycemia	Vascular factors
Diabetic ketoacidosis	Shock
Hypopituitarism	Pulmonary embolism
Myxedema	Gastrointestinal hemorrhage
Addison's disease	Dermatologic factors
Uremia	Burns
Malnutrition	Erythrodermas
Toxicologic factors	Iatrogenic factors
Alcohol	Cold fluid factors
Anesthetic agents	Exposure during treatment or
Barbiturates	postdelivery
Carbon monoxide	Prolonged extrications

▶ **TABLE 140–5. PRIMARY MECHANISMS OF HEAT DISSIPATION RELATED TO COLD ILLNESS**

Mechanism	Contribution to Heat Dissipation	Factors Influencing Rate of Loss
Radiation	Accounts for 55% to 65% of heat loss	Reduced by insulation (clothing/subcutaneous fat) Reduction in skin blood flow (vasoconstriction)
Conduction	Not a major route of heat loss under normal conditions but a major contributor in immersion incidents	Increased 5× in presence of wet clothing Increased 25–30× with submersion in cold water
Convection	Accounts for 15% of heat loss Heavily influenced by wind chill effect	Increased by wind currents Increased by bodily movement
Evaporation	Accounts for 20% to 25% of heat loss	Increased by wet skin

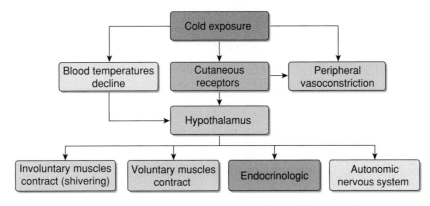

Figure 140–2. Physiologic responses in hypothermia. (With permission from Cooper MA, Danzl DF. Hypothermia. In: Hamilton GC, Sanders GR, Trott AT, (eds). *Emergency Medicine: An Approach to Clinical Problem-Solving.* Philadelphia, PA: W. B. Saunders; 1991:410.

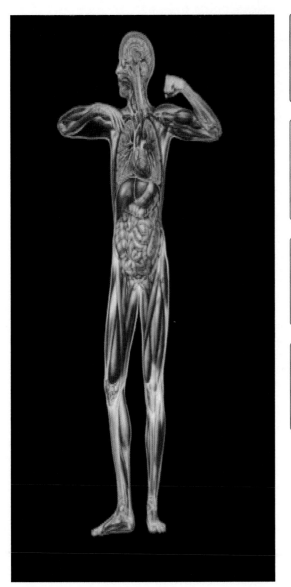

Central nervous effects
• Decrease cerebral metabolism
• Cerebral perfusion maintained until 25°C
• Electroencephalogram flat line 20°C

Respiratory effects
• Stimulation of respiratory drive (early)
• Decline in minute ventilation (as temperature falls)
• Bronchorrhea precipitating pulmonary edema

Cardiovascular effects
• Tachycardia (early)
• Bradycardia
• Decreased cardiac output
• Atrial dysrhythmias (32°C)
• Ventricular ectopy (<30°C)
• Osborn wave

Renal effects
• Vasoconstriction resulting in initial central hypovolemia
• Cold diuresis (enhanced by alcohol and cold water immersion)

Gastrointestinal effects
• Decreased gastrointestinal motility
• Ileus
• Constipation
• Poor rectal tone

Figure 140–3. A schematic showing the multisystem effects of hypothermia on the cardiovascular, central nervous, respiratory, renal, and gastrointestinal systems.

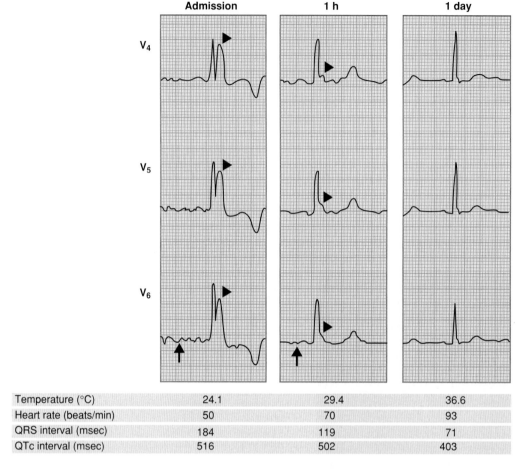

	Admission	1 h	1 day
Temperature (°C)	24.1	29.4	36.6
Heart rate (beats/min)	50	70	93
QRS interval (msec)	184	119	71
QTc interval (msec)	516	502	403

Figure 140–4. In severe hypothermia, the electrocardiogram (ECG) demonstrates the prominent elevation of the J deflection, so-called Osborn waves. The height of the J wave is proportionate to the degree of hypothermia, and this finding is usually most marked in the midprecordial leads. As the rewarming continues, the Osborn waves lessens in amplitude, and it disappears after 24 hours (With permission from Krantz MJ, Lowery CM. Giant Osborn waves in hypothermia. *N Eng J Med.* 2005;352(2):184.

below 32°C but are usually considered innocent because the ventricular response is slow. Ventricular ectopy is seen with temperatures <30°C and the risk of ventricular fibrillation is greatly increased. A J wave (Osborn wave) may be present at the junction of the QRS complex and ST segment (Fig. 140–4).[13,18] Although considered pathognomonic for hypothermia, the Osborn or J wave has no prognostic or predictive value in cases of hypothermia.[13] Asystole commonly occurs at 19°C.

As the core body temperature drops below 33°C, the patient becomes confused and ataxic. Brain enzymes are less functional with declining temperature, resulting in a linear decrease in cerebral metabolism. Cerebral perfusion is maintained until autoregulation fails at approximately 25°C. At 20°C, the electroencephalogram shows a flat line.

Cold initially stimulates the respiratory drive, but as temperature falls, a progressive decline in minute ventilation supervenes. Bronchorrhea, because of the local effect of cold air, can be severe, simulating pulmonary edema.[13,19]

Vasoconstriction in the extremities results in an initial central hypervolemia. The kidney responds rapidly, producing a large "cold diuresis" of dilute glomerular filtrate. Ethanol and immersion in cold water increase this early diuresis.

Gastrointestinal motility is decreased and gastric dilatation, ileus, constipation, and poor rectal tone commonly result. Inflammatory changes in the pancreas are also often found.

DIAGNOSIS

The diagnosis of hypothermia may be obvious when a history of exposure is known. However, hypothermia may develop insidiously because of causes other than exposure or to exposure in relatively warm environments.

The hypothermic patient is often not able to give an adequate history, and other sources of information should be sought. Family, friends, police, and paramedics are all valuable sources of information.

Once hypothermia is known or suspected, a history of exposure is sought, including the circumstances, location, and ambient temperature, the length of exposure, and presence or absence of submersion or wet skin and clothing.

▶ TABLE 140–6. PATHOPHYSIOLOGIC CHANGES DURING HYPOTHERMIA

Centigrade Temperature	Farenheit Temperature	Findings
37.6	99.6	Normal rectal temperature
37	98.6	Normal oral temperature
35	95.0	Maximal shivering Increased metabolic rate
33	91.4	Apathy Ataxia Anmesia Dysarthria
31	87.8	Decreased level of consciousness Bradycardia Hypotension Bradypnea Shivering stops
29	85.2	Dysrhythmias Insulin not effective Dilated pupils Poikilothermia
27	80.6	Areflexia No response to pain Comatose
25	77	Cerebral blood flow one-third normal Cardiac output one-half normal Significant hypotension
23	73.4	No corneal reflex Maximal ventricular fibrillation risk
19	66.2	Asystole Flat electroencephalogram
15	59.2	Lowest temperature survived from accidental hypothermia in an infant
9	48.2	Lowest temperature survived from therapeutic hypothermia

With permission from Cooper MA, Danzl DF. Hypothermia. In: Hamilton GC, Sanders AB, Strange GR, Trott AT, eds. *Emergency Medicine: An Approach to Clinical Problem-Solving.* Philadelphia, PA: WB Saunders; 1991:415.

If significant exposure is unlikely, an extensive history is required to search for clues for other causes of hypothermia (Table 140–4).

The key physical findings in patients with hypothermia, and the temperature level at which they occur, are depicted in Table 140–6. The core temperature defines the presence and severity of hypothermia. Most thermometers for routine clinical use will record a temperature down to only 34.4°C.[19] Special glass or electronic thermometers are required for accurate measurement of temperatures in hypothermic patients. Continuous monitoring of rectal, esophageal, or tympanic temperature is very useful during treatment.[13,18]

Shivering will often be present in the older child or adolescent but ceases by the time the temperature reaches 31°C. The skin is typically cold, firm, pale, or mottled. Localized damage due to frostbite may be present.[20] Shivering can increase heat production by four to five times. Behavioral responses, such as seeking a warm environment or putting on protective clothing, are major preventive mechanisms that are entirely absent in the infant. Shivering is also absent in neonates, making them entirely dependent on care from others, vasoconstriction, and heat generated by lipolysis.[16]

Early neurologic signs of hypothermia include confusion, apathy, poor judgment, slurred speech, and ataxia. Coma usually supervenes by the time the temperature reaches 27°C. Focal neurologic defects may be present. The Glasgow Coma Scale can serve as a useful quantitative means of following the patient's response to treatment, but it is not as useful with the nonverbal infant.

Since hypothermia affects multiple systems, other pathology can be masked. Signs of trauma, toxic ingestion, and endocrine disturbance should be sought, and the complete physical examination must be repeated at intervals during treatment to discover clues to problems that were initially masked by the hypothermia.

EVALUATION

For patients with hypothermia not related to exposure and in those exposure-related individuals who present with temperatures <32°C, extensive diagnostic testing may be indicated[14] (Table 140–7).

Arterial Blood Gases are useful for evaluation of oxygenation, ventilation, and acid–base status. In hypothermia, there is decreased tissue perfusion and the oxyhemoglobin dissociation curve is shifted to the left. Although some authorities have recommended correcting blood gas results for body temperature, correction can lead to false elevation of Po_2 and subsequent undertreatment. Metabolic acidosis is usually present and the buffering capacity of the blood is markedly reduced.

Complete Blood Count is useful for establishing a baseline. Typically, the hematocrit increases 2% for each 1°C drop in temperature. Hemoglobin may be decreased due to blood loss or chronic illness. The white blood count is reduced by sequestration and bone marrow depression. Even in the presence of severe infection, leukocytosis may not be seen.

Serum electrolytes should be monitored during the rewarming process to assess the need for intervention.

Renal function tests are useful for establishing baseline renal function but are poor indicators of fluid status in hypothermia. Acute tubular necrosis may develop after rewarming.

Serum glucose values may be elevated due to catecholamine effect and insulin inactivity below 30°C. Persistently elevated levels suggest pancreatitis or diabetic ketoacidosis. Hypoglycemia may develop due to inadequate glycogen stores in neonates and malnourished children.

Clotting studies, as well as platelet count and fibrinogen level, are indicated in cases of moderate-to-severe hypothermia. Cold induces thrombocytopenia and prolongs clotting times. Persistent changes after rewarming suggest the development of disseminated intravascular coagulation.

▶ **TABLE 140–7. KEY DIAGNOSTIC AND LABORATORY TESTING IN THE EVALUATION OF HYPOTHERMIA**

Diagnostic Test	Indication	Typical Findings	Caveats
Arterial blood gas (ABG)	Oxygenation Ventilation Acid base status	Metabolic acidosis	Avoid correction of results for body temperature. Can lead to false ↑ of P_{O_2}
Complete blood count (CBC)	Monitoring hemoglobin and white blood cell count Evaluation for sepsis	↓ Hemoglobin ↓ WBC secondary to sequestration and bone marrow depression	Hematocrit increases by 2% for each 1°C ↓ in temperature
Serum electrolytes	Monitoring during rewarming	Hypokalemia	No consistent effects on electrolyte concentrations.
Renal function tests	Useful for establishing baseline renal function	Acute tubular necrosis (w/rewarming)	Poor indicators of fluid status in hypothermia
Serum glucose	Monitoring to assess need for replacement or control	Elevated because of catecholamine effects and insulin activity below 30°C	Hypoglycemia may develop due to inadequate glycogen stores in neonates and malnourished children
Urinalysis	Monitoring of hydration status	Low-specific gravity secondary to a cold diuresis	No other consistent findings
Clotting studies	Monitoring in cases of moderate-to-severe hypothermia Evaluation for disseminated intravascular coagulation	Thrombocytopenia Prolonged clotting times	Persistent changes following rewarming suggest development of disseminated intravascular coagulation
Pancreatic enzymes	Monitoring for pancreatitis due to unreliability of abdominal examination	Elevated amylase and lipase	Pancreatitis in hypothermia is associated with a poor outcome
Electrocardiogram	Evaluation for myocardial ischemia Monitoring for dysrhythmias	The J wave is usually seen when the temperature falls below 32°C.	Indicated for all patients with a core temperature below 32°C
Cultures of body fluids	Monitoring in cases of moderate-to-severe hypothermia	-	Sepsis is a common cause of hypothermia in infants.
Radiologic imaging	Evaluation based upon history and clinical presentation	Chest radiograph indicated in all cases of hypothermia Cervical spine films for suspicion of trauma Cranial computed tomographic scanning for persistent mental status changes	Pulmonary edema may develop during rewarming and aspiration is relatively common

Amylase and lipase may be elevated and, because of the unreliability of the abdominal examination, may be the only indicators of the development of pancreatitis. Pancreatitis in hypothermia is associated with poor outcome.

Toxicologic studies are frequently indicated to detect causative or predisposing agents.

Urinalysis will demonstrate a low specific gravity due to cold diuresis.

Cultures of body fluids are indicated in all cases of moderate-to-severe hypothermia. Cultures from other body sites may also be indicated on the basis of the history and physical findings. Sepsis is a common cause of hypothermia in the infant and may also develop as a complication of hypothermia due to other causes.

Radiologic imaging should include a chest radiograph in all cases of significant hypothermia. Pulmonary edema may develop during rewarming and aspiration is relatively common. Cervical spine films may be indicated if there is suspicion of

trauma. Cranial computed tomographic scanning may be indicated in the setting of trauma or to search for other etiologic factors, especially when mental status does not clear along with rewarming.

Electrocardiogram is indicated for all patients with a core temperature <32°C to detect dysrhythmias or evidence of myocardial ischemia. The J wave (Osborn wave) (Fig. 140–4) is usually seen when the temperature falls below 32°C.

PREHOSPITAL CARE

A high index of suspicion is required to diagnose hypothermia in the field. Prehospital providers should presume hypothermia in situations where exposure, even at moderate temperatures, has occurred.[21]

Great caution is needed to prevent hypothermia or to initiate its early treatment in neonates. The neonate should immediately be dried and wrapped in warm blankets. Alternatively, the neonate can be placed against the body of the mother and then covered.

For other potentially hypothermic patients, wet clothing should be removed, and dry blankets applied. When prolonged extrications are required, hypothermia is particularly likely to develop. Protection should be provided whenever possible. Resuscitation fluids should be warmed whenever possible.

Ventilation should be supported as indicated and oxygenation maintained. Heated, humidified oxygen, if available, may minimize further core temperature loss and significantly add to other rewarming techniques. Cardiac monitoring is indicated to detect dysrhythmias. Because pulse and respiratory rates may be very slow in hypothermia, assessment for breathing and pulselessness is carried out over a 30- to 45-second period. If the patient is not breathing, ventilation is started immediately, using warmed humidified oxygen whenever possible. If there is no pulse, chest compressions are started immediately. Do not withhold basic life support while the patient is being rewarmed.

EMERGENCY DEPARTMENT MANAGEMENT

The initial approach to the patient with hypothermia is the same as that for any seriously ill patient, with evaluation and stabilization of the airway, breathing, and circulation before moving to other aspects of treatment.[18] The path of further management of hypothermia is directed by the results of the assessment of the patient's airway, breathing, and circulation (Fig. 140–5). Obtunded patients without protective airway reflexes require endotracheal intubation after preoxygenation. Endrotracheal intubation should be done as atraumatically as possible, but should not be withheld for fear of precipitating ventricular fibrillation. Intravenous lines are started and fluid resuscitation is guided by vital signs, urinary output, and pulmonary status. Cardiac monitoring is initiated. In addition, continuous monitoring of rectal, esophageal, or tympanic temperature is very helpful during treatment. A urinary catheter and a nasogastric tube are inserted. A bedside glucose determination is done to assess the need for glucose supplementation. If narcotic intoxication is a possibility, naloxone, 2 mg IV, is administered.

Cardiopulmonary resuscitation should be started in the pulseless patient, and interventions are guided by cardiac monitor findings. The cold myocardium may be resistant to defibrillation and to pharmacologic agents. If the initial, three defibrillation attempts fail to establish a rhythm, CPR is resumed and the patient is rewarmed to 30°C before defibrillation is repeated. Many patients spontaneously convert to an organized rhythm at a core temperature of 32°C to 35°C. During hypothermia, protein binding of drugs is increased, and most drugs will be ineffective in normal doses. Pharmacologic attempts to alter the pulse or blood pressure are to be avoided because drugs can accumulate in the peripheral circulation and subsequently lead to toxicity as rewarming occurs. It is important to remember that infants and children who have sustained prolonged hypothermic cardiac arrest have recovered with little or no neurologic impairment. In general, resuscitative efforts should continue until the hypothermic child is warmed to at least 30°C.[13,14,19]

In moderate-to-severe cases of hypothermia, active rewarming is started as soon as possible. Heated, humidified oxygen and intravenous fluids heated to 40°C have been shown to be safe and efficacious and are used from the beginning. Further heat loss is prevented by using radiant warmers for neonates and infants. The older child and adolescent should be covered with dry blankets. Active external rewarming, as with hot packs and electric blankets, can be dangerous. The rewarming of cold extremities can result in the mobilization of cold peripheral blood to the central circulation, resulting in core-temperature after-drop. Immersion in warm baths makes monitoring and resuscitation difficult. Cold, vasoconstricted skin is also very susceptible to thermal injury. Because of these concerns, active core rewarming is used in most cases of moderate-to-severe hypothermia.[13,14,18]

In addition to heated humidified oxygen and heated intravenous fluids, active core rewarming can be accomplished by irrigation of the stomach, bladder, and colon. Heat transfer by these techniques is somewhat limited. Rapid rewarming by irrigation of the mediastinum or pleural cavity via a thoracostomy tube is effective but very invasive. Peritoneal lavage with heated fluid (40°C–45°C) is probably a more effective method of active core rewarming. Extracorporeal rewarming is the most rapid method and is indicated in hypothermic cardiac arrest and with patients who present with completely frozen extremities. Using this technique, young, otherwise healthy people have survived deep hypothermia with no or minimal cerebral impairment.[13,14,18]

Forced air rewarming has recently been described as effective, noninvasive, and not associated with an after-drop phenomenon. Another noninvasive means of rewarming involves applying subatmospheric pressure to the hand and forearm, along with heat. This technique is described as immediately resulting in subcutaneous vasodilatation and rapid heat acquisition, rapidly eliminating shivering, and subjective improvement. Further studies of these techniques are needed.[13,22]

Previously healthy patients who are only mildly hypothermic (35°C–33°C) will usually reheat themselves safely if they are placed in a warm environment and given dry insulating coverings (passive external rewarming).

Beyond the neonatal period, sepsis is the most common cause of hypothermia in infants. All hypothermic patients should have a thorough evaluation to search for a source of infection and should have broad-spectrum antibiotics initiated early. An animoglycoside combined with ampicillin or a third-generation cephalosporin is generally recommended.

COLD WATER DROWNING

A special consideration in pediatric hypothermia is near drowning in cold water. This entity is discussed in Chapter 137.

FROSTBITE

Another special consideration is frostbite, which may occur in conjunction with hypothermia or as an isolated localized injury. Once primarily a military problem, frostbite is now more

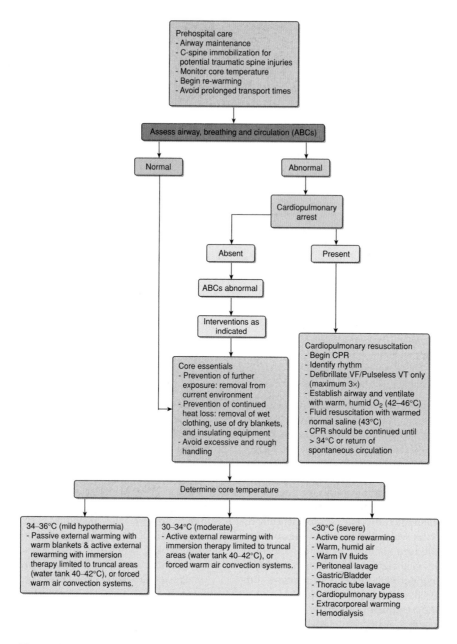

Figure 140–5. Approach to the patient with cold exposure. IV, intravenous; CPR, cardiopulmonary resuscitation. (With permission from McCullough L, Arora S. Diagnosis and treatment of hypothermia. *Am Fam Physician*. 2004;70(12):2329.)

prevalent in the civilian population as a result of occupational and recreational exposures. In frostbite, the body parts most susceptible are those areas farthest from the body's core; the earlobes, nose, hands, and feet. Predisposing factors to the development of frostbite include environmental, individual, behavioral, and occasion-linked factors[20,23] (Fig. 140–6).

Pathophysiology

The pathophysiology of frostbite includes three distinct pathways of tissue freezing: (1) extracellular formation of ice crystals, (2) hypoxia secondary to cold-induced local vasoconstriction, and (3) release of inflammatory mediators such as

prostaglandins PGF_2 and thromboxane A_2. All pathways can occur simultaneously thereby intensifying tissue damage. Cold exposure also increases blood viscosity, promotes vasospasm, and precipitates microthrombus formation. The release of inflammatory mediators has been shown to peak during the rewarming process and cycles of recurrent freezing and rewarming further increases the tissue levels.[13,24]

Classification of Frostbite Injuries

The clinical signs and symptoms of frostbite differ according to the depth of injury. Traditionally, frostbite has been classified by degree. First-degree frostbite is limited to the superficial

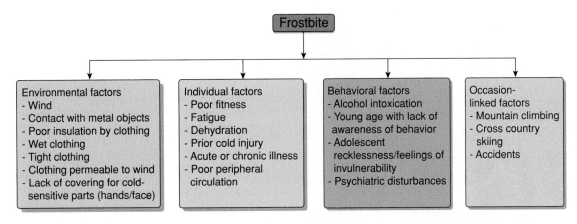

Figure 140–6. Predisposing factors for development of frostbite. (The environmental, individual, behavioral, and occasion-linked factors that may predispose individuals for the development of frostbite.)

epidermis. Erythema and edema occur and resolve without sequelae. Second-degree frostbite results in deeper epidermal involvement. Third-degree injury consists of full thickness skin injury. Recent studies have suggested that frostbite may be more usefully classified as superficial or deep[13,14,20,23] (Table 125–8). With superficial frostbite, the rewarmed skin develops clear blisters in contrast to the hemorrhagic blisters seen upon rewarming with deep frostbite (Figs. 140–7 and 140–8). Although no prognostic factors are entirely predictive, there are certain features that indict a favorable or unfavorable prognosis.[14]

Treatment

The treatment of frostbite is rapid rewarming. The preferred technique is immersion of the affected part in circulating warm water (40°C–42°C). Narcotic analgesics are often required to control pain during rewarming. A number of adjunctive therapies, such as vasodilators, thrombolytics, hyperbaric oxygen, and sympathectomy, have been recommended, but firm evidence for their effectiveness is not yet available.

It is very difficult to determine tissue viability after significant hypothermic injury. Debridement of nonviable tissue is best delayed for several days to weeks to preserve as much tissue as possible. However, recent improvements in radiologic assessment of tissue viability have led to the possibility of earlier surgery and more rapid rehabilitation times.[13,20]

Topical aloe vera cream and ibuprofen may be used for outpatient treatment after rewarming. More extensively injured patients will require continued inpatient treatment and pain control.

Rewarmed body parts are highly susceptible to refreezing, leading to even greater tissue loss. If exposure is anticipated, it is better not to rewarm the tissue.

Frostbite often results in sequelae that are persistent and may be permanent.

DISPOSITION

Most patients with hypothermia will require hospitalization for further treatment and evaluation. Those patients with a core temperature of <32°C will require cardiac monitoring. Profoundly, hypothermic patients with cardiac arrest and those with completely frozen extremities are candidates for extracorporeal rewarming and may require transfer to a tertiary care facility with this capability.

Patients with mild accidental hypothermia (35°C–32°C) may be rewarmed and discharged to a safe environment if there is no evidence of underlying disease.

▶ **TABLE 140–8. CLASSIFICATION OF FROSTBITE INJURIES**

Type of Frostbite	Area Affected	Appearance of Rewarmed Skin	Caveats
Superficial	Skin Subcutaneous tissue	Clear blisters Pale Waxy Numb Poor capillary refill	Extremity is very painful on rewarming
Deep	Bones Joints Tendons	Extremity lacks pain and feeling. With rewarming there is severe edema and blistering	

Favorable prognostic signs: Retained sensation, normal skin color, early appearance of clear blisters, warm tissues, edema.
Unfavorable prognostic signs: Lack of sensation, cold, cyanotic appearance, white "frozen" appearance, late appearance of hemorrhagic blisters, absence of edema.

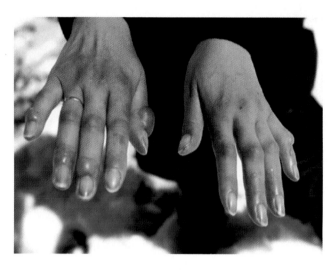

Figure 140–7. Clear blisters as commonly seen with superficial frostbite injuries.

PREVENTION

When used prior to the initiation of cold weather activities, proper planning can prevent most injuries. The first step is to be aware of cold risks. While little true acclimatization to the cold probably occurs, there is some value to practicing tasks that are to be performed in the cold and building up endurance before beginning a major cold activity. Good nutrition and hydration are helpful in resisting the stresses of cold weather activity. Sufficient clothing, either in layers or made of good insulating materials, is essential. Spare clothing is also essential, since it may be necessary to change into dry clothing if clothing becomes wet. Going slowly and avoiding exhaustion or exces-

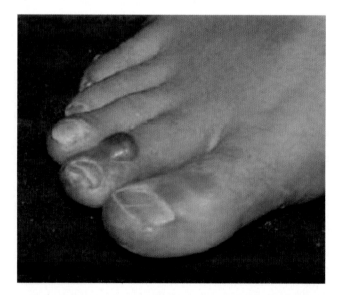

Figure 140–8. Hemorrhagic blister as commonly seen with deep frostbite injuries.

sive sweating is also helpful. Alcohol and tobacco should be strictly avoided, as should contact with metallic objects.

REFERENCES

1. Centers for Disease Control and Prevention. Heat-related deaths—United States, 1999–2003. *MMWR Morb Mortal Wkly Rep.* 2006;55:796–798.
2. Gaffin S, Moran D. Pathophysiology of heat-related illnesses. In: Auerbach PS, ed. *Wilderness Medicine.* 4th ed. St. Louis, Mo: Mosby; 2001:240–281.
3. American Academy of Pediatrics Committee on Sports Medicine and Fitness. Climatic heat stress and the exercising child and adolescent. *Pediatrics.* 2000;106:158–159.
4. Barrow M, Clark K. Heat related illnesses. *Am Fam Physician.* 1998;58:749–756.
5. Erickson T, Prendergast H. Procedures pertaining to hyperthermia. In: Roberts Jr, Hedges J, eds. *Clinical Procedures in Emergency Medicine.* 4th ed. WB Saunders; 2004:1358–1370.
6. Glazer J. Management of heatstroke and heat exhaustion. *Am Fam Physician.* 2005;71:2133–2140.
7. Howe A, Boden B. Heat-related illness in athletes. *Am J. Sports Med.* 2007;35:1384–1395.
8. Jardine D. Heat illness and heat stroke. *Pediatr Rev.* 2007;28: 249–258.
9. Noakes TD. A modern classification of the exercise-related heat illnesses. *J Sci Med Sport.* 2008;11:33–39.
10. O'Malley PG. Heat waves and heat-related illness: preparing for the increasing influence of climate on health in temperate areas. *JAMA.* 2007;298:917–919.
11. Hadad E, Rav-Acha M, Heled Y, et al. Heat stroke :a review of cooling methods. *Sports Med.* 2004;34:501–511.
12. Centers for Disease Control and Prevention. Hypothermia-related deaths—Philadelphia, 2001, and United States, 1999. *MMWR Morb Mortal Wkly Rep.* 2003;52:86–87.
13. Erickson T, Prendergast H. Procedures pertaining to hypothermia. In: Roberts, Hedges, ed. *Clinical Procedures in Emergency Medicine.* 4th ed. WB Saunders; 2004:1343–1357.
14. Biem J, Koehncke N, Classen D, et al. Out of the cold: management of hypothermia and frostbite. *CMAJ.* 2003;168:305–311.
15. Giesbrecht G. Cold stress, near drowning and accidental hypothermia: a review. *Aviat Space Environ Med.* 2000;71:733–752.
16. Reamy B. Disturbances due to cold. In: *Rakel RE, ed. Conn's Current Therapy.* 53rd ed. Philadelphia: WB Saunders; 2001:1171–1173.
17. Eddy V, Morris J, Cuullinane DC. Hypothermia, coagulopathy, and acidosis. *Surg Clin North Am.* 2000;30:845–854.
18. Giesbrecht G. Emergency treatment of hypothermia. *Emerg Med.* 2001;13:9–16.
19. Mccullough L, Arora S. Diagnosis and treatment of hypothermia. *Am Fam Physician.* 2004;70:2325–2332.
20. Murphy JV, Banwell PE, Roberts AH, et al. Frostbite: pathogenesis and treatment. *J Trauma.* 2000;48:171–178.
21. Giesbrecht G. Prehospital treatment of hypothermia. *Wilderness Med.* 2001;12:24–31.
22. Kornberger E, Schwarz B, Lindner KH, et al. Forced air surface rewarming in patients with severe accidental hypothermia. *Resuscitation.* 1999;41:105–111.
23. Cauchy E, Chetaille E, Marchand V, et al. Retrospective study of 70 cases of severe frostbite lesions: a proposed new classification scheme. *Wilderness Environ Med.* 2001;12:248–255.
24. Simon T, Soep J, Hollister J. Pernio in pediatrics. *Pediatrics.* 2005;116:e472–e475.

CHAPTER 141

High-Altitude Illness

Ira J. Blumen and Janis Tupesis

▶ HIGH-YIELD FACTS

- High-altitude illness often affects young and otherwise healthy individuals and there is a broad spectrum of disease. It progresses from the mildest form of acute mountain sickness (AMS) into the potentially life-threatening forms such as high-altitude pulmonary edema (HAPE) and high-altitude cerebral edema (HACE).
- A slow, graded ascent is the key to acclimatization. Acclimatization is generally defined as the body's physiologic adaptation to hypoxia at altitude. In the ideal setting, the first night's sleep occurs at <8000 ft, with the first day spent at rest.
- Pharmacologic agents may also be beneficial adjuncts to acclimatization. Acetazolamide (Diamox) has been shown to be very effective when staging is not possible or with individuals who are at an increased risk of high-altitude illness.
- Although normal acclimatization inhibits antidiuretic hormone (ADH) and aldosterone, resulting in a high-altitude–induced diuresis, the opposite is seen with AMS. Aldosterone, ADH, and renin–angiotensin increase, resulting in fluid retention and a leakage from the vascular space to the extravascular space.
- HACE is the most severe, life-threatening form of high-altitude illness. HACE is uncommon, affecting <1% to 2% of individuals who ascend without acclimatization.
- Definitive treatment of HACE is descent. High-flow oxygen is indicated as soon as symptoms are recognized and dexamethasone, at an initial dose of 1 to 2 mg/kg orally or intramuscularly, can produce dramatic improvement.
- HAPE is a life-threatening manifestation of high-altitude illness and represents a unique form of noncardiogenic pulmonary edema. It is estimated that HAPE affects 0.5% to 15% of those who ascend rapidly to high altitudes and is the leading cause of high-altitude death other than trauma.

▶ HIGH-ALTITUDE ILLNESS

Episodes of high-altitude illness have been documented for thousands of years, but these were relatively rare entities until the advent of modern travel. The increasing popularity of various recreational activities has led families and individuals to try to go higher (Fig. 141–1) and faster than ever before and on a more frequent basis. Hiking, mountain climbing, biking, skiing, hot air balloons, and gliders are among the various sports that can put individuals at risk of high-altitude illness. With modern modalities of travel, the incidence of high-altitude illness will continue to rise, putting more children and adults at risk (Fig. 141–2).

High-altitude illness, resulting from an individual's altered responses to hypoxia and decrease in barometric pressure,[1,2] often affects young and otherwise healthy individuals. There is a broad spectrum of disease, progressing from the mildest form of acute mountain sickness (AMS) to the potentially life-threatening forms of high-altitude pulmonary edema (HAPE) and high-altitude cerebral edema (HACE). Symptoms of high-altitude illness may develop within hours or days after ascent. In contrast, hypoxemia occurs within minutes to hours of arrival at altitude and results in the initiation of the cascade of physiologic events that lead to AMS, HAPE, and HACE.

There are a number of factors that influence the incidence, onset, and severity of high-altitude illness:

- Rate of ascent.
- Altitude achieved.
- Length of stay.
- Physical exertion.

Varying severity of high-altitude illness will occur when any of these factors or a combination of them exceeds the individual's ability to adapt to the new environment. Infants and children, because of their anatomical and physiologic differences, are at greater risk for developing both AMS and HAPE. This is primarily because of an increased risk of ventilation–perfusion mismatch resulting in hypoxia. Contributing factors[3] can include:

- Predisposition for paradoxical inhibition of respiratory drive (up to 1–2 months of age).
- More compliant rib cage.
- Reduced surfactant (preterm infants).
- Increased proportion of the pulmonary vascular bed with muscular arterioles in early infancy.
- Increased airway reactivity in response to hypoxia (infancy).
- Reduced upper and lower internal diameters of the airways.
- Fewer alveoli (early childhood).
- Presence of fetal hemoglobin until 4 to 6 months of age.

The highest incidence of AMS occurs between the ages of 1 and 20 years. The severity of symptoms decreases with increasing age.

High altitude is generally considered to be ≥8000 ft (2439 m). At this altitude, arterial oxygen saturation falls below 90% (Pao$_2$ 60%). Acclimatization is necessary to prevent illness. Although severe altitude illness is uncommon below 8000 ft,

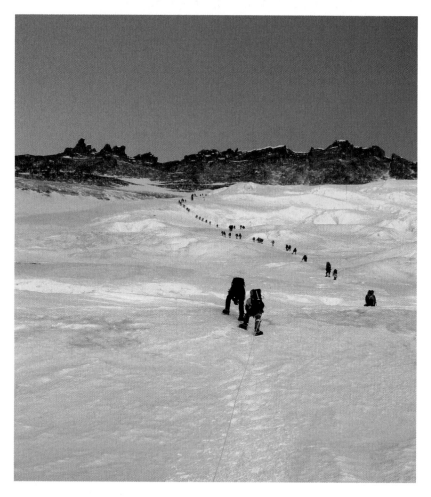

Figure 141–1. Climbing the Lhotse Face, Mt. Everest. Altitude 24,500 ft. (Photo courtesy of Gary Guller.)

medically compromised individuals may become symptomatic at *moderate altitude* (5000–8000 ft). At *extreme altitude*, which is generally greater than 18,000 ft (approximately 5500 m), acclimatization is not possible and altitude illness is inevitable (Fig. 141–3).

THE ATMOSPHERE AND PHYSICAL GAS LAWS

An understanding of the physical gas laws and the composition of the atmosphere is necessary to explain the occurrence of high-altitude illness. The atmosphere is a collection of gases with uniform percentage up to an altitude of approximately 70,000 ft. The largest percentage is nitrogen (78.08%), followed by oxygen (20.95%). At any given altitude, the force exerted can be represented as the barometric pressure or atmospheric pressure (Table 141–1).

Boyle's law states that the volume of a given mass of gas will vary inversely with its pressure ($P_1V_1 = P_2V_2$, where P_1 initial pressure, P_2 = final pressure, V_1 initial volume, and V_2 final volume). As an individual ascends, barometric pressure decreases and the volume of gas within an enclosed space expands. As the individual descends, the reverse is true.

Dalton's law of partial pressure describes the pressure exerted by gases at various altitudes. It states that the total pressure of a mixture of gases is the sum of the partial pressures of all the gases in the mixture. At sea level, barometric pressure is 760 mm Hg, and the percentage of oxygen in the atmosphere is equal to 20.95%. Therefore, the partial pressure of oxygen (P_{O_2}) at sea level is P_{O_2} = 20.95% × 760 mm Hg = 159.22 mm Hg.

As altitude increases and pressure decreases, gas expansion causes the available oxygen to decrease. At 10,000 ft, where the barometric pressure is 523 mm Hg, the percentage of oxygen *remains* 20.95%, but the partial pressure of oxygen will decrease to approximately 110 mm Hg and the alveolar P_{O_2} will drop to 60 mm Hg.

PHYSIOLOGIC RESPONSE

Several different physiologic responses are seen at high altitude. The response to hypoxia is the most significant. It includes increased cerebrospinal fluid (CSF) pressure, fluid retention, fluid shifts, and impaired gas exchange. Although no one is exempt from the effects of hypoxia, the onset and severity of symptoms will vary with individuals. The factors that

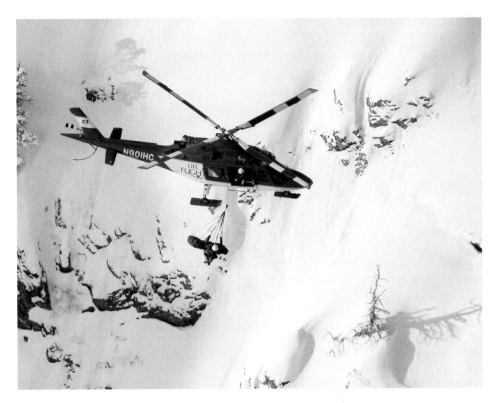

Figure 141–2. Airlift of injured hikers off the Mt. Olympus trail, near Salt Lake City, Utah. Elevation, 8600 ft. (Photo courtesy of Intermountain Life Flight.)

Figure 141–3. Hiking along Summit Ridge, Kilimanjaro, Tanzania. Altitude 19,340 ft. (Photo courtesy of Janis Tupesis, MD.)

► TABLE 141–1. **EFFECTS OF ALTITUDE**

Altitude (in ft)	Barometric Pressure		Po_2 (mm Hg)	Pao_2 (mm Hg)	$Paco_2$ (mm Hg)	Temp (F°)	Volume Ratio	O_2 Sat%
	mm Hg	PSI						
0	760	14.70	159.2	103.0	40.0	59.0	1.0	98
1000	733	14.17	153.6	98.2	39.4	55.4		
2000	706	13.67	147.9	93.8	39.0	51.8		
3000	681	13.17	142.7	89.5	38.4	48.4		
4000	656	12.69	137.4	85.1	38.0	44.8		
5000	632	12.23	132.5	81.0	37.4	41.2	1.2	
6000	609	11.78	127.6	76.8	37.0	37.6		
7000	586	11.34	122.8	72.8	36.4	34.0		
8000	565	10.92	118.4	68.9	36.0	30.4	1.3	93
9000	542	10.51	113.5	65.0	35.4	27.0		
10,000	523	10.11	109.6	61.2	35.0	23.4	1.5	87
11,000	503	9.72	105.4	57.8	34.4	19.8		
12,000	483	9.35	101.2	54.3	33.8	16.2		
13,000	465	8.98	97.4	51.0	33.2	12.6		
14,000	447	8.63	93.6	47.9	32.6	9.1		
15,000	429	8.29	89.9	45.0	32.0	5.5	1.8	84
16,000	412	7.97	86.3	42.0	31.4	1.9		
17,000	396	7.65	83.0	40.0	31.0	−1.7		
18,000	380	7.34	79.6	37.8	30.4	−5.2		72
19,000	364	7.04	76.3	35.9	30.0	−8.7		
20,000	349	6.75	73.1	34.3	29.4	−12.3	2.2	66
30,000	228	4.36	47.3			−47.9	3.3	
40,000	141	2.72	29.5			−62.7	5.4	
50,000	87	1.68	18.2			−62.7	8.7	

influence an individual's threshold for hypoxia include physical activity, sleep, physical fitness, metabolic rate, diet, nutrition, emotions, and fatigue. Alcohol ingestion and smoking act as respiratory depressants and will exacerbate the effects of hypoxia. Exposure to temperature extremes will increase a person's metabolic rate, increasing oxygen requirements and reducing the hypoxic threshold.

The body responds with both immediate and chronic physiologic adaptations to the hypoxic environment. Through acclimatization, a series of physiologic adjustments works to restore the tissue oxygen pressure to near its sea level value. Successful acclimatization will vary between individuals and cannot be predicted by physical conditioning, examination, or testing.

A slow, graded ascent is the key to acclimatization especially for individuals who have previously exhibited sensitivity to high-altitude changes.[4] In the ideal setting, the first night's sleep occurs at <8000 ft, with the first day spent at rest. If the altitude of the desired climb is between 10,000 and 14,000 ft, then the daily ascent is limited to 1000 ft. Beyond 14,000 ft, 2 days should be taken for each 1000-ft ascent (Fig. 141–4). Climbing to higher elevations during the day and descending to a lower altitude to sleep is one option to prevent AMS and facilitate acclimatization.

Pharmacologic agents may also be beneficial adjuncts to acclimatization. Acetazolamide (Diamox) has been shown to be very effective when staging is not possible or with individuals who are at an increased risk of high-altitude illness.[5]

Dexamethasone may also be effective in preventing AMS, but it is generally reserved for treatment.

Respiratory System

As an individual ascends, the hypoxic ventilatory response (HVR) will attempt to compensate for the decrease in arterial Po_2 through an increase in the ventilatory rate. An inadequate HVR, resulting in relative hypoventilation, has been suggested as the etiology for AMS and HAPE. Individuals with low tidal volumes and children are less able to respond to the hypoxic insult and therefore are more prone to AMS. HVR is genetically predetermined. It can be influenced by caffeine, alcohol, and numerous medications. Hypoxia from chronic heart or lung problems desensitizes this effect.

The threshold for increased ventilation is approximately 4000- to 5000-ft elevation. At an altitude of 8000 ft, an arterial oxygenation saturation of 93% is experienced. The maximum response occurs at 22,000 ft, at which point the minute volume will be nearly doubled.

The initial maximal effect of the HVR occurs at approximately 6 to 8 hours after arrival to altitude. A decline in the partial pressure of inspiratory oxygen (Pio_2) results in an increase in ventilation, and $Paco_2$ will decrease accordingly. The falling $Paco_2$ causes a mild respiratory alkalosis and a shift of the oxyhemoglobin dissociation curve to the left. The result is increased binding of oxygen with hemoglobin for transport to

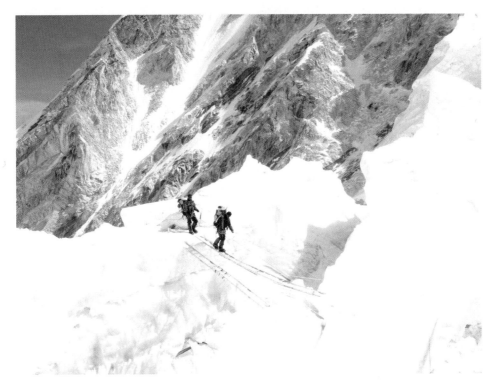

Figure 141–4. Hiking across Khumbu Icefall, Mt. Everest. Altitude 20,000 ft. (Photo courtesy of Gary Guller.)

the tissues. More importantly, the respiratory alkalosis provides negative feedback to the medulla, restricting the hypoxic ventilatory response. Further response is dependent on the renal excretion of bicarbonate, within 24 to 48 hours, to compensate for this respiratory alkalosis. Ventilation will slowly increase as the pH returns to normal. With no further ascent, this response can take 4 to 6 days. As an individual continues to higher elevation, subsequent acclimatization will be directed by the declining arterial P_{CO_2}.

Hypoxia and cold stressors will act as significant vasoconstrictors of the pulmonary vascular bed, resulting in an elevation of the pulmonary arterial pressure and an increased workload on the right side of the heart. The degree of pulmonary hypertension in response to a global hypoxia is thought to play an important role in the development of HAPE.

Cardiovascular System

The cardiovascular system is relatively resistant to hypoxia compared with the respiratory and central nervous systems. The cardiovascular system response to hypoxia may be observed in two phases. The heart rate will begin to increase at an altitude of 4000 ft. There will also be a slight increase in blood pressure secondary to increased catecholamines (induced from a diminished P_{aO_2}) and selective vasoconstriction. These increase the cardiac output. As acclimatization occurs, the heart rate will return to normal. If the individual fails to acclimatize, the heart rate will remain elevated, and the increase in cardiac activity will require more oxygen. The typical physiologic response of the cardiovascular system to altitude is to increase heart rate, blood pressure, peripheral vascular resistance, and cardiac output.

Hematopoietic System

The hematopoietic response to high altitude is a critical element in an individual's ability to acclimatize. All underlying changes within the hematopoietic system are geared toward increasing arterial oxygenation. Within hours of ascent, erythropoietin output is increased in response to the hypoxia. In approximately 4 to 5 days, there will be an increase in circulating red blood cells. This increase in red cell mass persists for 1 to 2 months after return to lower altitudes. At extreme altitudes, this hematopoietic response is detrimental. Oxygen transport is impeded by the increased blood viscosity, hemoconcentration, and increased red blood cell mass.

Increased 2,3-diphosphoglycerate (2,3-DPG) within the red blood cells is another hematopoietic response to hypoxemia. This shifts the oxyhemoglobin disassociation curve (Fig. 141–5) to the right, facilitating the release of oxygen from the blood to the tissues. With acclimatization, this shift to the right offsets the leftward shift of the oxyhemoglobin dissociation curve caused by hyperventilation and respiratory alkalosis.

Central Nervous System

Under normal conditions, cerebral blood flow is kept at a fairly constant rate. As a person's P_{O_2} falls, increased respiratory rate decreases the P_{CO_2}, eventually raising the pH of both the blood and the CSF. As the pH of CSF rises, chemoreceptors in the

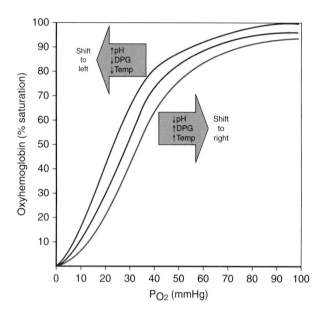

Figure 141–5. Oxygen/Dissociation curve.

brain case cerebral arterioles to dilate, resulting in increased cerebral blood flow. This response, which increases oxygen delivered to the brain, also increases intracranial pressure and can lead to HACE.

Renal System

As mentioned, the respiratory response to altitude is hyperventilation, resulting in respiratory alkalosis. Respiratory alkalosis stimulates renal excretion of bicarbonate, producing a compensatory metabolic acidosis. As the pH equalizes, ventilation may continue to increase. This ventilatory acclimatization subsides after 4 to 6 days at altitude.

During ascent, central blood volume will increase secondary to peripheral vasoconstriction. Antidiuretic hormone (ADH) and aldosterone are inhibited, resulting in a diuresis, decreased plasma volume, and hemoconcentration. Individuals without this diuretic response are at greater risk for fluid retention and high-altitude illness.

ACUTE MOUNTAIN SICKNESS

AMS is the most common and mildest form of high-altitude illness. Some individuals traveling to 8000 ft will become symptomatic, although nearly everyone who ascends to elevations between 11 000 and 20 000 ft will develop some clinical signs of AMS.

Clinical Presentation

The onset of AMS symptoms is usually within 4 to 8 hours of a rapid ascent, but it can be delayed for up to 4 days. Symptoms develop following strenuous activity or sleeping at high altitude. In most cases, symptoms peak in 24 to 48 hours and resolve by the third or fourth day. If the individual proceeds

to a higher altitude after the onset of AMS, symptoms may last considerably longer.

The clinical presentation of AMS includes the following symptoms, in order of prevalence:

- Headache.
- Sleep disturbance.
- Fatigue.
- Shortness of breath.
- Dizziness.
- Anorexia.
- Nausea.
- Vomiting.

AMS should be considered the etiology in any individual at altitude who develops at least three of these symptoms. Headache occurs in approximately two-thirds of individuals with AMS. It is throbbing in nature and worse after exercise, at night, or on awakening. Nausea and vomiting are common in children. In young children, however, signs of AMS are often less specific and include fussiness, as well as poor sleep, decreased appetite, and vomiting.[6]

Other symptoms associated with AMS include oliguria, mild peripheral edema, weakness, lassitude, malaise, irritability, decreased concentration, poor judgment, palpitations, deep inner chill, and a dull pain in the posterolateral chest wall.

On physical examination, vital signs may be normal or slightly elevated. Fluid retention is exhibited as fine rales or peripheral edema. Retinal hemorrhages may also be seen.

Sleep disturbance and periods of sleep apnea are common. Under normal sea level conditions, there is a mild decrease in oxygen saturation during sleep. This becomes more pronounced at altitude. While sleeping, the increased respiratory rate that accompanies high-altitude exposure causes a mild respiratory alkalosis that inhibits the respiratory drive, resulting in hypoventilation and periods of apnea. Brief episodes of hyperventilation occur next, increasing oxygen saturation while exacerbating the hypocapnia and further inhibiting ventilation. These episodes of periodic breathing (Cheyne–Stokes respirations), with apnea lasting up to 90 seconds, continue through the night, increasing the hypoxia associated with being at altitude.

The differential diagnosis of these symptoms includes an alcohol hangover, exhaustion, dehydration, and a viral syndrome. In addition, respiratory and CNS infections, exhaustion, hypothermia, gastritis, and carbon monoxide poisoning should be considered. However, if the symptoms occur shortly after arrival to altitude, they must be considered AMS until proved otherwise.

Pathophysiology

Although normal acclimatization inhibits ADH and aldosterone, resulting in a high-altitude-induced diuresis, the opposite is seen with AMS. Aldosterone, ADH, and renin–angiotensin increase, resulting in fluid retention and a leakage from the vascular space to the extravascular space.

There are two theories for the development of cerebral edema in AMS. The first theory is cytotoxic edema, which is induced by a deficiency in the ATP-dependent sodium pump caused by a hypoxic cellular injury, leading to an accumulation of intracellular fluid. The second is vasogenic edema. In this situation, hypoxia causes cerebral vasodilation, which in turn increases cerebral blood flow, capillary perfusion, and leakage through the blood–brain barrier.

The onset of AMS may be hastened by decreased vital capacity, increased CSF pressure, proteinuria, fluid retention, recent weight gain, or relative hypoventilation. It is postulated that children are more susceptible to AMS, as they are more sensitive to cerebral hypoxemia. Physical fitness does not impact on susceptibility to AMS.

Treatment

Treatment is initially directed toward prevention. Symptoms of AMS are most often mild and self-limiting, lasting only a few days. Once symptoms do occur, activity should be minimized, with no higher ascent until signs and symptoms have resolved. Proceeding to a lower altitude is indicated for any individual who shows no signs of improvement within 1 to 2 days or whose clinical condition worsens. Immediate descent is indicated if ataxia, decreased level of consciousness, confusion, dyspnea at rest, rales, or cyanosis are present. A descent of 1000 to 3000 ft is recommended. In some situations, as little as a 500-ft descent may result in improvement.

If descent is not an option, the use of supplementary oxygen will relieve most of the signs and symptoms of AMS. During sleep, 1 to 2 L/min can be of significant benefit.

A Gamow bag (Fig. 141–6) is a portable fabric hyperbaric bag that has been shown to relieve the central effects of AMS. Using a foot pump, it can be pressurized in excess of 100 torr for the physiologic equivalent of a 4000- to 5000-ft descent.

Symptomatic treatment for the headache is with acetaminophen, which will have no impact on the hypoxic ventilatory response. Victims of AMS are to refrain from using narcotics, which depress this response. Prochlorperazine, given for nausea and vomiting, is also effective in *increasing* the respiratory drive. The dosage of prochlorperazine for chil-

dren >10 kg in weight, or older than 2 years, is 0.1 to 0.15 mg/kg/dose IM, po, or PR.

The carbonic anhydrase inhibitor acetazolamide may be used in the treatment or prophylaxis of AMS. It decreases the reabsorption of bicarbonate, forcing a renal bicarbonate diuresis and resulting in a mild metabolic acidosis. This increases the ventilation rate and arterial Po_2. Low-dose acetazolamide is a particularly effective respiratory stimulant in the treatment of sleep apnea. The pediatric dosage for acetazolamide is 5 to 10 mg/kg/d, divided into two or three doses. Side effects include peripheral paresthesia, nausea, vomiting, polyuria, spoiling the taste of carbonated beverages, drowsiness, and confusion. Acetazolamide is contraindicated for those with sensitivities to sulfa drugs. When acetazolamide is used for prophylaxis, it should be started 48 hours before ascent and continued for at least 48 hours after arriving at the highest altitude. The dosage for older children and adults is 250 mg po q8 to 12 hours. When used to treat AMS, improvement is generally seen within 12 to 24 hours.

Dexamethasone is also used to treat AMS, although its mechanism of action is unknown.[7] Dexamethasone minimizes the symptoms of AMS but does not impact acclimatization. Its use is reserved for those with sulfa allergies or intolerance to acetazolamide. A loading dose of 4 mg po or IM is given, and improvement is generally noted within 2 to 6 hours. If there is no improvement after descent, a maintenance dose of 1 to 1.5 mg/kg/d (not to exceed 16 mg/d) divided q4 to 6 hours should be initiated for 5 days. The dose is then tapered for 5 days before it is discontinued. Rebound AMS may occur if the dexamethasone is discontinued at altitude.

Prevention

Prevention of AMS through acclimatization is not always possible for vacationing climbers, skiers (Fig. 141–7), and other sports enthusiasts. Prevention includes a slow, graded ascent and a diet high in carbohydrates, low in salt, and with adequate fluid intake. Alcohol and tobacco are to be avoided.

HIGH-ALTITUDE CEREBRAL EDEMA

HACE is the most severe, life-threatening form of high-altitude illness. HACE is uncommon, affecting <1% to 2% of individuals who ascend without acclimatization. It is rare below altitudes of 12 000 ft, but has resulted in death at elevations as low as 8200 ft. A common problem is the difficulty in differentiating between AMS and early HACE.

Clinical Presentation

HACE commonly begins with the symptoms of AMS and progresses to diffuse neurologic dysfunction. Onset of severe symptoms is 1 to 3 days after ascent to altitude, but early signs of AMS may rapidly deteriorate to severe HACE in as few as 12 hours. Evidence of HAPE may also be present.

Severe headaches, nausea, vomiting, and altered mental status are common symptoms associated with HACE. Truncal ataxia is the cardinal sign and this alone warrants immediate descent. If not recognized, HACE will proceed to include confusion, slurred speech, diplopia, hallucinations, seizures,

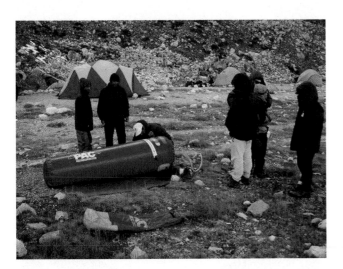

Figure 141–6. Treating and preparing a patient for medical evacuation using a Gamow Bag. (Photo courtesy of Gary Guller.)

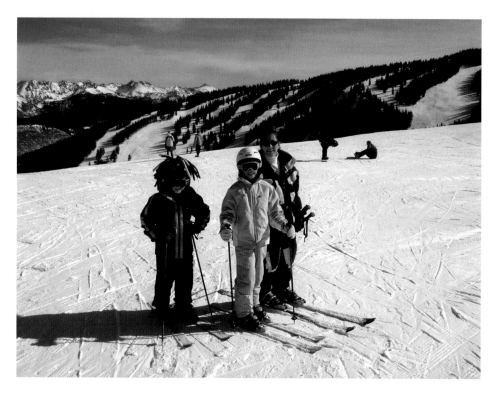

Figure 141–7. Ski vacations can expose children and adults to significant altitude changes from their baseline residential elevation. For example, the base of Vail village is at an elevation of 8120 ft and the summit is over 11 500 ft. (Photo courtesy of Vince and Liz Kellen.)

impaired judgment, cranial nerve palsies (third and sixth), abnormal reflexes, paresthesias, decreased level of consciousness, coma, and finally death. A 60% mortality is associated with HACE once coma is present.

The differential diagnosis includes head injury, subarachnoid hemorrhage, meningitis, encephalitis, carbon monoxide poisoning, transient ischemic attack, and cerebrovascular accident. Patients who become symptomatic at high altitude warrant a complete evaluation to rule out other etiologies.

Pathophysiology

HACE is the end-stage, severe form of AMS. HACE is thought to be associated with cytotoxic edema, vasogenic edema, or a combination of these two processes that cause cerebral edema. (Fig. 141–8) The time of onset for HACE would support the cytotoxic edema theory, whereas the response of HACE to corticosteroids would support the vasogenic edema theory.

Treatment

Definitive treatment of HACE is descent, and as quickly as possible. High-flow oxygen is indicated as soon as symptoms are recognized. Dexamethasone can produce dramatic improvement. An initial dose of 1 to 2 mg/kg po or IM (maximum dose 8 mg) is given followed by a maintenance dose of 1 to 1.5 mg/kg/d (not to exceed 16 mg/d) divided q4 to 6 hours for 5 days. The dose is then tapered for 5 days before it is

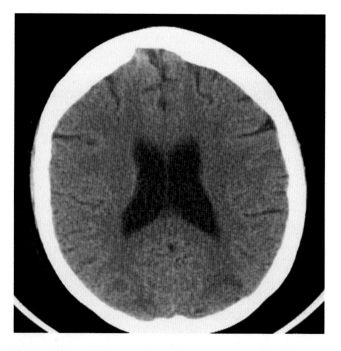

Figure 141–8. Diffuse cerebral edema consistent with HACE. (Photo courtesy of Christopher Straus, MD.)

discontinued. Acetazolamide has not been shown to be effective in the treatment of HACE. Hyperbaric therapy with the Gamow bag has been reported to be useful in mild HACE and may be life-saving if descent is impossible.

For severe cases, intubation and hyperventilation are indicated to decrease intracranial pressure. Furosemide and mannitol are second-line treatments.

Acute episodes of HACE may result in long-term neurologic deficits. Coma may persist for days. Persistent ataxia, impaired judgment, and behavioral changes have been reported to last as long as 1 year. For this reason, it is essential that any evidence of HACE be recognized and treated early and that other etiologies be ruled out if symptoms persist.

The key to prevention of HACE is acclimatization. However, cases of HACE have been reported in individuals who have limited their ascent to 1000 ft a day.

HIGH-ALTITUDE PULMONARY EDEMA

HAPE is a life-threatening manifestation of high-altitude illness and represents a unique form of noncardiogenic pulmonary edema. It is estimated that HAPE affects 0.5% to 15% of those who ascend rapidly to high altitudes. Other than trauma, it is the most common cause of death at altitude. While HAPE has occurred below 8000 ft,[8] it is more commonly associated with altitudes greater than 14 500 ft. HAPE is exacerbated by rapid ascent, cold stressors, a past history of HAPE, excessive exertion, and an inability to acclimatize. History of a recent upper respiratory tract infection has also been thought to be contributory.

Children and young adults are more susceptible to HAPE and individuals with a history of HAPE are at greater risk for recurrence. Children are also more susceptible to a special form of this high-altitude illness identified as *reentry HAPE*. This occurs in individuals who are living at higher altitudes and return to the set elevation after spending as little as 24 hours at lower altitude.

Clinical Presentation

The onset of HAPE usually occurs within 1 to 4 days after ascent to altitude, most commonly during the second night at altitude. However, initial symptoms may develop within hours following ascent.

Early in the course the victim will develop a dry cough, fatigue, and dyspnea on exertion. Symptoms of AMS often accompany these initial signs. A few localized rales may be audible in the right middle lobe auscultated over the right axilla. Rales increase with exercise (Fig. 141–9).

As HAPE progresses, the patient will have a productive clear cough, orthopnea, weakness, and altered mental status. This intensifies to severe dyspnea at rest, a cardinal sign of HAPE. The patient may be tachycardic, tachypneic, and febrile to 102°F. Rales become bilateral. Peripheral cyanosis advances to central cyanosis if treatment is not initiated. Dyspnea at rest, while at altitude, is HAPE until proved otherwise.

A chest radiograph reveals bilateral, fluffy, asymmetric infiltrates and dilated pulmonary arteries (Fig. 141–10). Cardiomegaly, a butterfly pattern of infiltrates, and Kerley-B lines, commonly seen in cardiogenic pulmonary edema, are not seen

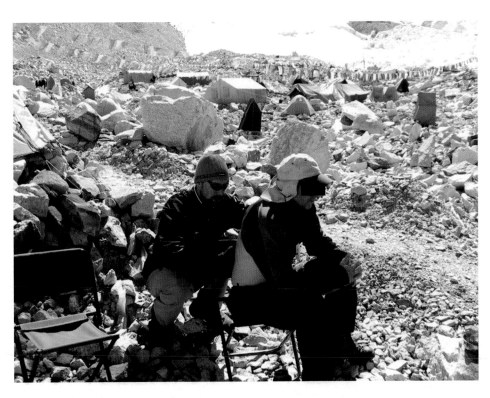

Figure 141–9. Evaluating a hiker for clinical signs of HAPE. Everest base camp. Altitude 17 600 ft. (Photo courtesy of Janis Tupesis, MD.)

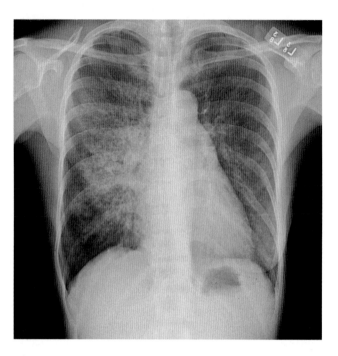

Figure 141–10. Noncardiogenic pulmonary edema consistent with HAPE. (Photo courtesy of Christopher Straus, MD.)

in HAPE. An electrocardiogram (ECG) may show sinus tachycardia, right ventricular strain, right axis deviation, P-wave abnormalities, prominent R waves in the right chest leads, and S waves in the left chest leads. Without treatment, florid pulmonary edema and respiratory failure will develop. Dysfunction of the CNS will ensue, leading to coma and death.

The differential diagnosis includes pneumonia, congestive heart failure, high-altitude bronchitis, pharyngitis, asthma, neurogenic pulmonary edema, pulmonary embolism, and adult respiratory distress syndrome. Hyperviscosity from dehydration and increased red blood cell mass results in a hypercoagulable state, which may play a role in the development of HAPE.

Pathophysiology

HAPE can affect individuals without prior history of cardiac or pulmonary disease. Pulmonary vasoconstriction secondary to the hypoxic stimuli elevates pulmonary artery pressures. The pulmonary hypertension is exacerbated by increased blood volume secondary to peripheral vasoconstriction and fluid retention. The end result is a noncardiogenic pulmonary edema.

Individuals with an elevated pulmonary artery pressure or with a blunted hypoxic ventilatory response have been shown to be at increased risk for HAPE. This is thought to be the reason why children and infants with pulmonary arterial hypertrophy are more prone to the development of HAPE. Congenital absence of a pulmonary artery may also predispose an individual to HAPE. It should be noted that not all individuals with pulmonary hypertension will develop HAPE. However, in a study involving ten children who had recovered from HAPE, all were found to have chronic pulmonary hypertension upon cardiac catheterization.[9]

Treatment

As with any form of high-altitude illness, immediate descent may be life-saving and is not to be delayed. There is a delicate balance, however, between rapid descent and the amount of energy the victim expends to descend quickly. Individuals may deteriorate from overexertion as they proceed to a lower altitude. Therefore, care must be taken to minimize the effort while maximizing the effect. A descent of 1000 to 2000 ft is usually adequate for symptomatic relief. In addition to rapid descent, bed rest, supplemental oxygen, and keeping the patient warm are necessary.

Physical activity and exposure to cold increase the catecholamine response, which increases pulmonary pressure. Supplemental oxygen effectively lowers pulmonary arterial pressure, which raises arterial oxygen saturation. As a result, heart rate and respiratory rate will decrease. High-flow oxygen at 6 to 8 L/min by mask is administered to anyone with significant symptoms. It may be possible to reverse symptoms with oxygen alone (without descent) over a period of 2 to 3 days.

An end-expiratory airway pressure (EPAP) mask that can deliver 5 to 10 cm H_2O of end-expiratory pressure can be used to improve oxygen delivery. When oxygen is not available and descent is not possible, the portable Gamow bag may be used for hyperbaric treatment and has been shown to be effective in patients with HAPE.

Pharmacologic agents play a limited role in the prevention and treatment of HAPE. Of note, the literature lacks specific mention regarding the use of preventative or therapeutic agents with children. Data suggests that acetazolamide may be useful in the prevention of HAPE. Newer agents, such as the β-adrenergic agonist salmeterol, have shown promising results in preventing pulmonary edema at high altitudes.[10] Salmeterol when administered at 125 μg every 12 hours was associated with a significant decrease in the incidence of HAPE.[10] Although early studies suggested that furosemide might be helpful,[11] it is now considered to have no role in the treatment of HAPE due, in part, to the prevalence of hypovolemia and dehydration. Slow-release nifedipine has been shown to be useful in treating HAPE by decrease pulmonary arterial pressure but may also cause hypotension. It remains the first line therapy and typically is administered as 10 mg orally, followed by 20 mg (sustained release) every 6 hours. Newer data suggests that some of the phosphodiesterase inhibitors, including sildenafil and tadalafil might be effective agents in treating HAPE. As opposed to nifedipine, tadalafil and dexamethasone were found to be beneficial without causing a drop in blood pressure.[12] Again, caution must be exercised in the use of a potentially hypovolemic dehydrated patient.

Rapid improvement and resolution of symptoms usually follow descent to a lower altitude. If oxygen saturation is <90%, hospitalization is indicated. In very severe cases of HAPE, intubation and ventilation with positive end-expiratory pressure may be needed.

The overall mortality of HAPE is 11%. Without treatment (descent or supplemental oxygen), the mortality increases to 44%.

An episode of HAPE is not a contraindication to further attempts to reach altitude. However, there is a higher incidence for recurrent symptoms with subsequent ascents.

ALTITUDE-RELATED SYNDROMES

High-Altitude Retinal Hemorrhage

It is estimated that 50% of individuals who ascend to 16,000 ft and 100% of those who ascend to 21,000 ft will develop high-altitude retinal hemorrhage (HARH) within 2 to 3 days after arrival to altitude. HARH presents with tortuous dilation of the retinal arteries and veins, retinal hemorrhages, and papilledema. The hemorrhages are most often throughout the fundus but spare the macula. It is painless and usually asymptomatic, with no visual disturbances noted. If the macula is involved, the victim may complain of cloudy or blurred vision. In these situations, descending to a lower altitude is indicated.

In most cases, HARH is self-limiting and usually resolves spontaneously within 2 to 3 weeks after descent. If the macula was involved, visual changes may be permanent. HARH may occur alone or in the presence of AMS, HAPE, or HACE. The incidence of HARH increases with strenuous activity and with a history of previous HARH.

Chronic Mountain Sickness

Chronic mountain sickness (CMS), also referred to as Monge's disease, is a rare complication of high-altitude illness. Some individuals will fail to acclimatize despite prolonged exposure or living at high altitude. Symptoms are similar to those of AMS and include headache, dyspnea, sleep disturbance, and fatigue.

CMS is associated with an inadequate hypoxic ventilatory response, resulting in persistent hypoxia and excessive erythropoietin production. Polycythemia follows, with the hematocrit often greater than 60. Congestive heart failure is seen.

Treatment for CMS includes descent to a lower altitude, oxygen, phlebotomy, and the use of respiratory stimulants such as acetazolamide.

Ultraviolet Keratitis

Snow blindness is caused by increased ultraviolet (UV) light exposure at higher altitudes secondary to the loss of the protective atmosphere and fewer pollutants. For every 1000 ft of ascent, UV exposure will increase by 5%. Patients develop a foreign body sensation or severe pain approximately 12 hours after exposure. They may also have periorbital edema, excessive tearing, photophobia, and conjunctival erythema. Treatment is with oral analgesics to alleviate the severe discomfort. Symptoms resolve within 24 hours. Sunglasses with polarized lenses and side blinders are preventative.

High-Altitude Pharyngitis and Bronchitis

High-altitude bronchitis and pharyngitis are common at altitudes >8000 ft, secondary to the excessive inhalation of dry, cold air that causes drying and cracking of the upper airway mucous membranes. Symptoms include a dry, hacking, and often painful cough. Symptoms are prevented or minimized by ensuring adequate hydration and salivation. Throat lozenges and hard candy help to maintain oral secretions. Inhaled steam, gargling, and oral fluids will also keep the mucous membranes moist. A cloth worn over the mouth and nose helps to warm the inspired air and trap moisture. Antibiotics are not helpful, whereas analgesics may be beneficial.

Preexisting Pulmonary Disease

Any pulmonary disease that affects breathing at sea level has the potential to cause further complications at high altitude. Supplemental oxygen may be necessary for any child with known hypoxemia, sleep disorder, or pulmonary hypertension. Neither asthma nor bronchospasm is known to be aggravated by high-altitude exposure. However, exposure to cold, dry air could worsen these problems.

Sickle Cell Disease

Patients with sickle cell disease are at increased risk for vasoocclusive crisis and hypoxemia over 5000 to 6500 ft. Patients with sickle cell trait are without risk for vasoocclusive crisis but are at increased risks for splenic infarction at increased altitudes. Patients with sickle cell disease are advised to use supplemental oxygen at elevations >5000 ft. Nonnarcotic analgesics and hydration are also indicated.

Pregnancy

Pregnancy is not a contraindication for women to participate in reasonable activities at reasonable altitude levels. There is no increase in complications, maternal or neonatal, associated with short-term exposure to high altitude. However, women who live at high altitude have been shown to have a higher incidence of low-birth-weight babies, maternal hypertension, and neonatal hyperbilirubinemia.

Peripheral Edema

Peripheral edema is a common complication at higher altitudes. Swelling of the face and distal extremities is most often noted and is more common in females. Although such edema responds spontaneously within 1 to 2 days, it should raise the suspicion of AMS.

Other Complications

Other syndromes associated with ascent to high altitude include altitude syncope and migraine headaches. Arterial or venous thrombosis (both peripheral and central) may develop secondary to increased viscosity, causing transient ischemic attacks. CNS tumors may be unmasked as a result of increased brain volume from the increased intracranial pressures. Seizures may be secondary to the hypoxia.

▶ SUMMARY

Each year larger numbers of individuals head toward higher elevations. As a result, physicians who practice in or near high-altitude regions must be familiar with the signs, symptoms, and management of altitude illnesses (Table 141–2). Poor judgment and inadequate training on the part of the victim should be anticipated. Adults who travel with children need to know that

▶ **TABLE 141–2. AN OVERVIEW OF HIGH-ALTITUDE ILLNESS**

	Acute Mountain Sickness (AMS)	High-Altitude Cerebral Edema (HACE)	High-Altitude Pulmonary Edema (HAPE)
Altitude	Rare below 8000 ft Affects nearly everyone who rapidly ascends to 11 000 ft	Rare below 12 000 ft	Rare below 8000 ft More commonly associated with altitudes >14 500 ft
Onset	Within 4–8 h of a rapid ascent but can be as long as 4 d Peaks within 24–48 h Usually resolves by the third or fourth day	Most often within 1–3 d after ascent to altitude	Usually within 1–4 d after ascent to altitude Most common during the second night at altitude
Symptoms	Most common: headache, sleep disturbance, fatigue, shortness of breath, dizziness, anorexia, nausea, vomiting, oliguria Other symptoms: mild peripheral edema, weakness, lassitude, malaise, irritability, decreased concentration, poor judgment, palpitations, deep inner chill, dull pain in the posterolateral chest wall	Severe headaches, nausea, vomiting, altered mental status Cardinal sign: truncal ataxia Will proceed to include confusion, slurred speech, diplopia, hallucinations, seizures, impaired judgment, cranial nerve palsies (third and sixth), abnormal reflexes, paresthesia, decreased level of consciousness, coma, death	Initial symptoms: dry cough, fatigue, dyspnea on exertion, few rales Symptoms of AMS may be present As symptoms progress: productive clear cough, orthopnea, weakness, altered mental status, tachycardia, tachypnea, fever, increased rales, cyanosis Cardinal sign: severe dyspnea at rest
Treatment	Rest Increase fluids No higher ascent until symptoms have resolved Proceed to a lower altitude if no improvement within 1–2 d or if symptoms worsen Supplemental oxygen, if available Symptomatic relief for headache, nausea Immediate descent is indicated for ataxia, decreased level of consciousness, confusion, dyspnea at rest, rales, or cyanosis Acetazolamide: adult, 250 mg bid; pediatric, 5–10 mg/kg/d bid Consider dexamethasone, 4 mg po/IM	Immediate descent High-flow oxygen Dexamethasone: Initial dose of 8 mg IM/IV Followed by 1–1.5 mg/kg/d divided qid to a maximum dose of 4 mg/dose Rest Hyperbaric therapy if descent is not possible	Mild-to-moderate HAPE: Bed rest, supplemental oxygen Observe closely Severe HAPE: Immediate descent, minimal exertion High-flow oxygen Nifedipine Hyperbaric therapy if descent is not possible
Prevention	Acclimatization: slow, graded ascent; first night's sleep should be at an altitude no greater than 8000 ft and the first day should be spent at rest; daily climb should then be limited to 1000 ft if the altitude is between 10 000 and 14 000 ft; beyond 14 000 climbers should take 2 d for each 1000-ft ascent. Avoid alcohol, sedatives, smoking Acetazolamide: start 48 h before ascent and continue for at least 48 h after arriving at the highest altitude; pediatric, 5–10 mg/kg/d bid; adult, 250 mg bid	Acetazolamide efficacy is unproved	Salmeterol, 125 μg every 12 h

children are more susceptible to high-altitude illness and to watch for symptoms.

In the high-altitude setting, any onset of symptoms that could represent high-altitude illness should be taken seriously. The mild symptoms of AMS can easily and quickly progress to the potentially deadly HACE or HAPE if not recognized, diagnosed, and treated promptly.

REFERENCES

1. Hackett PH, Roach RC. High-altitude illness. *N Engl J Med.* 2001;345:107.
2. Rodway GW, Hoffman LA, Sanders MH. High-altitude-related disorders—Part I: pathophysiology, differential diagnosis, and treatment. *Heart Lung.* 2003;32:353.

3. Samuels MP. The effects of flight and altitude. *Arch Dis Child.* 2004;89(5):448–455.

4. Dumont L, Mardirosoff C, Tramèr MR. Efficacy and harm of pharmacologic prevention of acute mountain sickness: quantitative systemic review. *BMJ.* 2000;321:267.

5. Basnyat B, Gertsch JK, Johson EW, et al. Efficacy of low dose acetazolamide for the prophylaxis of acute mountain sickness: a prospective double-blinded randomized, placebo controlled trial. *High Alt Med Biol.* 2003;4:45–52.

6. Carpenter TC, Niermeyer S, Durmowicz AG. Altitude-related illness in children. *Curr Probl Pediatr.* 1998;28:177.

7. Ferrazzini G, Maggiorini M, Kriemler S, et al. Successful treatment of acute mountain sickness with dexamethasone. *Br Med J (Clin Res Ed).* 1987;294:1380–1382.

8. Gabry AL, Ledoux X, Mozziconacci M, Martin C. High-altitude pulmonary edema at moderate altitude (alt; 2400 m; 7870 feet): a series of 52 patients. *Chest.* 2003;123:49.

9. Das BB, Wolfe RR, Chan KC, et al. High-altitude pulmonary edema in children with underlying cardiopulmonary disorders and pulmonary hypertension living at altitude. *Arch Pediatr Adolesc Med.* 2004;158:1170.

10. Sartori C, Allemann Y, Duplain H, et al. Salmeterol for the prevention of high-altitude pulmonary edema. *N Engl J Med.* 2002;346:1631.

11. Singh I, Kapila C, Khanna P, et al. High altitude pulmonary edema. *Lancet.* 1965;30:229–234.

12. Maggiorini M, Brunner-La Rocca HP, Peth S, et al. Both tadalafil and dexamethasone may reduce the incidence of high-altitude pulmonary edema: a randomized trial. *Ann Intern Med.* 2006;145:497.

CHAPTER 142

Dysbaric Injuries

Ira J. Blumen and Lisa Rapoport

▶ HIGH-YIELD FACTS

- An air embolism is the most serious dysbaric injury and requires aggressive care, which includes 100% oxygen, intravenous fluids, and hyperbaric treatment. Patients are placed in the Trendelenburg or left lateral decubitus position to minimize the passage of air emboli to the brain.
- Since nitrogen is not metabolized, it remains dissolved until the nitrogen gas pressure in the lungs decreases and the nitrogen can be removed. During a slow ascent, as the surrounding pressure decreases, the nitrogen that is absorbed into the tissues is released into the blood and the alveoli, but if the ascent is too quick, nitrogen levels do not have the opportunity to equalize among the tissues, blood, and alveoli, which results in the gas coming out of solution and forming gas bubbles in the blood or tissue.
- The treatment of choice for most air emboli and decompression illnesses is hyperbaric (recompression) therapy. This is initiated as soon as possible, ideally within 6 hours of the onset of symptoms.

▶ DYSBARIC INJURIES

Dysbaric injuries may be the result of several distinct events that expose an individual to a change in barometric pressure. The first possible etiology is an altitude-related event, which can be illustrated by the rapid ascent or descent during airplane transport or sudden cabin decompression at an altitude of 25 000 ft. The second type of dysbaric injury results from an underwater diving accident. A third dysbarism is caused by a blast injury that produces an *overpressure* effect. This section primarily discusses dysbaric diving injuries and, to a lesser extent, aviation-related dysbarisms. Blast injuries are beyond the scope of this chapter.

Scuba (self-contained underwater breathing apparatus) diving (Fig. 142–1) was developed in the mid-1940s and currently allows the sport diver to descend to depths >100 ft. There are an estimated 9 million certified scuba divers in the United States. Worldwide, the diving population continues to grow at a rate of 20% per year. There are a number of recreational diving organizations that have minimum age requirements for certifications. In general, candidates must be 15 or 16 years old for full certification. Pool-based divers may be certified at the age of 8 years, and some organizations will certify 10-year olds for ocean diving to 40 ft (12 m). However, certification is not required to dive. It is the untrained or poorly trained individual who is at greater risk for injury.

Scuba diving requires absolute adherence to safety rules and a modicum of common sense. Serious diving-related injuries and fatalities are rare and are often associated with unsafe behaviors or hazardous conditions. However, they can occur without apparent cause. On the average, each year, the Divers Alert Network receives more than 900 scuba diving injury notifications.[1] From 1995 to 2006, there has been an average of 85 diving fatalities annually in the United States and Canada.[2] On average, there were 16 diving injuries requiring hyperbaric recompression therapy in scuba divers aged 19 years and younger in North America between 1988 and 2002.[3] During this time period, the youngest diving fatality was 14 years old and the youngest injured diver was 11.[3]

Several terms are often used when discussing this topic. *Dysbarisms* represents the general topic of pressure-related injuries. *Barotrauma*, the most common diving injury, refers to the injuries that are a direct result of the mechanical effects of a pressure differential. The complications related to the partial pressure of gases and dissolved gases are called *decompression sickness*.

PHYSICAL GAS LAWS

Dysbarisms can best be explained through the physical gas laws and an understanding of pressure equivalents that cause these injuries. The amount of pressure exerted by air at sea level and at different altitudes or depths can be described in several different ways, as shown in Table 142–1.

Individuals and objects under water are exposed to progressively greater pressure due to the weight of the water. Small changes in the underwater depth result in large atmospheric pressure and volume changes. This is significantly different from the pressure and volume variation noted in air above sea level. *Boyle's law*, as previously described, explains this relationship. Under water, the largest proportionate change in the volume of a gas is seen close to the water surface. An air-filled cavity that is 33 ft below the water surface will double when it reaches the surface. In comparison, a volume of gas at sea level will need to rise to an altitude of 18,000 ft to double in volume.

Dalton's law of partial pressure, as previously presented, describes the pressure exerted by gases at various depths or altitudes. Each gas will exert a pressure equal to its proportion of the total gaseous mixture ($P_{total} = P_1 + P_2 + P_3 \ldots P_n$). Figure 142–2 depicts the gaseous composition of the atmosphere at sea level and the corresponding partial pressures.

Henry's law states that the quantity of gas dissolved in a liquid is proportional to the partial pressure of the gas in

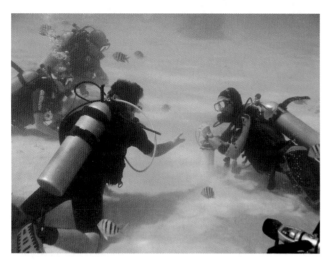

Figure 142–1. There are an estimated 9 million certified scuba divers in the United States. (Photo courtesy of Ron Lachman.)

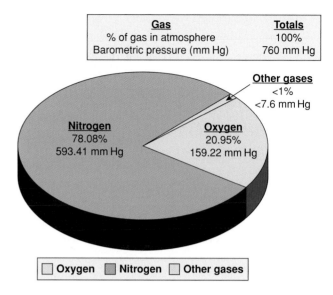

Gas	Totals
% of gas in atmosphere	100%
Barometric pressure (mm Hg)	760 mm Hg

Other gases
<1%
<7.6 mm Hg

Nitrogen
78.08%
593.41 mm Hg

Oxygen
20.95%
159.22 mm Hg

☐ Oxygen   ■ Nitrogen   ☐ Other gases

Figure 142–2. Atmospheric composition at sea level.

contact with the liquid. The partial pressure of a gas and the solubility of the gas determine the amount of gas that will dissolve into a liquid. This law will help explain the increased absorption of nitrogen during descent.

PATHOPHYSIOLOGY

The clinical findings of dysbaric injuries may be immediate or delayed in onset up to 36 hours. Most will occur during descent or in close proximity to ascent. A delayed presentation is possible, however, which may make diagnosis difficult.

▶ **TABLE 142–1. EFFECT OF ALTITUDE OR DEPTH ON AIR PRESSURE**

Altitude (ft) or Depth (ft of sea water [FSW])	Absolute Pressure (ATA)	Torr	PSI	Volume Ratio
Altitude				
40,000	0.19	141	2.72	5.39
30,000	0.30	228	4.36	3.33
20,000	0.46	349	6.75	2.18
10,000	0.69	523	10.11	1.45
5000	0.83	632	12.23	1.20
1000	0.97	733	14.17	1.04
Sea level	1	760	14.7	1
Depth				
33	2	1520	29.4	0.50
66	3	2280	44.1	0.33
99	4	3040	58.8	0.25
132	5	3800	73.5	0.20
165	6	4560	88.2	0.17
198	7	5320	102.9	0.14

Courtesy of Ira Blumen, M.D., Section of Emergency Medicine, Department of Medicine, University of Chicago Medical Center.

There are three mechanisms for dysbaric injuries. The first follows Boyle's law for trapped gas and changes in ambient pressure. The second follows Henry's law when gas dissolved in blood is released. The third deals with abnormal tissue concentrations of various gases.

BAROTRAUMA: DYSBARISMS FROM TRAPPED GASES

Barotrauma is the direct result of a pressure difference between the body's air-filled cavities, which are subject to the effects of Boyle's law, and the surrounding environment. While the individual is scuba diving, most symptoms will develop during a descent. On descent, a negative pressure develops within enclosed air spaces relative to the ambient surrounding pressure. If air is unable to enter these structures, equalization does not take place, and the air-filled cavities collapse. If the cavity is a rigid structure and unable to collapse, the negative pressure may result in fluid being displaced from the blood vessels of the surrounding mucosa into the intravascular space. The resulting injury pattern can include pain, hemorrhage, edema, vascular engorgement, and tissue damage.

If air is unable to escape on ascent, an expansion of gas within enclosed air spaces causes a positive pressure to develop. This may result in the rupture of such spaces or the compression of adjacent structures. Many of the symptoms of barotrauma in the human body result in a "squeeze" phenomenon. These trapped gas disorders are differentiated by the gas-filled part of the body that is affected.

Barotitis

Barometric pressure changes can result in disturbances of the external, middle, and inner ear. The tympanic membrane (TM) separates the middle ear from the outer ear. The eustachian tube functions as a valve allowing air pressure to equalize between the middle ear and ambient environment.

Barotitis media is the most common diving-related baro-trauma and involves the middle ear. It is commonly referred to as *middle ear squeeze* or *ear block*. Equalization via the eustachian tube will occur when there is a pressure differential of approximately 15 to 20 mm Hg. The diver becomes symptomatic if equalization is unsuccessful and the pressure differential reaches or approaches 100 mm Hg.

Middle ear squeeze commonly develops on descent between 10 and 20 ft below the surface. The symptoms include a fullness in the ears, severe pain, tinnitus, vertigo, nausea, disorientation, and transient, conductive hearing loss. Up to 10% of divers may have no pain during descent but will become symptomatic after the dive. If the diver is unable to equalize the pressure and continues to descend, symptoms may be exacerbated and the TM may rupture and bleed. With perforation, the caloric stimulation of cold water entering the middle ear can cause vertigo, nausea, and disorientation.

Physical examination may reveal erythema or retraction of the TM, blood behind the TM, a ruptured TM, or a bloody nasal discharge.

Treatment for middle ear squeeze should be directed toward its prevention before pain develops. Scuba divers should attempt to clear their ears every 2 to 3 ft during descent. Under normal situations, pressure in the middle ear is equalized without incidence by actively opening the eustachian tube, which opens and exposes the middle ear to ambient pressures. Divers must learn to open the eustachian tube through various maneuvers such as blowing the nose against pinched nostrils or repositioning the jaw (false yawning), while keeping a regulator in their mouth (Fig. 142–3). The Frenzel maneuver, another suggested treatment for barotitis, is performed by forcing closed the glottis and mouth while contracting the superior pharyngeal constrictors and the muscles of the floor of the mouth.

Equalization may be compromised if the eustachian tube is obstructed by swelling of the mucosa, the presence of

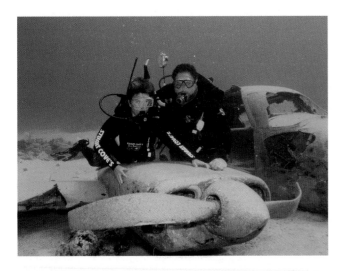

Figure 142–3. Low-volume scuba masks allow a diver to pinch his/her nose to open the eustachian tube to equalize pressure in the middle ear. They also allow for small amounts of air to be blown into the mask from the nose to prevent face mask squeeze. (Photo courtesy of Ron Lachman.)

polyps, previous trauma, allergies, upper respiratory infection, a sinus problem, or smoking. To decrease the incidence of ear discomfort and injury to the TM, a predive treatment of a topical vasoconstrictor nasal spray (oxymetazoline hydrochloride, 0.05%) may be beneficial when used approximately 15 minutes before beginning a dive. The recommended pediatric dosage for ages ≥6 years is two to three sprays in each nostril. Oxymetazoline hydrochloride is not recommended for children younger than 6 years. Pseudoephedrine may also be considered as a predive treatment. For ages 6 to 12, the recommended dose is 30 mg po. For children older than 12 years, the adult dose of 60 mg po may be used. If pain persists after the dive, analgesics may be used. If a predive decongestant was not used, it may be considered at this time.

Any patient with barotitis media is to be instructed to refrain from diving until all signs and symptoms have resolved. Erythema generally resolves within 1 to 3 days, whereas it will take 2 to 4 weeks when there is blood behind the TM. A perforated TM must heal before any further diving is attempted. A 10-day course of oral antibiotics and otic suspension is indicated if there is a perforation of the TM. ENT follow-up is given upon discharge from the emergency department. Barotrauma can occur during either descent or ascent. If air is unable to escape the middle ear through the eustachian tube during ascent, a diver may develop symptoms of *reverse ear squeeze*.

Alternobaric vertigo may develop during descent, but it is more common during ascent. A sudden change in middle ear pressure or asymmetrical middle ear pressure may result in decreased perfusion, affecting vestibular function. Symptoms include transient vertigo, tinnitus, nausea, vomiting, and fullness in the affected ear. Symptoms may last minutes to several hours after the completion of a dive. Decongestants, antiemetics, and medication for vertigo are recommended.

Barotitis externa occurs when the external auditory canal, which is normally a patent air-filled cavity that communicates with the surrounding environment, is occluded during descent. At the initiation of descent, the air would normally be replaced by water. If the external canal is obstructed, the enclosed air space will be subject to the increased ambient pressure, resulting in an *external ear squeeze* or *barotitis externa*. Obstruction can be caused by cerumen, ear plugs, or other foreign bodies. A diver may experience pain with or without bloody otorrhea.

Barotitis interna or *inner ear squeeze* is uncommon but may result in permanent injury to the structures of the inner ear. It often follows a vigorous Valsalva maneuver. In addition to sudden sensorineural hearing loss, symptoms include severe pain or pressure, vertigo, tinnitus, ataxia, nausea, vomiting, diaphoresis, and nystagmus. These patients must be seen emergently. The potential for recovery within a few months is very good in most patients treated conservatively. Others, however, may require surgical intervention.

Altitude-Related Barotitis

Barotitis media is the most common barotrauma of air travel. During ascent to altitude, gas will normally escape through the eustachian tube every 500 to 1000 ft to equalize pressures. As altitude decreases, the gas within the middle ear will contract. As with diving, equalization may be accomplished by yawning, swallowing, or performing the Valsalva maneuver. Children who are asleep should be awakened 5 minutes before descent and instructed to swallow more frequently. For infants, a bottle should be given during takeoff and landing. Although this may reduce the likelihood of barotitis media, it may increase the incidence of gastrointestinal distress after takeoff from swallowed air.

Barosinusitis

Normally, air can pass in and out of the sinus cavities without difficulty. However, if a person has a cold or sinus infection, air may be trapped and will be subject to the barometric pressure changes. Failure of the air-filled frontal or maxillary sinuses to equilibrate results in pain or pressure above, behind, or below the eyes, which is commonly referred to as *sinus squeeze*. Pain may persist for hours and may be accompanied by a bloody nasal discharge. The ethmoid and sphenoid sinuses rarely contribute to this type of barotrauma.

The treatment for barosinusitis is similar to the treatment of barotitis media. The most effective treatment involves the use of a vasoconstrictor nasal spray before initiating a dive or before starting a descent from altitude in an airplane. Antibiotics should be started and continued for 14 to 21 days.

Reverse sinus squeeze is felt during a diving ascent when an obstruction of the sinuses results in excessive pressure. A sharp pain will be felt in the affected sinus. Numbness may be felt along the infraorbital nerve if the maxillary sinus is affected. The diver should descend to a greater depth, relieving some of the discomfort, and then ascend at a slower rate.

Barodentalgia

Barodentalgia or *tooth squeeze* is often associated with recent dental extraction, dental fillings, periodontal infection, periodontal abscess, or tooth decay. Although this is a rare problem, individuals with preexisting dental or periodontal disease are more susceptible to this barotrauma. Treatment is directed toward preventative dental care and pain control. Following dental procedures, a minimum of 24 hours is advised before initiating a scuba dive.

Face Mask Squeeze

During descent, the increased ambient pressure will tend to exert increasing pressure against the air-filled face mask of a scuba diver. The diver may develop facial or eye pain, subconjunctival hemorrhages, subconjunctival edema, epistaxis, and periorbital edema. Face mask squeeze is commonly prevented by using a low-volume face mask that minimizes the amount of air and allows for additional small amounts of air to be blown into the mask from the nose (Fig. 142–3).

Aerogastralgia

Under normal circumstances, the stomach and intestines contain approximately 1 qt of gas. Ingesting carbonated beverage, chewing gum (and swallowing air), eating large meals, and preexisting gastrointestinal problems increase the amount of gas in the intestines. Gas expansion will cause discomfort, abdominal pain, belching, flatulence, nausea, vomiting, shortness of breath, or hyperventilation. Symptoms are prevented or re-lieved by belching or passing flatus. Wearing clothes that are loose and nonrestrictive is also of benefit. Although aerogastralgia is rarely a serious problem, significant distention of the abdominal contents may result in venous pooling and syncope. In addition, tachycardia, hypotension, and syncope may result from a vasovagal response to severe pain. Gastric rupture has also been reported.

Pulmonary Barotrauma

Pulmonary barotrauma follows drowning as the second most common cause of death among scuba divers. On descent, the air in the lungs can become compressed. If the lung volume were to decrease below residual volume, hemoptysis, hemorrhage, and pulmonary edema could occur. However, breathing from a compressed air source, this loss of volume will be prevented. Pulmonary overpressurization syndrome (POPS) is an example of the positive-pressure barotrauma that can be seen during ascent. The alveoli become overinflated and can rupture, causing a pneumothorax. Ruptured pulmonary veins allow air emboli to enter the systemic circulation. These can occur if the scuba diver fails to exhale adequately on ascent, or in the presence of predisposing lung disease. To reduce the risk of pulmonary barotrauma, divers are trained to not hold their breath. This is important not only during ascent but also in the event a diver is not aware of an unintended decrease of depth. This holds true for beginning-level divers who may not yet be skilled at managing depth regulation using a buoyancy device, or for children who may have smaller lungs and body mass making it more difficult to maintain a constant depth. Also at risk for pulmonary barotrauma are divers with obstructive airway diseases, including asthma and chronic obstructive pulmonary disease.

Air Embolism

An air embolism is the most serious dysbaric injury. Specific signs and symptoms will be determined by the final destination of air emboli. Because of the buoyancy of air and the fact that scuba divers are usually upright during ascent, the brain is most commonly affected. The onset of symptoms can be immediately on ascent, or within 10 to 20 minutes of surfacing. Neurologic symptoms that develop later than this are more likely caused by decompression sickness. A rapid onset and severe symptoms are suggestive of a poorer prognosis with both air embolism and decompression sickness. These patients require aggressive care, which includes 100% oxygen, intravenous fluids, and hyperbaric treatment. They are placed in the Trendelenburg or left lateral decubitus position (Durant's maneuver) to minimize the passage of air emboli to the brain. Air emboli affect the heart if they embolize to the coronary circulation, causing coronary artery occlusion, dysrhythmias, shock, and cardiac arrest. Although these complications are rare compared with other dysbaric injuries, they represent a significant risk to the victim.

Arterial air embolization to the brain is more common than to the heart or spinal cord. Neurologic symptoms are similar to those of a stroke and include numbness, dizziness, headaches, weakness, visual field deficits, confusion, behavioral changes, amnesia, paralysis, vertigo, blindness, aphasia, deafness, sensory deficit, seizures, focal deficits, and loss of consciousness. Because of the variety of neurologic presentations, a careful medical evaluation is warranted for the onset of any neurologic symptoms during or within a short time after the conclusion of a dive.

Pneumothorax and Emphysema

The patient with a confirmed or suspected pneumothorax, pneumopericardium, pneumomediastinum, or subcutaneous emphysema should not be exposed to any further barometric pressure changes. This is a significant problem if a pneumothorax develops during a dive. On ascent, a simple pneumothorax may progress to a tension pneumothorax, shock, and loss of consciousness. These complications may also occur during air transport in an unpressurized aircraft. Treatment of a scuba diving pneumothorax is no different than the treatment of other traumatic or nontraumatic pneumothoraxes. Hyperbaric (recompression) treatment is avoided since it can convert a simple pneumothorax to a tension pneumothorax. If hyperbaric treatment will be necessary, chest tubes must be placed before initiating recompression.

DECOMPRESSION SICKNESS: DYSBARISMS FROM EVOLVED GASES

Henry's law explains the formation of gas bubbles that separate from solution. Gases coming out of solution result in *decompression sickness*. A diver breathing compressed air is exposed to nitrogen, oxygen, and carbon dioxide. Approximately four-fifth of the air is nitrogen. Oxygen is metabolized, and the carbon dioxide is expelled. Under normal circumstances, additional nitrogen gas will not be absorbed by the body during inhalation. However, when the body is exposed to a varying ambient pressure, uptake or removal of nitrogen gas from the blood occurs. As ambient pressure increases, the positive-pressure gradient between the alveoli and the blood will result in more nitrogen being dissolved. As a dive progresses, the gas in the blood will equilibrate quickly with the gas in the alveoli. Nitrogen gas, however, is almost five times more soluble in fat. It will take longer to saturate these tissues. Therefore, the body will absorb more nitrogen gas at a rate that is dependent on the depth and duration of the dive. The longer and deeper the dive, the more nitrogen gas will be accumulated within the body.

Since nitrogen is not metabolized, it remains dissolved until the nitrogen gas pressure in the lungs decreases and the nitrogen can be removed. During a slow ascent, as the surrounding pressure decreases, the nitrogen that is absorbed into the tissues is released into the blood and the alveoli. If the ascent is too quick, nitrogen levels do not have the opportunity to equalize among the tissues, blood, and alveoli. The pressure outside the body will drop significantly below the sum of the partial pressures of the gases inside the body. This results in the gas coming out of solution and the formation of gas bubbles in the blood or tissue. Because of the increased dissolved nitrogen, it has a disproportionately higher partial pressure. Therefore, a significant difference in partial pressure occurs. It is the release of these nitrogen bubbles from solution that results in decompression sickness.

Diving tables are often used by scuba divers as a tool to minimize the risk of developing a decompression sickness. However, even if the dive tables are carefully followed, additional factors could precipitate a decompression sickness, such as increased physical activity during a dive, cold temperatures, obesity, alcohol ingestion, previous dives with inadequate surface time to equilibrate, and flying within 12 hours of a dive. Decompression sickness can be classified as follows:

- Type I that typically involves extravascular gas bubbles and causes joint pain, skin rashes, and lymphedema.
- Type II, which is the more severe form of decompression sickness that can lead to serious injury or death, is caused by intravascular nitrogen gas emboli. The presentation may be very similar to that of air emboli. Children are more prone to type II injuries.

Musculoskeletal Decompression Sickness

The term *bends* is often used to identify any form of decompression sickness. When used correctly, however, the term refers to the musculoskeletal syndrome involving the joints, which is a very common dysbarism. The bends occurs in up to 75% of all decompression injuries and is caused by the release of nitrogen gas bubbles from the blood into the tissues surrounding the joint.

Symptoms usually develop within 6 to 12 hours after the conclusion of a dive. A sharp, throbbing, or dull achy pain is a common presentation. There may also be associated numbness or tingling (paresthesia). The pain commonly is diffused in its origin but will become more localized as the intensity increases. The joints that are most often affected are the knees, shoulders, and elbows. Symptomatic relief may be obtained by splinting the extremity or by applying pressure over the affected joint. Massaging or moving the affected extremity often exacerbates the pain associated with the bends. The physical examination is usually unremarkable. On occasion, crepitus, edema, or tenderness are noted.

Cutaneous Decompression Sickness

The extravascular release of nitrogen gas bubbles from the blood into the skin usually results in benign dysbarisms. Rashes, with or without pruritus, can present with any of the following patterns: scarlatiniform, mottling (cutis marmorata), and erysipeloid. The release of nitrogen gas bubbles can cause subcutaneous emphysema, often involving the neck and other sites. When the neck is involved, the victim's voice may be altered, and the individual may complain of difficulty breathing or swallowing. In such a case when there is subcutaneous emphysema above the collarbone, there is concern for ruptured alveoli, a sign of more serious pulmonary barotrauma. Treatment of individuals with subcutaneous emphysema begins with 100% oxygen. The patient is then carefully examined for more serious dysbarisms and admitted.

Pulmonary Decompression Sickness

The decompression illness that affects the pulmonary system is referred to as the *chokes*. It is caused by arterial or venous nitrogen gas embolization that obstructs the pulmonary vasculature. The symptoms may begin immediately after a dive but often take up to 12 hours to develop. They last between 12 and 48 hours but can progress to a rapid deterioration. The classic triad of symptoms includes shortness of breath, cough, and substernal chest pain or chest tightness. The shortness of breath is described as a feeling of suffocation. The individual becomes tachycardiac and tachypneic. There is a nonproductive, often uncontrollable paroxysmal cough, which is exacerbated by deep inspiration. The chest pain is most frequently appreciated with deep inspiration, increased activity, and smoking. There is no radiation of the pain to the neck, arms, or abdomen.

Neurologic Decompression Sickness

Nitrogen gas embolism is the most serious decompression sickness. Venous gas emboli can result in venous obstruction, and arterial gas emboli can cause ischemia as a result of arterial obstruction or induced vasospasm. As with air embolus, the brain is most commonly affected. The onset of symptoms, however, will usually be delayed, with symptoms developing within 1 to 6 hours after a dive is concluded. These victims require aggressive care that includes 100% oxygen, intravenous fluids, and hyperbaric treatment. They are placed in the Trendelenburg or left lateral decubitus position to minimize the embolization to the brain.

Cerebral decompression injuries are more common with altitude-related decompression than with diving injuries. The symptoms are also similar to those of the air embolus. Common symptoms are headaches, visual field deficits, scintillating scotoma, confusion, behavioral changes, restlessness, amnesia, paralysis, blindness, deafness, hallucinations, sensory deficit, and seizures. Children primarily present with abnormal behavior, disorientation, and memory loss. The headache that develops is often dull and pulsating in nature. It may be unilateral and is often on the opposite side of the visual field deficits or scotoma. The mild-to-moderate pain will usually last for several hours. Scotoma may be peripherally or centrally located but often appear to move peripherally. They are appreciated with the eyes opened or closed and are unilateral or bilateral, singular or multiple. They appear as visual distortions or as colored lines that are horizontal or V-shaped.

Spinal cord complications are seen more often than cerebral decompression injuries as a result of diving accidents. An air embolism affects the spinal cord by blocking the venous return in the epidural vertebral venous system. This results in back pain, numbness in the extremities, weakness, paralysis, and urinary retention.

Decompression Shock

Decompression shock may be secondary to hypovolemia or due to vasovagal responses. Hypovolemia is caused by fluid loss and third spacing. The patient may become agitated, restless, cool to the touch, tachycardic, tachypneic, and finally hypotensive. If vasovagal symptoms dominate initially, the victim may present with diaphoresis, nausea, vomiting, bradycardia, light-headedness, and hypotension. Aggressive and timely management with intravenous fluids, 100% oxygen and recompression therapy should be initiated as quickly as possible.

Treatment of Decompression Sickness and Air Embolus

The morbidity and mortality for dysbaric injuries depends on the severity of the injury, rapid identification of the illness, and timely access to appropriate medical care. When the "system" works, the recovery rate is as high as 90%. Treatment begins with the administration of 100% oxygen, hydration, and rewarming.[4] In addition, the treatment of choice for most air emboli and decompression illnesses is hyperbaric (recompression) oxygen therapy (HBO). This is initiated as soon as possible, ideally within 6 hours of the onset of symptoms. Treatment of cerebral air emboli is less successful if HBO is delayed over 4 to 5 hours.[5] However, there is still benefit to providing delayed HBO treatment. In some cases of air emboli, hyperbaric therapy has been effective for patients who are not treated until 10 to 14 days after the onset of their symptoms.

The goal of treatment is to reduce the size of the liberated gas bubbles, facilitate the reabsorption of these air bubbles, prevent the formation of new bubbles, and improve oxygenation. The mechanism of HBO is complex, but by causing bubbles to decrease in size, hypoxia can be reduced downstream of blocked vessels. In addition, HBO removes the nidus for activation of the complement system.[4] Giving 100% oxygen also helps to replace undissolved nitrogen with oxygen, which is easier for tissues to utilize and eliminate from the body. In addition, HBO is postulated to provide additional benefit through delivering oxygen to tissues damaged by ischemic-reperfusion injury.[6]

Before hyperbaric treatment is initiated, certain procedures should be followed. Endotracheal tube cuffs and Foley catheter balloons should be filled with saline rather than air. It is essential to identify any pneumothorax and insert a chest tube prior to recompression. Some physicians have found Auralgan® otic drops beneficial to anesthetize the TM of smaller children who may have difficulty equalizing middle ear pressure during hyperbaric treatment.

The initiation of hyperbaric treatment is similar for types I and II decompression injuries. Victims are taken to a "depth" of 60 ft (FSW), which is equal to 2.8 atm. Supplemental oxygen at an F_{IO_2} of 100% is provided at 20-minute intervals, alternating with room air. The hyperbaric pressure will be reduced at a rate of 1 ft a minute to equal a depth of 30 ft for a period of time and then slowly brought back to "sea level."

Victims of an arterial air embolus will commonly be brought to an initial hyperbaric depth of 165 ft (6 atm). After 30 minutes, the patient will be brought slowly "up" to a depth of 60 and then 30 ft before returning to the normal ambient pressure.

Adjunctive therapies to HBO such as NSAIDs, glucocorticoids, lidocaine, aspirin, and heparin have been tried, but there is currently insufficient data to support their use. In addition to hyperbaric therapy, patients should be dried off immediately and kept warm to prevent hypothermia. A urine output should be maintained in the pediatric patient between 1 and 2 mL/kg/hr. Intravenous fluids that are in plastic bags should be used instead of glass bottles. Some individuals may experience neurologic deterioration after cessation of recompression therapy, possibly caused by (1) slow re-expansion of residual gas bubbles, (2) postischemic reperfusion, and (3) re-embolization from underlying pulmonary abnormality or injury.

Special precautions should also be taken for victims who must be transported by helicopter or airplane. In some cases, even the slightest elevation, which results in exposure to a decreased ambient pressure, may compromise the victim by causing further gas expansion. Helicopter transports should be done at as low an altitude as possible (less than 1000 ft), while ensuring the safety of the transport. Airplane transport should be conducted in aircraft that are capable of being pressurized to sea level.

Victims of type I decompression sickness are advised to abstain from any further scuba diving for at least 4 to 6 weeks and type II victims must wait at least 4 to 6 months. An air embolism or a second occurrence of any type II complications is serious enough to cease diving on a permanent basis.

DYSBARISMS CAUSED BY ABNORMAL GAS CONCENTRATION

Scuba diving is made possible through the use of compressed air tanks. As a diver descends, ambient pressure will increase causing a proportionate increase in the partial pressure of the compressed gases (Dalton's law). As a result, the partial pressure of the inhaled gas will increase at greater depths. The increased partial pressure of nitrogen represents the greatest concern to scuba divers. These symptoms are referred to as nitrogen narcosis.

Nitrogen Narcosis

The inhalation of nitrogen gas at elevated partial pressures may cause an interference with nerve conduction. As a result, nitrogen narcosis can produce a narcotic or intoxicating effect during a dive. Symptoms can include euphoria, uncontrollable laughter, impaired judgment, memory loss, light-headedness, hallucinations, loss of coordination, and impaired reflexes. The signs of nitrogen narcosis may become evident at depths beyond 80 ft. It is estimated that every 50 ft of depth during a dive can result in symptoms roughly equal to one martini on an empty stomach. The greatest risk of nitrogen narcosis is drowning. With any evidence or suspicion of confusion, disorientation, or altered mental status, the dive should be terminated. The affected diver should be escorted slowly to the surface by a second diver. No other treatment is required.

CONSIDERATIONS FOR DIVING IN CHILDREN

Practitioners of pediatric patients may be requested to screen a child for scuba diving. Medical and developmental considerations should be kept in mind for their increased predisposition of risk and injury to young divers. No concrete recommendations can be found in the medical literature for or against children participating in scuba diving.[3] However, considerations regarding the fitness to scuba dive have been addressed

Children with chronic sinusitis or otitis media should be adequately prophylaxed against congestion and potential diffi-

culty with equalization. Lung conditions that might cause blebs, such as cystic fibrosis, α_1-antitrypsin deficiency, or chronic obstructive pulmonary disease impart serious risk of pulmonary barotrauma. Children with active asthma exacerbations or cold- or exercise-induced asthma should be advised against diving. However, asthmatic children not currently experiencing an exacerbation are not at increased risk of pulmonary barotrauma. Any prior history of spontaneous pneumothorax or thoracic surgery is a contraindication, however, traumatic pneumothorax that is well healed may not preclude diving.[7]

Cardiac conditions, such as patent foramen ovale, or other situations creating a potential right-to-left shunt (e.g. ASD or VSD) cause increased risk of arterial embolism and decompression sickness. Furthermore, long QT syndrome may trigger fatal arrhythmias during swimming and diving.[7] Other conditions including claustrophobia, unrepaired inguinal hernias, and insulin-dependent diabetes mellitus are also considered contraindications. However, divers with sickle cell trait or Crohn's disease appear to be unaffected.

► SUMMARY

An understanding and awareness of the clinical signs and symptoms of dysbaric injuries is important for all emergency physicians. The diverse clinical findings of barotrauma and decompression illness may begin immediately upon ascent from a dive or can be delayed for days. A patient may present to the emergency department directly from the dive site, making the diagnosis evident. However, a patient may present up to 36 hours later after traveling hundreds or thousands of miles in returning home from a vacation.

Some patients will require only supportive care and can be safely discharged. Other patients, who may have limited complaints or physical findings, will require careful monitoring or aggressive and time-critical treatment. The increasing popularity of scuba diving makes it essential for the emergency physician to be able to differentiate the benign from the potentially serious dysbaric injuries.

For assistance with scuba diving-related injuries, contact:

Divers Alert Network (DAN)
- 24-Hour Diving Emergencies: 919–684–8111 or 1–919–684–4DAN (collect), 1–800–446–2671 (toll free), +1–919–684–9111 (Latin America Hotline)
- Information Line: 1–800–446.2671 or 1–919–684-2948, Mon-Fri, 9 AM to 5 PM (EST) http://www.diversalert network.org/

Other helpful Web sites:
- Scottish Diving Medicine. http://www.sdm.scot.nhs.uk/index.htm
- Scubadoc's Diving Medicine Online. http://www.scuba-doc.com

REFERENCES

1. Annual Divers Report 2006 Edition. Divers Alert Network. http://www.dan.org/medical/report/2006DANDivingReport.pdf. Accessed March 2008.
2. Annual Divers Report 2007 Edition. Divers Alert Network. http://www.dan.org/medical/report/2007DANDivingReport.pdf. Accessed March 2008.

3. Tsung JW, Chou KJ, Martinez CM, et al. An adolescent scuba diver with two episodes of diving-related injuries requiring hyperbasic oxygen recompression therapy: a case report with medical considerations for child and adolescent scuba divers. *Pediatr Emerg Care*. 2005;21(10):681–686.

4. Tetzlaff K, Shank ES, Muth CM. Evaluation and management of decompression illness–an intensivist's perspective. *Intensive Care Med*. 2003;29(12):2128–2136.

5. Hardy KR. Diving-related emergencies. *Emerg Med Clin North Am*. 1997;15:223.

6. Tibbles PM, Edelsberg JS. Hyperbaric oxygen therapy. *N Engl J Med*. 1996;334(25):1642–1648.

7. Godden D, Currie G, Denison D, et al. British Thoracic Society guidelines on respiratory aspects of fitness for diving. *Thorax*. 2003;58:3–13.

CHAPTER 143

Radiation Emergencies

Ira J. Blumen and James W. Rhee

▶ HIGH-YIELD FACTS

- Ionizing radiation is named for its ability to interact with matter, converting atoms to ions as a result of their gain or loss of electrons. Ionizing radiation is more dangerous than nonionizing radiation because such reactions lead to breaks in both DNA and RNA, damaging important biologic functions at the cellular metabolic level.
- The clinical effects of radiation exposure are related to the type of radiation involved, the amount of radiation and the nature of the exposure (continuous or intermittent). In addition, the harmful effects of ionizing radiation may be affected by the total time of the exposure, the distance from the radiation source, and the presence of any shielding (amount and type).
- There are two categories of radiation injuries with which the emergency physician should be familiar:
  - *Exposure* injury, which generally represents no threat to emergency care providers.
  - *Contamination*, which may represent a risk to emergency personnel.
- Radiation injury should be considered in the differential diagnosis for any patient who presents with a painless "burn," but who does not remember a thermal or chemical insult.
- *Acute radiation syndrome* may develop following a whole-body exposure of 100 rad or more that occurs over a relatively short period of time. Organ systems with rapidly dividing cells (bone marrow and gastrointestinal tract) are the most vulnerable to radiation injury.
- Although the effect of radiation on the hematopoietic system is characterized by pancytopenia, the absolute lymphocyte count represents the best way to estimate exposure hematologically. Leukocyte counts may be elevated initially because of demargination, but the lymphocyte portion of the differential will quickly start to decrease.
- Total-body irradiation with >1000 rad results in a neurovascular syndrome since, at such high radiation levels, even cells that are relatively resistant to injury are damaged. Ataxia and confusion quickly develop and there is direct vascular damage, with resultant circulatory collapse. The patient usually expires within hours.
- In the presence of contamination, if the patient's condition permits, decontamination should begin in the prehospital setting, which will reduce the potential spread of radioactive material and decrease the potential contamination of hospital workers or other rescuers. Fortunately, if appropriate management steps are taken, the radiation-contaminated patient should present little danger to hospital staff, even if decontamination was incomplete prior to arrival at the hospital.
- While both prehospital and hospital workers may be at risk, it is the prehospital personnel and other rescuers, who respond to the site of a radiation accident, who are more often exposed to significant radiation. A threshold of 5000 mrem (5 rem) should be the exposure limit, except to save a life. A once-in-a-lifetime exposure to 100 000 mrem (100 rem) to save a life has been established by the National Council on Radiation Protection as acceptable and will not result in any undue morbidity.
- The Joint Commission requires each emergency department to have a radiation accident plan. In the event of a medically significant radiation accident, a well-prepared and practiced plan will supply emergency care providers with an appropriate knowledge base, management protocols, and additional resources that can be called upon.

In May 2000, an Egyptian man found a shiny metal object along the roadside near his hometown. He took it home, where he lived with his wife, four children, and a sister. The object was placed on a cabinet near the front door and the father and his 9-year-old son frequently rubbed the object, believing it was a precious metal to be shined. One month later, the 9-year-old son died in a local hospital. Physicians diagnosed the boy with bone-marrow failure and skin inflammation. Within 2 weeks, the father and a daughter also died and the rest of the family was hospitalized, all with the same signs. The evidence suggested radiation sickness and was investigated by government authorities. The "precious metal" turned out to be iridium-192, a β–γ emitter, used like a portable radiography machine to check the quality of welds and perform other industrial scans. In addition to exposing this family, several hundred family associates, who gathered on a regular basis outside the home, were also exposed. Fortunately, the rest of the family recovered from their radiation-related illnesses.

Radiation accidents involving discarded medical and industrial sources get little attention compared to problems at nuclear power plants or weapons facilities. Unfortunately, these accidents occur around the world with surprising regularity and, in some instances, prove deadly.

According to the Radiation Emergency Assistance Center/Training Site (REAC/TS) Radiation Accident Registry, between 1944 and 2007, there have been 432 accidents worldwide. These accidents resulted in significant radiation exposure to 3082 individuals and in 127 deaths (Table 143–1).

	United States	Non-United States	Total	(FSU Data*)
Number of accidents	250	182	432	(137)
Number of persons involved	1358	132 453	133 811	(507)
Significant exposures[†]	796	2286	3082	(278)
Fatalities	26	101	127	(35)

*Not included in totals due to incomplete FSU (Former Soviet Union) Registry Data.
[†]DOE/NRC dose criteria.
Source: DOE/REAC/TS Radiation Accident Registry, Oak Ridge, TN, 2007.

Despite the relatively rare incidence of medically significant pediatric radiation accidents, our dependence on nuclear energy makes it necessary for today's emergency physician to understand its potential for disaster. Most obvious are the threats of sophisticated nuclear weaponry to individuals of all ages. However, the near disaster of Three Mile Island in Pennsylvania in 1979 and the Chernobyl Nuclear Power Station catastrophe in the former Soviet Union in 1986 serve as potent reminders of the severe underlying hazards to children and adults, even in peaceful nuclear energy utilization. A more probable predicament, however, is an isolated or limited exposure in a medical, industrial, or research accident, or during the transport of radionucleotides. Basic preparation for radiation emergencies is not difficult, but a thorough understanding of the pathophysiology and clinical presentation is a must in order to handle all aspects of these complex problems successfully.

Radiation accidents do not differentiate between children and adults. Therefore, all individuals are susceptible to radiation injury if the exposure is of significant dose and duration. Children, however, may suffer greater, short-, and long-term consequences of a significant radiation exposure for several reasons. Children are more susceptible to relatively greater internal exposure to inhaled radioactive gases given disproportionately higher minute ventilation.[1] Children are also at greater risk for developing subsequent malignancies when they are exposed to radiation.[2,3] Additionally, children are more likely than adults to experience psychological trauma leading to enduring psychological injury after a radiation disaster.[1,4]

▶ TYPES OF RADIATION

Radiation is a general term used to describe energy that is emitted from a source. The term encompasses the broad-wavelength microwave and extends through the ultra-high-frequency γ-rays. A radioactive substance, referred to as a radioisotope or radionucleotide, gives off radiation. A person exposed to external or remote radiation has been irradiated but does not become radioactive. The victim may give off radiation only if there was external or internal contamination caused by the presence of radioactive particles (α and β).

Radiation can be classified as either ionizing or nonionizing. In addition, radiation can be described either as nonparticulate (electromagnetic) or particulate. Electromagnetic radiation has no mass and no charge. It occurs in waveforms and is described by wavelengths. Examples of this nonparticulate/electromagnetic radiation can be found in both the ionizing and nonionizing radiation classifications. In contrast, particulate radiation has mass and can either be charged or uncharged ionizing radiation.

IONIZING RADIATION

Ionizing radiation is named for its ability to interact with matter. Atoms will convert to ions as a result of their gain or loss of electrons. Ionizing radiation is more dangerous than nonionizing radiation because such reactions lead to breaks in both DNA and RNA, damaging important biologic functions at the cellular metabolic level. Anomalies may be passed on to subsequent offspring or they may result in cell death or the inability to replicate. Ionized radiation has a high frequency, a short wavelength, and a billion times more energy than nonionizing radiation. Common sources of ionizing radiation are nuclear reactors, nuclear weapons, radioactive material, and radiography equipment. Material identified by the label radioactive produces ionizing radiation.

Types of ionizing radiation include α-particles, β-particles, and neutrons, which represent particulate radiation; and x-rays and γ-rays, which are nonparticulate forms of radiation. γ-Rays have the highest energy content of the nonparticulate and massless radiations. Their photon radiation originates in the atomic nucleus. They can penetrate deep into the tissue, depositing energy and interacting with the various layers they penetrate. Constant low-level exposure through cosmic radiation is a usual source. γ-Radiation is a common cause of acute radiation syndrome due to radioisotope decay and radiation from linear accelerators. A lead shield 1 to 2 in in depth or thick concrete would provide satisfactory protection from γ-rays. X-rays have the next highest energy content of the nonparticulate, massless radiations. Unlike the γ-ray, which is produced within the nucleus of the atom, x-rays originate from outside the nucleus and are emitted by excited electrons. Like the γ-ray, x-rays can also penetrate tissue and deposit energy deep within the cells. Their usual source is medical or industrial in nature. α-Particles are composed of two protons and two neutrons and possess a 2^+ electrical charge. They originate from the nucleus of the atom and, being relatively heavy radioactive emissions, can travel only inches from their source. In general, they cannot penetrate paper or epidermis because of their mass and size and are rarely harmful externally. Examples include plutonium, uranium, and radium. β-Particles have a small mass, composed of a single electron emitted from the atom's nucleus, and possess a 1 charge. They can disperse only a few feet from their source and penetrate tissues only a small amount (up to 8 mm), primarily causing thermal injuries. Clothing alone can often provide adequate protection from β-particles. Despite their inability to penetrate the skin to any significant depth, both α-particles and β-particles can be harmful if they are ingested or inhaled or if wounds are contaminated by these particles. The common research isotope tritium is an example, as is carbon[14] and phosphorous. Neutrons are the third type of particulate radiation. Without an electrical charge, they ionize by colliding with atomic nuclei within cells and tissues. They possess strong power to penetrate and represent the only form of radiation that can make previously stable atoms within the body radioactive. They can be more damaging than x-rays or γ-rays and are responsible for radioactive fallout. Nuclear reactors, nuclear weapons, and nuclear accelerators are common sources of neutron radiation. Specialized concrete is necessary to provide shielding from neutron radiation.

NONIONIZING RADIATION

Nonionizing radiation is relatively low energy in nature and does not result in acute radiation injuries or contamination. The adverse effects to humans are limited to local heat production. In order of decreasing energy content, the nonionizing forms of radiation include ultraviolet rays, visible light, infrared radiation, microwaves, and radio waves. These forms of nonionizing radiation also represent many of the electromagnetic radiations. Their energy content is less than that of γ-rays and x-rays, making them a less threatening form of radiation (Table 143–2).

▶ MEASURING RADIATION

Although radiation cannot be sensed by the human body, it can be detected and quantified by dosimeters or Geiger–Mueller tubes at levels far below those that result in any biologic significance. There are several units of measurement used in relation to radiation: *roentgen* is the unit of measurement used during the production of x-rays that measure the ion pairs produced in a given volume of air; *dose* represents the amount of energy deposited by radiation per unit of mass; and the *rad* (roentgen absorbed dose) is the basic unit of measurement. A rad can be defined as a unit of absorbed dose of radiant energy that is equal to 100 erg of energy deposited per gram of absorbing material. The gray (Gy) represents the standard international (SI) unit for dose:

$$1 \text{ Gy} = 100 \text{ rad}$$
$$1 \text{ cGy} = 1 \text{ rad}$$

Units of *rem* (roentgen equivalent in man) represent a calculated radiation unit of dose equivalent. The absorbed dose (rad) is multiplied by a factor to account for the relative biologic effectiveness (RBE) of the various types of radiation:

$$\text{rem} = \text{rad} \times \text{RBE}$$

▶ **TABLE 143–2. TYPES OF RADIATION**

Nonionizing
  Nonparticulate and electromagnetic*
    Ultraviolet rays
    Visible rays
    Infrared rays
    Microwaves
    Radio waves

Ionizing
  Nonparticulate and electromagnetic
    No mass
    No charge
    Penetrating
    Examples*
      γ-Rays
      X-rays
  Particulate
    Has mass
    Uncharged and penetrating
      Neutrons
      More damaging than x-rays or γ-rays
      No electrical charge
    Charged and nonpenetrating
      α-Rays
        2 Protons
        2 Neutrons
        2 + Charge
      β-Rays
        1 Electron
        1−Charge

*In order of decreasing energy content.

The *sievert* (Sv) is the SI unit for dose equivalent, where

$$1 \text{ Sv} = 100 \text{ rem}$$
$$1 \text{ cSv} = 1 \text{ rem}$$

Generally, the terms *rem* and *mrem* (millirem) are used when they refer to the exposure of biologic systems. For β-particles, x-rays, and γ-rays, the RBE = 1. Therefore, for these sources of radiation, 1 rad = 1 rem and 1 Gy = 1 Sv.

▶ RADIATION EXPOSURE

The clinical impact of radiation exposure depends on several factors. These factors are also important to properly coordinate the safety of both prehospital and hospital providers who may respond to a radiation incident.

The clinical effects of radiation exposure are related to the type of radiation involved, the amount of radiation and the nature of the exposure (continuous or intermittent). In addition, the harmful effects of ionizing radiation may be affected by the total time of the exposure, the distance from the radiation source, and the presence of any shielding (amount and type).

A radiation exposure over a prolonged period of time is less likely to be harmful to an individual than the same dose over a shorter time period. For example, an exposure of

100 rem in 1 second will be more harmful than an exposure of 100 rem over 1 year.

There is an inverse square relationship between distance from a radiation source and the resultant exposure, making increased distance an effective means to reduce the amount of exposure. An exposure can be reduced by a factor of 4 simply by doubling the distance from the radiation source. Tripling the distance will decrease the exposure by a factor of 9.

Shielding may be an effective method to reduce radiation exposure when one is dealing with low-energy radiation (x-rays). When dealing with medium- or high-energy radiation, shielding may become impractical due to the amount of lead or concrete that would be necessary.

In the United States, there are natural and technological radiation sources to which children and adults are commonly exposed (Fig. 143–1). Background radiation may represent an exposure between 300 and 360 mrem/y. Radon accounts for the largest amount of this background radiation (approximately 200 mrem/y). Consumer products (10 mrem/y), cosmic radiation (26 mrem/y), terrestrial radiation (28 mrem/y), nuclear medicine (14 mrem/y), other medical sources (39 mrem/y), and internal sources (40 mrem/y) account for the balance.[5]

Technological sources of radiation may represent a wide range of exposures to individuals. Color television may result in an exposure of 1 mrem/y; a round-trip, coast-to-coast jet flight may result in a 2 to 5 mrem exposure; and a chest x-ray causes an exposure between 5 and 10 mrem. The common radiation exposure to a patient during angiography may be 1000 mrem. As technology changes and new technologies are developed, we are likely to encounter additional sources of radiation in varying amounts.

▶ RADIATION INJURIES

There are two categories of radiation injuries with which the emergency physician should be familiar. The first type is an *exposure* injury, which generally represents no threat to emergency care providers. *Contamination*, the second type of radiation injury, may represent a potential risk to emergency personnel.

EXPOSURE

Exposure radiation injuries can be classified into two categories. A person may be the victim of a *localized radiation injury* or may have suffered a *whole-body exposure*.

Localized Radiation Injuries

A large dose of radiation exposure to a small part of the body will result in a local radiation injury. These injuries often occur over months or even years, but they may occur over a shorter amount of time.[6]

Localized radiation injuries most commonly affect the upper extremities, with the buttocks and thighs representing the next most common sites. Typically, these injuries occur in the occupational setting. In addition, adults and children may unknowingly come into contact with a radiation source by handling an unknown object and putting it into their pockets. Localized radiation accidents may also result from an inadvertent exposure to an intense radiation beam.

The dose of radiation that can result in a local radiation injury varies greatly. Larger doses are often better tolerated than a whole-body exposure. Accidental exposures from radioactive sources with a surface dose of nearly 20 000 rad/min have been reported to have caused localized radiation injuries.

The initial clinical picture of a localized radiation injury depicts a thermal injury to the skin. While thermal burns develop soon after an exposure, erythema from a local radiation injury is delayed.[7] Radiation injury should be considered in the differential diagnosis for any patient who presents with a painless "burn" but who does not remember a thermal or chemical insult.

Radiation source	Amount of experience (mrem/y)
Consumer products	111
Cosmic	26
Terrestrial	28
Nuclear medicine	14
Medical	19
Internal	40
Radon	200

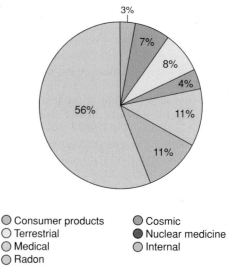

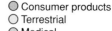

Figure 143–1. Common sources of natural and technological radiation exposure in the United States.

▶ TABLE 143–3. **LOCALIZED RADIATION INJURIES**

Type	Presentation	Exposure	Comments
Type I	Erythema only	600–1000 rad	Similar to a first-degree thermal burn. Erythema may be delayed up to 2–3 wk. A dose of 300 rad can result in a delayed hair loss (epilation). Dry desquamation or scaling may occur.
Type II	Transepidermal injury or wet desquamation	1000–2000 rad	Similar in severity to a second-degree partial-thickness thermal burn.
Type III	Dermal radionecrosis	>2000 rad	Severe pain with or without paresthesia. Resembles a severe chemical or scalding burn. Skin grafting may be necessary.
Type IV	Chronic radiation dermatitis	Recurrent exposure over several years	Can result in an eczematous appearance of the skin. Ulcerations and carcinoma are not uncommon.

Prolonged radiation exposure causes blood vessel fibrosis, leading to tissue necrosis. The outcome will be determined by the degree of blood vessel and tissue damage. Classification of these localized injuries can be divided into four types, differentiated by increasing epidermal and dermal injury. They are summarized in Table 143–3.

Whole-Body Exposure

Acute radiation syndrome may develop following a whole-body exposure of 100 rad or more that occurs over a relatively short period of time. Organ systems with rapidly dividing cells (bone marrow and gastrointestinal tract) are the most vulnerable to radiation injury. With greater doses of radiation, however, all organ systems may become involved, including the central nervous system.[8]

Estimating the exposure (in rads) of a whole-body radiation victim may be difficult when the patient presents to the emergency department. Dosimeters and Geiger counters are not standard equipment in many emergency departments and are often only able to identify radioactive contamination. Therefore, they are often of little help in determining the total radiation dose or duration of exposure. A mechanical dosimetry-monitoring device worn by the victim during the time of exposure would be helpful but is rarely available. Instead, the emergency physician's history and physical examination, along with baseline laboratory values, are essential in estimating the whole-body exposure. This technique is referred to as biologic dosimetry. For this purpose, the primary indicators include the time of onset of symptoms and depression of absolute lymphocyte count. The earlier signs and symptoms develop, the higher the dose of radiation exposure and the worse the prognosis. Table 143–4 identifies characteristic signs and symptoms with the radiation dose that can be anticipated following a whole-body exposure. A biologic dosimetry calculator is also available as a resource to clinicians through the Radiation Event Medical Management Website (http://www.remm.nlm.gov/ars_wbd.htm) maintained by the United States Department of Health and Human Services. The gold standard of radiation biodosimetry is cytogenetic biodosimetry, which identifies chromosomal aberrations. In the United States, this type of measurement is only available through the Armed Forces Radiobiology Research Institute (AFFRI) and REAC/TS. Consequently, the clinical symptoms and lymphocyte counts will still be the mainstay parameters for biologic dosimetry.

▶ TABLE 143–4. **BIOLOGICAL DOSIMETRY**

Indicator	Total-Body Dose	Comments
Nausea and vomiting		
Onset within 6 h	>100 rad (1 Gy)	Prodromal stage represents a good
Onset within 4 h	>200 rad (2 Gy)	clinical and biologic indicator to
Onset within 2 h	>400 rad (4 Gy)	estimate whole-body exposure
Onset within 1 h	>1000 rad (10 Gy)	
Lymphocyte count at 48 h		
>1200/mm³	100–200 rad (1–2 Gy)	Prognosis: good
300–1200/mm³	200–400 rad (2–4 Gy)	Prognosis: fair
<300/mm³	>400 rad (4 Gy)	Prognosis: poor
Diarrhea	>400 rad (4 Gy)	
Erythema of the skin	>600 rad (6 Gy)	Delayed onset
CNS symptoms (disorientation, ataxia, seizures, coma)	>1000 rad (10 Gy)	Rule out trauma Death within days

A progressive sequence of signs and symptoms following a whole-body exposure can be divided into four phases: prodromal, latent, manifest illness, and recovery or death.[8]

An individual's susceptibility and the dose of radiation, dose rate, and dose distribution will dictate the onset, duration, and character of symptoms in a predictable representation. The prodromal stage can begin within minutes to hours after exposure and is dose-dependent. The most common symptoms of this stage include nausea, vomiting, and fatigue. Exposure to <100 rad rarely causes symptoms and patients who do not exhibit nausea or vomiting within 6 hours of a radiation accident are unlikely to have been subject to a significant whole-body exposure. Prodromal markers beginning within 6 hours suggest an exposure in excess of 100 rad. Higher doses will result in a more rapid onset of these initial signs and symptoms, probably due to acute tissue injury and the subsequent release of vasoactive substances, including histamine and bradykinin.

A lower-dose exposure will yield a resolution of the prodromal symptoms over a period of days to weeks, during the latent stage. Progressively higher radiation doses will prolong the prodromal stage while limiting the latent period until a point is reached when it appears that the prodromal stage proceeds directly to the manifest illness stage without any resolution of the prodromal symptoms.

During the manifest illness stage, specific organ symptoms develop and the patient is at the greatest risk for infection and bleeding. Three syndromes may develop during this stage, depending on the total amount of radiation exposure: the hematopoietic syndrome (220–600 rad), the gastrointestinal syndrome (600–1000 rad), and the neurovascular syndrome (>1000 rad).

Although the effect of radiation on the hematopoietic system is characterized by pancytopenia, the absolute lymphocyte count represents the best way to estimate exposure hematologically.[9] Leukocyte counts may be elevated initially because of demargination, but the lymphocyte portion of the differential will quickly start to decrease. A 48-hour check will suggest the severity of the exposure. A lymphocyte count >1200/mm³ indicates a 100- to 200-rad exposure and most often a good prognosis. An absolute lymphocyte count of 300 to 1200/mm³ suggests a 200- to 400-rad exposure, which promises a fair outcome. Exposure to >400 rad is marked by a poor prognosis and is expected with counts <300/mm³. Pancytopenia may develop after a latent period lasting a few days to 3 weeks. The patient will subsequently suffer from dyspnea, malaise, purpura, bleeding, and opportunistic infection (Fig. 143–2).

Gastrointestinal illness will be most evident with total-body exposures of 600 to 1000 rad. The prodromal phase is abrupt and is marked by severe vomiting and diarrhea. The latent stage may be quite short and is followed by continued GI symptoms, leading to relentless fluid loss, fever, and prostration. The radiosensitive mucosal cells of the small bowel begin to slough, which, combined with the coexistent hematopoietic abnormalities, produces severe, bloody diarrhea. Even with intense supportive care, the patient rarely survives.[10]

Total-body irradiation with >1000 rad results in a neurovascular syndrome. At such high radiation levels, even cells that are relatively resistant to injury are damaged. Ataxia and confusion quickly develop and there is direct vascular dam-

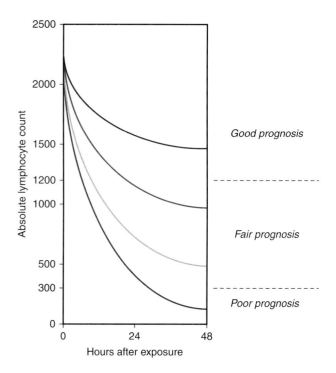

Figure 143–2. A 48-h check of the absolute lymphocyte count suggesting the severity of the exposure to radiation. Good prognosis: a lymphocyte count greater than 1200/mm³. A 100- to 200-rad exposure. Fair prognosis: an absolute lymphocyte count of 300 to 1200/mm³. A 200- to 400-rad exposure. Poor prognosis: lymphocyte count below 300/mm³. More than 400-rad exposure.

age, with resultant circulatory collapse.[10] The patient usually expires within hours.

Patients with lower levels of exposure and those patients fortunate enough to respond to aggressive supportive management will likely recover. Further management is guided by specific organ system insults. For these survivors, the long-term risks of exposure to ionizing radiation include cataracts, leukemia, and development of carcinomas. It should be noted that the median lethal dose of total-body irradiation is estimated at 400 rad (Table 143–5).

CONTAMINATION

Contamination is the second type of radiation accident. Radioactive particles, solid or liquid, may remain on the surface of the victim, resulting in an external contamination. Internal contamination may be the result of inhaled, ingested, or absorbed radioactive particles. Neutrons, β-particles, and α-particles are most commonly responsible for contamination. Unlike an exposure victim, the contaminated patient does represent an additional challenge and potential risk to hospital and prehospital personnel.

In most situations, if the patient's condition permits, decontamination should begin in the prehospital setting. This will reduce the potential spread of radioactive material and will decrease the potential contamination of hospital workers or

▶ TABLE 143–5. **WHOLE-BODY EXPOSURE**

Whole-Body Dose, Rad	Characteristics
5	Asymptomatic; normal blood studies
15	Chromosome abnormality may be detectable
50–75	Asymptomatic; minor depression of platelets and white cell count may be detectable
75–100	Nausea, vomiting, fatigue in 10%–15% of victims within 2 d
100–200	Prodrome: mild nausea, vomiting, and fatigue; onset within 6 h, lasting 3–6 h
	Latent stage: >2 wk
	Manifest illness stage
	Lymphocyte count >1200/mm^3 at 48 h
	Transient sterility in men
	Recovery: good prognosis with only symptomatic treatment
200–600	Prodrome: nausea and vomiting within 2–4 h, last <24 h
	Latent stage: 1–3 wk
	Manifest illness stage: hematopoietic
	@ 200–400 rad: lymphocyte count 300–1200/mm^3 at 48 h
	>400 rad: lymphocyte count <300/mm^3 at 48 h
	Pancytopenia may develop after a latent period of up to 3 wk: the patient will subsequently suffer from dyspnea, malaise, purpura, bleeding, and opportunistic infection
	Requires hospitalization, protective isolation, and support
	Upper dose range may require bone-marrow transplantation within 7–10 d of exposure
	Recovery:
	@ 200–400 rad: fair prognosis with supportive care and if the bone-marrow damage was not irreversible
	@ 400 rad: poor prognosis; lethal in approximately 50% of victims
600–1000	Prodrome: severe nausea, vomiting, and diarrhea within 1–2 h, lasting >48 h
	Latent stage: 0–7 d
	Manifest illness stage: gastrointestinal
	Recurrence of nausea and vomiting
	Fever, bloody diarrhea, dehydration, electrolyte imbalance, early sepsis, hemorrhage
	Leukocyte count drops to zero
	Recovery:
	Overall 90%–100% mortality within 30 d
	Lower-dose exposure with medical care has a 50% mortality
>1000	Prodrome: nausea and vomiting within 1 h
	Latent stage: none
	Manifest illness stage: neurovascular
	Dehydration, hypotension
	Disorientation, ataxia, confusion, seizures, coma
	Erythema and epilation (onset may be delayed)
	Recovery: 99%–100% incidence of death within days
>5000	Prodrome: almost immediate onset of nausea, vomiting
	Latent stage: none
	Manifest illness stage: cardiovascular, GI, and CNS.
	Hypotension, ataxia, cerebral edema, seizures (rapid onset)
	Recovery: death within 1–4 d

other rescuers. Fortunately, if appropriate management steps are taken, the radiation-contaminated patient should present little danger to hospital staff, even if decontamination was incomplete prior to arrival at the hospital.

▶ MANAGEMENT

It is important to realize that the general principles of patient care for radiation victims are no different than those for other medical problems. The initial assessment and management are directed toward the airway, breathing, and circulation. There are no acute, life-threatening complications of a survivable radiation injury that require immediate intervention. Emergency treatment should be supportive and directed toward the prevention of complications.

It will be important to determine, quickly, whether the patients are victims of a radiation exposure or a contamination. Radiation contamination requires that decontamination begin promptly after stabilization. The radiation exposure patient who is not contaminated represents no danger to the hospital staff or other patients. These victims can be managed

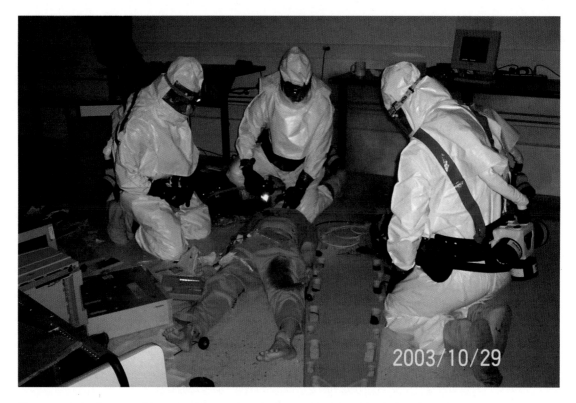

Figure 143–3. Care providers should wear appropriate personal protective equipment when treating hazmat victims in the field. The scene should be declared safe for level C personal protective equipment before providers are sent into the area. (Photo courtesy of Ken Williams, MD and the Rhode Island Disaster Initiative [RIDI].)

in the emergency department and require no immediate intervention related to the radiation exposure.

At all times, there must be a proper balance between patient care and the personal safety of rescuers and health care workers. Appropriate measures must be taken by both prehospital and hospital personnel to minimize their risk of exposure while managing either life-threatening injuries or the decontamination of the patients they serve.

While both prehospital and hospital workers may be at risk, it is the prehospital personnel and other rescuers who respond to the site of a radiation accident, who are more often exposed to significant radiation. A threshold of 5000 mrem (5 rem) should be the exposure limit, except to save a life. A once-in-a-lifetime exposure to 100 000 mrem (100 rem) to save a life has been established by the National Council on Radiation Protection as acceptable and will not result in any undue morbidity.

Hospital personnel are at a very low risk of significant radiation exposure when treating victims of a radiation accident. Off-site medical personnel who treated victims of the Three Mile Island and Chernobyl accidents were exposed to radiation doses of <14 mrem.

PREHOSPITAL MANAGEMENT

The history obtained by prehospital personnel is of paramount importance in management decisions regarding radiation vic-

tims. When possible, rescuers must gather details regarding the exact type, location, and duration of exposure. For internal exposure, the route of entry, type, and quantity of radioactive material should be determined. If the incident has occurred in an industrial or laboratory setting, initial decontamination procedures may be instituted by on-site personnel according to established protocols before EMS personnel arrive (Fig. 143–3). A quick response in decontamination will limit the exposure to the victim and decrease the amount of further contamination of both the ambulance and the emergency department. For unstable patients, the minimal action performed prior to rapid transport is the removal of contaminated clothing.

After transport of the patient to the hospital, EMS personnel and their vehicles must be inspected for the presence of radioactive contamination before they leave the facility. This must also be done at the scene for any ambulance and personnel who respond to the accident site and provide field assessment and stabilization without patient transport.

EMERGENCY DEPARTMENT MANAGEMENT

Few hospitals will be called on to treat victims of life-threatening radiation accidents. The exceptions are hospitals in close proximity to nuclear power plants or in the event of a nuclear war. It is more likely, however, that hospitals will be called on to attend victims of a minor industrial accident or an accident involving the transportation of radioactive materials. The end result will be a patient with "routine injuries," whose treatment may be complicated by an inadvertent radiation exposure with or without low-level radioactive contamination.

RADIATION ACCIDENT PLAN

The Joint Commission requires each emergency department to have a radiation accident plan. In the event of a medically significant radiation accident, a well-prepared and practiced plan will supply emergency care providers with an appropriate knowledge base, management protocols, and additional resources that can be called upon.

A major part of a well-prepared plan facilitates the identification of *significant* versus *perceived* radiation dangers. The incidence of significant radiation accidents may be rare for some hospitals, but the incidence of perceived radiation accidents may be much greater. A vehicular accident involving a truck or train carrying radioactive material near a school may send dozens (or hundreds) of anxious parents and their children to the emergency department. The staff of a well-prepared emergency department can assess the potential risks and, when appropriate, correct any misconceptions and ease the fears the general public may have.

A lack of experience, an incomplete knowledge base, and a significant degree of fear among health care providers often result in the mismanagement of radiation victims. Therefore, it is essential that an emergency department develop protocols for dealing with both the radiation exposure itself and the medical management of these victims.

The final component of an emergency department's resource plan for radiation emergencies is a list of "additional references." These resources include local, state, regional, and/or national agencies and their 24-hour telephone numbers that can be called for information or assistance. The U. S. Department of Energy is also available to coordinate a federal response and provide assistance through the radiological assistance program (RAP). RAP provides advice and radiological assistance to government agencies and to the private sector for incidents involving radioactive materials that pose a threat to the public health and safety or the environment. RAP can provide field deployable teams of health physics professionals equipped to conduct radiological monitoring and assessment. RAP is managed at eight regional coordinating offices across the country (Fig. 143–4).

The REAC/TS in Oak Ridge, Tennessee, is also available to provide treatment and medical consultation for injuries resulting from radiation exposure and contamination. REAC/TS can be contacted by calling 865–576-1005.

GENERAL PROCEDURES

Early notification of estimated time of arrival will allow the emergency department to implement its radiation accident plan

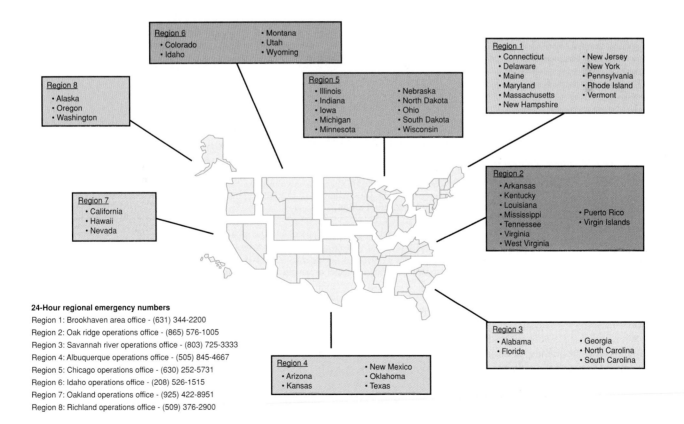

24-Hour regional emergency numbers
Region 1: Brookhaven area office - (631) 344-2200
Region 2: Oak ridge operations office - (865) 576-1005
Region 3: Savannah river operations office - (803) 725-3333
Region 4: Albuquerque operations office - (505) 845-4667
Region 5: Chicago operations office - (630) 252-5731
Region 6: Idaho operations office - (208) 526-1515
Region 7: Oakland operations office - (925) 422-8951
Region 8: Richland operations office - (509) 376-2900

Headquarters: Washington, DC- (202) 586-8100

Figure 143–4. U. S. Department of Energy Radiological Assistance Program Regional Coordinating Offices.

Emergency department preparation

Have appropriate contact with prehospital personnel to determine the following:
- Type of radiation accident
- Type, location, and duration of exposure
- Type of injuries (trauma and radiation)
- Number and condition of potential victims (contaminated and uncontaminated)
- Prehospital decontamination
- Radioactive material involved

Make the necessary preparation to receive, evaluate, and treat radiation victims:
- Notify appropriate individuals as outlined in radiation accident plan.
- Assure that adequate supplies and equipment are available for major resuscitation and decontamination.
- Prepare the designated separate entrance (if possible) to the emergency department for radiation victims.
- Establish separate contaminated and clean treatment areas that are clearly roped off.
- Assign separate staff (physicians, nurses, and technicians), if possible, to the clean and contaminated treatment areas.
  - Personnel assigned to either the clean or contaminated treatment areas must remain there.
  - If it becomes necessary to move within the treatment areas, it should be done only after appropriate monitoring for contamination.
- Assign staff to triage victims.
- Review treatment protocols and priorities with assigned staff.

Decontamination area

- Route from ambulance area to decontamination area and floor of decontamination area should be covered with plastic or paper secured with tape.
- Light switches, door handles, cabinet handles, etc. should be covered with tape.
- Assure that all staff are wearing film badges and protective and disposable clothing prior to initiating decontamination:
  - Surgical pants and shirt
  - Surgical cap
  - Waterproof shoe covers (taped to surgical pants)
  - Surgical gown
  - Surgical gloves (taped to surgical gown sleeves)
  - Second pair of surgical gloves, not taped
  - Surgical mask (respirators should be worn if airborne contaminants are suspected)
- Collect specimens for radiologic evaluation before and after decontamination.
- All waste should be captured in sealed containers labeled "Radioactive waste."
- Use a drainage table if available.
- Monitor patient for radiation contamination before and after decontamination procedures and record levels in patient's medical record.
- Individuals not directly involved in the evaluation or treatment of radiation victims must be kept away from the designated treatment areas.

Figure 143–5. Radiation accident plan: recommended emergency department procedures. (*continued*)

and to advise EMS personnel on initial prehospital decontamination.

When exposed solely to irradiation from γ-rays, x-rays, β-particles, and, frequently, neutrons, patients do not become radioactive. However, the radiation accident plan must assume that there will be external contamination. Figure 143–5 outlines an example of many of the procedures and actions that should be addressed in the radiation accident plan.

Separate contaminated and clean treatment areas must be established. When possible, prepare a separate entrance to the emergency department for radiation victims. The floor of the

contaminated treatment area and the ambulance receiving area must be covered with plastic or paper sheets to prevent the spread of contamination (Fig. 143–6). Devices must be immediately available to monitor both the patients and personnel for any evidence of radioactive contamination.

All personnel in the treatment area must wear protective clothing. This includes gowns, caps, masks, shoe covers, double gloves, and personal monitoring devices (film badges). If airborne contaminants are suspected, respirators must be worn. In most cases, decontamination begins during the prehospital stage, significantly reducing the risk of exposure to

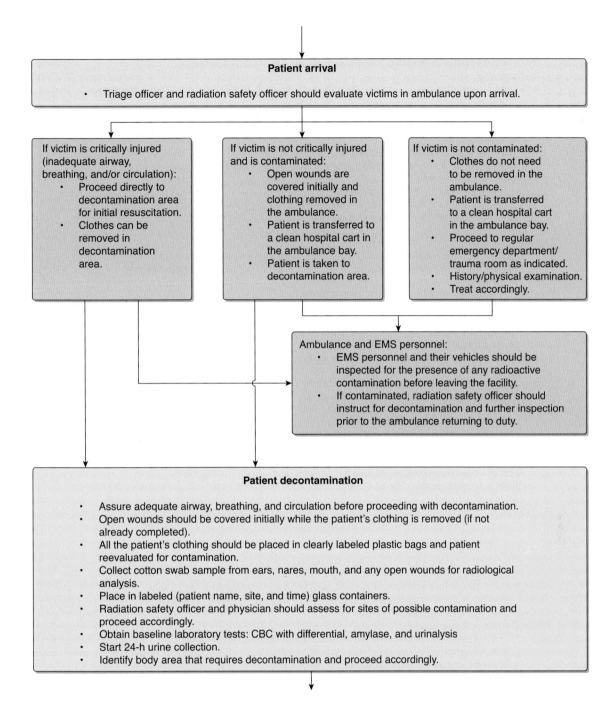

Patient arrival

- Triage officer and radiation safety officer should evaluate victims in ambulance upon arrival.

If victim is critically injured (inadequate airway, breathing, and/or circulation):
- Proceed directly to decontamination area for initial resuscitation.
- Clothes can be removed in decontamination area.

If victim is not critically injured and is contaminated:
- Open wounds are covered initially and clothing removed in the ambulance.
- Patient is transferred to a clean hospital cart in the ambulance bay.
- Patient is taken to decontamination area.

If victim is not contaminated:
- Clothes do not need to be removed in the ambulance.
- Patient is transferred to a clean hospital cart in the ambulance bay.
- Proceed to regular emergency department/ trauma room as indicated.
- History/physical examination.
- Treat accordingly.

Ambulance and EMS personnel:
- EMS personnel and their vehicles should be inspected for the presence of any radioactive contamination before leaving the facility.
- If contaminated, radiation safety officer should instruct for decontamination and further inspection prior to the ambulance returning to duty.

Patient decontamination

- Assure adequate airway, breathing, and circulation before proceeding with decontamination.
- Open wounds should be covered initially while the patient's clothing is removed (if not already completed).
- All the patient's clothing should be placed in clearly labeled plastic bags and patient reevaluated for contamination.
- Collect cotton swab sample from ears, nares, mouth, and any open wounds for radiological analysis.
- Place in labeled (patient name, site, and time) glass containers.
- Radiation safety officer and physician should assess for sites of possible contamination and proceed accordingly.
- Obtain baseline laboratory tests: CBC with differential, amylase, and urinalysis
- Start 24-h urine collection.
- Identify body area that requires decontamination and proceed accordingly.

Figure 143–5. (*Continued*)

emergency department staff. Despite this, fear of contamination may persist in poorly educated or ill-prepared hospital personnel.

Separate staff members are assigned to the clean and contaminated treatment areas. Staff assigned to the contaminated areas are provided appropriate personal protective equipment (Fig. 143–7). Medical staff is designated for triage and initial resuscitation, which must take place before decontamination.

A radiation safety officer should be assigned to monitor the treatment area and everyone within. This officer is given a Geiger–Mueller counter for detecting β- and γ-radiation or a scintillation detector, which offers a higher sensitivity in detecting α-, β-, γ-, and neutron particles. This designated individual oversees the decontamination procedures, the routing of patients, and the movement of hospital personnel. This is important to ensure adequate decontamination and to prevent the unintentional spread of contamination.

Treatment protocols and priorities should be reviewed with assigned staff. Established mechanisms to minimize their exposure, while not compromising patient care, should be reinforced. Ideally, several medical personnel should be assigned

- *Contaminated open wounds*
  - Open wound should be considered contaminated until proven otherwise.
  - Decontamination of open wounds should precede the irrigation of intact skin surfaces.
  - Protect uncontaminated surrounding areas by covering them with disposable adhesive surgical drapes.
  - Irrigate for 3 min with copious amounts of water or normal saline.
  - Sponges or cotton-tipped swabs should be used to further clean the orifices or wounds, as needed.
  - Carefully assess for and remove any foreign bodies.
  - Reevaluate for contamination and repeat the procedure as needed.
  - If contamination persists:
    - Wash with 3% hydrogen peroxide.
    - Consider surgical debridement (save all tissue).
    - Cover wounds following successful decontamination and proceed.

- *Contaminated eyes*
  - Protect uncontaminated areas around eyes by covering them with plastic drapes.
  - Irrigate eyes thoroughly with copious amounts of water or normal saline (proceed nose to temple).
  - Reevaluate for contamination and repeat as needed.

- *Contaminated ear canals*
  - Irrigate ear canal gently with small amounts of water.
  - Suction frequently.
  - Reevaluate for contamination and repeat as needed.

- *Contaminated nares and mouth* (*ingestion or inhalation*)
  - If patient's condition permits, turn head to side.
  - Irrigate gently with small amounts of water.
  - Suction frequently.
  - Prevent water from entering the stomach if possible.
  - Sponges or cotton-tipped swabs can be used to further clean the orifices or wounds, as needed.
  - Insert nasogastric tube into the stomach and monitor suctioned contents for contamination. If contaminated lavage with small amounts of water until clear of contamination.
  - If inhalation or ingestion is considered, initiate other measures to eliminate, neutralize, or block further contamination:
    - Ingestion: Activated charcoal, cathartics, specific chelating or blocking agents.
    - Inhalation: Bronchopulmonary lavage, specific blocking or chelating agents by nebulizer

- *Contaminated intact skin*
  - Decontaminate areas of the body with the highest radiation level.
  - If whole-body contamination:
    - Wash the entire body thoroughly with soap and copious amounts of water and rinse well.
    - Showering, if available, should be used only for patients with extensive body surface area contamination.
  - If localized contamination:
    - Protect uncontaminated areas by covering them with plastic drapes.
    - Wash the affected area thoroughly with soap and copious amounts of water and rinse well.
  - A scrub brush may be used, but do not abrade the skin.
  - Pay particular attention to skin folds, ears, and under fingernails.
  - Reevaluate for contamination and repeat the procedure as needed.
  - If contamination persists wash with Lava soap or a mixture of half cornmeal and half laundry detergent. If this fails to remove contamination, proceed with bleach (full strength for small areas or diluted for large areas).

- *Contaminated hair*
  - Protect uncontaminated areas by covering them with plastic drapes.
  - Do not shave hair, if necessary hair can be cut, but avoid abrading the skin.
  - Wash the affected area thoroughly with soap and copious amounts of water and rinse well.
- Reevaluate for contamination and repeat as needed.

Figure 143–5. (*Continued*)

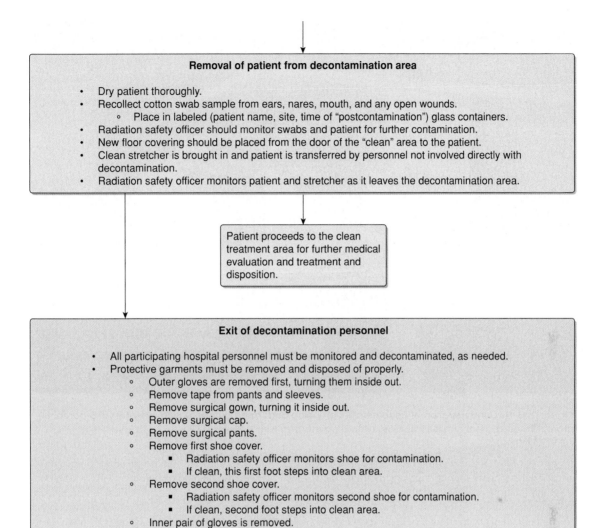

Removal of patient from decontamination area

- Dry patient thoroughly.
- Recollect cotton swab sample from ears, nares, mouth, and any open wounds.
  - Place in labeled (patient name, site, time of "postcontamination") glass containers.
- Radiation safety officer should monitor swabs and patient for further contamination.
- New floor covering should be placed from the door of the "clean" area to the patient.
- Clean stretcher is brought in and patient is transferred by personnel not involved directly with decontamination.
- Radiation safety officer monitors patient and stretcher as it leaves the decontamination area.

Patient proceeds to the clean treatment area for further medical evaluation and treatment and disposition.

Exit of decontamination personnel

- All participating hospital personnel must be monitored and decontaminated, as needed.
- Protective garments must be removed and disposed of properly.
  - Outer gloves are removed first, turning them inside out.
  - Remove tape from pants and sleeves.
  - Remove surgical gown, turning it inside out.
  - Remove surgical cap.
  - Remove surgical pants.
  - Remove first shoe cover.
    - Radiation safety officer monitors shoe for contamination.
    - If clean, this first foot steps into clean area.
  - Remove second shoe cover.
    - Radiation safety officer monitors second shoe for contamination.
    - If clean, second foot steps into clean area.
  - Inner pair of gloves is removed.
- Monitor hand, feet, and entire body for final time.
- Take a shower

Figure 143–5. (*Continued*)

to care for each contaminated patient. Individual exposure time can be decreased and a greater distance can be maintained from the patient when the health worker is not involved in direct decontamination or medical management. In cases of a highly radioactive contaminant or foreign body, a lead shield or apron is necessary to protect personnel (Fig. 143–6). However, in most situations, lead aprons are not effective protection against the most common contaminant, the medium-energy γ-ray.

Patients enter the emergency department through a separate entrance where radiation detection equipment is in place. Patients on ambulance stretchers are transferred to clean hospital carts in the ambulance bay.

The ideal decontamination site is an isolated room designed with a closed drainage and ventilation system and fully equipped for a major resuscitation. In many hospitals, the morgue is the only available isolation room meeting these criteria. Alternatively, the route from the ambulance area can be to an outside decontamination area. Resuscitation equipment and other emergency supplies should be relocated to this site

when the radiation accident plan is activated. Management of immediate life-threatening injuries remains the first priority for these patients. Following resuscitation, the radiation victim is carefully evaluated to determine if there is any surface contamination or if there is the possibility of inhaled or ingested radioactive material.

All burns and open wounds must also be evaluated for contamination. They must be irrigated with copious amounts of water and examined for foreign bodies. Highly contaminated foreign bodies, while rare, may represent the greatest single hazard to hospital personnel. These contaminants must be removed from the victim as safely and quickly as possible. Radiation burns may be delayed in their presentation. They are managed in the same way as non–radiation-induced partial- and full-thickness burns. Extensive β-particle burns often result in full-thickness injury and require skin grafting.

Individuals not directly involved in the evaluation or treatment of radiation victims must be kept away from the designated treatment areas. Personnel assigned to either the clean or contaminated treatment areas must remain there. If it becomes

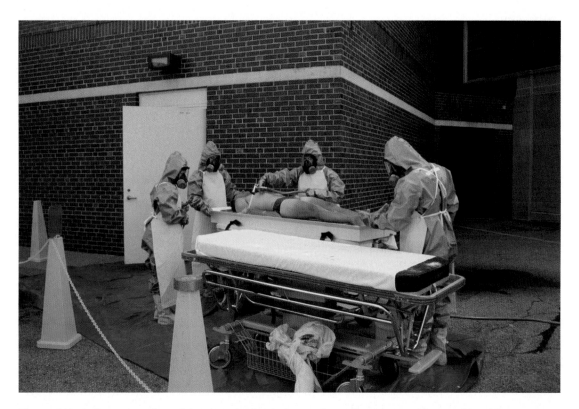

Figure 143–6. Demonstration of decontamination being performed outdoors with use of level B personal protective equipment and lead aprons. (Photo courtesy of Ken Williams, MD.)

necessary to move between the treatment areas, it should be done only after appropriate monitoring for contamination. Once the decontamination process for all victims has been completed, all participating hospital personnel must be reevaluated and decontaminated as needed. Their protective garments must be removed before they leave the treatment area and disposed of properly.

A baseline complete blood count, differential, platelet count, and electrolytes must be obtained. Patients who remain in the hospital should have blood for serial laboratory tests drawn at 12 and 24 hours. Patients who exhibit a decrease in absolute lymphocyte count will have to have a human leukocyte antigen (HL-A) typing performed in the event that a bone-marrow transplant should become necessary.

If there is any evidence of infection, it should be treated in the same way as other infections. Severely neutropenic patients should receive broad-spectrum prophylactic antimicrobial agents. Prophylaxis should include a fluoroquinolone with streptococcal coverage or a fluoroquinolone without streptococcal coverage plus penicillin or amoxicillin, antiviral drugs, and antifungal agents.[11]

Not all radiation victims will require hospitalization (Fig. 143–8), although, in general, exposures >100 rad may warrant inpatient care. If radiation victims exhibit severe vomiting, they should be admitted. Reverse isolation measures are used for all documented exposures of 200 to 1000 rem and for those patients with absolute lymphocyte counts <1200/mm³ or 50% of the baseline value. Treatment with colony-stimulating factors should be considered for those at risk for developing neutropenia.[8,12] For severely pancytopenic patients, stem cell transplantation is often necessary.[13]

In addition to the hematopoietic complications (infection and bleeding) that may be seen with whole-body radiation >200 to 600 rad, victims may develop significant fluid and electrolyte complications. Any indicated surgery must be performed without delay to avoid these additional problems.

Transfusion of selected blood products is based on the individual hematologic derangement encountered and should follow the usual guidelines for their use.

EXTERNAL CONTAMINATION

External contamination often presents a logistical problem for hospital workers. However, an organized radiation accident plan should facilitate both the logistical and medical management of these patients.[14] Victims of radiation exposure who show no signs of injury and are otherwise healthy may be best served at designated decontaminated facilities. In general, hospital resources should be used for radiation victims who also require medical management.

The process of decontamination, or cleaning the patient of particulate radioactive debris, should be initiated as soon as possible following the event. Rescue personnel must wear protective clothing, including rubber gloves, shoe covers, masks, and film badges. This protective clothing does not reduce the exposure to penetrating radiation. Rather, it serves to prevent any radioactive particles from coming in contact with the personnel or their clothing and to facilitate cleanup and disposal.

Initially, any open wounds are covered and the patient's clothing is removed; all articles are placed in clearly labeled plastic bags. Up to 70% to 90% of external contamination can

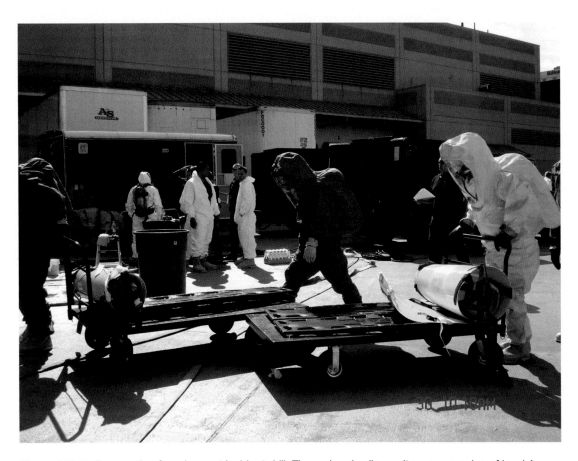

Figure 143-7. Preparation for a hazmat incident drill. The red and yellow suits are examples of level A personal protective equipment which would provide maximal skin and respiratory protection against an unknown hazard. Different colored suits can be used to signify different roles. (Photo courtesy of Ken Williams, MD.)

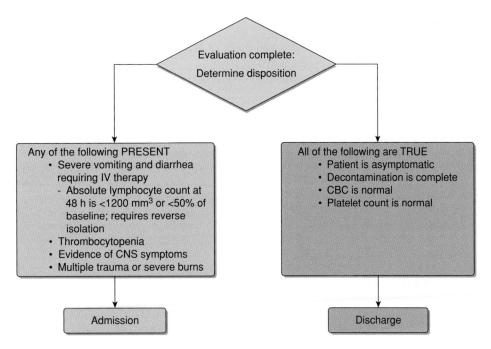

Figure 143-8. Patient Disposition.

be eliminated by this action alone. Any open wound is considered contaminated until proven otherwise, and decontamination should precede the irrigation of intact skin surfaces. The skin is then washed with copious amounts of water and soap, with particular attention to skin folds, ears, and fingernails. The use of damp washcloths, rather than rinsing with running water, may be more practical for some emergency departments. The disposal of contaminated washcloths in plastic bags may be easier than the collection of contaminated wash water. All waste must be captured in sealed containers labeled "Radioactive Waste."

Shaving of the patient's hair is to be avoided, along with excessive rubbing of the skin. Both of these maneuvers cause an increased risk of transdermal uptake. Open, uncontaminated wounds are covered with sterile dressings, and contaminated wounds are then cleaned aggressively, similar to other dirty wounds.

Whenever possible, a dosimeter should be used to determine the completeness of the decontamination. The goal is to get the radiation level "as low as reasonably achievable"; this is commonly referred to as the ALARA principle. When dealing with an external contamination, it is important to prevent it from becoming an internal contamination.

INTERNAL CONTAMINATION

Radioactive particles that are ingested or inhaled or that contaminate open wounds can cause significant cellular damage. These particles will continue to irradiate tissues until they are eliminated, neutralized, or blocked, or until they decay naturally. In general, there is a 1- to 2-hour window of time during which absorption of these particles occurs. Therefore, it is crucial that any interventions be performed during this period and as soon as possible.

At times, it may be difficult to determine the presence of an internal contaminant, especially if an external contaminant still clouds the picture. Clues may include the evidence of contamination around the mouth and nose. In addition, special treatment considerations will be determined by the type of radioactive material involved. Therefore, it is extremely important to identify the offending agent as early as possible, so that specific therapies may be started. These therapies include chelation and ion binding.

Diethylenetriaminepentaacetic acid (DTPA) administered as calcium-DTPA (Ca-DTPA) or zinc-DTPA (Zn-DTPA) are injectable chelators used for decorporation of plutonium and other transuranics (e.g., americium and curium) from the body. The United States Food and Drug Administration (FDA) approved both of these agents in 2004 for this indication.[15] Ca-DTPA should be given as the first dose as Ca-DTPA is more effective than Zn-DTPA during the first 24 hours after internal contamination. However, after the initial 24 hours, Ca-DTPA has no significant advantage over Zn-DTPA. If ongoing treatment is needed or if treatment is initiated over 24 hours after internal contamination, then Zn-DTPA is preferred as Ca-DTPA causes more loss of essential metals.[16]

In 2003, the FDA approved the use of Prussian blue (ferric ferrohexacyanate) for the treatment of known or suspected internal contamination with radioactive cesium and thallium. Thallium and cesium undergo enterohepatic circulation. Prus-

▶ **TABLE 143–6. POTASSIUM IODIDE DOSING**

Age	Daily Dose (mg)
>18 y	130
3–18 y	65
1 mo–3 y	32
Newborn—1 mo	16

Administration of potassium iodide should occur on a daily basis until risk of exposure has passed.

sian blue works by trapping thallium and cesium in the gastrointestinal tract, so that they cannot be reabsorbed. Instead they can be passed out of the body in the stool. By enhancing the elimination of these elements from the body, Prussian blue may reduce the risk of death and major illness from internal radioactive cesium or thallium contamination.[17] Inquiries for acquisition of any of DTPA agents or Prussian blue can be made to REAC/TS at 865–576-1005.

Other specific measures include the use of saturation and blocking. A blocking agent reduces radioactive uptake by saturating the tissues with a nonradioactive element. Potassium iodide (KI) is a blocking agent that reduces the uptake of radioactive iodine (^{131}I) by the thyroid gland. The administration of potassium iodide is most effective at blocking the uptake of radioactive iodine when given soon after exposure. One model demonstrates that potassium iodide would yield protective effects as high as 80% if administered 2 hours after exposure in individuals with an iodine-sufficient diets. However, this benefit would be reduced to 40% when potassium iodide was administered 8 hours after exposure.[18] An estimated thyroid exposure of 5 rad or more warrants the initiation of this treatment.[19] If the diagnosis has not yet been confirmed, there is little harm in administering a first dose of potassium iodine. Indeed, urgent consideration should be given to the administration of this agent to the pediatric population since they are especially vulnerable to radiation-induced thyroid disease.[2] The dose of KI is age dependent (Table 143–6).

A comprehensive list of radioactive agents and their respective treatments is beyond the scope of this text. Detailed and current information can be obtained from REAC/TS or through many poison control centers.

Ingestion

Initial stabilization and decontamination of radiation ingestions are the same as those for "routine" ingestions. In addition to supportive care measures, the goal is to prevent absorption and enhance elimination. Gastric decontamination procedures such as gastric emptying methods and activated charcoal are used in the usual manner. All bodily excretions (lavage fluid, emesis, urine, and feces) should be saved and labeled for radioactive evaluation and proper disposal.

Inhalation

Acute inhalation of radionucleotides is much less common than chronic low-level exposure. An acute inhalation contamination can occur in the event of a radioactive accident in conjunction with a fire or explosion. Radioactive iodine, for example, is highly volatile and likely to be inhaled.

When an inhalation contamination is suspected, a moistened cotton-tipped applicator can be used to swab the nasal passages and check for radioactivity. Bronchopulmonary lavage is performed for removal of particulate matter. Specific-blocking agents and chelating agents should be administered in this setting.

Open Wounds

Wounds that undergo successful decontamination can be surgically closed. Wounds that remain contaminated despite aggressive irrigation are left open for 24 hours. Debridement of these wounds may become necessary for further decontamination. Contaminated surgical instruments must be replaced to prevent further wound contamination.

Amputation of contaminated extremities is rarely indicated. Two situations may warrant this aggressive management. In the first, the amount of persistent contamination is so high that severe radiation-induced necrosis is anticipated. In the second, the degree of traumatic injury is so severe that functional recovery is doubtful.

EXPOSURE

Despite the significant illness and injury that can result from either a local radiation injury or a whole-body exposure, an emergency physician can offer only limited treatment. Aggressive supportive care is the mainstay of treatment for these patients—including fluid resuscitation for severe vomiting and diarrhea, standard trauma and burn care. Prophylactic antimicrobial agents, administration of cytokines, and stem cell transplants are other measures that may help decrease morbidity and mortality. The patient will face the greatest risks and management problems several days to several weeks later, at the onset of the manifest illness stage.

In some cases, nothing will alter the patient's outcome. Victims with a whole-body exposure of >1000 rad will likely die within 2 to 3 weeks.[20] For triage purposes, these patients should be classified as expectant or impending. Death ensues from the complications affecting the hematopoietic system as well as the gastrointestinal and central nervous systems. Emergency department management should consist of appropriate sedation, analgesics, and supportive care.

SPECIAL CONSIDERATION

A nuclear explosion presents logistic and patient care issues that may be difficult to manage effectively. Medical resources may be quickly depleted depending on the number of victims and the magnitude of injuries. To further complicate the situation, routine communications equipment, electronic equipment, and computers may be rendered useless by the electromagnetic pulse generated by the nuclear blast.

Victims of a nuclear explosion will be subject to three types of injury patterns. **Mechanical trauma** (blunt and penetrating) secondary to the blast effect of the explosion accounts for 50% of the released energy while **thermal injury** from heat dissipation represents 35% of the energy release. The remaining 15% of the thermonuclear energy release will cause **radiation injury**, 10% from radioactive fallout and only 5% as a result of the immediate release of γ-rays and neutrons.

▶ PROGNOSIS

The prognosis for survival and the concern for delayed complications, while important, are not of immediate concern to the emergency physician. The possibilities of leukemia, carcinoma, cataracts, accelerated aging, and secondary congenital defects are all issues that should be addressed at a later time, when personnel are available for counseling. Leukemia and delayed thyroid cancer and breast cancer are of significant concern in children <10 years of age.[2,3,21] In utero, exposure to as little as 5 to 10 rad can be associated with mental retardation or a small head circumference. Based on the presenting symptoms, patients can be classified into three major prognostic classifications: *survivor probable*, *survivor possible*, and *survivor improbable*.

SURVIVOR PROBABLE

This group includes individuals who are asymptomatic or who have minimal complaints that resolve within hours. Initial and subsequent leukocyte counts are not affected and estimated exposure is <200 rad (2 Gy). Following satisfactory decontamination, inpatient care is rarely needed.

SURVIVOR POSSIBLE

This group consists of patients with relatively brief gastrointestinal sequelae, usually lasting <48 hours. After initial presentation and the latent period, patients develop characteristic pancytopenia. Estimated exposure for this group is between 200 and 800 rad (2–8 Gy). An exposure of 400 rad represents the median lethal dose. Survival in this group is influenced by the aggressiveness of supportive therapy and hematologic intervention, antecedent health of the victim, and the response to bone-marrow transplantation (when indicated).

SURVIVOR IMPROBABLE

In these patients, the estimated whole-body exposure exceeds 800 rad (8 Gy). The prognosis is dismal despite aggressive supportive therapy and even the implementation of bone-marrow transplantation. If severe nausea, vomiting, and diarrhea begin within 1 hour of exposure and CNS symptoms appear early, a relatively early death can be expected.

REFERENCES

1. American Academy of Pediatrics Committee on Environmental Health. Radiation disasters and children. *Pediatrics.* 2003;111:1455–1466.
2. Astakhova LN, et al. Chernobyl-related thyroid cancer in children of Belarus: a case-control study. *Radiat Res.* 1998;150: 349–356.
3. Miller RW. Special susceptibility of the child to certain radiation-induced cancers. *Environ Health Perspect.* 1995;103 (suppl 6):41–44.

4. Somasundaram DJ, van de Put WACM. Management of trauma in special populations after a disaster. *J Clin Psychiatry.* 2006;67 (suppl 2):64–73.

5. Recommendations of the National Council on Radiation Protection and Measurements. Ionizing radiation exposure of the population of the United States. NCRP report; no. 93. Bethesda, MD; 1987.

6. Gottlöber P et al. The outcome of local radiation injuries: 14 years of follow-up after the Chernobyl accident. *Radiat Res.* 2001;155:409–416.

7. Chambers JA, Long JN. Radiation injury and the hand surgeon. *J Hand Surg.* 2008;33:601–611.

8. Waselenko JK et al. Medical management of the acute radiation syndrome: recommendations of the Strategic National Stockpile Radiation Working Group. *Ann Intern Med.* 2004;140: 1037–1051.

9. Goans RE et al. Early dose assessment in criticality accidents. *Health Phys.* 2001;81:446–449.

10. *Medical Management of Radiological Casualties Handbook.* 2nd ed. Bethesda, MD: Armed Forces Radiobiology Research Institute; 2003.

11. Jarrett D et al. Medical treatment of radiation injuries—current U. S. status. *Radiat Meas.* 2007;42:1063–1074.

12. Koenig K et al. Medical Treatment of radiological casualties: current concepts. *Ann Emerg Med.* 2005;45:643–652.

13. Dainiak N. The evolving role of haematopoietic cell transplantation in radiation injury: potentials and limitations. *Br J Radiol.* 2005;27:169–174.

14. Cone DC, Koenig KL. Mass casualty triage in the chemical, biological, radiological, or nuclear environment. *Europ J Emerg Med.* 2005;12:287–302.

15. US Food and Drug Administration, Center for Drug Evaluation and Research. FDA Approves Drugs to Treat Internal Contamination from Radioactive Elements. http://www.fda.gov/bbs/topics/news/2004/NEW01103.html. Accessed April 2008.

16. US Food and Drug Administration, Center for Drug Evaluation and Research. Calcium-DTPA and Zinc-DTPA Questions and Answers. http://www.fda.gov/Cder/drug/infopage/DTPA/QandA_DTPA.htm. Accessed April 2008.

17. US Food and Drug Administration, Center for Drug Evaluation and Research. Questions and Answers on Prussian Blue. http://www.fda.gov/cder/drug/infopage/prussian_blue/Q&A.htm. Accessed April 2008.

18. Zanzonico PB, Becker DV. Effects of time of administration and dietary iodine levels on potassium iodide (KI) blockade of thyroid irradiation by 131I from radioactive fallout. *Health Phy.* 2000;78:660–667.

19. US Food and Drug Administration, Center for Drug Evaluation and Research. Potassium Iodide as a Thyroid Blocking Agent in Radiation Emergencies. http://www.fda.gov/cder/guidance/4825fnl.htm. Accessed April 2008.

20. Mettler FA, Voelz GL. Major radiation exposure–what to expect and how to respond. *N Engl J Med.* 2002;346:1554–1561.

21. Prysyazhnyuk A et al. Twenty years after the Chernobyl accident: solid cancer incidence in various groups of the Ukrainian population. *Radiat Environ Biophys.* 2007;46:43–51.

SECTION XXI

PSYCHOSOCIAL EMERGENCIES

CHAPTER 144

Sexual Abuse

Sara L. Beers and Matthew Cox

▶ HIGH-YIELD FACTS

- Most sexual abuse examinations in children are normal even with known sexual abuse.
- The history is usually the most important piece of evidence in cases of suspected sexual abuse in children.
- All 50 states require reporting suspected child abuse including sexual abuse to a proper investigatory agency (child protective services and/or law enforcement).
- Sexually transmitted diseases are extremely rare in cases of pediatric sexual abuse.
- Screening for and empiric treatment of sexually transmitted diseases is not routinely recommended in cases of pediatric sexual abuse.
- Forensic evaluation is recommended by the American Academy of Pediatrics (AAP) when the abuse occurred within the previous 72 hours.
- Speculum examinations are not indicated in preadolescent female sexual abuse patients. A thorough external genital examination is sufficient.

▶ ETIOLOGY

The National Center on Child Abuse and Neglect defines child sexual abuse as "contact or interaction between a child and an adult when a child is being used for the sexual stimulation of that adult or another person. Sexual abuse may also be committed by another minor when that person is either significantly older than the victim or when the abuser is in a position of power or control over that child." Contact forms of child sexual abuse include fondling the child's genitals, getting the child to fondle an adult's genitals, mouth to genital contact, rubbing an adult's genitals on the child, or actually penetrating the child's vagina or anus. Noncontact forms of child sexual abuse include showing an adult's genitals to a child, showing the child pornographic material, or using the child as a model to make pornographic material.

Sexual abuse of children is a very real problem in our society. Children are most often abused by adults or older children who are known to them and who can exert power over them. The victim knows the offender in 8 out of 10 reported cases.[1] The offender can be a family member or a nonfamily member and is more frequently male.[2] The offender is frequently someone that the child trusts and will often persuade the child with bribes, tricks, or coercion to engage in sex or sexual acts. This can be followed by threats to the child if he or she tells.

Increased risk for sexual abuse of children is not related to socioeconomic status or race.[3] Family risk factors associated retrospectively with child sexual abuse include poor parent–child relationships, poor relationships between parents, absence of a protective parent, and presence of a nonbiologically related male in the house.[3]

▶ EPIDEMIOLOGY

Sexual abuse affects approximately 100,000 children each year in the United States.[4] Most abuse goes unreported during childhood. However, it is estimated that 20% of girls and 9% of boys are the victims of sexual abuse during childhood.[1,3] Children of all ages are the victims of sexual abuse, but are most likely to be abused sexually during preadolescence, that is, from ages 8 to 12 years.[3]

▶ PATHOGENESIS

The vast majority of children who are the victims of sexual abuse will have normal examinations without findings of injury. Studies have found that both normal-appearing genital tissues and nonspecific findings are seen in children known to be sexually abused.[5–7] Kellogg et al. found that of 36 adolescents who were pregnant at the time of or shortly before a sexual abuse examination, 22 (62%) had normal or nonspecific examination findings. Only 2 of these 36 girls (6%) had definitive findings consistent with penetration.[8]

There are many factors that contribute to the majority of examinations being normal even in the face of proven sexual abuse. Most sexual abuse of children occurs without the use of physical force and restraint. The perpetrator generally has no intent of harming the child physically because of a desire to reengage the child in the activities over time. A second point that contributes to the majority of children who are victims of sexual abuse having normal examinations is that fact that anogenital tissue heals very quickly. Studies of the healing process of the anogenital area consistently report that most injuries resulting from sexual abuse heal relatively quickly.[8–12] McCann et al. found that the healing of nonhymenal genital injuries in girls was as short as 24 hours for petechia, 2 days for bruising, 3 days for abrasions, and 5 days for edema.[12] Therefore, with frequent delays in disclosure of sexual abuse, injuries that may have been present at the time of the abuse will often have healed by the time the child undergoes a physical examination. Another factor that contributes to a lack of physical findings in children who are victims of sexual abuse is that genital tissues are mucosal tissues that are elastic in nature, well-vascularized, and heal quickly without scarring, making the tissues less prone to permanent tissue injury. This point is particularly pertinent to girls who are undergoing pubertal changes with the presence of estrogen that creates thicker and more redundant tissues, particularly thicker and more redundant hymenal tissue. A final note on the topic of "normal" examinations in children who have been sexually abused is specific to the anus. Because the anus can enlarge to large diameters to pass bowel movements, injuries to the anus from penetrating abuse are infrequent.[13]

When a child does have physical injuries from sexual abuse, the findings can involve the genitalia, anus, oral cavity, extragenital sites, or any combination of the above. These injuries might include superficial abrasions, bruises, tearing of the hymen, or deeper genital injury. In prepubertal girls, the most common genital injuries include superficial abrasions of the inner aspects of the labia minora, the periurethral area, and the posterior fourchette.[13] If an object such as a finger or penis has penetrated through the hymenal orifice, an interruption of the integrity of the hymenal edge may occur. If the hymenal tissue is thought of as the face of a clock (with the child in the supine position), the findings of the hymenal tissue from 3- to 9-o'clock positions are particularly noteworthy when assessing for injuries from abuse. Interruptions, lacerations, or injuries to the hymenal tissue may extend into the vagina or through the fossa navicularis, and in cases of extreme blunt force trauma, may extend onto the perineum.

Accidental straddle injuries on playground equipment, toys, furniture, etc., often result in physical injuries. Key in discerning such injuries from sexual abuse is that straddle injuries typically include injury to the clitoris, clitoral hood, mons pubis, and labia. Also important to note is that straddle injuries are usually asymmetric and do not involve the hymen.[3] Conversely, the posterior fourchette, fossa navicularis, and posterior hymen are the structures/area that are injured with penetrating traumatic events.[3]

Table 144–1 summarizes the guidelines and approach to interpreting physical and laboratory findings in suspected child abuse developed by a group of physician experts who met at child abuse conferences yearly between 2002 and 2005 and was published by Joyce Adams, MD, et al. in the *Journal of Pediatric and Adolescent Gynecology* in 2007. Figures 144–1 to 144–8 illustrate a variety of physical examination findings ranging from normal variants to findings diagnostic of trauma.

▶ RECOGNITION

Most of the time, when there is a concern of sexual abuse of a child presenting to a medical provider, the concern arises when a child discloses the abuse to an adult or a peer. Alternatively, the concern of sexual abuse arises when a parent or caregiver is concerned by an abnormal appearance of a child's anus or genitals, injury to a child's anus or genitals, or concern of bleeding or discharge from a child's anus or genitals. Behavior changes in a child may also alert a guardian or other caregiver of possible sexual abuse of a child. These may include sexual acting out behaviors, sleep disturbances, nightmares, enure-

sis and encopresis in previously potty-trained children, eating disturbances, and/or tantrums.

There will be a subset of sexually abused children that present to medical attention that do not come with a chief compliant of suspected sexual abuse. They may present with a variety of symptoms ranging from anogenital pain, itching, bleeding or discharge, abdominal pain, dysuria, constipation, and/or painful defecation. Much like physical abuse, sexual abuse must be included on the differential diagnosis of emergency medicine physicians and primary care providers who treat children. It is most important to remember that sexual abuse of children crosses all socioeconomic statuses and ethnicities.

In order to recognize abnormal genital findings on physical examination, medical providers must be able to recognize normal genital examinations. Familiarity with normal genital anatomy is an area of weakness of many physicians. Lentsch et al. reported surveys of pediatricians, family practitioners, and emergency department physicians that included photographs about genital anatomy. In the 1986 survey, only 59.1% of responding physicians correctly identified the hymen and 78.4% identified the urethra. Ten years later, the knowledge was not significantly improved, with only 61.7% identifying the hymen and 72.4% identifying the urethra.[14] In girls, it is important for the clinician to perform a detailed external genital examination noting the appearance of the genital structures including the labia majora, labia minora, urethral meatus, posterior fourchette, fossa navicularis, and the hymen (Fig. 144–9). The genital structures can have varied appearance based on the age and physical development of the patient. In both sexes, the examiner should externally visualize the anal opening, noting the anal folds and rectal tone.

Physician and medical providers who care for children must be able to identify other medical conditions in children that may present as possible sexual abuse. These conditions often cause anogenital pruritus and/or irritation. The genital area can be more susceptible to chemical and mechanical trauma compared to other areas of the body. Various soaps, shampoos, and lotions may cause chemical irritation. Restrictive clothing may lead to mechanical trauma. Poor hygiene can lead to fecal contamination and cause pruritus. Pinworms and scabies can present as pruritus of the anogenital area. Atopic dermatitis is rarely limited to the anogenital region, but can be part of a generalized eruption. Vulvar lichen sclerosus et atrophicus (LS) presents as hypopigmented, atrophic cutaneous tissue symmetrically distributed in an hourglass pattern around the vagina and anus. Its etiology is unknown but more commonly effects prepubertal and postmenopausal woman. Seborrheic dermatitis, presenting with waxy yellowish scales on an erythematous base, can involve the folds of the vulva in diapered infants. Psoriasis of the vulva is not uncommon and presents as erythematous, well-marginated patches with a red hue covered by grayish scales. Perianal streptococcal dermatitis is a bright red, sharply demarcated tender rash that affects children between 6 months and 10 years of age. It often follows a group A beta-hemolytic throat infection. Candidiasis is uncommon in healthy prepubertal girls, but can be associated with oral antibiotics, diabetes mellitus, and immunodeficiency. Peripubertal and pubertal girls can develop vaginal candidal infections that present with pruritus, inflammation, and a thick white discharge.

▶ TABLE 144–1. APPROACH TO INTERPRETING PHYSICAL AND LABORATORY FINDINGS IN SUSPECTED CHILD SEXUAL ABUSE

Normal Variants	Nonspecific Findings (Caused by Other Medical Conditions)	Indeterminate Findings*	Findings Diagnostic of Sexual Abuse or Trauma†
Periurethral or vestibular bands	Erythema of the vestibule, penis, scrotum, or perianal tissues	Deep notches or clefts in the posterior/inferior rim of the hymen in prepubertal girls	Acute lacerations of extensive bruising of labia, penis, scrotum, perianal tissues or perineum
Intravaginal ridges or columns	Increased vascularity of the vestibule and hymen	Deep notches or complete clefts in the hymen at 3- or 9-o'clock positions in adolescent girls	Fresh laceration of the posterior fourchette, not involving the hymen
Hymenal bumps or mounds	Labial adhesion	Smooth, noninterrupted rim of hymen between 4- and 8-o'clock positions, which appears to be less than 1-mm wide in the prone knee–chest position	Perianal scars
Hymenal tags or septal remnants	Vaginal discharge	Wart-like lesions in the genital or anal area	Scar of the posterior fourchette or fossa
Linea vestibularis (midline avascular area)	Friability of the posterior fourchette or commissure	Vascular lesions or ulcers in the genital or anal area	Laceration (tear, partial or complete) of the hymen, acute
Hymenal notch/cleft in the anterior (superior) half of hymenal rim (on or above the 3–9-o'clock positions)	Excoriations/bleeding vascular lesions	Marked immediate anal dilation to a diameter of 2 cm or more (in the absence of other predisposing factors: sedation, constipation, neuromuscular disorder)	Ecchymosis on the hymen (in the absence of known infectious process or coagulopathy)
Shallow/superficial notch or cleft in the inferior rim of the hymen (below 3–9-o'clock positions)	Perineal groove	Confirmed genital or anal Condyloma accuminata	Perianal lacerations extending deep to the external anal sphincter
External hymenal ridge	Anal fissures	Confirmed genital or anal herpes type 1 or 2	Hymenal transection (healed) between 4- and 8-o'clock positions on the rim of the hymen with virtually no hymen tissue left in this area
Congenital variants in the appearance of the hymen (crescent, annular, redundant, septate, cribriform, microperforate, and imperforate)	Venous congestion or venous pooling in the perianal area		Missing segment of hymenal tissue in the posterior (inferior) half of the hymen, wider than a transection
Diastasis ani (smooth area)	Flattening anal folds		Positive confirmed culture for gonorrhea (outside of neonatal period from genitals, anus, or throat)
Perianal skin tag	Partial or complete anal dilation to less than 2 cm with or without stool visible		Confirmed diagnosis of syphilis (if perinatal transmission ruled out)
Hyperpigmentation of the skin of labia minora or perianal tissues in children of color, i.e., African American			Tichomonas vaginalis (in child older than 1 y of age)

(continued)

▶ **TABLE 144–1. (CONTINUED) APPROACH TO INTERPRETING PHYSICAL AND LABORATORY FINDINGS IN SUSPECTED CHILD SEXUAL ABUSE**

Normal Variants	Nonspecific Findings (Caused by Other Medical Conditions)	Indeterminate Findings*	Findings Diagnostic of Sexual Abuse or Trauma†
Dilation of urethral opening with application of labial traction Thickened hymen			Positive culture for Chlamydia (in child older than 3 y of age using cell culture) Positive serology for HIV (if perinatal or transmission from blood products/needle contamination has been ruled out) Pregnancy Sperm identified in specimens taken directly from the child's body

*Findings may support a child's clear disclosure or sexual abuse, if one is given, but should be interpreted with caution with no disclosure.

†These anogenital findings support a disclosure of sexual abuse, if one is given, and are highly suggestive of abuse in the absence of a disclosure, unless the child and/or caretaker provide a clear timely plausible description of an accidental injury. Pregnancy and identified sperm are diagnostic of mucosal contact with infected genital secretions. In children, this contact is most likely to have been sexual.

▶ MANAGEMENT

The management of the child with suspected sexual abuse involves both medical management and legal management. All cases of suspected sexual abuse in children are required by law to be reported to child protective services (CPS) and law enforcement. Often a hospital's social worker is involved and helps with reporting the suspected abuse to law enforcement and CPS. The discussion in this chapter focuses on the medical management of suspected child sexual abuse.

All children should have an immediate medical evaluation if the abuse was within the previous 72 hours or there is bleeding or concern of acute injury. Many communities have designated child sexual abuse teams utilizing specialized nurses, nurse practitioners, and/or physicians that can be a resource for these evaluations. Otherwise, if the child is safe and without symptoms, an appointment can be made with at the next earliest convenience with the child's regular health care provider.

The emergency department evaluation should begin with an interview of the adult accompanying the child. This interview should take place away from the child. Key information to obtain includes why abuse is suspected, to whom did the child disclose to, what the child said, the type of contact the child described, the timing of the last possible abuse, behavior changes, medical concerns, who lives at home with the child, who cares for the child, and anything the adult has witnessed.

Next, the child should be interviewed. If possible, it is recommended that children with a developmental age of 3 or older should be interviewed alone.[15] Having the family leave the room for the interview will often allow the child to open up more without the fear of upsetting the family or getting into trouble. The interview of the child should take place in a child-friendly area that is free of distraction. Ideally the interviewer

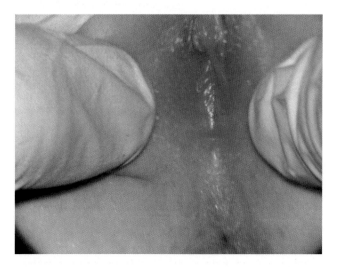

Figure 144–1. Labial adhesion; nonspecific finding.

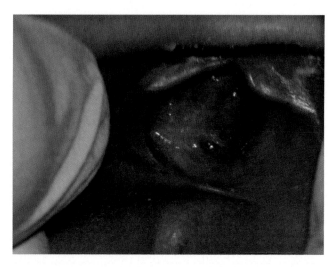

Figure 144–2. Imperforate hymen; congenital variant.

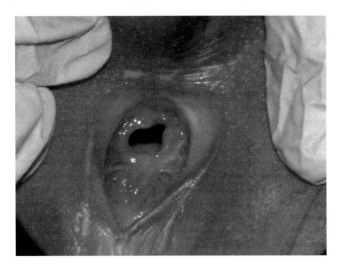

Figure 144–3. Cleft at 7-o'clock position with child in prone knee–chest position; indeterminate finding.

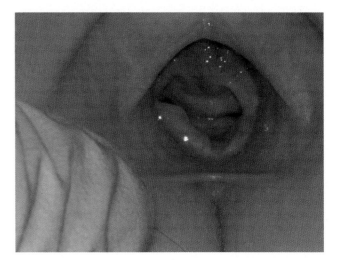

Figure 144–5. Healed hymenal transection at 6-o'clock position; diagnostic of trauma.

should use open-ended nonleading questions. "W" words (who, what, where, when, and how) are recommended. However, "why" questions should be avoided because they may imply blame on the child. If a skilled social worker has already obtained a detailed history from the child, the physician's interview can be abbreviated. Occasionally, further questioning of a child can be deleterious. The child may find repetitive questioning unpleasant or threatening, may infer that he or she is not believed, or may modify his or her history in response to repetitive questioning.[3] The history taken from the child is often the most important part of the overall evaluation. Great detail should be taken when documenting the history provided, with actual quotes from the child when possible. Upon finishing the interview, the child should be told that he or she did the right thing by telling.

Older children should be asked who they want to be in the room for the examination. This should be asked of the child without family members present. The examination should begin with a general physical examination. Prepubertal children

should not have a speculum examination. A detailed external genital examination is sufficient. There are several examination techniques when performing a genital examination. Younger children may be more comfortable and cooperative if seated in a caregiver's lap. Children 3 years of age and older usually tolerate being placed on an examination table.[16] The two most common examination techniques are the supine frog-leg position (the child lies with legs in full abduction and feet in apposition) and the prone knee–chest position (the child kneels on hands and knees and then places his or her head and chest on the examination table). In female patients, utilization of the labial separation and labial traction techniques allows complete visualization of the vulvar structures. This is done by gently grasping the labia majora and pulling the labia outward (toward the examiner) and laterally. Any abnormal finding noted in the supine position should be verified in the knee–chest position because the change in positioning can alter the appearance of the hymenal edge.[16] Male patients can

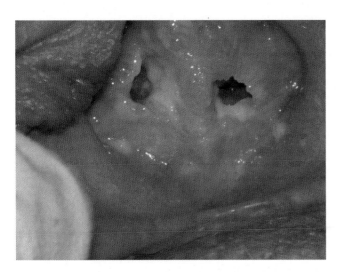

Figure 144–4. Septate hymen; congenital variant.

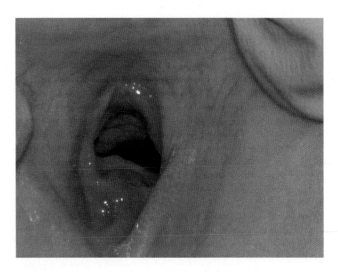

Figure 144–6. Same child as in Figure 144–5 in the prone knee–chest position.

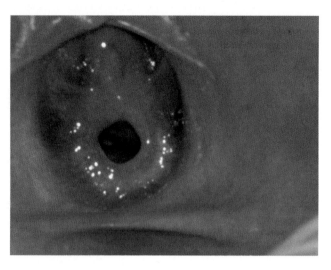

Figure 144–7. Periurethral bands and annular hymen; normal variant.

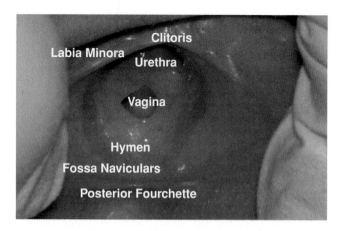

Figure 144–9. Normal anatomy with labels.

be examined in supine or prone positions. An examination of the perianal area is important in both female and male patients. This can be done in either the supine or lateral decubitus positions. The presence of stool in the vault or traction on the anus can cause the anus to dilate. Anal dilation of more than 2 cm without stool in the vault (this can be determined with direct visualization or less commonly a digital examination) may be concerning for possible abuse. As with the history, physical examination findings must be carefully and thoroughly documented in the medical record. Photographic documentation is strongly encouraged, particularly if the examination findings are thought to be abnormal.

In cases with suspected intravaginal injuries or active bleeding without an obvious external source, the internal vaginal examination should be performed only on prepubescent patients using general anesthesia and often requires consultation with a general surgeon who has expertise in examining and treating children.[17]

The AAP recommends forensic evidence collection if the evaluation is within 72 hours of the sexual abuse.[15] However, the yield from such evidence collection significantly drops off after 24 hours. In a study done by Christian et al., no swabs taken from a child's body were positive for blood after 13 hours or sperm/semen after 9 hours.[18] It is important that only medical providers who are experienced in the collection and preservation of forensic evidence perform a forensic evaluation. Part of a forensic evaluation requires that the child's clothing be collected and placed in a paper bag. Evidence must be collected and stored properly as it may be used as evidence in legal proceedings.

Universal screening for sexually transmitted diseases (STDs) is not necessary because the incidence of STDs among children who have been sexually abused is low. The Centers for Disease Control and Prevention (CDC) recommend testing for STDs in the following situations: when the child has had symptoms or signs of an STD, when a suspected assailant is known to have an STD or to be at high risk for STDs, when a sibling or another child or adult in the household or child's immediate environment has an STD, when the patient or parent requests testing, or when evidence of genital, oral, or anal penetration or ejaculation is present.[19] In nonacute evaluations, careful examinations without STD screening may be acceptable for asymptomatic, prepubertal children who lack clear history or physical examination findings indicative of penetrating sexual abuse.[3]

Enzyme-linked assays or DNA amplification tests, such as nucleic acid amplification tests (NAAT), for *Chlamydia trachomatis* and *Neisseria gonorrhoeae* can be utilized for noninvasive screening. Currently, the lack of sufficient clinical studies in prepubescent patients and the risk of false positive test results limit the utility of these tests for forensic purposes. Routine bacterial and cell cultures remain the gold standard for diagnosis of bacterial STDs. Swabs taken from the external genitalia are sufficient in prepubertal female patients. In adolescent female patients with history of rape, a speculum examination with cervical cultures is recommended. Again, while the vast minority of sexually abused children will not require STD screening, when cultures are warranted, cultures should also be taken from the throat and rectum. Blood tests for syphilis, HIV, hepatitis B and C should also be considered in high-risk cases.

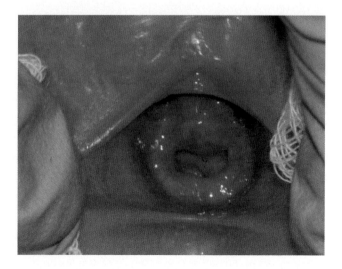

Figure 144–8. Crescentic hymen; normal variant.

Empiric treatment for STDs is usually not necessary. However, empiric treatment may be considered in cases of stranger assaults as well as in adolescent rape victims. Identified STDs should be treated with the appropriate regimens according to the published guidelines set by the CDC (see Chapter 97).

Treatment should include routine follow-up with a primary care provider. In cases with positive examination findings, close medical follow-up to assess healing of injuries is warranted. Follow-up visits can also provide opportunity to assess the need for further screening for STDs. Some infections may not have had time to manifest symptoms at the time of initial assessment. This follow-up with the child's pediatrician or outpatient child abuse clinic can also ensure that the child and family are receiving any needed counseling services.

▶ ANCILLARY STUDIES

Colposcopy provides a noninvasive method for visualizing the anogenital structures. It provides magnification and a light source, both of which can be helpful in identifying injury. The colposcope also allows a video or photograph to be taken for documentation. Photodocumentation of the anogenital examination can provide a means for quality enhancement programs (peer review) and help limit unnecessary repeat examinations.

Alternative light sources can be used during forensic evidence collection to guide collection of possible body fluids on victims. Alternative light sources include the Blue Max 6000 or a Wood's lamp. It is important to note though that material other than semen may also fluoresce with a Wood's lamp.

REFERENCES

1. American Academy of Pediatrics. *Child Abuse and Negl.* 2000. http://www.aap.org. Accessed March 2008.
2. Kellog N; Committee on Child Abuse and Neglect. AAP Clinical Report. *Pediatrics.* 2005;116(2):506–512.
3. Hymel K, Jenny C. Child sexual abuse. *Pediatr Rev.* 1996;17(7):236–249.
4. U.S. Department of Health and Human Services. *Natl Clgh Child Abuse Negl Inf.* 2004. http://www.hhs.gov. Accessed March 2008.
5. Adams JA, Harper K, Knudson S, et al. Examination findings in legally confirmed child sexual abuse: it's normal to be normal. *Pediatrics.* 1994;94(3):310–317.
6. Heger A, Ticson L, Velasquez O, et al. Children referred for possible sexual abuse: medical findings in 2384 children. *Child Abuse Negl.* 2002;26(6–7):645–659.
7. Botash AS. Examination for sexual abuse in prepubertal children: an update. *Pediatr Ann.* 1997;26(5):312–320.
8. Kellogg ND, Menard SW, Santos A. Genital anatomy in pregnant adolescents: "normal" does not mean "nothing happened." *Pediatrics.* 2004;3(1):67–69.
9. McCann J, Voris J, Simon M. Genital injuries resulting from sexual abuse; a longitudinal study. *Pediatrics.* 1992;89(2):307–317.
10. Finkel MA. Anogenital trauma in sexually abused children. *Pediatrics.* 1989;84(2):317–322.
11. Herger AH, McConnell G, Ticson L, et al. Healing patterns in anogenital injuries associated with sexual abuse, accidental injuries, or genital surgery in the preadolescent child. *Pediatrics.* 2003;112(4):829–837.
12. McCann J, Miyamoto S, Boyle C, Rogers K. Healing of non-hymenal genital injuries in prepubertal and adolescent girls: a descriptive study. *Pediatrics.* 2007;20(5):1000–1011.
13. Giardino A, Finkel M. Evaluating child sexual abuse. *Pediatr Ann.* 2005;34(5):382–394.
14. Lentsch KA, Johnson CF. Do physicians have adequate knowledge of child sexual abuse? The results of two surveys of practicing physicians, 1986 and 1996. *Child Maltreatment.* 2000;5:72–78.
15. American Academy of Pediatrics Committee on Child Abuse and Neglect. Guidelines for the evaluation of sexual abuse of children: subject review. *Pediatrics.* 1999;103(1):186–191.
16. Girardet R, Lahoti S, Parks D, et al. Issues in pediatric sexual abuse-what we know and where we need to go. *Curr Probl Pediatr Adolesc Health Care.* 2002;32:211–246.
17. Adams J, Kaplan R, Starling S, et al. Guidelines for medical care of children who may have been sexually abused. *J Pediatr Adolesc Gynecol.* 2007;20:163–172.
18. Christian C, Lavelle J, De Jong A, et al. Forensic evidence findings in prepubertal victims of sexual assault. *Pediatrics.* 2000;106(1):100–107.
19. Centers for Disease Control and Prevention. *Sexually Transmitted Diseases Treatment Guidelines 2006.* Atlanta, GA: Centers for Disease Control and Prevention. Department of Health and Human Services. 2006. http://www.cdc.gov/std/treatment/2006/sexual-assualt.htm. Accessed March 2008.

CHAPTER 145

Abuse and Neglect

Matthew Cox and Sara L. Beers

► HIGH-YIELD FACTS

- Identifying child abuse is challenging because the histories provided are typically inaccurate, nonspecific physical examination findings predominate, and physicians fail to include child abuse in their differential diagnosis.
- A careful, complete medical evaluation and detailed documentation are important components in cases of suspected child abuse.
- A key aspect in making a diagnosis of physical abuse is identifying the incompatibility of the history of trauma with the injuries identified.
- Skeletal injuries, such as metaphyseal corner fractures and posterior rib fractures, have a high specificity for inflicted injury and child abuse.
- Abusive head trauma encompasses a spectrum of abnormalities including subdural hematomas, skull fracture, and retinal hemorrhages.
- Neglect is the most common type of maltreatment reported. Neglect encompasses medical, supervisional, educational, physical, and nutritional forms.
- Physicians should *consider* child abuse in the differential diagnosis of all children presenting with injuries.

► EPIDEMIOLOGY

Child maltreatment is a serious cause of morbidity and mortality affecting young children in the United States and around the world. Child physical abuse is physical harm to a child at the hands of a caregiver that may encompass a single incident or repeated incidents.[1] Examples of physical abuse include abusive head trauma (the "shaken baby syndrome"), immersion burns, skeletal injuries, and inflicted, patterned bruises. According to recent data in *Child Maltreatment 2006*, there were 3.3 million referrals to child welfare agencies in the United States in 2006. Investigation into these referrals revealed abuse in 30% cases, involving nearly 1 million children. It is estimated that in 2006, there were more than 1500 deaths in the United States related to abuse and neglect.[2] Abuse is ranked as the third leading cause of homicide in children older than 1 year of age. The youngest children are most at risk for being abused. It is important to note that more than one-third of child abuse fatalities were involved with child welfare agencies prior to the child's death. This fact highlights the critical nature of a complete medical evaluation, thorough documentation, and communication with the child welfare system investigators. Children commonly present initially to an emergency department with injuries or medical problems caused by abuse and neglect. Thus, it is imperative that emergency health care professionals have knowledge of the function and mechanics of the child welfare system within their community, and have protocols for the evaluation and treatment of children suspected of being abused or neglected.

The spectrum of child abuse and neglect is broad and includes physical abuse (16%), sexual abuse (9%), emotional abuse (6.6%), and neglect (60%). There are many manifestations of neglect including medical, supervisional, physical, nutritional, and emotional forms. The broad spectrum of child abuse and neglect can range from clearly inflicted injuries pathognomonic for abuse to suspicious scenarios and injuries that warrant further investigation by the local child protection agency. The diagnosis of child abuse depends on information obtained from the medical history, physical examination, and injuries identified by ancillary studies. It is critical that a detailed medical record is kept in cases of suspected abuse, since this information would be frequently used by investigating agencies such as the police and child protection services. This chapter delineates the types of abuse most commonly seen in the emergency department, describes historical and physical indicators to help differentiate inflicted from noninflicted injuries, describes diagnostic studies useful in the medical evaluation, and discusses the legal obligations to report suspected abuse and neglect. It is vital that emergency medical care providers recognize, evaluate, and report suspected child abuse and neglect in order to facilitate the safety and well-being of children.

► ETIOLOGY

Child abuse and neglect is a complicated medical and social problem. It affects all aspects of society. A number of risk factors have been identified that are associated with child abuse, some more consistently than others; these are important when obtaining a history. Parental risk factors linked to child abuse are maternal age less than 19 years, single marital status, late or no prenatal care, parental depression, and lack of maternal education.[3] Other factors that are well documented to be associated with child maltreatment include parental substance abuse, parental mental illness, and domestic violence.

Risk factors for physical abuse involving children include male gender and young age. Prematurity, chronic illness, and congenital abnormalities are also considered to increase the child's risk of maltreatment. Children with physical disabilities and behavioral problems are at increased risk for abuse. Fatal child abuse is most common among children in the first year of life. Children who live in poverty are overrepresented in the child welfare and foster care systems.[4]

The environment in which a child resides may also place him or her at risk for abuse. There is a well-known and well-documented relationship between domestic violence and child abuse. Children sustain a wide range of physical injuries from family violence. Screening for domestic violence is an important aspect of the evaluation of child abuse. The American Academy of Pediatrics (AAP) supports universal screening of mothers for domestic violence as an active form of child abuse prevention.[5] Other environmental factors such as large family size and low family income have been identified as risk factors for physical abuse.

Risk factors should be considered as broadly defined markers rather than findings diagnostic of abuse and neglect. For physicians, it is imperative to consider child abuse in the differential diagnosis of any child who presents with injuries or illness that may have resulted from family violence or dysfunction regardless of race, socioeconomic class, or other perceived risk factors for abuse.

▶ RECOGNITION

Child physical abuse occurs when a caretaker inflicts an injury. Injuries can be manifested as cutaneous lesions, such as bruises, burns, whip marks, and bites, as musculoskeletal trauma, including fractures, as abusive head trauma, or as visceral trauma. In some cases, the patient may suffer an isolated injury. Unfortunately, many abused patients have been victimized repeatedly, resulting in numerous injuries of various ages.

MEDICAL HISTORY

One of the key elements in the evaluation of child abuse is the history provided by the caregiver and the child. An important diagnostic clue to the presence of child abuse is a discrepancy between the clinical findings and historical data supplied by the parents. The history provided by the adult accompanying the child is often inaccurate because the adult is either unaware of what happened to the child or is the perpetrator of the abuse, and is therefore unwilling to provide a truthful version of events. Victims of serious physical abuse are often too young or too ill to provide a history of their assault. Older victims may be too scared or intimidated to do so. A detailed history that is consistent with the child's injuries can help distinguish accidental from inflicted injury. Medical conditions that mimic abuse need to be considered in the differential diagnosis, so that proper treatment can be instituted and families are not inappropriately accused of malfeasance. Hettler and Greenes reviewed the diagnostic utility of certain historical features for identifying cases of abusive head trauma. They found some features to have high specificity and positive predictive value for diagnosing child abuse. These include a lack of history of trauma, a history of low-impact trauma in patients with persistent neurologic deficits, changing histories, and trauma blamed on home resuscitative efforts.[6]

In order to improve the identification of child abuse, it is important to consider inflicted injury in the differential diagnosis list of all pediatric injuries. There are some historical and

▶ **TABLE 145–1. HISTORICAL AND EXAMINATION FINDINGS SUGGESTIVE OF ABUSE**

Features suggestive of abuse
- History inconsistent with injuries
- History incompatible with child's development
- History that changes with time
- Contradictory histories
- Delay in seeking treatment
- Pathognomonic injuries (such as forced immersion burn, multiple fractures in different stages of healing)

physical examination features that offer clues to the diagnosis of inflicted injury (Table 145–1).

The history recorded should include the location, time, and mechanism of any injury. It is also important to identify the caretakers at the time of the injury and the composition of the household. Denial of trauma should also be carefully documented. If the child is verbal, the child should be interviewed separately from the parents.

PHYSICAL EXAMINATION

A thorough physical examination is vital in all cases of suspected child abuse. Findings indicative of abuse may be found incidentally during a routine physical examination or during an examination specifically intended to look for injuries.

The physical examination of a child with suspected inflicted injuries must be complete and all identified injuries should be carefully documented. The child should always be completely undressed. In older children, allow them to undress and put on a hospital gown while you step out of the room. In infants, subtle external injuries are often a clue to a more serious internal injury.[7] Approximately 50% of children intentionally injured will have injuries to the head and neck. These injuries include ecchymoses, abrasions, and oral injuries.[8] Bruises on the face and ears are highly concerning and warrant a detailed medical examination and evaluation. Oral injuries might include torn frenula, lacerations to the mucosal surfaces or palate, and dental trauma. Tears of the frenulum are highly suspicious in children who are not yet ambulatory. These injuries may occur from a blow to the face or from an object such as a pacifier, spoon, or bottle being forced into an infant's mouth. Bruises, burns, and scars should be measured, and their size, shape, location, and color carefully documented. Photographs are important adjuncts to the recorded physical examination and are not a substitute for accurate medical documentation. Verbal children should be asked about the cause of injuries, and physical findings should be discussed with family members. This will allow the family to explain the injury.

▶ CUTANEOUS INJURIES

The organ system with the highest number of inflicted injuries is the skin. These injuries include burns, bruises, lacerations, and abrasions. Burns are the most serious form of inflicted skin injury because they can be quite deep and involve large areas of a child's skin. Only a minority of pediatric burns are due

▶ TABLE 145–2. TEMPERATURES REQUIRED TO CAUSE FULL-THICKNESS BURNS

Temperature of Water in Degrees Celsius (Degrees Fahrenheit)	Duration of Exposure
44 (111)	360 min
45 (113)	180 min
47 (116)	40 min
48 (118)	15 min
49 (120)	10 min
51 (124)	6 min
53 (127)	30 s
55 (131)	30 s
60 (140)	3 s

to child abuse.[9] The most important aspect of evaluating suspected abusive burns is correlating the history with the physical examination findings. The clinician should ask the question: does the mechanism make sense? Other important factors to consider are the temperature of the substance that caused the burn and the duration of exposure. Water temperatures in excess of 120°F can result in burns within a few seconds, depending on the age of the patient and the location on the body. In this regard, investigation of the home environment is vital to ensure safety in the home (Table 145–2).

The etiology of burns includes scalds, flames, and contact with hot solids. Scald burns with hot tap water are the most frequent type of inflicted burns. The history of the injury must be carefully correlated with the observed pattern of injury, burn depth, and wound appearance. The immersion burn is a pathognomonic injury with involvement of the buttocks, posterior thighs, and feet, with relative sparing of the inguinal area. Immersion burns characteristically have uniform depth, an unvaried appearance, and distinct wound borders (Fig. 145–1).

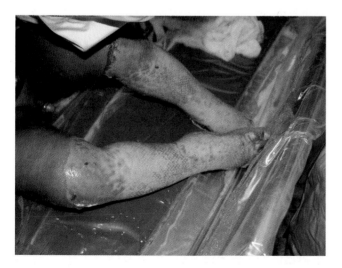

Figure 145–1. A 2-year-old boy presented to medical care with burns to both legs. Investigation revealed child was burned by mother's boyfriend in a bath tub after having a bowel movement in his pants. Burns are in a stocking-glove distribution consistent with immersion in a hot water.

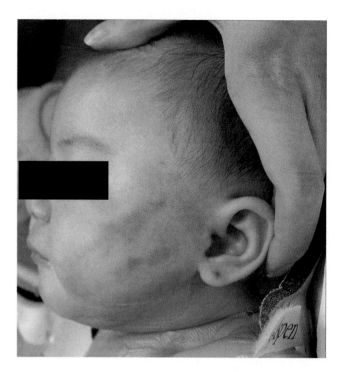

Figure 145–2. A 4-month-old girl presented with unresponsive episode at home. Examination revealed a patterned slap mark across her face. She was also identified to have severe brain injuries, bilateral retinal hemorrhages, and multiple rib fractures.

Bruises are a universal finding in ambulatory children; however, they are also among the most common injuries identified in abused children. Bruises in an unusual distribution or location are a cause for concern. The distribution of normal bruises varies by age and motor development.[7] For example, bruising is uncommon in nonambulatory children. In general, bruises to the extremities and over other bony prominences are common in normal children, and bruises centrally located, such as on the buttocks, chest, and abdomen, are less common. Estimating the age of a bruise is not recommended as it is fraught with multiple variables that affect accuracy. These include the depth of injury, baseline skin pigmentation, location of the injury, vascularity of the involved tissue, and the age of the patient.[10]

Patterned skin injuries, such as slap marks, loop marks, and bites, can be identified with careful examination. This type of injury is indicative of being struck with an object such as a belt, cord, or paddle. According to the AAP in 2002, inflicted injuries should be considered abusive if they leave a mark lasting more than 24 hours[11] (Fig. 145–2).

▶ MUSCULOSKELETAL TRAUMA

Examination of the skeletal system for physical abuse is an important component of the evaluation, especially for infants and toddlers. The physical examination may not always reveal skeletal deformity or tenderness. The AAP recommends that all children younger than 2 years with suspected abuse have a skeletal survey.[12] Leventhal and colleagues recognized that

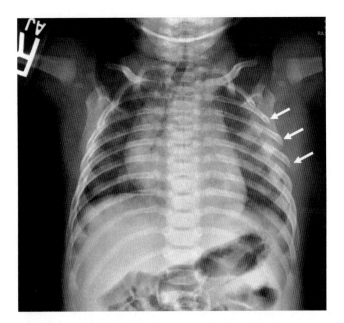

Figure 145–3. A 4-month-old boy presented with a chief complaint of respiratory distress and a clicking sensation in his chest. Multiple acute lateral rib fractures were identified. The mother confessed to forcibly squeezing the child's chest wall out of frustration.

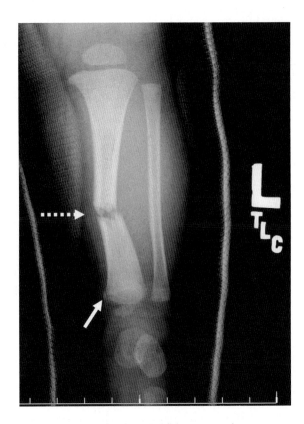

Figure 145–4. A 2-month-old child presented to a community hospital with a swollen leg. The history provided was that a 3-year-old child jumped on the infant. Radiographs revealed a transverse fracture of the left tibia and a metaphyseal corner fracture on the left distal tibia. In total, the child was identified to have 19 occult fractures.

24% of fractures in children younger than 3 years of age resulted from abuse; among children younger than 12 months, 39% were abuse related.[13] In battered infants, it is not uncommon to identify occult healing fractures indicating a pattern of repeated trauma.[14]

Skeletal injuries with a moderate to high specificity for child abuse include posterior rib fractures, especially when bilateral or multiple, metaphyseal fractures of the long bones, scapular fractures, fractures of the digits, and sternal fractures. Abusive skeletal injuries can be quite subtle with few, if any, presenting symptoms for many types of fractures, especially those involving ribs or a metaphysic of a long bone. In infants, lateral and/or posterior rib fractures are typically the result of compression of the chest wall (Fig. 145–3). Skeletal injuries in nonambulatory children should prompt medical evaluation for additional injuries (Fig. 145–4). Skeletal injuries with a low specificity for abuse include clavicular fractures, long bone fractures, and linear skull fractures. Evidence suggests that a follow-up skeletal survey approximately 2 weeks after the initial study increases the diagnostic yield, and should be considered when abuse is strongly suspected.[15]

▶ VISCERAL TRAUMA

Blunt trauma to the abdomen is a well-recognized but relatively infrequent manifestation of abuse, accounting for less than 1% of identified cases of child maltreatment. However, inflicted abdominal trauma is the second most common form of fatal inflicted injury, after neurotrauma. Abusive abdominal trauma may go unrecognized as it commonly results in nonspecific symptoms, and because external indicators of ab-

dominal trauma are often absent, even with severe injury. Reasons for seeking medical care range from severe signs and symptoms, such hypovolemic shock or peritonitis, to nonspecific complaints, such as abdominal pain or vomiting. Some children have asymptomatic injuries. Most abusive abdominal injury is caused by blunt trauma that results in solid organ injury, perforation of a hollow viscous, or shearing of mesenteric vessels. Most victims are young, generally between the ages of 6 months and 3 years. Injuries to the liver, pancreas, and small intestine predominate, but injuries to the spleen, kidneys, adrenal glands, bladder, and colon have been reported. Asymptomatic injuries may be discovered by routine screening of liver function tests and pancreatic enzymes or on abdominal computed tomography (CT) scans (Fig. 145–5). Maintaining an index of suspicion for abdominal injuries in children presenting with other inflicted injuries is important to assist in early recognition and potential treatment.[16]

▶ ABUSIVE HEAD INJURY

Abusive head injury is the leading cause of morbidity and mortality in physically abused children. Caffey, in a landmark article published in 1972, described the classic triad associated with inflicted neurotrauma: subdural hemorrhages, retinal

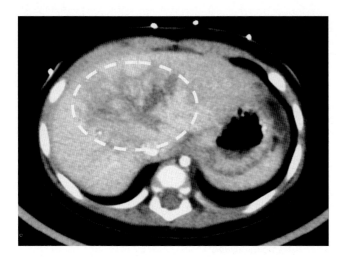

Figure 145–5. A 6-month-old boy presented with lethargy and multiple bruises. Liver enzymes were markedly elevated (ALT 19,232, AST 10,565). CT scan revealed severe liver contusion and lacerations.

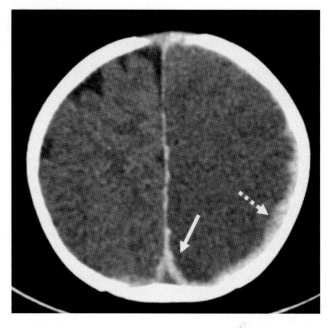

Figure 145–6. An 8-month-old child presented to medical care comatose after falling back from a seated position onto the carpeted floor. Examination revealed numerous bruises, severe retinal hemorrhages, and similar injuries in her twin brother.

hemorrhages, and metaphyseal fractures.[17] Since that time, much work has been done to enhance the recognition and to improve the understanding of the biomechanics and pathophysiology of inflicted head injury. Despite these efforts, controversy still exists regarding the mechanisms of injury, how patients present, and how specific certain injuries are for abuse. Over the years, many terms have been used to describe inflicted head injury, including shaken baby syndrome (SBS), shaken-impact syndrome, and abusive head injury. Because both shaking and blunt trauma to the head can result in the injuries described by Caffey, and because hypoxic ischemic injury is a recognized contributor to the brain injury seen in abused infants, the current recommendation is to refer to the injury with an inclusive term that does not specify the exact mechanism of injury, such as inflicted neurotrauma or abusive head trauma (AHT).

The etiology of AHT is rarely clear because an accurate history is almost always lacking, and the mechanisms of injury vary among patients. Victims of AHT are generally younger than 3 years; most are infants. Perpetrators tend to be men—fathers or a maternal boyfriend—although mothers and babysitters are frequently implicated.[18] The child's symptoms vary from mild lethargy, vomiting, or irritability to apnea and coma. Seizures are common in victims of abusive head injury and are reported in up to 80% of severely injured victims.[19]

Recognizing AHT is important; many cases are missed by physicians. Jenny et al. reported that 31% of patients with inflicted head injury had seen a physician with symptoms of their head injury an average of 2.8 times prior to identification of the abuse. Factors associated with missed diagnosis included age less than 6 months, Caucasian race, both parents living in the home, and presentation with mild, nonspecific symptoms such as vomiting, fever, and irritability.[20] Children with fatal or near-fatal injury are symptomatic immediately; evidence for prolonged lucid intervals in severely injured victims is lacking. In the case of fatal injury, death is usually caused by uncontrollable cerebral edema and increased intracranial pressure. Survivors of inflicted neurotrauma usually suffer moderate to severe disabilities, including cognitive delay, visual impairment, seizures, and overall poor developmental outcomes.

Features of AHT seen on physical examination include irritability, lethargy, soft tissue swelling of the scalp, full fontanelle, opisthotonic posturing, or coma. Vomiting is common; when it is accompanied by lethargy, it suggests the possibility of increased intracranial pressure. The hallmark feature of AHT is subdural hemorrhage, which may lie over one or both cerebral convexities but is often found in the posterior interhemispheric fissure (Fig. 145–6). The collection of blood is usually thin and resolves without neurosurgical intervention. CT scan is the first line modality in evaluating possible head injury. CT scan can be done quickly and is highly sensitive in identifying acute bleeding in all intracranial compartments. Magnetic resonance imaging (MRI) is a better means of detecting small subdural hematomas, subacute and chronic intracranial injuries, diffuse axonal injuries, cortical contusions, and posterior interhemispheric subdural hemorrhage (SDH). MRI is generally used in follow-up to further assess brain injury and secondary injury due to hypoxic ischemic events.

Injuries associated with AHT include retinal hemorrhages, skeletal injuries, cutaneous injuries, and visceral injuries. When identified, noncranial injuries provide support for the diagnosis of abuse. Approximately 80% of children with AHT have retinal hemorrhages. The hemorrhages may be unilateral or bilateral and may involve the preretinal, intraretinal, or subretinal layers. Dilated, indirect ophthalmoscopy performed by an ophthalmologist is preferred in the evaluation of suspected head injury to identify and document the extent of retinal involvement. All victims with AHT require a skeletal survey to evaluate for further injuries. Extracranial abnormalities are detected in 30% to 70% of abused children with head injuries. Skeletal injuries classically associated with inflicted neurotrauma include rib and metaphyseal fractures. The posterior rib injuries occur when there is compression of the chest wall causing the posterior rib to lever against the fulcrum of the transverse process. The metaphyseal fractures occur as the infant is held by the trunk and rotational forces are generated or when the extremities are used as handles.

▶ DIFFERENTIAL DIAGNOSIS OF CHILD ABUSE

The differential diagnosis of child abuse includes accidental trauma and many medical diseases that mimic abusive injuries (Table 145–3). Dermatologic findings that can be mistaken for bruises including "mongolian" spots, cultural practices such as coining, phytodermatitis, and connective tissue diseases such as Ehlers–Danlos syndrome. Conditions such as bullous impetigo, epidermolysis bullosa, and folk treatments may be confused with burns. Conditions that may mimic inflicted neurotrauma include accidental or birth-related trauma, hemorrhagic disease of the newborn, vascular malformations, and glutaric aciduria type I.

In evaluating a child with excessive or unusual bruises, it is important to include child abuse in the differential diagnosis along with isoimmune thrombocytopenic purpura (ITP), hemophilia, infection such as meningococcemia, Henoch–Schonlein purpura (HSP), and vitamin K deficiency. If a bleeding diathesis is suspected, recommended screening includes a complete blood count, platelet count, prothrombin time (PT), and partial thromboplastin time (PTT). Further studies would be directed by family history of disease processes and other clinical indicators.

▶ ANCILLARY STUDIES

Laboratory or radiographic testing in cases of suspected child abuse is guided by the age of the child, the injury pattern, the clinical condition of the child, and the consideration of differential diagnosis. For example, a coagulopathy screen is indicated for children who present with isolated bruising, and abdominal enzymes, including liver function enzymes, amylase, and lipase, are indicated for children with suspected abdominal trauma. Some children may present with an injury pattern that is pathognomonic for inflicted injury, and a search for an alternative diagnosis is unwarranted.

The skeletal survey is an important adjunct to the evaluation of abused infants and toddlers and is indicated for all children younger than 2 years with any suspicious injury. Skeletal surveys are generally not indicated for children older than 5 years of age since older children rarely have occult fractures. In patients between the ages of 2 and 5 years, there should be a high index of suspicion for abuse in order to justify a skeletal survey. Additional radiographic studies important in the evaluation of some abused children include radionuclide bone scans, ultrasound, CT scans, and MRI scans. In infants in whom physical injuries compatible with abuse are identified, strong consideration for neuroimaging is indicated; 30% of these cases have been reported to be associated with occult head injuries.[21]

▶ **TABLE 145–3. DIFFERENTIAL DIAGNOSIS OF INJURIES ASSOCIATED WITH CHILD ABUSE**

Bruises
1. Accidental injury
2. Dermatologic disorders
   Mongolian spots
   Erythema multiforme
   Phytodermatitis
3. Hematologic disorders
   Idiopathic thrombocytopenic purpura (ITP)
   Leukemia
   Hemophilia
   Vitamin K deficiency
   Disseminated intravascular coagulopathy (DIC)
4. Cultural practices
   Cao gio (coining)
   multiforme
   Quat sha (spoon rubbing)
5. Genetic diseases
   Ehlers–Danlos
   Familial dysautonomia (with congenital indifference to pain)
6. Vasculitis
   Henoch–Schonlein purpura

Burns
1. Accidental burns
2. Infection
   Staphylococcal scalded skin syndrome
   Impetigo
3. Dermatologic
   Phytodermatitis
   Stevens–Johnson reaction
   Fixed drug eruption
   Epidermolysis bullosa
   Severe diaper dermatitis
4. Cultural practices
   Cupping

Fractures
1. Accidental injury
2. Birth trauma
3. Metabolic bone disease
   Osteogenesis imperfecta
   Copper deficiency
   Rickets
4. Infection
   Congenital syphilis
   Osteomyelitis

Head Trauma
1. Accidental head injury
2. Hematologic disorders
   Vitamin K deficiency (hemorrhagic disease of the newborn)
   Hemophilia
3. Intracranial vascular abnormalities
4. Infection
5. Metabolic diseases
   Glutaric aciduria type I

► NEGLECT

Neglect is the inattention or omission on the part of the caregiver to provide for the needs of a child; it is the most common type of child maltreatment. Core needs include access to health care, appropriate shelter, proper nutrition, education, and emotional support. Neglect also includes failure to properly supervise and protect children from harm. Neglect must be differentiated from the manifestations of poverty. Poverty threatens a child's access to adequate nutrition, health care, and housing, but is a condition beyond the means of many parents to change. Neglect refers to omissions that are within the parent's control. Failure to thrive (FTT), medical neglect, drug-exposed newborns, and child abandonment are all examples of neglect.

FTT is the failure of a child to grow and develop adequately. The most common cause of FTT is inadequate nutrition. This diagnosis is achieved after eliminating primary organic diseases, carefully considering the infant's diet, and closely monitoring growth and development while paying strict attention to nutritional intake. Attention should be paid to the type of formula ingested, how the formula is prepared, and the velocity of growth since birth. The medical evaluation of an infant with FTT typically reveals sparse subcutaneous tissues, cachetic appearance, and poor/weak muscle tone (Fig. 145–7). All growth parameters should be plotted on an appropriate standardized growth curve. Diagnostic testing is done based on the clinical history, physical appearance, and medical findings.[22]

Medical neglect can range from a caretaker who refuses, denies, or fails to provide prescribed treatment for serious acute illness to the caretaker who fails to seek basic medical care for the child. A commonly encountered example of medical neglect is the child whose care provider is noncompliant with medications and medical follow-up for a readily treatable disease, which results in an increase in the severity of the disease that then requires escalating medical care.

Supervisional neglect includes child abandonment and lack of appropriate supervision. This type of neglect typically is diagnosed in the emergency department. Many cases of household trauma can be attributed to lack of appropriate supervision. Occasionally, children need to be admitted to the hospital for both medical indications and protection. The physician must serve as an advocate for the safety and well-being of the child.[23]

► MANAGEMENT

In all 50 states, child protection laws mandate all professions to notify their local child protection agency when there is a suspicion on child abuse or neglect. The term suspicion is defined as having a reasonable cause/concern that a child may be or has been harmed or neglected. All medical professionals working in the emergency department are mandated reports. Failure to report suspected abuse can result in criminal charges and loss of medical licensure. Medical reporters are typically protected from retribution when their report to child welfare agencies is made in good faith.

It is important for the physician to maintain communication with the family or care provider even when there is a concern of abuse or neglect. The alleged perpetrator may not be immediately known or be present in the hospital. As an advocate for the child, the physician must maintain objectivity and refrain from confrontational or accusatory statements when talking with the family. Specific discussions regarding mechanisms of injury and timing of injury should be avoided until investigators from law enforcement and child welfare agencies have had the opportunity to meet with the family.

Once a report of suspected abuse has been made, a child welfare worker will begin an investigation into the situation. In many communities, this investigation will be conducted along with a local law enforcement office. The investigating agencies will rely on medical information and information obtained during their investigation into the home and family environment to determine if there is enough evidence to substantiate the concern of child maltreatment. At times, the investigators will request written medical opinions or interviews with the medical care provider to assist in their investigation.

In cases of substantiated abuse, a physician may be asked to testify in both family and civil court proceedings. The family court proceedings help determine who has custody of the child. The criminal court proceedings deal with the criminal prosecution of cases. In either case, the emergency physician may be requested to formulate an opinion within a reasonable degree of medical certainty if a child has been abused. When available, the emergency physician should consult with a child abuse pediatrics specialist to aid in this assessment.

► CONCLUSION

A medical provider should have the ability to identify child abuse. Knowing the historical features and physical examination findings suggestive of abuse and utilizing appropriate diagnostic tests can increase recognition of this public health problem. Although child abuse cases are emotionally difficult

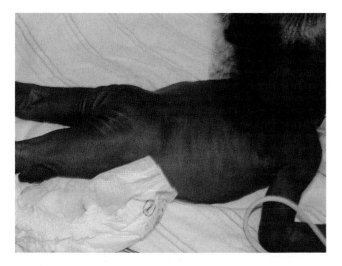

Figure 145–7. Failure to thrive. An 8-month-old boy presented to medical care weighing 10 lbs 3 oz. Birth weight had been 8 lbs. On examination he was cachetic, developmentally delayed, and had redundant skin folds. With a change in environment he readily gained weight.

and time consuming, physicians can help save or improve a child's life by identifying inflicted injuries and reporting the case to the appropriate authorities. Physicians can also play an important role in the prevention of child abuse by screening for risk factors, such as domestic violence and substance abuse, and providing appropriate anticipatory guidance.

REFERENCES

1. Kellogg N; and the Committee on Child Abuse and Neglect. American Academy of Pediatrics Clinical Report: evaluation of suspected child physical abuse. *Pediatrics*. 2007;119:1232.
2. U.S. Department of Health and Human Services, Administration on Children, Youth and Families. *Child Maltreatment 2006*. Washington, DC: U.S. Department of Health and Human Services; 2008. http://www.acf.hhs.gov/programs/cb/pubs/cm06/. Accessed March 2008.
3. Cadzow S, Armstrong K, Fraser J. Stressed parents with infants: reassessing physical abuse risk factors. *Child Abuse Negl*. 1999;23:845.
4. DiScala C, Sege R, Li G, et al. Child abuse and unintentional injuries: a 10-year retrospective. *Arch Pediatr Adolesc Med*. 2000;154:16.
5. American Academy of Pediatrics. The role of the pediatrician in recognizing and intervening on behalf of abused women. *Pediatrics*. 1998;101:1091.
6. Hettler J, Greenes D. Can the initial history predict whether a child with a head injury has been abused? *Pediatrics*. 2003;111:602.
7. Sugar N, Taylor J, Feldman K. Bruises in infants and toddlers: those who don't cruise rarely bruise. *Arch Pediatr Adolesc Med*. 1999;153:399.
8. Leavitt E, Pincus R, Bukachevsky R. Otolaryngologic manifestations of child abuse. *Arch Otolaryngol Head Neck Surg*. 1992;118:629.
9. Purdue G, Hunt J, Prescott P. Child abuse by burning—an index of suspicion. *J Trauma*. 1988;28:221.
10. Stephenson T, Bialas Y. Estimation of the age of bruising. *Arch Dis Child*. 1996;74:53.
11. Committee on Child Abuse and Neglect American Academy of Pediatrics. When inflicted injuries constitute child abuse. *Pediatrics*. 2002;110:644.
12. American Academy of Pediatrics. Diagnostic imaging of child abuse. *Pediatrics*. 2000;105:1345.
13. Leventhal J, Thomas S, Rosenfield S, et al. Fractures in young children: distinguishing child abuse from unintentional injuries. *Am J Dis Child*. 1993;147:87.
14. Kleinman P, Marks S, Richmond J, et al. Inflicted skeletal injury: a postmortem radiologic-histopathologic study in 31 infants. *AJR Am J Roentgenol*. 1995;165:647.
15. Kleinman P, Nimkin K, Spevak M, et al. Follow-up skeletal surveys in suspected child abuse. *AJR Am J Roentgenol*. 1996;167:893.
16. Coant P, Kornberg A, Brody A, et al. Markers for occult liver injury in cases of physical abuse in children. *Pediatrics*. 1992;89:274.
17. Caffey J. On the theory and practice of shaking infants. *Am J Dis Child*. 1972;124:161.
18. Starling S, Holden J, Jenny C. Abusive head trauma: the relationship of perpetrators to their victims. *Pediatrics*. 1995;95:259.
19. Jenny C, Hymel K, Ritzen A, et al. Analysis of missed abusive head trauma. *JAMA*. 1999;282:621.
20. Ewing-Cobbs L, Kramer L, Prasad M, et al. Neuroimaging, physical and developmental findings after inflicted and non-inflicted traumatic brain injury in young children. *Pediatrics*. 1998;102:300.
21. Rubin DM, Christian CW, Bianiuk LT, et al. Occult head injury in high-risk abused children. *Pediatrics*. 2003;111:1382.
22. Krugman SD, Dubowitz H. Failure to thrive. *Am Fam Physician*. 2003;68:879.
23. Hymel K; and the Committee on Child Abuse and Neglect. When is lack of supervision neglect? *Pediatrics*. 2006;118:196.

CHAPTER 146

Psychiatric Emergencies

Catherine Porter Moore

▶ HIGH-YIELD FACTS

- In all cases of psychiatric emergencies, organic disease etiology must be ruled out!
- The majority of adolescents are relieved to discuss psychiatric issues and actively seek treatment.
- It is essential to introduce community resources such as crisis lines, substance abuse resources and centers to patients and families.
- Suicide is common in adolescents: 20% to 25% of American adolescents have considered suicide seriously, 9% have attempted, and it is the third leading cause of death in 15- to 24-year-olds and fifth in 5- to 14-year-olds.
- Suicide National Hotline: 1-800-suicide.
- Psychosis is a *symptom*, not a *disease*.
- Schizophrenia tends to run in families.
- Any child that has been traumatized, by involvement or witness, can develop posttraumatic stress disorder (PTSD).
- PTSD may manifest in different ways in different developmental stages.
- PTSD occurs in 40% to 90% of sexually abused children and 11% to 50% in physically abused children.
- Children with burn injuries have over a 50% chance of having symptoms of PTSD.
- Conversion/somatization disorder is characterized by the presence of apparent physical disease that cannot be delineated organically and has pathologic origination in the psyche.
- Conversion/somatization disorder may present as abdominal pain, respiratory difficulty (paradoxical vocal cord dysfunction), pseudoseizures, and other somatoform disorders.

The first priority in evaluating and treating psychiatric patients in the emergency department (ED) is to determine the risk the patients pose to themselves and others. This assessment guides how best to care for the patient. Safe rooms that have no equipment and are highly visible to staff are optimal for psychiatric patients. Some patients may need one-on-one supervision by staff, others may need restraint. The provisions are made prior to other interventions.

Table 146–1 lists the historical information that should be obtained from a patient with psychiatric issues presenting to the ED. Emphasis should be placed on past psychiatric history with current medications taken, and a thorough social history to assess the home living condition, family and school relationship problems, and any history of substance abuse.

Examination of the psychiatric patient includes a full physical examination as well as complete neuro and mental status examination. The elements of a mental status examination can be reviewed in Table 146–2. When performing a mental status examination, particular attention should be paid to the caretakers as well as the patient. Assessment of the mental status of the caretaker can reveal much about the parent–child relationship and function.

▶ THE SUICIDAL PATIENT

ETIOLOGY/PATHOGENESIS

Biological correlations have been made with suicidal ideation. Low CSF levels of 5-hydroxy-indolacetic acid, low platelet imipramine binding, anomalies in the hypothalamic–pituitary–adrenal axis, sleep EEG abnormalities, and decreased REM sleep have been noted in patients with suicidal tendencies.[1] Most suicidal patients have psychiatric pathology with the most common being major depressive disorder (MDD)/dysthymia followed by disruptive behavior disorder, drug/alcohol abuse, and dependence and anxiety disorder.[1]

RECOGNITION

Many tools and psychiatric assessment modules have been designed to assess the suicidal patient. Usually patients present with a chief complaint of a suicide attempt that they confessed to or were confronted about. It is important to assess whether a patient with mental illness is at risk of suicide while in the ED. This can be ascertained in the interview. Horowitz and colleagues suggested a four-question screening tool to rapidly detect suicide risk. The four questions that yielded the highest sensitivity and negative predictive value consist of yes/no/I don't know questions addressing current and past suicidal ideation, past self-destructive behavior, and current stressors.[2]

1. Are you here because you tried to hurt yourself?
2. In the past week, have you been having thoughts about killing yourself?
3. Have you ever tried to hurt yourself in the past *other than this time*?
4. Has something very stressful happened to you in the past few weeks?

The more "yes" answers, the greater the risk of the patient posing a threat to themselves.

▶ **TABLE 146–1. THE PSYCHIATRIC HISTORY**

- Chief complaint
- History of present illness
- Past psychiatric history
- Birth and development history
- Past medical and surgical history, current medications, allergies
- Family history of medical and psychiatric issues
- Social history, living situation, school, grade, friends, history of abuse
- Substance abuse
- Medical and psychiatric system review

MANAGEMENT

In the initial management of patients with suicidal tendency, it is vital that the interviewer be compassionate. The interviewer should ascertain (1) the reason the patients desire to hurt themselves, (2) the plan to do so, (3) whether the patients have the means necessary to carry out the plan, and (4) the timing of the plan's execution. Admission is warranted if there are any medical issues or the patient is not deemed safe for discharge. Concerns for patient safety include the following

- Inability to maintain a safety (no-suicide) contract
- Active suicidal ideation (plan and intent)
- High intent or lethality of attempt
- Psychosis
- Volatile/unsafe family and home environment

Treatment of the patient with suicidal tendency may include both medical therapy and counseling. Multiple studies suggest that combining medical therapy (antidepressants such as a selective serotonin reuptake inhibitor [SSRI]) and cognitive behavioral therapy has the highest success rates.

Common treatment of depression with SSRI drugs has come under fire in recent years. In 2004, the Food and Drug Administration (FDA) issued a black box warning for all SSRIs,

▶ **TABLE 146–2. THE MENTAL STATUS EXAMINATION**

- ORIENTATION: Time, Place, Person, Why they are here?
- APPEARANCE: Neat? Well groomed? Caretaker's appearance?
- BEHAVIOR: Cooperative? Anxious? Agitated?
- PSYCHOMOTOR: Physical activity? Tics? Movements?
- MOOD: Happy? Angry? Sad? Depressed?
- AFFECT: Flat? Warm?
- THOUGHT PROCESS: Organized? Logical? Stray from topic to topic?
- THOUGHT CONTENT: Delusional? Hallucinating? Paranoid?
- SPEECH: Rambling? Tone? Volume?
- INSIGHT: Understanding of issues that prompted the visit?
- JUDGEMENT: Test of rational, clear thinking
- MEMORY: Short-term and delayed recall
- COGNITION: Reasoning, interpretation of complex ideas (calculations)

warning that "antidepressants increased the risk compared to placebo of suicidal thinking and behavior (suicidality) in children, adolescents, and young adults in short-term studies of major depressive disorder (MDD) and other psychiatric disorders."[3]

Bridge and colleagues published a meta-analysis that showed antidepressant use in children, adolescents, and young adults causes greater benefit than harm.[4] This study suggested close follow-up and evaluation on a case-by-case basis and that the patient on SSRIs is not at a greater risk in the ED than the one who is not on medications.

ANCILLARY STUDIES

If the patient's mental status is altered, a toxicology screen and ethanol level is warranted. Many intoxicated suicidal patients are no longer suicidal once the intoxicant wears off. Organic disease must be ruled out. Thyroid disease, autoimmune disease, and other organic disease states can cause or augment a patient's depression and tendency to commit suicide.

▶ THE PSYCHOTIC PATIENT

ETIOLOGY/PATHOGENESIS

Pediatric schizophrenia presents with psychosis at or before 12 years of age. DSM-IV-TR criteria include hallucinations (79%–82%), delusions (54%–63%), and thought disorder (40%–100%). Disorganized behavior, negative symptoms and impaired functioning, symptoms of later onset disease are not particularly diagnostic in children.[5]

Psychosis can be a feature of many other psychiatric diagnoses including MDD, bipolar disorder, and schizotoform disorder.

Most pediatric patients present with a chief complaint of auditory and/or visual hallucinations. Etiology can be basic psychiatric illness, but again it is essential that organic disease be ruled out. There are many medical conditions that produce psychosis including infection, rheumatic disease, especially lupus,[6] cerebral blood flow changes/hypoxia, temporal lobe epilepsy,[7] toxicological, vitamin deficiencies, metabolic and endocrine disorders, Reye syndrome, and Wilson's disease. Notable are encephalopathy with varied etiologies from infectious to Hashimoto encephalopathy.[8]

MANAGEMENT

Treatment of psychosis in the acute care setting is mostly pharmacological. Antipsychotics such as olanzapine, risperidone, and haloperidol have been used in pediatric ED settings.

ANCILLARY STUDIES

Ancillary studies are aimed at ruling out organic disease. As mentioned, many pathological processes can produce psychosis. It is vital that the patient with psychosis is cleared medically. In the ED, these patients should be assessed for altered mental status. This workup should include toxicology, electrolytes, kidney and liver functions, and ammonia level. Imaging including CT scan, MRI, and EEG may be necessary in selected cases. A lumbar puncture may be warranted to evaluate for meningitis and encephalitis.

▶ POSTTRAUMATIC STRESS DISORDER

ETIOLOGY/PATHOGENESIS

Posttraumatic stress disorder (PTSD) emerges after traumatic events that evoke intense fear, helplessness, or horror. The patient may have been involved in or been a witness to the trauma. The hypothalamic–pituitary–adrenal axis has been noted to be hyperactive in children and adolescents diagnosed with PTSD. Overall, these patients have elevated cortisol levels in urine and saliva.[9]

RECOGNITION

In the acute care setting, PTSD is something that should be recognized by its symptoms (detailed in the DSM-IV) of intrusive memories and/or dreams of the traumatizing event, avoidance of stimuli connected to the traumatic event, symptoms of excessive arousal/anxiety including inability to concentrate on tasks, exaggerated startle response, hypervigilance, insomnia, and inappropriate outbursts. These symptoms will manifest differently in different developmental stages.

Any trauma that warrants emergency evaluation can provoke a case of PTSD. It is at least 4 weeks of symptoms that distinguish PTSD from Acute Stress Disorder. Children with burn injuries have over a 50% chance of having symptoms of PTSD.[10]

MANAGEMENT

The Screening Tool for Early Predictors of PTSD (STEPP) questionnaire is a tool to screen for PTSD at the initial trauma presentation. It is composed of four questions for the patient, four questions for the parents, and four items from the medical record, which, based on previous studies, have shown to correlate with a greater likelihood of developing PTSD.[11]

Table 146–3 lists the items shown to increase risk of developing PTSD. More number of questions answered with a "yes" indicates a higher probability to develop PTSD. Treatment with counseling and pharmacotherapy should be determined on a case-by-case basis. It is important to facilitate long-term psychiatric evaluation and treatment for any child who is at risk.

Patients at greater risk of PTSD need ongoing follow-up to ensure that their pathology does not become more severe.

There is no laboratory or radiographic test to confirm or deny the existence of PTSD.

▶ THE PSYCHOPATHIC PATIENT: *WHEN JUNIOR KILLS FIDO*

American Heritage Dictionary defines psychopath as "a person with an antisocial personality disorder, manifested in aggres-

▶ TABLE 146–3. SCREENING FOR POSTTRAUMATIC STRESS DISORDER

Parental Questions
1. Did you see the incident in which your child got hurt?
2. Were you with your child in the ambulance/helicopter en route to the hospital?
3. When you first understood that your child had been hurt in the accident, did you feel really helpless?
4. Does your child have any problems paying attention or behavior problems?

Patient Questions
1. Was anyone else hurt/killed when you got hurt?
2. Was there a time when you didn't know where your parents were?
3. When you got hurt, or right afterwards, did you feel really afraid?
4. When you got hurt, or right afterwards, did you think you might die?

From the Medical Record
1. Suspected extremity fracture.
2. HR >104 if patient under 12 or >97 if 12 and older
3. 12 or older
4. Girl?

With permission from Ward-Begnoche WL, Aitken ME, Liggin R, et al. Emergency department screening for risk for post-traumatic stress disorder among injured children. *Inj Prev.* 2006;12:323–326.

sive, perverted, criminal, or amoral behavior without empathy or remorse."[12]

Antisocial personality disorder (APD) can only be diagnosed at 18 years of age or older. Children and adolescents often are diagnosed with oppositional defiant disorder (ODD) and conduct disorder (CD) prior to their diagnosis of APD. ODD is characterized by a pattern of negativity, hostility, and defiance lasting for at least 6 months during which four DSM-IV criteria are met. Diagnosis of CD is based on persistent history of "when a child seriously misbehaves with aggressive or nonaggressive behaviors against people, animals or property that may be characterized as belligerent, destructive, threatening, physically cruel, deceitful, disobedient, or dishonest. This may include stealing, intentional injury, and forced sexual activity."[13]

ETIOLOGY/PATHOGENESIS

It has been suggested that APD, CD, and ODD originate in poor bonding with the mother in the first five years of life. It is noted that these patients have deficits in fear recognition similar to patients with amygdala damage.[14]

Rarely does a case of ODD present in the ED. Certain behaviors of great concern to parents may present in the ED and can be characteristic of serious pathology. Fire starting and animal torture/killing are two such behaviors that deserve psychiatric evaluation. These patients may require intensive and long-term therapy, which should commence at the time of presentation to prevent worsening and progression to APD.

► CONVERSION/SOMATIZATION DISORDER

ETIOLOGY/PATHOGENESIS

Conversion/somatization disorder is thought to be triggered by psychosocial stressors. It is not understood how the stressor turns into somatic complaints. These complaints are not intentional, unlike factitious disorder and malingering. In one study, it was noted that boys with somatoform disorders had significantly poorer interpersonal relations and communications, whereas girls had higher rates of conflicts with family members.[15]

RECOGNITION

Once the possibility of organic disease has been excluded, psychiatric evaluation can make the diagnosis. In the case of paradoxical vocal cord dysfunction, the patient presents in refractory respiratory distress. Direct visualization of abnormal vocal cord movement (closing of the cords on inhalation) is the definite means of establishing the diagnosis.[16]

Nonepileptic seizures (NES) are associated with the DSM-IV diagnosis of conversion disorder and often take years to differentiate from epileptic seizures. Historically, NES occur more in stressful situations and not during sleep. They also register negative on the EEG.[17]

TREATMENT/MANAGEMENT

Often hospitalized for the somatic complaint, once diagnosed with conversion/somatizaion, these patients are treated with psychotherapy and often medical management (often SSRIs) to help the patients cope with the underlying stressor(s).

► THE AGGRESSIVE PATIENT

Aggressive patients are rare in the pediatric ED compared to the adult world, but they present a unique set of challenges. It is important to look for the etiology of the patient's aggression/discontent. If it can be easily removed from the patient's environment, it should be. Further, the aggressive patients need to be well supervised where they do not have the means to harm themselves or others. If verbal reassurance is ineffective in diffusing the aggression, escalation in care proceeds to seclusion and therapeutic holding. Therapeutic holding refers to at least two people physically restraining the patient.[18] In brief, the recommendations of the American Academy of Pediatrics are to (1) explain the necessity of restraint to the patient, (2) have specific physician orders including indication for and duration of restraint, (3) explain everything to the family, and (4) perform and document ongoing assessment of correct application of restraints, skin and neurovascular integrity, as well as efficacy of the restraints in meeting the indication for application.[18] Further, documentation for all restraints (physical/chemical) should mention what was done to protect the patient's well-being, best interest, rights, privacy, and self-respect.

Physical restraint is a good initial step in the stabilization of the aggressive patient. If care requires escalation from physical restraint/therapeutic holding, chemical restraint may be warranted. The goals of chemical restraint are to (1) decrease the patient's anxiety and discomfort, (2) minimize disruptive behavior, (3) prevent escalation of behavior, and (4) reverse the underlying cause.[19] Many agents have been employed, about half of which have FDA approval for indications in children. All chemical restraint use requires careful monitoring of the patient on cardiac apnea monitor and pulse oximetry. Several of the most common chemical restraints are detailed in Table 146–4. Lorazepam, midazolam and diazepam are benzodiazepines that work to sedate patients by activating GABA receptors and can, therefore, be helpful in aggressive behavior modification.

► TABLE 146–4. MEDICATION OPTIONS FOR ACUTE AGITATION

Generic Name	Brand Name(s)	Drug Class	Delivery	Onset of Action	Major/Common Side Effects
Lorazepam	Ativan	Benzodiazapine	IV/IM/po	5–10 min IV 20–40 min IM 20–30 min po	Respiratory depression
Haloperidol	Haldol	Typical antipsychotic	IM/po	5–10 min	EPS, Qtc ↑, NMS, hypotension
Chlorpromazine	Thorazine	Typical antipsychotic	IV/IM/po	15 min IM 30–60 min po	Altered cardiac conduction, esophageal dysmotility, EPS, NMS, hypotension
Droperidol	Inapsine	Typical antipsychotic	IV/IM	3–10 min	EPS, Qtc ↑, NMS, hypotension
Olanzapine	Zyprexa, Zydis	Atypical antipsychotic	IM/ODT/po	15–30 min IM 65 hours po	Bradycardia, few EPS, prolactin elevation, anticholinergic SE, orthostatic chypotension
Ziprastine	Geodon	Atypical antipsychotic	IM/po	30–43 min IM	Nausea/HA/dizziness few EPS, Qtc ↑, orthostatic hypotension, prolactin elevation
Hydroxyzine	Vistaril Atarax	Antihistamine (H1 receptor antagonist)	IM/po	15–30 min	Hypotension, SVT, hallucination, seizure, tremor

▶ TABLE 146–5. PSYCHIATRIC MEDICATIONS WITH SIDE EFFECTS OFTEN REQUIRING ED VISITS

Class	Examples	Side Effects
SSRI	Citalopram(Celexa), Fluoxetine (Prozac), Paroxetine (Paxil), Sertraline (Zoloft), Fluvoxamine (Luvox), Escitalopram (Lexapro)	SSRI-associated behavioral activation: Restlessness, agitation, hyperactivity Seratonin syndrome: Weakness, incoordination, hyper-reflexia, epistaxis
Tricyclic antidepressants	Amitriptyline (Elavil)	Arrhythmias, confusion, EPS, discoloration of urine, agranulocytosis, increased LFTs
Stimulants	Methylphenidate (Ritalin), Dexmethylphenidate (Focalin), Amphetamine (Adderall), Modafinil (Provigil)	Hypertension, induction of mania in bipolar activation, insomnia, decreased appetite and growth
Alpha adrenergic agonist	Clonidine	Raynaud's phenomenon, hypotension, bradycardia, sedation, water retention, parotid pain, constipation, anorexia. Abrupt discontinuation = hypertension and tachycardia
Benzodiazepines, antipsychotics, and atypical antipsychotics	See above	See above

Midazolam has the shortest duration of action of the three, followed by lorazepam and diazepam. Diazepam is available in a per rectum (PR) formulation as well. The major side effect is respiratory depression.

Neurolepic drugs, such as haloperidol, have been utilized extensively in treating the aggressive patient. The value of these medications in the acute care setting is owing to their sedating effects rather than their antipsychotic effect, as those usually take 7 to 10 days of treatment to have effect.

The rare incidence (1%) of extrapyramidal symptoms (EPS) can occur after one dose of neuroleptic drugs. Most commonly seen is dystonic reaction involving eyes, neck, and/or back. Rarely does EPS affect the airway. The treatment for EPS is diphenhydramine (IV or IM) and/or benzotropine (IV or IM).[19]

One also must be aware of neuroleptic malignant syndrome. This potentially fatal reaction is characterized by fever, sweating, hypertension, severe muscle rigidity, and delirium sometimes progressing to coma. Patients should be treated with dantroline and supportive care.

Droperidol is another neuroleptic drug used in the treatment of the aggressive patient. It alters the action of dopamine at subcortical levels to produce sedation and a dissociative state with a faster onset of action than haloperidol. Its use is controversial, as in 2001 the FDA issued a black box warning of fatal arrhythmias associated with its use. Subsequent studies have not corroborated this particular risk, but have confirmed the most common side effect of dystonia.[19]

Atypical psychotics, such as ziprasidone and olanzapine, are gaining favor in the acute management of aggressive patients. With a lower incidence of EPS, multiple routes of administration, and better tolerance, they are commonly used in the pediatric ED. Ziprasidone and olanzapine are recommended for the agitated schizophrenic patients. Olanzapine is also indicated for aggression/agitation associated with bipolar disorder.

Hydroxyzine is an antihistamine that has been used as an anxiolytic, can be administered IM, and has an onset of action comparable to that of lorazapam.

▶ PSYCHOTROPIC MEDICATIONS

Many medications are utilized in the management of psychiatric conditions in childhood and adolescence. It is important to understand the pharmacology of these medications in the context of the ED. Table 146–4 reviews agents used for acute agitation. Table 146–5 reviews agents used in the outpatient/long-term setting with potential side effects that could bring patients to the ED.

REFERENCES

1. Greydanus DE, Calles J Jr. Suicide in children and adolescents. *Prim Care Office Pract.* 2007;34:259–273.
2. Horowitz LM, Wang PS, Koocher GP, et al. Detecting suicide risk in a pediatric emergency department: development of a brief screening tool. *Pediatrics.* 2001;107:1133–1137.
3. Food and Drug Administration. *Anti Depressant Box Warning.* Beltsville, MD; May 2007. http://www.fda.gov/cder/drug/antidepressants/antidepressants_label_change_2007.pdf.
4. Bridge JA, Iyengar S, Salary CB, et al. Clinical response and risk for reported suicidal ideation and suicide attempts in pediatric antidepressant treatment: a meta-analysis of randomized controlled trials. *JAm Med Assoc.* 2007;297:1684–1696.
5. Pavuluri MN, Janicak PG, Naylor MW, et al. Early recognition and differentiation of pediatric schizophrenia and bipolar disorder. *Adolesc Psychiatry.* 2003;27:117–134.
6. Benseler SM, Silverman ED. Neuropsychiatric involvement in pediatric systemic lupus erythematosus. *Lupus.* 2007;16:564–571.

7. Oner O, Unal O, Deda G. A case of psychosis with temporal lobe epilepsy: SPECT changes with treatment. *Pediatr Neurol.* 2005;32:197–200.

8. Bismilla Z, Sell E, Donner E. Hashimoto encephalopathy responding to risperidone. *J Child Neurol.* 2007;22:855–857.

9. Pervanidou P, Chrousos GP. Post-traumatic stress disorder in children and adolescents: from Sigmund Freud's "trauma" to psychopathology and the (Dys)metabolic synndrome. *Horm Metab Res.* 2007;39:413–419.

10. Langeland W, Olff M. Psychobiology of posttraumatic stress disorder in pediatric injury patients: a review of the literature. *Neurosc Beh Rev.* 2008;32:161–174.

11. Ward-Begnoche WL, Aitken ME, Liggin R, et al. Emergency department screening for risk for post-traumatic stress disorder among injured children. *Inj Prev.* 2006;12:323–326.

12. *The American Heritage Dictionary of the English Language*, 4th ed. Boston, MA: Houghton Mifflin Company. http://www.bartleby.com/61/61/P0636100.html. Accessed December 4, 2006.

13. American Psychiatry Association. BehaveNet® Clinical Capsule. *APA Diagnostic Classification DSM-IV-TR.* Bellevue, WA: 2000. http:// www.behavenet.com/capsules/disorders/dsm4TRclassification.htm. Accessed January 10, 2005.

14. Dadds MR, Perry Y, Hawes DJ, et al. Attention to the eyes and fear-recognition deficits in child psychopathy. *Br J Psychiatry.* 2006;189:280–281.

15. Bisht J, Sankhyan N, Kaushal R, et al. Clinical profile of pediatric somatoform disorders. *Indian Pediatr.* 2008;45:111–115.

16. Loe RJ, Konakanchi R. Psychogenic respiratory distress: a case of paradoxical vocal cord dysfunction and literature review. *J Clin Psychiatry.* 1999;1:39–46.

17. Plioplys S, Asato MR, Bursch B, et al. Multidisciplinary management of pediatric nonepileptic seizures. *J Am Acad Child Adolesc Psychiatry.* 2007;46:1491–1495.

18. American Academy of Pediatrics, Committee on Pediatric Emergency Medicine. The use of physical restraint interventions for children and adolescents in the acute care setting. *Pediatrics.* 1997;99:497.

19. Sorrentino A. Chemical restraints for the agitated, violent, or psychotic pediatric patient in the emergency department: controversies and recommendations. *Curr Opin Pediatr.* 2004;16:201–205.

CHAPTER 147

Death of a Child in the Emergency Department

William R. Ahrens

▶ HIGH-YIELD FACTS

- The death of a child in an emergency department (ED) has profound effects on physicians as well as surviving family members.
- The language used when telling parents their child is dead should be direct and nonjudgmental.
- The dead child should always be referred to by name.
- Most parents would like a memento of their child.
- A miscarriage in the ED should be considered the loss of a child.

Informing family members and friends of a loved one's death is a fact of life for the emergency physician. Such deaths are often sudden and unexpected, and survivors are confronted with the loss of a loved one with no prior psychological preparation. They usually receive the news from strangers in a potentially chaotic and intimidating environment, and are required to make heart-wrenching decisions in a brutally short period of time. The situation is particularly difficult when the dead patient is a child. The interaction between the emergency physician and the ED staff and the dead child's family can be an important first step in recovery, or can have long-lasting destructive effects.

The majority of emergency physicians feel that managing the death of a child is far more difficult than managing the death of an adult; some consider it the most difficult aspect of their job. Many feel guilty or inadequate after a failed pediatric resuscitation, even if they realize that the patient had no chance of survival. Many feel impaired for the remainder of their shift. Few have had any formal training in how to tell parents that their child is dead. There is no information on how this particular traumatic experience affects emergency physicians or other members of the ED staff in the long term.[1]

The immediate reaction of family members to the sudden loss of a child is disbelief, even though many say that they knew before being told that their child had died. On the part of parents, a sense of failure or guilt is probably universal. Many describe the experience in the ED as one that is replayed in their minds "like a tape," thousands of times. They can often recall minute details of their experience and can remember verbatim exactly what they were told, and by whom. This is typical of how people process traumatic events.

▶ THE INTERVIEW

One of the most common complaints of families whose loved one died in an ED is that they were not kept informed of the progress of events. Given the reality that the vast majority of pediatric patients who arrive pulseless and apneac will die in the ED, the process of dealing with the patient's death should be considered part of the resuscitation; the family is the patient. Parents should be placed in a private, quiet room, with adequate seating. A staff member is designated to communicate with the family; ideally this is an individual who is experienced in delivering bad news. There are some families who will want to be present during the resuscitation. The decision to allow or invite family members into the resuscitation room depends largely on the comfort level of the ED staff. While there is no consensus regarding admitting family members into pediatric resuscitations, there is a growing movement in this direction. Recent publications have suggested that family members be at a minimum offered the opportunity to be present during the resuscitation.[2–4]

It is the responsibility of the attending physician to tell the parents that their child is dead. Every effort should be made to secure the department so that sufficient time can be spent with the family. If possible, the physician should be seated during the interview. The language used should be direct and nonjudgmental; it cannot be overemphasized that the dead child should be referred to by his or her name. Euphemisms for death are to be avoided; phrases like "the little guy didn't make it," or "the baby expired" can be deeply resented by parents, who perceive them as depersonalizing their child. "I am very sorry, but Brendon is dead," or "I am sorry to have to tell you that Becky has died," are two examples of acceptable terminology. Parents want to know why their child died, and that the staff did everything that could be done to save the child's life. The physician must reassure the family that they are not responsible for their child's death. Parents should be allowed time to ask questions. It is important that parents believe that the emergency physician and staff experience sorrow for the loss of the child.[5] If an interpreter is involved in the interview, they should stand behind the physician so that the physician can maintain eye contact with the parents during the discussion.

▶ AFTER THE INTERVIEW

Family members should be offered an opportunity to spend time with the dead child after the interview. Before this is done, resuscitation equipment is removed, the body is cleaned, and preferably wrapped in a blanket. Most but not all parents find that spending time with the child is helpful; some will want to hold the body, others will not. A reluctance to do so is a normal reaction for some people and does not signify child abuse. Parents should be allowed to stay until they are ready to leave.[5]

An integral part of the grieving process involves processing memories. The vast majority of family members who have a child die in an ED would like a physical memento of the patient. These include a lock of hair and/or an inkprint or plaster mold of a hand or foot. Clothing and other personal items should be returned. Mementos are concrete objects that allow survivors to maintain a sense of contact with their dead loved one. Unless one has lost a child, it is probably difficult to imagine how important they are.[5,6]

Because most pediatric arrests involve prolonged tissue asphyxia, organ donation is usually not possible. However, many patients are eligible to donate heart valves, skin, and corneas. While approaching family members about tissue donation immediately after the death of their child is extremely difficult, there are at least some family members who retrospectively wish they had been asked.[2] In some states all hospital deaths are reported to regional organ banks, where experts in asking families about donating organs are available to initiate the process.

Most cases of sudden death require an autopsy. It is important that this process be explained to family members. They must be told how to obtain the results. In some cases the family's personal physician may be available to discuss the findings; in many cases the local coroner will do so. In cases of suspected sudden infant death syndrome (SIDS), parents should not be told they will feel better if indeed the autopsy confirms SIDS as the cause of death; in many cases this is not true.[5] It is also important to realize that in situations where the cause of death of a previously healthy baby is unknown, as is the case with babies who die of SIDS, the local police will investigate the family's home as a potential crime scene. This obviously has the potential to further traumatize parents; at such a moment the ED staff must function as the family's advocate.

The long-term effects of the death of a child on family members are not well known and are difficult to study. Certainly losing a child is one of the most difficult experiences an individual can encounter in life. Spouses, grandparents, and surviving siblings will each experience the loss of the child in their own way. For children, the understanding of death largely depends on their developmental stage; young children in particular may have no concept of death, or may not perceive it as permanent. Older children develop an understanding that death is permanent, but can perceive it as evil or an entity that punishes people.[7] Parents will of course feel profound grief that is most intense during the first year after the loss of the child. Mothers may have a higher risk of pathologic grief re-

sponses than fathers. There may be an increase in psychiatric hospitalizations in parents who have lost a child.[8] It is often assumed that divorce is more common among spouses who have lost a child; there is no evidence to support this assumption, which is bitterly resented by many bereaved parents.[9]

A child's death can shatter the relationship of people with the everyday world, as well as their concepts of spirituality and their relationship with religion. The loss of a child can be perceived as unfair and senseless. An important aspect of recovery involves finding meaning and value in the dead child's life, however short it may have been. Maintaining a sense of contact with the child is important to many people; thus the value of physical mementos, which are the basis of memories. One mother is quoted, "I wanted her gown because it was the last thing she wore. I wanted the sheet from the bed. I wanted her bracelet from the hospital. They said they couldn't give us anything."[5,6] Sensing compassion on the part of the medical staff who attended the patient and family is important; parents want to know that their child was valued as an individual. Offering parents the opportunity to return to the hospital and discuss the child's death may in some cases be helpful; it is a chance to demonstrate to the family that the ED staff cared about their loved one.[10]

Bereaved parents will receive support from other family members, friends, and in many cases, clergy. There are also organized grief-support groups that have extensive experience and profound commitment to help parents cope with the death of a child. Often such groups become an important part of bereaved parents' lives. Parents should be made aware of their existence (see Table 147–1).

▶ MISCARRIAGE IN THE EMERGENCY DEPARTMENT

Miscarriage, or spontaneous abortion, is defined as the loss of pregnancy up to the 20th week of gestation. Between 10% and 20% of pregnancies will end in miscarriage. How many patients are diagnosed as having miscarried in an ED is unknown. Ironically, there is a large body of literature evaluating the effect of miscarriage on both mothers and fathers compared to that evaluating the effect of the loss of a born child. It is clear that miscarriage has profound psychological effects on both parents. Many people suffer from depression and anxiety after a miscarriage. Relationships between spouses are affected, as well as attitudes toward future pregnancies. Many people feel that the medical staff trivialized their loss; for most parents, the miscarriage was the loss of a baby. For some people, follow-up intervention can be helpful. While the death of a child is clearly different from a miscarriage, it is important for the emergency physician and the ED staff to acknowledge to patients who miscarry that a baby has been lost.[11]

► CARING FOR THE ED STAFF

Managing the death of a child in the ED will always be difficult and will affect all staff members. At least some emergency physicians and presumably other staff use counseling services after suffering traumatic events in the department, but they are by no means universally available. While critical incident stress debriefing is commonly used, there is limited data documenting its efficacy. It is likely that educating physicians and other staff members in the best way to communicate the death of a child or other bad news can benefit both staff and patients. At the very least, it creates a mutually supportive culture within the department regarding the management of death. There are multiple modalities that have been successfully used, including role-playing, hearing from parents whose child was pronounced dead in an ED, and incorporating "death-telling" into advanced life support courses.[12,13]

► FROM THE PARENTS

Some comments and suggestions from parents whose child died in an ED are as follows

- Just let the parents know you're sorry and that everything possible was done.
- Unless it has happened to you, don't say "I know how you feel," because you don't.
- Just be honest; say everything possible was done to save the child.
- Look the parents in the eyes. Explain that all attempts at resuscitation were performed.
- Tell them how sorry you are, that life isn't fair, and most importantly that it was not their fault.
- Allow your humanity to show. Our physician was very compassionate and he had tears in his eyes.

- Make sure you express how sorry you are and tell the loved ones how it affects the staff.
- It's okay to show emotion; don't be overly clinical.
- The doctor should say, "I'm sorry, we did all we could."
- As you well know, once your child is dead, you can never have enough mementos.

REFERENCES

1. Ahrens WA, Hart RG. Emergency physicians' experience with managing pediatric death. *Am J Emerg Med.* 1997;15:642.
2. Sachetti A. Acceptance of family member presence during pediatric resuscitation in the emergency department: effect of personal experience. *Pediatr Emerg Care.* 2000;16:85.
3. Eppich WJ, Arnold LD. Family member presence in the pediatric emergency department. *Curr Opin Pediatr.* 2003;15:294.
4. Henderson DP, Knapp JF. Report of the national consensus conference on family presence during pediatric cardiopulmonary resuscitation and procedures. *Pediatr Emerg Care.* 2005;21:787.
5. Ahrens WA, Hart RG. Pediatric death: managing the aftermath in the emergency department. *J Emerg Med.* 15:60,1997.
6. Meert KL, Thurston CS, Briller SH. The spiritual needs of parents at the time of their child's death in the pediatric intensive care unit and during bereavement: a qualitative study. *Pediatr Crit Care Med.* 2005;6:420.
7. Poltorak DY, Glazer JP. The development of children's understanding of death: cognitive and psychodynamic considerations. *Child Adolesc Psychiatr Clin North Am.* 2006;15:567.
8. Li J, Laursen T, Precht D, et al. Hospitalization for mental illness among parents after the death of a child. *NEJM.* 2005;352:1190.
9. When a child dies: a survey of bereaved parents; 1999. www.compassionatefriends.org/survey.shtml. Accessed April . . . 2008.
10. Meert KL, Eggly S, Plollack M, et al. Parents' perspectives regarding a physician-parent conference after their child's death in the pediatric intensive care unit. *J Pediatr.* 2007;151:50.
11. Badenhorst W, Hughes P. Psychological aspects of perinatal loss. *Best Pract Res Clin Obstet Gynaecol.* 2007;21:249.
12. Ahrens WA, Hart RG. Coping with pediatric death in the emergency department by learning from parental experience. *Am J Emerg Med.* 1998;16:67.
13. Greenberg LW, Ochsenshlager D, ODonell R, et al. Communicating bad news: a pediatric department's evaluation of a simulated interview. *Pediatrics.* 1999;103:1210.

SECTION XXII

EMERGENCY MEDICAL SERVICES AND MASS CASUALTY INCIDENTS

CHAPTER 148

Pediatric Prehospital Care

Craig J. Huang and Maeve Sheehan

▶ HIGH-YIELD FACTS

- The EMSC program is a federal program whose purpose is to improve the quality of pediatric emergency care using a variety of Internet resources and a multidisciplinary consortium of organizations.
- The first link in the chain of prehospital care is preparedness in the pediatrician's office and caregiver's knowledge of CPR and the 911 EMS system.
- The National EMS Education Standards is a blueprint for a proposed novel EMS education system comprising scope of practice, training curricula, and evolving standards of care.
- Appropriate specialized and pediatric-sized equipment and supplies are essential for prehospital providers and community emergency departments.
- Online medical direction of EMS is dependent on proper communication. Offline direction is dependent on readily identified, previously agreed-upon defined clinical scenarios.
- Minors cannot refuse treatment and transport in an emergency situation.
- Joint policies endorsed by the AAP and ACEP have been published regarding community hospital emergency department preparedness for emergency care for children.
- Particular attention must be focused on stabilizing the patient with suspected significant traumatic brain or cervical spine injuries.
- Special considerations must be taken into account in disaster management and terrorism conditions, children with special health care needs, situations where child maltreatment is suspected, and psychiatric emergencies.
- There are several controversial areas in pediatric prehospital care that deserve further research. Fortunately, there are resources, such as PECARN and NEDARC, which can assist those interested in conducting high-quality investigations.

▶ STATE OF PREHOSPITAL PEDIATRIC EMERGENCY CARE IN THE UNITED STATES

HISTORICAL PERSPECTIVE

Organized emergency medical services (EMS) had their beginning with the Department of Transportation (DOT), created

by the Highway Safety Act of 1966, which contributed to initial state development of regional EMS systems and training courses for emergency care providers. Federal guidelines and funding for specific components of EMS systems were established by the Emergency Medical Services Act of 1973.

EMS funding became more of the states' purview with the Omnibus Budget Reconciliation Act of 1981, which consolidated federal funding into the Preventive Health and Health Services block grant program of the Department of Health and Human Services (DHHS).

EMERGENCY MEDICAL SERVICES FOR CHILDREN

The Emergency Medical Services for Children (EMSC) Act of 1984 created the EMSC Program, which is administered by the U.S. DHHS's Health Resources and Services Administration (HRSA), along with the U.S. DOT's National Highway Traffic Safety Administration (NHTSA). The EMSC program is the only federal program whose purpose is to improve the quality of pediatric emergency care.

The Health Resources and Services Administration–Maternal and Child Health Bureau (HRSA–MCHB) funded the Institute of Medicine (IOM) Committee on Pediatric Emergency Medical Services, which produced a report on pediatric EMS, prehospital emergency care, and hospital-based emergency and trauma care in 1993, *Emergency Medical Services for Children*.[1] The IOM study was the first comprehensive investigation that helped delineate the state of pediatric emergency care, the shortcomings and deficiencies of the system, and an overall vision for overcoming the problems identified.

The IOM's Committee on the Future of Emergency Care in the United States Health System convened in 2003 to conduct a more exhaustive reexamination of the state of emergency care in the United States and to evaluate any progress accomplished since publication of the 1993 IOM report. The project included the 25-member main committee and three subcommittees.

Prehospital EMS, Pediatric Emergency Care, and Hospital-Based Emergency Department subcommittees were tasked with examining the challenges associated with providing integrated emergency services to pediatric patients within the context of the overall health system, as well as providing a specific assessment of prehospital EMS services and systems. The Pediatric Emergency Care Subcommittee reported their analysis in 2007 in *Emergency Care for Children: Growing Pains*,[2] regarding the unique role of pediatric emergency services, pediatric emergency care planning, preparedness, coordination, funding, professional training, and research.

Integration of EMSC within regional and state EMS systems is accomplished by a number of resource centers and grants, national and federal partnerships, and allied organizations:

- A new Web site hosted by NHTSA Office of EMS (OEMS), http://www.EMS.gov, has been developed to provide current background and updates on several federal EMS initiatives and programs such as EMSC, the National EMS Information System (NEMSIS), and the National EMS Advisory Council. It also serves as a single portal to other EMS Web sites, links, contact information, and trusted resources.
- The Web site of a national clearinghouse, the EMSC National Resource Center (NRC), in Washington, DC, http://www.ems-c.org, http://bolivia.hrsa.gov/emsc/, provides detailed information on EMSC resources and the EMSC program.
- The mission of an EMSC data center, the National EMSC Data Analysis Resource Center (NEDARC), in Salt Lake City, IL, is to help EMS agencies and EMSC projects develop their own resources to formulate and answer research questions, and to effectively convert available data into informative reports with appropriate statistical analyses (Web site: http://www.nedarc.org/nedarc/index.html).
- EMSC Partnership for Children (PFC) Stakeholder Group, formed in 2003, is a multidisciplinary consortium of 3 U.S. government agencies (NHTSA's Office of Emergency Medical Services, the Indian Health Service, and the Agency for Healthcare Research and Quality), 6 EMSC grantees, and 21 national and professional organizations that contribute to the EMSC program's strategic plan, which include the following:
  - Ambulatory Pediatric Association
  - American Academy of Family Physicians
  - American Academy of Pediatrics
  - American College of Emergency Physicians
  - American College of Osteopathic Emergency Physicians
  - American College of Surgeons
  - American Heart Association
  - American Pediatric Surgical Association
  - American Public Health Association
  - American Trauma Society
  - Emergency Nurses Association
  - Family Voices
  - National Association of Children's Hospitals and Related Institutions
  - National Association of EMS Physicians
  - National Association of Emergency Medical Technicians
  - National Association of EMS Educators
  - National Association of School Nurses
  - National Association of Social Workers
  - National Association of State EMS Officials
  - SAFE KIDS Worldwide
  - Society of Trauma Nurses.

► ANTICIPATORY GUIDANCE AND OFFICE PREPAREDNESS

Prehospital care begins in the pediatrician's office with anticipatory guidance to parents of all children, particularly parents of children with special health care needs. It is vital for physicians to encourage parents to have important phone numbers readily available, including the pediatrician's office, after-hour's call number, and poison control. Parents should know when to call 911 and how to initiate basic CPR. In a 1999 study from Houston, more than 60% of all cases of cardiopulmonary arrest in children took place in the home, and only 17% of family members initiated basic CPR.[3] According to an AAP policy statement in 2004, "The outcome from childhood out-of–hospital cardiac arrest is determined by timeliness of implementation of cardiopulmonary resuscitation." If a child suffers an out-of-hospital cardiac arrest, intact neurological survival is 4%.[4] Studies suggest survival in pediatric out-of-hospital cardiac arrest improves as much as 2.5 times with timely initiation of CPR.

The pediatrician's office is the first link in "the chain of survival" in the emergency care system; 82% of pediatricians' offices encounter one emergency per month.[5] It is important that the pediatrician's office is prepared to deal with these situations. This begins with anticipatory guidance to parents regarding when to bring a child straight to the emergency department. Triage personnel in the office should know when to direct parents to call 911.

If a child does come to the office suffering a medical emergency, personnel should have the training and equipment needed to attempt to stabilize the child until EMS arrives (Table 148–1).[6] The type of training and equipment is dependent on how long it usually takes for EMS personnel to arrive to the office. "In the setting of an emergency, primary care pediatricians must be able to provide basic airway management and initiate treatment of shock."[3]

The pediatrician should provide documentation to EMS personnel and hence the ED physician about interventions undertaken in the office, and more importantly, the child's response to the intervention provided.

When possible, as part of routine and emergency care, the pediatrician should provide parents with a problem list, vaccinations, and routine and emergency medications that their children need. This is particularly important for chronically ill children who may go to the emergency department directly. This is also a routine part of disaster preparedness.

► PREHOSPITAL PROFESSIONALS

TRAINING/EDUCATION

A national standard curricula (NSC) exists for emergency medical technician (EMT) basics, EMT intermediates, and EMT paramedics sponsored by NHTSA and the MCHB. These curricula outline comprehensive educational objectives for prehospital professionals (links available on NHTSA Web site, http://www.nhtsa.gov).

NHTSA and the HRSA entered into a cooperative agreement with the National Association of EMS Educators

► TABLE 148–1. RECOMMENDED EQUIPMENT FOR PEDIATRIC OFFICE EMERGENCIES

Office Emergency Equipment and Supplies	Priority*
Airway management	
Oxygen-delivery system	E
Bag-valve-mask (450 and 1000 mL)	E
Clear oxygen masks, breather and nonrebreather, with reservoirs (infant, child, adult)	E
Suction device, tonsil tip, bulb syringe	E
Nebulizer (or metered-dose inhaler with spacer/mask)	E
Oropharyngeal airways (sizes 00–5)	E
Pulse oximeter	E
Nasopharyngeal airways (sizes 12–30 Fr)	S
Magill forceps (pediatric, adult)	S
Suction catheters (sizes 5–16 Fr) and Yankauer suction tip	S
Nasogastric tubes (sizes 6–14 Fr)	S
Laryngoscope handle (pediatric, adult) with extra batteries, bulbs	S
Laryngoscope blades (0–2 straight and 2–3 curved)	S
Endotracheal tubes (uncuffed 2.5–5.5; cuffed 6.0–8.0)	S
Stylets (pediatric, adult)	S
Esophageal intubation detector or end-tidal carbon dioxide detector	S
Vascular access and fluid management	
Butterfly needles (19–25 gauge)	S
Catheter-over-needle device (14–24 gauge)	S
Arm boards, tape, tourniquet	S
Intraosseous needles (16 and 18 gauge)	S
Intravenous tubing, microdrip	S
Miscellaneous equipment and supplies	
Color-coded tape or preprinted drug doses	E
Cardiac arrest board/backboard	E
Sphygmomanometer (infant, child, adult, thigh cuffs)	E
Splints, sterile dressings	E
Automated external defibrillator with pediatric capabilities	S
Spot glucose test	S
Stiff neck collars (small/large)	S
Heating source (overhead warmer/infrared lamp)	S

Note that some offices are located at a distance from EMS services. Providers in offices that are located more than 10 min away from the nearest EMS service need equipment that may not be required in the initial minutes of a resuscitation but will be required as the resuscitation effort extends past 10 min.
*E, essential; S, strongly suggested (essential if EMS response time is 10 min).

(NAEMSE) to develop the National EMS Education Standards (the Standards), which will replace the current U.S. DOT's NSC. The Standards follow the system proposed by the *EMS Education Agenda for the Future: A Systems Approach*, which proposed several elements of model EMS education systems:

- National EMS Core Content National EMS Scope of Practice
- National EMS Education Standards
- National EMS Certification
- National EMS Program Accreditation

The National EMS Education Standards provide the framework for minimal learning objectives for the individual provider licensure/certification levels. In addition, the Standards also serve as a more dynamic and flexible guide for EMS educational systems, curricula, and instructional materials, allowing for continuing changes in evidence-based practice and evolving revised standards of care.

SUPPLEMENTAL EDUCATION RESOURCES FOR PREHOSPITAL PEDIATRIC EMERGENCY TRAINING

TRIPP

Teaching Resource for Instructors in Prehospital Pediatrics (TRIPP) is an older resource initially developed as an EMSC project by the New York City-Center for Pediatric Emergency Medicine (http://www.med.nyu.edu/pediatrics/emergency/

cpem/teaching/index.html), which was composed of health care providers from New York University Medical Center/Bellevue Hospital and Columbia University Medical Center/Harlem Hospital. Both TRIPP basic life support (BLS) and advanced life support (ALS) were designed to supplement and augment the information these providers received based on the NSC. Core sections were designed to help empower these professionals in recognizing and initiating the appropriate interventions for critically ill and injured children. Additional sections covered emergent clinical assessment and management issues unique to the pediatric population, using case-based scenarios with clearly defined objectives, student handouts, and supplemental resources and references lists.

PEPP

The National Pediatric Education for Paramedics (PEP) Task Force, funded by the Florida Emergency Medicine Foundation and the California EMS Authority, produced its first PEP course in 1995, utilizing the efforts of several state EMSC projects. The PEP course was restructured and expanded by a National Steering Committee established by the AAP in 1998 for all prehospital providers, thus the change to the Pediatric Education for Prehospital Professionals (PEPP) Course. The new PEPP course strives to use the most current evidence on pediatric prehospital interventions. It uses case-based lectures, live-action video, skill stations, and small group scenarios for a one-day BLS provider course and a 2-day ALS provider course. The PEPP course Web site (www.PEPPsite.com) provides information and links to course materials, a student manual, resource manual, live-action videotape, DVD and a CD-ROM toolkit of presentations, relevant images, and administrative forms.

► EQUIPMENT AND SUPPLIES

Proficient and appropriate prehospital care for children is dependent on pediatric-appropriate equipment and supplies. Pediatric BLS and ALS equipment and supply lists have been created by local EMS agencies and a collaborative effort of the Committee on Ambulance Equipment and Supplies and the National Emergency Medical Services for Children Resource Alliance (Tables 148–2 and 148–3).[7] Limited storage space, local/regional policies, as well as financial constraints ultimately dictate what particular supplies and equipment can be available for prehospital professionals on ambulances.

► MEDICAL DIRECTION AND PROTOCOLS

EMS medical direction can assume a variety of structures, from a single medical director to a physician advisory board, yet the founding principle of delegated practice is the same for any arrangement. Medical direction involves approving standards of care, policies, protocols, and procedures and assuring compliance with these standards with local and state regulations in order to assure quality patient care. The two categories of medical oversight are divided into direct or online medical control and indirect or offline medical control. Direct medical control consists of "real-time" supervision of EMS decisions and actions, which can occur directly on-scene or remotely

► **TABLE 148–2. BLS EQUIPMENT AND SUPPLIES FOR AMBULANCES**

Essential
Oropharyngeal airways: infant, child, adult (sizes 00–5)
Self-inflating resuscitation bag: child and adult sizes*
Masks for bag-valve-mask device: infant, child, and adult sizes†
Oxygen masks: infant, child, and adult sizes
Nonrebreathing mask: pediatric and adult sizes
Stethoscope
Backboard
Cervical immobilization device‡
Blood pressure cuff infant, child, and adult sizes
Portable suction unit with a regulator
Suction catheters: tonsil-tip and 6–14 Fr
Extremity splints: pediatric sizes
Bulb syringe
Obstetric pack
Thermal blanket§
Water-soluble lubricant

Desirable
Infant car seat‖
Nasopharyngeal airways: sizes 18–34 Fr, or 4.5–8.5 mm¶
Glasgow Coma Scale reference
Pediatric Trauma Score reference
Small stuffed toy

*A self-inflating resuscitation bag should be self-refilling, should have an oxygen reservoir, and should not have a pop-off valve. A child bag has a reservoir of 450 mL, whereas an adult bag has a reservoir of at least 1000 mL.
†A neonatal mask may be necessary for rescue units that may deliver a premature infant in the field.
‡Many types of cervical immobilization devices are available. These include wedges and collars. The type of device used will depend on local preference and policies and procedures. Whatever device is chosen should be stocked in a variety of sizes to fit infants, children, adolescents, and adults. The use of sandbags to meet this requirement is discouraged because they may cause injury if a patient must be turned.
§A thermal blanket may help minimize heat loss. Hypothermia will complicate many illnesses and injuries, particularly in infants and young children. The type of material used will depend on local preference, protocols, and procedures but may include Mylar, standard blankets, or aluminum foil for small infants.
‖Infants should be restrained in ambulances. Car seats may be used for medical emergencies or in trauma when the infant is already restrained in a seat and not critically injured. Traumatically injured infants should be restrained on a gurney if they are not already in a seat. Many types of seats are available to meet this guideline. A recently developed seat is collapsible and easy to store. The type of seat that is procured will be determined by local preference, policy, and procedure.
¶A nasopharyngeal airway may be useful when the upper airway compromises respiration and an oral airway cannot be secured. Providers must be trained in its use and know the contraindications for insertion of this device.

via radio or telephone. Medical oversight may be needed in these instances with regards to management decisions that are beyond the prehospital providers' scope of practice. Online medical control may also involve questions regarding field triage, transport issues, and refusals of and consent for care.

Indirect medical control often involves the development of standing orders and patient care protocols based on specific

▶ **TABLE 148-3. ALS EQUIPMENT AND SUPPLIES FOR AMBULANCES**

All ALS ambulances should carry everything on the BLS list, plus the following items.

Essential
Transport monitor
Defibrillator with adult and pediatric paddles*
Monitoring electrodes: pediatric sizes
Laryngoscope with straight blades 0–2, curved blades 2–4
Endotracheal tube stylets: pediatric and adult sizes
Endotracheal tubes: uncuffed sizes 2.5–6.0, cuffed sizes
Magill forceps: pediatric and adult
Nasogastric tubes: 8–16 Fr[†]
Nebulizer
IV catheters: 16–24 gauge
Intraosseous needles
Length/weight-based drug dose chart or tape[‡]
Needles: 20–25 gauge
Resuscitation drugs and IV fluids that meet the local standards of practice

Desirable
Blood glucose analysis system[§]
Disposable CO, detection device

*A defibrillator should be able to deliver 5–360 J. The addition of pediatric paddles may give the responding unit enhanced capabilities but is not essential for units that rarely use this equipment. The defibrillator may be equipped with only adult paddles/pads or pediatric paddles and adult paddles/pads. Units carrying only adult paddles/pads should ensure that providers are trained in the proper use of adult paddles in infants and children. When the defibrillator cannot deliver a low dose of joules for infants, shock at the lowest possible energy level.
[†]Nasogastric tubes may be useful when the transport time is greater than 30 min in patients who have abdominal distention that may impede respiration.
[‡]One example of a commercially available item that correlates length with weight to generate accurate drug doses and equipment needed for resuscitation is the Broselow tape. Other length/weight tapes or charts may be substituted for this device.
[§]Many EMS systems estimate blood glucose in the field. The accuracy of any one blood glucose test is influenced by many factors such as the shelf life of the particular strip used, how the blood sample was obtained, and the education of the providers performing the skill. Quality improvement is an important component of any laboratory analysis and should be applied to this field procedure. Universal precautions must always be followed when blood is handled.

predefined clinical scenarios that are readily identified by EMS personnel. A foundation of frequent, high-quality prehospital pediatric educational opportunities is necessary for meaningful offline medical direction and appropriate usage of protocols.

▶ LEGAL ISSUES

Minor patients cannot refuse treatment and transport in an emergency situation. If parents are present and refuse care for their children, they should be informed of the risks of not treating their child and asked to sign a form releasing the EMS service from responsibility. If there is a life-threatening emergency or suspected child abuse, a child must be treated and

transported regardless of consent. Communication with online medical control and documentation is of paramount importance in these situations. All prehospital providers should be aware of the existence of out-of-hospital do not resuscitate (DNR) documents in their state and their policies and protocols should include standard procedures that comply with state regulations. It is always important to remember that DNR orders can be revoked at any time based on the wishes of the legal guardian and/or parent.

▶ CARE IN THE COMMUNITY ED

Community hospital EDs provide the majority of emergency care for children and, consequently, emergency medicine providers have been asked to take a major role in advocating for essential equipment and supplies (Tables 148–4 and 148–5)[8] needed to stabilize and provide appropriate care for sick and injured children. In 2001, the AAP and American College of Emergency Physicians (ACEP) jointly released a policy statement suggesting a set of guidelines for pediatric preparedness of EDs by identifying a physician and nursing representatives to administrate and coordinate these objectives[9]:

- Staff education and training.
- Development of pediatric emergency treatment protocols, policies, and support services for the ED.
- Organization and maintenance of pediatric patient quality improvement initiatives.
- Establishment of transfer agreements and relationships with other local institutions that have the resources and personnel to provide a higher level of pediatric care.

Educational resources for providers in community EDs include the Pediatric Advanced Life Support (PALS) program sponsored by the American Heart Association, Advanced Pediatric Life Support (APLS) program supported by the AAP and ACEP, and the Emergency Nursing Pediatric Course (ENPC) developed by the Emergency Nurses Association. Regional specialized pediatric centers can also be an extremely helpful resource. Open communication and quality assurance feedback is essential.

▶ TRANSFER CONSIDERATIONS

Physicians in the ED should know the pediatric capabilities of the institution where they are working. It is also important to know when to transfer a patient and to whom. Many institutions choose to have transfer agreements with pediatric referral centers, particularly those institutions with pediatric trauma capabilities. In transferring a patient, the referring physician must contact the receiving physician, obtain acceptance, and also make arrangements for the transfer. The child must be stabilized to the full extent possible in the referring institution prior to the transfer.

▶ SPECIAL CONSIDERATIONS

PEDIATRIC TRAUMA

Traumatic injuries are leading cause of death in children. Unfortunately, significant differences from adults in the airway anatomy and cardiovascular and respiratory physiology of the

▶ TABLE 148-4. PEDIATRIC RESUSCITATION MEDICATIONS

Drug Name	How Supplied	Quantity per Container
Atropine	Prefilled syringe	10 mL (0.1 mg/mL), 5 mL (0.1 mg/mL)
Adenosine	Vial	1 mL (1 mg/mL)
Bretylium	Prefilled syringe	10 mL (50 mg/mL)
	Ampule	10 mL (50 mg/mL)
	Vial	20 mL (50 mg/mL)
Calcium chloride	Prefilled syringe	10 mL (100 mg/mL = 27.1 mg elemental calcium)
Dextrose	Prefilled syringe	10 mL (25% and 50%)
Dopamine	Vial	5 mL (40 mg/mL), 10 mL (40 mg/mL)
Dobutamine	Vial	10 mL (25 mg/mL), 20 mL (12.5 mg/mL)
Epinephrine	Prefilled syringe	1 mL, 2 mL
1:1000	Vial	30 mL (1 mg/mL)
Epinephrine 1:10,000	Prefilled syringe	10 mL (0.1 mg/mL), 3 mL (0.1 mg/mL)
Isoproterenol	Vial	5 mL (0.2 mg/mL)
Lidocaine	Prefilled syringe	5 mg/mL, 10 mg/mL, 15 mg/mL, 20 mg/mL
	Vial	40 mg/mL, 100 mg/mL, 200 mg/mL
	Ampule	5 mL (20 mg/mL)
Naloxone	Vial	1 mL, 10 mL (0.4 mg/mL), 1 mL, 10 mL (0.4 mg/mL)
Sodium bicarbonate	Prefilled syringe	50 mL (8.4%) (1 mEq/mL), 10 mL (8.4%) (1 mEq.mL), 10 mL (4.2%) (0.5 mEq/mL)

pediatric patient make evaluation and management of the traumatically injured child challenging. However, the treatment priorities in a child who is seriously injured are the same as those in an adult.

Critical management priorities should focus on the **ABCD**s: measures to maintain a patent **A**irway, ensure adequacy of **B**reathing and ventilation, support of **C**irculation with hemorrhage control, and minimizing any further **D**isability—with particular attention paid to those patients with a significant traumatic brain or cervical spine injury.

Advanced airway placement and control of ventilation, careful regulation of systemic blood pressure, and frequent assessment of neurologic status are paramount in the child with suspected significant traumatic brain injury. The Glasgow Coma Score (GCS) may be difficult to apply in younger children. Alternatively, the AVPU score may be used: **A**lert, responsive to **V**erbal stimulus, responsive to **P**ainful stimulus, or **U**nresponsive. Head injury is the leading cause of mortality in injured children; cervical spine injury, although rare, can lead to severe morbidity if not appropriately managed. Children may have spinal cord injury without apparent evidence on plain radiographs, therefore, proper spine immobilization should be maintained if an injury is suspected, if there are any neurological abnormalities, neck tenderness, or distracting injuries that would preclude a reliable physical examination until the child is calm and cooperative enough to allow a complete neck and back examination.

▶ DISASTER PREPAREDNESS

Children comprise one-third of the general population, but are frequently an afterthought in mass casualty incidents/disaster situations, despite being one of the segments of society more

at risk in the aftermath. The EMS continuum of resources and providers would be overrun by the large number of patients needing medical attention or an initial evaluation generated by the event—a current assessment of their responsiveness and preparedness is fundamental in improving their role in the disaster plan. The same issues necessitating pediatric-specific resources, equipment, and supplies would be multiplied severalfold. Disaster planning by federal, state, and local authorities *must* include pediatric-specific preparedness considerations. Health care advocates for children should proactively seek to provide expertise and advanced skills to enhance their community's mass casualty incident plans. Disaster preparedness is further discussed in the chapter on Mass Casualty Incidents.

▶ CHILDREN WITH SPECIAL HEALTH CARE NEEDS

Children with special health care needs constitute an extremely important subgroup of the pediatric patient population. Prehospital providers and often community hospitals are neither equipped nor experienced with dealing with these technology-dependent children. The AAP and ACEP jointly advocate the use of the Emergency Information Form (EIF) (Fig. 148–1) for Children with Special Health Care Needs (CSHCN) and have published a Joint Policy Statement on Emergency Preparedness for CSHCN initially in 1999 with links to a question-and-answer page, blank forms, instructions on how to use the form, multiple sample forms, and other resources available (http://www.aap.org/advocacy/emergprep.htm).[11] The AAP National Center of Medical Home Initiatives champions the idea of the "medical home" as a pediatric primary care delivery model for this population specifically (http://www.medicalhomeinfo.org/).

▶ **TABLE 148-5. GUIDELINES FOR MINIMUM EQUIPMENT AND SUPPLIES FOR CARE OF PEDIATRIC PATIENTS IN EDs**

Essential Equipment and Supplies

Monitoring
Cardiorespiratory monitor with strip recorder
Defibrillator (0–400 J capability) with pediatric and adult paddles (4.5 and 8 cm)
Pediatric and adult monitor electrodes
Pulse oximeter with sensors sizes newborn through adult
Thermometer/rectal probe*
Sphygmomanometer
Doppler blood pressure device
Blood pressure cuffs (neonatal, infant, child, adult, and thigh sizes)
Method to monitor endotracheal tube and placement[†]

Vascular access
Butterfly needles (19- to 25-gauge)
Catheter-over-needle devices (14- to 24-gauge)
Infusion device[‡]
Tubing for above
Intraosseous needles (16- and 18-gauge)[§]
Arm boards (infant, child, and adult sizes)
Intravenous fluid/blood warmers
Umbilical vein catheters (sizes 3.5 Fr and 5 Fr)[‖]
Seldinger technique vascular access kit (with pediatric sizes 3, 4, 5 Fr catheters)

Airway management
Clear oxygen masks (preterm, infant, child, and adult sizes)
Non-rebreathing masks (infant, child, and adult sizes)
Oral airways (sizes 00–5)
Nasopharyngeal airways (12–30 Fr)
Bag-valve-mask resuscitator, self-inflating (450 and 1000 mL sizes)
Nasal cannulae (infant, child, and adult sizes)
Endotracheal tubes: uncuffed (sizes 2.5–8.5) and cuffed (sizes 5.5–9)
Stylets (pediatric and adult sizes)
Laryngoscope handle (pediatric and adult)
Laryngoscope blades, curved (sizes 2 and 3) and straight (sizes 0–3)

Magill forceps (pediatric and adult)
Nasogastric tubes (sizes 6–14 Fr)
Suction catheters: flexible (sizes 5 to 16 Fr) and Yankauer suction tip
Chest tubes (sizes 8–40 Fr)
Tracheostomy tubes (sizes 00–6)[¶]

Resuscitation medications (Table 148–4)
Medication chart, tape, or other system to ensure ready access to information on proper per kilogram doses for resuscitation drugs and equipment sizes[#]

Miscellaneous
Infant and standard scales
Infant formula and oral rehydrating solutions
Heating source**
Towel rolls/blanket rolls or equivalent
Pediatric restraining devices
Resuscitation board
Sterile linen[††]

Specialized pediatric trays
Tube thoracotomy with water seal drainage capability
Lumbar puncture (spinal needle sizes 20-, 22-, and 25-gauge)
Urinary catheterization with pediatric Foley catheters (sizes 5–16 Fr)
Obstetric pack
Newborn kit
Umbilical vessel cannulation supplies
Meconium aspirator
Venous cutdown
Surgical airway kit[‡‡]

Fracture management
Cervical immobilization equipment (sizes child to adult)[§§]
Extremity splints
Femur splints (child and adult sizes)

Desirable equipment and supplies
Medical photography capability

*Suitable for hypothermic and hyperthermic measurements with temperature capability from 25° C to 44° C.
[†]May be satisfied by a disposable ETCO$_2$ detector, bulb, or feeding tube methods for endotracheal tube placement.
[‡]To regulate rate and volume.
[§]May be satisfied by standard bone marrow aspiration needles, 13- or 15-gauge.
[‖]Available within the hospital.
[¶]Ensure availability of pediatric sizes within the hospital.
[#]System for estimating medication doses and supplies may use the length-based method with color codes or other predetermined weight (kilogram)/dose method.
**May be met by infrared lamps or overhead warmer.
[††]Available within hospital for burn care.
[‡‡]May include any of the following items: tracheostomy tray, cricothyrotomy tray, ETJV (needle jet).
[§§]Many types of cervical immobilization devices are available. These include wedges and collars. The type of device chosen depends on local preference and policies and procedures. Whatever device is chosen should be stocked in sizes to fit infants, children, adolescents, and adults. The use of sandbags to meet this requirement is discouraged because they may cause injury if the patient has to be turned.

Emergency information form for children with special needs

American College of
Emergency Physicians*

American Academy
of Pediatrics

Date form	Revised	Initials
completed		
By whom	Revised	Initials

Name:		Birth date:	Nickname:
Home address:		Home/Work phone:	
Parent/guardian:		Emergency contact names & relationship:	
Signature/consent*:			
Primary language:		Phone number(s):	
Physicians:			
Primary care physician:		Emergency phone:	
		Fax:	
Current specialty physician: Specialty:		Emergency phone:	
		Fax:	
Current Specialty physician: Specialty:		Emergency phone:	
		Fax:	
Anticipated primary ED: Anticipated tertiary care center:		Pharmacy:	

Diagnoses/past procedures/physical exam:	
1.	Baseline physical findings:
2.	
3.	Baseline vital signs:
4.	
Synopsis:	
	Baseline neurological status:

*Consent for release of this form to health care providers

Figure 148–1. Emergency information form. (With permission from American College of Emergency Physicians and American Academy of Pediatrics.)

Diagnoses/past procedures/physical exam continued:	
Medications:	Significant baseline ancillary findings (lab, x-ray, ECG):
1.	
2.	
3.	
4.	Prostheses/appliances/advanced technology devices:
5.	
6.	

Management data:	
Allergies: Medications/foods to be avoided	and why:
1.	
2.	
3.	
Procedures to be avoided	and why:
1.	
2.	
3.	

Immunizations (mm/yy)

Dates						Dates					
DPT						Hep B					
OPV						Varice lla					
MMR						TB					
						status					
HIB						Other					

Antibiotic prophylaxis: Indication: Medication and dose:

Figure 148–1. (*Continued*)

ABUSE

In addition to inappropriate refusal of transport and care, prehospital providers may also encounter scenarios in which they observe or suspect child maltreatment or neglect. EMS personnel are mandated reporters of child abuse in almost every state. However, it is important that they do not confront those caregivers suspected of child abuse, but remember their primary responsibility is to stabilize and transport those patients safely to the ED. Careful documentation is a paramount in these situations.

PSYCHIATRIC CONSIDERATIONS

The floridly psychotic or aggressive pediatric patient presents a unique problem for prehospital providers. EMS personnel must not endanger their own safety, but must also efficiently

Common presenting problems/findings with specific suggested managements		
Problem Considerations	Suggested diagnostic studies	Treatment

Comments on child, family, or other specific medical issues:
Physician/provider signature: Print name:

Figure 148–1. (*Continued*)

evaluate, treat, stabilize, and transport these patients to the appropriate facility. Law enforcement assistance might be required and the use of physical and/or pharmaceutical restraints may also be necessary.

► AREAS FOR RESEARCH/ CONTROVERSIES

Research in pediatric prehospital provider care is important but difficult to accomplish. Problematic factors include the sometimes hazardous environment, the unpredictable nature of the patient's initial presentation, regional and local inconsistencies with protocols, and lack of current evidence to support specific management strategies. Innovations in pediatric-specific equipment for advanced airway management and vascular access have benefited the prehospital community. However, advanced airway issues, pain management control, out-of-hospital resuscitation, and proper spinal immobilization in trauma are only a few of the controversial topics that necessitate continued high-quality research. Fortunately, there are federally funded organizations that were created to help support the mission to conduct significant research in the field of pediatric emergency care.

► PECARN

PECARN (Pediatric Emergency Care Applied Research Network; http://www.pecarn.org/) originated from a cooperative agreement between the EMSC program and four academic medical centers to create the first federally funded pediatric emergency medicine research network. The PECARN consists of the following:

- A data coordinating center, the Central Data Management and Coordinating Center (CDMCC), at the University of Utah (http://www.pecarn.org/coordinating Center/index.html).
- 4 Research Node Centers (RNC).
- 21 Hospital Emergency Department Affiliates (HEDAs).

- A steering committee with equal representation from each RNC and CDMCC.

The PECARN's goal is to promote and facilitate high-priority, multi-institutional, collaborative research amongst EMSC investigators and providers.

► NEDARC

NEDARC is a national resource center and is funded by a cooperative agreement with HHS-MCHB, whose mission is to

- help develop data systems to evaluate state and national EMS system effectiveness.
- help enable EMSC grantees and state EMS office personnel develop proficiency in research and data utilization skills.
- provide technical, administrative, and research support to EMS agencies.

REFERENCES

1. Institute of Medicine, Committee on Pediatric Emergency Medical Services; Durch JS, Lohr KN, eds. *Emergency Medical Services for Children.* Washington, DC: National Academy Press; 1993.
2. Institute of Medicine, Committee on the Future of Emergency Care in the United States Health System. *Emergency Care for Children: Growing Pains.* Washington, DC: National Academy Press; 2007.
3. Donoghue A, Nadkarni V, Berg RA, et al. Out-of-hospital pediatric cardiac arrest: an epidemiologic review and assessment of current knowledge. *Ann Emerg Med.* 2005;46:512–522.
4. Committee on Pediatric Emergency Medicine. Role of pediatricians in advocating life support training courses for parents and the public. *Pediatrics.* 2004;114:1676.
5. Flores G, Weinstock DJ. The preparedness of pediatricians for emergencies in the office. *Arch Pediatr Adolesc Med.* 1996;150: 249–256.
6. Committee on Pediatric Emergency Medicine. Preparation for emergencies in the offices of pediatricians and pediatric primary care providers. *Pediatrics.* 2007;120:200–212.

7. Committee on Ambulance Equipment and Supplies, National Emergency Medical Service for Children Resource Alliance. Guidelines for pediatric equipment and supplies for basic and advanced life support ambulances. *Prehosp Emerg Care.* 1997; 1:286–287.

8. Committee on Pediatric Equipment and Supplies for Emergency Departments, National Emergency Medical Services for Children Resource Alliance. Guidelines for pediatric equipment and supplies for emergency departments. *Ann Emerg Med.* 1998;31:54–57.

9. American College of Emergency Physicians and the American Academy of Pediatrics. Care of children in the emergency department: guidelines for preparedness. *Ann Emerg Med.* 2001;37:423–427.

10. Committee on Pediatric Emergency Medicine. Consent for emergency medical services for children and adolescents. *Pediatrics.* 2003;111:703–706.

11. Committee on Pediatric Emergency Medicine. Emergency preparedness for children with special health care needs. *Pediatrics.* 1999;104:e53.

CHAPTER 149

Interfacility Transport

Maeve Sheehan and Craig J. Huang

▶ HIGH-YIELD FACTS

- Outcomes for critically ill and injured children improve when treatment is provided by skilled pediatric specialist transport teams.
- Appropriate medical care for any patient with an emergent condition should never be delayed because of inability to find a caregiver or guardian to give consent for treatment.
- The referring physician is responsible for stabilizing the patient's condition, within the capabilities of the referring institution, before the patient is transferred t another institution.
- Limitation of resuscitation orders (DNR) may be revoked at any time according to the parents or legal guardians' wishes.
- Composition of team personnel is driven by the needs of the patient being transported.
- A well-run communication system is vital for the safety of patients and transport personnel.
- All communications pertaining to transport should be recorded and saved.
- Transport personnel must be familiar with their protocols and the limitations and responsibilities of their specific profession's scope of practice.
- Safety training for the teams should be part of their initial training and ongoing competencies.
- Personal protective equipment is important to protect team members.
- Stresses of flight affect both the patient and crew members and should always be taken into consideration when transporting a patient.
- At high altitude, a child may become hypoxic and pneumothoraxes can expand.

▶ HISTORICAL PERSPECTIVES

Specialized transport systems have evolved from military conflicts; the earliest references date from the Napoleonic wars. The first reported transport of a patient via aircraft took place in 1915. Invented in 1942, the helicopter saw its first use in air medical transport in Burma in 1944.[1] Development of specialized pediatric transport teams began in the 1970s with the establishment of neonatal intensive care units. Outcomes for critically ill and injured children improve when treatment is provided by skilled pediatric specialists. The need for rapid and safe transport of such children has driven the formation of specialized pediatric transport teams.

▶ LEGAL CONSIDERATIONS

INTERFACILITY

Approximately 2%–3% of all children seeking treatment in an emergency department (ED) are not accompanied by a parent or legal guardian. All efforts should be made to obtain consent for treatment and transfer of a pediatric patient, but appropriate medical care for the patient with an urgent or emergent condition, including transport, should never be withheld or delayed because of problems obtaining consent. Appropriate documentation of these efforts is important.

Federal law under the Emergency Medical Treatment and Active Labor Act (EMTALA) mandates a medical screening for every patient seeking treatment in an ED of any hospital that participates in programs that seek federal funding, regardless of reimbursement considerations. If an emergency medical condition is identified, EMTALA mandates therapy up to and including surgical intervention.[2] If definitive care cannot be rendered at the local hospital, the patient should be transferred to a hospital that has the resources and capabilities to care for the patient. The referring physician is responsible for stabilizing the patient's condition, within the capabilities of the referring institution, before the patient is transferred to another facility. The referring physician is also responsible for initiating transport and selecting the mode of transfer. The receiving physician is responsible for ensuring that the receiving facility is able to deliver the necessary care and agrees to accept the transfer. They should also assist where possible in making arrangements for the transfer.[3] The transport team should be aware of any limitation of resuscitation orders that may be in place, especially in the case of a chronically ill child. Special state out-of-hospital "Do Not Resuscitate" orders (DNR) may exist, and these must be complied with. This information needs to be discussed with the medical control physician prior to transporting the child. DNR orders may be revoked at any time according to the wishes of the parent or legal guardian.

MEDICAL RESPONSIBILITY

One of the more complex legal issues in interfacility transport is regarding the legal responsibility for medical decisions and interventions at the referring facility. The specialty pediatric transport team may lead the process of preparing the child for transport, but the referring physician and other hospital personnel remain legally responsible for the patient. The referring physician chooses the transport service and the mode of transport most appropriate for the medical condition of the patient. If at any time the referring physician deems it in the best interest of the patient to intervene or cancel the transfer, the physician has a right and a duty to do so. The transport team has a duty to provide the best care possible to the patient. Although EMTALA states that the referring physician has legal responsibility, the transport service clearly assumes some liability when it begins rendering care. In reality, there is shared responsibility on the part of both parties.

▶ TEAM COMPOSITION AND TRAINING

Transport teams involve a variety of professional personnel, including physicians, nurses, respiratory care practitioners, paramedics, and emergency medical technicians. The ideal composition of the team is driven by the needs of the patient being transported[4] (Table 149–1). Team members should be dedicated to the transport program and trained to work as a team. The incidence of transport-related morbidity increases significantly when personnel without specialized train-

ing in pediatrics transport critically ill children. Only 10% of EMS transports involve pediatric patients, and many adult EMS providers lack all but basic training in the treatment of critically ill children, mainly owing to limited pediatric exposure. Specialized pediatric transport teams fill a needed void to help stabilize and transport critically ill and injured children to a tertiary care pediatric facility.[5] The presence of a physician on a team is variable. Transport literature indicates that non–physician-based transport team members are efficient and competent to perform advanced procedures, including intubations. It is essential that all transport team members have an opportunity to develop and maintain these skills on an ongoing basis.

▶ COMMUNICATION

Interfacility transports require coordination and communication between multiple care providers and facilities. A well-run communication system is vital for the safety of patients and transport personnel. The communication center should be staffed 24 hours a day, 7 days a week.

The transfer center coordinator receives initial communication and facilitates communication between the referring and receiving physician. The coordinator then notifies and

▶ **TABLE 149–1. POTENTIAL ADVANTAGES AND DISADVANTAGES OF VARIOUS PERSONNEL FOR NEONATAL PEDIATRIC TRANSPORT TEAMS**

Transport Personnel	Advantages	Disadvantages
Specialty-trained attending physician	Expertise; public relations; critical care training and skills	High salary cost; limited availability for full-time coverage; care and supervision limited to one patient at a time
Nonintensive care-, non-neonatology-, or nonemergency medicine-trained attending physician	Expertise; public relations	High salary cost; limited availability for full-time coverage; care and supervision limited to one patient at a time; critical care skill acquisition as needed
Fellow	Expertise; valuable training experience	Transport demands might overburden other aspects of training availability; availability might be limited by Accreditation Council for Graduate Medical Education (ACGME) work rules
Resident	Valuable training experience; salary cost may be built into the training program	Demands of transport compete with other aspects of training and education; limited clinical experience; availability might be limited by ACGME work rules
Advanced practice neonatal or pediatric nurse practitioner	Expertise; consistent quality of care	High salary costs; usually limited to discipline for which they are trained (e.g., neonatal nurse practitioner vs. pediatric nurse practitioner); acceptance as specialized provider by referring care team can be an issue if community expectations are for physician-led team
Critical care nurse	Availability; expertise with appropriate training; uniform quality of care	Initial acceptance by referring care team can be an issue; requires intensive training to function independently in the transport environment
Respiratory therapist	Focused respiratory assessments; knowledge of respiratory equipment; advanced airway and ventilator expertise	Focused airway training and experience; requires intensive training to expand to more global patient care
Paramedic or emergency medical technicians	Expertise in prehospital setting; availability; less costly than other team members	Less formal medical and pediatric training and perhaps experience; requires intensive training to assist with other areas of patient care

dispatches the appropriate team. The teams are in direct communication with the medical control physician via the transfer center. The transfer center coordinator tracks the location of the teams and can communicate with the referring hospital if delays because of weather or mechanical issues arise. The communication center can also coordinate follow-up information for referring facilities, while adhering to Health Insurance Portability and Accountability Act (HIPAA) regulations.

It is essential that all communications pertaining to transport are recorded and the recordings are preserved. Communication with outside facilities can be streamlined by having a contact number that is readily accessible. The transfer coordinator can have a standard set of basic questions that allow for easy identification of the appropriate receiving hospital unit, such as the ED or an intensive care unit. A transport outreach liaison can facilitate preparation for transport by communicating regularly with referring facilities, providing them with information on how to contact the transport service, and how best to prepare the child for transport.

▶ EQUIPMENT AND MEDICATION

Equipment and medication requirements for transport depend on the type of patient that the team encounters. The transport mission limitation policy should address the types of patients a facility has the capability to transport. Special equipment consideration is needed for basic life support (BLS) and advanced life support (ALS) transports, neonates, children, and adult-size patients. Pediatric equipment lists are available for EMS providers (see pediatric equipment list in Chapter 148). Specialized pediatric transport services possess a much more comprehensive list. This list should satisfy all city and state requirements, and be regularly updated by the transport medical director. Storage of medication should be addressed, since some medications need to be refrigerated. Multiple doses of medications and extra equipment need to be available for emergencies and long transports. Special regulations exist surrounding the use of narcotics. Medications should be checked daily, before and after each transport. The lists of equipment and supplies should be checked regularly to ensure that everything is present, in good working order, and within their expiration dates. Policies and procedures should be developed to ensure compliance with this standard.

▶ PROTOCOLS

Transport teams should have written protocols to direct patient care, under the authority of the transport medical director. These protocols need to be updated regularly by the medical director. Input should be sought from the teams utilizing the protocols, including legal counsel when necessary. Protocols should be easily accessible and straightforward. Protocols serve as a guideline for care until the teams can contact the medical control physician. Transport personnel must be familiar with the protocols, and the limitations and responsibilities of their specific profession's scope of practice. They need to seek help from their medical control physician or the physician on transport when they are outside their scope of practice

▶ MEDICAL DIRECTION

The medical director of the transport service is "a physician who is responsible for supervising and evaluating the quality of the medical care provided by the medical personnel."[6] He or she should be involved in all aspects of the care provided by the teams. This includes the hiring and education of the team members, including the transport medical control physicians, development of policies, procedures, and transport protocols, infection control principles, quality assurance, and overall safety of the program for the patients and staff. The medical director should "promote open communication with referring and accepting physicians and be accessible for concerns expressed by referring and accepting physicians regarding controversial issues and patient management."[6] The medical director of the transport team may be the medical control physician or he or she may have a designee.

The medical control physician is a physician who provides "on-line" medical advice to the teams on transport. The medical control physician is involved in giving advice to the referring physician with regard to stabilization of the patient prior to the team's arrival. He or she may help in selection of the most appropriate mode of transport. When the team arrives, report is usually given to the medical control physician, and a discussion ensues with regard to further stabilization and treatment during the transport. The medical control physician is available at all times to the teams if further advice is needed. All communication between the medical control physician and transport personnel should be recorded. The medical control physician should have the appropriate skill level regarding the patient population served by the transport service.

▶ REGULATORY REQUIREMENTS/ CERTIFICATION STANDARDS

Interfacility transport services must meet city and state requirements for ambulance services, as well as meet all hospital standards. If they have flight capabilities, they must also comply with FAA (Federal Aviation Administration) regulations. If they choose to do so, transport services may wish to become accredited by Commission on Accreditation of Medical Transport Systems (CAMTS). This organization was founded in 1990 as a response to a number of air-medical accidents in the 1980s. CAMTS is a nonprofit organization supported by 16 member organizations, including the American Academy of Pediatrics (AAP) and the American College of Emergency Physicians (ACEP). CAMTS offers a program to evaluate compliance with accreditation standards that demonstrate the ability of the transport service to deliver specific services to patients. Their focus is on quality of patient care and safety during transport. The Joint Commission on Accreditation of Healthcare Organizations (JCAHO) was developed in 1915 when the American College of Surgeons, based on a study that demonstrated dismal outcomes for hospitalized patients, allocated funds to establish standards for quality of patient care in hospitals. Both JCAHO and CAMTS are voluntary bodies which set minimum standards for quality of patient care and safety in the medical environment. In 1990, the AAP formed a Section of Transport

Medicine to address the interfacility transport of infants, children, and adolescents. In 1993, the AAP published Guidelines for Air and Ground Transport of Neonatal and Pediatric Patients. This manual is now in its third edition and serves as an invaluable resource for neonatal and pediatric transport services.[7]

▶ STABILIZATION FOR TRANSPORT

The goal of interfacility transport is to improve care provided to a patient. It is important that the child is as stable as possible for the transport. The accepting and/or medical control physician should give advice as needed to the referring facility on how to prepare the child for transport. Multiple interventions may need to be performed by the referring team and/or the transport team prior to the child leaving the referring facility. Attention must be paid to the basic concepts of medical care. If a child is in respiratory distress, he or she may need a stable airway prior to transport. Occasionally, a child may have an unexpectedly difficult airway or an airway that the primary medical team is uncomfortable attempting to intubate. The medical control physician should be involved in helping the referring physician in deciding what best options may exist in this situation. The transport team should have the necessary pediatric equipment to establish an airway, as well as adjuncts to help with a difficult airway. Some referring facilities will have anesthesia back-up should a problematic airway be encountered. Laryngeal mask airways (LMAs) are a temporizing measure, but are not considered stable airways for transport in many facilities.[8] It is also important to ensure that a child has adequate intravenous access prior to transport. Pneumothoraxes should be treated prior to flight. When the child reaches the accepting facility, the referring physician should get follow-up information about the patient he or she referred. It is important to address any quality assurance (QA) issues that may have arisen before or during the transport.

▶ MODES OF TRANSPORT

Children may be transported by ground ambulance, helicopter, or fixed-wing aircraft. Ground ambulance is the most common mode of transport. Advantages to transporting a child by ground ambulance include adequate space to perform emergency interventions and to permit transport of a family member. The truck can easily be halted to facilitate emergency interventions. There is no need for an airport or helicopter landing zone when transporting by ambulance, and ground transportation is less likely to be delayed owing to inclement weather. It is the safest mode of transport. The major disadvantage is the travel time needed to cover long distances, particularly if the child is critically ill.

Helicopter transport is becoming an increasingly popular method of medical transport. It is fast, and most hospitals have a space for a helicopter to land. It is often available for scene transports, particularly in remote and difficult terrain. Disadvantages include the stresses of flight, lack of space to perform emergency interventions, and unavailability in inclement weather. The distance a helicopter can travel depends on multiple factors (Table 149–2). Fixed-wing aircraft is usu-

ally reserved for long-distance interfacility transports. There is usually room on the plane to perform emergency interventions and to accommodate a parent. Problems include altitude considerations, weather limitations, and the need for an airport. Ground transportation needs to be arranged for pick up and return at each end of the transport. Determining the mode of transport ultimately depends on a number of factors. The main considerations involve the acuity of the child's illness, the resources available, the time of day, distance to be traveled, traffic, and weather. Whatever mode is chosen, it needs to be the safest possible for both the patient and the team.

▶ SAFETY/ALTITUDE PHYSIOLOGY AND AIR MEDICAL CONSIDERATIONS

VEHICLE SAFETY

Air and ground transports are not without risk. King and Woodward published a 5-year review of accidents involving pediatric and neonatal transports in 2002 and found that accident rates were approximately 1 per 1000 transports. Collisions where injury was sustained occurred at a rate of 0.546 per 1000 accidents. There were eight fatalities, all occurring with air transports.[9] According to the NTSB (National Transportation Safety Board), accident rates and the number of flight hours have increased substantially since this study was concluded.

Transport personnel must be familiar with safety features of the various transport vehicles in which they will be traveling. Safety considerations should be part of a team's initial and continuing training. Policies and procedures of the transport service should specifically address safety considerations, including considering weather, use of lights and sirens on the ambulance, use of restraints, weight limitations for flight, and vehicular maintenance. In the case of hazardous weather conditions, the final decision as to safety of travel should reside with the pilot or driver of the transport vehicle, and should be supported by the transport medical director. One must always err on the side of caution when it comes to patient and personnel safety.

PERSONNEL SAFETY

Personal protective equipment is important to protect the team members. The NTSB has stated that "helmets, flame-and-heat-resistant uniforms, and protective footwear can help reduce or prevent injury" in accidents.[10] Appropriate universal infectious disease precautions should be undertaken when dealing with all patients, not just those patients with known infections or who are bleeding. Gowns, gloves, and masks should be used whenever appropriate and possible, and transport policies should mirror the institutional-based policies in the case of accidental needle stick injuries or exposure to blood and/or body fluids.

It is important to provide appropriate equipment to personnel to prevent injury when lifting patients. Much media attention has focused on the growing problem of obesity in

▶ **TABLE 149-2. DETERMINING THE MODE OF TRANSPORT**

| Distance Traveled | Type of Transport Required* | | | |
	BLS	ALS 1	ALS 2	SCT
≤40 miles (ground)	GA	GA	GA	GA
40–100 miles	GA	GA	RWA	RWA
≥100 miles	GA/FWA	GA/FWA	FWA/RWA	FWA/RWA

Category	Transport Patient Classification System
BLS	Vital signs within normal limits upon arrival to referral
	No respiratory distress
	Trauma—Uncomplicated fractures
	IV access—None
	No medications anticipated
ALS 1	O$_2$ saturation >93% on 2 L/min or less via NC or 5 L/min by simple face mask
	Mild respiratory distress
	Stable tracheostomy
	Foreign body in esophagus without signs of respiratory distress
	Trauma
	Complicated fracture(s); stable, uncompromised neurovascular status
	Skull fracture(s) without loss of consciousness, altered mental status or closed head injury
	Burns <10% body surface area, no respiratory distress or facial involvement
	Mild dehydration
	Decreased glucose, vomiting, diarrhea or dehydration treated by referral
	Known seizure disorder on routine anticonvulsants without active seizure activity
	IV or central access
ALS 2	O$_2$ saturation >93% on ≥3 L/min or less via NC or ≥6 L/min by simple face mask
	Mild/moderate respiratory distress, requiring aerosol treatment
	Established tracheostomy, required ventilator support
	Foreign body in trachea or esophagus with respiratory distress
	Potential for hemodynamic instability/respiratory compromise
	Dehydration with increased heart rate, delayed capillary refill and/or decreased pulses, or requiring >1 fluid bolus by referral
	Any rule out sepsis with a rash
	Altered level of consciousness, Glasgow Coma Scale (GCS) >8
	Active seizure activity or anticonvulsants for undiagnosed seizures in the last 4 h
	Altered glucose levels with unknown etiology or diabetic ketoacidosis
	Trauma
	Single system trauma and fractures with potential for neurovascular compromise and/or hemodynamic instability
	Skull fracture with altered level of consciousness or closed head injury
	Burns >10% BSA or with potential airway compromise
	IV access—potential for fluid resuscitation
SCT	Inotropic support required
	Hemodynamic instability
	Moderate/severe respiratory distress
	Intubated patients
	GCS <8
	Trauma
	Multisystem
	Skull fracture with epidural bleed

BLS, basic life support; ALS1, advanced life support 1; ALS2, advanced life support 2; SCT, special care transport; GA, ground ambulance; RWA, rotor-wing aircraft; FWA, fixed-wing aircraft.
*Exceptions to consider: traffic delays; weather; no airport in proximal vicinity to referring facility; referral or accepting physician insisting on a specific mode of transport; transport mode first choice unavailable.

▶ **TABLE 149–3. STRESSES OF FLIGHT**

Stressor	Effects
Decreased partial pressure of oxygen	Hypoxia
Barometric pressure changes	Barotitis media, barosinusitis, barodontalgia, gastrointestinal changes
Thermal changes	Hypothermia, hyperthermia
Decreased humidity	Dehydration
Noise	Degradation of communication, fatigue, temporary or permanent hearing loss
Vibration	Motion sickness, fatigue, shortness of breath, abdominal or chest pain, increased metabolic rate, increased respirations, orthopedic problems
Fatigue	Impaired judgment, difficulty maintaining attention to details and tasks, lessened ability to communicate effectively; increased risk of error; diminished critical thinking skills
Gravitational forces	Exposure to positive and negative acceleration forces, decompression sickness
Spatial disorientation	Cannot interpret or process information being given by the senses
Flicker vertigo	Nausea, vomiting
Fuel vapors	Altered mental status, nausea, eye inflammation

children and equipment such as hydraulic stretchers should be available to the teams to minimize back injuries. Policies and procedures are also necessary to protect the teams from disruptive patients and parents. Psychiatric patients require special consideration, such as the need for restraint. Policies and procedures need to be in place and adhered to in order to protect the patient and crew when dealing with firearms and knives carried by family members.

MEDICAL SAFETY ISSUES AND ALTITUDE PHYSIOLOGY

There are multiple medical stresses that need to be taken into consideration when transporting critically ill and injured children by air. Stresses of flight affect both the patient and crew members. These include the changes in barometric pressure, hypoxia, temperature, dehydration, noise, vibration, g-forces, third spacing, and fatigue. Teams may suffer visual problems and spatial disorientation, particularly when flying at night. Teams and patients also need protection from potential toxic hazards in the air medical transport environment[11] (Table 149–3).

Changes in barometric pressure and hypoxia are perhaps the most significant stressor to the patient and crew. Three gas laws (Boyle's law, Dalton's law, and Henry's law) govern the behaviors of gases under conditions of changing pressure. During ascent, the barometric pressure falls, unless it is controlled by the aircraft. This has medical implications in multiple ways. Boyle's law states that the volume of a gas is inversely proportional to its pressure, when temperature is constant; therefore, as barometric pressure is reduced, gases expand. At 8000 feet, which is effective cabin altitude for most pressurized aircraft, gas expansion is approximately 30% greater than at sea level. This can result in a small clinically insignificant pneumothorax becoming a life-threatening tension pneumothorax during flight. Air in other body cavities can also expand. In the brain this can lead to intracranial hypertension. Air in the stomach can cause nausea and vomiting and gastric distension that can interfere with lung expansion. In the middle ear, it can cause significant pain if the Eustachian tube is blocked. Air in endotracheal (ET) tube cuffs can expand, resulting in compres-

sive forces on the inner trachia. Thus, preventive measures are undertaken to minimize the risk of gas expansion. Pneumothoraxes are drained prior to flight, nasogastric tubes inserted to decompress the stomach, and cuff pressures on ET tubes are monitored and decompressed as necessary. If a child is awake, he or she should be encouraged to suck on a pacifier and/or chew on descent. The aircraft should ascend and descend slowly, or may be able to fly at a lower altitude. A team member with a significant upper respiratory infection or blocked Eustachian tube may not be able to participate in an air transport. Another medical implication of altitude is the fact that the amount of gas dissolved in solution is directly proportional to the pressure of the gas over the solution (Henry's law). This means that as barometric pressure falls with altitude, less gas is dissolved in solution, so there is less oxygen dissolved in blood and the child can become hypoxic just by the change in altitude. At sea level, the percentage oxygen saturation in room air is 98%; at 8000 feet, this saturation falls to 93% based on barometric pressure alone. This has implications for patients who are already hypoxic or are very sensitive to oxygen content in the blood, such as children with pulmonary hypertension. Oxygen administration may be increased prior to ascent to prevent this from becoming clinically significant, or consideration may be given to flying at lower altitude.

As altitude increases the air cools and humidity drops. For each 1000-ft gain in altitude there is a 2°C drop in temperature. Ambient humidity in a pressurized aircraft after 1 hour of flying is <5%. Pumping additional gas into an airplane may cause the environment to be cooler and dryer. Patients and team members need warm light clothing. Temperature and hydration are monitored, particularly with neonates who are already more vulnerable to cold. Using a hat will reduce up to 60% of radiated heat loss. Transporting an infant in an isolette is also protective.

Teams and patients may need to wear ear protection to protect against noise stress. Hearing tests should be administered annually to transport team members who fly. Once a hearing loss occurs from noise-induced causes, the damage is permanent.

Vibration and G-forces may cause nausea and fatigue and should be minimized where possible (Table 149–4).[11]

▶ **TABLE 149–4. PREVENTION OF COMPLICATIONS DURING AIR TRANSPORT OF NEONATAL AND PEDIATRIC PATIENTS**

Gas expansion

1. Insert orogastric or nasogastric tubes open to air in every infant and child who may experience gastrointestinal symptoms or may be at risk for vomiting.
2. If a cuffed endotracheal or tracheostomy tube is in place, carefully monitor cuff pressure or consider replacement of air with water to prevent expansion of the cuff with altitude changes.
3. Ensure that chest tubes, endotracheal tubes, and other artificial vents are patent.
4. Suction airway well before and during transport, as needed.
5. Reevaluate frequently for presence of extrapulmonary air.
   a. Carry a portable transillumination device (for neonates)
   b. Have a needle thoracentesis set available
6. Request that, if possible, the pilot fly at a lower altitude or increase the cabin pressurization (to simulate a lower altitude) when transporting a patient with trapped gas (e.g., pneumothorax, pneumoperitoneum, or bowel obstruction).

Decreased P_{O_2}

1. Before leaving the referring hospital
   a. Ensure that the child is optimally oxygenated
   b. Correlate arterial P_{O_2} and P_{CO_2} measurements with cutaneous pulse oximetry and end-tidal carbon dioxide (ET_{CO_2})
   c. Check placement and stabilization of the endotracheal tube
2. En route
   a. Use a cutaneous oxygen saturation monitor for all patients requiring oxygen or assisted ventilation (along with frequent careful assessment of the color of skin and mucous membranes)
   b. Increase (fraction of inspired oxygen) F_{IO_2} as needed to maintain adequate oxygenation saturation
   c. The oxygen adjustment equation can be used to calculate the F_{IO_2} required at any cabin altitude or destination altitude as follows:
      $(F_{IO_2} \times BP_1$ (current barometric pressure) $= F_{IO_2}$ required $\times BP_2$ (destination or altitude barometric pressure)

▶ SPECIFIC CLINICAL TRANSPORT ISSUES

NEONATAL TRANSPORT

Special considerations need to be taken into account when transporting a neonate. Neonates, particularly if they are premature, are very vulnerable to environmental changes and it is essential that they be kept warm. Furthermore, neonates do not have extensive glucose stores, thus their blood glucose must be closely monitored. Special equipment needs to be available for the transport of neonates (small ET tubes, isolette, transwarmer, neonatal ventilator, etc.) A child weighing less than 10 kg should be transported in a transport isolette. In this they are protected from environmental hazards such as cold, noise, and turbulence. It is also important to secure the child within the isolette, as turbulence may arise during the transport.

ACTIVE CARDIAC ARREST

Interfacility transport teams are occasionally called to transport a child in active cardiac arrest that occurs at the referring institution. Policies and procedures should be in place to address this situation. The medical control physician should be actively involved in if and when to transport the patient. It is reasonable to deploy the transport team to the referring facility, but the child must be alive at the time the decision is made to transport. If the child has a stable airway, a pulse, and a manageable blood pressure, the transport may proceed, but the

parents or guardians of the child must be informed of the high risk of further cardiac arrest and death during transport. It is important to try and identify the cause of the arrest prior to transport, so necessary interventions may be implemented to prevent further arrest.

REFERENCES

1. IJ Blumen, H Rodenberg, eds. *Air Medical Physician Handbook.* Salt Lake City, UT: Air Medical Physician Association; 1999.
2. Committee on Pediatric Emergency Medicine. Consent for emergency medical services for children and adolescents. *Pediatrics.* 2003;111:703.
3. American College of Surgeons Committee on Trauma. *Advanced Trauma Life Support Manual.* 7th ed. Chicago, IL: American College of Surgeons; 2004.
4. Horowitz R, Rozenfeld R. Pediatric critical care interfacility transport. *Clin Pediatr Emerg Med.* 2007;8:190–202.
5. Ajizian S, Nakagawa T. Interfacility transport of the critically ill pediatric patient: *Chest.* 2007;132(4):1361–1367.
6. Commission on Accreditation of Medical Transport Systems. *Accreditation Standards.* 7th ed. Anderson, SC: Commission on Accreditation of Medical Transport Systems; 2007.
7. Woodward G, Insoft R, Pearson-Shaver , et al. The state of pediatric interfacility transport: Consensus of the Second National Pediatric and Neonatal Interfacility Transport Medicine Leadership Conference. *Pediatr Emerg Care.* 2002;18(1): 38–43.
8. Orenstein J. Prehospital pediatric airway management. *Clin Pediatr Emerg Med.* 2006;7:31–37.

9. King BR, Woodward GA. Pediatric critical care transport—the safety of the journey: a five-year review of vehicular collisions involving pediatric and neonatal transport teams. *Prehosp Emerg Care.* 2002;6:449–454.

10. National Transportation Safety Board. *Aviation Special Investigation Report: Special Investigation Report On Emergency Medical Service Operations.* Washington, DC: National Transportation Safety Board; 2006. http://www.ntsb.gov/publictn/2006/SIR0601.pdf. Accessed March 11, 2008.

11. American Academy of Pediatrics Task Force on Interhospital Transport; Woodware G, Insoft R, Kleinman M, eds. *Guidelines for Air and Ground Transport of Neonatal and Pediatric Patients.* Elk Grove Village, IL: American Academy of Pediatrics; 2007.

CHAPTER 150

Mass Casualty Management

Janet Lin

▶ HIGH-YIELD FACTS

- Few hospitals have disaster plans that specifically address pediatric patients.
- Differences in developmental capability, size, weight, and physiology are important considerations in mass casualty incidents involving children.
- Appropriate equipment and access to age- and weight-adjusted doses of medications in treating pediatric patients.
- Care must be taken during decontamination of children in order to avoid hypothermia.
- Children have age-dependent psychological issues that must be taken into account.

Recent history has reinforced the need for mass casualty event (MCE) preparedness. The effect of a disaster is nondiscriminatory, although certain populations are more vulnerable than others. Most MCE preparedness has been devoted to the population in general, which often assumes an adult patient. However, children are not simply small adults. Unique issues surround the care and clinical management of the child. This chapter discusses the unique issues involving the provision of care to children in an MCE.

▶ MASS CASUALTY EVENTS

A MCE is an event that is characterized by an imbalance between the needs and resources available within a health care system. There is no predetermined number of victims that designates an MCE; however, many programs consider an influx of ten patients as an MCE.[1] The inciting event can be owing to natural disasters, transportation-related failures, civil disturbances, war, or terrorist-related activities. Whether an event targets children, as was the case in Breslan, Russia, where in September 2004, Chechen terrorists took a school hostage in a situation that resulted in hundreds of child deaths,[2] or children are secondarily involved, pediatric patients have physiologic, developmental, and behavioral differences from adults that influence their management in an MCE.

▶ UNIQUE PEDIATRIC CONSIDERATIONS

AGE, SIZE, WEIGHT

While there is no consensus regarding what age defines a child, many consider the pediatric population to consist of patients from birth to 18 years of age.[3,4] However, treating an 18-year-old is obviously far different than treating an infant or child. An MCE involving pediatric victims demands a wide range of skills and the availability of equipment to accommodate a range of sizes and weights. In terms of clinical management, age is often considered a surrogate for size and weight. Medications like antibiotics, vaccines, or antidotes need to be dosed according to the age, size, and/or weight of a child. Because of the metabolic differences in children when compared to adults, response to medication treatment may vary.[4]

DEVELOPMENTAL AND BEHAVIORAL CONSIDERATIONS

The stage of motor and cognitive development of a child will influence a responder's ability to communicate with and care for a victim. Nonverbal children are not able to voice their complaints or injuries, and may not be able to cognitively distinguish between one who is trying to help them from one who may be trying to hurt them. Nonambulatory children will not be able to flee a dangerous situation and need to be carried and transported away. Depending on the age and cognitive development of a child, he/she may refuse to move or even run toward a threat.[5] They may lack self-preservation skills that tell them to run away from a dangerous situation, or lack the decisional capacity to follow directions from strangers who are trying to help. Children may suffer anxiety owing to separation from their family or primary caretakers during a disaster.[6] They are also very susceptible to the reactions and mental state of their caretakers.[7] Children rarely carry personal identification, which makes the process of identifying victims and later reuniting family with their children more difficult[8] (Table 150–1).

PHYSIOLOGIC DIFFERENCES

There are several unique physiological differences that make children potentially more vulnerable to exposures of agents that may be involved or released in an MCE. First, children have increased respiratory rates, which can lead to increased absorption of aerosolized chemicals, and thus more severe illness. Because of their small size children are generally closer to the ground, and so are potentially more vulnerable to agents that either settle on the ground or do not become airborne. Children also have an increased body surface area and thinner skin relative to adults, which can lead to increased absorption of toxic agents. They are more susceptible to hypothermia, especially if their skin is exposed, which may occur during

▶ **TABLE 150–1. SUMMARY OF PHYSIOLOGIC AND DEVELOPMENTAL DIFFERENCES IN THE PEDIATRIC POPULATION**

Differences	Implications
Physiologic differences	
Increased respiratory rate	Increased absorption of airborne agents
Increased surface area-to-volume ratio	Increased water loss
	Increased heat loss
Thinner skin	Increased absorption of dermatologic agents
	Increase water and heat loss
Smaller circulating volumes	Increased susceptibility to fluid loss: dehydration and/or circulatory collapse
Smaller stature	Closer to the ground
	Increased exposure to less volatile agents
Increased relative metabolism	Increased clearance of medications and agents
	Increased risk of hypoglycemia
Immunologic immaturity	Decreased ability to combat infectious agents
	Lack herd immunity
Developmental differences	
Limited verbal and motor skills	Inability to escape dangerous situations
	Inability to express symptoms or complaints
Lack self preservation skills	Run toward dangerous situation
	Fear of responders
Dependence on caretakers	Separation anxiety
	Inability to care for themselves
Lack coping skills	Increased susceptibility to PTSD or other psychological disturbances

decontamination. Children have smaller circulating blood volumes and they tend to preserve their hemodynamic function despite a relatively large volume loss; cardiovascular collapse can then occur suddenly. This translates into a narrow window for the recognition and treatment of hypovolemia and/or early shock, whether it is owing to vomiting and diarrhea, dehydration, or blood loss.[3] It is important to recognize these differences to allow for timely triage and identification of victims that may require immediate care (Table 150–1).

▶ CONSIDERATIONS FOR THE DELIVERY OF CARE TO THE PEDIATRIC POPULATION

PROVISION OF CARE

It has been recognized that a well-organized plan with community involvement can have positive effects on disaster response. However, many emergency medical services do not have pediatric-specific plans. In one study, only 248 out of 1808 preshospital emergency medical services surveyed had any specific plans for the care of children.[9] These plans can and should include recommendations for the use of a pediatric-specific mass casualty triage protocol, pediatric-sized equipment and supplies, proper decontamination guidelines, plans for reunification of children with their family, and for recognizing and addressing post-event mental health needs of the children and family.

Ideally, it is best to transport pediatric MCE victims to either a regional pediatric hospital or one that has extensive pediatric expertise. Logistically, this may be impossible, depending upon the type of disaster and the resources of the affected community. An MCE may involve both adults and their children. Separating a family may not be good or possible if there are an overwhelming number of victims. Because of this, hospitals need to think about providing care as a unit. That is, general hospitals need to be able to care for pediatric patients and pediatric hospitals need to be prepared to care for parent/adult victims as well.[10] It is essential that all health care workers and prehospital responders receive proper training and equipment to deal with children, often the most vulnerable victims.

TRIAGE

Adult mass casualty triage protocols cannot be universally used for pediatric patients. Most adult protocols rely on a victim's ability to verbalize and ambulate. Also, physiological differences between adults and children make the adult MCE triage protocols inappropriate for infants and children. Pediatric-specific triage protocols have been proposed. JumpSTART is a pediatric-specific protocol that has been suggested by Romig.[11] It is an adaptation of the existing adult MCE protocol, START (simple triage and rapid treatment). The JumpSTART method focuses on pediatric-specific parameters and places an emphasis on early airway intervention because respiratory failure usually precedes circulatory failure in children (Fig. 150–1). The Pediatric Assessment Triangle (PAT) has also been proposed as a potential MCE triage protocol (Fig. 150–2). The American Academy of Pediatrics (AAP) developed it in 2000 as part of an Emergency Medical Services for Children (EMS-C) project. The PAT relies on visual cues of appearance, work of breathing, and skin circulation to rapidly assess the acuity of a patient illness.[3,9]

EQUIPMENT

It is extremely important to have an array of infant-, child-, and adult-sized masks, airways, and endotracheal tubes available. One of the challenges in airway management is determining the proper endotracheal tube size. A pediatric emergency measuring tape, like a Broselow's tape (Fig. 150–3), is useful in estimating the proper equipment size without having to perform any time-consuming calculations or measurements. It is also useful for determining resuscitation medication doses, if required.

It can be anticipated that establishing intravenous access will be difficult and time consuming. Many victims will require access for fluid administration or medication administration. Alternative access sites (scalp, umbilical, central venous sites) and means (ultrasound aided, intraosseous (IO) access) must

JumpSTART pediatric MCI triage

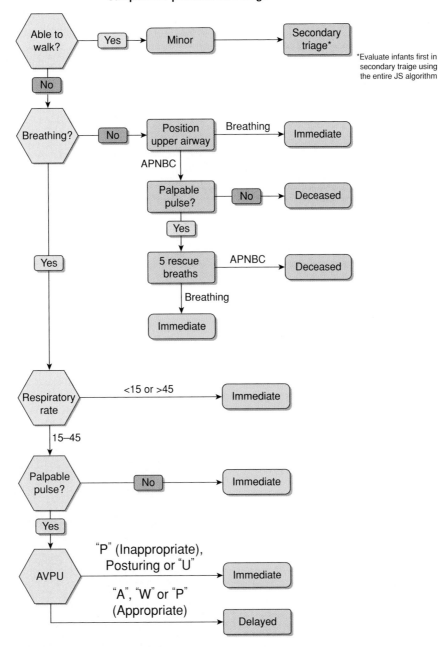

Figure 150–1. JumpSTART Triage algorithm. (With permission from developer, Lou E. Romig MD, FAAP, FACEP.)

be considered. Newer IO devices (EZ-IO®, Vidacare) function like a drill and can rapidly establish access, especially in a critical patient (Fig. 150–4).

MCE plans should include provisions for a minimum supply of appropriate pediatric-sized equipment and extra supplies. Some authors recommend having a 48-hour supply for the average daily pediatric patient census, plus enough for 100 extra patients available at all times in a hospital.[12] This equipment should be organized and stored in a designated area within the emergency department that is easily accessible in an MCE.

DECONTAMINATION

Decontamination needs to be performed in any MCE that involves suspected biological, chemical, or radiation exposures. Eighty-five to ninety-five percent of decontamination is accomplished simply by removing clothes and securing them in sealed bags or containers.[5] There are several key points to keep in mind about the decontamination of children. Most importantly, children are at higher risk for hypothermia than adults. It is important to ensure that water pressure is low (60 psi) and water temperature is 100°F (37.8°C). Skin exposure to wind and

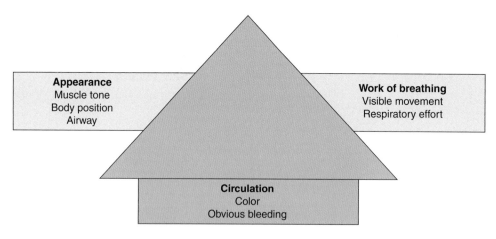

Figure 150–2. Pediatric assessment triangle.

air should be limited as much as possible and extra blankets and other warming equipment (mylar blankets, heating fans, etc.) be provided, especially after water decontamination. Ambient air should be kept warm to minimize evaporative heat loss. In general, it takes longer to decontaminate children. This may be because some children are hesitant to disrobe, unable to disrobe by themselves, or are frightened or anxious about being separated from parents or known caretakers. Patience and extra personnel may be required to perform decontamination and to maintain steady patient flow.[5] Because personal protective equipment (PPE) limits the dexterity of health care personnel, handling and decontaminating small children and infants require a higher degree of caution.[13]

MEDICATIONS

Appropriate medications and antidote administration can be difficult to determine in the pediatric population, especially in an MCE. The two main issues revolve around knowing which medications can be given to children, and determining the correct dose. Historically, many of the antibiotics that are used to treat illnesses caused by biological agents (i.e., ciprofloxacin and doxycycline) have not been used in children because of their potential toxic effects. However, newer recommendations support the use of these medications when indicated in a disaster or an MCE because the risks outweigh the benefits. The

Food and Drug Administration (FDA) recently approved the use of ciprofloxacin and doxycycline in children as prophylaxis against inhalational anthrax.[14]

Dose calculations can be cumbersome in an MCE because of the emergent need to initiate lifesaving treatment and the inability to obtain accurate weights. One strategy is to have medication names organized in an easy to read chart with pre-calculated doses that is located in a pediatric disaster kit and readily visible. Prepackaged medications, like MARK I autoinjectors containing atropine and pralidoxime, have the advantage of pre-filled medications in an easy-to-use device that does

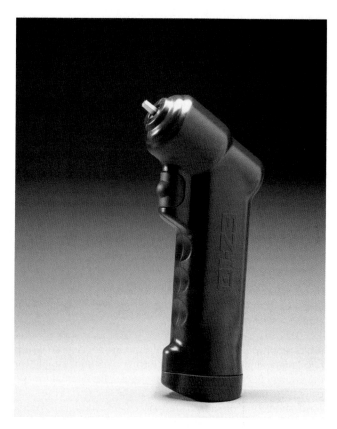

Figure 150–4. EZ-IO device. (Used with permission.)

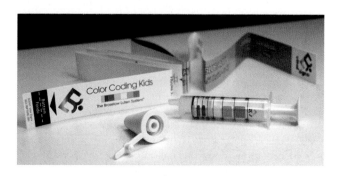

Figure 150–3. Broselow® pediatric emergency tape. (Used with permission.)

not require intravenous access. However, these have been developed primarily for military and/or adults. These devices can still be used in the pediatric population, but have to be dose adjusted.[14,15] The FDA approved pediatric-specific atropine autoinjectors in 2003.[16] The Broselow tape system has recently made available a new color-coded pediatric tape that contains doses for chemical treatment agents, including adult autoinjectors, thus decreasing the amount of time required to determine doses for victims. It is patterned after the original tape such that it can be used simultaneously.[17]

RECOVERY

Separation of children from family members and/or known caretakers can exacerbate an already traumatic situation. Every effort should be made to reunite family members with the child as soon as possible. Keeping and treating parent and child victims of an MCE together in the same facility is a logical strategy. This can help to allay the fears of the child and may also facilitate treating the child.[14] Taking photos or noting the clothing or personal articles on the child may be useful in helping parents identify their children.[18]

It is known that children suffer varying degrees of psychological disturbances after an MCE.[19–22] Long-term effects are not well understood.[20] Somatization is common, and many parents may not identify symptoms as psychological in nature. Physicians need to be vigilant about recognizing the signs and symptoms of children that are at risk for developing posttraumatic stress disorder (PTSD) after an MCE (Table 150–2). While

▶ **TABLE 150–2. POSTTRAUMATIC STRESS DISORDER AND RISK FACTORS ASSOCIATED WITH INCREASED RISK OF PSYCHOLOGICAL DISTURBANCES AFTER A DISASTER**

Posttraumatic stress disorder
Following an event, a victim has below symptoms that last greater than 1 month:
  1. Persistent reexperience of traumatic event.
  2. Avoidance behavior associated with traumatic event and generalized numbness to life.
  3. Hyperaroused or hypervigilant state.

Risk factors associated with increased risk of psychological disturbances
  • Children are victims.
  • Victims are close to the child, especially if death involved.
  • Witnessed the event, especially if graphic.
  • Indirect witnessing of event (i.e., graphic visual media).
  • Perception by child that his/her life was in danger at time of event.
  • Separation of child from parents or caretakers during event.
  • Loss of personal property during event.
  • Disruption of normal environment during event.
  • Prior history of traumatic experience.
  • Prior psychiatric history.
  • Parents have difficulty coping post event.
  • Lack of family social support.
  • Lack of community support or resources for children after event.

physicians may not feel qualified to treat these disorders, it is important to have mechanisms in place to help children address their reactions to disaster. The first step in addressing their reactions is to try to establish a safe environment. This may be accomplished simply by reuniting a child with his/her family. Second, children need to be reassured that their reactions are not as result of something right or wrong, but a normal reaction to an abnormal event. Mental health workers need to work with children and families immediately or soon after an event and intervene as necessary.[22,23]

REFERENCES

1. Waisman Y, Aharonson-Daniel L, Mor M, et al. The impact of terrorism on children: a two-year experience. *Prehosp Disaster Med.* Jul–Sep 2003;18(3):242–248.
2. McMahon MM. Preventing pediatric mass casualty events. *Disaster Manage Response.* Apr–Jun 2007;5(2):25–26.
3. Hohenhaus SM. Practical considerations for providing pediatric care in a mass casualty incident. *Nurs Clin North Am.* Sep 2005;40(3):523–533, ix.
4. Ginter PM, Wingate MS, Rucks AC, et al. Creating a regional pediatric medical disaster preparedness network: imperative and issues. *Matern Child Health J.* Jul 2006;10(4):391–396.
5. Chung S, Shannon M. Hospital planning for acts of terrorism and other public health emergencies involving children. *Arch Dis Child.* 2005 Dec;90(12):1300–7.
6. Gaines SK, Leary JM. Public health emergency preparedness in the setting of child care. *Fam Community Health.* Jul–Sep 2004;27(3):260–265.
7. Rassin M, Avraham M, Nasi-Bashari A, et al. Emergency department staff preparedness for mass casualty events involving children. *Disaster Manage Response.* Apr–Jun 2007;5(2):36–44.
8. Bernardo L, Veenema T. Pediatric emergency preparedness for mass gatherings and special events. *Disaster Manage Response.* 2004;2(4):118–122.
9. Shirm S, Liggin R, Dick R, Graham J. Prehospital preparedness for pediatric mass-casualty events. *Pediatrics.* Oct 2007;120(4):e756–761.
10. Markeson D, Reynolds S. The pediatrician and disaster preparedness. *Pediatrics.* 2006;117:560–565.
11. Romig L. Pediatric triage. A system to JumpSTART your triage of young patients at MCIs. *J Emerg Med Serv.* 2001;27:52–63.
12. Markenson D, Redlener I. Pediatric terrorism preparedness national guidelines and recommendations: findings of an evidenced-based consensus process. *Biosecur Bioterror.* 2004;2(4):301–319.
13. Agency for Healthcare Research and Quality. *The Decontamination of Children; Preparedness and Response for Hospital Emergency Departments* [05-0036-DVD]. Rockville, MD: US Department of Health and Human Services; Aug 2005.
14. Henretig F, Cieslak T, Eitzen E. Biological and chemical terrorism. *J Pediatr.* 2002;141:311–326.
15. Cieslak T, Henretig F. Ring-a-ring-a-roses: bioterrorism and its peculiar relevance to pediatrics. *Curr Opin Pediatrics.* 2003;15:107–111.
16. Shannon M, McMillan J. Chemical-biological terrorism and its impact on children. *Pediatrics.* 2006;118(3):1267–1278.
17. www.colorcodingkids.com. Accessed April 8, 2008.
18. Behney A, Breit M, Phillips C. Pediatric mass casualty: are you ready? *J Emerg Nurs.* Jun 2006;32(3):241–245.

19. Bernardo L. Pediatric implications in bioterrorism part 1: physiologic and psychosocial differences. *Int J Trauma Nurs.* 2001;7:14–16.

20. Hagan J. Psychosocial implications of disaster or terrorism on children: a guide for the pediatrician. *Pediatrics.* 2005;116:787–795.

21. Baker DR. A public health approach to the needs of children affected by terrorism. *J Am Med Womens Assoc.* Spring 2002;57(2):117–118, 121.

22. Coffman S. Children's reactions to disaster. *J Pediat Nurs.* 1998;13(6):376–382.

23. Gurwitch R, Kees M, Becker S, et al. When disaster strikes: responding to the needs of children. *Prehosp Disaster Med.* 2004;19(1):21–28.

SECTION XXIII

MEDICOLEGAL AND ADMINISTRATIVE ISSUES

CHAPTER 151

Medico-Legal Considerations

William R. Ahrens

► HIGH-YIELD FACTS

- The Emergency Medical Treatment and Labor Act (EMTALA) mandates a screening examination for all patients presenting to an ED—this essentially obviates the need for consent in a minor unaccompanied by a parent or guardian.
- The Health Insurance Portability and Accountability Act (HIPAA) mandates that all possible care be taken to ensure the confidentiality of a patient's medical records.
- Many states have "emancipated minor" statutes that permit adolescents to make their own health care decisions.
- When refusal of care becomes an issue, the "best interest" of the minor is the priority.
- Good forensic documentation is an important part of patient advocacy.
- Disclosure of medical errors is becoming increasing common and in the near future may become the law in many states.

The emergency medicine physician must work within the context of a society's laws as they apply to the emergency department (ED). He or she must also work within the framework of ethical paradigms as they apply to each patient; ethics is the branch of philosophy that deals with what is right and what is wrong. For the most part, laws will agree with what is considered to be ethical. However, in a multicultural and multireligious democracy, there will be occasions when a law is nonexistent, vague, or at odds with what may be considered ethical in a particular situation, and the physician must make a decision based on what is best for the patient. The chapter on "Ethical Considerations in the Emergency Department" explores the role of the emergency physician's ethical responsibility as an advocate for pediatric patients in situations where a law and ethics may collide. This chapter will discuss some basic legal issues as they pertain to the ED.

Laws in the United States can be divided into three categories: statutory, common, and administrative. Statutory law is codified by legislative bodies; an example is the requirement to report child abuse to authorities. Common law is based on case law; it has evolved over centuries, and is interpreted by judges as it applies to litigated cases. Common law applies to medical malpractice. Administrative laws are enabled by legislation and are issued by agencies in the form of regulations; an example is the Drug Enforcement Agencies regulations regarding the prescription of narcotics. U.S. law is also divided into state and federal law. Most laws applicable to emergency medicine are state laws. The federal statues that apply most directly to an ED are the Emergency Medical Treatment and Labor Act (EMTALA) and the Health Insurance Portability and Accountability Act (HIPAA).[1]

EMTALA was enacted by congress in 1986 as part of the Consolidated Omnibus Reconciliation Act of 1985 (COBRA) as a response to the refusal of some EDs to provide care to uninsured patients. One of the key provisions of EMALA is that when a patient requests care at an ED, "the hospital must provide an appropriate medical screening examination within the capability of the hospital's emergency department, including ancillary services routinely available to the emergency department, to determine whether an emergency medical condition (EMC) exists." If an EMC exists, the hospital must provide "with the staff and facilities available, for such further medical examination and such treatment as may be required to stabilize the medical condition or transfer the patient to another facility." The medical screening examination must be performed by a physician or someone accredited to do so by the medical staff. An EMC is a condition "manifesting itself by acute symptoms of sufficient severity, including severe pain, psychiatric disturbances, or symptoms of substance abuse, such that the absence of immediate medical attention could reasonably be expected to result in (a) placing the health of the individual in serious jeopardy, (b) serious dysfunction of any bodily organ or part."[2] Obviously, the definition of an EMC gives the emergency physician performing a legally required medical screening examination wide discretion to err on the side of caution, especially in the case of unaccompanied minors. Stabilization of the patient means that within reasonable clinical confidence, no material deterioration of the condition is likely to result from or occur during transfer. The receiving facility must agree to accept the transfer; all pertinent medical records must accompany the patient. The condition of the patient as well as the risks and potential benefit of the transfer must be documented.[2]

The Health Insurance Portability and Accountability Act (HIPAA) and the finalized version "Standards for Privacy of Individually Identifiable Health Information" (HIPAA Privacy Rule) require health care providers and institutions to provide a set of minimum standards to protect medical record privacy and confidentiality. The law reflects the fundamental ethical paradigm that all patients are entitled to privacy. Protecting privacy is within the code of ethics for emergency physicians, part of which states that "sensitive information may only be disclosed when such disclosure is necessary to carry out a stronger conflicting duty, such as a duty to protect an identifiable third party or to comply with a just law."[2] Confidentiality is closely related to privacy; in medicine, it refers to the duty not to disclose information conveyed to a health care provider without the patient's approval. Generally, HIPPA requires patient permission for information disclosure; consent is not required for disclosure of personal health information for purposes of treatment, payment, and health care operations.[3] Patient's consent is also not required for communication between consultants when threats to patient of public safety are involved, such as suicidal or homicidal ideation or terrorist threats, certain instances of abuse and neglect, and certain issues involving law enforcement. HIPPA confers a high degree of confidentiality or records pertaining to psychiatric treatment. A patient must approve the release of psychotherapy notes, unless they are being used for the purposes of treatment by the physician who originated them, or if they are necessary to avert an imminent threat to public health or safety.[2,3]

Confidentiality issues regarding minors, especially adolescents, are problematic. Adolescents are less likely to seek medical care if they feel that confidentiality will not be maintained, which has the potential to negatively impact their health. Thus, there needs to be a balance between the adolescent patient's inherent right of privacy and parents' right of access to information pertaining to the child for whom they are legally and morally responsible. The HIPPA Privacy Rule states that in most cases a parent is the "personal representative" of the child and thus has legal power to control the release of the minor's medical records. If the parent is not the personal representative of the child, state or other regulations apply. Examples where the parent is not the personal representative of the minor include situations where the minor can consent for their own medical care, when the parent agrees to a confidential relationship between the minor and physician, when the physician believes the child has been abused or that the parent is not acting in the child's best interest, and when a court-appointed guardian is the minor's personal representative. Laws regarding parents' right to access the medical records of adolescents who have received treatment for which they were able to consent vary from state to state.[2-4]

▶ CONSENT AND REFUSAL OF CARE

Informed consent is predicated on a patient or patient's representative demonstrating the intellectual capacity and emotional maturity to fully understand the information presented and the consequences of both acceding to medical treatment and refusing care. In most states the age at which a patient can consent for or refuse medical care is 18. However, states have increasingly recognized that a "bright-line rule" regarding who is an adult may not be appropriate, and many have adopted "mature minor" statutes.[5] Such statute presume that minors, in most cases beginning at age 14, have the cognitive and developmental capacity to comprehend the nature of the medical treatment offered and, therefore, the decisional capacity to accept or decline care. These statutes are case sensitive; consent relates to specific situations in which adolescents demonstrate the capacity to make decision related to their care. Almost all states have doctrines involving "emancipated minors"; laws vary, but most commonly include minors who are married, serving in the armed forces, are pregnant or parents, or who are self-sufficient as capable of making their own medical decisions. Most states have provisions that allow adolescents to seek psy-

chiatric care without the consent of their parents; the age at which they may do so varies from state to state. Other conditions that may preclude the need for consent in minors include treatment of sexually transmitted diseases, including HIV, contraceptive services, and treatment for substance abuse.[2-6]

Increasingly, minors who are not emancipated seek care in EDs. While every effort should be made to contact their parent or personal representative, EMTALA specifically requires a medical screening examination: this in essence obviates the issue of consent. The American College of Emergency Physicians states: "Under federal law, a minor can be examined, treated, stabilized, and even transferred to another hospital without consent ever being obtained from a parent or legal guardian." This applies to cases where the minor is brought to the ED with an emergency medical condition by a personal representative who for whatever reason may be impaired, and therefore incapable of informed consent, and who may not act in the best interests of the patient.[2]

Refusal of care is an issue that often involves a complex interaction between what is the law and what is perceived the patients' best interest, either by the patients themselves or their personal representative(s). There is no question that adults with adequate decisional capacity have the right to refuse medical care. When a conflict involving refusal of care for a minor arises, it is the best interest of the minor that is the priority. In cases involving a nonemancipated minor with an EMC, the physician has the obligation to use the legal system to protect the patient.

▶ FORENSIC DOCUMENTATION

The ED treats many victims of criminal assault. In the case of children, assault can be physical and/or sexual. Because most assaults entail some form of criminal activity, the examining physician has a high likelihood of becoming involved in the legal aftermath of the case. It can be argued that as a patient advocate as well as a member of society, the emergency physician has an ethical responsibility to develop expertise in documenting the history and physical findings pertinent to his or her patient so that the legal system can best provide justice for the victim, and potentially protect society from the perpetrator of the violence. In the pediatric patient who is a victim of maltreatment, careful and correct documentation can serve to protect the child from further harm; poor documentation can result in the child being returned to a potentially fatal environment.[7-9]

In cases that go to trial, the emergency physician may be asked to provide expert testimony. Despite this fact, most emergency physicians have no forensic training. Studies have found that documentation of violence-related injuries is often poor and that evidence is often mishandled.[9] In the case of child maltreatment, elements such as the explanation provided, whether witness were present, the developmental stage of the child, and a clear description of injuries are often absent from the documentation. Studies have also found that the extent of documentation of injuries is directly correlated with the filing of charges, conviction, and sentencing of perpetrators. Inaccurate interpretation of injuries, such as calling entrance wound an exit wound, can confuse and negatively impact subsequent litigation.[9]

▶ MEDICAL MALPRACTICE

The emergency physician works in a high-acuity environment, the very nature of which guarantees that there will inevitably be bad outcomes. In an increasingly litigious society, bad outcomes all but guarantee medical malpractice suits. The four requirements for malpractice are duty, a breach of duty, damages, and causation. A physician treating a patient in an ED has a "duty" to treat the patient. A breach of duty occurs when the physician does not treat the patient according to "the standard of care," or in a way that a reasonable physician practicing in a comparable setting would have done in a similar situation. Damages occur when a patient suffers an adverse outcome as a result of the care rendered. Causation means that the breach in care is shown to have caused the damages (some jurisdictions vary).[10]

A recent review of medical malpractice suits in the United States involving pediatric patients found that 49% of the cases involved children younger than 2 years. Diagnostic error was a factor in 39% of cases. The most common diagnoses involved were meningitis, fracture, appendicitis, and testicular torsion. Other factors cited were improper performance of procedure, failure to supervise staff, delay in treatment, failure to consult, failure to admit, and medication error. Most cases were settled out of court.[11]

Preventing, or at least minimizing, errors in the ED, and therefore medical malpractice suits, involves a combination of systems analysis, quality improvement, education, and teamwork. Despite all best efforts, however, mistakes will happen and patients will suffer. There is a rapidly growing and most likely unstoppable movement to inform patients when they have been the victim of a medical error. Studies have found that patients want to know when a mistake has happened; physicians are less likely to want to disclose an error. There is little information regarding error disclosure in the pediatric population. How error disclosure affects medical malpractice is as yet unknown—it may decrease the likelihood of a lawsuit. Many states have requirements for the standardized reporting of medical error. A few states require patient notification of medical error. Some states protect health care providers with "apology statues," where expressing remorse or apologizing for an error is not admissible in court as an admission of liability. Legislation in this area is constantly changing and will, no doubt, develop rapidly as public sentiment demanding full error disclosure grows. The standards set by Joint Commission on Accreditation of Healthcare Organizations require that patients and families be informed about medical errors.[12,13] The American College of Emergency Physicians policy on error disclosure is summarized in Table 151–1.[14]

▶ END-OF-LIFE CARE

Approximately 50 000 pediatric deaths occur annually in the United States. About 56% occur in the hospital; how many occur in EDs is unknown. It is likely that an emergency physician will someday be confronted with a pediatric patient suffering from a terminal illness who presents to the ED in a near-death situation. In most of these situations medical decision making is the responsibility of the parents of the patients, who are ex-

▶ **TABLE 151–1. ACEP POLICY ON DISCLOSURE OF MEDICAL ERRORS**

Health care institutions should develop polices and procedures for identifying and responding to medical errors and procedures for disclosing significant errors to patients.

Medical educators should develop and incorporate into their curricula programs on identifying and preventing medical errors and on communicating truthfully and sensitively with patients and their representatives about errors.

Emergency department directors . . . and other leaders in emergency medicine should play a leading role in developing institutional and ED policies for prompt error identification, responsible reporting, and proper remediation.

Society should adopt tort reforms and system changes that improve patient safety by encouraging disclosure of medical errors.

pected to act in the best interest of their child. As the concept of the emancipated minor expands and develops a stronger legal footing, more young patients will be able to make their own medical decisions, including refusing resuscitation. Legally and ethically, emergency physicians are not required to provide treatment that would be ineffective. However, futility is very difficult to define; situations involving resuscitative efforts are best guided by the parents, guardian, or patient, rather than the physician.[1] Parents who initially request aggressive treatment may later change their mind; withdrawing life support, including ventilation, is ethically and legally permissible even in the ED when it is no longer in the best interest of the patient.[15]

REFERENCES

1. Derse AR. Ethics and the law in emergency medicine. *Emerg Med Clin North Am.* 2006;24:547.
2. Teshome G, Closson FT. Emergency Medical Treatment and Labor Act: the basics and other medicolegal considerations. *Pediatr Clin North Am.* 2006;53:847.
3. Geiderman JM, Moskop JC, Derse AR. Privacy and confidentiality in emergency medicine: obligations and challenges. *Emerg Med Clin North Am.* 2006;24:633.
4. Baren JM. Ethical dilemmas in the care of minors in the emergency department. *Emerg Med Clin North Am.* 2006;24:619.
5. Campbell AT. Consent, competence, and confidentiality related to psychiatric conditions in adolescent medicine practice. *Adolesc Med Clin.* 2006;17:123.
6. Knapp JF, Dolan MA, Furnival RA, et al. Consent for emergency medical services for children and adolescents. *Pediatrics.* 2003;111:703.
7. Johnson TL. Updates and current trends in child protection. *Clin Pediatr Emerg Med.* 2004;5:270.
8. Jackson AM, Rucker A, Hinds T, et al. Let the record speak: medicolegal documentation in cases of child maltreatment. *Clin Pediatr Emerg Med.* 2006;7:181.
9. Wiler JL, Bailey H, Madsen TE. The need for emergency medicine resident training in forensic medicine. *Ann Emerg Med.* 2007;50:733.
10. Soloman RC. Ethical issues in medical malpractice. *Emerg Med Clin North Am.* 2006;24:733.
11. Selbst SM, Friedman M, Singh S. Epidemiology and etiology

of malpractice lawsuits involving children in US emergency departments and urgent care settings. *PEM Care.* 2005;21:165.

12. Straumanis JP. Disclosure of medical error: is it worth the risk? *Pediatr Crit Care Med.* 2007;8:538.

13. Moskop JC, Geiderman JM, Hobgood CD, et al. Emergency physicians and disclosure of medical errors. *Ann Emerg Med.* 2006;48:523.

14. American College of Emergency Physicians. *Disclosure of Medical Errors.* www.acep.org/portal/PracticeResources/PolicyResourcesByCategory/Ethics/DisclosureMedicalError. Accessed May 19, 2008.

15. Michelson KN, Steinhorn DM. Pediatric end-of-life issues and palliative care. *Clin Pediatr Emerg Med.* 2007;8:212.

CHAPTER 152

Ethical Considerations

Alan Johnson

► HIGH-YIELD FACTS

- Emergency medicine physicians provide medical care in a fiscally and ethically challenging environment. Care should be provided to anyone in need, regardless of immigration status or ability to pay.
- Physicians, patients, parents, and guardians share a common goal to protect the health and well-being of the child. In the event of a disagreement, every effort must be made to resolve conflicts to assure the best possible outcome for the child.
- No child should be denied medical care in the emergency department.
- Informed consent is the appropriate term for the process of reaching an agreement about medical care between a physician and a patient with full decision-making capacity and legal empowerment.
- Informed permission is the preferred term when a parent makes decisions for a patient lacking decision-making capacity or legal majority.
- Assent (or permission) of the patient is very important and should be sought whenever possible.
- Adolescents may be able to seek confidential and independent health care for a number of conditions defined by statute. Low-risk, high-benefit treatment may be provided if the physician believes the adolescent is as capable to consent as an adult.
- Treatment for an emergency medical condition should never be delayed if a patient is unable to provide informed consent or a parent or guardian is not present to provide permission.
- Family presence should be considered for all medical procedures and resuscitations.
- Despite a long history in medical education, practicing procedures on the newly dead is problematic. It should be done only with fully informed permission from a parent or guardian.

► INTRODUCTION

Medical ethics is a broad philosophical discipline that guides medical practitioners to act in the best interests of patients. Ethical conflicts may arise if there are differences of opinion about what those best interests might be. Many different approaches have been explored in detail, and many emergency medicine practitioners approach the discipline from different philosophical, moral, or religious viewpoints.[1,2]

Emergency medicine physicians are responsible for providing medical care in an increasingly fiscally and ethically challenging environment. Care is provided to anyone in need, regardless of immigration status or ability to pay. Emergency departments (ED) serve as an essential medical safety net; they are the only places in the United States where all patients are guaranteed medical care.[3] This fundamental dedication to provide care to those most in need or with no other health care options is a core ethical value of emergency medicine.[2]

In the practice of pediatric emergency medicine, patients, parents, guardians, and physicians generally have a common goal: to act in the best interests of the child. The physician has an obligation to diagnose and treat illness, alleviate discomfort, and provide for as rapid a recovery as possible. With effective communication, an agreement can usually be reached and a diagnostic, therapeutic, and follow-up plan can be implemented. Sometimes disagreements arise, which, if unresolved, could jeopardize the health and well-being of the child. Significant effort may be required to resolve conflicts in order to provide for the best possible outcome for the child from each party's perspective.

An emergency medicine physician needs to be familiar with current recommendations, policy statements, principles, and controversies that guide the practice of emergency medicine as they apply to the care of children. This section will focus on the ethical considerations at the intersection of emergency and pediatric medicine.

► TRIAGE AND OVERCROWDING

Pediatric patients make about 30 million visits to EDs in the United States each year, accounting for about 25% of all ED visits.[3] Ninety-two percent of these visits are to general community EDs. Although overcrowding of EDs is difficult to quantify, a reasonable definition is "the need for medical services exceeds available resources." More than 90% of academic EDs are overcrowded and 30% to 40% of emergency medicine directors report daily overcrowding.[4]

When resources are limited, a reasonable policy might consist of triaging less severely ill patients away from the ED to other health care resources in the community. However, in one trial of adult patients, 19% of patients met low-acuity criteria and were referred to a "help desk" for information about community resources. Unfortunately, the majority of the patients in the study either did not go to the "help desk" or did not seek further care. Application of the same low-acuity criteria to other sets of patients presenting for care have shown that a large proportion meeting low-risk criteria were ultimately found to be appropriate for an ED visit and a fair number were hospitalized.[5] Pediatric-specific triage protocols should be utilized at all EDs, but no triage protocol has been demonstrated to be ideal. Since differences exist between medical professionals' assessment of illness severity,[6] every effort must be made to provide care to all children presenting to an ED. It is a good practice to develop systems within the department and institution to provide a place to care for lower-acuity patients and to triage such patients to this area. In the event of an inappropriate triage, the patient can be re-triaged to the area providing a higher level of care. It might be appropriate to arrange an immediate appointment at and transportation to another off-site clinical area, but only if it were in the child's best interests, and if it would provide care equal to that in ED.[5] Since no triage system or protocol has demonstrated adequate sensitivity to identify all children requiring treatment, no child should be turned away or denied care based on an initial triage assessment that the complaint is low acuity.[7]

▶ MEDICALLY UNDERSERVED CHILDREN

Poor, immigrant, homeless, uninsured, and migrant children often do not have access to outpatient medical care. Many of the challenges they face make consistent and comprehensive medical care difficult if not impossible.[8] Poor children have higher rates of underimmunization, acute illnesses, asthma, injury, malnutrition, and mental health issues than the general population.[9] In addition to the problems associated with poverty, there may be significant cultural and linguistic barriers to obtaining effective care.[8] The Emergency Medicaid program was established in 1986 and provides coverage for uninsured documented and undocumented children with an emergency medical condition. Eligibility and benefits are set by the individual states.[10] These vulnerable children require not only excellent emergency medical care, but need to be connected to any federal, state, and community resources to help them access the Emergency Medicaid program and other support services to facilitate their overall health and well-being.[8]

Care should be provided for the presenting complaints and, whenever possible, a referral should be made to an accessible source of ongoing primary care in the community.[9] Policies requiring reporting of undocumented immigrants may deter them from seeking health care.[10] The American College of Emergency Physicians opposes federal and state initiatives that would require refusal of care to undocumented persons or reporting suspected undocumented persons to authorities.[11]

▶ CHILD ABUSE

When treating a patient that may have been abused, the physician must consider the best interests of the patient as the primary focus of the evaluation. A parent or caretaker may have conflicting interests, including wanting what is best for the child as well as protecting their own interest in avoiding investigation and prosecution. The treating physician needs to explain the process of investigation to the parent, assure the

parent that they are dedicated to the child's well-being, but also explain the legal mandate to report a suspected abusive situation to the local child protection agency. Even when a child is in protective custody, the parent may still remain in charge of medical decision making for the child. In the event that a parent does not seem to be acting in the child's best interests, a court proceeding to establish a guardian for medical decision making should be pursued.[12]

▶ INFORMED CONSENT, PARENTAL PERMISSION, AND ASSENT

The informed consent process is an ethical cornerstone of providing care to patients, since it balances the physician's desire to do what is best from a medical and scientific perspective with the patient's right to comprehensive information in order to decide what is best from their personal perspective. Informed consent is the appropriate term used for patients with full decision-making capacity and legal empowerment, and is the term commonly used when parents make decisions for their children. The American Academy of Pediatrics recommends the use of different terminology to clarify the unique interrelationships in the process of providing care to children. Informed consent remains the appropriate term for an adult or adolescent with decision-making capacity. Informed permission is the preferred term when a parent or other surrogate makes decisions for a patient lacking decision-making capacity. Assent (or agreement) of a patient lacking decision-making capacity is also very important and should be sought whenever possible and appropriate.[13]

In an emergency, a societal standard of presumed or implied consent exists that allows medical treatment to prevent harm based on the assumption that a person in danger would want to be saved. This standard applies if a patient is unconscious or seems to consent by cooperating with treatment. This same implied consent applies to the provision of care to a child in an emergency. Treatment for an emergency medical condition should never be delayed despite the inability of the patient to provide informed consent or the presence of a parent to provide permission.[2,7]

The process of obtaining parental permission and patient assent for nonemergency care is more complicated than the process of obtaining informed consent from an adult. The child's perspective needs to be considered and balanced with the perspective of the parent, the child's physicians, and societal standards of child welfare.[1,7,13] There has been a long struggle with these issues since it is recognized that usually, but not always, parents are strong and loving advocates for what they believe to be best for their children. Children, however, have rights independent of their parents. They have an evolving decision-making capacity that is dependent on psychological, emotional, and intellectual development and maturity that the physician must consider. Children should therefore participate in decision making as appropriate for their developmental status.[13]

An adult patient with appropriate decision-making capacity can provide consent for care; the generally accepted legal age of majority is 18 years.[14] Adolescents have a unique status, more like an adult than a child. State statutes reflect this and define the conditions for which adolescents may seek confidential and independent health care; these include sexually transmitted infections, pregnancy, psychiatric complaints, and substance abuse problems. Minors may also be legally "emancipated" or "mature" and able to consent for their own health care if they meet one of several conditions defined by the state as signifying independence, including marriage, pregnancy, parenthood, participation in military service, or financial independence.[14,15] Adolescents 14 and older have been shown to be able to make informed health care decisions as well as adults,[13] so for conditions not covered by statute, a "mature minor" approach allows low-risk, high-benefit treatments to be provided if the physician believes that the minor is as capable to consent for the treatment as an adult.[13,15]

▶ PARENTAL AND PATIENT REFUSAL

An adult patient with decision-making capacity may refuse medical treatment.[2,13] Refusal of recommended diagnostic testing and treatment for children is more problematic. In almost every circumstance, the child, the child's parents, and the child's physicians have in common the child's best interests, but there may be disagreement about what those interests are.[13] A parent refusing an invasive or painful diagnostic procedure may believe that they are acting in the best interests of the child—and the child may very well agree. Such a conflict can arise during the evaluation of a common complaint in a well-appearing patient with a symptom that suggests the possibility of a very serious disease, such as a fever in a neonate. Physicians consider painful and invasive tests to be routine, but they are often anything but routine from the perspective of the child and the parent. It is unusual for parents to refuse any testing at all, but sometimes they are concerned about a particular test, such as a lumbar puncture or a urethral catheterization. In the event that a parent refuses a diagnostic test, the physician needs to review the remaining options and make therapeutic decisions based on the available data in a similar manner to what must be done if a test is attempted but not successful. Therapy for a potentially dangerous or progressive condition should not be delayed or forgone for lack of a complete diagnostic evaluation.[13]

Providing emergency care to children requires a delicate balance of obtaining parental permission and the assent of the patient for care, while at the same time acknowledging the societal mandate that in a life-threatening situation the parent and patient cannot refuse life-saving therapy.[13] The most commonly discussed example is a child of the Jehovah's Witness faith needing a blood transfusion. Courts have consistently ruled that the child's welfare supercedes the religious practice.[16] In the case of an exsanguinating injury, the child should be transfused. If the child can be stabilized but is likely to need a transfusion in the near future, the local child protection agency should be involved and a judicial order mandating transfusion should be obtained. Only as a last resort should the child be taken from the parents' custody.

Adolescent refusal of care is more complicated. It is reasonable to respect an adolescent's refusal of care that would not subject them to a great risk of harm.[17]

▶ FAMILY PRESENCE FOR PROCEDURES AND RESUSCITATION

Traditionally, parents and families were excluded from the room for invasive procedures or when a critically ill or injured child was being resuscitated. This exclusion was justified by the fear that a parent might interfere with the procedure or resuscitation, might distract the caregivers from their primary focus, might be traumatized by the procedure or resuscitation, and might subject the physicians to physical harm or a higher degree of malpractice risk in the event of a bad outcome. Survey research reveals that families want to be given the choice about being present for an invasive procedure or resuscitation. Most choose to be present, and most feel that their presence is helpful to the child and to the health care team.[18]

Physician opinions vary and are influenced by institution, specialty, age, experience, and geographic area. There is a growing trend to support parental presence.[19] Family presence should be considered for all procedures and resuscitations. Assurance of safety for the patient and health care team is essential and may require exclusion of family members who are combative, threatening, intoxicated, mentally ill, or emotionally overwhelmed.[20]

▶ PRACTICING PROCEDURES ON THE NEWLY DEAD

Teaching and practicing procedures on the newly dead has a long history in medicine. It is practiced in about half of emergency medicine training programs. The most common procedure practiced is endotracheal intubation. More invasive procedures are performed, but less frequently. The consent or permission of a family member is rarely obtained.[21,22]

Compelling justifications for practicing procedures on the newly dead exist. It is argued that practicing certain procedures is an invaluable learning experience for the trainee and no harm can be inflicted on a corpse. A novice could learn an invasive but not disfiguring on a newly dead body in order to better serve the next living patient.[22] A more problematic approach is adopting the pretense of therapeutic intent prior to pronouncing a patient dead in order to practice invasive procedures that have no hope of benefiting the patient.[23]

Even if practicing procedures on the newly dead is an excellent way for a medical trainee to learn and many others will benefit from the physician's procedural skill in the future, it should only be done with permission from a parent. Such a conversation would be extremely difficult in such an emotionally charged situation, as are other discussions that occur near the end of life, including withdrawal of life support and organ donation. If teaching procedures on the newly dead is to be done, the teaching institution and program should have a policy covering this practice. Only those trainees requiring the skill should practice, and only after mastering the procedure on artificial models or donated cadavers. Only nonmutilating procedures should be performed and permission must be obtained in keeping with our standards of parental permission. Most families will agree to allow procedures to be practiced, but they want to be asked.[22–24]

► ADOLESCENT ISSUES

CONFIDENTIALITY

Adolescents may seek care in an ED alone or accompanied by a friend, sibling, or parent. In most cases, part of the history should be done alone with the adolescent to assure confidentiality and to discuss sensitive issues with medical implications. The adolescent must be assured that communications will be kept confidential, but the limits of confidentiality must also be discussed. Confidentiality may be breached in the event of a disclosure of abuse or homicidal or suicidal intent. Although every effort should be made to protect confidentiality, the adolescent needs to be aware that confidentiality may be breached by the parent's receipt of a detailed bill or statement from an insurer. An acceptable and confidential method to provide the patient with test results should also be explored at the time of the initial visit. Acceptable methods include the adolescent phoning back for their test results, discussing the situation with the patient's primary care physician, or calling the patient on their personal phone. If the patient is not available by phone, a message could be left for the patient to call for test results. A parent taking or hearing the message may want to know the results, but the confidentiality of the patient must be respected.[14,15]

CHAPERONES AND PHYSICAL EXAMINATION

A problem-focused physical examination of an adolescent may often be performed without discomforting or embarrassing the patient. When a breast, anorectal, genital, or pelvic examination is indicated, the examination should be clearly explained. The patient, parent, or physician may want to have a chaperone present for the more sensitive parts of the examination. The presence of the third party may protect the interests of both the patient and physician.[25]

EMERGENCY CONTRACEPTION

Although teen birth rates have been on the decline, 74% to 95% of adolescent pregnancies are unintended. Emergency contraception—the use of hormonal therapy up to 120 hours after unprotected sexual intercourse—may decrease the rate of unintended adolescent pregnancies. Education about and access to emergency contraception does not increase the frequency of protected or unprotected intercourse and should be offered to all adolescent women when sexuality issues are discussed. The American Academy of Pediatrics supports improved availability of emergency contraception, including full support of over-the-counter access.[26]

ABORTION

All adolescents need and deserve confidential care. Perhaps one of the most ethically challenging and controversial issues is providing confidential care to the pregnant adolescent con-sidering an abortion. Minors have the legal right to obtain an abortion without parental involvement or consent unless state law requires such involvement. If parental involvement is required, there must be a process to provide for judicial bypass. Most adolescents considering abortion actively involve their parents or other trusted adults in their decision-making process. Parental involvement in an adolescent's important life-changing decision might be desirable or even ideal, but legally required involvement may cause a delay in seeking care. The American Academy of Pediatrics recommends that an adolescent should involve a parent or other trusted adult in the decision-making process, but the adolescent's right to confidential care must be respected.[27]

DRUG USE AND DRUG SCREENING

Drug testing may need to be done as part of a diagnostic evaluation of a patient with an altered level of consciousness. Because such a patient would not be able to consent, testing with a clear medical indication would be covered by the community standard of presumed consent for emergency medical care.[15,28] Drug testing may also be required if a patient is in need of mental health services and needs to be aligned with the most appropriate treatment program or facility. Such testing should only be done with the consent of the patient, but might be permissible without consent if the patient is under an involuntary psychiatric hold. Sometimes drug testing may be required by law enforcement, but physicians should only participate in criminal investigations as required by law or court order.[29]

A parent may request drug testing if they suspect their child has been using drugs. There may be a conflict between the interests of the patient from the patient's and parent's perspective. It might be appropriate to test a young child without their assent but with a parent's permission, but an older adolescent should only be tested with full informed consent.[14,15]

Drug screening at home or as a condition of participation in sports or other school-related activities is also problematic. All tests have false-positives and false-negatives, and issues related to sensitivity, specificity, and pre-test probability require careful interpretation of a test result that might lead to misinterpretation of reality.[28] The cross-reactivity of prescription and over-the-counter medications and food products can cause additional problems with interpretation. A physician participating in a screening program would face conflicts regarding confidentiality, the therapeutic relationship, and the punitive result of such testing.[29] The American Academy of Pediatrics opposes involuntary screening of older adolescents on the basis of parental request. Until research demonstrates safety and efficacy, the Academy also opposes commercially available home drug testing or testing as a condition for participation in sports or any other school function.[29,30]

► CONCLUSION

Providing emergency medical care to children embodies many of the core ethical values of medicine, including providing care to anyone in need; despite their perceived need at presentation, immigration status, insurance, or ability to pay. Ethical challenges unique to pediatric emergency medicine present an opportunity and need for ongoing exploration and discussion with emergency medicine physicians and pediatricians. Children have an evolving capacity to take part in health care decisions, and by adolescence they may be able to make decisions as well as adults. Keeping the best interests of the child as the central focus should help guide physicians through the most challenging cases.

REFERENCES

1. Iserson KV. Ethical principles—emergency medicine. *Emerg Med Clin North Am.* 2006;24:513–545.

2. American College of Emergency Physicians Ethics Committee. American College of Emergency Physicians Ethics Manual. *Ann Emerg Med.* 1991;20:1153–1162.

3. American Academy of Pediatrics Committee on Pediatric Emergency Medicine. Overcrowding crisis in our nation's emergency departments: is our safety net unraveling? *Pediatrics.* 2004;114:878–888.

4. Hostetler MA, Mace S, Brown K, et al. Emergency department overcrowding and children. *Pediatr Emerg Care.* 2007;23:507–515.

5. Society for Academic Emergency Medicine Ethics Committee. Ethics of emergency department triage: SAEM position statement. *Acad Emerg Med.* 1995;2:990–995.

6. Maldonado T, Avner JR. Triage of the pediatric patient in the emergency department: are we all in agreement? *Pediatrics.* 2004;114:356–360.

7. American Academy of Pediatrics Committee on Pediatric Emergency Medicine. Consent for emergency medical services for children and adolescents. *Pediatrics.* 2003;111:703–706.

8. American Academy of Pediatrics Committee on Community Health Services. Providing care for immigrant, homeless, and migrant children. *Pediatrics.* 2005;115:1095–1100.

9. Morris DM, Gordon JA. The role of the emergency department in the care of homeless and disadvantaged populations. *Emerg Med Clin North Am.* 2006;24:839–848.

10. Young J, Flores G, Berman S. Providing life-saving health care to undocumented children: controversies and ethical issues. *Pediatrics.* 2004;114:1316–1320.

11. American College of Emergency Physicians. Delivery of care to undocumented persons. Dallas, TX: American College of Emergency Physicians; 2006. http://www.acep.org/practres.aspx?id=29168. Accessed February 25, 2008.

12. American Academy of Pediatrics Committee on Child Abuse and Committee on Bioethics. Forgoing life-sustaining medical treatment in abused children. *Pediatrics.* 2000;106:1151–1153.

13. American Academy of Pediatrics Committee on Bioethics. Informed consent, parental permission, and assent in pediatric practice. *Pediatrics.* 1995;95:314–317.

14. Jacobstein CR, Baren JM. Emergency department treatment of minors. *Emerg Med Clin North Am.* 1999;17:341–352.

15. Weddle M, Kokotailo P. Adolescent substance abuse. Confidentiality and consent. *Pediatr Clin North Am.* 2002;49:301–315.

16. Wooley S. Children of Jehovah's Witnesses and adolescent Jehovah's Witnesses: what are their rights? *Arch Dis Child.* 2005;90:715–719.

17. Elton A, Honig P, Bentovim A, et al. Withholding consent to lifesaving treatment: three cases. *Br Med J.* 1995;310:373–377.

18. Boudreaux ED, Francis JL, Loyacano T. Family presence during invasive procedures and resuscitation in the emergency department: a critical review and suggestions for future research. *Ann Emerg Med.* 2002;40:193–205.

19. Dingeman RS, Mitchell EA, Meyer EC, et al. Parent presence during complex invasive procedures and cardiopulmonary resuscitation: a systemic review of the literature. *Pediatrics.* 2007;120:842–854.

20. Henderson DP, Knapp JF. Report of the national consensus conference on family presence during pediatric cardiopulmonary resuscitation and procedures. *Pediatr Emerg Care.* 2005;21:787–791.

21. Fourre MW. The performance of procedures on the recently deceased. *Acad Emerg Med.* 2002;9:595–598.

22. Burns JP, Reardon FE, Truog RD. Using newly deceased patients to teach resuscitation procedures. *N Engl J Med.* 1994;331:1652–1655.

23. The Society of Academic Emergency Medicine Ethics Committee. Ethics seminars: the ethical debate on practicing procedures on the newly dead. *Acad Emerg Med.* 2004;11:962–966.

24. Moore GP. Ethics seminars: the practice of medical procedures in newly dead patients—is consent warranted? *Acad Emerg Med.* 2001;8:389–392.

25. American Academy of Pediatrics Committee on Practice and Ambulatory Medicine. The use of chaperones during the physical examination of the pediatric patient. *Pediatrics.* 1996;98:1202.

26. American Academy of Pediatrics Committee on Adolescence. Emergency contraception. *Pediatrics.* 2005;116:1026–1035.

27. American Academy of Pediatrics Committee on Adolescence. The adolescent's right to confidential care when considering abortion. *Pediatrics.* 1996;97:746–751.

28. Casavant MJ. Urine drug screening in adolescents. *Pediatr Clin North Am.* 2002;49:317–327.

29. American Academy of Pediatrics Committee on Substance Abuse. Testing for drugs of abuse in children and adolescents. *Pediatrics.* 1996 (Reaffirmed 2006);98:305–307.

30. American Academy of Pediatrics Committee on Substance Abuse. Testing for drugs of abuse in children and adolescents: addendum- testing in schools and at home. *Pediatrics.* 2007;119:627–630.

CHAPTER 153

Withholding or Terminating Resuscitation and Brain Death

Howard Hast

► HIGH-YIELD FACTS

- A patient with an advance directive to not resuscitate (a DNR order) may be treated but not resuscitated in the ED.
- Lacking advance directives, all children including those who are terminally ill must be provided with resuscitation. Rarely is there time or resources in the ED to initiate a conversation that would lead to a sound DNR order.
- There is no standard of care that dictates the duration of resuscitation for infants, children, or adolescents. The duration of resuscitation is at the discretion of the treating physicians.
- Brain death in infants and children typically cannot be determined in the ED because of the observation period required. To diagnose brain death, a set of criteria must be met that includes a compatible clinical history, a physical exam consistent with brain death, and may require supportive studies to definitively establish this diagnosis.

► WITHHOLDING OR TERMINATING RESUSCITATION

There are certain circumstances when resuscitation in the emergency department (ED) may be withheld. A terminally ill patient who presents to the ED with an advance directive such as a DNR order may be treated but not resuscitated. The order must be signed by the patient's attending physician and legal guardian and should be reviewed by the attending physician in the ED with the patient's guardian. The parents or legal guardian may withdraw the DNR order at any time, including shortly after arrival in the ED.

A terminally ill patient with no advance directives must be provided with advanced life support and resuscitation. Time and resources in the ED are insufficient to initiate the conversations that might result in a DNR order.

Termination of resuscitation and declaration of death is appropriate when there is no return of spontaneous circulation. There are no absolute standards of care that dictate the duration of resuscitation in the pediatric population. Survival after out-of-hospital arrest is poor and has been correlated to the number of doses of Epinephrine administered. In several studies, there were no survivors if more than one dose of epinephrine was administered, and a larger number of investigations revealed no survivors if more than two doses of epinephrine were administered. In terms of duration of resuscitation, multiple studies have demonstrated few survivors in resuscitations lasting more than 20 to 30 minutes, while other investigations have demonstrated intact survival only in patients who received less then 15 minutes of resuscitation.[1] Lacking universally accepted guidelines, the physician must determine the duration of resuscitation based upon the individual case. Certainly, hypothermic patients should have resuscitation continued until they have a body temperature of at least 35°C.

A number of studies have demonstrated that family members typically prefer to be present during resuscitation, and that their grieving is less problematic if they were present during the resuscitation. There should be one staff member assigned to be present with the family to answer questions and explain what is being done; the ED staff should be sensitive to the presence of family members during the resuscitation.[2]

► BRAIN DEATH

Brain death cannot be determined in the ED because of the observation period required. In some cases, particularly in normothermic children who have the return of spontaneous circulation after a prolonged resuscitation, the children will subsequently progress to brain death. Brain death is defined as a total and irreversible loss of cerebral function, including brain stem function. The most recent, widely accepted guidelines were penned in 1987 by The Task Force for the Determination of Brain Death in Children.[3] These guidelines were a consensus opinion regarding the necessary clinical history, physical examination criteria, observation periods, and confirmatory laboratory tests required to determine brain death in children. The guidelines are summarized below.

The *clinical history* must be consistent with the diagnosis of brain death. The cause of coma should be determined whenever possible. There must be no remediable or reversible conditions. Confounding factors such as toxic and metabolic disorders, the presence of sedative–hypnotic drugs, paralytic agents, hypothermia, hypotension, and surgically remediable conditions must be eliminated prior to establishing a diagnosis of brain death.

The *physical examination* is necessary to determine the failure of brain function. The physical examination criteria must consider the following:

- Coma and apnea must coexist
- A complete loss of consciousness, vocalization, and volitional activity

- Absent brain stem function
  - Fixed and dilated or midposition pupils
  - Absence of spontaneous eye movements
  - Absent oculocephalic and oculovestibular reflexes
  - Absent corneal reflexes
  - No cough or gag; no sucking or rooting reflexes
  - Respiratory movements absent without the ventilator
  - Flaccid tone and absence of spontaneous or induced movements, excluding spinal cord events such as reflex withdrawal or spinal myoclonus
  - After meeting these criteria, apnea testing may be performed.
- The examination results should remain consistent with brain death throughout the *observation and testing period.*

The observation period varies according to age:

- For children aged 7 days to 2 months, two examinations and EEGs separated by at least 48 hours.
- For children aged 2 months to 1 year, two examinations and EEGs separated by at least 24 hours. Repeat examination and EEG are not necessary if a concomitant cerebral radionuclide angiographic study demonstrates no visualization of cerebral arteries.
- For children older than 1 year, two examinations should be performed at least 12 hours apart. No corroborative laboratory studies are necessary. If hypoxic encephalopathy is present, observation for at least 24 hours is recommended. This may be reduced if an EEG shows electrocerebral silence or a radionuclide study is negative for cerebral blood flow.[3]

Although it is beyond the scope of this chapter, there are occasions when supportive studies are useful if not potentially essential, for example, in fulminant cases of acute peripheral neuropathies, such as acute inflammatory demyelinating polyradiculopathy or infant botulism, where the physical examination may be consistent with brain death.[4]

In many institutions, two examiners—typically from the pediatric neurology, pediatric neurosurgery, or pediatric critical care specialties—are necessary to complete a brain death determination. Corroborative studies such as EEG or a radionucleotide study are not mandatory in children older than 1 year of age when the physical examination and apnea testing are consistent with brain death. Following the 1987 guidelines, different institutions may vary in minor degree as to the specifics of how brain death is determined. Within each institution it is essential that the same protocol be followed for each infant or child to avoid uncertainty or error in this most important determination. Clinicians must devote the necessary time to explain the concept of brain death to the patient's family. Typically, multiple conversations during the observation and testing period are needed by most families to grasp and accept the concept that brain death is equivalent to cardiac death within our society. During this time, extended family and institutional support should be organized to assist the child's family in coping with this tragic diagnosis and their profound loss.

REFERENCES

1. Young KD, Seidel JS. Pediatric cardiopulmonary resuscitation: a collective review. *Ann Emerg Med.* 1999;33(2):195–205.
2. American Academy of Pediatrics, American Heart Association. *Pediatric Advanced Life Support Provider Manual.* Dallas, TX: American Heart Association; 2006:182–183.
3. Report of Special Task Force. Guidelines for the determination of brain death in children. *Pediatrics.* 1987;80:298–300.
4. Koszer S, Moshe SL. eMedicine: brain death in children. http://www.emedicine.com. Accessed May 5, 2008.

INDEX

Page numbers followed by f indicate figures; numbers followed by t indicate tables.

A

AAPCC (American Association of Poison Control Center), 982
Abdominal pain
    diagnostic tests, 596
        genital problems in males, 600
        gynecologic causes, 600
        history and examination, 595–596
    nonsurgical causes
        acute gastroenteritis, 598
        bleeding and pain, 599
        colic, 599
        constipation, 599
        inflammatory bowel disease, 599
        liver/pancreatic pain, 599
        urinary tract infections, 598–599
    obstruction, 597
    peritoneal irritation, 597
Abdominal injury, 274
Abdominal trauma
    evaluation, 277t
    management
        abdominal ultrasound, 278
        blunt abdominal trauma, 276
        computed tomography, 277
        diagnostic peritoneal lavage, 278
        general principles, 276
        laboratory evaluation, 277
        penetrating abdominal trauma, 276
    pathophysiology, 275
    patterns of injury
        bicycle crashes, 274
        child abuse, 274–275
        falls, 274
        motor vehicle collisions, 273–274
        sports injury, 274
    specific injuries
        abdominal wall, 279
        hollow organs, 279–280
        solid organs, 278–279
Abdominal ultrasound, 278, 610f
Abdominal wall, 279
Abetalipoproteinemia, 478
Abnormal chest auscultation, 262
Abortion, 1164
Abrasions, 334
Absolute lymphocyte, 1086t
Absolute neutrophil count (ANC), 843
Abuse and neglect
    abusive head injury, 1112–1114, 1113f
    ancillary studies, 1114
    child abuse, 1114, 1114t
    cutaneous injuries, 1110–1111
    epidemiology, 1109
    etiology, 1109–1110
    management, 1115
    musculoskeletal trauma, 1111–1112, 1112f

neglect, 1115
    recognition
        medical history, 1110
        physical examination, 1110
    visceral trauma, 1112
Abuse injuries, 1111f
Abusive head trauma (AHT), 1113
Accelerated idioventricular rhythm (AIVR), 448
ACE (angiotensin converting enzyme), 459
ACEP policy, 1159t
Acetabulum fractures, 323, 324f
Acetaminophen, 599
    acetaminophen toxicity
        gastrointestinal irritation, 888
        hepatic failure, 888
        latent period, 888
        recovery or deat, 888
        high-yield facts, 887
        laboratory studies, 888
        management
    antidote, 888
    gastrointestinal decontamination, 888
    pathophysiology, 887
Acetaminophen toxicity. See under Acetaminophen
Acetylcysteine, 889t
Acetylsalicylic acid (aspirin, ASA), 893
Acid burns, 908
Acid suppression, 610
Ackee (Blighia sapida), 986
Acquired coagulopathies. See under Bleeding disorders
Acquired immunodeficiency disease syndrome (AIDS). See under Sexually transmitted diseases (STD)
Acromioclavicular separation, 310
Activated thromboplastin time (aPTT), 811
Acute acetaminophen ingestion, 889t
Acute adrenal insufficiency, 642, 643t
Acute agitation medicatiom, 1121t
Acute asthma exacerbation, 363f, 367t
Acute ataxia, 478f
Acute bilirubin encephalopathy, 84
Acute blunt trauma, 757
Acute chest syndrome (ACS), 821, 822
Acute demyelinating encephalomyelitis (ADEM), 476
Acute depletion of energy (ATP), 195
Acute digoxin toxicity, 928t
Acute hemarthrosis, 827
Acute hemolytic transfusion reactions (AHTR), 834
Acute hemorrhage, 493
Acute leukemia, 837
Acute life-threatening event (ALTE), 609

Acute motor and sensory axonal neuropathy (ASMAN), 483
Acute myelogenous leukemia (AML), 837
Acute otitis externa. See under Nose Emergencies
Acute otitis media (mastoiditis). See under Nose emergencies
Acute pelvic pain, 791
Acute radiation syndrome, 1081, 1085
Acute renal failure, 696, 697, 1037
Acute respiratory distress syndrome (ARDS), 262, 383
Acute rheumatic fever (ARF), 442, 747, 861
Acute splenic sequestration crisis (ASSC), 825
Acute subdural hematomas, 238
Acute suppurative tenosynovitis, 856
Acute toxicity, 938
Acute traumatic diaphragmatic herniation, 267
Acute tubular necrosis, 1041
Acutely limping child, 98t
Adenovirus, 373, 772
ADH (anti-diuretic hormone), 660
Adnexae, 753–754
Adolescent pregnant patient
    deep vein thrombosis, 782
    eclampsia, 779–780
    ectopic pregnancy, 781
    emergency contraception, 783
    HELLP syndrome, 780
    hydatidiform mole, 783
    preeclampsia, 779
    Rh sensitization, 784
    trauma in pregnancy, 783
    vaginal bleeding
        placenta previa, 780
        placental abruption, 781
Adrenal insufficiency
    clinical presentation, 640
    differential diagnosis, 640
    disposition, 642
    management, 642
    epidemiology, 639
    etiology, 639
    laboratory findings, 640
    pathophysiology, 639
    signs and symptoms of, 641t
Adrenergic receptors, 201, 201t
Adrenoleukodystrophy (ALD), 639
Adult female deer tick, 548
Adult female dog tick, 548
Advanced life support (ALS), 1160
Advanced pediatric life support (APLS), 3
Advanced trauma life support (ATLS), 121
Aerogastralgia, 1076
Aeruginosa, 734
Afebrile pneumonia of infancy, 385

Afebrile seizure, 40–41
Africanized honeybees, 1013
Aggressive patient, 1120
AHA (American Heart Association), 203, 211, 429
AIDS. *See under* Sexually transmitted diseases (STD)
Air embolism, 1076–1077
Air transport of patients, 1147t
Airlift of injured hikers, 1061f
Airway and ventilation, 204
Airway injury, 265
Airway maintenance, 748
Airway management
  airway anatomy
    pediatric airway differences, 177
    recognizing conditions, 177
  clinical assessment, 177
  manual manipulation, 178–180
    bag-mask ventilation, 180
    oxygen administration, 180
    pharmacologic treatment, 180
    rescue breathing, 180
    tracheal intubation, 181
    ventilation bag types, 181
AIVR (accelerated idioventricular rhythm), 448
AKC (Atopic keratoconjunctivitis), 586
Alanine aminotransferase (ALT), 889
ALARA. *See* As low as reasonably achievable
Albendazole, 555
Albumin, 834
Alcohol solution 899f
Alkali burns, 907
Allergic conjunctivitis
  clinical presentation, 585–586
  differential diagnosis, 586
  pathophysiology, 585
  treatment, 586–587
  See also under Conjunctivitis in childhood
Allergic rhinitis
  pathophysiology, 585
  treatment, 587
Allergic transfusion reaction, 835
α-Adrenergic blocking agents, 923
Alpha-methylphenylethylamine, 955
ALTE (acute life-threatening event), 609
Altered mental status
  children coma scale, 34t
  congenital adrenal hyperplasia, 38
  diagnostic testing, 34
  disposition, 36
  etiology, 34t
  history, 33
  hypoglycemia, 38
  inborn errors of metabolism, 38
  intussusception, 37
  lead encephalopathy, 36
  mnemonic for coma, 35t
  pathophysiology, 33
  physical examination, 33
  special considerations, 36
  syndrome, 37
  therapy, 35
Altitude effects of, 1062t

Altitude-related syndromes. *See under* High-altitude illness
Alveolar gas exchange, 354
Amanita phalloides, 978f
American Academy of Pediatrics (AAA), 429, 1110
American Association of Poison Control Centers (AAPCC), 948
American college of chest physicians (ACCP), 505
American College of Rheumatology (ACR), 865
American Heart Association (AHA), 203, 211, 429
American mistletoe, 982
Aminobutyric acid (GABA), 149
Amperage, 1035
Amphetamines
  background, 955
  clinical manifestations, 955
  diagnostic testing, 956
  disposition, 957
  management, 956
  pharmacology, 955
Analgesia, 337, 742. *See also under* Procedural Sedation
Anaphylactic reactions, 1014
Anaphylaxis, 119
  allergens, 589
  ancillary tests, 590
  disposition, 591
  pathophysiology, 589
  presentation, 589
  special conditions, 590
  treatment, 590
Anaplasma phagocytophila, 552
Anaplastic large cell lymphoma (ALCL), 838
Anatomic snuffbox, 320
Anemia
  macrocytic anemia, 820
  microcytic anemia, 817
    iron deficiency, 818
    lead poisoning, 819
    thalassemia, 818–819
  normocytic anemia
    with high reticulocyte count, 819–820
    with low reticulocyte counts, 820
    peripheral smear interpretation, 818t
Ancillary tests, 416
Andersoni, 552
Anemia and dactylitis, 822f
Anemia of chronic disease (ACOD), 820
Anesthesia, 295–296, 337
Aneurysmal bone cyst (ABC), 872
Angiotensin converting enzyme (ACE), 459
Animal bite wounds, 1000
Ankle, 100
Ankle and foot fractures, 328–329
Anovulatory cycle, 809
Anoxic injury, 1041
Anterior cruciate ligament (ACL), 306
Anterior inferior iliac spine (AIIS), 305
Anterior inferior iliac spine (AIIS), 324f
Anterior pelvic fractures, 284
Anterior superior iliac spine (ASIS), 305
Anterior talofibular ligament (ATFL), 306

Anthrax, 575, 576, 577
Antibiotic prophylaxis, 398, 743
Antibiotic therapy, 12t
Antibiotics, 343–344, 909, 1000–1001
Anticholinergics, 368–369, 983
Anticoagulant rodenticides, 919t, 920t
Antidepressants
  atypical antidepressants, 932
  selective serotonin reuptake inhibitors, 931
  tricyclic antidepressants, 931
Antidiuretic hormone (ADH), 1069
Antidotal therapy, 921, 927, 938
Antidote, 888
Antiepileptic drug (AED), 43
Antigenic drift, 509
Antimicrobial therapy, 398, 408
Anti-nuclear antibodies (ANA), 865
Antireflux medications, 610
Antiretroviral (ARV) therapy, 540, 541t
Antisepsis and scrubbing, 338
Antistreptolysin (ASO), 693
Antivenom therapy
  crotalidae polyvalent antivenin, 1005–1007
  crotaline Fab antivenom, 1006
Antiviral medications, 515t
Antizole, 899f
Anus, 605
Aortic coarctation, 419, 420f
Aortic stenosis (AS), 420
Aortography, 231
Apgar Score, 213t
Aplastic crisis, 826
APLS (Advanced pediatric life support), 3
Apparent life-threatening event, 30t
Apparent life-threatening event. *See under* Sudden infant death syndrome
Appendicitis diagnosis, 598t
Appendix testis, torsion of
  diagnostic evaluation, 679
  management, 679
  signs and symptoms, 679
Aqueductal stenosis, 496f
Argyreia nervosa, 986
Aripiprazole, 936
Arrhythmias, 427
Arrhythmogenic right ventricular dysplasia (ARVD), 473
Arterial blood gases, 354–355, 1053
Arterial spasm and vasomotor instability, 1041
Arteriovenous malformation (AVM), 503
Arthropods. *See under* Parasitic infestations
As low as reasonably achievable (ALARA), 3, 171
Ascariasis, 554–555
Ascaris lumbricoides, 553
ASD (atrial septal defect), 419, 420f
Aspirin
  clinical presentation, 893
  laboratory studies, 893
  management, 894
  pathophysiology, 893
  pharmacokinetics, 893
Association of poison control centers (AAPCC), 969

Asthma
  clinical presentation, 362–366
  differential diagnosis, 366
  disposition/outcome, 370
  etiology/pathophysiology, 361–362
  exacerbation severity in emergency care
      setting, 364t, 365t
  radiographic findings, 366
  treatment,
      anticholinergics, 368–369
      corticosteroids, 369
      heliox, 369
      intubation, 370
      magnesium, 369
      mechanical ventilation, 370
      β-adrenergic agonists, 367–368
Asystole, 208
Ataxia
  acute ataxia
      acute cerebellar ataxia, 477
      acute postinfectious, 477
      chronic progressive ataxia, 477
      episodic ataxia, 469
      Guillain-Barr'e syndrome, 477
      intermittent, 477
      miller-fisher syndrome, 477
      myoclonic encephalopathy, 477
      myoclonus, 477
      opsoclonus, 477
      tumors, 477
  causes, 476
  chronic nonprogressive ataxia, 479
  chronic progressive ataxia, 477
  evaluation, 475
  pathophysiology, 475
  physical examination, 475
Atlantoaxial rotatory subluxation (AARS),
      251
Atlantooccipital dislocation (AOD), 250, 250f
Atlas fractures, 250
Atopic keratoconjunctivitis (AKC), 586
Atrial flutter and fibrillation. See under
      Dysrhythmias in children
Atrial septal defect (ASD), 419, 420f
Atrioventricular (AV) blocks, 445
Atrioventricular septal defect, 421
Atropa belladonna, 983
Atropine, 216, 340, 994
Attitude-related barotitis, 1075–1076
Atypical antidepressants, 932
Atypical antipsychotics. See under
      Neuroleptics
Atypical mycobacterial infection, 125f
Atypical pneumonia, 384
Automatic implantable cardiac defibrillators,
      451
AVPU method, 228
Avulsion fractures, 324
Avulsion injuries, 305
Axillary nerve damage, 310
Axis fractures, 252
Azathioprine, 138

B
B. pertussis infection. See Pertussis
Babesia microti, 559
Babesiosis, 551, 559

Bacillus anthracis (anthrax), 575
Back examination, 232
Backboard modifications, 248f
Bacterial conjunctivitis, 770, 772
Bacterial endocarditis, 442
Bacterial etiologies, 10
Bacterial tracheitis, 358
Bacterial vaginosis, 794
Bag versus rusch bag, 182
Bag-mask ventilation (BMV), 180
Bag-valve-mask (BVM) ventilation, 26, 357
Balanitis and balanoposthitis
  diagnostic evaluation, 685
  management, 685
  pathophysiology, 684
  signs and symptoms, 685
Balanoposthitis, 682, 684
Barbiturates, 151
Barodentalgia, 1076
Barosinusitis, 1076
Barotitis, 1074–1075
Barotraumas. See under Dysbaric injuries
Barrett's esophagus, 612
Bartholin abscess, 790
Bartholin's gland inflammation, 790f
Basilar skull fractures, 238
Beard distribution, 729
Bees and vespids
  management, 1014
  disposition, 1014
  pathophysiology, 1013–1014
Bell-clapper deformity, 678f
Bell's palsy, 485
Benign cardiac murmurs, 417t
Benzocaine, 990
Benzodiazepines, 39
β-adrenergic agonists, 367–368
β-Blockers, 435, 447
β-hemolytic Streptococcus, 793
Bicycle crashes, 274, 275f
Bilateral pelvic rami fractures, 324
Biliary atresia, 88
  ancillary studies, 623
  diagnosis, 623
  management, 623–624
Biliary tract disease. See under Liver and
      gallbladder
Bilirubin, 83, 86f
Biological dosimetry, 1085t
Bioterrorism
  anthrax, 575
  botulism, 580
  plague, 576
  smallpox, 579
Black widow spiders. See under Spider and
      arthropod bites
Bladder injuries, 276
Bleeding disorders
  acquired coagulopathies, 829
      hemolytic uremic syndrome, 830
      immune thrombocytopenic purpura,
          830–832
      intravascular coagulation, 829
      platelet disorders, 830
      hemophilia
          acute hemarthrosis, 827
          bleeding manifestations, 828

      intracranial hemorrhage, 828
      intramuscular bleeding, 827
      management, 828
  von Willebrand disease, 829
Bleeding manifestations, 828
Blepharoconjunctivitis, 774
Blood component therapy
  albumin, 834
  complications
      acute hemolytic transfusion reactions,
          834
      allergic transfusion reaction, 835
      delayed hemolytic transfusion
          reactions, 835
      febrile nonhemolytic transfusion
          reactions, 835
      infectious complications, 835
      massive transfusions, 835
  cryoprecipitate, 834
  factors, 834
  fresh frozen plasma, 833
  granulocyte concentrates, 833
  immune globulins, 834
  indications for transfusion, 834
  platelet concentrate, 833
  red blood cells, packed, 833
  whole blood, 833
Blood lead level (BLL), 963
Blood lead measurement, 964t
Blood pressure measurement, 455
Blood urea nitrogen (BUN), 693
Bloody diarrhea, 132f
Blue sheet, 565
blunt abdominal trauma, 276
Blunt aortic injury, 269
Blunt injury, 1039
Blunt ocular trauma, 757
Blunt thoracic trauma, 259–260
Blunt trauma, 259, 269
BMV, 181f
Bohler's angle, 330f
Bordatella pertussis, 12
Borrelia burgdorferi, 856
Borrelia burgdorferi, 545
Borrelia, 567
Botulism, 484, 580
Box jellyfish (sea wasp), 1018f
Boyle's law, 1060
BPD (bronchopulmonary dysplasia),
      376, 401
Brachial cleft cyst, 126f, 131
Brachioplexus injuries, 306–307
Brain death, 1167–1168
Brain dysfunction, 36t
Brain tumors and hydrocephalus, 493
Breast milk jaundice, 84
British antilewisite (BAL), 966
Brodifacoum, green-colored, 920f
Bronchodilators, 403
Bronchiolitis
  clinical presentation, 373
  differential diagnosis, 375
  disposition/outcome, 376
  etiology, 373
  pathophysiology, 373
  radiographic findings, 374
  treatment, 375

Bronchopneumonia (lobular) pneumonia, 388, 389f
Bronchopulmonary dysplasia (BPD), 376
  clinical presentation, 403
  differential diagnosis, 397
  disposition, 403
  etiology/pathophysiology
    infection, 402
    inflammation, 402
    malnutrition, 402
    mechanical ventilation, 401–402
    oxygen therapy, 402
  laboratory findings, 403
  treatment, 403
Brown recluse spiders. *See under* Spider and arthropod bites
Brudsinski sign, 521
Brugada syndrome, 472
B-type natriuretic peptide (BNP) assay, 424
Buccal hematoma, 828f
Buffers, 908
Bulla primary lesion, 118f
Burgdorferi, 545, 548
Buried stitch, 339–340, 340f
Burkitt's lymphoma, 838
Burn, 233, 403
Burn wounds, 1030f
Burner, 307
Button batteries, 910
BVM. *See* Bag-valve-mask

C

C. trachomatis, 797
Calcanofibular ligament (CF), 306
Calcification, 965f
Calcineurin inhibitors, 2
Calcium channel blockers, 459, 924
Calcium. *See under* Fluid and Electrolyte Disorders
Camphor, 989
Campylobacter, 571, 572t
Campylobacter gastroenteritis, 477
CA-MRSA (community acquired–methicillin resistant *Staphylococcus aureus*), 514
Cancer incidence, 838
Candida albicans, 794
Candida, 602
Candidal vaginitis. *See under* Vaginitis
Capnography, 24
Capsicum annuum, 982
Capsicum, 982
Carbon monoxide poisoning
  clinical presentation, 941
  disposition, 942
  laboratory studies, 942
  pathophysiology, 941
  toxicity, 942t
  treatment, 942
Carboxyhemoglobinemia, 23
Cardiac contusion, 268, 1041
Cardiac glycosides, 983
Cardiac lesions, 130t
Cardiac tamponade, 269
Cardiogenic shock, 229
Cardiopulmonary arrest in children, 207t

Cardiopulmonary resuscitation (CPR), 1027, 1054
  airway and ventilation, 204–205
  asystole and PEA, 208
  cardiopulmonary arrest, 209
  child's weight estimation, 205t
  dysrhythmias, 205, 208t
  life-support measures, 203
  paroxysmal supraventricular tachycardia, 207
  postresuscitation considerations, 209
  symptomatic bradycardia, 5–6
  vascular access priorities, 205
  ventricular fibrillation and PVT, 208
  ventricular tachycardia, 208
Cardiovascular injuries, 268
Carpal bones, fractures of, 320
Carpometacarpal dislocation, 320f
Carpometacarpal joint, 321
Cataracts, 1041
Caustic eye injuries, 909
Caustic injury, 758
Caustics
  button batteries, 910
  caustic eye injuries, 909
  hydrofluoric acid, 910
  laboratory studies, 908
    radiology studies, 908
    buffers, 908
    diluents, 908
    steroids, 909
    surgical intervention, 909
    wound care, 909
  management
    antibiotics, 909
    endoscopy, 909
    gastric decontamination, 909
  pathophysiology,
    acid burns, 908
    alkali burns, 907
  presentation and diagnosis, 908
Cavernous sinus thrombosis, 766
CBC. *See* Complete blood count
CDC (Clinical criteria for diagnosis), 525
Cellulitis, 765–767, 1001
Central nervous system (CNS), 837, 839, 846, 861, 895
Central venous pressure (CVP), 196
Centruroides envenomations, 1013
Cephalohematomas, 12
Cerebral palsy (CP), 499
  clinical presentation, 499
  complications, 500
  high-yield facts, 499
Cerebrospinal fluid (CSF), 495, 522
Cerebrovascular syndromes
  diagnosis, 503
    diagnostic evaluation, 504
    history, 503
    physical examination, 504
  disposition, 505
    high-yield facts, 501
    moyamoya, 505
    outcome, disability, 505
    postvaricella angiopathy, 506
    specific conditions

      transient cerebral, 506
    treatment, 505
Cervical spine, 231
Cervicitis, 804
Cervicothoracic sympathetic ganglionectomy, 451
Cestodes, 557
CFTR (cystic fibrosis transmembrane conductance regulator), 405
CHD (congenital heart disease), 9
Chemical conjunctivitis, 769
Chemical injuries to eye, 758
Chemical weapons
  nerve agents
    central, 994
    muscarinic, 993
    nicotinic, 993
  sulfur mustard, 994–995
Chemoprophylaxis, 564
Chest compressions, 214, 215f
Chest pain
  clinical presentation, 51
  diagnostic evaluation, 53–54
  differential diagnosis
    cardiac, 51
    gastrointestinal, 52
    idiopathic, 53
    musculoskeletal, 52
    psychogenic, 53
    respiratory, 51
  management, 54–55
  pneumonia, 53f
Chest radiograph (CXR), 261, 403, 416, 432, 440f, 441f, 463f
  Chest radiograph
    in aortic injury, 266
    in traumatic diaphragmatic hernia, 267
Chest roentgenogram, 388
Chest tube sizes, 264t
Chest wounds, 231
Chest x-ray, 366f
Child abuse, 274–275, 274f, 1162
Child death in ED
  caring for ED staff, 1125
  from parents, 1126
  interview, 1123
  interview, 1123–1124
  miscarriage IN ED, 1124–1125
Child in emergency department
  activity level, 6
  assessment and plan, 7
  developmental stages, 6
  history and physical, 7
  preparing for examination, 3
Child maltreatment, 1109
Children with special health care needs (CSHCN), 153, 1136t–1138t
Child's weight estimation, 205t
Chiropsalmus quadrumanus, 1017
Chlamydia, 822. *See also under* Sexually transmitted diseases (STD)
Chlamydia infections, 12
Chlamydia pneumonia, 386
Chlamydia trachomatis, 12, 679, 773, 859
Chlamydophila pneumoniae, 483
Chlamydophilia (chlamydia) pneumoniae, 386

Chlorophyllum molybdites, 979
Chloroquine, 990
Cholesteatoma, 736f
Choledochal cyst
   ancillary studies, 624
   diagnosis, 624
   management, 624
Cholelithiais and cholecystitis
   ancillary studies, 624
   diagnosis, 624
   management, 624
Cholinergic Crisis, 484
Chronic airway infection, 406
Chronic bilirubin encephalopathy, 84
Chronic cognitive impairments, 106
Chronic impetigo, 714f
Chronic mountain sickness (CMS), 1069
Chronic myelogenous leukemia (CML), 837
Chronic nonprogressive ataxia, 479
Chronic progressive ataxia, 477
Chronic Toxicity, 939
Chrysaora quinquecirrha, 1017
Cicuta maculate, 985f
Classic Lund and Browder chart, 1032
Clavicle, 855f
Clavicle and acromioclavicular joint, 309
Clitocybe dealbata, 978
Clostridia botulinum (botulism), 481, 575
Clostridium difficile, 74
Clostridium perfringens, 2t, 74
Clozapine, 935
Cluster headaches, 492
CMPA (Cow milk protein allergy), 77
Coagulation necrosis, 907, 908
Coccidia, 559–560
Cock-Robin deformity, 252f
Coelenterate nematocysts, 1018f
Coelenterates, 1017
Cognitive injury, 1041
Coin at thoracic inlet, 616f
Colchicine, 985
Colchicum autumnale, 985
Cold exposure, 1056t
Cold shock, 198
Colorado tick fever, 552
Coma. *See under* Altered Mental Status
Common radiological imaging, 596t
Compartment syndrome, 330
Complete blood count (CBC), 10, 87, 522,
   663, 821
Compression lacerations, 333
Computed tomography (CT), 39, 124, 277,
   964f
Concomitant abdominal injury, 260
Concussed athlete. *See under* Mild head
   injury
Concussion, 306
Concussion injuries, 743
Concussive brain injury (CBI), 105
Congenital adrenal hyperplasia (CAH), 131,
   639, 642f
Congenital anisocoria, 754
Congenital heart disease (CHD), 9
   classification, 416
   common presentations
      B-type natriuretic peptide assay, 424
      congestive heart failure, 423–424

      ductal-dependent lesions, 423
      Eisenmenger syndrome, 426
      hypertrophic cardiomyopathy, 425
      hypoxemic "TET" spells, 424
      isolated coronary artery anomalies,
         426
      presentations in older children and
         adults, 425
      undifferentiated sick infant, 421–423
   epidemiology, 413
   evaluation
      ancillary tests, 416
      history, 414
      hyperoxia test, 415
      physical examination, 414–415
   individual lesions, survey of
      aortic coarctation, 419, 420f
      aortic stenosis (AS), 420
      atrial septal defect (ASD),
         419, 420f
      atrioventricular septal defect, 421
      hypoplastic left heart syndrome
         (HLHS), 418, 419f
      patent ductus arteriosus (PDA), 420,
         421f
      pulmonic stenosis (PS), 419, 420f
      tetralogy of Fallot (TOF), 418, 419f
      total anomalous pulmonary venous
         return (TAPVR), 418, 419f
      transposition of great arteries (TGA),
         416, 418f
      tricuspid atresia, 416, 419f
      truncus arteriosus, 416, 418f
      ventricular septal defect (VSD), 420
   physiology
      fetal circulation, 413
      neonatal circulation, 413
   postcardiac surgery heart patient, care of
      cardiac transplant patients, 428
      categories of repair, 426
      infective endocarditis, prevention of,
         429
      outpatient referral, 429
      postoperative complications, 427
   syndromes, 414t
Congestive heart failure (CHF)
   acute decompensated heart failure,
      435
   compensated (chronic) CHF, 434f
   diagnostic studies
      chest radiograph (CXR), 432
      echocardiography (ECHO), 433
      electrocardiogram (EKG), 433
   etiologic basis, 432t
   future modalities in treatment, 435
   history, 431
   inotropic agents, 436t
   laboratory evaluation, 432
   load-altering agents, 436t
   oral dosing for digoxin, 434t
   pathophysiology, 431
   physical examination, 431
   signs and symptoms, 433t
   treatment, 434
Congenital masses, 125
Congenital short QT syndrome,
   472

Congenital vaginal obstruction
   clinical presentation, 788
   etiology, 787
   management, 788
Congestion, 767
Congestive heart failure (CHF), 423–424, 658,
   1041
Conjugated hyperbilirubinemia. *See under*
   Jaundice
Conjugated hyperbilirubinemia in newborn,
   causes of
   extrahepatic diseases, 88
   infectious causes, 88
   metabolic causes, 88
Conjugated neonatal hyperbilirubinemia
   ancillary studies, 621
   management/complications, 621
   recognition, 620
Conjunctiva and sclera, 754
Conjunctival and scleral lacerations, 757
Conjunctivitis, 767, 771t. *See also* Allergic
   conjunctivitis
Conjunctivitis in childhood, 771
   allergic conjunctivitis
      management, 774
      seasonal and perennial, 773
   bacterial conjunctivitis, 772
   herpes simplex and varicella-zoster, 773
      Chlamydia trachomatis, 773
      Neisseria gonorrhoeae, 773
   special forms
      blepharoconjunctivitis, 774
      Kawasaki disease, 774
      molluscum contagiosum, 774
      Perinaud oculoglandular syndrome,
         774
      Stevens–Johnson syndrome, 774
   vernal conjunctivitis, 774
   viral conjunctivitis, 772
Conocybe, 979
Contact dermatitis pattern, 708t
Contact potential, 1039
Continuous mattress stitch, 344f
Continuous positive airway pressure (CPAP),
   189, 198, 376, 401, 424
Continuous single lock stitch, 343f
Contractility, 434
Contrast media, 233
Contusions and hematomas, 334
Convallaria majalis, 983
Coprinus (antabuse), 978
Coprinus atramentarius, 978
Coral snakes. *See under* Snake
   envenomations
Corkscrew sign, 610f
Corneal abrasion, 756
Corneal and scleral foreign bodies, 757
Corpora cavernosum, 685
Corpora spongiosum, 685
Corticosteroids, 4, 356, 369, 715
Cow's milk protein allergy (CMPA), 77
CPAP (continuous positive airway pressure),
   180, 376
CPR. *See* Cardiopulmonary resuscitation
Crater peptic ulcer, 603
C-reactive protein (CRP), 11, 100, 852
Creatine kinase (CK), 54

Creatinine phosphokinase (CPK), 1005
Cricothyrotomy, 225, 265
Crohn's disease, 599
Cross-table lateral view (CTLV), 249
Crotalidae polyvalent antivenin, 1005–1007
Crotaline Fab antivenom, 1006
Crotaline snakebite wounds, 1005
Croup, 355–357
Cryoprecipitate, 834
Cryotherapy, 1005
CSHCN (children with special health care needs), 153
CSVT (cerebral sinovenous thrombosis), 501, 503t
CT scan, 292
    of abdomen, 233
    of head, 233
    scanner, 170f
Culex mosquito, 486
Cutaneous anthrax, 578
Cyanide antidotes, 974
Cyanide poisoning
    clinical presentation, 973
    cyanide antidotes, 974
    cyanide poisoning, 975f
    disposition, 975
    enzyme rhodanase, 973
    hydrogen sulfide toxicity, 975f
    hydroxocobalamin, 974
    hypoxia, 973
    laboratory evaluation, 974
    pathophysiology, 973
    smoke inhalation, 974
    sodium thiosulfate, 974
    Taylor kit, 974
    toxicokinetics, 973
    treatment
        cyanide antidotes, 974
        hydroxocobalamin, 974
        Taylor kit, 974
Cyanosis, 354
Cyclopeptide (Amanita phalloides), 977
Cystic fibrosis
    clinical presentation, 405
    differential diagnosis, 407
    etiology/pathophysiology, 405
    radiographic findings, 407
    treatment, 408
Cystic fibrosis transmembrane conductance regulator (CFTR), 405
Cytomegalovirus (CMV), 833

D
D. latum, 558
Darier's sign, 728, 729f
Datura stramonium, 983, 983f
Daucus carota, 983
Debridement, 339
Decontamination, 909
Deep (buried) sutures, 339
Deep sedation, 148
Deep vein thrombosis (DVT), 461, 462f, 782
Dehydration, 659
Delayed hemolytic transfusion reactions, 835
Delayed primary (tertiary) closure, 342
Delayed reactions, 1014

Delayed rupture, 1041
Delirium, 33
Dengue fever, 569
Dengue hemorrhagic fever (DHF), 570
Dental abscesses, 744
Dental anatomy, 741, 742f
Dental fracture terminology, 742t
Dental fractures, 741
Dentoalveolar infections, 743. See also under Oral cavity and neck emergency
Dentoalveolar trauma. See under Oral cavity and neck emergency
Dermacentor andersoni, 484
Dermacentor variabilis, 484, 545
Dermal melanosis, 728
Dexmedetomidine, 152
DFA (Direct fluorescent antibody), 397
Diabetes insipidus (DI), 660
Diabetic mother, 218
Diagnostic evaluation, 75
Diagnostic peritoneal lavage (DPL), 278
Diamond–Blackfan anemia, 820
Diaper dermatitis, 728, 728f
Diaphragmatic hernia, 217
Diaphyseal clavicle fractures, 309
Diaphyseal clavicle fractures, 309
Diaphyseal radius and ulnar fractures, 315–316
Diarrhea, 61f, 571. See also Vomiting
Diazepam, 994
Dieffenbachia, 981, 982, 982f
Dientamoeba fragilis, 558
Diethylenetriaminepentaacetic acid (DTPA), 1096
Difenoxin, 990
Differential diagnosis, 521
Diffuse brain swelling, 239
Diffuse cerebral edema, 1066f
Diffuse erythema and desquamation, 714f
Digital dermatomy, 1005
Digitalis, 447
Digitalis purpurea, 983
Digoxin, 926
Dihydroergotamine mesylate (DHE), 492
Diluents, 908
Direct anti-globulin test (DAT), 819
Direct fluorescent antibody (DFA) test, 384, 397
Direct strike, 1039
Disease Control and Prevention (CDC), 538
Diskitis, 856f
Dislocations, 305
Disseminated intravascular coagulation (DIC), 819, 829
Distal humeral physis fracture, 314
Distal interphalangeal (DIP) dislocation, 320
Distal interphalangeal (DIP) joint, 320
Distal phalanx, 319
Distal radius and ulna fractures, 316
Distal tibia, 872f
Distributive shock, 196
Diuretics, 459
Diving reflex, 1027
DNA, 1081
Dog-ears, correction of, 341
Domperidone, 610

Dopamine, 246
Dorsal dislocations, 320
Double-contrast CT scan, 233
DPL (diagnostic peritoneal lavage), 231, 278
Drowning, 1026t
    epidemiology, 1025
    management
        emergency department, 1027
        prehospital, 1027
        prognosis, 1028
    pathophysiology
        cardiovascular, 1026
        electrolytes, 1026–1027
        hematologic, 1027
        hypothermia, 1027
        neurologic, 1025–1026
        renal, 1027
Drug dosage parenteral, 392t
Drug use and drug screening, 1164
Drug-induced liver injury, 88
DUB. See Dysfunctional uterine bleeding
Duct cyst, 126f
Ductal-dependent lesions, 423
Ductus arteriosus, 413
Duodenum, 602
DVT (Deep vein thrombosis), 782
Dysbaric injuries
    barotrauma
        air embolism, 1076–1077
        attitude-related barotitis, 1075–1076
        barodentalgia, 1076
        barosinusitis, 1076
        barotitis, 1074–1075
        face mask squeeze, 1076
        pneumothorax and emphysema, 1077
        pulmonary barotrauma, 1076
    pathophysiology, 1074
    physical gas laws, 1073–1074
Dysfunctional uterine bleeding
    clinical presentation, 811
    definitions, 809
    diagnostic evaluation, 811–812
    etiology/risk factors, 810–811
    incidence, 809
    management, 812–813
    pathophysiology
        anovulatory cycle, 809
        ovulatory cycle, 809
    See also Dysmenorrhea
Dysmenorrhea, 600
    classification, 808t
    clinical presentation, 808
    definition, 807
    diagnostic evaluation, 808
    diagnostic modalities, 808t
    etiology/risk factors, 807
    incidence, 807
    management, 808–809
    pathophysiology, 807
    See also Dysfunctional uterine bleeding
Dysrhythmias, 206t
Dysrhythmias in children
    atrial flutter and fibrillation
        accelerated idioventricular rhythm (AIVR), 448

premature ventricular contractions (PVC), 448
ventricular fibrillation, 449
ventricular tachycardia (VT), 449
fast rates (paroxysmal supraventricular tachycardia), 446–447
hypertrophic cardiomyopathy, 452
long QT syndrome, 451
slow rates
atrioventricular blocks, 445
pacemakers in children, 446
sinus bradycardia, 445
systolic and diastolic blood pressures, 446t

E

E. Histolytica, 558
Ear lacerations, 347
Ears, 291
ECG (electrocardiogram), 52f, 417t
Echinococcus granulosus, 558
Echinoderms, 1021f
Echocardiography (ECHO), 433
Eclampsia, 779–780
Ectopic pregnancy, 600, 781
Eczema herpeticum, 723f
Edema, 605f
Ehrlichia chaffeensis, 551
Eikenella corrodens, 1001
Eisenmenger syndrome, 426
Elbow, 311
Elbow dislocation, 314
Electrical injury, 1037, 1037t
Electrical and lightning injuries
electrical injuries
anatomic sites of injury, 1036–1038
electrophysiology, 1035–1036
management, 1038
mechanisms of injury, 1036
prevention, 1038
lightning injuries
deposition, 1042
management, 1041–1042
mechanisms of injury, 1039
physics, 1039
prevention, 1042
sequelae, 1042
types of injuries, 1039–1041
management
emergency department care, 1038
prehospital care, 1038
Electrocardiogram (EKG), 433, 983, 1054
Electrolyte composition, 658f
Electrolyte disorders. *See* Fluid and electrolyte disorders
Elevated sweat electrolyte concentrations, 408t
ELISA. *See* Enzymelinked immunosorbent assay
Elliptocytosis, 820
Embedded sting ray barb, 1020f
emergency care for children, 1129
Emergency contraception (EC), 783, 1164
Emergency department (ED), child in. *See* Child in emergency department

Emergency department thoracotomy, 265, 270
Emergency medical services for children (EMSC), 1129
Emergency medical technician (EMT), 1130
Emergency Medical Treatment and Labor Act (EMTALA), 1157
Emergency physician (EP), 677
Empiric antibiotic therapy, 844t
Enchondroma, 871, 871f
Endocarditis, 427, 442
Endometriosis, 600
Endoscopy, 909
Endotracheal intubation, 212f, 214, 248
Endotracheal tube (ETT), 177, 190t, 214t, 370
Entamoeba, 567
Enterobiasis, 555
Enterobius vermicularis (pinworm), 553
Enterobius vermicularis, 794
Enteroviral infections, 772
Enteroviruses. *See under* Exanthems
Enthesitis-related arthritis, 864, 865
Environmental protection agency (EPA), 915
Enzyme rhodanase, 973
Enzymelinked immunosorbent assay (ELISA), 12, 572
Eosinophilia, 567
EPAP (expiratory positive airway pressure), 192
Epididymitis, 680t, 804
diagnostic evaluation, 680
management, 680
pathophysiology, 679
signs and symptoms, 679
Epidural hematoma, 239f, 240
Epiglottitis (supraglottitis), 357, 358f
Epinephrine, 216, 590, 1006
Epiphora, 754
Episcleritis, 767
Epistaxis. *See under* Nose Emergencies
Epstein–Barr virus, 428
Erythema infectiosum (fifth disease), 720
Erythema marginatum, 865
Erythema migrans, 549
Erythema multiforme, 711
Erythema toxicum, 727
Erythrocyte protoporphyrins (EP), 963
Erythrocyte sedimentation rate (ESR), 100, 852, 859
Escherichia coli, 87, 486, 679
Esmolol, 459
Esophageal coins, 617t
Esophageal detector device, 185f
Esophageal erythema and erosions, 611f
Esophageal mucosa, 602
Esophageal obstruction, 616t
Esophageal strictures, 612
Esophageal varices, 602
Esophagus, 602
Ethanol. *See under* Toxic alcohols
Ethical considerations
adolescent issues
abortion, 1164
chaperones and physical examination, 1164

confidentiality, 1164
drug use and drug screening, 1164
emergency contraception, 1164
child abuse, 1162
family presence, 1163
informed consent, parental permission, and assent, 1162
medically underserved children, 1162
parental and patient refusal, 1163
procedures on newly dead, 1163
triage and overcrowding, 1161–1162
Ethylene glycol poisoning, 900f
Ethylene glycol. *See under* Toxic alcohols
Etomidate, 152
ETT (endotracheal tube), 177, 190t
Ewing's sarcoma, 840
Exanthems
enteroviruses, 725
fifth disease (erythema infectiosum)
ancillary tests, 720
clinical findings, 720
complications, 720
epidemiology, 720
management, 720
pathophysiology, 720
herpes simplex
ancillary tests, 724
clinical findings, 722–724
complications, 724
epidemiology/pathophysiology, 722
management, 724
herpes zoster (shingles)
clinical findings, 721–722
complications, 722
pityriasis rosea
clinical findings, 725–726
roseola (exanthem subitum)
clinical findings, 719
complications, 719
epidemiology/pathophysiology, 719
management, 719
rubella (German measles)
ancillary tests, 719
clinical findings, 719
complications, 719
epidemiology, 718–719
management, 719
rubeola (measles)
ancillary tests, 717–718
clinical findings, 717
complications, 718
epidemiology/pathophysiology, 717
management, 718
scarlet fever
ancillary tests, 725
clinical findings, 725
complications, 725
management, 725
pathophysiology, 725
varicella (chicken pox)
ancillary tests, 720
clinical findings, 720
complications, 720–721
epidemiology, 720
management, 721
Exocrine pancreatic insufficiency, 407t
Exotic snakes, 1007

Expiratory positive airway pressure (EPAP), 192
Exposure management, 581
Extensor tendons, 318t
Extracorporeal membrane oxygenation (ECMO), 436, 376
Extrahepatic diseases 88, I.12.86
Extrapyramidal symptoms (EPS), 933
Extremity examination, 232
Eye discharge, 764
Eye emergency in childhood
    common eye complaints
        excessive tearing, 764
        eye discharge, 764
        eye pain, 763–764
        red eye, 763
    errors to avoid, 763
    nontraumatic eye disorders
        cellulitis, 765–767
        conjunctivitis, 767, 771t
        eyelid infections, 764–765
        ophthalmia neonatorum. *See* ophthalmia neonatorum, evaluation of *See also* conjunctivitis in childhood
        scleritis and episcleritis, 767
    physical examination, 761
        anterior segment, 762
        intraocular pressure, 763
        lids and orbit, 761–762
        posterior segment, 762–763
        pupils and extraocular movements, 762
        vision, 761
Eye pain, 763–764
Eye patching, 756
Eye trauma
    equipment, 755
    history, 753
    medications, 755
    physical examination
        adnexae, 753–754
        conjunctiva and sclera, 754
        fundoscopic examination and intraocular pressure, 755
        iris, 754
        lens, 754
        pupils, 754
        visual acuity, 753
    specific injuries
        chemical injuries to eye, 758
        conjunctival and scleral lacerations, 757
        corneal abrasion, 756
        corneal and scleral foreign bodies, 757
        foreign bodies in situ, 758
        hyphema, 756–757
        intraocular foreign body, 758
        lens injury, 757
        lid lacerations, 755
        retinal injury, 757
        retrobulbar hemorrhage, 757
        subconjunctival hemorrhage, 755
        thermal burns, 759
        traumatic iritis, 756
        ultraviolet keratitis, 759

Eyelid infections, 764–765
Eyelid lacerations, 346
Eyes, 290–291

F
Face mask squeeze, 1076
Facial lacerations, 292
Facial smallpox, 579
Factors influencing oxygen delivery, 196
Failure to thrive (FTT), 1115
Falciparum, 563, 567
Famotidin, 610
FAST (focused assessment sonography in trauma), 231
Fast antegrade conduction (Antidromic), 448f
Fast retrograde conduction (Orthodromic), 448f
Febrile appearing neonate. *See* Septic-appearing neonate
Febrile neonate, potential evaluation of, 10t
Febrile nonhemolytic transfusion reactions, 835
Febrile or nonhemolytic transfusion reactions (FNHTR), 835
Federal and drug administration (FDA), 581
Federal Insecticide Fungicide and Rodenticide Act (FIFRA), 915
Feeding disorders
    in infants, 77
    gastroesophageal reflux, 77
    high-yield facts, 77
    hypersensitivity, 78
    treatment, 77
Female black widow spider, 1010f
Femoral shaft fractures, 325
FFP and blood products, 921
Fibula fractures, tibia and, 327
Filarial nematodes, 557
Fingertip injuries, 348
Fire ants (*Solenopsis*), 1015
Fish tapeworm, 558
Flail chest, 267
Flatworms, 557
Flexion, abduction, and external rotation (FABER), 99
Flexor tendons, 318t
Flight stresses, 1146t
Fluid calculations, 659f
Fluid and electrolyte disorders
    calcium
        hypercalcemia, 666
        hypocalcemia, 667t
    fluids
        fluid compartments, 657
        fluid requirements, 659–660
        movement of fluid, 657–659
    potassium
        hyperkalemia, 663
        hypokalemia, 665
    sodium
        hypernatremia, 660
        hyponatremia, 662
Fluid resuscitation in shock, 229t, 230t
Flukes, 557
Focused assessment sonography in trauma (FAST), 231
Foley catheter, 221

Follicle stimulating hormone (FSH), 809
Food and drug administration (FDA), 171
Food-dependent exercise induced anaphylaxis (FDEIA), 590
Foot, 100
Foot fractures, 329–331
Forearm diaphyseal fractures, 315
Forehead lacerations, 346
Foreign body in situ, 758
Foreign body evaluation, 339
Foreign body obstruction, 359–360
Fournier's gangrene, 682
Foxglove (*Digitalis purpurea*) plant, 984f
Fracture terminology, 299
Francisella tularensis (tularemia), 551, 575
Fresh frozen plasma (FFP), 833, 915
Frontal sinus fractures, 293
Frostbite injuries, 1057, 1057t, 1058t
Frozen plasma, 834
Fulminant hepatic failure
    ancillary studies, 623
    management/complications, 623
    recognition, 623
Fundoscopy, 755, 757
Fungal infections, 844
Fungal orbital cellulites, 766

G
GABA (aminobutyric acid), 149
Galeazzi fracture, 316
Galeazzi test, 99f
Gamma-aminobutyric acid (GABA), 937, 995
Gamma-hydroxybutyrate (GHB), 995
    acute toxicity, 959
    diagnosis, 959
    high-yield facts, 959
    pathophysiology, 959
    pharmacology, 959
    treatment
        antidotal therapy, 960
        decontamination, 960
        disposition, 960
        enhanced elimination, 960
        stabilization, 960
Gamow bag, 1065f
Gardnerella vaginitis, 794. *See also under* Vaginitis
Gastric decontamination, 927
Gastric upset, 1041
Gastroenteritis, 71. *See also* Vomiting
Gastroesophageal reflux (GER)
    in children and adolescents
        clinical presentation, 611
        complications, 612
        differential diagnosis, 611
        evaluation, 611–612
    in children and adolescents (treatment)
        conservative therapy, 612
        pharmacologic therapy, 612
        surgical therapy, 612
    complications, 612t
    disease (GERD), 609
    in infants
        clinical presentation, 609
        differential diagnosis, 609–610
        evaluation, 610

in infants (treatment)
    acid suppression, 610
    conservative therapy, 610
    prokinetic agents, 610
  symptoms, 609t
Gastrointestinal foreign bodies
  anatomic sites for obstruction, 616–617
  colonic/rectal foreign bodies, 618
  diagnosis, 617
  procedural/surgical approaches, 618
  small bowel, 618
Gastrointestina irritants, 979
Gastrointestinal bleeding, 606
  lower gastrointestinal bleeding
    anus, 605
    intestine, 604
    rectum, 605
  upper gastrointestinal bleeding, 602
    duodenum, 602
    esophagus, 602
    stomach, 602
Gastrointestinal decontamination, 888, 920
Gastrointestinal emergencies, 846
Gastrointestinal infections, 76t
Gastrointestinal irritants, 979f
  American mistletoe, 982
  holly, 982
  poinsettia, 982
  pokeweed (*Phytolacca americana*), 982
Gastrointestinal irritation, 888
Gastroschisis, 217
GCS. *See* Glasgow coma scale
GDPP (gonadotropin-dependent precocious puberty), 789
Genital herpes, 803
Genital ulcers, 804
Genital warts. *See under* Sexually transmitted diseases (STD)
Genitourinary trauma
  assessment and management, 281
  bladder injuries, 276
  diagnostic studies, 286f
  pediatric sexual abuse, 285–286
  penile injuries, 284–285
  renal injuries, 281–282
  scrotal trauma, 284
  ureteral injuries, 282–284
  vulvar and vaginal injuries, 285
Gential morphology, 786f
GER. *See* Gastroesophageal reflux
GERD (gastroesophageal reflux disease), 609
Giant papillary conjunctivitis (GPC), 586
Giardia lamblia, 558–559, 567
Giardia trophozoite, 559f
Gilbert's syndrome, 85
GIPP (gonadotropin-independent precocious puberty), 789
Glasgow coma scale (GCS), 106, 233, 241t, 242
Glaucoma, 763
Glomerular filtration rate (GER), 696
Glomerulonephritis, 693
Gloriosa superba, 985
Glucose, 216
Glucose metabolism
  diabetic ketoacidosis, 629
    acidosis, 632

    cerebral edema, treatment, 633
    clinical manifestations, 630
    complications, 632
    disposition, 633
    epidemiology, 629
    fluid resuscitation, 631
    insulin therapy, 631
    management, 631
    pathophysiology, 629
    phosphate, 632
    potassium, 631
    precipitating factors, 630
    sodium, 631
  hypoglycemia
    adequate substrate, 636
    diagnostic evaluation, 634–635
    disposition, 637
    in infants and children, 635t
    management, 636
    pathophysiology, 634
    signs and symptoms, 634
Glucose-6-phosphate dehydrogenase (G6PD), 820
Goal-directed management, 201
Gonadotropin-dependent precocious puberty (GDPP), 789
Gonadotropin-independent precocious puberty (GIPP), 789
Gonococcal conjunctivitis, 773
Gonorrhea. *See under* Sexually transmitted diseases
Gonorrhoeae, 852
GPC (Giant papillary conjunctivitis), 586
Granulocyte concentrates, 833
Graves' disease, 645
Grief-support groups, 1124t
Griseofulvin, 715
Ground current injury, 1039
Group B streptococcus (GSB), 9
Growth plate, 299t
GU trauma. *See* Genitourinary trauma
Guillain Barrâê syndrome, 483, 514
Guinea worms, 557
Gunshot wounds, 276
Gymnopilus, 979
Gynecologic disorders
  acute pelvic pain, 791
  premenarcheal patients
    congenital vaginal obstruction, 787–788
    infant and toddler, 785
    labial adhesions, 788
    neonatal physiologic variants, 787
    older school-age children, 785
    physical examination, 785–787
    sexual development stages, 786t
    younger school-age children, 785
  of infancy and childhood
  pubertal vaginal bleeding
    Bartholin abcess, 790
    history and physical examination, 790
    ovarian torsion, 790
    precocious puberty, 789
    urethral prolapse, 788–789
    vaginal foreign body, 788
  of adolescence

Gyromitra spp, 977
Gyromitra, 977

H
H. influenzae type B pneumonia, 384
Haemophilus influenzae, 386, 519, 793, 822
Hair removal, 338
Hallucinogenic mushrooms, 979
Hamman sign, 266
Hand and wrist injuries, 317
HAPE clinical signs, 1067f
Hawaii five-O rule, 210t
Hazmat incident drill, 1095f
Head examination, 230
Head trauma
  anatomy, 237
  assessment, 242
  diagnostic studies, 242
  intracranial pressure, 239–241
  pathophysiology, 237
  specific injuries, 237–239
  treatment, 242–243
Headache
  algorithm, 490f
  etiology, 490t, 493
  evaluation, 489
  high-yield facts, 489
  laboratory studies, 490
  lumbar puncture, 491
  neuroimaging, 490
  primary headaches
    cluster headaches, 492
    migraine headaches, 491
    tension-type headaches, 492
    treatment, 492
  psychiatric, 486
  psychogenic, 494
  secondary headaches, 493
    acute hemorrhage, 493
    brain tumors and hydrocephalus, 493
    encephalitis, 493
    hypertensive encephalopathy, 493
    idiopathic intracranial hypertension, 493
    meningitis, 493
    pseudotumor cerebri, 493
Health Insurance Portability and Accountability Act (HIPAA), 1157
Health resources and services administration (HRSA), 1129
Heart rate (HR), 261
Heat dissipation, 1046t, 1050
Heat exposure, 1048t
Heat illness
  management, 1047–1050
  pathophysiology, 1045
  types
    heat cramps, 1046
    heat exhaustion, 1046
    heatstroke, 1046
Helicobacter pylori, 603
Heliox, 369
HELLP syndrome, 780
Hematemesis, 406
Hematochezia, 603
Hematologic complications, 842

Hematoma, 240, 279, 334
Hematomas, 334
Hematuria, 281
Hemiparesis, 499
Hemoglobin electrophoresis, 685
Hemolysis, 84
Hemolytic streptococcus, 861
Hemolytic uremic syndrome (HUS), 599, 696, 830
Hemophilia. *See under* Bleeding disorders
Hemophilus influenzae, 406, 483
Hemopneumothorax, 269
Hemorrhagic blister, 1058f
Hemorrhagic shock, 229t
Hemorrhagic stroke, 503t
Hemostasis, 338
Hemothorax, 261f
Hemothorax, 264
Hemotympanum, 291
Henoch–Schönlein purpura (HSP), 605. *See also under* Petechiae and purpura
Heparin-induced thrombocytopenia (HIT), 464
Hepatic enzymes, 888
Hepatic failure, 888
Hepatitis. *See under* Liver and gallbladder
Hereditary spherocytosis (HS), 820
Herpangina, 746
Herpes keratits, 773f
Herpes progenitalis in infant, 723f
Herpes simplex and varicella-zoster. *See under* conjunctivitis beyond neonatal period
Herpes simplex infection. *See under* Sexually transmitted diseases (STD)
Herpes simplex virus (HSV), 9, 770, 844. *See also under* Exanthems
Herpes zoster, 723f, 733. *See also under* Exanthems
Herpes zoster infection, 540
Herpetic gingivostomatitis, 744
Herpetic whitlow, 724f
High altitude cerebral edema (HACE). *See under* High altitude illness
High-altitude illness
  acute mountain sickness
    clinical presentation, 1064
    pathophysiology, 1064–1065
    prevention, 1065
    treatment, 1065
  altitude-related syndromes, 1069
    chronic mountain sickness(CMS), 1069
    peripheral edema, 1069
    pharyngitis and bronchitis, 1069
    preexisting pulmonary disease, 1069
    pregnancy, 1069
    retinal hemorrhage, 1069
    sickle cell disease, 1069
    ultraviolet keratitis, 1069
  atmosphere and physical gas laws, 1060
  high-altitude cerebral edema
    clinical presentation, 1065–1066
    pathophysiology, 1065
    treatment, 1066–1067
  high-altitude pulmonary edema
    clinical presentation, 1067–1068

    pathophysiology, 1068
    treatment, 1068
  physiologic response
    cardiovascular system, 1063
    central nervous system, 1063–1064
    hematopoietic system, 1063
    renal system, 1064
    respiratory system, 1062
High-altitude pharyngitis and bronchitis, 1069
High-frequency jet ventilation (HFJV), 402
High-frequency oscillatory ventilation (HFOV), 402
Hiking, 1061f, 1063f
Hindfoot injuries, 330
Hip dislocations, 324–325
Hip effusion, 853f
Hip joints, 99
Histolytica, 567
HIV and AIDS. *See under* Sexually transmitted diseases (STD)
HIV Infection, 538t
HIV. *See under* Sexually transmitted diseases (STD)
HIV-1 markers, 539t
Hobo spider. *See under* Spider and arthropod bites
Hodgkin disease, 837
Hollow organs, 279
Hollow visceral organs, 279
Holly, 982
Honeybees (*Apis mellifera*), 1013
Honey-crusted lesions of impetigo, 714f
Hookworms, 556–557
Hordeolum, 764
Horizontal mattress stitch, 344f
Hospital admission (pneumonia), 392
Human and animal bites
  antibiotics, 1000–1001
  history, 999
  physical examination, 999
  rabies prophylaxis, 1001–1002
  wound care, 999–1000
Human diploid cell vaccine (HDCV), 1001
Human granulocytic anaplasmosis (HGA), 552
Human immunodeficiency virus (HIV). *See under* Sexually transmitted diseases (STD)
Human metapneumovirus, 384
Human monocyte ehrlichiosis, 551
Human papillomavirus (HPV), 797, 800f
Human rabies immune globulin (HRIG), 1001
Human tetanus immune globulin (HTIG), 344
Humerus fractures. *See under* Upper extremities, injuries of
HUS. *See* Hemolytic uremic syndrome
Hydatidiform mole, 783
Hydralazine, 459
Hydrocarbons
  classification and properties, 913
  clinical presentation, 913
  disposition, 914
  high-yield facts, 913
  management, 914
  pathophysiology, 913

Hydrocolpos, 788
Hydrocephalus, 495, 496
Hydrofluoric acid, 758, 910
Hydrogen sulfide toxicity, 975f
Hydroxocobalamin, 974
Hydroxychloroquine, 990–991
Hymenoptera venoms, 1013
Hymenoptera. *See* Bees and vespids
Hypaque, 234
Hyperbaric oxygen (HBO), 941
Hyperbilirubinemia, 83, 87, 87f. *See also under* Liver and gallbladder
Hypercalcemia, 841
Hyperemia, 767
Hyperkalemia, 663, 665, 666, 842t
Hypernatremia, 660
  causes of, 660t
  treatment of, 661t
Hyperoxia test, 415
Hyperreflexia, 482
Hypersensitivity, I.78
Hyperstimulation of cholinergic receptors, 994
Hypertension, 455. *See also* Pediatric hypertension
Hypertensive encephalopathy, 493
Hyperthermia, 1049t
Hypertrophic cardiomyopathy (HC), 425, 452, 473
Hyperthyroidism
  clinical presentation, 647
  differential diagnosis, 647, 647t
  disposition, 648
  epidemiology, 645
  etiology, 645–647, 646t
  management, 647–648
  neonatal thyrotoxicosis, treatment of, 648
  pathophysiology, 645, 646t
Hypertrophic pyloric stenosis, 398
Hyperventilation, 40, 374
Hyphema, 756–757
Hypocalcemia, 667t, 910t
Hypoglycemia, 38, 41, 210, 210t
Hypokalemia, 665
Hyponatremia, 662, 663
Hypoplastic left heart syndrome (HLHS), 418, 419f
Hypoproteinemia, 405
Hypotension, 243
Hypothalamic–pituitary–gonadal axis, 789
Hypothermia, 23
  electrocardiogram (ECG), 1052t
  key diagnostic, 1054
  multisystem effects of, 1051f
  pathophysiologic changes, 1053t
Hypovolemic shock, 196, 216, 217
Hypoxia, 240, 375, 973
Hypoxic ventilatory response (HVR), 1062

I

IBD (inflammatory bowel disease), 599–600
Ibotenic acid, 978
ICP(intracranial pressure), 182, 222
Idiopathic epilepsy, 43f
Idiopathic intracranial hypertension, 493
Idiopathic thrombocytopenic pupura. *See under* Petechiae and purpura

Idiopathic ventricular tachycardia, 449
Ilex aquifolium, 982
Imidazoline decongestants, 991
Immune globulins, 834
Immune thrombocytopenic purpura (ITP), 830
Immune-mediated thrombocytopenia, 830f, 831t
Immunosuppressive state, 196
Imperforate hymen, 788
Impetigo contagiosa, 765
Imported diseases
   chemoprophylaxis, 564
   diagnostic studies, 566
   eosinophilia, 567
   immunizations, 564
   incubation periods, 564
   international travel-related diseases, 565
   laboratory investigations
   physical examination, 566
   risk factors, 566
   specific diseases
      dengue fever, 569
      diarrhea, 571
      malaria, 567
      paratyphoid enteric fevers, 571
      typhoid, 571
   travel locations 564
Imported fire ants. *See under* Spider and
   arthropod bites
Inborn errors of metabolism, 133t
   diagnostic testing, 670–672
   newborn screening, 672
   presentation, 669–670
   treatment, 672–673
Incidence rate, 520t
Incontinentia pigmenti, 728, 729f
Increased intracranial pressure (ICP), 181, 222
Individual lesions, survey of. *See under*
   Congenital heart disease
Indwelling venous access devices (IVAD), 843
Infantile botulism, 580
Infants and children, respiratory distress in, 24t
Infant rashes
   benign infant rashes, 727–728
   disorders of pigmentation, 728–729
   infancy vascular lesions of, 729–730
Infectious Diseases Society of America
   (IDSA), 429
Infectious musculoskeletal disorders
   acute suppurative tenosynovitis, 856
   intervertebral diskitis, 856
   Lyme disease, 856
   osteomyelitis
      clinical manifestations, 855
      diagnostic testing, 855
      etiology, 854
      pathophysiology, 854
      treatment, 855
   septic arthritis
      clinical presentation, 851
      diagnostic evaluation, 852–853
      differential diagnosis, 854

      etiology, 851
      treatment, 854
Infective endocarditis prevention, 429
Inferior vena cava (IVC), 413, 682
Inflammation, 402
Inflammatory and infectious heart disease
   acute rheumatic fever, 442
   endocarditis, 442
   myocarditis, 439
      clinical presentation, 440
      diagnosis, 441
      etiology, 440
      treatment, 441
   pericarditis, 439
Inflammatory bowel disease, 599, 864
Inflammatory musculoskeletal disorders
   rheumatic fever, 861–863
   spondyloarthropathies, 863
      enthesitis-related arthritis, 864
      inflammatory bowel disease, 864
      juvenile idiopathic arthritis, 865–866
      psoriatic arthritis, 864
      reactive arthritis, 864
   systemic lupus erythematosus, 860–861
   transient synovitis, 859
Influenza, 519
   clinical presentation, 513–514
   differential diagnosis, 514
   epidemiology and transmission, 510–513
   pathophysiology, 513
   prevention, 515t, 516t, 517
   radiographic findings, 514
   terms, 511t
   treatment, 514
Inguinal hernia, 681
   diagnostic evaluation, 681
   management, 681
   pathophysiology, 681
   signs and symptoms, 681
INH toxicity, 938t
Inhaled corticosteroids, 369
Initial antibiotic therapy, 578t
Injury severity measures, 234
Inocybe, 978
Inspiratory positive airway pressure (IPAP), 192
Insulin therapy, 631
Interfacility transport
   clinical transport issues
      active cardiac arrest, 1147
      neonatal transport, 1147
   communication, 1142–1143
   equipment and medication, 1143
   historical perspectives, 1141
   legal considerations, 1141–1142
      interfacility, 1141
      medical responsibility, 1141
   medical direction, 1143
   modes of transport, 1144, 1145t
   protocols, 1143
   regulatory requirements (certification
      standards), 1143–1144
   safety/altitude physiology (air medical
      consideration)
      personnel safety, 1144
      vehicle safety, 1144
      safety issues, 1146

      stabilization for transport, 1144
      team composition and training, 1142, 1142t
Interleukin-6, 402
Internet resources, 908t
Interstitial pneumonia, 388
Intervertebral diskitis, 856
Intestinal obstruction, 407f
Intestine, 604
Intra-abdominal injury in children, 277
Intracellular parasites, 569f, 570t
Intracranial hematoma, 41t
Intracranial pressure (ICP), 182, 222
Intramuscular bleeding, 827
Intraocular foreign body, 758
Intraoral lacerations, 343
Intraosseous (IO) infusion, 223
Intravascular coagulation, 829
Intravenous access, 214
Intravenous immunoglobulin (IVIG), 483, 534, 832
Intravenous pyelogram (IVP), 281, 690
Intubation, 370
Intubation depth, 214f
Invasive diagnostic testing, 388
Ionizing radiation, 1082–1083
Iontophoresis, 157
IPAP (inspiratory positive airway pressure), 192
Ipomea violacea, 986
Iron deficiency, 818
Iron poisoning
   clinical presentation, 969
   diagnosis, 970
   disposition, 971
   estimating risk, 969
   pathophysiology, 969
   toxicity, 969
   treatment, 970
Iron preparations, 970
Irrigation, 338–339
Ischemic stroke, 502t
Isolated coronary artery anomalies, 426
Isoniazid toxicity (INH), 937
   diagnosis, 938
   pathophysiology, 937
   pharmacology, 937
   treatment
      antidotal therapy, 938
      decontamination, 938
      disposition, 939
      enhanced elimination, 938
      stabilization, 938
Isopropanol. *See under* Toxic alcohols
Isotope cystography (IC), 690
Ixodes scapularis, 856
Ixodes scapularis, life cycle, 547
IVIG (intravenous gamma globulin), 483, 534, 832

J
Jaundice
   conjugated hyperbilirubinemia
      newborn. *See* conjugated
         hyperbilirubinemia in newborn,
      causes of older children, 88

Jaundice (*Contd.*)
  pathophysiology
    unconjugated hyperbilirubinemia
      newborns and young infants. *See*
        Jaundice in neonatal period
      older infants and children, 85–87
Jaundice in neonatal period
  differential diagnosis
    breast milk jaundice, 84
    increased hemolysis, 84
    physiologic jaundice, 83
  evaluation and management
    history and physical, 85
    laboratory evaluation, 85
    management approach, 85
  sequelae
    acute bilirubin encephalopathy, 84
    chronic bilirubin encephalopathy, 84
Jaw thrust maneuver, 179f
Jet ventilation setup, 186f
Joint fluid, 853t
Jones criteria, 747
Jones fracture, 330f
Jumper's knee, 306
JumpSTART Triage algorithm, 1152t
Juvenile ankylosing spondylitis, 864
Juvenile idiopathic arthritis (JIA), 866t

K
Kalmia latifolia, 983
Kawasaki disease, 118, 532f, 599
  ancillary data, 533
  clinical findings, 531
  complications, 534
  differential diagnosis 533
  etiology, 531
  high-yield facts, 531
  management, 534
  pathogenesis, 531
  phases
    acute or febrile phase, 532
    subacute phase, 533
  prognosis, 534
Kawasaki syndrome, 534t
Kernig sign, 521
Ketamine, 241
Ketamine toxicity. *See under* Phencyclidine
    (PCP)
Ketorolac, 159
Kiesselbach's plexus, 737
Kirschner-wire fixation, 319, 320
Knee, 100
Knee and patella dislocations, 327
Knee hemarthrosis, 828f
Knots for skin closure, 341
Koplik spots, 718f

L
Labetolol, 459
Labial adhesions, 788
Lacerations, 333
Laparotomy, 278, 279, 409
Laryngeal mask airway (LMA), 192, 214
Laryngoscope blades size, 178
Laryngotracheobronchitis, 355–357
Lateral clavicle injuries, 310
Lateral neck x-ray, 179f

Lateral spine, 249t
Latrodoctus genus, 1009
Lead encephalopathy, 966
Lead poisoning, 819
  clinical manifestations, 963–965
  high-yield facts, 963
  management, 965
  pathophysiology, 963
  pharmacokinetics, 963
  sources, 963
Lefort fractures, 294–295
Left parietal lobe, 505f
Lens injury, 757
Leptomeningeal cyst, 238
Lethal toxins in small doses
  benzocaine, 990
  camphor, 989
  chloroquine, 990
  hydroxychloroquine, 990–991
  imidazoline decongestants, 991
  lomotil, 990
  methyl salicylate, 991
Lethargy, 33
Levalalbuterol (Xopenex), 368
Levosimendan, 436
Lid lacerations, 755
Lidocaine devices and techniques, 157
Lidocaine-adrenaline-tetracaine (LAT), 337
Life-threatening event. *See under* Sudden
    infant death syndrome
Ligamentous injuries, 306
Lighting injuries, 1039, 1040f, 1040t
  prehospital care, 1041–1042
  emergency department care, 1042
Lightning injuries, 1039–1042
Limping child
  evaluation, 100
  high-yield facts, 97
  history, 97
  microbiology, 103
  physical examination, 97–99
    ankle, 100
    bone scan, 102
    CT scan/MRI, 102
    foot, 100
    hip joints, 99
    knee, 100
    radiographic analysis, 102
    sacroiliac joints, 99
    spine, 99
    ultrasound, 102
Linear nondepressed skull fractures, 238
Lionfish, 1020f
Lip lacerations, 347f, 348
Liquefaction necrosis, 907, 908
Lisfranc injury, 330f
Liver, 279
Liver and gallbladder
  biliary tract disease
    biliary atresia, 623–624
    choledochal cyst, 624
    cholelithiais and cholecystitis, 624
  hepatitis
    ancillary studies, 621
    diagnosis, 621
    management, 621
  hydrops of gallbladder, 624

  hyperbilirubinemia
    (conjugated) neonatal, 620–621, 621f
    (unconjugated) neonatal, 619–620,
      620f
    fulminant hepatic failure, 623
    post neonatal period, 621
LMA (laryngeal mask airway), 192
Lobar (alveolar), 388
Local anesthesia, 296
Lomotil, 990
Long QT syndrome, 451, 452f, 472
Loop diuretics, 460
Lopophora williamsii, 986
Lower airway, 353
Lower respiratory tract infections (LRTI), 386
Low-molecular-weight heparin (LMWH), 462,
    505
Low-volume fluid resuscitation (LVFR), 228
Loxosceles recluse, 1010f
LQTS (long QT syndrome), 472, 451, 452f
LRTI (Lower respiratory tract infections), 386
Ludwig's angina, 744
Lumbar puncture, 490, 158
Lumbar spine fracture, 275
Lupus erythematosus, 860
luxation injuries, 742t
LVFR (low-volume fluid resuscitation), 228
Lyme disease, 545, 550, 856
Lymph nodes, 122f
Lymphadenopathy, 121
Lymphnodular hyperplasia, 606f
Lymphoblastic lymphoma, 838
Lymphonodular hyperplasia, 605

M
Macrocytic anemia, 820
Macule/patch primary lesion, 116f
Magnesium, 369
Magnetic resonance imaging (MRI), 336, 483
Maintenance fluids, 660t
Malar fractures, 294
Malaria, 559, 567
Male genitourinary problems
  Fournier's gangrene, 682
  high-yield facts, 677
  penile emergencies
    balanitis and balanoposthitis, 683–684
    paraphimosis, 683
    phimosis, 682–683
    priapism, 685
  testicular pain (scrotal masses)
    epididymitis, 679
    Henoch–Scho nlein purpura, 682
    hydrocele, 682
    inguinal hernia, 681
    scrotal and testicular trauma, 680
    testicular torsion, 677
    testicular tumors, 681
    torsion of appendix testis. *See*
      Appendix testis, torsion of
    varicocele, 682
Malignant mediastinal tumors, 839
Mallampati score, 148
Mallet injuries, 319, 319f
Mallory–Weiss tears, 599
Malnutrition, 402
Malrotation, 317

Mammalian bite wounds, 344
Mandible fractures, 295
Mannitol, 243
Marine envenomations
    coelenterates
        clinical presentation, 1017–1018
        disposition, 1019
        management, 1018–1019
        pathophysiology, 1017
    echinoderms
        clinical presentation, 1021
        disposition, 1021
        management, 1021
        pathophysiology, 1021
    sea snakes
        clinical presentation, 1022
        disposition, 1022
        management, 1022
    venomous fish
        clinical presentation, 1020
        disposition, 1021
        management, 1020–1021
        pathophysiology, 1019–1020
Mass casualty events (MCE), 1149
Mass casualty management
    casualty events, 1149
    delivery of care
        decontamination, 1151–1152
        medications, 1151–1153
        provision of care, 1150
        recovery, 1153
        triage, 1150
    unique pediatric considerations
        age, size, weight, 1149
        developmental and behavioral
            consideration, 1149
        physiologic differences, 1149–1150
Massive hemoptysis, 406
Massive hemothorax, 264
Massive transfusions, 835
Material safety data sheets (MSDS) 908
Maternal and Child Health Bureau (MCHB),
    1129
Mattress stitches, 341
Maxillary central incisor, 741
Maxillary fractures, 294
Maxillofacial trauma
    associated injuries, 289–290
    emergency management, 290
    etiology, 289
    history, 290
    imaging studies, 292
    incidence, 289
    injuries, specific
        frontal sinus fractures, 293
        Lefort fractures, 294–295
        malar fractures, 294
        mandible fractures, 295
        maxillary fractures, 294
        nasal fractures, 293
        nasal ethmoidal orbital fractures,
            293
        orbital fractures, 293
        soft tissue injuries, 295
        supraorbital fractures, 293
    intraoral and mandibular examination,
        291–292

pain management and anesthesia,
    295–296
physical examination
    ears, 291
    eyes, 290–291
    facial lacerations, 292
    intraoral and mandibular examination,
        291
    midface, 291
    nose, 291
    physical examination, 290
McBurney's sign, 598t
McCune–Albright syndrome, 728
McGill forceps, 616f
MDMA (3,4-methylenedioxy-
        methamphetamine), 419f, 955
Mean BNP values, 424t
Mechanical trauma, 1097
Mechanical ventilation, 370, 401–402
Meconium, 216
Medial and lateral condyles, 313
Medial clavicle fractures, 309
Medial epicondylar fracture,
    313–314
Mediastinal syndrome (SMS) 845
Medical imaging
    algorithm, 166t
    computed tomography
        diagnostic and procedural
            considerations, 171
        physics and pathophysiology,
            170–171
        safety considerations, 171
    magnetic resonance imaging(MRI),
        172
        benefits and limitations, 172
        diagnostic and procedural
            considerations, 172
        physics and pathophysiology, 172
    ultrasound
        benefits and limitations, 1167
        diagnostic and procedural
            considerations, 167–168
        physics and pathophysiology,
            165–166
        safety considerations, 166–167
    x-rays, 168–169
        diagnostic and procedural
            considerations, 169
        physics and pathophysiology, 169
        safety considerations, 169
Medically underserved children, 1162
Medico-legal considerations
    consent and refusal of care, 1158
    end-of-life care, 1159
    forensic documentation, 1158
    medical malpractice, 1159
Meningitis, 520, 493
    management
        antibiotic treatment, 522
        corticosteroid treatment, 522
        stable patients, 522
        unstable patients, 521–522
    pathophysiology, 519
    presentation, 520
    sequelae, 522
Meningococcemia, 118

Menstrual cycle, 810f
Mental status examination, 1118t
Meperidine, 159
Metabolic disorders, 131
Metabolic emergencies, 842
    hypercalcemia, 841
    tumor lysis syndrome (TLS), 841
Metabolism cyclosporine, I.4t
Metabolism, inborn errors of, 131t
Metacarpal fractures, 320
Metacarpophalangeal joint, 320
Metallic staples, 336
Metaphyseal greenstick fracture, 328
Metaphyses, 842f
Metatarsal fractures, 329
Metered dose inhalers (MDIs), 368
Methanol. *See under* Toxic alcohols
Methemoglobinemia, 23, 156
Methicillin-resistant *Staphylococcus aureus*
    (MRSA), 713, 1001
Methyl salicylate, 991
Metoclopramide, 610
Metronidazole, 802
Microcytic anemia. *See under* Anemia
Microsomal ethanoloxidizing system
    (MEOS), 897
Middle and proximal phalanx, 319
Midface, 291
Midfoot fractures, 330
Midshaft clavicle fracture, 310
Migraine headaches, 491
Mild head injury
    anatomy, 105
    assessment, 106
    biomechanics, 105
    concussed athlete, 110
        recognition, 110
        response, 111
        rehabilitation (rest), 111
    disposition and discharge instructions,
        110
    ED management
        guidelines for imaging, 107
        hyperacute CT scan, 107
        imaging in children below 2 years,
            107
        imaging in preschool children, 107
        imaging in school-aged children, 107
        resuscitation, 107
    infant or toddler, 106
    pathophysiology, 105
    physical examination, 106
    return to play guidelines, 111
    school-aged child, 107
    special situations
        concussion in athlete, 108
        postconcussion syndrome, 109
        second impact syndrome, 108–109
Milia, 727
Miliaria, 727
Minor traumatic brain injuries (mTBI), 306
Miotic (pinpoint pupils), 947f
Mixed-function oxidase (MFO), 887
Moderate sedation, 338
Modified log-roll test., 100f
Mojave rattlesnake, 1006f
Molluscum contagiosum, 116, 774

Monomethylhydrazine-containing mushrooms, 977
Mononucleosis, 278
Monteggia fracture, 316
Morchella, 977
Morphine, 159
Mother-to-child transmission (MTCT), 537
Motor neuron findings, 482t
Motor vehicle collisions, 273–274
Mountain climbing, 1060f
Moyamoya, 505
MRSA (Methicillin-resistant *Staphylococcus aureus*), 713
Mucociliary apparatus, 383
Mucor, 766
Mucosal irritants, 981
Multiple doses of activated charcoal (MDAC), 894
Multiple hereditary exostoses (MHE), 871
Multiple trauma patient
    abdomen, 231–232
    additional treatment, 233
    back examination, 232
    burns, 233
    cervical spine, 231
    chest, 231
    disposition/transfer, 234
    head examination, 230–231
    imaging
        CT scan of abdomen, 233
        CT scan of head, 233
        ultrasonography, 233
        urologic studies, 233–234
    infant and adult airways, 222t
    injury severity measures, 234
    management guidelines
        airway, 225
        breathing, 227
        circulation, 227
        disability, 228
        exposure, 229
        primary survey, 223–225
    multisystem trauma, 224f
    nature of injuries, 221–223
    neurologic examination, 232
    pediatric trauma patient, 224t, 225t
    pediatric trauma systems, 223
    pediatric trauma, causes of, 222
    pediatric trauma, equipment sizes for, 226t
    pediatric vital signs, 225t
    prehospital care issues, 223
    resuscitation, 229–230
    skin, 232
    trauma activation, 224t
Munchausen's syndrome, 646
Mushroom poisoning, 977
    coprinus (antabuse), 978
    cyclopeptide-containing mushrooms, 977
    gastrointestina irritants, 979
    hallucinogenic mushrooms, 979
    ibotenic acid, 978
    monomethylhydrazine-containing mushrooms, 977
    muscarine-containing mushrooms, 978
    muscimol, 978
    renal toxins, 979

Multisystem trauma, 276
Multisystem trauma, 224t
Munchausen's syndrome, 646
Muromonab, 139
Muscarine-containing mushrooms, 978
Muscarinic actions, 993
Muscimol, 978
Muscle strength, 482t
Muscular dystrophies, 485
Musculoskeletal decompression sickness, 1077
Musculoskeletal tumors, 840
Myasthenia gravis, 484
Myasthenic crisis, 484
Mycophenolate mofetil (MMF), I.5, 861
Mycoplasma pneumoniae, 710
Mycoplasma pneumoniae, 735, 483, 373, 384, 387, 397
Mycoplasma tuberculosis, 772
Mycoplasma, 822
Myiasis, 561
Myocardial contusion, 268–269
Myocarditis. *See under* Inflammatory and infectious heart disease
Myoclonus, 477
Myoglobinuria, 1041
Myopathies, 485

N
N-acetylcysteine (NAC), 887
Naloxone, 216
Naloxone, 948f
Nasal fractures, 293
Nasal hematoma, 291f, 294f
Nasal foreign body, 737t
Nasal polyp, 739f
Nasal-ethmoidal-orbital (NEO) fractures, 293
Nasogastric tube insertion, 230
Nasotracheal intubation, 225
National high blood pressure education program (NHBPEP), 455
National highway traffic safety administration (NHTSA), 1129
National standard curricula (NSC), 1130
Natural and technological radiation, 1084
NEC (Necrotizing enterocolitis), 598
Neck masses, 122t, 123, 124
    anatomy, 121
    ancillary testing, 126
    differential diagnoses
        congenital masses, 125
        inflammatory conditions, 123–125
        neoplastic masses, 125
        traumatic conditions, 125
    disposition, 126
    high-yield facts, 121
    neck mass in no distress, 123
    respiratory distress, 121–123
Necrotizing enterocolitis (NEC), 598
Needle cricothyrotomy, 225
Needle thoracostomy, 270
Neisseria gonorrhoeae, 12, 770, 773, 679
Neisseria meningitidis, 519, 551
Nematodes (roundworms). *See under* Parasitic infestations
Neonatal bile pigment metabolism, 84
Neonatal cholestasis, 88

Neonatal emergencies
    cardiorespiratory presentations, 129
    endocrine, 131
    gastrointestinal, 132
    high-yield facts, 129
    metabolic disorders, 131
    seizures, 132
    surgical emergencies, 134
Neonatal myocardium, 413
Neonatal physiologic variants, 787
Neonatal pneumonia, 384
Neonatal pyoderma., 714f
Neonatal resuscitation, 212t
    High-yield facts, 211
    maternal risk factors, 211
    medications
        atropine, 216
        epinephrine, 216
        glucose, 216
        naloxone, 216
        sodium bicarbonate, 216
        volume expansion, 216
    newly born infant, assessment of, 212
    physiology newly born infant, 211
    requiring resuscitation, 212
    resuscitation
        chest compressions, 214
        endotracheal intubation, 214
        intravenous access, 214
        laryngeal mask airways, 214
        oxygen, 213
        positioning newborn, 213
        stimulation, 213
        temperature control, 213
        ventilation, 213
    special situations
        diabetic mother, 218
        diaphragmatic hernia, 217
        gastroschisis, 217
        meconium, 216
        omphalocele, 217
        pneumothorax, 218
        prematurity, 217
Neoplastic masses, 125
Nephroblastoma, 839
Nephrotic syndrome, 693, 695
Nerium oleander, 983
Nerve agents. *See under* Chemical weapons, nerve agents; Chemical weapons, vesicants
Nesiritide, 436
Neuroblastoma, 840, 840f
Neurocardiogenic, 469
Neurocutaneous syndromes, 41t
Neurofibromatosis, 728, 728f
Neurogenic shock, 229
Neuroimaging, 490
Neuroleptic agents, 934t
Neuroleptic malignant syndrome (NMS). *See under* Neuroleptics
Neuroleptics
    acute overdose
        clinical presentation, 933
        laboratory tests, 934
        management, 934
    atypical antipsychotics
        aripiprazole, 936

clozapine, 935
olanzapine, 935
paliperidone, 936
quetiapine, 935
resperidone, 935
ziprasidone, 936
dystonic reactions
clinical presentation, 933
management, 933
high-yield facts, 933
neuroleptic malignant syndrome
clinical presentation, 935
disposition, 935
management, 935
pharmacology, 933
pathophysiology, 933
Neurologic examination, 232
Neutrophil extracellular trap (NET), 383
Nevus flammus, 729
Newborns, respiratory distress in, 24t
Nexus, 247
Nicotinamideadenosine dinucleotide (NAD), 937
Nicotinic receptors, 993
NIPPV (noninvasive positive pressure ventilation), 193
Nitrous oxide, 149
Nomogram of bilirubin serum levels, 86
Nonaccidental head trauma, 239f
Nonaccidental trauma (NAT), 106, 239
Non-anticoagulant indoor rodenticides, 916t
Noncardiac syncope, 473
Non-Hodgkin lymphomas, 838
Noninvasive positive pressure ventilation (NIPPV), 193
Nonionizing radiation, 1083
Nonmalignant tumors of bone
aneurysmal bone cysts, 872
enchondromas, 871
high-yield facts, 869
nonossifying fibromas, 870
osteochondromas, 871
osteoid osteomas, 869
unicameral bone cysts, 871
Nonneutropenic oncology patient, 845
Nonossifying fibromas (NOF), 870
Nonparticulate (electromagnetic), 1082
Nonspecific vulvovaginitis. *See under* Vaginitis
Nonsteroidal anti-inflammatory drugs (NSAIDs), 601, 895, 895t, 808
clinical presentation, 895
laboratory studies, 895
management, 896
Nontraumatic eye disorders. *See under* Eye emergency in childhood
Norepinephrine-dopamine reuptake inhibitor (NDRI), 931
Normal atlantodental interval, 251f, 254f
Normal blood pressure for children, 4t
Normal heart rates for children, 4t
Normal respiratory rates, for children, I.4t
Normal saline (NS), 229
Normocytic anemia. *See under* Anemia
Nose, 291
Nose emergencies
acute otitis externa, 733

diagnosis, 677
differential diagnosis, 735
management, 734
pathophysiology, 733
acute otitis media(mastoiditis)
complications, 735
diagnosis 735
differential diagnosis, 735
management, 736
pathophysiology, 735
epistaxis
diagnostic findings, 737
etiology, 737
management, 738
foreign body, nose and ear
complications, 736
diagnostic findings, 736
management, 736
sinusitis
anatomy, 738
complications, 738
diagnostic findings, 738
differential considerations, 738
etiology, 738
management, 738
pathophysiology, 738
radiologic evaluation, 738
NSAID (Nonsteroidal anti-inflammatory drugs), 808

O

Obstructed nasolacrimal duct, 770
Obstructive shock, 197
Obtundation, 33
Obturator sign, 598t
Ocular herpes simplex, 773f
Ocular trauma. *See* Eye trauma
Oculoglandular syndrome, 121
Olanzapine, 935
Olecranon fractures, 315
Oligoanalgesia, 155
Omphalitis, 12
Omphalocele, 217
Omphalotus olearius, 979
Oncologic emergencies
childhood cancer, complications of
central nervous system emergencies, 846
gastrointestinal emergencies, 846
hematologic complications, 842
infectious complications
metabolic emergencies, 842
spinal cord compression, 845
superior mediastinal syndrome, 845
superior vena cava syndrome, 845
pediatric malignancies
acute leukemias, 837
central nervous system tumors, 839
Hodgkin disease, 837
musculoskeletal tumors, 840
neuroblastoma, 840
non-Hodgkin lymphomas, 838
retinoblastoma, 840
Wilms' tumor, 839
infectious complications, 843
fungal infections, 844
modifications to therapy, 844

nonneutropenic oncology patient, 845
parasitic infections, 844
viral infections, 844
Open pneumothorax, 265
Open safety pin in upper esophagus, 617f
Ophthalmia neonatorum, evaluation of, 767
bacterial conjunctivitis, 770
chemical conjunctivitis, 769
chlamydia trachomatis, 769
herpes simplex, 770
Neisseria gonorrhoeae, 770
noninfectious etiologies, 770
obstructed nasolacrimal duct, 770
viral etiologies (nonherpetic), 770
Opioids
age considerations, 945
developmental considerations, 945
with generic and trade names, 946
high-yield facts, 945
introduction, 945
pharmacology, 945
toxicokinetics, 945
Opsoclonus, 477
Optic neuritis, 763
Oral bronchodilators (albuterol), 376
Oral cavity and neck emergency
dentoalveolar infections, 743
complications, 744
diagnosis, 744
etiology, 744
management, 745
dentoalveolar trauma
complications, 742
diagnostic findings, 741
management, 742–743
oral and dental anatomy, 741, 742f
oral piercings, 748–749
oral soft tissue, infections of
diagnostic findings, 746
etiology, 745
management, 746
oropharyngeal trauma
complications, 743
diagnosis, 743
management, 743
peritonsillar abscess
complications, 747
diagnosis, 747
etiology, 747
management, 748
pharyngitis
complications, 747
diagnostic findings, 746
etiology, 746
management, 747
retropharyngeal abscess (RPA)
anatomy and physiology, 748
complications, 748
diagnostic findings, 748
etiology, 748
management, 748
Oral contraceptive pills (OCPs), 808, 812
Oral rehydration therapy (ORT), 76f
Oral soft tissue, infections of. *See under* Oral cavity and neck emergency
Orbital abscess, 766
Orbital cellulites, 765, 767f

Orbital fractures, 293
Orbital periosteum, 765
Organ donation, 271
Orofacial injuries, 1036
Oropharyngeal trauma. *See under* Oral
    cavity and neck emergency
Oropharynx examination, 747
Orotracheal intubation, 225
Orthopedic injuries
    clinical evaluation, 298
    high-yield facts, 297
    immature skeleton, 297
    physis injuries, 298
    special circumstances
        child abuse, 302
        nonaccidental trauma, 302
        birth trauma, fractures from, 302–303
    terminology, 297
Orthopedic referral, 320
Osgood-Schlatter disease, 306
Osgood-Schlatter disease, 327
Osmotic diuresis, 632
Osmotic pressure, 658f
Osteochondromas, 871
Osteoid osteomas, 869
Osteomyelitis, 852t. *See also under*
    Infectious musculoskeletal
    disorders
Osteosarcoma, 841
Otitis externa, 734
Otitis media., 735
Ottawa ankle rules, 329
Ovarian torsion, 790
Overzealous ventilations, 203
Ovulatory cycle, 809
Oximetry, 403
Oxycodone, 160
Oxygen delivery devices, 180f
Oxygen therapy, 402
Oxygen/dissociation curve., 1064t

P

PAC (perennial conjunctivitis), 585
pacemakers in children, 446
Packed red blood cells (PRBCS), 833
Pain management, 295–296
    analgesic agents, 159–160
    behavioral pediatric pain management
        behavioral interventions for infants,
          161
        preparation, 160
        procedural interventions, 161
    oligoanalgesia, 155
    pain assessment, 155–156
    procedural pain management
        abscess, 158
        fractures and burns, 158
        lacerations, 157
        lumbar puncture, 158
        penile procedures, 158
        urethral catheterization, 158
        venipuncture, 156–157
    sickle cell pain, 159
Paint chip ingestion, 966f
Palatal injury, 743
Paliperidone, 936
Pals guidelines, 204t

Panaeolus, 979
Pancreas, 279
Pancreatic exocrine insufficiency, 405
Pansinusitis, 739f
Papillae, 767
Papilledema, 495
Papule/plaque primary lesion, 117f
Paraphimosis, 683f, 684
    management, 683
    pathophysiology, 683
    reduction, 158
    signs and symptoms, 683
Parasitic infections, 844
Parasitic infestations, 553
    arthropods
        myiasis, 561
        pediculosis, 560–561
        scabies, 561
    cestodes, 557
    nematodes (roundworms)
        ascariasis, 554–555
        enterobiasis, 555
        filarial nematodes, 557
        hookworms, 556–557
        strongiloidiasis, 557
        trichinosis, 556
        trichuris trichiura, 556
    protozoa
        babesiosis, 559
        coccidia, 559–560
        dientamoeba fragilis, 558
        e. histolytica, 558
        giardia lamblia, 558–559
        malaria, 559
        pneumocystis, 559
        trypanosomes, 559
    symptoms, 554t
    trematodes (flukes), 557
Paratyphoid enteric fevers, 571
Parenchymal contusions, 238
Parenteral diuretics, 403
Parisitic vulvovaginitis. *See under* Vaginitis
Paroxysmal supraventricular tachycardia
    (PSVT), 446–447
Pastinaca sativa, 985
Patent ductus arteriosus (PDA), 420, 421f,
    401
Pathophysiology of drowning., 1026t
Patient with rash
    distribution, 115
    history, 113
    morphology, 113
        primary lesions, 114
        secondary lesions, 114
    physical examination, 113
    See also Pediatric dermatologic
        presentation
Patient-controlled analgesia (PCA), 822
PDA (patent ductus arteriosus), 420, 421f
PEA (pulseless electrical activity), 206
Pediatric advanced life support (PALS), 121,
    812
Pediatric anatomy and physiology, 260
Pediatric ankle injury, 328
Pediatric assessment triangle (PAT), 3, 4t,
    414, 1152t

Pediatric biological agent, 581
Pediatric burns
    clinical evaluation, 1031–1033
    disposition, 1033t, 1034
    epidemiology, 1029
    etiology
        child abuse, 1030
        flame, 1029
        flash, 1029
        thermal, 1029
    laboratory studies, 1033
    management, 1033
    pathophysiology
        first degree, 1030, 1031f
        fourth degree, 1030f, 1030–1031
        second degree, 1030, 1030f
        third degree, 1030, 1030f
Pediatric cervical spine injury
    analysis of radiographs, 249
    anatomy, 245
    epidemiology, 245
    evaluation and management, 246–249
    high-yield facts, 245
    injury patterns, 250
        atlantoaxial dislocation, 250
        atlantoaxial rotatory injury, 251
        atlantooccipital dislocation, 250
        atlas fractures, 250
        axis fractures, 252
        without radiographic abnormality, 255
        spinal cord injury, 255
        subaxial cervical spine injuries, 252
    physiology, 245
Pediatric dermatologic presentation
    anaphylaxis, 119
    Kawasaki disease, 118
    meningococcemia, 118
    purpura fulminans, 119
    staphylococcal scalded skin syndrome,
        118
    Stevens–Johnson syndrome (SJS), 117
    toxic epidermal necrolysis (TEN), 117
    toxic shock syndrome, 118
Pediatric drowning management of, 1028t
Pediatric dysrhythmias, 206t
Pediatric ECG, 418
Pediatric education for paramedics (PEP),
    1131
Pediatric elbow dislocations, 314
Pediatric emergency tape, 1152f
Pediatric Glasgow coma scale, 228. *See also*
    Glasgow coma scale
Pediatric hand injuries, 317
Pediatric HIV patient in ED
    clinical presentations, 538
    complications, 539
    diagnosis, 538
    epidemiology, 537
    highly active antiretroviral therapy
        (HAART), 537
    postexposure prophylaxis, 542
Pediatric hypertension
    assessment
        history, 456
        physical examination, 457
        testing, 457
    blood pressure measurement, 455

differential diagnosis, 456
hypertension, defining, 455
hypertensive emergency, 458t
individual agents
ace inhibitors, 459
α or β blockade, 459
calcium channel blockade, 459
diuretics, 459
hydralazine, 459
sodium nitroprusside, 457
treatment, 457
Pediatric obstructed airway, 25f
Pediatric pneumonia, 384
Pediatric prehospital care
anticipatory guidance, 1130
care in community ED, 1133
children with special health care needs
abuse, 1137
psychiatric, 1137
disaster preparedness, 1134
emergency care
historical perspective, 1129
medical services, 1129–1130
equipment and supplies, 1132, 1133t,
1135t
legal issues, 1132
medical direction and protocols, 1132
NEDARC, 1138
office preparedness, 1130
PECARN, 1138
pediatric trauma, 1133–1134
prehospital professionals
supplemental education, 1131–1132
training/education, 1130–1131
transfer considerations, 1133
Pediatric resuscitation medications, 1131,
1134
Pediatric septic shock, 199
Pediatric sexual abuse, 285–286
Pediatric sports injury
avulsions, 306
concussion and brachioplexus injuries,
306–307
dislocations, 305
fractures, 305
overuse syndromes, 306
return-to-play, 307
sprains and ligamentous injuries, 306
Pediatric thorax, 222
Pediatric trauma patient, 224t, 225t
Pediatric trauma score, 234, 234t
Pediatric trauma systems, 223
Pediatric trauma, equipment sizes for, 226t
Pediatric vital signs, 225t
Pediculosis, 560–561
Pediculosis capitis, 561f
Pediculosis humanus corporis, 561f
Pediculosis Phthirus pubis, 561f
Pediculus humanus capitus, 708
Pediculus humanus humanus, 708
Pedunculated polyp, 605f
PEEP (positive end-expiratory pressure), 189,
192, 198
Pelvic fractures, 323–324
Pelvic inflammatory disease (PID), 805
Pelvic ring, 323
Pelvis, 232

Pelvis and lower extremities, injuries of
ankle and foot fractures, 328–329
femoral shaft fractures, 325
foot fractures, 329–331
hip dislocations, 324–325
knee and patella dislocations, 327
knee and patella, 325–327
Osgood-Schlatter disease, 327
pelvic fractures, 323–324
proximal femur fractures, 325
tibia and fibula fractures, 327
Pelvis radiograph, 872f
Penetrating abdominal trauma, .276
Penetrating thoracic trauma, 260
Penile injuries, 284–285
Perennial conjunctivitis (PAC), 585
Peribronchial cuffing, 374
Pericardiocentesis, 270
Pericarditis, 439, 440t
Pericoronitis, 742
Perinaud oculoglandular syndrome, 774
Perineum/rectum, 232
Periodic paralysis, 485
Periodontal abscesses, 744
Periorbital infections, 765
Peripheral edema, 1069
Peritoneal irritation, 598t
Peritonsillar abscess (PTA), 359, 747. *See also
under* Oral cavity and neck
emergency
Permanent teeth, 743
Personal protective equipment, 1094f
Pertussis, 12
clinical presentation, 396
complications, 397
diagnostic evaluation
differential diagnosis, 397
laboratory diagnosis, 397
epidemiology, 395–396
hypertrophic pyloric stenosis, 398
microbiology, 395
oral dosages recommended, 398
pathophysiology, 395
prevention
postexposure prophylaxis, 398
vaccination, 399
treatment, 398
Petechiae and purpura
Henoch–Schonlein purpura
ancillary studies, 704
epidemiology, 703
etiology, 702–703
management, 704
pathophysiology, 703
recognition, 703
idiopathic thrombocytopenic purpura
etiology, 704
epidemiology, 704
pathophysiology, 704
recognition, 704
by sepsis
ancillary studies, 702
etiology, 701
management, 701–702
pathophysiology, 701
recognition, 701
Phagocytophilia, 552

Phalanges, fractures of. *See under* Upper
extremities, injuries of
Phalloides, 977
Pharmacologic agents, 201
Pharmacologic therapy, 434
Pharmacology, 933
Pharyngitis. *See under* Oral cavity and neck
emergency
Phencyclidine (PCP)
clinical findings, 953
disposition, 954
high-yield facts, 953
laboratory, 954
management, 954
pathophysiology, 953
Phenobarbital, 39
Philodendron, 981
Phimosis
diagnostic evaluation, 683
management, 683
pathophysiology, 682
signs and symptoms, 682
Phosphate, 632
Photo courtesy of CDC, 547f
Photophobia, 759
Phototherapy, 86t
Phylum Cnidaria, 1017
Physalia physalis, 1017
Physicians intent, 149
Physiologic jaundice, 83
Physis injuries, 299f
PID (pelvic inflammatory disease), 791
Pinworm, 553, 555–556, 555f, 794
Pit vipers. *See under* Snake envenomations
Pityriasis rosea. *See under* Exanthems
Placenta previa, 780
Placental abruption, 781
Plague, 576
Plasmodium, 567
Plastic deformation, 297
Platelet activating factor (PAF), 361
Platelet concentrate, 833
Pneumothorax and emphysema, 1077
Pneumocystis carinii, 844
Pneumocystis, 559
Pneumoniae, 519, 822
Pneumonia
atypical pneumonia, 384
causes of, 380t
clinical presentation, 380–382
differential diagnosis, 390
empiric therapy, 392–393
epidemiology/overview, 379
etiology, 383
infants (1 to 3 months), 385
infants (3 to 24 months), 386
laboratory studies, 387
management, 390–392
neonatal, 384
pathophysiology, 383
pediatric pneumonia (common
organisms), 384
radiographic evaluation, 388–390
risk factors, 382–383, 382t
school age and adolescents, 386
severe, life-threatening, 386
specific pathogens

Pneumonia (*Contd.*)
  Haemophilus influenzae, 386
  mycoplasma pneumoniae, 387
  respiratory syncytial virus, 387
  staphylococcus aureus, 386
  streptococcus pneumoniae, 386
  unusual causes, 387
  syndromes, 381t
  toddler/preschooler, 386
Pneumothorax, 54, 218, 262, 263f, 406
Poinsettia, 982
Poison hemlock (*Conium maculatum*), 984
Poisonous plants
  epidemiology, 981
  high-yield facts, 981
  identification of plants, 981
  psychoactive plants, 986
  specific toxic plants
    mucosal irritants, 981
    gastrointestinal upset. *See*
      Gastrointestinal irritants
    symptomatic plant ingestions. *See*
      Systemic toxins
Pokeweed (*Phytolacca americana*), 982
Polymerase chain reaction (PCR), 855
Polyvalent antivenin, 1006
Port wine stains, 729
Portuguese man-o'-war, 1018f
Positive end-expiratory pressure (PEEP), 189,
      192, 198, 262, 435
Positive pressure breaths (PPV), 213
Positive-pressure ventilation (PPV), 401
Post-auricular adenopathy, 719f
Postconcussion syndrome, 105, 109, 239
Postconcussive headaches, 1041
Posterior elbow dislocation, 314
Posterior fat pad sign, 312f8
Posteroanterior, 24
Postexposure prophylaxis, 542, 398
Postoperative wound care, 345
Poststreptococcal glomerulonephritis, 713
Posttransplant lymphoproliferative disease
      (PTLD), 4, 428
Posttraumatic stress disorder (PTSD), 1119t,
      1153, 1153t
Potassium, 631. *See also under* Fluid and
      Electrolyte Disorders
Potassium iodide dosing, 1096
Pott's puffy tumor, 739
PPI (proton pump inhibitors), 610
PPV (positive-pressure ventilation), 401
Pralidoxime chloride, 994
Preauricular lymphadenopathy, 773
Precocious puberty, 789
Preeclampsia, 779
Preexposure prophylaxis, 1001, 1002
Prehospital care of minor wounds, 334
Premature ventricular contractions (PVC),
      448, 926
Prematurity, 217
Premenarcheal patients. *See under*
      Gynecologic disorders
Prepubertal gonorrhea, 801f
Prepubertal herpes simplex, 803f
Priapism, 825
  diagnostic evaluation, 685
  management, 685

pathophysiology, 685
signs and symptoms, 685
Primary adrenal insufficiency, 641f
Primary brain injury, 237
Primary dysmenorrheal, 807
Primary headache, 491t
Primary HIV infection, 539f
Primary lesions, 114
Primary teeth, 746
Primary wound closure, 339
Primidone, 44t
Procalcitonin (PCT), 688
Procedural sedation
  analgesic agents, 149
  conscious sedation, 145
  deep sedation, 151–152
  equipment, 146
  health care needs, 153–12
  intravenous administration, 148
  minimal sedation/anxiolysis, 149
  moderate sedation, 149
  nonpharmacologic analgesia, 152
  oral administration, 148
  patient assessment, 145–4
  patient monitoring, 146
  PSA agents, 152
  sedative agents, 149
  subcutaneous (SQ), 148
  transmucosal drug, 148
Prognosis, 534
Prokinetic agents, 610
Prophylactic fasciotomy, 1005
Prophylaxis, 429
Propofol, 151
Propylthiouracil, 645
Proton pump inhibitors (PPIs), 610
Protozoa. *See under* parasitic infestations
Proximal femur fractures, 325
Proximal fibula, 873f
Proximal humerus, 871f
Proximal humerus fracture, 310–311
Proximal interphalangeal joint, 320
Proximal radius and ulna fractures, 315
Proximal tibia, 870f
Proximal tibial metaphysis, 328f
Pruritic rashes
  atopic dermatitis
    ancillary studies, 707
    etiology, 707, 708f
    management, 707
    pathophysiology, 707
    recognition, 707
  contact dermatitis
    ancillary studies, 708
    etiology, 708
    management, 708
    pathophysiology, 708
    recognition, 708
  erythema multiforme
    ancillary studies, 711
    etiology, 710
    management, 711
    pathophysiology, 710, 711f
    recognition, 710–711
  papular urticaria
    etiology, 709
    management, 710

pathophysiology, 709–710
recognition, 710
pediculosis
  etiology, 708
  management, 708
  pathophysiology, 708
  recognition, 708
scabies
  ancillary studies, 709
  etiology, 709, 709f
  management, 709
  pathophysiology, 709
  recognition, 709
urticaria
  etiology, 710
  management, 710
  pathophysiology, 710
  recognition, 710
Pseudomonas aeruginosa, 733
Pseudomonas, 772
Pseudosubluxation, 253f
Pseudotumor cerebri, 493
Psilocybe, 979
Psoas sign, 598t
Psoriatic arthritis, 864
PSVT (paroxysmal supraventricular
      tachycardia), 446–447, 207
Psychiatric emergencies
  aggressive patient, 1120
  conversion/somatization disorder
    etiology/pathogenesis, 1120
    recognition, 1120
    treatment/management, 1120
  posttraumatic stress disorder
    etiology/pathogenesis, 1119
    management, 1119
    recognition, 1119
  psychopathic patient:
    etiology/pathogenesis, 1119
  psychotic patient
    ancillary studies, 1118–1119
    etiology/pathogenesis, 1118
    management, 1118
  psychotropic medications, 1120
  suicidal patient
    ancillary studies, 1118
    etiology/pathogenesis, 1117
    management, 1118
    recognition, 1117–1118
Psychiatric history, 1118t
Psychiatric medications side effect, 1120t
Psychoactive plants, 986
Psychologic sequelae, 1041
Psychopathic patient, 1119
Psychotic patient, 1118
Psychotropic medications, 1121
PTLD (posttransplant lymphoproliferative
      disease), I.4
Pubertal vaginal bleeding. *See under*
      Gynecologic disorders
Pulled elbow, 314
Pulmonary barotrauma, 1076
Pulmonary contusion, 262, 268
Pulmonary embolism (PE), 463f, 782
Pulmonary emergencies, 130
Pulmonary hematoma, 262
Pulmonary injuries, 262

Pulmonary lacerations, 262
Pulmonic stenosis (PS), 419, 420f
Pulmozyme, 408
Pulseless electrical activity (PEA), 206
Pulseless ventricular tachycardia (PVT), 206
Puncture wounds, 348
Purified protein derivative (PPD), 127
Purpura fulminans, 119
Pustular melanosis, 727
PVC (premature ventricular contractions), 448
Pyloric stenosis Ultrasound, 168f
Pyomyositis, 486
Pyomyositis, 486
Pyridoxine, 977

Q

QRS axis, age-specific, 417t
Quetiapine, 935

R

Rabies prophylaxis, 1001–1002
Raccoon eyes, 238
Radial head subluxation, 314
Radiation accidents, 1082t, 1090–1093t
Radiation emergencies
    management
        emergency department management, 1088
        exposure, 1096
        external contamination, 1094–1096
        general procedures, 1089–1094
        internal contamination, 1096
        prehospital management, 1088
        radiation accident plan, 1089
    prognosis
        survivor improbable, 1097
        survivor possible, 1097
        survivor probable, 1097
    radiation exposure, 1083–1084
    radiation injuries
        contamination, 1086
        exposure, 1084–1086
    radiation measurement, 1083
    radiation, types of, 1082
        ionizing radiation, 1082–1083
        nonionizing radiation, 1083
Radiation exposure, 1083–1084
Radiation injuries, 1085t, 1097
    localized, 1085
    whole-body exposure, 1085
Radiation, type of, 1083t
Radiographic abnormality, 255
Radiographic findings, 965f
Radiographs, 318
Radiography in abdominal trauma, 277
Radioisotope, 1082
Radionucleotide, 1082
Radio-opaque foreign body X-ray, 170f
Ranitidine, 610
Rapid sequence induction, 241
Rapid sequence intubation (RSI), 184
Rapid viral antigen testing, 388
Reactive arthritis, 864
Recluse spider, 1010
Rectal gonorrhea, 801
Rectum, 605

Red blood cells, 569f
Red eye, 763
Reflux esophagitis, 611f
Regional nerve blocks, 338
Renal failure, 695t
Renal injuries, 281–282
Renal toxins, 979
Renal ultrasonography (RUS), 690
Resistance, 1035
Resperidone, 935
Respiratory distress, 121–123
    clinical presentation, 23
    differential diagnosis, 25
    disposition/outcome, 26
    in infants and children, 24t
    newborns, 24t
    laboratory and radiographic findings, 24
    pathophysiology, 23
    treatment, 25
Respiratory failure, 355
    advanced airway management
        mechanical ventilation, 192
        noninvasive mechanical ventilation, 192–193
    anatomy and physiology, 189
    assisted ventilation indications, 191
    laboratory studies, 190–191
    pertinent history, 189–190
    physical examination, 190
Respiratory fatigue, 374
Respiratory syncytial virus (RSV), 373, 387
Respiratory viruses, 512t
Resuscitation medications, 209t
Resuscitative thoracotomy, 227
Retained rock, 737f
Reticulocyte count, 819
Retinal injury, 757
Retinal vein obstruction, 763
Retinoblastoma, 840
Retrobulbar hemorrhage, 757
Retrograde amnesia, 1041
Retrograde urethrogram (RUG), 230
Retroperitoneal injuries, 231
Retropharyngeal abscess, 358–359, 359f.
        See also under Oral cavity and neck emergency
Retrophayngeal space, 124f
Return to play (RTP), 111
Reye's syndrome, 37
Rh sensitization, 784
Rhabdomyosarcoma, 840
Rheumatic fever, 859, 862t
Rheumatic heart disease (RHD), 861
Rhinitis. *See* Allergic rhinitis
Rhizopus, 766
Rhode island disaster initiative (RIDI), 1088f
Rhododendron, 983
Rhythm disturbances (arrhythmia), 197
Rib fracture, 54f, 267
Ricinus communis, 985, 985f
Rickets
    breast-feeding, 650
    decreased sunlight exposure, 650
    etiology, 649
    vitamin D deficiency, 649
Rickettsia rickettsii, 550
Right lower lobe infiltrate, 824f

Right testicle, torsion of, 678f
Right-axis deviation (RDA), 414
Ringer's lactate (LR), 229
Ritter's disease, 714
RMSF (Rocky mountain spotted fever), 550
RNA, 538, 1081
Rocky mountain spotted fever, 549
Rodenticides
    developmental considerations, 915
    disposition, 921
    high-yield facts, 915
    laboratory and diagnostic testing, 920
    management
        antidotal therapy, 921
        enhanced elimination, 920
        FFP and blood products, 921
        gastrointestinal decontamination, 920
        product identification, 920
    pathophysiology, 915–916
    pharmacology, 916
    toxicokinetics, 916
    unapproved, 917–918t
Roentgen, 168
Roseola (exanthem subitum). *See under* Exanthems
Rosving's sign, 598t
Round pneumonia, 389
Roundworms. *See under* Parasitic infestations
RSV (respiratory syncytial virus), 373, 387
Rubeola exanthema, 718f
Rubella (German measles). *See under* Exanthems
Rubeola (measles). *See under* Exanthems
Rumack-Matthew nomogram, 888
Running stitch, 341
RUS (renal ultrasonography), 690
Rusch bag and mask, 180f

S

S. aureus, 713
S. invicta, 1014
SAC (seasonal allergic conjunctivitis), 585
Sacroiliac joints, 99
Salicylates, 894t
Salmon patch, 729
Salmonella, 824
Salmonella enterica, 571
Salter-Harris classification system, 223
Salter-Harris fractures, 305, 311, 319f, 320, 326
Salter-Harris injury, 306
Salvia divinorum, 986
Sarcoptes scabiei (scabies), 561
SARS (severe acute respiratory syndrome), 387
SBI (Serious bacterial infection), 9
Scabies, 561
Scalp laceration, 336, 346
Scaphoid fractures, 320
Scapular fractures, 310
Scarlet fever, 725, 725f
SCIWORA (spinal cord injury without radiographic abnormality), 231
SCIWORA, 255
Scleral lacerations, 757
Scleritis and episcleritis, 767

Scorpions, 1012. *See also under* Spider and arthropod bites
Screw at thoracic inlet, 616f
Scrotal and testicular trauma, 680
Scrotal trauma, 284
Sea anemones, 1019f
Sea snakes, 1022f
Seasonal allergic conjunctivitis (SAC), 585
Seat belt sign, 275f
Seborrheic dermatitis, 713, 714f
Second impact syndrome (SIS), 108
Secondary closure technique, 341–342
Secondary lesions, 114
Secretory immunoglobulins, 383
Sedation and analgesic agents, 150
Seizures, 132
    algorithm, 42t
    anticonvulsant choice, 44t
    antiepilepsy drugs (AEDs), 44t, 45t
    classification, 39
    electroencephalogram, 4
    etiology of childhood, 41t
    febrile seizures
        disposition, 47
        laboratory evaluation, 46
        therapy, 46
    first afebrile seizure
        history, 40
        laboratory evaluation, 41
        physical examination, 41
        radiologic evaluation, 41
    neonatal epileptic syndromes
        laboratory evaluation, 44
        treatment, 45
    neonatal seizures, 43, 45t, 46t
    status epilepticus, 48
    therapeutic monitoring, 45t
Selective serotonin reuptake inhibitors (SSRI), 931
Self-inflating bag, 181f
Septic arthritis, 852t. *See also under* Infectious musculoskeletal disorders
Septic-appearing neonate
    bacterial etiologies, 10
    clinical presentation, 10
    evaluation, 11
    fever, 9
    specific conditions
        cephalohematomas, 12
        chlamydia infections, 12
        congenital heart disease, 12
        inborn errors of metabolism, 12
        omphalitis, 12
        pertussis, 12
    treatment, 11
    viral etiologies, 10
Sequelae, 522
Serious bacterial infection (SBI), 9
Seronegative enthesitis and arthritis (SEA), 864
Serum D-dimer test, 462
Serum electrolytes, 451, 1053
Serum glucose, 1053
Severe erosive disease, 611f
Severely dysmorphic atlas, 254f
Sexual assault, 541f

Sexually transmitted diseases (STD)
    chlamydia
        clinical manifestations, 797
        diagnosis, 797
        etiology, 797
        treatment, 798
    herpes simplex infection
        clinical manifestations, 803
        diagnosis, 803
        etiology, 803
        treatment, 804
    HIV and AIDS
        clinical manifestations, 804
        diagnosis, 804
        etiology, 804
        treatment, 804
    genital warts
        clinical manifestations, 800
        diagnosis, 800
        etiology, 798–800
        treatment, 800
    gonorrhea
        clinical manifestations, 801
        diagnosis, 801
        etiology, 800–801
        treatment, 801
    pelvic inflammatory disease, 805
    STD
        cervicitis, 804
        epididymitis, 804
        genital ulcers, 804
        urethritis, 804
    syphilis
        clinical manifestations, 802
        diagnosis, 802
        etiology, 802
        treatment, 803
    trichomoniasis
        clinical manifestation, 801
        diagnosis, 801
        etiology, 801
        treatment, 802
Shaken impact syndrome, 267
Shear injuries, 333
Sheep tapeworms, 558
Shigella, 567, 696
Shigella flexneri, 794
Shigella vaginitis. *See under* Vaginitis
Shingles (herpes zoster). *See under* Exanthems
Shock
    cardiogenic shock, 197
    causes, 196t
    distributive shock, 197
    hypovolemic shock, 196
    obstructive shock, 197
    pharmacologic agents, 201
    recognition, 197
    treatment/interventions, 198
Shoulder compression, 310
Shoulder dislocations, 310
Sickle cell disease (SCD) 821, 1069
    acute chest syndrome, 822
    aplastic crisis, 826
    high-yield facts, 821
    infection, 822–824

    priapism, 825
    splenic sequestration, 825
    stroke (cerebrovascular accidents), 824
    vasoocclusive crisis, 821
Sickle cell pain, 159
Side splash/flash, 1039
SIDS. *See* Sudden infant death syndrome
Simple continuous stitch, 343f
Simple interrupted stitch, 341, 343f
Sinding-Larsen-Johansson syndrome, 306
Single rescuer method of BMV, 181f
Sinus bradycardia, 445
Sinusitis. *See under* Nose Emergencies
Sirolimus, 139
Skin, 232
Skin anatomy, 333
Skin closure technique, 340
    correction of dog-ears, 341
    knots, 341
    mattress stitches, 341
    running stitch, 341
    simple interrupted stitch, 341
Skull radiographs, 242
Slipped capital femoral epiphysis (SCFE), 860
SLUGBAM, 978
Smallpox, 579, 580
Smithiana, 979
Smoke inhalation, 974
Snake envenomations
    coral snakes, 1007
        clinical presentation, 1007
        disposition, 1007
        management, 1007
    exotic snakes, 1007
    pit vipers
        anatomy, 1003
        antivenom therapy, 1005–1006
        clinical presentation, 1004
        diagnostic studies, 1005
        disposition, 1006
        hospital management, 1005
        pathophysiology, 1003
        prehospital management, 1004–1005
Sniffing position, 213f
Sodium, 631. *See also under* Fluid and electrolyte disorders
Sodium bicarbonate, 216
Sodium channel activators, 984
Sodium nitroprusside, 457
Sodium thiosulfate, 974
Soft tissue injury, 295
Soft tissue injury and wound repair
    history, 334
    management
        analgesia, 337
        anesthesia, 337
        antibiotic use, 343–344
        antisepsis and scrubbing, 338
        buried stitch, 339–340
        debridement, 339
        delayed primary (tertiary) closure, 342
        foreign body evaluation, 339
        hair removal, 338
        hemostasis, 338
        instruments, 335
        irrigation, 338–339

moderate sedation, 338
primary wound closure, 339
regional nerve blocks, 338
secondary closure, 341–342
skin closure, 340
Steri-strips, 337
surgical staples, 336
suture choice, 335, 336t
tissue adhesive, 337
wound cleaning, 338
wound closure technique, 335t
wound dressing, 342–343
See also Skin closure technique
minor injuries
abrasions, 334
contusions and hematomas, 334
lacerations, 333
physical examination, 334
postoperative wound care, 345
prehospital care, 334
selected injuries, management of
abrasions, 345
consultation guidelines, 348
ear lacerations, 347
eyelid lacerations, 346
fingertip injuries, 348
forehead lacerations, 346
lip lacerations, 348
puncture wounds, 348
scalp lacerations, 346
skin anatomy, 333
soft tissue anatomy, 333
Solanine, 983
Solanum dulcamara, 983
Solanum nigrum, 983
Solanum pseudocapsicum, 983
Solanum tuberosum, 983
Solid organs
liver, 279
pancreas, 279
spleen, 278
Specific absorption rate (SAR), 172
Specific renal syndromes
acute glomerulonephritis, 589
ancillary data, 693
diagnostic findings, 693
management, 693
acute renal failure, 696
diagnostic findings, 697
management, 698
diagnostic findings, 694
differential diagnosis, 695
hematuria, .694
hemolytic uremic syndrome, 696
management, 695
nephrotic syndrome, 693
proteinuria, 694t
Spider and arthropod bites
black widow spiders
anatomy, 1009
clinical presentation, 1009
disposition, 1010
management, 1009
pathophysiology, 1009
brown recluse spiders
anatomy, 1010

clinical presentation, 1010–1011
pathophysiology, 1010
hobo spider
disposition, 1011
management, 1011
hymenoptera. *See* Bees and vespids
imported fire ants, 1014
clinical presentation, 1015
management, 1015
pathophysiology, 1015
scorpions, 1012
anatomy, 1012
clinical presentation, 1013
pathophysiology, 1012
tarantulas, 1011–1012
Spinal cord compression, 845
Spinal cord injury, 248t, 255
Spine, 99
Spine injuries, 267–268
Spine, spinal cord injury without
radiographic abnormality
(SCIWORA), 245
Spironolactone (Aldactone), 436
Spleen, 278
Splenic sequestration, 825
Splenic sequestration, 825
Spondyloarthropathies. *See under*
Inflammatory musculoskeletal
disorders
Sports-related trauma, 274
SSRI (Selective serotonin reuptake
inhibitors), 931
SSSS (staphylococcal scalded skin
syndrome), 713
Standard laceration equipment, 335f
Staphylococcal scalded skin syndrome, 118
Staphylococcus, 124, 527
Staphylococcus aureus, 486, 514, 766, 851, 386, 406, 525, 707
Steri-strips, 337
Steroids, 909
Stevens–Johnson syndrome (SJS), 117, 774, 711, 711f
Sting ray, 1019f
Stinger, 307
Stomach, 602
Stone fish, 1020f
Stratum corneum, 707
Streptococcal toxic shock syndrome, 526
Streptococcus pneumoniae, 383, 386, 733, 5619, 821
Streptococcus, 124, 598, 519, 857, 693
Streptococcus pyogenes, 853, 707, 713
Stridor, algorithm for, 355
Stroke (cerebrovascular accidents), 824
Stroke volume, 261
Stroke diagnosis, .504t
Strongiloidiasis, 557
Sturge–Webber syndrome, 729
Subaxial cervical spine injuries, 252
Subconjunctival hemorrhage, 755
Subcutaneous emphysema, 291
Subcuticular stitch, 341f
Submandibular neck abscess, 124f
Subperiosteal abscess, 766
Subungual hematoma, 348

Sucking chest wound, 231, 265
Sudden infant death syndrome
apparent life-threatening event (ALTE), 29
disposition, 31
epidemiology, 29
etiology, 29
evaluation and management, 30
history, 29
initial assessment, 29
physical examination, 30
stabilization, 29
disposition, 28
epidemiology, 27
evaluation and management, 28
pathophysiology, 27
Suicidal patient, 1117
Sulfur mustard, 994
Superficial skin infections
fungal infections
ancillary studies, 715
etiology, 715
management, 715
pathophysiology, 715
recognition, 715
impetigo
ancillary studies, 713
etiology, 713
management, 713
pathophysiology, 713
recognition, 713
staphylococcal scalded skin syndrome (SSSS)
ancillary studies, 715
etiology, 713
management, 714
pathophysiology, 713
recognition, 714
Superior mediastinal syndrome, 845
Superior vena cava syndrome (SVCS), 845
Supination method, 315
Supracondylar fracture, 313f, 313t
Supracondylar humerus fractures, 312
Supraglottitis, 357
Supraorbital fractures, 293
Surface burns, 1036
Surgical emergencies, 134
Surgical staples, 336
Surgical thrombectomy, 464
Survivor, prognosis for. *See under* Radiation emergencies
Suture removal, 345
Suture types, 335, 336t
Symptomatic bradycardia, 207
Synchondrosis, 251f, 253f
Syncope
causes of, 470t
cardiac syncope
Brugada syndrome, 472
cardiomyoptahy, 473
congenital short qt syndrome, 472
hypertrophic cardiomyopathy, 473
long QT syndrome, 472
diagnostic approach, 471f
disposition, 473
high-yield facts, 469
history, 469
laboratory studies, 469

Syncope (*Contd.*)
  neurocardiogenic, 470
  pathophysiology, 469
  physical examination, 469
  syncope, etiologies of, 470
  treatment, 473
Syndrome of inappropriate antidiuretic
    hormone (SIADH), 662, 1039
Synovial hypertrophy, 827
Syphilis. *See under* Sexually transmitted
    diseases (STD)
Systemic analgesia, 296
Systemic inflammatory response syndrome
    (SIRS), 198
Systemic lupus erythematosus (SLE), 859
Systemic toxins
  ackee (*Blighia sapida*), 986
  anticholinergic substances, 983
  cardiac glycosides, 983
  colchicine, 985
  poison hemlock (*Conium maculatum*),
    984
  sodium channel activators, 984
  solanine, 983
  tobacco (*Nicotiana*), 984
  toxalbumins, 985
  water hemlock, 985
  yew, 984
Systolic and diastolic blood pressures, 446t

T
Tachyarrhythmia, 434f
Tachycardia algorithm, 450f
Tachypnea, 262, 381, 354
Tacrolimus, 138–139
Taenia solium, 558 *f*
Tapeworms, 557
TAPVR (total anomalous pulmonary venous
    return), 418, 419f
Tarantulas, 1011–1012
TBV (total blood volume), 279
Teaching resource for instructors in
    prehospital pediatrics (TRIPP)
Tearing, excessive, 764
Telecanthus, 290
Temperatures (full-thickness burns), 1111
Temporary transvenous pacemakers, 446
Tendon injury, 318
Tendon reflexes, 482t
Tension lacerations, 333
Tension pneumothorax, 231, 263–264
Tension-type headaches, 492
Terrain vehicle (ATV), 197
Tertiary closure technique, 342
Testicular appendix., 679f
Testicular detorsion, 679f
Testicular dislocation, 284
Testicular torsion
  diagnostic evaluation, 678
  management, 678
  pathophysiology, 677
  signs and symptoms, 678
Testicular tumors
  diagnostic evaluation, 681
  management, 681
  signs and symptoms 681
Tetanus immunization guidelines, 345f

Tetanus prophylaxis, 343–344
Tetracaine gel, 156
Tetracaine-adrenaline-cocaine (TAC), 337
Tetralogy of Fallot (TOF), 418, 419f
TGA (transposition of great arteries), 416,
    418f
Thalassemia, 818–819
Thermal burns, 759
Thermal injury 1097
Thevetia peruviana, 983
Thiazides, 460
Thoracic trauma
  epidemiology, 259
  injuries and management
    cardiac tamponade, 269
    cardiovascular injuries, 268
    flail chest, 267
    hemothorax, 264
    myocardial contusion, 268–269
    open pneumothorax, 265
    pneumothorax, 262
    pulmonary contusion, 262
    pulmonary lacerations, 262
    rib fractures, 267
    rupture of great vessels, 269
    spine injuries, 267–268
    tension pneumothorax, 263–264
    traumatic asphyxia, 265
    traumatic diaphragmatic hernia,
      266–267
    traumatic esophageal rupture, 266
    traumatic tracheal, 265
  law enforcement, 271
  mechanism of injury
    blunt thoracic trauma, 259–260
    pathophysiology, 260
    penetrating thoracic trauma, 260
    thoracic injury management, 260–262
  organ donation, 271
  procedures
    needle thoracostomy, 270
    tube thoracostomy, 270
Thoracostomy tubes, 265
Threadworm, 557
Thrombocytopenia, 820, 832, 846
Thromboembolic disease
  anticoagulant and thrombolytic dosing
  arterial thromboembolism (ATE), 461
  risk factors, 461
  venous thromboembolism, diagnosis of
    clinical presentation, 461
    complications, 464
    imaging, 462
    laboratory testing, 462
    treatment, 463
Thrombolytics, 464
Thrombotic thrombocytopenic purpura
    (TTP), 819
Thyrotoxicosis, 645
Thyrotropin receptor-stimulating antibodies
    (TRSAb), 645
Thumb spica, 301
Thyrotoxicosis, 645
TIBC (Total iron-binding capacity), 970
Tibia and fibula fractures, 327
Tibial spine avulsion fracture, 326f
Tibial tubercle avulsion fracture, 326f

Tick paralysis, 484
Tick-borne illnesses, 546f
Tick-borne infections
  babesiosis, 551
  Colorado tick fever, 552
  high-yield facts, 545
  human granulocytic anaplasmosis, 552
  human monocyte ehrlichiosis, 551
  Lyme disease, 545
  rocky mountain spotted fever, 549–551
  tularemia, 551
Tillaux fracture, 328f
Tinea capitis, 715
Tinea corporis, 715, 715f
Tissue adhesive, 337
Titratable acid, 907
TMP-SMX (Trimethoprimsulfamethoxazole),
    398
Tobacco (*Nicotiana*), 984
Toddler's fracture, 328
TOF (tetralogy of fallot), 418, 419f
Tongue (posterior portion), 178f
Tooth reimplantation, 743f
Topical anesthetics, 156
TORCH, 620
Torsion, 600
Torus fractures, 316
Total anomalous pulmonary venous return
    (TAPVR), 129, 418
Total body water (TBW), 657, 658
Total iron-binding capacity (TIBC), 970
Tourniquet injuries, 285
Toxalbumins, 985
Toxic alcohols, 901t
  ethanol
    clinical presentation, 897
    disposition, 898
    laboratory studies, 897
    management, 898
    pathophysiology, 897
    pharmacokinetics, 897
  ethylene glycol
    clinical presentation, 900
    laboratory studies, 900
    management, 900
    pharmacokinetics and
      pathophysiology, 900
  isopropanol
    clinical presentation, 901
    disposition, 901
    laboratory studies, 901
    management, 901
    pharmacokinetics and
      pathophysiology, 901
  methanol
    clinical presentation, 898
    disposition, 899
    laboratory studies, 898
    management, 899
    pharmacokinetics and
      pathophysiology, 898
Toxic epidermal necrolysis (TEN), 117, 711
Toxic megacolon, 604f
Toxic reactions, 1013
Toxic shock syndrome, 118
  clinical manifestations, 527
  differential diagnosis, 528

epidemiology, 526
etiology, 525
future, 528
high-yield facts, 525
pathogenesis, 525
recurrences, 528
Tracheostomy, 225
Trachomatis, 12
Transcutaneous devices (TcB), 85
Transfusion therapy, 835
Transfusion-related acute lung injury (TRALI), 835
Transient erythroblastopenia of childhood (TEC), 820
Transient paralysis and paresthesias, 1041
Transient synovitis, 859
Transphyseal fractures, 325
Transplant medicine, I.2t
Transplant patient in ED
    common complication, 2–4
    common complaints, 1–2
    with fever, 2t
    immunosupressive medications
        azathioprine, 4, 4t
        corticosteroids, 4
        cyclosporine, 4
        muromonab, 5
        mycophenolate mofetil, 5
        sirolimus, 5
        tacrolimus, 4–5
    infection prophylaxis, 5
Transposition of great arteries (TGA), 416, 418f
Transtentorial uncal herniation, 240
Transtracheal jet ventilation (TTJV), 225, 227, 227t
Transverse fracture of patella, 327f
Transverse myelitis, 483
Trauma activation, 224t
Trauma imaging algorithm, 166t
Trauma in children, 222t
Trauma in pregnancy, 783
Trauma patient x-ray, 170f
Trauma score, 234, 234t
Trauma-induced alteration, 239
Traumatic asphyxia, 265
Traumatic diaphragmatic hernia, 266–267
Traumatic esophageal rupture, 266
Traumatic head injuries, 238f
Traumatic injury, 245
Traumatic iritis, 756
Traumatic pancreatitis, 274, 279
Traumatic RUPTURE of great vessels, 269
Traumatic tibial apophysitis, 327
Traumatic tracheal, 265
Travel-related infectious, 566t, 565t
Trematodes (flukes), 557
Treponema pallidum, 802
Triage guidelines, 970t
Trichinella spiralis, 486, 556
Trichinosis, 486, 556
Trichobilharzia ocellata, 557
Trichomoniasis. *See under* Sexually transmitted diseases
Trichuris trichiura (whipworm), 553
Trichuris trichiura, 556

Tricuspid atresia, 416, 419f
Tricyclic antidepressants (TCAs), 931
Trifluorothymidine, 773
Trimethoprimsulfamethoxazole (TMP-SMX), 398
TRSAb (Thyrotropin receptorstimulating antibodies), 645
Truncus arteriosus, 416, 418f
Trypanosomes, 559
TSS (toxic shock syndrome) in children, 527
Tube thoracostomy
    emergency department thoracotomy, 270
    pericardiocentesis, 270
Tuberculosis (TB), 937
Tuberculosis skin testing, 388
Tuft fracture, 319f
Tularemia, 551
Tumor lysis syndrome (TLS), 841
Tumor necrosis factor (TNF), 575
Two-finger technique, 215f
Tympanic membrane, 735f, 1041
Typhoid, 571
Typhoid fever (TF), 563

U
UGI (upper gastrointestinal series), 610
Ulnar fractures, 315, 316
    diaphyseal radius, 315
    distal radius, 316
    proximal radius, 315
Ultrasonography, 167f, 233
Ultraviolet keratitis, 759, 1069
Undifferentiated sick infant, 421–423
Unfractionated heparin (UFH), 505
Unicameral bone cysts, 871
Unconjugated neonatal hyperbilirubinemia
    ancillary studies, 620
    management/complications, 620
    recognition, 619
Unilateral perched facet, 255
Upper airway emergencies
    foreign body obstruction, 359–360
    high-yield facts, 353
    management
        arterial blood gases, 354–355
        respiratory failure, 355
    pathophysiology
        lower airway considerations, 353
        upper airway considerations, 353
    specific clinical scenarios
        bacterial tracheitis, 358
        croup, 355–357
        epiglottitis (supraglottitis), 357
        peritonsillar abscess, 359
        retropharyngeal abscess, 358–359
    signs of distress, 353–354
Upper extremities, injuries of
    carpal fractures, 320
    clavicle and acromioclavicular joint, 309
    diaphyseal clavicle fractures, 309
    diaphyseal radius and ulnar fractures, 315–316
    dislocations
        carpometacarpal joint, 321
        distal interphalangeal joint, 320
        metacarpophalangeal joint, 320
        proximal interphalangeal joint, 320

distal radius and ulna fractures, 316
elbow dislocations, 314
fracture separation of distal humeral physis, 314
hand and wrist injuries, 317
humerus fractures
    elbow, 311
    humerus shaft fractures, 311
    proximal humerus fracture, 310–311
lateral clavicle injuries, 310
medial and lateral condyles, 313
medial clavicle fractures, 309
medial epicondylar fracture, 313–314
metacarpal fractures, 320
phalanges fractures
    distal phalanx, 319
    middle and proximal phalanx, 319
physical examination
    circulation, 317
    motor, 318
    observation, 317
    palpation, 317
    radiographs, 318
    sensation, 317
    tendon, 318
proximal radius, 315
radial head subluxation, 314
radius and ulna fractures, 315
supracondylar humerus fractures, 312
Upper gastrointestinal series (UGI), 610
Upward streamer/leader injury, 1039
Ureteral injuries, 282–284
Urethral catheterization, 158
Urethral prolapse, 788–789
Urethritis, 804
Uridine diphosphate glucuronosyltransferase (UGT), 83
Urinary output, 282t
Urinary tract diseases
    infection
        diagnostic evaluation, 688
        management and radiologic evaluation, 688–690
        pathophysiology, 687
        signs and symptoms, 687–688
    urolithiasis
        diagnostic evaluation, 691
        management, 691
        pathophysiology, 690
        signs and symptoms, 690–691
Urinary tract infections (UTI), 598–599. *See also under* Urinary tract diseases
Urine dipstick analysis, 281
Urolithiasis. *See under* Urinary tract diseases
Urologic studies, 233–234
Urticaria pigmentosa, 728
US storm deaths, 1039f
UTI (urinary tract infections), 598

V
Vaccination, 399
Vaccines (influenza), 516t
Vaginal bleeding. *See under* Adolescent pregnant patient
Vaginal foreign body, 788
Vaginal ulcer, 803f

Vaginitis
  candidal vaginitis
    clinical presentation, 794
    etiology, 794
    management, 794
  Gardnerella vaginitis
    clinical presentation, 794
    etiology, 794
  nonspecific vulvovaginitis
    causes of, 794t
    etiology, 793
    management, 793
    treatment, 794t
  shigella vaginitis
    clinical presentation, 794
    management, 794
  parisitic vulvovaginitis
    clinical presentation, 794
    management, 794
  vulvovaginitis, 793
Vancomycin, 393
Vanillylmandelic acid (VMA), 477
Vapotherm, 189
Varicella (chicken pox). *See under*
    Exanthems
Varicella rash, 721f
Varicella zoster virus (VZV), 773, 844
Variola virus (smallpox), 575
Vascular malformations, 729
Vasoactive agents, 202
Vasoactive agents, 202t
Vasoocclusive crisis, 821
Vasovagal, 469
Vaso-occlusive episode (VOE), 159
VCUG (voiding cystourethrogram), 690
Venipuncture pain, 156–157, 157f
  cold spray, 157
  lidocaine devices and techniques, 157
Venom immunotherapy, 1014
Venomous fish, 1019
Venous catheter, 215f
Venous thromboembolism (VTE), 461
Ventilation, 213
Ventilation-perfusion scan, 463f
Ventricular assist devices (VAD), 436
Ventricular fibrillation, 203, 449, 450f
Ventricular septal defect (VSD), 416, 420

Ventricular tachycardia (VT), 449, 450f
Ventriculoperitoneal shunt placement, 496f
Verapamil, 447
Vernal conjunctivitis, 586f, 774
Vernal keratoconjunctivitis (VKC), 585
Vesicant toxicity, 994
Vesicants. *See* Chemical weapons
Vesiculopustular and bullous lesions, 727t
Vin rose urine, 971f
Viral conjunctivitis, 772
Viral etiologies, I.10, 770
Viral hepatitis, 622t
Viral infections, 844
Viral myositis, 486
Viscum album, 982
Vision, 761
Visual acuity, 753
VKC (Vernal keratoconjunctivitis), 585
Volar dislocations, 320
Voltage, 1035
Vomiting, 73
  causes of, 74t
  diagnostic evaluation, 75
  gastroenteritis, 74
    etiology, 74
    pathophysiology, 74
  in infants, 610t
  prevention, 77
  treatment
    adjunctive therapy, 75
    oral rehydration therapy, 75
Von Willebrand disease, 829
VSD (ventricular septal defect), 416, 420
Vulvar and vaginal injuries, 285
Vulvovaginitis, 793

W

Waddel's triad, 274f, 275t
Warm shock, 197
Water hemlock, 985
Weakness (neurologic emergency)
  bell's palsy, 485
  cholinergic crisis, 484
  diagnosis, 482
    history, 476
    laboratory evaluation, 483
    physical examination, 482

disposition, 486
high-yield facts, 481
myasthenic crisis, 484
myopathies, 485
  muscular dystrophies, 485
  myopathies, 485
  periodic paralysis, 485
  poliomyelitis, 486
  pyomyositis, 486
  trichinosis, 486
  viral myositis, 486
  west nile virus, 486
pathophysiology, 481–2
weakness, causes of, 483
  botulism, 484
  Guillainâ Barrâê syndrome, 483
  myasthenia gravis, 484
  tick paralysis, 484
West Nile virus, 486
Whipworm, 553, 556, 556f
White blood cell count, 101t
Whole-body exposure, 1087t
Whole-bowel irrigation., 966f
Whooping cough. *See* Pertussis
Wide-complex tachycardia, 449
Wilms' tumor, 762, 839, 839f
Wolff–Parkinson–White (WPW) syndrome,
    205, 446
World Health Organization (WHO), 579
Wound
  care, 909, 999–1000
  cleaning, 338
  closure technique, 335t
  dressing, 342, 343

X

X-ray fluorometry (XRF), 965
X-ray machine, 169f

Y

Yersinia pestis (plague), 575
Yersinia, 486, 971
Yew, 984

Z

Zinc protoporphyrin (ZPP), 963, 965
Ziprasidone, 936